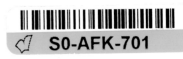

second edition

MOVEMENT DISORDERS

Neurologic Principles & Practice

Editors

Ray L. Watts, M.D.
John N. Whitaker Professor and Chairman
Department of Neurology
University of Alabama at Birmingham
School of Medicine
Birmingham, Alabama

William C. Koller, M.D., Ph.D.
Professor of Neurology
Director, Movement Disorders
Mount Sinai Medical Center
New York, New York

In memory of William C. Koller, M.D., Ph.D., 1945–2005

McGraw-Hill
Medical Publishing

New York   Chicago   San Francisco   Lisbon   London   Madrid   Mexico City   Milan
New Delhi   San Juan   Seoul   Singapore   Sydney   Toronto

The McGraw·Hill Companies

Movement Disorders: Neurologic Principles and Practice, Second Edition

1 2 3 4 5 6 7 8 9 0   CCI/CCI   0 9 8 7 6

ISBN 0-07-147654-7

NON-RETURNABLE

> **Notice**
>
> Medicine is an ever-changing science. As new research and clinical experience broaden our knowledge, changes in treatment and drug therapy are required. The authors and the publisher of this work have checked with sources believed to be reliable in their efforts to provide information that is complete and generally in accord with the standards accepted at the time of publication. However, in view of the possibility of human error or changes in medical sciences, neither the authors nor the publisher nor any other party who has been involved in the preparation or publication of this work warrants that the information contained herein is in every respect accurate or complete, and they disclaim all responsibility for any errors or omissions or for the results obtained from use of the information contained in this work. Readers are encouraged to confirm the information contained herein with other sources. For example and in particular, readers are advised to check the product information sheet included in the package of each drug they plan to administer to be certain that the information contained in this work is accurate and that changes have not been made in the recommended dose or in the contraindications for administration. This recommendation is of particular importance in connection with new or infrequently used drugs.

This book was set in Palatino by Keyword Publishing Services.
The editors were Marc Strauss and Michelle Watt.
The production supervisor was Sherri Souffrance.
Project management was provided by Keyword Publishing Services.
Courier Kendallville was printer and binder.
This book was printed on acid-free paper.

Library of Congress Cataloging-in-Publication Data
Movement Disorders : neurologic principles & practice / edited by Ray L. Watts, William
C. Koller.–2nd ed.
   p. ; cm.
Includes bibliographical references and index.
ISBN 0-07-137496-5
   1. Movement disorders. I. Watts, Ray L. (Ray Lannom), 1953- II, Koller, William C.,
1945-
   [DNLM: 1. Movement Disorders. 2. Neurodegenerative Diseases. 3. Neuromuscular
Diseases. WL 390 M9356 2004]
RC376.5.M69 2004
616.8'3–dc21
                                                                        2003054098

CONTENTS

CONTRIBUTORS *vii*
PREFACE *xiii*
COLOR PLATES *Fall between pages 402 and 403*

PART A

INTRODUCTION TO MOVEMENT DISORDERS

1. Approach to the Patient with a Movement Disorder and Overview of Movement Disorders *3*
   Ajit Kumar and Donald B. Calne

2. Neurobehavioral Aspects of Movement Disorders *17*
   Margaret M. Swanberg, Dean Foti, and Jeffrey Cummings

3. Neuroimaging of Movement Disorders *35*
   David J. Brooks

PART B

NEUROSCIENTIFIC FOUNDATIONS

4. Mitochondria in Movement Disorders *61*
   Claudia M. Testa

5. Functional Anatomy of Basal Ganglia and Motor Systems *87*
   Lhys Gombart, Jesus Soares, and Garrett E. Alexander

6. Physiology of the Basal Ganglia and Pathophysiology of Movement Disorders of Basal Ganglia Origin *101*
   Thomas Wichmann and Mahlon R. DeLong

7. Functional Neurochemistry of the Basal Ganglia *113*
   Jayaraman Rao

8. Neurotrophic Factors *131*
   Clifford W. Shults

9. Neuropathology of Movement Disorders: An Overview *143*
   Marla Gearing and Suzanne S. Mirra

PART C

CLINICAL DISORDERS

I. PARKINSONIAN STATES

PARKINSON'S DISEASE

10. Genetics of Parkinson's Disease and Parkinsonian Disorders *163*
    Zbigniew K. Wszolek, Katerina Markopoulou, and Bruce A. Chase

11. Epidemiology of Parkinson's Disease *177*
    Connie Marras and Caroline M. Tanner

12. Neurochemistry and Neuropharmacology of Parkinson's Disease *197*
    Federico Micheli, Maria G. Cersosimo and G. Frederick Wooten

13. Etiology of Parkinson's Disease *209*
    Yoshikuni Mizuno, Nobutaka Hattori and Hideki Mochizuki

14. Clinical Manifestations of Parkinson's Disease *233*
    Henry L. Paulson and Matthew B. Stern

15. Pharmacologic Treatment of Parkinson's Disease *247*
    Werner Poewe, Roberta Granata, and Felix Geser

16. Transplantation and Restorative Therapies for Parkinson's Disease *273*
    C. Warren Olanow, Thomas B. Freeman, and Jeffrey H. Kordower

17. Stereotaxic Surgery and Deep Brain Stimulation for Parkinson's Disease and Movement Disorders *289*
    Benjamin L. Walter and Jerrold L. Vitek

iii

18. Neurobehavioral Abnormalities in
Parkinson's Disease *319*
Ruth Djaldetti and Eldad Melamed

19. Parkinson's Disease: Neuropathology *327*
Bruce H. Wainer and Natividad P. Stover

20. Progressive Supranuclear Palsy *339*
Lawrence I. Golbe

21. Multiple-System Atrophy *359*
Lisa M. Shulman, Alireza Minagar, and William J. Weiner

OTHER PARKINSONIAN SYNDROMES

22. Infectious and Postinfectious
Parkinsonism *373*
Puiu Nisipeanu, Diana Paleacu, and Amos D. Korczyn

23. Toxin-Induced Parkinsonian Syndromes *383*
Rajesh Pahwa

24. Drug-Induced Parkinsonism *395*
Jean P. Hubble

25. Rare Degenerative Syndromes Associated
with Parkinsonism *403*
Wolfgang H. Oertel and J. Carsten Möller

26. Other Central Nervous System
Conditions *421*
Jacob I. Sage

II. TREMOR DISORDERS

27. Essential Tremor *431*
Maria Graciela Cersosimo and William C. Koller

28. Uncommon Forms of Tremor *459*
Bala V. Manyam

29. The Pathophysiology of Tremor *481*
Rodger J. Elble

III. DYSTONIC DISORDERS

IDIOPATHIC TORSION DYSTONIA

30. Childhood Dystonia *495*
Michele Tagliati, Alana Golden, and Susan B. Bressman

31. Adult-Onset Idiopathic Torsion
Dystonias *511*
Eduardo S. Tolosa and M. J. Marti

32. Treatment of Dystonia *527*
Joseph Jankovic

33. Symptomatic Dystonias *541*
Justo García de Yébenes, S. Cantarero, C. Tabernero, and A.V. Vázquez

IV. CHOREATIC DISORDERS

HUNTINGTON'S DISEASE

34. Genetics and Molecular Biology of
Huntington's Disease *571*
James F. Gusella and Marcy E. MacDonald

35. Clinical Features and Treatment of
Huntington's Disease *589*
Frederick J. Marshall

36. Neuropathology and Pathophysiology of
Huntington's Disease *603*
Steven M. Hersch, H. Diana Rosas, and Robert J. Ferrante

37. Tardive Dyskinesia *629*
Christopher G. Goetz and Stacy Horn

38. Other Choreatic Disorders *639*
Margery H. Mark

V. MYOCLONIC DISORDERS

39. Classification, Clinical Features, and
Treatment of Myoclonus *659*
Jose A. Obeso and Ivana Zamarbide

40. Pathophysiology of Myoclonic
Disorders *671*
Camilo Toro and Mark Hallett

VI. TIC DISORDERS

41. Tourette's Syndrome *685*
Roger Kurlan

42. Pathophysiology and Differential Diagnosis
of Tics *693*
Jorge L. Juncos

VII. ATAXIAS

43. The Molecular Genetics of the Ataxias *705*
George R. Wilmot and S.H. Subramony

44. Clinical Features and Treatment of
Cerebellar Disorders   *723*
Sid Gilman

45. Pathophysiology of
Cerebellar Disorders   *737*
*Scott E. Cooper, Darry S. Johnson,
and Erwin B. Montgomery, Jr.*

VIII. OTHER MOVEMENT DISORDERS

46. Corticobasal Degeneration   *763*
*Natividad P. Stover, Bruce H. Wainer,
and Ray L. Watts*

47. Wilson's Disease   *779*
Ronald F. Pfeiffer

48. Stiff-Person Syndrome   *799*
Oscar S. Gershanik

49. Gait Disorders   *813*
Lewis Sudarsky

IX. SPECIAL CONSIDERATIONS

50. Movement Disorders in Childhood   *825*
Leon S. Dure IV

51. Movement Disorders and Aging   *837*
Ali H. Rajput and Alex Rajput

52. Movement Disorders Specific to Sleep
and the Nocturnal Manifestations of
Waking Movement Disorders   *855*
David B. Rye and Donald L. Bliwise

53. Psychogenic Movement Disorders   *891*
*Daniel S. Sa, Néstor Gálvez-Jiménez, and
Anthony E. Lang*

54. Systemic Illnesses that Cause
Movement Disorders   *915*
Amy Colcher and Howard I. Hurtig

APPENDIX   *927*

INDEX   *945*

CONTRIBUTORS

Garrett E. Alexander, M.D., Ph.D.
Professor of Neurology
Emory University School of Medicine
Atlanta, Georgia

Donald L. Bliwise, Ph.D.
Professor of Neurology
Emory University School of Medicine
Atlanta, Georgia

Susan B. Bressman, M.D.
Chairman, Department of Neurology
Phillips Ambulatory Care Center
Beth Israel Medical Center
New York, New York

David J. Brooks, M.D., D.Sc., F.R.C.P., F.Med.Sci.
Hartnett Professor of Neurology, Imperial College, London
Chief Medical Officer, Imanet, Amersham Health,
and Clinical Director, Imaging Research Solutions Ltd
MRC Clinical Sciences Centre
Faculty of Medicine, Imperial College
Hammersmith Hospital
London, UK

Donald B. Calne, DM, F.R.S.C.
Professor Emeritus
Pacific Parkinsons Research Institute
University of British Columbia
Vancouver Hospital and Health Sciences Centre
Vancouver, British Columbia, Canada

S. Cantarero, M.D.
Servicio de Neurologia
Fundacion Jimenez Diaz
Madrid, Spain

Maria Graciela Cersosimo, M.D.
Program of Movement Disorders and
   Parkinson's Disease
University of Buenos Aires
Buenos Aires, Argentina

Bruce A. Chase, Ph.D.
Professor of Biology
University of Nebraska at Omaha
Omaha, Nebraska

Amy Colcher, M.D.
Clinical Assistant Professor of Neurology
Penn Neurological Institute
University of Pennsylvania
Philadelphia, Pennsylvania

Scott E. Cooper, M.D., Ph.D.
Movement Disorders Section
Department of Neurology
The Cleveland Clinic Foundation
Cleveland, Ohio

Jeffrey L. Cummings, M.D.
Augustus Rose Professor of Neurology
Professor of Psychiatry
David Geffen School of Medicine at UCLA
UCLA Alzheimer's Disease Center
Department of Neurology
Reed Neurological Research Center
UCLA School of Medicine
Los Angeles, California

Mahlon R. DeLong, M.D.
Professor and Director of Neuroscience Center
Department of Neurology
Emory University School of Medicine
Atlanta, Georgia

Ruth Djaldetti, M.D.
Department of Neurology
Rabin Medical Center
Petah Tiqva, Israel

Leon S. Dure IV, M.D.
William Bew White Professor of Pediatrics
Division Director of Pediatric Neurology
Department of Pediatrics
The University of Alabama at Birmingham
Birmingham, Alabama

Rodger J. Elble, M.D., Ph.D.
Professor and Chair
Department of Neurology and Center for Alzheimer Disease
   and Related Disorders
Southern Illinois University School of Medicine
Springfield, Illinois

Robert J. Ferrante, M.Sc., Ph.D.
Associate Professor
Departments of Neurology, Pathology, and Psychiatry
Boston University School of Medicine
Director, Experimental Neuropathology
Bedford Veterans Affairs Medical Center
Bedford, Massachusetts

Thomas B. Freeman, M.D.
Departments of Neurosurgery and Pharmacology
University of South Florida
Tampa, Florida

Dean Foti, M.D., FRCPC
Department of Medicine
University of British Columbia
Vancouver, British Columbia, Canada

Néstor Gálvez-Jiménez, M.D., FACP
Chief, Movement Disorders Program
Director, Neurology Residency Training Program
Department of Neurology
The Cleveland Clinic Florida
Weston, Florida

Justo García de Yébenes, M.D.
Servicio de Neurología
Fundación Jiménez Díaz
Madrid, Spain

Marla Gearing, Ph.D.
Center for Neurodegenerative Disease
Department of Pathology and Laboratory Medicine
Emory University
Atlanta, Georgia

Oscar S. Gershanik, M.D.
Professor and Chairman
Director, Extrapyramidal Diseases Section
Department of Neurology
Centro Neurologico-Hospital Frances
Buenos Aires, Argentina

Felix Geser, M.D.
Department of Neurology
University Hospital Innsbruck
Innsbruck, Austria

Sid Gilman M.D., F.R.C.P.
William J. Herdman Professor and Chair
Department of Neurology
University of Michigan Health System
Ann Arbor, Michigan

Christopher G. Goetz, M.D.
Professor of Neurological Sciences and Pharmacology
Rush Medical College
Rush University
Chicago, Illinois

Lawrence I. Golbe, M.D.
Professor and Acting Chairman
Department of Neurology
University of Medicine and Dentistry of
    NJ–Robert Wood Johnson Medical School
New Brunswick, New Jersey

Alana Golden, B.S.
Department of Neurology
Beth Israel Medical Center
New York, New York

Lhys Gombart, M.D., Ph.D.
Research Associate
Department of Neurology
Emory University School of Medicine
Atlanta, Georgia

Roberta Granata, M.D.
Department of Neurology
University Hospital Innsbruck
Innsbruck, Austria

James F. Gusella, Ph.D.
Molecular Neurogenetics Unit
Center for Human Genetic Research
Massachusetts General Hospital
Charlestown, Massachusetts

Mark Hallett, M.D.
Chief, Medical Neurology Branch
National Institute of Neurological
    Disorders and Stroke
National Institutes of Health
Bethesda, Maryland

Nobutaka Hattori, M.D., Ph.D.
Associate Professor of Neurology
Juntendo University School of Medicine
Bunkyo,Tokyo, Japan

Steven M. Hersch, M.D., Ph.D.
Associate Professor of Neurology
MassGeneral Institute for Neurodegenerative Disease
Massachusetts General Hospital and
    Harvard Medical School
Charlestown, Massachusetts

Stacy Horn, D.O.
Department of Neurological Sciences
Rush University
Rush-Presbyterian-St. Luke's Medical Center
Chicago, Illinois

Jean P. Hubble, M.D.
Medical Director, Neuroscience
Novartis Pharmaceuticals
East Hanover, New Jersey

Howard I. Hurtig, M.D.
Professor of Neurology
Penn Neurological Institute
University of Pennsylvania
Philadelphia, Pennsylvania

Joseph Jankovic, M.D.
Professor of Neurology
Director, Parkinson's Disease Center
    and Movement Disorders Clinic
Baylor College of Medicine
Houston, Texas

Darry S. Johnson, M.D.
Staff Neurologist
Arizona Medical Clinic, Ltd.
Peoria, Arizona

Jorge L. Juncos, M.D.
Associate Professor of Neurology
Movement Disorders Program
Emory University School of Medicine
Atlanta, Georgia

William C. Koller, M.D., Ph.D.
Professor of Neurology
Director, Movement Disorders
Mount Sinai Medical Center,
New York, New York

Amos D. Korczyn
Professor,
Sieratzki Chair of Neurology
Tel-Aviv University Medical School
Ramat Aviv, Israel

Jeffrey H. Kordower, Ph.D.
Department of Neurological Sciences
Rush-Presbyterian-St. Luke's Medical
    Center
Chicago, Illinois

Ajit Kumar DM
Pacific Parkinsons Research Institute
University of British Columbia
Vancouver Hospital and Health Sciences
    Centre
Vancouver, British Columbia, Canada

Roger Kurlan, M.D.
Professor of Neurology

University of Rochester School of
    Medicine and Dentistry
Rochester, New York

Anthony E. Lang, M.D.
Director, Division of Neurology
University of Toronto
Director, Movement Disorders Clinic
Toronto Western Hospital
Toronto, Ontario, Canada

Marcy E. MacDonald, Ph.D.
Molecular Neurogenetics Unit
Center for Human Genetic Research
Massachusetts General Hospital
Charlestown, Massachusetts

Bala V. Manyam, M.D.
Professor and Director,
    Plummer Movement Disorders Center
Department of Neurology
Scott & White Clinic and Memorial Hospital
Texas A&M University System Health Science
    Center College of Medicine
Temple, Texas

Margery H. Mark, M.D.
Associate Professor of Neurology
University of Medicine and Dentistry of
    NJ–Robert Wood Johnson Medical School
New Brunswick, New Jersey

Katerina Markopoulou, M.D., Ph.D.
Assistant Professor of Neurology
University of Nebraska Medical Center,
Omaha, Nebraska

Connie Marras, M.D.
The Parkinson's Institute
Sunnyvale, California

Frederick J. Marshall, M.D.
Assistant Professor of Neurology
University of Rochester School of
    Medicine and Dentistry
Rochester, New York

M.J. Marti, M.D.
Parkinson Disease and Movement Disorders Clinic
Assistant Professor
Faculty of Medicine
University of Barcelona
Barcelona, Spain

Eldad Melamed, M.D.
Professor of Neurology

Rabin Medical Center
Petah Tiqva, Israel

Federico Micheli, M.D., Ph.D.
Professor of Neurology
University of El Salvador and
    University of Buenos Aires, Argentina
Director of the Program of
    Movement Disorders and Parkinson's Disease
Institute of Applied Neurosciences
Hospital de Clinicas
Buenos Aires, Argentina

Alireza Minagar, M.D.
Assistant Professor of Neurology,
    Psychiatry and Anesthesiology
Louisiana State University Health
    Sciences Center
Shreveport, Louisiana

Suzanne S. Mirra, M.D.
Professor and Chair
Department of Pathology
SUNY Downstate Medical Center
Brooklyn, New York

Yoshikuni Mizuno, M.D.
Professor of Neurology
Juntendo University School of Medicine
Bunkyo, Tokyo, Japan

Hideki Mochizuki, M.D.
Associate Professor of Neurology
Jutendo University School of Medicine
Bunkyo, Tokyo, Japan

Jens Carsten Möller
Neurology Clinic
Philipps University of Marburg
Marburg, Germany

Erwin B. Montgomery, Jr., M.D.
Professor of Neurology
University of Wisconsin-Madison
Madison, Wisconsin

Puiu Nisipeanu, M.D.
Department of Neurology
Tel Aviv University Medical School
Ramat Aviv, Israel

Jose A. Obeso, M.D.
Professor and Consultant of Neurology
Clinica Universitaria and Medical School
University of Navarra
Pamplona, Spain

Wolfgang H. Oertel, M.D.
Director
Department of Neurology
Center of Nervous Disease
Philipps-University of Marburg
Marburg, Germany

C. Warren Olanow, M.D.
Professor and Chairman
Department of Neurology
Mount Sinai School of Medicine
New York, New York

Rajesh Pahwa, M.D.
Associate Professor of Neurology
Director, Parkinson Disease and
    Movement Disorder Center
University of Kansas Medical Center
Kansas City, Kansas

Diana Paleacu, M.D.
Department of Neurology
Tel Aviv University Medical School
Ramat Aviv, Israel

Henry L. Paulson, M.D., Ph.D.
Associate Professor of Neurology
University of Iowa Hospitals and Clinics
Iowa City, Iowa

Ronald F. Pfeiffer, M.D.
Professor and Vice Chair
Department of Neurology
University of Tennessee Health Science
    Center
Memphis, Tennessee

Werner Poewe, M.D.
Department of Neurology
University Hospital Innsbruck
Innsbruck, Austria

Ali. H. Rajput, M.B.B.S., F.R.C.P.C.
Professor Emeritus
Division of Neurology
University of Saskatchewan
Royal University Hospital
Saskatoon, Saskatchewan, Canada

Alex Rajput, M.D., F.R.C.P.C.
Associate Professor of Neurology
University of Saskatchewan
Royal University Hospital
Saskatoon, Saskatchewan, Canada

Jayaraman Rao, M.D.
Professor of Neurology and Neuroscience
Carl Baldridge Chair for Parkinson's Research
Director, Parkinson's Disease and
   Movement Disorders Center
Louisiana State University Health Sciences Center
New Orleans, Louisiana

H. Diana Rosas, M.D.
Department of Neurology
Massachusetts General Hospital
Center for Aging and
   Neurodegenerative Diseases (CAGN)
Charlestown, Massachusetts

David B. Rye, M.D., Ph.D.
Associate Professor of Neurology
Medical Director, Emory University Hospital
   Sleep Laboratory
Emory University School of Medicine
Atlanta, Georgia

Daniel S. Sa, M.D.
Movement Disorders Research Fellow
Movement Disorders Center
Toronto Western Hospital
Department of Medicine (Neurology)
University of Toronto
Toronto, Ontario, Canada

Jacob I. Sage, M.D.
Professor of Neurology
University of Medicine and Dentistry of NJ–Robert
   Wood Johnson Medical School
New Brunswick, New Jersey

Lisa M. Shulman, M.D.
Associate Professor of Neurology
Rosalyn Newman Distinguished
   Scholar in Parkinson's Disease
University of Maryland School of Medicine
Baltimore, Maryland

Clifford W. Shults, M.D.
Professor of Neurosciences
University of California, San Diego School
   of Medicine
San Diego, California

Jesus Soares, Ph.D.
Research Associate
Department of Neurology
Emory University School of Medicine
Atlanta, Georgia

Matthew B. Stern, M.D.
Parker Family Professor of Neurology
Director, Parkinson's Disease and
   Movement Disorders Center
University of Pennsylvania Health System
Penn Neurological Institute
Philadelphia, Pennsylvania

Natividad P. Stover, M.D.
Assistant Professor of Neurology
University of Alabama at Birmingham
Birmingham, Alabama

S.H. Subramony, M.D.
Professor and Vice-Chairman
Department of Neurology
University of Mississippi Medical Center
Jackson, Mississippi

Lewis Sudarsky, M.D.
Director, Movement Disorders
Brigham and Womens Hospital
Associate Professor of Neurology
Harvard Medical School
Brigham and Womens Hospital
Boston, Massachusetts

Margaret M. Swanberg, D.O.
Behavioural Neurology Service
Neurology Department
Walter Reed Army Medical Center
Washington, District of Columbia

C. Tabernero, M.D.
Servicio de Neurologia
Fundacion Jimenez Diaz
Madrid, Spain

Michele Tagliati, M.D.
Assistant Professor of Neurology
Beth Israel Medical Center
New York, New York

Caroline M. Tanner, M.D., Ph.D.
Director of Clinical Research
The Parkinson's Institute
Sunnyvale, California

Claudia M. Testa, M.D., Ph.D.
Assistant Professor of Neurology
Emory University School of Medicine
Atlanta, Georgia

Eduardo S. Tolosa, M.D.
Parkinson's Disease and Movement Disorders Clinic

Hospital Clinic i Provincial de Barcelona
Professor of Neurology, Faculty of Medicine
University of Barcelona
Barcelona, Spain

Camilo Toro, M.D.
Frederick Neurology LLC
Frederick, Maryland

A.V. Vázquez, M.D.
Servicio de Neurologia
Fundacion Jimenez Diaz
Madrid, Spain

Jerrold L. Vitek, M.D., Ph.D.
Professor of Neurology
Director, Functional and Stereotactic Neurology
Emory University School of Medicine
Atlanta, Georgia

Bruce H. Wainer, M.D., Ph.D.
Alice and Roy Richards Professor
Departments of Pathology and Neurology
Emory University School of Medicine
Atlanta, Georgia

Benjamin L. Walter, M.D.
Fellow, Functional and Stereotactic Neurology
Emory University School of Medicine
Atlanta, Georgia

Ray L. Watts, M.D.
John N. Whitaker Professor and Chairman
Department of Neurology
University of Alabama at Birmingham School
   of Medicine
Birmingham, Alabama

William J. Weiner, M.D.
Professor and Chairman of Neurology
Director, Maryland Parkinson's Disease
   and Movement Disorders Center
University of Maryland School
   of Medicine
Baltimore, Maryland

Thomas Wichmann, M.D.
Department of Neurology
Emory University School of Medicine
Atlanta, Georgia

George R. Wilmot, M.D., Ph.D.
Assistant Professor of Neurology
Director, Emory University Ataxia Center
Emory University School of Medicine
Atlanta, Georgia

G. Frederick Wooten, M.D.
Mary Anderson Harrison Professor and Chair
   of Neurology
University of VA Medical Center
Charlottesville, Virginia

Zbigniew K. Wszolek, M.D.
Professor of Neurology
Mayo Medical School
Jacksonville, Florida

Ivana Zamarbide
Fellow, Movement Disorders Unit
Clinica Universitaria and Medical School
University of Navarra
Pamplona, Spain

PREFACE

As we first considered writing a second edition of *Movement Disorders: Neurologic Principles and Practice* three years ago, we were not sure that there was sufficient new material to warrant it. As we reviewed the first edition in preparation for planning the contents of the second, however, we recognized clearly that very significant advances had occurred and that the field has continued to change at a rapid pace during the rewriting process. Examples of new advances include the discovery of several different genetic abnormalities that can cause familial parkinsonism (see Chapter 10); improved understanding of the molecular abnormalities in parkinsonian disorders (Synucleinopathies: PD, MSA; Tauopathies: PSP, Corticobasal degeneration, Pick's disease) (see Chapters 9 and 19); major advances in the treatment of Parkinson's disease (see Chapters 15 and 17); the emergence of gene therapy for PD (see Chapter 16); greater understanding of the molecular genetics of the inherited ataxias, necessitating the inclusion of a new chapter (see Chapter 43); and improved understanding of sleep disorders (see Chapter 52), just to name a few. A common theme now emerging from many lines of evidence is that a recurrent pathophysiologic mechanism of neurodegeneration consists of abnormal protein folding secondary to genetic mutations that leads to abnormal protein handling by the ubiquitin-proteasome system, resulting in significant neuronal dysfunction and eventual cell death. Mitochondrial dysfunction is another pathophysiologic mechanism common to a number of neurodegenerative movement disorders.

In this new edition we have kept the organization of sections based principally on clinical patterns of disease expression the same (phenotypic approach), but we have placed greater emphasis on the molecular bases where known (genetic approach). Future editions will likely change to be organized based on the molecular bases of disease as our knowledge advances.

As in the first edition, we have sought to present the material in a logical fashion beginning with Part I: Introduction to Movement Disorders (Chapters 1–3), followed by Part II: Neuroscientific Foundations (Chapters 4–9), and concluding with Part III: Clinical Disorders (Chapters 10–54, further segregated to address the major categories of movement disorders). We have included a large number of tables and figures that help present data more succinctly and are useful teaching aids. The Appendix contains an updated list of Patient Support Organizations.

Once again we are deeply appreciative for the support of our families and professional colleagues throughout the preparation of this second edition, and we are grateful for the assistance of the editorial and publishing staff of McGraw-Hill (especially Michelle Watt and Marc Strauss). Particular appreciation is extended to Tameka Ray, M.P.H., of Emory University (now of U.S. Centers for Disease Control), as well as Lisa Taylor and Aditi Sethi of the University of Alabama at Birmingham for their assistance with many aspects of the organizational, editorial, and publication processes that brought this second edition to fruition.

It is our hope that readers will find this second edition of even greater usefulness than the first.

Ray L. Watts, M.D.
Birmingham, Alabama

William C. Koller, M.D., Ph.D.
New York, New York

xiii

PART A
INTRODUCTION TO MOVEMENT DISORDERS

Chapter 1

APPROACH TO THE PATIENT WITH A MOVEMENT DISORDER AND OVERVIEW OF MOVEMENT DISORDERS

AJIT KUMAR and DONALD B. CALNE

HYPERKINETIC DISORDERS	3
Tremor	4
Chorea	6
Ballism	7
Dystonia	7
Athetosis	8
Myoclonus	8
Tics	9
Stereotypy	9
Akathisia	9
Periodic Leg Movements in Sleep (PLMS)	9
Restless Leg Syndrome (RLS)	10
Painful Legs and Moving Toes Syndrome (PLMT)	10
Phantom Dyskinesia	10
Paroxysmal Dyskinesias	10
Startle Disease or Hyperekplexia	10
Alien Limb	10
Hemifacial Spasm (HS)	11
Stiff Person Syndrome	11
HYPOKINETIC DISORDERS	11
Bradykinesia	11
Rigidity	11
Postural Disturbances	11
Parkinsonian Syndromes	11
Idiopathic Parkinsonism (IP)/Parkinson's Disease (PD)	11
Progressive Supranuclear Palsy (PSP)	12
Multisystem Atrophy (MSA)	12
Corticobasal Ganglionic Degeneration (CBGD)	12
Dementia with Lewy Bodies (DLBD)	12
Frontotemporal Dementias with Parkinsonism Linked to Chromosome 17 (FTDP-17)	12
APPROACH TO A PATIENT WITH A MOVEMENT DISORDER	12

The term "movement disorders" has been coined for diseases characterized by abnormal or excessive movements occurring in conscious patients. The term "extrapyramidal disorder" is an older classification of central motor disturbances not involving the corticospinal pathway.

Movement disorders is used in two contexts: (1) to describe a symptom or physical sign of abnormal or involuntary movement; (2) to describe a syndrome in which abnormal movements occur. Abnormal movements may be the only manifestation of a disease [e.g., essential tremor (ET), hemifacial spasm (HS)], or they can be part of a constellation of deficits [e.g., Parkinson's disease (PD), Huntington's disease (HD), progressive supranuclear palsy (PSP), Creutzfeldt-Jakob disease (CJD)]. Frequently, there may be more than one type of movement disorder associated with a disease [e.g., chorea, dystonia, and akinetic-rigid syndrome in HD and Wilson's disease (WD)] (see Table 1-1).

The first step when assessing a patient with a movement disorder is to establish its class and pattern, and this can often be difficult. The next step consists of determining whether the movement disorder appears in isolation or is associated with other neurological signs. Finally, one needs to determine the probable etiology (hereditary or sporadic; primary, or secondary to a known neurological disease). The differential diagnosis can be narrowed down by taking a careful history, with particular emphasis on birth and family history, and exposure to drugs and toxins, combined with a physical examination. Further investigations (Table 1-2) can be determined based on the differential diagnosis.

Some movement disorders are known to be associated with pathological changes in the basal ganglia (e.g., PD and HD), whereas the pathology in many others is still unclear [e.g., idiopathic torsion dystonia (ITD), tardive dyskinesia (TD) and Gilles de la Tourette syndrome (GTS)]. Movement disorders can be broadly classified into "hyperkinetic disorders," where there is excessive movement, and "hypokinetic disorders," where there is a paucity of movement (hypokinesias). The term "dyskinesia" can be applied to any type of involuntary movement. However, it is most frequently employed to describe the involuntary movements associated with levodopa treatment in patients with PD. The term "tardive dyskinesia" describes involuntary movements that can occur after treatment with neuroleptics.

ET is the commonest movement disorder, followed by PD, dystonia, and drug-induced movement disorders.

Hyperkinetic Disorders

In order to categorize abnormal movements (e.g., chorea, tremor, ballism, myoclonus), one must be able to recognize the type and pattern of the involuntary movements. This can be difficult when combinations of different movements occur in the same individual. Repeated examinations and video recordings over time can be helpful. Even so, it may be difficult to classify a particular abnormal movement.

TABLE 1-1 Overlapping Signs in Some Movement Disorders

	Parkinson's Disease	Progressive Supranuclear Palsy	Multisystem Atrophy	Huntington's Disease	Wilson's Disease	Essential Tremor	Drugs (dopaminergic receptor blockers)
Resting tremor	++	+	+	+	+	+	+
Postural tremor	+	+	+	+	+	++	+

There are certain characteristics, which can help one arrive at a diagnosis:

1. Topography: (distribution).
2. Symmetry: asymmetric or symmetric.
3. Nature: e.g., stereotyped or nonstereotyped.
4. Overflow to other body parts.
5. Velocity: slow, intermediate, or fast.
6. Rhythm: continuous or intermittent.
7. Relation to general voluntary movement.
8. Relation to specific tasks.
9. Relation to posture.
10. Relation to sleep.
11. Associated sensory symptoms.
12. Suppressibility.
13. Aggravating factors: e.g., stress, and anxiety.
14. Precipitating factors: e.g., stress, fatigue, alcohol, and caffeine.
15. Ameliorating factors: e.g., sleep, rest, and alcohol.
16. Distractibility and consistency: to distinguish functional movement disorders.

TREMOR

Tremor comprises involuntary oscillations of a body part produced by alternating or synchronous contractions of reciprocally innervated muscles.[1] It may be fast or slow, coarse or fine, uniplanar or biplanar. Resting tremor is seen with the body part completely at rest. Postural tremor appears while a limb is maintaining a posture. Tremor produced during movement is referred to as action tremor. Intentional tremor is also present during goal-directed activity but, in addition, worsens toward the completion of the activity. Tremor may involve the upper or lower limbs, lips, tongue, neck, or voice. True resting tremor has the following characteristics:

1. Occurs with the body part completely at rest.
2. Subsides with action.
3. Subsides with the assumption of a posture.

Postural tremor is seen immediately following the assumption of a posture. Some tremor can be seen both at rest and with action or the assumption of a posture; e.g., rubral tremors due to lesions of the cerebellar outflow pathways in the midbrain.

The rhythmic interruptions of involuntary sustained contractions in dystonia when the patient attempts to oppose them are referred to as dystonic tremor.[2]

PHYSIOLOGICAL TREMOR

Muscle fibers whose motor units are being recruited at subtetanic rates produce vibrations. This small amplitude tremor can be appreciated only by means of an accelometer or other system of amplification. When muscle contractions are maintained, as when the arms are held outstretched, the movement becomes visible to the naked eye.[3] This is referred to as enhanced physiological tremor. This can be caused or exacerbated by anxiety, fatigue, thyrotoxicosis, hypoglycemia, alcohol withdrawal, sympathomimetic drugs, lithium, sodium valproate, and methylxanthines such as caffeine. These causes should be excluded before arriving at a diagnosis of ET (see Chaps. 27–29).

ESSENTIAL TREMOR (ET)

ET, the commonest movement disorder, is typically a postural tremor, but may be accentuated by goal-directed activity. In some patients the tremor is only present when they assume certain postures or alter their posture. The upper limbs are most frequently involved and the tremor may initially be asymmetric. Some early PD patients may present with postural tremor, and this plus the asymmetry may confound a diagnosis.[4] The tremor is typically uniplanar with flexion-extension movements of the hand.

Abduction-adduction and pronation-supination movements of the hand are occasionally seen.[5] The other sites of involvement include the tongue, voice, head, lips, and trunk, alone or in combination.[6]

With the passage of time the frequency of the tremor decreases and the amplitude may increase.[7] Eventually there may be a resting tremor. In severe cases the tremor may interfere with nutrition and hydration and for these patients the term benign essential tremor is completely misplaced. Stress, anxiety, and central nervous system stimulants can all worsen the tremor. Alcohol in small quantities improves ET in most patients. Although this is a characteristic of ET, other forms of tremor may also respond.[8] Although the neurological examination is normal in the majority of patients with ET, soft signs such as mild abnormalities of tone, posture and balance may be seen.[4] ET can begin at any age, but is called senile tremor if it begins after the age of 65 years. ET is inherited in more than

TABLE 1-2 Approach to a Patient with a Movement Disorder

1. Careful history: With special attention to history of present illness; past medical history; current medications; prior history of medications, toxin exposure, infections; review of systems; family history (pedigree analysis if indicated); social and occupational history
2. Thorough physical examination: With special reference to the neurological and mental status examination. Of particular importance: Presence of involuntary movements; facial expression; eye movements and speech; motor examination of the limbs (strength, muscle tone and coordination); posture and gait, and reflexes
3. Ancillary studies
   a. Laboratory
      (1) Routine: Electrolytes (including calcium and phosphorus), BUN/creatinine, liver function tests (including bilirubin total/direct, transaminase levels, alkaline phosphatase), LDH, CPK, albumin and globulin levels, uric acid, complete blood counts (including RBC and WBC indices), platelet count, prothrombin time and partial thromboplastin time, thyroid function tests (thyroxine, T3 resin uptake (free T4 index), TSH), serum test for syphilis (FTA)
      (2) When indicated by history, examination and/or differential diagnosis:
         (a) Urine and/or serum toxin, and/or heavy metal screen
         (b) Urine collection (24-hour) for copper (together with creatinine and total protein)
         (c) Serum ceruloplasmin (+/− copper) level
         (d) Arterial blood gases
         (e) Peripheral blood smear examination for acanthocytes
         (f) Parathyroid hormone
         (g) Collagen vascular disease/antiphospholipid antibody work-up, including antinuclear antibodies, rheumatoid factor, lupus anticoagulant, and antiphospholipid antibodies
         (h) Antistreptolysin O titers (acute and convalescent)
         (i) Viral titers (acute and convalescent)
         (j) Lumbar puncture for pressure measurements and CSF analysis (with analyses for glucose, protein, and cell counts with differential counts, infectious agents and inflammatory conditions—IgG index, oligoclonal bands)
         (k) Serum folate, vitamin B_{12} levels, biopterin levels
         (l) Serum lactate and pyruvate
         (m) Serum and urine organic acids and amino acids
         (n) Antineuronal antibodies (serum and/or CSF)
   b. Lumbar puncture (see 3.a.(2)(j))
   c. Ophthalmologic: slit lamp examination for Kayser-Fleischer (KF) rings
   d. Genetic testing (also see Table 1-5)
   e. Electrophysiological
      (1) EEG
      (2) EMG/nerve conduction studies
      (3) Evoked responses (VEP, BAER, SSEP, P300)
      (4) Electronystagmography
      (5) Accelometric/electromyographic tremor and involuntary movement analysis
      (6) Cortical potentials/Bereitschaftpotential analysis
      (7) Electrical or magnetic transcranial stimulation for central motor pathway conduction studies
      (8) Movement time/reaction time analysis
      (9) Balance platform and gait laboratory assessment
      (10) Jerk locked EEG back-averaging for myoclonus
      (11) Polysomnography/sleep analysis
   f. Neuroimaging (see also Tables 1-7–1-9 and Chap. 3)
      (1) Computed tomographic (CT) scans: head and spine
      (2) Magnetic resonance imaging (MRI) scans: head and spine
      (3) Positron emission tomography (PET) and single-photon emission computed tomography (SPECT)
   g. Neuropsychological testing[79]
   h. Tissue biopsy
      (1) Muscle, nerve, skin, rectal mucosa, bone marrow: for storage/metabolic and inflammatory disorders
      (2) Muscle platelets: oxidative phosphorylation disorders
      (3) Brain: degenerative, infectious, and inflammatory disorders

BUN, blood urea nitrogen; LDH, lactate dehydrogenase; CPK, creatine phosphokinase; WBC, white blood cell; RBC, red blood cell; TSH, thyroid-stimulating hormone; FTA, free treponemal antibody; CSF, cerebrospinal fluid.

50 percent of patients and putative mapping of one causal gene has been linked to chromosome 2.[9] Apart from these features, essential, senile, and familial tremor are clinically the same.[10]

PARKINSONIAN RESTING TREMOR

Characteristically this is a slow, resting, biplanar, pill-rolling tremor in the 4–5 Hz frequency range. However, postural and kinetic tremors in a higher frequency range may also be seen. Onset of tremor is usually in one of the hands and is asymmetric.[11] Rarely it may begin in the legs. It may also involve the jaw and lips. A tremor of the perioral and nasal muscles (rabbit syndrome) can also occur as is sometimes observed with neuroleptic medication. The resting tremor (RT) may be intermittent early in the course of PD and can be precipitated by anxiety, stress, and contralateral hand clenching. RT is uncommon in other parkinsonian syndromes.[12] The appearance of RT in ET does not necessarily indicate an additional diagnosis of PD.[13] Resting tremor may be a prominent sign in drug-induced parkinsonism.

INTENTION TREMOR

This is seen in involvement of the cerebellum or its connections (see Chaps. 24, 44, 45). It is present during goal-directed movement and worsens terminally.

ORTHOSTATIC TREMOR

A variant of ET, orthostatic tremor is a typical postural tremor, which begins soon after standing up. There is a tremor of the lower limbs, which may cause the patellae to move up and down. Any other postures alleviate it. Most patients have a family history of ET.[14]

"WING-BEATING" TREMOR

This is large-amplitude, slow proximal tremor, causing the arms to be thrown up and down when extended. Changing the posture of the extended arm may alter the severity of the tremor. It is typically seen in WD (see Chap. 47).

PSYCHOGENIC TREMOR

Psychogenic tremor should be suspected when the clinical characteristics are not consistent with recognized forms of tremor. Good indicators include: sudden onset, inconsistent patterns, fluctuations in frequency and direction, distractibility, secondary gain, and dramatic response to placebo.

CONDITIONS RESEMBLING TREMOR

Rhythmic involuntary oscillations at a joint due to spontaneous clonus may resemble tremor. The presence of pyramidal signs helps to differentiate it from tremor. Distinguishing between high-amplitude action tremor and low-amplitude rhythmic myoclonus may be difficult.[15]

CHOREA

The word "chorea" derives from the Greek word for dance. Chorea consists of irregular, unpredictable brief, jerky movements that are usually of low amplitude. The term "semi-purposeful" is sometimes used to describe chorea to help to identify it.[15] Although choreatic movements are really purposeless, patients may incorporate them into a deliberate movement in order to make them less noticeable. The movements are usually distal, and range from mild chorea resembling fidgetiness in children to severe chorea interfering with speech, swallowing, maintaining posture and the ability to walk. Facial grimacing and abnormal respiratory sounds are other manifestations of chorea. Chorea may be associated with hypotonia of the limbs. The gait may resemble a waltz. Chorea can result in a "hung-up" tendon reflex due to muscle contraction immediately after the reflex contraction due to muscle stretch. Motor impersistence (e.g., inability to protrude the tongue in a sustained manner, sometimes referred to as "Jack-in-the-box tongue") and "milkmaid grip" due to contractions alternating with relaxations of grip may be seen.

Chorea may be the only neurological sign of disease, as in rheumatic chorea and thyrotoxicosis, or may be part of a constellation of other signs, as in HD or neuro-acanthocytosis (see Table 1-3 for causes). Keeping the wide differential diagnosis of chorea in mind, it is vital to take a detailed history, paying particular attention to the family and birth history, anoxic insult and exposure to drugs, in addition to looking for associated neurological signs.

TARDIVE DYSKINESIA

TD is defined as abnormal involuntary movement appearing after treatment with a neuroleptic drug for 3 or more months in a patient with no other identifiable causes for a movement disorder[16] (see Chap. 37). TD persists for long after the withdrawal of the offending drug and may indeed only appear for the first time after the drug is stopped. In addition, the movements may worsen briefly after the drug is withdrawn. The movements in TD are complex choreatic and dystonic movements that are classically orobuccolingual, resembling chewing movements, but may affect other body parts as well. They usually spare the forehead. TD may involve abdominal and pelvic muscles, producing truncal or thrusting movements, and may be associated with respiratory dyskinesias.[17] A distinctive feature of the choreatic movements in TD, as compared to chorea in other conditions, is their stereotyped appearance.[18] Rhythmic chewing movements, intermittent tongue protrusion and or pushing the inside of the cheek with the tongue (bon-bon sign) are common. The typical chorea in TD is brief but frequently may be associated with more sustained movements (tardive dystonia). In drug-induced tardive syndromes, the whole spectrum of chorea, dystonia, tics, and akathasia may be seen.

TABLE 1-3 Causes of Chorea

Hereditary-dominant	HD, PDS, DRPLA, neuroacanthocytosis, benign hereditary chorea, spinocerebellar ataxias
Hereditary-recessive	Wilson's disease, Niemann-Pick disease, Pelizaeus-Merzbacher disease, Hallervorden-Spatz disease, ataxia telangiectasia, Lesch-Nyhan disease
Maternal inheritance	Mitochondrial encephalopathies
Autoimmune	Rheumatic chorea, chorea gravidarum, systemic lupus erythematosus (SLE), polyarteritis nodosa, Behçet's disease
Metabolic	Hypo- or hypernatremia, hypocalcemia, hypo- or hyperglycemia, renal failure, hypoparathyroidism
Toxins	Mercury, carbon monoxide
Inflammatory	Encephalitis, acquired immune deficiency syndrome (AIDS)
Drugs	Neuroleptics, metoclopramide, L-dopa, anticonvulsants, steroids, oral contraceptives
Vascular	Infarcts

HD, Huntington's disease; PDS, paroxysmal dyskinesias; DRPLA, dentato-rubro-pallido-luysian atrophy.

BALLISM

Ballism is a proximal high-amplitude, sometimes flailing, movement related to chorea. As patients recover from ballism due to stroke, they often go through a phase of chorea. Ballism is usually limited to one side of the body (hemiballism). However, it may occur bilaterally (biballism) or confined to a single limb (monoballism). The cause of ballism is usually vascular, but other structural lesions and metabolic disturbances such as nonketotic hyperosmolar hyperglycemia can also produce it.

DYSTONIA

Dystonia is an abnormal movement characterized by sustained muscle contractions, frequently causing twisting and repetitive movements or abnormal postures.[19] Dystonic movements that are slow, twisting, and distal were formerly referred to as athetosis. Dystonia can be associated with fast rhythmic tremulous movements (dystonic tremor).[20] Dystonic movements can also be rapid resembling myoclonus (myoclonic dystonia). Electromyography (EMG) shows prolonged bursts typical of dystonia rather than the characteristic short duration bursts seen in myoclonus.[21]

Dystonia can involve any body part. According to the site of involvement, dystonia is classified as:

1. Focal: one body part involved (blepharospasm, oromandibular dystonia, spasmodic dysphonia, cervical dystonia, and occupational cramp).
2. Segmental dystonia: two or more contiguous parts are involved (Meige syndrome).
3. Multifocal dystonia: two or more noncontiguous parts are involved.
4. Hemidystonia: one side of the body is affected.
5. Generalized dystonia (crural with involvement of other parts).

RELATION TO ACTIVITY
Dystonia may occur when a body part is at rest or only when a body part is used to perform a voluntary activity (action dystonia). Also, a dystonia at rest may worsen on action. Idiopathic torsion dystonia (ITD) most often starts as a specific action dystonia, particularly inversion of the foot. As the disease progresses, dystonia occurs with nonspecific movements of other body parts (overflow dystonia) and ultimately at rest. Thus, any dystonia at rest represents a more severe form of dystonia than pure action dystonia. Dystonia may be task-specific (e.g., writer's or musician's cramp). Even in these conditions, as the disease progresses less specific actions provoke it. Some of these task-specific dystonias may be associated with an additional tremor or myoclonic component.[22] A subgroup of idiopathic dystonia with myoclonic spasms and responsiveness to alcohol is believed to be a variant of ITD.[23,24]

Dystonia can be aggravated by stress, anxiety, fatigue, specific postures, and action. It is frequently relieved by sleep and rest. A peculiar feature of dystonia is some patients' ability to relieve a movement by "sensory tricks" that are usually tactile or proprioceptive stimuli. For example, blepharospasm can sometimes be relieved by touching the area around the eyes. This phenomenon is unique to dystonia and can aid in the diagnosis. Dystonia can also be paroxysmal, as in the paroxysmal dyskinesias (see Chap. 38). Diurnal variation can be seen in dystonia as in "dopa-responsive dystonia" (DRD).[25,26] The onset is in the legs and usually begins in childhood. There can be problems with the gait and frequent falls. A characteristic worsening towards the end of the day is often observed. There may be associated features of parkinsonism, and the condition responds well to long-term small doses of L-dopa. DRD may be mistaken for cerebral palsy. Diagnosis is crucial because of the response to treatment. The inheritance is usually autosomal-dominant with variable penetrance and expression. Recently, the genetic defect has been mapped to chromosomes 14q (dominant) and 11p (recessive).[27,28]

PRIMARY VERSUS SECONDARY DYSTONIAS
Dystonia can be classified according to its etiology as idiopathic (primary) and symptomatic (secondary). Approximately 30 percent of dystonia is secondary. Both primary and

secondary dystonia can be familial or sporadic[29] (see Chaps. 30–33). In childhood, generalized dystonia may be primary or secondary. In adults, primary dystonia is usually focal. The age of onset of dystonia is important for prognosis, as young-onset dystonia tends to evolve into generalized dystonia, whereas adult-onset dystonia is likely to remain focal. Onset with dystonia at rest, early speech involvement (except spasmodic dysphonia), rapid course, and association with other neurological signs suggest a secondary dystonia. Hemidystonia is mostly symptomatic and calls for investigations for vascular or other structural lesions.[30,31]

Secondary dystonia may be associated with a variety of neurological signs other than dystonia. Dystonia in association with parkinsonism can occur in PD, PSP, multisystem atrophy (MSA), corticobasal ganglionic degeneration (CBGD), certain forms of spinocerebellar ataxia (Machado-Joseph disease), and the dystonia parkinsonism syndrome of the Philippines (lubag)[32] (see Chaps. 14, 15, 20, 21, 25, 33, 46, 47, 50).

Exposure to drugs (D2 dopamine receptor antagonists, chronic L-dopa therapy, anticonvulsants), anoxia, birth injury, toxic exposure (manganese, carbon monoxide (CO), carbon disulfide, methanol), head injury, stroke, and encephalitis can all cause dystonia (see Chap. 33). Metabolic and storage disorders such as WD, GM1 and GM2 gangliosidosis, Lesch-Nyhan syndrome, and dystonic lipidosis (Niemann-Pick type 3) can all be associated with dystonia (see Chaps. 25, 33). Of these, the diagnosis of WD is especially important, because it is treatable.

Acute dystonic reactions consist of sustained painful muscle spasms, with twisting and pulling movements occurring within minutes to hours of exposure to dopaminergic blocking drugs. Torticollis, retrocollis, trismus, blepharospasm, and ocular deviations may be seen. These idiosyncratic reactions to dopamine receptor (D2) blockers occur mainly in juveniles or young adults.

PSYCHOGENIC DYSTONIA

Psychogenic dystonia represents a major diagnostic challenge. Clinically inconsistent and incongruous postures and patterns of movement, give-away weakness, sensory complaints in the affected limb, multiple somatizations, presence of a psychiatric disorder, secondary gain, and amenability to suggestion are clues to this diagnosis.[33] However, some dystonias with an organic basis, such as cervical dystonia, remit spontaneously.[34]

ATHETOSIS

Athetosis was a term formerly used to describe distal, slow, writhing forms of dystonia. Pseudoathetosis refers to abnormal movements resembling athetosis due to proprioceptive sensory loss, most evident when visual compensation is removed. This occurs with lesions anywhere along the proprioceptive sensory pathways, including the parietal cortex, dorsal root ganglia, and peripheral nerve.[35]

Unlike dystonia, pseudoathetosis can be suppressed by supporting the limb.

MYOCLONUS

Myoclonus describes sudden shock-like movements due to muscle contractions or inhibition of ongoing muscle activity (negative myoclonus). Myoclonus is usually random and irregular in time as in chorea, but unlike chorea the spasm is more abrupt. On occasion myoclonus may be rhythmic or oscillatory. Tics may resemble myoclonus but they are voluntarily suppressible for short periods. Tics are also associated with an inner build-up of tension during the suppression. Myoclonus may be mild or sometimes severe enough to move the whole body. Topographically it may be focal, segmental, multifocal, or generalized. Myoclonus can occur spontaneously or it may be stimulus sensitive (light, touch, noise, etc.). Myoclonus can sometimes be precipitated by action, as in the Ramsay Hunt syndrome (see Chap. 39). The origin of myoclonus may be cortical or subcortical (brainstem or spinal) (see Chaps. 39, 46). Cortical myoclonus is an epileptic phenomenon, and the technique of back-averaging the electroencephalogram (EEG), using EMG activity as a trigger, will demonstrate the transient time-locked cortical event preceding the myoclonic jerk.

Myoclonus can be physiological and can occur after exercise, in excessive fatigue or when falling asleep (hypnagogic jerks). As in other movement disorders, myoclonus may be idiopathic (essential myoclonus). Onset of essential myoclonus can be at any age and there may be a positive family history. Epileptic (cortical) myoclonus is almost always associated with other forms of seizures and is more common in the younger age groups. Examples include juvenile myoclonic epilepsy of Janz, Rasmussen's encephalitis, and the progressive myoclonic epilepsy syndromes (PMEs). The PMEs are characterized by varying combinations of myoclonic and generalized seizures, ataxia, and dementia. The common causes are Lafora body disease, sialidosis, mitochondrial encephalopathy, neuronal ceroid lipofuscinosis (NCL), and dentatorubropallidoluysian atrophy (DRPLA). Myoclonus can also have a myriad of symptomatic causes. These include trauma, anoxia (Lance-Adams syndrome), post stroke, metabolic (hepatic and renal failure, hyponatremia, hypoglycemia, nonketotic hyperglycemia), subacute sclerosing panencephalitis, CJD, drugs (anticonvulsants), degenerative diseases (Alzheimer's, MSA), storage disorders (GM2 gangliosidosis, NCL, Tay-Sachs), WD, and spinal lesions.

FEATURES OF SOME SPECIFIC TYPES OF MYOCLONUS
The *Lance-Adams syndrome* comprises chronic action myoclonus after cerebral anoxia. It is often accompanied by cerebellar ataxia.[36] A dramatic response to 5-hydroxytryptophan (5-HTP) is a feature of this condition.

Spinal myoclonus is usually repetitive, in one limb. Spinal cord lesions such as those due to trauma, tumor, or inflammatory conditions may be responsible.[37]

Palatal myoclonus is characterized by rhythmic jerking of the soft palate, often in conjunction with the pharyngeal, laryngeal, and extraocular muscles and the diaphragm. These occur at a frequency of about 2 Hz and can persist in sleep. The site of the lesion is often the central tegmental tract (red nucleus to inferior olive), or occasionally the dentate nucleus. The cause is usually infarction, but the syndrome has been reported in neoplastic, inflammatory, and degenerative processes.[38] At autopsy, pathology has been found in the inferior olive.[39]

Asterixis (negative myoclonus) is due to brief lapses of tone in a limb held in a posture against gravity. EMG reveals irregular silent periods during these lapses. Asterixis is commonly seen in metabolic encephalopathies, as a reaction to general anesthesia, and during anticonvulsant therapy.

TICS

Tics are brief, involuntary, rapid, nonrhythmic movements (motor tics) or sounds (vocal tics) (see Chaps. 41, 42). They can be severe enough to be constantly present.[40] They occur against a background of normal motor activity. Tics can be classified into simple and complex. A simple motor tic is an abrupt, brief, isolated movement like an eye blink, shoulder shrug, facial grimace, or head jerk (clonic tic). The movement may also be slower and sustained, as in neck turning (tonic or dystonic tic). Complex motor tics include stereotyped facial expressions or patterned coordinated movements, such as touching or grooming behavior, smelling objects or body parts, shaking hands, scratching, kicking or obscene gesturing. The appearance of the complex motor tic may make it difficult to distinguish it from voluntary movement and many of these overlap with obsessive-compulsive behavior. Simple vocal tics usually consist of throat clearing, grunting, coughing, snorting or animal sounds such as hissing, barking, crowing, etc. Complex vocal tics comprise words, phrases, and, on occasion, obscene utterances or religious profanities. Tics are worsened by stress, anxiety, and fatigue. They are relieved by concentration on a task or absorbing activities such as reading or playing a musical instrument. Tics vary in frequency, amplitude, duration, and location. They are usually multifocal and can migrate from one body part to another. The common sites of occurrence are the face, neck, and shoulders. Tics are usually first noticed by others such as parents, teachers, and friends. Characteristic features of tics include:[41]

1. Occurrence of an irresistible urge to move before the tic. The tension that mounts before the tic is relieved by execution of the tic. In contrast to tics, the sensory urge to move in akathasia and restless leg syndrome (RLS) is constant. Also, the movements in akathasia tend to be more stereotyped.
2. Tics can be voluntarily suppressed for a short time; however, this leads to a build-up of tension and a rebound exacerbation.

Tics can be seen in the general population (habit spasms). Transient tic disorder occurs in up to 15 percent of children and usually takes the form of a simple motor or vocal tic. It usually remits within 1 year of occurrence, but may recur during periods of stress in adult life (see Chaps. 41, 42). Chronic tics persist throughout life. GTS represents the most severe form of the primary tic disorders. It has an hereditary basis, with the probable locus of the abnormal gene on chromosome 7.[42] The tics are chronic, multifocal, motor and vocal. TS is associated with attention-deficit hyperactivity disorder, obsessive-compulsive disorder, sleep disorders, echolalia (repeating sounds and words from an external source, usually the last sound), echopraxia (repeating movements of another person), palilalia (repeating own words or sounds with increasing speed and decreasing clarity), coprolalia (obscene utterances), and copropraxia (obscene gesturing) (see Chap. 41). A recently emphasized symptom of TS is the sensory tic.[43] These are uncomfortable somatic sensations such as tickle, touch and pressure, which are localized to specific body parts. Patients relieve these sensations by movements which are interpreted as voluntary (e.g., scratching a body part to relieve an itch). Tics can be due to secondary causes that include head injury, stroke, as part of neuroacanthocytosis, or dopaminergic receptor-blocking drugs where they may occur as a tardive syndrome.[44]

STEREOTYPY

Repetitive and continuous complex motor acts known as "stereotypies" occur in mental retardation, psychosis, Lesch-Nyhan syndrome, neuroacanthocytosis, and Rett's syndrome (RS). In RS, the movements are typically hand-wringing or hand-washing[45] (see Chaps. 25, 33, 37, 50).

AKATHISIA

Akathisia refers to motor activity as a voluntary effort to relieve continuous uncomfortable sensations. It usually takes the form of standing, pacing, trunk-rocking while standing, and sometimes marching on the spot. In severe cases the need for motor activity is irrepressible.[46] Akathisia is often seen in patients on neuroleptics. It can occur as an acute syndrome after administration of the first dose or after an increased dose, often in a young adult. It can also occur as a tardive syndrome more than 3 months after instituting treatment. Akathisia may also be seen in PD. When the lower limb movements in akathisia resemble choreatic movements, the patients' need to move differentiates akathisia from TD.

PERIODIC LEG MOVEMENTS IN SLEEP (PLMS)

PLMS, or nocturnal myoclonus, is distinct from the hypnagogic jerks experienced by normal people while falling asleep. It comprises repetitive, stereotyped extensions of the big toes and sometimes flexion of the ankles, knees, and hips.[47] Occasionally, the movements are unilateral. The movements occur in clusters lasting from 10 minutes to several hours and sometimes throughout sleep. PLMS can be associated with RLS, narcolepsy, or sleep apnea syndrome.[48,49]

RESTLESS LEG SYNDROME (RLS)

In RLS, or Ekbom's syndrome, patients experience sensory disturbances in the legs that are characteristically relieved by movement. The sensations are variously described as creeping, crawling, stretching or pulling, and are felt in the muscles, tendons, or bones. On occasion they may be felt in the upper limbs. The symptoms usually peak 15–20 minutes after lying down at night. Relief is obtained by moving the legs around or pacing. RLS differs from akathasia in that it occurs at night and is not associated with neuroleptic medication. RLS may be primary or occur in association with several conditions, including diabetes mellitus, uremia, carcinoma, pregnancy, malabsorption, and chronic obstructive airway disease. Many of these conditions are associated with sensory neuropathy and probably represent secondary RLS.[50]

PAINFUL LEGS AND MOVING TOES SYNDROME (PLMT)

In this disorder there is typically a deep boring pain in the lower limbs associated with continuous, stereotyped flexion-extension or abduction-adduction movements of the toes.[51] Involvement of the upper limbs has also been described.[52] The pain experienced may be mild to severe; immersing the feet in hot or cold water sometimes helps. The pain does not localize to any dermatome or peripheral nerve. In contrast to akathasia, movements do not relieve the sensation and there is no subjective desire to move the limbs. Indeed, patients often strive to stop the movements. The movements tend to disappear in sleep although they may occasionally persist. Some cases are associated with peripheral nerve or radicular lesions, but, in many, the neurological examination is normal. A similar disorder with moving toes but no associated pain has also been described.[53]

PHANTOM DYSKINESIA

This refers to involuntary movements of the stump associated with sensory phenomena such as paresthesiae and pain experienced by amputees. Phantom dyskinesia may occur spontaneously or as a result of neuroleptics.[54,55] Involuntary movements of the amputated stump without the associated sensory phenomena have also been described.[56]

PAROXYSMAL DYSKINESIAS

Paroxysmal dyskinesias are disorders characterized by episodes of involuntary movements lasting varying amounts of time with return to normality in between. Unlike seizures, there is no loss of consciousness, incontinence, or postical confusion. Three types of paroxysmal dyskinesias have been recognized[2]:

1. Paroxysmal kinesigenic dyskinesia (PKD).
2. Paroxysmal nonkinesigenic dyskinesia (PNKD).
3. Paroxysmal exertional dyskinesia (PED).

PKD is precipitated by sudden movements, startle, or hyperventilation. Stress or excitement worsen it. The attacks are brief, lasting less than 5 minutes, and occur several times a day. The attacks are mainly dystonic in nature and may be unilateral, alternating unilateral, or bilateral. In some patients the movements may be choreatic or ballistic.[57] Rest, or pressure on the affected limb may relieve the attack. Sensory symptoms may precede the attack.[58,59] The familial form is dominantly inherited. Unlike PNKD, both the familial and sporadic forms of PKD respond to anticonvulsants.

The attacks in PNKD occur spontaneously at rest but may be precipitated by stress, fatigue, caffeine, or alcohol. They are of longer duration than in PKD and may last many minutes to hours. They are also less frequent. When bilateral, they may be of sufficient magnitude to cause postural instability and falls. Orofacial dystonia can result in dysarthria. Attacks may be partially suppressed by rest, physical activity, or rubbing the limb.[60,61] Primary PNKD may be sporadic or familial. The familial cases show dominant inheritance (Mount-Reback syndrome, chromosome 2q). Secondary PNKD can occur due to a variety of conditions, including head trauma, multiple sclerosis, vascular events, and myelopathy.[62]

PED is triggered by prolonged exercise and the attacks are protracted. Inheritance is autosomal-dominant. Frontal lobe seizures are believed to be responsible for paroxysmal hypnogenic dyskinesias, particularly attacks of short duration.[63,64]

STARTLE DISEASE OR HYPEREKPLEXIA

Excessive startle or complex motor reactions in response to sudden unexpected stimuli occur in startle disease or hyperekplexia. When severe, there may be generalized muscle contraction resulting in postural instability and falls. After the fall, there is recovery of normal tone and control.[65] The attacks are worsened by stress and fatigue and ameliorated by central nervous system (CNS) depressants. Hyperekplexia may be sporadic or familial with dominant inheritance (chromosome 5q). Disorders such as the Jumping Frenchmen of Maine, Latah and Myriachit probably represent variants of startle disease. Abnormal startle and hyperekplexia have also been described in brainstem lesions.[66]

ALIEN LIMB

Alien limb is a term used to describe cases in which anterior corpus callosal lesions produce involuntary movements of a hand, associated with inability to distinguish the affected hand from the examiner's hand.[67] There is a feeling of foreignness about the affected limb or failure of the patient to recognize that it is their own limb that is moving.[68] Alien hand occurs in a nonparalyzed limb with intact sensation, in contrast to anosognosia. The movements are complex and may seem purposeful in spite of their involuntary nature. The movements may take the form of groping, pushing, clutching, or may be complex, such as picking up objects.[69] Alien hand occurs with structural lesions of the corpus callosum and medial frontal cortex.[70–72] It also occurs in corticobasal ganglionic degeneration (CBGD), where there may be associated features such as dyspraxia and cortical sensory loss (see Chap. 46).

HEMIFACIAL SPASM (HS)

HS is a condition in which there is contraction of the facial muscles, which is most often unilateral. It usually starts with eyelid twitching and can later involve the lower part of the face. It may be intermittent or continuous, and is precipitated by contraction of the facial muscles as in speaking or chewing. When bilateral, the facial contractions on both sides are asynchronous. The etiology is often any irritative lesion of the facial nerve, such as an aberrant intracranial blood vessel, tumor, or multiple sclerosis plaque.

STIFF PERSON SYNDROME

This is an unusual condition, with continuous isometric contraction of axial and proximal muscles resulting in pain and often ophistotonus (see Chap. 48). The disorder can be malignant, culminating in death.

Hypokinetic Disorders

BRADYKINESIA

Bradykinesia refers to slowness and poverty of movement. This typically manifests as hypomimia, micrographia, hypophonia, monotonous speech, reduced blink rate, and generalized motor slowness. A reduced arm swing while walking, one of the earliest signs in PD, is a manifestation of bradykinesia. Initiation of movement is often difficult. Repetitive hand and foot movements reveal a reduction in speed and amplitude, and there may be brief arrests of ongoing movement. Often it is the demeanor and overall gestalt that conveys the sense of bradykinesia in a parkinsonian syndrome.

RIGIDITY

Rigidity is an increase in muscle tone, which is equal in the flexors and extensors; it is elicited during passive movement.

Rigidity may be smooth (lead pipe) or ratchety (cogwheel). Assessment requires the patient to relax, and it is best detected in the more distal joints of a limb. Rigidity can be unmasked in mild cases by voluntary contralateral activation of the opposite limb (Froment's sign). Topographical distribution of rigidity may give a clue to diagnosis, as in the case of PSP, where axial rigidity is pronounced.

POSTURAL DISTURBANCES

In parkinsonian syndromes there can be significant postural disturbances. The trunk becomes flexed, resulting in a stooped posture, and the upper limbs may also assume a flexed posture. Marked flexion of the neck can be seen in MSA. In the majority of patients with PD, postural and gait abnormalities occur within the first 5 years.[73] There may be impairment of righting reflexes; this can be tested by asking the subject to balance with the feet together while the examiner pulls suddenly from behind. Postural instability is a major cause of falls.

PARKINSONIAN SYNDROMES

The tetrad of tremor, rigidity, bradykinesia, and postural disturbances constitutes parkinsonism. Although classically seen in PD (see Chap. 14), other degenerative diseases may present as a parkinsonian syndrome. These include PSP (see Chap. 20), MSA (see Chap. 21), CBGD (see Chap. 46), dementia with Lewy bodies (DLBD, see Chap. 25), Westphal variant of HD (see Chaps. 35, 50), DRD (see Chaps. 30, 32), pallidal degeneration (see Chap. 25) and neuroacanthocytosis (see Chaps. 3, 25). Symptomatic causes include WD (see Chap. 47), dopaminergic receptor-blocking drugs (see Chap. 24), toxins, 1-methyl-4-phenyl-1,2,3,6-tetrahydropyridine (MPTP), manganese, carbon disulfide vascular events, head injury, postencephalitic sequelae, and hydrocephalus.

IDIOPATHIC PARKINSONISM (IP)/PARKINSON'S DISEASE (PD)

PD is typically a disease of the elderly, but onset in the fourth or fifth decade is not unusual. The diagnosis can be considered when two of the three cardinal features of parkinsonism (i.e., tremor, rigidity, and bradykinesia) are present. Abnormal signs are usually asymmetric. Postural instability is best used as an adjunct to the diagnosis. Although postural instability may be seen early in a minority of PD patients, it can sometimes be seen in normal elderly subjects.[74,75] In addition to the motor abnormalities, there may be associated cognitive (bradyphrenia and dementia), autonomic, and mood (depression) abnormalities. Calne et al. have proposed stratifying patients into three groups of increasing diagnostic certainty: possible, probable, and definite.[76] Table 1-4 describes the exclusion criteria for IP.

TABLE 1-4 Exclusion Criteria for Idiopathic Parkinsonism

1. Neuroleptics, calcium channel-blocking drugs
2. Exposure to toxins: MPTP, CO inhalation, manganese, methanol, n-hexane
3. Definite encephalitis
4. Strokes, and stepwise deterioration
5. Repeated head injury
6. Early and severe dementia or autonomic dysfunction
7. Cerebellar signs, supranuclear gaze palsy, and negative response to high doses of L-dopa

1-methyl-4-phenyl-1,2,3,6-tetrahydropyridine (MPTP).

PROGRESSIVE SUPRANUCLEAR PALSY (PSP)

The characteristic features of PSP are a symmetrical akinetic-rigid syndrome with increased axial rigidity, impaired vertical gaze, early frequent falls, dysarthria, dysphagia, frontal lobe dementia, and poor response to L-dopa (see Chap. 20).

MULTISYSTEM ATROPHY (MSA)

MSA refers to parkinsonian syndromes with varying combinations of pyramidal, cerebellar, and autonomic involvement. Response to L-dopa is poor. When the parkinsonian component is most prominent it is referred to as striatonigral degeneration (MSA-SND). When the parkinsonian and cerebellar involvement are both prominent, it is referred to as sporadic olivopontocerebellar atrophy (MSA-OPCA) (see Chap. 21).

CORTICOBASAL GANGLIONIC DEGENERATION (CBGD)

CBGD is an asymmetric akinetic-rigid syndrome with cortical signs that include apraxia, cortical sensory loss, alien hand, stimulus-sensitive myoclonus, and poor response to L-dopa.[77]

DEMENTIA WITH LEWY BODIES (DLBD)

The characteristic features of DLBD are those of a parkinsonian syndrome with fluctuating dementia and psychosis. Hallucinations may be prominent.

FRONTOTEMPORAL DEMENTIAS WITH PARKINSONISM LINKED TO CHROMOSOME 17 (FTDP-17)

FTDP-17 comprises hereditary dementia, associated with parkinsonism.[78] The inheritance is autosomal-dominant and is due to mutations or deletions in the tau gene on chromosome 17. The clinical picture is heterogeneous, and varies depending on the type of deletion or mutation. Parkinsonian symptoms are often present. Response to L-dopa is poor.

Approach to a Patient with a Movement Disorder

Much of this book deals with how patients with specific movement disorders present to the clinician and how

TABLE 1-5 Molecular Genetics in Movement Disorders

Disease	Type of Inheritance	Chromosome	Ref(s)
Huntington's disease (HD)	AD	4p	80
Essential tremor (ET)	AD	2p	9
Neuroacanthocytosis	AD	9q	81
Lubag	X-linked	Xq	
Paroxysmal nonkinesigenic dyskinesia (PNKC)	AD	2q	2
Spinocerebellar ataxias (SCA)			
SCA-1	AD	6p	
SCA-2	AD	12q	
SCA-3	AD	14q	
SCA-4	AD	16q	
SCA-5	AD	11cent	
SCA-6	AD	19p	
Dopa-responsive dystonia (DRD)	AD	14q	27,28
Tourette's syndrome (TS)	AD	7q	42
Dentatorubropallidoluysian atrophy (DRPLA)	AD	12p	82
Wilson's disease (WD)	AR	13q	
Startle disease	AD	5q	2

AD, autosomal-dominant; AR, autosomal-recessive.

TABLE 1-6 Causes of Basal Ganglia Calcification

Hypo- and pseudohypoparathyroidism
Fahr's syndrome
Carbon monoxide (CO) intoxication
Birth anoxia
Tuberous sclerosis
Mitochondrial encephalopathies
Radiation, and methotrexate therapy
Acquired immune deficiency syndrome (AIDS)
Congenital folate deficiency, dihydropteridine reductase deficiency
Japanese B encephalitis, herpes simplex encephalitis
Down's syndrome
Cockayne syndrome

TABLE 1-7 Hyperintense MRI Signal in Basal Ganglia

Wilson's disease
Creutzfeldt-Jakob disease
Manganese toxicity
Hepatic encephalopathy
Calcified basal ganglia
AIDS
Normal aging

MRI, magnetic resonance imaging; AIDS, acquired immune deficiency syndrome.

they are managed. A systematic approach to the patient with a movement disorder will lead to a correct differential diagnosis and ultimately the correct diagnosis. The need for a comprehensive history with thorough and, if necessary, repeated physical examinations cannot be overemphasized. The clinical data thus obtained give direction

TABLE 1-8 Hypointense MRI Signal in Basal Ganglia

Wilson's disease (WD)
Leigh's disease
Carbon monoxide (CO) intoxication
Anoxia
Hallervorden-Spatz disease
Cyanide poisoning
Methanol intoxication
GM2 gangliosidosis
Hemolytic-uremic disease
Wasp-sting encephalopathy

MRI, magnetic resonance imaging.

to specific laboratory investigations when required. After this, a management protocol can be formulated, keeping in mind the unique characteristics of each patient. Table 1-2 provides a general framework for how to approach a patient with a movement disorder. Gene testing is now possible in several movement disorders, including HD, DRD, ITD, and the spinocerebellar ataxias. The modes of inheritance and gene loci for some movement disorders are given in Table 1-5. Tables 1-6 through 1-9 provide information about neuroimaging findings in various movement disorders. Chapter 3 covers neuroimaging in greater detail.

Acknowledgement

The authors thank Susan Calne for editorial assistance.

TABLE 1-9 PET Neuroimaging in Specific Movement Disorders

Movement Disorder	MRI	PET-FDG/FD	Ref(s)
Huntington's disease (HD)	Caudate atrophy	Hypometabolism in caudate and frontal lobes	83,84
Idiopathic distortion dystonia (ITD)	Normal	FD and FDG scans normal	85,86
Wilson's disease (WD)	Hypo- or hyperintensities in basal ganglia, thalamus, midbrain and frontal lobes	Hypometabolism in striatum, frontoparietal cortices and white matter	
		Reduced FD uptake	87
Idiopathic parkinsonism (IP)	Normal	Reduced FD uptake in striatum, especially putamen	88
		Hypermetabolism in pallidum in FDG scan	89
Progressive supranuclear palsy (PSP)	Midbrain atrophy	Reduced FD uptake in striatum	90
Multisystem atrophy/Shy-Drager Syndrome (MSA/SDS)	Cerebellar and brainstem atrophy	Reduced FD uptake in caudate and putamen	91,92
	Hyperintensity in dorsolateral putamen	Frontal and striatal hypometabolism in FDG scan	
Corticobasal ganglionic degeneration (CBGD)	Contralateral and later bilateral frontoparietal atrophy	Asymmetrical parietal and frontal hypometabolism in FDG scan	93
		Asymmetric reduction of striatal FD uptake	

MRI, magnetic resonance imaging; PET, positron emission tomography; FD, ^{18}F-dopa; FDG, ^{18}F-deoxyglucose.

References

1. Jankovic J, Fahn S: Physiological and pathological tremors: Diagnosis, mechanism and management. *Ann Intern Med* 93:460–465, 1980.
2. Fahn S: Involuntary movements, in Rowland LP (ed): *Merritt's Neurology*. Philadelphia: Lippincott Williams & Wilkins, 2000, pp 38–41.
3. Young RR, Weigner AW: Tremor, in Swash M, Kennard C (eds): *Scientific Basis of Clinical Neurology*. Edinburgh: Churchill Livingstone, 1985, pp 116–132.
4. Larsen TA, Calne DB: Essential tremor. *Clin Neuropharmacol* 6:185–206, 1983.
5. Critchley M: Observations on essential (heredofamilial) tremor. *Brain* 72:113–139, 1949.
6. Koller WC, Biary N: Metoprolol compared to propranolol in the treatment of essential tremor. *Arch Neurol* 41:171–172, 1984.
7. Elble RJ: Essential tremor frequency decreases with time. *Neurology* 55:1547–1551, 2000.
8. Rajput AH, Jamieson H, Hirsh S, et al: Relative efficacy of alcohol and propranolol in action tremor. *Can J Neurol Sci* 2:31–35, 1975.
9. Higgins JJ, Pho LT, Nee LE: A gene (*ETM*) for essential tremor maps to chromosome 2p22–. *Mov Disord* 12:859–864, 1997.
10. Findley LJ: Epidemiology and genetics of essential tremor. *Neurology* 54 (suppl 4):s8–s13, 2000.
11. Findley LJ, Gresty MA: Tremor. *Br J Hosp Med* 26:16–32, 1981.
12. Rajput AH, Rozdilsky B, Ang L, et al: Clinicopathological observations in essential tremor: Report of six cases. *Neurology* 41:1422–1424, 1991.
13. Rajput AH, Rozdilsky B, Ang L: Occurrence of resting tremor in Parkinson's disease. *Neurology* 41:1298–1299, 1991.
14. Fitzgerald PM, Jankovic J: Orthostatic tremor: An association with essential tremor. *Mov Disord* 1:60–64, 1991.
15. Kishore A, Calne DB: Involuntary movements: an overview, in Joseph AB, Young RR (eds): *Movement Disorders in Neurology and Neuropsychiatry*. Boston: Blackwell Scientific, 2000, pp 1–2.
16. Baldessarini RJ, Cole JO, Davis JM, et al: Tardive dyskinesia: Summary of a task force report of the American Psychiatric Association. *Am J Psychiatry* 137:1163–1172, 1980.
17. Faheem AD, Brightwell DR, Burton GC, et al: Respiratory dyskinesia and dysarthria from prolonged neuroleptic use: Tardive dyskinesia? *Am J Psychiatry* 139:517–518, 1982.
18. Shoulson I: On chorea. *Clin Neuropharmacol* 9(suppl 2):s85–s99, 1986.
19. Ad Hoc Committee (1984): Ad Hoc Committee of the Dystonia Medical Research Foundation meeting in February 1984.
20. Jedynak CP, Bonnet AM, Agid Y: Tremor and idiopathic dystonia. *Mov Disord* 6:230–236, 1991.
21. Obeso JA, Rothwell JC, Lang AE, Marsden CD: Myoclonic dystonia. *Neurology* 33:825–830, 1983.
22. Ravits J, Hallet M, Baker M, et al: Primary writing tremor and myoclonic writer's cramp. *Neurology* 35:1387–1391, 1985.
23. Kurlan R, Behr J, Medved L, et al: Myoclonus and dystonia: A family study. *Adv Neurol* 50:385–389, 1988.
24. Quinn NP, Rothwell JC, Thompson PD, Marsden CD: Hereditary myoclonic dystonia, hereditary torsion dystonia and hereditary essential myoclonus: An area of confusion. *Adv Neurol* 50:391–401, 1988.
25. Segawa M, Hosaka A, Miyagawa F, et al: Hereditary progressive dystonia with marked diurnal variation. *Adv Neurol* 14:215–233, 1976.
26. Nygaard TG, Marsden CD, Duvoisin RC: Dopa responsive dystonia. *Adv Neurol* 50:377–384, 1988.
27. Tanaka H, Endo K, Tsuji S, et al: The gene for hereditary progressive dystonia with marked diurnal fluctuation maps to chromosome 14q. *Ann Neurol* 37:405–408, 1995.
28. Ichinose H, Suzuki T, Inagaki H, et al: Molecular genetics of dopa-responsive dystonia. *Biol Chem* 380:1355–1364, 1999.
29. Fahn S: Concept and classification of dystonia. *Adv Neurol* 50:1–8, 1988.
30. Pettigrew LC, Jankovic J: Hemidystonia: A report of 22 patients and a review of the literature. *J Neurol Neurosurg Psychiatry* 48:650–657, 1985.
31. Marsden CD, Obeso JA, Zarranz JA, Lang AE: The anatomical basis of symptomatic hemidystonia. *Brain* 108:463–484, 1985.
32. Lee LV, Kupke KG, Caballar-Onazaga F, et al: The phenotype of the X-linked dystonia-parkinsonism syndrome—an assessment of 42 cases in the Philippines. *Medicine* 70:179–187, 1991.
33. Fahn S, Williams DT: Psychogenic dystonia. *Adv Neurol* 50:431–455, 1988.
34. Friedman A, Fahn S: Spontaneous remissions in spasmodic torticollis. *Neurology* 36:398–400, 1986.
35. Sharp FR, Rando TA, Greenberg SA, et al: Pseudochoreoathetosis: Movements associated with loss of proprioception. *Arch Neurol* 51:1103–1109, 1994.
36. Lance JW, Adams RD: The syndrome of action myoclonus as a sequel to hypoxic encephalopathy. *Brain* 86:111–136, 1963.
37. Frenken CWGM, Notermans SLH, Korten JJ, et al: Myoclonic disorders of spinal origin. *Clin Neurol Neurosurg* 79:107–118, 1978.
38. Lapresle J: Palatal myoclonus. *Adv Neurol* 43:265–273, 1986.
39. Ronthal M, Greenstein P: Myoclonus and asterixis, in Joseph AB, Young RR (eds): *Movement Disorders in Neurology and Neuropsychiatry*. Boston: Blackwell Scientific, 1999, pp 449–456.
40. Kurlan R: Tic disorders: An overview, in Joseph AB, Young RR (eds): *Movement Disorders in Neurology and Neuropsychiatry*. Boston: Blackwell Scientific, 1999, pp 437–441.
41. Jankovic J: The neurology of tics, in Marsden CD, Fahn S (eds): *Movement Disorders* 2. London: Butterworth, 1987, pp 383–405.
42. Kroisel PM, Petek E, Emberger N, et al: Candidate region for Gilles de la Tourette syndrome at 7q31. *Am J Med Genet* 101:259–261, 2001.
43. Kurlan R, Lichter D, Hewitt D: Sensory tics in Tourette's syndrome. *Mov Disord* 6:248–252, 1991.
44. Klawans HL, Falk DK, Nausieda PA, et al: Gilles de la Tourette syndrome after long-term chlorpromazine therapy. *Neurology* 28:1064–1068, 1978.
45. Dure IV LS, Percy AK: Rett syndrome: A clinical and neurobiologic review, in Joseph AB, Young RR (eds): *Movement Disorders in Neurology and Neuropsychiatry*. Boston: Blackwell Scientific, 1999, pp 613–622.
46. Gibb WRG, Lees AJ: The clinical phenomenon of akathasia. *J Neurol Neurosurg Psychiatry* 49:881–886, 1986.
47. Coleman RM: Periodic movements in sleep (nocturnal myoclonus) and restless leg syndrome, in Guilleminault C (ed): *Sleeping and Waking Disorders: Indications and Techniques*. Menlo Park, CA: Addison Wesley, 1982, pp 265–296.
48. Lugaresi E, Cirignotta F, Coccagna GP, et al: Nocturnal myoclonus and restless leg syndrome. *Adv Neurol* 43:295–307, 1986.
49. Wetter TC, Pollmacher T: Restless legs and periodic leg movements in sleep syndromes. *J Neurol* 244(suppl 1):S37–S45, 1997.

50. Ekbom KA: Restless legs, in Vinken PJ, Bruyn GW (eds): *Handbook of Clinical Neurology: Diseases of Nerves.* Amsterdam: Elsevier Science, 1970, pp 311–320.

51. Spillaine JD, Nathan PW, Kelly RE, Marsden CD: Painful legs and moving toes. *Brain* 94:541–556, 1971.

52. Montagna P, Cirignotta F, Sacqugna T, et al: 'Painful legs and moving toes' associated with polyneuropathy. *J Neurol Neurosurg Psychiatry* 46:399–403, 1983.

53. Dressler D, Thompson PD, Gledhill RF, et al: The syndrome of painful legs and moving toes. *Mov Disord* 9:13–21, 1994.

54. Barnes TRE, Braude WM: Akathasia variants and tardive dyskinesia. *Arch Gen Psychiatry* 42:874–878, 1985.

55. Jankovic J, Glass JP: Metoclopramide-induced phantom dyskinesia. *Neurology* 35:432–435, 1985.

56. Kulisevsky J, Marti-Fabregas J, Grau JM: Spasms of amputation stumps. *J Neurol Neurosurg Psychiatry* 55:626–627, 1992.

57. Pryles CV, Livingston S, Ford FR: Familial paroxysmal choreoathetosis of Mount and Reback. *Pediatrics* 9:44–47, 1952.

58. Stevens H: Paroxysmal choreoathetosis—a form of reflex epilepsy. *Arch Neurol* 14:415–420, 1966.

59. Jung S, Chen KM, Brody JA: Paroxysmal choreoathetosis. *Neurology* 23:749–755, 1973.

60. Weber MB: Familial paroxysmal dystonia. *J Nerv Ment Dis* 145:221–226, 1967.

61. Walker ES: Familial paroxysmal dystonic choreoathetosis: A neurologic disorder simulating psychiatric illness. *Johns Hopkins Med J* 148:108–113, 1981.

62. Bennet DA, Goetz CG: Acquired paroxysmal dyskinesias, in Joseph AB and Young RR (eds): *Movement Disorders in Neurology and Neuropsychiatry.* Boston: Blackwell Scientific, 1992, pp 540–556.

63. Oguni M, Oguni H, Kosaza MY, et al: A case with nocturnal paroxysmal unilateral dystonia and interictal right frontal epileptic EEG focus: A lateralized variant of nocturnal paroxysmal dystonia. *Brain Dev* 14:412–416, 1992.

64. Meierkord H, Fish DR, Smith SJ: Is nocturnal paroxysmal dystonia a form of frontal lobe epilepsy? *Mov Disord* 7:38–41, 1992.

65. Andermann F, Andermann E: Startle disease or hyperekplexia (letter). *Ann Neurol* 16:367–368, 1984.

66. Gambardella A, Valention P, Annesi G, et al: Hyperekplexia in a patient with a brainstem anomaly. *Acta Neurol Scand* 99:255–259, 1999.

67. Bundick T Jr, Spinella M: Subjective experience, involuntary movement and posterior alien hand syndrome. *J Neurol Neurosurg Psychiatry* 68:83–85, 2000.

68. Levine DN: The alien hand, in Joseph AB, Young RR (eds): *Movement Disorders in Neurology and Neuropsychiatry.* Boston: Blackwell Scientific, 1992, pp 691–695.

69. Riley DE, Lang AE, Lewis A, et al: Cortico-basal ganglionic degeneration. *Neurology* 40:1203–1212, 1990.

70. Bogen JE: The callosal syndrome, in Heiman KM, Valenstein E (eds): *Clinical Neuropsychology.* New York: Oxford University Press, 1979, pp 308–359.

71. Goldenberg G, Mayer NH, Toglia JV: Medial frontal cortex and the alien hand sign. *Arch Neurol* 36: 683–686, 1981.

72. Levine DN, Rinn WE: Opticosensory ataxia and alien hand syndrome after posterior cerebral artery infarction. *Neurology* 36:1094–1097, 1986.

73. Martilla R, Rinn UK: Disability and progression of Parkinson's disease. *Acta Neurol Scand* 56:159–169, 1977.

74. Jankovic J, McDermott M, Carter J, et al: Variable expression of Parkinson's disease: A baseline assessment of the DATATOP cohort. *Neurology* 40:1529–1534, 1990.

75. Weiner WJ, Nora LM, Glantz RH: Elderly inpatients: Postural reflex impairment. *Neurology* 34:945–947, 1984.

76. Calne DB, Snow BJ, Lee CS: Criteria for diagnosing Parkinson's disease. *Ann Neurol* 32:S125–S127, 1992.

77. Lang AE: Parkinsonism in corticobasal degeneration. *Adv Neurol* 82:83–89, 2000.

78. Reed LA, Wszolek ZK, Hutton M: Phenotypic correlations in FTDP-17. *Neurobiol Aging* 22:89–107, 2001.

79. Pillon B, Dubois B, Agid Y: Testing cognition may contribute to the diagnosis of movement disorders. *Neurology* 46:329–334, 1996.

80. Cudkowicz ME, Martin TB, Koroshetz WJ: The neurology of Huntington's disease, in Joseph AB, Young RR (eds): *Movement Disorders in Neurology and Neuropsychiatry.* Boston: Blackwell Scientific, 1999, pp 147–154.

81. Rubio JP, Danek A, Stone C, et al: Choreoacanthocytosis: Genetic linkage to chromosome 9q21. *Am J Hum Genet* 61:899–908, 1997.

82. Ikeuchi T, Koide K, Onodera R, et al: Dentatorubropallidoluysian atrophy (DRPLA): Molecular basis for wide clinical features of DRPLA. *Clin Neurosci* 3:23–27, 1995.

83. Hayden MR, Martin WRW, Stoessl AJ, et al: Positron emission tomography in the early diagnosis of Huntington's disease. *Neurology* 36:888–894, 1986.

84. Martin WRW, Cark CM, Amman W, et al: Cortical glucose metabolism in Huntington's disease. *Neurology* 42:223–229, 1992.

85. Leenders KL, Quinn N, Frackowiak RSJ, Marsden CD: Brain dopaminergic system studied in patients with dystonia using positron emission tomography. *Adv Neurol* 50:243–247, 1988.

86. Stoessl AJ, Martin WRW, Clark CM, et al: PET studies in cerebral glucose metabolism in idiopathic torticollis. *Neurology* 36:653–657, 1986.

87. Snow BJ, Bhatt MH, Martin WRW, Calne DB: Dopaminergic metabolism in Wilson's disease studied with positron emission tomography. *J Neurol Neurosurg Psychiatry* 53:12–17, 1990.

88. Leenders KL, Salmon EP, Tyrell P, et al: The nigrostriatal dopaminergic system assessed *in vivo* by positron emission tomography in healthy volunteer subjects and patients with Parkinson's disease. *Arch Neurol* 47:1290–1298, 1990.

89. Martin WRW, Stoessl JA, Adam MJ, et al: Positron emission tomography in Parkinson's disease: Glucose and DOPA metabolism. Parkinson's disease. *Adv Neurol* 45:95–101, 1986.

90. Bhatt MH, Snow BJ, Martin WRW, et al: Positron emission tomography in progressive supranuclear palsy. *Arch Neurol* 48:389–391, 1991.

91. Bhatt MH, Snow BJ, Martin WRW, Calne DB: Positron emission tomography in Shy-Drager syndrome. *Ann Neurol* 28:101–103, 1990.

92. Eidelberg D, Takikawa S, Moeller JR, et al: Striatal hypometabolism distinguishes striatonigral degeneration from Parkinson's disease. *Ann Neurol* 33:518–527, 1993.

93. Sawle GV, Brooks DJ, Marsden CD, et al: Corticobasal ganglionic degeneration. *Brain* 114:541–556, 1991.

NEUROBEHAVIORAL ASPECTS OF MOVEMENT DISORDERS

MARGARET M. SWANBERG, DEAN FOTI, and
JEFFREY CUMMINGS

FRONTAL SUBCORTICAL CIRCUITS   17
NEUROPSYCHIATRIC DISTURBANCES   18
    Depression   19
    Mania   20
    Psychosis   21
    Personality Alterations   21
    Obsessive-Compulsive Disorder (OCD)   22
    Anxiety   23
    Sleep and Sexual Disturbances   24
COGNITIVE DISTURBANCES   24
    Executive Function   25
    Memory   25
    Speech and Language   26
    Visuospatial Function   26
    Praxis   27
DEMENTIA   27
COMMENT   29

Behavioral changes accompany most movement disorders and were frequently acknowledged in the initial reports of basal ganglia diseases. Kinnier Wilson used the term "psychical" in reference to the behavior of 8 of the 12 patients he reported with "Wilson's disease" in 1912.[1] Similarly, George Huntington referred to "insanity with a tendency to suicide" as an essential feature of the disease that bears his name.[2] James Parkinson's essay on the shaking palsy refers to the "unhappy sufferer," but his comment "the senses and intellect remain uninjured" was considerably less accurate.[3] However, an appreciation of the shared substrate of behavior and movement disorders was not fully understood for many years, and a multitude of psychodynamic and "reactive" theories were proposed,[4–6] or cognitive and emotional disorders were simply ignored and left unstudied. A compelling argument for common neurophysiological processes underlying motion and emotion is the high frequency of intellectual impairment, depression, and personality changes in diseases of the basal ganglia, as well as the common occurrence of motor disorders seen in schizophrenia, affective disorders, and obsessive-compulsive disorder.[7] The psychosocial aspects of movement disorders play a role in behavioral and affective changes of basal ganglia

disease, but animal experiments,[8] progress in understanding frontal subcortical circuits,[9–12] and evidence from focal lesions of the basal ganglia[13,14] have clarified the anatomic substrate of behavior changes in conditions with subcortical dysfunction.

The principal theme developed in this chapter is that behavioral changes are common to a number of movement disorders and are an expression of the interruption of specific components of frontal subcortical circuits. Summary of the relevant frontal subcortical circuits as they apply to behavior is presented, followed by an overview of neurobehavioral aspects of movement disorders, divided into the various behavioral "domains" of the basal ganglia: neuropsychiatric symptoms, mild cognitive changes, and dementia.

Frontal Subcortical Circuits

There are five circuits linking the frontal lobes and subcortical structures: motor, oculomotor, dorsolateral prefrontal, lateral orbitofrontal, and anterior cingulate.[9–11] The latter three originate in the prefrontal cortex and are responsible for distinct neurobehavioral syndromes involving cognition and emotion.[9] All circuits share common structures and organization, originating in the frontal lobe with sequential projections to the striatum, globus pallidus (GP)/substantia nigra (SN), and thalamus, ultimately linking back to the frontal lobe (Fig. 2-1). Each circuit has a direct and an indirect (via GP external and subthalamic nucleus) pathway from the striatum to the GP interna (GPi)/SN. The circuits adjacent to each other remain anatomically segregated. The inputs to the circuits are broad and may involve functionally related structures outside of the circuit, whereas the output is more specific to localized cortical areas. The original concept of five major circuits proposed by Alexander in 1986 has recently been modified, with some circuits composed of several parallel segregated circuits.[15,16] The fundamental idea of two limbic circuits and a dorsolateral prefrontal executive circuit is preserved.

The dorsolateral prefrontal circuit originates in the frontal lobe convexity and projects to the dorsolateral head of the caudate, with subsequent projections to the more lateral dorsomedial GP and rostral SN.[11,12] These neurons then project to the ventral anterior (VA) and medial dorsal (MD) thalamic nuclei, which connect back to the dorsolateral prefrontal cortex. Disruption of this circuit results in a dorsolateral prefrontal syndrome with deficits in executive function and motor programming.[9,12] These patients exhibit difficulties in maintaining or shifting set, generating organizational strategies, and retrieving memories, and they have reduced verbal and nonverbal fluency.[17,18] Functional aspects of this area are assessed by the Wisconsin Card Sort Test (WCST), Trails A and B, proverb interpretation, odd-man-out, sequencing tests such as the tower of Hanoi, and tests requiring alternating or withholding of motor responses.[19]

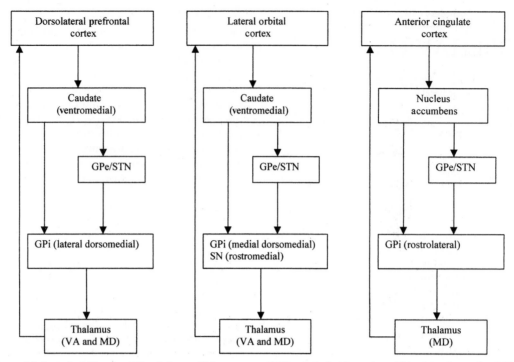

FIGURE 2-1 Frontal Subcortical Circuits. GPe, globus pallidus externa; STN, subthalamic nucleus; VA, ventral anterior; MD, medial dorsal; GPi, globus pallidus interna.

The lateral orbitofrontal circuit (Fig. 2-1) originates in the inferolateral prefrontal cortex and projects to the ventromedial caudate nucleus, which then projects to the dorsomedial GP and rostromedial SN. These projections are to areas similar to the dorsolateral frontal circuit, but more medial in all the involved structures. The return path is via the VA and MD thalamic nuclei, which project back to the orbitofrontal cortex. The integrity of this circuit is important in the inhibition of interference from external cues and in self-monitoring. Disturbance of the orbitofrontal circuit results in significant personality alterations consisting primarily of disinhibition and irritability.

The third behavioral circuit is the anterior cingulate circuit (Fig. 2-1), originating in the anterior cingulate gyrus and projecting to the ventral striatum. The latter includes the nucleus accumbens, olfactory tubercle, and parts of the ventromedial caudate and putamen. There are multiple additional limbic inputs to the ventral striatum. The ventral striatum then connects to the ventral and rostrolateral GP and rostrodorsal SN, which in turn project to the paramedian part of the MD nucleus of the thalamus, which ultimately projects back to the anterior cingulate cortex. Dysfunction in this circuit results in the medial frontal-anterior cingulate syndrome with apathy and reduced initiative. The integrity of this circuit is critical for drive and motivation.

Disruption of multiple frontal subcortical circuits by basal ganglia disease results in the frequent occurrence of personality and mood disorders, as well as cognitive dysfunction in patients with movement disorders. Thus, movement disorders can be considered markers of disease affecting structural and neurochemical components of frontal subcortical circuits. Movement abnormalities occur primarily with disease affecting caudate, putamen, and subthalamic nucleus, whereas disorders of prefrontal cortex and thalamus have less effect on motility.

Neuropsychiatric Disturbances

Degenerative diseases of the basal ganglia are associated with movement disorders and neuropsychiatric syndromes. Behavioral changes also are noted in focal disease of the basal ganglia. The nature of neuropsychiatric symptoms found in movement disorders is similar to that seen in primary psychiatric disease, and there is support from neuroimaging studies that identical regions may be involved. The neuropsychiatric symptoms include depression, mania, personality change, psychosis, obsessive-compulsive disorder, anxiety, apathy, sexual behavior changes, and sleep disturbance.

TABLE 2-1 Movement Disorders with Depression

Parkinson's disease
Dementia with Lewy bodies
Huntington's disease
Corticobasal degeneration
Idiopathic calcification of the basal ganglia
Wilson's disease
Vascular parkinsonism
Progressive supranuclear palsy
Neuroacanthocytosis
Spinocerebellar degenerations
Gilles de la Tourette syndrome

DEPRESSION

Depression refers to an alteration in mood, with significant sadness, hopelessness, and anhedonia, and is often associated with change in appetite, loss of sexual drive, sleep disturbances, psychomotor retardation, and fatigue.[7] Depression occurs in a number of movement disorders (Table 2-1). Difficulties in assessing the prevalence of depression in movement disorders arise primarily from variability in assessment techniques. Recent studies have used standardized questionnaires such as the Geriatric Depression Rating Scale (GDS),[20] Beck Depression Inventory (BDI),[21] Hamilton Rating Scale for Depression (HAMD),[22] Montgomery-Asberg Scale for Depression,[23] and the Neuropsychiatric Inventory (NPI).[24] There is also the variability of selection criteria and referral biases. Finally, depression in hypokinetic movement disorders such as Parkinson's disease (PD) can be more complicated to assess, as psychomotor slowing is an integral aspect of the motor manifestations.

Dysfunction in either the orbitofrontal or the dorsolateral frontal circuit is associated with depression.[9] In particular, the caudate appears to have a key role in mediating mood, as disorders of the caudate nucleus have a high rate of depression.[25] Depression has been associated with orbital and caudate hypometabolism on positron emission tomography (PET) in both PD and Huntington's disease (HD).[26,27]

PARKINSON'S DISEASE

Depression is common in patients with PD. The frequency of depression overall is approximately 40 percent. The motor manifestations of PD confound the use of standardized inventories in PD. The BDI has been found to have variable sensitivity and may be useful as a screening instrument;[28] the HAMD-17 and the Montgomery-Asberg Depression Rating Scales are very useful in differentiating depressed from nondepressed PD patients.[29] The severity of the depression is sufficient to meet criteria for a major depressive episode in slightly more than 20–50 percent of those with mood disorders, with the others manifesting dysthymia or minor depression.[25]

The relationships of depression with motor impairment, age of onset, disease duration and severity, and degree of cognitive impairment continue to be areas of debate. Some authors suggest that those meeting criteria for a major depressive episode are likely to have more advanced disease, higher akinesia scores, greater cognitive impairment, and higher incidence of falls.[30] A prospective study by Giladi et al.[31] found an association between disease severity and presence of depression and dementia in an older age-of-onset subgroup of PD patients, but not in younger age-of-onset patients. Depression was associated with younger age-of-onset, regardless of disease severity. Other studies have shown that depression prevalence is independent of age, disease duration, or severity. In nearly 25 percent of PD patients who are depressed, the depression precedes the onset of motor symptoms.[31,32] Depression may be a prodromal symptom in a subgroup of patients with younger age-of-onset, decreased severity, and stronger family history.[33]

Clinical manifestations of depression in PD include apathy, psychomotor retardation, memory impairment, pessimism, irrationality, and suicidal ideation without significant suicidal behavior. Psychotic depression is rare. However, anxiety is seen more often among elderly depressed than younger depressed patients and may not be specific to PD. The nature of the depression of PD is not identical to that seen in idiopathic depression; there is more sadness without significant guilt or self-blame, and a high rate of anxiety.[25,34,35]

Depression is associated with greater cognitive dysfunction in PD. Those with depression perform more poorly on executive function tasks, such as the WCST, verbal fluency, and trail-making. Longitudinal follow-up of depressed versus non-depressed PD patients over a 4-year period by Starkstein and coworkers showed a significantly greater decline in cognitive function in depressed patients.[36] The presence of depression and dementia are significantly associated.[37]

The etiology of depression in PD is not fully determined. The contributions of reactive versus endogenous factors remain to be identified.[38–40] Depression often predates motor disabilities,[33] and PD patients are more depressed than other disabled patients matched for severity of functional impairment.[41] These findings argue against a predominant psychosocial model. There is a serotonergic deficit in PD, which may be important in mediating depression. Studies of nondepressed versus depressed PD patients showed lower cerebrospinal fluid (CSF) 5-hydroxyindoeacetic acid (5-HIAA) in the depressed group, but severity of depression did not correlate with the level, nor did all depressed patients have low CSF 5-HIAA.[40,42] Depressed patients also have been found to have lower levels than those diagnosed with dysthymia. Pathologically, greater reduction of dorsal raphe nuclei serotonergic neurons have been found in the brains of depressed PD patients compared to nondepressed patients.[43] The role of dopamine in PD with depression is not clear. Decreased levels of dopamine in PD may confer an increased risk of depression; many patients evidenced increased severity of depressive symptomatology during the "off" state. However, treatment with dopamine-containing agents does not alleviate depression. Alterations in norepinephrine levels have been variably associated with depression in PD. Differences in neurotransmitter changes because of variable cell loss in subcortical nuclei in PD may explain why only a subgroup of patients become depressed.

Imaging has shown regional metabolic differences between depressed and nondepressed PD patients. Using PET, Ring and colleagues have shown a selective decrease in medial frontal metabolism in both depressed PD patients as well as in those with idiopathic depression, whereas these changes were not present in nondepressed PD patients.[26] Berg et al., using magnetic resonance imaging (MRI) and transcranial sonography, have shown that there are alterations in the signal of the midline brainstem nuclei, including the raphe nuclei, in depressed PD patients when compared to nondepressed patients matched for age and disease duration.[44]

A model has been proposed by Cummings for the pathogenesis of depression in PD that hinges on biochemical abnormalities in the cortex and basal ganglia, resulting in the behaviors of decreased reward mediation, environmental dependency, and inadequate stress response.[24] These behavioral deficiencies result in symptoms of apathy, worthlessness, helplessness, hopelessness, and dysphoria.

HUNTINGTON'S DISEASE

Depression is common in HD, with approximately half of patients affected and 30 percent meeting criteria for major depressive episode.[45–48] It is the second most common neuropsychiatric disorder in HD (after dementia) and may precede the neurological symptoms by 2–20 years. Depression is a frequent early finding in HD. A large study examining over 1200 individuals with HD found that 40 percent endorsed depression within 12 months of disease onset.[49] Suicide is four to six times more common in HD than in other depressed patients, and up to 20 times higher in the age group 50–69 years.[45,50] Increased impulsivity because of associated dysfunction of the orbitofrontal circuit may result in the higher rate of suicide. Interruption of the anterior cingulate circuit by dysfunction in the ventral striatum may result in diminished motivation in combination with reduced reinforcement of reward-oriented behavior, behavioral changes that manifest in the symptoms of worthlessness, hopelessness, and apathy. PET studies reveal that depression in HD is associated with reduced glucose metabolism in the orbitofrontal and inferior prefrontal regions similar to that found in depressed patients without a primary neurologic disorder.[51]

OTHER MOVEMENT DISORDERS

Depression is the second most common psychiatric manifestation in Wilson's disease (WD), occurring in 20–30 percent.[49,52–54] Only personality alterations are more common. Depression is unlikely to be purely reactive, as it frequently presents before diagnosis or disability. However, it is generally poorly responsive to treatment of the copper disorder. In addition, depression is common in dementia with Lewy bodies (DLBD), with a frequency approximating or greater than that seen in Alzheimer's disease.[55,56] Depression also occurs frequently in corticobasal degeneration.[57]

Other movement disorders in which depression occurs include progressive supranuclear palsy (PSP), neuroacanthocytosis, idiopathic calcification of the basal ganglia (ICBG), and Tourette's syndrome (TS).[49,58–61]

MANIA

Mania seen in the course of primary bipolar disorder frequently has an associated movement disorder of hyperkinesis. Similarly, classic movement disorders have been associated with mania (Table 2-2). Secondary mania is characterized by elated and/or irritable mood for at least 1 week, with three of the associated features of hyperactivity, pressured speech, flight of ideas, grandiosity, decreased sleep, distractibility, and lack of judgment in the absence of delirium or dementia. Hypomania has similar diagnostic criteria but with shorter duration of at least 4 days, and milder symptoms producing less interference with functioning. Secondary mania has been associated with a wide variety of neurological, metabolic, and toxic etiologies.

The movement disorder most commonly associated with mania is HD.[45–47,62] Approximately 10 percent of HD patients develop hypomania with increased energy, elevated mood, decreased sleep, pressured speech, and sometimes associated hypersexuality. While the majority of HD patients with an affective disorder will manifest depression, approximately 25 percent will actually meet criteria for bipolar disorder. Hypomania is more common than mania, but the latter may occur. There are reports of hypomania and mania in WD,[52–54] postencephalitic parkinsonism,[63] and Gerstmann-Straussler-Scheinker disease, a familial prion disease with cerebellar symptoms and dementia. Mania and hemiballismus have been described following right thalamic infarction, and the majority of focal lesions producing mania occur on the right side of the brain.[64,65] Although mania does not occur in untreated PD, drug-induced mania, hypomania, and euphoria occur in 1.5–12 percent of patients treated

TABLE 2-2 Movement Disorders with Hypomania/Mania

Huntington's disease
Wilson's disease
Parkinson's disease
Postencephalitic parkinsonism
Sydenham's chorea
Gerstmann-Straussler-Scheinker disease
Idiopathic calcification of the basal ganglia

with L-dopa or dopamine agonists. Mania has been reported with selegiline. The risk of these drug-induced behaviors is higher in PD patients with a past history of hypomania or mania.[66]

The pathogenesis of secondary mania is uncertain, but evidence from focal lesions suggests that the region abutting the third ventricle near the hypothalamus in the midline as well as the right basotemporal or inferofrontal region[65] are of importance in the mediation of manic symptoms.

PSYCHOSIS

Psychosis is a loss of reality testing resulting from the inability to accurately evaluate perceptions or thought, leading the patient to make incorrect inferences about external reality. Like mania, there are a number of secondary causes of psychosis. The anatomic correlates of secondary psychosis involve subcortical structures, as well as cortex, particularly temporoparietal cortex.[67] However, the relationship of a schizophreniform psychosis to the basal ganglia is specifically linked to diseases that affect the caudate nucleus. The etiologies of the degenerative basal ganglia disorders with psychosis also support involvement of the caudate. Schizophreniform psychosis (with disordered thought content and form) is more common in HD and ICBG, which affect predominantly the caudate.[49,62,68] In contrast, WD, Hallervorden-Spatz's disease, and idiopathic PD are associated less commonly with psychosis and have minimal structural effects on the caudate.[48,52,53] The psychosis in the caudate disorders tends to be refractory to management.

Psychosis occurs in 6–25 percent of HD patients, although the number presenting with psychosis is less clear. A large analysis of 1238 patients with HD found that within 1 year of onset of disease nearly 12 percent suffered from suspiciousness and paranoia and 5 percent had delusions or hallucinations. Over the course of disease 37 percent demonstrated paranoia, and 30 percent demonstrated delusions.[49]

The neuropathology of psychosis in HD is not well understood. Theories include a relative hyperdopaminergic state superimposed on abnormal subcortical circuits.[69] The early occurrence of behavioral changes in the absence of movement disorder may relate to the preferential early loss of spiny neurons in the medial caudate. Utilizing functional neuroimaging, there appears to be bihemispheric decreased metabolism in psychotic HD patients with a reduction in the number of striatal D2 receptors.[70] Psychosis has been linked to a higher number of trinucleotide repeats.[71]

Psychosis may be seen in ICBG at an early age before the emergence of the movement disorder, and in a variety of other disorders (Table 2-3). WD is associated with many behavioral changes; however, reviews note that schizophreniform psychosis is uncommon.[54,72] Schizophreniform states with delusions, hallucinations, and catatonia were often seen in postencephalitic parkinsonism, and patients were susceptible to recurrence of psychosis when treated with L-dopa.

TABLE 2-3 Movement Disorders with Psychosis

Huntington's disease
Idiopathic calcification of the basal ganglia
Sydenham's chorea
Postencephalitic parkinsonism
Parkinson's disease
Vascular parkinsonism
Dementia with Lewy bodies
Wilson's disease
Thalamic degenerations
Prion diseases
    Creutzfeldt-Jakob disease
    Gerstmann-Straussler-Scheinker disease

Drug-associated psychosis is common in PD. It occurs most often in the setting of a clear sensorium, with primarily visual hallucinations, but a confusional psychosis can occur with dementia or anticholinergic use. The majority of the hallucinations consist of normal-sized, stationary people with a variable duration.[73] More recent studies have found that use of dopamine-containing agents alone cannot account for the prevalence of psychosis in PD.[74,75] Hallucinations are present in approximately 23–30 percent of PD patients. Several other factors, including disease severity, dementia, depression, poor visual acuity, and altered sleep-wake cycle, are risk factors for the occurrence of psychosis.[73,76]

Hallucinations, a core feature of the diagnosis of DLB, and delusions, a supportive feature, are common, with a prevalence of 20–80 percent.[77] These delusions and hallucinations are more complex and bizarre, with more frequent misidentifications; this aids in distinguishing DLB from Alzheimer's.[78]

The relationship between movement disorders and psychosis is found in the disruption of structures of the limbic striatum. The structures are either affected directly, as in HD, or disturbed functionally, as in the thalamic degenerations. Dopamine also plays a role, as psychosis is rarely seen in dopamine-deficient disorders such as idiopathic PD but is prominent in HD, in which there is relative preservation of dopamine. The variety of motor abnormalities that occurs in schizophrenia may reflect similar dysfunction in frontal subcortical circuits.

PERSONALITY ALTERATIONS

Personality refers to a behavioral style: one's feelings, attitudes, predominant mood, and pattern of behavior. The disturbances noted in movement disorders include apathy, irritability, lability, impulsivity, aggression, agitation, and sometimes even violence. The presentation of personality changes before the appearance of the movement disorder argues for a neuroanatomic substrate for the behavioral alterations. Similar behaviors occur in the setting of frontal lobe injuries, and disruption of prefrontal projections is essential in the production of personality change in movement disorders.

Apathy is frequently reported in globus pallidus lesions resulting from carbon monoxide (CO) poisoning, with concomitant "psychic akinesia." This can often be reversed by external stimuli, an observation also made with postencephalitic parkinsonism. Similarly, patients with HD have early loss of spontaneity but will engage in tasks when external stimuli are supplied. Once the stimulation is removed, inertia returns. These deficits are likely mediated by disruption of the medial frontal-anterior cingulate subcortical circuit.

Early personality change with irritability, indifference, and lability of mood is described in progressive supranuclear palsy (PSP). Apathy and disinhibition are found more frequently in PSP than in PD.[58]

The rate of personality changes in WD ranges from 20 to 46 percent; irritability with anger, lack of appropriate emotion, apathy, compulsive behaviors, hostile feelings, and reduced sexual interest have been described.[53] There is a tendency for patients with WD to underreport their symptoms.

Personality changes in HD are ubiquitous, with apathy, irritability, lability, and impulsivity frequently described. Aggression in HD can occur in the setting of personality disorders, psychosis, or depression, with a frequency of approximately 60 percent. Folstein found that 30 percent of 182 HD patients met criteria for intermittent explosive disorder and 6 percent for antisocial personality disorder. Irritability and lability occur early in HD when the ventromedial caudate is preferentially affected, disrupting connections to the orbitofrontal cortex.[79] Risky decision-making has been reported in HD, further implicating the frontal subcortical circuits, particularly those with connections to the orbitofrontal cortex.[80]

Aggressive behavior, hyperactivity or temper outbursts are described in 60–70 percent of patients with TS,[61,81] and, in one large study, 49 percent met criteria for attention deficit disorder with hyperactivity. There is no clear relationship between the severity of the tics and behavioral difficulties, and the extent of the genetic connection between TS and attention deficit disorder continues to be debated.

PARKINSON'S DISEASE PERSONALITY

The issue of personality in PD has been much discussed, and no definitive conclusions have been reached. Fifty years ago, PD was considered by some to be a consequence of disordered personality.[5,6] Sands believed that the suppression of emotions ultimately resulted in the symptoms of PD. Although our current understanding of neuropharmacology and neuropathology may dismiss such considerations, the issue of a "premorbid personality" of PD remains contentious. Some have found that PD patients have reduced risk-taking behavior with decreased novelty-seeking, but others have not confirmed this finding.[82] They are often described as rigid, frugal, and contemplative; these characteristics represent diminished novelty-seeking behavior

possibly related to dopamine dysfunction. These interpretations of "personality" may reflect decreased mental flexibility from underlying cognitive impairment.

Studies by Riklan et al.[83] and Smythies[84] found no evidence for a PD personality using standardized personality questionnaires. Others showed that PD patients were morally rigid, cautious, less flexible, and exhibit less novelty-seeking compared to others with similar disability produced by rheumatoid arthritis or orthopedic conditions. Hubble et al. found PD patients to be quieter, less flexible, and more cautious than controls in a retrospective survey of current and premorbid personality.[85] The assessment of current status did not correlate with degree of motor disability but did correlate with depression scores. Twin studies also support a distinctive premorbid personality style, with the affected twin being more introverted. Other reported premorbid traits to include industriousness, punctuality, inflexibility, and cautiousness. PD patients may also have lower lifetime risk of cigarette smoking, coffee drinking, and alcohol consumption,[86,87] and these behaviors may reflect personality-based lifestyle decisions.

Hubble and Koller summarized four potential interpretations of a PD personality: personality contributes to the development of PD; PD causes the personality (the change represents a preclinical phase of disease); personality type and PD may develop in the same at risk population; and, finally, the personality may reflect the early expression of a depressed mood in patients who are at risk for both depression and PD. Until means of detecting PD at a very early presymptomatic state are developed, this issue will remain unresolved.

OBSESSIVE-COMPULSIVE DISORDER (OCD)

OCD is characterized by recurrent obsessions and/or compulsions that interfere significantly with normal routine and are experienced as distressing. Obsessions may be thoughts, images, or impulses and frequently include ideas of dirt, disease, or aggressive or sexual acts. Compulsions are repetitive behaviors or mental acts and typically involve hand-washing, checking, counting, touching, and avoiding. The compulsive behaviors are aimed at reducing stress or preventing a dreaded situation. However, they are often excessive or not connected in a realistic fashion with what they were designed to neutralize or prevent.

The relationship between movement disorders and OCD is most strongly exemplified in consideration of the high association between TS and OCD.[61,81] The frequency of obsessive-compulsive behavior in TS varies from 30 to 60 percent, depending on biases in referral population, diagnostic criteria, and method of data acquisition. Family studies demonstrate that OCD is seen more frequently in close relatives of patients with TS than in controls.[81] Larger studies, which used standardized evaluation techniques, found an overall frequency of obsessive-compulsive behavior in 50 percent of TS patients. Similarly, one sees a higher rate of tics in primary OCD, with 20 percent of children meeting criteria for TS after 2–7 years of follow-up in a study of primary OCD (TS excluded). Family pedigrees are suggestive of gender-specific phenotypic expression within TS families, with females predominantly developing OCD and males TS. There are many overlapping features of OCD and TS, including waxing and waning course, repetitive behaviors and complex movements/rituals, preoccupation with sexual and aggressive content, and partial voluntary suppressibility.[88] The severity of OCD in TS is generally milder than classic OCD and may be more suitably considered as obsessive-compulsive behavior. The nature of the behaviors differs somewhat from primary OCD, with more touching and aligning rituals in TS, as opposed to a higher number of germ-related cleaning rituals in primary OCD. In TS, the OCD symptoms begin in early adolescence and continue or increase, whereas the tics may decrease.

A relationship between OCD and the basal ganglia is suggested by clinical and neurobiological information.[81,89–92] Focal lesions of the basal ganglia have produced symptoms typical of OCD, although the anxiety or distress from withholding compulsions is frequently lacking. OCD has been reported in many movement disorders (Table 2-4). Postencephalitic parkinsonism produces some of the most striking examples, with attacks of compulsive counting and forced thinking frequently associated with oculogyric crises. Sometimes, forced grunting or shouting similar to tics of TS occurred at the same time. OCD has been reported in PSP and in PD, particularly when the right hemisphere is preferentially involved. Clinical manifestations typically include checking, doubting, and cleaning behaviors. OCD symptoms may be more closely linked to severity of disease, with prevalence increasing with greater disease severity.[93] OCD also occurs in choreiform disorders, such as Sydenham's chorea and HD. OCD has been infrequently reported in HD, perhaps because repetitive behaviors were misinterpreted as perseverative rather than recognized as obsessional features associated with the behaviors. Italian researchers have identified a HD pedigree with a 34 percent lifetime prevalence of OCD. They also propose that the incidence of OCD in HD may be higher than reported due to underreporting by

TABLE 2-4 Movement Disorders with Obsessive-Compulsive Disorder

Gilles de la Tourette syndrome
Postencephalitic parkinsonism
Parkinson's disease
Vascular parkinsonism
Progressive supranuclear palsy
Huntington's disease
Sydenham's chorea
Meige's syndrome

patients during screening evaluations as was found in their study.[94]

The neurobiological mechanisms of OCD appear to involve a disturbance in the ventral striatum or pallidum with disruption of the orbitofrontal subcortical circuit. Volumetric MRI studies in TS have shown reduced size of the left caudate, putamen, and pallidum. A small number of PET studies in primary OCD demonstrate increased metabolism in either the orbitofrontal cortex bilaterally, the basal ganglia (particularly caudate), or the thalamus. Cerebral metabolic and perfusion changes are noted following treatment with selective serotonin reuptake inhibitors, with decreases in bilateral caudate nuclei, orbitofrontal cortex, and thalamus.[81,95] The failure of the basal ganglia to suppress or inhibit overlapping motor, cognitive, and limbic circuits may result in recurrent excitation, producing these stereotyped behaviors or movement disorder. Baxter et al. proposed that loss of gating function of the basal ganglia is responsible for the release of ritualistic behavior.[96] The eventual identification of the TS gene will contribute significantly to the understanding of OCD.

ANXIETY

Anxiety is a feeling of worry, uneasiness, dread, or foreboding in the absence of an appropriately threatening stimulus. Anxiety occurs in the setting of a number of psychiatric disorders, including depression, mania, OCD, and schizophrenia. Thus, anxiety may occur in a number of conditions discussed earlier in the chapter. Movement disorders that may initially present with prominent anxiety include WD and HD.[46,47,54] Dewhurst et al. reported that anxiety was present on admission in 12 of 102 patients with HD.[97] As noted, depression in PD is often associated with significant anxiety, and anxiety may predate the onset of motor symptoms.[33] In one large study examining 139 patients utilizing the Neuropsychiatric Inventory,[98] apathy and anxiety were found to cluster together.[75] Anxiety is a common side-effect of medication, occurring in 20 percent of advanced PD patients treated with selegiline. Falling dopamine levels during "off" periods are usually associated with significant anxiety, as well as mood changes, and should prompt readjustment of medications. Fluctuations in mood and anxiety levels can occur independent of motor disability.[99]

Just as anxiety occurs commonly in the setting of movement disorders, anxiety syndromes often have abnormal motor activity, usually associated with the autonomic arousal. There is often pacing, increased respiration, widening of palpebral fissures, raising of eyebrows, and rigid posturing of the body.

It is likely that in anxiety disorders parallel circuits are activated via the limbic striatal circuits, and multiple neurotransmitters, including gamma-aminobutyric acid, norepinephrine, dopamine, and serotonin, are involved.

SLEEP AND SEXUAL DISTURBANCES

Movement disorders can be associated with prominent alterations in sleep and sexual behavior either alone or as part of a dysautonomic state. Pathologic changes in the locus ceruleus and raphe nuclei have been implicated in the autonomic changes in PD.[100] Presynaptic dopamine depletion has been linked to the sleep alterations in PD.[101,102] The projections between the ventral striatum and hypothalamus are also essential in these basic life functions. A few pertinent relationships will be highlighted, but complete discussion is beyond the scope of this chapter.

Sleep disorders can be divided into hypersomnias, insomnias, and parasomnias (sleep-related conditions that do not affect the total amount of sleep).[7] Hypersomnias with increased total sleep time and excessive daytime sleepiness have been reported in patients with focal basal ganglia lesions. Postencephalitic parkinsonism is associated with persisting disturbances in sleep, including sleep-wake reversal and drowsiness alternating with insomnia. Whipple's disease, a disorder with hypersomnalence, diarrhea, cognitive deficits, and supranuclear gaze palsy, is associated with the unique movement disorder oculomasticatory myorhythmia.[103] Excessive daytime sleepiness may be associated with neurogenic sleep apnea that can occur in the multisystem atrophies because of autonomic dysfunction.

Parasomnias are commonly related to the side-effects of dopaminergic agents, with sleep fragmentation, vivid dreams, nightmares, and night terrors. They may occur in basal ganglia disorders independent of dopamine therapy. Rapid eye movement (REM) sleep behavior disorder may occur early in the course of DLBD, and in some reports preceded the onset of the dementia syndrome.[104] Machado-Joseph disease, an autosomal-dominant degenerative disorder that presents with a mixture of cerebellar and extrapyramidal signs, has sleep disturbances in 50 percent of patients with nocturnal cries, nightmares, and disrupted REM sleep.

Sleep disturbances are common in PD. Questionnaire surveys indicate that up to 98 percent of PD patients experienced at least one symptom causing sleep problems since the onset of their disease. Polysomnographic studies in PD have revealed disturbances in sleep macrostructure (reduced sleep efficiency, increased amounts of wakefulness, decreased amounts of REM sleep, and increased REM latency) and disturbances in microstructure (decreased sleep spindles, increased arousals, poorly formed K-complexes, and excessive muscle activity during REM sleep).[105–107] Motor disturbances are numerous, including increased periodic leg movements, reduced turning in bed, and L-dopa-induced myoclonus. REM behavioral disorder is frequent in PD, and in some cases precedes the onset of typical PD symptoms. Reduced REM sleep latency has been associated with hallucinations.[108]

Dopaminergic agents have been implicated as a causative factor in the sleep disturbances seen in PD. Dopamine agonists such as pramipexole and ropinirole have been associated with daytime sleep attacks;[109] however, this has been reported with use of L-dopa and cabergoline.[110,111] Increasing age, advanced disease, and higher dose are important factors contributing to an increased frequency of this side-effect.

Sexual behavior may be similarly divided into hypersexuality, hyposexuality, and sexual deviations.[7] Hypersexuality and hyposexuality are commonly seen in primary psychiatric disease and are frequently a consequence of drugs used in their treatment. Hypersexuality occurs as a side-effect of dopaminergic medication in 0.9–3 percent of PD patients and may occur either with or without mania or psychosis; however, reduced interest and function are much more common.[112,113]

Sexual deviations, including inappropriately disrobing and masturbating in public, have been reported in WD. Changes in sexuality are well documented in HD. Reduced libido and inhibited orgasm are frequently reported.[46,114] Other sexual alterations include increased incidence of sexual assault, promiscuity, incest, exhibitionism, and voyeurism. Paraphilias are also seen in HD and may be more common in male patients with inhibited orgasm and increased sexual interest. Compulsive sexual touching and exhibitionism may occur in the spectrum of behavioral changes associated with TS.

Disturbances in sexual behavior have been linked to pathological involvement of structures in the brainstem and diencephalon. Gorman and Cummings suggest that the inferior frontal cortex, hypothalamus, amygdaloid nuclei, and medial striatal/septal region are relevant areas in the production of sexual dysfunction.[115] The medial striate region in HD is affected early and may underlie the changes in sexual behavior. The similarity of these abnormal sexual behaviors to those seen in frontal lobe injury suggests that the disruption of the orbitofrontal-ventral striatal circuit may be mediating the behavioral change.

Cognitive Disturbances

There has been extensive investigation of the cognitive disturbances associated with movement disorders, particularly PD and HD. Many studies have been hampered by the comorbid motor deficits that interfere with neuropsychological evaluation, but great strides have been made in isolating individual cognitive domains. Other confounding aspects have been the inclusion of groups of patients with both early cognitive decline and advanced dementia, variable severity of motor deficits among subjects, and lack of control for the effects of medication and mood disorders. Cognitive disturbance can occur because of the isolated effects of subcortical pathology, but many movement disorders have additional cortical pathology, which further confounds the characterization of the cognitive deficits. This part of the chapter will summarize pertinent aspects of cognitive dysfunction in the absence of overt dementia. A discussion of dementia follows in the final section of this chapter.

EXECUTIVE FUNCTION

Executive function can be broadly defined as the ability to plan and carry out complex, goal-directed behavior. These functions include planning, organizing, sequencing, and abstracting. The frontal lobes and their connections to subcortical structures are critical for executive function. Many cognitive domains are affected by disturbances of executive function. Impaired executive function is the core early deficit in disorders of the basal ganglia and results in difficulties in the generation, maintenance, shifting, and blending of set. The interruption of the striatal-pallidothalamic-dorsolateral frontal circuit is likely the underlying basis for the disturbance in executive function.

Executive dysfunction can be shown in focal lesions of the basal ganglia in the absence of any other coexisting pathology. However, these disturbances are generally milder than those seen in the degenerative subcortical diseases, such as PD, HD, or PSP. Patients with focal caudate lesions showed impairment on the WCST; fewer concepts were found than by controls.

PARKINSON'S DISEASE

Deficits of executive function in early PD have been consistently demonstrated and may result from dopaminergic and cholinergic deficits alone or in combination.[116,117] Nondemented PD patients showed decreased generation and maintenance of set, and slowness in shifting set in new learning situations without impairments in overlearned tasks.[118] In general, PD patients benefit from external cues and structure. The deficits can result from either perseverative errors or from difficulty shifting attention to a novel stimulus. Deficits in maintaining set, partially by disengaging from infrequent cues more easily and an inability to ignore irrelevant stimuli, may contribute to apparent bradyphrenia when attempting to solve problems. A significant effect of age on cognition with a worsening performance on the WCST in this subset of PD patients who were older has been found.[119] Deficits have been noted in the temporal ordering of events within a procedural task. Executive dysfunction has also been found to contribute to the memory impairment seen in PD and may be more prominent in sporadic PD than in familial PD.[117]

HUNTINGTON'S DISEASE

HD patients often complain early in their course of organizational difficulties, such as scheduling daily activities, organizing their work, and following recipes. Early on they may have impaired planning but intact decision-making.[120] They have particular difficulties in changing mental set, making multiple perseverative errors on tests such as the WCST.

Executive dysfunction and cognitive impairment may predict development of the disease in asymptomatic gene carriers, and is believed by some to be diagnostic even in the absence of the typical motor and affective changes.[121] In addition, assessment of executive function is adequate to monitor disease progression in the early stages.[122] These deficits tend to be more severe than in PD and interfere substantially with evaluation of other domains of cognitive function.

OTHER MOVEMENT DISORDERS

Executive dysfunction can be seen in many other movement disorders, usually in the setting of a subcortical dementia. Few studies have investigated executive tasks in the early course of basal ganglia disease in patients without dementia. However, a study by Pillon et al. showed that PSP patients in the early stages of cognitive decline were more impaired than HD and PD patients on frontal lobe testing.[123] Most of the multisystem atrophies produce only mild intellectual impairment. Robbins and coworkers found executive deficits in striatonigral degeneration in the absence of significant intellectual impairment. Deficits in set shifting and working memory were qualitatively different from those of PSP and PD patients, more closely resembling errors made by patients with frontal lobe dysfunction.[161]

MEMORY

Memory can be divided into the domains of declarative and procedural.[124,125] Declarative memory involves items or episodes that are accessible to conscious recollection, whereas procedural memory involves perceptual or motor skills not readily accessible to conscious recall. The hippocampal memory system is essential in the storage of new information, whereas frontal subcortical circuits are strategic in the organized recall of information. The basal ganglia are important in procedural memory. Thus, it is not surprising that the memory deficits encountered in movement disorders consist of a retrieval deficit for declarative memory, and abnormalities in procedural memory.

Impaired declarative memory has been demonstrated in focal lesions of the caudate, with poor retrieval rather than a storage deficit.[14] Memory defects in HD and PD are similar in character, but they are more severe in HD. The deficits parallel those seen in focal caudate lesions, with impaired retrieval of declarative memories.[126] Disordered executive function may contribute to the memory retrieval deficit, as both HD and PD patients show poor learning strategies, and impaired temporal sequencing of memories.[116,117]

Procedural memory has been studied extensively in early HD. Impairment in motor learning with sparing of declarative memory has been shown reliably in some HD patients. However, variations occur in early HD, with deficits in declarative memory in some and in procedural memory in others. Impaired procedural learning has been demonstrated in a serial reaction-time paradigm in PSP.[127]

Examination of remote memory in HD has shown defective recall with a flat temporal gradient. Beatty et al. showed a deficit of equal severity in recalling information from sequentially more remote decades, which differs significantly from the patterns seen in early Alzheimer's disease or Korsakoff patients.[128] This pattern supports the role of the basal ganglia in "accessing" stored declarative information.

SPEECH AND LANGUAGE

Aphasia is not commonly seen in disorders restricted to the basal ganglia, but speech disorders with altered verbal output are common. Disorders of verbal output include reiterative speech disorders and dysarthria.

Aphasia from focal subcortical lesions is usually associated with damage to the white matter pathways and is thus generally not seen in degenerative diseases of the basal ganglia. Aphasia occurs in movement disorders when there is concomitant cortical pathology. Aphasia has been reported in corticobasal ganglionic degeneration (CBGD) in 21 percent of cases, and several autopsy-confirmed cases of CBGD presented with progressive aphasia.[129–131] The nature of the aphasia is usually characterized as nonfluent, with impaired naming and decreased verbal fluency.[129] Creutzfeldt-Jakob disease frequently has associated aphasia during its course, and it may present with a mixed transcortical aphasia and echolalia with a movement disorder.

More subtle language deficits in sentence comprehension, especially with syntactically embedded questions, have been described in early PD. In demented PD patients, deficits were noted in phrase length, speech melody, information content of spontaneous speech, and comprehension of verbal and written commands when compared to nondemented PD. Verbal fluency is reduced in both PD and HD and less of what is said is considered to be informative.[132] In addition, reduced word retrieval on confrontational naming is found. Reduction in the expression and comprehension of prosody have been noted in PD and HD, hypothesized to reflect decreased emotional cognition, although more recent literature suggests a link between emotional prosody and impaired executive function.[133]

Reiterative speech patterns occur in movement disorders and can be echolalic (the tendency to repeat words and phrases just addressed to the patient) or palilalic (the involuntary repetition of words or phrases initiated by the patient). Echolalia has been reported in HD, neuroacanthocytosis, catatonia, postencephalitic parkinsonism, TS, and startle disease (hyperekplexia). McPherson et al. have postulated that echolalia may be a result of involvement of frontal subcortical circuits, with interruption of "inhibiting" responses and the presence of environmental dependency.[134] Palilalia occurs in movement disorders such as postencephalitic parkinsonism and ICBG. In a recent prospective study of repetitive speech disturbances in PD, two types of disturbances were characterized: hyperfluent forms resembling palilalia, and dysfluent forms resembling stuttering. These types of speech alterations

were more frequent in advanced disease states but did not always correlate with cognitive impairment.[135]

Disturbed rate, volume, and initiation of speech are commonly seen with focal lesions of the basal ganglia.[136] Degenerative diseases of the basal ganglia show similar speech abnormalities. Dysarthric speech frequently occurs in HD, sometimes to the point of unintelligibility. Perseverative features, decreased initiation, and respiratory dyskinesias may further impair articulation. Hypokinetic movement disorders often produce dysarthria, hypophonia, and occasionally mutism.

VISUOSPATIAL FUNCTION

Visuospatial function encompasses a number of aspects: sensory perception, motor, attention, cognition, and body-spatial orientation. Tests for these different categories have been devised in an attempt to understand visuospatial function in health and disease. There have been extensive studies on the integrity of visuospatial function in movement disorders. As in other areas of cognition, methodological issues have hampered definitive conclusions. These include the interference of motor disability, inconsistent assessment or organizational (executive) dysfunction, and inadequate attention to the presence of dementia or depression. However, clever paradigms with minimal motor components have been devised to try to account for some of these issues.

PARKINSON'S DISEASE

Visuospatial dysfunction is reported frequently in PD, but conclusions as to whether it is an integral part of the disorder are mixed.[137–140] Cummings and Huber reviewed the reported abnormalities in the subcategories of visuospatial function, identifying abnormalities in PD in all areas except visual sensory abilities, and visual recognition (right-left orientation, recognition of familiar faces and places).[137] A progressive pattern of increasing deficit with advancing disease has been noted: early impairment on rod orientation tests, followed by difficulties with line orientation, block design, and picture arrangement, and, finally, deficits in nonfamiliar-face discrimination. Some deficits, such as copying complex figures, recognition of embedded figures, and performance of a task requiring spatial updating, can be accounted for by confounding impairment in executive or motor function. However, the consistency of results across many studies, lack of correlation within tests to severity of motor disability, and lack of improvement with L-dopa argue in favor of visuospatial deficit in PD.

OTHER MOVEMENT DISORDERS

Visuospatial function has been less extensively evaluated in HD. HD patients with only mild intellectual decline performed poorly on tests of egocentric orientation, such as determining direction or position based on an internal representation of space (i.e., one's own position). Lawrence et al.

demonstrated that HD patients had deficits on pattern and spatial recognition, and delayed visual search times.[141] Deficits of visuospatial function have been described in olivopontocerebellar atrophy, perhaps implicating cerebello-cortical loops in mediating visuospatial organization. In striatonigral degeneration, mixed results have been reported, with most investigations identifying deficits similar to those of PD. Finally, severe visuospatial and constructional disturbances secondary to parietal lobe involvement are common in CBGD.

PRAXIS

Apraxia is the inability to perform a motor act despite intact comprehension, motor and sensory skills, and cooperation. Ideomotor apraxia is the inability to carry out an action to command despite retained spontaneous ability to carry out a sequence of actions, especially when handling actual objects.[142,143] The main movement disorder with abnormal praxis is CBGD, which frequently presents with asymmetric ideomotor limb apraxia. Apraxia was reported in 71 percent of cases in one series and may lead to complete loss of limb function. Apraxia of gaze, eyelid opening, and speech can occur. The disorder is attributed primarily to neuronal loss in the frontoparietal cortex, although a role for the basal ganglia cannot be excluded.

PD was reported to have increased apraxia by Grossman et al. and more recently ideomotor apraxia was found to occur in 25 percent of PD patients in a study by Leiguarda,[142] but others have not confirmed this in early, nondemented PD patients.

The only other movement disorder with frequent apraxia is Creutzfeldt-Jakob disease, where it forms a component of the dementia and may appear early in the course in association with extrapyramidal or cerebellar signs.

Dementia

Dementia is an acquired syndrome of intellectual impairment as a consequence of brain dysfunction. The clinical criteria for dementia are varied, accounting for differing reported rates of dementia in movement disorders. Many studies have used criteria from the DSM-IV[144] for defining dementia, which requires a decline in intellectual function of sufficient severity to interfere with social and occupational function. The degree to which functioning is impaired because of intellectual, as opposed to motor, disability is sometimes difficult to determine in movement disorders.

Dementia in disorders of the basal ganglia is predominantly of the subcortical type. The cardinal features include psychomotor slowing, memory retrieval deficits, abnormal executive function with an impaired ability to manipulate knowledge, alterations in mood or personality, and abnormalities in speech. Dilapidation in cognition has been used to describe

the intellectual impairment, referring to the executive function deficits. Patients may perform individual aspects of a task properly but fail at integrating all necessary sequences. Mood and behavioral changes most frequently consist of depression and a lack of motivation or initiative. Although the division of dementia into cortical and subcortical types has been challenged, based on a lack of corresponding anatomic specificity, it remains a useful clinical phenomenological distinction. Perhaps more accurate terminology would use "frontal subcortical systems dementia," as it is the disruption of the three behavioral circuits that produces the cardinal manifestations. Table 2-5 lists the movement disorders more commonly associated with dementia.

PARKINSON'S DISEASE

The reported frequency of dementia in PD varies from 4 to 93 percent, with an overall frequency of 39.9 percent based on a review of 27 studies.[145] The variability arises from differing methods of cognitive assessment, definition of dementia, and study populations. The best current prevalence data from the general population suggests that dementia in PD occurs in 40 percent. The rate of dementia in PD is higher than in the general population matched for age and sex, with an estimated 6-fold increased risk in those with PD.[146] Risks for dementia include parkinsonism with predominant rigidity and greater disability. Progression of disability and mortality is also higher in demented PD patients, compared with that in nondemented PD. A prospective study examining the incidence of and risk factors for dementia in PD found that age of onset and disease duration did not confer an increased risk.[147]

There are clinical subtypes of dementia within PD, and these may correlate with different underlying pathologies. Mild cognitive deficits in PD are ubiquitous, as discussed in the section on cognitive disturbances. The dementia in PD is most commonly mild to moderate in severity, with bradyphrenia, memory retrieval deficits, impaired set shifting and maintenance, impaired problem-solving, poor visuospatial function, decrease word list generation, and prominent mood disorder. However, more severe dementia in PD occurs and is usually but not invariably associated with Alzheimer's disease-type neuritic plaques and cortical Lewy bodies.[148] Dementia tends to have mixed cortical and subcortical features.[149]

HUNTINGTON'S DISEASE

Dementia in HD is considered one of the cardinal features of the disease, although the reported cross-sectional prevalence has varied from 15 to 95 percent, depending on diagnostic criteria.[150] The characteristics of the dementia conform to a subcortical type, with early changes in personality and mood with or without psychosis, followed by cognitive deficits primarily in the realms of memory retrieval deficits, executive dysfunction, and slowing of cognition. Higher cortical

TABLE 2-5 Movement Disorders with Dementia

Subcortical Pattern	Cortical Pattern
Parkinsonism	Corticobasal ganglionic degeneration
Parkinson's disease	Creutzfeldt-Jakob disease
Progressive supranuclear palsy	Gerstmann-Straussler-Scheinker disease
Hallervorden-Spatz disease	Parkinson's disease + Alzheimer's disease
Idiopathic calcification of the basal ganglia	Dementia with Lewy bodies
Corticobasal ganglionic degeneration	
Dementia with Lewy bodies	
Postencephalitic parkinsonism	
Parkinsonism-dementia/ALS of Guam	
Olivopontocerebellar atrophy	
Dentatorubropallidoluysian atrophy	
Spinocerebellar degenerations	
Vascular	
Lacunar state	
Binswanger disease	
Thalamic degenerations	
Hydrocephalus	
Whipple disease	
Dementia pugilistica	
Hyperkinetic	
Huntington's disease	
Wilson's disease	
Neuroacanthocytosis	

ALS, amyotrophic lateral sclerosis.

deficits, such as aphasia, agnosia, and apraxia, are typically lacking. There appears to be little relationship between the extent of psychopathology and the severity of cognitive deficits. The intellectual impairment progresses as the disease advances and has been variably correlated with duration of illness, with some authors finding cognitive changes, including memory loss as a middle- to late-stage finding, whereas others find that subtle cognitive changes may be a predictive factor.[122,151] Degree of caudate atrophy and number of trinucleotide repeats may be associated with intellectual impairment.

The nature of the behavioral and neuropsychological deficits in HD is similar to that seen in patients with frontal lobe lesions. The dementia in HD is attributed to striatal degeneration and interruption of frontal subcortical circuits, although some authors feel that the inconsistent neuropathological changes reported in the cerebral cortex may be relevant.

PROGRESSIVE SUPRANUCLEAR PALSY

PSP is an example of a disorder with pure subcortical neuropathological changes manifesting with dementia. Personality change with apathy may occur early along with mild cognitive deficits; the cognitive impairment usually progresses to moderate intellectual impairment with deficits in memory retrieval and slowing of information processing and manipulation. Dementia has been found in the later stages by the majority of authors and may be more rapidly progressive than in PD patients.[152] Hypometabolic changes in the dorsal frontal lobe on PET support a relationship between dementia and interruption of frontal subcortical circuits.

MULTISYSTEM ATROPHIES

The multisystem atrophies include olivopontocerebellar atrophy (OPCA), striatonigral degeneration (SND), and Shy-Drager syndrome (SDS). These disorders have both familial and sporadic forms. Dementia has been found frequently in certain subgroups of OPCA but is not present until the very late stages in some families.[153] Classification of these disorders continues to be problematic, and it is difficult to establish any clear profiles of dementia across all subgroups.

Patients with sporadic versus familial OPCA were compared by Berciano, who found dementia in 35 percent of the former and 57 percent of the latter, mostly in the middle-to-late stages of the disease.[154] Dementia may occur early and was a dominant feature in 11–22 percent of cases. For the most part, the dementias have the subcortical pattern of cognitive impairment, with gradually progressive cognitive decline involving slowness of information processing, apathy, frontal/executive dysfunction, and impaired visuoconstructional skills. Deficits of cortical function, such as aphasia, apraxia, and agnosia, have generally been absent, although two members of one family reported with OPCA type V (as classified by Konigsmark and

Weiner[155]) were described with aphasia. The occurrence of aphasia may relate to cortical neuronal loss described in this subgroup.

Cognitive impairment in SND and SDS is usually mild, with impairments predominantly involving executive function. Patients generally do not meet criteria for dementia. The deficits are milder than in PSP and similar to those observed in the early stages of PD, although the limited number of studies have produced conflicting results.

WILSON'S DISEASE

Intellectual impairment has been reported in WD, but the deficits are mild in severity compared with those seen in PSP and HD. As noted earlier in the chapter, personality alterations may occur early in the disease and often predate cognitive or neurological decline. Failure to progress in school may be an early sign in juvenile-onset cases. Neuropsychological changes include retrieval deficits on the Wechsler Memory Scale, decline in full-scale IQ, and poor concentration.[156] Dening and Berrios classified only 11 of 45 patients suspected of cognitive deficits as being intellectually impaired in a retrospective review.[72] The cognitive deficits may respond to a reduction in copper. The relationship between cognitive, neuropathological, and radiological changes in WD has not been systematically assessed.

RARER MOVEMENT DISORDERS WITH PROMINENT DEMENTIA

Dementia is a prominent feature of some less common basal ganglia disorders. ICBG is a familial disorder with extensive calcification of the basal ganglia, despite normal serum calcium and phosphate. It presents with chorea or parkinsonian-type extrapyramidal disorder. The younger-onset form of ICBG presents primarily with psychosis, whereas the later-onset variety (mean age 50 years) presents with dementia and movement disorder.[60,157] Dementia typical of a subcortical process, with memory retrieval deficits and poor concentration, is characteristic.

Hallervorden-Spatz disease is a rare familial disorder with deposition of iron-containing pigment in the globus pallidus and ventral substantia nigra. The dementia syndrome includes psychomotor slowing, poor memory, impaired attention and concentration, and diminished intellectual function. The movement disorder is heterogeneous, with rigidity, dystonic posturing, and chorea predominating.

Parkinsonism-dementia/ALS complex of Guam presents with early, often severe, dementia, which may be the most prominent disability. The mental status changes are inexorably progressive with personality changes in mental slowing, poor memory, and frequent mood disorders.

CBGD is another rare neurodegenerative disorder that may present with dementia or manifest cognitive complaints as the disease progresses. It typically presents as an L-dopa-resistant asymmetric akinetic-rigid syndrome associated with apraxia, cortical sensory loss, and alien limb syndromes. In a retrospective review of all cases of pathologically confirmed CBGD, investigators found that 9 of 13 cases presented with behavioral changes and/or memory loss and were erroneously diagnosed as either Alzheimer's disease or frontotemporal dementia.[158] They concluded that cognitive symptoms, behavioral changes, memory loss, and language alterations are common in CBGD.

Finally, thalamic degenerations are a heterogeneous group of rare disorders in which there are cognitive and behavioral changes, consisting of amnesia, confusion, apathy, and labile affect in association with a variety of motor disorders such as involuntary movements, chorea, ataxia, and myoclonus.[159,160] Akinetic mutism may occur. The amnestic quality of the memory defects is in contrast to the more typical retrieval deficit seen in subcortical dementias, and reflects involvement of the hippocampal-thalamic memory storage system.

Comment

The interruption of the three frontal subcortical circuits mediating behavior results in neuropsychiatric and cognitive disturbances in most movement disorders. These neurobehavioral changes can occur with both focal basal ganglia lesions and degenerative diseases involving subcortical structures. Early behavioral changes are common, and awareness of the association with movement disorders may allow earlier diagnosis and potentially more efficacious therapy.

Acknowledgments

This project was supported by a National Institute on Aging Alzheimer's Disease Research Center grant (AG 16570), an Alzheimer's Disease Research Center of California grant, and the Sidell-Kagan Foundation. Dr. Swanberg is supported by the United States Army.

References

1. Wilson SAK. Progressive lenticular degeneration: A familial nervous disease associated with cirrhosis of the liver. *Brain* 34:295–507, 1912.
2. Huntington G: On chorea. *Med Surg Rep* 26:317–321, 1872.
3. Parkinson J: *An Essay on the Shaking Palsy*. London: Sherwood, Neely and Jones, 1817.
4. Booth G: Psychodynamics in parkinsonism. *Psychosom Med* 10:1–4, 1948.
5. Lit AC: Man behind a mask: An analysis of the psychomotor phenomena of Parkinson's disease. *Acta Neurol Belg* 68:863–874, 1968.

6. Sands I: The type of personality susceptible to Parkinson's disease. *Mt Sinai J Med* 9:792–794, 1942.

7. Cummings JL: *Clinical Neuropsychiatry*. New York: Grune & Stratton, 1985.

8. Denny-Brown D: *The Basal Ganglia and Their Relationship to Disorders of Movement*. Oxford: Oxford University Press, 1962.

9. Cummings JL: Frontal-subcortical circuits and human behavior. *Arch Neurol* 50:873–880, 1993.

10. Alexander GE, Crutcher MD: Functional architecture of basal ganglia circuits: Neural substrates of parallel processing. *Trends Neurosci* 13:266–271, 1990.

11. Alexander GE, De Long MR, Strick PL: Parallel organization of functionally segregated circuits linking basal ganglia and cortex. *Annu Rev Neurosci* 9:357–381, 1986.

12. Alexander GE, Crutcher MD, DeLong MR: Basal ganglia-thalamocortical circuits: Parallel substrates for motor, oculomotor, prefrontal and limbic functions. *Prog Brain Res* 85:119–146, 1990.

13. Dubois B, Defontaines B, DeWeer B, et al: Cognitive and behavioral changes in patients with focal lesions of the basal ganglia. *Adv Neurol* 65:29–41, 1995.

14. Mendez MF, Adams NL, Lewandowski KS: Neurobehavioral changes associated with caudate lesions. *Neurology* 39:349–354, 1989.

15. Middleton FA, Strick PL: A revised neuroanatomy of frontal-subcortical circuits, in Cummings JL, Lichter DG (eds): *Frontal-Subcortical Circuits in Psychiatric and Neurologic Disorders*. New York: Guilford Press, 2001, pp 44–58.

16. Middleton FA, Strick PL: Basal ganglia output and cognition: Evidence from anatomical, behavioral and clinical studies. *Brain Cogn* 42:183–200, 2000.

17. Stuss DT, Benson DF: *The Frontal Lobes*. New York: Raven Press, 1986.

18. Benton AL: Differential behavioral effects in frontal lobe disease. *Neuropsychologia* 6:53–60, 1968.

19. Lezak, MD: *Neuropsychological Assessment*. Oxford: Oxford University Press, 1995.

20. Yesavage JA, Brink TL, Rose TL, et al: Development and validation of a geriatric depression screening: A preliminary report. *J Psychiatr Res* 17:37–49, 1982.

21. Beck AT, Ward CH, Mendelson M, et al: An inventory for measuring depression. *Arch Gen Psychiatry* 4:561–571, 1961.

22. Hamilton M: A rating scale for depression. *J Neurol Neurosurg Psychiatr* 23:56–62, 1960.

23. Montgomery SA, Asberg M: A new depression scale, designed to be sensitive to change. *Br J Psychiatr* 134:382–389, 1979.

24. Aarsland D, Litvan I, Larsen JP: Neuropsychiatric symptoms in patients with progressive supranuclear palsy and Parkinson's disease. *J Neuropsychiatry Clin Neurosci* 13:42–49, 2001.

25. Cummings JL: Depression and Parkinson's disease: A review. *Am J Psychiatry* 149:443–454, 1992.

26. Ring HA, Bench CJ, Trimble MR, et al: Depression in Parkinson's disease: A positron emission study. *Br J Psychiatry* 165:333–339, 1994.

27. Mayberg HS, Starkstein SE, Sadzot B, et al: Selective hypometabolism in the inferior frontal lobe in depressed patients with Parkinson's disease. *Ann Neurol* 28:57–64, 1990.

28. Leentjens AF, Verhey FR, Luijckx GJ, Troost J: The validity of the Beck Depression Inventory as a screening and diagnostic instrument for depression in patients with Parkinson's disease. *Mov Disord* 15:1221–1224, 2000.

29. Leentjens AF, Verhey FR, Lousberg R, et al: The validity of the Hamilton and Montgomery-Asberg Depression rating scales as screening and diagnostic tools for depression in Parkinson's disease. *Int J Geriatr Psychiatry* 15:644–649, 2000.

30. Schrag A, Jahanshahi M, Quinn NP: What contributes to depression in Parkinson's disease? *Psychol Med* 31:65–73, 2001.

31. Giladi N, Treves TA, Paleacu D, et al: Risk factors for dementia, depression and psychosis in long standing Parkinson's disease. *J Neural Transm* 107:59–71, 2001.

32. Cooper JA, Sagar HJ, Jordan N, et al: Cognitive impairment in early, untreated Parkinson's disease and the relationship to motor disability. *Brain* 114:2095–2122, 1991.

33. Shiba M, Bower JH, Maraganore DM, et al: Anxiety disorders and depressive disorders preceding Parkinson's disease: A case-control study. *Mov Disord* 15:669–677, 2000.

34. Santamaria J, Tolosa E, Valles A: Parkinson's disease with depression: A possible subgroup of idiopathic parkinsonism. *Neurology* 36:1130–1133, 1986.

35. Gotham AM, Brown RG, Marsden CD: Depression in Parkinson's disease: A quantitative and qualitative analysis. *J Neurol Neurosurg Psychiatry* 49:381–389, 1986.

36. Schiffer RB, Kurlan R, Rubin A, et al: Evidence for atypical depression in Parkinson's disease. *Am J Psychiatry* 145:1020–1022, 1988.

37. Starkstein SE, Bolduc PL, Mayberg HS, et al: Cognitive impairments and depression in Parkinson's disease: A follow-up study. *J Neurol Neurosurg Psychiatry* 53:597–602, 1990.

38. MacCarthy B, Brown R: Psychosocial factors in Parkinson's disease. *Br J Clin Psychol* 28:41–52, 1989.

39. Mayberg HA, Solomon DH: Depression in Parkinson's disease: A biochemical and organic viewpoint. *Adv Neurol* 65:49–60, 1995.

40. Sano M, Stern Y, Cote L, et al: Depression in Parkinson's disease: A biochemical model. *J Neuropsychiatry Clin Neurosci* 2:88–92, 1990.

41. Ehmann TS, Beninger RJ, Gawel MJ, et al: Depressive symptoms in Parkinson's disease: A comparison with disabled control subjects. *J Geriatr Psychiatry Neurol* 2:3–9, 1990.

42. Mayeux R, Stern Y, Sano M, et al: The relationship of serotonin to depression in Parkinson's disease. *Mov Disord* 3:237–244, 1988.

43. Paulus W, Jellinger K: The neuropathologic basis of different clinical subgroups of Parkinson's disease. *J Neuropathol Exp Neurol* 50:743–755, 1991.

44. Berg D, Supprian T, Hofmann E, et al: Depression in Parkinson's disease: Brainstem midline alteration on transcranial sonography and magnetic resonance imaging. *J Neurol* 246:1186–1193, 1999.

45. Cummings JL: Behavioral and psychiatric symptoms associated with Huntington's disease. *Adv Neurol* 65:179–186, 1995.

46. Caine ED, Shoulson I: Psychiatric syndromes in Huntington's disease. *Am J Psychiatry* 140:728–733, 1983.

47. Rosenblatt A, Leroi I: Neuropsychiatry of Huntington's disease and other basal ganglia disorders. *Psychosomatics* 41:24–30, 2000.

48. Lauterbach ED, Cummings JL, Duffy J, et al: Neuropsychiatric correlates and treatment of lenticulostriatal diseases: A review of the literature and overview of research opportunities in Huntington's, Wilson's, and Fahr's diseases. *J Neuropsychiatry Clin Neurosci* 10:249–266, 1998.

49. Kirkwood SC, Su JL, Conneally PM, Foroud T: Progression of symptoms in the early and middle stages of Huntington's disease. *Arch Neurol* 58:273–278, 2001.

50. Schoenfeld M, Myers RH, Cupples LA, et al: Increased rate of suicide among patients with Huntington's disease. *J Neurol Neurosurg Psychiatry* 47:1283–1287, 1984.

51. Mayberg HS, Starkstein SE, Sadzot B, et al: Selective hypometabolism in the inferior frontal lobe in depressed patients with Huntington's disease. *Ann Neurol* 28:57–64, 1989.

52. Akil M, Schwartz JA, Dutchak D, et al: The psychiatric presentations of Wilson's disease. *J Neuropsychiatry Clin Neurosci* 3:377–382, 1991.

53. Akil M, Brewer GJ: Psychiatric and behavioral abnormalities in Wilson's disease. *Adv Neurol* 65:171–178, 1995.

54. Portala K, Westermark K, von Knorring L, Ekselius L: Psychopathology in treated Wilson's disease determined by means of CPRS expert and self-ratings. *Acta Psychiatr Scand* 101:104–109, 2000.

55. McKeith I, Perry E, Perry R: Report of the Second Dementia with Lewy Body International Workshop: Diagnosis and treatment. *Neurology* 53:902–905, 1999.

56. Swanberg M, Cummings JL: Risk-benefit considerations in the treatment of dementia with Lewy bodies. *Drug Saf* 25:511–523, 2003.

57. Cummings JL, Litvan I: Neuropsychiatric aspects of corticobasal degeneration, in Litvan I, Goetz CG, Lang AE (eds): *Corticobasal Degeneration*. Philadelphia: Lippincott Williams & Wilkins, 2000, pp 147–151.

58. Litvan I, Mega M, Cummings JL, Fairbanks L: Neuropsychiatric aspects of progressive supranuclear palsy. *Neurology* 47:1184–1189, 1996.

59. Wyszynski B, Merriam A, Medalia A, et al: Choreoacanthocytosis: Report of a case with psychiatric features. *Neuropsychiatry Neuropsychol Behav Neurol* 2:137–144, 1989.

60. Cummings JL, Gosenfeld LF, Houlihan JP, McCaffrey T: Neuropsychiatric disturbances associated with idiopathic calcification of the basal ganglia. *Biol Psychiatry* 18:591–601, 1983.

61. Coffey BJ, Park KS: Behavioral and emotional aspects of Tourette syndrome. *Neurol Clin* 15:277–289, 1997.

62. DeMarchi N, Mennella R: Huntington's disease and its association with psychopathology. *Harvard Rev Psychiatry* 7:278–289, 2000.

63. Fairweather DS: Psychiatric aspects of the post-encephalitic syndrome. *J Ment Sci* 93:201–254, 1947.

64. Mendez MF: Mania in neurologic disorders. *Curr Psychiatry Rep* 2:440–445, 2000.

65. Kulisevsky J, Berthier ML, Pujol J: Hemiballismus and secondary mania following a right thalamic infarction. *Neurology* 43:1422–1424, 1993.

66. Factor SA, Molho ES, Podskalny GD, Brown D: Parkinson's disease: Drug-induced psychiatric states. *Adv Neurol* 65:115–138, 1995.

67. Cummings JL: Psychosis in neurologic disease: Neurobiology and pathogenesis. *Neuropsychiatr Neuropsychol Behav Neurol* 5:144–150, 1992.

68. Beckson M, Cummings JL: Psychosis in basal ganglia disorders. *Neuropsychiatr Neuropsychol Behav Neurol* 5:126–131, 1992.

69. Cummings JL: Behavioral and psychiatric symptoms associated with HD, in Weiner WJ, Lang AE (eds): *Advances in Neurology*. New York: Raven Press, 1995, pp 179–186.

70. Leslie WD, Greenberg CR, Abrams DN, Hobson D: Clinical deficits in Huntington's disease correlate with reduced striatal uptake on iodine-123 epidepride single-photon emission tomography. *Eur J Nucl Med* 26:1458–1464, 1999.

71. Tsuang D, Almqvist EW, Lipe H, et al: Familial aggregation of psychotic symptoms in Huntington's disease. *Am J Psychiatry* 157:1955–1959, 2000.

72. Dening TR, Berrios GE: Wilson's disease: Psychiatric symptoms in 195 cases. *Arch Gen Psychiatry* 46:1126–1134, 1989.

73. Holroyd S, Currie L, Wooten GF: Prospective study of hallucinations and delusions in Parkinson's disease. *J Neurol Neurosurg Psychiatry* 70:734–738, 2001.

74. Aarsland D, Cummings JL, Larsen JP: Neuropsychiatric differences between Parkinson's disease with dementia and Alzheimer's disease. *Int J Geriatr Psychiatry* 16:184–191, 2001.

75. Aarsland D, Larsen JP, Lim NG, et al: Range of neuropsychiatric disturbances in patients with Parkinson's disease. *J Neurol Neurosurg Psychiatry* 67:494–496, 1999.

76. Fenelon G, Mahieux F, Huon R, Ziegler M: Hallucinations in Parkinson's disease: Prevalence, phenomenology and risk factors. *Brain* 123:733–745, 2000.

77. Morris SK, Olichney JM, Corey-Bloom J: Psychosis in dementia with Lewy bodies. *Semin Clin Neuropsychiatry* 3:51–60, 1998.

78. Hirono N, Cummings JL: Neuropsychiatric aspects of dementia with Lewy bodies. *Curr Psychiatry Rep* 1:85–92, 1999.

79. Folstein SE: *Huntington's Disease: A Disorder of Families*. Baltimore: Johns Hopkins University Press, 1989, pp 49–64.

80. Stout JC, Rodawalt WC, Siemers ER: Risky decision making in Huntington's disease. *J Int Neuropsychol Soc* 7:92–101, 2001.

81. Swerdlow NR: Obsessive-compulsive disorder and tic syndromes. *Med Clin North Am* 85:122–134, 2001.

82. Jacobs H, Heberlein I, Vieregge A, Vieregge P: Personality traits in young patients with Parkinson's disease. *Acta Neurol Scand* 103:82–87, 2001.

83. Riklan M, Weiner H, Diller L: Somato-psychologic studies in Parkinson's disease. I. An investigation into the relationship of certain disease factors to psychological functions. *J Nerv Ment Dis* 129:263–272, 1959.

84. Smythies JR: The previous personality in parkinsonism. *J Psychosom Res* 11:169–171, 1967.

85. Hubble JP, Venkatesch R, Hassanein RES, et al: Personality and depression in Parkinson's disease. *J Nerv Ment Dis* 181:657–662, 1993.

86. Benedetti MD, Bower JH, Maraganore DM, et al: Smoking, alcohol, and coffee consumption preceding Parkinson's disease. *Neurology* 55:1350–1358, 2000.

87. Menza M: The personality associated with Parkinson's disease. *Curr Psychiatry Rep* 2:421–426, 2000.

88. Miguel EC, Baer L, Coffey BJ, et al: Phenomenological differences appearing with repetitive behaviors in obsessive-compulsive disorder and Gilles de la Tourette syndrome. *Br J Psychiatry* 170:140–145, 1997.

89. Saxena S, Rauch SL: Functional neuroimaging and the neuroanatomy of obsessive-compulsive disorder. *Psychiatr Clin North Am* 23:563–586, 2000.

90. Garcia-Cairasco N, Miguel EC, Rauch SL, Leckman JF: Current controversies and future directions in basal ganglia research. *Psychiatr Clin North Am* 20:945–962, 1997.

91. Rauch SL, Savage CR: Neuroimaging and neuropsychology of the striatum. *Psychiatr Clin North Am* 20:741–768, 1997.

92. Anderson KE, Louis ED, Stern Y, Marder KS: Cognitive correlates of obsessive and compulsive symptoms in Huntington's disease. *Am J Psychiatry* 158:799–801, 2001.

93. Alegret M, Junque C, Valldeoriola F, et al: Obsessive-compulsive symptoms in Parkinson's disease. *J Neurol Neurosurg Psychiatry* 70:394–396, 2001.

94. De Marchi N, Morris M, Mennella R, et al: Association of obsessive-compulsive disorder and pathological gambling with Huntington's disease in an Italian pedigree: Possible association with Huntington's disease mutation. *Acta Psychiatr Scand* 97:62–65, 1998.

95. Saxena S, Brody AL, Maidment JM, et al: Localized orbitofrontal and subcortical metabolic changes and predictors of response to paroxetine treatment in obsessive-compulsive disorder. *Neuropsychopharmacology* 21:683–693, 1999.

96. Baxter LR, Schwartz JM, Bergmann KS, et al: Caudate glucose metabolic rate changes with drug and behavior therapy for obsessive-compulsive disorder. *Arch Gen Psychiatry* 49:681–690, 1992.

97. Dewhurst K, Oliver J, Trick KLK, McKnight AL: Neuropsychiatric aspects of Huntington's disease. *Confin Neurol* 31:258–268, 1969.

98. Cummings JL, Mega M, Gray K, et al: The Neuropsychiatric Inventory: Comprehensive assessment of psychopathology in dementia. *Neurology* 44:2308–2314, 1994.

99. Richard I, Justus A, Kurlan R: Relationship between mood and motor fluctuations in Parkinson's disease. *J Neuropsychiatry Clin Neurosci* 13:35–41, 2001.

100. Rub U, Braak H, Sandmann-Keil D, Braak E: The nuclei of the gain setting system in the human brain are severely affected by Parkinson's specific changes. *Mov Disord* 15:286–292, 2000.

101. Arnulf I, Bonnet AM, Damier P, et al: Hallucinations, REM sleep and Parkinson's disease: A medical hypothesis. *Neurology* 55:281–288, 2000.

102. Wetter TC, Collado-Seidel V, Pollmacher T, et al: Sleep and periodic leg movement patterns in drug-free patients with Parkinson's disease and multiple system atrophy. *Sleep* 23:361–367, 2000.

103. Schwartz MA, Selhorst JB, Ochs AL, et al: Oculomasticatory myorhythmia: A unique movement disorder occurring in Whipple's disease. *Ann Neurol* 20:677–683, 1986.

104. Turner RS, D'Amato CJ, Chervin RD, Claivas M: The pathology or REM sleep behavior disorder with comorbid Lewy body dementia. *Neurology* 55:1730–1732, 2000.

105. Wetter TC, Collado-Seidel V, Trenkwalder C: Polysomnagraphic investigation of patients with Parkinson's disease in comparison with healthy subjects. *Somnology* 3:300–306, 1999.

106. Hogl B, Gomex A, Garcia S, et al: A clinical, polysomnagraphic and pharmacologic study of sleep benefit in Parkinson's disease. *Neurology* 50:1332–1339, 1998.

107. Poewe W, Hogl B: Parkinson's disease and sleep. *Curr Opin Neurol* 13:423–426, 2000.

108. Rye DB, Bliwise DL, Dihenia B, Gurecki P: Fast track: Daytime sleepiness in Parkinson's disease. *J Sleep Res* 9:63–69, 2000.

109. Frucht S, Rogers JD, Greene PE, et al: Falling asleep at the wheel: Motor vehicle mishaps in persons taking pramipexole and ropinirole. *Neurology* 52:1908, 1999.

110. Pal S, Bhattacharya KF, Agapito C, Chaudhuri KR: A study of excessive daytime sleepiness and its clinical significance in three groups of Parkinson's disease patients taking pramipexole, cabergoline and levodopa mono and combination therapy. *J Neural Transm* 108:71–77, 2001.

111. Clarenbach P: Parkinson's disease and sleep. *J Neurol* 247:20–23, 2000.

112. Welsh M, Hung L, Waters CH: Sexuality in women with Parkinson's disease. *Mov Disord* 12:923–927, 1997.

113. Lambert D, Waters CH: Sexual dysfunction in Parkinson's disease. *Clin Neurosci* 5:73–77, 1998.

114. Federoff JP, Peyser C, Franz ML, et al: Sexual disorders in Huntington's disease. *J Neuropsychiatry Clin Neurosci* 6:147–153, 1994.

115. Gorman DG, Cummings JL: Hypersexuality following septal injury. *Arch Neurol* 49:308–310, 1992.

116. Fournet N, Moreaud O, Roulin JL, et al: Working memory functioning in medicated Parkinson's disease patients and the effect of withdrawal of dopaminergic medications. *Neuropsychology* 14:247–253, 2000.

117. Dujardin K, Defebvre L, Grundberg C, et al: Memory and executive function in sporadic and familial Parkinson's disease. *Brain* 124:389–398, 2001.

118. Levin BE, Tomer R, Rey G: Clinical correlates of cognitive impairments in Parkinson's disease, in Huber SJ, Cummings JL (eds): *Parkinson's Disease: Behavioral and Neuropsychological Aspects*. New York: Oxford University Press, 1992, pp 97–106.

119. Canavan AGM: The performance on learning tasks of patients in the early stages of Parkinson's disease. *Neuropsychologia* 27:141–156, 1989.

120. Watkins LH, Rogers RD, Lawrence AD, et al: Impaired planning but intact decision making in early Huntington's disease: Implications for specific fronto-striatal pathology. *Neuropsychologia* 38:1112–1125, 2000.

121. Hahn-Barma V, Deweer B, Durr A, et al: Are cognitive changes the first symptoms of Huntington's disease? A study of gene carriers. *J Neurol Neurosurg Psychiatry* 64:172–177, 1998.

122. Bachoud-Levi AC, Maison P, Bartolomeo P, et al: Retest effects and cognitive decline in longitudinal follow-up of patients with early HD. *Neurology* 56:1052–1058, 2001.

123. Pillon B, Dubois B, Ploska A, Agid Y: Severity and specificity of cognitive impairment in Alzheimer's, Huntington's, and Parkinson's diseases and progressive supranuclear palsy. *Neurology* 41:634–643, 1991.

124. Bright P, Kopelman MD: Learning and memory: Recent findings. *Curr Opin Neurol* 14:449–455, 2001.

125. Siegel DJ: Memory: An overview, with emphasis on developmental, interpersonal, and neurobiological aspects. *J Am Acad Child Adolesc Psychiatry* 40:997–1011, 2001.

126. Rohrer D, Salmon DP, Wixted JT, Paulsen JS: The disparate effects of Alzheimer's disease and Huntington's disease on semantic memory. *Neuropsychology* 13:381–388, 1999.

127. Grafman N: Frontal lobe function in progressive supranuclear palsy. *Arch Neurol* 47:533–558, 1990.

128. Beatty WW, Salmon DP, Butters N, et al: Retrograde amnesia in patients with Alzheimer's disease or Huntington's disease. *Neurobiol Aging* 9:181–186, 1988.

129. Kertesz A, Martinez-Lage P, Davidson W, Munoz DG: The corticobasal degeneration syndrome overlaps progressive aphasia and frontotemporal dementia. *Neurology* 55:1368–1375, 2000.

130. Mimura M, Oda T, Tsuchiya K, Kato M, et al: Corticobasal degeneration presenting with nonfluent primary progressive

aphasia: A clinicopathological study. *J Neurol Sci* 183:19–26, 2001.

131. Litvan I, Grimes DA, Lang DA, et al: Clinical features differentiating patients with postmortem confirmation of progressive supranuclear palsy and corticobasal degeneration. *J Neurol* 246:1–5, 1999.

132. Murray LL: Spoken language production in Huntington's and Parkinson's diseases. *J Speech Lang Hear Res* 43:1350–1366, 2000.

133. Breitenstein C, Van Lancker D, Daum I, Waters CH: Impaired perception of vocal emotions in Parkinson's disease: Influence of speech time processing and executive function. *Brain Cogn* 45:277–314, 2001.

134. McPherson SE, Kuratani JD, Cummings JL, et al: Creutzfeldt-Jacob disease with mixed transcortical aphasia: Insights into echolalia. *Behav Neurol* 7:197–203, 1994.

135. Benke T, Hohenstein C, Poewe W, Butterworth B: Repetitive speech phenomena in Parkinson's disease. *J Neurol Neurosurg Psychiatry* 69:319–324, 2000.

136. Alexander M, Naeser MA, Palumbo CL: Correlations of subcortical CT lesions sites and aphasia profiles. *Brain* 110:961–991, 1987.

137. Cummings JL, Huber SJ: Visuospatial abnormalities in Parkinson's disease, in Huber SJ, Cummings JL (eds): *Parkinson's Disease: Behavioral and Neuropsychological Aspects*. New York: Oxford University Press, 1992, pp 59–73.

138. Levin BE, Llabre MM, Reisman S, et al: Visuospatial impairment in Parkinson's disease. *Neurology* 41:365–369, 1991.

139. Mohr E, Litvan I, Williams J, et al: Selective deficits in Alzheimer and parkinsonian dementia: Visuospatial function. *Can J Neurol Sci* 17:292–297, 1990.

140. Stelmach GE, Phillips JG, Chau AW: Visuo-perceptual processing in parkinsonians. *Neuropsychologia* 27:485–493, 1989.

141. Lawrence AD, Hodges JR, Rosser AE, et al: Evidence for specific cognitive deficits in preclinical Huntington's disease. *Brain* 121:1329–1341, 1998.

142. Leiguarda R: Limb apraxia: Cortical or subcortical. *Neuroimage* 14:137–141, 2001.

143. Leiguarda RC, Marsden CD: Limb apraxias higher order disorders of sensorimotor integration. *Brain* 123:860–879, 2000.

144. American Psychiatric Association: *Diagnostic and Statistical Manual of Mental Disorders (DSM-IV)*, 4th ed. Washington, DC: American Psychiatric Press, 1997.

145. Cummings JL: Intellectual impairment in Parkinson's disease: Clinical, pathologic, and biochemical correlates. *J Geriatr Psychiatry Neurol* 1:24–36, 1988.

146. Aarsland D, Andersen K, Larsen JP, et al: Risk of dementia in Parkinson's disease: A community-based, prospective study. *Neurology* 56:730–736, 2001.

147. Hughes TA, Ross HF, Musa S, et al: A 10-year study of the incidence of and factors predicting dementia in Parkinson's disease. *Neurology* 54:1596–1602, 2000.

148. Hurtig HI, Trojanowski JQ, Galvin J, et al: Alpha-synuclein cortical Lewy bodies correlate with dementia in Parkinson's disease. *Neurology* 54:1916–1921, 2000.

149. Ross GW, Mahler ME, Cummings JL: The dementia syndromes of Parkinson's disease: Cortical and subcortical features, in Huber SJ, Cummings JL (eds): *Parkinson's Disease: Behavioral and Neuropsychological Aspects*. New York: Oxford University Press, 1992, pp 132–148.

150. Morris M: Dementia and cognitive changes in Huntington's disease. *Adv Neurol* 65:187–200, 1995.

151. Jason Gregor W, Suchowersky O, Pajurkova E, et al: Cognitive manifestations of Huntington disease in relations to genetic structure and clinical onset. *Arch Neurol* 54:1081–1088, 1997.

152. Soliveri P, Monza D, Paridi D, et al: Neuropsychological follow-up in patients with Parkinson's disease, striatonigral-type multisystem atrophy, and progressive supranuclear palsy. *J Neurol Neurosurg Psychiatry* 69:313–318, 2000.

153. Cohen S, Freedman M: Cognitive and behavioral changes in the parkinson-plus syndromes. *Adv Neurol* 65:139–157, 1995.

154. Berciano J: Olivopontocerebellar atrophy: A review of 117 cases. *J Neurol Sci* 53:253–272, 1982.

155. Konigsmark BW, Weiner LP: The olivopontocerebellar atrophies: A review. *Medicine* 49:227–241, 1970.

156. Medalia A, Issacs-Glabermann K, Scheinberg H: Neuropsychological impairment in Wilson's disease. *Arch Neurol* 45:502–504, 1988.

157. Francis AF: Familial basal ganglia calcification and schizophreniform psychosis. *Br J Psychiatry* 135:360–362, 1979.

158. Grimes DA, Lang AE, Bergeron CB: Dementia as the most common presentation of cortico-basal ganglionic degeneration. *Neurology* 53:1969–1974, 1999.

159. Moossy J, Martinez AJ, Hanin I, et al: Thalamic and subcortical gliosis with dementia. *Arch Neurol* 44:510–513, 1987.

160. Janssen JC, Lantos PL, Al-Sarraj S, Rossor MN: Thalamic degeneration with negative prion protein immunostaining. *J Neurol* 247:48–51, 2000.

161. Robbins TW, James M, Owen AM, et al: Cognitive deficits in progressive supranuclear palsy, Parkinson's disease, and multiple system atrophy in tests sensitive to frontal lobe function. *J Neurol Neurosurg Psychiatry* 57:79–88, 1994.

Chapter 3

NEUROIMAGING OF MOVEMENT DISORDERS

DAVID J. BROOKS

PARKINSON'S DISEASE   36
    The Presynaptic Dopaminergic System   36
    Detection of Preclinical PD   37
    Microglial Activation in PD   38
    Modifying Progression of PD   39
    Restorative Approaches in PD   40
    Fluctuations and Dyskinesias in PD   42
    Dementia and PD   43
    Brain Activation in PD   44
ATYPICAL PARKINSONIAN SYNDROMES   46
    Multisystem Atrophy (MSA)   46
    Progressive Supranuclear Palsy (PSP)   47
    Corticobasal Degeneration (CBD)   47
INVOLUNTARY MOVEMENT DISORDERS   48
    Huntington's Disease (HD) and Other Choreas   48
    Transplantation of HD   49
    Dystonia   49
    Dopa-Responsive Dystonia (DRD) and
        Dystonia-Parkinsonism   51
CONCLUSIONS   51

With the advent of high-field magnetic resonance imaging (MRI), volumetric acquisitions, and more sophisticated sequences, the role of structural imaging in the diagnosis of parkinsonian disorders is becoming more important. MRI can be helpful in a number of ways. First, structural lesions can be excluded. Basal ganglia tumors, hemorrhages, small vessel disease, and calcification have all been associated with parkinsonism, as has hydrocephalus. There is still debate concerning whether vascular parkinsonism is a distinct entity, although 5 percent of parkinsonian cases have no other evident pathology.[1] Second, high-field MRI utilizing gray and white matter signal-suppressing inversion recovery sequences show abnormal signal from the substantia nigra compacta in the majority of idiopathic Parkinson's disease (PD) patients.[2,3]

The striatum appears normal on T_2-weighted MRI in PD, but in striatonigral degeneration and multisystem atrophy (MSA) the putamen characteristically shows reduced signal running up the lateral extent due to iron deposition and this may be covered by a rim of increased signal due to gliosis[4-6] (Fig. 3-1). If concomitant pontocerebellar degeneration is also present, the lateral as well as longitudinal pontine fibers become evident as high signal on T_2 MRI, manifesting as the "hot cross bun" sign. Cerebellar and pontine atrophy may be visually obvious with increased signal evident in the cerebellar peduncles. Formal MR volumetry detects putamen and brainstem atrophy in most established cases.[7] Patients with progressive supranuclear palsy (PSP) do not show the putamen signal changes characteristic of MSA but may show third ventricular widening and midbrain atrophy. In corticobasal degeneration (CBD), asymmetric hemispheric atrophy may be present and MRI can usefully exclude multi-infarct disease and multifocal leukoencephalopathy.

MRI findings in nondegenerative movement disorders, such as idiopathic dystonia and Tourette's syndrome, tend to be normal, although cases of acquired dystonia may show structural lesions in the lentiform nucleus or posterior thalamus.[8] MRI signal changes, generally manifested as raised T_2-weighted signal, can be found in the lentiform nucleus and other gray matter areas in established neurological Wilson's disease, although the sensitivity of this modality for detecting subclinical cerebral involvement in the hepatic form is unclear.[9] Altered striatal T_2-weighted MRI signal and later caudate atrophy are visually evident in clinically affected cases of Huntington's disease (HD).[10] Asymptomatic adult HD gene carriers generally have normal MRI findings on inspection but formal MR volumetry can often detect subclinical caudate and putamen atrophy.[11]

Functional imaging provides a robust means of detecting and characterizing the regional changes in brain metabolism and receptor binding associated with movement disorders. It can be of diagnostic value and also help to throw light on the pathophysiology underlying parkinsonian syndromes and involuntary movements. Functional imaging also provides a sensitive means of detecting subclinical disease in subjects at risk for degenerative disorders and of objectively following disease progression.

There are four main approaches to functional imaging. Positron emission tomography (PET) has the highest sensitivity, being able to detect femtomolar levels of

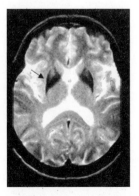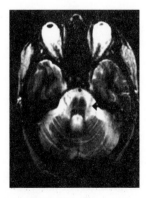

FIGURE 3-1 MRI findings in MSA. Reduced lateral putamen signal and the pontine "hot cross bun" sign can be seen on T_2-weighted images.

positron-emitting radioisotopes at a spatial resolution of 2–3 mm. It allows quantitative in vivo examination of alterations in regional cerebral blood flow (rCBF), glucose, oxygen, and dopa metabolism, and brain receptor binding. Single photon emission tomography (SPECT) is a less-sensitive modality, but it is more widely available and provides measures of rCBF and receptor binding. Magnetic resonance spectroscopy (MRS) has lower sensitivity and spatial resolution than the two radioisotope imaging approaches, detecting millimolar metabolite levels (N-acetylaspartate, lactate, phospholipids, ATP) at a spatial resolution of around 1 cm. Finally, MRI can detect activation-induced changes in oxygenation of venous blood draining from brain regions when subjects perform tasks—the BOLD technique.

The changes in regional cerebral function that characterize different movement disorders can be examined in two main ways. First, focal changes in resting levels of regional cerebral metabolism, blood flow, and neuroreceptor availability can be measured. Second, abnormal patterns of brain activation or levels of neurotransmitter release can be detected when patients with movement disorders perform motor and cognitive tasks or are exposed to drug challenges. The majority of functional imaging research into brain function in movement disorders has, to date, concerned PET and SPECT, so this chapter will concentrate on these techniques but will address functional MRI and proton MRS findings where relevant.

Parkinson's Disease

The pathology of Parkinson's disease (PD) targets the dopamine cells in the substantia nigra in association with the formation of intraneuronal Lewy inclusion bodies.[12] Serotonergic cells in the median raphe and noradrenergic cells in the locus ceruleus are also involved, as are other pigmented and brainstem nuclei. Loss of cells from the substantia nigra in PD results in profound dopamine depletion in the striatum, lateral nigral projections to putamen being most affected.[13,14] Lewy bodies are also found in the anterior cingulate and frontal, parietal, and temporal association cortex of nondemented PD cases at autopsy.[15] It remains uncertain whether dementia of Lewy body type and PD represent opposite ends of a spectrum. Dementia of Lewy body type has overlapping features with Alzheimer's disease (AD), which is twice as prevalent in PD, although it is associated with a higher prevalence of fluctuating confusion, hallucinations, early-onset rigidity, and gait difficulties.[16]

THE PRESYNAPTIC DOPAMINERGIC SYSTEM

The function of dopamine terminals in PD can be examined in vivo in several ways. First, terminal dopa decarboxylase activity can be measured with ^{18}F-dopa PET.[17,18] Second, the availability of presynaptic dopamine transporters can be assessed with tropane-based PET and SPECT tracers.[19–23] Third, vesicle monoamine transporter density in dopamine terminals can be examined with ^{11}C-dihydrotetrabenazine (DHTBZ) PET.[24] In early hemiparkinsonian cases, ^{18}F-dopa PET shows bilaterally reduced putamen tracer uptake, activity being most depressed in the putamen contralateral to the affected limbs[25] (Fig. 3-2). ^{18}F-dopa PET can, therefore, detect subclinical disease evidenced as involvement of the "asymptomatic" putamen contralateral to clinically unaffected limbs.

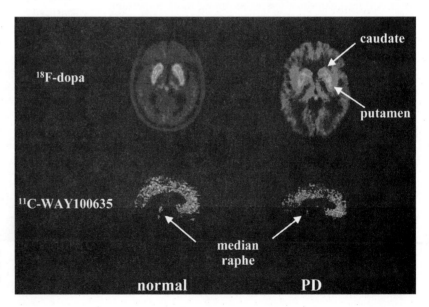

FIGURE 3-2 Dopamine terminal and serotonin HT$_{1A}$ function in PD. ^{18}F-dopa and ^{11}C-WAY100635 PET images for a normal subject and a PD patient. There is a selective loss of putamen dopamine storage and median raphe HT$_{1A}$ binding in PD. (*Courtesy of M. Doder.*) See Color Plate Section.

On average, PD patients show a 60% loss of specific putamen ^{18}F-dopa uptake in life compared to a 60–80 percent loss of ventrolateral nigra compacta cells and 95 percent loss of putamen dopamine at autopsy.[26] These findings suggest that striatal dopamine terminal dopa decarboxylase activity may be relatively upregulated in PD, presumably to boost dopamine turnover by remaining neurons. Cases of early PD (Hoehn and Yahr stage 1) show a 30–40 percent loss of ^{18}F-dopa uptake in the putamen contralateral to the affected limbs, suggesting that this loss of dopa decarboxylase activity may represent the threshold for onset of symptoms.

It is known that the pathology of PD is not uniform, ventrolateral nigral dopaminergic projections to the dorsal putamen being more affected than dorsomedial projections to the head of caudate.[14] ^{18}F-dopa PET reveals that, in patients with unilateral PD (Hoehn and Yahr stage 1), contralateral dorsal posterior putamen dopamine storage is first reduced.[27] As all limbs become clinically affected, ventral and anterior putamen and dorsal caudate dopaminergic function also become involved. Finally, when PD is well advanced, ventral head of caudate ^{18}F-dopa uptake starts to fall.

Not all dopamine fibers degenerate in early PD. Nigrostriatal projections comprise the densest dopamine pathway, but there is a lesser nigro-internal pallidal pathway.[28] The striatum is the main input and the globus pallidus interna (GPi) the main output nucleus of the basal ganglia, and dopamine release modulates the function of both these structures. While putamen ^{18}F-dopa uptake is reduced by 30–40 percent at the onset of parkinsonian rigidity and bradykinesia, GPi ^{18}F-dopa uptake is increased by 30–40 percent, but subsequently falls as the disease advances.[29] This coincides with the presence of treatment complications, such as fluctuating responses to levodopa, suggesting that both putamen and pallidus require tonic dopamine release to facilitate efficient fluent movements.

There are now many radiotracers, mainly tropane-based, that are available for measuring dopamine transporter binding on nigrostriatal terminals and so providing a measure of integrity of dopaminergic function in PD. PET tracers include ^{11}C-CFT[20] and ^{18}F-CFT,[19] ^{11}C-RTI-32,[30] ^{11}C-nomifensine,[31] and ^{11}C-phenylethylamine,[32] which bind to both dopamine and noradrenaline reuptake sites. Available SPECT tracers include the tropane analogues ^{123}I-beta-CIT,[21] ^{123}I-FP-CIT,[22] ^{123}I-altropane,[33] and ^{99m}Tc-TRODAT-1.[34] ^{123}I-beta-CIT gives the highest striatal:cerebellar uptake ratio of these SPECT tracers, but this reflects low cerebellar nonspecific, rather than high striatal specific, uptake and so this tracer provides a potentially noisy reference signal. Additionally, it binds nonselectively to dopamine, noradrenaline, and serotonin transporters and has the disadvantage that it takes 24 hours to equilibrate throughout the brain following intravenous injection, so scanning has to be delayed until the following day. For this reason, SPECT tracers such as ^{123}I-FP-CIT and ^{123}I-altropane have come into vogue because, despite their lower and time-dependent striatal:cerebellar uptake ratios, a diagnostic scan can be performed within 2–3 hours of tracer injection. More recently a technetium-based tropane tracer, ^{99m}Tc-TRODAT-1, has been developed. This gives a lower (2:1) striatal:cerebellar uptake ratio than the ^{123}I-based tracers and is less well extracted by the brain, but it has the advantage that it is readily available in kit form. All the above PET and SPECT tracers appear to differentiate clinically probable early PD from normal subjects or essential tremor patients with a sensitivity of around 90 percent.[21,35,36] A positive PET or SPECT scan can thus be valuable for supporting a diagnosis of PD where there is diagnostic doubt. It is not clear, however, whether a negative PET or SPECT scan fully excludes this diagnosis.

Putamen uptake of PET and SPECT dopaminergic tracers shows an inverse correlation with degree of locomotor disability in PD, reflecting limb bradykinesia and rigidity rather than rest tremor severity.[22,37] Relative to the dopamine vesicle transporter marker, ^{11}C-DHTBZ, it has been shown that putamen ^{18}F-dopa uptake is relatively upregulated and binding of the dopamine transporter marker ^{11}C-methylphenidate relatively downregulated in PD.[32] This finding makes physiological sense, as increased dopamine turnover and decreased reuptake in a dopamine-deficiency syndrome should help to preserve synaptic transmitter levels.

In PD there is loss not only of dopamine but also of serotonin projections. Median raphe serotonin HT_{1A} binding in the midbrain, measured with ^{11}C-WAY100635 PET, reflects the functional integrity of serotonergic cell bodies. In PD there is a mean 25 percent loss of median raphe HT_{1A} binding (Fig. 3-2) and, interestingly, severity of rest tremor correlates significantly with individual levels of median raphe ^{11}C-WAY100635 binding.[38] This suggests that midbrain tegmentum pathology involving serotonin projections rather than nigral cell loss may be relevant to the etiology of PD tremor.

DETECTION OF PRECLINICAL PD

It has been estimated from postmortem studies that, for every patient who presents with clinical PD, there may be 10–15 subclinical cases with incidental brainstem Lewy body disease in the community.[39] Subjects likely to be at risk of developing Parkinson's disease include relatives of patients with the disorder.[40] Piccini et al.[41] used ^{18}F-dopa PET to study 32 asymptomatic adult relatives in 7 kindreds with familial PD, each of which contained at least 2 affected individuals with L-dopa-responsive parkinsonism. In 5 of these kindreds the pathology was unknown; the sixth kindred was subsequently found to have *parkin* gene mutations, while the seventh kindred was known to have diffuse Lewy body disease (DLBD). Affected individuals from the 6 non-*parkin* kindreds all showed the typical pattern of reduced striatal ^{18}F-dopa uptake associated with sporadic PD: putamen tracer uptake was more severely reduced than caudate. The *parkin*

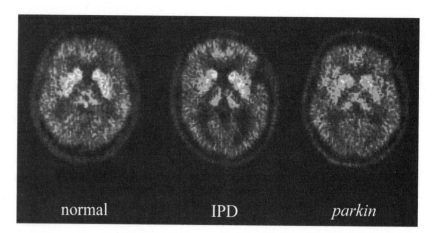

FIGURE 3-3 F-dopa uptake in PD. ^{18}F-dopa PET in idiopathic (IPD) and *parkin*-associated PD. There is a selective loss of putamen dopamine storage in IPD but uniform striatal involvement in *parkin* disease. (*Courtesy of N. Khan.*) See Color Plate Section.

normal   IPD   *parkin*

cases showed a severe loss of both caudate and putamen dopamine storage (Fig. 3-3).

Of the asymptomatic adult relatives scanned, 25 percent showed levels of putamen ^{18}F-dopa uptake reduced more than 2.5 SD (standard deviation) below the normal mean. Three of the 8 asymptomatic relatives with reduced putamen ^{18}F-dopa uptake subsequently developed clinical parkinsonism. Based on clinical surveys, a 15 percent prevalence is normally quoted for the presence of a positive family history in PD, although this approaches 40 percent if a fully informative history is available.[40] ^{18}F-dopa PET findings indicate that 25 percent of asymptomatic adult relatives of index cases with familial parkinsonism (i.e., 50 percent of the at-risk population) have evidence of subclinical dopaminergic dysfunction.

[18]F-dopa PET findings for 34 asymptomatic and two clinically concordant co-twins of idiopathic sporadic PD patients aged 23–67 years have also been reported.[42] Eighteen co-twins were monozygotic (MZ), while 16 were dizygotic (DZ); 10 (55 percent) of the 18 MZ and 3 (18 percent) of the 16 DZ co-twins had levels of putamen ^{18}F-dopa uptake that were reduced more than 2.5 SD below the normal mean. The finding of a significantly higher concordance (55 percent versus 18 percent, $P = 0.03$) for dopaminergic dysfunction in MZ compared with DZ PD co-twins supports a genetic contribution towards this apparently sporadic disorder. Interestingly, when a subgroup of these co-twins was scanned serially, all 10 of the asymptomatic MZ co-twins scanned showed a decrease in putamen ^{18}F-dopa uptake on repeat scanning 4.0 ± 1.7 years after the first scan; the mean rate of the loss of putamen ^{18}F-dopa uptake was 4.5 percent per year. On the basis of their follow-up scans, 3 more MZ co-twins were classified as having subclinical PD. Nine asymptomatic DZ co-twins (mean age 56.7 ± 15.2 years) were also scanned twice over a period of 4.3 ± 2.2 years but showed no significant change in putamen ^{18}F-dopa uptake. The percentage annual loss in putamen ^{18}F-dopa uptake for MZ and DZ co-twins was significantly different ($P = 0.001$).

Over the 7 years of follow-up, 2 MZ co-twins and 1 DZ co-twin died without developing symptoms, while 4 MZ co-twins became clinically concordant for PD (at 65, 70, 72, and 78 years of age, 14, 2, 9, and 20 years after the onset of PD in their co-twin), resulting in a clinical concordance of 22.2 percent at follow-up. The clinical concordance within the MZ pairs over 60 years of age was higher (50 percent, 4 of 8). None of the DZ twin pairs became clinically concordant, and the difference in clinical concordance between the MZ and DZ twin pairs in the 60–70 age group of age was significant ($P = 0.04$; Fisher exact test).

It has long been recognized that PD patients perform poorly on the University of Pennsylvania Smell Identification Test (UPSIT) olfactory test battery. A recent survey scanned 25 hyposmic and 23 normosmic relatives of PD patients with beta-CIT SPECT in order to screen them for the presence of subclinical dopaminergic dysfunction. Four subclinical cases were found and these are now being followed.[43]

MICROGLIAL ACTIVATION IN PD

Microglia constitute 10–20 percent of white cells in the brain and form its natural defence mechanism. They are normally in a resting state, but local injury causes them to activate and swell, expressing HLA antigens on the cell surface and releasing cytokines. The mitochondria of activated but not resting microglia express peripheral benzodiazepine sites which may have a role in preventing apoptosis via membrane stabilization. ^{11}C-PK11195 is an isoquinoline which binds selectively to peripheral benzodiazepine sites and so provides an in vivo PET marker of glial activation.

Loss of substantia nigra neurons in PD is known to be associated with microglial activation.[44] ^{11}C-PK11195 PET has been used to study microglial activation in PD and has detected increased signal in both the nigra and pallidum (Fig. 3-4).[45] The nigral ^{11}C-PK11195 uptake reflects

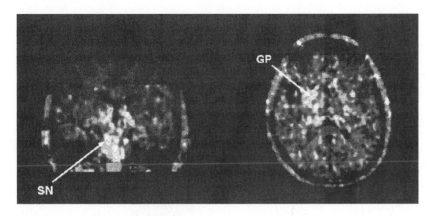

FIGURE 3-4 ^{11}C-PK11195 PET images for a PD patient showing microglial activation in the midbrain and pallidum. SN, substantia nigra; GP, globus pallidus. (*Courtesy of A. Gerhard.*) See Color Plate Section.

local degeneration, while the pallidal signal may result from excess glutamate release from subthalamic projections as a consequence of dopamine deficiency.

MODIFYING PROGRESSION OF PD

There are a number of difficulties that arise when attempting to assess the progression of PD clinically as rating scales are subjective, nonlinear, consider multiple aspects of the disorder, and are biased towards particular symptoms—bradykinesia in the case of the Unified Parkinson's Disease Rating Scale (UPDRS). More importantly, symptomatic therapy can mask disease progression and it is difficult to achieve a full washout. PET and SPECT imaging and, potentially, MRI of the nigra provide complementary biological markers for objectively monitoring disease progression in vivo in PD. They are limited, however, to providing information concerning particular aspects of the disorder, such as dopamine terminal function or changes in nigral water environment.

Striatal ^{18}F-dopa uptake has been shown to correlate with subsequent postmortem dopaminergic cell densities in the substantia nigra and striatal dopamine levels of patients and of 1-methyl-4-phenyl-1,2,3,6-tetrahydropyridine (MPTP) lesioned monkeys.[46,47] It is also highly reproducible and, at least in subjects with an intact dopamine system, does not appear to be influenced by dopaminergic medication.[48,49] ^{18}F-dopa PET can, therefore, be used as a marker of dopamine terminal function in PD, although it may overestimate terminal density due to a relative upregulation of dopa decarboxylase in remaining neurons as a response to nigral cell loss. Striatal ^{123}I-beta-CIT uptake has also been shown to be unaffected by several weeks of exposure to L-dopa[50] and dopamine agonists.[51] In contrast to ^{18}F-dopa, ^{123}I-beta-CIT uptake may underestimate terminal density due to a relative downregulation of dopamine transporters in remaining neurons as a response to nigral cell loss.

Several series have now shown that loss of striatal ^{18}F-dopa uptake occurs more rapidly in PD than in age-matched controls.[52–54] On average, in early L-dopa-treated PD, putamen ^{18}F-dopa uptake has been reported to decline by around 10 percent per annum while caudate uptake falls at about half that rate. Parallel rates of loss of putamen dopamine transporter binding have been reported with ^{18}F-CFT PET[55] and ^{123}I-beta-CIT,[56] ^{123}I-FP-CIT,[57] and ^{123}I-IPT SPECT.[58] In one series, striatal ^{123}I-beta-CIT uptake in early PD correlated with initial levels of striatal transporter binding, suggesting an exponential disease process.[59]

As functional imaging can objectively follow loss of dopamine terminal function in PD, it provides a potential means of monitoring the efficacy of putative neuroprotective agents. Dopamine agonists are one such possible class as they suppress endogenous dopamine production in vivo, so attenuating its oxidative metabolism with potential free radical formation. They are also weak antioxidants and free radical scavengers in their own right, and may also act as mitochondrial membrane stabilizers, so blocking the apoptotic cascade. Two different trials have examined the relative rates of loss of dopamine terminal function in early PD in patients randomized to a dopamine agonist or L-dopa.

In the REAL PET 2-year double-blind multinational study, 186 de novo PD patients were randomized (1:1) to ropinirole or L-dopa.[60] The primary endpoint was change in putamen ^{18}F-dopa uptake (Ki, influx constant) measured with PET. Scan data from six PET centers were transformed into standard stereotactic space at one center in order to normalize brain position and shape. Parametric Ki images were then generated and sampled with a standard region-of-interest (ROI) template. Ki images were also interrogated with statistical parametric mapping (SPM99) to localize voxel clusters where significant between-group differences in rates of loss of dopaminergic function were occurring; 74 percent of the ropinirole group and 73 percent of the L-dopa group completed the study. Mean (SD) daily doses of double-blind medication after 2 years were 12.2 (6.1) mg ropinirole and 558.7 (180.8) mg L-dopa. Only 14 percent of the ropinirole group and 8 percent of the L-dopa group required open supplementary L-dopa. Interestingly, 11 percent of the untreated patients thought to have PD were found to have normal caudate and putamen ^{18}F-dopa uptake at entry (identified by blinded review) and this group was analyzed separately. The ROI analysis found that loss of putamen Ki was significantly slower over 2 years with ropinirole (−13.4 percent) than with L-dopa (−20.3 percent; $P = 0.022$). SPM revealed that falls in Ki were significantly slower in both putamen and substantia nigra with ropinirole compared with L-dopa (putamen: ropinirole, −14.1 percent; L-dopa, −22.9 percent; $P < 0.001$; substantia nigra: ropinirole, +4.3 percent; L-dopa, −7.5 percent; $P = 0.025$). Clinically, the incidence of dyskinesia was 26.7 percent with L-dopa but only 3.4 percent with ropinirole ($P < 0.001$). Improvements in mean UPDRS motor scores while taking medication were, however, superior (by 6.34 points) for the L-dopa cohort.

The other trial comprised a subgroup of the CALM-PD study in which a cohort of 82 early PD patients were randomized 1:1 to the dopamine agonist pramipexole (0.5 mg tds) or L-dopa (100 mg tds) and had serial ^{123}I-beta-CIT SPECT over a 4-year period.[61] Open supplementary L-dopa was allowed if there was lack of therapeutic effect. Patients treated initially with pramipexole ($n = 42$) showed a significantly slower mean relative decline of striatal beta-CIT uptake compared to subjects treated initially with L-dopa ($n = 40$) at 2 (47 percent), 3 (44 percent), and 4 (37 percent) years. Again, the incidence of complications was significantly reduced in the pramipexole cohort, but improvement in UPDRS score while taking medication was greater in the L-dopa cohort.

These two trials, therefore, produced parallel findings, both suggesting that treatment with an agonist in early PD slows loss of dopamine terminal function by around one-third and delays treatment-associated complications. A difficulty is that the functional imaging findings favoring use of ropinirole and pramipexole as early treatment were not paralleled by a better clinical outcome in the PD agonist cohorts as judged by UPDRS motor scores while receiving medication. Additionally, one cannot rule out differential chronic pharmacological effects of the treatments on the imaging modalities though long-term exposure to L-dopa does not appear to effect striatal ^{18}F-dopa or ^{123}I-beta-CIT uptake in subjects with normal dopaminergic function. The real test will be whether early use of agonists delays the need for institutional care in the long term.

RESTORATIVE APPROACHES IN PD

HUMAN FETAL CELL IMPLANTATION TRIALS

As well as providing a means of following natural disease progression and monitoring the effects of putative neuroprotective agents, functional imaging provides a means of examining the efficacy of restorative approaches to PD. Possible approaches include striatal implants of human and porcine fetal mesencephalic cells, retinal cells that release L-dopa/dopamine, and transformed cells that secrete dopamine, nerve growth factors, or express antiapoptotic genes, neural progenitor cells, and direct intrastriatal infusions of nerve growth factors.

There have now been several open series detailing clinical and ^{18}F-dopa PET findings in advanced PD patients after implantation of fetal mesencephalic cells or tissue into striatum.[62] The Lund group have reported serial clinical and ^{18}F-dopa PET findings over a period of 10 years on 2 PD patients following implantation of fetal midbrain cells into the putamen contralateral to their more affected limbs. Both of these patients have maintained a clinical improvement, particularly in "on" time, which went from 40 percent to all of the day in 1 unilaterally grafted case whose ^{18}F-dopa uptake into the implanted putamen reached the lower end of the normal range. It was subsequently demonstrated that the graft released normal synaptic levels of dopamine after an amphetamine challenge (Fig. 3-5).[63]

Another 4 unilaterally transplanted PD patients showed ^{18}F-dopa PET evidence of graft function 1 year following surgery and 3 responded clinically to transplantation, but the fourth deteriorated and now has signs suggestive of MSA.[64] In a subsequent series of 4 bilaterally transplanted patients, a mean 50 percent improvement in UPDRS scores was demonstrated at 2 years, associated with a 60 percent increase in putamen and 30 percent increase in caudate ^{18}F-dopa uptake.[65]

Clinically successful transplantation of fetal tissue with corroborative serial ^{18}F-dopa PET findings has also been reported for 5 PD patients in a 2-year open follow-up French study,[66] and for 6 PD patients in a 2-year follow-up series from Tampa, Florida.[67] In the French study, grafted putamen Ki values correlated with percentage time "on" during the day and finger dexterity while in an "off" state. Two of the transplanted PD patients in the Florida series died from unrelated causes and viable tyrosine hydroxylase-staining graft tissue forming connections with host neurons was found at autopsy.[68]

Given the encouraging findings of these pilot open series, two major double-blind controlled trials on the efficacy of implantation of human fetal cells in PD were sponsored by the NIH in the US. The first of these involved 40 patients who were 34–75 years of age and had severe PD (mean duration 14 years).[69] These were randomized to receive either an implant of human fetal mesencephalic tissue or undergo sham surgery, and were followed for 1 year with a subsequent extension to 3 years. In the transplant recipients, mesencephalic tissue from four embryos cultured for up to 1 month was implanted into the putamen bilaterally (two embryos per side) via a frontal approach. In the patients who underwent sham surgery, holes were drilled in the skull but the dura was not penetrated. No immunotherapy was used. The transplanted patients showed no significant improvement in the primary endpoint, clinical global impression, at 1 year but there was a significant mean 18 percent improvement in mean UPDRS motor score compared with the sham surgery group when tested in the morning before receiving medication ($P = 0.04$). This improvement was more evident for patients under 60 years of age (34 percent improvement; $P = 0.005$). At 3 years, mean total UPDRS score was improved

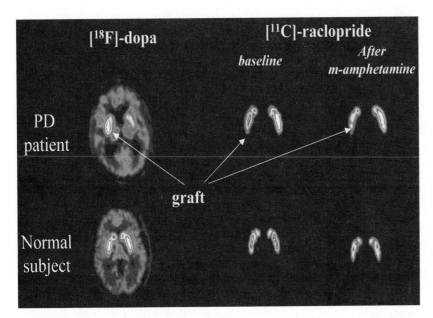

FIGURE 3-5 Dopamine release from nigral transplants visualized *in vivo* in Parkinson's disease. ^{18}F-dopa and ^{11}C-raclopride PET images before and after amphetamine for a normal subject and a PD patient. It can be seen that the PD patient takes up normal levels of striatal ^{18}F-dopa on the unilaterally grafted side and that striatal ^{11}C-raclopride falls normally after amphetamine. (*Courtesy of P. Piccini.*) See Color Plate Section.

38 percent in the younger and 14 percent in the older transplanted groups (both $P < 0.01$); 16 out of 19 transplanted patients individually showed an increase in putamen ^{18}F-dopa uptake (group mean increase 40 percent), and increases were similar in the younger and older cohorts.[70] A drawback was that "off" dystonia and dyskinesias developed in 15 percent of the patients who received transplants in this series, even after reduction or discontinuation of L-dopa.

More recently, the second trial NIH trial has reported.[71] Here, 34 patients were randomized to receive bilateral implants of fetal mesencephalic tissue from four fetuses per side or from one fetus per side into posterior putamen, or had sham surgery (a partial burr hole without penetration of the dura). Fetal tissue was cultured for less than 48 hours before transplantation and all patients received immunosuppression for 6 months after surgery. The trial duration was 2 years and the primary outcome variable was the UPDRS motor score and quality of life. Putamen ^{18}F-dopa uptake was assessed with PET in a subset of patients; 31 patients completed and 2 patients died during the trial, while another 3 died subsequently from unrelated causes. At autopsy the transplanted patients showed significantly higher tyrosine hydroxylase staining in the putamen relative to the sham-grafted treated patients with graft innervation evident. Putamen ^{18}F-dopa uptake was unchanged in the control patients but showed a one-third increase in patients receiving tissue from four fetuses. Unfortunately, no significant differences were seen between the groups in clinical rating scores. The mean UPDRS motor score off medication for the controls deteriorated by 9.4, 3.5, and -0.7 points over 2 years for the controls, one fetus, and four fetus groups (four fetus versus controls $P = 0.096$). Additionally, no significant differences in "on" time without dyskinesias, total

"off" time, ADL (activities of daily living) scores, or L-dopa dose required were evident between the groups. Interestingly, those patients with lowest UPDRS scores responded significantly better to transplantation than to sham surgery. "Off" period dyskinesias were evident in 13 of 23 implanted patients but were not seen in the control arm.

In summary, despite both histological and ^{18}F-dopa PET evidence of graft function, neither of these controlled trials demonstrated clinical efficacy with their primary endpoints, and in both "off" period dyskinesias were problematic. There were indications, however, that younger, more severely affected patients benefited from intrastriatal implantation of human fetal dopamine cells.

INTRAPUTAMINAL GLIAL CELL LINE-DERIVED NEUROTROPHIC FACTOR (GDNF) INFUSION

GDNF is a potent neurotrophic factor known to prevent the degeneration of dopamine neurons in rodent and primate models of PD where nigral degeneration is toxically induced with 6-hydroxydopamine or MPTP. The safety and efficacy of infusing GDNF directly into the posterior putamen has been recently studied in a small open trial.[72] Five PD patients had in-dwelling catheters inserted and all have tolerated continuous GDNF delivery at a final level of 14 μg/day (6 μL/hour) for over 1 year, unilaterally in 1 patient and bilaterally in 4 patients, without serious side-effects. Significant improvements were reported in UPDRS subscores: 39 percent and 61 percent improvements in the off-medication motor III and ADL II subscales, respectively, at 12 months. No change in cognitive status was detected on a battery of behavioral tests. Regions of interest sited in the vicinity of the catheter tip showed 18–24 percent increases in putaminal ^{18}F-dopa Ki, which were confirmed with statistical parametric mapping. Additionally, SPM detected 16–26 percent increases in nigral dopamine storage, suggesting that retrograde transport of GDNF may have occurred. These findings imply that putamen GDNF infusion is safe and may represent a potential restorative approach for PD.

FLUCTUATIONS AND DYSKINESIAS IN PD

PD patients with fluctuating responses to L-dopa show lower putamen ^{18}F-dopa uptake than those with early disease and sustained therapeutic responses. A confounder, however, when trying to compare presynaptic dopamine terminal function in these groups is that the former tend to have an earlier age of disease onset, more severe disease, longer disease duration, and a greater cumulative exposure to L-dopa. By using ANCOVA to factor out effects of age at onset and disease duration in groups of fluctuators and nonfluctuators and also matching subgroups of these patients for age of onset and disease duration, De La Fuente-Fernandez et al. concluded that mean putamen ^{18}F-dopa uptake was 28 percent lower in PD patients with motor complications than in those without, but that there was considerable overlap of the two individual ranges.[73] While loss of putamen dopamine terminal function predisposes PD patients towards development of L-dopa-associated complications, it cannot be solely responsible for determining the timing of onset of fluctuations and involuntary movements. Dopamine receptors broadly fall into D1 (D1, D5) and D2 (D2, D3, D4) classes. The striatum contains mainly D1 and D2 receptor subtypes, and these both play a role in modulating locomotor function. PET with spiperone-based tracers and ^{123}I-IBZM SPECT studies have both reported normal levels of striatal D2 binding in untreated PD, while ^{11}C-raclopride PET has shown 10–20 percent increases in putamen D2 site availability.[74,75] In chronically treated PD, ^{11}C-methylspiperone PET and ^{123}I-IBZM SPECT studies have reported normal or mildly reduced striatal D2 binding.[74] Serial ^{11}C-raclopride PET has shown that, after 6 months of exposure to L-dopa, the mildly increased putamen ^{11}C-raclopride binding seen in de novo PD patients normalizes.[76] Chronically L-dopa-exposed PD cases continue to show normal levels of putamen D2 binding, explaining their good locomotor response to L-dopa, while caudate D2 binding becomes 20 percent reduced.[77] ^{11}C-SCH23390 PET, a marker of D1 site binding, shows normal striatal uptake in de novo PD,[78] while patients who have been exposed to L-dopa for several years show a 20 percent reduction in striatal binding.[77] These findings are in good agreement with in vitro reports of striatal dopamine D1 and D2 receptor binding based on autopsy material from endstage patients.

As previously discussed, a confounder when trying to compare postsynaptic dopamine receptor function in PD patients with and without motor complications is that the former tend to have an earlier age of onset, more severe

disease, longer disease duration, and a greater cumulative exposure to L-dopa. Striatal dopamine D1 and D2 receptor availability has been examined in age-matched subgroups of 8 L-dopa-exposed dyskinetic patients and 10 nondyskinetic patients with similar clinical disease duration, disease severity, and daily L-dopa dosage.[77] Mean caudate and putamen D1 and putamen D2 binding were normal for both the dyskinetic and the nondyskinetic PD subgroups, while caudate D2 binding was reduced in each by around 15 percent.

Other series have also noted similar striatal dopamine D1 and D2 binding in fluctuating and dyskinetic PD patients compared with sustained responders.[79] These findings therefore suggest that onset of motor complications in PD is not primarily associated with alterations in striatal dopamine receptor availability.

[11]C-raclopride PET allows changes in levels of striatal dopamine release to be monitored. A challenge with an intravenous bolus of 0.3 mg/kg metamphetamine caused a 24 percent reduction in putamen ^{11}C-raclopride binding in normal subjects due to competition with the dopamine released for D2 receptor binding.[63] When early nonfluctuating PD patients are given 3 mg/kg of L-dopa as an intravenous bolus, they show a mean 10 percent fall in posterior putamen ^{11}C-raclopride binding, while advanced cases with fluctuations show a 23 percent fall.[80] These reductions in putamen ^{11}C-raclopride binding correlate with disease severity assessed off medication with the UPDRS and indicate that, as loss of dopamine terminals in PD increases, striatal buffering of dopamine fails when clinical doses of exogenous L-dopa are administered. This failure reflects a combination of upregulation of striatal dopamine synthesis and release from L-dopa by the remaining terminals along with severe loss of dopamine transporters preventing reuptake. It is this phenomenon, rather than changes in postsynaptic dopamine D1 and D2 receptor binding, that is likely to be the explanation for the more rapid response of advanced PD patients to oral L-dopa. This process will also result in high nonphysiological swings in synaptic dopamine levels, which may lead to excessive dopamine receptor internalization, again promoting fluctuating treatment responses.

De La Fuente-Fernandez et al. have examined changes in ^{11}C-raclopride binding after an oral L-dopa challenge in advanced PD and shown that "off" episodes do not necessarily coincide with low synaptic dopamine levels.[81] This finding is again in favor of fluctuations occurring either due to inappropriate levels of dopamine receptor internalization at times, making them unpredictably unavailable at the cell surface for stimulation, or due to aberrant downstream changes in basal ganglia transmission making them refractory, rather than due to a lack of dopaminergic tone at postsynaptic D2 receptors.

Medium spiny projection neurons in the caudate and putamen release opioids and substance P along with gamma-aminobutyric acid (GABA) into external and

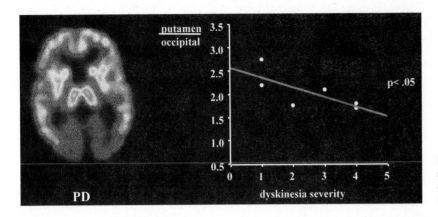

FIGURE 3-6 ^{11}C-Diprenorphine binding in PD, showing an inverse correlation between levels of putamen uptake and dyskinesia severity. (*Courtesy of P. Piccini.*) See Color Plate Section.

internal pallidum.[82] Striatal projections to external pallidum (GPe) contain enkephalin, which binds mainly to delta opioid sites and inhibits GABA release in the GPe. Striatal projections to internal pallidum (GPi) transmit dynorphin, which binds to kappa opioid sites and inhibits glutamate release from STN afferents to the GPi, and substance P which binds to NK1 receptors. It is thought that phasic firing of striatopallidal projection neurons results primarily in GABA release, while sustained tonic firing causes additional modulatory opioid and substance P release. The caudate and putamen also contain high densities of mu, kappa, and delta opioid sites. These receptors are located both presynaptically on dopamine terminals, where they regulate dopamine release, and postsynaptically on interneurons and medium spiny projection neurons to pallidum terminals. There is now strong evidence supporting the presence of deranged opioid and substance P transmission in the basal ganglia of PD patients both from postmortem studies and lesion animal models of this disorder.[83,84] At autopsy, endstage treated PD patients show raised levels of pallidal preproenkephalin. In rats lesioned with the nigral toxin 6-OHDA (6-hydroxydopamine) there are raised levels of striatal enkephalin and preproenkephalin expression while prodynorphin expression is suppressed.[82] When such animals are made hyperkinetic or frankly dyskinetic after chronic exposure to pulsatile doses of l-dopa, further overexpression of striatal preproenkephalin is seen along with raised expression of prodynorphin and substance P. l-Dopa-naïve MPTP-lesioned monkeys have also been reported to show raised striatal enkephalin and reduced substance P mRNA expression.[85] Exposure to l-dopa for 1 month failed to normalize striatal preproenkephalin mRNA expression while substance P mRNA expression became elevated.

[11]C-Diprenorphine PET is a nonselective marker of mu, kappa, and delta opioid sites, and its binding is sensitive to levels of endogenous opioids. If raised basal ganglia levels of enkephalin and dynorphin are associated with levodopa-induced dyskinesias (LIDs) then PD patients with motor complications would be expected to show reduced binding of ^{11}C-diprenorphine compared to those with sustained treatment responses. Piccini et al. have reported significant reductions in ^{11}C-diprenorphine binding in caudate, putamen, thalamus, and anterior cingulate in dyskinetic patients compared with sustained responders (Fig. 3-6).[86] Individual levels of putamen ^{11}C-diprenorphine uptake correlated inversely with severity of dyskinesia. ^{18}F-L829165 PET is a selective marker of NK1 site availability. In a preliminary study, thalamic NK1 availability has been shown to be reduced in dyskinetic PD patients but normal in nondyskinetic cases.[87] These in vivo findings support the presence of elevated levels of endogenous peptides in the basal ganglia of dyskinetic PD patients and suggest that this, rather than a primary alteration in dopamine receptor binding, may in part be responsible for the appearance of involuntary movements.

DEMENTIA AND PD

RESTING BRAIN METABOLISM

PET studies have shown increased levels of resting oxygen and glucose metabolism in the contralateral lentiform nucleus of hemiparkinsonian patients with early disease, while PD patients with established bilateral involvement have normal levels of lentiform metabolism.[88,89] Covariance analysis reveals an abnormal profile of relatively raised resting lentiform nucleus and lowered frontal metabolism in PD patients with established disease even when absolute values are normal.[90] The degree of expression of this profile correlates with clinical disease severity.

Nondemented PD patients show normal cortical metabolism, while [18]FDG (^{18}F-deoxyglucose) PET scans of frankly demented PD patients show an Alzheimer pattern of impaired brain glucose utilization, posterior parietal and temporal association areas being most affected.[91,92] It remains unclear whether the pattern of glucose hypometabolism in demented PD patients reflects coincidental Alzheimer's disease (AD), cortical Lewy body disease, loss of cholinergic projections, or some other degenerative process. Clinicopathological series suggest that there is considerable overlap in the cortical FDG PET findings of coincidental AD and cortical Lewy body disease, but that cortical Lewy body disease cases show a greater reduction in resting glucose metabolism of the primary visual cortex.[93] Interestingly, in one series, one-third of nondemented PD patients with established disease showed subclinical resting temporoparietal cortical metabolic dysfunction with both [18]FDG PET and ^{31}P-NMR spectroscopy.[94] Whether these are cases that will go on to become demented is still unclear.

DOPAMINERGIC FUNCTION

The prevalence of dementia is raised 2-fold in Parkinson's disease; possible causes include direct cortical involvement by diffuse Lewy body disease (DLBD), coincident AD, small vessel disease, and loss of cholinergic projections.[95] Additionally, DLBD is thought to be the pathological diagnosis in around 20 percent of cases with the clinical picture of AD. Whether DLBD and PD represent opposite ends of a spectrum is unclear, but DLBD patients show not only cerebral cortical neuronal loss, with Lewy bodies in surviving neurons, but also loss of nigrostriatal dopaminergic neurons. In contrast, nigral pathology is mild in AD. Using ^{123}I-FP-CIT SPECT, Walker et al.[96] have examined striatal dopamine transporter binding in 27 patients with clinically presumed DLBD, 17 with AD, 19 drug-naive patients with PD, and 16 controls. The presumed DLBD and PD patients had significantly lower uptake of caudate and putamen ^{123}I-FP-CIT than patients with AD ($P < 0.001$) and controls ($P < 0.001$). A problem, however, with the interpretation of this finding is that the DLBD and PD patient groups had equivalent parkinsonism on their UPDRS and Hoehn and Yahr ratings, while the AD patients and controls had slight or no rigidity. The SPECT findings could, therefore, simply have reflected clinical selection bias. The authors, however, were able subsequently to correlate their SPECT findings with 10 postmortem examinations. Nine of these 10 cases were thought to have DLBD in life but only 4 had this diagnosis at autopsy. All 4 had reduced striatal ^{123}I-FP-CIT uptake. Five of the 10 cases had AD pathology and 4 of these 5 had normal ^{123}I-FP-CIT SPECT. These clinicoimaging correlations suggest that ^{123}I-FP-CIT SPECT may be helpful in discriminating DLBD from AD, but its role in patients with isolated dementia without parkinsonism remains unproven.

BRAIN ACTIVATION IN PD

While studies of resting CBF and metabolism provide insight into the cerebral dysfunction underlying movement disorders, measuring changes in rCBF while patients perform motor or cognitive tasks can be more revealing. When normal subjects move a joystick in freely selected directions with their right hand paced by a regular tone, $H_2^{15}O$ PET detects associated rCBF increases in contralateral sensorimotor cortex (SMC) and lentiform nucleus, and bilaterally in anterior cingulate, supplementary motor area (SMA), lateral premotor cortex (PMC), and dorsolateral prefrontal cortex (DLPFC).[97] Self-paced extensions of the index finger result in a similar pattern of activation.[98] When PD patients, scanned after stopping L-dopa for 12 hours, perform the same motor tasks, normal activation of SMC, PMC, and lateral parietal association areas are seen, but there is impaired activation of the contralateral lentiform nucleus and the anterior cingulate, SMA, and DLPFC—i.e., of those frontal areas that receive direct input from the basal ganglia. It is well recognized that, while patients with PD can perform isolated limb movements efficiently, attempts to perform repetitive or sequences of movements results in a fall in amplitude, and motor arrest. Using $H_2^{15}O$ PET, Samuel et al. demonstrated underactivity of mesial frontal areas and deactivation of dorsolateral prefrontal areas when patients perform prelearned sequential opposition finger-thumb movements with one or both hands.[99] Lateral premotor and parietal areas were relatively overactivated, suggesting adaptive recruitment of a network normally used to facilitate externally cued rather than freely chosen movements (Fig. 3-7). The cerebellum plays a primary role in coordination and accurate tracking. Rascol et al.[100] reported abnormally raised levels of cerebellar regional CBF when PD patients perform sequential finger-thumb opposition movements. Functional MRI has also demonstrated underactivity of the anterior supplementary motor area and DLPFC, and overactivity of lateral premotor and parietal areas in PD during sequential finger movements.[101] Additionally, overactivity of motor cortex and caudal SMA was also noted. The detection of motor area overactivity by these workers may, in part, reflect greater sensitivity of MRI compared with PET for activation studies, but may also reflect the more complex design of the paradigm employed. Here, the subjects had to perform fist-clenching in between sequential finger-thumb opposition movements. In support of the presence of primary motor cortex overactivation in PD, a second group has reported this finding when patients performed an externally cued reaching task.[102]

It has been proposed that: (1) dorsal prefrontal cortex plays a crucial role in motor decision-making; (2) the supplementary motor area prepares and optimizes volitional motor programs once selected;[103] (3) lateral premotor cortex has a primary role in facilitating motor responses to external visual and auditory stimuli. An inability to activate DLPFC and SMA during freely selected and sequential movements could explain the difficulty that PD patients experience in initiating such actions. In contrast, their ability to overactivate lateral premotor and primary motor cortex allows them to respond well to visual and auditory cues, such as stepping over lines on the floor to aid their walking.

EFFECTS OF TREATMENT

If loss of dopamine is responsible for the impaired activation of striatofrontal projections in PD, it should be possible to restore it by administering dopaminergic medication.

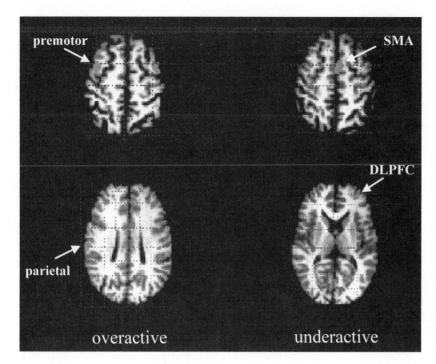

premotor

SMA

DLPFC

parietal

overactive

underactive

FIGURE 3-7 Statistical parametric maps showing the location of reduced and increased activation during sequential finger movements in PD. SMA, supplementary motor area; DLPFC, dorsolateral prefrontal cortex. (*Courtesy of M. Samuel.*) See Color Plate Section.

Reduction of bradykinesia when PD patients performed paced joystick movements in freely chosen directions after subcutaneous injection of the nonselective dopamine D1 and D2 agonist, apomorphine, was associated with significant increases in both SMA and dorsolateral prefrontal cortex blood flow.[104,105] [133]Xe SPECT rCBF and event-related functional MRI studies have also demonstrated improvement in SMA flow during finger movements after PD patients are treated with apomorphine[106] and L-dopa.[107] Functional MRI was also able to detect a reduction in the overactivity of motor and lateral premotor cortex during joystick movements after L-dopa administration.[108]

The effects of striatal fetal dopaminergic cell implantation on movement-related premotor and prefrontal activation in PD has been studied. Four PD patients who received bilateral human fetal mesencephalic transplants into caudate and putamen were studied with $H_2^{15}O$ PET at baseline and over the 2 years following surgery. Six months after transplantation, mean striatal dopamine storage capacity, measured with ^{18}F-dopa PET, was significantly elevated in these patients (putamen 78 percent, caudate 27 percent).[109] This was associated with a mean 12-point clinical improvement on the UPDRS but no significant change in cortical activation. By 18 months postsurgery there was a 24-point reduction in UPDRS score despite no further increase in striatal ^{18}F-dopa uptake. SMA and DLPFC activation during performance of joystick movements in freely chosen directions had now significantly improved. These findings suggest that the function of the graft goes beyond that of a simple dopamine

delivery system and that functional integration of the grafted neurons into the host brain is necessary in order to produce substantial clinical recovery and restore cortical activation in PD.

Loss of striatal dopamine in PD leads to reduced inhibition of the GPi by striatum, resulting in excessive inhibitory pallidal output to the ventral thalamus and cortex and aberrant burst firing. By inhibiting motor GPi, either by lesioning or high-frequency electrical deep brain stimulation (DBS), this excessive inhibition is reduced, so aiding volitional movement and improving frontal activation in PD patients. An alternative approach is to reduce the excitatory glutamatergic input to GPi from the subthalamic nucleus (STN) with high-frequency DBS. A number of series have now established that pallidotomy, pallidal and STN DBS all improve rigidity and bradykinesia in PD.

Grafton et al.[110] examined the regional cerebral activation in 6 PD patients associated with reaching out to grasp lighted targets before and after pallidotomy while withdrawn from medication. Surgery resulted in significantly increased SMA and lateral premotor activation despite little change in patient performance. Significantly increased activation of SMA, lateral premotor cortex, and dorsal prefrontal cortex after pallidotomy has also been demonstrated in PD patients off medication when performing joystick movements in freely selected directions.[111]

There have been several $H_2^{15}O$ PET reports on the functional effects of DBS in PD. GPi stimulation improves contralateral bradykinesia and rigidity in association with increased resting levels of SMA and lentiform rCBF,[112] and increased contralateral sensorimotor, mesial premotor, and anterior cingulate cortex activation during performance of a visually guided reaching task.[113] STN DBS improves rostral SMA, lateral premotor, and dorsolateral prefrontal cortex activation in PD during performance of joystick movements in freely chosen directions.[114,115] In contrast to pallidotomy, however, STN stimulation also results in increases in resting thalamic and decreases in resting motor cortex and caudal SMA rCBF, and reduced motor cortex activation. The decreased motor cortex activation may be a consequence of antidromic stimulation of direct projections to STN.

Atypical Parkinsonian Syndromes

MULTISYSTEM ATROPHY (MSA)

This condition is characterized pathologically by argyrophilic, alpha-synuclein-positive, inclusions in glia and neurons in substantia nigra, striatum, brainstem, and cerebellar nuclei, and intermediolateral columns of the cord. It manifests as a parkinsonian syndrome with autonomic failure and ataxia, and includes striatonigral degeneration (SND), progressive autonomic failure (PAF), and olivopontocerebellar atrophy (OPCA) within its spectrum. Patients are often L-dopa-nonresponsive (see Chap. 22). [18]FDG PET studies in patients with clinically probable SND show reduced levels of striatal glucose metabolism in 80–100 percent of cases, in contrast to PD where striatal metabolism is preserved.[116–118] Eidelberg et al. reported that parkinsonian patients with low levels of striatal glucose metabolism, irrespective of their L-dopa response, show little improvement after pallidotomy.[119] Patients with the full syndrome of MSA have reduced mean levels of cerebellar, along with putamen and caudate, glucose hypometabolism. [18]FDG PET, therefore, provides a sensitive means of detecting the presence of striatal dysfunction where atypical parkinsonism is suspected.

Proton MRS can also help discriminate SND from PD.[120] N-Acetylaspartate (NAA) is a metabolic marker of neuronal integrity present in millimolar concentrations. Reduced NAA:creatine proton MRS signal ratios were reported from the lentiform nuclei in 6 out of 7 clinically probable SND cases, while 8 out of 9 probable PD cases showed normal levels of putamen NAA.

The function of both the pre- and postsynaptic dopaminergic systems is impaired in patients with SND. As in PD, putamen ^{18}F-dopa uptake is asymmetrically reduced, and individual levels of putamen ^{18}F-dopa uptake correlate with disability.[121] Patients with the full syndrome of MSA show a significantly greater reduction in mean caudate ^{18}F-dopa uptake than equivalently rigid PD patients, although individual ranges overlap and a greater involvement of caudate only discriminates SND from PD with 70 percent specificity.[122] [18]FDG PET and proton MRS appear to be more robust than ^{18}F-dopa PET for discriminating

typical from atypical parkinsonsm. Pirker et al. recently examined striatal dopamine transporter binding in PD and MSA patients, and concluded that, while ^{123}I-beta-CIT SPECT reliably discriminates PD and MSA from normal, it cannot reliably discriminate between these two parkinsonian conditions.[123]

SND patients show mild, but significant, reductions in their mean putamen ^{11}C-SCH23390 (D1) and ^{11}C-raclopride (D2) uptake, while this remains preserved in PD.[124–126] Again, there is an overlap between SND, normal, and PD ranges, so striatal D1 and D2 binding does not provide a sensitive discriminator of SND from PD. In support of this viewpoint, ^{123}I-IBZM SPECT found reduced striatal D2 binding in only two-thirds of de novo parkinsonian patients who showed a negative apomorphine response.[127] Given that a significant number of parkinsonian patients who respond poorly to L-dopa show normal levels of striatal D2 binding, it seems likely that degeneration of pallidal and brainstem rather than striatal projections is responsible for their refractory status. Seppi et al.[128] used ^{123}I-IBZM SPECT to follow striatal degeneration longitudinally in a group of early MSA cases. They found an annual 10 percent loss of striatal D2 binding in their 18-month study and concluded that ^{123}I-IBZM SPECT provides a valid future approach for testing the efficacy of putative neuroprotective agents in MSA.

The basal ganglia are rich in opioid peptides and binding sites and these are differentially affected in SND and PD. ^{11}C-diprenorphine is a nonspecific opioid antagonist binding with equal affinity to mu, kappa, and delta sites. In nondyskinetic PD patients, caudate and putamen ^{11}C-diprenorphine uptake is preserved, whereas putamen uptake is reduced in 50 percent of patients thought to have SND.[129] ^{123}I-MIBG SPECT can be used to study functional integrity of cardiac sympathetic innervation in PD and MSA. Both these conditions show a reduction in mediastinal ^{123}I-MIBG signal, but this is significantly greater in PD, even in cases where no clinical evidence of autonomic failure is present.[130] This finding suggests a greater involvement of postganglionic sympathetic innervation of the myocardium in PD compared with MSA.

[11]C-PK11195 PET, an in vivo marker of microglial activation, has been used to study glial activation in MSA. More widespread subcortical increases in ^{11}C-PK11195 uptake are seen compared with PD, targeting nigra, putamen, pallidum, thalamus, and brainstem.[131] It remains to be determined whether striatal ^{11}C-PK11195 uptake will provide a sensitive discriminator of MSA and PD.

In order to determine the overlap between pure autonomic failure, OPCA, and SND, groups of these patients have been studied with PET and proton MRS. Two out of 7 PAF patients showed reduced putamen ^{18}F-dopa uptake in one series, suggesting that subclinical nigral dysfunction was present.[121] One of these patients subsequently developed MSA. In a series of 10 sporadic OPCA patients with autonomic failure but no rigidity, 7 showed reduced

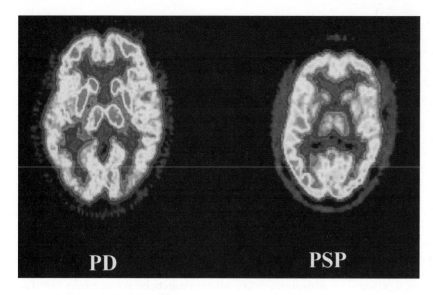

FIGURE 3-8 [18]FDG PET showing reduced resting basal ganglia glucose metabolism in PSP. (*Courtesy of P. Piccini.*) **See Color Plate Section.**

putamen ^{18}F-dopa uptake and 4 had reduced putamen ^{11}C-diprenorphine binding indicative of the presence of subclinical SND.[132] Reduced levels of striatal ^{18}F-dopa uptake,[133] striatal glucose hypometabolism,[134] and reduced lentiform NAA:creatine signal have also been reported in other series of sporadic OPCA cases.[120] In summary, the majority of sporadic OPCA cases with autonomic failure show functional imaging evidence of subclinical striatonigral dysfunction.

PROGRESSIVE SUPRANUCLEAR PALSY (PSP)

PSP is characterized pathologically by neurofibrillary tangle formation and neuronal loss in the substantia nigra, pallidum, superior colliculi, brainstem nuclei, and the periaqueductal gray matter. There is a lesser degree of cortical involvement (see Chap. 21). A number of series have reported changes in resting regional cerebral glucose metabolism in patients with clinically probable PSP, several of whom have later had the diagnosis confirmed at autopsy.[135–140] Cortical metabolism is globally depressed, and frontal areas are particularly targeted, levels of metabolism correlating with disease duration and performance on psychometric tests of frontal function. Hypofrontality is not specific for PSP; it can be seen in PD, SND, Pick's disease, HD, and depression. One case of clinically probable PSP with appropriate [18]FDG PET findings was subsequently reported to show progressive subcortical gliosis at autopsy.[141] Basal ganglia, cerebellar, and thalamic resting glucose metabolism are also depressed in PSP, so distinguishing it from PD where metabolism is preserved (Fig. 3-8). Proton MRS studies also show reduced lentiform nucleus NAA:creatine ratios in PSP, in contrast to PD.[142] While [18]FDG PET and proton MRS will discriminate at least 80 percent of PSP cases from PD, they are unable to reliably discriminate PSP from SND as striatal and frontal hypometabolism

can be a feature of both these disorders. The pathology of PSP uniformly targets nigrostriatal dopaminergic projections and so, in contrast to PD, putamen and caudate ^{18}F-dopa uptake are equivalently reduced in PSP, levels correlating inversely with disease duration.[17,143,144] In one series, ^{18}F-dopa PET was able to discriminate 90 percent of PSP from PD cases on the basis of uniform caudate and putamen involvement in the former.[122] Messa et al. have also reported equivalent loss of putamen ^{123}I-beta-CIT uptake in PD and PSP but significantly greater caudate involvement in the latter.[145] Pirker et al., however, found ^{123}I-beta-CIT SPECT less useful for discriminating PD from PSP.[123] There is no clear correlation between levels of striatal ^{18}F-dopa uptake in PSP and the degree of disability.[17] Unlike PD and SND, where locomotor impairment appears to correlate with loss of dopaminergic fibres, loss of mobility in PSP is probably determined by degeneration of nondopaminergic pallidal and brainstem projections. Striatal D2 binding in PSP has been studied with both PET and SPECT; reductions have been consistently reported, although only 50–70 percent of patients individually show significant receptor loss.[126,146–148] It is likely that degeneration of downstream pallidal and brainstem projections is responsible for the poor L-dopa responsiveness of PSP rather than loss of dopamine receptors alone. Striatal ^{11}C-diprenorphine is also reduced in PSP,[129] as is striatal acetylcholine esterase activity.[149]

CORTICOBASAL DEGENERATION (CBD)

This condition classically presents with an akinetic-rigid, apraxic limb which may exhibit alien behavior. Cortical sensory loss, dysphasia, myoclonus, supranuclear gaze problems, and bulbar dysfunction are also features, while intellect is spared until late. Eventually, all four limbs become involved and the condition is invariably poorly L-dopa-responsive. The pathology consists of collections of swollen, achromatic, tau-positive-staining Pick cells in the absence of argyrophilic Pick bodies which target the posterior frontal, inferior parietal, and superior temporal lobes, the substantia nigra, and the cerebellar dentate nuclei [219] (see Chap. 48).

PET and SPECT studies on patients with the clinical syndrome of CBD show greatest reductions in resting cortical oxygen and glucose metabolism in posterior frontal, inferior parietal, and superior temporal regions.[150–153] The thalamus and striatum are also involved. The metabolic reductions are strikingly asymmetrical, being most severe contralateral to the more affected limbs. This contrasts with PD patients, who have preserved and symmetrical levels of striatal and thalamic glucose metabolism.

Striatal ^{18}F-dopa uptake is also reduced in CBD in an asymmetrical fashion, being most depressed contralateral to the more affected limbs.[150] Like PSP, but in contrast to PD, caudate and putamen ^{18}F-dopa uptake are similarly depressed in CBD. ^{123}I-beta-CIT SPECT also shows an asymmetrical reduction in striatal dopamine transporter binding in CBD,[123] while ^{123}I-IBZM SPECT shows a severe asymmetrical reduction of striatal D2 binding.[154]

The above imaging findings may help discriminate CBD from Pick's disease where inferior frontal hypometabolism predominates, from PD where striatal metabolism is preserved and caudate ^{18}F-dopa uptake is relatively spared, and from PSP where frontal and striatal metabolism tend to be more symmetrically involved.[155] Having said that, both Pick's and PSP pathology have been subsequently reported in clinically apparent CBD cases.

Involuntary Movement Disorders

HUNTINGTON'S DISEASE (HD) AND OTHER CHOREAS

HD is an autosomal-dominantly transmitted disorder associated with an excess of CAG triplet repeats (>38) in the IT15 gene on chromosome 4. The function of this gene is still uncertain, but the pathology of HD targets medium spiny projection neurons in the striatum causing intranuclear and cytoplasmic inclusions to form (see Chaps. 34–36). Patients with predominant chorea show a selective loss of striatal-external globus pallidal projections which express GABA and enkephalin, while those with a predominant akinetic-rigid syndrome (the Westphal variant) show additional severe loss of striatal-internal pallidal fibres containing GABA and dynorphine.[156,157] A number of other degenerative disorders are also associated with chorea, including neuroacanthocytosis (NA), dentatorubropallidoluysian atrophy (DRPLA), and benign familial chorea (BFC) (see Chap. 38).

The inflammatory disorders systemic lupus erythematosus (SLE) and Sydenham's chorea are also associated with chorea, as is chronic neuroleptic exposure. The mechanism underlying tardive dyskinesia (TD) is uncertain; postmortem studies have found low levels of subthalamic and pallidal glutamate decarboxylase,[158] while neurochemical studies on a primate TD model have reported severe depletion of subthalamic and pallidal GABA.[159] These findings suggest that TD, like HD, may be associated with deranged GABA transmission.

Clinically affected HD patients show severely reduced levels of resting glucose and oxygen metabolism of their caudate and lentiform nuclei.[160–162] Levels of resting putamen metabolism correlate with locomotor function and caudate metabolism with performance on executive tests sensitive to frontal lobe function.[163,164] In early HD, cortical metabolism is preserved but as the disease progresses and dementia becomes prominent it also declines, the frontal cortex being targeted.[165] Caudate hypometabolism is not specific to HD, also being seen in NA, DRPLA, and some cases of BFC.[166–169] In contrast, striatal glucose metabolism is normal or elevated in inflammatory choreas, and tardive dyskinesia.[170–172]

Regional cerebral metabolism in HD has also been studied with proton MRS. NAA levels in the basal ganglia are reduced in affected patients, whereas lactate levels in the basal ganglia and cortex are elevated, suggesting that mitochondrial dysfunction is a feature of this disorder.[173] If the pathology of HD arises due to mitochondrial dysfunction, raised lactate levels in asymptomatic adult gene carriers should be expected. To date, lactate levels have been reported to be normal in asymptomatic gene carriers, more in favor of mitochondrial dysfunction representing an associated phenomenon rather than being causative. The medium spiny striatal neurons that degenerate in HD express D1, D2, opioid, and benzodiazepine receptors. PET and SPECT studies with benzamide- and spiperone-based tracers have all confirmed that striatal D2 binding is reduced by at least 30 percent in clinically affected HD patients.[11,148,174–176] ^{11}C-SCH23390 PET studies in HD have demonstrated reduced D1 binding in both striatum and temporal cortex.[177] Turjanski et al.[175] used ^{11}C-SCH23390 and ^{11}C-raclopride PET to study both D1 and D2 binding in HD. They found a parallel reduction in striatal binding to these receptor subtypes irrespective of phenotype, levels of D1 and D2 binding correlating with severity of rigidity rather than chorea. Striatal opioid[178] and benzodiazepine[179] binding have also been shown to be reduced in clinically affected HD patients. Reductions are relatively small (20 percent), however, compared with the mean 60 percent loss of dopamine D1 and D2 receptor binding.

The finding of reduced striatal dopamine receptor binding in patients with HD is, however, not specific for this cause of chorea: a mean 70 percent reduction of striatal ^{11}C-raclopride binding has also been reported in neuroacanthocytosis.[180] In contrast, normal striatal D2 binding has been reported in SLE chorea[175] and tardive dyskinesia.[181–183] This finding argues against the hypothesis that TD results from striatal D2 receptor supersensitivity following prolonged exposure

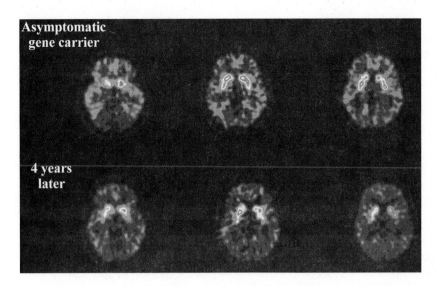

Asymptomatic gene carrier

4 years later

FIGURE 3-9 Dopamine D1 binding in HD. Serial ^{11}C-SCH23390 PET scans in a HD gene carrier, showing loss of striatal binding over 4 years. (*Courtesy of T. Andrews.*) See Color Plate Section.

to neuroleptics and suggests that the postmortem reports of downstream reductions in pallidal and subthalamic GABA levels are of greater relevance.

As clinically affected HD patients show at least a 30 percent loss of striatal glucose metabolism and dopamine receptor binding, [18]FDG, ^{11}C-SCH23390, and ^{11}C-raclopride PET should all be capable of detecting subclinical dysfunction, if present, in asymptomatic HD gene carriers. Reduced caudate glucose metabolism has been reported in 9 out of 12 and 3 out of 8 asymptomatic adult HD gene carriers in two different series,[184,185] while Weeks et al. showed a significant parallel loss of striatal D1 and D2 binding in 4 out of 8 asymptomatic adults with the HD mutation.[186]

The rate of progression of HD has also been followed with PET. Grafton et al. found that caudate glucose metabolism declined annually by 3.1 percent in their cohort of HD patients,[187] while Antonini et al. reported an annual 6 percent change in striatal D2 binding.[188] Andrews et al. have reported an annual fall in striatal D1 and D2 binding of 3–4 percent in symptomatic HD gene carriers and 6 percent in asymptomatic HD gene carriers with active subclinical disease (Fig. 3-9).[189] Pavese et al.[190] found a linear 5 percent annual decline in striatal D2 binding in early HD measured serially on three occasions over 5 years. These workers were also able to detect early loss of frontal D2 binding with ^{11}C-raclopride PET. These findings all suggest that functional imaging provides an objective means of following HD progression in the event of effective neuroprotective or restorative interventions being found.

TRANSPLANTATION OF HD

Transplantation of embryonic striatal tissue into the degenerated striatum of rat and primate models of HD has been shown to be safe, and has demonstrated good graft survival with differentiation and integration of striatal grafts into host striatum. Recovery of striatal dopamine D2 binding in rats and marmosets lesioned with ibotenic acid after implantation of fetal striatal tissue has been detected with ^{11}C-raclopride PET.[191–193] In primate models, recovery of skilled motor and cognitive performance has been reported within 2 months, and improvements in dystonia scores within 4–5 months of grafting.[194] Physiological, neurochemical, and anatomical studies have shown that a partial restoration of striatal input and output circuitry by implanted striatal neurons does occur, but the time course of this in primates and humans remains unclear.

Clinical studies of the possible therapeutic effects of striatal allografts in patients with HD are now running in the US, France, and England. Bachoud-Levi et al.[195,196] reported that 3 of 5 HD patients implanted with striatal cells from 8–9 week gestation fetuses improved over the course of 12 months, while two deteriorated. In the 3 that clinically improved, it was possible to detect striatal graft function, as evidenced by loci of increased glucose utilization seen with [18]FDG PET, but not in the 2 cases that subsequently deteriorated.

DYSTONIA

Dystonia is characterized by involuntary posturing, and muscle spasms. The primary torsion dystonias (PTD) range from severe, young-onset, generalized disorders to late-onset focal disease. The most common familial form of generalized PTD, DYT1 dystonia, is an autosomal-dominant disorder with around 40 percent penetrance and generally early-onset starting in a lower limb (see Chap. 32). All cases of DYT1 dystonia identified have a common mutation: a GAG deletion within the coding region of the DYT1 gene on chromosome 9q34 which codes for torsin A, an ATP-binding protein of unknown function. A second generalized PTD locus has been mapped to chromosome 8p (DYT6); affected individuals have adult-onset generalized dystonia with craniocervical disease or focal dystonia. A third PTD gene (DYT13) has been mapped to chromosome 1p and has a phenotype of cranial-cervical and upper limb involvement with occasional generalization. Postmortem studies have shown that DYT1 mRNA is highly expressed in dopaminergic neurons of the substantia nigra pars compacta. This could conceivably result in abnormal dopaminergic neurotransmission in dystonia, although histopathological studies have failed to identify consistent structural or neurotransmitter abnormalities in idiopathic torsion dystonia (ITD). Regions affected in acquired dystonia include caudate, putamen, globus pallidus, and posterior thalamus.[8] It has been suggested that ITD arises due to a reduced inhibitory output from the basal ganglia to ventral thalamus and premotor areas causing these to become inappropriately overactive. There have been a number of [18]FDG PET studies on resting levels of regional cerebral glucose metabolism in dystonia. A problem in interpreting the findings of early studies arises due to the heterogeneity of the patient groups recruited: familial, sporadic, and acquired dystonia have all been considered together and patients with focal or hemidystonia have been favored in order to provide side-to-side comparisons of basal ganglia function. As a consequence, the relevance of some of these PET findings to PTD is uncertain. Additionally, some of these patients were clearly experiencing active muscular spasms while reportedly at rest. Resting lentiform nucleus metabolism in dystonia has been variously reported to be increased,[197,198] normal,[199–201] and decreased.[202]

Covariance analysis of [18]FDG PET findings in DYT1 carriers has produced more consistent and interpretable findings. In a series of reports, Eidelberg et al.[203] have shown an abnormal resting metabolic profile in DYT1 carriers, levels of lentiform nucleus glucose metabolism being relatively reduced and frontal metabolism raised. This pattern is seen whether DYT1 gene carriers are clinically affected or asymptomatic and is a pattern opposite to that seen in PD. A study on DYT1 dystonic patients while asleep has also shown preservation of this abnormal pattern of resting glucose metabolism and confirmed that it is not movement-related. More recently, the same profile has been reported by these workers in other genetic mutations (e.g. DYT6) causing dystonia[183] and in essential blepharospasm.[204] These findings suggest a common imbalance of basal ganglia-frontal function may underlie the dystonias.

Cerebral activation studies in PTD have suggested an imbalance between sensorimotor and premotor cortex function. If dystonia patients perform paced joystick movements with their right hands in freely selected directions, they show significantly increased levels of contralateral putamen, rostral supplementary motor area, lateral premotor cortex, and dorsolateral prefrontal area activation.[205] In contrast,

activation of contralateral sensorimotor cortex and caudal SMA is impaired; these are the motor cortical areas that send direct pyramidal tract projections to the spinal cord. Tempel and Perlmutter[206,207] also noted attenuation of sensorimotor cortex and caudal SMA activation in PTD, and focal dystonia during vibrotactile stimulation. The pattern of activation in dystonia is, therefore, very different from the pattern associated with PD, where striatal, SMA, and prefrontal areas underfunction while primary motor cortex activation is either normal or increased.

It would seem, therefore, that dystonic limb movements in PTD are associated with inappropriate overactivation of basal ganglia-premotor area projections. Patients with acquired hemi- or focal dystonia due to basal ganglia and thalamic lesions also show increased levels of mesial and lateral premotor cortex, and dorsolateral prefrontal area activation during arm movement.[208] In contrast to PTD patients, however, acquired dystonia patients with basal ganglia lesions show raised rather than reduced primary motor cortex activation. This finding suggests that the pathology of PTD may have a direct inhibitory effect on primary sensorimotor cortex function not seen in secondary cases with focal basal ganglia lesions.

The question then arises: what is the significance of the frontal association area overactivity that is evident in both idiopathic and acquired dystonia? Three possibilities can be envisaged. First, the overactivity represents a primary dysfunction of motor planning circuitary. Second, the functional deficit in dystonia is at an executive level, and the prefrontal cortex becomes overactive in a conscious attempt to try and suppress the unwanted movements. Third, the frontal overactivity simply represents a secondary phenomenon reflecting primary basal ganglia overactivity.

Against the first hypothesis is the observation that ITD patients and normal subjects activate dorsolateral prefrontal and rostral supplementary motor areas equivalently when simply imagining joystick movements in freely chosen directions, but not performing them.[209] This suggests that the primary functional deficit in idiopathic dystonia must lie at an executive rather than planning level. Whether the frontal association area overactivity is simply secondary to primary basal ganglia overactivity or represents an adaptive phenomenon in a conscious attempt to suppress the syndrome, however, still remains unclear. In order to investigate this further, writer's cramp patients were studied while writing before and after treatment with botulinus toxin. These patients again demonstrated premotor overactivity and sensorimotor underactivity while writing continuously, and this pattern did not reverse after relief of the associated forearm cramp with botulinus toxin.[210] This would suggest that the frontal overactivity seen in dystonia during limb movement is part of the pathophysiology of the syndrome and is not simply an adaptive phenomenon to the presence of involuntary muscle spasms.

PET reports on dopaminergic function in dystonia have been confounded by inclusion of heterogeneous groups of patients. The only study to assess striatal ^{18}F-dopa uptake in purely familial PTD was by Playford et al. These workers found that 8 out of 11 PTD patients had normal striatal dopamine storage but that the 3 with most severe disease and taking high doses of anticholinergics showed mild impairment of putamen ^{18}F-dopa uptake.[211] The authors concluded that dopamine terminal function was normal in the majority of PTD cases. Two asymptomatic obligate gene carriers were studied and both had normal striatal ^{18}F-dopa uptake. Martin et al.[212] examined 3 PTD dystonic subjects with ^{18}F-dopa PET. One of these had normal and 2 reduced striatal ^{18}F-dopa uptake. In contrast, Otsuka et al. found a mildly raised level of mean striatal ^{18}F-dopa uptake in 8 patients with idiopathic dystonia.[201] Most recently, a ^{123}I-beta-CIT SPECT study has reported normal striatal uptake in 10 patients with torticollis.[213] Combining the findings of these studies, it would appear likely that striatal dopamine terminal function is normal in the majority of PTD cases.

Striatal D2 binding has also been studied in idiopathic dystonia. An ^{18}F-spiperone PET study reported a mean 20 percent reduction putamen D2 binding in a collection of patients with either Meige syndrome or writer's cramp, but there was a wide overlap with the normal binding range.[214] A similar finding was reported in a ^{123}I-epidepride SPECT study involving 10 torticollis cases.[213] Reduced striatal D2 availability could conceivably result in decreased activity of the indirect striatopallidal pathway and breakthrough involuntary movements.

DOPA-RESPONSIVE DYSTONIA (DRD) AND DYSTONIA-PARKINSONISM

Dominantly inherited DRD is related to GTP-cyclohydrolase 1 deficiency in the majority of cases, the genetic defect being located on chromosome 14 (see Chap. 32). This enzyme constitutes part of the tetrahydrobiopterin synthetic pathway, the cofactor for tyrosine hydroxylase. Patients are unable to manufacture L-dopa, and hence dopamine, from endogenous tyrosine but can still convert exogenous L-dopa to dopamine. DRD cases generally present in childhood with diurnally fluctuating dystonia and later develop background parkinsonism. Occasionally, the condition presents as pure parkinsonism in adulthood. ^{18}F-dopa PET and ^{123}I-beta-CIT SPECT findings are normal in the majority of DRD patients, so distinguishing this condition from early-onset dystonia-parkinsonism where severely reduced putamen ^{18}F-dopa and ^{123}I-beta-CIT uptake is found.[215-218]

Conclusions

Functional imaging:

- Provides a sensitive and objective means of detecting dopamine terminal dysfunction in PD where clinical doubt exists.

- May be helpful in demonstrating striatal hypometabolism or reduced D2 binding in suspected atypical variants.
- Can detect subclinical functional abnormalities when present in asymptomatic relatives at risk for PD and HD gene carriers.
- Enables PD and HD progression to be objectively monitored and the efficacy of putative neuroprotective and restorative approaches to be evaluated.
- Shows a common abnormal profile of resting glucose metabolism in the genetic dystonias.
- Can detect microglial activation in subcortical degenerations.

Blood flow and ligand activation studies have:

- Established that the akinesia of PD is associated with selective underfunctioning of the supplementary motor area and dorsal prefrontal cortex while inappropriate overactivity of these areas is associated with dystonia.
- Found that parkinsonian "off" periods do not correlate well with basal ganglia synaptic dopamine levels, suggesting a postsynaptic contribution.
- Shown that implants of fetal midbrain tissue can release normal amounts of dopamine after amphetamine challenges.

References

1. Hughes AJ, Daniel SE, Kilford L, Lees AJ: The accuracy of the clinical diagnosis of Parkinson's disease: A clinicopathological study of 100 cases. *J Neurol Neurosurg Psychiatry* 55:181–184, 1992.
2. Hutchinson M, Raff U: Structural changes of the substantia nigra in Parkinson's disease as revealed by MR imaging. *Am J Neuroradiol* 21:697–701, 2000.
3. Hu MT, White SJ, Herlihy AH, et al: A comparison of (18)F-dopa PET and inversion recovery MRI in the diagnosis of Parkinson's disease. *Neurology* 56:1195–1200, 2001.
4. Savoiardo M, Girotti F, Strada L, Ciceri E: Magnetic resonance imaging in progressive supranuclear palsy and other parkinsonian disorders. *J Neural Transm Suppl* 42:93–110, 1994.
5. Schrag A, Kingsley D, Phatouros C, et al: Clinical usefulness of magnetic resonance imaging in multiple system atrophy. *J Neurol Neurosurg Psychiatry* 65:65–71, 1998.
6. Schrag A, Good CD, Miszkiel K, et al: Differentiation of atypical parkinsonian syndromes with routine MRI. *Neurology* 54:697–702, 2000.
7. Schulz JB, Skalej M, Wedekind D, et al: Magnetic resonance imaging-based volumetry differentiates idiopathic Parkinson's syndrome from multiple system atrophy and progressive supranuclear palsy. *Ann Neurol* 45:65–74, 1999.
8. Bhatia KP, Marsden CD: The behavioural and motor consequences of focal lesions of the basal ganglia in man. *Brain* 117:859–876, 1994.

9. Starosta-Rubinstein S, Young AB, Kluin K, et al: Clinical assessment of 31 patients with Wilson's disease: Correlations with structural changes on magnetic resonance imaging. *Arch Neurol* 44:365–370, 1987.

10. Savoiardo M, Strada L, Oliva D, et al: Abnormal MRI signal in the rigid form of Huntington's disease. *J Neurol Neurosurg Psychiatry* 54:888–891, 1991.

11. Antonini A, Leenders KL, Spiegel R, et al: Striatal glucose metabolism and dopamine D-2 receptor binding in asymptomatic gene carriers and patients with Huntington's disease. *Brain* 119:2085–2095, 1996.

12. Jellinger K: The pathology of parkinsonism, in Marsden CD, Fahn S (eds): *Movement Disorders 2*. London: Butterworths, 1987, pp 124–165.

13. Fearnley JM, Lees AJ: Ageing and Parkinson's disease: Substantia nigra regional selectivity. *Brain* 114:2283–2301, 1991.

14. Kish SJ, Shannak K, Hornykiewicz O: Uneven pattern of dopamine loss in the striatum of patients with idiopathic Parkinson's disease. *N Engl J Med* 318:876–880, 1988.

15. Braak H, Tredici KD, Rub U, et al: Staging of brain pathology related to sporadic Parkinson's disease. *Neurobiol Aging* 24:197–211, 2003.

16. McKeith IG, Galasko D, Kosaka K, et al: Consensus guidelines for the clinical and pathologic diagnosis of dementia with Lewy bodies (DLB): Report of the consortium on DLB international workshop. *Neurology* 47:1113–1124, 1996.

17. Brooks DJ, Ibañez V, Sawle GV, et al: Differing patterns of striatal ^{18}F-dopa uptake in Parkinson's disease, multiple system atrophy and progressive supranuclear palsy. *Ann Neurol* 28:547–555, 1990.

18. Tedroff J, Aquilonius S-M, Hartvig P, et al: Cerebral uptake and utilisation of therapeutic [β-^{11}C]-L-DOPA in Parkinson's disease measured by positron emission tomography. Relations to motor response. *Acta Neurol Scand* 85:95–102, 1992.

19. Rinne JO, Bergman J, Ruotinnen H, et al: Striatal uptake of a novel PET ligand, [^{18}F]β-CFT, is reduced in early Parkinson's disease. *Synapse* 31:119–124, 1999.

20. Frost JJ, Rosier AJ, Reich SG, et al: Positron emission tomographic imaging of the dopamine transporter with ^{11}C-WIN 35,428 reveals marked declines in mild Parkinson's disease. *Ann Neurol* 34:423–431, 1993.

21. Marek K, Seibyl JP, Zoghbi SS, et al: [I-123] beta-CIT SPECT imaging demonstrates bilateral loss of dopamine transporters in hemiparkinsons disease. *Neurology* 46:231–237, 1996.

22. Benamer HTS, Patterson J, Wyper DJ, et al: Correlation of Parkinson's disease severity and duration with I-123-FP-CIT SPECT striatal uptake. *Mov Disord* 15:692–698, 2000.

23. Seibyl JP, Marek KL, Quinlan D, et al: Decreased single-photon emission computed tomographic [^{123}I]β-CIT striatal uptake correlates with symptom severity in Parkinson's disease. *Ann Neurol* 38:589–598, 1995.

24. Frey KA, Koeppe RA, Kilbourn MR, et al: Pre-synaptic monoaminergic vesicles in Parkinson's disease and normal aging. *Ann Neurol* 40:873–884, 1996.

25. Nahmias C, Garnett ES, Firnau G, Lang A: Striatal dopamine distribution in Parkinsonian patients during life. *J Neurol Sci* 69:223–230, 1985.

26. Leenders KL, Salmon EP, Tyrrell P, et al: The nigrostriatal dopaminergic system assessed in vivo by positron emission tomography in healthy volunteer subjects and patients with Parkinson's disease. *Arch Neurol* 47:1290–1298, 1990.

27. Morrish PK, Sawle GV, Brooks DJ: Clinical and [^{18}F]dopa PET findings in early Parkinson's disease. *J Neurol Neurosurg Psychiatry* 59:597–600, 1995.

28. Lindvall O, Bjorklund A: Dopaminergic innervation of the globus pallidus by collaterals from the nigrostriatal pathway. *Brain Res* 172:169–173, 1979.

29. Whone AL, Moore RY, Piccini P, Brooks DJ: Plasticity in the nigropallidal pathway in Parkinson's disease: An ^{18}F-dopa PET study. *Ann Neurol* 53:206–213, 2003 (abstract).

30. Guttman M, Burkholder J, Kish SJ, et al: [^{11}C]RTI-32 PET studies of the dopamine transporter in early dopa-naive Parkinson's disease: Implications for the symptomatic threshold. *Neurology* 48:1578–1583, 1997.

31. Tedroff J, Aquilonius S-M, Laihinen A, et al: Striatal kinetics of [11C]-(+)-nomifensine and 6-[18F]fluoro-L-dopa in Parkinson's disease measured with positron emission tomography. *Acta Neurol Scand* 81:24–30, 1990.

32. Lee CS, Samii A, Sossi V, et al: In vivo positron emission tomographic evidence for compensatory changes in presynaptic dopaminergic nerve terminals in Parkinson's disease. *Ann Neurol* 47:493–503, 2000.

33. Fischman AJ, Bonab AA, Babich JW, et al: [C-11,I-127] altropane: A highly selective ligand for PET imaging of dopamine transporter sites. *Synapse* 39:332–342, 2001.

34. Mozley PD, Schneider JS, Acton PD, et al: Binding of [Tc-99m]TRODAT-1 to dopamine transporters in patients with Parkinson's disease and in healthy volunteers. *J Nucl Med* 41:584–589, 2000.

35. Brooks DJ, Playford ED, Ibanez V, et al: Isolated tremor and disruption of the nigrostriatal dopaminergic system: An ^{18}F-dopa PET study. *Neurology* 42:1554–1560, 1992.

36. Benamer TS, Patterson J, Grosset DG, et al: Accurate differentiation of parkinsonism and essential tremor using visual assessment of [^{123}I]-FP-CIT imaging: The [^{123}I]-FP-CIT Study Group. *Mov Disord* 15:503–510, 2000.

37. Vingerhoets FJG, Schulzer M, Caine DB, Snow BJ: Which clinical sign of Parkinson's disease best reflects the nigrostriatal lesion? *Ann Neurol* 41:58–64, 1997.

38. Doder M, Rabiner EA, Turjanski N, et al: Tremor in Parkinson's disease and serotonergic dysfunction: An ^{11}C-WAY 100635 PET study. *Neurology* 60:601–605, 2003.

39. Golbe LI: The genetics of Parkinson's disease: A reconsideration. *Neurology* 40 (suppl 3):7–16, 1990.

40. Lazzarini AM, Myers RH, Zimmerman TRJ, et al: A clinical genetic study of Parkinson's disease: Evidence for dominant transmission. *Neurology* 44:499–506, 1994.

41. Piccini P, Morrish PK, Turjanski N, et al: Dopaminergic function in familial Parkinson's disease: A clinical and ^{18}F-dopa PET study. *Ann Neurol* 41:222–229, 1997.

42. Piccini P, Burn DJ, Ceravalo R, et al: The role of inheritance in sporadic Parkinson's disease: Evidence from a longitudinal study of dopaminergic function in twins. *Ann Neurol* 45:577–582, 1999.

43. Berendse HW, Booij J, Francot CMJE, et al: Subclinical dopaminergic dysfunction in asymptomatic Parkinson's disease patients' relatives with a decreased sense of smell. *Ann Neurol* 50:34–41, 2001.

44. McGeer PL, Itagaki S, Boyes BE, McGeer EG: Reactive microglia are positive for HLA-DR in the substantia nigra of Parkinson's and Alzheimer's disease brains. *Neurology* 38:1285–1291, 1988.

45. Gerhard A, Banati RB, Cagnin A, Brooks DJ: In vivo imaging of activated microglia with [C-11]PK11195 positron emission tomography (PET) in idiopathic and atypical Parkinson's disease. *Neurology* 56 (suppl 3):A270, 2001 (abstract).

46. Snow BJ, Tooyama I, McGeer EG, et al: Human positron emission tomographic [^{18}F]fluorodopa studies correlate with dopamine cell counts and levels. *Ann Neurol* 34:324–330, 1993.

47. Pate BD, Kawamata T, Yamada T, et al: Correlation of striatal fluorodopa uptake in the MPTP monkey with dopaminergic indices. *Ann Neurol* 34:331–338, 1993.

48. Ceravolo R, Piccini P, Bailey DL, et al: 18F-dopa PET evidence that tolcapone acts as a central COMT inhibitor in Parkinson's disease. *Synapse* 43:201–207, 2002.

49. Turjanski N, Lees AJ, Brooks DJ: Striatal dopaminergic receptor dysfunction in patients with restless legs syndrome: ^{18}F-dopa and ^{11}C-raclopride PET studies. *Neurology* 52:932–937, 1999.

50. Innis RB, Marek KL, Sheff K, et al: Effect of treatment with L-dopa/carbidopa or L-selegiline on striatal dopamine transporter SPECT imaging with [I-123]beta-CIT. *Mov Disord* 14:436–442, 1999.

51. Ahlskog JE, Uitti RJ, O'Connor MK, et al: The effect of dopamine agonist therapy on dopamine transporter imaging in Parkinson's disease. *Mov Disord* 14:940–946, 1999.

52. Vingerhoets FJG, Snow BJ, Lee CS, et al: Longitudinal fluorodopa positron emission tomographic studies of the evolution of idiopathic parkinsonism. *Ann Neurol* 36:759–764, 1994.

53. Morrish PK, Rakshi JS, Sawle GV, Brooks DJ: Measuring the rate of progression and estimating the preclinical period of Parkinson's disease with [^{18}F]dopa PET. *J Neurol Neurosurg Psychiatry* 64:314–319, 1998.

54. Nurmi E, Ruottinen HM, Bergman J, et al: Rate of progression in Parkinson's disease: A 6-[18F]fluoro-L-dopa PET study. *Mov Disord* 16:608–615, 2001.

55. Nurmi E, Ruottinen HM, Kaasinen V, et al: Progression in Parkinson's disease: A positron emission tomography study with a dopamine transporter ligand. *Ann Neurol* 47:804–808, 2000.

56. Marek K, Innis R, van Dyck C, et al: [123I]beta-CIT SPECT imaging assessment of the rate of Parkinson's disease progression. *Neurology* 57:2089–2094, 2001.

57. Winogrodzka A, Bergmans P, Booij J, et al: [123I]FP-CIT SPECT is a useful method to monitor the rate of dopaminergic degeneration in early-stage Parkinson's disease. *J Neural Transm* 108:1011–1019, 2001.

58. Schwarz J, Tatsch K, Linke R, et al: Measuring the decline of dopamine transporter binding in patients with Parkinson's disease using 123I-IPT and SPECT. *Neurology* 48 (suppl 2):A208, 1997 (abstract).

59. Marek KL, Innis R, Seibyl J: β-CIT/SPECT assessment of determinants of variability in progression of Parkinson's disease. *Neurology* 52 (suppl 2):A91–A92, 1999 (abstract).

60. Whone AL, Watts RL, Stoessl J, et al: Slower progression of PD with ropinirol versus L-dopa: The REAL-PET study. *Ann Neurol* 54:403–414, 2003.

61. Parkinson Study Group: Dopamine transporter brain imaging to assess the effects of pramipexole vs levodopa on Parkinson disease progression. *JAMA* 287:1653–1661, 2002.

62. Lindvall O: Cerebral implantation in movement disorders: State of the art. *Mov Disord* 14:201–205, 1999.

63. Piccini P, Brooks DJ, Bjorklund A, et al: Dopamine release from nigral transplants visualised in vivo in a Parkinson's patient. *Nat Neurosci* 2:1137–1140, 1999.

64. Wenning GK, Odin P, Morrish PK, et al: Short- and long-term survival and function of unilateral intrastriatal dopaminergic grafts in Parkinson's disease. *Ann Neurol* 42:95–107, 1997.

65. Hagell P, Schrag AE, Piccini P, et al: Sequential bilateral transplantation in Parkinson's disease: Effects of the second graft. *Brain* 122:1121–1132, 1999.

66. Remy P, Samson Y, Hantraye P, et al: Clinical correlates of [^{18}F]fluorodopa uptake in five grafted parkinsonian patients. *Ann Neurol* 38:580–588, 1995.

67. Hauser RA, Freeman TB, Snow BJ, et al: Long-term evaluation of bilateral fetal nigral transplantation in Parkinson disease. *Arch Neurol* 56:179–187, 1999.

68. Kordower JH, Freeman TB, Chen EY, et al: Fetal nigral grafts survive and mediate clinical benefit in a patient with Parkinson's disease. *Mov Disord* 13:383–393, 1998.

69. Freed CR, Greene PE, Breeze RE, et al: Transplantation of embryonic dopamine neurons for severe Parkinson's disease. *N Engl J Med* 344:710–719, 2001.

70. Nakamura T, Dhawan V, Chaly T, et al: Blinded positron emission tomography study of dopamine cell implantation for Parkinson's disease. *Ann Neurol* 50:181–187, 2001.

71. Olanow CW, Goetz CG, Kordower JH, et al: A double-blind controlled trial of bilateral fetal nigral transplantation in Parkinson's disease. *Ann Neurol* 54:403–414, 2003.

72. Gill SS, Patel NK, Hotton GR, et al: Direct brain infusion of glial cell line-derived neurotrophic factor (GDNF) in Parkinson's disease. *Nat Med* 9:589–595, 2003.

73. De la Fuente-Fernandez R, Pal PK, Vingerhoets FJG, et al: Evidence for impaired presynaptic dopamine function in parkinsonian patients with motor fluctuations. *J Neural Transm* 107:49–57, 2000.

74. Playford ED, Brooks DJ: In vivo and in vitro studies of the dopaminergic system in movement disorders. *Cerebrovasc Brain Metab Rev* 4:144–171, 1992.

75. Rinne UK, Laihinen A, Rinne JO, et al: Positron emission tomography demonstrates dopamine D2 receptor supersensitivity in the striatum of patients with early Parkinson's disease. *Mov Disord* 5:55–59, 1990.

76. Antonini A, Schwarz J, Oertel WH, et al: [^{11}C]Raclopride and positron emission tomography in previously untreated patients with Parkinson's disease: Influence of L-dopa and lisuride therapy on striatal dopamine D$_2$-receptors. *Neurology* 44:1325–1329, 1994.

77. Turjanski N, Lees AJ, Brooks DJ: PET studies on striatal dopaminergic receptor binding in drug naive and L-dopa treated Parkinson's disease patients with and without dyskinesia. *Neurology* 49:717–723, 1997.

78. Rinne JO, Laihinen A, Nagren K, et al: PET demonstrates different behaviour of striatal dopamine D1 and D2 receptors in early Parkinson's disease. *J Neurosci Res* 27:494–499, 1990.

79. Kishore A, De la Fuente-Fernández R, Snow BJ, et al: Levodopa-induced dyskinesias in idiopathic parkinsonism (IP): A simultaneous PET study of dopamine D1 and D2 receptors. *Neurology* 48:A327, 1997 (abstract).

80. Torstenson R, Hartvig P, Långström B, et al: Differential effects of levodopa on dopaminergic function in early and advanced Parkinson's disease. *Ann Neurol* 41:334–340, 1997.

81. De la Fuente-Fernandez R, Lu JQ, Sossi V, et al: Biochemical variations in the synaptic level of dopamine precede motor fluctuations in Parkinson's disease: PET evidence of increased dopamine turnover. *Ann Neurol* 49:298–303, 2001.

82. Henry B, Brotchie JM: Potential of opioid antagonists in the treatment of levodopa-induced dyskinesias in Parkinson's disease. *Drugs Aging* 9:149–158, 1996.

83. Nisbet AP, Foster OJF, Kingsbury A, et al: Preproenkephalin and preprotachykinin messenger-RNA expression in normal human basal ganglia and in Parkinson's disease. *Neuroscience* 66:361–376, 1995.

84. Jolkkonen J, Jenner P, Marsden CD: L-Dopa reverses altered gene expression of substance P but not enkephalin in the caudate-putamen of common marmosets treated with MPTP. *Mol Brain Res* 32:297–307, 1995.

85. Lavoie B, Parent A, Bedard PJ: Effects of dopamine denervation on striatal peptide expression in parkinsonian monkeys. *Can J Neurol Sci* 18:373–375, 1991.

86. Piccini P, Weeks RA, Brooks DJ: Opioid receptor binding in Parkinson's patients with and without levodopa-induced dyskinesias. *Ann Neurol* 42:720–726, 1997.

87. Whone AL, Rabiner EA, Arahata Y, et al: Reduced substance P binding in Parkinson's disease complicated by dyskinesias: An F-18-L829165 PET study. *Neurology* 58(suppl 3):A488–A489, 2002.

88. Miletich RS, Chan T, Gillespie M, et al: Contralateral basal ganglia metabolism is abnormal in hemiparkinsonian patients. An FDG-PET study. *Neurology* 38:S260, 1988.

89. Wolfson LI, Leenders KL, Brown LL, Jones T: Alterations of regional cerebral blood flow and oxygen metabolism in Parkinson's disease. *Neurology* 35:1399–1405, 1985.

90. Eidelberg D, Moeller JR, Dhawan V, et al: The metabolic topography of parkinsonism. *J Cereb Blood Flow Metab* 14:783–801, 1994.

91. Peppard RF, Martin WRW, Guttman M, et al: The relationship of cerebral glucose metabolism to cognitive deficits in Parkinson's disease. *Neurology* 38(suppl 1):364, 1988.

92. Kuhl DE, Metter EJ, Benson DF: Similarities of cerebral glucose metabolism in Alzheimer's and Parkinsonian dementia. *J Cereb Blood Flow Metab* 5:S169–S170, 1985.

93. Bohnen NI, Minoshima S, Giordani B, et al: Motor correlates of occipital glucose hypometabolism in Parkinson's disease without dementia. *Neurology* 52:541–546, 1999.

94. Hu MTM, Taylor-Robinson SD, Chaudhuri KR, et al: Cortical dysfunction in non-demented Parkinson's disease patients: A combined ^{31}Phosphorus MRS and ^{18}FDG PET study. *Brain* 123:340–352, 2000.

95. Korczyn AD. Dementia in Parkinson's disease: *J Neurol* 248 (suppl 3):III1–4, 2001.

96. Walker Z, Costa DC, Walker RW, et al: Differentiation of dementia with Lewy bodies from Alzheimer's disease using a dopaminergic presynaptic ligand. *J Neurol Neurosurg Psychiatry* 73:134–140, 2002.

97. Playford ED, Jenkins IH, Passingham RE, et al: Impaired mesial frontal and putamen activation in Parkinson's disease: A PET study. *Ann Neurol* 32:151–161, 1992.

98. Jahanshahi M, Jenkins IH, Brown RG, et al: Self-initiated versus externally-triggered movements: Measurements of regional cerebral blood flow and movement-related potentials in normals and Parkinson's disease. *Brain* 118:913–933, 1995.

99. Samuel M, Ceballos-Baumann AO, Blin J, et al: Evidence for lateral premotor and parietal overactivity in Parkinson's disease during sequential and bimanual movements: A PET study. *Brain* 120:963–976, 1997.

100. Rascol O, Sabatini U, Fabre N, et al: The ipsilateral cerebellar hemisphere is overactive during hand movements in akinetic parkinsonian patients. *Brain* 120:103–110, 1997.

101. Sabatini U, Boulanouar K, Fabre N, et al: Cortical motor reorganization in akinetic patients with Parkinson's disease: A functional MRI study. *Brain* 123:394–403, 2000.

102. Thobois S, Dominey P, Decety J, et al: Overactivation of primary motor cortex is asymmetrical in hemiparkinsonian patients. *Neuroreport* 11:785–789, 2000.

103. Mushiake H, Inase M, Tanji J: Selective coding of motor sequence in the supplementary motor area of the monkey cerebral cortex. *Exp Brain Res* 82:208–210, 1990.

104. Jenkins IH, Fernandez W, Playford ED, et al: Impaired activation of the supplementary motor area in Parkinson's disease is reversed when akinesia is treated with apomorphine. *Ann Neurol* 32:749–757, 1992.

105. Brooks DJ, Jenkins IH, Passingham RE: Positron emission tomography studies on regional cerebral control of voluntary movement, in Mano N, Hamada I, DeLong MR (eds): *Role of the Cerebellum and Basal Ganglia in Voluntary Movement.* Amsterdam: Excerpta Medica, 1993, pp 267–274.

106. Rascol O, Sabatini U, Chollet F, et al: Supplementary and primary sensory motor area activity in Parkinson's disease. Regional cerebral blood flow changes during finger movements and effects of apomorphine. *Arch Neurol* 49:144–148, 1992.

107. Rascol O, Sabatini U, Chollet F, et al: Normal activation of the supplementary motor area in patients with Parkinson's disease undergoing long-term treatment with levodopa. *J Neurol Neurosurg Psychiatry* 57:567–571, 1994.

108. Haslinger B, Erhard P, Kampfe N, et al: Event-related functional magnetic resonance imaging in Parkinson's disease before and after levodopa. *Brain* 124:558–570, 2001.

109. Piccini P, Lindvall O, Bjorklund A, et al: Delayed recovery of movement-related cortical function in Parkinson's disease after striatal dopaminergic grafts. *Ann Neurol* 48:689–695, 2000.

110. Grafton ST, Waters C, Sutton J, et al: Pallidotomy increases activity of motor association cortex in Parkinson's disease: A positron emission tomographic study. *Ann Neurol* 37:776–783, 1995.

111. Samuel M, Ceballos-Baumann AO, Turjanski N, et al: Pallidotomy in Parkinson's disease increases SMA and prefrontal activation during performance of volitional movements: An $H_2^{15}O$ PET study. *Brain* 120:1301–1313, 1997.

112. Davis KD, Taub E, Houle S, et al: Globus pallidus stimulation activates the cortical motor system during alleviation of parkinsonian symptoms. *Nat Med* 3:671–674, 1997.

113. Fukuda M, Mentis M, Ghilardi MF, et al: Functional correlates of pallidal stimulation for Parkinson's disease. *Ann Neurol* 49:155–164, 2001.

114. Limousin P, Greene J, Polak P, et al: Changes in cerebral activity pattern due to subthalamic nucleus or internal pallidum stimulation in Parkinson's disease. *Ann Neurol* 42:283–291, 1997.

115. Ceballos-Baumann AO, Boecker H, Bartenstein P, et al: A positron emission tomographic study of subthalamic nucleus stimulation in Parkinson disease: Enhanced movement-related activity of motor-association cortex and decreased motor cortex resting activity. *Arch Neurol* 56:997–1003, 1999.

116. De Volder AG, Francard J, Laterre C, et al: Decreased glucose utilisation in the striatum and frontal lobe in probable striatonigral degeneration. *Ann Neurol* 26:239–247, 1989.

117. Otsuka M, Ichiya Y, Hosokawa S, et al: Striatal blood flow, glucose metabolism, and ^{18}F-dopa uptake: Difference in Parkinson's disease and atypical parkinsonism. *J Neurol Neurosurg Psychiatry* 54:898–904, 1991.

118. Eidelberg D, Takikawa S, Moeller JR, et al: Striatal hypometabolism distinguishes striatonigral degeneration from Parkinson's disease. *Ann Neurol* 33:518–527, 1993.

119. Eidelberg D, Moeller JR, Ishikawa T, et al: Regional metabolic correlates of surgical outcome following unilateral pallidotomy for Parkinson's disease. *Ann Neurol* 39:450–459, 1996.

120. Davie CA, Wenning GK, Barker GJ, et al: Differentiation of multiple system atrophy from idiopathic Parkinson's disease using proton magnetic resonance spectroscopy. *Ann Neurol* 37:204–210, 1995.

121. Brooks DJ, Salmon EP, Mathias CJ, et al: The relationship between locomotor disability, autonomic dysfunction, and the integrity of the striatal dopaminergic system, in patients with multiple system atrophy, pure autonomic failure, and Parkinson's disease, studied with PET. *Brain* 113:1539–1552, 1990.

122. Burn DJ, Sawle GV, Brooks DJ: The differential diagnosis of Parkinson's disease, multiple system atrophy, and Steele-Richardson-Olszewski syndrome: Discriminant analysis of striatal 18F-dopa PET data. *J Neurol Neurosurg Psychiatry* 57:278–284, 1994.

123. Pirker W, Asenbaum S, Bencsits G, et al: [I-123]beta-CIT SPECT in multiple system atrophy, progressive supranuclear palsy, and corticobasal degeneration. *Mov Disord* 15:1158–1167, 2000.

124. Shinotoh H, Aotsuka A, Yonezawa H, et al: Striatal dopamine D$_2$ receptors in Parkinson's disease and striato-nigral degeneration determined by positron emission tomography, in Nagatsu T, Fisher A, Yoshida M (eds): *Basic, Clinical, and Therapeutic Advances of Alzheimer's and Parkinson's Diseases.* New York: Plenum Press, 1990, vol 2, pp 107–110.

125. Shinotoh H, Inoue O, Hirayama K, et al: Dopamine D$_1$ receptors in Parkinson's disease and striatonigral degeneration: A positron emission tomography study. *J Neurol Neurosurg Psychiatry* 56:467–472, 1993.

126. Brooks DJ, Ibanez V, Sawle GV, et al: Striatal D$_2$ receptor status in Parkinson's disease, striatonigral degeneration, and progressive supranuclear palsy, measured with ^{11}C-raclopride and PET. *Ann Neurol* 31:184–192, 1992.

127. Schwarz J, Tatsch K, Arnold G, et al: ^{123}I-iodobenzamide-SPECT predicts dopaminergic responsiveness in patients with de-novo parkinsonism. *Neurology* 42:556–561, 1992.

128. Seppi K, Donnemiller E, Riccabona G, et al: Disease progression in PD vs MSA: A SPECT study using 123-I IBZM. *Parkinsonism and related disorders.* 7:S24, 2001 (abstract).

129. Burn DJ, Rinne JO, Quinn NP, et al: Striatal opioid receptor binding in Parkinson's disease, striatonigral degeneration, and Steele-Richardson-Olszewski syndrome: An ^{11}C-diprenorphine PET study. *Brain* 118:951–958, 1995.

130. Druschky A, Hilz MJ, Platsch G, et al: Differentiation of Parkinson's disease and multiple system atrophy in early disease stages by means of I-123-MIBG-SPECT. *J Neurol Sci* 175:3–12, 2000.

131. Gerhard A, Banati RB, Goerres GB, et al: [11C](R)PK11195 PET imaging of microglial activation in multiple system atrophy. *Neurology* 61:686–689, 2003.

132. Rinne JO, Burn DJ, Mathias CJ, et al: PET studies on the dopaminergic system and striatal opioid binding in the olivopontocerebellar atrophy variant of multiple system atrophy. *Ann Neurol* 37:568–573, 1995.

133. Otsuka M, Ichiya Y, Kuwabara Y, et al: Striatal ^{18}F-dopa uptake and brain glucose metabolism by PET in patients with syndrome of progressive ataxia. *J Neurol Sci* 124:198–203, 1994.

134. Gilman S, Koeppe RA, Junck L, et al: Patterns of cerebral glucose metabolism detected with positron emission tomography differ in multiple system atrophy and olivopontocerebellar atrophy. *Ann Neurol* 36:166–175, 1994.

135. D'Antona R, Baron JC, Samson Y, et al: Subcortical dementia: Frontal cortex hypometabolism detected by positron tomography in patients with progressive supranuclear palsy. *Brain* 108:785–800, 1985.

136. Blin J, Baron JC, Dubois P, et al: Positron emission tomography study in progressive supranuclear palsy. *Arch Neurol* 47:747–752, 1990.

137. Goffinet AM, De Volder AG, Gillain C, et al: Positron tomography demonstrates frontal lobe hypometabolism in progressive supranuclear palsy. *Ann Neurol* 25:131–139, 1989.

138. Foster NL, Gilman S, Berent S, et al: Cerebral hypometabolism in progressive supranuclear palsy studied with positron emission tomography. *Ann Neurol* 24:399–406, 1988.

139. Otsuka M, Ichiya Y, Kuwabara Y, et al: Cerebral blood flow, oxygen and glucose metabolism with PET in progressive supranuclear palsy. *Ann Nucl Med* 3:111–118, 1989.

140. Goffinet A, DeVolder AG, Gillain C, et al: Positron tomography demonstrates frontal lobe hypometabolism in progressive supranuclear palsy. *Ann Neurol* 25:131–139, 1989.

141. Foster NL, Gilman S, Berent S, et al: Progressive subcortical gliosis and progressive supranuclear palsy can have similar clinical and PET abnormalities. *J Neurol Neurosurg Psychiatry* 55:707–713, 1992.

142. Davie CA, Barker GJ, Machado C, et al: Proton magnetic resonance spectroscopy in Steele-Richardson-Olszewski syndrome. *Mov Disord* 12:767–771, 1997.

143. Leenders KL, Frackowiak RS, Lees AJ: Steele-Richardson-Olszewski syndrome. Brain energy metabolism, blood flow and fluorodopa uptake measured by positron emission tomography. *Brain* 111:615–630, 1988.

144. Bhatt MH, Snow BJ, Martin WRW, et al: Positron emission tomography in progressive supranuclear palsy. *Arch Neurol* 48:389–391, 1991.

145. Messa C, Volonte MA, Fazio F, et al: Differential distribution of striatal ^{123}I]β-CIT in Parkinson's disease and progressive supranuclear palsy, evaluated with single-photon emission tomography. *Eur J Nucl Med* 25:1270–1276, 1998.

146. Baron JC, Maziere B, Loc'h C, et al: Progressive supranuclear palsy: Loss of striatal dopamine receptors demonstrated in vivo by positron tomography and 76Br-bromospiperone. *Lancet* ii:1–7, 1983.

147. Wienhard K, Coenen HH, Pawlik G, et al: PET studies of dopamine receptor distribution using [18F]fluoroethylspiperone: Findings in disorders related to the dopaminergic system. *J Neural Transm* 81:195–213, 1990.

148. Brucke T, Podreka I, Angelberger P, et al: Dopamine D2 receptor imaging with SPECT: Studies in different neuropsychiatric disorders. *J Cereb Blood Flow Metab* 11:220–228, 1991.

149. Pappata S, Traykov L, Tavitian B, et al: Striatal reduction of acetylcholinesterase in patients with progressive supranuclear

palsy (PSP) as measured in vivo by PET and ^{11}C-physostigmine (^{11}C-PHY). *J Cereb Blood Flow Metab* 17 (suppl 1):S687, 1997.

150. Sawle GV, Brooks DJ, Marsden CD, Frackowiak RSJ: Corticobasal degeneration: A unique pattern of regional cortical oxygen metabolism and striatal fluorodopa uptake demonstrated by positron emission tomography. *Brain* 114:541–556, 1991.

151. Eidelberg D, Dhawan V, Moeller JR, et al: The metabolic landscape of cortico-basal ganglionic degeneration: Regional asymmetries studied with positron emission tomography. *J Neurol Neurosurg Psychiatry* 54:856–862, 1991.

152. Blin J, Vidhailhet M-J, Pillon B, et al: Corticobasal degeneration: Decreased and asymmetrical glucose consumption as studied by PET. *Mov Disord* 7:348–354, 1992.

153. Markus HS, Lees AJ, Lennox G, et al: Patterns of regional cerebral blood flow in corticobasal degeneration studied using HMPAO SPECT: Comparison with Parkinson's disease and normal controls. *Mov Disord* 10:179–187, 1995.

154. Frisoni GB, Pizzolato G, Zanetti O, et al: Corticobasal degeneration: Neuropsychological assessment and dopamine D-2 receptor SPECT analysis. *Eur Neurol* 35:50–54, 1995.

155. Nagahama Y, Fukuyama H, Turjanski N, et al: Cerebral glucose metabolism in corticobasal degeneration: Comparison with progressive supranuclear palsy and normal controls. *Mov Disord* 12:691–696, 1997.

156. Albin RL, Qin Y, Young AB, et al: Preproenkephalin messenger RNA-containing neurons in striatum of patients with symptomatic and presymptomatic Huntington's disease: An in situ hybridisation study. *Ann Neurol* 30:542–549, 1991.

157. Albin RL, Reiner A, Anderson KD, et al: Striatal and nigral neuron subpopulations in rigid Huntington's disease: Implications for the functional anatomy of chorea and rigidity-akinesia. *Ann Neurol* 27:357–365, 1990.

158. Andersson U, Haggstrom J-E, Levin ED, et al: Reduced glutamate decarboxylase activity in the subthalamic nucleus of patients with tardive dyskinesia. *Mov Disord* 4:37–46, 1989.

159. Gunne LM, Haggstrom J-E, Sjoquist B. Association with persistent neuroleptic-induced dyskinesia of regional changes in brain GABA synthesis. *Nature* 309:347–349, 1984.

160. Kuhl DE, Phelps ME, Markham CH, et al: Cerebral metabolism and atrophy in Huntington's disease determined by 18FDG and computed tomographic scans. *Ann Neurol* 12:425–434, 1982.

161. Hayden MR, Martin WRW, Stoessl AJ, et al: Positron emission tomography in the early diagnosis of Huntington's disease. *Neurology* 36:888–894, 1986.

162. Leenders KL, Frackowiak RSJ, Quinn N, Marsden CD: Brain energy metabolism and dopaminergic function in Huntington's disease measured in vivo using positron emission tomography. *Mov Disord* 1:69–77, 1986.

163. Young AB, Penney JB, Starosta-Rubinstein S, et al: PET scan investigations of Huntington's disease: Cerebral metabolic correlates of neurological features and functional decline. *Ann Neurol* 20:296–303, 1986.

164. Berent S, Giordani B, Lehtinen S, et al: Positron emission tomographic scan investigations of Huntington's disease: Cerebral metabolic correlates of cognitive function. *Ann Neurol* 23:541–546, 1988.

165. Kuwert T, Lange HW, Langen KJ, et al: Cortical and subcortical glucose consumption measured by PET in patients with Huntington's disease. *Brain* 113:1405–1423, 1990.

166. Dubinsky RM, Hallett M, Levey R, Di Chiro G: Regional brain glucose metabolism in neuroacanthocytosis. *Neurology* 39:1253–1255, 1989.

167. Hosokawa S, Ichiya Y, Kuwabara Y, et al: Positron emission tomography in cases of chorea with different underlying diseases. *J Neurol Neurosurg Psychiatry* 50:1284–1287, 1987.

168. Kuwert T, Lange HW, Langen KJ, et al: Normal striatal glucose consumption in two patients with benign hereditary chorea as measured by positron emission tomography. *J Neurol* 237:80–84, 1990.

169. Suchowersky O, Hayden MR, Martin WRW, et al: Cerebral metabolism of glucose in benign hereditary chorea. *Mov Disord* 1:33–45, 1986.

170. Guttman M, Lang AE, Garnett ES, et al: Regional cerebral glucose metabolism in SLE chorea: Further evidence that striatal hypometabolism is not a correlate of chorea. *Mov Disord* 2:201–210, 1987.

171. Weindl A, Kuwert T, Leenders KL, et al: Increased striatal glucose consumption in Sydenham chorea. *Mov Disord* 8:437–444, 1993.

172. Pahl JJ, Mazziotta JC, Cummings J, et al: Positron emission tomography in tardive dyskinesia and Huntington's disease. *J Cereb Blood Flow Metab* 7:1253–1255, 1987.

173. Jenkins BG, Koroshetz WJ, Beal MF, Rosen BR: Evidence for impairment of energy metabolism in vivo in Huntington's disease using localised ^{1}H NMR spectroscopy. *Neurology* 43:2689–2695, 1993.

174. Hägglund J, Aquilonius S-M, Eckernäs S, et al: Dopamine receptor properties in Parkinson's disease and Huntington's chorea evaluated by positron emission tomography using [11C]-N-methyl-spiperone. *Acta Neurol Scand* 75:87–94, 1987.

175. Turjanski N, Weeks R, Dolan R, et al: Striatal D_1 and D_2 receptor binding in patients with Huntington's disease and other choreas: A PET study. *Brain* 118:689–696, 1995.

176. Pirker W, Asenbaum S, Wenger S, et al: Iodine-123-epidepride-SPECT: Studies in Parkinson's disease, multiple system atrophy and Huntington's disease. *J Nucl Med* 38:1711–1717, 1997.

177. Karlsson P, Lundin A, Anvret M, et al: Dopamine D1 receptor number: A sensitive PET marker for early brain degeneration in Huntington's disease. *Eur Arch Psychiatry Clin Neurosci* 243:249–255, 1994.

178. Weeks RA, Cunningham VJ, Piccini P, et al: ^{11}C-Diprenorphine binding in Huntington's disease: A comparison of region of interest analysis and statistical parametric mapping. *J Cereb Blood Flow Metab* 17:943–949, 1997.

179. Holthoff VA, Koeppe RA, Frey KA, et al: Positron emission tomography measures of benzodiazepine receptors in Huntington's disease. *Ann Neurol* 34:76–81, 1993.

180. Brooks DJ, Ibanez V, Playford ED, et al: Presynaptic and postsynaptic striatal dopaminergic function in neuroacanthocytosis: A positron emission tomographic study. *Ann Neurol* 30:166–171, 1991.

181. Andersson U, Eckernas SA, Hartvig P, et al: Striatal binding of ^{11}C-NMSP studied with positron emission tomography in patients with persistent tardive dyskinesia: No evidence for altered dopamine receptor binding. *J Neural Transm* 79:215–226, 1990.

182. Blin J, Baron JC, Cambon H, et al: Striatal dopamine D2 receptors in tardive dyskinesia: PET study. *J Neurol Neurosurg Psychiatry* 52:1248–1252, 1989.

183. Trost M, Carbon M, Edwards C, et al: Primary dystonia: Is abnormal functional brain architecture linked to genotype? *Ann Neurol* 52:853–856, 2002.

184. Grafton ST, Mazziotta JC, Pahl JJ, et al: A comparison of neurological, metabolic, structural, and genetic evaluations in persons at risk for Huntington's disease. *Ann Neurol* 28:614–621, 1990.

185. Hayden MR, Hewitt J, Martin WRW, et al: Studies in persons at risk for Huntington's disease. *N Engl J Med* 317:382–383, 1987.

186. Weeks RA, Piccini P, Harding AE, Brooks DJ: Striatal D_1 and D_2 dopamine receptor loss in asymptomatic mutation carriers of Huntington's disease. *Ann Neurol* 40:49–54, 1996.

187. Grafton ST, Mazziotta JC, Pahl JJ, et al: Serial changes of cerebral glucose metabolism and caudate size in persons at risk for Huntington's disease. *Arch Neurol* 49:1161–1167, 1992.

188. Antonini A, Leenders KL, Eidelberg D: [C-11]Raclopride-PET studies of the Huntington's disease rate of progression: Relevance of the trinucleotide repeat length. *Ann Neurol* 43:253–255, 1998.

189. Andrews TC, Weeks RA, Turjanski N, et al: Huntington's disease progression: PET and clinical observations. *Brain* 122:2353–2363, 1999.

190. Pavese N, Rosser AE, Brooks DJ, et al: Cortical dopamine D_2 receptor dysfunction in Huntington's disease. *Mov Disord* 17:P1050, 2002

191. Fricker RA, Torres EM, Hume SP, et al: The effects of donor stage on the survival and function of embryonic striatal grafts in the adult rat brain. II. Correlation between positron emission tomography and reaching behaviour. *Neuroscience* 79:711–722, 1997.

192. Kendall L, Rayment D, Aigbirhio F, et al: In vivo PET analysis of the status of striatal allografts in the common marmoset. *Eur J Neurosci* 10:15604, 1998.

193. Torres EM, Fricker RA, Hume SP, et al: Assessment of striatal graft viability in the rat in vivo using a small diameter PET scanner. *Neuroreport* 6:2017–2021, 1995.

194. Brasted PJ, Watts C, Torres EM, et al: Behavioural recovery following striatal transplantation: Effects of postoperative training and P-zone volume. *Exp Brain Res* 128:535–538, 1999.

195. Bachoud-Levi AC, Bourdet C, Brugieres P, et al: Safety and tolerability assessment of intrastriatal neural allografts in five patients with Huntington's disease. *Exp Neurol* 161:194–202, 2000.

196. Bachoud-Levi A, Remy P, Nguyen JP, et al: Motor and cognitive improvements in patients with Huntington's disease after neural transplantation. *Lancet* 356:1975–1979, 2000.

197. Chase T, Tamminga CA, Burrows H: Positron emission studies of regional cerebral glucose metabolism in idiopathic dystonia. *Adv Neurol* 50:237–241, 1988.

198. Eidelberg D, Dhawan V, Cedarbaum J, et al: Contralateral basal ganglia hypermetabolism in primary unilateral limb dystonia. *Neurology* 40 (suppl 1):399, 1990.

199. Gilman S, Junck L, Young AB, et al: Cerebral metabolic activity in idiopathic dystonia studied with positron emission tomography. *Adv Neurol* 50:231–236, 1988.

200. Stoessl AJ, Martin WRW, Clark C, et al: PET studies of cerebral glucose metabolism in idiopathic torticollis. *Neurology* 36:653–657, 1986.

201. Otsuka M, Ichiya Y, Shima F, et al: Increased striatal ^{18}F-dopa uptake and normal glucose metabolism in idiopathic dystonia syndrome. *J Neurol Sci* 111:195–199, 1992.

202. Karbe H, Holthoff VA, Rudolf J, et al: Positron emission tomography demonstrates frontal cortex and basal ganglia hypometabolism in dystonia. *Neurology* 42:1540–1544, 1992.

203. Eidelberg D, Moeller JR, Antonini A, et al: Functional brain networks in DYT1 dystonia. *Ann Neurol* 44:303–312, 1998.

204. Hutchinson M, Nakamura T, Moeller JR, et al: The metabolic topography of essential blepharospasm: A focal dystonia with general implications. *Neurology* 55:673–677, 2000.

205. Ceballos-Baumann AO, Passingham RE, Warner T, et al: Overactivity of rostral and underactivity of caudal frontal areas in idiopathic torsion dystonia: A PET activation study. *Ann Neurol* 37:363–372, 1995.

206. Tempel LW, Perlmutter JS: Abnormal vibration-induced cerebral blood flow responses in idiopathic dystonia. *Brain* 113:691–707, 1990.

207. Tempel LW, Perlmutter JS: Abnormal cortical responses in patients with writer's cramp. *Neurology* 43:2252–2257, 1993.

208. Ceballos-Baumann AO, Passingham RE, Marsden CD, Brooks DJ: Overactivity of primary and accessory motor areas after motor reorganisation in acquired hemi-dystonia: A PET activation study. *Ann Neurol* 37:746–757, 1995.

209. Ceballos-Baumann AO, Marsden CD, Passingham RE, et al: Cerebral activation with performing and imagining movement in idiopathic torsion dystonia (ITD): A PET study. *Neurology* 44 (suppl 2):A338, 1994 (abstract).

210. Ceballos-Baumann AO, Sheean G, Marsden CD, et al: Botulinum toxin does not reverse the cortical dysfunction associated with writer's cramp. *Brain* 120:571–582, 1997.

211. Playford ED, Fletcher NA, Sawle GV, et al: Integrity of the nigro-striatal dopaminergic system in familial dystonia: An ^{18}F-dopa PET study. *Brain* 116:1191–1199, 1993.

212. Martin WRW, Stoessl AJ, Palmer M, et al: PET scanning in dystonia. *Adv Neurol* 50:223–229, 1988.

213. Naumann M, Pirker W, Reiners K, et al: Imaging the pre- and postsynaptic side of striatal dopaminergic synapses in idiopathic cervical dystonia: A SPECT study using [^{123}I]Epidepride and [^{123}I]β-CIT. *Mov Disord* 13:319–323, 1998.

214. Perlmutter JS, Stambuk MK, Markham J, et al: Decreased [F-18] spiperone binding in putamen in idiopathic focal dystonia. *J Neurosci* 17:843–850, 1997.

215. Sawle GV, Leenders KL, Brooks DJ, et al: Dopa-responsive dystonia: [^{18}F]Dopa positron emission tomography. *Ann Neurol* 30:24–30, 1991.

216. Snow BJ, Nygaard TG, Takahashi H, Calne DB: Positron emission tomography studies of dopa-responsive dystonia and early-onset idiopathic parkinsonism. *Ann Neurol* 34:733–738, 1993.

217. Turjanski N, Bhatia K, Burn DJ, et al: Comparison of striatal ^{18}F-dopa uptake in adult-onset dystonia-parkinsonism, Parkinson's disease, and dopa-responsive dystonia. *Neurology* 43:1563–1568, 1993.

218. Naumann M, Pirker W, Reiners K, et al: [123I]beta-CIT single-photon emission tomography in DOPA-responsive dystonia. *Mov Disord* 12:448–451, 1997.

219. Feaney MB, Dickson DW: Widespread cytoskeletal pathology characterizes corticobasal degeneration. *Am J Pathol* 146:1388–1396, 1995.

PART B

NEUROSCIENTIFIC FOUNDATIONS

MITOCHONDRIA IN MOVEMENT DISORDERS

CLAUDIA M. TESTA

MITOCHONDRIAL STRUCTURE AND FUNCTION	61
Mitochondria as Organelles Within Cells	61
Mitochondrial Genetics	62
Oxidative Phosphorylation	65
Apoptosis in Normal Development	67
Reactive Oxygen Species (ROS) and Normal	
Mitochondria	67
Calcium Regulation	68
CONSEQUENCES OF MITOCHONDRIAL	
DYSFUNCTION	68
Decreased ATP Production	68
Apoptosis in Disease	68
Toxic Levels of ROS	69
Disruption of Calcium Regulation	70
MITOCHONDRIA AND AGING	71
MITOCHONDRIAL DYSFUNCTION IN	
MOVEMENT DISORDERS	72
Parkinson's Disease (PD)	72
Huntington's Disease (HD)	73
THERAPEUTICS	74
Antioxidants	75
Creatine (Cr)	77
CONCLUSIONS	78

Classical mitochondrial disorders include maternally inherited diseases caused by mutations in mitochondrial DNA (mtDNA), and diseases due to nuclear mutations that directly affect mitochondrial proteins. These disorders encompass a wide range of clinical phenotypes, and can manifest at any stage of life. Many include basal ganglia pathology and movement disorder symptoms in their phenotype, suggesting a broader role for mitochondria in extrapyramidal disease. Now, in addition to considering movement disorder symptoms as part of mitochondrial disease phenotypes, neurologists are actively examining mitochondrial defects that may contribute to neurodegenerative movement disorders such as Parkinson's disease (PD) and Huntington's disease (HD).

Neurodegenerative disorders are chronic, slowly progressive conditions that cause loss of specific neuronal cell types over time. This group includes movement disorders such as PD, HD, Wilson's disease and Friedreich's ataxia, as well as Alzheimer's disease and amyotrophic lateral sclerosis (ALS). These disorders are heterogeneous with respect to the predominant cell types involved, inheritance, and symptoms, but share key characteristics such as selective cell vulnerability in the setting of widely expressed disease genes. They likely have interrelated pathophysiologies as well as therapeutic strategies. Mitochondrial dysfunction has been proposed as one such unifying factor underlying cell loss in neurodegenerative disorders. Mitochondria are now thought to contribute to the genetic and environmental events that culminate in a chronic progressive movement disorder.

It is still unclear if mitochondrial dysfunction is a primary cause or a secondary step in the pathogenic process. Elucidating the extent and exact nature of mitochondrial involvement in movement and other neurodegenerative disorders is a major contemporary scientific and clinical challenge. A working knowledge of the basic mitochondrial physiology underpinning recent scientific and clinical trial advances is therefore becoming essential to understanding and treating movement disorders. This chapter reviews relevant aspects of mitochondrial genetics, oxidative phosphorylation biochemistry, types and consequences of damage to mitochondrial function, and evidence for mitochondrial dysfunction in movement disorders such as PD and HD. Finally, current information on new potential therapeutics based on enhancing mitochondrial function is discussed.

Mitochondrial Structure and Function

MITOCHONDRIA AS ORGANELLES WITHIN CELLS

Mitochondria are membrane-bound cytoplasmic organelles[1,2] (Fig. 4-1) that vary considerably in size, shape, number, and exact intracellular location between different cell types. Mitochondria have two lipid bilayer plasma membranes. The outer membrane is permeable to most small molecules, making the intermembrane space, between the outer and inner membranes, similar to the cell's cytoplasm. The highly folded, and thus much larger, inner membrane is impermeable to nearly all molecules, but contains specific transporters to move molecules back and forth. Protein complexes embedded in the inner membrane comprise the oxidative phosphorylation pathway discussed below. Contained within the inner membrane is the matrix, a concentrated aqueous space that contains mitochondrial DNA (mtDNA), transcription and translation machinery, and metabolic pathway components.

Mitochondria have many functions. For example, the mitochondrial matrix houses most of the citric acid cycle and fatty acid oxidation pathways. This chapter concentrates on some of the mitochondrial functions currently relevant to movement disorders: adenosine triphosphate (ATP) production, involvement in cell death pathways, reactive oxygen

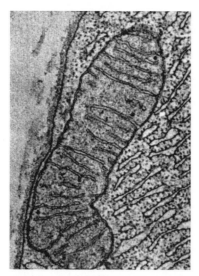

FIGURE 4-1 Electron micrograph of a mitochondrion.
(From Berg et al.[1] Used with permission.)

species production, and calcium regulation. All of these functions are influenced by mitochondrial genetics and genotype-to-phenotype interactions. Mitochondrial genetics is driven by the particular evolutionary role of mitochondria in cells.

Mitochondria are probably derived from previously independent aerobic bacteria that became symbiotic components of ancient eukaryotic cells.[3] New mitochondria are made by simple fission from existing mitochondria, as in bacterial reproduction, and each mitochondrion contains its own DNA, RNA, and ribosomes. Over the course of evolution, genes that were probably part of the original symbiotic bacterial DNA moved to the host cell nuclear DNA, so that mitochondria no longer contain all the DNA needed to manufacture their proteins. Instead, nuclear DNA in the host cell now encodes most mitochondrial proteins. This mix of intrinsic and host DNA contributes to the range of etiologies for mitochondrial dysfunction.

MITOCHONDRIAL GENETICS

Classical mitochondrial diseases vary between families, within families, and between tissues within an individual. Widely expressed causative mutations can generate either widespread damage or discrete neuronal loss. How mitochondrial dysfunction causes such a range of disease is in part a function of mitochondrial genetics. The unique impact of mitochondrial genetics on disease is based on several concepts: maternal transmission of mtDNA; distinct mitochondrial and nuclear genomes; inherited versus somatic mtDNA mutations; heteroplasmy; replicative segregation; and threshold for phenotype.

INHERITANCE OF MITOCHONDRIAL AND NUCLEAR GENOMES

Each human mitochondrion contains its own DNA, a double-stranded 16,569-base-pair circular genome encoding 13 proteins, small and large ribosomal RNAs, and sufficient tRNAs to translate all of its own codons[4] (Fig. 4-2). Human mitochondria, with their mtDNA, are transmitted to an embryo from the oocyte cytoplasm, while sperm mitochondria are eliminated from the fertilized egg, probably via ubiquitination.[5,6] Thus, unlike nuclear DNA, which undergoes biparental inheritance, mtDNA is inherited through the maternal line.[7] There are, however, reports of low levels of paternal transmission of mitochondria in mice,[8,9] and the possibility of an extremely low level of paternal mtDNA inheritance in humans is an ongoing debate.[10] There is a recent case report of a paternal mtDNA haplotype background in a patient with a sporadic single large disease-causing mtDNA mutation.[11]

While mtDNA is essential to mitochondrial function, most proteins needed by a mitochondrion are encoded on nuclear DNA. This means that mitochondrial function and contribution to disease are regulated by two distinct genomes, which can have separate or interacting effects. For example, complex I of the mitochondrial respiration chain, discussed in the next section, is composed of 43 proteins, 7 encoded by mtDNA and the rest encoded by nuclear genes,[12] including at least one located on the X chromosome.[13] Thus, defects in complex I may arise from maternally inherited mtDNA mutations, X-linked defects, or autosomal-dominant or -recessive mutations.

Inherited mutations help determine disease severity. A mutation that has a large impact on mitochondrial function results in widespread early problems. For example, subacute necrotizing encephalopathy (Leigh's disease) is a severe pediatric mitochondrial disorder characterized by symmetric necrosis of the basal ganglia, as well as thalamus, brainstem regions, cerebellum, and spinal cord posterior columns.[14] Leigh's disease is caused by a variety of inherited mutations with large impact on mitochondrial functioning,[14] including complex I activity.[15,16] In contrast, more moderate mutations may have no noticeable impact early in life, but combine with other factors to produce late-onset symptoms. Over time, an individual may be exposed to exogenous toxins or accumulate somatic mtDNA mutations. A person with normal genes or very mild inherited mtDNA and nuclear mutations may withstand accumulating somatic mtDNA damage, whereas someone with inherited mutations of moderate functional impact could have less tolerance for toxic exposures and somatic mutations, experience decreased mitochondrial function, and more easily acquire a chronic neurodegenerative disorder.[17,18]

ACQUIRED mtDNA MUTATIONS

The interaction of inherited mtDNA and nuclear DNA mutations with somatic mtDNA mutations is thought to

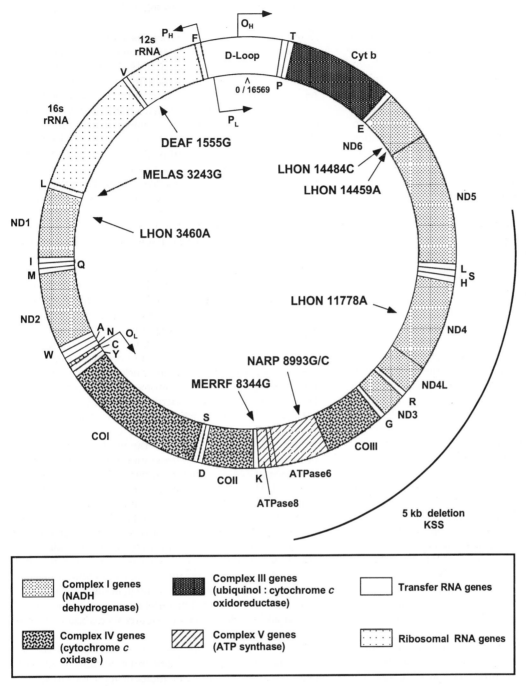

FIGURE 4-2 Genome map of human mitochondrial DNA (mtDNA). mtDNA is a circular 16,569-base genome. The D-loop region directs replication and transcription. The origins of H-strand (O_H) and L-strand (O_L) replication, and promoters for both strands (P_H, P_L) are indicated. Shaded areas represent coding regions for subunits of complexes I, III, IV and V, as well as ribosomal ribonucleic acids (rRNA). Coding regions for transfer RNAs (tRNA) are indicated by the standard one-letter codes for the corresponding amino acids. Locations of some identified disease-causing mutations are labeled by phenotype. DEAF, maternally inherited deafness; KSS, Kearns-Sayre syndrome; LHON, Leber's hereditary optic neuropathy; MELAS, mitochondrial encephalopathy, lactic acidosis, and stroke-like episodes; MERFF, myoclonic epilepsy with ragged-red fibers; NARP, neuropathy, ataxia, retinitis pigmentosa. (*From Wallace DC, Lott MT: MITOMAP: A Human Mitochondrial Genome Database, http://www.mitomap.org, 2003.*)

contribute to the complexity of mitochondrial disorder phenotypes, and the appearance of highly variable diseases later in life. mtDNA is highly susceptible to somatic mutations.[19] The mtDNA point mutation rate is ten times that of nuclear DNA.[19,20] In addition to point mutations, mtDNA often sustains large deletions, rearrangements, and other mutations.[17,21] Several factors contribute to the high mtDNA mutation rate.[18,19,21] mtDNA does not have histones to protect against damage, and mitochondria have more limited DNA repair mechanisms than the nucleus. In addition, mtDNA is exposed to damaging oxygen radicals, natural by-products of oxidative phosphorylation which is housed by mitochondria, as discussed below.

The accumulation of somatic mutations over time may have an impact on the brain in general and the basal ganglia in particular, as demonstrated by relative mtDNA mutation rates. Mutation rates can be estimated by measuring levels of specific mtDNA mutations, or screening for multiple large-scale deletions.[21] A commonly used mutation rate marker, a 5-kilobase mtDNA deletion (mtDNA^{4977}), accumulates in brain to a higher degree than in heart.[22–24] Within brain, the highest mtDNA^{4977} levels are in substantia nigra, caudate, and putamen, with lower levels in cerebral cortex and negligible levels in cerebellum.[22,24] The mtDNA^{4977} mutation level is also higher in HD cortex than in age-matched control brains.[25] Neurons may accumulate mtDNA mutations because they acquire more new mtDNA mutations through heavy use of oxidative phosphorylation or other means. Mechanisms of changing mtDNA mutation levels over time may also work against neurons.

mtDNA MUTATION LEVELS CHANGE OVER TIME

Levels of both inherited and acquired mtDNA mutations change over time with the formation of new mtDNA copies and new cells. There are several hundred mitochondria in each human cell, each containing two to ten mtDNA copies.[26] Although the total amount of mtDNA is usually less than 1 percent of total cellular DNA, there are thousands of copies of mtDNA per cell. Replication of mtDNA is under relaxed control, so unlike nuclear DNA it is not bound to replicate only once per cell cycle.[18] The phenomenon of many mtDNA copies able to replicate between cell cycles creates key distinctions between mtDNA and nuclear DNA genetics. For example, mtDNA mutation levels may increase within a cell by preferential replication of mutated mtDNAs. Possible mechanisms for such intracellular selection include faster, more frequent, replication of shorter mtDNAs with large deletions. Paradoxical replication of small mtDNA mutations may also occur.[10,27] This means that a point mutation that causes decreased protein activity may be replicated more often, providing more mtDNA copies and higher protein levels in an effort to overcome the lower protein activity within that cell.[10]

The burden of mtDNA mutations can also change between cells, through cell division. A given mutation may occur in any or all mtDNA copies within a cell. Homoplasmy occurs when all the mtDNAs in a cell contain the same mutation. A mother with oocytes homoplasmic for a given mutation transmits only mutated mtDNA to her children, generating a stable level of inherited mutation between siblings and continued inheritance of the mutation through the maternal line.[18] The existence within one cell of both wild-type and affected mtDNAs for a given specific mutation is called heteroplasmy. In somatic cells, heteroplasmy combines with the rate of cell replication to create variation in mtDNA mutation levels, and therefore phenotype, between tissues or cells within one individual patient.[14,17,18]

As a heteroplasmic cell divides, its mitochondria are distributed into the daughter cells via a sorting process that has only recently been detailed and is still not clearly understood.[10,28] Wild-type and mutant mtDNA copies can segregate by chance during cell division, so that each daughter cell may get a different total number of mtDNAs, and a different percentage of mutant mtDNA copies.[10] Over many cell divisions, the percentage of wild-type or mutated mtDNA will drift. For example, when a cell divides, one daughter cell may get few mutated mtDNAs, while the other gets many. The daughter cell with a low number of mtDNAs divides, sending a small percentage of its mutated mtDNAs to one new daughter cell, and a higher percentage to the other. A series of divisions placing a small percentage of mutated mtDNAs into daughter cells will eventually generate a cell line with very few or no mutated mtDNAs. Conversely, sequential divisions in which most of the mutated mtDNA goes into one daughter cell will lead to a cell line with most or all mutated mtDNA; thus, some cell lines derived from the initial parent cell will be homoplasmic, with all or no mutated mtDNA. Cell lines in between the two extremes will also exist. This process of sorting out wild-type and mutated mtDNA over a series of cell divisions is called replicative segregation. Tissues that generate new cells frequently will therefore have a large range of mutated mtDNA levels as they create many cell lines from a progenitor cell.[18] This affords the tissue a rescue mechanism for generating cells without accumulated somatic mtDNA mutations. Cells with low replication rates or postmitotic tissues, such as neurons, cannot use replicative segregation to sort out mtDNA mutations.[18] Instead, neurons accumulate somatic mtDNA mutations over time.

Heteroplasmy also contributes to the variability in mtDNA genotype and phenotype between individuals in the same family. Germ cell line generation differs from somatic cell replication in some respects: meiotic replicative segregation can be very rapid;[17] there is a large amplification of mtDNA during oogenesis, creating sampling errors;[17,18] and it is possible that only a small proportion of oocyte mtDNA is transmitted to the fetus.[18] A similar heteroplasmy principle does apply. If each oocyte contains a different percentage of wild-type versus mutated mtDNA, then a mother heteroplasmic for a mutation may transmit different levels of mutated mtDNA to each child. Daughters will repeat the process, producing a large variation in mutation levels between individuals in one family.[18]

MULTIPLE PROCESSES CONTRIBUTE TO THE OVERALL MITOCHONDRIAL GENOTYPE

In summary, an individual starts with an mtDNA mutation level determined by maternal germ cell line heteroplasmy and maternal mtDNA inheritance. Because nuclear DNA encodes most mitochondrial proteins, the inherited nuclear genome plus inherited mtDNA comprises the initial mitochondrial genetic background. In addition to this inherited baseline, mtDNA susceptibility to mutagenesis creates a combination of acquired and inherited mtDNA mutations. Some tissues may accumulate somatic mtDNA mutations at a higher rate than others. Levels of established mtDNA mutations can change as mtDNA replicates within a cell. Heteroplasmic mtDNA mutation levels also alter over time through replicative segregation (or lack thereof) within an individual's different cell lines. The combined inherited and acquired mtDNA and inherited nuclear mutations together produce mitochondrial dysfunction and resulting phenotype over time.

GENOTYPE TO PHENOTYPE CONSIDERATIONS

How does the burden of each individual mutation and the total mutation level translate into phenotype? One process that affects the genotype to phenotype interaction is the threshold effect of mitochondrial function.[15,29] In a heteroplasmic cell, protein products from wild-type mtDNAs may be able to compensate for mutated products. Higher percentages of mutated mtDNA have a greater impact on mitochondrial functioning. The point when wild-type proteins cannot overcome the impact of mutated mtDNA products, allowing some phenotype to occur, is the threshold mutation level. Past this threshold, the drop-off of function can be very steep. The specific threshold level varies between tissues and cells, according to their dependence on a particular protein's specific activity, and their relative reliance on basic mitochondrial functions.

Together, the threshold effect and mitochondrial genetics allow systemic mitochondrial defects to cause very specific tissue or cell damage. Neurons are heavily dependent on mitochondria for ATP production and survival; thus, neurons may be more sensitive than other cells to a given mtDNA mutation level and mitochondrial protein activity loss. Neurons also acquire more mtDNA mutations, through higher exposure to mutating conditions and lack of replicative segregation decreases in mtDNA mutation levels. The combination of low mtDNA mutation level threshold for functional impact in neurons with the high neuronal mtDNA mutation burden could help explain why neurons are particularly susceptible to mitochondrial disease.

Even with the concepts discussed above, the complex relationship of mitochondrial genotype to phenotype is not well understood. Different mtDNA or nuclear DNA mutations can result in the same "mitochondrial" phenotype, and a single mtDNA mutation can produce different phenotypes. Leigh's disease, a disorder with prominent basal ganglia involvement, is caused by a wide range of mutations affecting several different nuclear and mtDNA genes, as mentioned above. Threshold effect explains some but not all of the genotype to phenotype conversion for Leigh's disease.[15,29] Leigh's disease is a severe pediatric disorder associated with different types of high functional impact mutations, but the same variable genotype phenomenon occurs in adult-onset diseases. Leber's hereditary optic neuropathy (LHON) presents in adulthood with subacute, painless visual loss in both eyes due to optic nerve degeneration. LHON is caused by point mutations in genes encoding mitochondrial proteins ND4[30] and ND6[31] among others.[15,16] ND4 and ND6 are both subunits of complex I, discussed below.

LHON illustrates both how multiple genotypes can create the same phenotype, and how a given genotype can cause highly variable clinical pictures. Point mutations in ND6 and ND4 that cause LHON also cause familial movement disorders. The 11778 ND4 mutation, the most common cause of LHON, can also cause parkinsonism and multisystem degeneration.[32] The ND6 mutation can present as generalized dystonia early in life in some family members, while other family members develop LHON.[31,33,34] The differences may be due in part to heteroplasmic mutation level variation between family members and threshold effect, but how one particular form of mitochondrial dysfunction, in this case decreased complex I activity, can cause such distinct phenotypes remains unclear.

OXIDATIVE PHOSPHORYLATION

Mitochondria are often referred to as the cell's "power generators" because mitochondria are the site of oxidative phosphorylation (oxphos),[35] the final pathway of energy-producing metabolism in aerobic cells.[1,2,12] Varied fuel sources, such as carbohydrates, fats, and amino acids, are catabolized via oxidative metabolic pathways. Oxidation is the loss of electrons from a compound; thus, as fuel sources are broken down, electrons are released by oxidation. Electrons are collected by specific enzymes from the multitude of different oxidation reactions and moved to a small number of universal electron acceptor molecules, such as nicotinamide adenine dinucleotide (NAD^+). Metabolic pathways converge when these electron acceptor molecules in turn donate electrons to oxphos. Oxphos is the process by which movement of electrons from donor molecules, or oxidation, is coupled to phosphorylation of ADP to ATP, producing "energy" for use by the cell. In oxphos, electrons move from donor molecules through a sequence of complexes, the electron transport chain, ultimately to molecular oxygen. Metabolic processes that consume oxygen are called respiration; thus, mitochondrial consumption of oxygen in oxphos is called mitochondrial respiration, and the oxphos machinery that consumes oxygen, the

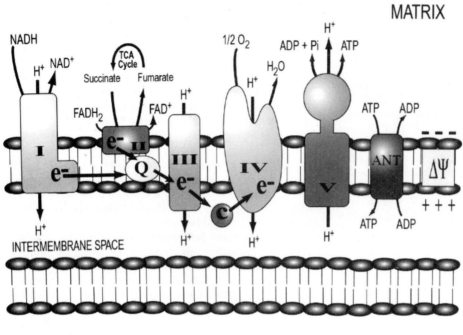

FIGURE 4-3 Oxidative phosphorylation. Electrons (e⁻) enter the mitochondrial electron transport chain from donors such as reduced nicotinamide adenine dinucleotide (NADH) and reduced flavin adenine dinucleotide (FADH₂). The electron donors leave as their oxidized forms, NAD⁺ and FAD⁺. Electrons move from complex I (I), complex II (II), and other donors to coenzyme Q₁₀ (Q). Coenzyme Q₁₀ transfers electrons to complex III (III). Cytochrome *c* (c) transfers electrons from complex III to complex IV (IV). Complexes I, III, and IV use the energy from electron transfer to pump protons (H⁺) out of the mitochondrial matrix, creating a chemical and electrical (Δψ) gradient across the mitochondrial inner membrane. Complex V (V) uses this gradient to add a phosphate (Pᵢ) to adenosine diphosphate (ADP), making adenosine triphosphate (ATP). Adenosine nucleotide transferase (ANT) moves ATP out of the matrix. (*From D. Wolf. Used with permission.*)

electron transport chain, is also called the mitochondrial respiratory chain. The protein complexes that transfer electrons from donor molecules to oxygen, and that phosphorylate ADP, are embedded in the inner mitochondrial membrane.

Oxphos begins with electron transfer from a donor molecule such as NADH (the reduced, or electron-carrying, form), which then leaves as NAD⁺ (the oxidized form, electrons lost), ready to accept electrons again from cellular metabolic pathways (Fig. 4-3). Electrons from NADH are transferred via complex I, also called NADH:ubiquinone oxyreductase, a very large multiprotein enzyme. Complex I moves electrons from NADH to ubiquinone, which is also called coenzyme Q. This reaction is coupled to movement by complex I of protons from the matrix to the intermembrane space. Thus complex I uses the energy released by electron transfer (as electrons move down an activation energy gradient) to pump protons across the inner mitochondrial membrane. Energy from the electron transfer reaction, originally "stored" in NADH, is now "stored" as the potential across the

inner mitochondrial membrane created by pumping protons in one direction, out of the matrix.

Complex II, also called succinate dehydrogenase, transfers electrons from a different initial donor, succinate, to coenzyme Q. Complex II, like complex I, is a multisubunit protein complex in the inner mitochondrial membrane, but it is much smaller, and it does not contain a proton pump. In addition to complex II and complex I, coenzyme Q also receives electrons from other sources, such as glycerol 3-phosphate. Coenzyme Q is a lipid-soluble molecule that can diffuse through the lipid bilayer inner mitochondrial membrane. Coenzyme Q, a key electron transporter in mitochondrial respiration, also functions as an antioxidant and as a major source of reactive oxygen species, roles discussed in the sections below.

Reduced (electron-carrying) coenzyme Q moves electrons from multiple sources to complex III. This huge complex is a dimer of two identical multisubunit monomers. Complex III transfers electrons from coenzyme Q to cytochrome *c*. Like complex I, complex III uses energy released in electron transfers to pump protons across the inner mitochondrial membrane, from the matrix to the intermembrane space, adding to the proton gradient across the inner membrane.

Finally, cytochrome *c* diffuses through the intermembrane space from complex III to complex IV. Cytochrome *c* is a small molecule that normally stays in the intermembrane space as part of the mitochondrial electron transport chain, but in pathologic conditions it may be released into the cytoplasm, triggering a form of programmed cell death, discussed below. Complex IV, or cytochrome oxidase, the final large inner membrane multisubunit complex in the electron transport chain, transfers electrons from cytochrome *c* to molecular oxygen. Complex IV, like complexes I and III, also pumps protons across the inner membrane. Molecular oxygen is consumed in this final step of mitochondrial respiration as it is reduced (gains electrons) to water (H_2O).

Overall, the components of the electron transport chain, complex I through complex IV and the electron carriers coenzyme Q and cytochrome *c*, act together to move electrons from cellular metabolic pathways to oxygen. The energy released in the process drives proton pumps that create a proton gradient across the inner mitochondrial membrane. This is both a chemical (pH) gradient, as the concentration of protons is higher in the intermembrane space than the matrix, and an electrical gradient ($\Delta\psi_m$), as positively charged protons are in the intermembrane space and negatively charged molecules are left in the matrix. The combined force of these chemical and electrical gradients is used by complex V to make ATP.[36,37] Complex V, or ATP synthase, has a proton pore that allows protons to flow back passively into the matrix, providing complex V with the energy to add a phosphate to adenosine diphosphate (ADP), creating ATP and completing the oxphos process.

In addition to oxphos, mitochondria play several other important roles within the cell. Individual parts of the oxphos machinery, such as coenzyme Q and cytochrome *c*, have discrete functions outside of oxphos. Mitochondrial dysfunction may therefore impact several important cell processes, and individual therapeutic compounds targeted at oxphos function can have multiple mitochondrion-related effects.

APOPTOSIS IN NORMAL DEVELOPMENT

Apoptosis is an active, complex, specific programmed pattern of cell death. Programmed cell death is an important component of normal development, including development of the nervous system.[38] Mitochondrial involvement in apoptosis was first demonstrated in a cell-free experimental system;[39] since then, extensive research has detailed the role of mitochondria as the linchpin of many complex programmed cell death pathways.[40–43] When activated by cellular damage, proapoptotic signaling molecules from the Bcl-2 protein family move to the mitochondrial membrane, where antiapoptosis regulators already reside.[42] Proapoptotic signals cause mitochondrial release

of cytochrome *c*[44] and other apoptogenic molecules from the intermembrane space into the cytosol. Cytochrome *c* then activates an aspartate-specific cysteine protease (caspase), caspase-3, a major effector of apoptosis in neurons.[45] Loss of this mitochondrion-based mechanism blocks normal neuronal development, as seen in transgenic mouse strains with knockouts of caspase-3 or proteins downstream of activated caspase-3. These mice have brain overgrowth and early death.[38]

REACTIVE OXYGEN SPECIES (ROS) AND NORMAL MITOCHONDRIA

Reactive oxygen species (ROS) are a subset of "free radicals," a term for all molecules with an unpaired electron in an outer orbital.[46] ROS are molecules that contain oxygen with an unpaired electron, making them highly chemically reactive; ROS will aggressively nonenzymatically donate electrons to other compounds, or take up protons from other molecules, in order to form an electron pair. Formation of an electron pair between an ROS and another compound can create a chemical bond, altering, and potentially damaging, the compound.[46] There are several sources of ROS in normal cells.[46–50] For example, exposure to ultraviolet or ionizing radiation can convert water and molecular oxygen (O_2) to ROS or a related reactive species, singlet oxygen.[46] Some specialized cells, such as neutrophils, produce high levels of ROS via enzymatic pathways in response to particular stimuli.[50,51] Apart from these special cases, the major source of ROS in nearly all cells is mitochondria.

Most O_2 consumed by mitochondrial respiration is converted to water. O_2 has a very high affinity for electrons, making it a good final electron acceptor for oxphos, but this characteristic also makes it liable to accept unpaired electrons from reactive intermediates in the course of oxphos. Respiratory chain complexes reduce or oxidize electron carriers in steps, and tightly constrain electron carriers to prevent release of partially reduced intermediates. The major example is coenzyme Q, which is reduced by complex I in two steps.[1,2] The first step, which adds one electron, creates the free radical semiquinone species ($Q^{\bullet-}$). The second creates the fully reduced ubiquinol (QH_2). At complex III, QH_2 goes through a series of steps, the Q cycle, to transfer electrons to cytochrome *c*. $Q^{\bullet-}$ is generated in the Q cycle as QH_2 is oxidized. At both complexes, electrons usually proceed through the respiratory chain, but some $Q^{\bullet-}$ does escape to donate an unpaired electron to O_2 during normal oxphos.[52–56] About 2 percent of O_2 used by mitochondrial respiration is converted to superoxide anion ($O_2^{\bullet-}$) in this way.[57]

This normal "leak" of electrons during oxphos has several consequences. Normal levels of ROS act as signals to the cell and to the mitochondrion. ROS can regulate activity of proteins via changes in cysteinyl residue oxidation state. Key protein targets include transcription factor families such as AP-1 and NF-kappaB, so ROS can alter gene expression levels. Enzymes such as protein kinases are also targets, so ROS influence posttranslational protein modifications.[48,58,59] On the other hand, even normal levels of ROS may damage nearby structures; for example, ROS from mitochondrial oxphos may contribute to the high rate of mtDNA mutations, as discussed above.

CALCIUM REGULATION

With normal neuronal functioning, large local increases in cytosolic calcium (Ca^{2+}) can occur as Ca^{2+} enters the cytoplasm through voltage-gated Ca^{2+} channels, ion-permeable neurotransmitter receptors, and endoplasmic reticulum stores released by second messenger systems. Mitochondria act as a Ca^{2+} "sink" or buffer, preventing sustained high peaks of cytosolic Ca^{2+}.[60–62] When cytosolic Ca^{2+} rises, mitochondrial Ca^{2+} also increases.[63] Mitochondria take up Ca^{2+} through a passive Ca^{2+} uniporter using the proton gradient ($\Delta\psi_m$) generated by oxphos for energy, and extrude calcium mainly via an active sodium (Na^+)/Ca^{2+} exchanger.[64] Calcium entering a mitochondrion can activate further ATP production via activation of Ca^{2+}-sensitive enzymes.[64] Thus, normal mitochondria both help regulate and respond to changes in cytosolic Ca^{2+}.

Consequences of Mitochondrial Dysfunction

DECREASED ATP PRODUCTION

Severe defects in any of the oxphos components can result in decreased ATP synthesis. Inability to maintain ATP production will profoundly disturb cell homeostasis, eventually leading to necrotic cell death. Neurons are particularly susceptible to loss of oxphos ATP production, because they are critically dependent on glycolysis for energy and cannot compensate with ATP production by other means.

Decreases in ATP production may interact with other insults to create conditions for neuronal damage. An estimated 40 percent of neuronal ATP production is used by Na^+/potassium (K^+)-ATPase for maintaining ion gradients and the neuronal membrane potential.[65,66] Decreasing mitochondrial oxphos ATP production may therefore create ion gradient disturbances and changes in neuronal membrane potential, which in turn alter baseline cell function and possibly increase cell vulnerability to damage.[67] For example, glutamate excitotoxicity occurs when sustained glutamate input activates Ca^{2+}-permeable *N*-methyl-D-aspartate (NMDA) receptors, which then let large influxes of Ca^{2+} into the cell. Membrane depolarization due to lower Na^+/K^+-ATPase function releases the voltage-dependent magnesium blockade of NMDA receptors,[68] so that glutamate can more easily activate NMDA receptors.[69] This allows greater glutamate-induced Ca^{2+} influx into the cell, and greater glutamate toxicity at lower levels of glutamate activity.[67]

Excitotoxicity has long been implicated in movement disorder pathology. Understanding and repairing mitochondrial oxphos may provide a way to act on excitotoxicity pathways and other cell damage mechanisms that react to changing ATP production.

APOPTOSIS IN DISEASE

Mitochondria can also participate in apoptotic cell death. The interaction of Bcl-2 family proteins with mitochondria, and how mitochondrial release of cytochrome *c* can trigger apoptosis, is discussed above. While apoptosis is essential to normal development, abnormally regulated apoptosis can cause early cell loss and contribute to disease. The final pathway of cell damage and death after mitochondrial dysfunction may depend on the exact type and degree of insult.[43,64] For example, extreme Ca^{2+} or oxidative stress loads lead to necrosis, while lower intensity versions of the same insults can cause apoptosis.[70–72] This makes mitochondrial apoptosis intriguing in terms of neurodegenerative pathophysiology, a chronic process that probably involves multiple, interacting low-level insults. Because of the difficulty of finding and studying apoptotic cells in humans,[73,74] the role of apoptosis in neurodegenerative disorders is controversial, but it remains a topic of debate and study as apoptosis pathways present tempting targets for therapeutics to "rescue" failing cells.

The dual role of cytochrome *c* in oxphos and apoptosis points to the complex interaction between oxphos and other mitochondrial functions. Defects in oxphos may impact cell death pathways or other functions in addition to ATP production. Another example of this link between oxphos components and apoptosis is complex I, which may have additional functions beyond its primary role in the mitochondrial electron transport chain.[16] A new complex I subunit in bovine heart mitochondria is the bovine homolog of GRIM-19.[75] GRIM-19 is the protein product of a cell death regulatory gene induced by beta-interferon and retinoic acid.[75] This finding suggests a direct role for complex I in apoptosis signaling pathways. In addition, complex I may interact with apoptosis pathways via regulation of permeability transition (PT) pore opening.[16]

THE PT PORE

A large, not yet completely defined, mitochondrial protein complex, the PT pore may be the end site at which several different external insults and consequences of pathological mitochondrial dysfunction come together to trigger apoptosis.[76] The PT pore is a large Ca^{2+}-dependent complex that creates an opening in the mitochondrial inner membrane. PT pore opening allows diffusion of low molecular weight solutes, including charged ions, out of the mitochondrion, causing mitochondrial depolarization and calcium release.[64] Increased calcium, increased ROS, and loss of ATP can all trigger PT pore opening.[43,77] The flow of electrons through complex I may also directly regulate PT pore activity.[78,79] Widespread PT pore activation can cause massive mitochondrial depolarization and subsequent necrosis, but more limited PT pore opening may release mitochondrial proapoptotic molecules and start the apoptosis cascade,[43,80] or participate in Ca^{2+} regulation. A role for PT pore complex components in regulating apoptosis signaling molecules closely associated with the mitochondrion has also been proposed.[43] Overall, understanding mitochondrial involvement in apoptosis, including triggers for mitochondrial release of apoptosis signals, alternative roles of oxphos components, and the role of the PT pore, may provide avenues for rescuing neurons at a final common stage of damage and disease.

TOXIC LEVELS OF ROS

Transfer of one electron to O_2, as happens at a low rate during normal oxphos, creates superoxide ($O_2^{\cdot-}$). Excessive $O_2^{\cdot-}$ can be damaging by itself, and its breakdown drives formation of other even more damaging ROS. $O_2^{\cdot-}$ reacts with iron-sulfur-containing proteins, releasing ferrous iron (Fe^{2+}). The superoxide dismutase (SOD) enzymes catalyze conversion of $O_2^{\cdot-}$ to hydrogen peroxide (H_2O_2) (Fig. 4-4).[81] H_2O_2 reacts with Fe^{2+} to form hydroxyl ion (OH^-) and the highly reactive hydroxyl radical ($OH^{\cdot}$) via the Fenton reaction.[55,82,83] $O_2^{\cdot-}$ can also react with nitric oxide to form highly reactive peroxynitrite.[84,85] Increases in ROS that overwhelm the cells normal biochemical antioxidants and reducing enzymes cause "oxidative stress."

As the major source of ROS in normal cellular states, the mitochondrion is the key site for abnormally increased ROS production. Excessive physiologic ROS production can be caused by greatly increasing O_2, as in reperfusion, making more O_2 available to react with $Q^{\cdot-}$ and form $O_2^{\cdot-}$. Increased cellular Ca^{2+} may generate a similar consequence. As Ca^{2+} rises, mitochondria take up Ca^{2+}, depleting the inner membrane proton gradient ($\Delta\psi_m$). As $\Delta\psi_m$ decreases, mitochondrial respiration increases to compensate, with a parallel increase in ROS production.[58]

Mitochondrial dysfunction also leads to increased ROS. Blockade of complex I or complex III at the coenzyme Q electron transfer steps, by intrinsic defects in complex proteins or exogenous toxins, can create a "pile-up" of increased, unused $Q^{\cdot-}$ available to react with O_2, thus increasing $O_2^{\cdot-}$ production.[55,86] Increased mitochondrial ROS production may trigger increased apoptosis,[21,87] possibly by activating PT pore opening and cytochrome *c* release, as discussed above. Excess ROS also damages mitochondria and other cellular components, with potentially widespread impact on cellular functions.

OXIDATIVE DAMAGE

ROS can damage all types of macromolecules in the cell. ROS interact with polyunsaturated fatty acids, a major component of lipid bilayer membranes, to cause lipid peroxidation.[46,88] This chain reaction generates lipid peroxide radicals, which go on to react with other fatty acids, and hydroperoxides, which are not reactive but are unstable and can fragment. Lipid breakdown products such as malondialdehyde and 4-hydroxynonenal accumulate as membranes become progressively damaged and fragmented. Aldehyde breakdown products can react with protein sulfhydryl groups to form carbonyls.[89] Direct ROS oxidation of amino acids can also produce carbonyls, as well as tyrosine and cysteine crosslinking, and specific oxidized amino acid residues.[89-91] Oxidative modification of proteins can alter conformation and function, and mark proteins for degradation.[89] It can also promote protein aggregation and make proteins more resistant to normal clearance.[90,92] Protein aggregates are a pathologic hallmark of many movement disorders. Finally, ROS can attack DNA, causing a variety of lesions, including formation of specific oxidized bases such as 8-hydroxyguanine.[93] Oxidized bases render DNA more susceptible to general lesions such as strand breaks and crosslinking.[48,93,94] Repair mechanisms in the cell such as lipases, proteases, and ribonucleases break down ROS-modified compounds. These systems are a final check against ROS damage, dealing with the consequences of ROS that get by cellular antioxidant defenses.

As the source of most ROS in the cell, the mitochondrion is also a major target for ROS damage. Mitochondrial membranes, oxphos components and other proteins, and mtDNA are all affected by ROS. mtDNA is particularly vulnerable to oxidative damage, as discussed above. Damage to oxphos components can lead to decreased complex I and complex III function and increased ROS production, creating a vicious cycle of ROS-induced damage and further ROS release.

CELLULAR ANTIOXIDANT SYSTEMS

Cells normally control ROS levels with a variety of antioxidant enzyme systems.[46,83] For example, SOD converts $O_2^{\cdot-}$ to H_2O_2, as mentioned above (Fig. 4-4). The mammalian SOD family includes a mitochondrial manganese-dependent SOD (MnSOD), and both extracellular and cytosolic copper/zinc SODs (Cu/ZnSOD).[85] H_2O_2 is then converted to water by glutathione peroxidase (GPX) and catalse, completing the transition from an ROS, $O_2^{\cdot-}$, to a nontoxic molecule.[55,83,85]

In addition to enzyme systems, cells contain antioxidant compounds. Antioxidants are molecules that can safely convert ROS to nonreactive species (i.e., compounds without unpaired electrons). An antioxidant either accepts unpaired electrons from an ROS, leaving a reduced form of the antioxidant and an inactive oxygen compound, or donates electrons to an ROS, leaving an oxidized form of the antioxidant molecule along with the inactive oxygen compound. Either way, a new free radical form of the antioxidant compound is created. This molecule has an unpaired electron carried by a much less reactive molecule than the original ROS.[46,95] The new free radical molecule must then be recycled back to its initial antioxidant form via interaction with other

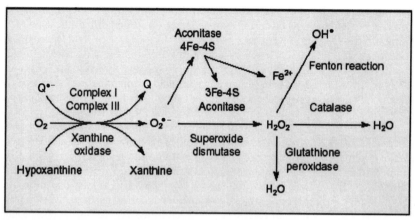

FIGURE 4-4 Antioxidant systems produce and remove reactive oxygen species (ROS) in the cell. Molecular oxygen (O_2) is converted to superoxide anion ($O_2^{\bullet-}$) by mitochondrial electron transport chain components via reaction with free radical semiquinone forms ($Q^{\bullet-}$) of coenzyme Q (Q). Some specialized cells generate $O_2^{\bullet-}$ with xanthine oxidase or other systems. For most cells, mitochondria are the major source of $O_2^{\bullet-}$. $O_2^{\bullet-}$ is converted to hydrogen peroxide (H_2O_2) by superoxide dismutase (SOD). Glutathione peroxidase and catalase convert H_2O_2 to water (H_2O), completing the transition from $O_2^{\bullet-}$ to nonreactive molecules. H_2O_2 can also interact with ferrous ions (Fe^{2+}), generating the highly reactive hydroxyl radical ($OH^{\bullet}$). $O_2^{\bullet-}$ can contribute to Fe^{2+} and $OH^{\bullet}$ formation by attacking iron-containing enzymes such as aconitase, releasing Fe^{2+}. (*Modified from Raha and Robinson.[55] Used with permission.*)

compounds, such as physiologic electron donors (reducing agents) or other free radicals.[95]

Antioxidants may act as part of an enzyme system or alone. The major water-soluble antioxidant, glutathione, is part of the GPX system.[83,96] Glutathione is used by GPX to convert H_2O_2 to water. Reduced glutathione (GSH) becomes oxidized (GSSG) in this reaction.[46,48,55] GSSG is recycled back to GSH by glutathione reductase, using NADPH. Measurement of the ratio of GSH to GSSG is a key method of determining the overall ROS level and redox state of a cell; low GSH and high GSSG may reflect high H_2O_2 conversion, and high $O_2^{\bullet-}$ producing H_2O_2.[96]

Important lipid-soluble antioxidants include alpha-tocopherol and coenzyme Q. alpha-Tocopherol, a vitamin E compound, halts the chain of lipid peroxidation by donating an electron to lipid peroxide radicals, leaving a low reactivity alpha-tocoperoxyl radical.[97] Phenoxyl radicals can be recycled by the reduced (QH_2) form of coenzyme Q,[95] which also itself directly blocks lipid peroxidation. In normal cells, these enzyme systems and antioxidant compounds maintain a balance between useful ROS production and damaging oxidative stress.

Mitochondrial damage by ROS can set up a cycle of impaired cellular antioxidants and increasing mitochondrial dysfunction. For example, QH_2 is produced during mitochondrial respiration. Therefore, mitochondrial dysfunction can directly reduce the supply of antioxidants and compounds that recycle antioxidants, thus depleting defenses against ROS.[97] In this potential feed-forward loop, abnormal mitochondria produce increased ROS, ROS attack mitochondrial components and decrease mitochondrial function, decreased mitochondrial function leaves cells less able to regenerate antioxidants, and lower antioxidant levels allow more ROS to damage mitochondria.[97]

DISRUPTION OF CALCIUM REGULATION

Defects in the mitochondrial respiration chain may impact proton pumping across the inner membrane, so that $\Delta\psi_m$ decreases, and the inner membrane becomes relatively depolarized. Inability to maintain $\Delta\psi_m$ impairs calcium regulation, and the mitochondrion no longer has the energy needed to take up cytosolic Ca^{2+}.[98] Increased free cytosolic Ca^{2+} leads to cell death through multiple pathways.[99] Lack of mitochondrial Ca^{2+} buffering may interact with glutamate-induced Ca^{2+} influxes to enhance excitotoxic damage to neurons, as discussed above.

Sustained excessive increases in mitochondrial Ca^{2+} concentration, whether from glutamate activity or other means, contribute to neuronal damage and cell death.[60] Increased mitochondrial Ca^{2+} is thought to combine with multiple other factors, including increased ROS and decreased ATP, to trigger PT pore opening, leading to necrosis or apoptosis, as discussed above. Glutamate increases cytosolic Na^+ as well as Ca^{2+}.[100] Glutamate excitotoxicity may therefore exacerbate toxic mitochondrial Ca^{2+} loads by two methods: direct increases in cytosolic and thus mitochondrial Ca^{2+}; and decreased activity of the Na^+/Ca^{2+}-ATPase used to reduce intramitochondrial Ca^{2+}.[67] In fact, mitochondrial Ca^{2+} uptake is required for glutamate-induced neuronal death in cell culture.[101] In summary, disruption of mitochondrial Ca^{2+} regulation may be a primary event, worsening the cell's ability to handle Ca^{2+} loads and increase ATP production based on Ca^{2+} signals, or a secondary event, as increasing mitochondrial calcium contributes to PT pore opening and further mitochondrial and neuronal damage.

Mitochondria and Aging

Age is a major risk factor for many movement disorders, particularly neurodegenerative disorders.[102,103] Mitochondria are thought to play a key role in normal aging. Changes in mitochondrial function with age may interact with other disease processes to create chronic, degenerative disorders later in life.

Mitochondria are probably the major source of free radicals in aging through their production of ROS. The free radical theory of aging proposes that cumulative free radical damage to cell components is the basis of aging.[104,105] In fact, maximum lifespan in many species is inversely related to the mitochondrial respiration rate and to levels of oxidative damage.[92,106] The correlations between aging, oxidative damage, and decreased mitochondrial function are extensive and well studied. Oxidative stress is widely accepted as at least a contributing factor to aging. Still, definitive evidence for a direct causal mechanism linking mitochondria, oxidative stress, and aging remains elusive,[92,107] in part due to the inherent individual variation in ROS production and the results of oxidative damage.[92]

A second factor linking mitochondrial dysfunction to aging is that mtDNA is susceptible to continued somatic mutations over time, as discussed above. Accumulating mtDNA mutations can gradually affect mitochondrial function, so extensive work has focused on mtDNA mutation rates and the association of mtDNA mutation rates with mitochondrial changes in function in the course of aging.[21,108] Increases in particular mtDNA mutations with age are well established, but many are modest.[21] Because mtDNA mutations vary widely in location and type, one challenge is to detect the range of possible mutations and achieve a good estimate of the mutation rate. Capturing the full range of mtDNA mutations may reveal a threshold mutation level that can result in a clear functional impact.[109,110]

Either as a consequence of accumulated mtDNA mutations or other factors, mitochondrial respiration function decreases with age.[14,21,111,112] Complex IV-deficient muscle fibers (cytochrome *c* oxidase negative) increase with age in human heart, ocular muscles, and skeletal muscle.[113–115] Complex IV loss correlates with increasing mtDNA mutation levels.[115] Isolated mitochondria from human liver and skeletal muscle show declining respiratory function with age.[111,112,116] More general measures of oxphos function also decline with age.[21] For example, the mitochondrial membrane potential generated by oxphos and used to drive ATP production decreases with age.[21,117,118]

In addition to a decline in normal mitochondrial function, there is also an increase in mitochondrial ROS production and ROS-induced mitochondrial damage with age. Superoxide and H_2O_2 production both increase with age.[106,107] Oxidative damage to mtDNA, a consequence of as well as possible cause of high ROS, increases in brain and other tissues with age.[21,119] Protein oxidation and lipid peroxidation in mitochondria also occur with age,[21] although studies yield different results in different tissue and cell types.[103] The general redox state in mitochondria may change with age-related ROS increases, as reflected by increased mitochondrial GSSG.[120] The combination of decreasing mitochondrial oxphos function and increasing ROS is presumed to lead to downstream consequences of mitochondrial dysfunction such as apoptosis,[21] as discussed in preceding sections.

There is a proposed vicious cycle of decreased mitochondrial function with age, increased ROS production, and further mitochondrial damage. How direct this cycle is, and what triggers it to start, is still being investigated. Animal models with known mutations that result in premature aging are one avenue of investigation closely related to studies of disease pathology.[21] For example, complex II gene mutation in *Caenorhabditis elegans* causes increased oxidative stress and decreased lifespan.[121] Treatment of these worms with SOD/catalase mimetics normalizes lifespan.[122] This model demonstrates one way in which an initial genetic defect could affect mitochondrial respiration, starting the cycle of mitochondrial dysfunction, ROS production, and aging.

Oxidative damage to the whole cell, not just mitochondria, occurs in the brain with age.[103] Although mtDNA has higher mutation rates than nuclear DNA, oxidative DNA damage also increases in brain nuclear DNA with age, as measured by 8-hydroxyguanine levels.[123,124] Lipofuscin, a compound formed by the reaction of proteins and lipid peroxidation products,[125] increases with age in brain.[126] Studies of lipid peroxidation products in brain have yielded mixed results, with age-related increases in some cells but only disease-related increases in others,[127,128] making it so far unclear if brain lipid peroxidation is a significant feature of normal aging or a phenomenon of late-onset disease.[103,128]

Protein oxidation in brain increases with aging, as a function of increased ROS, decreased ability to repair or degrade damaged proteins, or both.[89,92,129] Oxidative modification has several effects on proteins, as discussed above, including alterations in conformation and activity. Indeed, activity of enzymes susceptible to oxidation decreases with age.[92,129] Oxidative modification of proteins may therefore be an important aging factor.

Antioxidant systems work to maintain a normal balance of ROS and other free radicals in the cell. Age-related changes in antioxidant defenses would render the mitochondrion, and the cell, less able to cope with increasing oxidative stress. While an increase in ROS with aging is generally accepted, controversy exists over whether antioxidant systems change with age. Compared to the wealth of correlative data on ROS and aging, data for any change in antioxidant levels is relatively weak.[107] For example, there is no change in antioxidant enzyme activities in brain in aging mice despite increases in oxidative DNA damage.[124] Many studies take the approach of boosting antioxidant activity in order to prolong normal lifespan. In addition to restoring normal lifespan to complex II mutation *C. elegans* strains, SOD/catalase mimetics extend lifespan in wild-type worms.[122] Overexpression of both Cu/ZnSOD and catalase in transgenic *Drosophila melanogaster* flies does increase lifespan and decrease oxidative stress,[130] but the same effects are not seen in flies overexpressing only one of these two antioxidant enzyme genes, or in transgenic mice.[103] Supplementation with various antioxidant molecules has been reported to increase lifespan in different animals, but thus far human clinical trials have not shown a change in mortality rates.[107,131] The role of antioxidant defenses in aging remains unclear.

Mitochondrial Dysfunction in Movement Disorders

mtDNA mutations cause a range of movement disorders, including ataxias and dystonia, as discussed above. A nuclear DNA mutation altering a mitochondrial protein causes the deafness dystonia syndrome.[132,133] Mutations in the vitamin E binding protein gene cause an ataxia syndrome,[134] and Friedreich's ataxia is thought to be a nuclear-encoded mitochondrial genetic disorder.[135,136] A role for mitochondrial dysfunction is also postulated for neurodegenerative movement disorders that are not associated with a single inherited mutation, such as PD, and disorders whose genetic mutation does not clearly affect a mitochondrial protein, such as HD. This section reviews evidence for mitochondrial involvement in PD and HD. The two diseases provide an illustration of how underlying mitochondrial dysfunction can create movement disorder pathology in either primarily idiopathic or fully inherited diseases.

PARKINSON'S DISEASE (PD)

There is increasing evidence that mitochondrial dysfunction may be a key pathological mechanism in PD. PD is a chronic, slowly progressive disease characterized by tremor, bradykinesia, rigidity, and gait disturbance. The incidence of disease increases with age, with as many as 1 percent of people over age 65 affected.[102] Five to 10 percent of cases are clearly familial; these include mutations of alpha-synuclein,[137,138] *parkin*,[139] DJ-1,[140] and ubiquitin C-terminal hydrolase L1 (UCH-L1).[141] The cause of disease in the majority sporadic cases is unknown, but is likely to involve a combination of genetic predisposition and long-term environmental exposures.[102] Current medical and surgical symptomatic therapies have greatly improved functional capacity

and survival in PD, but many patients still develop disabling motor complications on escalating treatment regimens, and there is no proven therapy to delay onset or slow progression of disease.

Mitochondrial dysfunction in PD was first suggested by an outbreak of parkinsonism caused by a synthetic opiate contaminant, 1-methyl-4-phenyl-1,2,3,6-tetrahydropyridine (MPTP).[142,143] MPTP induces acute, permanent parkinsonism after its metabolite, 1-methyl-4-phenylpyridinium (MPP+), is actively, specifically taken up into dopaminergic neurons,[144,145] where it inhibits complex I.[146,147] Given the striking clinical and pathological similarities between MPTP-induced parkinsonism and idiopathic PD, several groups investigated complex I defects in PD. Complex I activity is decreased in PD brain.[148–150] Complex I is also decreased in platelets, muscle, and fibroblasts in PD patients, suggesting a systemic mitochondrial defect underlying this specific neurodegeneration.[151,152]

The selectivity of MPTP's action is based on its specific uptake into dopaminergic cells via the dopamine transporter,[144] but, if PD patients have a systemic dysfunction of complex I, then a systemic complex I inhibitor should also cause parkinsonism even without the selective uptake mechanism of MPTP. Rotenone, an organic pesticide, is highly lipophilic, so it easily crosses the blood-brain barrier to bind to complex I in neuronal mitochondria without using an active selective uptake system. Chronic systemic infusion of rotenone in rats causes selective degeneration of the nigrostriatal pathway, even in the presence of global partial complex I inhibition.[153,154]

It is unclear if complex I inhibition in PD is entirely due to environmental exposures, or a combination of acquired and genetic insults. Studies with cytoplasmic hybrid (cybrid) cells suggest there is some contributing mtDNA defect in PD. Cybrid cells are created by fusing cells depleted of all mtDNA with platelets, which contain mtDNA but do not have nuclei. When cybrids are made with platelets from PD patients, the cybrid cells have decreased complex I activity compared to cybrids made with control platelets, suggesting a defect in the PD mtDNA.[155,156] Despite these results, causative mtDNA mutations in PD have not yet been identified, so the exact nature of the proposed mitochondrial defect in PD is as yet unknown. On the other hand, a complementary approach is to look for mtDNA mutations associated with reduced, rather than increased, risk of PD. One recent study found that some mtDNA haplogroups, and one specific single nucleotide polymorphism in a complex I component, were associated with a reduced risk of PD compared to other haplogroups.[157]

Does a partial inhibition of complex I in PD have any of the effects predicted for mitochondrial dysfunction? Rotenone increases H_2O_2 production by isolated brain mitochondria using NADH-linked substrates,[158] demonstrating how blockage of mitochondrial respiration at complex I can lead to more $Q^{\cdot-}$ and increased production of ROS, as discussed in the sections above. Complex I is just one possible site of ROS production, but it may be an essential site for pathophysiologic effects. In in vitro isolated nerve terminal preparations, complex III and complex IV inhibition have high thresholds for ROS formation followed by big increases in ROS once inhibition levels are over threshold, but complex I defects lead to ROS formation even at low levels of complex I dysfunction.[159] Thus, the low levels of complex I defect seen in PD may be physiologically significant.

There is growing evidence of increased oxidative stress and ROS damage in PD and its experimental models.[160] Increased lipid peroxidation[161,162] and oxidative damage of DNA[163,164] and proteins[165] have been observed in PD substantia nigra. There is a decreased level of GSH in substantia nigra of PD brains,[166] suggesting that increased H_2O_2 and ROS levels are present. MPTP increases free radical and ROS production in vitro,[167,168] and mice treated with MPTP have increased brain levels of lipid peroxidation[169] and 3-nitrotyrosine,[170] along with decreased GSH.[171]

Overall, extensive evidence suggests the involvement of oxidative stress in PD pathophysiology, although the mechanisms by which complex I defects and oxidative stress lead to specific PD pathology remain unclear. Dopaminergic cells may be particularly vulnerable to oxidative stress because dopamine catabolism itself creates ROS.[73,172,173] The combination of high baseline ROS plus a secondary, in itself nontoxic, ROS increase might explain damage to dopaminergic neurons.

Familial PD cases may have unique links between oxidative stress and cell death. For example, cybrids of platelets from familial PD patients with alpha-synuclein mutations show increased evidence of oxidative stress, implying that mitochondrial damage may accumulate in cells in these patients.[174] Also, there is an interaction between alpha-synuclein expression and oxidative damage. Cells expressing mutant alpha-synuclein have an increased sensitivity to cell death caused by oxidative stress,[175,176] and wild-type alpha-synuclein that has been damaged by free radicals may be more prone to aggregation.[177] As alpha-synuclein is found in Lewy bodies in idiopathic as well as familial PD cases, an interaction between alpha-synuclein and oxidative damage could be important in general PD pathophysiology.

In addition to increased ROS, other downstream consequences of mitochondrial dysfunction may be important in PD. One study has found increased activated caspase-3 in substantia nigra pars compacta (SNc) neurons in PD compared to controls.[178] While there is some evidence that SNc neurons die by apoptosis in PD, the role of apoptosis in PD remains controversial, in part because it is technically difficult to find solid morphologic evidence for apoptosis in postmortem human brain.[73,74] Models of PD may strengthen the case for apoptosis in PD. MPTP induces apoptosis[179] and increased activated caspase-3[180] in mouse SNc. If apoptosis, triggered by mitochondrial dysfunction or other factors, is the final step in SNc cell death, knowledge of the specific cellular pathways involved could point to ways to prolong neuronal survival.

HUNTINGTON'S DISEASE (HD)

Huntington's disease (HD) is an autosomal-dominant disorder characterized by progressive chorea, dystonia, loss of coordination, psychiatric symptoms, dementia, and weight loss. The responsible genetic mutation is an expanded triplet repeat of CAG (glutamine) in the coding region of huntingtin, a protein of unknown function.[181] In HD, huntingtin fragments form intraneuronal aggregates of unclear pathologic significance.[182] Affected individuals are rapidly disabled by early functional decline, and require close care for another 10–20 years before succumbing to the effects of severe physical and mental deterioration.

The pathogenesis of HD is still unclear, but increasing evidence indicates that defects in mitochondrial energy production contribute to the process. Progressive weight loss in HD patients despite high caloric intake has long suggested the presence of an underlying metabolic defect.[183] Cortical biopsy specimens from HD patients show morphologically abnormal mitochondria.[184] There is a decrease in glucose utilization, revealed by positron emission tomography, in the caudate nucleus and putamen in HD, which appears early and precedes bulk tissue loss.[185] Magnetic resonance spectroscopy of HD brain shows in vivo lactate elevations in cerebral cortex and basal ganglia.[186,187] This suggests greater use of anaerobic metabolism in those regions, or an inability to use the end-products of glycolysis. There is evidence for decreased complex II/III activity, more so than complex IV activity, in striatum from postmortem HD brains,[188–191] and decreased complex I activity in HD platelets and muscle.[192,193]

Consequences of mitochondrial dysfunction are also observed in HD, including evidence for oxidative stress and apoptosis. Lipofuscin, a putative marker of oxidative stress, is increased in HD neurons, especially those most vulnerable to degeneration.[194,195] A marked increase in mitochondrial DNA deletions occurs in the cerebral cortex of HD patients (Mecocci, 1993 #153). Markers of oxidative damage to lipids, proteins, and DNA are elevated in HD striatum and cortex.[189,196] DNA strand breaks accumulate in brain tissue specimens from HD patients, suggesting ongoing apoptosis.[197] Crossbreeding caspase-1-dominant negative mice with transgenic HD mice slows disease progression, as does intraventricular administration of caspase inhibitors.[198]

An hypothesis involving mitochondrial dysfunction in HD must relate to the huntingtin mutation in this autosomal-dominant fully penetrant disease. Huntingtin is ubiquitously expressed in human tissues,[199] so a mitochondrial defect related to mutant huntingtin could be systemic. Lymphocytes from HD patients have abnormal mitochondrial Ca^{2+} handling.[200] The HD mitochondria depolarize at lower Ca^{2+} loads,[200] implying that the mitochondria are unable to tolerate Ca^{2+} increases, putting cells at greater risk of losing ATP production when stressed by Ca^{2+} increases or other means. In an in vitro system, fusion proteins containing long CAG repeats caused mitochondria to depolarize at lower Ca^{2+} loads, relating CAG repeat length to this potential HD-specific mitochondrial defect.[201]

This work builds on an earlier study in which HD lymphoblast mitochondria underwent greater depolarization after cyanide stress (damage to complex IV function) compared to controls, an effect blocked by inhibiting PT pore opening.[202] The level of this effect correlated with the CAG repeat length. HD lymphoblasts in this study were also more susceptible to staurosporine-induced apoptosis, associated with increased caspase-3 activation.[202] Thus a mitochondrial dysfunction specific to HD cells and related to CAG repeat length was associated with increased apoptosis.

One theory of polyglutamine toxicity proposes that long CAG segments can form pores in cell membranes with a selective high conductance for H^+ and K^+.[203] Mutant huntingtin associated with mitochondria has been observed by electron microscopy,[200,204] and huntingtin is observed in mitochondrial fractions by western blot.[205] A pore formed by large CAG repeat length huntingtin in mitochondrial membranes would allow protons to flow down the electrochemical gradient built up by mitochondrial respiration, causing the mitochondrion to depolarize. Alternatively, instead of forming a new kind of mitochondrial membrane pore, huntingtin could interact with PT pore components to promote PT pore opening with loss of $\Delta\psi_m$.[201] Overall, an association between mutant huntingtin and mitochondria may lead to an increased propensity for mitochondrial depolarization. As a mitochondrion depolarizes, it can no longer use its proton gradient to regulate Ca^{2+} fluxes, potentially rendering cells more vulnerable to glutamate excitotoxicity and other stressors. Loss of the proton gradient also depletes the driving force for oxphos ATP synthesis. Finally, mitochondrial depolarization increases PT pore opening, and can trigger apoptosis via cytochrome *c* release and caspase-3 activation, leading to early cell death.

Additional insights into how a systemic mitochondrial defect can lead to HD-like selective neuronal loss come from HD model systems. The complex II inhibitors 3-nitropropionic acid (3-NPA) and malonate cause striatal lesions in rodents that resemble the selective striatal medium spiny neuronal loss seen in HD, even when 3-NPA is administered systemically.[206–210] These experimental lesions can be blocked with the same agents that lower brain lactate levels in HD.[211,212] Thus, as in PD, systemic mitochondrial respiration inhibitors are used to create animal models that help study selective cell vulnerability in HD, although the exact nature of any mitochondrial defect in HD may differ from that proposed for PD or other disorders. These studies will be important in resolving potential differences in the current literature: lymphocyte,[200–202] platelet,[193] and muscle[192] studies demonstrate possible systemic mitochondrial changes in HD, whereas decreased complex II/III activity is observed specifically in postmortem HD striatum, emphasizing change in a particular cell type.[189,191]

HD animal models also help examine the interaction of mitochondrial dysfunction with huntingtin expression and CAG repeat length. Several different HD transgenic models exist, which use different constructs, full-length or truncated human huntingtin, and varying CAG repeat lengths.[213] N-Acetylaspartate, which is synthesized by mitochondria, is decreased in vivo in HD transgenic mice at young ages prior to neuronal loss, suggesting impaired mitochondrial function.[214,215] The study discussed above which found abnormal mitochondrial Ca^{2+} handling in human HD lymphoblasts showed the same abnormality in brain mitochondria from HD transgenic mice expressing full-length mutant huntingtin with 72 CAG repeats, but not huntingtin with 18 CAG repeats.[200] The defect in Ca^{2+} handling preceded neuronal degeneration and motor abnormalities in the mice by months, and so may represent an early step in HD pathogenesis.

Human and animal model data are coming together to support a key role for mitochondria in HD pathophysiology, although the exact nature of the mitochondrial dysfunction, and the connection of mitochondria to huntingtin, remains the subject of much ongoing work. There is evidence for mitochondrial dysfunction and its downstream consequences in HD patients, toxin models of HD, and transgenic models. Theories of mitochondrial involvement in HD address evidence for systemic versus local mitochondrial defects, the existence of the widely expressed disease gene, CAG repeat length effects, and specific neuronal degeneration. In addition to ongoing basic research, theories of mitochondrial dysfunction in HD are behind current neuroprotective clinical trials, as discussed below.

Therapeutics

This is an exciting time in mitochondrial research as new therapeutics aimed at improving mitochondrial dysfunction undergo preliminary trials in movement disorder populations. Some therapeutic approaches related to mitochondria are aimed at potential consequences of unknown primary pathophysiologic processes. For example, apoptosis may represent a final common pathway of multiple interacting insults, including mitochondrial dysfunction, so inhibiting apoptosis pathways could improve neuronal survival.[216] Minocycline, a compound now in clinical trials for HD treatment, is thought to inhibit caspase-1 and caspase-3,[217] as well as mitochondrial release of cytochrome *c*.[218]

Other therapies exploit interactions between mitochondrial dysfunction and other processes. Decreased mitochondrial Ca^{2+} regulation could increase cell vulnerability to the high Ca^{2+} loads associated with glutamate excitotoxicity or even normal glutamate neurotransmission, as discussed above. Glutamate receptor antagonists that decrease glutamate-stimulated calcium influx, or intracellular Ca^{2+} buffers, could protect cells from this consequence of mitochondrial dysfunction.[60]

This section reviews some of the new therapeutics that directly interact with mitochondria, particularly agents that have some movement disorders clinical trial data available. Also, many of these compounds are available in over-the-counter forms and are already widely used by patients, making an understanding of their actions and potential best usage important for practicing physicians. Creatine is one example of a widely used supplement that may have direct effects on mitochondrial oxphos energetics, and is therefore under active clinical trial study in movement disorders. Antioxidants protect from a consequence of mitochondrial dysfunction, but many are either intrinsic mitochondrial components or rely directly on mitochondria for regulation. Although increasing antioxidant levels has not been shown to increase normal lifespan or otherwise alter normal aging[107] as discussed above, antioxidants may still be helpful in pathologic states. Use of small antioxidant compounds and manipulation of antioxidant enzyme systems is discussed below. A wider range of approaches, such as enhancing repair mechanisms to "rescue" macromolecules damaged by ROS,[107] are likely to emerge in the near future in this rapidly changing field.

ANTIOXIDANTS

GENERAL CONSIDERATIONS

Antioxidants are molecules that can safely convert ROS to nonreactive species, as discussed above. Based on the growing evidence of mitochondrial dysfunction and oxidative stress in neurodegenerative disorders, antioxidants are now under active investigation as therapeutics. This section concentrates on a small number of currently available antioxidants, and some general categories of antioxidants important in new drug design. Many more synthetic and dietary agents are under investigation, and more compounds will undoubtedly become important in basic research and clinical trials in the near future.

Bioavailability, metabolism, absorption, and food sources are all important factors in the use of common antioxidants as therapeutics.[219] Specificity of action is also a consideration. An antioxidant may react with many free radical species, or may be designed as a selective scavenger, to target a specific ROS. Also, an effective antioxidant would both react with a specific target and make a low reactivity species that is easily reused.[46] Some phenolic compounds such as vitamin E are good antioxidants because they inactivate ROS but only generate low-reactivity free radical vitamin E forms that are readily recycled. Others, such as etoposide, still inactivate lipid peroxide radicals but at the expense of creating new highly active free radicals that themselves damage cells. The free radical products of antioxidant compounds are therefore a consideration in designing new antioxidant therapeutics.[95]

Finally, the availability of most antioxidant compounds as over-the-counter nutritional supplements that are not regulated for content, efficacy or side-effects presents a special challenge to their therapeutic use. Many patients and unaffected people are already taking antioxidants in dietary supplements without consistent dosing and despite the lack of information on long-term effects or actual benefit. Often patients take several supplements in combination, although interactions between different antioxidants make the results of their combined use unclear. More accurate information on these compounds is essential to advise patients properly about dietary supplements, in terms both of their best impact on disease and their interactions with other medications and long-term health.

COENZYME Q_{10}

Coenzyme Q (2,3-dimethoxy-5-methyl-6-multiprenyl-1,4-benzoquinone) is a lipophilic molecule with a quinone group plus a variable number of isoprene units. Coenzyme Q_{10}, with 10 isoprene units, is the form found in humans, as well as many other species.[220] Coenzyme Q moves electrons through the mitochrondrial electron transport chain in oxphos.[52] Because it accepts electrons from complex II and other sources as well as from complex I, coenzyme Q may help compensate for partial complex I inhibition (as hypothesized to occur in PD) by moving electrons into oxphos from other sources. In addition, coenzyme Q is the major source of ROS in the cell; conversely, coenzyme Q can also act as an antioxidant. Partially reduced coenzyme Q ($Q^{\cdot-}$, semiquinone) is produced during normal mitochondrial respiration, and may occur in excess if oxphos is blocked, as discussed above. $Q^{\cdot-}$ contributes to ROS formation and cell dysfunction.[52-56] In contrast, fully reduced coenzyme Q (QH_2) has the opposite effect. QH_2 is an important antioxidant that directly blocks lipid peroxidation and other ROS damage.[52,221,222] QH_2 can also recycle alpha-tocopherol back to its antioxidant state.[95,221] The action of coenzyme Q therefore depends on the energy state of oxphos and the mitochondrion, and the exact (reduced or partially reduced) state of coenzyme Q.

Coenzyme Q_{10} has a long therapeutic history. Numerous clinical trials over the past 30 years have investigated the role of coenzyme Q_{10} in the treatment of congestive heart failure, hypertension, and other forms of cardiovascular disease,[223,224] although the benefits so far have not been large or consistent enough to develop clear recommendations for its use in these diseases. Open-label studies of coenzyme Q_{10} have been conducted for such varied indications as migraine prevention,[225] and primary biliary cirrhosis.[226]

Clinical trials of coenzyme Q_{10} in mitochondrial disorders with underlying mtDNA mutations, natural clinical targets for this agent, have produced mixed results. Despite encouraging case reports, particularly in mitochondrial myopathy, encephalopathy, lactic acidosis, and stroke-like episodes (MELAS),[227-229] double-blind trials of coenzyme Q_{10} in mitochondrial encephalomyopathies show only a trend of improvement[230] or no clinical benefit,[231] even when changes in biochemical measures do occur. Difficulties in designing and interpreting such trials include the large phenotypic variability in these diseases, the short duration of trials compared to the chronic nature of the disorders, and small numbers of patients in each trial.

The effectiveness of coenzyme Q_{10} in mitochondrial encephalomyopathies may also be hampered by its bioavailability in the brain. Coenzyme Q_{10} is lipophilic, so controversy exists over the level of absorption of orally administered coenzyme Q_{10}, and the ability to achieve therapeutic levels in the brain. Some studies in rodents assert increases in brain homogenate and brain mitochondrial levels of coenzyme Q_{10} after administration in the diet.[232,233] Levels of absorption as well as interactions with other antioxidants and the varied functions of coenzyme Q may all contribute to the mixed clinical trial data for coenzyme Q_{10} in movement disorders to date.

A recent pilot study of coenzyme Q_{10} in PD suggested there was a slower change in the United Parkinson Disease Rating Scale (UPDRS) score, particularly part II (activities of daily living) in the highest dose treatment group compared to placebo.[234] The 80 patients enrolled in this multicenter double-blind placebo-controlled trial were randomized to 300, 600 or 1200 mg total a day of coenzyme Q_{10} for 16 months. All groups, including placebo, received 1200 IU a day of vitamin E. There was a positive trend in the primary outcome measure, the relationship between drug dose and mean change in the total UPDRS. This encouraging result will form the basis for a larger phase III trial, necessary to confirm and detail any effect of coenzyme Q_{10} in PD before it can be recommended as a PD treatment. Of note, study patients receiving coenzyme Q_{10} had increased mitochondrial electron transport chain activity in plasma by one measure, an NADH to cytochrome *c* reductase assay (complex I to III activity). Also of interest is that a vitamin E plus coenzyme Q_{10} regimen had an increased effect over vitamin E alone. The clinical effect of coenzyme Q_{10} observed in this trial may therefore be due to the action of coenzyme Q_{10} as a "bridge" past partial complex I dysfunction, as an antioxidant, as an agent to boost vitamin E antioxidant activity via increased vitamin E recycling, or some combination of functions.

Prior to the PD trial, a multicenter randomized double-blind clinical trial of coenzyme Q_{10} and a glutamate receptor antagonist, remacemide, was conducted in early HD:[235] 347 patients were treated for 30 months with either, both, or neither agent. This study used a 600 mg total daily dose of coenzyme Q_{10}. There was no significant change in the primary outcome measure, the patients total functional capacity, in any group, although coenzyme Q_{10} groups showed a trend (13 percent) toward slower decline after the first year of treatment. In addition, a trend toward improvement was seen in coenzyme Q_{10}-treated patients in secondary measures of functional decline, cognitive tests, and a behavioral scale. The HD trial was powered to identify a larger change, so a larger trial group or different dose range design may still uncover a significant benefit for coenzyme Q_{10} in HD.[235] The recent PD trial also opens the door to renewed consideration of coenzyme Q_{10} in HD and other movement disorders, as it suggests

that the disparity between the PD and HD trials could be due to different coenzyme Q_{10} doses rather than intrinsic differences between the two diseases.

The HD and PD clinical trial results stand in contrast to prior positive research data on coenzyme Q_{10} in humans and rodent models. The increase in lactate found in human HD brains in vivo and the neuronal damage caused by complex II inhibitors in rats both respond to coenzyme Q_{10} administration.[212,233] This agrees with data in PD mitochondrial toxin models, that coenzyme Q_{10} also attenuates MPTP toxicity in mice.[236] One study of HD transgenic mice observed improved survival with coenzyme Q_{10} in the diet, alone or with remacemide,[237] to a degree similar to the trend to improvement seen in the human HD clinical trial. Another study did not find a change in survival in transgenic HD mice given coenzyme Q_{10} and remacemide, but did observe transient improvements in motor skills.[238] At the moment, there is no clear recommendation for coenzyme Q_{10} use in HD or PD, although many patients continue to take it, and its use has been proposed for several other neurodegenerative disorders, including ALS[136] and Friedreich's ataxia.[135] Further basic research studies and clinical trials are needed to clearly define the role of coenzyme Q_{10} in the treatment of movement disorders.

ESSENTIAL NUTRIENTS AND DIETARY ANTIOXIDANTS

Essential nutrients, meaning nutrients that are not synthesized by cells but which must be consumed in the diet, include many antioxidant compounds.[239] "Vitamin E" refers to a group of naturally occurring compounds, the tocopherols and tocotrienols.[50,219] Of these, the most extensively studied specific compound is alpha-tocopherol, although others are also antioxidants.[59] Vitamin C (ascorbic acid) and beta-carotene are also essential nutrients.[219] These compounds can all directly interact with ROS. They also interact with each other; for example, vitamin C can recycle alpha-tocopherol back to its reduced state.[239] Other essential nutrients contribute to antioxidant enzyme function. Zinc, copper, selenium, manganese, and iron are all parts of antioxidant enzymes: zinc, manganese, and copper are components of SOD enzymes; GPX contains selenium; and the heme compound catalase contains iron.[83] The existence of essential nutrient antioxidants has inspired considerable research into the impact of diet on different diseases, and the usefulness of general diet modification or specific nutrient supplementation as disease treatment.[47,59]

Dietary antioxidants such as vitamin E and vitamin C have been tested extensively in many disease groups, including cancer and cardiovascular disease,[50] but have shown little effect in treatment trials as opposed to observational trials. This is so far the case for movement disorders as well. A small (15 patients) open-label trial of high-dose alpha-tocopherol and ascorbate found a delay to L-dopa use of 2.5 years with the combined antioxidant treatment compared to other unrelated PD patient groups not taking antioxidants.[240] In contrast, a large (800 patients) prospective double-blind placebo-controlled trial of alpha-tocopherol at 2000 IU total per day and the monoamine oxidase B (MAO-B) inhibitor deprenyl showed no significant effect for alpha-tocopherol.[241] This study focused on early PD, using a primary endpoint of initiation of L-dopa therapy. Treatment with alpha-tocopherol also did not affect other measures, including cognitive performance, freezing of gait, and mortality.[241,242]

A small (18 patients) double-blind placebo-controlled crossover study of alpha-tocopherol in tardive dyskinesia showed no benefit overall, but did find a mild positive effect on the Abnormal Involuntary Movement Scale (AIMS) score in a subgroup of patients with tardive dyskinesia for 5 years or less.[243] A prospective double-blind placebo-controlled trial of alpha-tocopherol in HD patients yielded disappointing but still intriguing results:[244] 73 patients received 3000 IU total daily alpha-tocopherol or placebo for 1 year. Although there was no significant impact on primary outcome measures in the treatment group, on post hoc analysis there was a significant gain on a quantified neurologic exam in treated patients early in the course of HD compared to more advanced HD patients. Thus, if alpha-tocopherol is at all effective in movement disorders, it may have its best impact earlier in the course of disease, although this stands in contrast to the larger PD trial result. In addition, all patients in the HD trial also received vitamin C and vitamin A. Use of these antioxidants in both alpha-tocopherol and placebo groups may have biased against finding a treatment effect.

In addition to essential nutrients, there are numerous other dietary sources of antioxidants. For example, polyphenols such as flavinoids are found in fruit, vegetables, wine, tea, grains, and flowers.[219,245] Often one dietary source contains a mix of potential antioxidants. Flavenoids are also taken in over-the-counter supplements. Gingko biloba, a complex plant extract and popular supplement, is rich in flavenoids, and other potential antioxidants.[245,246] Gingko biloba may protect against lipid peroxidation and other oxidative damage.[247] Treatment of AD with a gingko biloba extract yielded a modest beneficial effect on cognition in a double-blind, placebo-controlled trial.[248]

Research studies of dietary sources use whole foods, non-specific extracts of whole foods, or individual identified flavinoids to test antioxidant actions.[245] Green tea extracts attenuate damage in a mouse model of PD and in an in vitro PD system.[249,250] Rats fed dried extracts of strawberries, blueberries, or spinach have less age-related decline of various neuronal and cognitive function markers.[251] How multiple compounds are delivered in a food source, and how they then interact in the body, may have a complex influence on the efficacy of dietary antioxidants.

It is unclear if there is a greater benefit from consumption of whole foods compared to isolated antioxidants from the same foods. A prospective observational study of two large cohorts (76,890 women and 47,331 men) found no change in risk for PD with use of vitamin E, vitamin C, or multivitamin supplements; however, there was a reduced risk for PD with consumption of foods high in vitamin E.[252] This result illustrates how the sources, mix, and duration of use (lifelong dietary habits versus relatively recent supplements) of these compounds might combine to affect disease, and how these factors make studying the effects of dietary antioxidants a challenge.

ANTIOXIDANT ENZYMES

Treatment with a specific antioxidant molecule may help decrease oxidative stress and damage in disease. Another approach to altering cellular redox states and ROS levels is to modify antioxidant enzyme function. For example, boosting SOD activity could reduce $O_2^{\cdot-}$ levels and provide protection against neuronal damage in PD or HD. Indeed, overexpression of human MnSOD[253] or Cu/ZnSOD[254] in transgenic mice attenuates MPTP toxicity. Cu/ZnSOD transgenic mice are also more resistant to 3-NPA, possibly via reduction of free radicals.[255] Bovine Cu/ZnSOD has been tested in clinical trials against acute and chronic inflammation such as osteoarthritis and side-effects of chemotherapy and radiation, with promising but mixed results.[256] Its use was limited in part by immunologic reaction to the bovine source. Also, native SOD is too large to easily penetrate the blood-brain barrier. Modified, synthesized forms of SOD that can scavenge $O_2^{\cdot-}$ and cross the blood-brain barrier[257] may prove useful as therapeutic agents in the future.

Understanding the full consequences of changing antioxidant enzyme function will be important to tailoring drug use to desired antioxidant effects. Increased SOD activity decreases $O_2^{\cdot-}$ levels, but creates more H_2O_2 that could form excess $OH^{\cdot}$ (Fig. 4-4). The Cu/ZnSOD mutation that causes a familial form of ALS is thought to create a toxic gain of function, possibly by increasing SOD production of $OH^{\cdot}$.[258,259] Increased $OH^{\cdot}$ production was observed in one study of transgenic mice overexpressing normal human Cu/ZnSOD.[260] This could have functional consequences. As mentioned earlier, overexpression of Cu/ZnSOD alone in a transgenic *Drosophila* model does not improve lifespan or ability to withstand oxidative stressors,[261] but concomitant catalase and SOD overexpression can increase lifespan,[130] suggesting the catalase is necessary to compensate for increased SOD-driven H_2O_2 production in this model. While overexpression of SOD in transgenic mice protects against some oxidative stressors, it can increase susceptibility to other stressors, such as paraquat,[260] and infections.[262] This kind of tradeoff could complicate therapeutic use of SOD and other antioxidant enzymes.[55,83]

CREATINE (Cr)

Creatine (Cr) is an example of a "bioenergetic" therapy, or a compound that enhances cellular use of the mitochondrial oxphos ATP production system. Cr is a guanidino compound that is both taken up in food and synthesized de novo in cells from arginine, glycine, and methionine.[247,263] It is converted to phosphocreatine (PCr) by any of several creatine kinase (CK) isoenzymes. PCr is a form of energy storage for cells; as ATP is depleted at high-energy sites in the cell, PCr is used to regenerate more ATP from ADP.[263] To create this storage system, mitochondrial CK (mtCK) catalyzes new PCr synthesis from Cr using oxphos-generated ATP. The Cr/PCr system greatly increases cellular capacity for phosphate energy storage. This "PCr shuttle" hypothesis[264,265] of how Cr contributes to cellular energetics highlights the close ties between mitochondrial oxphos and Cr function.

A larger range of potential Cr actions is still being uncovered.[247,263] Cr may attenuate oxidative stress through indirect antioxidant effects,[247] and recent work suggests that Cr can also act as a direct antioxidant.[266] Cr increases synaptic vesicle glutamate uptake,[267] and so could protect cells with mitochondrial dysfunction, and presumed poor Ca^{2+} regulation, from high glutamate loads.[268] In addition, mtCK inhibits PT pore opening when in its octameric form.[269] Cr and PCr help regulate free radical dimerization and inactivation of mtCK, and subsequent PT pore opening.[270,271]

More than 90 percent of Cr in humans is in muscle, where PCr helps provide energy for muscle contraction. Cr has therefore become a popular ergogenic dietary supplement for athletes, from professionals to young adolescents, in addition to the usual intake of Cr in normal diet. However, primary defects of Cr function have a larger impact on the nervous system than on muscle, suggesting an important role for Cr in brain metabolism. Transgenic mice with knockouts of the brain CK isoform have a complex phenotype, including decreases in learning and memory, grooming behavior, weight gain, and life-expectancy.[263] Very rare human inborn errors of metabolism yield little to no Cr in brain, even if serum concentrations are normal.[272] The heterogeneous phenotypes include severe neurologic symptoms, predominantly developmental delay but including extrapyramidal symptoms.[263,273]

Oral Cr supplementation in these rare patients improves neurologic symptoms.[274,275] It can also alter brain Cr levels, but only slowly, after months of treatment, and not up to normal levels despite more easily achieved levels in serum and muscle.[276] These observations suggest limited blood-brain barrier penetration by Cr. Use of Cr supplementation for nervous system disorders may therefore require long-term high-dose treatment protocols, and measurement of cerebrospinal fluid Cr or its breakdown product, creatinine, instead of serum concentrations.[263]

Animal studies provide increasing evidence supporting Cr use in neuroprotection.[247,263] Cr decreased MPTP toxicity in a mouse PD model.[277] Cr has been tested in several different HD animal models. It attenuated malonate[278,279] and 3-NPA[278,280] toxicity in rat, and improved animal survival and delayed brain pathology in HD transgenic mice.[281,282] The accumulated animal data has led to ongoing clinical trials in HD and PD, as well as in ALS and other neurologic disorders.[247,263]

Ongoing clinical trials will help address both questions of efficacy in movement disorders and issues of safety. Controversy exists over the importance of theoretical long-term consequences of Cr use, particularly effects on renal function through multiple potential mechanisms.[263] Commercial Cr is made by chemical synthesis, so products may include contaminants with unclear safety profiles. Because Cr is currently distributed as a food supplement, quality and purity of different preparations are not established, an important consideration in tracking long-term benefits and side-effects.

Conclusions

Mitochondria play an important role in movement disorders. Syndromes with prominent movement disorder components such as Leigh's disease and some dystonias illustrate basic principles of mitochondrial genetics and mitochondrial genotype-to-phenotype interactions. The unique properties of mitochondria as mtDNA-containing organelles within neurons contribute to disorders with causative mtDNA and nuclear DNA mutations. Such mutations directly affect oxphos components and other key mitochondrial proteins, emphasizing the close association between mitochondrial dysfunction and movement disorders. Mitochondrial dysfunction and its consequences, including disruption of oxphos, changes in ROS production, impaired calcium regulation, and pathologic triggering of cell death pathways, are also increasingly recognized as part of the larger picture of overlapping functional defects contributing to chronic progressive neurodegenerative disorders.

Current research continues to work forward from toxin exposure and transgenic models of disease, and backwards from observations of neuroprotection by mitochondria-related agents, to detail the mechanisms of mitochondrial involvement in movement disorders. Even with the growing body of work discussed in this chapter, basic questions remain unanswered, particularly regarding neurodegenerative movement disorders such as PD and HD. It is still unclear if and how mtDNA mutations or normal polymorphisms interact with exogenous factors and nuclear genetic backgrounds to produce primary disease, or if normal mitochondrial function becomes damaging in the context of a particular cell or tissue as a secondary pathologic process. Either way, mitochondria will be critical to understanding disease process, treatment, and prevention in these devastating neurologic disorders.

Acknowledgments

This work was supported by NIH/NINDS grant K08NS44267-01, and a Cotzias Fellowship from the American Parkinson Disease

Association. The author thanks T.B. Sherer and J.T. Greenamyre for helpful discussions.

References

1. Berg JM, Tymoczko J, Stryer L: *Biochemistry.* New York, W.H. Freeman, 2001.
2. Nelson DL, Cox MM: *Lehninger Principles of Biochemistry.* New York: Worth, 2000.
3. Gray MW, Burger G, Lang BF: Mitochondrial evolution. *Science* 283:1476–1481, 1999.
4. Anderson S, Bankier AT, Barrell BG, et al: Sequence and organization of the human mitochondrial genome. *Nature* 290:457–465, 1981.
5. Cummins JM, Wakayama T, Yanagimachi R: Fate of micro-injected spermatid mitochondria in the mouse oocyte and embryo. *Zygote* 6:213–222, 1998.
6. Sutovsky P, Moreno RD, Ramalho-Santos J, et al: Ubiquitin tag for sperm mitochondria. *Nature* 402:371–372, 1999.
7. Giles RE, Blanc H, Cann HM, et al: Maternal inheritance of human mitochondrial DNA. *Proc Natl Acad Sci U S A* 77:6715–6719, 1980.
8. Gyllensten U, Wharton D, Josefsson A, et al: Paternal inheritance of mitochondrial DNA in mice. *Nature* 352:255–257, 1991.
9. Shitara H, Hayashi J-I, Takahama S, et al: Maternal inheritance of mouse mtDNA in interspecific hybrids: Segregation of the leaked paternal mtDNA followed by the prevention of subsequent paternal leakage. *Genetics* 148:851–857, 1998.
10. Birky CW: The inheritance of genes in mitochondria and chloroplasts: Laws, mechanisms, and models. *Annu Rev Genet* 35:125–148, 2001.
11. Schwartz M, Vissing J: Paternal inheritance of mitochondrial DNA. *N Engl J Med* 347:576–580, 2002.
12. Hatefi Y: The mitochondrial electron transport and oxidative phosphorylation system. *Annu Rev Biochem* 54:1015–1069, 1985.
13. Smeitink J, van den Heuvel L: Human mitochondrial complex I in health and disease. *Am J Hum Genet* 64:1505–1510, 1999.
14. Shoffner JM: Oxidative phosphorylation diseases and movement disorders, in Watts RL, Koller WC (eds): *Movement Disorders: Neurologic Principles and Practice.* New York: McGraw-Hill, 1997, pp 51–71.
15. DiMauro S, Andreu AL, De Vivo DC: Mitochondrial disorders. *J Child Neurol* 17 (suppl 3):S35–S45, 2002.
16. Greenamyre JT, Sherer TB, Betarbet R, et al: Complex I and Parkinson's disease. *IUBMB Life* 52:135–141, 2001.
17. Wallace DC: Mitochondrial DNA sequence variation in human evolution and disease. *Proc Natl Acad Sci U S A* 91:8739–8746, 1994.
18. Larsson NG, Clayton DA: Molecular genetic aspects of human mitochondrial disorders. *Annu Rev Genet* 29:151–178, 1995.
19. Richter C, Park JW, Ames BN: Normal oxidative damage to mitochondrial and nuclear DNA is extensive. *Proc Natl Acad Sci U S A* 85:6465–6467, 1988.
20. Brown WM, George M Jr, Wilson AC: Rapid evolution of animal mitochondrial DNA. *Proc Natl Acad Sci U S A* 76:1967–1971, 1979.

21. Wei YH, Lee HC: Oxidative stress, mitochondrial DNA mutation, and impairment of antioxidant enzymes in aging. *Exp Biol Med* 227:671–682, 2002.
22. Corral-Debrinski M, Horton T, Lott MT, et al: Mitochondrial DNA deletions in human brain: Regional variability and increase with advanced age. *Nat Genet* 2:324–329, 1992.
23. Corral-Debrinski M, Shoffner JM, Lott MT, et al: Association of mitochondrial DNA damage with aging and coronary atherosclerotic heart disease. *Mutat Res* 275:169–180, 1992.
24. Soong NW, Hinton DR, Cortopassi G, et al: Mosaicism for a specific somatic mitochondrial DNA mutation in adult human brain. *Nat Genet* 2:318–323, 1992.
25. Horton TM, Graham BH, Corral-Debrinski M, et al: Marked increase in mitochondrial DNA deletion levels in the cerebral cortex of Huntington's disease patients. *Neurology* 45:1879–1883, 1995.
26. Bogenhagen D, Clayton DA: The number of mitochondrial deoxyribonucleic acid genomes in mouse L and human HeLa cells. Quantitative isolation of mitochondrial deoxyribonucleic acid. *J Biol Chem* 249:7991–7995, 1974.
27. Yoneda M, Chomyn A, Martinuzzi A, et al: Marked replicative advantage of human mtDNA carrying a point mutation that causes the MELAS encephalomyopathy. *Proc Natl Acad Sci U S A* 89:11164–11168, 1992.
28. Yaffe MP: The machinery of mitochondrial inheritance and behavior. *Science* 283:1493–1497, 1999.
29. Wallace DC: Mitochondrial diseases in man and mouse. *Science* 283:1482–1488, 1999.
30. Wallace DC, Singh G, Lott MT, et al: Mitochondrial DNA mutation associated with Leber's hereditary optic neuropathy. *Science* 242:1427–1430, 1988.
31. Jun AS, Brown MD, Wallace DC: A mitochondrial DNA mutation at nucleotide pair 14459 of the NADH dehydrogenase subunit 6 gene associated with maternally inherited Leber hereditary optic neuropathy and dystonia. *Proc Natl Acad Sci U S A* 91:6206–6210, 1994.
32. Simon DK, Pulst SM, Sutton JP, et al: Familial multisystem degeneration with parkinsonism associated with the 11778 mitochondrial DNA mutation. *Neurology* 53:1787–1793, 1999.
33. Shoffner JM, Brown MD, Stugard C, et al: Leber's hereditary optic neuropathy plus dystonia is caused by a mitochondrial DNA point mutation. *Ann Neurol* 38:163–169, 1995.
34. Novotny EJ Jr, Singh G, Wallace DC, et al: Leber's disease and dystonia: A mitochondrial disease. *Neurology* 36:1053–1560, 1986.
35. Kennedy EP, Lehninger AL: Oxidation of fatty acids and tricarboxylic acid cycle intermediates by isolated rat liver mitochondria. *J Biol Chem* 179:957–972, 1949.
36. Mitchell P, Moyle J: Chemiosmotic hypothesis of oxidative phosphorylation. *Nature* 213:137–139, 1967.
37. Stock D, Gibbons C, Arechaga I, et al: The rotary mechanism of ATP synthase. *Curr Opin Struct Biol* 10:672–679, 2000.
38. Vaux DL, Korsmeyer SJ: Cell death in development. *Cell* 96:245–254, 1999.
39. Newmeyer DD, Farschon DM, Reed JC: Cell-free apoptosis in *Xenopus* egg extracts: Inhibition by Bcl-2 and requirement for an organelle fraction enriched in mitochondria. *Cell* 79:353–364, 1994.
40. Green DR, Reed JC: Mitochondria and apoptosis. *Science* 281:1309–1312, 1998.

41. Desagher S, Martinou JC: Mitochondria as the central control point of apoptosis. *Trends Cell Biol* 10:369–377, 2000.

42. Gross A, McDonnell JM, Korsmeyer SJ: Bcl-2 family members and the mitochondria in apoptosis. *Genes Dev* 13:1899–1911, 1999.

43. Crompton M: Mitochondrial intermembrane junctional complexes and their role in cell death. *J Physiol* 529 (Pt 1):11–21, 2000.

44. Liu X, Kim CN, Yang J, et al: Induction of apoptotic program in cell-free extracts: Requirement for dATP and cytochrome *c*. *Cell* 86:147–157, 1996.

45. Schulz JB, Weller M, Moskowitz MA: Caspases as treatment targets in stroke and neurodegenerative diseases. *Ann Neurol* 45:421–429, 1999.

46. Del Maestro RF: An approach to free radicals in medicine and biology. *Acta Physiol Scand Suppl* 492:153–168, 1980.

47. Ames BN, Shigenaga MK, Hagen TM: Oxidants, antioxidants, and the degenerative diseases of aging. *Proc Natl Acad Sci U S A* 90:7915–7922, 1993.

48. Janssen YM, Van Houten B, Borm PJ, et al: Cell and tissue responses to oxidative damage. *Lab Invest* 69:261–274, 1993.

49. Cross CE, Halliwell B, Borish ET, et al: Oxygen radicals and human disease. *Ann Intern Med* 107:526–545, 1987.

50. Lindsay DG, Astley SB: European research on the functional effects of dietary antioxidants: EUROFEDA. *Mol Aspects Med* 23:1–38, 2002.

51. Babior BM: Oxygen-dependent microbial killing by phagocytes (first of two parts). *N Engl J Med* 298:659–668, 1978.

52. Beyer RE: An analysis of the role of coenzyme Q in free radical generation and as an antioxidant. *Biochem Cell Biol* 70:390–403, 1992.

53. Boveris A, Cadenas E, Stoppani AO: Role of ubiquinone in the mitochondrial generation of hydrogen peroxide. *Biochem J* 156:435–444, 1976.

54. Turrens JF, Alexandre A, Lehninger AL: Ubisemiquinone is the electron donor for superoxide formation by complex III of heart mitochondria. *Arch Biochem Biophys* 237:408–414, 1985.

55. Raha S, Robinson BH: Mitochondria, oxygen free radicals, disease and ageing. *Trends Biol Sci* 25:502–508, 2000.

56. Cadenas E, Boveris A, Ragan CI, et al: Production of superoxide radicals and hydrogen peroxide by NADH-ubiquinone reductase and ubiquinol-cytochrome *c* reductase from beef-heart mitochondria. *Arch Biochem Biophys* 180:248–257, 1977.

57. Chance B, Sies H, Boveris A: Hydroperoxide metabolism in mammalian organs. *Physiol Rev* 59:527–605, 1979.

58. Dalton TP, Shertzer HG, Puga A: Regulation of gene expression by reactive oxygen. *Annu Rev Pharmacol Toxicol* 39:67–101, 1999.

59. Jackson MJ, Papa S, Bolanos J, et al: Antioxidants, reactive oxygen and nitrogen species, gene induction and mitochondrial function. *Mol Aspects Med* 23:209–285, 2002.

60. Krieger C, Duchen MR: Mitochondria, Ca(2+) and neurodegenerative disease. *Eur J Pharmacol* 447:177–188, 2002.

61. Nicholls DG, Budd SL: Mitochondria and neuronal survival. *Physiol Rev* 80:315–359, 2000.

62. Duchen MR: Contributions of mitochondria to animal physiology: From homeostatic sensor to calcium signaling and cell death. *J Physiol* 516(Pt 1):1–17, 1999.

63. Peng TI, Greenamyre JT: Privileged access to mitochondria of calcium influx through N-methyl-D-aspartate receptors. *Mol Pharmacol* 53:974–980, 1998.

64. Crompton M: The mitochondrial permeability transition pore and its role in cell death. *Biochem J* 341(Pt 2):233–249, 1999.

65. Astrup J, Sorensen PM, Sorensen HR: Oxygen and glucose consumption related to Na+-K+ transport in canine brain. *Stroke* 12:726–730, 1981.

66. Ritchie JM, Straub RW: Oxygen consumption and phosphate efflux in mammalian non-myelinated nerve fibres. *J Physiol* 304:109–121, 1980.

67. Greene JG, Greenamyre JT: Bioenergetics and glutamate excitotoxicity. *Prog Neurobiol* 48:613–634, 1996.

68. Nowak L, Bregestovski P, Ascher P: Magnesium gates glutamate-activated channels in mouse central neurones. *Nature* 307:462–465, 1984.

69. Albin RL, Greenamyre JT: Alternative excitotoxic hypotheses. *Neurology* 42:733–738, 1992.

70. Ankarcrona M, Dypbukt JM, Bonfoco E, et al: Glutamate-induced neuronal death: A succession of necrosis or apoptosis depending on mitochondrial function. *Neuron* 15:961–973, 1995.

71. Bonfoco E, Krainc D, Ankarcrona M, et al: Apoptosis and necrosis: Two distinct events induced, respectively, by mild and intense insults with N-methyl-D-aspartate or nitric oxide/superoxide in cortical cell cultures. *Proc Natl Acad Sci U S A* 92:7162–7166, 1995.

72. Leist M, Single B, Castoldi AF, et al: Intracellular adenosine triphosphate (ATP) concentration: A switch in the decision between apoptosis and necrosis. *J Exp Med* 185:1481–1486, 1997.

73. Blum D, Torch S, Lambeng N, et al: Molecular pathways involved in the neurotoxicity of 6-OHDA, dopamine and MPTP: Contribution to the apoptotic theory in Parkinson's disease. *Prog Neurobiol* 65:135–172, 2001.

74. Burke RE, Kholodilov NG: Programmed cell death: Does it play a role in Parkinson's disease? *Ann Neurol* 44:S126–S133, 1998.

75. Fearnley IM, Carroll J, Shannon RJ, et al: GRIM-19, a cell death regulatory gene product, is a subunit of bovine mitochondrial NADH:ubiquinone oxidoreductase (complex I). *J Biol Chem* 276:38345–38348, 2001.

76. Marzo I, Brenner C, Zamzami N, et al: The permeability transition pore complex: A target for apoptosis regulation by caspases and Bcl-2-related proteins. *J Exp Med* 187:1261–1271, 1998.

77. Bernardi P, Petronilli V: The permeability transition pore as a mitochondrial calcium release channel: A critical appraisal. *J Bioenerg Biomembr* 28:131–138, 1996.

78. Chauvin C, De Oliveira F, Ronot X, et al: Rotenone inhibits the mitochondrial permeability transition-induced cell death in U937 and KB cells. *J Biol Chem* 276:41394–41398, 2001.

79. Fontaine E, Eriksson O, Ichas F, et al: Regulation of the permeability transition pore in skeletal muscle mitochondria. Modulation by electron flow through the respiratory chain complex I. *J Biol Chem* 273:12662–12668, 1998.

80. Schild L, Keilhoff G, Augustin W, et al: Distinct Ca2+ thresholds determine cytochrome *c* release or permeability transition pore opening in brain mitochondria. *FASEB J* 15:565–567, 2001.

81. McCord JM, Fridovich I: Superoxide dismutase. An enzymic function for erythrocuprein (hemocuprein). *J Biol Chem* 244:6049–6055, 1969.

82. Fridovich I: The biology of oxygen radicals. *Science* 201:875–880, 1978.

83. Mates JM: Effects of antioxidant enzymes in the molecular control of reactive oxygen species toxicology. *Toxicology* 153:83–104, 2000.

84. Beckman JS, Beckman TW, Chen J, et al: Apparent hydroxyl radical production by peroxynitrite: Implications for endothelial injury from nitric oxide and superoxide. *Proc Natl Acad Sci U S A* 87:1620–1624, 1990.

85. Fridovich I: Superoxide radical and superoxide dismutases. *Annu Rev Biochem* 64:97–112, 1995.

86. Robinson BH: Human complex I deficiency: Clinical spectrum and involvement of oxygen free radicals in the pathogenicity of the defect. *Biochim Biophys Acta* 1364:271–286, 1998.

87. Jacobson MD: Reactive oxygen species and programmed cell death. *Trends Biochem Sci* 21:83–86, 1996.

88. Farber JL, Kyle ME, Coleman JB: Mechanisms of cell injury by activated oxygen species. *Lab Invest* 62:670–679, 1990.

89. Stadtman ER: Protein oxidation and aging. *Science* 257:1220–1224, 1992.

90. Dean RT, Fu S, Stocker R, et al: Biochemistry and pathology of radical-mediated protein oxidation. *Biochem J* 324(Pt 1):1–18, 1997.

91. Griffiths HR, Moller L, Bartosz G, et al: Biomarkers. *Mol Aspects Med* 23:101–208, 2002.

92. Stadtman ER: Importance of individuality in oxidative stress and aging. *Free Radic Biol Med* 33:597–604, 2002.

93. Shigenaga MK, Ames BN: Assays for 8-hydroxy-2'-deoxyguanosine: A biomarker of in vivo oxidative DNA damage. *Free Radic Biol Med* 10:211–216, 1991.

94. Halliwell B, Aruoma OI: DNA damage by oxygen-derived species. Its mechanism and measurement in mammalian systems. *FEBS Lett* 281:9–19, 1991.

95. Kagan VE, Tyurina YY: Recycling and redox cycling of phenolic antioxidants. *Ann N Y Acad Sci* 854:425–434, 1998.

96. Dickinson DA, Forman HJ: Glutathione in defense and signaling: Lessons from a small thiol. *Ann N Y Acad Sci* 973:488–504, 2002.

97. Augustin W, Wiswedel I, Noack H, et al: Role of endogenous and exogenous antioxidants in the defence against functional damage and lipid peroxidation in rat liver mitochondria. *Mol Cell Biochem* 174:199–205, 1997.

98. Gunter TE, Pfeiffer DR: Mechanisms by which mitochondria transport calcium. *Am J Physiol* 258:C755–786, 1990.

99. Choi DW: Glutamate neurotoxicity and diseases of the nervous system. *Neuron* 1:623–634, 1988.

100. Kiedrowski L, Costa E: Glutamate-induced destabilization of intracellular calcium concentration homeostasis in cultured cerebellar granule cells: Role of mitochondria in calcium buffering. *Mol Pharmacol* 47:140–147, 1995.

101. Stout AK, Raphael HM, Kanterewicz BI, et al: Glutamate-induced neuron death requires mitochondrial calcium uptake. *Nat Neurosci* 1:366–373, 1998.

102. Tanner CM, Goldman SM: Epidemiology of Parkinson's disease. *Neurol Clin* 14:317–335, 1996.

103. Floyd RA, Hensley K: Oxidative stress in brain aging. Implications for therapeutics of neurodegenerative diseases. *Neurobiol Aging* 23:795–807, 2002.

104. Harman D: Free radical theory of aging. *Mutat Res* 275:257–266, 1992.

105. Harman D: Aging: A theory based on free radical and radiation chemistry. *J Gerontol* 11:298–300, 1956.

106. Sohal RS, Weindruch R: Oxidative stress, caloric restriction, and aging. *Science* 273:59–63, 1996.

107. Sohal RS, Mockett RJ, Orr WC: Mechanisms of aging: An appraisal of the oxidative stress hypothesis. *Free Radic Biol Med* 33:575–586, 2002.

108. Linnane AW, Marzuki S, Ozawa T, et al: Mitochondrial DNA mutations as an important contributor to ageing and degenerative diseases. *Lancet* 1:642–645, 1989.

109. Hayakawa M, Katsumata K, Yoneda M, et al: Age-related extensive fragmentation of mitochondrial DNA into minicircles. *Biochem Biophys Res Commun* 226:369–377, 1996.

110. Nagley P, Wei YH: Ageing and mammalian mitochondrial genetics. *Trends Genet* 14:513–517, 1998.

111. Cooper JM, Mann VM, Schapira AH: Analyses of mitochondrial respiratory chain function and mitochondrial DNA deletion in human skeletal muscle: Effect of ageing. *J Neurol Sci* 113:91–98, 1992.

112. Yen TC, Chen YS, King KL, et al: Liver mitochondrial respiratory functions decline with age. *Biochem Biophys Res Commun* 165:944–1003, 1989.

113. Muller-Hocker J: Cytochrome-*c*-oxidase deficient cardiomyocytes in the human heart – an age-related phenomenon. A histochemical ultracytochemical study. *Am J Pathol* 134:1167–1173, 1989.

114. Muller-Hocker J: Cytochrome *c* oxidase deficient fibres in the limb muscle and diaphragm of man without muscular disease: An age-related alteration. *J Neurol Sci* 100:14–21, 1990.

115. Muller-Hocker J, Seibel P, Schneiderbanger K, et al: Different in situ hybridization patterns of mitochondrial DNA in cytochrome *c* oxidase-deficient extraocular muscle fibres in the elderly. *Virchows Arch A Pathol Anat Histopathol* 422:7–15, 1993.

116. Trounce I, Byrne E, Marzuki S: Decline in skeletal muscle mitochondrial respiratory chain function: Possible factor in ageing. *Lancet* 1:637–639, 1989.

117. Harper ME, Monemdjou S, Ramsey JJ, et al: Age-related increase in mitochondrial proton leak and decrease in ATP turnover reactions in mouse hepatocytes. *Am J Physiol* 275:E197–206, 1998.

118. Hagen TM, Yowe DL, Bartholomew JC, et al: Mitochondrial decay in hepatocytes from old rats: Membrane potential declines, heterogeneity and oxidants increase. *Proc Natl Acad Sci U S A* 94:3064–3069, 1997.

119. Barja G, Herrero A: Oxidative damage to mitochondrial DNA is inversely related to maximum life span in the heart and brain of mammals. *FASEB J* 14:312–318, 2000.

120. de la Asuncion JG, Millan A, Pla R, et al: Mitochondrial glutathione oxidation correlates with age-associated oxidative damage to mitochondrial DNA. *FASEB J* 10:333–338, 1996.

121. Ishii N, Fujii M, Hartman PS, et al: A mutation in succinate dehydrogenase cytochrome *b* causes oxidative stress and ageing in nematodes. *Nature* 394:694–697, 1998.

122. Melov S, Ravenscroft J, Malik S, et al: Extension of lifespan with superoxide dismutase/catalase mimetics. *Science* 289:1567–1569, 2000.

123. Nakae D, Akai H, Kishida H, et al: Age and organ dependent spontaneous generation of nuclear 8-hydroxydeoxyguanosine in male Fischer 344 rats. *Lab Invest* 80:249–261, 2000.

124. Hamilton ML, Van Remmen H, Drake JA, et al: Does oxidative damage to DNA increase with age? *Proc Natl Acad Sci U S A* 98:10469–10474, 2001.

125. Brunk UT, Terman A: Lipofuscin: Mechanisms of age-related accumulation and influence on cell function. *Free Radic Biol Med* 33:611–619, 2002.

126. Kato Y, Maruyama W, Naoi M, et al: Immunohistochemical detection of dityrosine in lipofuscin pigments in the aged human brain. *FEBS Lett* 439:231–234, 1998.

127. Yoritaka A, Hattori N, Uchida K, et al: Immunohistochemical detection of 4-hydroxynonenal protein adducts in Parkinson disease. *Proc Natl Acad Sci U S A* 93:2696–2701, 1996.

128. Montine TJ, Neely MD, Quinn JF, et al: Lipid peroxidation in aging brain and Alzheimer's disease. *Free Radic Biol Med* 33:620–626, 2002.

129. Smith CD, Carney JM, Starke-Reed PE, et al: Excess brain protein oxidation and enzyme dysfunction in normal aging and in Alzheimer disease. *Proc Natl Acad Sci U S A* 88:10540–10543, 1991.

130. Orr WC, Sohal RS: Extension of life-span by overexpression of superoxide dismutase and catalase in *Drosophila melanogaster*. *Science* 263:1128–1130, 1994.

131. Herbert V: The antioxidant supplement myth. *Am J Clin Nutr* 60:157–158, 1994.

132. Jin H, Kendall E, Freeman TC, et al: The human family of deafness/dystonia peptide (DDP) related mitochondrial import proteins. *Genomics* 61:259–267, 1999.

133. Koehler CM, Leuenberger D, Merchant S, et al: Human deafness dystonia syndrome is a mitochondrial disease. *Proc Natl Acad Sci U S A* 96:2141–2146, 1999.

134. Ouahchi K, Arita M, Kayden H, et al: Ataxia with isolated vitamin E deficiency is caused by mutations in the alpha-tocopherol transfer protein. *Nat Genet* 9:141–145, 1995.

135. Lodi R, Rajagopalan B, Bradley JL, et al: Mitochondrial dysfunction in Friedreich's ataxia: From pathogenesis to treatment perspectives. *Free Radic Res* 36:461–466, 2002.

136. Beal MF: Coenzyme Q10 administration and its potential for treatment of neurodegenerative diseases. *Biofactors* 9:261–266, 1999.

137. Kruger R, Kuhn W, Muller T, et al: Ala30pro mutation in the gene encoding alpha-synuclein in Parkinson's disease. *Nat Genet* 18:106–108, 1998.

138. Polymeropoulos MH, Lavedan C, Leroy E, et al: Mutation in the α-synuclein gene identified in families with Parkinson's disease. *Science* 276:2045–2047, 1997.

139. Kitada T, Asakawa S, Hattori N, et al: Mutations in the parkin gene cause autosomal recessive juvenile parkinsonism. *Nature* 392:605–608, 1998.

140. Bonifati V, Rizzu P, van Baren MJ, et al: Mutations in the DJ-1 gene associated with autosomal recessive early-onset parkinsonism. *Science* 299:256–259, 2003.

141. Leroy E, Boyer R, Auburger G, et al: The ubiquitin pathway in Parkinson's disease. *Nature* 395:451–452, 1998.

142. Langston JW, Ballard PA, Tetrud JW, et al: Chronic parkinsonism in humans due to a product of meridine-analog synthesis. *Science* 219:979–980, 1983.

143. Langston JW, Forno LS, Tetrud J, et al: Evidence of active nerve cell degeneration in the substantia nigra of humans years after 1-methyl-4-phenyl-1,2,3,6-tetrahydropyridine exposure. *Ann Neurol* 46:598–605, 1999.

144. Javitch JA, D'Amato RJ, Strittmatter SM, et al: Parkinsonism-inducing neurotoxin, *N*-methyl-4-phenyl-1,2,3,6-tetrahydropyridine: Uptake of the metabolite *N*-methyl-4-phenylpyridine by dopamine neurons explains selective toxicity. *Proc Natl Acad Sci U S A* 82:2173–2177, 1985.

145. Chiba K, Trevor AJ, Castagnoli N Jr: Metabolism of the neurotoxic tertiary amine, MPTP, by brain monoamine oxidase. *Biochem Biophys Res Commun* 120:574–578, 1984.

146. Nicklas WJ, Heikkila RE: Inhibition of NADH-linked oxidation in brain mitochondria by 1-methyl-4-phenylpyridine, a metabolite of the neurotoxin 1-methyl-4-phenyl-1,2,3,6-tetrahydropyridine. *Life Sci* 36:2503–2508, 1985.

147. Higgins DS, Greenamyre JT: [^{3}H]Dihydrorotenone binding to NADH:ubiquinone reductase (complex I) of the electron transport chain: An autoradiographic study. *J Neurosci* 16:3807–3816, 1996.

148. Hattori N, Tanaka M, Ozawa T, et al: Immunohistochemical studies on complexes I, II, III, and IV of mitochondria in Parkinson's disease. *Ann Neurol* 30:563–571, 1991.

149. Schapira AHV, Cooper JM, Dexter D, et al: Mitochondrial complex I deficiency in Parkinson's disease. *Lancet* i:1269, 1989.

150. Schapira AHV, Mann VM, Cooper JM, et al: Anatomic and disease specificity of NADH CoQ$_1$ reductase (complex I) deficiency in Parkinson's disease. *J Neurochem* 55:2142–2145, 1990.

151. Haas RH, Nasirian F, Nakano K, et al: Low platelet mitochondrial complex I and complex II/III activity in early untreated Parkinson's disease. *Ann Neurol* 37:714–722, 1995.

152. Parker WD, Boyson SJ, Parks JK: Abnormalities of the electron transport chain in idiopathic Parkinson's disease. *Ann Neurol* 26:719–723, 1989.

153. Betarbet R, Sherer TB, MacKenzie G, et al: Chronic systemic pesticide exposure reproduces features of Parkinson's disease. *Nat Neurosci* 3:1301–1306, 2000.

154. Sherer TB, Kim JH, Betarbet R, et al: Subcutaneous rotenone exposure causes highly selective dopaminergic degeneration and alpha-synuclein aggregation. *Exp Neurol* 179:9–16, 2003.

155. Gu M, Cooper JM, Taanman J-W, et al: Mitochondrial DNA transmission of the mitochondrial defect in Parkinson's disease. *Ann Neurol* 44:177–186, 1998.

156. Swerdlow RH, Parks JK, Miller SW, et al: Origin and functional consequences of the complex I defect in Parkinson's disease. *Ann Neurol* 40:663–671, 1996.

157. Van Der Walt JM, Nicodemus KK, Martin ER, et al: Mitochondrial polymorphisms significantly reduce the risk of Parkinson disease. *Am J Hum Genet* 72:804–811, 2003.

158. Cino M, Del Maestro RF: Generation of hydrogen peroxide by brain mitochondria: The effect of reoxygenation following post-decapitative ischemia. *Arch Biochem Biophys* 269:623–638, 1989.

159. Sipos I, Tretter L, Adam-Vizi V: Quantitative relationship between inhibition of respiratory complexes and formation of reactive oxygen species in isolated nerve terminals. *J Neurochem* 84:112–118, 2003.

160. Zhang Y, Dawson VL, Dawson TM: Oxidative stress and genetics in the pathogenesis of Parkinson's disease. *Neurobiol Dis* 7:240–250, 2000.

161. Dexter DT, Carter CJ, Wells FR, et al: Basal lipid peroxidation in substantia nigra is increased in Parkinson's disease. *J Neurochem* 52:381–389, 1989.

162. Jenner P: Oxidative stress as a cause of Parkinson's disease. *Acta Neurol Scand* 84:6–15, 1991.

163. Sanchez-Ramos JR, Övervik E, Ames BN: A marker of oxyradical-mediated DNA damage (8-hydroxy-2'-deoxyguanosine) is increased in the nigro-striatum of Parkinson's disease brain. *Neurodegeneration* 3:197–204, 1994.

164. Zhang J, Perry G, Smith MA, et al: Parkinson's disease is associated with oxidative damage to cytoplasmic DNA and RNA in substantia nigra neurons. *Am J Pathol* 154:1423–1429, 1999.

165. Floor E, Wetzel MG: Increased protein oxidation in human substantia nigra pars compacta in comparison with basal ganglia and prefrontal cortex measured with an improved dinitrophenylhydrazine assay. *J Neurochem* 70:268–275, 1998.

166. Sian J, Dexter DT, Lees AJ, et al: Alterations in glutathione levels in Parkinson's disease and other neurodegenerative disorders affecting basal ganglia. *Ann Neurol* 36:348–355, 1994.

167. Hasegawa E, Takashige K, Oishi T, et al: 1-Methyl-4-phenylpyridinium (MPP+) induces NADH-dependent superoxide formation, and enhances NADH-dependent lipid peroxidation in bovine heart submitchondrial particles. *Biochem Biophys Res Commun* 170:1049–1055, 1990.

168. Kitamura Y, Kosaka T, Kakimura JI, et al: Protective effects of the antiparkinsonian drugs talipexole and pramipexole against 1-methyl-4-phenylpyridium-induced apoptotic death in human neuroblastoma SH-SY5Y cells. *Mol Pharmacol* 54:1046–1054, 1998.

169. Rios C, Tapia R: Changes in lipid peroxidation induced by 1-methyl-4-phenyl-1,2,3,6-tetrahydropyridine and 1-methyl-4-phenylpyridinium in mouse brain homogenates. *Neurosci Lett* 77:321–326, 1987.

170. Pennathur S, Jackson-Lewis V, Przedborski S, et al: Mass spectrometric quantification of 3-nitrotyrosine, *ortho*-tyrosine, and *o,o'*-dinitrotyrosine in brain tissue of 1-methyl-4-phenyl-1,2,3,6-tetrahydropyridine-treated mice, a model of oxidative stress in Parkinson's disease. *J Biol Chem* 274:34621–34628, 1999.

171. Desole MS, Esposito G, Fresu L, et al: Correlation between 1-methyl-4-phenylpyridinium ion (MPP+) levels, ascorbic acid oxidation and glutathione levels in striatal synaptosomes of the 1-methyl-4-phenyl-1,2,3,6-tetrahydropyridine (MPTP)-treated rat. *Neurosci Lett* 161:121–123, 1993.

172. Hirsch EC, Faucheux B, Damier P, et al: Neuronal vulnerability in Parkinson's disease. *J Neural Transm* 50 (suppl):79–88, 1997.

173. Uhl GR: Hypothesis: The role of dopaminergic transporters in selective vulnerability of cells in Parkinson's disease. *Ann Neurol* 43:555–560, 1998.

174. Swerdlow RH, Parks JK, Cassarino DS, et al: Biochemical analysis of cybrids expressing mitochondrial DNA from contursi kindred Parkinson's subjects. *Exp Neurol* 169:479–485, 2001.

175. Kanda S, Bishop JF, Eglitis MA, et al: Enhanced vulnerability to oxidative stress by α-synuclein mutations and C-terminal truncation. *Neuroscience* 97:279–284, 2000.

176. Ko L, Mehta ND, Farrer M, et al: Sensitization of neuronal cells to oxidative stress with mutated human α-synuclein. *J Neurochem* 75:2546–2554, 2000.

177. Souza JM, Giasson BI, Chen Q, et al: Dityrosine cross-linking promotes formation of stable α-synuclein polymers. *J Biol Chem* 275:18344–18349, 2000.

178. Hartmann A, Hunot S, Michel PP, et al: Caspase-3: A vulnerability factor and final effector in apoptotic death of dopaminergic neurons in Parkinson's disease. *Proc Natl Acad Sci U S A* 97:2875–2880, 2000.

179. Spooren WP, Gentsch C, Wiessner C: Tunel-positive cells in the substantia nigra of C57Bl/6 mice after a single bolus of 1-methyl-4-phenyl-1,2,3,6-tetrahydropyridine. *Neuroscience* 85:649–651, 1998.

180. Viswanath V, Larson J, Andersen JK: Attenuation of 1-methyl-4-phenyl-1,2,3,6-tetrahydropyridine toxicity in mice expressing the baculoviral caspase inhibitor p35. *Soc Neurosci Abstr* 26:2000.

181. The Huntington's Disease Collaborative Research Group: A novel gene containing a trinucleotide repeat that is expanded and unstable on Huntington's disease chromosomes. *Cell* 72:971–983, 1993.

182. DiFiglia M, Sapp K, Chase K, et al: Aggregation of huntingtin in neuronal intranuclear inclusions and dystrophic neurites in brain. *Science* 277:1990–1993, 1997.

183. O'Brien C, Miller C, Goldblatt D, et al: Extraneural metabolism in early Huntington's disease. *Ann Neurol* 28:300–301, 1990.

184. Goebel H, Heipertz R, Scholz W, et al: Juvenile Huntington chorea: Clinical, ultrastructural, and biochemical studies. *Neurology* 28:23–31, 1978.

185. Kuhl D, Phelps M, Markham C, et al: Cerebral metabolism and atrophy in Huntington's disease determined by 18FDG and computed tomographic scan. *Ann Neurol* 12:425–434, 1990.

186. Jenkins BG, Koroshetz WJ, Beal MF, et al: Evidence for impairment of energy metabolism in vivo in Huntington's disease using localized 1H NMR spectroscopy. *Neurology* 43:2689–2695, 1993.

187. Harms L, Meierkord H, Timm G, et al: Decreased *N*-acetyl-aspartate/choline ratio and increased lactate in the frontal lobe of patients with Huntington's disease: A proton magnetic resonance spectroscopy study. *J Neurol Neurosurg Psychiatry* 62:27–30, 1997.

188. Brennan WA Jr, Bird ED, Aprille JR: Regional mitochondrial respiratory activity in Huntington's disease brain. *J Neurochem* 44:1948–1950, 1985.

189. Browne SE, Bowling AC, MacGarvey U, et al: Oxidative damage and metabolic dysfunction in Huntington's disease: Selective vulnerability of the basal ganglia. *Ann Neurol* 41:646–653, 1997.

190. Gu M, Gash M, Mann V, et al: Mitochondrial defect in Huntington's disease caudate nucleus. *Ann Neurol* 39:385–389, 1996.

191. Tabrizi SJ, Cleeter MWJ, Xuereb J, et al: Biochemical abnormalities and excitotoxicity in Huntington's disease brain. *Ann Neurol* 45:25–32, 1999.

192. Arenas J, Campos Y, Ribacoba R, et al: Complex I defect in muscle from patients with Huntington's disease. *Ann Neurol* 43:397–400, 1998.

193. Parker WD Jr, Boyson SJ, Luder AS, et al: Evidence for a defect in NADH:ubiquinone oxidoreductase (complex I) in Huntington's disease. *Neurology* 40:1231–1234, 1990.

194. Braak H, Braak E: Allocortical involvement in Huntington's disease. *Neuropathol Appl Neurobiol* 18:539–547, 1992.

195. Tellez-Nagel I, Johnson AB, Terry RD: Studies on brain biopsies of patients with Huntington's chorea. *J Neuropathol Exp Neurol* 33:308–332, 1973.

196. Browne S, Ferrante R, Beal M: Oxidative stress in Huntington's disease. *Brain Pathol* 9:147–163, 1999.

197. Portera-Cailliau C, Hedreen JC, Price DL, et al: Evidence for apoptotic cell death in Huntington disease and excitotoxic animal models. *J Neurosci* 15:3775–3787, 1995.

198. Ona VO, Li M, Vonsattel JP, et al: Inhibition of caspase-1 slows disease progression in a mouse model of Huntington's disease. *Nature* 399:263–267, 1999.

199. Gutekunst CA, Levey AI, Heilman CJ, et al: Identification and localization of huntingtin in brain and human lymphoblastoid

cell lines with anti-fusion protein antibodies. *Proc Natl Acad Sci U S A* 92:8710–8714, 1995.

200. Panov AV, Gutekunst CA, Leavitt BR, et al: Early mitochondrial calcium defects in Huntington's disease are a direct effect of polyglutamines. *Nat Neurosci* 5:731–736, 2002.

201. Panov AV, Burke JR, Strittmatter WJ, et al: In vitro effects of polyglutamine tracts on Ca2+-dependent depolarization of rat and human mitochondria: Relevance to Huntington's disease. *Arch Biochem Biophys* 410:1–6, 2003.

202. Sawa A, Wiegand GW, Cooper J, et al: Increased apoptosis of Huntington disease lymphoblasts associated with repeat length-dependent mitochondrial depolarization. *Nat Med* 5:1194–1198, 1999.

203. Monoi H, Futaki S, Kugimiya S, et al: Poly-L-glutamine forms cation channels: Relevance to the pathogenesis of the polyglutamine diseases. *Biophys J* 78:2892–2899, 2000.

204. Gutekunst CA, Li SH, Yi H, et al: The cellular and subcellular localization of huntingtin-associated protein 1 (hap1): Comparison with huntingtin in rat and human. *J Neurosci* 18:7674–7686, 1998.

205. Wellington CL, Leavitt BR, Hayden MR: Huntington disease: New insights on the role of huntingtin cleavage. *J Neural Transm Suppl* 1–17, 2000.

206. Brouillet E, Hantraye P, Ferrante RJ, et al: Chronic mitochondrial energy impairment produces selective striatal degeneration and abnormal choreiform movements in primates. *Proc Natl Acad Sci U S A* 92:7105–7109, 1995.

207. Beal MF, Brouillet E, Jenkins B, et al: Neurochemical and histologic characterization of striatal excitotoxic lesions produced by the mitochondrial toxin 3-nitropropionic acid. *J Neurosci* 13:4181–4192, 1993.

208. Brouillet E, Jenkins BG, Hyman BT, et al: Age-dependent vulnerability of the striatum to the mitochondrial toxin 3-nitropropionic acid. *J Neurochem* 60:356–359, 1993.

209. Greene J, Porter R, Eller R, et al: Inhibition of succinate dehydrogenase by malonic acid produces an "excitotoxic" lesion in rat striatum. *J Neurochem* 61:1151–1154, 1993.

210. Henshaw R, Jenkins B, Schulz J, et al: Malonate produces striatal lesions by indirect NMDA receptor activation. *Brain Res* 647:161–166, 1994.

211. Koroshetz WJ, Jenkins BG, Rosen BR, et al: Energy metabolism defects in Huntington's disease and effects of coenzyme Q_{10}. *Ann Neurol* 41:160–165, 1997.

212. Beal MF, Henshaw DR, Jenkins BG, et al: Coenzyme Q_{10} and nicotinamide block striatal lesions produced by the mitochondrial toxin malonate. *Ann Neurol* 36:882–888, 1994.

213. Menalled LB, Chesselet MF: Mouse models of Huntington's disease. *Trends Pharmacol Sci* 23:32–39, 2002.

214. Bates TE, Strangward M, Keelan J, et al: Inhibition of N-acetylaspartate production: Implications for ^{1}H MRS studies *in vivo*. *Neuroreport* 7:1397–1400, 1996.

215. Jenkins BG, Klivenyi P, Kustermann E, et al: Nonlinear decrease over time in N-acetyl aspartate levels in the absence of neuronal loss and increases in glutamine and glucose in transgenic Huntington's disease mice. *J Neurochem* 74:2108–2119, 2000.

216. Wellington CL, Hayden MR: Caspases and neurodegeneration: On the cutting edge of new therapeutic approaches. *Clin Genet* 57:1–10, 2000.

217. Chen M, Ona VO, Li M, et al: Minocycline inhibits caspase-1 and caspase-3 expression and delays mortality in a transgenic mouse model of Huntington disease. *Nat Med* 6:797–801, 2000.

218. Zhu S, Stavrovskaya IG, Drozda M, et al: Minocycline inhibits cytochrome c release and delays progression of amyotrophic lateral sclerosis in mice. *Nature* 417:74–78, 2002.

219. Stahl W, van den Berg H, Arthur J, et al: Bioavailability and metabolism. *Mol Aspects Med* 23:39–100, 2002.

220. Battino M, Ferri E, Gorini A, et al: Natural distribution and occurrence of coenzyme Q homologues. *Membr Biochem* 9:179–190, 1990.

221. Frei B, Kim MC, Ames BN: Ubiquinol-10 is an effective lipid-soluble antioxidant at physiological concentrations. *Proc Natl Acad Sci U S A* 87:4879–4883, 1990.

222. Castilho RF, Kowaltowski AJ, Meinicke AR, et al: Oxidative damage of mitochondria induced by Fe(II)citrate or t-butyl hydroperoxide in the presence of Ca2+: Effect of coenzyme Q redox state. *Free Radic Biol Med* 18:55–59, 1995.

223. Langsjoen PH, Langsjoen AM: Overview of the use of CoQ10 in cardiovascular disease. *Biofactors* 9:273–284, 1999.

224. Tran MT, Mitchell TM, Kennedy DT, et al: Role of coenzyme Q10 in chronic heart failure, angina, and hypertension. *Pharmacotherapy* 21:797–806, 2001.

225. Rozen TD, Oshinsky ML, Gebeline CA, et al: Open label trial of coenzyme Q10 as a migraine preventive. *Cephalalgia* 22:137–141, 2002.

226. Watson JP, Jones DE, James OF, et al: Case report: Oral antioxidant therapy for the treatment of primary biliary cirrhosis: A pilot study. *J Gastroenterol Hepatol* 14:1034–1040, 1999.

227. Ihara Y, Namba R, Kuroda S, et al: Mitochondrial encephalomyopathy (MELAS): Pathological study and successful therapy with coenzyme Q10 and idebenone. *J Neurol Sci* 90:263–271, 1989.

228. Bresolin N, Bet L, Binda A, et al: Clinical and biochemical correlations in mitochondrial myopathies treated with coenzyme Q10. *Neurology* 38:892–899, 1988.

229. Abe K, Fujimura H, Nishikawa Y, et al: Marked reduction in CSF lactate and pyruvate levels after CoQ therapy in a patient with mitochondrial myopathy, encephalopathy, lactic acidosis and stroke-like episodes (MELAS). *Acta Neurol Scand* 83:356–359, 1991.

230. Chen RS, Huang CC, Chu NS: Coenzyme Q10 treatment in mitochondrial encephalomyopathies. Short-term double-blind, crossover study. *Eur Neurol* 37:212–218, 1997.

231. Bresolin N, Doriguzzi C, Ponzetto C, et al: Ubidecarenone in the treatment of mitochondrial myopathies: A multi-center double-blind trial. *J Neurol Sci* 100:70–78, 1990.

232. Kwong LK, Kamzalov S, Rebrin I, et al: Effects of coenzyme Q(10) administration on its tissue concentrations, mitochondrial oxidant generation, and oxidative stress in the rat. *Free Radic Biol Med* 33:627–638, 2002.

233. Matthews RT, Yang L, Browne S, et al: Coenzyme Q10 administration increases brain mitochondrial concentrations and exerts neuroprotective effects. *Proc Natl Acad Sci U S A* 95:8892–8897, 1998.

234. Shults CW, Oakes D, Kieburtz K, et al: Effects of coenzyme Q10 in early Parkinson disease: Evidence of slowing of the functional decline. *Arch Neurol* 59:1541–1550, 2002.

235. The Huntington Study Group: A randomized, placebo-controlled trial of coenzyme Q10 and remacemide in Huntington's disease. *Neurology* 57:397–404, 2001.

236. Beal MF, Matthews RT, Tieleman A, et al: Coenzyme Q10 attenuates the 1-methyl-4-phenyl-1,2,3,6-tetrahydropyridine

(MPTP) induced loss of striatal dopamine and dopaminergic axons in aged mice. *Brain Res* 783:109–114, 1998.

237. Ferrante RJ, Andreassen OA, Dedeoglu A, et al: Therapeutic effects of coenzyme Q10 and remacemide in transgenic mouse models of Huntington's disease. *J Neurosci* 22:1592–1599, 2002.

238. Schilling G, Coonfield ML, Ross CA, et al: Coenzyme Q10 and remacemide hydrochloride ameliorate motor deficits in a Huntington's disease transgenic mouse model. *Neurosci Lett* 315:149–153, 2001.

239. Machlin LJ, Bendich A: Free radical tissue damage: Protective role of antioxidant nutrients. *FASEB J* 1:441–445, 1987.

240. Fahn S: An open trial of high-dosage antioxidants in early Parkinson's disease. *Am J Clin Nutr* 53:380S–382S, 1991.

241. The Parkinson Study Group: Effects of tocopherol and deprenyl on the progression of disability in early Parkinson's disease. *N Engl J Med* 328:176–183, 1993.

242. Shoulson I: Datatop: A decade of neuroprotective inquiry. Parkinson study group. Deprenyl and tocopherol antioxidative therapy of parkinsonism. *Ann Neurol* 44:S160–166, 1998.

243. Egan MF, Hyde TM, Albers GW, et al: Treatment of tardive dyskinesia with vitamin E. *Am J Psychiatry* 149:773–777, 1992.

244. Peyser CE, Folstein M, Chase GA, et al: Trial of D-alpha-tocopherol in Huntington's disease. *Am J Psychiatry* 152:1771–1775, 1995.

245. Esposito E, Rotilio D, Di Matteo V, et al: A review of specific dietary antioxidants and the effects on biochemical mechanisms related to neurodegenerative processes. *Neurobiol Aging* 23:719–735, 2002.

246. Kleijnen J, Knipschild P: Ginkgo biloba. *Lancet* 340:1136–1139, 1992.

247. Tarnopolsky MA, Beal MF: Potential for creatine and other therapies targeting cellular energy dysfunction in neurological disorders. *Ann Neurol* 49:561–574, 2001.

248. Le Bars PL, Katz MM, Berman N, et al: A placebo-controlled, double-blind, randomized trial of an extract of ginkgo biloba for dementia. North American EGB Study Group. *JAMA* 278:1327–1332, 1997.

249. Levites Y, Weinreb O, Maor G, et al: Green tea polyphenol (−)-epigallocatechin-3-gallate prevents *N*-methyl-4-phenyl-1,2,3,6-tetrahydropyridine-induced dopaminergic neurodegeneration. *J Neurochem* 78:1073–1082, 2001.

250. Levites Y, Youdim MB, Maor G, et al: Attenuation of 6-hydroxydopamine (6-OHDA)-induced nuclear factor-kappaB (NF-kappaB) activation and cell death by tea extracts in neuronal cultures. *Biochem Pharmacol* 63:21–29, 2002.

251. Joseph JA, Shukitt-Hale B, Denisova NA, et al: Reversals of age-related declines in neuronal signal transduction, cognitive, and motor behavioral deficits with blueberry, spinach, or strawberry dietary supplementation. *J Neurosci* 19:8114–8121, 1999.

252. Zhang SM, Hernan MA, Chen H, et al: Intakes of vitamins E and C, carotenoids, vitamin supplements, and PD risk. *Neurology* 59:1161–1169, 2002.

253. Klivenyi P, St Clair D, Wermer M, et al: Manganese superoxide dismutase overexpression attenuates MPTP toxicity. *Neurobiol Dis* 5:253–258, 1998.

254. Przedborski S, Kostic V, Jackson-Lewis V, et al: Transgenic mice with increased Cu/Zn-superoxide dismutase activity are resistant to *N*-methyl-4-phenyl-1,2,3,6-tetrahydropyridine-induced neurotoxicity. *J Neurosci* 12:1658–1667, 1992.

255. Beal MF, Ferrante RJ, Henshaw R, et al: 3-Nitropropionic acid neurotoxicity is attenuated in copper/zinc superoxide dismutase transgenic mice. *J Neurochem* 65:919–922, 1995.

256. Flohe L: Superoxide dismutase for therapeutic use: Clinical experience, dead ends and hopes. *Mol Cell Biochem* 84:123–131, 1988.

257. Wengenack TM, Curran GL, Poduslo JF: Postischemic, systemic administration of polyamine-modified superoxide dismutase reduces hippocampal ca1 neurodegeneration in rat global cerebral ischemia. *Brain Res* 754:46–54, 1997.

258. Wiedau-Pazos M, Goto JJ, Rabizadeh S, et al: Altered reactivity of superoxide dismutase in familial amyotrophic lateral sclerosis. *Science* 271:515–518, 1996.

259. Yim MB, Kang JH, Yim HS, et al: A gain-of-function of an amyotrophic lateral sclerosis-associated Cu,Zn-superoxide dismutase mutant: An enhancement of free radical formation due to a decrease in Km for hydrogen peroxide. *Proc Natl Acad Sci U S A* 93:5709–5714, 1996.

260. Peled-Kamar M, Lotem J, Wirguin I, et al: Oxidative stress mediates impairment of muscle function in transgenic mice with elevated level of wild-type Cu/Zn superoxide dismutase. *Proc Natl Acad Sci U S A* 94:3883–3887, 1997.

261. Orr WC, Sohal RS: Effects of Cu-Zn superoxide dismutase overexpression of life span and resistance to oxidative stress in transgenic *Drosophila melanogaster*. *Arch Biochem Biophys* 301:34–40, 1993.

262. Golenser J, Peled-Kamar M, Schwartz E, et al: Transgenic mice with elevated level of CuZnSOD are highly susceptible to malaria infection. *Free Radic Biol Med* 24:1504–1510, 1998.

263. Wyss M, Schulze A: Health implications of creatine: Can oral creatine supplementation protect against neurological and atherosclerotic disease? *Neuroscience* 112:243–260, 2002.

264. Bessman SP, Geiger PJ: Transport of energy in muscle: The phosphorylcreatine shuttle. *Science* 211:448–452, 1981.

265. Saks VA, Rosenshtraukh LV, Smirnov VN, et al: Role of creatine phosphokinase in cellular function and metabolism. *Can J Physiol Pharmacol* 56:691–706, 1978.

266. Lawler JM, Barnes WS, Wu G, et al: Direct antioxidant properties of creatine. *Biochem Biophys Res Commun* 290:47–52, 2002.

267. Xu CJ, Klunk WE, Kanfer JN, et al: Phosphocreatine-dependent glutamate uptake by synaptic vesicles. A comparison with ATP-dependent glutamate uptake. *J Biol Chem* 271:13435–13440, 1996.

268. Brewer GJ, Wallimann TW: Protective effect of the energy precursor creatine against toxicity of glutamate and beta-amyloid in rat hippocampal neurons. *J Neurochem* 74:1968–1978, 2000.

269. Brdiczka D, Beutner G, Ruck A, et al: The molecular structure of mitochondrial contact sites. Their role in regulation of energy metabolism and permeability transition. *Biofactors* 8:235–242, 1998.

270. Stachowiak O, Dolder M, Wallimann T, et al: Mitochondrial creatine kinase is a prime target of peroxynitrite-induced modification and inactivation. *J Biol Chem* 273:16694–16699, 1998.

271. O'Gorman E, Beutner G, Dolder M, et al: The role of creatine kinase in inhibition of mitochondrial permeability transition. *FEBS Lett* 414:253–257, 1997.

272. Stockler S, Holzbach U, Hanefeld F, et al: Creatine deficiency in the brain: A new, treatable inborn error of metabolism. *Pediatr Res* 36:409–413, 1994.

273. van der Knaap MS, Verhoeven NM, Maaswinkel-Mooij P, et al: Mental retardation and behavioral problems as presenting signs of a creatine synthesis defect. *Ann Neurol* 47:540–543, 2000.

274. Leuzzi V, Bianchi MC, Tosetti M, et al: Brain creatine depletion: Guanidinoacetate methyltransferase deficiency (improving with creatine supplementation). *Neurology* 55:1407–1409, 2000.

275. Stockler S, Isbrandt D, Hanefeld F, et al: Guanidinoacetate methyltransferase deficiency: The first inborn error of creatine metabolism in man. *Am J Hum Genet* 58:914–922, 1996.

276. Schulze A, Ebinger F, Rating D, et al: Improving treatment of guanidinoacetate methyltransferase deficiency: Reduction of guanidinoacetic acid in body fluids by arginine restriction and ornithine supplementation. *Mol Genet Metab* 74:413–419, 2001.

277. Matthews RT, Ferrante RJ, Klivenyi P, et al: Creatine and cyclocreatine attenuate MPTP neurotoxicity. *Exp Neurol* 157:142–149, 1999.

278. Matthews RT, Yang L, Jenkins BG, et al: Neuroprotective effects of creatine and cyclocreatine in animal models of Huntington's disease. *J Neurosci* 18:156–163, 1998.

279. Malcon C, Kaddurah-Daouk R, Beal MF: Neuroprotective effects of creatine administration against NMDA and malonate toxicity. *Brain Res* 860:195–198, 2000.

280. Shear DA, Haik KL, Dunbar GL: Creatine reduces 3-nitropropionic-acid-induced cognitive and motor abnormalities in rats. *Neuroreport* 11:1833–1837, 2000.

281. Ferrante RJ, Andreassen OA, Jenkins BG, et al: Neuroprotective effects of creatine in a transgenic mouse model of Huntington's disease. *J Neurosci* 20:4389–4397, 2000.

282. Andreassen OA, Dedeoglu A, Ferrante RJ, et al: Creatine increase survival and delays motor symptoms in a transgenic animal model of Huntington's disease. *Neurobiol Dis* 8:479–491, 2001.

FUNCTIONAL ANATOMY OF BASAL GANGLIA AND MOTOR SYSTEMS

LHYS GOMBART, JESUS SOARES, and GARRETT E. ALEXANDER

CORTICAL MOTOR AREAS   88
   Corticospinal System   88
   Primary Motor Cortex (MC)   90
   Lateral Premotor Fields   90
   Medial Premotor Fields   90
FUNCTIONAL ORGANIZATION OF THE BASAL
  GANGLIA   91
   Motor Circuitry of the Basal Ganglia   91
   Functionally Segregated Circuits   94
   Role of Dopamine   95
   Functional Models of Basal Ganglia Organization   95

While the neuronal substrates for many reflexes and basic movement synergies are present at spinal levels, it is the complex system of cortical and subcortical motor circuits that provides the flexible control over segmental mechanisms necessary for adaptive and skilled motor acts. Our knowledge of this suprasegmental motor system has evolved rapidly over the past decade. Not too long ago, it was generally agreed that there were three distinct motor fields within the cerebral cortex; we now know of at least eight. Over the past few years, we have also come to appreciate that the motor system's functional organization is highly distributed. This is evident not only in the parallel, descending connections that arise from the various cortical motor areas, but also in the families of long-loop, reentrant pathways that pass through the basal ganglia and cerebellum before returning, by way of the thalamus, to the cortical motor fields.

As indicated schematically in Fig. 5-1, the segmental circuitry associated with the motor nuclei of the spinal cord is influenced by two principal categories of descending pathways: those originating from the cerebral cortex, and those arising from various brainstem nuclei, many of which are themselves recipients of descending cortical influences. The cortical motor fields, whose descending projections serve, both directly and indirectly, to modulate the output of the segmental motor apparatus, are influenced in turn by other cortical areas (sensory and associative) and by outputs from the basal ganglia and the cerebellum.

These last two structures can each be viewed as parallel, reentrant processing stations that receive separate, but largely similar, inputs from widespread cortical areas (including motor, premotor, and somatosensory cortex) and return their own respective influences to specific, and largely separate, portions of the precentral motor fields via basal ganglia- and cerebellar-specific connections within the ventrolateral ("motor") thalamus. As indicated in Fig. 5-1, both the basal ganglia and the cerebellum also direct some of their outflow to brainstem descending systems.

While motor circuits that engage the basal ganglia are the principal focus of this chapter, it is worth noting that the parallel features of cerebellar circuitry are at least as impressive as those of the basal ganglia. For example, the "vestibular/oculomotor," "spinal," and "cerebral" subdivisions of cerebellar cortex (so designated because of their characteristic sources of input) project their corresponding downstream influences via separate, though parallel, channels passing through the various output nuclei of the cerebellum. Within the cerebral subdivision alone, multiple parallel, long-loop cerebellothalamocortical pathways

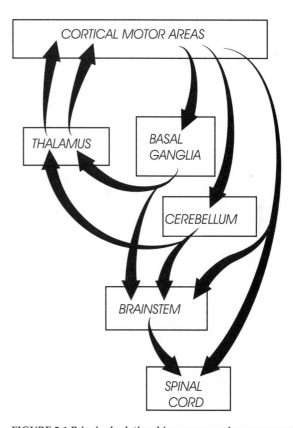

FIGURE 5-1 Principal relationships among major components of the motor system. Note that the basal ganglia and cerebellum may be viewed as key elements in two parallel, reentrant systems that return their influences to cortical motor areas through separate portions of the ventrolateral thalamus. This figure also emphasizes the parallel projections of the cortical motor fields to multiple levels of the motor system.

have been demonstrated. These loops exhibit maintained segregation of functionally diverse inputs,[1] each centered on a different group of functionally related cortical fields. For example, a closed cerebellar motor loop centered on motor cortex, premotor cortex, and cingulate motor area engages separate thalamic and deep cerebellar nuclear territories from those included in a parallel, cerebellar associative loop centered on frontal and parietal association cortex.[2]

Cortical Motor Areas

In humans and other primates, motor control depends critically upon the integrity of various precentral motor fields distributed throughout much of the frontal lobe. Most are located within frontal agranular cortex, comprising Brodmann's areas 4 and 6. However, recent studies have shown that some of the cortical motor fields are actually located within bordering regions of cingulate cortex, areas that traditionally had been considered part of the limbic system. Even so, all of the known motor fields can properly be termed precentral, as each lies within or rostral to the rostral bank of the central sulcus.

The frontal lobes of nonhuman primates contain no less than eight (and by some reckonings as many as ten) discrete motor fields, six of which send direct projections to spinal levels. The latter include primary motor cortex (MC; area 4) and five nonprimary motor fields or "premotor" areas. Until the early part of this decade, it was still customary to distinguish but two nonprimary motor fields within the human brain: premotor cortex on the lateral convexity, and the supplementary motor area (SMA) on the medial wall. However, advances in functional brain imaging have shown that each of the cortical motor fields identified earlier in nonhuman primates has its counterpart in humans. Moreover, all ten of the putative motor fields identified thus far in monkeys and humans have been identified as well in prosimian galagos, indicating that this complex and highly differentiated network of cortical motor fields emerged early in the course of primate evolution.[3]

Locations of the known cortical motor fields are indicated for the monkey in Fig. 5-2. The four motor fields of the lateral convexity include MC, the dorsal (PMd) and ventral (PMv) premotor areas, and the newly identified pre-PMd. Those of the medial wall include SMA and pre-SMA, and the rostral (CMAr) and caudal (CMAc) cingulate motor areas. Each of the nonprimary areas with direct corticospinal projections—PMd, PMv, SMA, CMAr, CMAc—shares reciprocal connections with MC and, like MC, each contains a complete somatotopic map.[4–6] These six precentral motor fields also share other important characteristics:[7] each is reciprocally connected with a portion of the motor thalamus;[8–10] each receives a characteristic set of inputs from the parietal lobe;[11–13] and each sends substantial projections to basal ganglia and cerebellum.[14–16] Both pre-SMA and pre-PMd,

motor fields that lack direct connections with MC and do not project directly to spinal levels, each receive input from both frontal and parietal association cortex, share reciprocal connections with each other, and are connected in turn with their respective namesakes.[17–21]

CORTICOSPINAL SYSTEM

The motor fields with corticospinal projections innervate the ventral horn of the spinal cord at both cervical and lumbar levels.[6,22–24] These projections are glutamatergic[25] and excitatory, although they facilitate both inhibitory and excitatory circuitry at spinal levels. In many respects, the corticospinal projections, originating in different cortical areas can properly be construed as comprising multiple parallel, but functionally differentiated, descending systems. The corticospinal (or "pyramidal") tract comprises efferent projections, not only from multiple motor areas, but also from several somatosensory areas. The latter include primary somatosensory fields (areas 3, 1, and 2) and the somatosensory association area within adjacent area 5.[26]

In the human, approximately 1 million corticospinal fibers pass through each medullary pyramid, with 70–90 percent crossing in the motor decussation to form the lateral corticospinal tract, and the remainder passing uncrossed into the ventral corticospinal tract. Corticospinal fibers descending in the lateral corticospinal tract terminate on interneurons of almost all categories, but especially on those related to motoneurons of distal muscles of the limb. In primates, the direct monosynaptic corticospinal projections to motoneurons are likewise concentrated upon the cells related to the distal extremity musculature. In addition, some corticospinal fibers descending ipsilaterally in the ventral corticospinal tract make connections on both sides of the cord with interneurons related to motoneurons of axial and girdle muscles. In higher primates, the corticospinal tract increases enormously in size, and the distribution of terminals within the spinal gray matter shifts ventrally to include the motoneuron pools, reflecting increased direct control over segmental output. The terminal fields of corticospinal fibers that project to interneurons and propriospinal neurons in the intermediate zone are topographically organized. In the monkey, for example, those parts of area 4 that represent the distal limb musculature project to the interneurons and short propriospinal neurons in the dorsolateral portions of the intermediate zone, while those that represent the proximal musculature project to the interneurons and long propriospinal neurons of the ventromedial portion of the spinal intermediate zone.

Comparative studies indicate that corticospinal projections have emerged and been selectively strengthened in various species (especially primates) roughly in accordance with an increasing capacity for the execution of movements that are highly fractionated (i.e., in which closely approximated structures, such as fingers, are moved in relative independence).[16,27] Selective lesions of the corticospinal

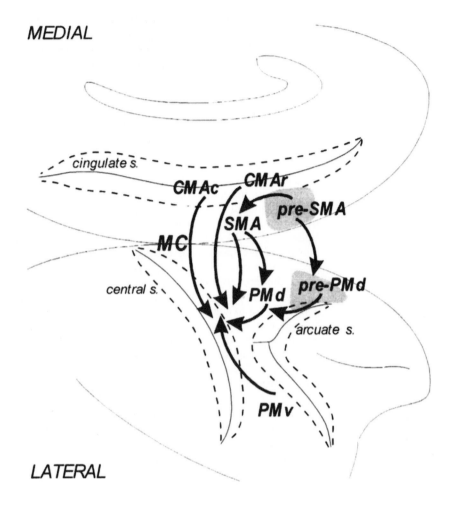

FIGURE 5-2 Locations of eight precentral motor fields in the monkey. Indicated in light stipple are the six motor fields with direct projections to spinal levels, including MC and the five premotor fields with which it shares reciprocal connections. Indicated by dark stipple are the two premotor fields without direct connections either to MC or to spinal levels. CMAc, caudal cingulate motor area; CMAr, rostral cingulate motor area; MC, primary motor cortex; PMd, dorsal premotor area; PMv, ventral premotor area; SMA, supplementary motor area; s., sulcus.

pathway lead to the specific loss of ability to perform movements of this type. The capacity for making fractionated movements is not based on simple point-to-point mappings of corticomotoneurons onto spinal motoneurons.[28] Instead, there is substantial convergence and divergence of connections between these two sets of neurons.

Injection of individual corticospinal axons with anatomical tracers has shown that each axon can give rise to a surprisingly large number of terminal branches that diverge to innervate multiple separate spinal motor nuclei.[29] Conversely, the ventral horn at a given level of the spinal cord receives somatotopically specific corticospinal inputs from several different cortical motor fields.[5,23,24,30] Electrophysiological studies indicate that most corticospinal neurons have direct, presumably monosynaptic, connections with more than one muscle.[31-34] The "muscle field" of a given corticospinal neuron is usually restricted to a relatively small number of functionally related muscles. Corticospinal neurons that influence a particular muscle are often clustered together, but their individual muscle fields may differ significantly.

How, then, can somatotopic specificity and the capacity for fractionated movements be explained in the face of the striking convergence and divergence of descending corticospinal projections from the various cortical motor fields? The answer to this question is not yet known with any certainty. However, evidence from other systems would suggest that much of the gross topography/somatotopy within the motor system may be genetically determined, while the fine-tuning (e.g., in terms of the response properties of individual neurons) may depend significantly upon experience and associated activity-dependent changes in local synaptic strengths. Convergent corticospinal inputs to a given motor unit might be differentially strengthened (or weakened) by experience according to activity-dependent synaptic learning rules. As discussed below in connection with the basal ganglia, such processes could lead to the coordination of functionally related but spatially distributed corticospinal neurons, or clusters of such neurons, and thereby account for movement fractionation despite the absence of one-to-one mapping between cortical and spinal motoneurons.

PRIMARY MOTOR CORTEX (MC)

MC is coextensive with Brodmann's area 4, the agranular cortex within and immediately rostral to the anterior bank of the central sulcus that contains giant layer V pyramidal neurons. In addition to its corticospinal output, MC also contributes substantial projections to each of the premotor areas and to several somatosensory areas (including areas 3a, 1, 2, and 5), as well as to the ventrolateral thalamus (VPLo, VLo, VLc), basal ganglia (putamen), and cerebellum (via the various precerebellar nuclei).[14,35] These additional outputs presumably serve to inform the target areas of the intended movement ("corollary discharge"), and to exert some influence over the outputs from these areas.[36] Evidence in monkeys suggests that these noncorticospinal projections from the MC are derived largely from separate populations of non-pyramidal tract neurons (non-PTNs), rather than from PTN collaterals.

Single-neuron recordings in MC of monkeys reveal somatotopic organization and typically strong directional tuning of movement-related discharge, with the activity of most cells depending also on the movement's force, whether the movement is isotonic or isometric.[31] Many MC neurons show selective activation during the preparation for a planned movement, and such preparatory activity is often directionally tuned as well.[37,38] Functional imaging of MC in humans—with positron emission spectroscopy (PET) and with functional magnetic resonance imaging (fMRI)—has shown analogous somatotopic activations, unconditionally related to passive or active movements of particular body parts.[21,39–43] During the planning or imagery of a movement that is merely rehearsed but not executed, increases in blood flow are seen within SMA and within premotor cortex on the lateral surface of the hemisphere, but not within MC.[44–46]

LATERAL PREMOTOR FIELDS

Many neurons in PMd discharge selectively during the preparation of goal-directed limb movements,[47,48] particularly those based on visual instructions.[49–51] Lesions and reversible inactivation of this area impair performance of tasks where there are arbitrary linkages between visual instructions and instructed movements. Functional imaging studies in humans have shown activation of PMd with similar tasks.[46,52,53] The more rostral pre-PMd can be differentiated from PMd proper both anatomically and functionally, based on the predominance of visual and associative inputs in pre-PMd and the corresponding prevalence of visual and behaviorally contingent activations of neurons in this region.[11,17,19,54,55]

Neurons in PMv show preferential activation in association with visually guided reaching and grasping movements, and lesions of this region result in corresponding functional impairments.[56] There is some controversy over the extent to which activity in this area involves sensory representations of visual space versus gaze effects, but much of the reaching-related activity in this region is encoded in extrinsic rather than intrinsic (i.e., body-centered) coordinates.[57]

Studies in humans have suggested several roles for the premotor cortex of the lateral convexity, without necessarily distinguishing between dorsal and ventral subfields. One such role is the control of proximal limb musculature and interlimb coordination. Patients with premotor lesions manifest proximal weakness, and their apraxic deficits are often confined to movements involving proximal musculature.[58] Such proximal limb-kinetic apraxia contrasts sharply with the bimanual—and notably distal—apraxic deficits associated with lesions of SMA (see below).

Studies in humans have shown maximal increases in regional cerebral blood flow (rCBF) in lateral premotor areas during voluntary movements that require sensory guidance.[53,59] Patients with premotor lesions have been shown to have specific impairments in using sensory cues (visual, auditory or tactile) to recall previously learned movements, though they have no difficulty in retrieving the same movements on the basis of spatial cues.[60] Such observations have led to suggestions that lateral premotor cortex in humans may serve as a higher motor association area and play an important role in the preparation for movement.[61] Both are consistent with studies of the preparatory discharges of monkey PMd neurons, which appear to encode salient task contingencies that the subject must take into account in planning an appropriate motor response.[47,50,62] Both lateral and medial premotor areas show preferential increases in rCBF during motor tasks that require the subject to select among several possible arm movements.[53,63]

MEDIAL PREMOTOR FIELDS

Until relatively recently, SMA was considered synonymous with mesial area 6, the entire expanse of agranular cortex on the medial wall of the hemisphere. However, there is now general agreement that the most rostral portion, the newly designated pre-SMA, should be distinguished from SMA proper because pre-SMA—unlike SMA proper—lacks direct connections with MC and does not project directly to spinal levels but does receive direct input from frontal and posterior parietal association cortex.[5,30,64] Nevertheless, SMA and pre-SMA do share strong, reciprocal connections with each other, indicating that pre-SMA is likely to play a significant role in high-level motor control. Neurons in both SMA and pre-SMA show clear involvement in the preparation and execution of limb movements, but pre-SMA neurons tend to show stronger relationships to visual and visuomotor processing than their counterparts in SMA.[65,66] Functional imaging of SMA and pre-SMA have shown motor activations with complex behavioral contingencies.[67–69]

SMA lesions in humans may lead to a severe poverty of movement (akinesia), and mutism.[70] It is noteworthy in this regard that a major output of the basal ganglia is directed (via the thalamus) to SMA. It remains uncertain, however, whether the akinesia and mutism associated with lesions of

SMA can be explained simply in terms of the loss of basal ganglia influences on the cerebral cortex. Nevertheless, reduced movement-related activation of SMA has been demonstrated in Parkinson's disease by PET measures of rCBF. This deficit is largely corrected in parallel with improved motor function following stereotaxic posteromedial pallidotomy.[71,72]

Participation of SMA in complex motor functions is supported by single-cell recordings in SMA of monkeys, which have revealed changes in neuronal activity related not only to movement execution but also to the preparation for movement and motor set.[73] Many SMA neurons show selective, sustained activation following an instruction that permits the subject to prepare for an upcoming movement, and then cease firing as the movement begins. Such findings are consistent with the results of human studies of event-related potentials and functional brain imaging,[46,74–76] which have implicated SMA in neural processes underlying the preparation for movement. What has yet to be determined is precisely how the lateral and medial premotor areas differ in respect to their respective contributions to the processes underlying movement preparation.

Lesions of SMA are associated with impaired control of bimanual movements in both humans and monkeys.[77] This may be related to the fact that even unilateral limb movements tend to result in bilateral activation of SMA. Nevertheless, in single-cell recording studies in monkeys, the large majority of SMA neurons show restricted, contralateral sensorimotor fields, and microstimulation of SMA results in focal movements of contralateral body parts (in accordance with a clearly evident somatotopy).[73] However, studies have also shown that both SMA[78] and MC[79] contain select populations of neurons that discharge exclusively during coordinated, bilateral movements of the digits and not during movements of either hand by itself. Taken together, these findings suggest that SMA may play a special role in the coordination of movements involving both sides of the body.

SMA has also been implicated in the control of sequential movements. Disruption of activity in this area in humans and other primates interferes with the capacity to learn or reproduce remembered sequences of movements.[80,81] Single-cell recordings in monkeys[82] have shown that neurons in SMA—but not in MC—discharge selectively during or in anticipation of a particular sequence of movements (and not in relation to the same components executed in a different sequence), and similar results have been obtained with functional imaging.[83] Numerous functional imaging studies in humans have shown changes in rCBF in the region of SMA associated with the learning of motor sequences.[84–86]

The cingulate motor areas have come to be recognized as such only relatively recently. In monkeys, at least two can be identified within the cingulate sulcus: CMAr in Brodmann's area 23c, and CMAc in area 24c. Both of these premotor fields project directly to the spinal cord and to the basal ganglia.[87,88] CMAr receives strong connections from dorsolateral prefrontal cortex and from the pre-SMA.[89–91]

Studies in monkeys have demonstrated movement-related and preparatory activity in neurons in CMAr and in CMAc,[92,93] with the caudal area containing a higher proportion of neurons discharging selectively in relation to self-initiated rather than stimulus-triggered movements.[94] CMAr appears to be uniquely involved in the selection of appropriate movements conditioned by the quality of associated reward, as demonstrated both by muscimol inactivation and by characterization of behavior-correlated neuronal activity.[95] Functional imaging studies in humans have demonstrated activation of cingulate motor areas in association with a range of simple and more complex motor behaviors,[36,59] including learned movement sequences[85] and vibration-induced illusory limb movement (in CMAc).[68]

Functional Organization of the Basal Ganglia

The basal ganglia comprise the striatum (including the putamen and caudate nucleus, which together constitute the neostriatum, and the ventral striatum—also known as the limbic striatum), the globus pallidus, the substantia nigra and the subthalamic nucleus, all of which are functionally subdivided into skeletomotor, oculomotor, associative, and limbic territories based on their physiological properties and on their interconnections with cortical and thalamic territories of the same functionalities.[96] As indicated in Fig. 5-3, the large-scale organization of the basal ganglia can be viewed as a family of reentrant loops that are organized in parallel, each taking its origin from a particular set of functionally related cortical fields (skeletomotor, oculomotor, etc.), passing through the functionally corresponding portions of the basal ganglia, and returning to parts of those same cortical fields by way of specific basal ganglia-recipient zones in the dorsal thalamus.

Due to maintained segregation along each of these corticobasal ganglia-thalamocortical circuits, there is little direct communication among the separate functional domains, except by way of corticocortical interactions. While virtually the entire cortical mantle is mapped topographically onto the striatum, often considered the "input" portion of the basal ganglia, the cortically directed signals from the basal ganglia output nuclei (internal pallidum, and substantia nigra pars reticulata) are returned exclusively to foci within the frontal lobe (after first passing through the corresponding portions of the thalamus). Because of their parallel organization, it is generally suspected that the operations performed at corresponding stations along each of these loops are quite similar.

MOTOR CIRCUITRY OF THE BASAL GANGLIA

The skeletomotor circuitry of the basal ganglia includes several noteworthy features, some of which may be important in shaping the specific contributions that these structures

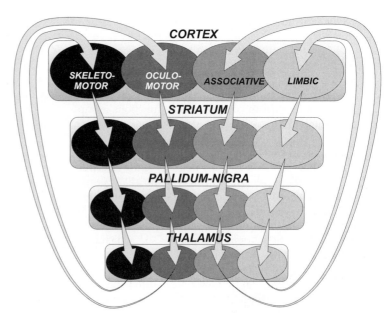

FIGURE 5-3 Parallel, functionally segregated, basal ganglia-thalamocortical loops. Each of these partially closed reentrant pathways engages a separate portion of cortex, basal ganglia, and thalamus.

make to the control of movement. The broad outlines of basal ganglia motor circuitry are depicted in Fig. 5-4.

CORTICAL INPUTS

Like the cerebellum, the basal ganglia receive topographic inputs from most of the sensorimotor territories of the cerebral cortex, including primary and secondary somatosensory areas, MC, and all premotor areas.[14,15,97–99] Directed toward the sensorimotor portion of the neostriatum, these coordinated corticostriatal inputs impose a well-defined somatotopic organization upon their target nucleus, which, in primates, coincides roughly with the putamen. The majority of the putamen-projecting sensorimotor areas also send topographic projections to the subthalamic nucleus.[88,100,101] Both the corticostriatal and the corticosubthalamic projections are excitatory, and probably glutamatergic.[102]

STRIATUM

In the putamen, as in the rest of the striatum, the large majority of neurons are of the medium spiny type (MSN). MSNs are gamma-aminobutyric acid (GABA)-ergic projection neurons,[103] and in primates they comprise two distinct populations: one expressing dopamine D2 receptors and projecting to the external segment of the globus pallidus (GPe), and the other projecting either to the internal segment of the globus pallidus (GPi) or to the substantia nigra pars reticulata (SNr).[104,105] At rest, putamen projection neurons are nearly silent, although most have well-defined sensorimotor fields and discharge selectively in relation to specific parameters of movement or specific aspects of the preparation for movement.[106–108]

The other type of putamen neuron that has been well studied is the large, aspiny interneuron.[109,110] Unlike MSNs, the large interneurons are spontaneously active and do not discharge in relation to specific parameters of movement preparation or execution. Rather, they discharge briefly (only one or two spikes) and synchronously following the presentation of a conditioned sensory stimulus that signifies the imminent delivery of a reward.[111] In this respect, their behavior is similar to that of dopamine neurons (see below). The spontaneously active interneurons appear to be cholinergic, but their synaptic influence on neighboring MSNs has remained uncertain.[112] Electron-microscopic studies have shown that cholinergic synapses on the somata and dendritic shafts and spines of MSNs are mainly of the symmetric type,[113] indicating that the direct synaptic effects of aspiny interneurons on MSNs are largely inhibitory. In primates, two types of muscarinic receptors, m1 and m2, are differentially localized within MSNs and aspiny interneurons, respectively.[114] Moreover, m1 receptors have been shown to reside mainly within MSN spines that bear asymmetric synapses formed by corticostriatal and extrinsic monoaminergic axons, while m2 receptors are confined to cholinergic axons of aspiny interneurons forming synapses with MSNs that are overwhelmingly of the symmetric type.[114] These results suggest there are at least two functionally distinct types of cholinergic actions within the striatum: (1) modulation of excitatory (glutamatergic) corticostriatal inputs to MSNs via m1 receptors; and (2) modulation of acetylcholine release from aspiny interneurons via m2 receptors.

GLOBUS PALLIDUS AND SUBSTANTIA NIGRA

Those portions of GPi and SNr that receive input from the putamen constitute the sensorimotor output nuclei

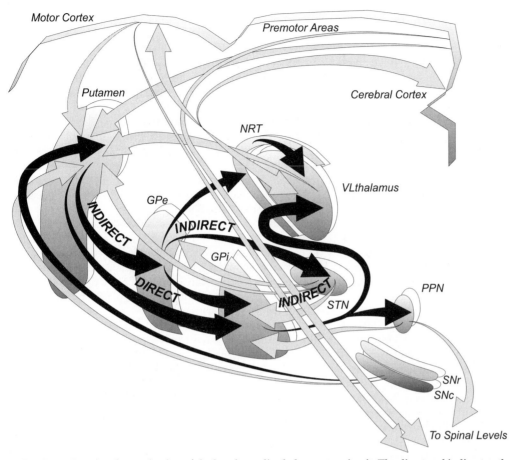

FIGURE 5-4 Functional organization of the basal ganglia skeletomotor circuit. The direct and indirect pathways through the basal ganglia are indicated. Excitatory pathways are indicated by light shading, inhibitory pathways by dark shading. Connections between thalamus and cortex are reciprocal. Connections to and from SNr (which parallel those of GPi) are not shown. A further simplification shows the thalamostriate projection arising from VL thalamus rather than from the centromedian nucleus. GPe, external segment of globus pallidus; GPi, internal segment of globus pallidus; NRT, thalamic reticular nucleus; PPN, pedunculopontine nucleus; SNc, substantia nigra pars compacta; SNr, pars reticulata; STN, subthalamic nucleus; VLthalamus, ventrolateral thalamus.

of the basal ganglia, sending GABAergic projections to their respective targets in both the ventrolateral thalamus (nucleus ventralis lateralis, and nucleus ventralis anterior), and the centromedian nucleus of the thalamus.[9,115–117] Anatomically, GPi and SNr share many common features, and from a functional standpoint they can be viewed as two subdivisions of a single basal ganglia output nucleus.[118] Neurons in the sensorimotor territories of GPi/SNr have movement-related receptive fields that are similar to those of the putamen's MSNs, but GPi/SNr neurons differ from MSNs in having relatively high spontaneous discharge rates (60–80 Hz) that are modulated both upwards and downwards depending on their particular sensorimotor response fields.[119,120] Neurons in the sensorimotor territory of GPe have discharge properties and sensorimotor fields that are comparable to those in GPi/SNr.

DIRECT AND INDIRECT PATHWAYS

The basal ganglia output nuclei (GPi/SNr) receive not only direct inputs from the striatum via the GPi- and SNr-projecting MSNs, but also an important converging source of information via what has come to be termed the indirect pathway through the basal ganglia.[105,121,122] The direct and indirect pathways are illustrated in Fig. 5-3. The indirect pathway takes its origin from the GPe-projecting MSNs. In turn, the GABAergic neurons of GPe project mainly to the subthalamic nucleus,[123] whose excitatory, glutamatergic neurons send feedforward connections to GPi/SNr, completing one arm of the indirect pathway, and feedback connections to GPe.[102,124]

A second arm of the indirect pathway is formed by GPe projections that pass directly to GPi/SNr.[105,121] A remarkable consequence of this is that activation of MSNs associated with either arm of the indirect pathway should increase basal ganglia output by increasing neuronal activity at the level of GPi/SNr: in one case, by disinhibiting the subthalamic nucleus with its excitatory projections to GPi/SNr; in the other, by directly disinhibiting GPi/SNr. In contrast, activation of MSNs associated with the direct pathway should decrease basal ganglia output by directly suppressing activity at the level of GPi/SNr. Given the reentrant nature of basal ganglia-thalamocortical connections, cortically initiated activation of the direct pathway might therefore be expected to result in positive feedback at cortical levels, with corresponding activation of the indirect pathway giving rise, conversely, to negative feedback.

THALAMIC RETICULAR NUCLEUS

GPe sends an inhibitory, feedforward projection to the nucleus reticularis of the thalamus (NRT),[125,126] which in turn imposes a robust, GABAergic modulation upon the basal ganglia-recipient nuclei of the ventrolateral thalamus. There appears to be a functional consistency among the various GPe projections, in that cortically induced activations of GPe-projecting MSNs should have the net effect of producing negative feedback at cortical levels, based on the functional effects of each of the known GPe projections—including both arms of the indirect pathway, and the GPe projections to the NRT.

On the other hand, the role of NRT in basal ganglia operations may be much more complicated. It is generally accepted that NRT plays an important role in gating thalamocortical transmission from the dorsal thalamus, and that it does so in a roughly topographic manner that links specific portions of NRT with specific thalamic nuclei and their cortical target zones.[127] NRT receives collateral, excitatory inputs from corticothalamic as well as thalamocortical fibers, which must pass through this nucleus en route to their respective termination zones in cortex and thalamus.

PEDUNCULOPONTINE NUCLEUS (PPN)

While the PPN, located in the dorsolateral pontomesencephalic tegmentum, is not generally considered part of the basal ganglia, this structure has strong, reciprocal connections with the basal ganglia output nuclei and with the subthalamic nucleus, and it also sends unreciprocated glutamatergic projections to the dopaminergic neurons of the substantia nigra pars compacta (SNc; see below), as well as to the putamen and caudate nucleus.[128,129] PPN is somatotopically organized in primates, receiving corticotegmental inputs from MC, SMA, pre-SMA, PMd, and PMv that converge in topographic fashion to represent each body part.[130] Despite this somatotopic segregation, there is compelling anatomical evidence that functionally segregated GPi outflow from motor, associative and limbic territories overlaps within PPN to provide functionally integrated input to the target neurons, which are limited to the noncholinergic projection neurons of PPN.[131]

Lesions, chemical inactivation or high-frequency stimulation of PPN in primates results in akinesia.[132–134] It has been suggested that the akinesia of Parkinson's disease might result from excessive GABAergic inhibitory outflow from GPi/SNr to PPN in this condition. This is supported by a recent demonstration in primates that the akinesia of 1-methyl-4-phenyl-1,2,3,6-tetrahydropyridine (MPTP)-induced parkinsonism can be reversed by injection of the GABA antagonist bicuculline into PPN.[135] PPN contains two populations of neurons: cholinergic and noncholinergic.[129,136] The noncholinergic neurons send excitatory, glutamatergic projections to GPi/SNr, SNc, and the subthalamic nucleus. The cholinergic neurons project to thalamus, and to GPi/SNr.

As with GPi/SNr, there is a convergence of inputs from both the direct and indirect pathways at the level of the PPN. In this case, however, activation of either pathway at the level of the MSNs leads to the same polarity of response within the PPN (i.e., activation of PPN by disinhibited subthalamic inputs, or direct disinhibition of PPN by inputs from GPe or from GPi/SNr).

Until recently, descending projections of the basal ganglia output nuclei have received relatively little attention, it having been generally assumed that directly descending basal ganglia influences on the skeletomotor system extended no further caudally than the PPN. Studies in cats and rats revealed substantial PPN outflow to the reticulospinal system.[137,138] These findings have not yet been extended to primates.

FUNCTIONALLY SEGREGATED CIRCUITS

One of the remarkable features of basal ganglia circuitry is that functionally discrete channels of information processing are maintained throughout the various corticobasal ganglia-thalamocortical pathways in the face of layer-to-layer connectivity that is highly convergent. In the case of the skeletomotor pathways, for example, basal ganglia neurons have been shown to have highly refined sensorimotor fields that are comparable in their somatotopic and behavioral specificity to the sensorimotor fields of neurons at cortical levels. Yet the convergence ratio along the corticostriatal pathway, for instance, has been estimated to be 10^3–10^4:1. Recent quantitative studies of layer-to-layer connectivity within basal ganglia circuits have begun to explain this apparent paradox.

Detailed analysis of corticostriatal synaptic organization has shown that even MSNs with overlapping dendritic fields (on the order of 2500 neighboring striatal neurons lie within the dendritic arbor of a single MSN) have few presynaptic cortical axons in common, and, conversely, corticospinal neurons with overlapping axons seldom innervate the same striatal neurons.[139] In other words, the apparently massive convergence of presynaptic inputs is, in fact, highly focused and selective, in accordance with the observed finely tuned response fields of individual striatal neurons that are often sharply differentiated from those of neighboring MSNs.[140]

Much of this organization may be genetically determined, but experience-dependent synaptic modification may also play a role. The correlative nature of this type of learning might be expected to strengthen preferentially those connections that link neurons with similar functional properties.

ROLE OF DOPAMINE

An important feature of basal ganglia organization is the pervasive role of dopamine. The functionality of dopamine in basal ganglia operations appears to be complex and multifaceted.[141] Dopaminergic inputs to the putamen and caudate nucleus comprise mesostriatal projections from SNc.[142] GP and subthalamic nucleus have also been shown to receive dopaminergic inputs from SNc. Separate mesocortical projections from the ventral tegmental area provide dopaminergic innervation to most of the neocortex, including all of the cortical motor fields.[143] Collaterals of the mesostriatal system were shown recently in primates to constitute mesothalamic system that provides dopaminergic input to motor and limbic-related nuclei of the thalamus.[144] There is abundant indirect evidence suggesting that dopamine may have differential effects on the direct and indirect pathways, tending to activate striatal MSNs that project directly to GPi while suppressing those that project to GPe.[105] Such differential effects would suggest in turn that the overall influence of dopamine on basal ganglia operations may include the enhancement of positive feedback, and suppression of negative feedback, returned to the various cortical areas that receive basal ganglia influences. This scenario is complicated by a variety of evidence indicating that dopamine may have a more subtle, neuromodulatory effect on MSN activity rather than the conventional excitatory and inhibitory synaptic effects posited in the most current models of the direct and indirect pathways.[141]

Dopamine has also been shown to have a role in synaptic plasticity within the striatum, being implicated in both long-term potentiation (LTP) and long-term depression (LTD).[145,146] The nigrostriatal pathway provides an extraordinarily dense dopaminergic input to each MSN, which is comparable in magnitude to the 5000 or so corticostriatal synapses that individual MSNs receive.[147–149] The behavioral correlates of dopamine neurons have been studied in considerable depth.[150,151] Unlike nearly all the other basal ganglia motor circuit neurons, except perhaps the large, aspiny interneurons of the striatum,[111] dopamine neurons do not show activity changes in relation to movement per se, but discharge instead in relation to conditions involving the probability and imminence of behavioral reinforcement.[152]

The newly discovered facts that dopamine may play a crucial role in the cellular mechanisms of LTD and LTP within the striatum, and that dopamine neurons discharge selectively in relation to specific reward contingencies, combine to suggest the intriguing hypothesis that dopamine

neurons may play an important role in determining when striatal synapses should be strengthened or weakened. In this respect, dopamine neurons might be seen as playing a role in striatal information-processing analogous to that played by an "adaptive critic" in certain types of connectionist networks that are capable of autonomous learning.[151]

FUNCTIONAL MODELS OF BASAL GANGLIA ORGANIZATION

Disinhibition plays an important role in many current models of basal ganglia operation.[105] In the case of the oculomotor pathways of the basal ganglia, for example, there is compelling evidence that striatally induced, phasic inhibition of SNr neurons leads to the generation of saccadic eye movements through the release of command neurons in the superior colliculus from the tonic, GABAergic inhibition they receive via the nigrotectal pathway.[153] The elegant simplicity of this model has helped to motivate similar models of how the basal ganglia's skeletomotor circuitry may contribute to movement control, the chief difference being the emphasis in most skeletomotor models on disinhibition at the level of the thalamus rather than the brainstem.[122]

These models of the basal ganglia's skeletomotor circuitry assume that voluntary movements are facilitated in the context of focused disinhibition of the basal ganglia-recipient portions of the ventrolateral thalamus. This focused thalamic disinhibition is thought to be generated either by phasic enhancement of transmission through the direct pathway, by phasic suppression of transmission through the indirect pathway, or by a combination of these two processes. Conversely, according to this same scheme, decreased transmission through the direct pathway, or increased transmission through the indirect pathway, would have the effect of suppressing voluntary movements.

With the steady accumulation of more detailed analyses of the microarchitecture of basal ganglia circuitry,[105] the functional models have become increasingly refined. It has been shown, for instance, that, in addition to medium spiny projection neurons, the striatum also contains GABAergic interneurons that provide feedforward inhibition of the MSNs.[121] That substance P-containing striatal MSNs of the direct pathway share reciprocal local feedback connections with their enkephalin-positive counterparts of the indirect pathway has also been demonstrated.[154] While there had previously been little electrophysiological evidence of local interactions among MSNs giving rise to surround inhibition, such effects are now known to be prominent.[155]

Certain issues are still unresolved. It remains to be determined whether the demonstrated convergence of inputs from direct and indirect pathways onto individual neurons in GPi/SNr[156] results in a functional interaction that is antagonistic or complementary. One possibility is an antagonistic, push/pull system that would scale or brake an intended movement (e.g., with flexion-activated inputs from the two pathways being superimposed and thereby tending to cancel one another out). Another possibility is a center-surround system that could facilitate an intended movement pattern while suppressing potentially conflicting ones. Some recent evidence from functional imaging studies lends support to this latter alternative.[157]

Certain observations are difficult to reconcile with simple models of basal ganglia function based primarily on the concept of thalamic disinhibition. For example, contrary to the models' prediction, lesions of basal ganglia output nuclei generally do not result in dyskinesias; in fact, one of the most reliable benefits of the medial pallidotomy procedure has been the reduction or elimination of L-dopa-induced dyskinesias.[158,159] Possible explanations for the apparent paradox have been suggested.[160,161]

A related difficulty for thalamic disinhibition theories is that lesions of the ventrolateral thalamus do not result in akinesia, and yet according to such theories parkinsonian akinesia is generally attributed to increased basal ganglia outflow that results in excessive inhibition at the level of the ventrolateral thalamus. One possible explanation for this discrepancy is that we may have underestimated the functional significance of descending basal ganglia outflow to the PPN (and from there to the reticulospinal system), in which case lesions of the thalamus that block only the reentrant (cortically projected) influences of the basal ganglia may leave intact those descending influences that are conveyed more directly to the segmental motor apparatus. Nevertheless, the range of issues such as these that remain as yet unresolved makes it difficult to accept any of the prevailing theories of basal ganglia function as definitive and complete.

References

1. Middleton FA, Strick PL: Cerebellar output channels. *Int Rev Neurobiol* 41:61–82, 1997.
2. Dum RP, Strick PL: An unfolded map of the cerebellar dentate nucleus and its projections to the cerebral cortex. *J Neurophysiol* 89:634–639, 2003.
3. Wu CW, Bichot NP, Kaas JH: Converging evidence from microstimulation, architecture, and connections for multiple motor areas in the frontal and cingulate cortex of prosimian primates. *J Comp Neurol* 423:140–177, 2000.
4. Picard N, Strick PL: Motor areas of the medial wall: A review of their location and functional activation. *Cereb Cortex* 6:342–353, 1996.
5. He SQ, Dum RP, Strick PL: Topographic organization of corticospinal projections from the frontal lobe: Motor areas on the medial surface of the hemisphere. *J Neurosci* 15:3284–3306, 1995.
6. He SQ, Dum RP, Strick PL: Topographic organization of corticospinal projections from the frontal lobe: Motor areas on the lateral surface of the hemisphere. *J Neurosci* 13:952–980, 1993.
7. Geyer S, Matelli M, Luppino G, et al: Functional neuroanatomy of the primate isocortical motor system. *Anat Embryol (Berl)* 202:443–474, 2000.

8. Sakai ST, Inase M, Tanji J: Pallidal and cerebellar inputs to thalamocortical neurons projecting to the supplementary motor area in *Macaca fuscata*: A triple-labeling light microscopic study. *Anat Embryol (Berl)* 199:9–19, 1999.
9. Hoover JE, Strick PL: The organization of cerebellar and basal ganglia outputs to primary motor cortex as revealed by retrograde transneuronal transport of herpes simplex virus type 1. *J Neurosci* 19:1446–1463, 1999.
10. Matelli M, Luppino G: Thalamic input to mesial and superior area 6 in the macaque monkey. *J Comp Neurol* 372:59–87, 1996.
11. Tanne-Gariepy J, Rouiller EM, Boussaoud D: Parietal inputs to dorsal versus ventral premotor areas in the macaque monkey: Evidence for largely segregated visuomotor pathways. *Exp Brain Res* 145:91–103, 2002.
12. Johnson PB, Ferraina S, Bianchi L, et al: Cortical networks for visual reaching: Physiological and anatomical organization of frontal and parietal lobe arm regions. *Cereb Cortex* 6:102–119, 1996.
13. Luppino G, Murata A, Govoni P, et al: Largely segregated parietofrontal connections linking rostral intraparietal cortex (areas AIP and VIP) and the ventral premotor cortex (areas F5 and F4). *Exp Brain Res* 128:181–187, 1999.
14. Tokuno H, Inase M, Nambu A, et al: Corticostriatal projections from distal and proximal forelimb representations of the monkey primary motor cortex. *Neurosci Lett* 269:33–36, 1999.
15. Inase M, Tokuno H, Nambu A, et al: Corticostriatal and corticosubthalamic input zones from the presupplementary motor area in the macaque monkey: Comparison with the input zones from the supplementary motor area. *Brain Res* 833:191–201, 1999.
16. Nudo RJ, Sutherland DP, Masterton RB: Variation and evolution of mammalian corticospinal somata with special reference to primates. *J Comp Neurol* 358:181–205, 1995.
17. Fujii N, Mushiake H, Tanji J: Rostrocaudal distinction of the dorsal premotor area based on oculomotor involvement. *J Neurophysiol* 83:1764–1769, 2000.
18. Matelli M, Luppino G: Parietofrontal circuits for action and space perception in the macaque monkey. *Neuroimage* 14:S27–S32, 2001.
19. Luppino G, Rozzi S, Calzavara R, et al: Prefrontal and agranular cingulate projections to the dorsal premotor areas F2 and F7 in the macaque monkey. *Eur J Neurosci* 17:559–578, 2003.
20. Fink GR, Frackowiak RS, Pietrzyk U, et al: Multiple nonprimary motor areas in the human cortex. *J Neurophysiol* 77:2164–2174, 1997.
21. Mayer AR, Zimbelman JL, Watanabe Y, et al: Somatotopic organization of the medial wall of the cerebral hemispheres: A 3 Tesla fMRI study. *Neuroreport* 12:3811–3814, 2001.
22. Dum RP, Strick PL: Spinal cord terminations of the medial wall motor areas in macaque monkeys. *J Neurosci* 16:6513–6525, 1996.
23. Maier MA, Armand J, Kirkwood PA, et al: Differences in the corticospinal projection from primary motor cortex and supplementary motor area to macaque upper limb motoneurons: An anatomical and electrophysiological study. *Cereb Cortex* 12:281–296, 2002.
24. Galea MP, Darian-Smith I: Multiple corticospinal neuron populations in the macaque monkey are specified by their unique cortical origins, spinal terminations, and connections. *Cereb Cortex* 4:166–194, 1994.
25. Valtschanoff JG, Weinberg RJ, Rustioni A: Amino acid immunoreactivity in corticospinal terminals. *Exp Brain Res* 93:95–103, 1993.

26. Galea MP, Darian-Smith I: Postnatal maturation of the direct corticospinal projections in the macaque monkey. *Cereb Cortex* 5:518–540, 1995.

27. Bortoff GA, Strick PL: Corticospinal terminations in two new-world primates: Further evidence that corticomotoneuronal connections provide part of the neural substrate for manual dexterity. *J Neurosci* 13:5105–5118, 1993.

28. Maier MA, Illert M, Kirkwood PA, et al: Does a C3-C4 propriospinal system transmit corticospinal excitation in the primate? An investigation in the macaque monkey. *J Physiol* 511 (Pt 1):191–212, 1998.

29. Shinoda Y, Yamaguchi T, Futami T: Multiple axon collaterals of single corticospinal axons in the cat spinal cord. *J Neurophysiol* 55:425–448, 1986.

30. Luppino G, Matelli M, Camarda R, et al: Corticospinal projections from mesial frontal and cingulate areas in the monkey. *Neuroreport* 5:2545–2548, 1994.

31. McKiernan BJ, Marcario JK, Karrer JH, et al: Correlations between corticomotoneuronal (CM) cell postspike effects and cell-target muscle covariation. *J Neurophysiol* 83:99–115, 2000.

32. Fetz EE: Are movement parameters recognizably coded in activity of single neurons? *Behav Brain Sci* 15:679–690, 1992.

33. Olivier E, Baker SN, Nakajima K, et al: Investigation into non-monosynaptic corticospinal excitation of macaque upper limb single motor units. *J Neurophysiol* 86:1573–1586, 2001.

34. Lemon RN, Maier MA, Armand J, et al: Functional differences in corticospinal projections from macaque primary motor cortex and supplementary motor area. *Adv Exp Med Biol* 508:425–434, 2002.

35. Takada M, Tokuno H, Nambu A, et al: Corticostriatal projections from the somatic motor areas of the frontal cortex in the macaque monkey: Segregation versus overlap of input zones from the primary motor cortex, the supplementary motor area, and the premotor cortex. *Exp Brain Res* 120:114–128, 1998.

36. Blakemore SJ, Rees G, Frith CD: How do we predict the consequences of our actions? A functional imaging study. *Neuropsychologia* 36:521–529, 1998.

37. Shen L, Alexander GE: Neural correlates of a spatial sensory-to-motor transformation in primary motor cortex. *J Neurophysiol* 77:1171–1194, 1997.

38. Crammond DJ, Kalaska JF: Prior information in motor and premotor cortex: Activity during the delay period and effect on pre-movement activity. *J Neurophysiol* 84:986–1005, 2000.

39. Mima T, Sadato N, Yazawa S, et al: Brain structures related to active and passive finger movements in man. *Brain* 122 (Pt 10):1989–1997, 1999.

40. Kawashima R, Inoue K, Sugiura M, et al: A positron emission tomography study of self-paced finger movements at different frequencies. *Neuroscience* 92:107–112, 1999.

41. Sadato N, Ibanez V, Campbell G, et al: Frequency-dependent changes of regional cerebral blood flow during finger movements: Functional MRI compared to PET. *J Cereb Blood Flow Metab* 17:670–679, 1997.

42. Jenkins IH, Bain PG, Colebatch JG, et al: A positron emission tomography study of essential tremor: Evidence for overactivity of cerebellar connections. *Ann Neurol* 34:82–90, 1993.

43. Goodman MM, Chen P, Plisson C, et al: Synthesis and characterization of iodine-123 labeled 2beta-carbomethoxy-3beta-(4'-((Z)-2-iodoethenyl)phenyl)nortropane. A ligand for in vivo imaging of serotonin transporters by single-photon-emission tomography. *J Med Chem* 46:925–935, 2003.

44. Thobois S, Dominey PF, Decety PJ, et al: Motor imagery in normal subjects and in asymmetrical Parkinson's disease: A PET study. *Neurol* 55:996–1002, 2000.

45. Stephan KM, Fink GR, Passingham RE, et al: Functional anatomy of the mental representation of upper extremity movements in healthy subjects. *J Neurophysiol* 73:373–386, 1995.

46. Deiber MP, Ibanez V, Sadato N, et al: Cerebral structures participating in motor preparation in humans: A positron emission tomography study. *J Neurophysiol* 75: 233–247, 1996.

47. Hoshi E, Tanji J: Contrasting neuronal activity in the dorsal and ventral premotor areas during preparation to reach. *J Neurophysiol* 87:1123–1128, 2002.

48. Boussaoud D, Kermadi I: The primate striatum: neuronal activity in relation to spatial attention versus motor preparation. *Eur J Neurosci* 9:2152–2168, 1997.

49. Ochiai T, Mushiake H, Tanji J: Effects of image motion in the dorsal premotor cortex during planning of an arm movement. *J Neurophysiol* 88:2167–2171, 2002.

50. Shen L, Alexander GE: Preferential representation of instructed target location versus limb trajectory in dorsal premotor area. *J Neurophysiol* 77:1195–1212, 1997.

51. Bussey TJ, Wise SP, Murray EA: Interaction of ventral and orbital prefrontal cortex with inferotemporal cortex in conditional visuomotor learning. *Behav Neurosci* 116:703–715, 2002.

52. Simon SR, Meunier M, Piettre L, et al: Spatial attention and memory versus motor preparation: Premotor cortex involvement as revealed by fMRI. *J Neurophysiol* 88:2047–2057, 2002.

53. Grafton ST, Fagg AH, Arbib MA: Dorsal premotor cortex and conditional movement selection: A PET functional mapping study. *J Neurophysiol* 79:1092–1097, 1998.

54. Wang Y, Shima K, Isoda M, et al: Spatial distribution and density of prefrontal cortical cells projecting to three sectors of the premotor cortex. *Neuroreport* 13:1341–1344, 2002.

55. Fogassi L, Raos V, Franchi G, et al: Visual responses in the dorsal premotor area F2 of the macaque monkey. *Exp Brain Res* 128:194–199, 1999.

56. Rizzolatti G, Fogassi L, Gallese V: Motor and cognitive functions of the ventral premotor cortex. *Curr Opin Neurobiol* 12:149–154, 2002.

57. Mushiake H, Tanatsugu Y, Tanji J: Neuronal activity in the ventral part of premotor cortex during target-reach movement is modulated by direction of gaze. *J Neurophysiol* 78:567–571, 1997.

58. Freund H-J, Hummelsheim H: Lesions of premotor cortex in man. *Brain* 108:697–773, 1985.

59. Inoue K, Kawashima R, Satoh K, et al: PET study of pointing with visual feedback of moving hands. *J Neurophysiol* 79:117–125, 1998.

60. Halsband U, Freund H-J: Premotor cortex and conditional motor learning in man. *Brain* 113:207–222, 1990.

61. Freund H-J: Premotor area and preparation of movement. *Rev Neurol (Paris)* 146:543–547, 1990.

62. Kurata K, Hoshi E: Movement-related neuronal activity reflecting the transformation of coordinates in the ventral premotor cortex of monkeys. *J Neurophysiol* 88:3118–3132, 2002.

63. Dagher A, Owen AM, Boecker H, et al: Mapping the network for planning: A correlational PET activation study with the Tower of London task. *Brain* 122(Pt 10):1973–1987, 1999.

64. Zilles K, Schlaug G, Matelli M, et al: Mapping of human and macaque sensorimotor areas by integrating architectonic, transmitter receptor, MRI and PET data. *J Anat* 187:515–537, 1995.

65. Fujii N, Mushiake H, Tanji J: Distribution of eye- and arm-movement-related neuronal activity in the SEF and in the SMA and pre-SMA of monkeys. *J Neurophysiol* 87:2158–2166, 2002.

66. Shima K, Mushiake H, Saito N, et al: Role for cells in the pre-supplementary motor area in updating motor plans. *Proc Natl Acad Sci USA* 93:8694–8698, 1996.

67. Jenkins IH, Jahanshahi M, Jueptner M, et al: Self-initiated versus externally triggered movements. II. The effect of movement predictability on regional cerebral blood flow. *Brain* 123 (Pt 6):1216–1228, 2000.

68. Naito E, Ehrsson HH, Geyer S, et al: Illusory arm movements activate cortical motor areas: A positron emission tomography study. *J Neurosci* 19:6134–6144, 1999.

69. Humberstone M, Sawle GV, Clare S, et al: Functional magnetic resonance imaging of single motor events reveals human presupplementary motor area. *Ann Neurol* 42:632–637, 1997.

70. Nagao S, Kitazawa H: Subdural applications of NO scavenger or NO blocker to the cerebellum depress the adaptation of monkey post-saccadic smooth pursuit eye movements. *Neuroreport* 11:131–134, 2000.

71. Grafton ST, Waters C, Sutton J, et al: Pallidotomy increases activity of motor association cortex in Parkinson's disease: A positron emission tomographic study. *Ann Neurol* 37:776–783, 1995.

72. Samuel M, Ceballos-Baumann AO, Turjanski N, et al: Pallidotomy in Parkinson's disease increases supplementary motor area and prefrontal activation during performance of volitional movements: An H2(15)O PET study. *Brain* 120:1301–1313, 1997.

73. Tanji J: New concepts of the supplementary motor area. *Curr Opin Neurobiol* 6:782–787, 1996.

74. Strik WK, Fallgatter AJ, Brandeis D, et al: Three-dimensional tomography of event-related potentials during response inhibition: evidence for phasic frontal lobe activation. *Electroencephalogr Clin Neurophysiol* 108:406–413, 1998.

75. Neshige R, Lüders H, Shibasaki H: Recording of movement-related potentials from scalp and cortex in man. *Brain* 111:719–736, 1988.

76. Ikeda A, Luders HO, Collura TF, et al: Subdural potentials at orbitofrontal and mesial prefrontal areas accompanying anticipation and decision making in humans: a comparison with Bereitschaftspotential. *Electroencephalogr Clin Neurophysiol* 98:206–212, 1996.

77. Kermadi I, Liu Y, Tempini A, et al: Effects of reversible inactivation of the supplementary motor area (SMA) on unimanual grasp and bimanual pull and grasp performance in monkeys. *Somatosens Mot Res* 14:268–280, 1997.

78. Tanji J, Okano K, Sato KC: Neuronal activity in cortical motor areas related to ipsilateral, contralateral, and bilateral digit movements of the monkey. *J Neurophysiol* 60:325–343, 1988.

79. Aizawa H, Mushiake H, Inase M, et al: An output zone of the monkey primary motor cortex specialized for bilateral hand movement. *Exp Brain Res* 82:219–221, 1990.

80. Gerloff C, Corwell B, Chen R, et al: Stimulation over the human supplementary motor area interferes with the organization of future elements in complex motor sequences. *Brain* 120:1587–1602, 1997.

81. Nakamura K, Sakai K, Hikosaka O: Effects of local inactivation of monkey medial frontal cortex in learning of sequential procedures. *J Neurophysiol* 82:1063–1068, 1999.

82. Tanji J, Shima K: Role for supplementary motor area cells in planning several movements ahead. *Nature* 371:413–416, 1994.

83. Picard N, Strick PL: Activation on the medial wall during remembered sequences of reaching movements in monkeys. *J Neurophysiol* 77:2197–2201, 1997.

84. Boecker H, Dagher A, Ceballos-Baumann AO, et al: Role of the human rostral supplementary motor area and the basal ganglia in motor sequence control: Investigations with H2 15O PET. *J Neurophysiol* 79:1070–1080, 1998.

85. Grafton ST, Hazeltine Elvry RB: Abstract and effector-specific representations of motor sequences identified with PET. *J Neurosci* 18:9420–9428, 1998.

86. Honda M, Deiber MP, Ibanez V, et al: Dynamic cortical involvement in implicit and explicit motor sequence learning. A PET study. *Brain* 121(Pt 11):2159–2173, 1998.

87. Morecraft RJ, Louie JL, Schroeder CM, et al: Segregated parallel inputs to the brachial spinal cord from the cingulate motor cortex in the monkey. *Neuroreport* 8:3933–3938, 1997.

88. Takada M, Tokuno H, Hamada I, et al: Organization of inputs from cingulate motor areas to basal ganglia in macaque monkey. *Eur J Neurosci* 14:1633–1650, 2001.

89. Morecraft RJ, Van Hoesen GW: Convergence of limbic input to the cingulate motor cortex in the rhesus monkey. *Brain Res Bull* 45:209–232, 1998.

90. Lu M-T, Preston JB, Strick PL: Interconnections between the prefrontal cortex and the premotor areas in the frontal lobe. *J Comp Neurol* 341:375–392, 1994.

91. Bates JF, Goldman-Rakic PS: Prefrontal connections of medial motor areas in the rhesus monkey. *J Comp Neurol* 336:211–228, 1993.

92. Akkal D, Bioulac B, Audin J, et al: Comparison of neuronal activity in the rostral supplementary and cingulate motor areas during a task with cognitive and motor demands. *Eur J Neurosci* 15:887–904, 2002.

93. Russo GS, Backus DA, Ye S, et al: Neural activity in monkey dorsal and ventral cingulate motor areas: Comparison with the supplementary motor area. *J Neurophysiol* 88:2612–2629, 2002.

94. Shima K, Aya K, Mushiake H, et al: Two movement-related foci in the primate cingulate cortex observed in signal-triggered and self-paced forelimb movements. *J Neurophysiol* 65:188–202, 1991.

95. Tanji J, Shima K, Matsuzaka Y: Reward-based planning of motor selection in the rostral cingulate motor area. *Adv Exp Med Biol* 508:417–423, 2002.

96. Alexander GE, Crutcher MD, DeLong MR: Basal ganglia-thalamocortical circuits: Parallel substrates for motor, oculomotor, 'prefrontal' and 'limbic' functions. *Prog Brain Res* 85:119–146, 1990.

97. Cavada C, Goldman-Rakic PS: Topographic segregation of corticostriatal projections from posterior parietal subdivisions in the macaque monkey. *Neuroscience* 42:683–696, 1991.

98. Flaherty AW, Graybiel AM: Corticostriatal transformations in the primate somatosensory system. Projections from physiologically mapped body-part representations. *J Neurophysiol* 66:1249–1263, 1991.

99. Yeterian EH, Pandya DN: Striatal connections of the parietal association cortices in rhesus monkeys. *J Comp Neurol* 332:175–197, 1993.

100. Nambu A, Tokuno H, Inase M, et al: Corticosubthalamic input zones from forelimb representations of the dorsal and ventral divisions of the premotor cortex in the macaque monkey: Comparison with the input zones from the primary motor cortex and the supplementary motor area. *Neurosci Lett* 239:13–16, 1997.

101. Nambu A, Takada M, Inase M, et al: Dual somatotopical representations in the primate subthalamic nucleus: Evidence for ordered but reversed body-map transformations from the primary motor cortex and the supplementary motor area. *J Neurosci* 16:2671–2683, 1996.

102. Nambu A, Tokuno H, Hamada I, et al: Excitatory cortical inputs to pallidal neurons via the subthalamic nucleus in the monkey. *J Neurophysiol* 84:289–300, 2000.

103. Smith Y, Charara A, Paquet M, et al: Ionotropic and metabotropic GABA and glutamate receptors in primate basal ganglia. *J Chem Neuroanat* 22:13–42, 2001.

104. Aubert I, Ghorayeb I, Normand E, et al: Phenotypical characterization of the neurons expressing the D1 and D2 dopamine receptors in the monkey striatum. *J Comp Neurol* 418:22–32, 2000.

105. Smith Y, Bevan MD, Shink E, et al: Microcircuitry of the direct and indirect pathways of the basal ganglia. *Neuroscience* 86:353–387, 1998.

106. Crutcher MD, Alexander GE: Movement-related neuronal activity selectively coding either direction or muscle pattern in three motor areas of the monkey. *J Neurophysiol* 64:151–163, 1990.

107. Alexander GE, Crutcher MD: Preparation for movement: Neural representations of intended direction in three motor areas of the monkey. *J Neurophysiol* 64:133–150, 1990.

108. Graybiel AM, Aosaki T, Flaherty AW, et al: The basal ganglia and adaptive motor control. *Science* 265:1826–1831, 1994.

109. Aosaki T, Tsubokawa H, Ishida A, et al: Responses of tonically active neurons in the primate's striatum undergo systematic changes during behavioral sensorimotor conditioning. *J Neurosci* 14:3969–3984, 1994.

110. Kawaguchi Y, Wilson CJ, Augood SJ, et al: Striatal interneurones: Chemical, physiological and morphological characterization. *Trends Neurosci* 18:527–535, 1995.

111. Kimura M: The role of primate putamen neurons in the association of sensory stimuli with movement. *Neurosci Res* 3:436–443, 1986.

112. Kawaguchi Y, Wilson CJ, Augood SJ, et al: Striatal interneurones: Chemical, physiological and morphological characterization. *Trends Neurosci* 18:527–535, 1995.

113. Phelps PE, Houser CR, Vaughn JE: Immunocytochemical localization of choline acetyltransferase within the rat neostriatum: A correlated light and electron microscopic study of cholinergic neurons and synapses. *J Comp Neurol* 238:286–307, 1985.

114. Alcantara AA, Mrzljak L, Jakab RL, et al: Muscarinic m1 and m2 receptor proteins in local circuit and projection neurons of the primate striatum: Anatomical evidence for cholinergic modulation of glutamatergic prefronto-striatal pathways. *J Comp Neurol* 434:445–460, 2001.

115. Sakai ST, Inase M, Tanji J: The relationship between MI and SMA afferents and cerebellar and pallidal efferents in the macaque monkey. *Somatosens Mot Res* 19:139–148, 2002.

116. Francois C, Tande D, Yelnik J, et al: Distribution and morphology of nigral axons projecting to the thalamus in primates. *J Comp Neurol* 447:249–260, 2002.

117. Kultas-Ilinsky K, Reising L, Yi H, et al: Pallidal afferent territory of the *Macaca mulatta* thalamus: Neuronal and synaptic organization of the VAdc. *J Comp Neurol* 386:573–600, 1997.

118. Hardman CD, Henderson JM, Finkelstein DI, et al: Comparison of the basal ganglia in rats, marmosets, macaques, baboons, and humans: Volume and neuronal number for the output, internal relay, and striatal modulating nuclei. *J Comp Neurol* 445:238–255, 2002.

119. Inase M, Li BM, Takashima I, et al: Pallidal activity is involved in visuomotor association learning in monkeys. *Eur J Neurosci* 14:897–901, 2001.

120. Turner RS, Anderson ME: Pallidal discharge related to the kinematics of reaching movements in two dimensions. *J Neurophysiol* 77:1051–1074, 1997.

121. Bolam JP, Hanley JJ, Booth PA, et al: Synaptic organisation of the basal ganglia. *J Anat* 196(Pt 4):527–542, 2000.

122. Alexander GE, Crutcher MD: Functional architecture of basal ganglia circuits: Neural substrates of parallel processing. *Trends Neurosci* 13:266–271, 1990.

123. Shink E, Bevan MD, Bolam JP, et al: The subthalamic nucleus and the external pallidum: Two tightly interconnected structures that control the output of the basal ganglia in the monkey. *Neuroscience* 73:335–357, 1996.

124. Sato F, Parent M, Levesque M, et al: Axonal branching pattern of neurons of the subthalamic nucleus in primates. *J Comp Neurol* 424:142–152, 2000.

125. Kayahara T, Nakano K: The globus pallidus sends axons to the thalamic reticular nucleus neurons projecting to the centromedian nucleus of the thalamus: A light and electron microscope study in the cat. *Brain Res Bull* 45:623–630, 1998.

126. Hazrati L-N, Parent A: Projection from the external pallidum to the reticular thalamic nucleus in the squirrel monkey. *Brain Res* 550:142–146, 1991.

127. Jones EG: *The Thalamus*. New York: Plenum Press, 1985.

128. Charara A, Smith Y, Parent A: Glutamatergic inputs from the pedunculopontine nucleus to midbrain dopaminergic neurons in primates: *Phaseolus vulgaris*-leucoagglutinin anterograde labeling combined with postembedding glutamate and GABA immunohistochemistry. *J Comp Neurol* 364:254–266, 1996.

129. Nakano K, Hasegawa Y, Tokushige A, et al: Topographical projections from the thalamus, subthalamic nucleus and pedunculopontine tegmental nucleus to the striatum in the Japanese monkey, *Macaca fuscata. Brain Res* 537:54–68, 1990.

130. Matsumura M, Nambu A, Yamaji Y, et al: Organization of somatic motor inputs from the frontal lobe to the pedunculopontine tegmental nucleus in the macaque monkey. *Neuroscience* 98:97–110, 2000.

131. Shink E, Sidibe M, Smith Y: Efferent connections of the internal globus pallidus in the squirrel monkey: II. Topography and synaptic organization of pallidal efferents to the pedunculopontine nucleus. *J Comp Neurol* 382:348–363, 1997.

132. Nandi D, Liu X, Winter JL, et al: Deep brain stimulation of the pedunculopontine region in the normal non-human primate. *J Clin Neurosci* 9:170–174, 2002.

133. Matsumura M, Kojima J: The role of the pedunculopontine tegmental nucleus in experimental parkinsonism in primates. *Stereotact Funct Neurosurg* 77:108–115, 2001.

134. Kojima J, Yamaji Y, Matsumura M, et al: Excitotoxic lesions of the pedunculopontine tegmental nucleus produce contralateral hemiparkinsonism in the monkey. *Neurosci Lett* 226:111–114, 1997.

135. Nandi D, Aziz TZ, Giladi N, et al: Reversal of akinesia in experimental parkinsonism by GABA antagonist microinjections in the pedunculopontine nucleus. *Brain* 125:2418–2430, 2002.

136. Lavoie B, Parent A: Pedunculopontine nucleus in the squirrel monkey: Cholinergic and glutamatergic projections to the substantia nigra. *J Comp Neurol* 344:232–241, 1994.

137. Nakamura Y, Kudo M, Tokuno H: Monosynaptic projection from the pedunculopontine tegmental region to the reticulospinal neurons of the medulla oblongata: An electron microscopic study in the cat. *Brain Res* 524:353–356, 1990.

138. Rye DB, Lee HJ, Saper CB, et al: Medullary and spinal efferents of the pedunculopontine tegmental nucleus and the adjacent mesopontine tegmentum in the rat. *J Comp Neurol* 269:315–341, 1988.

139. Kincaid AE, Zheng T, Wilson CJ: Connectivity and convergence of single corticostriatal axons. *J Neurosci* 18:4722–4731, 1998.

140. Nambu A, Kaneda K, Tokuno H, et al: Organization of corticostriatal motor inputs in monkey putamen. *J Neurophysiol* 88:1830–1842, 2002.

141. Calabresi P, Centonze D, Bernardi G: Electrophysiology of dopamine in normal and denervated striatal neurons. *Trends Neurosci* 23:S57–S63, 2000.

142. Smith Y, Kieval JZ: Anatomy of the dopamine system in the basal ganglia. *Trends Neurosci* 23:S28–S33, 2000.

143. Lewis DA, Melchitzky DS, Sesack SR, et al: Dopamine transporter immunoreactivity in monkey cerebral cortex: Regional, laminar, and ultrastructural localization. *J Comp Neurol* 432:119–136, 2001.

144. Freeman A, Ciliax B, Bakay R, et al: Nigrostriatal collaterals to thalamus degenerate in parkinsonian animal models. *Ann Neurol* 50:321–329, 2001.

145. Calabresi P, Gubellini P, Centonze D, et al: Dopamine and cAMP-regulated phosphoprotein 32 kDa controls both striatal long-term depression and long-term potentiation, opposing forms of synaptic plasticity. *J Neurosci* 20:8443–8451, 2000.

146. Watanabe K, Kimura M: Dopamine receptor-mediated mechanisms involved in the expression of learned activity of primate striatal neurons. *J Neurophysiol* 79:2568–2580, 1998.

147. Descarries L, Watkins KC, Garcia S, et al: Dual character, asynaptic and synaptic, of the dopamine innervation in adult rat neostriatum: A quantitative autoradiographic and immunocytochemical analysis. *J Comp Neurol* 375:167–186, 1996.

148. Hersch SM, Ciliax BJ, Gutekunst CA, et al: Electron microscopic analysis of D1 and D2 dopamine receptor proteins in the dorsal striatum and their synaptic relationships with motor corticostriatal afferents. *J Neurosci* 15:5222–5237, 1995.

149. Doucet G, Descarries L, Garcia S: Quantification of the dopamine innervation in adult rat neostriatum. *Neuroscience* 19:427–445, 1986.

150. Hollerman JR, Schultz W: Dopamine neurons report an error in the temporal prediction of reward during learning. *Nat Neurosci* 1:304–309, 1998.

151. Schultz W, Dayan P, Montague PR: A neural substrate of prediction and reward. *Science* 275:1593–1599, 1997.

152. Schultz W, Romo R: Dopamine neurons of the monkey midbrain: Contingencies of responses to stimuli eliciting immediate behavioral reactions. *J Neurophysiol* 63:607–624, 1990.

153. Hikosaka O, Wurtz RH: Modification of saccadic eye movements by GABA-related substances. II. Effects of muscimol in monkey substantia nigra pars reticulata. *J Neurophysiol* 53:292–308, 1985.

154. Yung KK, Smith AD, Levey AI, et al: Synaptic connections between spiny neurons of the direct and indirect pathways in the neostriatum of the rat: Evidence from dopamine receptor and neuropeptide immunostaining. *Eur J Neurosci* 8:861–869, 1996.

155. Tunstall MJ, Oorschot DE, Kean A, et al: Inhibitory interactions between spiny projection neurons in the rat striatum. *J Neurophysiol* 88:1263–1269, 2002.

156. Bolam JP, Smith Y: The striatum and the globus pallidus send convergent synaptic inputs onto single cells in the entopeduncular nucleus of the rat: A double anterograde labelling study combined with postembedding immunocytochemistry for GABA. *J Comp Neurol* 321:456–476, 1992.

157. Brooks DJ: Imaging basal ganglia function. *J Anat* 196(Pt 4):543–554, 2000.

158. Samuel M, Caputo E, Brooks DJ, et al: A study of medial pallidotomy for Parkinson's disease: Clinical outcome, MRI location and complications. *Brain* 121:59–75, 1998.

159. Baron MS, Vitek JL, Bakay RA, et al: Treatment of advanced Parkinson's disease by posterior GPi pallidotomy: 1-year results of a pilot study. *Ann Neurol* 40:355–366, 1996.

160. Vitek JL, Giroux M: Physiology of hypokinetic and hyperkinetic movement disorders: Model for dyskinesia. *Ann Neurol* 47:S131–S140, 2000.

161. Krack P, Pollak P, Limousin P, et al: Opposite motor effects of pallidal stimulation in Parkinson's disease. *Ann Neurol* 43:180–192, 1998.

Chapter 6

PHYSIOLOGY OF THE BASAL GANGLIA AND PATHOPHYSIOLOGY OF MOVEMENT DISORDERS OF BASAL GANGLIA ORIGIN

THOMAS WICHMANN and MAHLON R. DELONG

ANATOMY OF THE BASAL GANGLIA   101
FUNCTIONAL CONSIDERATIONS   102
    Motor Functions of the Basal Ganglia   102
    Segregation Versus Convergence   102
    "Scaling" versus "Focusing"   103
    Motor Subcircuits   103
MOVEMENT DISORDERS   104
    Hypokinetic Movement Disorders   104
    Hyperkinetic Movement Disorders   106
CONCLUSION   108

The basal ganglia are implicated in the pathophysiology of a wide spectrum of movement disorders. In recent years, significant advances have led to major insights into the anatomy and function of the basal ganglia and into the pathophysiology of disorders that involve these structures. In this chapters the anatomy and physiology of the basal ganglia and the pathophysiologic mechanisms underlying hypo- and hyperkinetic movement disorders are considered.

Anatomy of the Basal Ganglia

Anatomic and physiologic studies indicate that the basal ganglia are components of larger segregated circuits, which also involve parts of the cortex and thalamus.[1–3] These circuits appear to be similarly organized in anatomical terms, and have been named according to the presumed functions of their cortical areas of origin. In the monkey, functionally segregated "motor," "oculomotor," "associative," and "limbic" circuits have been identified. Each of these circuits originates in a specific cortical area, passes through separate portions of the basal ganglia and thalamus, and then projects back onto the original cortical area. In each of these circuits, the striatum functions as the "input" stage of the basal ganglia, whereas the internal segment of the globus pallidus (GPi) and the pars reticulata of the substantia nigra (SNr) serve as output stations.

The motor manifestations of movement disorders appear to result from disturbances in the "motor" circuit. This circuit comprises pre- and postcentral sensorimotor fields, motor territories of the basal ganglia, and portions of the thalamus. Cortical projections from the sensorimotor fields terminate largely in the postcommissural putamen, the motor portion of the striatum (Fig. 6-1). Putamenal output is in turn directed towards motor portions of GPi/SNr via two pathways: a "direct," monosynaptic, pathway from the putamen to motor portions of GPi/SNr, and an "indirect" pathway passing through the motor areas of the external pallidal segment (GPe) and the subthalamic nucleus (STN). Although it appears that different populations of neurons in STN innervate GPi and SNr (e.g., Ref.[4]), these connections are generally considered functionally similar. There are also direct reciprocal connections between GPe and GPi/SNr that circumvent the STN (e.g., Ref.[5]). GPi/SNr motor output is in large part directed towards the ventral anterior (VA) and ventrolateral (VL) nucleus of the thalamus and the intralaminar nuclei of the thalamus (i.e., the centromedian and parafascicular nuclei), where it influences the activity of thalamocortical projection neurons. Additional movement-related projections reach midbrain nuclei, in particular the pedunculopontine nucleus (PPN), which may offer direct access of basal ganglia output to bulbar and spinal cord centers, circumventing the cortex. With the exception of the excitatory (glutamatergic) projection between STN and GPi/SNr, the intrinsic connections of the basal ganglia, as well as their output to thalamus, superior colliculus and midbrain are all inhibitory and GABAergic.

Release of dopamine from terminals of the nigrostriatal projection, which arises from the substantia nigra pars compacta (SNc), appears to facilitate transmission over the direct pathway via activation of D1 receptors and to inhibit transmission over the indirect pathway via activation of D2 receptors (e.g., Ref.[6,7]). Both D1 and D2 receptors are located on dendritic spines of striatal output neurons which receive cortical input. This location enables dopamine released in the striatum to modulate corticostriatal transmission. The overall effect of dopamine released in the striatum appears to be a reduction of basal ganglia output, leading, by disinhibition, to increased activity of thalamocortical projection neurons, and a facilitation of movement. Conversely, reduction of striatal dopamine, as occurs in parkinsonism, should increase basal ganglia outflow and inhibit movement. In addition, basal ganglia output may be modulated by extrastriatal release of dopamine. For example, SNc sends dopaminergic projections to STN, GPi, and thalamus,[8] and dopamine may reach the SNr via dendritic release (e.g., Refs.[9–11]). In these nuclei, dopamine may act presynaptically on striatal efferents or postsynaptically on output neurons.

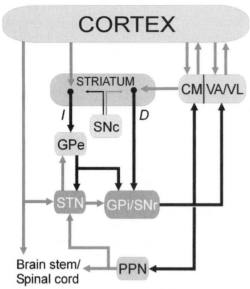

FIGURE 6-1 Schematic diagram of the basal ganglia-thalamocortical circuitry under normal conditions. Inhibitory connections are shown as filled arrows, excitatory connections as open arrows. D, direct pathway; I, indirect pathway; GPe, external segment of the globus pallidus; GPi, internal segment of the globus pallidus; SNr, substantia nigra, pars reticulata; SNc, substantia nigra, pars compacta; STN, subthalamic nucleus; VA, ventral anterior thalamus; VL, ventrolateral thalamus, CM, centromedian nucleus; PPN, pedunculopontine nucleus.

Functional Considerations

By virtue of their anatomical connections, the basal ganglia are likely involved in the modulation and fine-tuning of the activity of large portions of the frontal cortex, having a role in the control of movements, and in limbic and associative functions. The anatomic similarities between the different cortical-basal ganglia-thalamocortical circuits suggest that the function of the basal ganglia in the different circuits is also similar. Among the circuits passing through the basal ganglia, the motor circuit has been studied most extensively because of its possible involvement in the pathophysiology of movement disorders.

MOTOR FUNCTIONS OF THE BASAL GANGLIA

Although the basal ganglia have been implicated in a wide variety of motor functions, including the planning, initiation and execution of movements, the evidence from behavioral studies in animals and man for a specific role of the basal ganglia in the control of movement is not entirely conclusive. Many speculations regarding the role of the basal ganglia in the control of normal behavior have been based on the study of deficits arising from functional or structural abnormalities affecting the basal ganglia. For instance, a role of the

basal ganglia in initiation of movement is suggested by the severe disturbance of this in Parkinson's disease (PD) (i.e., akinesia), although support for this from animal experiments is lacking. Similarly, a role of the basal ganglia in movement execution as suggested by the development of bradykinesia in parkinsonian subjects is not firmly established because data from lesions in animals and man are inconsistent regarding this point (see, e.g., Refs.[12–19]). A role of the basal ganglia in the control of sequential or simultaneous movements has been inferred from the fact that parkinsonian patients do poorly in motor tasks that involve such movements.[20–25] More recently, it was shown that such patients appear to rely more on external cues when performing these movements than normal controls. This led to the hypothesis that the basal ganglia-thalamocortical circuitry may have a role in the generation or use of internally cued sequential or simultaneous movements.[21–23] Similarly, observations of deficits in parkinsonian patients have also been used to argue for a role of the basal ganglia in the execution of learned movements (e.g., Refs.[26,27]).

While these findings clearly establish a role of the basal ganglia in the development of movement disorders, they do not by themselves constitute evidence for a role of these structures in the control of normal movement, because abnormal basal ganglia output may simply disrupt cortical activity nonspecifically. For instance, it has always been puzzling that lesions of the basal ganglia outflow nuclei have relatively minor long-term effects on motor performance.[12,13,19,28,29] Although this finding may be explainable by the action of compensatory mechanisms, and thus may not negate a "motor function" of the basal ganglia, it indicates that these structures are not essential in motor control.

More direct evidence for involvement of these structures in the control of normal movement comes from electrophysiologic studies recording the discharge of single basal ganglia neurons. Such studies have indeed shown that many neurons in the basal ganglia exhibit discharge correlated with certain parameters of limb movements, such as amplitude, velocity, or direction (e.g., Refs.[30–33]). Although mostly correlative and thus inadequate to establish a causal relationship between basal ganglia discharge and aspects of behavior, these studies still provide the best available insights into basal ganglia function, and the considerations outlined below therefore largely focus on results from these experiments.

SEGREGATION VERSUS CONVERGENCE

The apparent parallel organization of basal ganglia-thalamocortical pathways and the paucity of interneurons or axon collaterals in the basal ganglia nuclei (e.g., Refs.[34–37]) suggest that the flow of information in the different circuits remains largely segregated. Indeed, electrophysiologic recording studies have shown that the discharge of individual neurons in the basal ganglia in a wide variety of behavioral paradigms does not appear to contain new information or extract features that were not already apparent in the discharge of the respective cortical source regions. On the other hand, it is almost certain that integration of inputs takes place within the basal ganglia, because the number of striatal neurons receiving cortical afferents is much smaller than the number of cortical neurons sending these projections, and the number of output neurons in the striatum in turn is larger than the number of target neurons in GP/SN. Pallidal neurons have large dendritic fields which are traversed by a multitude of striatal efferent fibers,[35,38] an arrangement that may form the anatomical basis for convergence. This "funneling" of information may permit recombination of cortical inputs which may serve as an important mechanism of modulation of cortical activity.

Under physiologic conditions, most neurons in the basal ganglia output nuclei appear to respond to a narrow range of input stimuli, which suggests that convergence may not play an important role in normal basal ganglia function. This view is further supported by crosscorrelation studies that show that the discharge of neighboring pallidal neurons is not correlated.[39,40] Recording in monkeys depleted of dopamine supply to the basal ganglia, however, has shown that, compared to the normal state, motor-related neurons in both segments of the GP and in STN lose some specificity for individual movements, and that the degree of synchrony between neighboring neurons is increased.[39,41–44] This suggests that dopamine may help to maintain segregation between the different circuits passing through the basal ganglia. Segregation of basal ganglia circuits, as well as channels within individual circuits, may thus be a dynamic rather than static phenomenon with dopamine playing a gatekeeper role in maintaining specificity. It is unknown whether this role is restricted to striatal dopamine, or may extend to extrastriatal dopamine or even to other neuromodulators in the basal ganglia (such as serotonin).

"SCALING" VERSUS "FOCUSING"

Tonic high-frequency inhibitory output of motor areas of the basal ganglia to the thalamus is thought to restrain the overall amount of movements to the appropriate amount. Facilitation of a particular desired movement is likely the result of phasic reduction of basal ganglia output, leading to a (brief) disinhibition of thalamocortical neurons (e.g., Ref.[45]). Given the polarities of connections in the motor circuit, this disinhibition should primarily be the result of the transmission of phasic cortical inputs to striatal neurons that give rise to the direct pathway (e.g., Ref.[46]). In contrast, phasic activity over the indirect pathway should lead to increased GPi/SNr discharge,[46] and to further suppression of thalamocortical neurons and movement.

The temporal interplay between the activity of direct and indirect inputs to the basal ganglia output nuclei may give the basal ganglia a role in influencing characteristics of movements as they are carried out. The basal ganglia may thus act

to scale certain movement parameters such as amplitude or velocity ("scaling" hypothesis). The motor circuit may also act to compare phasic neuronal responses, that reflect processed efferent copies of motor commands from precentral motor areas, with proprioceptive feedback. A signal from this comparator would then be projected back to the precentral motor areas via the thalamus. In this case the motor circuit would scale movements by constraining motor commands within desired limits.

In addition, basal ganglia output may act to focus the cortical selection of movements ("focusing" hypothesis; see, e.g., Refs.[19,47,48]) by facilitation of intended movements, and inhibition of related but unwanted ones involving the same or nearby joints. A potential anatomic substrate for such a "center-surround" mechanism has been proposed[49] based on the finding that STN efferents to GPi may terminate broadly, whereas the direct putamen-GPi projection may terminate more specifically on individual pallidal cells. More recent data, however, argue in favor of a more specific manner of arborization of subthalamopallidal efferents.[50,51] By amplifying phasic activity both in the direct and in the indirect pathway (i.e., by providing a "gain" higher than 1), the contribution of the basal ganglia in the "focusing" model would be to sharpen the contrast in activity between cortical areas that govern wanted and unwanted movements, and thereby to stabilize and select individual movements. It is clear, however, that the vast majority of neurons in the basal ganglia do *not* alter their discharge during initiation or execution of individual movements. For instance, with intended elbow flexion, neurons related to orofacial or leg movements are not likely to discharge. This implies that the "focusing" action (if it exists) would be limited to a rather small number of neurons that are concerned with the particular motor activity under way.

MOTOR SUBCIRCUITS

Combined single-cell/behavioral studies in primates have shown that discharge of basal ganglia neurons in the motor territory of the basal ganglia in relation to movement is heterogeneous, primarily with regard to the timing of discharge in relation to behavioral events. This may not only be due to technical or species differences, but may also be explainable by the observation from recent anatomic and physiologic studies[52–58] that the motor circuit encompasses several segregated subcircuits, that emanate from different cortical areas (such as supplementary motor area (SMA), and arcuate premotor area). The function of these cortical areas, and thus the function of the associated motor subcircuits, may differ, and such differences may determine discharge characteristics of individual associated basal ganglia neurons, such as the timing of neuronal discharge in relation to movement. Neuronal activity related to execution or termination of movement may be more commonly found in neurons belonging to a subcircuit originating in the primary motor cortex.[58] In contrast, discharge of basal ganglia neurons that discharge long prior to onset of movement and EMG activity ("preparatory discharge")[59–63] may predominate in basal ganglia neurons that belong to a subcircuit that originates in SMA or other mesial motor areas. Such preparatory or "set"-related activity may encode certain characteristics of the upcoming movement, such as the direction, amplitude, or target location, or may be related to spatial memory, attention, or other factors.

It should be clear from these considerations that a role of the basal ganglia in motor control is likely, but that most evidence for specific functions is indirect, allowing no firm conclusions regarding the precise role of these structures in planning, execution or termination of movement.

Movement Disorders

In recent years, significant progress has been made in understanding the pathophysiologic mechanisms underlying the major movement disorders of basal ganglia origin. This group of disorders involves disruption of the delicate balance between the activity of the direct and the indirect pathways which appears to characterize the normal state. *Hypokinetic* movement disorders are thought to arise from a relative preponderance of activity of the indirect pathway, leading to an increase of (inhibitory) basal ganglia output to the thalamus. Conversely, *hyperkinetic* disorders are likely due to a shift of the balance towards the direct pathway, leading to reduced basal ganglia output.

HYPOKINETIC MOVEMENT DISORDERS

GENERAL PATHOPHYSIOLOGIC MODEL

Parkinson's disease (PD) is the prototypic hypokinetic movement disorder. Clinically, parkinsonism is characterized by the tetrad of akinesia, bradykinesia, rigidity, and tremor. The term "akinesia" is defined as poverty of movement, secondary to impaired movement initiation. "Bradykinesia" refers to slowness of movement, and "rigidity" to increased resistance to passive stretch. Parkinsonian tremor consists of low-frequency oscillations, mainly occurring at rest. Pathologically, it is characterized by degeneration of the dopaminergic nigrostriatal projection. Study of the pathophysiologic mechanisms resulting from degeneration of nigrostriatal fibers has been greatly facilitated by the introduction of an animal model that reproduces many of the pathologic and behavioral abnormalities of human parkinsonism—i.e., the primate treated with 1-methyl-4-phenyl-1,2,3,6-tetrahydropyridine (MPTP).[2,42,64,65]

Recent electrophysiologic experiments and studies of the metabolic activity in the basal ganglia of such monkeys suggest that loss of dopaminergic input to the striatum leads to overall increased activation of the indirect pathway, and decreased activity in the direct pathway (Fig. 6-2). Both changes result in increased basal ganglia output to the thalamus, leading to increased inhibition of thalamocortical neurons. In accordance with this, microelectrode recording has shown that the tonic activity in GPe is decreased, whereas the neuronal activity in STN and GPi[41–43,66] is increased relative to pre-MPTP levels. In support of the concept that increased output from the basal ganglia motor circuit is important in

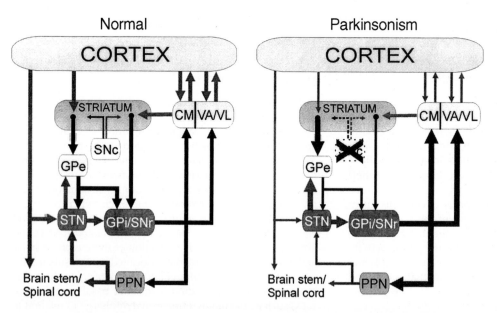

FIGURE 6-2 Activity changes in the basal ganglia-thalamocortical circuitry in Parkinson's disease. Degeneration of the nigrostriatal pathway leads to differential changes in the two striatopallidal projections, indicated by the thickness of the connecting arrows (cf. Fig. 6-1). Basal ganglia output to the thalamus is increased. For abbreviations see legend to Fig. 6-1.

parkinsonian pathophysiology, inactivation of motor portions of STN or GPi markedly ameliorates parkinsonian motor signs.[64,67–70]

In addition to the above-mentioned changes in overall basal ganglia activity, phasic neuronal responses to joint manipulation in STN, GPi and thalamus[41–43,71] occur more often, are more pronounced and show widened receptive fields after treatment with MPTP. There is also a marked change in the synchrony of discharge in the basal ganglia. Crosscorrelation studies have revealed that a substantial proportion of neighboring neurons in globus pallidus and STN discharge in unison in MPTP-treated primates.[43] This is in contrast to the virtual absence of synchronized discharge of such neurons in normal monkeys (e.g., Ref.[40]).

Following the encouraging results of lesions of the basal ganglia output structures on parkinsonian signs in MPTP-treated primates, stereotactic lesioning of these nuclei has recently been reintroduced as a treatment for PD.[72–77] This has offered an opportunity to directly study some of the abnormalities as they occur in the human disorder. Thus, electrophysiologic recording during these procedures has revealed that neuronal discharge rates in GPi are increased relative to GPe and are characterized by frequent burst discharges and a high degree of synchronous discharge of neighboring neurons (although studies in normal controls are not feasible, of course).[78,79]

The clinical results of these new lesioning strategies also support the concept that Parkinson's disease is characterized by increased basal ganglia output. For instance, GPi lesions have been shown to be remarkably effective in the amelioration of parkinsonian signs as well as drug-induced dyskinesias and motor fluctuations.[72–77] Positron emission tomography (PET) studies have demonstrated that the decreased cortical activation seen in parkinsonian patients is at least partially resolved after stereotactic pallidotomy, concomitant to recovery of motor function.[75,80,81]

AKINESIA, BRADYKINESIA, RIGIDITY

Akinesia, usually the earliest signs of parkinsonism in MPTP-treated primates, is seen after doses of the neurotoxin small enough to damage almost exclusively the dopamine supply to the striatum, making it very likely that most parkinsonian abnormalities result from dopamine loss in the basal ganglia. In all stages of parkinsonism, most importantly in the earliest, dopamine depletion is consistently greatest in the sensorimotor territory of the striatum, the putamen, which implicates abnormalities in the motor circuit in the development of parkinsonism. This is further supported by recent PET studies of preclinical and clinical parkinsonian patients,[82] in which reduced putaminal ^{18}F-dopa uptake has consistently been the earliest sign of striatal dopamine deficiency, with relative sparing of the dopaminergic innervation to other striatal areas. The involvement of the motor circuit is also supported by the finding that lesions or inactivation of the motor territory within the GP and the STN strikingly ameliorate

parkinsonian signs, including akinesia, bradykinesia, and rigidity.[64,67,72–76,80,81,83,84]

The changes in tonic and phasic activity of basal ganglia output (see above) are probably transmitted via cortical motor areas to result in akinesia, bradykinesia, and rigidity. Increased tonic inhibition of thalamocortical neurons by excessive output from GPi/SNr may reduce the responsiveness of cortical mechanisms involved in motor control and may prevent the faithful transmission to the cortex of superimposed phasic reductions in activity that occur during movement execution, which may interfere with the normal scaling of movement. Increased *tonic* inhibition of thalamocortical neurons by increased basal ganglia output in parkinsonism may also render precentral motor areas less responsive to other inputs normally involved in initiating movements or may interfere with "set" functions that have been shown to be highly dependent on the integrity of basal ganglia pathways.[85] Increased gain in the feedback from proprioceptors, reflected by increased *phasic* activity in the basal ganglia, may signal excessive movement or velocity to precentral motor areas, leading to a slowing or premature arrest of ongoing movements, and to greater reliance upon external clues during movement.

Some evidence for the involvement of abnormal activity in cortical areas that belong to the motor circuit and are presumably related to motor planning comes from studies of the Bereitschaftspotential (readiness potential), a slow negative cortical potential that precedes self-paced movements and is thought to reflect the neural activity in SMA.[86] The early portion of the Bereitschaftspotential is smaller in parkinsonian patients than in age-matched controls,[86,87] suggesting a deficit in the normal function of the SMA in the early stages of preparation for self-initiated movements. PET studies of cerebral blood flow in human patients have revealed that dopamine loss in the striatum leads to decreased blood flow (thus, by inference, reduced synaptic activity) in the SMA, motor cortex, and dorsolateral prefrontal cortex (e.g., Refs.[75,80–82,88–91]).

Although the pathophysiologic changes in basal ganglia discharge that underlie akinesia, bradykinesia and rigidity are thought to be the same in general terms (i.e., changes of tonic or phasic basal ganglia output), the expression of these signs may depend on abnormalities in different motor subcircuits. Conceivably, akinesia, a defect in movement preparation and initiation, may be related to abnormal discharge in the subcircuit whose activity is mostly "preparatory" (i.e., the subcircuit emanating from SMA, and mesial cortical motor areas). In contrast, bradykinesia and rigidity may result from abnormalities in the subcircuit arising from primary motor cortex (see, e.g., discussion in Refs.[54,55]).

The concept that increased inhibition of thalamocortical neurons by increased output from GPi/SNr will ultimately result in akinesia is probably too simplistic, because lesions of the areas of the thalamus that receive basal ganglia input (VL/VA) do not result in akinesia (e.g., Refs.[92–94]). Abnormal basal ganglia output to targets other than the thalamus (e.g., the PPN) may therefore also play a role in the development of akinesia.

TREMOR

Although tremor in PD has been largely considered as a result of thalamic oscillatory discharge, it has more recently been linked to abnormal discharge in the basal ganglia (e.g., Ref.[95]). This possibility is in large part based on the observation that surgical interruption of pallidal outflow either by disruption of pallidal efferents or by lesions of GPi can produce lasting relief of tremor in parkinsonian patients,[83,96,97] and that lesions of the STN in MPTP-treated African green monkeys reduce tremor significantly.[64] This may be explainable by increased tonic basal ganglia output to the thalamus, which may promote oscillatory activity through increased hyperpolarization in that nucleus.[98,99] This tendency for rhythmic oscillations of thalamocortical neurons may be further enhanced by periodic bursting in reticular thalamus during moments of immobility. Alternatively, loss of dopamine in the basal ganglia output nuclei (GPi/SNr) rather than the striatum may be important in the generation of tremor (discussed in Refs.[68,100,101]). Loss of dopamine in the basal ganglia may lead to unmasking of pacemaker-like properties in the basal ganglia nuclei which have been demonstrated by intracellular recordings from GP in brain slices from adult guinea pigs when the recorded cells were abruptly depolarized from a hyperpolarized membrane potential.[102] Internuclear interactions, such as the 'GPe- STN' pacemaker[103] may also contribute to the generation of oscillatory activity in the basal ganglia (see also discussion in Ref.[104]). Bursts of spikes synchronous with visible tremor have also been recorded in the STN and GPi of MPTP-treated monkeys[41,43] and in parkinsonian patients undergoing pallidotomy (e.g., Refs.[78,79]). Interestingly, oscillatory discharge is not a prominent feature of striatal discharge in parkinsonian animals, suggesting that the oscillations seen in the basal ganglia output pathways may result from abnormalities of the extrastriatal basal ganglia themselves, or may reach the basal ganglia via the corticosubthalamic pathway. Oscillatory activity in motor areas of the basal ganglia output nuclei or the thalamus will eventually lead to rhythmic activity in thalamocortical cells, which in turn may lead to oscillations in corticospinal projection neurons. In parkinsonian patients undergoing stereotactic thalamotomy, neurons discharging at the parkinsonian tremor frequency have indeed been detected in areas of the thalamus that receive basal ganglia input (discussed in Ref.[105]).

NONMOTOR PHENOMENA

PD clearly encompasses more than motor phenomena. Although a detailed discussion of the pathogenesis of nonmotor signs of parkinsonism is beyond the scope of this chapter, it is likely that these abnormalities rely on abnormal discharge in nonmotor circuits of the basal ganglia which may be affected by dopamine loss in much the same way as the motor circuit. For instance, oculomotor abnormalities appear to be the result of dopaminergic loss in the "oculomotor" basal ganglia-thalamocortical circuit.[106] Similarly, some of the cognitive and psychiatric disturbances seen in parkinsonian patients are reminiscent of syndromes seen after lesions of the dorsolateral prefrontal cortex (problems with executive functions) or of the anterior cingulate (apathy, personality changes). These symptoms may be the result of loss of dopamine in the dorsolateral or ventral caudate nucleus, respectively.[107] Finally, disturbance of the normal function of cortical-basal ganglia-thalamocortical circuits has also been implicated in the occurrence of obsessive-compulsive symptoms in some parkinsonian patients, as well as in patients with other diseases of presumed basal ganglia origin, such as Tourette's disease.[108–111]

HYPERKINETIC MOVEMENT DISORDERS

In general, hyperkinetic disorders are thought to arise from pathophysiologic changes that are opposite from those seen in PD. The main hyperkinetic symptoms (chorea, ballismus, and dystonia) may all be characterized by reduced basal ganglia output to the thalamus, leading to disinhibition of thalamocortical neurons, which in turn leads to the development of involuntary movements. The term chorea refers to discrete involuntary arrhythmic jerky movements, whereas ballismus refers to more proximal involuntary movements, resembling throwing motions of larger amplitude. The term dystonia refers to slower, more sustained movements and abnormal postures with co-contraction of antagonist muscles.

HEMIBALLISM

In the majority of cases hemiballism results from lesions involving the STN.[112–117] In terms of the anatomic model outlined above, such lesions interrupt the indirect pathway, leaving activity along the direct pathway unopposed (Fig. 6-3). This leads to the development of involuntary movements. Electrophysiologic experiments have directly demonstrated that fiber-sparing STN lesions result in reduced activity in both GPi and GPe, concomitant with the development of chorea, and that the proportion of cells that respond to somatosensory examination with increases in discharge is dramatically reduced in both nuclei under these conditions.[118]

HUNTINGTON'S DISEASE (HD)

HD is the classic basal ganglia disorder characterized by chorea. Pathologically, striatal projection neurons degenerate in this disorder. This process, however, is not random, but follows a sequence in most patients, which allows chorea to develop. It is postulated that striatal output neurons projecting to GPe are preferentially affected, leading to reduced inhibition of neurons in that nucleus, and, subsequently, increased inhibition of STN neurons, resulting in decreased GPi output, the hallmark of hyperkinetic disorders. In later

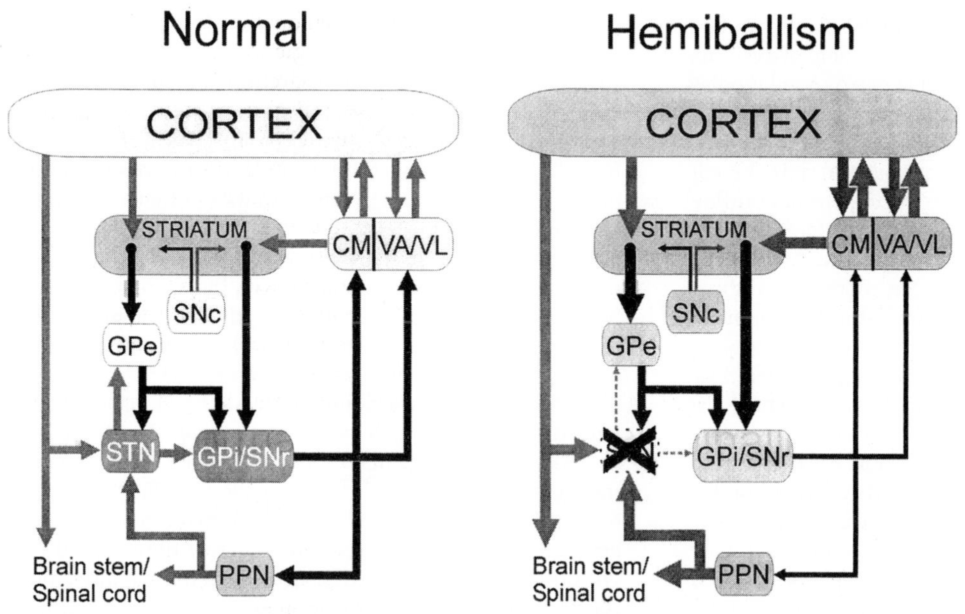

Normal   Hemiballism

FIGURE 6-3 Activity changes in the basal ganglia-thalamocortical circuitry in hemiballism. Hemiballism, as all other hyperkinetic movement disorders, is characterized by a net reduction in basal ganglia output to the thalamus. For abbreviations see legend to Fig. 6-1.

stages of the disease, inhibitory striatal output neurons to GPi also degenerate, which results in disinhibition of GPi neurons. Increased activity of GPi neurons will reduce the amount of chorea, and may later even lead to the development of parkinsonian features.

DRUG-INDUCED DYSKINESIAS

Chronic administration of dopaminergic drugs to parkinsonian patients may lead to the development of dyskinesias by shifting the balance between direct and indirect pathway towards the direct pathway, resulting in decreased basal ganglia output. Dopamine receptor activation may result in activation of the direct pathway (via dopamine D1 receptors), and inhibition of the putamen-GPe connection (part of the indirect pathway, via D2 receptors). Both changes will again lead to reduced basal ganglia output, and presumably to increased activity of thalamocortical neurons. It has been shown in MPTP-treated primates that dopaminergic drugs reduce pallidal discharge, and that drug-induced dyskinesias appear when pallidal activity is reduced to very low levels.[119,120] It is unknown why this phenomenon occurs predominantly after previous damage to the nigrostriatal system (PD) and prolonged exposure to dopaminergic agonists. Compensatory changes in dopamine receptor number or binding characteristics in response to dopamine depletion may be essential for this phenomenon.[121]

DYSTONIA

The pathophysiology of dystonia is less well understood than the pathophysiology of chorea. This is in part due to the fact that the term dystonia describes a symptom which may arise from a variety of probably unrelated disease processes, such as basal ganglia diseases, but also cerebellar[122–124] or brainstem disorders.[124,125] Dystonia of basal ganglia origin often develops after focal striatal lesions, particularly of the putamen, often weeks or months after the inciting basal ganglia lesion, suggesting that it results from secondary changes rather than from the primary lesion. Thus, compensatory changes in the affinity or number of dopamine receptors in the remainder of the striatum, or a reorganization of striatal topography may eventually lead to changes in the activity of the other basal ganglia structures. Dystonia is often seen in the context of parkinsonism, and a subgroup of patients with dystonia will respond to treatment with L-dopa (e.g., Refs.[126,127]). In most cases, however, damage to the nigrostriatal tract is probably not necessary for the development of dystonia (see, e.g., discussion in Ref.[128]). Rather, dystonia appears to develop frequently in individuals who have been exposed to dopaminergic drugs. There is no consensus whether stimulation of D1 receptors, D2 receptors, or both, is needed for dystonia to occur. In cases in which dystonia results from lesions affecting the striatum or its dopaminergic supply (see, e.g., Ref.[129]), such lesions may affect the affinity or number of dopamine receptors in the unlesioned portion of the striatum, or may lead to reorganization of striatal topography, resulting eventually in altered activity in the basal ganglia output structures.

Metabolic studies in dystonic primates have suggested that dystonia may be associated with reduction of activity along the putamen-GPe connection, and increased inhibition of STN and GPi by GPe efferents.[130,131] Pharmacologic studies suggest that abnormalities in both the indirect and the direct pathway are important in the development of dystonia. For instance, it has been shown that D2 receptor antagonists have a substantial potential of inducing dystonia, presumably by increasing striatal outflow to GPe via the indirect pathway, whereas D1 receptor antagonists may be beneficial in this regard, presumably by reducing striatal outflow to GPi along the direct pathway.[132,133] By inference, these data suggest that a relative increase in the activity along the direct pathway (compared to that along the indirect pathway) may strongly contribute to dystonia. Supporting this concept, recent recording studies in patients undergoing pallidotomy as treatment of dystonia demonstrated lowered average discharge rates in both pallidal segments,[134] in contrast to parkinsonian patients in whom discharge rates in GPi are increased.[135–137] The reduction of discharge in GPe alone would lead to increased GPi discharge. The fact that discharge rates in GPi are, in fact, reduced, argues for additional overactivity of the direct (inhibitory) pathway. The phasic responsiveness of pallidal neurons to somatosensory stimuli in both parkinsonism and dystonia is similar, with increased responses in both cases and with greater synchronicity between neighboring pallidal neurons.

Recent PET studies in dystonic patients have demonstrated widespread changes in the activity of prefrontal areas.[138–141] Physiologic studies have also provided considerable evidence that dystonia is associated with increased excitability of motor areas (particularly the SMA), likely due to widespread decrease in cortical inhibition.[142–145]

These findings suggest that parkinsonism and dystonia differ with regard to the level of activity in the direct pathway, but have in common increased activity along the indirect pathway, as well as increased phasic responsiveness and synchronization of pallidal discharge. From these considerations, it appears that the pathophysiology of dystonia may represent a combination of features of hyper- and hypokinetic disorders.

Conclusion

Although the evidence from animal experiments and ablative procedures in man has lent support to a model of normal function and the pathophysiologic considerations outlined above, the models clearly fall short of "explaining" the role of the basal ganglia in voluntary movement and movement disorders. The reason for this lies in the unavailability of feasible methods to clearly establish the physiologic function of the basal ganglia in motor control. As mentioned above, the most powerful tool for studies of this kind, single-cell recording studies in behaving primates, helps to support anatomical concepts of the basal ganglia circuitry, but cannot establish a clear motor function because they are correlative. The study of deficits that result from basal ganglia abnormalities also fails in this regard, because studies on individuals

with such disorders demonstrate merely that altered basal ganglia output disturbs motor performance, but not that these structures are important for normal movement. Furthermore, movement disorders such as PD affect not only the basal ganglia, but also cortical and other subcortical regions (e.g., Refs.[146–148]), rendering the reduction of the pathophysiology of movement disorders to abnormalities in the basal ganglia alone too simplistic.

In fact, lesions of these structures often lead to results that are difficult to understand given the current models of basal ganglia function. For instance, the models predict that reduced basal ganglia output should lead to excess movement, as it is seen, for instance, after lesions of the STN (e.g., Ref.[118]). Pallidal lesions in normal or parkinsonian monkeys or in parkinsonian patients, however, have not been associated with involuntary movement other than occasional transient dyskinesias[29,83,149] (but see Ref.[19]). Furthermore, if the basal ganglia have an important role in motor control, as is generally believed, it is expected that reduction of basal ganglia output should lead to disturbances of normal movement. As mentioned above, however, neither GPi nor STN lesions in man or experimental animals lead to significant long-term abnormalities of voluntary movement.[29,64,68,149] It appears that voluntary movement can be controlled with reduced or absent GPi/SNr activity. Basal ganglia output may therefore be either relatively unimportant for movement initiation or execution, or its loss can be rapidly and readily compensated for by other parts of the motor system. In contrast, increased basal ganglia output, as seen in PD appears to severely disrupt motor performance on a more permanent basis.

Overall, our understanding of the contribution of the basal ganglia to movement and behavior lags far behind our understanding of the pathophysiology of PD and other movement disorders. Although impressive advances in the understanding and treatment of these disorders have been made in recent years, more comprehensive knowledge of normal basal ganglia functioning will ultimately be necessary to maximize therapeutic outcome for patients affected by basal ganglia disorders.

References

1. Alexander GE, DeLong MR, Strick PL: Parallel organization of functionally segregated circuits linking basal ganglia and cortex. *Ann Rev Neurosci* 9:357–381, 1986.
2. Albin RL, Young AB, Penney JB: The functional anatomy of basal ganglia disorders. *Trends Neurosci* 12:366–375, 1989.
3. Alexander GE, Crutcher MD, DeLong MR: Basal ganglia-thalamocortical circuits: Parallel substrates for motor, oculomotor, 'prefrontal' and 'limbic' functions. *Prog Brain Res* 85:119–146, 1990.
4. Parent A, Smith Y: Organization of efferent projections of the subthalamic nucleus in the squirrel monkey as revealed by retrograde labeling methods. *Brain Res* 436:296–310, 1987.

5. Hazrati LN, Parent A, Mitchell S, et al: Evidence for interconnections between the two segments of the globus pallidus in primates: A PHA-L anterograde tracing study. *Brain Res* 533:171–175, 1990.

6. Gerfen CR, Engber TM, Mahan LC, et al: D1 and D2 dopamine receptor-regulated gene expression of striatonigral and striatopallidal neurons. *Science* 250:1429–1432, 1990.

7. Gerfen CR: Molecular effects of dopamine on striatal-projection pathways. *Trends in Neurosci* 23:S64–70, 2000.

8. Freeman A, Ciliax B, Bakay R, et al: Nigrostriatal collaterals to thalamus degenerate in parkinsonian animal models. *Ann Neurol* 50:321–329, 2001.

9. Lavoie B, Smith Y, Parent A: Dopaminergic innervation of the basal ganglia in the squirrel monkey as revealed by tyrosine hydroxylase immunohistochemistry. *J Comp Neurol* 289:36–52, 1989.

10. Cheramy A, Leviel V, Glowinski J: Dendritic release of dopamine in the substantia nigra. *Nature* 289:537–542, 1981.

11. Gauchy C, Desban M, Glowinski J, et al: NMDA regulation of dopamine release from proximal and distal dendrites in the cat substantia nigra. *Brain Res* 635:249–256, 1994.

12. DeLong MR, Coyle JT: Globus pallidus lesions in the monkey produced by kainic acid: Histologic and behavioral effects. *Appl Neurophysiol* 42:95–97, 1979.

13. Horak FB, Anderson ME: Influence of globus pallidus on arm movements in monkeys. I. Effects of kainic acid-induced lesions. *Journal of Neurophysiol* 52:290–304, 1984.

14. Hore J, Villis T: Arm movement performance during reversible basal ganglia lesions in the monkey. *Exp Brain Res* 39:217–228, 1980.

15. MacLean PD: Effects of lesions of globus pallidus on species-typical display behavior of squirrel monkeys. *Brain Res* 149:175–196, 1978.

16. Ranson SW, Berry C: Observations on monkeys with bilateral lesions of the globus pallidus. *Arch Neurol Psychiatry* 46:504–508, 1941.

17. Strub RL: Frontal lobe syndrome in a patient with bilateral globus pallidus lesions. *Arch Neurol* 46:1024–1027, 1986.

18. Kato M, Kimura M: Effects of reversible blockade of basal ganglia on a voluntary arm movement. *Journal of Neurophysiol* 68:1516–1534, 1992.

19. Mink JW, Thach WT: Basal ganglia motor control. III. Pallidal ablation: Normal reaction time, muscle cocontraction, and slow movement. *J Neurophysiol* 65:330–351, 1991.

20. Bennett KM, Marchetti M, Iovine R, et al: The drinking action of Parkinson's disease subjects. *Brain* 118:959–970, 1995.

21. Cunnington R, Iansek R, Bradshaw JL, et al: Movement-related potentials in Parkinson's disease. Presence and predictability of temporal and spatial cues. *Brain* 118:935–950, 1995.

22. Martin KE, Phillips JG, Iansek R, et al: Inaccuracy and instability of sequential movements in Parkinson's disease. *Exp Brain Res* 102:131–140, 1994.

23. Georgiou N, Bradshaw JL, Iansek R, et al: Reduction in external cues and movement sequencing in Parkinson's disease. *J Neurol Neurosurg Psychiatry* 57:368–370, 1994.

24. Benecke R, Rothwell JC, Dick JPR, et al: Disturbances of sequential movements in patients with Parkinson's disease. *Brain* 110:361–379, 1987.

25. Benecke R, Rothwell JC, Dick JPR, et al: Simple and complex movements off and on treatment in patients with Parkinson's disease. *J Neurol Neurosurg Psychiatry* 50:296–303, 1987.

26. Rolls ET: Neurophysiology and cognitive functions of the striatum. *Rev Neurol* 150:648–660, 1994.

27. Marsden CD: Which motor disorder in Parkinson's disease indicates the true motor function of the basal ganglia?, in *Ciba Found Symp* 107:225–241, 1984.

28. Trouche E, Beaubaton D, Amato G, et al: Changes in reaction time after pallidal or nigral lesion in the monkey. *Adv Neurol* 40:29–38, 1984.

29. DeLong MR, Georgopoulos AP: Motor functions of the basal ganglia, in Brookhart JM, Mountcastle VB, Brooks VB, Geiger SR (eds): *Handbook of Physiology. The Nervous System. Motor Control,* Sect 1, Vol II, Pt 2. Bethesda, American Physiological Society, 1981, pp 1017–1061.

30. Inase M, Buford JA, Anderson ME: Changes in the control of arm position, movement, and thalamic discharge during local inactivation in the globus pallidus of the monkey. *J Neurophysiol* 75:1087–1104, 1996.

31. Turner RS, Grafton ST, Votaw JR, et al: Motor subcircuits mediating the control of movement velocity: A PET study. *J Neurophysiol* 80:2162–2176, 1998.

32. Anderson ME, Turner RS: A quantitative analysis of pallidal discharge during targeted reaching movement in the monkey. *Exp Brain Res* 86:623–632, 1991.

33. DeLong MR: The neurophysiologic basis of abnormal movements in basal ganglia disorders. *Neurobehav Toxicol & Teratol* 5:611–616, 1983.

34. Yelnik J, Percheron G, Francois C: A golgi analysis of the primate globus pallidus. II. Quantitative morphology and spatial orientation of dendritic arborizations. *J Comp Neurol* 227:200–213, 1984.

35. Francois C, Percheron G, Yelnik J, et al: A golgi analysis of the primate globus pallidus. I. Inconstant processes of large neurons, other neuronal types, and afferent axons. *J Comp Neurol* 227:182–199, 1984.

36. Francois C, Yelnik J, Percheron G: Golgi study of the primate substantia nigra. II. Spatial organization of dendritic arborizations in relation to the cytoarchitectonic boundaries and to the striatonigral bundle. *J Comp Neurol* 265:473–493, 1987.

37. Yelnik J, Francois C, Percheron G, et al: Golgi study of the primate substantia nigra. I. Quantitative morphology and typology of nigral neurons. *J Comp Neurol* 265:455–472, 1987.

38. Percheron G, Yelnik J, Francois C: A golgi analysis of the primate globus pallidus. III. Spatial organization of the striato-pallidal complex. *J Comp Neurol* 227:214–227, 1984.

39. Nini A, Feingold A, Slovin H, et al: Neurons in the globus pallidus do not show correlated activity in the normal monkey, but phase-locked oscillations appear in the MPTP model of parkinsonism. *J Neurophysiol* 74:1800–1805, 1995.

40. Wichmann T, Bergman H, DeLong MR: The primate subthalamic nucleus. I. Functional properties in intact animals. *J Neurophysiol* 72:494–506, 1994.

41. Filion M, Tremblay L, Bedard PJ: Abnormal influences of passive limb movement on the activity of globus pallidus neurons in parkinsonian monkeys. *Brain Res* 444:165–176, 1988.

42. Miller WC, DeLong MR: Altered tonic activity of neurons in the globus pallidus and subthalamic nucleus in the primate MPTP model of parkinsonism, in Carpenter MB, Jayaraman A (eds): *The Basal Ganglia II.* New York: Plenum Press, 1987, pp 415–427.

43. Bergman H, Wichmann T, Karmon B, et al: The primate subthalamic nucleus. II. Neuronal activity in the MPTP model of parkinsonism. *J Neurophysiol* 72:507–520, 1994.

44. Vitek JL, Ashe J, DeLong MR, et al: Altered somatosensory response properties of neurons in the 'motor' thalamus of MPTP treated parkinsonian monkeys. *Soc Neurosci Abstr* 16:425, 1990.

45. Chevalier G, Deniau JM: Disinhibition as a basic process in the expression of striatal functions. *Trends Neurosci* 13:277–280, 1990.

46. Kita H: Physiology of two disynaptic pathways from the sensorimotor cortex to the basal ganglia output nuclei, in Percheron G, McKenzie JS, Feger J (eds): *The Basal Ganglia IV. New Ideas and Data on Structure and Function.* New York: Plenum Press, 1994, pp 263–276.

47. Mink JW, Thach WT: Basal ganglia motor control. I. Nonexclusive relation of pallidal discharge to five movement modes. *J Neurophysiol* 65:273–300, 1991.

48. Mink JW, Thach WT: Basal ganglia motor control. II. Late pallidal timing relative to movement onset and inconsistent pallidal coding of movement parameters. *J Neurophysiol* 65:301–329, 1991.

49. Hazrati LN, Parent A: Convergence of subthalamic and striatal efferents at pallidal level in primates: An anterograde double-labeling study with biocytin and PHA-L. *Brain Res* 569:336–340, 1992.

50. Smith Y, Bevan MD, Shink E, et al: Microcircuitry of the direct and indirect pathways of the basal ganglia. *Neuroscience* 86:353–387, 1998.

51. Shink E, Bevan MD, Bolam JP, et al: The subthalamic nucleus and the external pallidum: Two tightly interconnected structures that control the output of the basal ganglia in the monkey. *Neuroscience* 73:335–357, 1996.

52. Middleton FA, Strick PL: Basal-ganglia 'projections' to the prefrontal cortex of the primate. *Cereb Cortex* 12:926–935, 2002.

53. Hoover JE, Strick PL: The organization of cerebellar and basal ganglia outputs to primary motor cortex as revealed by retrograde transneuronal transport of herpes simplex virus type 1. *J Neurosci* 19:1446–1463, 1999.

54. Middleton FA, Strick PL: New concepts about the organization of basal ganglia output. *Advances in Neurology* 74:57–68, 1997.

55. Hoover JE, Strick PL: Multiple output channels in the basal ganglia. *Science* 259:819–821, 1993.

56. Nambu A, Yoshida S-I, Jinnai K: Discharge patterns of pallidal neurons with input from various cortical areas during movement in the monkey. *Brain Res* 519:183–191, 1990.

57. Yoshida S, Nambu A, Jinnai K: The distribution of the globus pallidus neurons with input from various cortical areas in the monkeys. *Brain Res* 611:170–174, 1993.

58. Jinnai K, Nambu A, Yoshida S, et al: The two separate neuron circuits through the basal ganglia concerning the preparatory or execution processes of motor control, in Mamo N, Hamada I, DeLong MR (eds): *Role of the Cerebellum and Basal Ganglia in Voluntary Movement.* Elsevier Science, 1993, pp 153–161.

59. Schultz W, Romo R: Role of primate basal ganglia and frontal cortex in the internal generation of movements. I. Preparatory activity in the anterior striatum. *Exp Brain Res* 91:363–384, 1992.

60. Romo R, Schultz W: Role of primate basal ganglia and frontal cortex in the internal generation of movement. III. Neuronal activity in the supplementary motor area. *Exp Brain Res* 91:396–407, 1992.

61. Alexander GE, Crutcher MD: Neural representations of the target (goal) of visually guided arm movements in three motor areas of the monkey. *J Neurophysiol* 64:164–178, 1990.

62. Alexander GE, Crutcher MD: Preparation for movement: Neural representations of intended direction in three motor areas of the monkey. *J Neurophysiol* 64:133–150, 1990.

63. Jaeger D, Gilman S, Aldridge JW: Primate basal ganglia activity in a precued reaching task: Preparation for movement. *Exp Brain Res* 95:51–64, 1993.

64. Bergman H, Wichmann T, DeLong MR: Reversal of experimental parkinsonism by lesions of the subthalamic nucleus. *Science* 249:1436–1438, 1990.

65. DeLong MR: Primate models of movement disorders of basal ganglia origin. *Trends Neurosci* 13:281–285, 1990.

66. Filion M, Tremblay L: Abnormal spontaneous activity of globus pallidus neurons in monkeys with MPTP-induced parkinsonism. *Brain Res* 547:142–151, 1991.

67. Aziz TZ, Peggs D, Sambrook MA, et al: Lesion of the subthalamic nucleus for the alleviation of 1-methyl-4-phenyl-1,2,3,6-tetrahydropyridine (MPTP)-induced parkinsonism in the primate. *Mov Disord* 6:288–292, 1991.

68. Wichmann T, Bergman H, DeLong MR: The primate subthalamic nucleus. III. Changes in motor behavior and neuronal activity in the internal pallidum induced by subthalamic inactivation in the MPTP model of parkinsonism. *J Neurophysiol* 72:521–530, 1994.

69. Baron MS, Wichmann T, Ma D, et al: Effects of transient focal inactivation of the basal ganglia in parkinsonian primates. *J Neurosci* 22:592–599, 2002.

70. Guridi J, Herrero MT, Luquin R, et al: Subthalamotomy improves MPTP-induced parkinsonism in monkeys. *Stereotact Func Neurosurg* 62:98–102, 1994.

71. Vitek JL, Ashe J, DeLong MR, et al: Altered somatosensory response properties of neurons in the 'motor' thalamus of MPTP treated parkinsonian monkeys. *Soc Neurosci Abstr* 16:425, 1990.

72. Laitinen LV, Bergenheim AT, Hariz MI: Leksell's posteroventral pallidotomy in the treatment of Parkinson's disease. *J Neurosurg* 76:53–61, 1992.

73. Baron MS, Vitek JL, Bakay RAE, et al: Treatment of advanced Parkinson's disease by GPi pallidotomy: 1 year pilot-study results. *Ann Neurol* 40:355–366, 1996.

74. Iacono RP, Lonser RR: Reversal of Parkinson's akinesia by pallidotomy. *Lancet* 343:418–419, 1994.

75. Dogali M, Fazzini E, Kolodny E, et al: Stereotactic ventral pallidotomy for Parkinson's disease. *Neurology* 45:753–761, 1995.

76. Laitinen LV: Pallidotomy for Parkinson's disease. *Neurosurg Clinics North Amer* 6:105–112, 1995.

77. Sutton JP, Couldwell W, Lew MF, et al: Ventroposterior medial pallidotomy in patients with advanced Parkinson's disease. *Neurosurgery* 36:1118–1125, 1995.

78. Vitek JL, Ashe J, Kaneoke Y: Spontaneous neuronal activity in the motor thalamus: Alteration in pattern and rate in parkinsonism. *Neuroscience* 20, Part 1:561, 1994.

79. Hutchison WD, Lozano AM, Davis K, et al: Differential neuronal activity in segments of globus pallidus in Parkinson's disease patients. *Neuroreport* 5:1533–1537, 1994.

80. Ceballos-Bauman AO, Obeso JA, Vitek JL, et al: Restoration of thalamocortical activity after posteroventrolateral pallidotomy in Parkinson's disease. *Lancet* 344:814, 1994.

81. Samuel M, Ceballos-Baumann AO, Turjanski N, et al: Pallidotomy in Parkinson's disease increases supplementary motor area and prefrontal activation during performance of volitional

movements: An H2(15)O PET study. *Brain* 120:1301–1313, 1997.

82. Brooks DJ: Detection of preclinical Parkinson's disease with PET. *Neurology* 41(suppl 2):24–27, 1991.

83. Svennilson E, Torvik A, Lowe R, et al: Treatment of parkinsonism by stereotactic thermolesions in the pallidal region. A clinical evaluation of 81 cases. *Acta Psychiat Neurol Scand* 35:358–377, 1960.

84. Bakay RAE, DeLong MR, Vitek JL: Posteroventral pallidotomy for Parkinson's disease (letter). *J Neurosurg* 77:487–488, 1992.

85. Alexander GE, Crutcher MD: Functional architecture of basal ganglia circuits: Neural substrates of parallel processing. *Trends Neurosci* 13:266–271, 1990.

86. Deecke L: Cerebral potentials related to voluntary actions: Parkinsonism and normal subjects, in Delwaide PJ and Agnoli A (eds): *Clinical Neurophysiology in Parkinsonism.* Amsterdam and Oxford: Elsevier, 1985, pp 91–105.

87. Dick JPR, Rothwell JC, Day BL, et al: The Bereitschaftspotential is abnormal in Parkinson's disease. *Brain* 112:233–244, 1989.

88. Calne D, Snow BJ: PET imaging in Parkinsonism. *Adv Neurol* 60:484, 1993.

89. Eidelberg D: Positron emission tomography studies in Parkinsonism. *Neurol Clin* 10:421, 1992.

90. Eidelberg D: The metabolic landscape of Parkinson's disease. *Adv Neurol* 80:87–97, 1999.

91. Brooks DJ: Positron emission tomography studies in movement disorders. *Neurosurgery Clinics of North America* 9:263–282, 1998.

92. Narabayashi H: Surgical treatment in the levodopa era, in Stern G (ed): *Parkinson's Disease.* London: Chapman & Hall, 1990, pp 597–646.

93. Narabayashi H: Sterotaxic Vim thalamotomy for treatment of tremor. *Eur Neurol* 29:S29–S32, 1989.

94. Hassler R, Mundinger F, Riechert T: *Stereotaxis in Parkinsonian Syndromes.* Berlin-Heidelberg: Springer-Verlag, 1979.

95. Vitek JL, Wichmann T, DeLong MR: Current concepts of basal ganglia neurophysiology with respect to tremorgenesis, in Findley LJ and Koller W (eds): *Handbook of Tremor Disorders.* New York: Marcel Dekker Inc., 1994, pp 37–50.

96. Spiegel EA, Wycis HT: Ansotomy in paralysis agitans. *Arch Neurol Psychiat* 71:598–614, 1954.

97. Hassler R, Reichert T, Mundinger F, et al: Physiological observations in stereotaxic operations in extrapyramidal motor disturbances. *Brain* 83:337–350, 1960.

98. Buzsaki G, Smith A, Berger S, et al: Petit mal epilepsy and parkinsonian tremor: Hypothesis of a common pacemaker. *Neuroscience* 36(1):1–14, 1990.

99. Llinas RR: The intrinsic electrophysiological properties of mammalian neurons: Insights into central nervous system function. *Science* 242:1654–1664, 1988.

100. Dacko S, Smith MG, Schneider JS: Immunohistochemical study of the pallidal complex in symptomatic and asymptomatic MPTP-treated monkeys, normal human, and Parkinson's disease patients. *Soc Neurosci Abstr* 16:428, 1990.

101. Bernheimer H, Birkmayer W, Hornykiewicz O, et al: Brain dopamine and the syndromes of Parkinson and Huntington. *J Neurol Sci* 20:415–455, 1973.

102. Nambu A, Llinas R: Electrophysiology of globus pallidus neurons in vitro. *J Neurophysiol* 72:1127–1139, 1994.

103. Plenz D, Kitai S: A basal ganglia pacemaker formed by the subthalamic nucleus and external globus pallidus. *Nature* 400:677–682, 1999.

104. Bevan MD, Magill PJ, Terman D, et al: Move to the rhythm: Oscillations in the subthalamic nucleus-external globus pallidus network. *Trends in Neurosci* 25:525–531, 2002.

105. Pare D, Curro'Dossi R, Steriade M: Neuronal basis of the parkinsonian resting tremor: A hypothesis and its implications for treatment. *Neuroscience* 35:217–226, 1990.

106. Miyashita N, Hikosaka O, Kato M: Visual hemineglect induced by unilateral striatal dopamine deficiency in monkeys. *Neuroreport* 6:1257–1260, 1995.

107. Cummings JL: Frontal-subcortical circuits and human behavior. *Arch Neurol* 50:873–880, 1993.

108. Hollander E, Cohen L, Richards M, et al: A pilot study of the neuropsychology of obsessive-compulsive disorder and Parkinson's disease: Basal ganglia disorders. *J Neuropsychiatry Clini Neurosci* 5:104–107, 1993.

109. Rauch SL, Whalen PJ, Curran T, et al: Probing striato-thalamic function in obsessive-compulsive disorder and Tourette syndrome using neuroimaging methods. *Adv Neurol* 85:207–224, 2001.

110. Kulisevsky J, Litvan I, Berthier ML, et al: Neuropsychiatric assessment of Gilles de la Tourette patients: Comparative study with other hyperkinetic and hypokinetic movement disorders. *Mov Disord* 16:1098–1104, 2001.

111. Saba PR, Dastur K, Keshavan MS, et al: Obsessive-compulsive disorder, Tourette's syndrome, and basal ganglia pathology on MRI [letter]. *J Neuropsychiatry Clini Neurosci* 10:116–117, 1998.

112. Carpenter MB, Whittier JR, Mettler FA: Analysis of choreoid hyperkinesia in the rhesus monkey: Surgical and pharmacological analysis of hyperkinesia resulting from lesions in the subthalamic nucleus of Luys. *J Comp Neurol* 92:293–332, 1950.

113. Whittier JR, Mettler FA: Studies of the subthalamus of the rhesus monkey. II. Hyperkinesia and other physiologic effects of subthalamic lesions with special references to the subthalamic nucleus of Luys. *J Comp Neurol* 90:319–372, 1949.

114. Crossman AR, Sambrook MA, Jackson A: Experimental hemichorea/hemiballismus in the monkey. Study on the intracerebral site of action in a drug-induced dyskinesia. *Brain* 107:579–596, 1984.

115. Hammond C, Feger J, Bioulac B, et al: Experimental hemiballism in the monkey produced by unilateral kainic acid lesion in corpus Luysii. *Brain Res* 171:577–580, 1979.

116. Kase CS, Maulsby GO, deJuan E, et al: Hemi-chorea-hemiballism and lacunar infarction in the basal ganglia. *Neurology* 31:452–455, 1981.

117. Hamada I, DeLong MR: Excitotoxic acid lesions of the primate subthalamic nucleus result in transient dyskinesias of the contralateral limbs. *J Neurophysiol* 68:1850–1858, 1992.

118. Hamada I, DeLong MR: Excitotoxic acid lesions of the primate subthalamic nucleus result in reduced pallidal neuronal activity during active holding. *J Neurophysiol* 68:1859–1866, 1992.

119. Papa SM, Desimone R, Fiorani M, et al: Internal globus pallidus discharge is nearly suppressed during levodopa-induced dyskinesias. *Ann of Neurol* 46:732–738, 1999.

120. Lozano AM, Lang AE, Levy R, et al: Neuronal recordings in Parkinson's disease patients with dyskinesias induced by apomorphine. *Ann of Neurol* 47:S141–146, 2000.

121. Gerfen CR: Dopamine receptor function in the basal ganglia. *Clini Neuropharmacol* 18:S162–S177, 1995.

122. Tranchant C, Maquet J, Eber AM, et al: Angiome caverneux cerebelleux, dystonie cervicale et diaschisis cortical croise. *Rev of Neurol* 147:599–602, 1991.

123. Gille M, Jacquemin C, Kiame G, et al: Myelinolyse centropontine avec ataxie cerebelleuse et dystonie. *Rev of Neurol* 149:344–346, 1993.

124. Janati A, Metzer WS, Archer RL, et al: Blepharospasm associated with olivopontocerebellar atrophy. *J Clini Neuro-Ophthalmol* 9:281–284, 1989.

125. Krauss JK, Mohadjer M, Braus DF, et al: Dystonia following head trauma: A report of nine patients and review of the literature. *Mov Disord* 7:263–272, 1992.

126. Nygaard TG: Dopa-responsive dystonia. *Current Opinion in Neurology* 8:310–313, 1995.

127. Patel K, Roskrow T, Davis JS, et al: Dopa responsive dystonia. *Arch Dis Child* 73:256–257, 1995.

128. Playford ED, Fletcher NA, Sawle GV, et al: Striatal [18F]dopa uptake in familial idiopathic dystonia. *Brain* 116:1191–1199, 1993.

129. Perlmutter JS, Tempel LW, Black KJ, et al: MPTP induces dystonia and parkinsonism. Clues to the pathophysiology of dystonia. *Neurology* 49:1432–1438, 1997.

130. Mitchell IJ, Luquin R, Boyce S, et al: Neural mechanisms of dystonia: Evidence from a 2-deoxyglucose uptake study in a primate model of dopamine agonist-induced dystonia. *Mov Disord* 5:49–54, 1990.

131. Hantraye P, Riche D, Maziere M, et al: A primate model of Huntington's disease: Behavioral and anatomical studies of unilateral excitotoxic lesions of the caudate-putamen in the baboon. *Exp Neurol* 108:91–104, 1990.

132. Gerlach J, Hansen L: Clozapine and D1/D2 antagonism in extrapyramidal functions. *Br J Pychiatry* 17(Suppl):34–37, 1997.

133. Casey DE: Dopamine D1 (SCH23390) and D2 (haloperidol) antagonists in drug-naive monkeys. *Psychopharmacology* 107:18–22, 1992.

134. Vitek JL, Zhang J, Evatt M, et al: GPi pallidotomy for dystonia: Clinical outcome and neuronal activity, in Fahn S, Marsden CD and DeLong MR (eds): *Dystonia 3*. Philadelphia: Lippincott-Raven, 1998, pp 211–220.

135. Lozano A, Hutchison W, Kiss Z, et al: Methods for microelectrode-guided posteroventral pallidotomy. *J Neurosurg* 84:194–202, 1996.

136. Vitek JL, Kaneoke Y, Turner R, et al: Neuronal activity in the internal (GPi) and external (GPe) segments of the globus pallidus (GP) of parkinsonian patients is similar to that in the MPTP-treated primate model of parkinsonism. *Soc Neurosci Abstr* 19:1584, 1993.

137. Sterio D, Beric A, Dogali M, et al: Neurophysiological properties of pallidal neurons in Parkinson's disease. *Ann Neurol* 35:586–591, 1994.

138. Eidelberg D, Moeller JR, Ishikawa T, et al: The metabolic topography of idiopathic torsion dystonia. *Brain* 118:1473–1484, 1995.

139. Galardi G, Perani D, Grassi F, et al: Basal ganglia and thalamo-cortical hypermetabolism in patients with spasmodic torticollis. *Acta Neurol Scand* 94:172–176, 1996.

140. Playford ED, Passingham RE, Marsden CD, et al: Increased activation of frontal areas during arm movement in idiopathic torsion dystonia. *Mov Disord* 13:309–318, 1998.

141. Karbe H, Holthoff VA, Rudolf J, et al: Positron emission tomography demonstrates frontal cortex and basal ganglia hypometabolism in dystonia. *Neurology* 42:1540–1544, 1992.

142. Hallett M and Toro C: Dystonia and the supplementary sensorimotor area. *Adv Neurol* 70:471–476, 1996.

143. Ikoma K, Samii A, Mercuri B, et al: Abnormal cortical motor excitability in dystonia. *Neurology* 46:1371–1376, 1996.

144. Hallett M: The neurophysiology of dystonia. *Arch Neurol* 55:601–603, 1998.

145. Berardelli A, Rothwell JC, Hallett M, et al: The pathophysiology of primary dystonia. *Brain* 121:1195–1212, 1998.

146. Forno LS, Langston JW, DeLanney LE, et al: Locus ceruleus lesions and eosinophilic inclusions in MPTP-treated monkeys. *Ann Neurol* 20:449–455, 1986.

147. Forno LS, DeLanney LE, Irwin I, et al: Similarities and differences between MPTP-induced parkinsonism and Parkinson's disease. *Adv Neurol* 60:600–608, 1993.

148. Gibb WR: Neuropathology of Parkinson's disease and related syndromes. *Neurol Clin* 10:361–376, 1992.

149. Laitinen LV, Bergenheim AT and Hariz MI: Ventroposterolateral pallidotomy can abolish all parkinsonian symptoms. *Stereotact Funct Neurosurg* 58:14–21, 1992.

Chapter 7 _____

FUNCTIONAL NEUROCHEMISTRY OF THE BASAL GANGLIA

JAYARAMAN RAO

OVERVIEW OF THE CIRCUITS OF THE
  BASAL GANGLIA   113
NEUROCHEMICAL ORGANIZATION OF THE
  DOPAMINERGIC SYSTEM IN THE BASAL
  GANGLIA   114
    Source of Dopamine in the Basal Ganglia   114
    Molecular Diversity of Dopamine Receptors and
      Their Signal Transduction   115
    Dopamine Receptor Distribution in the
      Basal Ganglia   115
    Functions of Dopamine Receptor Subtypes   115
NEUROCHEMICAL ORGANIZATION OF THE
  ACETYLCHOLINERGIC SYSTEM IN THE
  BASAL GANGLIA   116
    Source of Acetylcholine in the Basal Ganglia   116
    Molecular Diversity of Cholinergic Receptors and
      Their Signal Transduction   117
    Cholinergic Receptor Distribution in the
      Basal Ganglia   117
    Functions of the Acetylcholinergic Receptors   119
NEUROCHEMICAL ORGANIZATION OF THE
  GLUTAMATERGIC SYSTEM IN THE
  BASAL GANGLIA   119
    Source of Glutamate in the Basal Ganglia   119
    Molecular Diversity of Glutamate Receptors and
      Their Signal Transduction   120
    Glutamatergic Receptor Distribution in the
      Basal Ganglia   120
    Functions of the Glutamatergic Receptors   122
NEUROCHEMICAL ORGANIZATION OF THE
  SEROTONERGIC SYSTEM IN THE
  BASAL GANGLIA   123
    Source of Serotonin in the Basal Ganglia   123
    Molecular Diversity of Serotonin Receptors and
      Their Signal Transduction   123
    Serotonergic Receptor Distribution in the
      Basal Ganglia   123
    Functions of the Serotonergic Receptors   124
SUMMARY   125

Progressive degeneration of neurons of the various nuclei of the basal ganglia leads to many clinical disorders manifesting in severe disabling motor, autonomic, and cognitive problems. The different nuclei of the basal ganglia, especially the striatum, are the sites of actions of diverse neurotransmitters and neuropeptides.[1] Classic and modern neuroanatomical and neurochemical studies have facilitated us in drawing a working model of the circuits of the basal ganglia.[2–4] Experimental exploitation of these circuits with molecular biological techniques has advanced our understanding of the molecular circuitries that are involved in their actions and interactions as well as the role played by the individual neurotransmitters and neuropeptides in the functions of the basal ganglia.

This chapter reviews the information relevant to the patterns of organization of four major neurotransmitters, viz., dopamine, acetylcholine, glutamate and serotonin, and their receptors in the basal ganglia and briefly relates to the changes that occur in the diseases of the basal ganglia.

Overview of the Circuits of the Basal Ganglia

The basal ganglia, especially the striatum, based on its converging inputs from functionally diverse cortical regions and their subcortical afferents, may be divided into many functional subcompartments. The putamen processes the motor component of basal ganglia-thalamocortical circuits, whereas caudate and nucleus accumbens mediate cognitive, emotive, and limbic inputs.[5] The spiny neurons, the principal input and output cells accounting for more than three-quarters of the total striatal neuronal population, receive the excitatory synaptic inputs from neocortex as well as thalamus and the dopaminergic input from substantia nigra pars compacta (SNc).[6] Two neurochemically and anatomically distinct populations of spiny neurons of the striatum project downstream to the globus pallidus internal segment (GPi) and substantia nigra pars reticulata (SNr), which are the basal ganglia output nuclei (GPi/SNr). A specific subpopulation of gamma-aminobutyric acid (GABA)- and substance P-containing spiny neurons that project directly to the GPi and SNr form the direct pathway. The indirect pathway arises from a separate subpopulation of spiny neurons that coexpress GABA and enkephalin and project to the external segment of globus pallidus (GPe).[7] GPe sends a GABAergic projection to the subthalamus (STN), which in turn provides glutamatergic innervations of GPi/SNr. The high basal discharge of the GABAergic GPi neurons, the major output nucleus of the basal ganglia circuit, results in tonic inhibitory control over the nonmotor and motor thalamus, and the mesopontine tegmentum.

This working model of basal ganglia circuits (Fig. 7-1) suggests that the basal activity of the pallidal neurons is kept in check by a balance of the direct inhibitory pathway tending to reduce basal ganglia output and the excitatory indirect pathway tending to increase the output. During normal movement, changes in the balance of the direct and

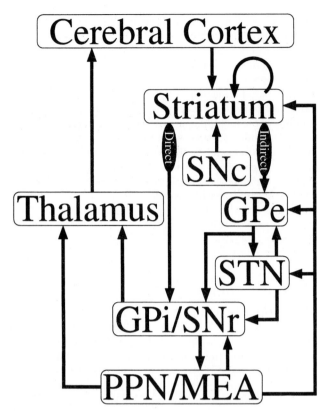

FIGURE 7-1 Schematic of basal ganglia circuitry model.
Direct and indirect pathways originating from striatum are
named according to the immediacy of their regulation of the basal
ganglia output nuclei, GPi/SNr. The projections from each region
are color coded by their major neurotransmitters in the Color
Gallery. GPe, globus pallidus external segment; GPi/SNr, globus
pallidus internal segment/substantia nigra pars reticulata;
PPN/MEA, pedunculopontine nucleus/midbrain extrapyramidal
area; SNc, substantia nigra pars compacta; STN, subthalamic
nucleus.

indirect pathways reduce GPi/SNr inhibition of thalamus, allowing engagement of thalamocortical circuits necessary for the speed and guidance of movements. An imbalance of activity, however, in the direct and indirect pathways can perturb the normal degree of GPi/SNr inhibition of thalamocortical activity, producing either hypokinetic or hyperkinetic movement disorders.[8,9] For example, in Parkinson's disease (PD), models suggest that activity is reduced in the direct pathway and increased in the indirect pathway, both leading to enhanced GPi/SNr activity and excessive inhibition of thalamus.[8,9]

The remainder of the chapter focuses on the receptor gene families for dopamine, acetylcholine (ACh), and glutamate, and summarizes relevant information about the patterns of organization of four major neurotransmitters and their receptors in the basal ganglia.

Neurochemical Organization of the Dopaminergic System in the Basal Ganglia

SOURCE OF DOPAMINE IN THE BASAL GANGLIA

About 80 percent of the total brain dopamine is in the striatum, with the next highest level in the substantia nigra followed by the GP and STN. Even within the striatum, dopamine levels are uneven. The caudal head and the rostral body of the caudate contain more dopamine than the rostral head, the caudal regions, and the tail of the caudate nucleus. Within the putamen, the caudal regions have more dopamine than the rostral regions. Dopamine levels in SNc are three times more than in SNr, and GPe has more dopamine than GPi.[10]

Dopaminergic innervations of the nucleus accumbens arise from the ventral tegmental area (A8) group of dopaminergic neurons of the mesencephalon and that of the caudate nucleus and the putamen from the A9 cell group in SNc.[11] The dopaminergic neurons of SNc are organized into dorsal and ventral tiers.[12] The ventral tier of SNc neurons projects to the dorsolateral motor striatum; the dorsal tier projects to the associative striatum. The different subdivisions of the ventral tegmental area (VTA) project to the nucleus accumbens, and the fundus striatum.[13] Dopamine release from SNc neurons is further regulated by cholecystokinin and neurotensin, two neuropeptides that are colocalized within these midbrain dopaminergic neurons.[14] The tyrosine hydroxylase (TH)-immunopositive fibers from the midbrain dopaminergic neurons are distributed throughout the striatum, but in a heterogeneous pattern[15,16] that is consistent with the fact that levels of dopamine vary in different regions of the striatum.[10] TH-immunoreactive fibers are more dense in the dorsal and ventral caudate nucleus and the nucleus accumbens than in the dorsolateral striatum. Throughout the striatum there are many TH-poor patches intermixed with TH-rich matrix regions.

Another important source of dopamine to the human striatum is the two types of TH-immunopositive neurons that reside within the striatum.[15] These neurons express mRNA for dopamine transporter, suggesting that dopamine is actively transported into these neurons.[17,18] The number of these neurons increases in 1-methyl-4-phenyl-1,2,3,6-tetrahydropyridine (MPTP) models of PD in primates, thereby suggesting that these striatal dopaminergic neurons are generated as a consequence of striatal dopamine denervation.[15]

Collaterals from the nigrostriatal fibers also innervate GPi and GPe, and STN densely.[15] GPi has more dense dopaminergic innervation than GPe. The SNc cells that project to the pallidal segments are resistant to MPTP.[19,20]

Dopaminergic terminals synapse predominantly on dendritic shafts and spines of striatal medium spiny neurons,[21,22] where they appear to regulate responsiveness to cortical and thalamic excitatory drive.[23,24] Distinct subpopulations of dopaminergic neurons project to the patch and matrix compartments.[25] These compartments represent separate subchannels of afferent and efferent circuits through basal ganglia. Based on corticostriatal connections, the striatal patch compartment processes limbic information, whereas the striatal matrix processes sensorimotor information.[25] SNc neurons also extend dendrites into pars reticulata, where they release dopamine, modulating GABA release, neuronal activity in pars reticulata and, subsequently, basal ganglia output to thalamus.[26] In primates, dopaminergic neurons are separated into dorsal and ventral groups, which project to ventral and dorsolateral striatum, respectively.[27] The ventrally located dopaminergic neurons in primates projecting to motor striatum are the most vulnerable in PD, in MPTP and rotenone toxicity.[28–33]

MOLECULAR DIVERSITY OF DOPAMINE RECEPTORS AND THEIR SIGNAL TRANSDUCTION

The diverse effects of dopamine are mediated by D1 and D2 subfamilies of dopamine receptors, which are defined by pharmacological, anatomic, and biochemical criteria.[34–38] All dopamine receptors identified to date are members of the superfamily of G protein-coupled receptors (GPCR).[39] All GPCRs have a seven transmembrane spanning structure linked by three alternating extracellular and intracellular domains, an extracellular N-terminal, and a cytoplasmic C-terminal. More than 1000 GPCRs, accounting for more than 1 percent of the total human genome, have been identified. On the basis of their structure, the GPCRs are classified into families A, B, and C.[39] Besides the well-established role of triggering the second messenger functions, activation of G proteins may also trigger molecular cascades that are responsible for cell survival, cell death, and neoplasia.[40] Dopamine receptors have structural and functional similarities to G protein receptors of other monoamines and rhodopsin, and belong to the A family of GPCRs. The genes coding for the D1 subfamily are intronless, and have a shorter third cytoplasmic loop, but have an intracellular C-terminal, which is seven times longer than in D2 receptors.[38]

The D1 subclass consists of D1 and D5 receptors. They are coupled to the G proteins Gs and Golf, resulting in an increase in adenylyl cyclase and cyclic AMP levels postsynaptically. Dopamine has 10 times more affinity to D5 receptor than for D1, but pharmacologically D1 and D5 are otherwise indistinguishable.[38]

The D2 subclass consists of D2, D3, and D4 receptors, which are coupled to the inhibitory Gi, Go class of G proteins, result in a decrease in adenylyl cyclase and cyclic AMP levels, and modulate ion channels. The D2 receptors are further divided into D2S and D2L, but both receptors have similar pharmacology and distribution patterns.[38] The D4 receptors show polymorphism,[41] but the significance of the polymorphic variants remains to be explored.

The classification of the dopamine receptor gene family, including binding properties, selective agonists and antagonists, and general distributions in brain are summarized in Table 7-1.

DOPAMINE RECEPTOR DISTRIBUTION IN THE BASAL GANGLIA

All the dopamine receptor subtypes have been localized to different nuclei of the basal ganglia.[42] The striatum shows the maximum expression of D1 receptors in the human brain.[38,43,44] D1 receptor mRNA is found throughout the nucleus accumbens, caudate nucleus, and the putamen. The labeling for D1 receptor mRNA is more dense in the nucleus accumbens and the medial caudate than in the lateral regions of the putamen, thereby suggesting a pattern of decreasing intensity from a medial to a lateral direction.[44] The mRNA for D1 receptor is expressed in the GABA- and substance P-containing neurons that project directly to GPi and SNr; accordingly, the D1 receptor protein, but not mRNA, for D1 receptor is highly expressed in GPi and SNr.[25] D1 receptors are also expressed highly in the prefrontal cortex,[45] in contrast to barely detectable levels of D2 binding in these cortical areas.

D2 receptor mRNA is highly expressed in spiny neurons that express GABA and enkephalin and project to GPe and indirectly to GPi through STN.[46] GPe shows significant D2 immunoreactivity. The D2 receptor protein is localized to the dendrites and spine heads more than to the soma of these striatal input-output neurons. The D1 and D2 receptors are expressed mostly in different subpopulations of the striatal spiny neurons, but D1 and D2 receptors may be colocalized in a small but significant group of neurons.[47,48] The dendrites of SNc cells contain D2 autoreceptors.

The nucleus accumbens shows the highest concentration of D3 receptors of all brain regions. D3 mRNA is localized in the spiny neurons of nucleus accumbens that show colocalization of neurotensin and substance P.[49–51]

The D4 receptors are expressed in the soma, dendritic shaft, and spines of the medium spiny neurons of the striatum, more so in the striosomes than in the matrix.[52,53] D4 receptor labeling was more dense in the dorsolateral compartment than in the ventromedial caudate nucleus and the nucleus accumbens, a pattern that is opposite to that of D1 distribution in the striatum. The external and internal segments of GP and SNr demonstrate labeling for D4 receptors.[52,53]

D5 receptor mRNAs have been localized within the medium spiny neurons as well as in the large cholinergic interneurons of the striatum and in the terminals of the GABA/striatopallidal neurons. Dense labeling of D5 receptors is also noted in SNc and SNr.[54]

FUNCTIONS OF DOPAMINE RECEPTOR SUBTYPES

Pharmacological, behavioral, and gene manipulation (knockout) techniques have recently begun to unravel the role

TABLE 7-1 Dopamine Receptor Subtypes

Receptor Subtype	Pharmacological Class	Isoforms	Second Messenger	Selective Agonists	Selective Antagonists	Localization
D1 Subfamily			Increase cyclic AMP	SKF 38393 CY 208-243 (partial agonists) A 77636 SKF 82958 (full agonists)	SCH 23390 (some 5-HT effects) SCH-39166 (no 5-HT effects)	
D1 (DIA)	D1					Striatal spiny neurons (direct pathway)
D5 (DIB)	D1	Pseudogenes on chromosomes 1 and 2 polymorphisms				Cortex, thalamus, cholinergic striatal neurons, SNc
D2 Subfamily			Decrease cyclic AMP	Bromocriptine Quinpirole	Spiroperidol (some 5-HT effects) Raclopride	
D2 (D2A)	D2	Short/long splice variants, 6 introns				Striatal spiny neurons (indirect pathway)
D3 (D2B)	D2	2 splice variants (truncated), 5 introns		7-OH-DPAT PD 128,907		SNc (autoreceptor) Ventral striatum, limbic regions
D4 (D2C)	D2	Polymorphisms (2–10 repeats)			Clozapine (some muscarinic + 5-HT effects) L 745870 U 101958	Poorly understood

7-OH-DPAT, 7-hydroxy-N, N-di-n-propyl-2-aminotetralin; SNc, substantia nigra pars compacta.

played by the individual subtypes of several neurotransmitters, including dopamine and serotonin.[38,55,56] These studies suggest that D1 receptors may be involved in: locomotor activity in novel environment; spatial and working memory, especially cortical D1 receptors; and locomotor responses to psychostimulant drugs.[56–58] D2 receptors play a major role in initiating and maintaining normal locomotor behavior.[56] D2 autoreceptors when activated by agonists cause a decreased release of dopamine and resultant decrease in motor activity, whereas agonists of postsynaptic D2 receptors induce hyperactivity.[56] Mice lacking D2 receptors have a prominent hunched posture and delay in initiating movements, as well as other locomotor and postural features of PD.[59] D2 receptors, when co-activated with D1 receptors, play a major role in locomotor responses to drugs of abuse. D3 receptors, located mostly in the limbic striatum, when stimulated specifically, induced hypolocomotion, and antagonists of D3 receptors induced hyperlocomotion.[38,55,56] D3 receptors may also have a role in drug-seeking behavior.[60] The D4 receptor has been speculated to play a role in novelty-seeking behavior.[61] The D5 receptors may inhibit locomotor behavior.[55,56]

Neurochemical Organization of the Acetylcholinergic System in the Basal Ganglia

SOURCE OF ACETYLCHOLINE IN THE BASAL GANGLIA

The dense cholinergic input to the different subnuclei of the basal ganglia is from two different sources. The striatum contains exceptionally high levels of acetylcholine (Ach), and acetylcholinesterase.[6] Striatal ACh is derived almost exclusively from giant aspiny interneurons, which constitute 2 percent of total striatal neurons.[62] These cholinergic neurons are tonically active, and fire at about 5 Hz; they pause their tonic firing on conditioned motor task, facilitating dopamine release during this pause.[62,63] The cholinergic terminals derived from these neurons ramify densely and extensively and synapse predominantly on spiny neurons,[64] where ACh modulates, postsynaptically, the responsiveness of the spiny neurons to the excitatory cortical and thalamic inputs located on the spine heads.[65] These large cholinergic interneurons receive mostly glutamatergic input from the cerebral cortex

Constant,[66] and less-prominent dopaminergic input from SN and VTA.[67]

The GP, STN, SN, and thalamus receive significant cholinergic projections from the ascending outputs of the pedunculopontine nucleus (PPN).[68–70] The PPN projection to the GPi is less dense than its projection to the SN and STN. The PPN, representing the Ch5 subgroup of cholinergic neurons of the brain, is located in the mesopontine tegmentum, and contains both cholinergic and glutamatergic components. The PPN itself receives direct projections from GPi[71] and SNr, and projects caudally to motor structures in brainstem.[72] The pallido-PPN projections may terminate preferentially in the cholinergic subdivision of PPN.[73,74] In PD, there is pathological involvement of the PPN.[75] Moreover, there is a dramatic increase (>200 percent) in muscarinic binding sites in GPi in this disease, possibly reflecting compensatory upregulation of the receptors in the face of reduced cholinergic activity.[76] Thus, in addition to the intrinsic cholinergic system in striatum, the PPN mediates cholinergic effects on other extrastriatal sites of the basal ganglia.

MOLECULAR DIVERSITY OF CHOLINERGIC RECEPTORS AND THEIR SIGNAL TRANSDUCTION

The cholinergic effects are mediated by the ligand-gated ion channel nicotinic acetylcholinergic receptor family (nAChR),[77,78] and the G protein-coupled muscarinic acetylcholinergic (mAChR) family.[79,80] Both classes of receptors are abundant in the brain and basal ganglia structures.

NICOTINIC RECEPTORS

The ionotropic nAChR has a pentameric structure consisting of two copies of one of the many subtypes of α subunits, separated by a copy of one of the β subunits and/or γ subunit and a δ subunit. Eight α (α2–α10) and three β subunits (β2–β4) of the nAChRs have been cloned. Different combinations of these α and β subunits form varieties of functional nAChRs with pharmacological and physiological properties that are distinct to each of them.[77,78] The α4-β2-containing nAChR, a receptor with very high binding affinity to nicotine, is the most common type observed in the brain and in some nuclei

of the basal ganglia. The mRNA for α4-β2 nAChR is very densely expressed in SNc, and these receptors are found on the dopaminergic terminals in the striatum.[78]

MUSCARINIC RECEPTORS

The five distinct subtypes of mAChRs are members of the A family group of the GPCR superfamily. The m1, m3, and m5 receptors are functionally related and are coupled to Gαq11 and Gα13 subtypes of G proteins, which lead to activation of phospholipase C and phospholipase D. m2 and m4 couple to the inhibitory Gi and Go proteins, leading to inhibition of adenylyl cyclase and decrease in cyclic AMP levels.[79,80]

The classification of the mAChR gene family, including binding properties, signal transduction mechanisms, and distributions in brain, is summarized in Table 7-2.

CHOLINERGIC RECEPTOR DISTRIBUTION IN THE BASAL GANGLIA

NICOTINIC RECEPTORS

The α4 and β2 subunits containing nAChR are the most common in the brain, and the basal ganglia. Bungarotoxin-binding α7 is the next most commonly found subunit of nAChR. The mRNA for α 3, 4, 5, 6, and 7 subunits and β 2, 3, and 4 subunits has been localized to the SN and VTA. α7 expression may be more prominent in VTA than in SN. β2 is expressed in all the neurons of VTA and SN. mRNA for nAChRs has not been localized convincingly in any of the striatal neurons. The α4-β2 nAChR is very densely expressed in SNc, and the protein for these receptors is found on the dopaminergic terminals in the striatum. Nicotinic receptors in the basal ganglia appear to be mostly located in the presynaptic nerve terminals and facilitate the release of dopamine in the striatum.[77,78]

MUSCARINIC RECEPTORS

All mAChR mRNAs and proteins have been detected in basal ganglia.[81–90] The m1, m2, and m4 receptors account for the vast majority of striatal muscarinic binding sites,[83–85] and are distributed heterogeneously in the patch and matrix compartments of the striatum.[86] The m4 subtype (see Figs. 7-2 and 7-3)

TABLE 7-2 Muscarinic Acetylcholine Receptor Subtypes

Molecular Subtype	Pharmacological Subclass	Isoforms	Second Messenger	Basal Ganglia Localization
m1	M1	None	Increase PI hydrolysis	Striatal spiny neurons (direct and indirect pathways)
m2	M2	None	Decrease cyclic AMP	Cholinergic striatal interneurons, PPN, cortex, thalamus
m3	M3 > M1 > M2	None	Increase PI hydrolysis	Subthalamus and widespread regions outside striatum
m4	M1 and M2	None	Decrease cyclic AMP	Striatal spiny neurons (direct pathway)
m5	M1 > M2	None	Increase PI hydrolysis	SNc (nigrostriatal terminals?)

PI, phosphatidylinositol; PPN, pedunculopontine nucleus; SNc, substantia nigra pars compacta.

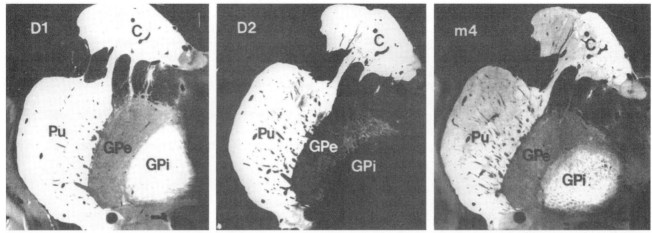

FIGURE 7-2 Immunocytochemical localization of dopaminergic (D1 and D2) and muscarinic cholinergic (m4) receptor subtypes in monkey basal ganglia. Low-power darkfield micrograph of immunoperoxidase-stained brain tissue sections through neostriatum and globus pallidus. Note intense staining (white areas) of all three receptors in caudate (C) and putamen (Pu), and selective localization to either globus pallidus interna (GPi) for D1 and m4 or globus pallidus externa (GPe) for D2, suggesting selective expression of the subtypes in the striatofugal neurons and terminals of the direct or indirect pathways, respectively. Coronal sections; lateral portion positioned on the left and medial on the right; scale bars = 100 μm.

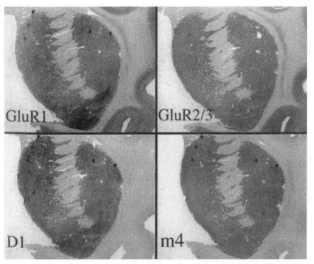

FIGURE 7-3 Comparison of the distributions of GluR1, GluR2/3, D1, and m4 proteins in human striatum. Note that GluR1, D1, and m4 are all enriched in patches (arrows), but GluR2/3 is not.

FIGURE 7-4 Immunocytochemical localization of muscarinic cholinergic m2 receptor subtype in large striatal interneurons. Several examples of human striatal interneurons expressing m2. These neurons have the same frequency, size, and morphology as giant aspiny interneurons, and m2 colocalizes with choline acetyltransferase immunoreactivity, a marker for cholinergic neurons.

is the most abundant mAChR in neostriatum, accounting for 50 percent of total mAChR, and may be the key target for anticholinergic drugs used in movement disorders. The m4 immunoreactivity is dense in patches and corresponds to patches high in D1 and glutamate receptor subunit GluR1 (Fig. 7-3). The other muscarinic receptor proteins do not show such differential localization in patch and matrix divisions. The m4 mRNA and protein are present in about 70 percent of spiny neurons of striatum,[81,86,87] particularly those that express substance P,[88] and, thus, probably project via the direct pathway to basal ganglia output nuclei. Fig. 7-2 shows intense m4 immunoreactivity in the caudate and putamen, and in the terminal zone of the direct pathway projection neurons in GPi. m4 mRNA is also noted in 50 percent of D2/enkephalin spiny neurons of the striatum, which contribute to the indirect pathway. This finding suggests the possibility that m4, like D1, is localized on the terminals of direct pathway projection neurons. The m1 subtype is expressed in all of the spiny projection neurons, whereas the m2 receptor (Fig. 7-4) is expressed in the cholinergic interneurons only.[87,88]

The m1 subtype is mostly postsynaptic on the dendrites and spines of all spiny neurons; m4 is postsynaptic in the spines of a subset of spiny neurons, as well as presynaptically localized in axon terminals, many of which appear to be GABAergic and are probably from the axon collaterals of the direct pathway projection neurons.[86] In contrast, m2 is abundant in cholinergic nerve terminals, where the presynaptic receptor controls transmitter release. Thus, differential expression and trafficking of the mAChR subtypes allows ACh to have different effects on direct and indirect pathway spiny neurons, as well as on interneurons.

Among other basal ganglia structures, the m4 receptor protein is highly enriched in GPi (Fig. 7-2). Because mAChR mRNAs are not detected in GPi,[81] the protein is probably synthesized and transported to the GABAergic terminals of the striatal projection neurons, which express m4 mRNA[81] and protein.[87] Another possibility, however, is that m4 is present on glutamatergic terminals derived from subthalamus, which also expresses the m4 mRNA.[81] The mAChR binding sites in GPi are upregulated substantially in PD, perhaps secondary to reduced cholinergic transmission from PPN.[76] The subthalamus also expresses relatively high levels of m3 mRNA[81] and protein.[84] The PPN expresses high levels of m2 protein,[29] where it probably functions as an autoreceptor. Finally, the dopaminergic neurons in SN are one of few sites in the brain with m5 mRNA[81] and with no other reported receptor subtypes. Although there are only very low levels of m5 protein (e.g., where detectable, accounting for less than 2 percent of total mAChR), this receptor might be localized on nigrostriatal terminals, because dopamine release in striatum is known to be regulated by a muscarinic receptor.[90]

FUNCTIONS OF THE ACETYLCHOLINERGIC RECEPTORS

The central cholinergic system has been speculated to play a role in reward and reinforcement,[91] memory,[92] attention mechanisms,[92] neuroprotection,[93] locomotor activity, analgesia, and neurotransmitter release.[94] The cholinergic system of the central nervous system (CNS) may be classified broadly into two major subdivisions: the rostral division, consisting of the septohippocampal system, the nucleus basalis of Meynert, and related nuclei; and the caudal group of cholinergic neurons in the PPN, and lateral dorsal tegmental nucleus. While the rostral group plays a prominent role in memory and attention mechanisms, the caudal PPN group has a role in locomotor, reward and reinforcement behavior, and in arousal and alerting phenomenon.[92] These diverse functions of the cholinergic system are mediated by both nAChR and mAChR. In the absence of specific agonists and antagonists, our understanding of the roles of these individual AChRs in the functions of basal ganglia is derived from knockout studies.[95–108]

NICOTINIC RECEPTORS

The most important function of presynaptic nAChR in the basal ganglia is to modulate neurotransmitter release.[94]

However, knockout studies have provided additional information of the specific role that the individual subunits may play in other functions of nAChR.[95,96] The β2 subunit appears to play a major role in many of the speculated effects of nicotine. Mice lacking the β2 subunit not only lose high-affinity nicotine binding but also nicotine-induced dopamine but not acetylcholine release, as well as the reinforcing properties of nicotine, suggesting that the β2 subunit is critical for nicotine, and possibly cocaine, addiction.[96–99] The α5-deficient mice demonstrate significant decrease in the short-term effects of nicotine.[100]

MUSCARINIC RECEPTORS

m1 mAChR plays a facilitatory role in the striatum.[101–103] In m1-deficient mice, there is an increased extracellular dopamine level, and consequently increased locomotor activity.[103,104] The increased dopamine level in the striatum has been speculated to be due to decreased inhibition of the nigrostriatal dopaminergic neurons by the m1-deficient striatonigral direct pathway.[103]

Almost all D1 receptor-expressing medium spiny striatal projection neurons that send direct pathway to GPi also express M4 (as well as M1) muscarinic receptors, whereas less than half of the D2 receptor-expressing striatal projection neurons that send efferents to GPe and form part of the indirect pathway express the M4 subtype. m4 nAChR-deficient mice have an increased spontaneous locomotor activity and, when D1 receptor is stimulated with agonists, the hyperactivity is further enhanced, suggesting that the D1 receptor and m4 mAChR have opposing effects on the direct pathway.[105] This is reflected at the cellular level by the fact that D1 receptor stimulation leads to an increase in adenylyl cyclase, whereas m4 stimulation decreases adenylyl cyclase, within the spiny neurons.[105]

The m5 nAChRs, which are prominently expressed in the dopaminergic neurons of SN and VTA, regulate the release of dopamine in the striatum, and may play an active role in drug-seeking behavior, especially reward and withdrawal of opiates.[106]

The M2 and M3 receptors, which are not expressed prominently in the basal ganglia, may mediate analgesia,[107] salivary gland secretion, food intake, and weight gain,[108] respectively.

Neurochemical Organization of the Glutamatergic System in the Basal Ganglia

SOURCE OF GLUTAMATE IN THE BASAL GANGLIA

Glutamate is the principal excitatory neurotransmitter in the brain. Within the basal ganglia circuitry, it plays a prominent role in the physiology of the cortex, striatum, GP, STN, SN, and thalamus. The striatum receives a massive glutamatergic projection from virtually all areas of the neocortex.[109,110] In addition, the centromedian and parafascicular thalamic nuclei send glutamatergic projections to the striatum.[111] Terminals from cortex synapse almost exclusively on heads of dendritic spines, whereas those from thalamus synapse mostly with dendrites and, less frequently, with spines.[111] Individual dendritic spines of striatal neurons receive convergent input from cortical glutamatergic afferents and dopaminergic nigrostriatal cells. Cortical glutamatergic neurons also send projections to STN, SN, and thalamus. Other regions of the basal ganglia (GPe, GPi, and SNc/SNr) receive excitatory glutamatergic input from the STN.[111] In short, all nuclei of the basal ganglia either receive and/or send glutamatergic projections. There are significant alterations in glutamatergic neurotransmission in disorders of the basal ganglia, and the glutamate system is an important target for therapeutic intervention as well as for potential neuroprotective agents.[112]

MOLECULAR DIVERSITY OF GLUTAMATE RECEPTORS AND THEIR SIGNAL TRANSDUCTION

Glutamate receptors are classified into ionotropic receptors (iGluR), and metabotropic receptors (mGluR).[113] The cation-specific iGluRs are named for the agonist compounds that elicit specific physiological response, and are called *N*-methyl-D-aspartate (NMDA), alpha-amino-3-hydroxy-5-methyl-4-isoxazole-propionic acid (AMPA), and kainate (KA) receptors.

NMDA RECEPTORS

Most NMDA receptors are heteromeric, with distinct pharmacological and physiological properties. They are classified further into two subdivisions.[113–118] The NMDAR 1 subunit exists in at least eight alternatively spliced variants (NMDAR 1a-h), which differ in their properties and distribution. Homomeric NMDAR 1 receptors contain each of the regulatory sites found on native NMDA receptors, but agonist-induced current flow is greatly reduced compared to that of native NMDA receptors. The other family of NMDA receptor subunits, NMDAR 2A-D, shows a much more restricted anatomic distribution. Each of these subunits can combine with the NMDAR 1 subunit to form NMDA receptors, which have large current fluxes, and distinctive pharmacological and physiological properties.

AMPA/KA RECEPTORS

The AMPA receptor subunits were the first of the glutamate receptors to be cloned.[119,120] Like other ligand-gated ion channels, the AMPA receptors are multimeric heteromers composed of several distinct subunits. GluR1-4 (also known as GluR A-D) are AMPA receptor subunits, which can assemble in various combinations to form functional receptors.[113] The specific subunit composition of a given AMPA receptor determines its precise physiological, and pharmacological properties. The permeability of AMPA receptors to Ca^{2+} is determined by receptor subunit composition. GluR1 and GluR3 can form homomeric or heteromeric receptor channels that are permeable to Ca^{2+}. The inclusion of a GluR2 subunit in the receptor assembly, however, prevents Ca^{2+} permeability.[121] Alternative splicing of the RNA of each of the four AMPA receptor subunits (GluR1-4), termed "flip" and "flop," add further to the complexity in the composition of AMPA receptors.[122] KA is a powerful agonist of the AMPA receptors, but recent studies have shown that it activates several distinct groups of ionotropic receptors. There are five subtypes of KA receptors (GluR5-7, KA1, and KA2). The functions of KA receptors are being established.[113]

METABOTROPIC RECEPTORS

The metabotropic receptors are coupled to G proteins and belong to the family C type of GPCRs. Characteristic of this family of GPCRs, mGluRs have an exceptionally long N-terminal. Molecular cloning studies have demonstrated the existence of at least eight distinct metabotropic receptor genes (mGluR1-8), at least six of which (mGluR1-5, and mGluR7) are expressed in the brain.[113,123] mGluRs are further divided into three groups. Group I mGluRs, consisting of mGluR1 and mGluR5, stimulate phospholipase C, and increase levels of inositol triphosphate and intracellular calcium. In contrast, groups II (mGluR2, and mGluR3) and III (mGluR4-8) inhibit adenylyl cyclase and thus decrease cyclic AMP levels.

GLUTAMATERGIC RECEPTOR DISTRIBUTION IN THE BASAL GANGLIA

NMDA RECEPTORS

Receptor binding studies indicate that NMDA receptors are found throughout the basal ganglia but are most abundant in striatum.[124,125] Lower levels are seen in GP, STN, SN, and thalamus. Within the striatum, NMDA receptors are preferentially enriched in striatonigral projection neurons.[124] Among the different subtypes, the NMDAR 1 gene product shows an extremely widespread distribution, with moderate to intense staining in striatum, and lower but detectable levels in GP, STN, SNc/SNr, and thalamus.[126,127] An example of this immunoreactivity in SNc/SNr is shown in Fig. 7-5; staining is particularly prominent in dendrites in SNr. The NMDAR 1 mRNA is expressed prominently in the enkephalin-positive medium spiny neurons of the striatum.

The mRNAs for the NMDAR 2 family of subunits are differentially distributed in basal ganglia structures.[127] In the striatum, NMDAR 2B is the predominant species, but NMDAR 2A is also detectable. Elsewhere, in the GP, STN, and SN, NMDAR 2D is most abundant. Interestingly, NMDAR 2C, generally considered a cerebellar subunit, is relatively enriched in SNc. Within the striatum, differences in cellular expression of NMDA receptor subunit genes and isoforms have been described.[128] Enkephalin-positive projection neurons have higher levels of NMDAR 1 and NMDAR 2B

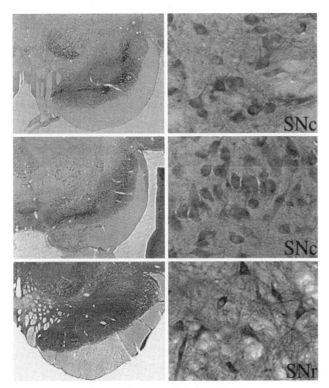

FIGURE 7-5 Immunocytochemistry of glutamate receptor subunits in monkey substantia nigra. GluR1(top) and GluR2/3(middle) immunoreactive neurons are relatively concentrated in the SNc. In contrast, the NMDAR 1(bottom) subunit is more abundant in SNr, where much of the immunoreactivity is found in dendrites.

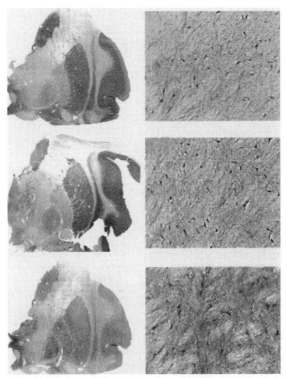

FIGURE 7-6 Distribution of GluR1, GluR2/3, and GluR4 in human basal ganglia; panels on right show higher magnification of cells in the GPi. Note that each of the subunits shows both cellular and neuropil staining in this nucleus.

message than intrinsic somatostatin and cholinergic neurons. In contrast, these interneurons express NMDAR 2D mRNA, but the enkephalin-positive neurons do not. Thus, there is evidence that different populations of striatal neurons express distinct heteromeric forms of the NMDA receptor.[129]

AMPA RECEPTORS

Antibodies recognizing GluR1 label medium spiny, medium aspiny, and large aspiny, neurons of the striatum.[130,131] Moreover, the GluR1 subunit appears to be enriched in striosomes corresponding to substance P-enriched and calbindin-poor regions. In addition, in the human striatum, GluR1 patches colocalize with dopamine D1 receptor patches (Fig. 7-3). In contrast, antibodies that recognize GluR2/3 and GluR4 do not show differential striosomal versus matrix staining. GluR2/3 antibodies primarily label medium spiny neurons, and GluR4 antibodies do not label striatal neurons. In the rat striatum, GluR1 does not colocalize with striatopallidal or striatonigral projection neurons, but it does colocalize with parvalbumin-positive interneurons.[130] In contrast, GluR2/3 is localized to most projection neurons.

GluR1 is also found in GPe, GPi, STN, and SNc/SNr.[132] Fig. 7-6 shows GluR1 immunoreactivity in striatum and

GPe/GPi in the human brain, and demonstrates stained neurons in the GPi. Fig. 7-7 shows the intense GluR1 immunoreactivity in monkey STN, and Fig. 7-5 shows labeled neurons in SN.[133] Neurons enriched in GluR2/3 are found in GPi (Fig. 7-6), and in SNc/SNr (Fig. 7-5), and there are GluR4-immunoreactive neurons in SNr. Finally, it should be noted that GluR4 and, to a lesser extent, GluR1 may be located in glial cells in some brain regions.[132]

METABOTROPIC RECEPTORS

Analysis of the regional and cellular distributions of mGluR message in the basal ganglia reveals that these receptors have distinct localizations.[134–137] Both substance P- and enkephalin-containing medium-sized projection neurons and the large interneurons of the striatum express mRNA and proteins for mGluR1 and mGluR5.[135] mGluR1 and mGluR5 are immunolabeled strongly in both pallidal segments, as well as preferentially in the glutamatergic subthalamopallidal synapses.[136] Among the group II mGluRs, mGluR2 mRNA is expressed mostly in the large striatal interneurons, and mGluR3 mRNA in most striatal neurons.[137] This group of mGluRs is absent in the pallidal segments. Only low levels of the group III family members are expressed in the striatum and the pallidal segments, but proteins of these receptors

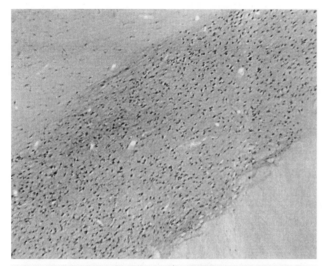

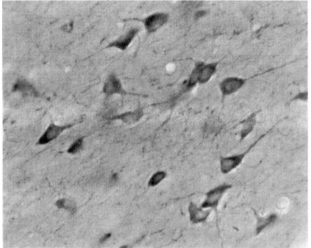

FIGURE 7-7 GluR1 immunoreactivity in the monkey subthalamic nucleus (top panel). Bottom panel shows a higher magnification (×40).

TABLE 7-3 Glutamate Receptor Subtypes in the Basal Ganglia

Receptor Type	Basal Ganglia Localization
NMDA	
NMDAR 1	Striatum: *projection neurons > intrinsic neurons; GPe; GPi; STN; SNc; SNr*
NMDAR 2A	Striatum
NMDAR 2B	Striatum: *projection neurons > intrinsic neurons*
NMDAR 2C	SNc
NMDAR 2D	Striatum: *intrinsic neurons ≫ projection neurons; GPe; GPi; STN; SNc; SNr*
AMPA	
GluR1	Striatum: *patch > matrix; intrinsic neurons ≫ projection neurons?; medium spiny, medium aspiny & large aspiny neurons; GPe; GPi; STN; SNc; SNr*
GluR2/3	Striatum: *medium spiny neurons; GPi; SNc*
GluR4	GPi; SNr; glia
Metabotropic	
mGluR1	Striatum < GPe < GPi < STN < SNc < SNr
mGluR2	STN
mGluR3	Striatum; glia
mGluR4	Striatum
mGluR5	Striatum: *projection neurons ≫ intrinsic neurons; ≫ GPe; GPi; STN; SNc; SNr*

acquisition, formation, consolidation, and recall.[140,141] The different glutamate receptors may have individual, but overlapping, contributions to these different components of memory mechanisms.

NMDA RECEPTORS

NMDA receptors mediate excitatory neurotransmission. The NMDA receptors play a critical role in very important steps of memory mechanisms. They are highly permeable to Ca^{2+}. The entry of Ca^{2+} is important to the initiation of several molecular events in the synapse.[113] The influx of Ca^{2+} is an early and critical step towards the formation of LTP in the CA1 region of the hippocampus, an area of the brain which plays an important role in memory in humans and other animals.[140,141] Lesions of CA1 or blocking NMDA receptors lead to memory dysfunctions. NMDAR 1 knockouts demonstrate significant loss of memory,[142,143] while enhancement of this receptor improves memory.[144] While lack of entry of Ca^{2+} through NMDA receptors leads to memory dysfunctions, too much of Ca^{2+} entering the cells leads to excitotoxic cell death. NMDA antagonists prevent cell death in various models of excitotoxic damage.[113]

AMPA RECEPTORS

Activation of AMPA receptors by glutamate mediate most of the fast, excitatory neurotransmission in the CNS.[113] The binding of glutamate or AMPA to the receptor is associated with influx of Na^+ from the extracellular space to

are strongly expressed in the glutamatergic corticostriate and GABAergic striatopallidal terminals.

The distributions of glutamate receptors in the basal ganglia are summarized in Table 7-3.

FUNCTIONS OF THE GLUTAMATERGIC RECEPTORS

Glutamate provides the excitatory input to almost the entire CNS. It has been proposed to play a major role in neuronal excitability, synaptic plasticity related to learning and memory, epileptogenesis, and excitotoxic cell death.[113,138,139] Most of our understanding of the role of glutamate receptors in learning and memory is derived from studies in the hippocampal region. The cellular mechanisms of long-term potentiation (LTP) and long-term depression (LTD) are critical for synaptic plasticity that is related to memory the intracellular compartment, although some native AMPA receptors are highly permeable to Ca^{2+}. Unlike NMDA receptors, AMPA receptors demonstrate less permeability to Ca^{2+} than the NMDA receptors, but a higher permeability to Na^+ and K^+. Since blocking of AMPA receptors with pharmacological agents completely blocks fast transmission at the synapse, the true nature of the function of the individual AMPA receptors must be derived from other methods, including studies using gene manipulation, and knockout techniques. Knockouts of GluR1 and GluR2 show memory dysfunctions. These studies suggest that, along with NMDA receptors, activation of AMPA receptors is equally important for LTP, and more so for LTD, mechanisms.

METABOTROPHIC GLUTAMATE RECEPTORS

mGluRs may play a role in both LTP and LTD, but evidence for its role in LTD is more significant. Among the eight different mGluRs, the family I type of GluRs, those associated with phosphatidylinositol turnover may have an important role in facilitating NMDA receptor activation-mediated LTP in the hippocampus. Most of the studies establishing a major role for glutamate in memory mechanisms have involved the hippocampal CA1 region, and it is clear that similar mechanisms also exist in different subdivisions of striatum,[145–147] amygdala,[148] and, for that matter, wherever glutamate is present.

Neurochemical Organization of the Serotonergic System in the Basal Ganglia

SOURCE OF SEROTONIN IN THE BASAL GANGLIA

The serotonin-producing neurons, based on their anatomic locations and connectivity, are grouped into nine (B1-B9) subdivisions.[149,150] The basal ganglia receive dense serotonergic innervations (B5) from the dorsal raphe nucleus (DRN).[151] About 35 percent of DRN neurons located in project to the striatum and 80–90 percent of these projections arise from the rostral and dorsomedial region of DRN.[151] The DRN neurons that project to the basal ganglia are functionally distinct and belong to a group of neurons that respond physiologically to altered muscle tone and sleep-wake and arousal states.[152] In contrast, the caudal "autonomic" subdivision of DRN projects to the hypothalamic-pituitary axis, and plays a role in the neuroendocrine response to stress.[153]

The different subnuclei of the basal ganglia receive varying densities of serotoninergic innervations. Earlier neurochemical studies suggested that serotonin levels are higher in the SN and GP than in the striatum.[154] Immunocytochemical studies confirm that the SN receives the heaviest serotonergic innervation.[151,155] Axons from DRN terminate more densely in the caudal and lateral third than in the rostral and medial substantia nigra. The dense region of serotonergic innervations of caudal and lateral nigra may correspond to the region

of SN that degenerates the earliest in PD, and is vulnerable to the mitochondrial toxins MPTP and rotenone.[12,31–33] The serotonergic fibers terminate mostly in SNr, where the dendrites of the dopaminergic neurons of SNc reside. The DRN neurons that project to the SN also project to the striatum by axon collaterals.

Within the GP, the medial pallidal segment stains more intensely for serotonin-immunopositive terminals than the lateral pallidal segment. The STN receives moderately dense serotonergic innervations from the dorsal raphe.[155]

The caudate and putamen receive less-dense serotonergic innervations than the SN and GP, and the distribution pattern of the serotonergic terminals is heterogeneous. The nucleus accumbens and the ventro- and dorsomedial limbic striatum receive denser serotonergic innervations than the associative striatum and the dorsolateral motor striatum.[155]

There are many significant patches of dorsolateral striatum which stain poorly for serotonergic terminals, and these serotonin-poor patches correspond to TH-poor patches and striosomes. The matrix areas of the striatum receive significantly more dense serotonin immunostaining, and correspond to TH-rich matrix compartment of the striatum. These findings suggest that the limbic and nonlimbic compartments of the striatum may be influenced by different serotonergic mechanisms.[155] The serotonergic terminals terminate predominantly on the dendritic spines or the shaft of the output neurons of the striatum, GP, and SN.[155]

MOLECULAR DIVERSITY OF SEROTONIN RECEPTORS AND THEIR SIGNAL TRANSDUCTION

Modern molecular biological and pharmacological techniques have identified seven different families of serotonin (5-HT) receptors (5-HT_1 to 5-HT_7), and 14 different 5-HT receptors.[156,157] All but one family, the 5-HT_3 family, which is a ligand-gated cation channel, are G protein-linked metabotropic receptors. Members of the 5-HT_1 family, consisting of 5-HT_{1A}, 5-HT_{1B}, 5-HT_{1D}, 5-HT_{1E}, and 5-HT_{1F} subtypes, are coupled mostly to Gi/o/z proteins, and, when activated, inhibit adenylyl cyclase activity, decrease cyclic AMP postsynaptically, and open K^+ channels. The 5-HT_2 family members (5-HT_{2A}, 5-HT_{2B}, 5-HT_{2C}) are coupled to Gq/11 proteins, and result in an increase in phospholipase C activity, an increase in inositol trisphosphate and diacylglycerol levels postsynaptically, and also close K^+ channels. The rest of the members of 5-HT receptor families, 5-HT_3 to 5-HT_7, are coupled to Gs proteins, and, when activated, stimulate adenylyl cyclase activity and lead to increased levels of cyclic AMP postsynaptically.

SEROTONERGIC RECEPTOR DISTRIBUTION IN THE BASAL GANGLIA

The various 5-HT receptors are distributed throughout the various nuclei of the basal ganglia.[157] Most are found

TABLE 7-4 Serotonergic Receptor Subtypes in the Basal Ganglia

Receptor Family	Type of Receptor	Effector Mechanisms	Subtypes	Location in the Basal Ganglia	Speculated Function in
5-HT$_1$	G protein-linked	Inhibits adenylyl cyclase Opens K$^+$ channels	5-HT$_{1A}$	Caudate-putamen Subthalamic nucleus	Anxiety, depression
			5-HT$_{1B}$	Caudate-putamen Substantia nigra Globus pallidus	Locomotion
			5-HT$_{1D\,alpha}$ 5-HT$_{1D\,beta}$	Substantia nigra	
			5-HT$_{1E}$	Caudate-putamen	
			5-HT$_{1F}$	Caudate-putamen	
5-HT$_2$	G protein-linked	Stimulation of phospholipase C Closing of K$^+$ channels	5-HT$_{2A}$	Nucleus accumbens Caudate-putamen	
			5-HT$_{2B}$	None detected in the basal ganglia	
			5-HT$_{2C}$	Nucleus accumbens Caudate-putamen Substania nigra	
5-HT$_3$	Ligand-gated cation channel			GABAergic projections neurons of caudate-putamen	Anxiety, depression Emesis
5-HT$_4$	G protein-linked	Stimulation of adenylyl cyclase		GABAergic projections neurons of caudate-putamen	Anxiety, depression
5-HT$_{5A}$	G protein-linked	Inhibits adenylyl cyclase		Caudate-putamen	
5-HT$_{5B}$	G protein-linked			Caudate-putamen	
5-HT$_6$	G protein-linked	Stimulation of adenylyl cyclase		Dendrites of GABAergic striatopallidal and strlatonigral neurons	Dopamine transmission
5-HT$_7$	G protein-linked	Stimulation of adenylyl cyclase		None detected in the basal ganglia	Circadian rhythms

postsynaptically at the target site of different nuclei of the basal ganglia. The 5-HT$_{1B/1D}$ receptors are localized to the soma, dendrite, and axon terminals of the DRN neurons as autoreceptors, and, when stimulated, decrease the firing rate and/or decrease release of serotonin at their terimals.[157,158]

The different subtypes of the 5-HT receptor family have been identified in the caudate-putamen, SN, and the pallidal segments.[157] mRNA for several of these receptors (5-HT$_{1A,1B/1D}$, 5-HT$_{2A,2C}$, 5-HT$_3$, 5-HT$_4$, 5-HT$_5$) are localized predominantly postsynaptically in the GABAergic output neurons of the striatum, and the proteins of these receptors are found in the target sites of the terminals of the striatal output neurons, namely GPe and SNr.[157] The 5-HT$_{2C}$ subtype is more dense in the medial GP than in any other basal ganglia structure, and this receptor is upregulated in PD.[159] The 5-HT$_{2C}$ receptor mRNA is localized to the GABAergic output neurons of GPi. Of the most recently identified 5-HT$_6$ and 5-HT$_7$ families, the 5-HT$_6$ family of receptors, located in the dendrites of the GABAergic striatopallidal and striatonigral output neurons, appear to have significant interaction with the dopaminergic system. The 5-HT$_{2B}$ and 5-HT$_7$ receptors have not yet been localized to any nucleus of the basal ganglia.[157]

FUNCTIONS OF THE SEROTONERGIC RECEPTORS

Serotonin plays an important role in neurobiological mechanisms of anxiety, sleep-wake cycle, mood regulation, neuroendocrine and locomotor response to stress, and pain. Recently, gene knockout technology has been used to understand the specific role played by individual 5-HT receptor subtypes in various functions of the serotonergic system.[160,161] The 5-HT$_{1A}$ knockouts exhibit a heightened anxiety response,[161] and pharmacological studies suggest that 5-HT$_{1A}$ agonists have anxiolytic and antidepressant properties, thereby suggesting a role of 5-HT$_{1A}$ in anxiety response.[157] The 5-HT$_{1B}$ knockouts have increased locomotor activity, increased aggressiveness, and a tendency to self-administer cocaine.[161] This behavior has been speculated to be due to a lack of expression of 5-HT$_{1B}$ receptor in the inhibitory GABAergic output neurons of the striatum, so that the mesencephalic neurons go unchecked, resulting in increased release of dopamine and leading to a heightened addictive behavior.[161] The 5-HT$_{1B/D/F}$ receptor agonists, the triptans, cause vasoconstriction, and reduce inflammatory response and pain of migraine attacks.[162] Several atypical and typical antipsychotic drugs have high affinity to 5-HT$_{2C/A}$ receptors.[157] The 5-HT$_3$ receptors facilitate dopamine transmission, and antagonsits of these receptors are anxiolytics and antiemetics.[157] The recently identified 5-HT$_6$ receptor may interact significantly with the GABAergic medium spiny neurons of the striatum,[157] and the 5-HT$_7$ receptor may play a role in circadian rhythms.[157]

The pioneering biochemical studies of Hornykiewicz et al. clearly demonstrated that brain serotonin levels are decreased (40 percent) in human PD.[163] Subsequent studies by several other groups showed that serotonin levels are indeed decreased in PD, more so in the depressed PD patients than in the nondepressed patients.[163] Neuropathological studies using traditional techniques, and immunocytochemical methods using antibodies specific to phenylalanine hydroxylase, have confirmed that DRN neurons do degenerate in PD.[164,165] The DRN neuron counts may be normal in the early stages of PD, but the loss is significant in patients in late stages of PD, although not as severe as the dopaminergic neurons of SN. The 5-HT neuronal loss in multisystem atrophies may be more predominant in raphe magnus, raphe pallidus, and raphe obscurus, which send descending serotonergic projections to the autonomic and motor nuclei of the brainstem and spinal cord.[166]

Despite these advancements, the role played by serotonin in the functions of the basal ganglia remains to be explored. The observation that there is a more significant decrease of serotonin in depressed PD patients and patients in later stages of the disease than in the nondepressed PD patients suggests that serotonin may be involved in the locomotor and/or cognitive responses to anxiety and mood.

Summary

The striatum, the entry point of all major information to the basal ganglia, receives converging inputs from several neurotransmitter systems. Of these, dopamine is the predominant neurotransmitter, as supported by the observation that 80 percent of all brain dopamine is found in the striatum. Dopamine provides an input to almost every striatal neuron. The limbic and associative cortical areas send excitatory glutamatergic input to the striatum. The intralaminar and other thalamic nuclei also convey their information through the glutamatergic projections to the striatum. Along with the cortical and thalamic glutamatergic afferents, the serotonergic inputs converge onto the dendritic spines and shafts of the same medium spiny input-output neuron of the striatum where the dopaminergic terminals also terminate. The activity of the medium spiny neuron is further modified by the giant cholinergic and other interneurons. Dopamine, as the predominant neurotransmitter, is in a position to reinforce, either positively or negatively, learning, initiating, consolidating, memorizing, and retrieving the information provided by the glutamatergic and serotonergic systems[167] (Fig. 7-8). This basic structural and neurochemical unit of the striatum is preserved in both the ventral and dorsal striatum.[168] There is

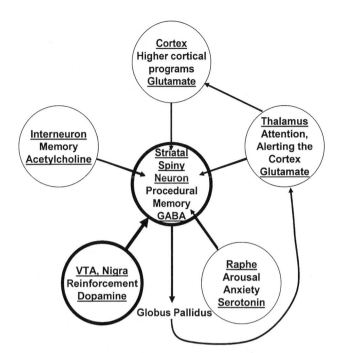

FIGURE 7-8 Schematics of pattern of convergence of major afferents to the striatum and their neurotransmitters. VTA: ventral tegmental area; GABA: Gamma-aminobutyric acid.

overwhelming evidence from clinical and basic science literature that hyper- and hypodopaminergic states in the striatum manifest in hyper- or hypokinetic syndromes. Dysfunctions of this basic neurochemical unit in the motor compartment of the striatum may be responsible for the spectrum of abnormal movements that are noted in disorders of the basal ganglia. However, it must be emphasized that, besides their role in locomotor behavior, the basal ganglia have been speculated to be involved in procedural memory,[169–172] attentional mechanisms,[173,174] learning, and addictive behavior.[174,175] The next wave of information relating to the molecular cascades that are responsible for interactions between dopamine and other neurotransmitters and neuropeptides will further consolidate our understanding of the functions of the basal ganglia.

Acknowledgment

Supported by Dr. Carl Baldridge Parkinson's Disease Research Fund.

References

1. Graybiel A: Neurotransmitters and neuromodulators in the basal ganglia. *Trends Neurosci* 13:244–254, 1990.

2. Alexander G, Delong M, Strick P: Parallel organization of functionally segregated circuits linking basal ganglia and cortex. *Annu Rev Neurosci* 9:357–381, 1986.

3. Albin RL, Young AB, Penney JB: The functional anatomy of basal ganglia disorders. *Trends Neurosci* 12:366–375, 1989.

4. Alexander GE, Crutcher MD: Functional architecture of basal ganglia circuits: Neural substrates of parallel processing. *Trends Neurosci* 13:266–271, 1990.

5. Jayaraman A: Functional compartments of the cat striatum. *Neurosci Abstr* 11:199, 1985.

6. Smith Y, Bevan MD, Shink E, et al: Microcircuitry of the direct and indirect pathways of the basal ganglia. *Neuroscience* 86:353–387, 1998.

7. Reiner A, Anderson KD: The patterns of neurotransmitter and neuropeptide co-occurrence among striatal projection neurons: Conclusions based on recent findings. *Brain Res Rev* 15:251–265, 1990.

8. Penney JBJ, Young AB: Striatal inhomogeneities and basal ganglia function. *Mov Disord* 1:3–15, 1986.

9. DeLong MR: Primate models of movement disorders of basal ganglia origin. *Trends Neurosci* 13:281–285, 1990.

10. Hornykiewicz O: Chemical neuroanatomy of the basal ganglia—normal and in Parkinson's disease. *J Chem Neuroanat* 22:3–12, 2001.

11. Bjorklund A, Lindvall O: Dopamine-containing systems in the CNS, in Bjorklund A, Hokfelt T (eds): *Classical Transmitters in the CNS: Handbook of Chemical Neuroanatomy*. New York: Elsevier, 1984, part 1, pp 55–122.

12. Hassler R: Zur Pathologie der Paralysis Agitans und des postencephalitischen Parkinsonismus. *J Psychol Neurol* 48:387–455, 1938.

13. Parent A, Mackey A, De Bellefeuille L: The subcortical afferents to caudate nucleus and putamen in primate: A fluorescence retrograde double labeling study. *Neuroscience* 10:1137–1150, 1983.

14. Jayaraman A, Nishimori T, Dobner P, et al: Cholecystokinin and neurotensin mRNAs are differentially expressed in subnuclei of the ventral tegmental area. *J Comp Neurol* 296:291–302, 1990.

15. Prensa L, Cossette M, Parent A: Dopaminergic innervation of human basal ganglia. *J Chem Neuroanat* 20:207–213, 2000.

16. Holt DJ, Graybiel AM, Saper CB: Neurochemical architecture of the human striatum. *J Comp Neurol* 384:1–25, 1997.

17. Betarbet R, Turner R, Chockkan V, et al: Dopaminergic neurons intrinsic to the primate striatum. *J Neurosci* 17:6761–6768, 1997.

18. Betarbet R, Greenamyre JT: Differential expression of glutamate receptors by the dopaminergic neurons of the primate striatum. *Exp Neurol* 159:401–408, 1999.

19. Parent A, Lavoie B, Smith Y, Bedard P: The dopaminergic nigropallidal projection in primates: distinct cellular origin and relative sparing in MPTP-treated monkeys. *Adv Neurol* 53:111–116, 1990.

20. Schneider JS, Dacko S: Relative sparing of the dopaminergic innervation of the globus pallidus in monkeys made hemiparkinsonian by intracarotid MPTP infusion. *Brain Res* 556:292–296, 1991.

21. Pickel VM, Beckley SC, Joh TH, Reis DJ: Ultrastructural immunocytochemical localization of tyrosine hydroxylase in the neostriatum. *Brain Res* 225:373–385, 1981.

22. Arluison M, Dietl M, Thibault J: Ultrastructural morphology of dopaminergic nerve terminals and synapses in the striatum of the rat using tyrosine hydroxylase immunocytochemistry: A topographical study. *Brain Res Bull* 13:269–285, 1984.

23. Bouyer JJ, Park DH, Joh TH, Pickel VM: Chemical and structural analysis of the relation between cortical inputs and tyrosine hydroxylase-containing terminals in rat neostriatum. *Brain Res* 302:267–275, 1984.

24. Wilson CJ: Basal ganglia, in GM Shepherd (ed): *The Synaptic Organization of the Brain*. New York: Oxford University Press, 1990, pp 279–316.

25. Gerfen C: The neostriatal mosaic: Multiple levels of compartmental organization in the basal ganglia. *Annu Rev Neurosci* 15:285–320, 1992.

26. Gauchy C, Kemel ML, Desban M, et al: The role of dopamine released from distal and proximal dendrites of nigrostriatal dopaminergic neurons in the control of GABA transmission in the thalamic nucleus ventralis medialis in the cat. *Neuroscience* 22:935–946, 1987.

27. Lynd-Balta E, Haber SN: The organization of midbrain projections to the striatum in the primate: Sensorimotor-related striatum versus ventral striatum. *Neuroscience* 59:625–640, 1994.

28. German DC, Dubach M, Askari S, et al: 1-Methyl-4-phenyl-1,2,3,6-tetrahydropyridine-induced parkinsonian syndrome in *Macaca fascicularis*: Which midbrain dopaminergic neurons are lost? *Neuroscience* 24:161–174, 1988.

29. Hirsch EC, Graybiel AM, Agid Y: Selective vulnerability of pigmented dopaminergic neurons in Parkinson's disease. *Acta Neurol Scand Suppl* 126:19–22, 1989.

30. German DC, Manaye KF, Sonsalla PK, Brooks BA: Midbrain dopaminergic cell loss in Parkinson's disease and MPTP-induced parkinsonism: Sparing of calbindin-D28k-containing cells. *Ann N Y Acad Sci* 648:42–62, 1992.

31. Graybiel AM, Moratalla R, Quinn B, et al: Early-stage loss of dopamine uptake-site binding in MPTP-treated monkeys. *Adv Neurol* 60:34–39, 1993.

32. Hirsch E, Graybiel AM, Agid YA: Melanized dopaminergic neurons are differentially susceptible to degeneration in Parkinson's disease. *Nature* 334:345–348, 1988.

33. Betarbet R, Sherer TB, MacKenzie G, et al: Chronic systemic pesticide exposure reproduces features of Parkinson's disease. *Nat Neurosci* 3:1301–1306, 2000.

34. Kebabian JW, Calne DB: Multiple receptors for dopamine. *Nature* 277:93–96, 1979.

35. Civelli O, Bunzow JR, Grandy DK: Molecular diversity of the dopamine receptors. *Annu Rev Pharmacol Toxicol* 33:281–307, 1993.

36. Jackson DM, Westlind-Danielsson A: Dopamine receptors: Molecular biology, biochemistry and behavioural aspects. *Pharmacol Ther* 64:291–370, 1994.

37. Hartman DS, Civelli O: Dopamine receptor diversity: Molecular and pharmacological perspectives. *Prog Drug Res* 48:173–194, 1997.

38. Missale C, Nash SR, Robinson SW, et al: Dopamine receptors: from structure to function. *Physiol Rev* 78:189–225, 1998.

39. Gether U: Uncovering molecular mechanisms involved in activation of G protein-coupled receptors. *Endocr Rev* 21:90–113, 2000.

40. Marinissen MJ, Gutkind JS: G-protein-coupled receptors and signalling networks: Emerging paradigms. *Trends Pharmacol Sci* 22:368–376, 2001.

41. Van Tol HHM, Wu CM, Guan H-C, et al: Multiple dopamine D4 receptor variants in the human population. *Nature* 358:149–152, 1992.

42. Meador-Woodruff JH, Damask SP, Wang J, et al: Dopamine receptor mRNA expression in human striatum and neocortex. *Neuropsychopharmacology* 15:17–29, 1996.

43. Dearry A, Gingrich JA, Falardeau P, et al: Molecular cloning and expression of the gene for a human D1 dopamine receptor. *Nature* 347:72–76, 1990.

44. Hurd YL, Suzuki M, Sedvall GC: D1 and D2 dopamine receptor mRNA expression in whole hemisphere sections of the human brain. *J Chem Neuroanat* 22:127–137, 2001.

45. Lidow MS, Koh PO, Arnsten AF: D1 dopamine receptors in the mouse prefrontal cortex: Immunocytochemical and cognitive neuropharmacological analyses. *Synapse* 47:101–108, 2003.

46. Khan ZU, Gutierrez A, Martin R, et al: Differential regional and cellular distribution of dopamine D2-like receptors: An immunocytochemical study of subtype-specific antibodies in rat and human brain. *J Comp Neurol* 402:353–371, 1998.

47. Lester J, Fink S, Aronin N, et al: Colocalization of D1 and D2 dopamine receptor mRNAs in striatal neurons. *Brain Res* 621:106–110, 1993.

48. Surmeier DJ, Eberwine J, Wilson CJ, et al: Dopamine receptor subtypes colocalize in rat striatonigral neurons. *Proc Natl Acad Sci U S A* 89:10178–10182, 1992.

49. Landwehrmeyer B, Mengod G, Palacios JM: Dopamine D3 receptor mRNA and binding sites in human brain. *Brain Res Mol Brain Res* 18:187–192, 1993.

50. Murray AM, Ryoo HL, Gurevich E, et al: Localization of dopamine D3 receptors to mesolimbic and D2 receptors to mesostriatal regions of human forebrain. *Proc Natl Acad Sci U S A* 91:11271–11275, 1994.

51. Gurevich EV, Joyce JN: Distribution of dopamine D3 receptor expressing neurons in the human forebrain: Comparison with D2 receptor expressing neurons. *Neuropsychopharmacology* 20:60–80, 1999.

52. Mrzljak L, Bergson C, Pappy M, et al: Localization of dopamine D4 receptors in GABAergic neurons of the primate brain. *Nature* 381:245–248, 1996.

53. Rivera A, Cuellar B, Giron FJ, et al: Dopamine D4 receptors are heterogeneously distributed in the striosomes/matrix compartments of the striatum. *J Neurochem* 80:219–229, 2002.

54. Khan ZU, Gutierrez A, Martin R, et al: Dopamine D5 receptors of rat and human brain. *Neuroscience* 100:689–699, 2000.

55. Sibley DR: New insights into dopaminergic receptor function using antisense and genetically altered animals. *Annu Rev Pharmacol Toxicol* 39:313–341, 1999.

56. Glickstein SB, Schmauss C: Dopamine receptor functions: Lessons from knockout mice [corrected]. *Pharmacol Ther* 91:63–83, 2001.

57. El-Ghundi M, Fletcher PJ, Drago J, et al: Spatial learning deficit in dopamine D(1) receptor knockout mice. *Eur J Pharmacol* 383:95–106, 1999.

58. Williams GV, Goldman-Rakic PS: Modulation of memory fields by dopamine D1 receptors in prefrontal cortex. *Nature* 376:572–575, 1995.

59. Baik JH, Picetti R, Saiardi A, et al: Parkinsonian-like locomotor impairment in mice lacking dopamine D2 receptors. *Nature* 377:424–428, 1995.

60. Caine SB, Koob GF: Modulation of cocaine self-administration in the rat through D-3 dopamine receptors. *Science* 260:1814–1816, 1993.

61. Dulawa SC, Grandy DK, Low MJ, et al: Dopamine D4 receptor-knock-out mice exhibit reduced exploration of novel stimuli. *J Neurosci* 19:9550–9556, 1999.

62. Zhou FM, Wilson CJ, Dani JA: Cholinergic interneuron characteristics and nicotinic properties in the striatum. *J Neurobiol* 53:590–605, 2002.

63. Pisani A, Bonsi P, Picconi B, et al: Role of tonically-active neurons in the control of striatal function: Cellular mechanisms and behavioral correlates. *Prog Neuropsychopharmacol Biol Psychiatry* 25:211–230, 2001.

64. Izzo PN, Bolam JP: Cholinergic synaptic input to different parts of spiny striatonigral neurons in the rat. *J Comp Neurol* 269:219–234, 1988.

65. Kemp JM, Powell TPS: The termination of fibres from the cerebral cortex and thalamus upon dendritic spines in the caudate nucleus: A study with the Golgi method. *Philos Trans R Soc Lond Biol Sci* 262:429–439, 1971.

66. Contant C, Umbriaco D, Garcia S, et al: Ultrastructural characterization of the acetylcholine innervation in adult rat neostriatum. *Neuroscience* 71:937–947, 1996.

67. Kubota Y, Inagaki S, Shimada S, et al: Neostriatal cholinergic neurons receive direct synaptic inputs from dopaminergic axons. *Brain Res* 413:179–184, 1987.

68. Mesulam M-M, Mash D, Hersh L, et al: Cholinergic innervation of the human striatum, globus pallidus, subthalamic nucleus, substantia nigra, and red nucleus. *J Comp Neurol* 323:252–268, 1992.

69. Rye DB, Saper CB, Lee HJ, Wainer BH: Pedunculopontine tegmental nucleus of the rat: Cytoarchitecture, cytochemistry, and some extrapyramidal connections of the mesopontine tegmentum. *J Comp Neurol* 259:483–528, 1987.

70. Pahapill PA, Lozano AM: The pedunculopontine nucleus and Parkinson's disease. *Brain* 123(Pt 9):1767–1783, 2000.

71. Kim R, Nakano K, Jayaraman A, et al: Projections of the globus pallidus and adjacent structures: An autoradiographic study in the monkey. *J Comp Neurol* 169:263–290, 1976.

72. Rye DB, Lee HJ, Saper CB, Wainer BH: Medullary and spinal efferents of the pedunculopontine tegmental nucleus and adjacent mesopontine tegmentum in the rat. *J Comp Neurol* 269:315–341, 1987.

73. Rye D, Thomas J, Levey A: Distribution of molecular muscarinic (m1-m4) receptor subtypes and choline acetyltransferase in the pontine reticular formation of man and non-human primates. *Sleep Res Abstr* 24:59, 1995.

74. Shink E, Sidibe M, Smith Y: Efferent connections of the internal globus pallidus in the squirrel monkey: II. Topography and synaptic organization of pallidal efferents to the pedunculopontine nucleus. *J Comp Neurol* 382:348–363, 1997.

75. Zweig RM, Jankel WR, Hedreen JC, et al: The pedunculopontine nucleus in Parkinson's disease. *Ann Neurol* 26:41–46, 1989.

76. Griffiths PD, Sambrook MA, Perry R, Crossman AR: Changes in benzodiazepine and acetylcholine receptors in the globus pallidus in Parkinson's disease. *J Neurol Sci* 100:131–136, 1990.

77. Changeux JP, Bertrand D, Corringer PJ, et al: Brain nicotinic receptors: Structure and regulation, role in learning and reinforcement. *Brain Res Brain Res Rev* 26:198–216, 1998.

78. Klink R, de Kerchove d'Exaerde A, Zoli M, et al: Molecular and physiological diversity of nicotinic acetylcholine receptors in the midbrain dopaminergic nuclei. *J Neurosci* 21:1452–1463, 2001.

79. Caulfield MP, Birdsall NJ: International Union of Pharmacology. XVII. Classification of muscarinic acetylcholine receptors. *Pharmacol Rev* 50:279–290, 1998.

80. van Koppen CJ, Kaiser B: Regulation of muscarinic acetylcholine receptor signaling. *Pharmacol Ther* 98:197–220, 2003.

81. Weiner DM, Levey AI, Brann MR: Expression of muscarinic acetylcholine and dopamine receptor mRNAs in rat basal ganglia. *Proc Natl Acad Sci U S A* 87:7050–7054, 1990.

82. Vilaro MT, Mengod G, Palacios JM: Advances and limitations of the molecular neuroanatomy of cholinergic receptors: The example of multiple muscarinic receptors. *Prog Brain Res* 98:95–101, 1993.

83. Levey A, Kitt C, Simonds W, et al: Identification and localization of muscarinic acetylcholine receptor proteins in brain with subtype-specific antibodies. *J Neurosci* 11:3218–3226, 1991.

84. Levey AI, Edmunds SM, Heilman CJ, et al: Localization of muscarinic m3 receptor protein and m3 receptor binding in rat brain. *Neuroscience* 63:207–221, 1994.

85. Flynn D, Ferrari-DiLeo G, Mash D, Levey A: Differential regulation of molecular subtypes of muscarinic receptors in Alzheimer's disease. *J Neurochem* 64:1888–1891, 1995.

86. Hersch SM, Gutekunst CA, Rees HD, et al: Distribution of m1-m4 muscarinic receptor proteins in the rat striatum: Light and electron microscopic immunocytochemistry using subtype-specific antibodies. *J Neurosci* 14:3351–3363, 1994.

87. Bernard V, Normand E, Bloch B: Phenotypical characterization of the rat striatal neurons expressing muscarinic receptor genes. *J Neurosci* 12:3591–3600, 1992.

88. Yan Z, Flores-Hernandez J, Surmeier DJ: Coordinated expression of muscarinic receptor messenger RNAs in striatal medium spiny neurons. *Neuroscience* 103:1017–1024, 2001.

89. Rye D, Thomas J, Levey A: Distribution of molecular muscarinic (m1-m4) receptor subtypes and choline acetyltransferase in the pontine reticular formation of man and non-human primates. *Sleep Res Abstr* 24:59, 1995.

90. Yasuda RP, Ciesla W, Flores LR, et al: Development of antisera selective for m4 and m5 muscarinic cholinergic receptors: Distribution of m4 and m5 receptors in rat brain. *Mol Pharmacol* 43:149–157, 1993.

91. Kitabatake Y, Hikida T, Watanabe D, et al: Impairment of reward-related learning by cholinergic cell ablation in the striatum. *Proc Natl Acad Sci U S A* 100:7965–7970, 2003.

92. Everitt BJ, Robbins TW: Central cholinergic systems and cognition. *Annu Rev Psychol* 48:649–684, 1997.

93. Belluardo N, Mudo G, Blum M, et al: Neurotrophic effects of central nicotinic receptor activation. *J Neural Transm Suppl* 60:227–245, 2000.

94. Dani JA: Overview of nicotinic receptors and their roles in the central nervous system. *Biol Psychiatry* 49:166–174, 2001.

95. Cordero-Erausquin M, Marubio LM, Klink R, et al: Nicotinic receptor function: New perspectives from knockout mice. *Trends Pharmacol Sci* 21:211–217, 2000.

96. Picciotto MR, Caldarone BJ, King SL, et al: Nicotinic receptors in the brain. Links between molecular biology and behavior. *Neuropsychopharmacology* 22:451–465, 2000.

97. Picciotto MR, Caldarone BJ, Brunzell DH, et al: Neuronal nicotinic acetylcholine receptor subunit knockout mice: Physiological and behavioral phenotypes and possible clinical implications. *Pharmacol Ther* 92:89–108, 2001.

98. Marubio LM, Gardier AM, Durier S, et al: Effects of nicotine in the dopaminergic system of mice lacking the alpha4 subunit of neuronal nicotinic acetylcholine receptors. *Eur J Neurosci* 17:1329–1337, 2003.

99. Zachariou V, Caldarone BJ, Weathers-Lowin A, et al: Nicotine receptor inactivation decreases sensitivity to cocaine. *Neuropsychopharmacology* 24:576–589, 2001.

100. Salas R, Orr-Urtreger A, Broide RS, et al: The nicotinic acetylcholine receptor subunit alpha 5 mediates short-term effects of nicotine in vivo. *Mol Pharmacol* 63:1059–1066, 2003.

101. Bymaster FP, McKinzie DL, Felder CC, et al: Use of M1-M5 muscarinic receptor knockout mice as novel tools to delineate the physiological roles of the muscarinic cholinergic system. *Neurochem Res* 28:437–442, 2003.

102. Zhang W, Yamada M, Gomeza J, et al: Multiple muscarinic acetylcholine receptor subtypes modulate striatal dopamine release, as studied with M1-M5 muscarinic receptor knock-out mice. *J Neurosci* 22:6347–6352, 2002.

103. Hamilton SE, Nathanson NM: The M1 receptor is required for muscarinic activation of mitogen-activated protein (MAP) kinase in murine cerebral cortical neurons. *J Biol Chem* 276:15850–15853, 2001.

104. Gerber DJ, Sotnikova TD, Gainetdinov RR, et al: Hyperactivity, elevated dopaminergic transmission, and response to amphetamine in M1 muscarinic acetylcholine receptor-deficient mice. *Proc Natl Acad Sci U S A* 98:15312–15317, 2001.

105. Gomeza J, Zhang L, Kostenis E, et al: Enhancement of D1 dopamine receptor-mediated locomotor stimulation in M(4) muscarinic acetylcholine receptor knockout mice. *Proc Natl Acad Sci U S A* 96:10483–10488, 1999.

106. Basile AS, Fedorova I, Zapata A, et al: Deletion of the M5 muscarinic acetylcholine receptor attenuates morphine reinforcement and withdrawal but not morphine analgesia. *Proc Natl Acad Sci U S A* 99:11452–11457, 2002.

107. Wess J, Duttaroy A, Gomeza J, et al: Muscarinic receptor subtypes mediating central and peripheral antinociception studied with muscarinic receptor knockout mice: A review. *Life Sci* 72:2047–2054, 2003.

108. Yamada M, Miyakawa T, Duttaroy A, et al: Mice lacking the M3 muscarinic acetylcholine receptor are hypophagic and lean. *Nature* 410:207–212, 2001.

109. Divac I, Fonnum F, Storm-Mathisen J: High affinity uptake of glutamate in terminals of corticostriatal axons. *Nature* 266:377–378, 1977.

110. Young A, Bromberg M, Penney J: Decreased glutamate uptake in subcortical areas deafferented by sensorimotor cortical ablation in the cat. *J Neurosci* 1:241–249, 1981.

111. Parent A: Extrinsic connections of the basal ganglia. *Trends Neurosci* 13:254–258, 1990.

112. Blandini F, Porter R, Greenamyre J: Glutamate and Parkinson's disease. *Mol Neurobiol* 12:73–94, 1996.

113. Ozawa S, Kamiya H, Tsuzuki K: Glutamate receptors in the mammalian central nervous system. *Prog Neurobiol* 54:581–618, 1998.

114. Ishii T, Moriyoshi K, Sugihara H, et al: Molecular characterization of the *N*-methyl-D-aspartate receptor subunits. *J Biol Chem* 268:2836–2843, 1993.

115. Kutsuwada T, Kashiwabuchi N, Mori H, et al: Molecular diversity of the NMDA receptor channel. *Nature* 358:36–41, 1992.

116. Meguro H, Mori H, Araki K, et al: Functional characterization of a heteromeric NMDA receptor channel expressed from cloned cDNAs. *Nature* 357:70–74, 1992.

117. Monyer H, Sprengel R, Schoepfer R, et al: Heteromeric NMDA receptors: Molecular and functional distinction of subtypes. *Science* 256:1217–1221, 1992.

118. Moriyoshi K, Masu M, Ishii T, et al: Molecular cloning and characterization of the rat NMDA receptor. *Nature* 354:31–37, 1991.

119. Keinanen K, Wisden W, Sommer B, et al: A family of AMPA-selective glutamate receptors. *Science* 249:556–560, 1990.

120. Hollmann M, O'Shea-Greenfield A, Rogers S, Heinemann S: Cloning by functional expression of a member of the glutamate receptor family. *Nature* 342:643–648, 1989.

121. Hollmann M, Hartley M, Heineman S: Ca2+ permeability of KA-AMPA-gated glutamate receptor channels depends on subunit composition. *Science* 252:851–853, 1991.

122. Sommer B, Keinanen K, Verdoorn T, et al: Flip and flop: A cell specific functional switch in glutamate-operated channels. *Science* 249:1580–1585, 1990.

123. Pin J-P, Duvoisin R: The metabotropic glutamate receptors: Structure and functions. *Neuropharmacology* 34:1–26, 1995.

124. Albin RL, Makowiec RL, Hollingsworth ZR, et al: Excitatory amino acid binding sites in the basal ganglia of the rat: A quantitative autoradiographic study. *Neuroscience* 46:35–48, 1992.

125. Ravenscroft P, Brotchie J: NMDA receptors in the basal ganglia. *J Anat* 196(Pt 4):577–585, 2000.

126. Petralia R, Yokotani N, Wenthold R: Light and electron microscope distribution of the NMDA receptor subunit NMDAR1 in the rat nervous system using a selective antipeptide antibody. *J Neurosci* 14:667–696, 1994.

127. Nash N, Heilman C, Rees H, Levey A: Novel human NMDA receptor subunits: Cloning and immunological characterization of exon 5 containing isoforms. *Soc Neurosci Abstr* 21:1111, 1995.

128. Standaert D, Testa C, Young A, Penney J: Organization of *N*-methyl-D-aspartate glutamate receptor gene expression in the basal ganglia of the rat. *J Comp Neurol* 343:1–16, 1994.

129. Landwehrmeyer G, Standaert D, Testa C, et al: NMDA receptor subunit mRNA expression by projection neurons and interneurons in rat striatum. *J Neurosci* 15:5297–5307, 1995.

130. Martin LJ, Blackstone CD, Levey AI, et al: AMPA glutamate receptor subunits are differentially distributed in rat brain. *Neuroscience* 53:327–358, 1993.

131. Petralia RS, Wenthold RJ: Light and electron immunocytochemical localization of AMPA-selective glutamate receptors in the rat brain. *J Comp Neurol* 318:329–354, 1992.

132. Paquet M, Smith Y: Differential localization of AMPA glutamate receptor subunits in the two segments of the globus pallidus and the substantia nigra pars reticulata in the squirrel monkey. *Eur J Neurosci* 8:229–233, 1996.

133. Paquet M, Tremblay M, Soghomonian JJ, et al: AMPA and NMDA glutamate receptor subunits in midbrain dopaminergic neurons in the squirrel monkey: An immunohistochemical and in situ hybridization study. *J Neurosci* 17:1377–1396, 1997.

134. Testa C, Standaert D, Young A, Penney J: Metabotropic glutamate receptor mRNA expression in the basal ganglia of the rat. *J Neurosci* 14:3005–3018, 1994.

135. Testa C, Standaert D, Landwehrmeyer G, et al: Differential expression of mGluR5 metabotropic glutamate receptor mRNA by rat striatal neurons. *J Neurosci* 354:241–252, 1995.

136. Hubert GW, Paquet M, Smith Y: Differential subcellular localization of mGluR1a and mGluR5 in the rat and monkey substantia nigra. *J Neurosci* 21:1838–1847, 2001.

137. Smith Y, Charara A, Hanson JE, et al: GABA(B) and group I metabotropic glutamate receptors in the striatopallidal complex in primates. *J Anat* 196(Pt 4):555–576, 2000.

138. Riedel G, Platt B, Micheau J: Glutamate receptor function in learning and memory. *Behav Brain Res* 140:1–47, 2003.

139. Shimizu E, Tang YP, Rampon C, et al: NMDA receptor-dependent synaptic reinforcement as a crucial process for memory consolidation. *Science* 290:1170–1174, 2000.

140. Malenka RC, Nicoll RA: Long-term potentiation: A decade of progress? *Science* 285:1870–1874, 1999.

141. Mayford M, Kandel ER: Genetic approaches to memory storage. *Trends Genet* 15:463–470, 1999.

142. McHugh TJ, Blum KI, Tsien JZ, et al: Impaired hippocampal representation of space in CA1-specific NMDAR1 knockout mice. *Cell* 87:1339–1349, 1996.

143. Tsien JZ, Huerta PT, Tonegawa S: The essential role of hippocampal CA1 NMDA receptor-dependent synaptic plasticity in spatial memory. *Cell* 87:1327–1338, 1996.

144. Tang YP, Shimizu E, Dube GR, et al: Genetic enhancement of learning and memory in mice. *Nature* 401:63–69, 1999.

145. Gubellini P, Saulle E, Centonze D, et al: Selective involvement of mGlu1 receptors in corticostriatal LTD. *Neuropharmacology* 40:839–846, 2001.

146. Gubellini P, Saulle E, Centonze D, et al: Corticostriatal LTP requires combined mGluR1 and mGluR5 activation. *Neuropharmacology* 44:8–16, 2003.

147. Thomas MJ, Malenka RC: Synaptic plasticity in the mesolimbic dopamine system. *Philos Trans R Soc Lond B Biol Sci* 358:815–819, 2003.

148. Chapman PF, Ramsay MF, Krezel W, et al: Synaptic plasticity in the amygdala: Comparisons with hippocampus. *Ann N Y Acad Sci* 985:114–124, 2003.

149. Dahlstrom A, Fuxe K: Localization of monoamines in the lower brain stem. *Experientia* 20:398–399, 1964.

150. Tork I: Anatomy of the serotonergic system. *Ann N Y Acad Sci* 600:9–34; discussion 34–35, 1990.

151. Steinbusch HW, Nieuwenhuys R, Verhofstad AA, et al: The nucleus raphe dorsalis of the rat and its projection upon the caudatoputamen. A combined cytoarchitectonic, immunohistochemical and retrograde transport study. *J Physiol (Paris)* 77:157–174, 1981.

152. Jacobs BL, Fornal CA: Serotonin and motor activity. *Curr Opin Neurobiol* 7:820–825, 1997.

153. Lowry CA: Functional subsets of serotonergic neurones: Implications for control of the hypothalamic-pituitary-adrenal axis. *J Neuroendocrinol* 14:911–923, 2002.

154. Bacopoulos NG, Redmond DE, Roth RH: Serotonin and dopamine metabolites in brain regions and cerebrospinal fluid of a primate species: Effects of ketamine and fluphenazine. *J Neurochem* 32:1215–1218, 1979.

155. Lavoie B, Parent A: Immunohistochemical study of the serotonergic innervation of the basal ganglia in the squirrel monkey. *J Comp Neurol* 299:1–16, 1990.

156. Hoyer D, Clarke DE, Fozard JR, et al: International Union of Pharmacology classification of receptors for 5-hydroxytryptamine (serotonin). *Pharmacol Rev* 46:157–203, 1994.

157. Barnes NM, Sharp T: A review of central 5-HT receptors and their function. *Neuropharmacology* 38:1083–1152, 1999.

158. Gothert M: Presynaptic serotonin receptors in the central nervous system. *Ann N Y Acad Sci* 604:102–112, 1990.

159. Fox SH, Brotchie JM: 5-HT2C receptor binding is increased in the substantia nigra pars reticulata in Parkinson's disease. *Mov Disord* 15:1064–1069, 2000.

160. Gingrich JA, Hen R: The broken mouse: The role of development, plasticity and environment in the interpretation of phenotypic changes in knockout mice. *Curr Opin Neurobiol* 10:146–152, 2000.

161. Gingrich JA, Hen R: Dissecting the role of the serotonin system in neuropsychiatric disorders using knockout mice. *Psychopharmacology (Berl)* 155:1–10, 2001.

162. Tepper SJ, Rapoport AM, Sheftell FD: Mechanisms of action of the 5-HT1B/1D receptor agonists. *Arch Neurol* 59:1084–1088, 2002.

163. Kish SJ: Biochemistry of Parkinson's disease: Is a brain serotonergic deficiency a characteristic of idiopathic Parkinson's disease? *Adv Neurol* 91:39–49, 2003.

164. Paulus W, Jellinger K: The neuropathologic basis of different clinical subgroups of Parkinson's disease. *J Neuropathol Exp Neurol* 50:743–755, 1991.

165. Halliday GM, Blumbergs PC, Cotton RG, et al: Loss of brainstem serotonin- and substance P-containing neurons in Parkinson's disease. *Brain Res* 510:104–107, 1990.

166. Kovacs GG, Kloppel S, Fischer I, et al: Nucleus-specific alteration of raphe neurons in human neurodegenerative disorders. *Neuroreport* 14:73–76, 2003.

167. Schultz W: Predictive reward signal of dopamine neurons. *J Neurophysiol* 80:1–27, 1998.

168. Nicola SM, Malenka RC: Modulation of synaptic transmission by dopamine and norepinephrine in ventral but not dorsal striatum. *J Neurophysiol* 79:1768–1776, 1998.

169. Phillips AG, Carr GD: Cognition and the basal ganglia: A possible substrate for procedural knowledge. *Can J Neurol Sci* 14:381–385, 1987.

170. Knowlton BJ, Mangels JA, Squire LR: A neostriatal habit learning system in humans. *Science* 273:1399–1402, 1996.

171. Squire LR, Zola SM: Structure and function of declarative and nondeclarative memory systems. *Proc Natl Acad Sci U S A* 93:13515–13522, 1996.

172. Squire LR: Memory systems. *CR Acad Sci III* 321:153–156, 1998.

173. Jayaraman A: The basal ganglia and cognition: An interpretation of anatomical connectivity pattern, in Schneider JS, and Lidsky T (eds): *Basal Ganglia and Behavior: Sensory Aspects of Motor Functioning*. Toronto: Hans Huber Publications, 1987, pp 149–160.

174. Nieoullon A: Dopamine and the regulation of cognition and attention. *Prog Neurobiol* 67:53–83, 2002.

175. Nestler EJ: Common molecular and cellular substrates of addiction and memory. *Neurobiol Learn Mem* 78:637–647, 2002.

Chapter 8 _____

NEUROTROPHIC FACTORS

CLIFFORD W. SHULTS

TRANSFORMING GROWTH FACTOR-β FAMILY   131
    Glial Cell Line-Derived Neurotrophic Factor   131
    Other Members of the GDNF Family   132
    TGF-β1, 2, and 3   133
    Alternate Methods for Administration of GDNF
       and Other Members of the GDNF Family   133
NEUROTROPHINS   135
    BDNF   135
    NT-3   136
    NT-4/5   136
FIBROBLAST GROWTH FACTORS   136
CILIARY NEUROTROPHIC FACTOR   137
EPIDERMAL GROWTH FACTOR/TRANSFORMING
    GROWTH FACTOR-α   137
INSULIN   137
SUMMARY   137

The initial concept of neurotrophic factors was shaped by the original studies of nerve growth factor (NGF), which was the first neurotrophic factor to be identified.[1] These early studies indicated that neurotrophic factors are produced in the target tissue and retrogradely transported to the neurons, which are dependent on exposure to the trophic factor for survival. For example, a trophic factor that is supportive of the survival of the dopaminergic neurons in the substantia nigra pars compacta (SNc) would be produced in the striatum and retrogradely transported to the neurons in the SNc. Subsequent studies have expanded our understanding of modes of actions of neurotrophic factors.[2] Neurotrophic factors can be produced not only by targets of the neurons but also by adjacent cells, such as glia and ensheathing cells of peripheral nerves, and act on the nearby neurons. Neurotrophic factors can also be produced by neurons and act in a paracrine, autocrine and, perhaps, even an intracrine fashion. In addition, neurotrophic factors can be transported antegradely and released.[3]

A trophic factor could be important in a neurological disorder by virtue of a role in the pathogenesis, or as a treatment, of the disorder. Although there is, as yet, no example in which a deficiency of a specific neurotrophic factor is the unequivocal cause of a neurological disorder, it is plausible that a deficiency of a neurotrophic factor could be the cause or a contributing factor in the development of a disorder. In fact, a recent study has demonstrated that in certain cases of familial Parkinson's disease (PD), the affected subjects carry a mutation in the gene for Nurr1, which is a protein important in the differentiation of nigral dopaminergic neurons.[4] Also, there appears to be a relative deficiency in fibroblast growth factor-2 (FGF-2) and brain-derived neurotrophic factor (BDNF) in the nigral dopaminergic neurons in parkinsonian brains (see below).

Trophic factors hold great promise in the treatment of neurological disorders, and could potentially act by a number of mechanisms. Because PD is the movement disorder in which neurotrophic factors have been studied most extensively, it is discussed here as a model for the ways in which neurotrophic factors could be used. First, a trophic factor could slow the progressive loss of dopaminergic neurons in the SNc, which underlies PD. Second, a trophic factor could enhance the activity of remaining nigral dopaminergic neurons. Third, a trophic factor could stimulate remaining dopaminergic neurons in the SNc and their axons projecting to the striatum to sprout collateral axons and reinnervate the striatum. Fourth, trophic factors could also be indirectly useful in the treatment of PD, when used in conjunction with transplantation of dopaminergic neurons, or other catecholaminergic cells, to the striatum in parkinsonian patients. Finally, investigators have discovered that certain trophic factors can cause proliferation and/or differentiation of embryonic neuronal progenitor cells in vitro. This discovery raises the possibility that trophic factors could be used to promote the proliferation of progenitor cells and differentiation into relatively pure cultures of dopaminergic neurons, which could later be transplanted in parkinsonian patients.[5,6] Because most of the work directed towards a possible role for trophic factors in pathogenesis or treatment of movement disorders has been directed towards PD, most of the studies discussed will be related to PD.

Transforming Growth Factor-β Family

The TGF-β superfamily is a large family of trophic factors that include TGF-β1-5, glial cell line-derived neurotrophic factor (GDNF), neurturin, artemin/neublastin/enovin and persephin, and distantly related factors such as activins/inhibins, and bone morphogenic proteins.[7-9]

GLIAL CELL LINE-DERIVED NEUROTROPHIC FACTOR

GDNF was purified from a rat glial cell line on the basis of its ability to promote dopamine uptake in cultures of embryonic mesencephalic cells.[10] In Lin's initial study,[10] GDNF was also demonstrated to increase the survival of dopaminergic neurons, but not of serotonergic or gamma-aminobutyric acid (GABAergic) neurons, in embryonic midbrain cultures, as well as to increase the neurite outgrowth and the average size of the dopaminergic neurons. During development of the nigrostriatal dopaminergic system in the rat, the message for GDNF is sequentially expressed in the midbrain, then in the striatum.[11] At embryonic day 15.5, a time at which nigral dopaminergic neurons have undergone their final division and the initial innervation of the striatum by nigral dopaminergic axons is occurring, abundant message for GDNF is found in the midbrain, but little message for GDNF is expressed in the developing striatum. At postnatal day 1, as connections between the nigral dopaminergic neurons and their targets in the striatum mature, message for GDNF is reduced in the midbrain but is conspicuously increased in the striatum. This pattern of expression of message for GDNF suggests that it acts first as a locally derived trophic factor and then as a target-derived trophic factor. Nakajima et al. recently reported that lesioning of the nigrostriatal dopaminergic system by injection of 6-hydroxydopamine (6-OHDA) into the substantia nigra increased the trophic activity in the striatum ipsilateral to the lesion for cultured dopaminergic neurons and that a major component to the trophic activity is GDNF and a minor component is FGF-2.[12] The message for GDNF is also expressed in many other regions of the nervous system and in nonneural tissue, including muscle.[13–18] For example, the message for GDNF has been found in the striatum, hippocampus, cortex, and spinal cord in the adult rat and human brain.[15] The widespread distribution of GDNF suggests that it is also a trophic factor for nondopaminergic neurons, and a number of studies have shown this to be the case. Both in vitro and in vivo, GDNF has been shown to support the survival of motor neurons.[19–22] GDNF has also been reported to attenuate the convulsions and loss of hippocampal neurons in kainic acid-treated rats[23] and to promote the survival of cultured neurons from peripheral autonomic ganglia.[24]

The original study of Lin et al. directed the focus of the first in vivo studies of GDNF toward its effects on the nigrostriatal dopaminergic system.[10] Studies have indicated that GDNF may be useful in the treatment of PD by a number of the mechanisms discussed in the introduction to this chapter. Early studies indicated that GDNF can support the survival of injured nigral dopaminergic neurons. Tomac et al. found that supranigral or intrastriatal injection of GDNF in mice before or after treatment with l-methyl-4-phenyl-l,2,3,6-tetrahydropyridine (MPTP) exerted protective or reparative effects on the mesostriatal dopaminergic system.[25] Beck et al. found that daily supranigral injections of GDNF in rats with transection of the medial forebrain bundle increased the survival of the axotomized nigral dopaminergic neurons.[26] Kearns and Gash reported that intranigral administration of GDNF decreased the loss of tyrosine hydroxylase (TH)-immunoreactive neurons in the SNc that occurred after intranigral or intrastriatal administration of 6-OHDA.[27]

Implicit in the studies mentioned above is the ability of GDNF to increase the activity of nigral dopaminergic neurons. This has been directly studied in intact rats and monkeys. Hudson et al. reported that a single unilateral intranigral injection of GDNF in intact rats induced an increase in motor activity, sprouting of TH-immunoreactive fibers toward the injection site, increased TH immunoreactivity in the ipsilateral striatum, and an increase in the level of dopamine in the SNc.[28]

The report by Tomac et al.[25] suggests that GDNF can cause regeneration of the mesostriatal dopaminergic system. Hoffer et al. reported that, in rats with nearly complete unilateral lesions of the nigrostriatal dopaminergic system, a single injection of GDNF into the lesioned SNc resulted in attenuation of apomorphine-induced rotation and an increase in the levels of dopamine in the lesioned SNc. Interestingly, despite the improvement in rotational behavior, reinnervation of the striatum by dopaminergic axons from the SNc did not occur.[29]

Recent studies have shown that, even when administered a number of weeks after lesioning of the nigrostriatal dopaminergic system, GDNF can have a restorative effect. Aoi et al. reported that a single intrastriatal injection of GDNF 4 weeks after lesioning of the nigrostriatal dopaminergic system by injection of 6-OHDA into the striatum reduced apomorphine-induced rotation and increased dopaminergic cell bodies and fibers.[30] Interestingly, Kirik et al. reported that intraventricular infusion was more effective than intrastriatal infusion of GDNF in rats that had received intrastriatal injection of 6-OHDA.[31]

The work discussed above led to a clinical trial of GDNF in patients with PD. Nutt et al. conducted a multicenter, randomized, double-blind, placebo-controlled, sequential cohort study to compare the effects of monthly intracerebroventricular (ICV) administration of placebo and 25, 75, 150, 300, and 500 to 4000 µg of GDNF in 50 subjects with PD for 8 months with an open-label study of extended exposure up to an additional 20 months and maximum single doses of up to 4000 µg in 16 subjects.[32] The total score and score on the motor portion of the Unified Parkinson Disease Rating Scale during clinically defined "on" and "off" periods were not improved by GDNF at any dose. Common adverse events included nausea, anorexia, vomiting, and weight loss. Paresthesias, which were often described as electric shocks (Lhermitte's sign), were common in GDNF-treated subjects and were not dose-related, and the paresthesias resolved on discontinuation of GDNF. Asymptomatic hyponatremia occurred in over half of subjects receiving 75 µg or larger doses of GDNF, and it was symptomatic in several subjects. The open-label portion of the extension study had similar adverse events and lack of therapeutic efficacy. The authors concluded that GDNF administered by ICV injection was biologically active, as evidenced by the adverse events encountered in their study. Nutt et al. hypothesized that GDNF did not improve parkinsonism, possibly because that it did not reach the target tissues: putamen and substantia nigra.[32]

OTHER MEMBERS OF THE GDNF FAMILY

Relatively soon after the discovery of GDNF, three other members of this family were discovered: neurturin,[33] artemin/neublastin/enovin,[34–36] and persephin.[37] All of the more recently discovered members of the GDNF family have been shown to have trophic effects for mesencephalic dopaminergic neurons. The GDNF family ligands signal through a multicomponent complex composed of Ret tyrosine kinase and the glycosylphosphatidylinositol (GPI)-anchored coreceptors GFRalpha1–4, which are the preferred coreceptors of GDNF, neurturin, artemin/neublastin/enovin, and persephin, respectively.[38,39] Message for GFRalpha1, 2, and 4 has been found in the SNc of the mouse.[40,41] Like GDNF, these other members of the GDNF family have been shown to affect a variety of neural systems and nonneural tissues.[38,42] For example, receptors for GDNF and neurturin are separate in the dorsal root ganglia, and receptors for artemin/neublastin/enovin are found in overlapping neurons,[43,44] and artemin/neublastin/enovin appears to be important in the development of sympathetic axons.[45]

Neurturin has been studied more extensively in regards to PD than have artemin/neublastin/enovin, and persephin. Neurturin is first expressed in the ventral mesencephalon and then in the striatum, and the message persists in the striatum of the adult mouse.[42,46] Åkerud et al. reported that neurturin is regulated differently in the developing striatum from GDNF; it increases in the striatum as GDNF is decreasing.[47] Lesion of the nigrostriatal system with 6-OHDA in the rat results in increase in the messages for GDNF, artemin/enovin/neublastin, and persephin but not for neurturin in the striatum during a period of 3–9 weeks following the injury.[48] Supranigral administration of both GDNF and neurturin protected the nigral dopaminergic neurons in rats treated with 6-OHDA, but only GDNF induced sprouting and hypertrophy of the dopaminergic neurons.[47] Similarly, Rosenblad et al. reported that intrastriatal administration of GDNF was more protective of the nigrostriatal dopaminergic system than intrastriatal administration of neurturin in rats treated with intrastriatal injection of 6-OHDA.[49] Novel means of administration of artemin/neublastin/enovin and persephin are discussed below.

TGF-β1, 2, AND 3

Other members of the TGF-β superfamily have also been shown to be trophic for mesencephalic dopaminergic neurons in vitro. Krieglstein and Unsicker reported that TGF-β1, 2, and 3 promoted survival of dopaminergic neurons isolated from the embryonic rat midbrain.[50] TGF-β1, 2, and 3 also protected the dopaminergic neurons against toxicity of N-methyl-4-phenylpyridinium (MPP+). Poulsen et al. demonstrated that TGF-β2, and 3, but not TGF-β1, supported the survival of dopaminergic neurons from the embryonic rat midbrain.[11] Poulsen et al. also studied the distribution of the message for TGF-β1, 2, and 3 and GDNF in the developing rat brain.[11] At embryonic day 15.5, message for TGF-β2 and GDNF are present in close proximity to the dopaminergic neurons in the developing midbrain. At postnatal day 1, the

message for GDNF is present in the striatum, the message for TGF-β2 is present in the frontal, entorhinal, perirhinal, and piriform cortices, and the message for TGF-β3 is present in the olfactory bulb. The differences in the distributions of mRNA for TGF-β2 and 3, and GDNF suggests that members of the TGF-β superfamily may be associated with different parts of the mesencephalic dopaminergic system. GDNF appears to be associated with the nigrostriatal system, and TGF-β2 appears be associated with the mesocortical system.

ALTERNATE METHODS FOR ADMINISTRATION OF GDNF AND OTHER MEMBERS OF THE GDNF FAMILY

The promising preclinical work but the disappointing results of ICV injection in PD patients led researchers to begin to develop alternative means for administration of GDNF and other members of the GDNF family so that the nigrostriatal dopaminergic system could be targeted.

DIRECT INFUSION

The recognition that administration of trophic factors will need to be targeted to specific regions of the nervous system and delivered in a controllable fashion has resulted in the development of innovative techniques for delivery. Because of the substantial preclinical data indicating that GDNF might have a beneficial effect in PD, I will use GDNF as the prototype and discuss novel methods of administration. Grondin et al. reported that, in MPTP-treated hemiparkinsonian monkeys, infusion of GDNF into both putamen or into the right ventricle resulted in behavioral improvement and increases in striatal dopamine, the density of TH-IR axons in the striatum, and the size of nigral dopaminergic neurons.[51] Oiwa et al. reported that intrastriatal injection of neurturin 3 days prior to intrastriatal injection of 6-OHDA significantly increased the number of TH-immunoreactive neurons in the substantia nigra ipsilateral to the lesion at 2 and 8 weeks later, as well as density of TH-immunoreactive axons and concentration of dopamine in the lesioned striatum.[52] When the neurturin was given 12 weeks after the 6-OHDA lesion, it significantly reduced methamphetamine-induced rotation, significantly increased the density of TH-immunoreactive fiber density in the striatum, and caused a nonsignificant increase in number of nigral TH-immunoreactive neurons. A recent, preliminary study suggests that continuous infusion of GDNF into the putamen in PD subjects may be beneficial.[53] Five PD patients with a previous good response to L-dopa underwent unilateral or bilateral insertion of cannulae into the dorsal putamen through which recombinant human GDNF was chronically infused via indwelling pumps. Chronic GDNF infusion resulted in improved motor function in all 5 of the patients with reduction in off-time duration and severity, reduction in dyskinesia duration and severity, and an increase in on-time duration. The chronic infusion of GDNF was reported to be well tolerated.

A variation of direct infusion is the implantation of microspheres that release GDNF. Gouhier et al. reported that such microspheres implanted into the striatum of rats at the same time as injection of 6-OHDA into the striatum attenuated injury to the nigrostriatal dopaminergic system.[54] The applicability of this technique to a chronic neurodegenerative disease, which progresses over decades, is uncertain.

VIRAL VECTORS

Kordower et al. performed a series of studies using a lentivirus that had been genetically engineered to express GDNF.[55] In the first study in aged monkeys, lentivirus that had been genetically engineered to express GDNF or a control protein was injected into both the striatum and the substantia nigra, and the animals were sacrificed 3 months later.

Immunohistochemical studies revealed substantial production of GDNF at the injection sites, and antegrade and retrograde transport of the protein. Fluorodopa uptake in the striatum ipsilateral to the injections of GDNF lentivirus but not control virus showed an increase at 3 months after injection. Similarly, there was an increase in the levels of dopamine and its metabolites, and TH-immunoreactivity in the caudate and putamen ipsilateral to the injection sites.

Other viral vectors are being explored. Connor et al. reported intrastriatal injection of adenovirus that had been engineered to express preproGDNF (Ad GDNF).[56] In aged (20 months) Fischer 344 rats, Ad GDNF was injected either near dopaminergic cell bodies in the SNc or within the dopaminergic terminals in the striatum. One week following gene delivery, the neurotoxin 6-OHDA was injected unilaterally into the striatum to cause progressive degeneration of the dopaminergic neurons. Injection of Ad GDNF into either the striatum or the SNc provided significant cell protection against 6-OHDA. However, only striatal injection of Ad GDNF protected against the development of behavioral and neurochemical changes.

Mandel et al. reported that perinigral injection of adeno-associated virus (AAV) that had been engineered to express GDNF in rats 3 weeks prior to intrastriatal injection of 6-OHDA protected most of the dopaminergic neurons in the SNc.[57] McGrath et al. reported on intranigral administration of AAV that had been engineered to express GDNF into rats 5 weeks after lesioning of the nigrostriatal dopaminergic system with 6-OHDA.[58] They found that within 4 weeks of administration the animals exhibited significant behavioral recovery, which correlated with increased expression of dopaminergic markers in the substantia nigra, the medial forebrain bundle, and the striatum. Similarly, Wang et al. reported that injection of AAV expressing GDNF into the striatum even 4 weeks after injection of 6-OHDA into the striatum resulted in greater level of TH-immunoreactive fibers and levels of dopamine in the striatum, dopaminergic neurons in the substantia nigra, and significant behavioral recovery.[59]

Although studies of administration of GDNF have focused on its effects on the nigrostriatal dopaminergic system, recent work has indicated that GDNF delivered via intrastriatal injection of a lentiviral vector increased the number of TH-immunoreactive neurons present in the striatum of aged monkeys. Interestingly, MPTP treatment in young monkeys increased the number of these TH-IR neurons 8-fold, and treatment with GDNF delivered via a lentiviral vector further increased the number 7-fold.[60]

CELL-BASED VECTORS

Shingo et al. genetically engineered baby hamster kidney cells to express GDNF, and encapsulated them in a polymer.[61] The encapsulated cells were implanted unilaterally into the striatum of rats either before or after injection of 6-OHDA into the striatum. Animals that received the encapsulated cells showed preservation of the nigrostriatal dopaminergic system and reduction in rotational symmetry. Ostenfeld et al. treated neural precursor cells with a lentivirus to express GDNF; these GDNF-expressing precursor cells increased the density of TH-immunoreactive neurites when cocultured with embryonic mesencephalic cells.[62] However, when the GDNF-expressing precursor cells were cotransplanted with embryonic mesencephalic cells into the striatum in hemiparkinsonian rats, there was no effect on behavior and GDNF expression could not be detected at 8 weeks after implantation.

Persephin is another member of the GDNF family, which has been demonstrated to have trophic effects on the nigrostriatal system. Åkerud et al. engineered neural stem cells to overexpress persephin.[63] The persephin-expressing neural stem cells were implanted into the striatum; they distributed widely and gave rise to neurons, astrocytes, and oligodendrocytes. In unlesioned mice they enhanced dopaminergic function, and in mice lesioned with 6-OHDA they reduced the damage to the nigrostriatal system.

Alternate cellular sources of trophic factors have also been explored. Espejo et al. reported that intrastriatal grafts of extra-adrenal chromaffin cells of Zuckerkandl's organ, which expressed GDNF and TGF-β1, induced a gradual improvement of functional deficits in parkinsonian rats, striatal dopaminergic reinnervation, and enhancement of dopamine levels in grafted striatum.[64]

USE WITH PROGENITOR CELLS

A number of investigators have reported that GDNF can be used in conjunction with other trophic factors to drive the proliferation and differentiation of neural progenitor cells to a dopaminergic phenotype. Leé et al. reported that treatment of mouse embryonic stem cells with specific mitogen and specific signaling factors, including FGF-8, resulted in high yields of dopaminergic and serotonergic neurons.[5] Similarly, Chung et al. found that treatment with sonic hedgehog, FGF-8, and ascorbic acid increased the formation of TH-immunoreactive cells in Nurr-1-transduced embryonic stem cells.[6] Carvey et al. reported that progenitor cells from the embryonic mesencephalon could be expanded by treatment first with epidermal growth factor (EGF), then interleukin 1 (IL-1) and then IL-1, IL-11, leukemia inhibitory factor, and GDNF to establish a line of cells of which approximately 75 percent had a dopaminergic phenotype.[65]

Neurotrophins

NGF was the first neurotrophic factor to be characterized.[1] In 1989, Liebrock et al. determined the structure of a second protein that is trophic for neurons, BDNF.[66] Recognition that BDNF and NGF share approximately 50 percent homology in amino acid sequence suggest they might be members of a larger family of neurotrophic molecules. Soon after this homology was reported, five groups identified a third molecule that is similar in amino acid sequence to NGF and BDNF.[67-71] The family of trophic factors was named the neurotrophins, and the third member to be recognized was designated neurotrophin-3 (NT-3). Shortly thereafter, neurotrophin-4/5 (NT-4/5) was identified in vipers and humans.[72,73] Neurotrophin-6 and neurotrophin-7 (NT-6, NT-7) were subsequently discovered in fish.[74,75] Members of the neurotrophin family exist naturally as homodimers. They act through the Trk family of receptors, which are tyrosine kinases,[76] and p75^{NTR}, which can act as a proapoptotic signal or in concert with Trk as a prosurvival signal.[77] NGF binds to Trk-A; BDNF and NT-4/5 act through Trk-B; and NT-3 acts primarily through Trk-C. Trk-B and Trk-C exist both as full-length and truncated forms that lack the tyrosine kinase domain. The full-length forms of Trk-B are found in the central nervous system (CNS) on neurons, and the truncated forms are found on nonneuronal cells, such as astrocytes, and ependyma. Trk-C appears to be found exclusively on neurons and blood vessels.[78]

There is, as yet, no evidence that a deficit of any of the neurotrophins is the cause of a specific movement disorder, but deficiencies of BDNF have been reported in the SNc in parkinsonian brains (see below). One study of three families with autosomal-dominant inherited parkinsonism found no linkage with polymorphic markers linked to the BDNF gene.[79] A subsequent study reported a linkage to homozygosity for the V66M polymorphism.[80] Mutant mice lacking BDNF were found to have severe degeneration in several sensory ganglia, but midbrain dopaminergic neurons did not appear to be affected.[81,82]

BDNF

Despite the finding that BDNF appears not to be necessary for the development of mesencephalic dopaminergic neurons,[81,82] anatomic studies of the distribution of the message of both BDNF and Trk-B suggest that BDNF plays a role(s) in function of the basal ganglia. In vitro and in vivo studies have supported this notion. Hofer et al. found a small but detectable level of mRNA for BDNF in the striatum of the adult rat,[83] and Okazawa et al. reported that oral administration of L-dopa increased expression of BDNF mRNA in the striatum of mice.[84] The message for Trk-B is present in the SNc, but also is present in the striatum.[78,85] BDNF injected into the striatum diffuses a short distance, and some is retrogradely transported to the SNc.[86,87] Production of BDNF in the target, the striatum, and the retrograde transport of the trophic factor to the dependent cells, dopaminergic neurons in the SNc, are consistent with established mechanisms for the effect of a trophic factor.[2] BDNF has also been shown to be transported from the substantia nigra to the striatum.[3] In addition, BDNF has been shown to be responsible for inducing normal expression of the dopamine D3 receptor in nucleus accumbens both during development and in adulthood, and to trigger D3 overexpression in the striatum of hemiparkinsonian rats.[88] There are alternative mechanisms by which BDNF might have an effect on the dopaminergic neurons of the SNc. Studies have indicated that BDNF may serve autocrine or paracrine functions for the neurons.[89,90] Gall et al. reported that the message for BDNF is expressed in cells in the dopaminergic neurons in the medial SNc and ventral tegmental area (VTA) as well as in adjacent regions in the mesencephalon.[91] Mogi et al. reported significant reduction in BDNF-immunoreactive material in the caudate, putamen, and substantia nigra in PD brains.[92] Parain et al. reported decreased numbers melanized neurons immunoreactive for BDNF in SNc in the PD brains.[93] Howells et al. reported the presence of message for BDNF in human SNc and a loss in the SNc in PD brains, which exceeded the loss of nigral cells, suggesting reduced expression of BDNF in the remaining cells.[94] Howells et al. hypothesized that in the SNc it plays an autocrine/paracrine role and that loss of BDNF-expressing neurons may compromise adjacent neurons.[94]

A role for BDNF in the function of the nigrostriatal dopaminergic system is further supported by in vitro studies. Hyman et al. and Knüsel et al. reported that BDNF supported the survival of dopaminergic neurons and promoted dopamine uptake in cultures of fetal mesencephalic cells.[95-97] Of considerable interest were the further observations that BDNF promoted survival in vitro of fetal dopaminergic neurons treated with MPP$^+$ and 6-OHDA, toxins that are relatively selective for dopaminergic neurons.[95,98,99]

A number of in vivo studies have indicated that BDNF may be useful in the treatment of PD by virtue of its ability to protect and enhance the activity of nigral dopaminergic neurons. Early studies in rats with transection of the nigrostriatal dopaminergic axons did not demonstrate ability of BDNF to protect the nigral dopaminergic neurons.[100] Frim et al. reported that implantation into the mesencephalic tegmentum of fibroblasts, which had been genetically engineered to produce BDNF, reduced the loss of nigral neurons caused by intrastriatal infusion of MPP$^+$.[101] Shults et al. demonstrated in rats that intrastriatal injections of BDNF reduced the apomorphine-induced rotation, and the loss of striatal dopaminergic axons and nigral neurons caused by intrastriatal injection of 6-OHDA.[102]

BDNF has also been shown to enhance the activity of nigral dopaminergic neurons in vivo. Altar et al. reported that chronic supranigral infusion of BDNF in rats resulted in amphetamine-induced rotation contraversive to the side of BDNF infusion (the pattern of rotation is consistent with increased activity of the dopaminergic system on the side of infusion), and increased the ratio of homovanillic acid to dopamine, which is an index of dopamine turnover.[103,104] Shults et al. reported that a single, unilateral injection of BDNF into the mesencephalon of rats resulted in an increase in amphetamine-induced, contraversive rotation that persisted for a number of months after the single treatment.[105] Shen et al. reported that chronic supranigral infusions of BDNF increased the number of active dopaminergic neurons, the average firing rate, and the number of action potentials contained within bursts of the dopaminergic neurons.[106]

Investigators have yet to demonstrate that BDNF can support sprouting of collateral axons from residual dopaminergic neurons in animal models of PD. However, Lucidi-Phillipi et al. reported that fibroblasts genetically engineered to produce BDNF, when implanted in the SNc in intact rats, induced sprouting of dopaminergic fibers into the grafted fibroblasts.[107] BDNF may be useful when used in conjunction with transplanted fetal nigral dopaminergic neurons. Sauer et al. reported that BDNF enhanced the function but not the survival of fetal nigral neurons grafted to the striatum in rats.[108] Yurek et al. reported that the optimal effect of exogenous BDNF on the development of dopaminergic neurons in fetal nigral cells transplanted to the striatum in rats occurred at a postnatal age when endogenous dopamine and BDNF show the greatest increases during the normal development of the striatum.[109]

NT-3

The role of NT-3 in the mesostriatal dopaminergic system has been less thoroughly studied than that of BDNF. The message for NT-3 is present in the dopaminergic neurons of the medial SNc, VTA, and retrorubral nucleus in the rat.[91] In fact, more of the dopaminergic neurons of the ventral mesencephalon appeared to contain message for NT-3 than contained message for BDNF. Hyman et al. reported that NT-3 supported survival of dopaminergic and GABAergic cells in cultures of mesencephalic cells from rat embryos.[96] However, Knüsel et al. reported that, unlike BDNF, NT-3 did not increase dopamine uptake in cultured mesencephalic cells.[97] Altar et al. reported that both BDNF and NT-3 reversed rotational behavior deficits and augmented striatal dopaminergic and serotonergic metabolism in a model of PD in which there is a partial lesion of the nigrostriatal dopaminergic system.[110]

NT-4/5

NT-4/5 has been studied less extensively than BDNF and NT-3. Because both it and BDNF act through Trk-B, it is not surprising that the effects of NT-4/5 in studies in the basal ganglia have been similar.[104,111] In explants of E14 mesencephalon, Meyer et al. reported that NT-4/5 had an additive trophic effect with GDNF on the number of TH-immunoreactive cells and dopamine release.[112] In addition to their effects on the nigrostriatal dopaminergic system, BDNF and NT-4/5 have been shown to be protective of striatal neurons in vitro.[111,113,114] This effect may be a result of an increase in calcium-binding proteins, such as calbindin and calretinin. However, implantation into the striatum of fibroblasts that had been genetically engineered to produce NGF, but not those engineered to produce BDNF, reduced the size of the lesion caused by excitotoxins.[115] These results suggest that neurotrophins may be useful in degenerative disorders of the striatum such as Huntington's disease (HD). In addition to its effects on the basal ganglia, BDNF has been shown to have a protective effect on a number of other neuronal types, including motor neurons.[116–120]

Fibroblast Growth Factors

A number of pieces of data have accumulated to indicate that FGF-l (acidic FGF, or aFGF) and FGF-2 (basic FGF, or bFGF) can have trophic effects on mesencephalic dopaminergic cells.[121] FGF-l and FGF-2 were the first members of the FGF family of trophic factors to be isolated and are the most thoroughly characterized.[121] Twenty-three members of the FGF family have been identified.[122] A number of anatomic studies have demonstrated the presence of FGF-l and FGF-2 message and protein in the dopaminergic neurons in the ventral mesencephalon.[123–126] Tooyama et al. extended the anatomic studies to parkinsonian brains.[127] This group reported that, in brains from patients without neurological disease, approximately 94 percent of the pigmented neurons in the SNc were immunoreactive for FGF-2. In parkinsonian brains, both the number of pigmented neurons and the number of FGF-2-immunoreactive cells were severely depleted, but the reduction in FGF-2-immunoreactive neurons (4.7 percent of that of control brains) was even greater than that of pigmented neurons (30.3 percent that of control brains). In the parkinsonian brains, only 8.2 percent of the remaining pigmented neurons contained FGF-2-immunoreactive material. This group also reported that in HD there is an increase in FGF-l-immunoreactive material in the striatum, which appears to accompany the gliosis.[128] FGF-8 appears to be crucial to the development of the dopaminergic neurons in the midbrain.[129]

Four high-affinity FGF receptors have been identified.[121] There appears to be overlapping recognition and specificity among the four known high-affinity FGF receptors: one high-affinity receptor may bind with similar affinity to several of the known FGFs, and one FGF may bind with similar affinity to several of the high-affinity receptors. Wanaka et al. carried out in situ hybridization studies and found a wide distribution of the message for FGF-l in receptor rat brain.[130] The neurons of the SNc and VTA showed moderate binding. Little signal for the bFGF receptor could be detected in the striatum.

A number of groups have demonstrated that FGF-2 increases dopamine uptake and/or survival of dopaminergic neurons in cultures of fetal mesencephalic cells,[131–135] and a number of the studies have indicated that the effects of FGF-2 require the presence of glia. Also, a number of studies have indicated that FGF-2 has a trophic effect on the nigrostriatal dopaminergic system in vivo. Otto and Unsicker reported that implantation of Gelfoam, which had been soaked in bFGF, into one striatum in MPTP-treated mice increased the levels of dopamine and TH activity in the striatum bilaterally.[136] Implantation of the Gelfoam also increased the density of TH-immunoreactive axons in the striatum, but only in the side of Gelfoam implantation. The effect of FGF-2 was noted if it was administered at the time of MPTP administration, or 8 days later. A subsequent study from this group indicated that treatment with FGF-2 did not induce greater gliosis than did treatment with cytochrome *c*, suggesting that increased gliosis was not the cause of the benefit from FGF-2 treatment.[137] Date et al. noted a similar phenomenon in young mice that received intrastriatal injections of FGF-l at 2, 7, and 12 days after administration of MPTP.[138] However, administration of FGF-l in aged mice treated with MPTP had no effect. Matsuda et al. reported that addition of FGF-2 to grafts of fetal dopaminergic neurons transplanted into the striatum of hemiparkinsonian rats, at a dose of 5 ng but not 50 ng, enhanced the reduction in rotational asymmetry.[139] Gage's group reported that grafting of fibroblasts genetically engineered to produce FGF-2 with fetal nigral dopaminergic neurons in hemiparkinsonian rats substantially increased the number of dopaminergic neurons surviving in the grafted striatum.[140]

Ray et al. reported that treatment of embryonic neurons from the hippocampus could cause proliferation and perpetuation of the neurons.[141] This finding raises the possibility that dopaminergic neurons could be grown and purified in vitro and later transplanted to patients with PD.

Ciliary Neurotrophic Factor

Hagg and Varon reported that, in rats with transection of the nigrostriatal axons, infusion of ciliary neurotrophic factor (CNTF) into the rostral SNc reduced the loss of neurons in the SNc.[142] Although treatment with CNTF prevented death of the dopaminergic neurons, it did not prevent loss of TH, the rate-limiting enzyme in the synthesis of dopamine, from the neurons. These data suggest that CNTF has a general neuroprotective effect, but the ability to protect or induce recovery of function within the nigrostriatal dopaminergic system remains to be established.

Epidermal Growth Factor/Transforming Growth Factor-α

EGF and TGF-α are structurally similar, and both bind with high affinity to, and appear to mediate, their effects through a common receptor, the EGF receptor.[143] Mogi et al. reported that levels of EGF-like and TGF-α-like material, as well as IL-1β-like and IL-6-like material, were significantly higher in the striatum from parkinsonian brains than from control brains.[144] They commented that the increase in these cytokines, which can be trophic for neurons, in the parkinsonian striatum could be a compensatory, neurotrophic response to degeneration in the nigrostriatal system. Although this hypothesis is quite plausible, the cytokines could also play a role in the degenerative process.

EGF has been reported to have trophic effects on mesencephalic dopaminergic neurons both in vitro and in vivo, but appears to exert its effect through stimulation of proliferation of glia.[145] Törnqvist et al. reported that implantation of rods that released EGF into the striatum in hemiparkinsonian rats that also received transplantation of fetal mesencephalic cells increased the outgrowth of dopaminergic fibers, but FGF-2 was more effective.[146] Alexi and Hefti reported that TGF-α increased the number of surviving dopaminergic neurons and dopamine uptake in cultures of embryonic dopaminergic neurons, but the effect may have been mediated by glia.[147]

Insulin

Moroo et al. reported the loss of insulin receptor-immunoreactive material in neurons of the SNc, but not oculomotor nucleus, in parkinsonian brains.[148] Such loss was not noted in brains from patients who had suffered from Alzheimer's disease or amyotrophic lateral sclerosis. This observation provides support for the hypothesis that reduction in trophic support to the dopaminergic neurons in the SNc may contribute to degeneration of the SNc found in PD.

Summary

Only within the past 15 years has the number of neurotrophic factors identified, our understanding of the actions of neurotrophic factors, and our appreciation of the relevance of neurotrophic factors to movement disorders increased enormously. Studies have suggested that deficiencies in neurotrophic factors may contribute to the pathogenesis of certain movement disorders. Numerous in vitro and in vivo studies have indicated that neurotrophic factors may be useful in the treatment of PD through a number of mechanisms. GDNF currently appears to be the most promising trophic factor to become useful in the treatment of PD. However, in the first clinical trial of GDNF, PD patients did not benefit and adverse events were common. This trial underscored the fact that trophic factors typically affect a number of neural systems and ICV infusion will likely not be effective. Investigators have begun to develop alternate methods to deliver trophic factors to selected regions of the nervous system and to be able to control the delivery.

A limited number of studies have also indicated that neurotrophic factors may also be useful in the treatment of degenerative disorders of the striatum, such as HD. Despite the challenges, trophic factors hold promise for treatment of PD and other degenerative neurological disorders through a number of mechanisms.

References

1. Levi-Montalcini R: The nerve growth factor 35 years later. *Science* 237:1154–1162, 1987.
2. Korsching S: The neurotrophic factor concept: A reexamination. *J Neurosci* 13:2739–2748, 1993.
3. Altar CA, DiStefano PS: Neurotrophin trafficking by anterograde transport. *Trends Neurosci* 21:433–437, 1998.
4. Le WD, Xu P, Jankovic J, et al: Mutations in NR4A2 associated with familial Parkinson disease. *Nat Genet* 33:85–89, 2003.
5. Lee SH, Lumelsky N, Studer L, et al: Efficient generation of midbrain and hindbrain neurons from mouse embryonic stem cells. *Nat Biotechnol* 18:675–679, 2003.
6. Chung S, Sonntag KC, Andersson T, et al: Genetic engineering of mouse embryonic stem cells by Nurr1 enhances differentiation and maturation into dopaminergic neurons. *Eur J Neurosci* 16:1829–1838, 2002.
7. Miyazono K, Ichijo H, Heldin C-H: Transforming growth factors: Latent forms, binding proteins and receptors. *Growth Factors* 8:11–22, 1993.
8. Flanders KC, Ren RF, Lippa CF: Transforming growth factor-betas in neurodegenerative disease. *Prog Neurobiol* 54:71–85, 1998.
9. Kulkarni AB, Thyagarajan T, Letterio JJ: Function of cytokines within the TGF-beta superfamily as determined from transgenic and gene knockout studies in mice. *Curr Mol Med* 2:303–327, 2002.
10. Lin L-FH, Doherty DH, Lile JD, et al: GDNF: A glial cell line-derived neurotrophic factor for midbrain dopaminergic neurons. *Science* 260:1130–1132, 1993.
11. Poulsen KT, Armanini MP, Klein RI, et al: TGFβ2 and TGFβ3 are potent survival factors for midbrain dopaminergic neurons. *Neuron* 13:1245–1252, 1994.
12. Nakajima K, Hida H, Shimano Y, et al: GDNF is a major component of trophic activity in DA-depleted striatum for survival and neurite extension of DAergic neurons. *Brain Res* 916:76–84, 2001.
13. Strömberg I, Björklund L, Johansson M, et al: Glial cell line-derived neurotrophic factor is expressed in the developing but not adult striatum and stimulates developing dopamine neurons in vivo. *Exp Neurol* 124:401–412, 1993.
14. Schaar DG, Sieber B-A, Dreyfus CF, et al: Regional and cell-specific expression of GDNF in rat brain. *Exp Neurol* 124:368–371, 1993.
15. Springer JE, Mu X, Bergmann LW, et al: Expression of GDNF mRNA in rat and human nervous tissue. *Exp Neurol* 127:167–170, 1994.
16. Suter-Crazzolara C, Unsicker K: GDNF is expressed in two forms in many tissues outside the CNS. *Neuroreport* 5:2486–2488, 1994.
17. Springer JE, Seeburger JL, He J, et al: cDNA sequence and differential mRNA regulation of two forms of glial cell line-derived neurotrophic factor in Schwann cells and rat skeletal muscle. *Exp Neurol* 131:47–52, 1995.
18. Choi-Lundberg DL, Bohn MC: Ontogeny and distribution of glial cell line-derived neurotrophic factor (GDNF) mRNA in rat. *Dev Brain Res* 85:80–88, 1995.
19. Henderson CE, Phillips HS, Pollock RA, et al: GDNF: A potent survival factor for motoneurons present in peripheral nerve and muscle. *Science* 266:1062–1064, 1994.
20. Zurn AD, Baetge EE, Hammang JP, et al: Glial cell line-derived neurotrophic factor (GDNF), a new neurotrophic factor for motoneurones. *Neuroreport* 6:113–118, 1994.
21. Yan Q, Matheson C, Lopez O: In vivo neurotrophic effects of GDNF on neonatal and adult facial motor neurons. *Nature* 373:341–344, 1995.
22. Oppenheim RW, Houenou L, Johnson JE, et al: Developing motor neurons rescued from programmed and axotomy induced cell death by GDNF. *Nature* 373:344–346, 1995.
23. Martin I, Miller G, Rosendahl M, et al: Potent inhibitory effects of glial derived neurotrophic factor against kainic acid mediated seizures in the rat. *Brain Res* 683:172–178, 1995.
24. Ebendal T, Tomac A, Hoffer BJ, et al: Glial cell line-derived neurotrophic factor stimulates fiber formation and survival in cultured neurons from peripheral autonomic ganglia. *J Neurosci Res* 40:276–284, 1995.
25. Tomac A, Lindqvist E, Lin L-F H, et al: Protection and repair of the nigrostriatal dopaminergic system of GDNF in vivo. *Nature* 373:335–339, 1995.
26. Beck KD, Valverde J, Alexi R, et al: Mesencephalic dopaminergic neurons protected by GDNF from axotomy-induced degeneration in the adult brain. *Nature* 373:339–341, 1995.
27. Kearns CM, Gash DM: GDNF protects nigral dopamine neurons against 6-hydroxydopamine in vivo. *Brain Res* 672:104–111, 1995.
28. Hudson J, Granholm A-C, Gerhardt GA, et al: Glial cell line-derived neurotrophic factor augments midbrain dopaminergic circuits in vivo. *Brain Res Bull* 36:425–432, 1995.
29. Hoffer BJ, Hoffman A, Bowenkamp K, et al: Glial cell line-derived neurotrophic factor reverses toxin-induced injury to midbrain dopaminergic neurons in vivo. *Neurosci Lett* 182:107–111, 1994.
30. Aoi M, Date I, Tomita S, et al: Single administration of GDNF into the striatum induced protection and repair of the nigrostriatal dopaminergic system in the intrastriatal 6-hydroxydopamine injection model of hemiparkinsonism. *Restor Neurol Neurosci* 17:31–38, 2001.
31. Kirik D, Georgievska B, Rosenblad C, et al: Delayed infusion of GDNF promotes recovery of motor function in the partial lesion model of Parkinson's disease. *Eur J Neurosci* 13:1589–1599, 2001.
32. Nutt JG, Burchiel KJ, Comella CL, et al. and ICV GDNF Study Group. Implanted intracerebroventricular. Glial cell line-derived neurotrophic factor. Randomized, double-blind trial of glial cell line-derived neurotrophic factor (GDNF) in PD. *Neurology* 60:69–73, 2003.

33. Kotzbauer PT, Lampe PA, Heuckeroth RO, et al: Neurturin, a relative of glial-cell-line-derived neurotrophic factor. *Nature* 384:467–470, 1996.

34. Baloh RH, Tansey MG, Lampe PA, et al: Artemin, a novel member of the GDNF ligand family, supports peripheral and central neurons and signals through the GFRalpha3-RET receptor complex. *Neuron* 21:1291–1302, 1998.

35. Rosenblad C, Grønborg M, Hansen C, et al: In vivo protection of nigral dopamine neurons by lentiviral gene transfer of the novel GDNF-family member neublastin/artemin. *Mol Cell Neurosci* 15:199–214, 2000.

36. Masure S, Geerts H, Cik M, et al: Enovin, a member of the glial cell-line-derived neurotrophic factor (GDNF) family with growth promoting activity on neuronal cells. Existence and tissue-specific expression of different splice variants. *Eur J Biochem* 266:892–902, 1999.

37. Milbrandt J, de Sauvage FJ, Fahrner TJ, et al: Persephin, a novel neurotrophic factor related to GDNF and neurturin. *Neuron* 20:245–253, 1998.

38. Baloh RH, Enomoto H, Johnson EM Jr, et al: The GDNF family ligands and receptors: Implications for neural development. *Curr Opin Neurobiol* 10:103–110, 2000.

39. Saarma M: GDNF: a stranger in the TGF-beta superfamily? *Eur J Biochem* 267:6968–6971, 2000.

40. Golden JP, Baloh RH, Kotzbauer PT, et al: Expression of neurturin, GDNF, and their receptors in the adult mouse CNS. *J Comp Neurol* 398:139–150, 1998.

41. Masure S, Cik M, Hoefnagel E, et al: Mammalian GFRalpha-4, a divergent member of the GFRalpha family of coreceptors for glial cell line-derived neurotrophic factor family ligands, is a receptor for the neurotrophic factor persephin. *J Biol Chem* 275:39427–39434, 2000.

42. Golden JP, DeMaro JA, Osborne PA, et al: Expression of neurturin, GDNF, and GDNF family-receptor mRNA in the developing and mature mouse. *Exp Neurol* 158:504–528, 1999.

43. Baudet C, Mikaels A, Westphal H, et al: Positive and negative interactions of GDNF, NTN and ART in developing sensory neuron subpopulations, and their collaboration with neurotrophins. *Development* 127:4335–4344, 2000.

44. Orozco OE, Walus L, Sah DW, et al: GFRalpha3 is expressed predominantly in nociceptive sensory neurons. *Eur J Neurosci* 13:2177–2182, 2001.

45. Honma Y, Araki T, Gianino S, et al: Artemin is a vascular-derived neurotrophic factor for developing sympathetic neurons. *Neuron* 35:267–282, 2002.

46. Horger BA, Nishimura MC, Armanini MP, et al: Neurturin exerts potent actions on survival and function of midbrain dopaminergic neurons. *J Neurosci* 18:4929–4937, 1998.

47. Åkerud P, Alberch J, Eketjäll S, et al: Differential effects of glial cell line-derived neurotrophic factor and neurturin on developing and adult substantia nigra dopaminergic neurons. *J Neurochem* 73:70–78, 1999.

48. Zhou J, Yu Y, Tang Z, et al: Differential expression of mRNAs of GDNF, 2000. *Neuroreport* 11:3289–3293, 2000.

49. Rosenblad C, Kirik D, Björklund A: Neurturin enhances the survival of intrastriatal fetal dopaminergic transplants. *Neuroreport* 10:1783–1787, 1999.

50. Krieglstein K, Unsicker K: Transforming growth factor-β promotes survival of midbrain dopaminergic neurons and protects them against *N*-methyl-4-phenylpyridinium ion toxicity. *Neuroscience* 63:1189–1196, 1994.

51. Grondin R, Zhang Z, Yi A, et al: Chronic, controlled GDNF infusion promotes structural and functional recovery in advanced parkinsonian monkeys. *Brain* 125(Pt 10):2191–2201, 2002.

52. Oiwa Y, Yoshimura R, Nakai K, et al: Dopaminergic neuroprotection and regeneration by neurturin assessed by using behavioral, biochemical and histochemical measurements in a model of progressive Parkinson's disease. *Brain Res* 947:271–283, 2002.

53. Gill SS, Patel NK, O'Sullivan KO, et al: Chronic intraputaminal infusion of GDNF in the treatment of advanced Parkinson's disease. *Soc Neurosci (Abstr)* 691.8, 2002.

54. Gouhier C, Chalon S, Aubert-Pouessel A, et al: Protection of dopaminergic nigrostriatal afferents by GDNF delivered by microspheres in a rodent model of Parkinson's disease. *Synapse* 44:124–131, 2002.

55. Kordower JH, Emborg ME, Bloch J, et al: Neurodegeneration prevented by lentiviral vector delivery of GDNF in primate models of Parkinson's disease. *Science* 290:767–773, 2000.

56. Connor B, Kozlowski DA, Schallert T, et al: Differential effects of glial cell line-derived neurotrophic factor (GDNF) in the striatum and substantia nigra of the aged Parkinsonian rat. *Gene Ther* 6:1936–1951, 1999.

57. Mandel RJ, Spratt SK, Snyder RO, et al: Midbrain injection of recombinant adeno-associated virus encoding rat glial cell line-derived neurotrophic factor protects nigral neurons in a progressive 6-hydroxydopamine-induced degeneration model of Parkinson's disease in rats. *Proc Natl Acad Sci U S A* 94:14083–14088, 1997.

58. McGrath J, Lintz E, Hoffer BJ, et al: Adeno-associated viral delivery of GDNF promotes recovery of dopaminergic phenotype following a unilateral 6-hydroxydopamine lesion. *Cell Transplant* 11:215–227, 2002.

59. Wang L, Muramatsu S, Lu Y, et al: Delayed delivery of AAV-GDNF prevents nigral neurodegeneration and promotes functional recovery in a rat model of Parkinson's disease. *Gene Ther* 9:381–389, 2002.

60. Palfi S, Leventhal L, Chu Y, et al: Lentivirally delivered glial cell line-derived neurotrophic factor increases the number of striatal dopaminergic neurons in primate models of nigrostriatal degeneration. *J Neurosci* 22:4942–4954, 2002.

61. Shingo T, Date I, Yoshida H, et al: Neuroprotective and restorative effects of intrastriatal grafting of encapsulated GDNF-producing cells in a rat model of Parkinson's disease. *J Neurosci Res* 69:946–954, 2002.

62. Ostenfeld T, Tai YT, Martin P, et al: Neurospheres modified to produce glial cell line-derived neurotrophic factor increase the survival of transplanted dopamine neurons. *J Neurosci Res* 69:955–965, 2002.

63. Åkerud P, Holm PC, Castelo-Branco G, et al: Persephin-overexpressing neural stem cells regulate the function of nigral dopaminergic neurons and prevent their degeneration in a model of Parkinson's disease. *Mol Cell Neurosci* 21:205–222, 2002.

64. Espejo EF, Gonzalez-Albo MC, Moraes JP, et al: Functional regeneration in a rat Parkinson's model after intrastriatal grafts of glial cell line-derived neurotrophic factor and transforming growth factor beta1-expressing extra-adrenal chromaffin cells of the Zuckerkandl's organ. *J Neurosci* 21:9888–9895, 2001.

65. Carvey PM, Ling ZD, Sortwell CE, et al: A clonal line of mesencephalic progenitor cells converted to dopamine neurons by hematopoietic cytokines: A source of cells for transplantation in Parkinson's disease. *Exp Neurol* 171:98–108, 2001.

66. Leibrock J, Lottspeich F, Hohn A, et al: Molecular cloning and expression of brain-derived neurotrophic factor. *Nature* 341:149–152, 1989.

67. Ernfors F, Ibáñez CF, Ebendal T, et al: Molecular cloning and neurotrophic activities of a protein with structural similarities to nerve growth factor: Developmental and topographical expression in the brain. *Proc Natl Acad Sci U S A* 87:5454–5458, 1990.

68. Hohn A, Leibrock J, Bailey K, et al: Identification and characterization of a novel member of the nerve growth factor/brain-derived neurotrophic factor family. *Nature* 344:339–341, 1990.

69. Kaisho Y, Yoshimura K, Nakahama K: Cloning and expression of a cDNA encoding a novel human neurotrophic factor. *FEBS Lett* 266:187–191, 1990.

70. Maisonpierre PC, Belluscio L, Squinto S, et al: Neurotrophin3: A neurotrophic factor related to NGF and BDNF. *Science* 247:1446–1451, 1990.

71. Rosenthal A, Goeddel DV, Nguyen T, et al: Primary structure and biological activity of a novel human neurotrophic factor. *Neuron* 4:767–773, 1990.

72. Ip NY, Ibáñez CF, Nye SH, et al: Mammalian neurotrophin-4: Structure, chromosomal localization, tissue distribution, and receptor specificity. *Proc Natl Acad Sci U S A* 89:3060–3064, 1992.

73. Berkemeier LY, Winslow JW, Kaplan DR, et al: Neurotrophin-5: A novel neurotrophic factor that activates trk and trkB. *Neuron* 7:857–866, 1991.

74. Gotz R, Koster R, Winkler C, et al: Neurotrophin-6 is a new member of the nerve growth factor family. *Nature* 372:266–269, 1994.

75. Lai KO, Fu WY, Ip FC, et al: Cloning and expression of a novel neurotrophin, NT-7, from carp. *Mol Cell Neurosci* 11:64–76, 1998.

76. Barbacid M: The Trk family of neurotrophin receptors. *J Biol* 25:1386–1403, 1994.

77. Miller FD, Kaplan DR: Neurotrophin signalling pathways regulating neuronal apoptosis. *Cell Mol Life Sci* 58:1045–1053, 2001.

78. Altar CA, Siuciak JA, Wright P, et al: In situ hybridization of trkB and trkC receptor mRNA in rat forebrain and association with high-affinity binding of [^{125}I]BDNF, [^{125}I]NT~4/5 and [^{125}I]NT-3. *Eur J Neurosci* 6:1389–1405, 1994.

79. Gasser T, Wszolek ZK, Trofatter J, et al: Genetic linkage studies in autosomal dominant parkinsonism: Evaluation of seven candidate genes. *Ann Neurol* 36:387–396, 1994.

80. Momose Y, Murata M, Kobayashi K, et al: Association studies of multiple candidate genes for Parkinson's disease using single nucleotide polymorphisms. *Ann Neurol* 51:133–136, 2002 [erratum in: *Ann Neurol* 51:534, 2002].

81. Ernfors P, Lee K-F, Jaenisch R: Mice lacking brain-derived neurotrophic factor develop with sensory deficits. *Nature* 368:147–149, 1994.

82. Jones KR, Farifias I, Backus C, et al: Targeted disruption of the BDNF gene perturbs brain and sensory neuron development but not motor neuron development. *Cell* 76:989–999, 1994.

83. Hofer M, Pagliusi SR, Hohn A, et al: Regional distribution of brain-derived neurotrophic factor mRNA in the adult mouse brain. *EMBO J* 9:2459–2464, 1990.

84. Okazawa H, Murata M, Wantanabe M, et al: Dopaminergic stimulation up-regulates the in vivo expression of brain derived neurotrophic factor (BDNF) in the striatum. *FEBS Lett* 3123:138–142, 1992.

85. Lindsay RM, Altar CA, Cedarbaum JM, et al: The therapeutic potential of neurotrophic factors in the treatment of Parkinson's disease. *Exp Neurol* 124:103–118, 1993.

86. Anderson KD, Alderson RF, Altar CA, et al: The differential distributions of exogenous BDNF, NGF and NT-3 in the brain corresponds to the relative abundance and distribution of high- and low-affinity neurotrophin receptors. *J Comp Neurol* 357:1–22, 1995.

87. Mufson EJ, Kroin IS, Sobreviela T, et al: Intrastriatal infusions of brain-derived neurotrophic factor: Retrograde transport and colocalization with dopamine containing substantia nigra neurons in rat. *Exp Neurol* 129:15–26, 1994.

88. Guillin O, Diaz J, Carroll P, et al: BDNF controls dopamine D3 receptor expression and triggers behavioural sensitization. *Nature* 411:86–89, 2001.

89. Schecterson LC, Bothwell M: Novel roles for neurotrophins are suggested by BDNF and NT-3 mRNA expression in developing neurons. *Neuron* 9:449–463, 1992.

90. Acheson A, Conover IC, Fandl JP, et al: A BDNF autocrine loop in adult sensory neurons prevents cell death. *Nature* 374:450–453, 1995.

91. Gall CM, Gold SI, Isackson PJ, et al: Brain-derived neurotrophic factor and neurotrophin-3 mRNAs are expressed in ventral midbrain regions containing dopaminergic neurons. *Mol Cell Neurosci* 3:56–63, 1992.

92. Mogi M, Togari A, Kondo T, et al: Brain-derived growth factor and nerve growth factor concentrations are decreased in the substantia nigra in Parkinson's disease. *Neurosci Lett* 270:45–48, 1999.

93. Parain K, Murer MG, Yan Q, et al: Reduced expression of brain-derived neurotrophic factor protein in Parkinson's disease substantia nigra. *Neuroreport* 10:557–561, 1999.

94. Howells DW, Porritt MJ, Wong JY, et al: Reduced BDNF mRNA expression in the Parkinson's disease substantia nigra. *Exp Neurol* 166:127–135, 2000.

95. Hyman C, Hofer M, Barde Y-A, et al: BDNF is a neurotrophic factor for dopaminergic neurons of the substantia nigra. *Nature* 350:230–232, 1991.

96. Hyman C, Juhasz M, Jackson C, et al: Overlapping and distinct actions of the neurotrophins BDNF, NT-3, and NT-4/5 on cultured dopaminergic and GABAergic neurons of the ventral mesencephalon. *J Neurosci* 14335–14347, 1994.

97. Knüsel B, Winslow JW, Rosenthal A, et al: Promotion of central cholinergic and dopaminergic neuron differentiation by brain-derived neurotrophic factor but not neurotrophin 3. *Proc Natl Acad Sci U S A* 88:961–965, 1991.

98. Spina MB, Squinto SP, Miller J, et al: Brain-derived neurotrophic factor protects dopamine neurons against 6-hydroxydopamine and N-methyl-4-phenylpyridinium ion toxicity: Involvement of the glutathione system. *J Neurochem* 59:99–106, 1992.

99. Beck KD, Knusel B, Winslow JW, et al: Pretreatment of dopamineric neurons in culture with brain-derived neurotrophic factor attenuates toxicity of 1-methyl-4-phenyl-pyridinium. *Neurodegeneration* 1:27–36, 1992.

100. Knusel B, Beck KD, Winslow JW, et al: Brain-derived neurotrophic factor administration protects basal forebrain cholinergic but not nigral dopaminergic neurons from degenerative changes after axotomy in the adult rat brain. *J Neurosci* 12:4391–4402, 1992.

101. Frim DM, Uhier TA, Galpern WR, et al: Implanted fibroblasts genetically engineered to produce brain-derived neurotrophic

factor prevent 1-methyl-4-phenylpyridinium toxicity to dopaminergic neurons in the rat. *Proc Natl Acad Sci U S A* 91:5104–5108, 1994.

102. Shults C, Kimber T, Altar CA: BDNF attenuates the effects of intrastriatal injection of 6-hydroxydopamine. *Neuroreport* 6:1109–1112, 1995.

103. Altar CA, Boylan CB, Jackson C, et al: Brain-derived neurotrophic factor augments rotational behavior and nigrostriatal dopamine turnover in vivo. *Proc Natl Acad Sci U S A* 89:11347–11351, 1992.

104. Altar CA, Boylan CB, Fritsche M, et al: The neurotrophins NT4/5 and BDNF augment serotonin, dopamine, and GABAergic systems during behaviorally effective infusions to the substantia nigra. *Exp Neurol* 130:31–40, 1994.

105. Shults CW, Matthews RT, Altar CA, et al: A single intramesencephalic injection of brain-derived neurotrophic factor induces persistent rotational asymmetry in rats. *Exp Neurol* 125:183–194, 1994.

106. Shen R-Y, Altar CA, Chiodo LA: Brain-derived neurotrophic factor increases the electrical activity of pars compacta dopamine neurons in vivo. *Proc Natl Acad Sci U S A* 91:8920–8924, 1994.

107. Lucidi-Phillipi CA, Gage FH, Shults CW, et al: Brain-derived neurotrophic factor-transduced fibroblasts: Production of BDNF and effects of grafting to the adult rat brain. *J Comp Neurol* 354:361–376, 1995.

108. Sauer H, Fischer W, Nikkhah G, et al: Brain-derived neurotrophic factor enhances function rather than survival of intrastriatal dopamine cell-rich grafts. *Brain Res* 626:37–44, 1993.

109. Yurek DM, Hipkens SB, Wiegand SJ, et al: Optimal effectiveness of BDNF for fetal nigral transplants coincides with the ontogenic appearance of BDNF in the striatum. *J Neurosci* 18:6040–6047, 1998.

110. Altar CA, Boylan CB, Fritsche M, et al: Efficacy of brain-derived neurotrophic factor and neurotrophin-3 on neurochemical and behavioral deficits associated with partial nigrostriatal dopamine lesions. *J Neurochem* 63:1021–1032, 1994.

111. Widmer IR, Hefti F: Neurotrophin-4/5 promotes survival and differentiation of rat striatal neurons developing in culture. *Eur J Neurosci* 6:1669–1679, 1994.

112. Meyer M, Matarredona ER, Seiler RW, et al: Additive effect of glial cell line-derived neurotrophic factor and neurotrophin-4/5 on rat fetal nigral explant cultures. *Neuroscience* 108:273–284, 2001.

113. Mizuno K, Camahan J, Nawa H: Brain-derived neurotrophic factor promotes differentiation of striatal GABAergic neurons. *Dev Biol* 165:243–256, 1994.

114. Nakao N, Kokaia Z, Odin P, et al: Protective effects of BDNF and NT-3 but not PDGF against hypoglycemic injury to cultured striatal neurons. *Exp Neurol* 131:1–10, 1995.

115. Frim DM, Uhier TA, Short MP, et al: Effects of biologically delivered NGF, BDNF and bFGF on striatal excitotoxic lesions. *Neuroreport* 4:367–370, 1993.

116. Yan Q, Elliott J, Snider WD: Brain-derived neurotrophic factor rescues spinal motor neurons from axotomy-induced cell death. *Nature* 360:753–755, 1992.

117. Ip NY, Li Y, Yancopoulos GD, et al: Cultured hippocampal neurons show responses to BDNF, NT-3, and NT-4, but not NGF. *J Neurosci* 13:3394–3405, 1993.

118. Yan Q, Matheson C, Lopez OT, et al: The biological responses of axotomized adult motoneurons to brain-derived neurotrophic factor. *J Neurosci* 14:5281–5291, 1994.

119. Cheng B, Goodman Y, Begley JG, et al: Neurotrophin-4/5 protects hippocampal and cortical neurons against energy deprivation and excitatory amino acid-induced injury. *Brain Res* 650:331–335, 1994.

120. Friedman B, Kleinfeld D, Ip NY, et al: BDNF and NT-4/5 exert neurotrophic influences on injured adult spinal motor neurons. *J Neurosci* 15:1044–1056, 1995.

121. Baird A: Fibroblast growth factors: Activities and significance of non-neurotrophin growth factors. *Curr Opin Neurobiol* 4:78–86, 1994.

122. Ford-Perriss M, Abud H, Murphy M: Fibroblast growth factors in the developing central nervous system. *Clin Exp Pharmacol Physiol* 28:493–503, 2001.

123. Bean AJ, Elde R, Cao X, et al: Expression of acidic and basic fibroblast growth factors in the substantia nigra of rat, monkey, and human. *Proc Natl Acad Sci U S A* 88:10237–10241, 1991.

124. Stock A, Kuzis K, Woodward WR, et al: Localization of acidic fibroblast growth factor in specific subcortical neuronal populations. *J Neurosci* 12:4688–4700, 1992.

125. Cintra A, Cao Y, Oellig C, et al: Basic FGF is present in dopaminergic neurons of the ventral midbrain of the rat. *Neuroreport* 2:597–600, 1991.

126. Bean AJ, Oellig C, Pettersson RF, et al: Differential expression of acid and basic FGF in the rat substantia nigra during development. *Neuroreport* 3:993–996, 1992.

127. Tooyama I, Kawamata T, Walker D, et al: Loss of basic fibroblast growth factor in substantia nigra neurons in Parkinson's disease. *Neurology* 43:372–376, 1993.

128. Tooyama I, Kremer HPH, Hayden MR, et al: Acidic and basic fibroblast growth factor-like immunoreactivity in the striatum and midbrain in Huntington's disease. *Brain Res* 610:1–7, 1993.

129. Ye W, Shimamura K, Rubenstein JLR, et al: FGF and Shh signals control dopaminergic and serotonergic cell fate in the anterior neural plate. *Cell* 93:755–766, 1998.

130. Wanaka A, Johnson EM, Milbrandt J: Localization of FGF receptor mRNA in the adult rat central nervous system by in situ hybridization. *Neuron* 5:267–281, 1990.

131. Ferrari G, Minozzi M-C, Toffano G, et al: Basic fibroblast growth factor promotes the survival and development of mesencephalic neurons in culture. *Dev Biol* 133:140–147, 1989.

132. Knüsel B, Michel PP, Schwaber JS, et al: Selective and non-selective stimulation of central cholinergic and dopaminergic development in vitro by nerve growth factor, basic fibroblast growth factor, epidermal growth factor, insulin and the insulin-like growth factors I and II. *J Neurosci* 10:558–570, 1990.

133. Engele J, Bohn MC: The neurotrophic effects of fibroblast growth factors on dopaminergic neurons in vitro are mediated by mesencephalic glia. *J Neurosci* 11:3070–3078, 1991.

134. Hartikka J, Staufenbiel M, Lubbert H: Cyclic AMP, but not basic FGF, increases the in vitro survival of mesencephalic dopaminergic neurons and protects them from MPP+-induced degeneration. *J Neurosci Res* 32:190–201, 1992.

135. Park TH, Mytilineou C: Protection from 1-methyl-4-phenylpyridinium (MPP+) toxicity and stimulation of regrowth of MPP+ damaged dopaminergic fibers by treatment of mesencephalic cultures with EGF and basic FGF. *Brain Res* 599:83–97, 1992.

136. Otto D, Unsicker K: Basic FGF reverses chemical and morphological deficits in the nigrostriatal system of MPTP-treated mice. *J Neurosci* 10:1912–1921, 1990.

137. Otto D, Unsicker K: FGF-2 in the MPTP model of Parkinson's disease: Effects on astroglial cells. *Glia* 11:47–56, 1994.

138. Date I, Notter MFD, Felten SY, et al: MPTP-treated mice but not aging mice show partial recovery of the nigrostriatal dopaminergic system by stereotaxic injection of acidic fibroblast growth factor (aFGF). *Brain Res* 526:156–160, 1990.

139. Matsuda S, Saito H, Nishiyama N: Basic fibroblast growth factor ameliorates rotational behavior of substantia nigral-transplanted rats with lesions of the dopaminergic nigrostriatal neurons. *Jpn J Pharmacol* 59:365–370, 1992.

140. Takayama H, Ray J, Raymon HK, et al: Basic fibroblast growth factor increases dopaminergic graft survival and function in a rat model of Parkinson's disease. *Nat Med* 1:53–58, 1995.

141. Ray J, Peterson D, Schinstine M, et al: Proliferation, differentiation, and long-term culture of primary hippocampal neurons. *Proc Natl Acad Sci U S A* 90:3602–3606, 1993.

142. Hagg T, Varon S: Ciliary neurotrophic factor prevents degeneration of adult rat substantia nigra dopaminergic neurons in vivo. *Proc Natl Acad Sci U S A* 90:6315–6319, 1993.

143. Adamson ED: Developmental activities of the epidermal growth factor receptor. *Curr Top Dev Biol* 24:1–29, 1990.

144. Mogi M, Harada M, Kondo T, et al: Interleukin-1β, interleukin-6, epidermal growth factor and transforming growth factor-α are elevated in the brain from parkinsonian patients. *Neurosci Lett* 180:147–150, 1994.

145. Shults CW: Neurotrophic factors-potential therapies, in Koller WC, Paulson E (eds): *Therapy of Parkinson's Disease*, 2nd ed. New York: Marcel Dekker, 1994, pp 559–570.

146. Törnqvist N, Björklund L, Almqvist P, et al: Implantation of bioactive growth factor-secreting rods enhances fetal dopaminergic graft survival, outgrowth density, and functional recovery in a rat model of Parkinson's disease. *Exp Neurol* 164:130–138, 2000.

147. Alexi T, Hefti F: Trophic actions of transforming growth factors on mesencephalic dopaminergic neurons developing in culture. *Neuroscience* 55:903–918, 1993.

148. Moroo I, Yamada T, Makino H, et al: Loss of insulin receptor immunoreactivity from the substantia nigra pars compacta neurons in Parkinson's disease. *Acta Neuropathol* 87:343–348, 1994.

Chapter 9

NEUROPATHOLOGY OF MOVEMENT DISORDERS: AN OVERVIEW

MARLA GEARING and SUZANNE S. MIRRA

GROSS NEUROPATHOLOGIC EXAMINATION IN
   MOVEMENT DISORDERS   143
MICROSCOPIC EXAMINATION OF THE BRAIN IN
   MOVEMENT DISORDERS   144
SYNUCLEINOPATHIES   145
   Idiopathic Parkinson's Disease (PD)   145
   Dementia with Lewy Bodies (DLB)   146
   Multisystem Atrophy (MSA)   148
TAUOPATHIES   149
   Progressive Supranuclear Palsy (PSP)   149
   Corticobasal Degeneration (CBD)   150
   Frontotemporal Dementia and Parkinsonism
      with Linkage to Chromosome 17 (FTDP-17)   152
SUMMARY   152

The diagnosis and assessment of movement disorders present special challenges to neuropathologists and clinicians alike. Clinicopathological studies affirm diagnostic problems in assessing patients with parkinsonism.[1-3] In 1992, Hughes et al.[4] found that only 76 of 100 patients clinically diagnosed as having idiopathic Parkinson's disease (PD) exhibited nigral Lewy bodies at autopsy; neuropathologic diagnoses on the remaining 24 cases included progressive supranuclear palsy (PSP), multisystem atrophy (MSA), and Alzheimer's disease (AD). By 1997, diagnostic accuracy had improved to 84 percent.[5] Two different groups reviewed the literature and proposed the establishment of levels of probability for the clinical diagnosis of PD,[6,7] analogous to those widely adopted for the clinical diagnosis of AD.[8] A recent study comparing various clinical criteria for the diagnosis of idiopathic PD reported diagnostic accuracy as high as 90 percent.[9] In comparison, for AD, the accuracy of the clinical diagnosis was 87 percent for 106 subjects enrolled in the multicenter longitudinal study CERAD (Consortium to Establish a Registry for Alzheimer's Disease)[10] and assessed using standard clinical[11] and neuropathologic[12] batteries. Standard criteria have been proposed for the neuropathologic diagnosis of PSP[13,14] and corticobasal degeneration (CBD);[15] additional work is warranted, however, to further standardize and refine criteria for the neuropathologic diagnosis of PD and other movement disorders. As the clinical diagnosis of movement disorders may be problematic, neuropathologists examining autopsy brains derived from such individuals must evaluate the material in a manner sufficiently comprehensive as to encompass a broad range of diagnostic possibilities. We believe that many neurodegenerative disorders or overlapping pathologies remain undetected at autopsy if a complete assessment is not carried out.

Gross Neuropathologic Examination in Movement Disorders

Gross examination of the brains of individuals with movement disorders is often informative and may guide additional microscopic studies. Many of the same principles governing the gross and even microscopic assessment of brains derived from individuals with AD and non-AD dementias pertain to movement disorders. The reader is referred to two publications in which guidelines with color illustrations are provided for nonspecialist pathologists.[16,17]

In all cases, the convexity should be carefully evaluated before cutting the brain for the presence and distribution of cortical atrophy, exemplified by narrowing of the gyri and widening of the sulci. Perirolandic atrophy (i.e., involvement of the precentral and postcentral gyri), often asymmetric, is characteristic, although not pathognomonic of CBD (as depicted in Chap. 46), and the pathologist may wish to sample cortex from both hemispheres for comparison of microscopic features. When feasible, it is advisable to have a pathologist examine the entire brain prior to any dissection for research or other purposes. Otherwise, significant asymmetry may be overlooked.

Evaluation of the base of the brain includes assessment of the circle of Willis for atherosclerosis or other changes. In addition, degeneration of the brainstem and cerebellum, such as that seen in olivopontocerebellar atrophy (OPCA), a form of multisystem atrophy (MSA), may be appreciated when the base of the pons, the cerebellar peduncles, the inferior olivary nuclei or the cerebellar hemispheres or vermis exhibit external evidence of atrophy (see Chap. 21).

Sections through the cerebral hemispheres, cut in either coronal or other planes for comparison with neuroimaging studies, may also be revealing. On these sections, cortical atrophy is exemplified by narrowing of the cortical ribbon, widening of sulci, enlarged Sylvian fissures, reduction in the volume of underlying white matter of the centrum semiovale or corpus callosum, and ventricular enlargement. Asymmetrical atrophy, such as that seen in the frontoparietal cortex in CBD or in the frontal, temporal or, rarely, the parietal lobe in Pick's disease, may be apparent. Enlargement of the temporal horn of the lateral ventricle often reflects narrowing of the entorhinal cortex, a very common feature in AD. The hippocampus is involved in a broad range of neurodegenerative disorders and other conditions and should always be examined; it is often atrophic in AD, a condition that frequently coexists with PD and other disorders. The amygdala, too, is virtually always involved and is often atrophic in AD. The amygdala is also a common site for detection of Lewy bodies in dementia with Lewy bodies (DLB).

Gross examination of subcortical gray matter, especially the basal ganglia, also provides clues to the underlying pathology. For example, variable atrophy with flattening of the normally convex contour of the head of the caudate nucleus is seen in Huntington's disease[18] (see also Chap. 36), and in some cases of Pick's disease[19] or CBD.[15] Brownish discoloration and atrophy of the putamen are characteristic features of striatonigral degeneration (SND), a form of MSA.[20] Atrophy of the bilateral globus pallidus may be appreciated in PSP when there is extensive neuronal loss and gliosis in this region (see Chap. 20). Rusty discoloration of the pallidum and nigra are seen in Hallervorden-Spatz disease, although the associated iron deposits and ovoids or swollen axons are observed to variable degrees in these regions in other more common neurodegenerative disorders. Necrosis and cystic degeneration of the globus pallidus may be seen in carbon monoxide poisoning, although bilateral and symmetrical lacunes caused by cerebrovascular disease occur in the pallidum as well. The subthalamic nucleus is often narrowed and, occasionally, is barely discernible in PSP.

The midbrain often displays enlargement of the aqueduct in PSP. Pallor of the substantia nigra occurs not only in idiopathic PD, where it may be asymmetric, but also in a number of movement disorders, including PSP, CBD, and MSA. Nigral pallor is also observed in about 25–30 percent of individuals with neuropathologically confirmed AD in whom there is concomitant PD pathology (defined by CERAD as nigral degeneration and Lewy bodies at any site). Such cases would also be classified as DLB according to consensus criteria.[21] The cerebral peduncles may be reduced in size in CBD, and this change may be asymmetrical, reflecting Wallerian degeneration secondary to degeneration of motor cortex or underlying white matter.

Sections through the brainstem and cerebellum may reveal grossly apparent loss of myelinated fibers or atrophy of the base of the pons, along with reduction in size of the middle cerebellar peduncles in OPCA. The fourth ventricle may be enlarged in long-standing or severe cases of PSP, as well as in MSA. Pallor of the locus ceruleus is seen with idiopathic PD, PSP, and AD.[17] The inferior olivary nuclei may appear atrophic in OPCA; although these nuclei are often involved at a microscopic level in PSP, this change is rarely detected grossly. Cerebellar cortical atrophy, such as that associated with OPCA, may be appreciated if the cerebellar folia are widely separated from one another and firmer than normal. The dentate nucleus may appear discolored or have a distorted contour in several disorders, including PSP, particularly when there is underlying grumose degeneration.

Microscopic Examination of the Brain in Movement Disorders

Adequate histopathologic assessment of movement disorder cases requires extensive sampling of potentially involved regions of the brain and spinal cord. In addition, because cognitive dysfunction, neurobehavioral problems, and speech abnormalities are frequently observed in patients with movement disorders, the neuropathologic workup should include an assessment of those changes associated with dementia. A reasonable workup, in our view, would involve sampling the following structures. Focal regions of cerebral cortical atrophy should be examined along with representative sections from frontal, temporal, parietal, occipital, anterior cingulate, and insular cortex similar to those recommended for AD.[12,17] Perirolandic cortex, if possible bilateral, should be examined whenever CBD or atypical parkinsonism is considered, even if this cortex appears grossly normal. Hippocampus, entorhinal cortex, and amygdala—sites that exhibit a spectrum of neurodegenerative changes, including Lewy bodies and Lewy neurites—should also be examined in all cases. In addition, sections of basal ganglia, substantia innominata, thalamus, subthalamic nucleus, hypothalamus, midbrain, pons, medulla, and cerebellum—including hemisphere, vermis, deep white matter, and dentate nucleus—should be taken. These subcortical sections may be crucial for making the diagnosis of such disorders as PSP, which can be easily overlooked if structures such as the subthalamic or inferior olivary nuclei are not examined. Spinal cord, when available, should be sampled at all levels (e.g., cervical, thoracic, and lumbar).

Routine staining of preparations with hematoxylin-eosin, along with a battery of special stains, is recommended. These include silver stains such as Bielschowsky and Sevier Munger preparations for detection of neurofibrillary tangles seen in PSP, AD, and other disorders, as well as senile plaques, neuropil threads, and Pick bodies. The Gallyas silver stain is preferred by some for use in staging of neurofibrillary degeneration as proposed by Braak and Braak,[22] and is considered the stain of choice for glial and neuronal inclusions in MSA, PSP, CBD, and Pick's disease (see Chin et al,[23] and Burn and Jaros[24] for reviews).

Immunohistochemistry is an important adjunct for the neuropathologic assessment of many neurodegenerative disorders, including those associated with parkinsonism and/or dementia.[25] Use of tau antibodies will reveal tau-positive inclusions in CBD, PSP, AD, Pick's disease, and frontotemporal dementia with parkinsonism linked to chromosome 17 (FTDP-17; see Feany and Dickson[26] and Dickson et al.[15] for reviews). Ubiquitin or alpha-synuclein immunohistochemistry enhances the detection of cortical Lewy bodies,[27–29] highlights the intriguing immunoreactive neurites within CA2-3 of the hippocampus and other sites in a spectrum of cases exhibiting cortical and nigral Lewy bodies,[27,30–34] and labels the glial and neuronal cytoplasmic inclusions associated with all forms of MSA.[35–38]

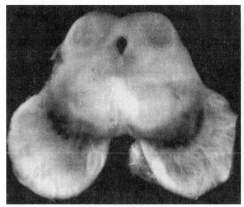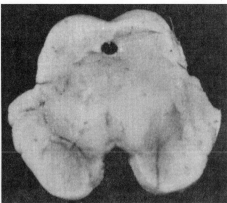

FIGURE 9-1 In contrast to the normally pigmented substantia nigra on the left, marked pallor is appreciated in the nigra of an individual with idiopathic Parkinson's disease (*right*).

Ubiquitin immunohistochemistry also highlights the neuronal inclusions of amyotrophic lateral sclerosis[39,40] and frontal lobe dementia with motor neuron disease.[41,42] The ballooned achromatic neurons characteristic of CBD but seen in many other disorders label intensely with antibodies to neurofilament protein[43] and alpha-B-crystallin.[44,45] Antibodies to beta-amyloid peptide are useful in estimating the extent and distribution of amyloid deposition in senile plaques and blood vessels, not only in AD but also in all neurodegenerative disorders.

We believe that neuropathologists must balance their responsibility to provide diagnoses, thorough assessment, and correlation with clinical, neuropsychological, neuroimaging, and genetic and molecular data with the practical considerations of reducing costs in the laboratory. Evaluations similar to those described above are expensive, and, unless additional support for the autopsy is available, such neuropathology assessments are difficult to implement outside of the scope of funded research investigations.

In the following pages of this chapter, we briefly highlight the neuropathologic hallmarks of selected movement disorders and related conditions. A current trend in the field of neuropathology is to group neurodegenerative diseases according to their major protein abnormalities. Thus, PD, DLB, and MSA all fall under the category of "synucleinopathies." CDB, PSP, FTDP-17, and Pick's disease are all considered "tauopathies." As each movement disorder is described in detail in the chapters that follow, we have not attempted to be totally comprehensive but rather have stressed key differential features. We have also emphasized the commonality, heterogeneity, and overlap among movement disorders and other neurodegenerative disorders.

Synucleinopathies

The "synucleinopathies" are characterized by the aggregation of alpha-synuclein, a 140 amino acid protein normally localized to presynaptic terminals in brain.[46,47] In PD and DLB, aggregates of alpha-synuclein are found primarily in neurons in the form of Lewy bodies and Lewy neurites. In contrast, in MSA, aggregates of alpha-synuclein are most prominent in oligodendrocytes in the form of glial cytoplasmic inclusions. There is, however, overlap among these diseases; similar glial inclusions have been reported in PD and DLB,[48–51] and neuronal inclusions are common in MSA.[52] Thus, some investigators have proposed that MSA and Lewy body disease may represent different ends of a spectrum of diseases.[53]

IDIOPATHIC PARKINSON'S DISEASE (PD)

A detailed description of the neuropathology and anatomic basis of PD is provided in Chap. 20. The reader is also referred to Forno's excellent review on the neuropathology of PD.[54]

The major gross finding in idiopathic PD is pallor of the substantia nigra (Fig. 9-1), the result of loss of pigmented dopaminergic neurons, most prominently within the ventral lateral cell groups.[55] Occasionally, the pallor and nigral degeneration are asymmetric. Microscopic examination of the nigra in idiopathic PD reveals variable neuronal loss and gliosis, along with evidence of "pigmentary incontinence" exemplified by the finding of neuromelanin within macrophages or free within the neuropil.

The presence of single or multiple Lewy bodies within pigmented neurons of the nigra, as depicted in Fig. 9-2, is characteristic, although not pathognomonic, of idiopathic PD and DLB, and most, but not all, cases of familial PD.[56] Lewy bodies are concentric eosinophilic cytoplasmic inclusions with peripheral halos and dense cores (see Pollanen et al.[57] for review). Ultrastructurally, they are composed of a dense osmiophilic core surrounded by radiating 8–10 nm filaments.[58,59] Lewy bodies label with antibodies to neurofilament protein,[60–62] ubiquitin,[29] and alpha-synuclein.[27,63] They are widely distributed within cortical and subcortical sites and, as reviewed by Forno,[54] may be found in the locus

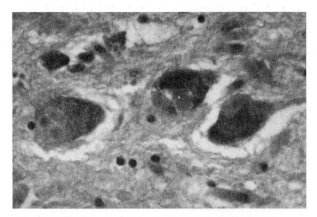

FIGURE 9-2 Three pigmented neurons from the substantia nigra contain multiple Lewy bodies within their cytoplasm. Macrophages filled with neuromelanin are seen at top left. Hematoxylin-eosin stain.

ceruleus, nucleus basalis of Meynert, dorsal motor nucleus of the vagus, hypothalamus, Edinger-Westphal nucleus, raphe nuclei, olfactory bulb, and autonomic ganglia. Lewy bodies are also found in the cerebral cortex in most cases of idiopathic PD.[4,64,65] Cortical Lewy bodies assume a more amorphous appearance than their subcortical counterparts (Fig. 9-3) and may be difficult to detect on standard stains. Their detection may be enhanced by ubiquitin or alpha-synuclein immunohistochemistry.[27,29,63]

In her review, Forno[54] adopted the operational definition of PD as a "distinctive progressive disorder characterized by tremor, rigidity, and bradykinesia, and pathologically by nerve cell loss in the substantia nigra and the presence of Lewy's intraneuronal inclusion bodies." Yet, as Forno and others point out, the presence of similar neuropathologic

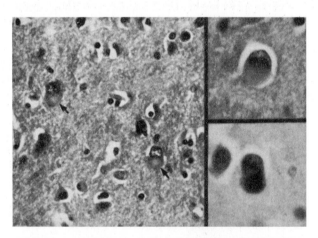

FIGURE 9-3 Cortical Lewy bodies, indicated by arrows, are seen in two neurons (*left*, hematoxylin-eosin stain). Single cortical Lewy bodies are depicted at higher magnification (*upper right*, hematoxylin-eosin stain; *lower right*, alpha-synuclein immunohistochemistry).

features in primary dementia cases reinforces the notion that there is no absolute gold standard for the neuropathologic diagnosis of PD. As emphasized by Koller,[66] the specificity and sensitivity of PD pathology is not clearly established, and the spectrum of pathology underlying dementia in PD is poorly understood. At least some cases of PD with dementia show concomitant AD neuropathology.[4,67,68] In addition, cell loss, gliosis, and Lewy body formation may be seen in the nucleus basalis of Meynert, but these changes apparently do not distinguish cases of PD with and without dementia. Additional longitudinal clinicopathological studies are needed to understand the underpinnings of dementia and other features of idiopathic PD.

DEMENTIA WITH LEWY BODIES (DLB)

The brains of individuals presenting with primary dementia may exhibit neuropathologic features virtually indistinguishable from those described above in idiopathic PD. Regardless of nosologic considerations, given the differences in clinical presentation, it is amazing but true that making a distinction between idiopathic PD and DLB, based upon current neuropathologic approaches alone, is a difficult if not impossible task.

As reviewed by Hansen and Crain,[16] numerous names have been applied to DLB. Some reflect the frequent coexistence of AD neuropathology (e.g., "AD + PD"[69] or "Lewy body variant of AD"[70]). In fact, in multicenter clinicopathological studies of patients diagnosed as having AD, CERAD autopsy findings revealed PD changes in at least one-fifth of AD cases.[10,12] Although extrapyramidal signs in AD are not invariably accompanied by PD pathology,[71] a prospective CERAD study revealed that extrapyramidal dysfunction occurs more frequently in AD patients with coexistent PD pathology than in those with "pure AD" pathology.[72] Many of these AD + PD cases show fewer neurofibrillary tangles than "pure" AD cases;[73] a significant subset, however, show a full range of neurofibrillary degeneration.[74] The term "diffuse Lewy body disease" has also been widely used for DLB,[75] although some investigators reserved this term for dementia associated with Lewy bodies in the absence of significant AD changes (in our hands, such cases are quite rare). Indeed, clinical, neuropathologic, and neurobiological distinctions between diffuse Lewy body disease and AD have been suggested.[28,30,70,76–79]

Several sets of criteria have been proposed for the clinical diagnosis of DLB (for review, see Papka et al.[80]). The Consortium on Dementia with Lewy bodies formulated consensus criteria for the clinical and pathological diagnosis of DLB.[21] In addition to progressive cognitive decline, the conferees agreed that features necessary for the clinical diagnosis of probable DLB should include at least two of the following: fluctuating cognition with pronounced variations in attention and alertness, recurrent visual hallucinations that are typically well formed and detailed, and spontaneous motor features of parkinsonism. Supportive features

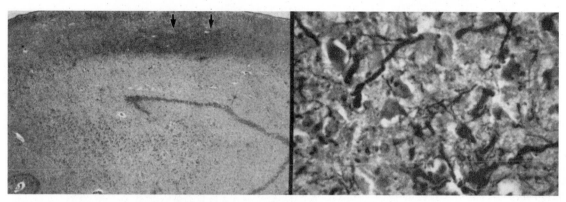

FIGURE 9-4 CA2-3 neurites in hippocampus in a case of AD with concomitant PD pathology (nigral degeneration, and Lewy bodies in cortical and subcortical sites). Ubiquitin-immunoreactive neurites (arrows) are seen in a low power view of Ammon's horn of hippocampus (*left*) and at a higher magnification (*right*). Ubiquitin immunohistochemistry.

included repeated falls, syncope, transient loss of consciousness, and neuroleptic sensitivity. Subsequent evaluations of these criteria have supported their utility, but suggest that additional improvements may be needed to optimize the balance between specificity and sensitivity.[28,81,82] Not unexpectedly, the essential neuropathologic feature required by the Consortium for the diagnosis of DLB was the presence of Lewy bodies.[21] Associated but not essential histopathologic features included "Lewy-related neurites,"[30,33] and microvacuolization or spongiform change,[83] plaques, neurofibrillary tangles, and regional neuronal loss, especially in nigra, locus ceruleus, and nucleus basalis of Meynert. Given the extensive overlap between AD and DLB, however, Lowe and Dickson[84] have advocated using a descriptive approach to the neuropathologic evaluation of DLB cases.

Dickson et al. first reported ubiquitin-immunoreactive neurites in CA2-3 of Ammon's horn of the hippocampus (Fig. 9-4) in diffuse Lewy body disease,[30,31] but not in patients with "pure AD." Subsequently, these "Lewy neurites" were shown to be alpha-synuclein-positive.[27,34] We examined a series of 120 cases of diverse neurodegenerative disease[33] and found that these Lewy neurites were present not only in cases of AD with concomitant PD changes but also in two cases of idiopathic PD and two cases of PSP, all of which had concomitant cortical Lewy bodies. Thus, this neuritic change coexists with cortical Lewy bodies but is independent of other pathologies, such as AD. Nor are these neurites observed in disorders with nigral degeneration without Lewy bodies (e.g., SND). Ubiquitin- and alpha-synuclein-immunoreactive neurites have been observed in brainstem nuclei, and in the nucleus basalis of Meynert in idiopathic PD.[32,34,85] More investigation is needed to understand the significance of these changes.

Another feature linking AD, DLB, and PD is pathologic changes in the amygdala. Some studies point to the amygdala as a site of early and high-density Lewy body development in DLB.[86,87] Hamilton[88] reported finding Lewy bodies in the amygdala in 60 percent of patients with AD, regardless of the

presence or absence of Lewy bodies in other brain regions. Finally, the amygdala has been identified as a site exhibiting significant pathology in PD. In one recent study of nondemented PD patients, investigators reported alpha-synuclein- and ubiquitin-positive Lewy bodies and Lewy neurites in the amygdala, along with a 20 percent reduction in amygdala volume relative to age-matched controls.[89]

A third intriguing feature prominent in some cases of AD with coexistent PD pathology (AD + PD) is that of spongiform change in the gray matter mimicking that of Creutzfeldt-Jakob disease (CJD) (Fig. 9-5). Unlike CJD, however, this vacuolization occurs in a stereotypical distribution, predominantly involving the entorhinal, superior temporal, and insular cortices as well as the amygdala.[83] The spongy change in these regions is usually interspersed with

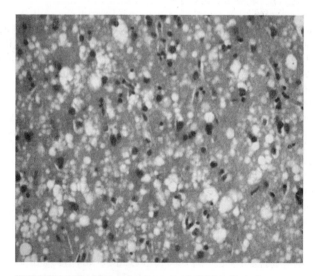

FIGURE 9-5 Florid spongy change mimicking that of Creutzfeldt-Jakob disease is appreciated in entorhinal cortex in a case of AD with concomitant PD pathology (nigral degeneration, and Lewy bodies in cortical and subcortical sites).

typical AD changes and Lewy bodies. To our knowledge, similar spongiform changes have not been observed in idiopathic PD.

MULTISYSTEM ATROPHY (MSA)

The nonfamilial forms of MSA include OPCA, SND, and Shy-Drager syndrome (see Chap. 21). This group of conditions is characterized clinically by parkinsonism, autonomic dysfunction, and pyramidal and cerebellar symptoms or signs. Given that virtually all cases of MSA exhibit autonomic dysfunction, Gilman et al.[90] proposed that this family of disorders be classified according to predominant symptomatology; thus patients with motor features dominated by parkinsonism would be classified as having MSA-P, while those with predominantly cerebellar signs would be classified as having MSA-C. In practice, SND can be difficult to distinguish from other "Parkinson's plus" syndromes, as these are sometimes complicated by cerebellar signs or autonomic dysfunction.[91,92] Advances in our understanding of the neuropathology of MSA, particularly the detection of ubiquitin- and alpha-synuclein-positive glial cytoplasmic inclusions in both forms of MSA, have affirmed the notion that the disorders included under the rubric of MSA have common pathogenetic links and represent a unified group of disorders.[93] Indeed, it is the presence of alpha-synuclein-positive glial cytoplasmic inclusions (GCI) that places sporadic OPCA in this group and differentiates it neuropathologically from the hereditary spinocerebellar disorders associated with trinucleotide repeat expansions[94,95].

The neuropathologic features of OPCA include atrophy of the pons, middle cerebellar peduncles, and inferior olivary nuclei. The cerebellum exhibits variable loss of Purkinje cells in the cortex; the dentate nucleus displays gliosis, but its neurons are generally well preserved. The spinal cord may exhibit degeneration of the posterior columns and spinocerebellar tracts. In Shy-Drager syndrome, where autonomic dysfunction is a prominent feature, loss of neurons in the intermediolateral cell column of the thoracic spinal cord and Onuf's nucleus in the sacral cord may be observed.

SND, which may coexist with OPCA, is generally characterized clinically by bradykinesia and rigidity unresponsive to L-dopa therapy. At autopsy, the brain exhibits bilateral brownish discoloration and atrophy of the putamen (Fig. 9-6), with extensive neuronal loss and, often, florid gliosis. The globus pallidus may also be involved to a lesser extent. The substantia nigra exhibits pallor with loss of neurons and generally mild-to-moderate gliosis, but, with rare exceptions, Lewy bodies are not seen.

A major advance in our understanding of MSA was the finding of GCI (Fig. 9-7) by Papp et al.;[93] this was subsequently confirmed by many groups (see Lantos[96] for review). Currently, cytoplasmic inclusions, found in neurons and glial cells, are well recognized as a key feature of MSA pathology and are found in OPCA, SND, and Shy-Drager syndrome.

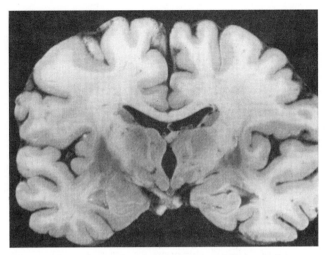

FIGURE 9-6 Multisystem atrophy. Atrophy of the lenticular nuclei with marked discoloration of the bilateral putamen is appreciated in an individual with striatonigral degeneration.

The GCI preferentially involve small cells resembling oligodendroglia in the white matter, whereas the neuronal inclusions tend to involve cells in the pons, basal ganglia, and other sites. Despite differences in gross pathology, SND and OPCA do not exhibit any significant differences in the distribution of GCI.[97] GCI are slightly eosinophilic, stain black on silver stains and label consistently with antibodies to alpha-synuclein, ubiquitin and alpha-B-crystallin; they also label to varying degrees with antibodies to alpha- and beta-tubulin and microtubule-associated proteins (MAP), such as MAP5 and tau.[96] Ultrastructurally, GCI consist of non-membrane-bound cytoplasmic aggregates of coated filaments 20–40 nm in diameter;[53] uncoated filaments have a diameter

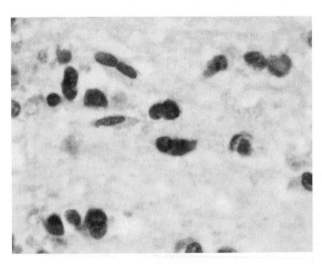

FIGURE 9-7 Alpha-synuclein immunohistochemistry reveals glial cytoplasmic inclusions in the putamen in a case of multisystem atrophy. See Color Plate Section.

of approximately 5–10 nm, on the order of that of filaments of recombinant alpha-synuclein fibrillized in vitro.[37,98,99] The GCI in MSA are immunohistochemically distinct from the glial inclusions in other neurodegenerative diseases and appear relatively specific to MSA, although, as mentioned earlier, occasional GCI have been reported in Lewy body disease. Thus, GCI are currently accepted as a hallmark of MSA. This suggests, then, that a fundamental aspect of the disease pathogenesis may involve abnormalities in oligodendrocyte function rather than neuronal degeneration per se.[24,100]

Tauopathies

The "tauopathies" are characterized by the aggregation of the MAP tau. In PSP, CBD, Pick's disease, argyrophilic grain disease, and FTDP-17, both neurons and glia show aggregates of tau, although the distribution and specific types of changes differ among these disorders. In the discussion that follows, we will focus on three major tauopathies that can present as movement disorders, namely PSP, CBD, and FTDP-17.

PROGRESSIVE SUPRANUCLEAR PALSY (PSP)

The gross changes in the brain of an individual with PSP, however subtle, may provide clues to the underlying pathology. The globus pallidus, a site of predilection, may be shrunken in cases with extensive neuronal loss and gliosis (Fig. 9-8). Atrophy of the subthalamic nucleus is more commonly observed. Examination of the midbrain usually reveals pallor of the substantia nigra which is, of course, not specific for PSP. However, when accompanied by enlargement of the aqueduct of Sylvius, PSP should be suspected. The aqueduct is variably enlarged secondary to involvement of the periaqueductal gray matter and superior colliculi. In long-standing cases, the third and fourth ventricles, too, may be dilated.

The histopathology and the distribution of changes in PSP, as originally described by Steele et al.,[101] are relatively stereotypical. Globose neurofibrillary tangles within neurons of subcortical nuclei are the major neuropathologic hallmark (Fig. 9-9), along with variable neuronal loss and gliosis. These changes are most commonly encountered in the globus pallidus, substantia nigra, subthalamic nucleus, colliculi, red nucleus, inferior olivary nucleus, and dentate nucleus. Cortical tangles may also be encountered[13] and are more frequent in cases exhibiting cognitive deficits.[102] Unlike the tangles in AD, which are comprised of paired helical filaments, the tangles in PSP are composed of straight filaments 15–18 nm in diameter.[103]

There has been increasing recognition of glial tangle pathology in PSP (for reviews, see Chin and Goldman,[23] and Dickson[104]). Several major morphological types have been described and are best appreciated on Gallyas silver and tau immunohistochemical preparations: tufted astrocytes, thorn-shaped astrocytes, coiled bodies, and interfascicular threads. Although none of these changes is absolutely specific for PSP, the tufted astrocytes (Fig. 9-9) are particularly characteristic. They consist of tufts of radiating fibers, often surrounding a central astrocytic nucleus, and are most prominent in the putamen and in the precentral and premotor cortices.[105]

Another interesting histopathologic feature strongly associated with but not pathognomonic for PSP is grumose degeneration, an eosinophilic granular change in the dentate nucleus attributed to clusters of distended axon terminals and preterminals with accumulations of organelles.[106,107] Grumose degeneration is associated most commonly with PSP,[107] but has also been described in Ramsay Hunt syndrome,[108] dentatorubropallidoluysial atrophy,[106,109] Machado-Joseph disease,[110,111] and early-onset AD.[112] We have observed grumose degeneration in two cases of CBD:[113] one with combined PSP-CBD features, and the other with typical clinical and neuropathologic features of CBD.

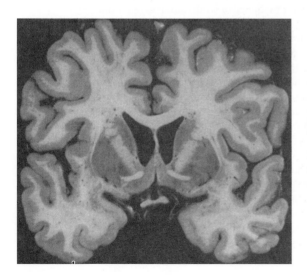

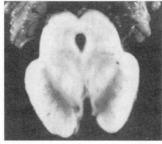

FIGURE 9-8 Progressive supranuclear palsy. Atrophy and slight discoloration of bilateral globus pallidus are appreciated on this coronal section (*left*). The midbrain exhibits characteristic enlargement of the aqueduct of Sylvius and pallor of the substantia nigra (*right*).

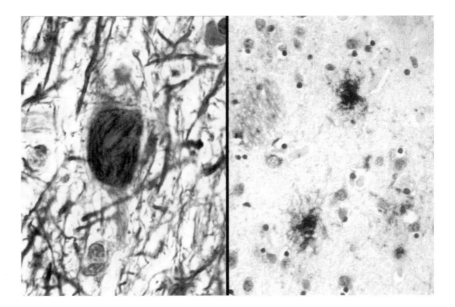

FIGURE 9-9 Progressive supranuclear palsy. A neuron in the globus pallidus contains a characteristic globose neurofibrillary tangle (*left*, Bielschowsky silver preparation). Tau immunohistochemistry reveals tufted astrocytes in the putamen (*right*). See Color Plate Section.

In a study of 20 patients of neuropathologically diagnosed PSP,[114] we found that PSP exhibits remarkable neuropathologic and clinical heterogeneity. The clinical diagnosis of PSP was made in 10 of these individuals, whereas probable AD was the primary diagnosis in another 7. In addition to PSP neuropathology, 12 of the 20 patients (60 percent) showed concomitant pathological changes of AD, PD, or both disorders. Other coexisting pathologies included CBD (two patients), and hippocampal sclerosis. Our observations indicate that AD and PD changes coexist with PSP neuropathology in a substantive proportion of patients. Moreover, our results suggest that PSP may be underdiagnosed and deserves more prominence in the differential diagnosis of dementing illness.

Other investigators, too, have observed heterogeneity of clinical and neuropathologic features in PSP and overlap among PSP, CBD, DLB, FTDP-17, and Pick's disease.[104,115–119] Indeed, this overlap has been a confounding factor as investigators have sought to formulate clinical and neuropathologic criteria for the diagnosis of PSP.[13,14,120] Both clinical markers and neuropathologic features are required for diagnosis; neither alone is considered sufficient to differentiate CBD, PSP, Pick's disease, and postencephalitic parkinsonism.[14,15]

AD and PD features have also been observed by others in PSP. Clinically, PSP patients may present with dementia,[121] and many develop dementia during the course of their disease.[101,122] On neuropathologic exam, senile plaques have been observed in this disorder, as well as in other neurodegenerative diseases.[123–126] Lewy bodies have been noted in brainstem nuclei and cerebral cortex in PSP.[127,128]

While PSP was traditionally thought to be nonfamilial, several reports suggest that familial PSP is more common than previously thought.[129,130] In several pedigrees, neuropathologic evaluation revealed pathology typical of PSP.[129–131]

In at least one pedigree, a mutation in the tau gene on chromosome 17 has been documented.[132]

CORTICOBASAL DEGENERATION (CBD)

The neuropathologic features of CBD are illustrated and described in Chapter 46. CBD is characterized by cortical atrophy involving the frontoparietal lobe, often asymmetrical and predominantly involving perirolandic cortex.[15] In some cases, especially those with atypical clinical presentation, we find that the atrophy involves more rostral frontal cortex.[113] Loss of volume of the centrum semiovale and thinning of the corpus callosum reflect the loss of cortical neurons, often accompanied by destruction of underlying white matter. Degeneration of motor cortex and subcortical white matter may lead to ipsilateral atrophy of the cerebral peduncle or other evidence of wallerian degeneration.

Microscopic examination of regions of cortical degeneration reveal neuronal loss and gliosis and, often, striking loss of myelin and axons in underlying white matter. A characteristic histopathologic feature of CBD, seen on routine hematoxylin-eosin preparations or with neurofilament[43] or alpha-B-crystallin immunohistochemistry,[44,45] is the ballooned or achromatic neuron (Fig. 9-10). These abnormal neurons are prominent in areas of cortical degeneration, usually in the deeper layers, but they may be observed in subcortical regions as well. As discussed elsewhere in this chapter, they are not specific for CBD and occur in a variety of disorders.[43] Degeneration of the substantia nigra is usually pronounced in CBD, although involvement of other subcortical structures, such as basal ganglia and dentate nucleus, is much more variable.

Neurofibrillary tangles within neurons and glial cells and abundant tau pathology are increasingly recognized

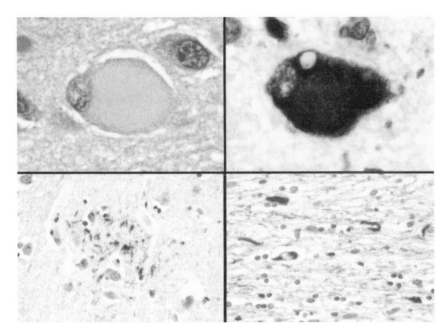

FIGURE 9-10 Corticobasal degeneration. Ballooned neurons are present in multiple regions of neocortex (*top left*, hematoxylin-eosin stain; *top right*, alpha-B-crystallin immunohistochemistry). Tau immunohistochemistry reveals astrocytic plaques in neocortical gray matter (*bottom left*), and coiled bodies and threads in the white matter (*bottom right*). See Color Plate Section.

features of CBD, best seen with Gallyas silver stain and tau immunohistochemistry (see Chin and Goldman,[23] and Dickson et al.[15]). Unlike the inclusions in MSA, those in CBD are generally ubiquitin-negative. The neuronal tangles occur in the basal ganglia and brainstem, and their ultrastructure has been variously reported as composed of 15-nm straight tubules versus twisted filaments with a long periodicity.[133–136] Cortical neurons may show diffuse cytoplasmic tau immunoreactivity, small dense profiles resembling small neurofibrillary tangles, or delicate skein-like neurofibrillary inclusions. Two major types of glial inclusions are described: coiled bodies in oligodendroglia, similar to those seen in PSP, and so-called "astrocytic plaques" (Fig. 9-10), described by Feany and Dickson.[137] These "plaques" consist of loose annular clusters of distended tau-positive distal astrocyte processes without central nuclei or amyloid. Some investigators have suggested that astrocytic plaques represent the most specific pathologic feature of CBD,[15,137,138] although we observed such astrocytic plaques in a tauopathy resembling CBD with a P301L mutation in tau.[139] The enormous extent of tau histopathology in both white and gray matter in CBD, as observed by Feany et al.[116,137] is remarkable. These investigators found that large numbers of tau-positive neuropil threads, mostly consisting of astrocytic processes, distinguish CBD from PSP and Pick's disease. These threads are more numerous in CBD, particularly in the white matter, where the number of threads and oligodendroglial inclusions is very high, compared with that in other disorders.

In a study of 11 cases of neuropathologically diagnosed CBD, we found considerable clinical and neuropathologic heterogeneity.[113] Of the 11 patients in our series, 7 presented with unilateral limb dysfunction, although the remaining

4 patients had less typical presentations, including memory loss, behavioral changes, and difficulties with speech or gait. All 11 patients eventually developed extrapyramidal signs, as well as cortical features, most commonly, apraxia. Neuropathologic study revealed predominant neuronal loss and gliosis of perirolandic cortex in 7 of 11 patients; degeneration of more rostral frontal cortex was observed in 3 of the 4 patients with atypical clinical presentations. All cases displayed ballooned neurons, tau-positive neuronal and glial inclusions, threads and grains, and nigral degeneration. Of the 11 patients, 6 manifested overlapping neuropathologic features of one or more disorders, including AD, PSP, PD, and hippocampal sclerosis. Interestingly, these 6 patients had all exhibited memory loss early in the course of their illness. Our findings suggest that CBD is a pathologically and clinically heterogeneous disorder with substantial overlap with other neurodegenerative disorders.

Given the lack of universally accepted standard diagnostic criteria and the diversity of clinical presentations, the clinical diagnosis of CBD may be difficult.[2,113,140–143] As reviewed by Schneider et al.,[113] CBD and Pick's disease have overlapping clinical features. For example, not only is dementia common in CBD, but at least one report found it to be the most common presenting symptom in CBD.[141] Extensive clinicopathological overlap between CBD and PSP has also been observed. Patients with both disorders can present with dementia[144] or with an extrapyramidal syndrome that usually fails to respond to dopaminergic agents.[2,118] Moreover, eye movement abnormalities, dystonic posturing, and gait imbalance occur in both PSP and CBD;[2] the evolution and predominance of these signs differ in classic cases. This clinical overlap is not surprising given that there is some overlap in the distribution of subcortical pathology in both conditions.

Hauw and coworkers[13,14] examined the validity and reliability of neuropathologic diagnoses of PSP and related disorders, and they proposed criteria for CBD. Exclusion criteria proposed by Litvan et al.,[14] however, would eliminate patients with coexisting PD, AD, or certain other pathologies. Our findings suggest that a substantial proportion of otherwise typical CBD patients would be excluded on the basis of these exclusion criteria. More recently proposed criteria[15] emphasize tau-immunoreactive lesions; cases with coexisting changes of other neurodegenerative disorders are considered mixed cases according to these criteria. In our view and according to the Office of Rare Diseases criteria,[15] it is the compendium of neuropathologic findings, often in concert with clinical features, which allows the diagnosis of CBD. Each of the neuropathologic features, in and of itself, is nonspecific. Ballooned neurons have been seen in a variety of central nervous system disorders,[43] including Pick's disease,[145] argyrophilic grain disease,[146,147] CJD,[148] PSP,[149] amyotrophic lateral sclerosis (ALS),[150] and AD.[43] Moreover, tau-positive neuronal and glial inclusions occur in Pick's disease, PSP, and FTDP-17,[15,116,139,151] although there are distinctions as described above, and tau-positive neurofibrillary tangles are a prominent feature in AD. Similarly, focal or asymmetric cortical degeneration occurs in other disorders (e.g., Pick's disease, frontal lobe dementia, and ALS with frontal lobe dementia).

There is particularly striking pathological overlap among CBD, PSP, and Pick's disease.[15] In addition to focal and often asymmetric cortical degeneration, Pick's disease and CBD show ballooned neurons, variable degeneration of the substantia nigra and basal ganglia, and tau-positive inclusions. Yet, Pick's bodies, typically numerous in Pick's disease, are absent or infrequently noted in CBD and PSP. Moreover, the hippocampus, a principal site of pathology in Pick's disease, is typically spared in the other two disorders. Neurofibrillary tangles, glial inclusions, and tau-related pathology are more prominent in Pick's disease than was previously appreciated.[15,23] Yet the distribution, severity, and specific types of changes differ among CBD, Pick's disease, and PSP. While Pick's disease exhibits primarily neuronal tau pathology, PSP and CBD exhibit significant glial pathology, which predominates in the cortex in CBD and in the basal ganglia and brainstem in PSP.

FRONTOTEMPORAL DEMENTIA AND PARKINSONISM WITH LINKAGE TO CHROMOSOME 17 (FTDP-17)

FTDP-17 presents a particular diagnostic challenge to clinicians and neuropathologists alike, as FTDP-17 cases may show clinical and/or pathologic features indistinguishable from those of CBD, PSP, or Pick's disease. Clinically, FTDP-17 cases may present with dementia or disinhibition, suggesting frontotemporal pathology, or with motor symptoms such as dopa-unresponsive parkinsonism (for review, see Foster et al.[152]), and members of the same pedigree may show

markedly different presentations.[153] Oculomotor problems such as supranuclear gaze palsy may also develop in some patients. Neuropathologically, FTDP-17 cases show frontotemporal atrophy, and most kindreds also show atrophy of the basal ganglia and pallor of the substantia nigra. Microscopically, most cases show neuronal loss, gliosis, and tau pathology in neurons and glia.[151] However, the specific features of the tau pathology may vary substantially among pedigrees, with some families showing pathology resembling that of PSP,[154] Pick's disease,[155,156] CBD,[139] or progressive subcortical gliosis,[157] one family showing features of both CBD and PSP,[119] and still other families showing a unique distribution of tau pathology.[151,152] Two families have been reported as showing no distinctive pathologic features such as plaques, tangles, Lewy bodies, or Pick bodies;[158,159] at least one of these has subsequently been shown to exhibit tau deposits in neurons and glia.[160] A recent study by Miyasaka et al.,[161] using antibodies specific for mutant or wild-type tau, demonstrated that the tau deposits in FTDP-17 are composed exclusively of mutant tau.

Family history is an important consideration in distinguishing between FTDP-17 and other tauopathies, and genetic testing for mutations in the tau gene on chromosome 17 is needed to confirm the diagnosis.[15] In addition to genetic testing and careful examination of the compendium of neuropathologic changes, biochemical analysis of insoluble tau may be a useful adjunct in distinguishing among the various "tauopathies." Alternative splicing of exon 10 of the tau gene gives rise to isoforms with either 3 or 4 repeat sequences in the microtubule-binding domain. The insoluble tau in CBD and PSP is comprised of primarily 4-repeat isoforms, while in Pick's disease it is predominantly 3-repeat isoforms. In comparison, the insoluble tau in AD is composed of a mixture of 3- and 4-repeat isoforms.[151,162]

Summary

The extensive overlap observed among movement disorders and other neurodegenerative disorders suggests common pathophysiological mechanisms. The increasing recognition of widespread tau-associated and glial pathology in these disorders, discussed earlier in this chapter and in two excellent reviews by Feany and Dickson[26] and Chin and Goldman,[23] highlights the potential relationship of disorders such as CBD, Pick's disease, FTDP-17, and PSP and provokes questions about their relationship to AD. Ultrastructural and molecular studies in these disorders have shown both similarities and differences regarding the morphology of the inclusions and biochemical properties of the tau polypeptides.[15] Similarly, the recognition of alpha-synuclein in PD, DLB, and MSA raises the question of how these disorders may be related to one another and to AD, in which approximately one-third of cases exhibit concomitant Lewy body pathology.

The apolipoprotein E (ApoE) ε4 allele is recognized as a major risk factor for familial and sporadic AD,[163,164] and may also play a role in the development of Lewy body disease, at least when the latter is accompanied by Alzheimer-type pathology.[165–169] Whether the ApoE ε4 allele plays a role in the development of other neurodegenerative diseases remains unclear. Some investigators have noted an increased frequency of the ApoE ε4 allele in those disorders characterized by tau cytoskeletal pathology (i.e., CBD, PSP, and Pick's disease);[170–173] others have not observed this trend.[174–176] Still other investigators report an effect of the ε2 allele of ApoE in the development of various tauopathies.[177–179] Neither the ε2 nor the ε4 allele has been reported to have any effect on the development of multisystem atrophy.[173,180]

In summary, there is considerable overlap among the movement disorders and other neurodegenerative disorders. As emphasized throughout this chapter, common clinical features may lead to diagnostic problems. Furthermore, for a patient in whom one disorder (e.g., PSP) has been diagnosed, a physician might be reluctant to assign a second diagnosis (e.g., AD). Although standard clinical and neuropathologic diagnostic criteria have been developed for several of the disorders discussed in this chapter, further testing and refinement of these criteria is needed.

Acknowledgments

The authors thank Robert Baul and Dayna McDermott for assistance with histopathology. This work was supported by NIH Grants AG10130, ES12068-01, and AG00959.

References

1. Bower JH, Dickson DW, Taylor L, et al: Clinical correlates of the pathology underlying parkinsonism: A population perspective. *Mov Disord* 17:910–916, 2002.
2. Litvan I, Agid Y, Goetz C, et al: Accuracy of the clinical diagnosis of corticobasal degeneration: A clinicopathological study. *Neurology* 48:119–125, 1997.
3. Rajput AH, Rozdilsky B, Rajput A: Accuracy of clinical diagnosis in parkinsonism: A prospective study. *Can J Neurol Sci* 18:275–278, 1991.
4. Hughes AJ, Daniel SE, Kilford L, Lees AJ: Accuracy of clinical diagnosis of idiopathic Parkinson's disease: A clinico-pathological study of 100 cases. *J Neurol Neurosurg Psychiatry* 55:181–184, 1992.
5. Hughes AJ: Clinicopathological aspects of Parkinson's disease. *Eur Neurol* 38(suppl 2):13–20, 1997.
6. Gelb DJ, Oliver E, Gilman S: Diagnostic criteria for Parkinson disease. *Arch Neurol* 56:33–39, 1999.
7. Larsen JP, Dupont E, Tandberg E: Clinical diagnosis of Parkinson's disease: Proposal of diagnostic subgroups classified at different levels of confidence. *Acta Neurol Scand* 89:242–251, 1994.
8. McKhann G, Drachman D, Folstein M, et al: Clinical diagnosis of Alzheimer's disease: Report of the NINCDS-ADRDA Work Group under the auspices of Department of Health and Human Services Task Force on Alzheimer's Disease. *Neurology* 34:939–944, 1984.
9. Hughes AJ, Daniel SE, Lees AJ: Improved accuracy of clinical diagnosis of Lewy body Parkinson's disease. *Neurology* 57:1497–1499, 2001.
10. Gearing M, Mirra SS, Hedreen JC, et al: The Consortium to Establish a Registry for Alzheimer's Disease (CERAD). Part X. Neuropathology confirmation of the clinical diagnosis of Alzheimer's disease. *Neurology* 45:461–466, 1995.
11. Morris JC, Heyman A, Mohs RC: The Consortium to Establish a Registry for Alzheimer's Disease (CERAD). Part I. Clinical and neuropsychological assessment of Alzheimer's disease. *Neurology* 39:1159–1165, 1989.
12. Mirra SS, Heyman A, McKeel D, et al: The Consortium to Establish a Registry for Alzheimer's Disease (CERAD). Part II. Standardization of the neuropathologic assessment of Alzheimer's disease. *Neurology* 41:479–486, 1991.
13. Hauw JJ, Daniel SE, Dickson D, et al: Preliminary NINDS neuropathologic criteria for Steele-Richardson-Olszewski syndrome (progressive supranuclear palsy). *Neurology* 44:2015–2019, 1994.
14. Litvan I, Hauw JJ, Bartko JJ, et al: Validity and reliability of the preliminary NINDS neuropathologic criteria for progressive supranuclear palsy and related disorders. *J Neuropathol Exp Neurol* 55:97–105, 1996.
15. Dickson DW, Bergeron D, Chin SS, et al: Office of Rare Diseases neuropathologic criteria for corticobasal degeneration. *J Neuropathol Exp Neurol* 61:935–946, 2002.
16. Hansen LA, Crain BJ: Making the diagnosis of mixed and non-Alzheimer's dementias. *Arch Pathol Lab Med* 119:1023–1031, 1995.
17. Mirra SS, Hart MN, Terry RD: Making the diagnosis of Alzheimer's disease: A primer for practicing pathologists. *Arch Pathol Lab Med* 117:132–144, 1993.
18. Vonsattel JP, Myers RH, Stevens TJ, et al: Neuropathological classification of Huntington's disease. *J Neuropathol Exp Neurol* 44:559–577, 1985.
19. Kosaka K, Ikeda K, Kobayashi K, Mehraein P: Striatopallidonigral degeneration in Pick's disease: A clinicopathological study of 41 cases. *J Neurol* 238:151–160, 1991.
20. Takei Y, Mirra SS: Striatonigral degeneration: A form of multiple system atrophy with clinical parkinsonism. *Prog Neuropathol* 2:60–77, 1973.
21. McKeith IG, Galasko D, Kosaka K, et al: Consensus guidelines for the clinical and pathologic diagnosis of dementia with Lewy bodies (DLB): Report of the Consortium on DLB International Workshop. *Neurology* 47:1113–1124, 1996.
22. Braak H, Braak E: Neuropathological stageing of Alzheimer-related changes. *Acta Neuropathol* 82:239–259, 1991.
23. Chin SS-M, Goldman JE: Glial inclusions in CNS degenerative diseases. *J Neuropathol Exp Neurol* 55:499–508, 1996.
24. Burn DJ, Jaros E: Multiple system atrophy: Cellular and molecular pathology. *Mol Pathol* 54:419–426, 2001.
25. Dickson DW, Feany MB, Yen SH, et al: Cytoskeletal pathology in non-Alzheimer degenerative dementia: New lesions in diffuse Lewy body disease, Pick's disease, and corticobasal degeneration. *J Neural Transm Suppl* 47:31–46, 1996.
26. Feany MB, Dickson DW: Neurodegenerative disorders with extensive tau pathology: A comparative study and review. *Ann Neurol* 40:139–148, 1996.

27. Dickson DW, Farrer MJ, Mehta ND, et al: Antibodies to non-amyloid component of plaques (NACP) specifically label Lewy bodies and Lewy neurites, but not other inclusions in neurodegenerative diseases. *J Neuropathol Exp Neurol* 57:516, 1998 [abstract].

28. Gomez-Isla T, Growdon WB, McNamara M, et al: Clinicopathologic correlates in temporal cortex in dementia with Lewy bodies. *Neurology* 53:2003–2009, 1999.

29. Lennox G, Lowe J, Morrell K, et al: Anti-ubiquitin immunocytochemistry is more sensitive than conventional techniques in the detection of diffuse Lewy body disease. *J Neurol Neurosurg Psychiatry* 52:67–71, 1989.

30. Dickson DW, Ruan D, Crystal H, et al: Hippocampal degeneration differentiates diffuse Lewy body disease (DLBD) from Alzheimer's disease: Light and electron microscopic immunocytochemistry of CA2-3 neurites specific to DLBD. *Neurology* 41:1402–1409, 1991.

31. Dickson DW, Schmidt ML, Lee VM-Y, et al: Immunoreactivity profile of hippocampal CA2/3 neurites in diffuse Lewy body disease. *Acta Neuropathol* 87:269–276, 1994.

32. Irizarry MC, Growdon W, Gomez-Isla T, et al: Nigral and cortical Lewy bodies and dystrophic nigral neurites in Parkinson's disease and cortical Lewy body disease contain α-synuclein immunoreactivity. *J Neuropathol Exp Neurol* 57:334–337, 1998.

33. Kim H, Gearing M, Mirra SS: Ubiquitin-positive CA2/3 neurites in hippocampus coexist with cortical Lewy bodies. *Neurology* 45:1768–1770, 1995.

34. Spillantini MG, Crowther RA, Jakes R, et al: α-Synuclein in filamentous inclusions of Lewy bodies from Parkinson's disease and dementia with Lewy bodies. *Proc Natl Acad Sci U S A* 95:6469–6473, 1998.

35. Arima K, Uéda K, Sunohara N, et al: NACP/α-synuclein immunoreactivity in fibrillary components of neuronal and oligodendroglial cytoplasmic inclusions in the pontine nuclei in multiple system atrophy. *Acta Neuropathol* 96:439–444, 1998.

36. Kato S, Nakamura H, Hirano A, et al: Argyrophilic ubiquitinated cytoplasmic inclusions of Leu-7-positive glial cells in olivopontocerebellar atrophy (multiple system atrophy). *Acta Neuropathol* 82:488–493, 1991.

37. Spillantini MG, Crowther RA, Jakes R, et al. Filamentous α-synuclein inclusions link multiple system atrophy with Parkinson's disease and dementia with Lewy bodies. *Neurosci Lett* 251:205–208, 1998.

38. Wakabayashi K, Hayashi S, Kakita A, et al: Accumulation of α-synuclein/NACP is a cytopathological feature common to Lewy body disease and multiple system atrophy. *Acta Neuropathol* 96:445–452, 1998.

39. Kato T, Katagiri T, Hirano A, et al: Lewy body-like hyaline inclusions in sporadic motor neuron disease are ubiquitinated. *Acta Neuropathol* 77:391–396, 1989.

40. Lowe J, Aldridge F, Lennox G, et al: Inclusion bodies in motor cortex and brainstem of patients with motor neurone disease are detected by immunocytochemical localisation of ubiquitin. *Neurosci Lett* 105:7–13, 1989.

41. Anderson VE, Cairns NJ, Leigh PN: Involvement of the amygdala, dentate and hippocampus in motor neuron disease. *J Neurol Sci* 129:75–78, 1995.

42. Wightman G, Anderson VE, Martin J, et al: Hippocampal and neocortical ubiquitin-immunoreactive inclusions in amyotrophic lateral sclerosis with dementia. *Neurosci Lett* 139:269–274, 1992.

43. Dickson DW, Yen S-H, Suzuki KI, et al: Ballooned neurons in select neurodegenerative diseases contain phosphorylated neurofilament epitopes. *Acta Neuropathol* 71:216–223, 1986.

44. Kato S, Hirano A, Umahara T, et al: Comparative immunohistochemical study on the expression of alpha B crystalline, ubiquitin and stress-response protein 27 in ballooned neurons in various disorders. *Neuropathol Appl Neurobiol* 18:335–340, 1992.

45. Lowe J, Errington DR, Lennox G, et al: Ballooned neurons in several neurodegenerative disorders and stroke contain alpha B crystalline. *Neuropathol Appl Neurobiol* 18:341–350, 1992.

46. Irizarry MC, Kim T-W, McNamara M, et al: Characterization of the precursor protein of the non-Aβ component of senile plaques (NACP) in the human central nervous system. *J Neuropathol Exp Neurol* 55:889–895, 1996.

47. Iwai A, Masliah E, Yoshimoto M, et al: The precursor protein of non-Aβ component of Alzheimer's disease amyloid is a presynaptic protein of the central nervous system. *Neuron* 14:467–475, 1995.

48. Arai T, Uéda K, Ikeda K, et al: Argyrophilic glial inclusions in the midbrain of patients with Parkinson's disease and diffuse Lewy body disease are immunopositive for NACP/α-synuclein. *Neurosci Lett* 259:83–86, 1999.

49. Hishikawa N, Hashizume Y, Yoshida M, Sobue G: Widespread occurrence of argyrophilic glial inclusions in Parkinson's disease. *Neuropathol Appl Neurobiol* 27:362–372, 2001.

50. Mochizuki A, Komatsuzaki Y, Shoji S: Association of Lewy bodies and glial cytoplasmic inclusions in the brain of Parkinson's disease. *Acta Neuropathol* 104:534–537, 2002.

51. Piao YS, Wakabayashi K, Hayashi S, et al: Aggregation of α-synuclein/NACP in the neuronal and glial cells in diffuse Lewy body disease: A survey of six patients. *Clin Neuropathol* 19:163–169, 2000.

52. Arima K, Murayama S, Mukoyama M, Inose T: Immunocytochemical and ultrastructural studies of neuronal and oligodendroglial cytoplasmic inclusions in multiple system atrophy. 1. Neuronal cytoplasmic inclusions. *Acta Neuropathol* 83:453–460, 1992.

53. Dickson DW, Lin W-I, Liu W-K, Yen S-H: Multiple system atrophy: A sporadic synucleinopathy. *Brain Pathol* 9:721–732, 1999.

54. Forno LS: Neuropathology of Parkinson's disease. *J Neuropathol Exp Neurol* 55:259–272, 1996.

55. Fearnley JM, Lees AJ: Ageing and Parkinson's disease: Substantia nigra regional selectivity. *Brain* 114:2283–2301, 1991.

56. Gasser T: Molecular advances in Parkinson's disease. *Adv Neurol* 86:23–32, 2001.

57. Pollanen MS, Dickson DW, Bergeron C: Pathology and biology of the Lewy body. *J Neuropathol Exp Neurol* 52:183–191, 1993.

58. Duffy P, Tennyson V: Phase and electron microscopic observations of Lewy bodies and melanin granules in the substantia nigra and locus ceruleus in Parkinson's disease. *J Neuropathol Exp Neurol* 24:398–414, 1965.

59. Pappolla MA: Lewy bodies of Parkinson's disease: Immune electron microscopic demonstration of neurofilament antigens in constituent filaments. *Arch Pathol Lab Med* 110:1160–1163, 1986.

60. Goldman JE, Yen S-H, Chiu F-C, Peress NS: Lewy bodies of Parkinson's disease contain neurofilament antigens. *Science* 221:1082–1084, 1983.

61. Hill WD, Lee VM-Y, Hurtig HI, et al: Epitopes located in spatially separate domains of each neurofilament subunit are present in Parkinson's disease Lewy bodies. *J Comp Neurol* 309:150–160, 1991.

62. Schmidt ML, Murray J, Lee VM-Y, et al: Epitope map of neurofilament protein domains in cortical and peripheral nervous system Lewy bodies. *Am J Pathol* 139:53–65, 1991.

63. Gomez-Tortosa E, Irizarry MC, Gomez-Isla T, Hyman BT: Clinical and neuropathological correlates of dementia with Lewy bodies. *Ann N Y Acad Sci* 920:9–15, 2000.

64. DeVos RA, Jansen EN, Stam FC, et al: 'Lewy body disease': Clinico-pathologic correlations in 18 consecutive cases of Parkinson's disease with and without dementia. *Clin Neurol Neurosurg* 97:13–22, 1995.

65. Mattila PM, Roytta M, Torikka H, et al: Cortical Lewy bodies and Alzheimer-type changes in patients with Parkinson's disease. *Acta Neuropathol* 95:576–582, 1998.

66. Koller WC: How accurately can Parkinson's disease be diagnosed? *Neurology* 42(1 suppl 1):6–16, 1992.

67. Jellinger KA: Morphological substrates of dementia in parkinsonism. A critical update. *J Neural Transm Suppl* 51:57–82, 1997.

68. Perl DP, Olanow CW, Calne D: Alzheimer's disease and Parkinson's disease: Distinct entities or extremes of a spectrum of neurodegeneration? *Ann Neurol* 44(3 suppl 1):S19–S31, 1998.

69. Ditter SM, Mirra SS: Neuropathologic and clinical features of Parkinson's disease in Alzheimer's disease patients. *Neurology* 37:754–760, 1987.

70. Hansen L, Salmon D, Galasko D, et al: The Lewy body variant of Alzheimer's disease: A clinical and pathologic entity. *Neurology* 40:1–8, 1990.

71. Morris JC, Drazner M, Fulling K, et al: Clinical and pathological aspects of parkinsonism in Alzheimer's disease. A role for extranigral factors? *Arch Neurol* 46:651–657, 1989.

72. Hulette C, Mirra S, Wilkinson, Heyman A, et al: The Consortium to Establish a Registry for Alzheimer's Disease (CERAD). Part IX. A prospective cliniconeuropathologic study of Parkinson's features in Alzheimer's disease. *Neurology* 45:1991–1995, 1995.

73. Hansen LA, Masliah E, Galasko D, Terry RD: Plaque-only Alzheimer disease is usually the Lewy body variant, and vice versa. *J Neuropathol Exp Neurol* 52:648–654, 1993.

74. Gearing M, Lynn M, Mirra SS: Neurofibrillary pathology in Alzheimer's disease with Lewy bodies. Two subgroups. *Arch Neurol* 56:203–208, 1999.

75. Dickson DW, Davies P, Mayeux R, et al: Diffuse Lewy body disease: Neuropathological and biochemical studies of six patients. *Acta Neuropathol* 75:8–15, 1987.

76. Bergeron C, Pollanen M: Lewy bodies in Alzheimer disease: One or two diseases? *Alzheimer Dis Assoc Disord* 3:197–204, 1989.

77. Crystal HA, Dickson DW, Lizardi JE, et al: Antemortem diagnosis of diffuse Lewy body disease. *Neurology* 40:1523–1528, 1990.

78. Del Ser T, Hachinski V, Merskey H, Munoz DG: Clinical and pathologic features of two groups of patients with dementia with Lewy bodies: Effect of coexisting Alzheimer-type lesion load. *Alzheimer Dis Assoc Disord* 15:31–44, 2001.

79. Perry RH, Irving D, Blessed G, et al: Senile dementia of Lewy body type: A clinically and neuropathologically distinct form of Lewy body dementia in the elderly. *J Neurol Sci* 95:119–139, 1990.

80. Papka M, Rubio A, Schiffer RB: A review of Lewy body disease: An emerging concept of cortical dementia. *J Neuropsychiatry Clin Neurosci* 10:267–279, 1998.

81. Luis CA, Barker WW, Gajaraj K, et al: Sensitivity and specificity of three clinical criteria for dementia with Lewy bodies in an autopsy-verified sample. *Int J Geriatr Psychiatry* 14:526–533, 1999.

82. McKeith IG, Ballard CG, Perry RH, et al: Prospective validation of consensus criteria for the diagnosis of dementia with Lewy bodies. *Neurology* 54:1050–1058, 2000.

83. Hansen LA, Masliah E, Terry RD, Mirra SS: A neuropathological subset of Alzheimer's disease with concomitant Lewy body disease and spongiform change. *Acta Neuropathol* 78:194–201, 1989.

84. Lowe J, Dickson D: Pathological diagnostic criteria for dementia associated with cortical Lewy bodies: Review and proposal for a descriptive approach. *J Neural Transm Suppl* 51:111–120, 1997.

85. Gai WP, Blessing We, Blumbergs PC: Ubiquitin-positive degenerating neurites in the brainstem in Parkinson's disease. *Brain* 118:1447–1459, 1995.

86. Marui W, Iseki E, Nakai T, et al: Progression and staging of Lewy pathology in brains from patients with dementia with Lewy bodies. *J Neurol Sci* 195;153–159, 2002.

87. Rezaie P, Cairns N, Chadwick A, Lantos PL: Lewy bodies are located preferentially in limbic areas in diffuse Lewy body disease. *Neurosci Lett* 212:111–114, 1996.

88. Hamilton RL: Lewy bodies in Alzheimer's disease: A neuropathological review of 145 cases using α-synuclein immunohistochemistry. *Brain Pathol* 10:378–384, 2000.

89. Harding AJ, Stimson E, Henderson JM, Halliday GM: Clinical correlates of selective pathology in the amygdala of patients with Parkinson's disease. *Brain* 125:2431–2445, 2002.

90. Gilman S, Low PA, Quinne N, et al: Consensus statement on the diagnosis of multiple system atrophy. *J Auton Nerv System* 74:189–192, 1998.

91. Golbe LI: Progressive supranuclear palsy, in Stern MB, Koller WC (eds): *Parkinsonian Syndromes.* New York: Marcel Dekker, 1993, pp 227–247.

92. Koike Y, Takahashi A: Autonomic dysfunction in Parkinson's disease. *Eur Neurol* 38(suppl 2):8–12, 1997.

93. Papp MI, Kahn JE, Lantos PL: Glial cytoplasmic inclusions in the CNS of patients with multiple system atrophy (striatonigral degeneration, olivopontocerebellar atrophy and Shy-Drager syndrome). *J Neurol Sci* 94:79–100, 1989.

94. Gilman S, Quinn NP: The relationship of multiple system atrophy to sporadic olivopontocerebellar atrophy and other forms of idiopathic late-onset cerebellar atrophy. *Neurology* 46:1197–1199, 1996.

95. Koeppen AH: The hereditary ataxias. *J Neuropathol Exp Neurol* 57:531–543, 1998.

96. Lantos PL: The definition of multiple system atrophy: A review of recent developments. *J Neuropathol Exp Neurol* 57:1099–1111, 1998.

97. Dickson DW, Liu W, Hardy J, et al: Widespread alterations of alpha-synuclein in multiple system atrophy. *Am J Pathol* 155:1241–1251, 1999.

98. Crowther RA, Jakes R, Spillantini MG, Goedert M. Synthetic filaments assembled from C-terminally truncated α-synuclein. *FEBS Lett* 436:309–312, 1998.

99. Giasson BI, Uryu K, Trojanowski JQ, Lee VM. Mutant and wild type human α-synucleins assemble into elongated filaments with distinct morphologies in vitro. *J Biol Chem* 274:7619–7622, 1999.

100. Castellani R: Multiple system atrophy: Clues from inclusions. *Am J Pathol* 153:671–676, 1998.

101. Steele JC, Richardson JC, Olszewski J: Progressive supranuclear palsy: A heterogeneous degeneration involving the brain-stem, basal ganglia and cerebellum with vertical gaze and pseudo-bulbar palsy, nuchal dystonia and dementia. *Arch Neurol* 10:333–359, 1964.

102. Bigio EH, Brown DF, White CL III: Progressive supranuclear palsy with dementia: Cortical pathology. *J Neuropathol Exp Neurol* 58:359–364, 1999.

103. Tellez-Nagel I, Wisniewski HM: Ultrastructure of neurofibrillary tangles in Steele-Richardson-Olszewski syndrome. *Arch Neurol* 29:324–327, 1973.

104. Dickson DW: Neuropathologic differentiation of progressive supranuclear palsy and corticobasal degeneration. *J Neurol* 246(suppl 2):II6–15, 1999.

105. Matsusaka H, Ikeda K, Akiyama H, et al: Astrocytic pathology in progressive supranuclear palsy: Significance for neuropathological diagnosis. *Acta Neuropathol* 96:248–252, 1998.

106. Arai N: "Grumose degeneration" of the dentate nucleus. A light and electron microscopic study in progressive supranuclear palsy and dentatorubropallidoluysial atrophy. *J Neurol Sci* 90:131–145, 1989.

107. Mizusawa H, Yen S-H, Hirano A, Llena JF: Pathology of the dentate nucleus in progressive supranuclear palsy: A histological, immunohistochemical and ultrastructural study. *Acta Neuropathol* 78:419–428, 1989.

108. Kobayashi K, Morikawa K, Fukutani Y, et al: Ramsay Hunt syndrome: Progressive mental deterioration in association with unusual cerebral white matter change. *Clin Neuropathol* 13:88–96, 1994.

109. Yamashita S, Iwamoto H, Hara M, et al: Sisters with early onset hereditary dentatorubral-pallidoluysian atrophy of childhood: DNA analysis and clinicopathological findings [title translated from Japanese]. *No To Hattatsu* 27:473–479, 1995.

110. Iwabuchi K, Nagatomo H, Tanabe T, et al: An autopsied case of type 2 Machado-Joseph's disease or spino-pontine degeneration [title translated from Japanese]. *No To Shinkei* 45:733–740, 1993.

111. Kogure T, Oda T, Katoh Y: Autopsy cases of hereditary ataxia pathologically diagnosed as the Japanese type of Joseph disease: Cliniconeuropathological findings [title translated from Japanese]. *Seishin Shinkeigaku Zasshi* 92:161–183, 1990.

112. Hattori H, Tanaka S, Kondoh H, et al: A case of juvenile Alzheimer's disease with various neurological features such as myoclonus, showing grumose degeneration in the dentate nucleus [title translated from Japanese]. *Rinsho Shinkeigaku* 30:647–653, 1990.

113. Schneider JA, Watts RL, Gearing M, et al: Corticobasal degeneration: Neuropathologic and clinical heterogeneity. *Neurology* 48:959–969, 1997.

114. Gearing M, Olson DA, Watts RL, Mirra SS: Progressive supranuclear palsy: Neuropathologic and clinical heterogeneity. *Neurology* 44:1015–1024, 1994.

115. Brett FM, Henson C, Staunton H: Familial diffuse Lewy body disease, eye movement abnormalities, and distribution of pathology. *Arch Neurol* 59:464–467, 2002.

116. Feany MB, Mattiace LA, Dickson DW: Neuropathologic overlap of progressive supranuclear palsy, Pick's disease, and corticobasal degeneration. *J Neuropathol Exp Neurol* 55:53–67, 1996.

117. Jendroska K, Rossor MN, Mathias CJ, Daniel SE: Morphological overlap between corticobasal degeneration and Pick's disease: A clinicopathological report. *Mov Disord* 10:111–114, 1995.

118. Litvan I, Agid Y, Jankovic J, et al: Accuracy of clinical criteria for the diagnosis of progressive supranuclear palsy (Steele-Richardson-Olszewski syndrome). *Neurology* 46:922–930, 1996.

119. Reed LA, Schmidt ML, Wszolek ZK, et al: The neuropathology of a chromosome 17-linked autosomal dominant parkinsonism and dementia ("pallido-ponto-nigral degeneration"). *J Neuropathol Exp Neurol* 57:588–601, 1998.

120. Collins SJ, Ahlskog JE, Parisi JE, Maraganore DM: Progressive supranuclear palsy: Neuropathologically based diagnostic clinical criteria. *J Neurol Neurosurg Psychiatry* 58:167–173, 1995.

121. Kleinschmidt-DeMasters BK: Early progressive supranuclear palsy: Pathology and clinical presentation. *Clin Neuropathol* 8:79–84, 1989.

122. Verny M, Jellinger KA, Hauw JJ, et al: Progressive supranuclear palsy: A clinicopathological study of 21 cases. *Acta Neuropathol* 91:427–431, 1996.

123. Mann DMA, Jones D: Deposition of amyloid (A4) protein within the brains of persons with dementing disorders other than Alzheimer's disease and Down's syndrome. *Neurosci Lett* 109:68–75, 1990.

124. Sasaki S, Maruyama S, Toyoda C: A case of progressive supranuclear palsy with widespread senile plaques. *J Neurol* 238:345–348, 1991.

125. Tsuboi Y, Josephs KA, Cookson N, Dickson DW: APOE E4 is a determinant for Alzheimer type pathology in progressive supranuclear palsy. *Neurology* 60:240–245, 2003.

126. Urasaki K, Kuriki K, Namerikawa M, et al: An autopsy case of Alzheimer's disease with a progressive supranuclear palsy overlap. *Neuropathology* 20:233–238, 2000.

127. Judkins AR, Forman MS, Uryu K, et al: Co-occurrence of Parkinson's disease with progressive supranuclear palsy. *Acta Neuropathol* 103:526–530, 2002.

128. Mori H, Oda M, Komori T, et al: Lewy bodies in progressive supranuclear palsy. *Acta Neuropathol* 104:273–278, 2002.

129. de Yébenes JG, Sarasa JL, Daniel SE, Lees AJ: Familial progressive supranuclear palsy. Description of a pedigree and review of the literature. *Brain* 118:1095–1103, 1995.

130. Rojo A, Pernaute RS, Fontan A, et al: Clinical genetics of familial progressive supranuclear palsy. *Brain* 122:1233–1245, 1999.

131. Brown J, Lantos P, Stratton M, et al: Familial progressive supranuclear palsy. *J Neurol Neurosurg Psychiatry* 56:473–476, 1993.

132. Stanford PM, Halliday GM, Brooks WS, et al: Progressive supranuclear palsy pathology caused by a novel silent mutation in exon 10 of the tau gene: Expansion of the disease phenotype caused by tau gene mutations. *Brain* 123:880–893, 2000.

133. Ksiezak-Reding H, Morgan K, Mattiace LA, et al: Ultrastructure and biochemical composition of paired helical filaments in corticobasal degeneration. *Am J Pathol* 145:1496–1508, 1994.

134. Takahashi T, Amano N, Hanihara T, et al: Corticobasal degeneration: Widespread argentophilic threads and glia in addition to neurofibrillary tangles. Similarities of cytoskeletal abnormalities in corticobasal degeneration and progressive supranuclear palsy. *J Neurol Sci* 138:66–77, 1996.

135. Tracz E, Dickson DW, Hainfeld JF, Ksiezak-Reding H: Paired helical filaments in corticobasal degeneration: The fine fibrillary structure with NanoVan. *Brain Res* 773:33–44, 1997.

136. Wakabayashi K, Oyanagi K, Makifuchi T, et al: Corticobasal degeneration: Etiopathological significance of the cytoskeletal alterations. *Acta Neuropathol* 87:545–553, 1994.

137. Feany MB, Dickson DW: Widespread cytoskeletal pathology characterizes corticobasal degeneration. *Am J Pathol* 146:1388–1396, 1995.

138. Komori T, Arai N, Oda M, et al: Astrocytic plaques and tufts of abnormal fibers do not coexist in corticobasal degeneration and progressive supranuclear palsy. *Acta Neuropathol* 96:401–408, 1998.

139. Mirra SS, Murrell JR, Gearing M, et al: Tau pathology in a family with dementia and a P301L mutation in tau. *J Neuropathol Exp Neurol* 58:335–345, 1999.

140. Bergeron C, Pollanen MS, Weyer L, et al: Unusual clinical presentations of cortical-basal ganglionic degeneration. *Ann Neurol* 40:893–900, 1996.

141. Grimes DA, Lang AE, Bergeron CB: Dementia as the most common presentation of cortical-basal ganglionic degeneration. *Neurology* 53:1969–1974, 1999.

142. Kertesz A, Martinez-Lage P, Davidson W, Munoz DG: The corticobasal degeneration syndrome overlaps progressive aphasia and frontotemporal dementia. *Neurology* 55:1368–1375, 2000.

143. Stover NP, Watts RL: Corticobasal degeneration. *Semin Neurol* 21:49–58, 2001.

144. Bergeron C, Davis A, Lang AE: Corticobasal ganglionic degeneration and progressive supranuclear palsy presenting with cognitive decline. *Brain Pathology* 8:355–365, 1998.

145. Dickson DW: Neuropathology of Pick's disease. *Neurology* 56(suppl 4):S16–S20, 2001.

146. Braak H, Braak E: Cortical and subcortical argyrophilic grains characterize a disease associated with adult onset dementia. *Neuropathol Appl Neurobiol* 15:13–26, 1989.

147. Jellinger KA: Dementia with grains (argyrophilic grain disease). *Brain Pathol* 8:377–386, 1998.

148. Nakazato Y, Hirato J, Ishida Y, et al: Swollen cortical neurons in Creutzfeldt-Jakob disease contain a phosphorylated neurofilament epitope. *J Neuropathol Exp Neurol* 49:197–205, 1990.

149. Mackenzie IRA, Hudson LP: Achromatic neurons in the cortex of progressive supranuclear palsy. *Acta Neuropathol* 90:615–619, 1995.

150. Manetto V, Sternberger NH, Perry G, et al: Phosphorylation of neurofilaments is altered in amyotrophic lateral sclerosis. *J Neuropathol Exp Neurol* 47:642–653, 1986.

151. Spillantini MG, Bird TD, Ghetti B: Frontotemporal dementia and parkinsonism linked to chromosome 17: A new group of tauopathies. *Brain Pathol* 8:387–402, 1998.

152. Foster NL, Wilhelmsen K, Sima AA, et al: Frontotemporal dementia and parkinsonism linked to chromosome 17: A consensus conference. *Ann Neurol* 41:706–715, 1997.

153. Bugiani O, Murrell JR, Giaccone G, et al: Frontotemporal dementia and corticobasal degeneration in a family with a P301S mutation in tau. *J Neuropathol Exp Neurol* 58:667–677, 1999.

154. Reed LA, Grabowski TJ, Schmidt ML, et al: Autosomal dominant dementia with widespread neurofibrillary tangles. *Ann Neurol* 42:564–572, 1997.

155. Murrell JR, Spillantini MG, Zolo P, et al: Tau gene mutation G389R causes a tauopathy with abundant Pick body-like inclusions and axonal deposits. *J Neuropathol Exp Neurol* 58:1207–1226, 1999.

156. Rizzini C, Goedert M, Hodges JR, et al: Tau gene mutation K257T causes a tauopathy similar to Pick's disease. *J Neuropathol Exp Neurol* 59:990–1001, 2000.

157. Goedert M, Spillantini MG, Crowther RA, et al: Tau gene mutation in familial progressive subcortical gliosis. *Nat Med* 5:454–457, 1999.

158. Lynch T, Sano M, Marder KS, et al: Clinical characteristics of a family with chromosome 17-linked disinhibition-dementia-parkinsonism-amyotrophy complex. *Neurology* 44:1878–1884, 1994.

159. Yamaoka LH, Welsh-Bohmer KA, Hulette CM, et al: Linkage of frontotemporal dementia to chromosome 17: Clinical and neuropathological characterization of phenotype. *Am J Hum Genet* 59:1306–1312, 1996.

160. Hulette CM, Pericak-Vance MA, Roses AD, et al: Neuropathological features of frontotemporal dementia and parkinsonism linked to chromosome 17q21–22 (FTDP-17): Duke family 1684. *J Neuropathol Exp Neurol* 58:859–866, 1999.

161. Miyasaka T, Morishima-Kawashima M, Ravid R, et al: Selective deposition of mutant tau in the FTDP-17 brain affected by the P301L mutation. *J Neuropathol Exp Neurol* 60:872–884, 2001.

162. Buee L, Delacourte A: Comparative biochemistry of tau in progressive supranuclear palsy, corticobasal degeneration, FTDP-17 and Pick's disease. *Brain Pathol* 9:681–693, 1999.

163. Corder EH, Saunders AM, Strittmatter WJ, et al: Gene dose of apolipoprotein E type 4 allele and the risk of Alzheimer's disease in late onset families. *Science* 261:921–923, 1993.

164. Strittmatter WJ, Saunders AM, Schmechel D, et al: Apolipoprotein E: High-avidity binding to β-amyloid and increased frequency of type 4 allele in late-onset familial Alzheimer disease. *Proc Natl Acad Sci U S A* 90:1977–1981, 1993.

165. Benjamin R, Leake A, Edwardson JA, et al: Apolipoprotein E genes in Lewy body and Parkinson's disease [letter]. *Lancet* 343:1565, 1994.

166. Galasko D, Saitoh T, Xia Y, et al: The apolipoprotein E allele ε4 is overrepresented in patients with the Lewy body variant of Alzheimer's disease. *Neurology* 44:1950–1951, 1994.

167. Gearing M, Schneider JA, Rebeck GW, et al: Alzheimer's disease with and without coexisting Parkinson's disease changes: Apolipoprotein E genotype and neuropathologic correlates. *Neurology* 45:1985–1990, 1995.

168. Pickering-Brown SM, Mann DA, Bourke JP, et al: Apolipoprotein E4 and Alzheimer's disease pathology in Lewy body disease and in other β-amyloid-forming diseases [letter]. *Lancet* 343:1155, 1994.

169. St. Clair D, Norrman J, Perry R, et al: Apolipoprotein E ε4 allele frequency in patients with Lewy body dementia, Alzheimer's disease and age-matched controls. *Neurosci Lett* 176:45–46, 1994.

170. Farrer LA, Abraham CR, Volicer L, et al: Allele ε4 of apolipoprotein E shows a dose effect on age at onset of Pick disease. *Exp Neurol* 136:162–170, 1995.

171. Ingelson M, Fabre SF, Lilius L, et al: Increased risk for frontotemporal dementia through interaction between tau polymorphisms and apolipoprotein E ε4. *Neuroreport* 12:905–909, 2001.

172. Kalman J, Juhasz A, Majtenyi K, et al: Apolipoprotein E polymorphism in Pick's disease and in Huntington's disease. *Neurobiol Aging* 21:555–558, 2000.

173. Schneider JA, Gearing M, Robbins RS, et al: Apolipoprotein E genotype in diverse neurodegenerative disorders. *Ann Neurol* 38:131–135, 1995.

174. Morris HR, Vaughan JR, Datta SR, et al: Multiple system atrophy/progressive supranuclear palsy: α-Synuclein, synphilin, tau and APOE. *Neurology* 55:1918–1920, 2000.

175. Pickering-Brown SM, Owen F, Isaacs A, et al: Apolipoprotein E ε4 allele has no effect on age at onset or duration of disease in cases of frontotemporal dementia with Pick- or microvacuolar-type histology. *Exp Neurol* 163:452–456, 2000.

176. Tabaton M, Rolleri M, Masturzo P, et al: Apolipoprotein E ε4 allele frequency is not increased in progressive supranuclear palsy. *Neurology* 45:1764–1765, 1995.

177. Ghebremedhin E, Schultz C, Thal DR, et al: Genetic association of argyrophilic grain disease with polymorphisms in alpha-2 macroglobulin and low-density lipoprotein receptor-related protein genes. *Neuropathol Appl Neurobiol* 28:308–313, 2002.

178. Sawa A, Amano N, Yamada N, et al: Apolipoprotein E in progressive supranuclear palsy in Japan. *Mol Psychiatry* 2:341–342, 1997.

179. Verpillat P, Camuzat A, Hannequin D, et al: Association between the extended tau haplotype and frontotemporal dementia. *Arch Neurol* 59:935–939, 2002.

180. Cairns NJ, Atkinson PF, Kovacs T, et al: Apolipoprotein E ε4 allele frequency in patients with multiple system atrophy. *Neurosci Lett* 221:161–164, 1997.

PART C
CLINICAL DISORDERS

I. PARKINSONIAN STATES

PARKINSON'S DISEASE

Chapter 10 _____

GENETICS OF PARKINSON'S DISEASE AND PARKINSONIAN DISORDERS

ZBIGNIEW K. WSZOLEK, KATERINA MARKOPOULOU, and BRUCE A. CHASE

HISTORICAL BACKGROUND: PRE-L-DOPA ERA   164
L-DOPA ERA: PHENOTYPIC CHARACTERIZATION
   OF KINDREDS WITH FAMILIAL PARKINSONISM   164
     Kindreds with a "Typical" PD Phenotype (Type I)   164
     Kindreds with a PPS Phenotype (Type II)   164
     Kindreds with a Neurodegenerative Phenotype
       and Some Parkinsonian Features (Type III)   166
     Kindreds with Juvenile Parkinsonism (Type IV)   166
MOLECULAR GENETIC ANALYSIS OF KINDREDS
   WITH FAMILIAL PARKINSONISM   166
     Kindreds with the IP Phenotype (Type I)   166
     Molecular Genetic Analysis of Kindreds with the
       PPS Phenotype (Type II)   167
     Kindreds with a Neurodegenerative Phenotype
       and Some Parkinsonian Features (Type III)   168
     Molecular Genetic Analysis of Kindreds with a
       Juvenile Parkinsonism Phenotype (Type IV)   168
SUMMARY   171

The etiology of idiopathic parkinsonism/Parkinson's disease (PD) remains unknown (see Chaps. 11 and 13). Approximately 75 percent of cases seen in specialized movement disorders clinics fulfill the standard diagnostic criteria for PD. The remaining 25 percent of patients with parkinsonian symptoms either have secondary parkinsonism due to identifiable causes (e.g., trauma, infection, tumor, stroke, medication, illicit drug use, or toxin exposure), or their parkinsonism is a part of a well-defined parkinsonism-plus syndrome (PPS) (e.g., progressive supranuclear palsy (see Chap. 20), multisystem atrophy (see Chap. 21), corticobasal degeneration (see Chap. 46), Wilson's disease (see Chap. 47), cerebellar disorders (see Chaps. 43 and 44), or others).[1]

Environmental factors have long been thought to play an important role in the pathogenesis of PD (see Chap. 11). In recent years, however, the identification of familial forms of parkinsonism has underscored the importance of genetic factors in the pathogenesis of PD.

The familial forms of parkinsonism can be subdivided into two types: those with a PD phenotype and those with a PPS phenotype.[2–4] Individuals with a PD phenotype exhibit a combination of symptoms, including bradykinesia, rigidity, resting tremor, and postural instability. These symptoms respond to L-dopa therapy. Furthermore, these patients do not exhibit cerebellar or lower motoneuron deficits, conjugate gaze paresis (except mildly impaired upward gaze), autonomic failure, or pyramidal dysfunction.[5] The neuropathologic findings include neuronal loss and gliosis in the substantia nigra (SN) and locus ceruleus (LC), and the presence of Lewy bodies in surviving neurons.[6]

Individuals affected with PPS are usually younger than those affected with PD. In PPS patients, the disease follows a more aggressive course, and death often occurs at a younger age. Parkinsonian symptoms show either no improvement with L-dopa or the improvement is short-lived. Affected patients may present with the cardinal features of parkinsonism, but frequently resting tremor is absent and rigidity is more pronounced in axial rather than appendicular muscles. Pyramidal signs, eye movement abnormalities, sensory disturbances, sphincter incontinence, autonomic dysfunction, respiratory difficulties, dementia, personality changes, depression, lower motoneuron involvement, and other signs frequently occur in PPS, either alone or in combination. Pathologic findings of PPS also differ from those of PD. Neuronal loss and gliosis typically involve not only the SN and LC but also many other subcortical and brainstem nuclei, as well as cerebral and cerebellar cortices. The LC, however, may be spared. Lewy bodies may not be present in surviving SN neurons, or, alternatively, they may have a widespread distribution. Frequently, neurofibrillary tangles (NFT), senile plaques, amyloid deposits, and ballooned neurons are seen.[1]

Familial forms of PPS have been difficult to classify based solely on clinical criteria. A review of the literature has shown that extrapyramidal features, including cardinal parkinsonian signs, are frequently seen in kindreds predominantly presenting with dementia, personality changes, amyotrophy, and dystonia. In fact, the possibility that PD, Alzheimer's disease (AD), and amyotrophic lateral sclerosis (ALS) have a common etiology has been raised previously.[7,8]

Much like the spinocerebellar ataxias (see Chaps. 43 and 44), where molecular genetic analysis has led to a rational classification based on mutations in genes for known proteins, the recent progress of molecular genetic analysis of familial parkinsonism has also led to a more rational classification of these syndromes. For example, some familial parkinsonism forms can now be classified as alpha-synucleinopathies or tauopathies. In a number of familial forms, the phenotype has been linked to a particular chromosomal region, but the molecular genetic defect has not yet been identified. It is likely, therefore, that this type of classification will evolve as new molecular genetic information becomes available. A summary of the molecular genetic characterization of the different forms of familial parkinsonism will be discussed more extensively later in this chapter.

Historical Background: Pre-L-Dopa Era

In his original monograph published in 1847, James Parkinson did not implicate hereditary factors in the pathogenesis of PD.[9] However, in his classic 1888 textbook, Gowers stated that an hereditary basis can be "traced" in up to 15 percent of PD cases.[10] Bell and Clark, in a review of the literature in 1926, described 10 kindreds with "shaking palsy" in which hereditary factors were thought to play a role, and provided 20 references of earlier accounts of familial paralysis agitans.[11] Allen, in 1937, described 25 kindreds with inherited parkinsonism and speculated that in approximately two-thirds of these kindreds the inheritance was autosomal-dominant and due to a "single autosomal gene."[12] Van Bogaert, in 1954, described a kindred whose members were affected with ALS, parkinsonism, or a combination of the two.[13] Mjönes, in his extensive monograph published in 1949, provided detailed description of 8 pedigrees with inherited parkinsonism, some of which exhibited atypical features.[14] Biemond and Sinnege, in 1955, reported a multigenerational kindred with early-onset atypical parkinsonism with 6 affected individuals and pathologic findings that included nigral depigmentation, astrocytic gliosis, and "phagocytosing microglia."[15] Biemond and Beck reported another smaller kindred in 1955.[16] Šercl and Kovarìk in 1963 reported several kindreds with an ALS phenotype, one of which exhibited extrapyramidal features.[17] Two additional kindreds were initially described in the pre-L-dopa era, but have subsequently been re-examined and are discussed below.[18,19]

L-Dopa Era: Phenotypic Characterization of Kindreds with Familial Parkinsonism

Kindreds with parkinsonism published since the introduction of L-dopa can be classified into four major categories utilizing clinical, genealogical, and pathological criteria.

KINDREDS WITH A "TYPICAL" PD PHENOTYPE (TYPE I)

In kindreds with a "typical" PD phenotype, affected individuals usually present with cardinal parkinsonian signs such as bradykinesia, rigidity, postural instability, resting tremor, and positive response to L-Dopa. Neuropathologic findings include neuronal loss, gliosis, and Lewy bodies in the SN. The parkinsonian phenotype is inherited as an autosomal-dominant trait. A number of kindreds have been described in which the clinical presentation consists of more or less of these typical PD features.[3,4,18,20–29] Neuropathologic findings in affected members of these kindreds include neuronal loss, gliosis, and Lewy body formation in the SN. In some of the kindreds, widespread NFT are seen in addition to gliosis and Lewy bodies in the SN, while, in others, widespread distribution of Lewy bodies is observed. The Italian-American

(Contursi) kindred described by Golbe et al.[21] is characterized clinically by typical PD features, but without resting tremor and with a relatively young age of onset and rapid disease course.

KINDREDS WITH A PPS PHENOTYPE (TYPE II)

Affected members of these kindreds usually display more than two, if not all, cardinal parkinsonian signs, as well as additional features that include amyotrophy, dementia, dystonia, ataxia, or eye movement abnormalities. L-Dopa responsiveness is usually absent or short-lived. Neuropathologic findings are more widespread than those seen in PD kindreds with involvement, not only of the SN, LC, and other brainstem nuclei, but also the cerebral cortex, thalamus, striatum, and hippocampus. Lewy bodies, both typical and atypical, are usually absent. If present they have a more widespread distribution. NFT, senile plaques, amyloid deposits, and ballooned neurons are also frequently seen. The phenotype is inherited as an autosomal-dominant trait. Molecular genetic analysis has demonstrated that a number of these kindreds are associated with mutations in the tau gene.

A large number of kindreds with the PPS phenotype have been described.[4,19,20,26,30–69] Families in this category exhibit clinical features of parkinsonism but also a variety of other neurologic abnormalities. The nonparkinsonian features can be used to aid in the classification of these syndromes. It should be noted, however, that this classification may be misleading for two reasons. First, different kindreds frequently overlap in their clinical features. Second, some kindreds may display multiple nonparkinsonian findings. Widespread pathologic abnormalities, with or without Lewy body formation, are also characteristic of this group of kindreds. Brief descriptions of the subtypes of PPS are provided below.

PPS-AMYOTROPHY

A number of kindreds with parkinsonism and amyotrophy have been reported.[4,26,31,41,44,65,66] The parkinsonism in all of these kindreds is characterized by bradykinesia and rigidity; typical parkinsonian resting tremor has been described in only some of the kindreds, whereas in others a variety of other nonparkinsonian features have been described. Some but not all kindreds demonstrate consistent L-dopa responsiveness. Adequate autopsy information is available for only some of the kindreds. The neuropathological findings include depigmentation, gliosis, and neuronal loss in the SN, Lewy body formation in some kindreds, and axonal spheroids in anterior horn cells in others. In most of the kindreds the phenotype is inherited as an autosomal-dominant trait.

PPS-DEMENTIA

A number of kindreds that predominantly exhibit parkinsonism also display progressive dementia as a part of their clinical picture.[19,30,32,33,36,41,46,48,50,57,58,62,65,66,68] In the majority of the kindreds, the parkinsonism is characterized by brady-kinesia. Rigidity and resting tremor are less commonly seen. L-Dopa responsiveness has been noted in some kindreds. Once again, a variety of other nonparkinsonian features are present in these kindreds, including amyotrophy. Neuronal loss and gliosis in the SN is seen in the majority of the kindreds for which autopsy findings have been reported. Lewy bodies are present in some kindreds. They are either limited to brain-stem nuclei or exhibit a widespread distribution in both the brainstem and cortex. NFT, senile plaques, ballooned neurons, amyloid plaques, and spongiform changes, occurring alone or in combination, are also seen in some of the kindreds. In the majority of these kindreds the phenotype is inherited as an autosomal-dominant trait, although in some it is inherited as an autosomal-recessive trait.

PPS-PSYCHIATRIC DISTURBANCES

A relatively large number of kindreds have been described with predominant parkinsonism in which psychiatric dys-function also develops.[32–35,37–40,47–49,52–54,56–58,60,62,65,66,69] Depression is rather prevalent, while manic-depressive disorder, psychosis, and personality changes are less common. Bradykinesia and rigidity are present in the majority of these kindreds, and resting tremor is less prevalent. L-Dopa respon-siveness has been noted in some of the kindreds. As with the previous subgroups, a variety of other nonparkinsonian features are present in these kindreds. Autopsy information available for some kindreds reveals depigmentation, neu-ronal loss, and gliosis in the SN. In some of the kindreds, Lewy bodies are confined to the brainstem structures, whereas they are widespread in other kindreds. Ballooned neurons and spongiform changes are seen in some kindreds, whereas NFT and senile plaques are absent. In the majority of these kin-dreds the phenotype is inherited as an autosomal-dominant trait.

PPS-DYSTONIA

A number of kindreds with predominant parkinsonism also include dystonia as part of their clinical picture.[45,50,51,57–59,67] Bradykinesia and rigidity are present in most affected mem-bers of the kindreds, and resting tremor is less common. The presence of resting tremor does not serve as a predictor of L-Dopa responsiveness. As with other subgroups, a variety of other nonparkinsonian features are present. In the neuro-pathological findings that have been reported for some of these kindreds, Lewy bodies are absent. The phenotype is usually inherited as an autosomal-dominant trait, but, in some kindreds, it is inherited as an autosomal-recessive trait.

PPS-EYE MOVEMENT ABNORMALITIES

A number of kindreds have been reported that display a variety of eye movement or visual difficulties, including vertical gaze paresis, strabismus, nystagmus, "jerky" ocular pursuit, apraxia of eyelid opening and closing, oculogyric crises, slow saccades, and "visual difficulties" of an unspec-ified nature.[31,36,42–45,48,51,57–59,61,65,66,68] The most frequently described abnormalities are vertical gaze paresis, and nys-tagmus. While affected members of all kindreds display bradykinesia and rigidity, resting tremor is less common. The neuropathologic findings may include Lewy bodies that are either confined to the brainstem or have a widespread dis-tribution. In the majority of the kindreds the phenotype is inherited as an autosomal-dominant trait, but in some kin-dreds it is inherited as an autosomal-recessive or X-linked trait.

PPS-POSTURAL TREMOR

Postural tremor associated with parkinsonism has been described in a number of kindreds.[31,34,36–40,45,49,50,62] Bradykinesia and rigidity are present in affected members of the majority of the kindreds, but resting tremor is less com-monly seen. Neuropathologic findings include Lewy bodies confined to the brainstem or with a more widespread dis-tribution. In the majority of the kindreds the phenotype is inherited as an autosomal-dominant trait, but in some it is inherited as an autosomal-recessive trait.

PPS-MYOCLONUS/SEIZURES

Some kindreds with a predominantly parkinsonian pheno-type also exhibit myoclonus or seizures as part of their clinical phenotype.[19,30,42,43,48,52,53,61,62] In these kindreds, bradykine-sia and rigidity are very common, whereas resting tremor is less common. In the majority of the kindreds there is no L-Dopa responsiveness. Neuropathologic findings include Lewy bodies with a widespread distribution. Ballooned neu-rons are also seen in affected members of some kindreds. In the majority of the kindreds the phenotype is inherited as an autosomal-dominant trait.

PPS-RESPIRATORY ABNORMALITIES

A number of kindreds with a combination of depres-sion, hypoventilation, and parkinsonism have been reported.[32–34,47,56,69] All display bradykinesia and some have resting tremor. The kindreds with resting tremor also have L-Dopa responsiveness. Lewy bodies are present in the brain-stem in affected members of some, but not all, kindreds. In these kindreds, the phenotype is inherited as an autosomal-dominant trait.

PPS-MISCELLANEOUS ABNORMALITIES

A variety of other neurologic features have been described in PPS kindreds. These include ataxia, pyramidal signs, choreo-athetosis, tourettism, sleep disorders, dysarthria, dysphagia, anorexia, mutism, urinary incontinence, scoliosis, sensory abnormalities, and "encephalopathy."

KINDREDS WITH A NEURODEGENERATIVE PHENOTYPE AND SOME PARKINSONIAN FEATURES (TYPE III)

A number of other kindreds have been described that are characterized primarily by neurodegenerative features such as dementia, personality changes, ALS, or dystonia, but which also may include some parkinsonian signs as a part of their clinical syndrome.[66,70–106] In these kindreds, affected individuals usually present with dementia, personality changes, amyotrophy, pyramidal signs, and dystonia, alone or in combination. Affected individuals may exhibit extrapyramidal signs, including one or more of the parkinsonian cardinal features. For some of these kindreds there is no information available regarding L-Dopa responsiveness. Neuropathologic findings may include neuronal loss in the SN. Lewy bodies, typical and atypical, have been reported.

KINDREDS WITH JUVENILE PARKINSONISM (TYPE IV)

Juvenile parkinsonism that is inherited as an autosomal-recessive trait (ARJP) was initially reported in the Japanese population.[63] The phenotype of ARJP is in some aspects indistinguishable from that of typical sporadic PD. There is L-dopa responsiveness that is usually long-lasting. In addition to the typical parkinsonian features, however, ARJP is characterized by early disease onset (< 30 years), the presence of dystonia, and prominent diurnal fluctuation of symptoms. The neuropathologic findings include neuronal loss and gliosis in the SN but Lewy bodies are absent. Since the original description of ARJP in the Japanese population, a number of kindreds with a similar phenotype and worldwide distribution have been reported. The majority of the ARJP kindreds have been associated with mutations in the parkin gene.

Molecular Genetic Analysis of Kindreds with Familial Parkinsonism

Since the publication of the first edition of this book, significant progress has occurred in our understanding of molecular genetic aspects of familial parkinsonism.

KINDREDS WITH THE IP PHENOTYPE (TYPE I)

Molecular genetic characterization of these kindreds has implicated a number of different chromosomal regions. In some of these regions the relevant genetic lesion has been identified, whereas in others a genetic abnormality has not yet been identified.

An Italian-American (Contoursi) kindred and a number of Greek and Greek-American kindreds are associated with the presence of a point mutation in exon 4 (G209A) of the coding region of the alpha-synuclein gene (PARK1).[107,108]

A small German kindred has been associated with mutations in exon 3 (G88C) of the alpha-synuclein gene.[109] These mutations exhibit autosomal dominant inheritance with reduced penetrance. Alpha-synuclein has been identified in cytoplasmic aggregates in different neurodegenerative disorders, including amyloid plaques in AD, in Lewy bodies in both familial and sporadic PD, and in Lewy bodies of diffuse Lewy body disease (DLBD), in glial cytoplasmic inclusions in multisystem atrophy (MSA), and in motoneurons and glial cells in ALS.[110,111] Mutations in the alpha-synuclein gene to date have been only identified in familial and sporadic forms of PD, but not in AD, DLBD, MSA, or ALS. The formation and role of the intracytoplasmic aggregates in parkinsonian syndromes and in neurodegenerative diseases in general remain unclear. The aggregates themselves may be toxic to neurons, be associated with the beneficial sequestration of abnormal proteins or interfere with normal cellular protein turnover. Furthermore, within the different multigenerational kindreds, there are a number of phenotypic differences such as disease severity, age of onset, and neuropathologic findings, even though the primary genetic defect is nominally the same (i.e., a mutation in the coding region of alpha-synuclein). This phenotypic variability suggests that other genetic and/or environmental factors may contribute to the parkinsonian phenotype in these kindreds.

Interestingly, an analysis of the expression of the alpha-synuclein gene in a large Greek-American kindred with familial parkinsonism (Family H)[108] demonstrated that, in contrast to the Italian-American Contursi kindred,[21,107] the G209A allele is either *not* expressed, or its expression is significantly reduced in lymphoblastoid cell lines established from affected individuals. In addition, the G209A allele is not expressed in asymptomatic at-risk individuals whose age is older than the mean age of onset for their generation, whereas it is expressed in an at-risk individual who is younger than the age of disease onset for their generation. In some families with the G209A mutation, the differential expression of the G209A allele at both the mRNA and protein level has been confirmed using real-time quantitative RT-PCR (reverse transcriptase polymerase chain reaction) methods and mass spectrometry.[112] These findings indicate that there is differential expression of the G209A allele relative to the normal allele at the alpha-synuclein gene and support the hypothesis that levels of alpha-synuclein or altered ratios of normal to mutant alpha-synuclein expression are important for disease pathogenesis. Furthermore, these findings implicate for the first time the mechanism of haploinsufficiency, the deleterious effect of one copy of the wild-type allele at a particular locus[113] in neurodegeneration. Haploinsufficiency has been associated with an autosomal-dominant mode of inheritance, a mode usually associated with a gain-of-function mutational mechanism. Interestingly, abnormal levels of huntingtin expression have been also implicated in the pathogenesis of Huntington's disease, the prototype of a neurodegenerative disorder associated with a gain-of-function mutation and a dominant mode of inheritance.[114] Finally, they raise the possibility of an age-dependent downregulation of gene expression as a potential mechanism underlying disease pathogenesis. At this point, the relationship between the presence of the point mutation in the coding region of alpha-synuclein and the lack of expression remains unclear.

In addition to the mutations in the alpha-synuclein gene, a point mutation (I93M) has been identified in the gene for ubiquitin C-terminal hydrolase L1 (UCH-L1, PARK5) in a family with a presumed autosomal-dominant mode of inheritance, reduced penetrance, and a PD phenotype.[115] The function of UCH-L1 is unknown, but it is highly expressed in the brain. It is presumed to act in the ubiquitin-proteasome pathway and hydrolyze ubiquitinated proteins, thus leading to the recycling of ubiquitin.[116]

Since the description of the two mutations in the alpha-synuclein gene, a number of American kindreds traced genealogically to northern Europe [26] and some European kindreds have been associated with a susceptibility locus on the short arm of chromosome 2 (2p13, PARK3). The relevant gene has not yet been identified.[117] Another region on chromosome 4 (4p15, PARK 4) has been associated with a large kindred with an early-onset PD phenotype with some instances of dementia.[19,30,118] More recently, chromosomal regions 1p35-36 (PARK 6) and 1p36 (PARK7) have been associated with kindreds with a PD phenotype.[119,120] In a large Japanese family with an autosomal-dominant mode of inheritance, the PD phenotype has been linked to a region on chromosome 12p11.2-q13p.1 (PARK8).[121] Another locus on chromosome 1p32 for late-onset PD was identified in Iceland.[122]

A genome-wide screen using 174 families with multiple cases of PD showed evidence of linkage to six distinct chromosomal regions: 3q, 5q, 6q (parkin), 8p, 9q, and 17q (tau).[123] Finally, the tau gene (17q21-22) has been implicated as a susceptibility gene for PD.[124] A summary of the known mutations associated with a PD phenotype to date is shown in Table 10-1. A summary of all genes or loci associated with parkinsonism to date is shown in Table 10-2. Future clinical and pathological studies of families with these genetic loci/mutations are needed to determine if their phenotype is similar to this one observed in sporadic form of PD.

MOLECULAR GENETIC ANALYSIS OF KINDREDS WITH THE PPS PHENOTYPE (TYPE II)

Since the first edition of this book, there has also been considerable progress in the molecular analysis of kindreds with a PPS phenotype. The discovery that families with a wide range of clinical presentations, including PD, Pick's disease, and ALS features, are linked to a locus on chromosome 17q21-22 led to the description of new syndrome of frontotemporal dementia and parkinsonism linked to chromosome 17 (FTDP-17).[125] Further molecular genetic studies have identified the presence of tau mutations in almost the entire original and subsequently described families.

TABLE 10-1 Mutations Associated with Kindreds with the PD Phenotype

Chromosomal Region	Gene	Mutation	Mutant Allele Expression
4q21-23	Alpha-synuclein	G209A/A53Thr	Present in some kindreds, absent in others
		G88C/30P	Level of expression of mutant allele correlates with phenotypic severity
4p15	Ubiquitin C-terminal hydrolase L1	I193M	NA

NA, not available.

The tau gene is alternatively spliced and contains 16 exons that encode 6 isoforms of a microtubule-associated protein expressed predominantly in axons in the central nervous system.[126] The 6 isoforms range in length from 352 to 441 amino acids and result from amino-acid sequence differences at the C- and N-termini of tau. At the C-terminus are microtubule binding motifs that contain repeats. These consist of either three (3R-tau) or four (4R-tau) tandemly repeated sequences of 31 amino acids. At the N-terminus, 29 or 58 amino acid inserts can be present or absent. The amino acid sequence differences result from alternative splicing of exons 2, 3, and 10. The inclusion of exon 10 and the 31 amino acid repeat it encodes gives rise to the 4R isoforms, whereas its exclusion gives rise to the 3R isoforms. The 4R-tau isoforms are thought to promote microtubule assembly more efficiently than the 3R-tau isoforms. The alternative splicing of exons 2 and 3 leads to the formation of isoforms without a 29 amino acid insert (0N), with a 29 amino acid insert (1N) or with a 58 amino acid insert (2N). In the normal brain, the ratio of 3R- to 4R-tau is approximately 1:1.[127] The ratio of the N isoforms varies with the 1N isoform being the most prevalent and the 2N being the least prevalent. The alternative splicing of tau is developmentally regulated with the 3R-0N isoform being present in the fetal brain. In the postnatal period all isoforms are present.[126] Finally, tau isoforms can be phosphorylated, and the phosphorylation is also developmentally regulated. Hyperphosphorylated tau isoforms form the paired helical filaments that are present in NFT.

Since 1998, when the first tau mutations were identified,[128-130] a large number of other tau mutations have been described.[131] The majority of these mutations are missense and intronic point mutations, but deletion mutation has also been reported. Missense mutations have been identified in exons 1, 9, 10, 12, and 13, and intronic mutations have been found between exons 9 and 10 and exons 10 and 11.[128-167] Interestingly, it appears that the vast majority of mutations involve exon 10 and its flanking introns. These mutations appear to affect the alternative splicing of exon 10 and consequently alter the ratio of 3R- to 4R-tau.

TABLE 10-2 Familial Parkinsonism Associated with Known Gene Mutations or Loci

Name	Chromosomal Region	Gene	Range (Mean) of Age of Disease Onset (Years)	Phenotype	Response to L-Dopa
Autosomal-dominant					
PARK 1	4q21	Alpha-synuclein (2 mutations)	20–85 (46)	PD, some cases with dementia	Good
PARK 3	2p13	Unknown	36–89 (58)	PD, some cases with dementia	Good
PARK 4	4p15	Unknown	24–48 (30+)	PD, some cases with dementia	Good
PARK 5	4p14-15	UCH-L1	49–51 (50)	PD	Good
PARK 8	12p11.2-q13.11	Unknown	38–68 (51)	PD	Good
	1p	Unknown	NA (late-onset)	PD	Good
	3q	Unknown	Late-onset	PD	None
	5q	Unknown	Late-onset	PD	Good
	8p	Unknown	Late-onset	PD	Good
	9q	Unknown	Late-onset	PD	None
SCA 2	12q23-24.1	SCA2 (ataxin-2)	19–61 (39)	PD	Fair
SCA 3	14q32.1	SCA3 (ataxin-3)	31–57 (42)	PD	Good
FTDP-17	17q21-22	Tau (multiple mutations)	25–76 (49)	FTD, PD, PSP, CBD, ALS	Poor
DYT12	19q13	Unknown	12–45 (23)	Rapid-onset dystonia-parkinsonism	Poor
Autosomal-recessive					
PARK 2	6q25.22-27	Parkin (multiple mutations)	6–58 (26)	PD	Good
PARK 6	1p35-36	Unknown	32–48 (41)	PD	Good
PARK 7	1p36	Unknown	27–40 (33)	PD	Good
X-Linked-recessive					
DYT3	Xq13.1	Unknown	12–48 (35)	Dystonia-parkinsonism	Poor
Mitochondrial					
	Complex 1	ND4	(31)	PD with dementia, dystonia, and ophthalmoplegia	Fair
	Complex 1	Unknown	35–79 (42)	PD	Good

UCH-L1, ubiquitin carboxyterminal hydrase L1; PD, idiopathic parkinsonism/Parkinson's disease; FTDP-17, frontotemporal dementia and parkinsonism linked on chromosome 17; FTD, frontotemporal dementia; PSP, progressive supranuclear palsy; CBD, corticobasal degeneration; ALS, amyotrophic lateral sclerosis; NA, not available.

This is clinically relevant, since biochemical studies from the brains of affected members of FTDP-17 kindreds indicate that only 4R-tau is present. Mutations in exons 12 and 13 affect the microtubule binding domain. The extensive genetic and biochemical analysis of the mutations associated with FTDP-17 has allowed for the emergence of a correlation between an abnormal tau genotype and a phenotypic manifestation.[131] Details of the identified mutations and their phenotypes are shown in Table 10-3.

KINDREDS WITH A NEURODEGENERATIVE PHENOTYPE AND SOME PARKINSONIAN FEATURES (TYPE III)

The molecular analysis of kindreds assigned to this category based on clinical criteria revealed that they have a rather diverse genetic basis and have implicated at least three different genes: GTPCH I, parkin, and tau. For example, dopa-responsive dystonia (DRD) kindreds have been associated with mutations in the gene for guanosine triphosphate cyclohydrolase I (GTPCH I). GTPCH I is the rate-limiting enzyme in the production of tetrahydrobiopterin, which is a cofactor for tyrosine hydroxylase. Reported mutations include missense, nonsense, and splice-site mutations, small deletions, as well as mutations in the presumed GTPCH I regulatory regions.[168] Interestingly, some of the DRD kindreds have been associated with homozygous and heterozygous deletions in the parkin gene.[169] Locus on chromosome 19q13 (DYT12) has been implicated for rapid-onset dystonia-parkinsonism families,[59,170] and locus on chromosome Xq13 (DYT3) for dystonia-parkinsonism (Lubag disease).[171] SCA2 and SCA3 mutations have been described in families with ataxia associated with parkinsonism.[172,173] Finally, mitochondrial complex 1 dysfunction has been reported in PD families[174,175] (see Table 10-2).

MOLECULAR GENETIC ANALYSIS OF KINDREDS WITH A JUVENILE PARKINSONISM PHENOTYPE (TYPE IV)

The molecular analysis of kindreds with an ARJP phenotype revealed that mutations in the parkin gene underlie

TABLE 10-3 Mutations in Tau and Clinical Features Associated with Kindreds with the PPS Phenotype

	Mutations not in Exon 10				Mutations in Exon 10	Exon 10 5′ Splice-site Mutations
	Exon 1	Exon 9	Exon 12	Exon 13		
Age at onset (years)						
<30					P301S	−2
31–40				G389R	delN296	+3, +11, +14, +16
41–50		G272V	E342V		N279K P301L	+12, +13
51<	R5H		V337M K369I	R406W	L284L S305S del280K	−2
Duration (years)						
<5	R5H			G389R	del280 delN296	−1, +11, +12
6–10		G272V	E342V K369I		N279K L284L P301L P301S	+3, +14, +16
11–15			V337M			−1, +3, +11
15<				R406W		+3, +12
First sign						
Parkinsonism	R5H	G272V	V337M E342V K369I		N279K P301L delN296	−2, −1, +12, +14, +16
Dementia	R5H			R406W	L284L delN296	−1, +11
Personality change		G272V			P301L	+3, +12, +14, +16
Parkinsonism						
Early-prominent					N279K delN296	−2
Late-prominent					P301S	
Rare-minimal		G272V			P301L	
Dementia						
Early-prominent		G272V	V337M K369I	R406W	del280K L284L P301L P301S	−1, +12, −2, +3, +11, +13
Late-prominent					N279K	
Rare-minimal						
Personality change						
Early-prominent		G272V	V337M K369I	R406W	del280K L284L P301L P301S	−2, −1, +12, +14, +16
Eye movement abnormalities					N279K P301S delN296	−1, +3
Epilepsy			V337M		P301S	
Myoclonus					P301S	+11
Pyramidal signs					N279K	−1, +3, +12
Amyotrophy					P301L	+14

Modified from Ghetti B, Hutton ML, Wszolek ZK. Frontotemporal dementia and parkisonism linked to chromosome 17 associated with tau gene mutations (FTDB-17T) In: D. Dickson, ed. Neurodegeneration: the molecular pathology of dementia and movement disorders. Basel: ISN Neuropath Press, 2003, pp 86–102.

TABLE 10-4 Parkin Mutations Associated with ARJP or Early-Onset PD

Type of Mutation	Exon	Domain	Identified in
Deletion			
	2	Ubiquitin	Heterozygote
	3	Ubiquitin	Homozygote/heterozygote
	4		Homozygote/heterozygote
	5		Heterozygote
	6–7	RING	Heterozygote
	8		Heterozygote
	7–9	RING/IBR	Heterozygote
	3–9	Ubiquitin, RING/IBR	Heterozygote
202-203delAG	2	Ubiquitin	Homozygote/heterozygote
255delA	2	Ubiquitin	Homozygote
871delG	7	RING	Homozygote
Duplication			
	3	Ubiquitin	Homozygote/heterozygote
	6	RING	Heterozygote
	7	RING	Heterozygote
	11	RING	Heterozygote
Triplication			
	2	Ubiquitin	Heterozygote
Missense/nonsense			
Arg33Stop	2		
Arg42Pro	2	Ubiquitin	Homozygote
321-322insGT	3	Ubiquitin	Homozygote
Lys161Asn	4		Homozygote
Lys211Asn	6		Homozygote
Arg256Cys	7	RING	Heterozygote
Cys268Stop	7	RING	Homozygote
Arg275Trp	7	RING	Heterozygote
Asp280Asn	7	RING	Homozygote
Cys289Gly	7	RING	Homozygote
Gly328Glu	9		Homozygote
Arg334Cys	9	IBR	Homozygote
1142-1143delGA	9	IBR	Homozygote
Thr415Asn	11		Homozygote
Gly430Asp	12	RING	Homozygote
Cys431Phe	12	RING	Homozygote
Trp453Stop	12	RING	Homozygote
Compound heterozygotes			
Lys161Asn; 202-203delAG		Ubiquitin	Heterozygote
Ex4; G1292T		Ubiquitin	Heterozygote
Ex3; Arg275Trp	7	RING	

IBR, in between RING finger domain.

the kindred phenotype. The parkin gene is located on chromosome 6 (6q25.2-q27) and is rather large. It is 500 kilobase long, contains 12 exons and encodes a 465 amino acid protein. This protein has interesting features that include a homology to ubiquitin at its N-terminus and a RING-finger motif at its C-terminus. Parkin has been recently shown to function as an ubiquitin protein ligase (E3) and to interact with the ubiquitin-conjugating enzyme E2. It can ubiquitinate itself and promote its own degradation.[169,176,177] It also interacts with glycosylated forms of alpha-synuclein.

All of these findings clearly link parkin to the ubiquitin-proteasome pathway, a pathway that normally functions to eliminate cellular proteins that are destined for destruction.

At least 60 different mutations have been reported in the parkin gene (Table 10-4). The majority of these mutations have been associated with ARJP and early-onset PD. They include point mutations, deletions, exon duplications, and triplications, as well as compound heterozygotes.[178–180] Interestingly, the phenotypic spectrum of parkin mutations is continuing to expand and includes cases with late-disease onset, cerebellar signs, and dystonia.[169]

The mechanism(s) by which the different mutations lead to the particular phenotypes are under active investigation. An emerging hypothesis is that these mutations lead to a loss of function of parkin as an E3 enzyme, resulting in failure of the proteolysis mediated by the ubiquitin-proteasome system and the accumulation of as yet unidentified proteins. This leads to neuronal cell death in the substantia nigra without the formation of Lewy bodies.

Summary

This chapter documents that there is a large number of familial parkinsonian syndromes with a wide phenotypic spectrum. A classification of parkinsonian kindreds based on their clinical and neuropathologic criteria has been rather difficult, and made more complicated by the fact that the phenotype associated with a single kindred may vary. The information obtained to date from molecular genetic analysis has led to the emergence of different disease categories based on the type of genetic defect and suggested multiple, different hypotheses about the underlying mechanisms of neurodegeneration. The terms alpha-synucleinopathies and tauopathies have become widely accepted, although the precise mechanism by which abnormalities in alpha-synuclein and tau lead to neurodegeneration is not fully understood. Indeed, both gain-of-function and loss-of-function mechanisms have been implicated in the neurodegeneration seen in these syndromes.

The majority of the currently described familial parkinsonian syndromes deviate significantly in their clinical and pathological characteristics from the typical features of sporadic PD. Interestingly, however, the genes identified in these syndromes have also been directly implicated in the pathogenesis of the sporadic form of PD, even though mutations in these genes have not yet been described in sporadic PD. All genes implicated to date in PD pathogenesis have been shown to be expressed in the brain,[181] and interact either directly or indirectly with each other.[182] For example, the protein product of the alpha-synuclein gene binds with protein product of the tau gene,[183] and parkin ubiquitinates a glycosylated form of alpha-synuclein.[184] To date, no interaction has been reported between tau and parkin.

There is clearly much to discover from molecular genetic analyses, as a number of loci in which the relevant genetic defect has yet to be identified (see Table 10-2) do seem to play a role in PD pathogenesis. Therefore, it is likely that the progress in the molecular genetic analysis of these loci will lead to further elucidation of the genetic pathways underlying neurodegeneration, and potentially provide a handle to analyze the interaction of genetic pathways with environmental factors that contribute to PD pathogenesis and neurodegeneration.

References

1. Jankovic J: Parkinsonism-plus syndromes. *Mov Disord* 4:S95, 1989.
2. Duvoisin RC: Research on the genetics of Parkinson's disease: Will it lead to the cause and a cure, in Stern MB (ed): *Beyond the Decade of the Brain*. Chapel Place: Wells Medical Limited, 1994, p 95.
3. Lazzarini AM, Myers RH, Zimmerman TR Jr, et al: A clinical genetic study of Parkinson's disease: Evidence for dominant transmission. *Neurology* 44:499, 1994.
4. Denson MA, Wszolek ZK: Familial parkinsonism: Our experience and review. *Parkinsonism Related Disord* 1:35, 1995.
5. Calne DB: Is idiopathic parkinsonism the consequence of an event or a process? *Neurology* 44:5, 1994.
6. Fearnley J, Lees A: Pathology of Parkinson's disease, in Calne DB (ed): *Neurodegenerative Diseases*. Philadelphia: WB Saunders, 1994, p 545.
7. Calne DB, Eisen A: The relationship between Alzheimer's disease, Parkinson's disease and motor neuron disease. *Can J Neurol Sci* 16:547, 1989.
8. Uitti RJ, Calne DB: Pathogenesis of idiopathic parkinsonism. *Eur Neurol* 33:6, 1993.
9. Parkinson J: *An Essay on the Shaking Palsy*. London: Whittingham and Rowland for Sherwood, Neely and Jones, 1817.
10. Gowers WR: *Diseases of the Nervous System*. Philadelphia: P Blakiston, 1988.
11. Bell J, Clark AJ: A pedigree of paralysis agitans. *Ann Eugenics* 1:455, 1926.
12. Allen W: Inheritance of the shaking palsy. *Arch Intern Med* 60:424, 1937.
13. Van Bogaert L, Radermecker MA: Scléroses latérales amyotrophiques typiques et paralysies agitantes héréditaires, dans une méme famille, avec une forme de passage possible entre les deux affections. *Mschr Psychiatr Neurol* 185, 1954.
14. Mjönes H: Paralysis agitans: A clinical and genetic study. *Acta Psychiatr Neurol Scand Suppl* 54:1, 1949.
15. Biemond A, Sinnege JLM: Tabes of Friedreich with degeneration of the substantia nigra, a special type of hereditary parkinsonism. *Confin Neurol* 15:129, 1955.
16. Biemond A, Beck W: Neural muscle atrophy with degeneration of the substantia nigra. *Confin Neurol* 15:142, 1955.
17. Šercl M, Kovarík J: On the familial incidence of amyotrophic lateral sclerosis. *Acta Neurol Scand* 39:169, 1963.
18. Branger F: Une forme familiale de paralysie agitante dans une souche des grisons. *J Genet Hum* 5:261, 1956.
19. Spellman GG: Report of familial cases of parkinsonism. *JAMA* 179:372, 1962.
20. Otto FG: Ein Beitrag zu familiär gehäuft Auftretenden fällen von Parkinsonismus. *Nervenarzt* 54:423, 1983.
21. Golbe LI, Di Iorio G, Bonavita V, et al: A large kindred with autosomal dominant Parkinson's disease. *Ann Neurol* 27:276, 1990.
22. Mauri JA, Asensio M, Jimenez A, et al: [Familial Parkinson disease]. *Neurologia* 5:45, 1990.
23. Maraganore DM, Harding AE, Marsden CD: A clinical and genetic study of familial Parkinson's disease. *Mov Disord* 6:205, 1991.
24. Sawle GV, Wroe SJ, Lees AJ, et al: The identification of presymptomatic parkinsonism: Clinical and [18F]dopa positron emission tomography studies in an Irish kindred. *Ann Neurol* 32:609, 1992.

25. Petelin LS: Clinical aspects and treatment of parkinsonism. *Neurology* 43:9, 1993.

26. Wszolek ZK, Cordes M, Calne DB, et al: Hereditärer Morbus Parkinson: Bericht über drei Familien mit autosomal-dominanten Erbgang. *Nervenarzt* 64:331, 1993.

27. Waters CH, Miller CA: Autosomal dominant Lewy body parkinsonism in a four-generation family. *Ann Neurol* 35:59, 1994.

28. Bonifati V, Vanacore N, Meco G: Anticipation of onset age in familial Parkinson's disease. *Neurology* 44:1978, 1994.

29. Wszolek ZK, Pfeiffer B, Fulgham JR, et al: Western Nebraska family (family D) with autosomal dominant parkinsonism. *Neurology* 45:502, 1995.

30. Muenter MD, Forno LS, Hornykiewicz O, et al: Hereditary form of parkinsonism-dementia. *Ann Neurol* 43:768, 1998.

31. Ziegler DK, Schimke RN, Kepes JJ, et al: Late onset ataxia, rigidity, and peripheral neuropathy. A familial syndrome with variable therapeutic response to levodopa. *Arch Neurol* 27:52, 1972.

32. Perry TL, Wright JM, Berry K, et al: Dominantly inherited apathy, central hypoventilation, and Parkinson's syndrome: clinical, biochemical, and neuropathologic studies of 2 new cases. *Neurology* 40:1882, 1990.

33. Perry TL, Bratty PJ, Hansen S, et al: Hereditary mental depression and Parkinsonism with taurine deficiency. *Arch Neurol* 32:108, 1975.

34. Purdy A, Hahn A, Barnett HJ, et al: Familial fatal Parkinsonism with alveolar hypoventilation and mental depression. *Ann Neurol* 6:523, 1979.

35. Tune LE, Folstein M, Rabins P, et al: Familial manic-depressive illness and familial Parkinson's disease: A case report. *Johns Hopkins Med J* 151:65, 1982.

36. Mata M, Dorovini-Zis K, Wilson M, et al: New form of familial Parkinson-dementia syndrome: Clinical and pathologic findings. *Neurology* 33:1439, 1983.

37. Roy M, Boyer L, Barbeau A: A prospective study of 50 cases of familial Parkinson's disease. *Can J Neurol Sci* 10:37, 1983.

38. Barbeau A: Parkinson's disease: Clinical features and etiopathology, in Vinken PJ, Bruyn GW, Klawans HL (eds): *Handbook of Clinical Neurology.* New York: Elsevier Science, 1986, p 87.

39. Barbeau A, Roy M: Familial subsets in idiopathic Parkinson's disease. *Can J Neurol Sci* 11:144, 1984.

40. Barbeau A, Roy M, Boyer L: Genetic studies in Parkinson's disease. *Adv Neurol* 40:333, 1984.

41. Schmitt HP, Emser W, Heimes C: Familial occurrence of amyotrophic lateral sclerosis, parkinsonism, and dementia. *Ann Neurol* 16:642, 1984.

42. Laxova R, Brown ES, Hogan K, et al: An X-linked recessive basal ganglia disorder with mental retardation. *Am J Med Genet* 21:681, 1985.

43. Gregg RG, Metzenberg AB, Hogan K, et al: Waisman syndrome, a human X-linked recessive basal ganglia disorder with mental retardation: Localization to Xq27.3-qter. *Genomics* 9:701, 1991.

44. Spitz MC, Jankovic J, Killian JM: Familial tic disorder, parkinsonism, motor neuron disease, and acanthocytosis: A new syndrome. *Neurology* 35:366, 1985.

45. Nygaard TG, Duvoisin RC: Hereditary dystonia-parkinsonism syndrome of juvenile onset. *Neurology* 36:1424, 1986.

46. Giménez-Roldán S, Mateo D, Escalona-Zapata J: Familial Alzheimer's disease presenting as L-dopa-responsive parkinsonism. *Adv Neurol* 45:431, 1986.

47. Roy EP 3rd, Riggs JE, Martin JD, et al: Familial parkinsonism, apathy, weight loss, and central hypoventilation: Successful long-term management. *Neurology* 38:637, 1988.

48. Inose T, Miyakawa M, Miyakawa K, et al: Clinical and neuropathological study of a familial case of juvenile parkinsonism. *Jpn J Psychiatry Neurol* 42:265, 1988.

49. Degl'Innocenti F, Maurello MT, Marini P: A parkinsonian kindred. *Ital J Neurol Sci* 10:307, 1989.

50. Rosenberg RN, Green JB, White CL 3rd, et al: Dominantly inherited dementia and parkinsonism, with non-Alzheimer amyloid plaques: A new neurogenetic disorder. *Ann Neurol* 25:152, 1989.

51. Ishikawa A, Tanaka K, Koyama A, et al: A patient presenting mainly dystonia in a family with juvenile parkinsonism, in Nagatsu T (ed): *Basic Clinical and Therapeutic Aspects of Alzheimer's and Parkinson's Diseases.* New York: Plenum Press, 1990, pp 227.

52. Sage JI, Miller DC, Golbe LI, et al: Clinically atypical expression of pathologically typical Lewy-body parkinsonism. *Clin Neuropharmacol* 13:36, 1990.

53. Duvoisin RC: The genetics of Parkinson's disease: A review, in Rinne UK, Nagatsu T, Horowski R (eds): *International Workshop Berlin Parkinson's Disease.* The Netherlands: Medicom Europe, 1991, p 38.

54. Takei A, Chiba S, Sato Y, et al: Familial Parkinson's disease and familial manic-depressive illness, in Nagatsu T (ed): *Basic Clinical and Therapeutic Aspects of Alzheimer's and Parkinson's Diseases.* New York: Plenum Press, 1990, p 201.

55. Tanaka H, Ishikawa A, Ginns EI, et al: Linkage analysis of juvenile parkinsonism to tyrosine hydroxylase gene locus on chromosome 11. *Neurology* 41:719, 1991.

56. Lechevalier B, Schupp C, Fallet-Bianco C, et al: [Familial parkinsonian syndrome with athymhormia and hypoventilation]. *Rev Neurol* 148:39, 1992.

57. Wszolek ZK, Pfeiffer RF, Bhatt MH, et al: Rapidly progressive autosomal dominant parkinsonism and dementia with pallido-ponto-nigral degeneration. *Ann Neurol* 32:312, 1992.

58. Wszolek ZK, Pfeiffer RF: Rapidly progressive autosomal dominant parkinsonism and dementia with pallidopontonigral degeneration, in Stern MB, Koller WC (eds): *Parkinsonian Syndromes.* New York: Marcel Dekker, 1993, p 297.

59. Dobyns WB, Ozelius LJ, Kramer PL, et al: Rapid-onset dystonia-parkinsonism. *Neurology* 43:2596, 1993.

60. Bhatia KP, Daniel SE, Marsden CD: Familial parkinsonism with depression: A clinicopathological study. *Ann Neurol* 34:842, 1993.

61. Golbe LI, Lazzarini AM, Schwarz KO, et al: Autosomal dominant parkinsonism with benign course and typical Lewy-body pathology. *Neurology* 43:2222, 1993.

62. Mizutani T, Inose T, Nakajima S, et al: Familial parkinsonism and dementia with "ballooned neurons". *Adv Neurol* 60:613, 1993.

63. Yamamura Y, Arihiro K, Kohriyama T, et al: [Early-onset parkinsonism with diurnal fluctuation: Clinical and pathological studies]. *Rinsho Shinkeigaku* 33:491, 1993.

64. Nisipeanu P, Kuritzky A, Korczyn AD: Familial levodopa-responsive parkinsonian-pyramidal syndrome. *Mov Disord* 9:673, 1994.

65. Lynch T, Sano M, Marder KS, et al: Clinical characteristics of a family with chromosome 17-linked disinhibition-dementia-parkinsonism-amyotrophy complex. *Neurology* 44:1878, 1994.

66. Wilhelmsen KC, Lynch T, Pavlou E, et al: Localization of disinhibition-dementia-parkinsonism-amyotrophy complex to 17q21-22. *Am J Hum Genet* 55:1159, 1994.

67. Sasaki R, Kuzuhara S, Taniguchi A, et al: [A family of parkinsonism in which the clinical feature of constituents varied with the age of onset]. *Rinsho Shinkeigaku* 34:736, 1994.

68. Najim al-Din AS, Wriekat A, Mubaidin A, et al: Pallidopyramidal degeneration, supranuclear upgaze paresis and dementia: Kufor-Rakeb syndrome. *Acta Neurol Scand* 89:347, 1994.

69. Tsuboi Y, Wszolek ZK, Kusuhara T, et al: Japanese family with parkinsonism, depression, weight loss, and central hypoventilation. *Neurology* 58:1025, 2002.

70. Moya G, Miranda-Nieves G, Perez Sotelo M: [A familial case of progressive spinal amyotrophy showing clinically inapparent, histologic manifestations of the pallidum, locus niger, corpus Luysii and fasciculus gracilis]. *Acta Neurol Psychiatr Belg* 69:1002, 1969.

71. Arnould G, Tridon P, Weber M, et al: [Familial form of subacute spinal amyotrophy. Anatomo-clinical study]. *Rev Neurol (Paris)* 126:70, 1972.

72. Finlayson MH, Martin JB: Cerebral lesions in familial amyotrophic lateral sclerosis and dementia. *Acta Neuropathol (Berl)* 26:237, 1973.

73. Alter M, Schaumann B: Hereditary amyotrophic lateral sclerosis. A report of two families. *Eur Neurol* 14:250, 1976.

74. Lee LV, Pascasio FM, Fuentes FD, et al: Torsion dystonia in Panay, Philippines. *Adv Neurol* 14:137, 1976.

75. Kupke KG, Lee LV, Viterbo GH, et al: X-Linked recessive torsion dystonia in the Philippines. *Am J Med Genet* 36:237, 1990.

76. Kupke KG, Lee LV, Muller U: Assignment of the X-linked torsion dystonia gene to Xq21 by linkage analysis. *Neurology* 40:1438, 1990.

77. Lee LV, Kupke KG, Caballar-Gonzaga F, et al: The phenotype of the X-linked dystonia-parkinsonism syndrome. An assessment of 42 cases in the Philippines. *Medicine (Baltimore)* 70:179, 1991.

78. Graeber MB, Muller U: The X-linked dystonia-parkinsonism syndrome (XDP): Clinical and molecular genetic analysis. *Brain Pathol* 2:287, 1992.

79. Kupke KG, Graeber MB, Muller U: Dystonia-parkinsonism syndrome (XDP) locus: Flanking markers in Xq12- q21.1. *Am J Hum Genet* 50:808, 1992.

80. Graeber MB, Kupke KG, Muller U: Delineation of the dystonia-parkinsonism syndrome locus in Xq13. *Proc Natl Acad Sci U S A* 89:8245, 1992.

81. Waters CH, Takahashi H, Wilhelmsen KC, et al: Phenotypic expression of X-linked dystonia-parkinsonism (lubag) in two women. *Neurology* 43:1555, 1993.

82. Waters CH, Faust PL, Powers J, et al: Neuropathology of lubag (X-linked dystonia parkinsonism). *Mov Disord* 8:387, 1993.

83. Muller U, Haberhausen G, Wagner T, et al: DXS106 and DXS559 flank the X-linked dystonia-parkinsonism syndrome locus (DYT3). *Genomics* 23:114, 1994.

84. Allen N, Knopp W: Hereditary parkinsonism-dystonia with sustained control by L-DOPA and anticholinergic medication. *Adv Neurol* 14:201, 1976.

85. Nygaard TG, Marsden CD, Duvoisin RC: Dopa-responsive dystonia. *Adv Neurol* 50:377, 1988.

86. Segawa M, Hosaka A, Miyagawa F, et al: Hereditary progressive dystonia with marked diurnal fluctuation. *Adv Neurol* 14:215, 1976.

87. Segawa M, Ohmi K, Itoh S, et al: Childhood basal ganglia disease with remarkable response to L-dopa, "hereditary basal ganglia disease with marked diurnal fluctuation". *Shinryo* 24:667, 1971.

88. Segawa M, Nomura Y, Kase M: Hereditary progressive dystonia with marked diurnal fluctuation: Clinicopathophysiological identification in reference to juvenile Parkinson's disease. *Adv Neurol* 45:227, 1987.

89. Segawa M, Nomura Y, Kase M: Diurnally fluctuating hereditary progressive dystonia, in Vinken PJ, Bruyn GW, Klawans HL (eds): *Handbook of Clinical Neurology*. New York: Elsevier Science Publishers, 1986, p 529.

90. Segawa M, Nomura Y, Tanaka S, et al: Hereditary progressive dystonia with marked diurnal fluctuation: Consideration on its pathophysiology based on the characteristics of clinical and polysomnographical findings. *Adv Neurol* 50:367, 1988.

91. Ujike H, Nakashima M, Kuroda S, et al: [Two siblings of juvenile Parkinson's disease dystonic type (Yokochi type 3) and hereditary progressive dystonia with marked diurnal fluctuation (Segawa)]. *Rinsho Shinkeigaku* 29:890, 1989.

92. Nygaard TG, Takahashi H, Heiman GA, et al: Long-term treatment response and fluorodopa positron emission tomographic scanning of parkinsonism in a family with dopa-responsive dystonia. *Ann Neurol* 32:603, 1992.

93. Nygaard TG: Dopa-responsive dystonia. Delineation of the clinical syndrome and clues to pathogenesis. *Adv Neurol* 60:577, 1993.

94. Segawa M, Nomura Y: Hereditary progressive dystonia with marked diurnal fluctuation. Pathophysiological importance of the age of onset. *Adv Neurol* 60:568, 1993.

95. Nygaard TG, Wilhelmsen KC, Risch NJ, et al: Linkage mapping of dopa-responsive dystonia (DRD) to chromosome 14q. *Nat Genet* 5:386, 1993.

96. Ichinose H, Ohye T, Takahashi E, et al: Hereditary progressive dystonia with marked diurnal fluctuation caused by mutations in the GTP cyclohydrolase I gene. *Nat Genet* 8:236, 1994.

97. Tanaka H, Endo K, Tsuji S, et al: The gene for hereditary progressive dystonia with marked diurnal fluctuation maps to chromosome 14q. *Ann Neurol* 37:405, 1995.

98. Kim RC, Collins GH, Parisi JE, et al: Familial dementia of adult onset with pathological findings of a "non-specific" nature. *Brain* 104:61, 1981.

99. Khoubesserian P, Davous P, Bianco C, et al: [Familial dementia of the Neumann type (subcortical gliosis)]. *Rev Neurol* 141:706, 1985.

100. Jankovic J, Kirkpatrick JB, Blomquist KA, et al: Late-onset Hallervorden-Spatz disease presenting as familial parkinsonism. *Neurology* 35:227, 1985.

101. Constantinidis J: [A familial syndrome: A combination of Pick's disease and amyotrophic lateral sclerosis]. *Encephale* 13:285, 1987.

102. Bird TD, Lampe TH, Nemens EJ, et al: Familial Alzheimer's disease in American descendants of the Volga Germans: Probable genetic founder effect. *Ann Neurol* 23:25, 1988.

103. Bird TD, Sumi SM, Nemens EJ, et al: Phenotypic heterogeneity in familial Alzheimer's disease: A study of 24 kindreds. *Ann Neurol* 25:12, 1989.

104. Nygaard TG, Trugman JM, de Yebenes JG, et al: Dopa-responsive dystonia: The spectrum of clinical manifestations in a large North American family. *Neurology* 40:66, 1990.

105. Lanska DJ, Currier RD, Cohen M, et al: Familial progressive subcortical gliosis. *Neurology* 44:1633, 1994.

106. Campion D, Brice A, Hannequin D, et al: A large pedigree with early-onset Alzheimer's disease: Clinical, neuropathologic, and genetic characterization. *Neurology* 45:80, 1995.

107. Polymeropoulos MH, Lavedan C, Leroy E, et al: Mutation in the alpha-synuclein gene identified in families with Parkinson's disease. *Science* 276:2045, 1997.

108. Markopoulou K, Wszolek ZK, Pfeiffer RF, et al: Reduced expression of the G209A alpha-synuclein allele in familial Parkinsonism. *Ann Neurol* 46:374, 1999.

109. Kruger R, Kuhn W, Muller T, et al: Ala30Pro mutation in the gene encoding alpha-synuclein in Parkinson's disease. *Nat Genet* 18:106, 1998.

110. Spillantini MG, Schmidt ML, Lee VM, et al: Alpha-synuclein in Lewy bodies [letter]. *Nature* 388:839, 1997.

111. Mezey E, Dehejia A, Harta G, et al: Alpha synuclein in neuro-degenerative disorders: Murderer or accomplice? *Nat Med* 4:755, 1998.

112. Kobayashi H, Krüger R, Markopoulou K, et al: Haploinsufficiency at the α-synuclein gene underlies phenotypic severity in familial Parkinson's disease. *Brain* 126:32, 200.

113. Fisher E, Scambler P: Human haploinsufficiency: One for sorrow, two for joy. *Nat Genet* 7:5, 1994.

114. Cattaneo E, Rigamonti D, Goffredo D, et al: Loss of normal huntingtin function: New developments in Huntington's disease research. *Trends Neurosci* 24:182, 2001.

115. Leroy E, Boyer R, Auburger G, et al: The ubiquitin pathway in Parkinson's disease. *Nature* 395:451, 1998.

116. Maraganore DM, Farrer MJ, Hardy JA, et al: Case-control study of the ubiquitin carboxy-terminal hydrolase L1 gene in Parkinson's disease. *Neurology* 53:1858, 1999.

117. Gasser T, Muller-Myhsok B, Wszolek ZK, et al: A susceptibility locus for Parkinson's disease maps to chromosome 2p13. *Nat Genet* 18:262, 1998.

118. Farrer M, Gwinn-Hardy K, Muenter M, et al: A chromosome 4p haplotype segregating with Parkinson's disease and postural tremor. *Hum Mol Genet* 8:81, 1999.

119. Valente EM, Bentivoglio AR, Dixon PH, et al: Localization of a novel locus for autosomal recessive early-onset parkinsonism, PARK6, on human chromosome 1p35-p36. *Am J Hum Genet* 68:895, 2001.

120. van Duijn CM, Dekker MC, Bonifati V, et al: Park7, a novel locus for autosomal recessive early-onset parkinsonism, on chromosome 1p36. *Am J Hum Genet* 69:629, 2001.

121. Funayama M, Hasegawa K, Kowa H, et al: A new locus for Parkinson's disease (PARK8) maps to chromosome 12p11.2-q13.1. *Ann Neurol* 51:296, 2002.

122. Hicks A, Petursson H, Jonsson T, et al: A susceptibility gene for late-onset idiopathic Parkinson disease successfully mapped. *Am J Hum Genet* 69:200, 2001.

123. Scott WK, Nance MA, Watts RL, et al: Complete genomic screen in Parkinson disease: Evidence for multiple genes. *JAMA* 286:2239, 2001.

124. Martin ER, Scott WK, Nance MA, et al: Association of single-nucleotide polymorphisms of the tau gene with late-onset Parkinson disease. *JAMA* 286:2245, 2001.

125. Foster NL, Wilhelmsen K, Sima AA, et al: Frontotemporal dementia and parkinsonism linked to chromosome 17: A consensus conference. *Ann Neurol* 41:706, 1997.

126. Goedert M, Spillantini MG, Serpell LC, et al: From genetics to pathology: Tau and alpha-synuclein assemblies in neurodegenerative diseases. *Philos Trans R Soc Lond B Biol Sci* 356:213, 2001.

127. Lee VM, Goedert M, Trojanowski JQ: Neurodegenerative tauopathies. *Annu Rev Neurosci* 24:1121, 2001.

128. Poorkaj P, Bird TD, Wijsman E, et al: Tau is a candidate gene for chromosome 17 frontotemporal dementia. *Ann Neurol* 43:815, 1998.

129. Hutton M, Lendon CL, Rizzu P, et al: Association of missense and 5'-splice-site mutations in tau with the inherited dementia FTDP-17. *Nature* 393:702, 1998.

130. Clark LN, Poorkaj P, Wszolek Z, et al: Pathogenic implications of mutations in the tau gene in pallido-ponto-nigral degeneration and related neurodegenerative disorders linked to chromosome 17. *Proc Natl Acad Sci U S A* 95:13103, 1998.

131. Reed LA, Wszolek ZK, Hutton M: Phenotypic correlations in FTDP-17. *Neurobiol Aging* 22:89, 2001.

132. Dumanchin C, Camuzat A, Campion D, et al: Segregation of a missense mutation in the microtubule-associated protein tau gene with familial frontotemporal dementia and parkinsonism. *Hum Mol Genet* 7:1825, 1998.

133. Spillantini MG, Crowther RA, Kamphorst W, et al: Tau pathology in two Dutch families with mutations in the microtubule-binding region of tau. *Am J Pathol* 153:1359, 1998.

134. Spillantini MG, Murrell JR, Goedert M, et al: Mutation in the tau gene in familial multiple system tauopathy with presenile dementia. *Proc Natl Acad Sci U S A* 95:7737, 1998.

135. Bird TD, Nochlin D, Poorkaj P, et al: A clinical pathological comparison of three families with frontotemporal dementia and identical mutations in the tau gene (P301L). *Brain* 122:741, 1999.

136. Bugiani O, Murrell JR, Giaccone G, et al: Frontotemporal dementia and corticobasal degeneration in a family with a P301S mutation in tau. *J Neuropathol Exp Neurol* 58:667, 1999.

137. Delisle MB, Murrell JR, Richardson R, et al: A mutation at codon 279 (N279K) in exon 10 of the tau gene causes a tauopathy with dementia and supranuclear palsy. *Acta Neuropathol (Berl)* 98:62, 1999.

138. D'Souza I, Poorkaj P, Hong M, et al: Missense and silent tau gene mutations cause frontotemporal dementia with parkinsonism-chromosome 17 type, by affecting multiple alternative RNA splicing regulatory elements. *Proc Natl Acad Sci U S A* 96:5598, 1999.

139. Iijima M, Tabira T, Poorkaj P, et al: A distinct familial presenile dementia with a novel missense mutation in the tau gene. *Neuroreport* 10:497, 1999.

140. Goedert M, Spillantini MG, Crowther RA, et al: Tau gene mutation in familial progressive subcortical gliosis. *Nat Med* 5:454, 1999.

141. Houlden H, Baker M, Adamson J, et al: Frequency of tau mutations in three series of non-Alzheimer's degenerative dementia. *Ann Neurol* 46:243, 1999.

142. Murrell JR, Spillantini MG, Zolo P, et al: Tau gene mutation G389R causes a tauopathy with abundant pick body-like inclusions and axonal deposits. *J Neuropathol Exp Neurol* 58:1207, 1999.

143. Nasreddine ZS, Loginov M, Clark LN, et al: From genotype to phenotype: A clinical pathological, and biochemical investigation of frontotemporal dementia and parkinsonism (FTDP-17) caused by the P301L tau mutation. *Ann Neurol* 45:704, 1999.

144. Rizzu P, Van Swieten JC, Joosse M, et al: High prevalence of mutations in the microtubule-associated protein tau in a population study of frontotemporal dementia in the Netherlands. *Am J Hum Genet* 64:414, 1999.

145. Yasuda M, Kawamata T, Komure O, et al: A mutation in the microtubule-associated protein tau in pallido-nigro-luysian degeneration. *Neurology* 53:864, 1999.

146. Mirra SS, Murrell JR, Gearing M, et al: Tau pathology in a family with dementia and a P301L mutation in tau. *J Neuropathol Exp Neurol* 58:335, 1999.

147. Sperfeld AD, Collatz MB, Baier H, et al: FTDP-17: An early-onset phenotype with parkinsonism and epileptic seizures caused by a novel mutation. *Ann Neurol* 46:708, 1999.

148. Spillantini MG, Yoshida H, Rizzini C, et al: A novel tau mutation (N296N) in familial dementia with swollen achromatic neurons and corticobasal inclusion bodies. *Ann Neurol* 48:939, 2000.

149. Arima K, Kowalska A, Hasegawa M, et al: Two brothers with frontotemporal dementia and parkinsonism with an N279K mutation of the tau gene. *Neurology* 54:1787, 2000.

150. Kodama K, Okada S, Iseki E, et al: Familial frontotemporal dementia with a P301L tau mutation in Japan. *J Neurol Sci* 176:57, 2000.

151. Lippa CF, Zhukareva V, Kawarai T, et al: Frontotemporal dementia with novel tau pathology and a Glu342Val tau mutation. *Ann Neurol* 48:850, 2000.

152. Ghetti B, Murrell JR, Zolo P, et al: Progress in hereditary tauopathies: A mutation in the tau gene (G389R) causes a Pick disease-like syndrome. *Ann N Y Acad Sci* 920:52, 2000.

153. Stanford PM, Halliday GM, Brooks WS, et al: Progressive supranuclear palsy pathology caused by a novel silent mutation in exon 10 of the tau gene: Expansion of the disease phenotype caused by tau gene mutations. *Brain* 123:880, 2000.

154. Tanaka R, Kobayashi T, Motoi Y, et al: A case of frontotemporal dementia with tau P301L mutation in the Far East. *J Neurol* 247:705, 2000.

155. Yasuda M, Takamatsu J, D'Souza I, et al: A novel mutation at position +12 in the intron following exon 10 of the tau gene in familial frontotemporal dementia (FTD-Kumamoto). *Ann Neurol* 47:422, 2000.

156. Yasuda M, Yokoyama K, Nakayasu T, et al: A Japanese patient with frontotemporal dementia and parkinsonism by a tau P301S mutation. *Neurology* 55:1224, 2000.

157. Tsuboi Y, Baker M, Hutton M, et al: Families with N279K mutation on the tau gene. Clinical, molecular, genetic and pathological studies. *Neurology* 56(suppl 3):A126, 2001.

158. Rizzini C, Goedert M, Hodges JR, et al: Tau gene mutation K257T causes a tauopathy similar to Pick's disease. *J Neuropathol Exp Neurol* 59:990, 2000.

159. Miyamoto K, Kowalska A, Hasegawa M, et al: Familial frontotemporal dementia and parkinsonism with a novel mutation at an intron 10+11-splice site in the tau gene. *Ann Neurol* 50:117, 2001.

160. Neumann M, Schulz-Schaeffer W, Crowther RA, et al: Pick's disease associated with the novel tau gene mutation K369I. *Ann Neurol* 50:503, 2001.

161. Pastor P, Pastor E, Carnero C, et al: Familial atypical progressive supranuclear palsy associated with homozygosity for the delN296 mutation in the tau gene. *Ann Neurol* 49:263, 2001.

162. Hayashi S, Toyoshima Y, Hasegawa M, et al: Late-onset frontotemporal dementia with a novel exon 1 (Arg5His) tau gene mutation. *Ann Neurol* 51:525, 2002.

163. Janssen JC, Warrington EK, Morris HR, et al: Clinical features of frontotemporal dementia due to the intronic tau 10(+16) mutation. *Neurology* 58:1161, 2002.

164. Lantos PL, Cairns NJ, Khan MN, et al: Neuropathologic variation in frontotemporal dementia due to the intronic tau 10(+16) mutation. *Neurology* 58:1169, 2002.

165. Pickering-Brown SM, Richardson AM, Snowden JS, et al: Inherited frontotemporal dementia in nine British families associated with intronic mutations in the tau gene. *Brain* 125:732, 2002.

166. Rosso SM, van Herpen E, Deelen W, et al: A novel tau mutation, S320F, causes a tauopathy with inclusions similar to those in Pick's disease. *Ann Neurol* 51:373, 2002.

167. Saito Y, Geyer A, Sasaki R, et al: Early-onset, rapidly progressive familial tauopathy with R406W mutation. *Neurology* 58:811, 2002.

168. Tassin J, Durr A, Bonnet AM, et al: Levodopa-responsive dystonia. GTP cyclohydrolase I or parkin mutations? *Brain* 123:1112, 2000.

169. Klein C, Pramstaller PP, Kis B, et al: Parkin deletions in a family with adult-onset, tremor-dominant parkinsonism: Expanding the phenotype. *Ann Neurol* 48:65, 2000.

170. Kramer PL, Mineta M, Klein C, et al: Rapid-onset dystonia-parkinsonism: Linkage to chromosome 19q13. *Ann Neurol* 46:176, 1999.

171. Haberhausen G, Schmitt I, Kohler A, et al: Assignment of the dystonia-parkinsonism syndrome locus, DYT3, to a small region within a 1.8-Mb YAC contig of Xq13.1. *Am J Hum Genet* 57:644, 1995.

172. Gwinn-Hardy K, Chen JY, Liu HC, et al: Spinocerebellar ataxia type 2 with parkinsonism in ethnic Chinese. *Neurology* 55:800, 2000.

173. Gwinn-Hardy K, Singleton A, O'Suilleabhain P, et al: Spinocerebellar ataxia type 3 phenotypically resembling parkinson disease in a black family. *Arch Neurol* 58:296, 2001.

174. Simon DK, Mayeux R, Marder K, et al: Mitochondrial DNA mutations in complex I and tRNA genes in Parkinson's disease. *Neurology* 54:703, 2000.

175. Swerdlow RH, Parks JK, Davis JN 2nd, et al: Matrilineal inheritance of complex I dysfunction in a multigenerational Parkinson's disease family. *Ann Neurol* 44:873, 1998.

176. Shimura H, Hattori N, Kubo S, et al: Familial Parkinson disease gene product, parkin, is a ubiquitin-protein ligase. *Nat Genet* 25:302, 2000.

177. Mizuno Y, Hattori N, Mori H, et al: Parkin and Parkinson's disease. *Curr Opin Neurol* 14:477, 2001.

178. Lucking CB, Durr A, Bonifati V, et al: Association between early-onset Parkinson's disease and mutations in the parkin gene. French Parkinson's Disease Genetics Study Group. *N Engl J Med* 342:1560, 2000.

179. Abbas N, Lucking CB, Ricard S, et al: A wide variety of mutations in the parkin gene are responsible for autosomal recessive parkinsonism in Europe. French Parkinson's Disease Genetics Study Group and the European Consortium on Genetic Susceptibility in Parkinson's Disease. *Hum Mol Genet* 8:567, 1999.

180. Hedrich K, Kann M, Lanthaler AJ, et al: The importance of gene dosage studies: Mutational analysis of the parkin gene in early-onset parkinsonism. *Hum Mol Genet* 10:1649, 2001.

181. Imai Y, Soda M, Takahashi R: Parkin suppresses unfolded protein stress-induced cell death through its E3 ubiquitin-protein ligase activity. *J Biol Chem* 275:35661, 2000.

182. Solano SM, Miller DW, Augood SJ, et al: Expression of alpha-synuclein, parkin, and ubiquitin carboxy-terminal hydrolase L1 mRNA in human brain: Genes associated with familial Parkinson's disease. *Ann Neurol* 47:201, 2000.

183. Lansbury PT, Brice A: Genetics of Parkinson's disease and biochemical studies of implicated gene products. *Curr Opin Genet Dev* 12:299, 2002.

184. Shimura H, Schlossmacher MG, Hattori N, et al: Ubiquitination of a new form of alpha-synuclein by parkin from human brain: Implications for Parkinson's disease. *Science* 293:263, 2001.

Chapter 11

EPIDEMIOLOGY OF PARKINSON'S DISEASE

CONNIE MARRAS and CAROLINE M. TANNER

DIAGNOSTIC CONSIDERATIONS 177
CONSIDERATIONS IN RISK FACTOR ASSESSMENT 178
DISEASE FREQUENCY AND DISTRIBUTION 178
    Incidence 178
    Prevalence 179
    Mortality 179
    Age-Specific Distribution 184
    Gender-Specific Distribution 184
    Race-Specific Distribution 184
    Temporal Trends 185
    Geographic Distribution 185
RISK FACTORS 186
    Methodologic Considerations 186
    Factors Directly Associated with PD 186
    Factors Inversely Associated with PD 189
    Conclusions from Risk Factor Assessment 190
CONCLUSION 190

In the 1950s, Kurland[1] and his colleagues in Rochester, Minnesota, and Gudmundsson[2] in Iceland provided the first community-based estimates of Parkinson's disease (PD) prevalence, finding it to be one of the most common neurodegenerative disorders of the elderly. Epidemiologic investigation plays an important role in health planning, by providing estimates of disease frequency, including regional and temporal variations. This chapter reviews the worldwide incidence and prevalence of PD, and provides the reader with tools for interpreting such studies.

Epidemiology is also a powerful method for investigating disease etiology. Observational studies have revealed numerous factors that are associated, positively or negatively, with the occurrence of PD. These associations include both environmental and genetic factors. Prevailing thought as to whether genetic or environmental factors are more important in causing PD has fluctuated back and forth multiple times since the disease was first described in 1817.[3] The etiology remains unknown, and this may reflect a complex interaction of environmental and genetic factors which combine to cause disease. These factors could also vary from individual to individual or population to population. Epidemiologic studies thus continue to be a cornerstone of our search for the determinant(s) of PD.

Here, we review the associations, both direct and indirect, of PD with demographic and environmental factors. We also consider familial factors, as these have been revealed using observational study designs. First, we emphasize some methodologic considerations important to the interpretation of this rapidly expanding literature.

Diagnostic Considerations

Because there is no antemortem biologic marker for PD, the diagnosis in living subjects is based entirely on the neurologic examination. The cardinal signs of Parkinson's disease (bradykinesia, resting tremor, cogwheel rigidity, and postural reflex impairment) are not unique to PD, but are seen in several possibly related but clinically distinct disorders such as progressive supranuclear palsy, multisystem atrophy, or diffuse Lewy body disease. Particularly early in the course, clinical distinction among these disorders is difficult. The overlap in clinical features between multiple disorders which do not have premortem biological markers creates a challenge for epidemiologic studies. Estimates of disease frequency will vary according to the diagnostic criteria used. For example, a study using the presence of parkinsonism as the only diagnostic criterion for PD will likely include many persons with other disorders. Attempts to discover the determinants of disease will be confounded if samples of "cases" include patients with clinically similar disorders but with different risk factors. Strict diagnostic criteria, therefore, are desirable to ensure homogeneity of a study sample, but often they are difficult to employ, particularly in a retrospective fashion.

While diagnostic criteria are not uniformly applied in contemporary studies of PD, differences in case ascertainment and diagnosis were even greater in the past. These differences may profoundly affect comparisons and study conclusions. Pooled analyses of epidemiologic studies are not likely to be meaningful, due to variations in diagnostic criteria or lack of specific criteria. Studies including secondary cases of parkinsonism, such as postencephalitic, vascular or drug-induced parkinsonism, were common in the past.[4–7] Potential erroneous outcomes include overestimation of disease frequency, loss of power in assessing risk factors, and overestimation of the role of genetics by inclusion of persons with other heritable movement disorders.[8]

Since the diagnosis of PD is dependent entirely on the neurologic history and examination, some subjects may be misclassified despite the use of clear diagnostic criteria. In one series, 20 percent of cases diagnosed in life as having PD had some other diagnosis, usually some form of atypical parkinsonism, at autopsy.[9] Since cases in which the clinical diagnosis is in question are more likely to be referred for autopsy, this rate is likely higher than would be found if all cases could be evaluated pathologically.[10] Nonetheless, these results highlight the possibility that some cases of atypical parkinsonism may be erroneously diagnosed as PD. Inclusion of these cases in risk factor studies may lessen the likelihood that a variable associated with PD can be clearly identified. Also, their inclusion in genetic studies may lead to erroneous conclusions about the contribution of heredity. As PD is a relatively uncommon disorder, and most studies are based on relatively small numbers of cases, the error introduced by misclassification can be significant.

As genetic factors associated with the development of parkinsonism are elucidated, further challenges in classification arise. In recent years, gene mutations associated with classical mendelian inheritance of phenotypes very similar to, and in some cases indistinguishable from, classical PD have been identified.[11–13] In the case of mutations of the gene encoding alpha-synuclein, the associated pathology is consistent with classical PD.[14] However, in patients with mutations of the parkin gene, the characteristic Lewy bodies of Parkinson's disease are not found.[15,16] This creates a challenging problem of classification, as the degree to which this genetically defined subset is distinct from the original clinically defined disorder is unclear. To date, these mutations have been found to be very uncommon causes of PD. Multiple studies of patients with both sporadic and familial PD have failed to find mutations in the alpha-synuclein gene in over 800 patients.[17–23] Studies examining the frequency of parkin gene mutations among patients with PD have demonstrated that it is common only in the very young-onset (younger than 20 years) patients. Only 2 of 64 patients with sporadic PD and onset between ages 30 and 45 had *parkin* mutations.[13] No *parkin* mutations were found in a sample of 118 patients with typical later-onset (over 45 years of age) PD. Twenty-three of these subjects reported a family history suggestive of autosomal-recessive inheritance.[24] Since at least 95 percent of parkinsonism in the community has onset after age 50,[25] *parkin* mutations remain a rare cause of parkinsonism.

Genetic testing is not a routine part of epidemiologic studies examining nongenetic determinants of PD or disease frequency. As the genetic heterogeneity of "PD" is revealed, however, epidemiologic studies can be targeted to specific genetically defined entities, and the epidemiology of PD will become more complex. Environmental factors influencing the penetrance and/or expression of each disorder may be different. Thus, genetic differences between patients may determine susceptibility to individual environmental factors, or may influence clinical features such as age of onset or severity. As our investigations can be targeted to more genetically homogeneous subsets of patients, associations of each subset with environmental or genetic modifying factors which were previously obscured could become evident. Alternatively, if major determinants are environmental and not genetic, studying genetically homogeneous populations would be unnecessary.

Considerations in Risk Factor Assessment

Risk factor assessment can be affected by the diagnostic difficulties mentioned above, additionally by the uncertain length of a presymptomatic period, and by the fact that PD is a disorder of late life. The clinical manifestations of PD may be preceded by a long "latent" stage.[26] The existence of presymptomatic PD is suggested by the finding of reduced striatal fluorodopa uptake consistent with degeneration of nigrostriatal pathways in asymptomatic individuals who later have developed symptoms of PD.[27,28] The finding of Lewy bodies in the brains of persons not known to have clinical evidence of PD during life lends further support. "Incidental Lewy bodies" and clinical Parkinson's disease are both age-related phenomena.[29,30] If these incidental Lewy body cases and asymptomatic striatal dopamine depletion represent subclinical PD, then many persons with the identical pathologic process will be missed using current diagnostic methods in which biological disease markers are lacking. This makes the identification of environmental risk factors difficult for several reasons. An uncertain proportion of exposed but as yet not clinically manifest cases may be "misclassified" as unaffected, reducing the ability to detect associations. Also, a long latent period implies that environmental influences are active in the distant past, and accurate exposure history is more difficult to acquire for more remote events. A latent period of uncertain length makes it impossible to target exposure histories to a specific period, and potential measurement error is further increased.

The inability to obtain accurate risk factor or family histories is further worsened by the fact that PD is a disorder of late life. The identification of familial patterns of disease is difficult if pathologically affected family members die before clinical signs are apparent. Even once families are identified, clinical information and diagnostic accuracy is limited for ancestral generations. Even more scarce is blood and tissue for thorough molecular genetic investigations. In addition to the epidemiologic challenges presented by PD, ascertaining exposures is a difficult task in any setting. These issues will be addressed in the specific sections on risk factors to which they apply.

Despite the challenges outlined in the preceding paragraphs, epidemiologic investigations have added considerably to our understanding of PD and serve as an impetus to future study. These results will be summarized in the remainder of this chapter.

Disease Frequency and Distribution

INCIDENCE

Incidence is the most accurate estimate of disease frequency as it is the measure of the number of new cases occurring in a given time period for a specific location. It is relatively unaffected by factors affecting disease survival. This is particularly important for a slowly progressive disorder such as PD. It is, however, affected by the age and gender distribution of a population from which the sample is derived when considering a disorder whose frequency is age-dependent. Therefore crude total incidence rates must be compared with caution.

Incidence rates are comparable across populations when age-adjusted to a reference population, or when compared within small age strata. Most populations have relatively similar proportions of men and women, but when study methods bias the sample in favor of men or women this must be taken into account when comparing incidence rates across studies. Crude incidence rates of idiopathic PD in studies which consider the entire age range and both sexes range from 4.5 to 19 per 100,000 population per year, reflecting, at least in part, variations in study design such as ascertainment methods, case definition, and age distribution of the sample population.[31–42] More uniform rates (9.7 to 13.8 per 100,000 population per year) are obtained when the results are age-adjusted to a reference population (Table 11-1). Higher values, ranging from 14.8 to 23.8 per 100,000 population per year were obtained in earlier studies which did not distinguish secondary parkinsonism from PD.[4–7] Some studies made the diagnosis of parkinsonism based solely on medical record,[43] and may have included persons with other disorders, such as essential tremor. In fact, a study conducted in Finland found that 201 of 775 patients who carried the diagnosis of PD on the basis of medical records were considered to have essential tremor when examined.[6] Even considering only examination-verified cases consistent with idiopathic PD, estimates of incidence and prevalence can vary significantly by minor alterations in diagnostic criteria.[44]

PREVALENCE

Most persons with PD live many years before death. Consequently, the prevalence of the disease is much higher than incidence. More precise estimates can be obtained with a similar sample size and, because prevalence can be obtained in a cross-sectional fashion without longitudinal observation, it is also easier to obtain. The cases identified in prevalence studies are not necessarily representative of all patients with PD, however, as long-surviving cases are more likely to be identified. Interpretations of observations on disease characteristics or risk factors based on prevalence data must take this into account.

Three approaches have been used to estimate the prevalence of PD. The first method estimates prevalence based on clinic populations, most often at an academic referral center. This technique is inherently inaccurate as social or economic factors may determine who seeks medical care at a given clinical site. In addition there may be an over-representation of midstage disease cases with mildly affected individuals not requiring or seeking care at a referral center and end-stage patients being unable to travel to the clinic. The second approach estimates prevalence from health service records, and is subject to similar biases as the first method, although larger, more diverse clinical populations can be surveyed. In settings where health care is universally available and uniformly delivered, good estimates can be obtained using this method. The third method estimates prevalence based on door-to-door screening of a target population, followed

by a physician examination of screen-positive individuals. This method is the most accurate, but the time and expense involved limit its widespread application.

Crude estimates of PD prevalence have been reported to vary from 18 per 100,000 persons in a Shanghai, China, population survey[45] to 328 per 100,000 in a door-to-door survey of the Parsi community in Bombay, India (a population in which 44 percent of persons are aged 50 years or older).[46] As seen for incidence, a more restricted range is seen when results can be age-adjusted to a reference population (72–258.8, age-adjusted to the 1990 US census; Tables 11-2 through 11-5). Most estimates of overall crude prevalence (males and females, entire age range) fall between 100 and 200 per 100,000 people, although, as might be predicted, the prevalence estimates derived by door-to-door methods are greater than those derived by other methods for comparable populations (see Tables 11-2–11-5).[6,31–34,36,38,41,46–74]

Variations in case ascertainment and diagnostic criteria can only account for some of the variability in disease frequency observed. For example, studies of PD prevalence between the Island of Als and the Faroe Islands, two geographically and genetically distinct areas of Denmark, found a 2-fold higher disease prevalence in the Faroe Islands despite use of the same study methods. Differences in genetic and/or environmental risk factors are suggested.[48] Further study, therefore, would be warranted to examine for unique environmental exposures on the Faroe Islands which may have caused a disease cluster, or to look for differences in allelic frequencies of candidate susceptibility genes between the two populations. Such follow-up studies could give important clues to the determinants of PD.

MORTALITY

In the case of PD, mortality rates are more readily available than other measures of disease frequency (incidence and prevalence); nevertheless, death rates do not accurately reflect the true distribution of disease. The reason is that PD is not a direct cause of death; it is recorded on half or less of the death certificates of known cases.[75,76] Mortality rates are also influenced by variability in diagnostic accuracy, temporal and geographic differences in death statistics reporting, and the age distribution of the source population. Also, reported rates vary depending on whether PD must be noted on the death certificate as an underlying cause of death or can be a contributing cause for inclusion. Nonetheless, mortality rate represents a unique population-based statistic because the information is accrued over long time periods in virtually all communities. Although of limited usefulness for estimating absolute values of disease frequency, comparisons of mortality rates between subgroups of patients and over time may show important trends, when mortality statistics have been collected using similar methods.

In general, higher mortality rates have been reported for the US and Northern Europe.[75,77–86] Mortality rates for PD increase with age in all reports, rising sharply after age 60

TABLE 11-1 Age-Adjusted Total[a] and Age-Specific Incidence of PD per 100,000 Person-Years

Reference	Population Studied	Total Age-Adjusted[a] Incidence (Person-Years of Observation)	<40	40–44	45–49	50–54	55–59	60–64	65–69	70–74	75–79	80–84	≥85
Mayeux et al., 1995[34]	New York City, US	10.4 (639,294)	0				10.7		54.2		132.6		212.8
Kusumi et al., 1996[33]	Yonago City, Japan	11.7 (526,814)	0	0	4.2	2.3	16.7	27.2	51.5	81.1	76.8	113.7	26.0
Fall et al., 1996[32]	Ostergotland County, Sweden	9.7 (85,331)	1.6	3.3			9.0		22.4		59.4	79.5	
Bower et al., 1999[35]	Olmsted County, Minnesota, US	13.8 (1,424,474)		0.44			17.4		52.5		93.1	79.1	
Baldereschi et al., 2000[100]	Italy	NA (12,152)				NA			221	239	353	678	NA
MacDonald et al., 2000[42]	United Kingdom	NA (150,345)		0	20			50	37	222	100	0	.116
Chen et al., 2001[31]	Taiwan	11.3[b] (49,830)	NA	0		18.5			47.4		100.2	0	0

a To 1990 US Census.
b Assumes no cases below age 40.
NA, not available.

180

TABLE 11-2 Age-Adjusted Total[a] and Age-Specific Prevalence of PD per 100,000 in Europe

Reference	Location	Age-Adjusted[a] Prevalence (Denominator)	Age Strata										
			<40	40–44	45–49	50–54	55–59	60–64	65–69	70–74	75–79	80–84	≥85
Marttila and Rinne, 1976[6]	Finland	118.1 (402,988)	0.8	27.8			136.2		503.5	736.1		464.8	
Rosati et al., 1980[39]	Italy	72.1 (1,473,800)	3.3	38.6			204.5		342.1	311.3		82.6	
Sutcliffe et al., 1985[62]	England	102.1 (208,000)	0	3			4.0		277.0	702.0		1136	
Mutch et al., 1986[63]	Scotland	135.1 (151,616)	0	46.6			77.9		254.0	839.6		1925	
Morgante et al., 1992[66b]	Italy	258.8 (24,496)	NA	0			115.6		621.4	1978.3		3055	
Dias et al., 1994[57]	Portugal	112.6 (219,928)	0	0	36			169	652			890	
Tison et al., 1994[67b]	France	NA (3149)			NA			500		400	1800	2200	4800
de Rijk et al., 1995[74b]	Netherlands	NA (6969)			NA			300		1000	3100		4300
Sutcliffe and Meara, 1995[41]	England	107.1 (302,500)	0.6	4	10	76	111	159	343	664	856	1400	1044
Trenkwalder et al., 1995[69b]	Germany	NA (982)			NA	NA					713		
de Rijk et al., 1997[124b]	Europe, 5 countries	NA (17,205)			NA	NA			600	100	2800	3600	3400
Chio et al., 1998[52]	Italy	106.5 (61,830)		0			115.3		288.2	835.1		894.0	
Errea et al., 1999[51]	Spain	128.4 (60,724)	3.3	16.5			100.2		435.6	953.3		892.9	
de Rijk et al., 2000[73b]	Europe, 7 countries	NA (18,506)			NA				600	1000	2400	3000	2580
Schrag et al., 2000[49]	England	131.2 (121,608)	NA	12			109		342	961		1265	

[a] Adjusted to 1990 US Census.
[b] Door-to-door surveys or random sample from population registers.
NA, not available.

TABLE 11-3 Age-Adjusted Total[a] and Age-Specific Prevalence of PD per 100,000 in Asia

Reference	Location	Age-Adjusted[a] Prevalence (Denominator)	<40	40–44	45–49	50–54	55–59	60–64	65–69	70–74	75–79	80–84	≥85
								Age Strata					
Harada et al., 1983[38]	Japan	94.1 (125,291)	4.7	39.9		85.8		245.1		698.4		752.7	
Li et al., 1985[95b]	China	NA (63,195)		NA			92		145		615		
Okada et al., 1990[64]	Japan	76.9 (80,639)	23.2		19.6		63.6		338.6	478.7		335.7	
Wang et al., 1994[97b]	China	NA (2,205)		NA			0		780.0		1750	2500	
Kusumi et al., 1996[33]	Japan	104.7 (132,315)	0		41.84	23.29	71.52	210.01	457.93	669.1	850.48	750.0	
Wang et al., 1996[70]	Taiwan	NA (3915)		NA		273		535		565		1839	
Chen et al., 2001[31]	Taiwan	168 (10,058)[c]	NA		37.8	122.5		546.7		819.7		2197.8	

[a] Adjusted to 1990 US Census.
[b] Door-to-door surveys or random sample from population registers.
[c] Assumes no cases under 40 years of age.
NA, not available.

TABLE 11-4 Age-Adjusted Total[a] and Age-Specific Prevalence of PD per 100,000 in North and South America

Reference	Location	Age-Adjusted[a] Prevalence (Denominator)	<40	40-44	45-49	50-54	55-59	60-64	65-69	70-74	75-79	80-84	≥85
Svensen, 1991[71]	Alberta, Canada	NA (2,400,000)	NA		46.6		77.9	254.0		839.6		1925	
Mayeux et al., 1992[65]	New York, USA	87.0 (179,941)		23		45.7		234.8		525.6		1145	
Mayeux et al., 1995[34]	New York, USA	85.4 (213,302)	1.3				99.3		509.5		1192.9		823.8
Chouza et al., 1996[54b]	Uruguay	NA (4468)	NA			163			270			2703	
Melcon et al., 1997[44b]	Argentina	NA (7765)	NA		0		152.9	636.9		1727.0		3385.4	

[a] Adjusted to 1990 US Census.
[b] Door-to-door survey or random sample from population registers.
NA, not available.

TABLE 11-5 Age-Adjusted Total[a] and Age-Specific Prevalence of PD per 100,000 in New Zealand and Australia

Reference	Location	Age-Adjusted[a] Prevalence (Denominator)	<40	40-44	45-49	50-54	55-59	60-64	65-69	70-74	75-79	80-84	≥85
Caradoc-Davies et al., 1992[58]	New Zealand	109.6 (105,075)			3.7			91.1		476.0		999	1994.6
McCann et al., 1998[72b]	Australia	NA (1207)				414						NA	
Chan et al., 2001[110b]	Australia	NA (527)			NA					3600			

[a] Adjusted to 1990 US Census.
[b] Door-to-door survey or random sample from population registers.
NA, not available.

to rates of 100 per 100,000 or more in those aged 80 or greater at death. Mortality rates, like incidence and prevalence, are slightly higher for men than for women. Reported PD mortality increased from the early 1920s to the 1950s in all countries studied.[87] In subsequent years, rates increased in the older age groups, but were decreased or stable at younger ages at death. Longer survival, fewer cases of postencephalitic parkinsonism, as well as improved ascertainment likely contribute to these trends. Compared with persons without PD, mortality is increased approximately 2-fold after adjusting for age.[88–91]

Examination of mortality rates by state within the US found as much as 2-fold variation from state to state, with a significant south to north increasing gradient, which was particularly evident in whites.[92] Regional variation in mortality from PD has also been reported in other countries.[86,93] If this does not reflect variation in ascertainment or reporting practices for cause of death, then these patterns may provide clues to environmental or other risk factors for PD.

AGE-SPECIFIC DISTRIBUTION

Both the incidence and the prevalence of PD increase with increasing age of the population surveyed (Tables 11-1–11-5). The disease is rare before age 50, and incidence and prevalence increase steadily until approximately the ninth decade for incidence or the tenth decade for prevalence, when rates appear to decline. This apparent decline among the most elderly likely represents an artifact resulting from poor ascertainment and the very few people in these age groups. It may also reflect diagnostic uncertainty separating PD from other types of parkinsonism, particularly in persons with coexisting dementia.[8]

GENDER-SPECIFIC DISTRIBUTION

In most studies, PD appears to be slightly more common in men than in women.[6,37–40,46,58,59,62–65,71,94–97] Most dramatic is the finding of a more than 3-fold increased prevalence in men compared to women in China.[98] More typically, prevalence rates in men are elevated, but less than twice the rates in women. The observed male preponderance is less robust than the association with increasing age, and there is some variability across studies. The male preponderance is consistent in incidence studies and across the age range,[34–36,99,100] with only one exception.[33] Therefore, the association does not appear to be due to differences in survival or in the underlying age composition of the populations sampled. However, differences in access to health care, diagnostic practices or attitudes toward seeking health care may contribute to this apparent increased risk of PD for men.

RACE-SPECIFIC DISTRIBUTION

The prevalence of PD appears to vary internationally (Tables 11-2–11-5). The differences in disease frequency may reflect variations in risk determined by the genetic composition of the populations surveyed, and/or exposure to environmental risk factors. Alternatively, differences in study methods, diagnostic patterns or survival with disease may account for the differences. Caucasians in Europe and North America are usually reported to have a higher prevalence, while rates are intermediate for Orientals in Japan and China and lowest for blacks in Africa. These data have been interpreted as an indication that whites have a higher risk for PD. However, more recent studies from Asia do not show striking differences in disease prevalence compared with studies in Caucasians (Tables 11-2–11-5). Whether this reflects an actual change in the frequency of disease, improved survival with disease or improved identification of cases is not known. As shown in Table 11-6, several hospital-based studies conducted in the US and Africa found lower rates of PD in blacks.[101–105] These observations are subject to biases, including those resulting from differences in utilization of health care, differences in perception of disease, and differences in survival. In support of the importance of such factors, a more recent study of PD frequency in New York City found similar *incidence* rates across white, black and Hispanic patients despite significantly lower prevalence in blacks.[34]

Estimates of prevalence vary so widely, even within ethnically similar populations, that any conclusions regarding a racial (or genetic) basis to differences in PD prevalence across studies should be made with caution. For example, Chio et al. compared age- and sex-adjusted prevalence figures derived from nine Italian studies and found a 2-fold variation in prevalence rates. Methodologic differences between studies may account for some of the variation.[106] However, insight into the relative importance of

TABLE 11-6 Crude Prevalence of PD Based on Race and Gender: Hospital-Based Surveys

Location	Prevalence (per 100,000)		
	Men	Women	Total
Johannesburg, South Africa[101]			
Whites			159
Blacks			4
Baltimore, US[102]			
Whites	128	121	
Blacks	31	9	
Mississippi, US[103]			
Whites			159
Blacks			103
New Orleans, US[104]			
Whites			146
Blacks			22
Harare, Zimbabwe[105]			
Whites			94
Blacks			21

genetic and environmental factors can be obtained by comparing disease frequency in genetically similar populations separated geographically, being careful to use comparable sampling methods. Such studies suggest a stronger environmental than genetic contribution to variations in disease frequency by race. For example, using the same case ascertainment methods and with standardized training, Schoenberg et al. demonstrated a 5-fold greater age-standardized prevalence among African-Americans in Copiah County, Mississippi, than in Ibadan, Nigeria.[107] This is in keeping with the similar prevalence of PD between whites and African-American blacks found in their door-to-door survey in Copiah County, Mississippi.[96] The same pattern of findings is seen in a study by Morens et al., who found an incidence of PD in a cohort of Japanese-American men[88] more in keeping with other American frequency studies than Asian studies. This pattern would suggest that racial differences are due to environmental factors affecting incidence or survival.

In contrast, a prevalence study simultaneously comparing Bulgarian gypsies to Bulgarian Caucasians and using more intensive methods to ascertain gypsy PD cases found a considerably lower prevalence of PD in gypsies (16.2 versus 136.7), albeit with wide confidence intervals.[50] Gypsies are thought to be of North Indian descent, with genetic background closer to Asians than to Europeans. This is consistent with a genetic origin to racial differences in prevalence estimates, as the two groups had no identified differences in environmental exposures; however, it is impossible to be certain that all relevant exposures were considered. Apparently contradictory results regarding the influence of race on the distribution of disease could reflect variable contributions of genetic and environmental factors in determining the occurrence of PD across different ethnic groups. The clarification of the true differences in disease risk associated with race require confirmation in prospective incidence studies in racially diverse populations, similar to the studies conducted in New York City[34] or in Northern California.[108] Ideally, these would be conducted using survey methods that identify all members of a population, such as door-to-door survey, to minimize bias due to healthcare-related factors and obtain more accurate estimates of disease frequency. It must be recognized, however, that the resources needed for such intensive ascertainment restrict investigations to the study of small populations. This limits the precision of the estimates that can be obtained.

TEMPORAL TRENDS

Whether the incidence of PD has changed since 1817 is unknown due to the paucity of longitudinal data. In general, studies show slightly increasing or stable incidence and prevalence over time. PD incidence was studied in Olmsted County, Minnesota, during the period 1935–1988.[109] To minimize variability resulting from differences in diagnostic criteria over time, all cases were classified by a single neurologist using existing diagnostic criteria. Estimated incidence increased from 9.2 per 100,000 annually for the interval 1935–1944 to 16.3 per 100,000 for the interval 1975–1984. More recently, a comparison of age-adjusted prevalence rates in Finland between 1971 and 1992 using comparable methods showed an increased overall prevalence (139 to 166) which was entirely accounted for by a significant increase in the prevalence among men (138 to 228). Incidence rates followed the same trends.[36] In a door-to-door survey in Australia, at least a 42.5 percent higher prevalence estimated in 2001 compared to a 1966 survey, when methodologic differences between the studies were taken into account.[110] Using comparable methods based on identification of cases through general practitioners in Northampton, England, a moderate increase in prevalence (108 to 121 per 100,000) was found between 1982 and 1990.[41] These results could be attributed to changing awareness of the symptoms of PD, changing attitudes toward making a diagnosis of the disorder, as well as evolving diagnostic criteria. In contrast, other studies have shown stable disease frequency. A prospective cohort study of Japanese-American men in Hawaii found no significant trends in prevalence at three time points between 1982 and 1992. Another study comparing prevalence and incidence in Yonago City, Japan, between 1980 and 1992 found stable disease frequency.[33] Similarly, using health service records, the incidence of PD was found to be relatively stable over 15 years in Minnesota.[99] It is possible that the time intervals considered are too short to reasonably expect changes in disease frequency, particularly the prevalence of a disorder of relatively long duration such as PD. In a meta-analysis using age- and gender-adjustment for comparison purposes, Zhang and Roman found no significant temporal fluctuations in the incidence and prevalence in Europe and the US over the past 50 years.[111] Yet, because the studies included employed a broad range of methods and diagnostic criteria, many including atypical cases or postencephalitic cases, conclusions drawn from this analysis may be misleading. Whether or not the incidence and prevalence of PD is increasing or stable is not clear.

GEOGRAPHIC DISTRIBUTION

The reported rates of PD show marked geographic variation. For comparison, Zhang and Roman adjusted reported rates to the 1970 US population.[111] Age-adjusted incidence rates varied worldwide from 1.9 per 100,000 in China to 22.1 per 100,000 in Rochester, Minnesota. Age-adjusted prevalence ranged from 18 per 100,000 in China to 234 per 100,000 in Montevideo, Uruguay. Similar variation is seen in the age-adjusted prevalence rates of Tables 11-2–11-5. Even within the same country, epidemiologic studies have documented significant regional variation in the mortality[86,92,93] and prevalence[48] rates of patients with PD. In the US, for example, higher mortality rates with increasing latitude has been suggested.[92] Any of the reported differences in PD frequency could be artifacts of differences in study design, including diagnostic criteria and case ascertainment. Socioeconomic factors likely have a greater impact on the estimated prevalence than on the incidence of PD. Lower prevalence rates may simply reflect poor socioeconomic conditions and consequently shortened survival. Since most reported rates are of prevalence, rather than incidence, this qualification is important. However, if these differences represent true variations in disease frequency, they likely reflect differences in the distribution of genetic and environmental risk factors for PD between the populations studied. Identification of these would provide important direction for clinical and basic scientists investigating PD etiology.

Risk Factors

METHODOLOGIC CONSIDERATIONS

Many studies have investigated factors associated with the occurrence of PD, and numerous environmental exposures, behavioral factors, and demographic factors have been identified as being directly or indirectly associated with the disease. Those directly associated may be related to the cause of PD, while those inversely associated could be protective factors. These studies are invaluable for the clues to disease etiology that they provide; however, there are limitations to the conclusions that can be drawn from them. The vast majority of these studies have been case-control studies collecting retrospective information on exposures, often over the lifetime of the participants. This method generates a measure of association between an exposure and disease, but causality cannot be proven.

Retrospective studies are limited by uncertainty and bias in measurement due to several factors. Because of the retrospective nature of the data collection it is not always clear that the exposure preceded the onset of the disease. Even when the proper temporal relationship seems obvious, such as a childhood exposure and late-life onset of symptoms, or in a prospective study of disease incidence, the suspected presymptomatic period is of unknown duration (as discussed earlier), making it impossible to know whether or not an exposure has predated the beginning of the pathological process. The retrospective nature of the data collection also makes the exposure difficult to confirm. This is particularly true for a late-life disorder when the timing of the determining events is unknown. Early life exposures can rarely be verified. Even most midlife exposures are obtained by self-report, and are rarely confirmed by written records or biological assays such as blood tests for environmentally persistent chemicals or metals. Case-control studies are susceptible to recall bias, where affected individuals are more likely to think about and recall unusual exposures than controls as they search themselves for reasons that they have PD. This potential bias is particularly important when the exposures cannot be objectively confirmed. It is also important to remember that case-control studies of PD most often sample prevalent cases, which are only a subset of the population of interest. Also of interest are those already deceased with PD and those who were destined to develop disease. Therefore, these studies may be detecting factors associated with long survival with disease, or early onset of disease. Lastly, in observational studies, there is no way to distinguish the influential evironmental factor from among several that are usually found together. An example of this is rural living and well-water consumption, or the many chemicals found in cigarette smoke. For all of these reasons, complementary investigations to support causality must be performed. This includes collaboration with basic scientists to confirm biological plausibility, looking for dose-response relationships between exposure and disease frequency or severity, and consistency of association across studies.

FACTORS DIRECTLY ASSOCIATED WITH PD

DEMOGRAPHIC FACTORS

Increasing age is the factor most consistently associated with an increased risk of PD (Tables 11-1–11-5). When considered as a clue to the cause of PD, this association may reflect age-related neuronal vulnerability. However, other time-dependent factors such as duration of exposure to a toxicant or the accumulation of a genetically determined biologic defect cannot easily be separated from age-related changes. Overall, men appear to be at slightly greater risk (about 1.5 times) of developing PD than women (see section on gender-specific distribution). Whether these reported differences reflect differences in ascertainment, inherent biologic differences in susceptibility, or gender-associated behavioral differences resulting in greater toxicant exposures is unknown.

FAMILIAL FACTORS

Epidemiologic studies of familial patterns of disease can provide valuable clues to the importance of genetic factors to PD. It must be remembered, however, that, since families also share behaviors and environments, familial clustering may sometimes have nongenetic causes. Multiple case-control studies have implicated a genetic component to PD by finding that cases more frequently have affected family members than controls (Table 11-7). The odds ratio for PD associated with having a family member affected with the disease versus not has ranged from 3.5 to 14.6 using patients identified at specialty clinics.[112–120] Community-based studies have also shown an increased risk, but of lower magnitude (odds ratios 2.3–3.7).[121–123] In a single prospective community-based study, the relative risk of developing PD over a mean follow-up time of 2 years was 2.5 in those with an affected first-degree relative compared with those without. Among persons with at least two affected relatives, the relative risk was 10.4, although the confidence interval was wide (1.2–89.2).[124]

The population of Iceland provides a unique means for investigating the role of genetics in PD because of their

TABLE 11-7 Risk of PD Associated with a Family History of Disease: Case-Control Studies

Study	Cases/Controls	Odds Ratio (95% Confidence Interval)	Study Population Characteristics
Semchuck et al., 1993[122]	130/260	2.4 (1.03, 5.4)[b] 3.7 (1.7, 7.9)[c]	Population-based
Morano et al., 1994[112]	74/148	3.9 (1.3, 11.6)	Movement disorders clinic
Payami et al., 1994[114]	114/114	3.5 (1.3, 9.4)[b]	Movement disorders clinic
Bonifati et al., 1995[113]	100/100	4.9 (2.0, 11.9)[a]	Movement disorders clinic
Vieregge et al., 1995[115]	66/72	7.1 (0.35, 25.2)[c]	Movement disorders clinic
Marder et al., 1996[121]	233/1172	2.3 (1.3, 4.0)[b]	Population-based
De Michele et al., 1996[116]	116/232	14.6 (7.2, 29.6)[a]	Movement disorders clinic
Elbaz et al., 1999[123]	175/481	3.2 (1.6–6.6)[b]	Population-based
Taylor et al., 1999[118]	140/147	3.9 (1.7, 8.9)[a]	Movement disorders clinic
Werneck and Alvarenga, 1999[119]	92/110	14.5 (2.98, 91.38)[a]	Hospital neurology clinic
Preux et al., 2000[120]	140/280	10.1 (2.9–35.0)[b]	Hospital clinic
Autere et al., 2000[117]	268/210	2.9 (1.3–6.4)[b]	Hospital neurology clinic

[a] Any relative.
[b] First-degree relatives.
[c] First- and second-degree relatives.

longstanding database of genealogic information in a relatively genetically and environmentally isolated population. After identifying 772 living and dead persons with parkinsonism over the preceding 50 years, genealogic information over 11 centuries was used to determine relatedness of those with parkinsonism and a control group.[125] PD cases were more closely related than the controls, and PD risk was increased most in siblings, less so in offspring. This pattern supports a role for a common early environmental factor or, alternatively, recessively inherited modifying genes. Analysis of familial patterns of PD in Finland, a similarly isolated population, also concluded that genetic factors were important in the pathogenesis of the disease, more so in early-onset disease, and that contributing genetic factors were likely to be heterogeneous.[126] One of the significant limitations of studies in such isolated populations is uncertain generalizability. If susceptibility to PD is determined by a combination of genetic and environmental factors, then genetic risk factors identified in a genetically isolated population may not be relevant to other populations.

A genetic contribution to PD is also suggested by the discovery of families with parkinsonism inherited in an autosomal-dominant or autosomal-recessive pattern. The clinical or pathological features of at least some of the cases in most of these families are not fully consistent with those of typical PD. However, in many individual cases the disorder is indistinguishable from idiopathic PD. Genetic linkage analysis has revealed causative mutations in only a few of the families, and these mutations have been found to be rare causes of PD. The pathologic mechanisms of these mutations may provide important avenues of research, however.

Twin studies have also been used to test the hypothesis of a genetic contribution to the etiology of PD, with their results failing to support a major effect. Intra-pair concordance rates should be much higher in monozygotic (MZ) twins than in dizygotic (DZ) twins if a genetic factor is an important causative component of PD. Twin studies have shown similar rates of concordance in MZ and DZ twin pairs.[127–132] The overall similarity in concordance in MZ and DZ pairs is not consistent with a significant genetic contribution to PD. Yet, in a late life disorder with a potentially long presymptomatic period it is possible that a cross-sectional study underestimates twin concordance by failure to identify presymptomatic individuals and individuals that have already died but were destined to manifest the disease. Discrepancies of up to 28 years in age of onset between MZ twins has been reported.[132] In a small number of twin pairs discordant for PD clinically, many of the asymptomatic co-twins had significantly decreased putamenal ^{18}F-dopa uptake measured by positron emission tomography,[133,134] suggesting concordance for dopamine system deficits. Additionally, a pattern of higher dopamine deficit concordance in MZ than DZ twin pairs has been found in one study.[28] Longitudinal clinical follow-up in such cohorts will be important to confirm the relevance of such findings. One twin study found that concordance rates were much higher when symptoms began before the age of 50.[132] This has suggested that the importance of genetic factors is not uniform across the age range, and that, in the less common young-onset parkinsonism, genetic factors appear to be primary.

Associations between PD and other diseases can give clues to common pathogenesis. A family history of essential tremor has also been found to be more common in patients with PD than in controls.[116,118] This observation is also susceptible to bias in that persons with PD are likely to be particularly observant of tremor in others. If there truly is a positive association between PD and essential tremor, it suggests shared determinants between the two diseases.

CHEMICAL EXPOSURE

Following the description of a cluster of toxicant-induced parkinsonism strikingly similar to PD,[135] interest in an environmental cause of PD burgeoned. The responsible compound, the pyridine 1-methyl-4-phenyl-1,2,3,6-tetrahydropyridine (MPTP), induces clinical, pathological, and biochemical changes in humans and primates remarkably like those of PD.[136–138] While MPTP is unlikely to be environmentally present in sufficient quantities to cause most cases of PD, chemically similar compounds more commonly present might theoretically be causative. For example, the herbicide paraquat is a structural analogue of MPTP, and the pesticide rotenone shares with MPTP the common function of inhibiting mitochondrial complex 1. In rats, chronic exposure to rotenone results in a progressive nigral lesion,[139] and paraquat depletes dopamine in frogs.[140] Such observations complement epidemiologic studies of associations between pesticides and PD.

Multiple case-control studies have investigated the association between pesticide exposure and PD. Most have found positive associations. A meta-analysis of 19 such studies from North America, Europe and Asia until 1999 found a combined odds ratio of 1.94 (95% confidence interval, CI, 1.49–2.53) for PD in the presence of a positive history of pesticide exposure.[141] Across studies, a dose-response relationship was also suggested. A population-based study of PD mortality found a significantly higher rate in California counties using pesticides than in counties with negligible pesticide use.[142] To date, most studies have investigated occupational pesticide use; however, one study has also implicated home pesticide and herbicide use (odds ratio 1.9, 95% CI 1.3–2.9).[143] It is interesting that rural living, drinking well-water, and farming have also been identified as associated with the occurrence of PD in multiple studies.[144] It is possible that these findings represent co-occurrence with pesticide exposure or other as yet unidentified pathogenic factors.

Most epidemiological studies have not investigated associations between individual agents or even classes of agents and PD. Pesticides have different, often poorly defined, mechanisms of toxicity and it is not clear which mechanisms are relevant to PD. If there truly is a causative association between some pesticides or herbicides and PD, then the odds ratios reported thus far are likely an underestimation of the effect of the pathogenic agent(s). Among the classes or agents that have been studied, organochlorines,[145] alkylated phosphate,[145] carbamates,[145,146] paraquat,[147] and dieldrin[148] have been implicated as increasing the risk for PD. Despite the consistency of the association with pesticide exposure and the supporting laboratory evidence, case-control studies are still unable to unequivocally demonstrate causality, for the reasons discussed above. The findings to date await replication in unselected, prospectively followed cohorts. Once specific agents are identified, further investigation in the laboratory will be essential to identifying mechanisms of injury.

Pesticides are not the only chemicals to be implicated. Studies have detected positive associations between PD and history of exposure to "any chemicals,"[119,149] industrial exposure,[150,151] solvents,[145,149] wood preservatives,[145] glues, paints or lacquers,[145] carbon monoxide,[145] and general anesthesia.[145] Most of these observations await confirmation in other studies and the associations remain tentative at present.

METAL EXPOSURE

Exposure to metals has been investigated as a risk factor for PD, prompted in part by the long-known ability of manganese toxicity to produce parkinsonism,[152] the finding of elevated iron levels in the substantia nigra of patients with PD,[153] and epidemiologic associations between industrial activities involving metal exposure and elevated rates of PD.[151,154] The results of studies of specific metal exposure have been inconsistent,[155] although some studies have suggested a positive association between manganese and mercury exposure.[155] Variations in methods of determining exposure status, as well as frequency and levels of exposure in the population studied, may contribute to the inconsistencies. For example, in one case-control study, positive associations with multiple exposures elicited by subjective assessment could not be confirmed by a more objective job exposure matrix method.[145] This could be because subjective assessments are prone to recall bias. On the other hand, job exposure matrices are unable to individualize exposure assessment beyond that usual for the stated occupation, so such assessments tend to be imprecise, even though more objective. Further complicating the study of risk factors is the finding that certain exposure combinations may be associated with increased risk, yet each single exposure at similar levels is not. This may be the case for exposure to combinations of lead-copper, lead-iron, and iron-copper.[155] Similarly, the combination of maneb and paraquat causes more injury in animals than either agent alone.[156]

DIETARY FACTORS

A number of foods and nutrients have been investigated for their association, both direct and indirect, with PD. Increased risk with total fat,[157,158] in particular animal fat,[158,159] has been found in several studies. This has been hypothesized to be due to oxidative stress, as lipids are a source of oxygen radicals through peroxidation. Other dietary factors have not yet been consistently associated with PD. The imprecise nature of estimating food intake over long periods (as in the period before the onset of PD) makes the accurate study of dietary risk factors very difficult. The challenges are compounded by the fact that any one of a number of components of each food may be the factor of interest.

OTHER POTENTIAL RISK FACTORS

Because infection (probably viral) resulted in an epidemic of parkinsonism following encephalitis early in this century, the belief that PD was the result of infection persisted for decades, despite the clear differences clinically and pathologically in the postencephalitic disease and PD.[160] While an infectious agent has never been identified in PD,[161–165] and the insidious onset and slowly progressive course make traditional agents unlikely, the ubiquitous soil pathogen *Nocardia asteroides* has been reported to cause a nigral lesion in animals and has been proposed as a cause of PD.[166] Evidence supporting this hypothesis was not found in a serological study in humans.[167] An inverse association between childhood measles infection and PD has been found in one study.[168] Whether this finding represents a protective effect, an adverse effect of previous measles infection in adulthood causing reduced survival or reduced recognition of PD, or an association between measles and another factor cannot be determined from the present data.

Several factors related to life experience or behavioral factors have been associated with the occurrence of PD. Emotional stress, which may cause increased dopamine turnover resulting in increased risk of oxidative nerve cell death,[169,170] has been associated with an increased disease risk in two studies of persons surviving extreme emotional and physical hardship.[171–173] A positive association with head trauma has been reported in several studies,[116,118,119,145,149,174] and heavy physical work has also been implicated.[175]

A particular personality type has been identified as more common before the onset of PD than among controls in multiple studies, including twin studies.[176] The features of this personality include shyness, cautiousness, inflexibility, punctuality, and depressiveness. Whether this represents the earliest feature of the neurochemical changes of PD, or an association between such a personality and causative environmental exposures or genetic factors, is not known.

Various occupational risk factors have also been proposed. The types of work identified are diverse, and a common underlying factor is not obvious. Among the occupations associated with increased risk in at least one study are construction work,[177] working in healthcare,[178] occupation in social sciences, law and library,[178] teaching,[178] carpentry,[179] and cleaning.[179] As with many other proposed risk factors, the associations await confirmation in other studies. Regarding clues to etiology that these associations provide, exposures inherent in the type of work must be considered. It is also possible, however, that certain occupations are chosen based upon suitability to the personality type that is associated with PD. Therefore, not all occupational associations may represent clues to etiology.

Putative risk factors for PD lead to important hypotheses regarding disease etiology and pathophysiology, which may launch large efforts of investigation by basic and clinical researchers. With the numerous associations that have been observed, it is important to find ways to focus attention for further investigation on those most likely to be genuine and relevant. Thus, attention to biological plausibility, dose-response relationships, and consistency of association are important considerations.

FACTORS INVERSELY ASSOCIATED WITH PD

CIGARETTE SMOKING

The inverse association between cigarette smoking and PD, a long-standing puzzle, has been reported in the majority of case-control studies.[116,118–120,145,147,149,175,177,179–193] Twin studies also support this inverse association. Cigarette smoking was less frequent in the affected twins of discordant MZ twin pairs in three studies.[194,195] MZ twins are particularly powerful for investigating environmental factors as genetic factors influencing disease occurrence are eliminated. When twins have lived together much of their lives many environmental factors are controlled as well.

A dose-response relationship has been confirmed in a large prospective study,[196] and a case-control study.[197] The relationship may be age-dependent, with a much greater inverse association in younger-onset cases.[192] In addition, an interaction between smoking status (in pack-years) and monoamine oxidase B (MAO-B) genotype has been found in one study. The inverse relationship between smoking and the occurrence of PD was smaller for those with the G allele of the dopamine-metabolizing enzyme MAO-B than for those with the A allele. Observing such interactions may provide clues to the mechanisms by which cigarette smoking and PD are related; however, the significance of the inverse association still remains elusive.

Earlier mortality in smokers (thus dying before manifesting PD) has been proposed as an explanation for the observed inverse association. However, a large cohort study demonstrated a reduced incidence of PD in cigarette smokers even at young ages when mortality from any cause is low, and found insufficient mortality differences between smokers and nonsmokers to account for the reduction in incident PD cases.[198] Direct protective effects of nicotine may contribute,[199,200] or nicotine or other components of cigarette smoke may induce xenobiotic metabolizing enzymes, enabling more rapid detoxification of a parkinsonism-causing toxicant.[201,202] Alternatively, the so-called "parkinsonian personality," which is proposed to be a reflection of an underlying dopamine deficiency, may result in the avoidance of novelty seeking behaviors such as smoking,[203] or in a lack of propensity for addiction.

COFFEE CONSUMPTION AND OTHER DIETARY FACTORS

A lack of propensity for addiction in people with PD is also suggested by the finding of an inverse relationship between coffee consumption and PD, independent of smoking status. This relationship has now been seen in two prospective cohorts and three case-control studies.[179,204–207] This relationship does not appear to extend to decaffeinated coffee, and extends to caffeine from noncoffee sources, suggesting that caffeine is the determining factor in the relationship.[205,206]

An inverse association between PD and the amount of antioxidants consumed in the diet, including vitamin E, has been a topic of particular interest among dietary factors. Such an association would support a role for oxidative stress in the degeneration of nigral neurons, and has potential implications for disease prevention. Several case-control studies have suggested an inverse association, but most recent studies have not supported this.[157,158,208–214] To date, coffee consumption, likely reflecting caffeine intake, is the only dietary factor consistently inversely associated with PD.

CONCLUSIONS FROM RISK FACTOR ASSESSMENT

In summary, among environmental factors, exposure to pesticides as a risk factor, and cigarette smoking and caffeine consumption as factors associated with decreased risk, have the most support in the literature thus far. There is also support for the role of genetic factors in determining susceptibility to PD, as the presence of disease in a family member has also been consistently found to be a risk factor. The role of genetic susceptibility in PD is a rapidly expanding field, and genetic factors may modify the effect of environmental and demographic factors on the risk of disease. Such interactions represent an additional challenge to understanding the various contributions to the cause of PD. The roles of specific genes in the susceptibility to PD are discussed in Chapter 10.

Conclusion

Epidemiologic investigations of the patterns of disease occurrence have given many clues to the cause(s) of PD. Multiple associations with genetic and environmental factors have been identified, and various studies have also suggested interactions between the environment and genes in the process leading to PD. The challenge over the coming years will be to discern which associations are etiologically relevant. This will involve important reciprocal communication between clinical and basic scientists. The biological plausibility of associations identified through epidemiologic studies can be tested in the laboratory. Contributions from basic science about mechanisms of toxicity of compounds or insights from animal models can guide future epidemiologic studies to confirm relevance to human disease. Such collaboration will be essential given the evolving picture of multiple contributing factors to the cause of PD.

References

1. Kurland L: Epidemiology: Incidence, geographic distribution and genetic considerations, in Field W (ed): *Pathogenesis and Treatment of Parkinsonism*. Springfield: Charles C Thomas, 1958.
2. Gudmundsson K: A clinical survey of parkinsonism in Iceland. *Acta Neurol Scand* 43:1–61, 1967.
3. Parkinson J. *An Essay on the Shaking Palsy*. London: Sherwood, Neeley, and Jones, 1817.
4. Kurland LT. Epidemiology: Incidence, geographic distribution and genetic considerations, in Fields WS (ed): *Pathogenesis and Treatment of Parkinsonism*. Springfield: Charles C Thomas, 1958, pp 5–43.
5. Gudmundsson KR: A clinical survey of parkinsonism in Iceland. *Acta Neurol Scand* 33:9–61, 1967.
6. Marttila RJ, Rinne UK: Epidemiology of Parkinson's disease in Finland. *Acta Neurol Scand* 53:81–102, 1976.
7. Rajput AH, Offord KP, Beard CM, Kurland LT: Epidemiology of parkinsonism: Incidence, classification and mortality. *Ann Neurol* 16:278–282, 1984.
8. Bower JH, Maraganore DM, McDonnell SK, Rocca WA: Influence of strict, intermediate, and broad diagnostic criteria on the age- and sex-specific incidence of Parkinson's disease. *Mov Disord* 15:819–825, 2000.
9. Hughes AJ, Daniel SE, Kilford L, Lees AJ: Accuracy of clinical diagnosis of idiopathic Parkinson's disease: A clinicopathological study of 100 cases. *J Neurol Neurosurg Psychiatry* 55:181–184, 1992.
10. Maraganore D, Anderson D, Bower H, et al: Autopsy patterns for Parkinson's disease and related disorders in Olmsted County, Minnesota. *Neurology* 53:1342–1344, 1999.
11. Polymeropoulos M, Lavedan C, Leroy E, et al: Mutation in the α-synuclein gene identified in families with Parkinson's disease. *Science* 276:2045–2047, 1997.
12. Kitada T, Asakawa S, Hattori N, et al: Mutations in the parkin gene cause autosomal recessive juvenile parkinsonism. *Nature* 392:605–608, 1998.
13. Lucking CB, Durr A, Bonifati V, et al: Association between early-onset Parkinson's disease and mutations in the parkin gene. French Parkinson's Disease Genetics Study Group. *N Engl J Med* 342:1560–1567, 2000.
14. Langston JW, Sastry S, Chan P, et al: Novel alpha-synuclein-immunoreactive proteins in brain samples from the Contursi kindred, Parkinson's, and Alzheimer's disease. *Exp Neurol* 154:684–690, 1998.
15. Yamamura Y, Hattori N, Matsumine H, et al: Autosomal recessive early-onset parkinsonism with diurnal fluctuation: Clinicopathologic characteristics and molecular genetic identification. *Brain Dev* 22(suppl 1):S87–91, 2000.
16. Takahashi H, Ohama E, Suzuki S, et al: Familial juvenile parkinsonism: Clinical and pathologic study in a family. *Neurology* 44:437–441, 1994.
17. Farrer M, Destee T, Becquet E, et al: Linkage exclusion in French families with probable Parkinson's disease. *Mov Disord* 15:1075–1083, 2000.
18. Farrer M, Wavrant-De Vrieze F, Crook R, et al: Low frequency of alpha-synuclein mutations in familial Parkinson's disease. *Ann Neurol* 43:394–397, 1998.
19. Vaughan J, Durr A, Tassin J, et al: The alpha-synuclein Ala53Thr mutation is not a common cause of familial Parkinson's disease: A study of 230 European cases. European Consortium on Genetic Susceptibility in Parkinson's Disease. *Ann Neurol* 44:270–273, 1998.
20. Vaughan JR, Farrer MJ, Wszolek ZK, et al: Sequencing of the alpha-synuclein gene in a large series of cases of familial Parkinson's disease fails to reveal any further mutations. The European Consortium on Genetic Susceptibility in Parkinson's Disease (GSPD). *Hum Mol Genet* 7:751–753, 1998.

21. Lin JJ, Yueh KC, Chang DC, Lin SZ: Absence of G209A and G88C mutations in the alpha-synuclein gene of Parkinson's disease in a Chinese population. *Eur Neurol* 42:217–220, 1999.

22. Nagar S, Juyal RC, Chaudhary S, et al: Mutations in the alpha-synuclein gene in Parkinson's disease among Indians. *Acta Neurol Scand* 103:120–122, 2001.

23. Chan DK, Mellick G, Cai H, et al: The alpha-synuclein gene and Parkinson disease in a Chinese population. *Arch Neurol* 57:501–503, 2000.

24. Oliveri RL, Zappia M, Annesi G, et al: The parkin gene is not involved in late-onset Parkinson's disease. *Neurology* 57:359–362, 2001.

25. Nelson L, Van Den Eeden S, Tanner C, et al: Incidence of idiopathic Parkinson's disease (PD) in a health maintenance organization (HMO): Variations by age, gender and race/ethnicity. *Neurology* 48:A334, 1997.

26. Koller WC, Langston JW, Hubble JP, et al: Does a long preclinical period occur in Parkinson's disease. *Neurology* 41(suppl 2): 8–13, 1991.

27. Sawle GV, Wroe SJ, Lees AJ, et al: The identification of presymptomatic parkinsonism: Clinical and [^{18}F]dopa positron emission tomography studies in an Irish kindred. *Ann Neurol* 32:609–617, 1992.

28. Piccini P, Burn DJ, Ceravolo R, et al: The role of inheritance in sporadic Parkinson's disease: Evidence from a longitudinal study of dopaminergic function in twins. *Ann Neurol* 45:577–582, 1999.

29. Forno LS. Concentric hyalin intraneuronal inclusions of Lewy type in brains of elderly persons (60 incidental cases): Relationships to parkinsonism. *J Am Geriatr Soc* 17:557–575, 1969.

30. Gibb WRG, Lees AJ: The relevance of the Lewy body to the pathogenesis of idiopathic Parkinson's disease. *J Neurol Neurosurg Psychiatry* 51:745–752, 1988.

31. Chen RC, Chang SF, Su CL, et al: Prevalence, incidence, and mortality of PD: A door-to-door survey in Ilan County, Taiwan. *Neurology* 57:1679–1686, 2001.

32. Fall PA, Axelson O, Fredriksson M, et al: Age-standardized incidence and prevalence of Parkinson's disease in a Swedish community. *J Clin Epidemiol* 49:637–641, 1996.

33. Kusumi M, Nakashima K, Harada H, et al: Epidemiology of Parkinson's disease in Yonago City, Japan: Comparison with a study carried out 12 years ago. *Neuroepidemiology* 15:201–207, 1996.

34. Mayeux R, Marder K, Cote LJ, et al: The frequency of idiopathic Parkinson's disease by age, ethnic group, and sex in northern Manhattan, 1988–1993. *Am J Epidemiol* 142:820–827, 1995.

35. Bower JH, Maraganore DM, McDonnell SK, Rocca WA: Incidence and distribution of parkinsonism in Olmsted County, Minnesota, 1976–1990. *Neurology* 52:1214–1220, 1999.

36. Kuopio AM, Marttila RJ, Helenius H, Rinne UK: Changing epidemiology of Parkinson's disease in southwestern Finland. *Neurology* 52:302–308, 1999.

37. Ashok P, Radhakrishan K, Sridharan R, Mousa M: Epidemiology of Parkinson's disease in Benghazi, North-East Libya. *Clin Neurol Neurosurg* 88:1109–113, 1986.

38. Harada H, Nishikawa S, Takahashi K: Epidemiology of Parkinson's disease in a Japanese city. *Arch Neurol* 40:151–154, 1983.

39. Rosati G, Granieri E, Pinna L, et al: The risk of Parkinson disease in Mediterranean people. *Neurology* 30:250–255, 1980.

40. Granieri E, Carreras M, Casetta I, et al: Parkinson's disease in Ferrara, Italy, 1967 through 1987. *Arch Neurol* 48:854–857, 1991.

41. Sutcliffe RL, Meara JR: Parkinson's disease epidemiology in the Northampton District, England, 1992. *Acta Neurol Scand* 92:443–450, 1995.

42. MacDonald BK, Cockerell OC, Sander JW, Shorvon SD: The incidence and lifetime prevalence of neurological disorders in a prospective community-based study in the UK. *Brain* 123:665–676, 2000.

43. Brewis M, Poskanzer MD, Rolland H, Miller H: Neurological disease in an English city. *Acta Neurol Scand* 42(suppl 24):1–89, 1966.

44. Melcon MO, Anderson DW, Vergara RH, Rocca WA: Prevalence of Parkinson's disease in Junin, Buenos Aires Province, Argentina. *Mov Disord* 12:197–205, 1997.

45. Shi YM: Parkinson's disease in Hong Koy district, Shanghai. *Chin J Epidemiol* 8:205–209, 1987.

46. Bharucha NE, Bharucha EP, Bharucha AE, et al: Prevalence of Parkinson's disease in the Parsi community of Bombay, India. *Arch Neurol* 45:1321–1323, 1988.

47. Milanov I, Kmetska K, Karakolev B, Nedialkov E: Prevalence of Parkinson's disease in Bulgaria. *Neuroepidemiology* 20:212–214, 2001.

48. Wermuth L, von Weitzel-Mudersbach P, Jeune B: A two-fold difference in the age-adjusted prevalences of Parkinson's disease between the island of Als and the Faroe Islands. *Eur J Neurol* 7:655–660, 2000.

49. Schrag A, Ben-Shlomo Y, Quinn NP: Cross sectional prevalence survey of idiopathic Parkinson's disease and parkinsonism in London. *BMJ* 321:21–22, 2000.

50. Milanov I, Kmetski TS, Lyons KE, Koller WC: Prevalence of Parkinson's disease in Bulgarian gypsies. *Neuroepidemiology* 19:206–209, 2000.

51. Errea J, Ara J, Aibar C, dePedroCuesta J: Prevalence of Parkinson's disease in Lower Aragon, Spain. *Mov Disord* 14:596–604, 1999.

52. Chio A, Magnani C, Schiffer D: Prevalence of Parkinson's disease in Northwestern Italy: Comparison of tracer methodology and clinical ascertainment of cases. *Mov Disord* 13:400–405, 1998.

53. Wermuth L, Joensen P, Bunger N, Jeune B: High prevalence of Parkinson's disease in the Faroe Islands. *Neurology* 49:426–432, 1997.

54. Chouza C, Ketzoian C, Caamano JL, et al: Prevalence of Parkinson's disease in a population of Uruguay. Preliminary results. *Adv Neurol* 69:13–17, 1996.

55. Tandberg E, Larsen JP, Nessler EG, et al: The epidemiology of Parkinson's disease in the county of Rogaland, Norway. *Mov Disord* 10:541–549, 1995.

56. Menniti-Ippolito F, Spila-Alegiani S, Vanacore N: Estimate of parkinsonism prevalence through drug prescription histories in the Province of Rome, Italy. *Acta Neurol Scand* 92:49–54, 1995.

57. Dias JA, Felgueiras MM, Sanchez JP, et al: The prevalence of Parkinson's disease in Portugal. A population approach. *Eur J Epidemiol* 10:763–767, 1994.

58. Caradoc-Davies TH, Weatherall M, Dixon GS, et al: Is the prevalence of Parkinson's disease in New Zealand really changing? *Acta Neurol Scand* 86:40–44, 1992.

59. Acosta J. Epidemiology of Parkinson's disease: Record of patients in our rural medium: Verjel de la Frontera. *9th International Symposium on Parkinson's Disease.* Jerusalem, 1988; p 57.

60. Rocca W, Morgante L, Grigoletto F, et al: Prevalence of Parkinson's disease (Parkinson's disease) and other parkinsonisms: A door-to-door survey in two Sicilian communities. *Neurology* 40(suppl 1):422, 1990.

61. Rosati G, Granieri L, Aiello I, et al: The risk of Parkinson's disease in Mediterranean people. *Neurology* 30:250–255, 1980.

62. Sutcliffe RLG, Prior R, Mawby B, McQuillan WJ: Parkinson's disease in the district of Northampton Health Authority, United Kingdom. A study of prevalence and disability. *Acta Neurol Scand* 72:363–379, 1985.

63. Mutch W, Dingwall-Fordyce I, Downie A, et al: Parkinson's disease in a Scottish city. *BMJ* 292:534–536, 1986.

64. Okada K, Kobayashi S, Tsunematsu T: Prevalence of Parkinson's disease in Izumo City, Japan. *Gerontology* 36:340–344, 1990.

65. Mayeux R, Denaro J, Hemenegildo N, et al: A population-based investigation of Parkinson's disease with and without dementia: Relationship to age and gender. *Arch Neurol* 49:492–497, 1992.

66. Morgante L, Rocca WA, di Rosa AE, et al: Prevalence of Parkinson's disease and other types of parkinsonism: A door-to-door survey in three Sicilian municipalities. *Neurology* 42:1901–1907, 1992.

67. Tison F, Dartigues JF, Dubes L, et al: Prevalence of Parkinson's disease in the elderly: A population study in Gironde, France. *Acta Neurol Scand* 90:111–115, 1994.

68. de Rijk MC, Tzourio C, Breteler MMB, et al: Prevalence of parkinsonism and Parkinson's disease in Europe: The EUROPARKINSON collaborative study. *J Neurol Neurosurg Psychiatry* 62:10–15, 1997.

69. Trenkwalder C, Schwarz J, Gebhard J, et al: Starnberg trial on epidemiology of parkinsonism and hypertension in the elderly. *Arch Neurol* 52:1017–1022, 1995.

70. Wang SJ, Fuh JL, Teng EL, et al: A door-to-door survey of Parkinson's disease in a Chinese population in Kinmen. *Arch Neurol* 53:66–71, 1996.

71. Svensen LW: Regional disparities in the annual prevalence rates of Parkinson's disease in Canada. *Neuroepidemiology* 10:205–210, 1991.

72. McCann SJ, LeCouteur DG, Green AC, et al: The epidemiology of Parkinson's disease in an Australian population. *Neuroepidemiology* 17:310–317, 1998.

73. de Rijk MC, Launer LJ, Berger K, et al: Prevalence of Parkinson's disease in Europe: A collaborative study of population-based cohorts. Neurologic Diseases in the Elderly Research Group. *Neurology* 54:S21–23, 2000.

74. de Rijk MC, Breteler MMB, Graveland GA: Prevalence of Parkinson's disease in the elderly: The Rotterdam study. *Neurology* 45:2143–2146, 1995.

75. Imaizumi Y, Kaneko R: Rising mortality from Parkinson's disease in Japan, 1950–1992. *Acta Neurol Scand* 91:169–176, 1995.

76. Beyer MK, Herlofson K, Arsland D, Larsen JP: Causes of death in a community-based study of Parkinson's disease. *Acta Neurol Scand* 103:7–11, 2001.

77. Lilienfeld DE, Chan E, Ehland J, et al: Two decades of increasing mortality from Parkinson's disease among the US elderly. *Arch Neurol* 47:731–734, 1990.

78. Williams GR: Morbidity and mortality with parkinsonism. *J Neurosurg* 24:138–143, 1966.

79. Svenson LW: Geographic distribution of deaths due to Parkinson's disease in Canada: 1979–1986. *Mov Disord* 5:322–324, 1990.

80. Riggs JE: Longitudinal Gompertzian analysis of Parkinson's disease mortality in the US, 1955–1986: The dramatic increase in overall mortality since 1980 is the natural consequence of deterministic mortality dynamics. *Mech Age Dev* 55:221–233, 1990.

81. Kurtzke JF, Goldberg ID: Parkinsonism death rates by race, sex, and geography. *Neurology* 38:1558–1561, 1988.

82. Treves TA, de Pedro-Cuesta J: Parkinsonism mortality in the US, 1. Time and space distribution. *Acta Neurol Scand* 84:389–397, 1991.

83. Vanacore N, Bonifati V, Bellatreccia A, et al: Mortality rates for Parkinson's disease and parkinsonism in Italy (1969–1987). *Neuroepidemiology* 11:65–73, 1992.

84. Clarke CE: Mortality from Parkinson's disease in England and Wales 1921–89. *J Neurol Neurosurg Psychiatry* 56:690–693, 1993.

85. Chió A, Magnani C, Tolardo G, Schiffer D: Parkinson's disease mortality in Italy, 1951 through 1987: Analysis of an increasing trend. *Arch Neurol* 50:149–153, 1993.

86. Bonifati V, Vanacore N, Bellatreccia A, Meco G: Mortality rates for parkinsonism in Italy (1969 to 1987). *Acta Neurol Scand* 87:9–13, 1993.

87. Chandra V, Bharucha NE, Schoenberg BS: Mortality data for the US for deaths due to and related to twenty neurologic diseases. *Neuroepidemiology* 3:149–168, 1984.

88. Morens D, Davis J, Grandinetti A, et al: Epidemiologic observations on Parkinson's disease: Incidence and mortality in a prospective study of middle-aged men. *Neurology* 46:1044–1050, 1996.

89. Louis ED, Marder K, Cote L, et al: Mortality from Parkinson disease. *Arch Neurol* 54:260–264, 1997.

90. Morgante L, Salemi G, Meneghini F, et al: Parkinson disease survival: A population-based study. *Arch Neurol* 57:507–512, 2000.

91. Di Rocco A, Molinari SP, Kollmeier B, Yahr MD: Parkinson's disease: Progression and mortality in the L-DOPA era. *Adv Neurol* 69:3–11, 1996.

92. Lanska DJ: Comparison of utilization of Sinemet and Parkinson's disease mortality as surrogate indicators of Parkinson's disease in the United States. *J Neurol Sci* 145:105–108, 1997.

93. Imaizumi Y: Geographical variations in mortality from Parkinson's disease in Japan, 1977–1985. *Acta Neurol Scand* 91:311–316, 1995.

94. D'Alessandro R, Gamberini G, Granieri E, et al: Prevalence of Parkinson's disease in the Republic of San Marino. *Neurology* 37:1679–1682, 1987.

95. Li S, Schoenberg B, Wang C, et al: A prevalence survey of Parkinson's disease and other movement disorders in the People's Republic of China. *Arch Neurol* 42, 1985.

96. Schoenberg B, Anderson D, Haerer A: Prevalence of Parkinson's disease in the biracial population of Copiah County, Mississippi. *Neurology* 35:841–845, 1985.

97. Wang SJ, Fuh JL, Liu CY, et al: Parkinson's disease in Kin-Hu, Kinmen: A community survey by neurologists. *Neuroepidemiology* 13:69–74, 1994.

98. Li SC, Schoenberg BS, Wang CC, et al: A prevalence survey of Parkinson's disease and other movement disorders in the people's republic of China. *Arch Neurol* 42:655–657, 1985.

99. Rocca WA, Bower JH, McDonnell SK, et al: Time trends in the incidence of parkinsonism in Olmsted County, Minnesota. *Neurology* 57:462–467, 2001.

100. Baldereschi M, Di Carlo A, Rocca WA, et al: Parkinson's disease and parkinsonism in a longitudinal study: Two-fold higher incidence in men. ILSA Working Group. Italian Longitudinal Study on Aging. *Neurology* 55:1358–1363, 2000.

101. Reef HE: Prevalence of Parkinson's disease in a multiracial community, in Jage HWA, Bruyn GW, Heihstee APJ (eds): *Eleventh World Congress of Neurology* (International Congress Series 427). Amsterdam: Excerpta Medica, 1977, p 125.

102. Kessler II: Epidemiologic studies of Parkinson's disease. III. A community-based survey. *Am J Epidemiol* 96:242–254, 1972.

103. Schoenberg BS, Anderson DW, Haerer AF: Prevalence of Parkinson's disease in the biracial population of Copiah County, Mississippi. *Neurology* 35:841–845, 1985.

104. Paddison RM, Griffith RP: Occurrence of Parkinson's disease in black patients at Charity Hospital in New Orleans. *Neurology* 24:688–690, 1974.

105. Lombard A, Gelfand M: Parkinson's disease in the African. *Cent Afr J Med* 24:5–8, 1978.

106. Chio A, Magnani C, Schiffer D: Prevalence of Parkinson's disease in northwestern Italy: Comparison of tracer methodology and clinical ascertainment of cases. *Mov Disord* 13:400–405, 1998.

107. Schoenberg BS, Osuntokun BO, Adeuja AOG, et al: Comparison of the prevalence of Parkinson's disease in the rural United States and in rural Nigeria: Door-to-door community studies. *Neurology* 38:645–646, 1988.

108. Van Den Eeden SK, Tanner CM, Bernstein AL, et al: Incidence of Parkinson's disease: Variation by age, gender and race/ethnicity. *Am J Epidemiol* 157:1015–1022, 2003.

109. Tanner CM, Thelen JA, Offord KP, et al: Parkinson's disease incidence in Olmsted County, MN: 1935–1988. *Neurology* 42:194–194, 1992.

110. Chan DK, Dunne M, Wong A, et al: Pilot study of prevalence of Parkinson's disease in Australia. *Neuroepidemiology* 20:112–117, 2001.

111. Zhang Z, Roman G: Worldwide occurrence of Parkinson's disease: An updated review. *Neuroepidemiology* 12:195–208, 1993.

112. Morano A, Jimenez-Jimenez FJ, Molina JA, Antolin MA: Risk-factors for Parkinson's disease: Case-control study in the province of Caceres, Spain. *Acta Neurol Scand* 89:164–170, 1994.

113. Bonifati V, Fabrizio E, Vanacore N, et al: Familial Parkinson's disease: A clinical genetic analysis. *Can J Neurol Sci* 22:272–279, 1995.

114. Payami H, Larsen K, Bernard S, Nutt JG: Increased risk of Parkinson's disease in parents and siblings of patients. *Ann Neurol* 36:659–661, 1994.

115. Vieregge P, Heberlein I: Increased risk of Parkinson's disease in relatives of patients. *Ann Neurol* 37:685, 1995.

116. De Michele G, Filla A, Volpe G, et al: Environmental and genetic risk factors in Parkinson's disease: A case-control study in Southern Italy. *Mov Disord* 11:17–23, 1996.

117. Autere JM, Moilanen JS, Myllyla VV, Majamaa K: Familial aggregation of Parkinson's disease in a Finnish population. *J Neurol Neurosurg Psychiatry* 69:107–109, 2000.

118. Taylor CA, Saint-Hilaire MH, Cupples LA, et al: Environmental, medical, and family history risk factors for Parkinson's disease: A New England-based case control study. *Am J Med Genet* 88:742–749, 1999.

119. Werneck AL, Alvarenga H: Genetics, drugs and environmental factors in Parkinson's disease. A case-control study. *Arq Neuropsiquiatr* 57:347–355, 1999.

120. Preux PM, Condet A, Anglade C, et al: Parkinson's disease and environmental factors. Matched case-control study in the Limousin region, France. *Neuroepidemiology* 19:333–337, 2000.

121. Marder K, Tang M, Mejia H, et al: Risk of Parkinson's disease among first-degree relatives: A community-based study. *Neurology* 47:155–160, 1996.

122. Semchuk K, Love E, Lee R: Parkinson's disease: A test of the multifactorial etiologic hypothesis. *Neurology* 43:1173–1180, 1993.

123. Elbaz A, Grigoletto F, Baldereschi M, et al: Familial aggregation of Parkinson's disease: A population-based case-control study in Europe. EUROPARKINSON Study Group. *Neurology* 52:1876–1882, 1999.

124. de Rijk MC, Breteler MM, van der Meche FG, Hofman A: The risk of Parkinson's disease among persons with a family history of Parkinson's disease or dementia: The Rotterdam study. *Neurology* 48:A333, 1997.

125. Sveinbjornsdottir S, Hicks AA, Jonsson T, et al: Familial aggregation of Parkinson's disease in Iceland. *N Engl J Med* 343:1765–1770, 2000.

126. Moilanen JS, Autere JM, Myllyla VV, Majamaa K: Complex segregation analysis of Parkinson's disease in the Finnish population. *Hum Genet* 108:184–189, 2001.

127. Marsden CD: Parkinson's disease in twins. *J Neurol Neurosurg Psychiatry* 50:105–106, 1987.

128. Marttila RJ, Kaprio J, Koskenvuo M, Rinne UK: Parkinson's disease in a nationwide twin cohort. *Neurology* 3817:1217–1219, 1988.

129. Vieregge P, Schiffke KA, Friedrich HJ, et al: Parkinson's disease in twins. *Neurology* 42:1453–1461, 1992.

130. Ward C, Duvoisin R, Ince S, et al: Parkinson's disease in 65 pairs of twins and in a set of quadruplets. *Neurology* 33:815–824, 1983.

131. Zimmerman TR Jr, Bhatt M, Calne DB, Duvoisin RC: Parkinson's disease in monozygotic twins: A follow-up study. *Neurology* 41(suppl 1):255, 1991.

132. Tanner CM, Ottman R, Goldman SM, et al: Parkinson disease in twins: An etiologic study. *JAMA* 281:341–346, 1999.

133. Burn DJ, Mark MH, Playford ED, et al: Parkinson's disease in twins studied with ^{18}F-dopa and positron emission tomography. *Neurology* 42:1894–1900, 1992.

134. Holthoff VA, Vieregge P, Kessler J, et al: Discordant twins with Parkinson's disease: Positron emission tomography and early signs of impaired cognitive circuits. *Ann Neurol* 36:176–182, 1994.

135. Langston JW, Ballard PA, Tetrud JW, Irwin I: Chronic parkinsonism in humans due to a product of meperidine analog synthesis. *Science* 219:979–980, 1983.

136. Forno LS, Langston JW, DeLanney LE, et al: Locus ceruleus lesions and eosinophilic inclusions in MPTP-treated monkeys. *Ann Neurol* 20:449–455, 1986.

137. Ricaurte GA, DeLanney LE, Irwin I, Langston JW: Older dopaminergic neurons do not recover from the effects of MPTP. *Neuropharmacology* 26:97–99, 1987.

138. Davis GC, Williams AC, Markey SP, et al: Chronic parkinsonism secondary to intravenous injection of meperidine analogues. *Psychiatr Res* 1:249–254,1979.

139. Betarbet R, Sherer TB, MacKenzie G, et al: Chronic systemic pesticide exposure reproduces features of Parkinson's disease. *Nat Neurosci* 3:1301–1306, 2000.

140. Barbeau A, Dallaire L, Buu NT, et al: Comparative behavioral, biochemical and pigmentary effects of MPTP, MPP+ and paraquat in *Rana pipiens*. *Life Sci* 37:1529–1538, 1985.

141. Priyadarshi A, Khuder SA, Schaub EA, Shrivastava S: A meta-analysis of Parkinson's disease and exposure to pesticides. *Neurotoxicology* 21:435–440, 2000.

142. Ritz B, Yu F: Parkinson's disease mortality and pesticide exposure in California 1984–1994. *Int J Epidemiol* 29:323–329, 2000.

143. Nelson LM, Van Den Eeden SK, Tanner CM, et al: Home pesticide exposure and the risk of Parkinson's disease. *Neurology* 54:A472–473, 2000.

144. Priyadarshi A, Khuder SA, Schaub EA, Priyadarshi SS: Environmental risk factors and Parkinson's disease: A metaanalysis. *Environ Res* 86:122–127, 2001.

145. Seidler A, Hellenbrand W, Robra BP, et al: Possible environmental, occupational, and other etiologic factors for Parkinson's disease: A case-control study in Germany. *Neurology* 46:1275–1284, 1996.

146. Semchuk KM, Love EJ, Lee RG: Parkinson's disease and exposure to agricultural work and pesticide chemicals. *Neurology* 42:1328–1335, 1992.

147. Liou HH, Tsai MC, Chen CJ, et al: Environmental risk factors and Parkinson's disease: A case-control study in Taiwan. *Neurology* 48:1583–1588, 1997.

148. Fleming L, Mann JB, Bean J, et al: Parkinson's disease and brain levels of organochlorine pesticides. *Ann Neurol* 36:100–103, 1994.

149. Smargiassi A, Mutti A, De Rosa A, et al: A case-control study of occupational and environmental risk factors for Parkinson's disease in the Emilia-Romagna region of Italy. *Neurotoxicology* 19:709–712, 1998.

150. Tanner CM: The role of environmental toxins in the etiology of Parkinson's disease. *Trends Neurosci* 12:49–54, 1989.

151. Rybecki BA, Johnson CC, Uman J, Gorell JM: Parkinson's disease mortality and the industrial use of heavy metals in Michigan. *Mov Disord* 8:87–92, 1993.

152. Anthony JC, LeResche L, Niaz U, et al: Limits of the "Mini-Mental State" as a screening test for dementia and delirium among hospital patients. *Psychol Med* 12:397–408, 1982.

153. Sofic E, Paulus W, Jellinger KA, et al: Selective increase of iron in substantia nigra zona compacta of Parkinsonian brains. *J Neurochem* 56:978–982, 1991.

154. Aquilonius S, Hartvig P: A Swedish county with unexpectedly high utilization of anti-parkinsonian drugs. *Acta Neurol Scand* 74:379–382, 1986.

155. Gorell JM, Rybicki BA, Cole Johnson C, Peterson EL: Occupational metal exposures and the risk of Parkinson's disease. *Neuroepidemiology* 18:303–308, 1999.

156. Thiruchelvam M, Richfield EK, Baggs RB, et al: The nigrostriatal dopaminergic system as a preferential target of repeated exposures to combined paraquat and maneb: Implications for Parkinson's disease. *J Neurosci* 20:9207–9214, 2000.

157. Johnson CC, Gorell JM, Rybicki BA, et al: Adult nutrient intake as a risk factor for Parkinson's disease. *Int J Epidemiol* 28:1102–1109, 1999.

158. Logroscino G, Marder K, Cote L, et al: Dietary lipids and antioxidants in Parkinson's disease: A population-based, case-control study. *Ann Neurol* 39:89–94, 1996.

159. Anderson KC, Checkoway L, Franklin G, et al: Dietary factors in Parkinson's disease: The role of food groups and specific foods. *Mov Disord* 14:21–27, 1999.

160. Poskanzer DC, Schwab RS, Fraser DW: Further observations on the cohort phenomenon in Parkinson's syndrome, in Barbeau A, Brunette JR (eds): *Progress in Neurogenetics*. Amsterdam: Excerpta Medica, 1969, pp 497–505.

161. Mattock C, Marmot MG, Stern GM: Could Parkinson's disease follow intra-uterine influenza: A speculative hypothesis. *J Neurol Neurosurg Psychiatry* 51:753–756, 1988.

162. Ehmeier KP, Mutch WJ, Calder SA, et al: Does idiopathic parkinsonism in Aberdeen follow intrauterine influenza? *Neurol Neurosurg Psychiatry* 52:911–913, 1989.

163. Elizan TS, Casals J: The viral hypothesis in Parkinson's disease and Alzheimer's disease: A critique, in Kurstak E, Lipowski ZJ, Morozov PV (eds): *Viruses, Immunity, and Mental Disorders*. New York: Plenum Medical, 1987, pp 47–59.

164. Marttila R, Halonen P, Rinne U: Influenza virus antibodies in parkinsonism. *Arch Neurol* 34:99–100, 1977.

165. Fazzini E, Fleming J, Fahn S: Cerebrospinal fluid antibodies to coronaviruses in patients with Parkinson's disease. *Neurology* 40(suppl 1):169, 1990.

166. Kobbata S, Beaman BL: L-Dopa-responsive movement disorder caused by *Norcardia asteroides* localized in the brains of mice. *Infect Immun* 59:181–191, 1991.

167. Hubble JP, Cao T, Kjelstrom JA, et al: *Nocardia* species as an etiologic agent in Parkinson's disease: Serological testing in a case-control study. *J Clin Microbiol* 33:2768–2769, 1995.

168. Sasco A, Paffenberger R Jr: Measles infection and Parkinson's disease. *Am J Epidemiol* 122:1017–1031, 1985.

169. Snyder A, Stricker E, Zigmond M: Stress-induced neurological impairments in an animal model of parkinsonism. *Ann Neurol* 18:544–551, 1985.

170. Spina M, Cohen G: Dopamine turnover and glutathione oxidation: Implications for Parkinson's disease. *Proc Natl Acad Sci U S A* 86:1398–1400, 1989.

171. Treves T, Rabey J, Korczyn A: Case-control study, with use of temporal approach, for evaluation of risk factors for Parkinson's disease. *Mov Disord* 5:11, 1990.

172. Gibberd FB, Simmonds JP: Neurological disease in ex-far-east prisoners of war. *Lancet* ii:135–137, 1980.

173. Page WF, Tanner CM: Parkinson's disease and motor-neuron disease in former prisoners-of-war. *Lancet* 355:843, 2000.

174. Lees AJ: Trauma and Parkinson disease. *Rev Neurol (Paris)* 153:541–546, 1997.

175. Kuopio AM, Marttila RJ, Helenius H, Rinne UK: Environmental risk factors in Parkinson's disease. *Mov Disord* 14:928–939, 1999.

176. Menza M: The personality associated with Parkinson's disease. *Curr Psychiatry Rep* 2:421–426, 2000.

177. Herishanu YO, Medvedovski M, Goldsmith JR, Kordysh E: A case-control study of Parkinson's disease in urban population of southern Israel. *Can J Neurol Sci* 28:144–147, 2001.

178. Tsui JK, Calne DB, Wang Y, et al: Occupational risk factors in Parkinson's disease. *Can J Public Health* 90:334–337, 1999.

179. Fall PA, Fredrikson M, Axelson O, Granerus AK: Nutritional and occupational factors influencing the risk of Parkinson's disease: A case-control study in southeastern Sweden. *Mov Disord* 14:28–37, 1999.

180. Zayed J, Ducic S, Campanella G, et al: Environmental factors in the etiology of Parkinson's disease. *Can J Neurol Sci* 17:286–291, 1990.

181. Hertzman C, Wiens M, Bowering D, et al: Parkinson's disease: A case-control study of occupational and environmental risk factors. *Am J Indust Med* 17:349–355, 1990.

182. Sterm M, Dulaney E, Gruber S, et al: The Epidemiology of Parkinson's disease: a case-control study of young-onset and old-onset patients. *Arch Neurol* 48:903–907, 1991.

183. Rajput A, Offurd K, Beard C, Kurland L: A case-control study of smoking habits, dementia, and other illnesses in idiopathic Parkinson's disease. *Neurology* 37:226–232, 1987.

184. Kahn HA. The Dorn study of smoking and mortality among U.S. veterans: report on eight and one-half years of observation, in Haenszel W (ed): *Epidemilogic Approaches to the Study of Cancer and other Diseases* 19:1–125, 1966.

185. Baumann R, Jameson H, McKean H, et al: Cigarette smoking and Parkinson's disease: I. A comparison of cases with matched neighbors. *Neurology* 30:839–843, 1980.

186. Burch P: Cigarette smoking and Parkinson's disease. *Neurology* 31:500, 1981.

187. Godwin-Austin R, Lee P, Marmot M: Smoking and Parkinson's disease. *J Neurol Neurosurg Psychiatry* 45:577–581, 1982.

188. Haack D, Baumann R, McKean H: Nicotine exposure and Parkinson's disease. *Am J Epidemiol* 114:119–200, 1981.

189. Kessler I, Diamond E: Epidemiologic studies of Parkinson's disease. I. Smoking and Parkinson's disease: A survey and explanatory hypothesis. *Am J Epidemiol* 94:16–25, 1971.

190. Nefzinger M, Quadfasel F, Karl V: A retrospective study of smoking and Parkinson's disease. *Am J Epidemiol* 88:149–158, 1968.

191. Tanner C, Koller W, Gilley D, et al: Cigarette smoking, alcohol drinking and Parkinson's disease: Cross-cultural risk assessment. *Mov Disord* 5:11, 1990.

192. Tzourio C, Rocca WA, Breteler MM, et al: Smoking and Parkinson's disease. An age-dependent risk effect? The EUROPARKINSON Study Group. *Neurology* 49:1267–1272, 1997.

193. Hellenbrand W, Seidler A, Boeing H, et al: Diet and Parkinson's disease. I: A possible role for the past intake of specific foods and food groups. Results from a self-administered food-frequency questionnaire in a case-control study. *Neurology* 47:636–643, 1996.

194. Tanner CM, Goldman SM, Aston DA, et al: Smoking and Parkinson's disease in twins. *Neurology* 58:581–588, 2002.

195. Bharucha N, Stokes L, Schoenberg B, et al: A case-control study of twin pairs discordant for Parkinson's disease: A search for environmental risk factors. *Neurology* 36:284–288, 1986.

196. Grandinetti A, Morens DM, Reed D, MacEachern D: Prospective study of cigarette smoking and the risk of developing idiopathic Parkinson's disease. *Am J Epidemiol* 139:1129–1138, 1994.

197. Gorell JM, Rybicki BA, Johnson CC, Peterson EL: Smoking and Parkinson's disease: A dose-response relationship. *Neurology* 52:115–119, 1999.

198. Morens DM, Grandinetti A, Davis JW, et al: Evidence against the operation of selective mortality in explaining the association between cigarette smoking and reduced occurrence of idiopathic Parkinson disease. *Am J Epidemiol* 144:400–404, 1996.

199. Jansson B, Jankovic J: Low cancer rates among patients with Parkinson's disease. *Ann Neurol* 17:505–509, 1985.

200. Maggio R, Riva M, Vaglini F, et al: Nicotine prevents experimental parkinsonism in rodents and induces striatal increase of neurotrophic factors. *J Neurochem* 71:2439–2446, 1998.

201. Kirch DG, Alho AM, Wyatt RJ: Hypothesis: A nicotine-dopamine interaction linking smoking with Parkinson's disease and tardive dyskinesia. *Cell Mol Neurobiol* 8:285–291, 1988.

202. Soto-Otero R, Mendez-Alvarez E, Riguera-Vega R, et al: Studies on the interaction between 1,2,3,4-tetrahydro-beta-carboline and cigarette smoke: A potential mechanism of neuroprotection for Parkinson's disease. *Brain Res* 802:155–162, 1998.

203. Menza MA, Forman NE, Goldstein HS, Golbe LI: Parkinson's disease, personality, and dopamine. *J Neuropsychiat Clin Neurosci* 2:282–287, 1990.

204. Benedetti MD, Bower JH, Maraganore DM, et al: Smoking, alcohol, and coffee consumption preceding Parkinson's disease: A case-control study. *Neurology* 55:1350–1358, 2000.

205. Ascherio A, Zhang SM, Hernan MA, et al: Prospective study of caffeine consumption and risk of Parkinson's disease in men and women. *Ann Neurol* 50:56–63, 2001.

206. Ross GW, Abbott RD, Petrovitch H, et al: Association of coffee and caffeine intake with the risk of Parkinson disease. *JAMA* 283:2674–2679, 2000.

207. Hellenbrand W, Boeing H, Robra B, et al: Diet and Parkinson's Disease II: A possible role for the past intake of specific nutrients. Results form a self-administered food-frequency questionnaire in a case-control study. *Neurology* 47:644–650, 1996.

208. Scheider WL, Hershey LA, Vena JE, et al: Dietary antioxidants and other dietary factors in the etiology of Parkinson's disease. *Mov Disord* 12:190–196, 1997.

209. Anderson C, Checkoway H, Franklin GM, et al: Dietary factors in Parkinson's disease: The role of food groups and specific foods. *Mov Disord* 14:21–27, 1999.

210. Hellenbrand W, Boeing H, Robra BP, et al: Diet and Parkinson's disease. II: A possible role for the past intake of specific nutrients. Results from a self-administered food-frequency questionnaire in a case-control study. *Neurology* 47:644–650, 1996.

211. de Rijk MC, Breteler MB, den Breeijen JH, et al: Dietary antioxidants and Parkinson disease. *Arch Neurol* 54:762–765, 1997.

212. Golbe LI, Farrell TM, Davis PH: Follow-up study of early-life protective and risk factors in Parkinson's disease. *Mov Disord* 5:66–70, 1990.

213. Golbe LI, Farrell TM, Davis PH: Case-control study of early life dietary factors in Parkinson's disease. *Arch Neurol* 45:1350–1353, 1988.

214. Vieregge P, Maravic C, Friedrich H-J: Life-style and dietary factors early and late in Parkinson's disease. *Can J Neurol Sci* 19:170–173, 1992.

Chapter 12

NEUROCHEMISTRY AND NEUROPHARMACOLOGY OF PARKINSON'S DISEASE

FEDERICO MICHELI, MARIA G. CERSOSIMO, and
G. FREDERICK WOOTEN

DOPAMINE	198
General Metabolism	198
Disposition of Dopamine Neurons in Brain	198
Role of Dopamine in Parkinson's Disease (PD)	199
Dopamine Receptors	200
NOREPINEPHRINE	200
SEROTONIN	201
GAMMA-AMINOBUTYRIC ACID	201
ACETYLCHOLINE	201
NEUROPEPTIDES	201
ENDOGENOUS FREE RADICAL SCAVENGERS AND GENERATORS	202
MITOCHONDRIAL FUNCTION	203
IN VIVO NEUROCHEMISTRY: POSITRON EMISSION TOMOGRAPHY IN PARKINSON'S DISEASE	203
NEUROCHEMICAL ANALYSIS OF LEWY BODIES	204
SIGNIFICANCE OF NEUROCHEMICAL STUDIES OF PARKINSON'S DISEASE	205

The motor signs and symptoms of Parkinson's disease (PD) result primarily from dysfunction of the basal ganglia. The central mechanism for the physiological dysfunction of the basal ganglia in PD is a progressive decline in the concentration of dopamine. In the past 25 years, much progress has been made in identifying the anatomic connections and in characterizing the regional neurochemistry of the basal ganglia. The major intrinsic and extrinsic connections of the several cell groups that comprise the basal ganglia and identified neurotransmitters for each pathway are summarized in Fig. 12-1. Probably the first findings to support the relationship between PD and the basal ganglia were the clinicopathological correlations of Wilson,[1] coupled with the observations made by neuropathologists of neuronal loss and depigmentation of the substantia nigra in the brains of parkinsonian patients.[2] The subsequent discovery of profound reductions in the concentration of the monoamine neurotransmitter dopamine in the caudate nucleus and putamen of parkinsonian patients,[3] and the recognition that pigmented neurons of the substantia nigra project to the striatum and provide it with dopaminergic input, strengthened the evidence that PD

is primarily a disease of the basal ganglia.[4] Later observations that the neurotoxic opiate derivative 1-methyl-4-phenyl-1,2,3,6-tetrahydropyridine (MPTP) produced parkinsonism in humans and other primates, with resultant neuropathological changes restricted primarily to the substantia nigra and large decrements in the striatal concentration of dopamine, provided further substantiation for the pathophysiological basis of PD.[5]

The following structures are considered to comprise the basal ganglia: the putamen, caudate, globus pallidus (external and internal segments), subthalamic nucleus, and substantia nigra (pars reticulata, and pars compacta). The major sources

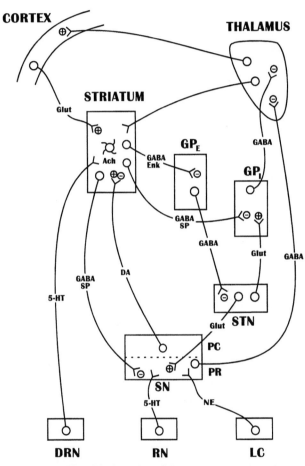

FIGURE 12-1 Simplified version of the major anatomic pathways within the basal ganglia, including identification of known neurotransmitters, when such information is available. Names and initials in large type identify anatomically distinct nuclear groups within the basal ganglia; abbreviations and contractions in small type denote neurotransmitters. GP$_E$, globus pallidus external segment; GP$_I$, globus pallidus internal segment; STN, subthalamic nucleus; SN, substantia nigra (PC, pars compacta; PR, pars reticulata); DRN, dorsal raphe nucleus; RN, raphe nuclei; LC, locus ceruleus; Glut, glutamate; Ach, acetylcholine; Enk, enkephalin; GABA, gamma-aminobutyric acid; SP, substance P; 5-HT, serotonin; NE, norepinephrine.

of afferents to basal ganglia structures arising from extrinsic neuronal groups include the neocortex to the caudate and putamen (collectively referred to as the striatum), the non-specific nuclei of the thalamus to the striatum, the locus ceruleus to the substantia nigra, and the raphe nuclei to the substantia nigra and the striatum. The major efferent pathways from the basal ganglia structures to the extrinsic neuronal groups include the substantia nigra pars reticulata, and the globus pallidus internal segment to the thalamus, as well as the substantia nigra pars reticulata to the deep layers of the superior colliculus, the brainstem reticular formation, and the spinal cord. The various nuclear groups of the basal ganglia are intimately interconnected. The striatum and substantia nigra have prominent reciprocal connections. The striatum also projects to both segments of the globus pallidus. The subthalamic nucleus receives afferents from the external segment of the globus pallidus and projects to both the substantia nigra pars reticulata and the internal segment of the globus pallidus. In addition, the striatum contains numerous interneurons that do not project outside the striatum. (For an extensive review of basal ganglia anatomy, see Ref. 6.)

The neurotransmitters that have been identified for each projection pathway are depicted in Fig. 12-1, but the entirety of a particular projection may not be represented. For example, glutamate is used as a transmitter by neurons projecting from the neocortex to the stratum, but other as yet unidentified neurotransmitters may also be present in this extensive projection. The neurotransmitters used by many of the basal ganglia projection pathways are known; this provides the potential for selective modification of activity in specific basal ganglia circuits by drugs.

Dopamine

GENERAL METABOLISM

Dopamine is synthesized in the brain from the amino acid L-tyrosine via the intermediate compound L-3,4-dihydroxyphenylalanine (L-dopa). Tyrosine hydroxylase (TH), the enzyme that catalyzes the conversion of L-tyrosine to L-dopa, is the rate-limiting step in dopamine synthesis. Because TH is highly localized in catecholamine neurons, it is often used by investigators as a specific marker for dopamine neurons. L-Aromatic amino acid decarboxylase (L-AAAD), the enzyme that catalyzes the conversion of L-dopa to dopamine, has a relatively low substrate specificity and is thought to be present not only in dopamine neurons but also in other cells not specialized to synthesize catecholamines. Once synthesized, dopamine is concentrated in storage vesicles; the membranes of these cytoplasmic organelles contain a high-affinity, energy-dependent, carrier-mediated transport system that concentrates dopamine within the vesicle against a concentration gradient.

Under physiological conditions, dopamine is released from dopaminergic neurons by a calcium-dependent mechanism. Dopamine thus released into the synaptic cleft is inactivated primarily by a high-affinity, stereospecific, carrier-mediated reuptake process. After reuptake, dopamine may be sequestered again in storage vesicles for re-release. Released dopamine in the synaptic cleft may bind to specific cell-surface dopamine receptors on the same neuron from which it is released (autoreceptor) or on another neuron (postsynaptic receptor). Some dopamine receptors are linked positively to a dopamine-sensitive adenylate cyclase enzyme activity. When dopamine occupies this receptor, the rate of synthesis of cyclic adenosine monophosphate (cyclic AMP) is increased. Other cell-surface dopamine receptors appear to be linked negatively to adenylate cyclase. When these receptors are occupied by dopamine, there is a reduction in the rate of cyclic AMP synthesis.[7] At least 5 different dopamine receptors have been cloned and sequenced, each fitting into one of two large families, based on the nature of the linkage to adenylate cyclase (see Chap. 8).

Dopamine is inactivated enzymatically by the action of both monoamine oxidase (MAO), an enzyme associated with mitochondria and present in two forms (MAO-A, and MAO-B), and catechol-*O*-methyltransferase (COMT), an enzyme localized primarily in glial cells in the brain. The resultant deamination and 3-*O*-methylation of dopamine produces homovanillic acid (HVA), the principal metabolite of dopamine (Fig. 12-2).

DISPOSITION OF DOPAMINE NEURONS IN BRAIN

Several dopaminergic neuronal cell groups have been identified in the central nervous system.[8] The most prominent group is the mesotelencephalic group. This group is composed of: the nigrostriatal system, with cell bodies in the substantia nigra pars compacta that project primarily to the striatum, and the mesocortical system, with cell bodies in the ventral tegmental area that project to the mesial frontal, anterior cingulate, and entorhinal cortices; olfactory bulb; anterior olfactory nucleus; olfactory tubercle; piriform cortex; nucleus accumbens; and amygdaloid complex. The tuberohypophysial system projects from the arcuate and periventricular hypothalamic nuclei to the intermediate lobe of the pituitary gland and the median eminence. The incertohypothalamic system projects from the zona incerta and posterior hypothalamus to the dorsal hypothalamic area and septum. Finally, the periventricular system contains cell bodies in the periventricular region of the medulla that project to the periventricular and periaqueductal gray, tegmentum, tectum, thalamus, and hypothalamus. The regional "fallout" of dopaminergic neurons in the subsantia nigra of patients with PD appears to be rather specific and selective.[9] Loss of pigmented neurons appears to be greatest in the lateral ventral tier, followed by the medial ventral tier, and the dorsal tier. This contrasts dramatically with the pattern of pigmented neuron loss during normal aging in the substantia nigra.

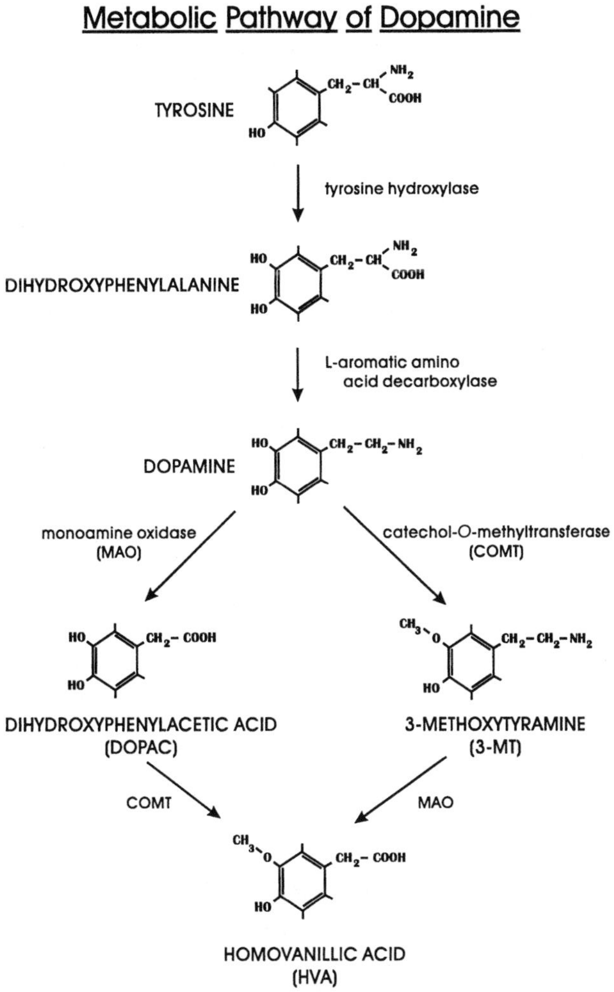

Metabolic Pathway of Dopamine

TYROSINE

↓ tyrosine hydroxylase

DIHYDROXYPHENYLALANINE

↓ L-aromatic amino acid decarboxylase

DOPAMINE

monoamine oxidase (MAO) / \ catechol-O-methyltransferase (COMT)

DIHYDROXYPHENYLACETIC ACID (DOPAC)   3-METHOXYTYRAMINE (3-MT)

COMT \ / MAO

HOMOVANILLIC ACID (HVA)

FIGURE 12-2 Enzymatic synthesis and inactivation of dopamine.

In normal aging, the lateral ventral tier is relatively spared, compared to the cell loss in other regions of the substantia nigra.

ROLE OF DOPAMINE IN PARKINSON'S DISEASE (PD)

The first findings to suggest a role for dopamine in PD were the observations that reserpine treatment produced both the clinical and pathophysiological (i.e., depletion of striatal dopamine) pictures of parkinsonism.[10] Subsequently, Carlsson et al.[10] showed that treatment with the dopamine precursor L-dopa reversed the behavioral effects of reserpine and partially restored brain dopamine levels in laboratory animals. These observations, coupled with early histofluorescence data showing very high concentrations of dopamine in the striatum, led Hornykiewicz to study the concentration of dopamine in postmortem brain material from patients who had died with PD.[3]

The discovery of marked reductions in the concentration of dopamine and HVA in the caudate, putamen, and substantia nigra of parkinsonian patients opened the door to a new era in the diagnosis and treatment of brain disease (Table 12-1).[3,11–13] Furthermore, there was a strong positive correlation between the severity of the premorbid parkinsonian clinical syndrome and the degree of dopamine depletion in the striatum. The data, which are summarized in Table 12-1, showed a reduction in dopamine concentration in all basal ganglia structures. A more recent study of the postmortem striatal dopamine deficit in subregions of the parkinsonian basal ganglia found nearly complete depletion of dopamine in all segments of the putamen.[14] The greatest reduction was found in the caudal portion of the putamen, where dopamine levels were less than 1 percent of those in control postmortem brains.

Interestingly, the degree of reduction in dopamine concentration was much greater than the reduction in HVA concentration in brains of parkinsonian patients (see Table 12-1). Thus, the ratio of dopamine to HVA was much lower in these brains than in those of controls. Similar changes in the dopamine to HVA ratio have been noted following partial lesions of the nigrostriatal pathway in experimental animals, and as a consequence of treatment with dopamine antagonist drugs. These changes in the dopamine to HVA ratio may reflect both an increase in the metabolic activity of the few remaining dopamine neurons and a reduced capacity for reuptake and storage of released dopamine.[15]

Another postmortem study focused on enzymatic markers of dopamine neurons and dopamine metabolism (Table 12-2). This study revealed marked reductions in the activities of TH and L-AAAD in the caudate, putamen, and substantia

TABLE 12-1 Dopamine (DA) and HVA Concentrations in Discrete Brain Regions from Controls and PD Patients

Brain Region	DA (µg/g wet wt)	HVA (µg/g wet wt)	DA/HVA
Putamen[a]			
Control	5.06 ± 0.39(17)	4.92 ± 0.32(16)	1.03
Parkinsonian patient	0.14 ± 0.13(3)	0.54 ± 0.13(3)	0.26
Caudate nucleus[a]			
Control	4.06 ± 0.47(18)	2.92 ± 0.37(19)	1.39
Parkinsonian patient	0.20 ± 0.19(3)	1.19 ± 0.10(3)	0.17
Substantia nigra[b,c]			
Control	0.46(13)[b]	2.32(7)[c]	0.20
Parkinsonian patient	0.07(10)[b]	0.41(9)[c]	0.17
Nucleus accumbens[d]			
Control	3.79 ± 0.82(8)	4.38 ± 0.64(8)	0.86
Parkinsonian patient	1.61 ± 0.28(4)	3.13 ± 0.13(3)	0.51

Results are expressed as mean ± SEM. Number in parentheses is number of cases.
[a]Ref. 11.
[b]Ref. 3.
[c]Ref. 12.
[d]Ref. 13.

TABLE 12-2 Activities of TH, L-AAAD, COMT, and MAO in Discrete Brain Regions from Controls and PD Patients

Brain Region	TH (nmol CO_2/30 min/100 mg protein)	L-AAAD (nmol CO_2/2h/100 mg protein)	COMT (nmol NMN/h/100 mg protein)	MAO (nmol PPA/30 min/100 mg protein)
Putamen				
Control	$17.4 \pm 2.4(3)$	$432 \pm 109(18)$	$24.1 \pm 2.5(11)$	$1520 \pm 127(11)$
Parkinsonian patient	$3.1 \pm 1.2(3)^a$	$32 \pm 7(13)^b$	$19.8 \pm 3.7(9)$	$1648 \pm 128(10)$
Caudate nucleus				
Control	$18.7 \pm 2.0(3)$	$364 \pm 95(19)$	$25.4 \pm 2.8(10)$	$1726 \pm 149(10)$
Parkinsonian patient	$3.2 \pm 0.5(2)^a$	$54 \pm 14(13)^b$	$17.8 \pm 3.8(9)$	$1742 \pm 197(10)$
Substantia nigra				
Control	$17.4(1)$	$549 \pm 294(15)$	$26.4 \pm 4.7(5)$	$1828 \pm 200(5)$
Parkinsonian patient	$6.1 \pm 1.5(3)$	$21 \pm 6(10)$	$21.7 \pm 10.2(9)$	$1477 \pm 284(4)$

Results are expressed as mean $\pm$ SEM. Number in parentheses is number of patients.
[a]Differs from control $P < 0.02$.
[b]Differs from control $P < 0.01$.
Source: Data derived from Ref. 11.

nigra of patients with PD, but no changes were found in the levels of activity of MAO and COMT. These results reflect the high degree of localization of TH and L-AAAD in dopamine neurons in the striatum, compared to the more general distribution of MAO and nonneuronal distribution of COMT activities.

Radiolabeled cocaine has been used as a ligand marker for the neuronal membrane transport site responsible for the reuptake of catecholamines into catecholaminergic neurons. The binding of cocaine to striatal membranes in patients who died with PD was greatly reduced, compared to that of controls.[16] Similar findings have been obtained with ligands more selective for the dopamine reuptake site, such as GBR-12935.[17] These results support previous evidence of a large reduction in all measurable neuronal markers for nigrostriatal dopaminergic neurons in the brains of patients with PD.

DOPAMINE RECEPTORS

The principal molecular site of action of dopamine in the brain is at dopamine receptors. Dopamine receptors are divided into two main families or categories: D1-like (positively linked to adenylate cyclase), and D2-like (negatively linked to adenylate cyclase).[7] Five different dopamine receptors have now been cloned and sequenced, but each of the 5 falls into one of the two main "families." Thus, D1-like receptors include D1 and D5, whereas D2, D3, and D4 are D2-like receptors. The D1 and D2 types are expressed predominantly in the basal ganglia, whereas D3, D4, and D5 have a low level of expression in this structure (see Chap. 8).

D1 receptors in the basal ganglia appear to be expressed predominantly by striatonigral and striatopallidal (to medial pallidum) neurons that are GABAergic and also express substance P and dynorphin. In contrast, D2 receptors appear to be expressed primarily by substantia nigra dopaminergic neurons (autoreceptors), cholinergic interneurons in the striatum (i.e., some large aspiny neurons), and striatopallidal neurons projecting to the lateral segment of the globus pallidus that are GABAergic and coexpress enkephalin. Physiologically, the striatonigral and striatomedial pallidal pathways appear to be activated by the action of dopamine, whereas the striatolateral pallidal pathway appears to be tonically inhibited by the action of dopamine. However, the capacity of dopamine to reverse optimally the bradykinesia, rigidity, and tremor caused by dopamine depletion appears to require the action of dopamine at both receptor types. (For a brief review of this subject, see Ref. 18.)

Numerous studies on dopamine receptor number and density have been carried out in the brains of patients with PD and in experimental animal models of the disease. So far, these studies have contributed little to our understanding of the mechanism of side-effects of L-dopa and dopamine agonists such as psychosis and dyskinesia, nor have they yet resulted in improvement in the management of patients with PD.

As both D1 and D2 receptors are involved in the motor response to exogenous L-dopa, a recent focus of interest has been centered in studying whether polymorphisms of the genes coding for these receptors could be implicated in the genetic susceptibility to PDD.

Certain alleles of the short tandem repeat polymorphism of the dopamine receptor D2 gene have been found to reduce the risk of developing peak-of-dose dyskinesias and may contribute to decreased susceptibility to such induced dyskinesias.[19]

Norepinephrine

The principal source of noradrenergic afferents to the forebrain is the locus ceruleus.[20] The locus ceruleus is one of the pigmented brainstem nuclei that is characteristically abnormal in the brains of parkinsonian patients. Specifically, these brains show depigmentation and loss of neurons, with Lewy bodies in the locus ceruleus. Several investigators have described reductions of norepinephrine concentration and dopamine-beta-hydroxylase activity (a specific enzymatic marker of noradrenergic neurons) in forebrain regions. [21,22] Data are conflicting about whether norepinephrine levels are affected in the hypothalamus of patients with PD.[21,23] Studies of dopamine-beta-hydroxylase activity in the A1 and A2 noradrenergic areas of the brainstem of parkinsonian patients did not reveal any changes, suggesting that these nuclear groups, which also have rostral projections, are spared in PD.[24] Because levels of norepinephrine were rarely below 50 percent of those of controls in the brains of parkinsonian patients, and, apparently, because certain noradrenergic cell groups of the lower brainstem were spared completely, it is unlikely that PD is associated with a generalized central catecholaminergic deficiency. The consequences of reduced norepinephrine levels in the adult brain are not clear, although evidence for both motor and cognitive functions of noradrenergic systems has been presented.[20]

Serotonin

The principal locations of cell bodies of serotonergic neurons are the raphe nuclei of the brainstem. There is no neuropathological evidence to suggest that these cell groups are specifically affected in PD. Nevertheless, serotonin levels were reduced throughout the forebrain in patients with PD, particularly in the striatum, substantia nigra, and hippocampus.[22,25] The mechanism and significance of the reduction in brain serotonin levels are not known; however, reduced serotonin levels may represent regulation of serotonergic neuronal activity in response to reduced activity of dopaminergic and/or noradrenergic neurons.

Gamma-Aminobutyric Acid

Gamma-aminobutyric acid (GABA) is a neurotransmitter found in several prominent basal ganglia projection pathways. There are probably GABA-releasing interneurons in the striatum, as well as GABAergic striatopallidal, striatonigral, nigrocollicular, and pallidothalamic projections.[6] No studies have suggested that these neurons are affected primarily by the pathological process in PD. It is possible, however, that up- or downregulation of GABA activity might occur as a consequence of dopamine depletion in the striatum.

Two specific markers for GABAergic neurons have been studied in postmortem brain material from patients with PD. These include direct measurement of brain GABA levels and assay of the activity of glutamic acid decarboxylase (GAD), the enzyme that catalyzes the conversion of glutamic acid to GABA. Perry et al. found that GABA levels were elevated significantly in the putamen of parkinsonian patients,[26] whereas

Laaksonen et al. found reduced GABA levels in cerebral and cerebellar cortices but no change in GABA levels in any other brain region.[27] Lloyd and Hornykiewicz found reduced GAD activity (approximately 50 percent of that of controls) in the striatum, globus pallidus, and substantia nigra,[28] a finding confirmed by Laaksonen.[27] Subsequently, Perry et al. reported, however, that GAD activity in the putamen of parkinsonian patients did not differ from that in controls.[26]

Thus, there is controversy about whether GAD activity is altered in the brains of patients with PD. Nevertheless, the critical issue is whether GABA turnover is altered and, if so, in which neuronal groups. The development of pharmacological means to manipulate GABA neurotransmission is a potential avenue for new therapeutic strategies in the management of Parkinson's disease.

Acetylcholine

The principal site of action of cholinergic neurons in basal ganglia circuitry is thought to be the numerous cholinergic interneurons identified in the striatum.[6] Measurement of the activity of choline acetyltransferase (ChAT), the enzyme that catalyzes the one-step synthesis of acetylcholine, is the most frequently used marker for the cholinergic neurons. Lloyd et al. reported a significant reduction in ChAT activity in the putamen, caudate nucleus, globus pallidus, and substantia nigra in the brains of parkinsonian patients.[29] These changes in activity, again, may reflect regulation in response to reduced dopamine levels, rather than primary pathological involvement. Ruberg et al. found reduced ChAT activity in cerebral cortex and hippocampus in brains of patients with PD, which perhaps relates to the dementing process in these patients.[30]

Neuropeptides

Several of the neuropeptides regarded as neurotransmitters or neuromodulators are present in rather high concentrations in some nuclear groups of the basal ganglia. Their distribution has been mapped by immunocytochemical techniques, and radioimmunoassays have been used to quantify regional concentrations of various neuropeptides.

Motor signs of Parkinson's disease have been ascribed in part to overinhibition of the external globus pallidus secondary to hyperactivity of striatopallidal GABA/enkephalinergic neurons.[31]

Inhibition of pallidal GABA release following a dopamine-depleting lesion suggests that enkephalin may attenuate such release in the globus pallidus, specifically after striatal dopamine loss in PD animal models.[31]

Recently Fernandez et al.[32] measured the levels of the neuropeptides Met- and Leu-enkephalin, substance P, and neurotensin by a combined high-performance liquid chromatography-radioimmunoassay method in autopsy samples of basal ganglia from PD patients, incidental Lewy body disease patients (presymptomatic PD) and matched controls. Dopamine levels were reduced in the caudate nucleus and putamen in PD, but were unaltered in incidental Lewy body disease, while Met-enkephalin values were reduced in the caudate nucleus, putamen, and substantia nigra in PD. Whereas Met-enkephalin levels were reduced in the caudate nucleus and in the putamen in incidental Lewy body disease, Leu-enkephalin levels were decreased in the putamen and undetectable in the substantia nigra in PD. Leu-enkephalin levels were unchanged in incidental Lewy body disease, although there was a trend to reduction in putamen. Substance P levels were reduced in the putamen in PD, but no significant changes were observed in incidental Lewy body disease. Neurotensin levels were increased in the substantia nigra in PD, but were not altered significantly in incidental Lewy body disease, tending to parallel the changes in PD. The changes in basal ganglia peptide levels in incidental Lewy body disease generally followed a trend similar to those seen in PD, but were less marked, suggesting that they are integral part of the disease pathology rather than secondary to dopaminergic neuronal loss or long-term drug therapy.

De Ceballos and Lopez-Lozano[33] assessed Met-enkephalin substance P, and TH immunostaining in caudate nucleus biopsies from 15 PD patients who underwent surgical procedures, amd found that low Met-enkephalin immunostaining tended to correlate with disease severity. The different patterns of abnormalities found suggest that a variety of neurochemical phenotypes may exist among PD patients.

Changes in preproenkephalin gene expression in the caudate and putamen have been associated to striatal damage, but their role in the pathogenesis of L-DOPA-induced dyskinesias remains controversial.[34]

Functional interactions between somatostatinergic and dopaminergic transmitter systems have been well documented, supporting a role of somatostatin in several neuropsychiatric disorders, including PD.[35]

Some investigators have suggested that cholecystokinin-8 (CCK-8) coexists with dopamine in dopaminergic neurons.[36] However, using radioimmunoassay methods, Studler et al. found reduced CCK-8 levels in the substantia nigra but not in striatal or corticolimbic areas innervated by dopaminergic neurons.[37] These results from postmortem brains of parkinsonian patients cast doubt on the coexistence of dopamine and CCK-8 in nigral neurons.

Somatostatin levels in the basal ganglia of nondemented patients with PD failed to differ from those of controls.[38] However, somatostatin levels in the frontal cortex, hippocampus, and entorhinal cortex of demented parkinsonian patients were reduced, compared to levels in nondemented parkinsonian patients.[38]

As more information is accumulated about the cellular localization and physiological function of neuropeptides, the significance of these various changes in PD may be elucidated.

Endogenous Free Radical Scavengers and Generators

Oxidative stress appears to play a leading role in the pathogenesis of PD[39–41] (see Chap. 13). Studies aimed at elucidating the mechanism of MPTP- induced neuronal toxicity mainly focused much attention on the possibility that oxidative MPTP metabolism generates cytotoxic free radical species. Cohen speculated that the generation of free radical species by MAO activity may contribute to dopaminergic neuronal death in PD.[42] In primates, the dopaminergic nigrostriatal neurons contain high concentrations of the pigment neuromelanin. Graham argued that PD may result from cytotoxicity of the products of catecholamine and melanin oxidation.[43] Furthermore, the concentration of iron is now known to be increased, and that of ferritin reduced, in the brains of patients with PD.[44] Iron catalyzes the production of hydroxyl radicals from hydrogen peroxide. Thus, the higher concentrations of free iron in the parkinsonian brain may predispose this disease state to a high rate of free radical production.[44]

Recently, disturbances in brain iron metabolism have been linked to synucleinopathies. Iron binding to alpha-synuclein accumulated in Lewy bodies was investigated by Golts et al., who found that the conformation of alpha-synuclein may be modulated by metals, with iron stimulating aggregation and magnesium inhibiting.[45]

In a similar study, it was found that free radical generators such as dopamine and hydrogen peroxide also stimulate the production of intracellular aggregates of alpha-synuclein and ubiquitin.[46] Sangchot et al. documented that abnormal iron accumulation decreased cell viability, and increased lipid peroxidation. In addition, morphological studies disclosed that iron altered mitochondrial morphology, disrupted the nuclear membrane, and translocated alpha-synuclein from perinuclear regions into the disrupted nucleus.[47] Recently, Borie et al. investigated the association between iron-related gene polymorphisms and PD and found a significantly higher frequency of G258S transferrin polymorphisms in PD patients, particularly in cases with onset after age 60 and negative family history. Such findings suggest that genetic variations in the control of iron metabolism may contribute to the pathogenesis of PD.[48]

Free radicals are generated constantly in all living tissue, and, when their intracellular concentrations become too high, damage to cellular elements (e.g., lipid, protein, DNA) may occur. Such damage is minimized by endogenous agents such as glutathione, ascorbate, beta-carotene, and tocopherol,[49] which are free radical "scavengers." Also, enzymatic defenses exist that "scavenge" free radicals; these enzymes include superoxide dismutase, catalase, and glutathione peroxidase (which requires reduced glutathione).[49] Kunikowska and Jenner studied the regional distribution in rat basal ganglia of messenger ribonucleic acid (mRNA) for the antioxidant enzymes Cu-Zn superoxide dismutase (SOD), MnSOD, and glutathione peroxidase. mRNA levels were significantly higher in substantia nigra pars compacta than in other regions of the basal ganglia, suggesting that substantia nigra pars compacta would be vulnerable to oxidative stress without the high antioxidant capacity provided by these cytoprotective enzymes.[50]

Interestingly the substantia nigra of early PD patients has dramatically decreased levels of the thiol tripeptide glutathione.[40] Perry et al. reported that reduced glutathione levels were lower in the substantia nigra than in any other human brain region, and that reduced glutathione levels were absent virtually from the substantia nigra of patients dying with PD.[51] Because reduced glutathione is an important endogenous antioxidant, as well as a cofactor for the free radical-scavenging enzyme glutathione peroxidase, it is interesting to speculate that the substantia nigra may be the region of the brain most susceptible to the toxic effects of free radicals. In vitro studies have demonstrated that the reduction in cellular glutathione is associated with a decrease in ubiquitin-protein conjugate levels, and such inhibition of the ubiquitin proteosome protein degradation pathway may contribute to protein build-up and subsequent cell death.[52] Furthermore, it was shown that glutathione depletion results in selective inhibition of mitochondrial complex I activity.[39]

The activity of catalase has also been reported to be reduced in the brains of patients with PD.[53]

Increased products of lipid peroxidation have been found in the substantia nigra in the parkinsonian brain, and this was associated with a decrease in polyunsaturated fatty acids, which are the substrates for lipid peroxidation.[54] A 10-fold increase in lipid hydroperoxides in the parkinsonian brain has also been documented.[55]

Each of the above observations provides circumstantial evidence to support a role for excessive free radical production in the pathogenesis of PD.

Mitochondrial Function

Over the last few years the mitochondrion has been regarded as the link for signaling pathways involved in degenerative processes. The mitochondrion seems to play a major role in the cellular decision-making that leads, irreversibly, toward the execution phase of cellular death processes[56] (see Chaps. 5 and 14). Mitochondria are the major source of superoxide, and are responsible for activating apoptosis and oxidative damage during acute neuronal cell death and neurodegenerative disorders such as Alzheimer's disease and PD.[57]

In 1989, Parker et al. reported a selective reduction in the activity of complex I of the mitochondrial electron transport chain in platelets of patients with PD,[58] a finding confirmed by several research teams (e.g., Benecke et al,[59]). Subsequently, a selective reduction in NADH-coenzyme Q1 reductase activity (specific for complex I) was reported in the substantia nigra, but not in other areas of the brain, including

the globus pallidum and cerebral cortex,[60] of patients with PD.[61] Furthermore, such abnormality was not found in postmortem material from patients with multisystem atrophy. It is thus a remarkable coincidence that MPP^+, the active toxic metabolite of MPTP, appears to exert its cytotoxic effects by inhibiting complex I of the mitochondrial electron transport chain.

Recently, a family of Sephardic Jews with progressive external ophthalmoparesis, skeletal muscle weakness, and parkinsonism with an autosomal-recessive inheritance suggesting a novel mitochondrial disorder of intergenomic communication has been reported.[62]

Experimental work with animal models chronically exposed to the pesticide rotenone, a complex I inhibitor which mimics the complex I deficit in PD, caused retrograde degeneration of the substantia nigra over several months.[63,64] In addition, recent studies showed that abnormal accumulation of alpha-synuclein could lead to mitochondrial alterations liable to result in oxidative stress and, eventually, cell death.[65]

Preliminary studies suggest that coenzyme Q10, an essential cofactor of the electron transport gene as well as a major antioxidant, which is particularly effective within mitochondria, appears to slow down the progressive deterioration of function in PD,[66] while blocking the apoptotic cascade, has been proposed as a target of neuroprotective therapy.[67]

Again, whether these changes in complex I activity are primary or secondary and whether they are genetically transmitted or acquired remains to be shown. Hopefully, a deeper understanding of mitochondrial dysfunction in PD will afford clues to develop novel therapeutic efforts.

In Vivo Neurochemistry: Positron Emission Tomography in Parkinson's Disease

Positron emission tomography (PET) techniques have provided the first reliable in vivo marker for neurochemical deficit in PD (see Chap. 3).

PET may be useful to assess disease progression and the efficacy of diverse neuroprotective therapies, as well as the impact of functional neurosurgery on PD patients.[68–70] More recently, PET techniques have been employed to assess subclinical dopaminergic dysfunction in asymptomatic (parkin) mutation carriers.[71,72]

Using ^{18}F-fluorodeoxyglucose and PET imaging techniques, it is possible to estimate in vivo the regional rate of glucose utilization in brains of parkinsonian patients.

Martin et al. found increased glucose utilization in the inferomedial portion of the basal ganglia, probably corresponding to the globus pallidus, in patients with PD.[73] Similar changes were also reported using [15]O imaging with PET techniques in parkinsonian patients.[74] Such an increase in glucose utilization in the globus pallidus was seen in experimental animals with lesions of the substantia nigra, and may represent increased physiological activity in striatal efferents to the globus pallidus as a consequence of reduced dopamine neurotransmission in the striatum.[75]

Another advance in the field of in vivo neurochemistry using PET technology was the development of a method to image dopamine neurons, using radiolabeled L-dopa.[76]

To date, ^{18}F-dopa has been the gold standard to measure presynaptic dopaminergic function. Striatal uptake of ^{18}F-dopa is markedly decreased in PD, more in putamen than in caudate nucleus, and inversely correlates with the severity of motor signs and disease duration.[77]

The uptake of this tracer depends not only on the density of dopaminergic terminals in the striatum but also on dopamine turnover, which in early-stage PD is increased as a result of compensatory mechanisms of surviving dopaminergic terminals. Therefore, ^{18}F-dopa uptake may be upregulated in early PD. [78,79] The density of dopaminergic terminals may be assessed using new dopamine ligands such as [76]Br-Fe-CBT. Riveiro et al. compared the striatal uptake of ^{18}F-dopa and [76]Br-Fe-CBT in patients with early and advanced PD. They found that reduction in [76]Br-Fe-CBT uptake was more severe than reduction of ^{18}F-dopa uptake in early stages. Interestingly, no significant differences were found in the reduction of both tracers in advanced PD patients, suggesting that compensatory mechanisms are only present in early PD and that ^{18}F-dopa, but not [76]Br-Fe-CBT, is upregulated in early disease.[78]

Nummi et al., using ^{18}F-dopa PET scan, found that the disease process in PD first affects posterior putamen, followed by the anterior putamen, and caudate nucleus but, once started, the absolute rate of decline is the same.[68]

Finally, the use of PET for the differential diagnosis of movement disorders is gaining clinical relevance since new tracers are becoming available, as well as objective techniques for the interpretation of PET images in order to achieve an operator-independent analysis.[80] Unfortunately, these methods are extremely expensive and only available as a research tool.

Neurochemical Analysis of Lewy Bodies

These intraneuronal cytoplasmic inclusions were found first in neurons of the substantia innominata and dorsal motor nucleus of the vagus.[81] Subsequently, Lewy bodies were also detected in pigmented cells of the substantia nigra, as well as in the hypothalamus, locus ceruleus, raphe nuclei of the midbrain and rostral pons, sympathetic ganglia, and spinal cord.[82] The dense core of Lewy bodies is composed of tightly packed aggregates of filaments, vesicular profiles, and other granular material; at the periphery, filamentous structures emerge radially and are mixed with granular and vesicular material. Immunocytochemical studies using polyclonal antibodies to neurofilament polypeptides have demonstrated specific staining of Lewy bodies.[83]

Recently, intracytoplasmic inclusions consisting of alpha-synuclein, a brain presynaptic protein, have been shown to be characteristic of neurodegenerative Lewy body disorders, and an unprecedented and extensive burden of alpha-synuclein pathology in the striatum has been described.[84,85] Alpha-synuclein is a major component of Lewy bodies and Lewy neurites, intraneuronal inclusions that are regarded as neuropathological hallmarks of PD.[86] These findings have provided important clues about the pathogenesis of PD.

Two missense mutations of the alpha-synuclein gene (A30P and A53T) have been described in several families with an autosomal dominant form of PD, but alpha-synuclein also constitutes one of the main components of Lewy bodies in sporadic cases of PD.[87] Moreover, it has been shown that glial cells, both astrocytes and oligodendrocytes, are also affected by alpha-synuclein pathology.[88] However, the pathogenic relationship between alterations in the biology of alpha-synuclein and PD-associated neurodegeneration remains speculative. Protein aggregation appears to be the common denominator in a series of distinct neurodegenerative diseases, although its role in the associated neuronal pathology in these various conditions is still elusive. The accumulation of alpha-synuclein, ubiquitin, and other proteins in Lewy bodies in degenerating dopaminergic neurons in substantia nigra in idiopathic PD suggests that inhibition of normal/abnormal protein degradation may contribute to neuronal death. However, although it appears likely that aggregation of alpha-synuclein may interfere with its normal function in the cell, this is not the primary cause of the related neurodegeneration.[89]

In support, in vitro models of proteasomal dysfunction that replicate the two cardinal pathological features of Lewy body diseases (namely, neuronal death, and the formation of cytoplasmic ubiquitinated inclusions) suggest that inclusion body formation and cell death may be dissociated from one another.[90]

Recent evidence that inhibition of the ubiquitin-proteasome pathway leads to altered protein handling and Lewy body formation suggests that this dysfunction may be responsible for degeneration of the nigrostriatal pathway in idiopathic PD.[91] Parkin mutations can also cause familial PD and parkin is also found in Lewy bodies. Interestingly, the absence of Lewy bodies in patients with parkin mutations suggests that parkin might be necessary for the formation of Lewy bodies.[92]

Recently, it has been shown that parkin interacts with and ubiquitinates the alpha-synuclein-interacting protein, synphilin-1, a novel protein that interacts with alpha-synuclein.[88,93] Coexpression of alpha-synuclein, synphilin-1, and parkin results in the formation of Lewy-body-like ubiquitin-positive cytosolic inclusions.[92]

Although little is known about its normal function, alpha-synuclein appears to interact with a variety of proteins and membrane phospholipids, and may therefore participate in a number of signaling pathways. In particular, it may play a role in regulating cell differentiation, synaptic plasticity, cell survival, and dopaminergic neurotransmission.[11]

It should be noted, however, that Lewy bodies may simply represent a cellular response to some other primary insult (see also Chap. 20).

Significance of Neurochemical Studies of Parkinson's Disease

Selective degeneration of the dopaminergic nigrostriatal pathway is the central pathological process in PD. The resulting reduction in striatal dopamine concentration is a condition sufficient for the emergence of the signs and symptoms of parkinsonism. The development of L-dopa therapy and newer direct-acting dopamine agonists in the treatment of PD grew out of the recognition of this relationship between dopamine deficiency and parkinsonian symptoms.

The changes in levels of other neurotransmitters, in neuronal markers, and in regional brain metabolism probably represent regulatory responses to the decrement in striatal dopamine neurotransmission. Future neurochemical studies holding the greatest promise of benefit to parkinsonian patients may be divided into two categories: studies aimed at understanding the effects of dopamine depletion on other neurons, and neurotransmitter systems that allow the symptoms of parkinsonism to emerge, may form the basis for new therapeutic strategies to supplement dopamine replacement; studies aimed at identifying the source of the selective vulnerability of dopamine neurons in patients with PD could result in therapeutic strategies to arrest the progression of, or actually prevent, PD.

References

1. Wilson SAK: Progressive lenticular degeneration: A familial nervous disease associated with cirrhosis of the liver. *Brain* 34:295–489, 1912.
2. Hassler R: Zur Pathologie der Paralysis Agitans und des postenzephalitischen Parkinsonismus. *J Psychol Neurol* 48:387–476, 1938.
3. Hornykiewicz O: Die topische Lokalisation und das Verhalten von Noradrenalin und Dopamin (3-Hydroxytyramin) in der Substantia Nigra des normalen und parkinsonkranken Menschen. *Wien Klin Wochenschr* 75:309–312, 1963.
4. Hornykiewicz O: Dopamine (3-hydroxytyramine) and brain function. *Pharmacol Rev* 18:925–962, 1966.
5. Langston JW, Ballard P, Tetrud JW, Irwin I: Chronic parkinsonism in humans due to a product of meperidine-analog synthesis. *Science* 291:979–980, 1983.
6. Carpenter MB: Anatomy of the corpus striatum and brainstem integrating systems, in Brooks VB (ed): *Handbook of Physiology.* Bethesda, MD: American Physiological Society, 1981, pp 947–995.

7. Stoof JC, Kebabian JW: Two dopamine receptors: Biochemistry, physiology and pharmacology. *Life Sci* 35:2281–2296, 1984.
8. Moore RY, Bloom FE: Central catecholamine neuron systems: Anatomy and physiology of the dopamine systems. *Annu Rev Neurosci* 1:129–169, 1976.
9. Fearnley JM, Lees AJ: Aging and Parkinson's disease: Substantia nigra regional selectivity. *Brain* 114: 2283–2301, 1991.
10. Carlsson A, Lindquist M, Magnusson T: 3,4-Dihydroxyphenylalanine and 5-hydroxytryptophan as reserpine antagonists. *Nature* 180:1200–1201, 1957.
11. Lloyd KG, Davidson L, Hornykiewicz O: The neurochemistry of Parkinson's disease: Effect of L-dopa therapy. *J Pharmacol Exp Ther* 195:453–464, 1975.
12. Bernheimer H, Hornykiewicz O: Herabgesetzte Konzentration der Homovanillinsäuure im Gehirn von parkinsonkranken Menschen als Ausdruck des Stöurung des zentralen Opaminstofwechsels. *Klin Wochenschr* 43:711–715, 1965.
13. Price KS, Farley IJ, Hornykiewicz O: Neurochemistry of Parkinson's disease: Relation between striatal and limbic dopamine. *Adv Biochem Psychopharmacol* 19:293–300, 1978.
14. Kish SJ, Shannak K, Hornykiewicz O: Uneven pattern of dopamine loss in the striatum of patients with idiopathic Parkinson's disease. *N Engl J Med* 318:876–880, 1988.
15. Zigmond MJ, Stricker EM: Parkinson's disease: Studies with an animal model. *Life Sci* 35:5–18, 1984.
16. Pimoule C, Schoemaker H, Javoy-Agid F, et al: Decrease in [^{3}H] cocaine binding to the dopamine transporter in Parkinson's disease. *Eur J Pharmacol* 95:145–146, 1983.
17. Maloteaux J-M, Vanisberg M-A, Laterre C, et al: [^{3}H]GBR 12935 binding to dopamine uptake sites: Subcellular localization and reduction in Parkinson's disease and progressive supranuclear palsy. *Eur J Pharmacol* 156:331–340, 1988.
18. Trugman JM, Leadbetter R, Zolis ME, et al: Treatment of severe axial tardive dystonia with clozapine: Case report and hypothesis. *Mov Disord* 9:441–4464, 1994.
19. Oliveri RL, Annesi G, Zappia M, et al: Dopamine D2 receptor gene polymorphism and the risk of levodopa induced dyskinesias in PD. *Neurology* 53:1425–1430, 1999.
20. Moore RY, Bloom FE: Central catecholamine neuron systems: Anatomy and physiology of the norepinephrine and epinephrine systems. *Annu Rev Neurosci* 2:113–168, 1979.
21. Farley IJ, Hornykiewicz O: Noradrenaline in subcortical brain regions of patients with Parkinson's disease and control subjects, in Birkmayer W, Hornykiewicz O (eds): *Advances in Parkinsonism.* Basel: Editiones Roche, 1976, pp 178–185.
22. Scatton B, Javoy-Agid F, Rouquier L, et al: Reduction of cortical dopamine, noradrenaline, serotonin, and their metabolites in Parkinson's disease. *Brain Res* 275:321–328, 1983.
23. Javoy-Agid F, Rubert M, Taquet H, et al: Biochemical neuropathology of Parkinson's disease. *Adv Neurol.* 40:189–198, 1984.
24. Kopp N, Denoroy L, Thomasi M, et al: Increase in noradrenaline-synthesizing enzyme activity in medulla oblongata in Parkinson's disease. *Acta Neuropathol* 56:17–21, 1982.
25. Bernheimer H, Birkmayer W, Hornykiewicz O: Verteilung des 5-Hydroxytryptamin (Serotonin) in Gehirn des Menschen und sein Verhalten bei Patienten mit Parkinson-Syndrom. *Klin Wochenschr* 39:1056–1059, 1961.
26. Perry TL, Javoy-Agid F, Agid Y, Fibiger HC: Striatal gabaergic neuronal activity is not reduced in Parkinson's disease. *J Neurochem* 40:1120–1123, 1983.

27. Laaksonen H, Rinne UK, Sonninen V, Riekkinen P: Brain GABA neurons in Parkinson's disease. *Acta Neurol Scand* 57 (suppl 67):282–283, 1978.

28. Lloyd KG, Hornykiewicz O: L-Glutamic acid decarboxylase in Parkinson's disease: Effect of L-dopa therapy. *Nature* 243: 521–523, 1973.

29. Lloyd KG, Möhler H, Hertz P, Bartholini G: Distribution of choline acetyltransferase and glutamate decarboxylase within the substantia nigra and in other brain regions from control and parkinsonian patients. *J Neurochem* 25:789–795, 1975.

30. Ruberg M, Ploska A, Javoy-Agid F, Agid Y: Muscarinic binding and choline acetyltransferase activity in parkinsonian subjects with reference to dementia. *Brain Res* 232:129–139, 1982.

31. Schroeder JA, Schneider JS: GABA-opioid interactions in the globus pallidus: [D-Ala2]-Met-enkephalinamide attenuates potassium-evoked GABA release after nigrostriatal lesion. *J Neurochem* 82:666–673, 2002.

32. Fernandez A, de Ceballos ML, Rose S, et al: Alterations in peptide levels in Parkinson's disease and incidental Lewy body disease. *Brain* 119:823–830, 1996.

33. De Ceballos ML, Lopez-Lozano JJ: Subgroups of parkinsonian patients differentiated by peptidergic immunostaining of caudate nucleus biopsies. *Peptides* 20:249–257, 1999.

34. Quik M, Police S, Langston JW, Di Monte DA: Increases in striatal preproenkephalin gene expression are associated with nigrostriatal damage but not L-DOPA-induced dyskinesias in the squirrel monkey. *Neuroscience* 113:213–220, 2002.

35. Lu JQ, Stoessl AJ: Somatostatin modulates the behavioral effects of dopamine receptor activation in parkinsonian rats. *Neuroscience* 112:261–266, 2002.

36. Hökfelt T, Skirboll L, Rehfeld JF, et al: A subpopulation of mesencephalic dopamine neurons projecting to limbic areas contains a cholecystokinin-like peptide: Evidence from immunohistochemistry combined with retrograde tracing. *Neuroscience* 5:2093–2124, 1980.

37. Studler JM, Javoy-Agid F, Cesselin F, et al: CCK-8-immunoreactivity distribution in human brain: Selective decrease in the substantia nigra from parkinsonian patients. *Brain Res* 243:176–179, 1982.

38. Epelbaum J, Ruberg M, Moyse E, et al: Somatostatin and dementia in Parkinson's disease. *Brain Res* 278:376–379, 1983.

39. Jha N, Jurma O, Lalli G, et al: Glutathione depletion in PC12 results in selective inhibition of mitochondrial complex I activity. Implications in Parkinson's disease. *J Biol Chem* 275:26096–26101, 2000.

40. Mytilineou C, Kramer BC, Yabut JA: Glutathione depletion and oxidative stress. *Parkinsonism Relat Disord* 8:385–387, 2002.

41. Yoshioka M, Tanaka K, Miyazaki I, et al: The dopamine agonist cabergoline provides neuroprotection by activation of the glutathione system and scavenging free radicals. *Neurosci Res* 43:259–267, 2002.

42. Cohen G: The pathobiology of Parkinson's disease: Biochemical aspects of dopamine neuron senescence. *J Neural Trans* 19(suppl):89–103, 1983.

43. Graham DG: Catecholamine toxicity: A proposal for the molecular pathogenesis of manganese neurotoxicity and Parkinson's disease. *Neurotoxicology* 5:83–96, 1984.

44. Fahn S, Cohen G: The oxidant stress hypothesis in Parkinson's disease: Evidence supporting it. *Ann Neurol* 32:804–812, 1992.

45. Golts N, Snyder H , Frasier M, et al: Magnesium inhibits spontaneous and iron induced aggregation of alpha synuclein. *J Biol Chem* 277:16116–16123, 2002.

46. Ostretova-Golts N, Petrucelli L, Hardy J, et al: The A53T alpha synuclein mutation increases iron dependent aggregation and toxicity. *J Neurosci* 20:6048–6054, 2002.

47. Sangchot P, Sharma S, Chetsawang B, et al: Deferoxamine attenuates iron-induced oxidative stress and prevents mitochondrial aggregation and alpha-synuclein translocation in SK-N-SH cells in culture. *Dev Neurosci* 24:143–153, 2002.

48. Borie C, Gasparini F, Verpillat P, et al: French Parkinson's Disease Genetic Study Group. Association study between iron-related genes polymorphisms and Parkinson's disease. *J Neurol* 249: 801–804, 2002.

49. Freeman BA, Crapo JD: Biology of disease: Free radicals and tissue injury. *Lab Invest* 47:412–426, 1982.

50. Kunikowska G, Jenner P: The distribution of copper, zinc and manganese superoxide dismutase, and glutathione peroxidase messenger ribonucleic acid in rat basal ganglia. *Biochem Pharmacol* 63:1159–1164, 2002.

51. Perry TL, Godin DV, Hansen S: Parkinson's disease: A disorder due to nigral glutathione deficiency? *Neurosci Lett* 33:305–310, 1982.

52. Jha N, Kumar MJ, Boonplueang R, Andersen JK: Glutathione decreases in dopaminergic PC12 cells interfere with the ubiquitin protein degradation pathway: Relevance for Parkinson's disease? *J Neurochem* 80:555–561, 2002.

53. Ambani LM, Van Woert MH, Murphy S: Brain peroxidase and catalase in Parkinson's disease. *Arch Neurol* 32:114–118, 1975.

54. Dexter DT, Carter CJ, Wells FR: Basal lipid peroxidation in substantia nigra is increased in Parkinson's disease. *J Neurochem* 52:381–389, 1989.

55. Jenner P: Oxidative stress as a cause of Parkinson's disease. *Acta Neurol Scand* 84:6–15, 1991.

56. Tornero D, Ce a V, Gonzalez Garcia C, Jordan J: The role of the mitochondrial permeability transition pore in neurodegenerative processes. *Rev Neurol* 35:354–361, 2002.

57. Tornero D, Ce a V, Gonzalez Garcia C, Jordan J: The role of the mitochondrial permeability transition pore in neurodegenerative processes. *Rev Neurol* 35:354–361,2002.

58. Parker WD, Boyson SJ, Parks JK: Abnormalities of the electron transport chain in idiopathic Parkinson's disease. *Ann Neurol* 26:719–723, 1989.

59. Benecke R, Strumper P, Weiss H: Electron transfer complexes I and IV of platelets are abnormal in Parkinson's disease but normal in Parkinson-plus syndromes. *Brain* 116:1451–1463, 1993.

60. Ebadi M, Govitrapong P, Sharma S, et al: Ubiquinone (coenzyme Q10) and mitochondria in oxidative stress of Parkinson's disease. *Biol Signals Recept* 10:224–253, 2001.

61. Schapira AH, Mann VM, Cooper JM: Anatomic and disease specificity of NADH CoQ1 reductase (complex I) deficiency in Parkinson's disease. *J Neurochem* 55:2142–2145, 1990.

62. Casali C, Bonifati V, Santorelli FM, et al: Mitochondrial myopathy, parkinsonism, and multiple mtDNA deletions in a Sephardic Jewish family. *Neurology* 56:802–805, 2001.

63. Greenamyre JT, MacKenzie G, Peng TI, Stephans SE: Mitochondrial dysfunction in Parkinson's disease. *Biochem Soc Symp* 66:85–97, 1999.

64. Greenamyre JT, Sherer TB, Betarbet R, Panov AV: Complex I and Parkinson's disease. *IUBMB Life* 52:135–141, 2001.

65. Hsu LJ, Sagara Y, Arroyo A, et al: Alpha-synuclein promotes mitochondrial deficit and oxidative stress. *Am J Pathol* 157: 401–410, 2000.

66. Lamensdorf I, Graeme E, Harvey-White J, et al: 3,4-Dihydroxyphenylacetaldehyde potentiates the toxic effects of metabolic stress in PC12 cells. *Brain Res* 868:191–201, 2000.

67. Naoi M, Maruyama W, Akao Y, Yi H: Mitochondria determine the survival and death in apoptosis by an endogenous neurotoxin, *N*-methyl(*R*)salsolinol, and neuroprotection by propargylamines. *J Neural Transm* 109:607–621, 2002.

68. Nurmi E, Ruottinen HM, Bergman J, et al: Rate of progression in Parkinson's disease: A 6-[18F]fluoro-L-dopa PET study. *Mov Disord* 16:608–615, 2001.

69. Dagher A: Functional imaging in Parkinson's disease. *Semin Neurol* 21:23–32, 2001.

70. Brooks DJ, Samuel M: The effects of surgical treatment of Parkinson's disease on brain function: PET findings. *Neurology* 55:S52–59, 2000.

71. Khan NL, Valente EM, Bentivoglio AR, et al: Clinical and subclinical dopaminergic dysfunction in PARK6-linked parkinsonism: An 18F-dopa PET study. *Ann Neurol* 52:849–853, 2002.

72. Khan NL, Brooks DJ, Pavese N, et al: Progression of nigrostriatal dysfunction in a parkin kindred: An [18F]dopa PET and clinical study. *Brain* 125:2248–2256, 2002.

73. Martin WRW, Beckman JH, Calne DB, et al: Cerebral glucose metabolism in Parkinson's disease. *Can J Neurol Sci* 11:169–173, 1984.

74. Leenders K, Wolfson L, Gibbs J, et al: Regional cerebral blood flow and oxygen metabolism in Parkinson's disease and their response to L-dopa. *J Cereb Blood Flow Metab* 3:S488–S489, 1983.

75. Wooten GF, Collins RC: Metabolic effects of unilateral lesion of the substantia nigra. *J Neurosci* 1:285–291, 1981.

76. Garnett ES, Firnau G, Nahmias C: Dopamine visualized in the basal ganglia of living man. *Nature* 305:137–138, 1983.

77. Thobois S, Guillouet S, Broussolle E: Contributions of PET and SPECT to the understanding of the pathophysiology of Parkinson's disease. *Neurophysiol Clin* 31:321–340, 2001.

78. Ribeiro MJ, Vidailhet M, Loc'h C, et al: Dopaminergic function and dopamine transporter binding assessed with positron emission tomography in Parkinson disease. *Arch Neurol* 59:580–586, 2002.

79. Sossi V, de La Fuente-Fernandez R, Holden JE, et al: Increase in dopamine turnover occurs early in Parkinson's disease: Evidence from a new modeling approach to PET 18F-fluorodopa data. *J Cereb Blood Flow Metab* 22:232–239, 2002.

80. Lucignani G, Gobbo C, Moresco RM, et al: The feasibility of statistical parametric mapping for the analysis of positron emission tomography studies using 11C-2-beta-carbomethoxy-3-beta-(4-fluorophenyl)-tropane in patients with movement disorders. *Nucl Med Commun* 23:1047–1055, 2002.

81. Lewy FH: Paralysis agitans. I. Pathologische Anatomie, in Lewandowski M (ed): *Handbuck der Neurologie*. Berlin: Springer, 1912, pp 920–933.

82. Greenfield JG, Bosanquet FD: The brainstem lesion in parkinsonism. *J Neurol Neurosurg Psychiatry* 16:213–226, 1953.

83. Goldman JE, Yen S-H, Chiu F-C, Peress NS: Lewy bodies of Parkinson's disease contain neurofilament antigens. *Science* 221:1082–1084, 1983.

84. Duda JE, Giasson BI, Mabon ME, et al: Novel antibodies to synuclein show abundant striatal pathology in Lewy body diseases. *Ann Neurol* 52:205–210, 2002.

85. Cole NB, Murphy DD: The cell biology of alpha-synuclein: A sticky problem? *Neuromol Med* 1:95–109, 2002.

86. Lo Bianco C, Ridet JL, Schneider BL, et al: Alpha-synucleinopathy and selective dopaminergic neuron loss in a rat lentiviral-based model of Parkinson's disease. *Proc Natl Acad Sci U S A* 99: 10813–10818, 2002.

87. Lee MK, Stirling W, Xu Y, et al: Human alpha-synuclein-harboring familial Parkinson's disease-linked Ala-53->Thr mutation causes neurodegenerative disease with alpha-synuclein aggregation in transgenic mice. *Proc Natl Acad Sci U S A* 99:8968–8973, 2002.

88. Takahashi H, Wakabayashi K: The cellular pathology of Parkinson's disease. *Neuropathology* 21:315–322, 2001.

89. Rajagopalan S, Andersen JK: Alpha synuclein aggregation: Is it the toxic gain of function responsible for neurodegeneration in Parkinson's disease? *Mech Ageing Dev* 122:1499–1510, 2001.

90. Rideout HJ, Larsen KE, Sulzer D, Stefanis LJ: Proteasomal inhibition leads to formation of ubiquitin/alpha-synuclein-immunoreactive inclusions in PC12 cells. *Neurochem* 78: 899–908, 2001.

91. McNaught KS, Jenner P: Proteasomal function is impaired in substantia nigra in Parkinson's disease. *Neurosci Lett* 297: 191–194, 2001.

92. Chung KK, Zhang Y, Lim KL, et al: Parkin ubiquitinates the alpha-synuclein-interacting protein, synphilin-1: Implications for Lewy-body formation in Parkinson disease. *Nat Med* 7:1144–1150, 2001.

93. Wakabayashi K, Engelender S, Yoshimoto M, et al: Synphilin-1 is present in Lewy bodies in Parkinson's disease. *Ann Neurol* 47:521–523, 2000.

Chapter 13

ETIOLOGY OF PARKINSON'S DISEASE

YOSHIKUNI MIZUNO, NOBUTAKA HATTORI, and
HIDEKI MOCHIZUKI

HISTORICAL ASPECTS   209
THE MODERN ERA   209
    MPTP and Parkinsonism   210
    Environmental Neurotoxins   210
    Smoking   211
    Endogenous Neurotoxins   212
    Genetic Predisposition   212
    Genetic Association Studies   212
    Familial PD   217
    Mitochondria in PD   218
    Oxidative Stress in PD   218
    Cytokines   219
    Other Factors Contributing to Nigral
       Neurodegeneration   221
    PD and Apoptosis   221
SUMMARY AND CONCLUSION   223

Historical Aspects

The etiology of Parkinson's disease (PD) has long been discussed since the original description of this disease by James Parkinson in 1817.[1] Parkinson mentioned the possibility of chronic injury to the cervical cord, which gives rise to nerves to the upper extremities, because the disease often starts in the upper extremities. But he did not make any definite statement on the etiology and pathogenesis of the disease.

As parkinsonism was the frequent sequel of Von Economo's encephalitis, it had been postulated that virus infection might have been a cause of nigral degeneration in PD. Von Economo's encephalitis started with the epidemics in Vienna in 1916,[2] and resulted in worldwide pandemics until 1926, with a high morbidity of up to 80 percent.[3] The incidence of parkinsonism among recovered patients was up to 80 percent or more by the tenth year after the acute episode of encephalitis.[4] The pathologic hallmark of postencephalitic parkinsonism is the presence of Alzheimer's neurofibrillary tangles in the remaining neurons of the substantia nigra (SN).[5,6] It is unlikely that Von Economo's encephalitis plays any etiologic role in the pathogenesis of PD.[7]

Parkinsonism may occur as a sequel of various kinds of encephalitis other than Von Economo's encephalitis, such as Japanese B encephalitis,[8] western equine encephalitis,[9,10]

Coxsackie B type 2 encephalitis,[11] and central European tickborne encephalitis.[12] But parkinsonism after these encephalitides is usually nonprogressive, and it is unlikely that these infections play any etiologic role in PD.

As herpes simplex viruses have affinity to monoamine neurons in the brainstem,[13] being able to stay in the nervous system for a long period without causing inflammation or symptoms,[14] it was postulated that a specific form of infection with herpes simplex viruses might cause PD. Increases in antibody titers against herpes simplex virus components have been reported in the literature.[15,16] However, herpes simplex virus particles[17] or herpes simplex DNA[18] have never been found in the brains of patients who died of PD. Influenza virus infection was also considered. As an influenza pandemic occurred simultaneously with Von Economo's encephalitis between 1918 and 1919,[19] a possible association of influenza virus infection and PD was investigated by many workers;[17,18,20,21] however, none of them could demonstrate any causal association between influenza infection and PD. Recently, Borna virus has been implicated as an etiologic agent in PD. Ikuta et al. found the Borna virus genome in the SN in 4 out of 9 patients with PD (personal communication).

Another possibility that was once postulated is chronic metal intoxication. Chronic manganese intoxication produces parkinsonism,[22,23] and the manganese and aluminum contents of water consumed by Guamanian people who developed parkinsonism-dementia complex were high.[24] However, the clinical picture and pathologic changes in chronic manganese intoxication are different from those of PD.[22,23] Pathologic changes are most prominent in the internal segment of the globus pallidus and subthalamic nucleus.[25] Furthermore, brain manganese level is not elevated in PD.[26] Thus, it seems unlikely that chronic exogenous metal intoxication plays a role in the etiology and pathogenesis of PD.

Another possibility once discussed is the MIF (melnocyte-stimulating hormone (MSH)-release inhibiting factor) deficiency theory.[27] MIF is a tripeptide synthesized in the hypothalamus and released into pituitary portal vessels, inhibiting the release of MSH from the anterior pituitary gland.[28] This theory was postulated because serum MSH levels were elevated in PD patients,[29] MSH aggravated parkinsonism,[30] and MIF showed marginal improvement in parkinsonism.[31,32] However, disturbance of MIF secretion or degeneration of MIF-producing neurons has never been proved in the brain of patients with PD, and it is unlikely that MIF plays any etiologic role.

The Modern Era

The modern era started with the discovery of the specific nigral neurotoxin 1-methyl-4-phenyl-1,2,3,6-tetrahydropyridine (MPTP). Today, many PD specialists believe that nigral neuronal death is initiated by the interaction of environmental

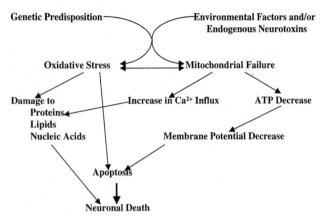

FIGURE 13-1 Pathogenesis of Nigral Neuronal Death in Parkinson's Disease.

neurotoxins, and that genetic predisposition induces mitochondrial dysfunction and oxidative damage in nigral neurons,[33-36] which are believed to die of apoptosis[37-39] (see Fig. 13-1). In this chapter, we review recent progress in the etiology and pathogenesis of PD.

MPTP AND PARKINSONISM

Modern research on the etiology and pathogenesis of PD began with the discovery of MPTP. In 1979, Davis et al.[40] reported a patient who developed severe parkinsonism after injecting a home-made illicit narcotic. This patient was examined by neurologists at the National Institutes of Health and showed marked improvement after treatment with L-dopa and bromocriptine. However, 18 months later he was dead. Postmortem examination revealed extensive degeneration and loss of pigmented neurons in the SN.[40] Only one Lewy body-like inclusion was said to have been found in the SN.

In 1982, several young adults in northern California developed a parkinsonian syndrome after intravenous use of what was purported to be "synthetic heroin."[41,42] Langston et al.[41] analyzed those drug samples and identified MPTP as the probable toxin responsible for their parkinsonism. MPTP-induced parkinsonism is usually nonprogressive, but recently Langston et al.[43] reported evidence to suggest active nerve cell degeneration in the SN years after MPTP exposure. They studied three subjects exposed to MPTP for 3-16 years before their deaths. In addition to moderate to severe depletion of pigmented neurons in the SN without Lewy bodies, they found gliosis and clustering of microglia around nerve cells. They interpreted these findings as indicative of active ongoing nerve cell loss.

MPTP is taken up into astrocytes in the brain, and oxidized to MPP+ (1-methyl-4-phenylpyridinium ion) by monoamine oxidase B (MAO-B).[44] Then MPP+ is actively taken up into nigrostriatal neurons[45] through dopamine transporters,[46] with marked concentration within dopaminergic neurons.[47] MPP+ is actively taken up into mitochondria of nigral neurons, depending on the electrical potential gradient between the inside and the outside of the mitochondrial inner membrane.[48] Within the mitochondria, MPP+ inhibits mitochondrial complex I and NADH-linked state 3 respiration.[48-50] The reason why MPP+ can inhibit complex I is probably due to its structural similarity to NAD+. The inhibition of mitochondrial respiration results in loss of oxidative phosphorylation and a rapid fall in the ATP level.[51] Ramsay et al.[52] estimated that MPP+ would be concentrated up to 800-fold within mitochondria compared to the external medium.

In addition to the inhibition of complex I, MPP+ also inhibits the alpha-ketoglutarate dehydrogenase complex of the tricarboxylic acid cycle.[53] This dual inhibition of complex I and the alpha-ketoglutarate dehydrogenase complex by MPP+ accounts for the marked inhibition of mitochondrial state 3 respiration by MPP+. The alpha-ketoglutarate dehydrogenase complex provides NADH for complex I and catalyzes the oxidation of alpha-ketoglutarate to succinate; the latter becomes a substrate for complex II. Thus inhibition of the alpha-ketoglutarate dehydrogenase complex would impair electron transfer via complex II because of an insufficient supply of succinate for complex II.

In addition to ATP depletion and energy crisis, MPP+ induces apoptotic cell death at lower concentrations.[54,55] Recently, Vila et al.[56] showed upregulation of Bax, a proapoptotic protein, and downregulation of Bcl-2 in the SN of mice treated with MPTP. Furthermore, they showed that mutant mice lacking Bax were significantly more resistant to MPTP than their wild-type littermates. In addition, Turmel et al.[57] reported caspase activation at days 1 and 2 after the end of MPTP intoxication in mice.

Although MPTP-induced parkinsonism is the best model of PD currently available, it probably has nothing to do with the etiology of PD. Goodwin and Kite[58] addressed the question of whether or not MPTP is present in the environment. They analyzed soot formed from partial combustion of coal by a sensitive gas chromatography-mass spectrometry method and were unable to detect MPTP.

ENVIRONMENTAL NEUROTOXINS

As this subject has been discussed in detail in Chapter 11, only pertinent points will be discussed here. Environmental factors that have been reported to increase the risk of developing PD include rural living,[59-64] use of well-water,[59-63,65] exposure to pesticides and herbicides,[59-63,66-69] industrial chemicals,[70] and head trauma.[71] The mean interval between the first head trauma and the onset of PD was reported as 36.5 years.[71] Much controversy exists as to the role of environmental factors in the etiology of PD,[61,64,69,71-73] but it is interesting to note that herbicides and pesticides, and some agricultural products, may contain substances that inhibit mitochondrial complex I activity. Recently, Betarbet et al.[74]

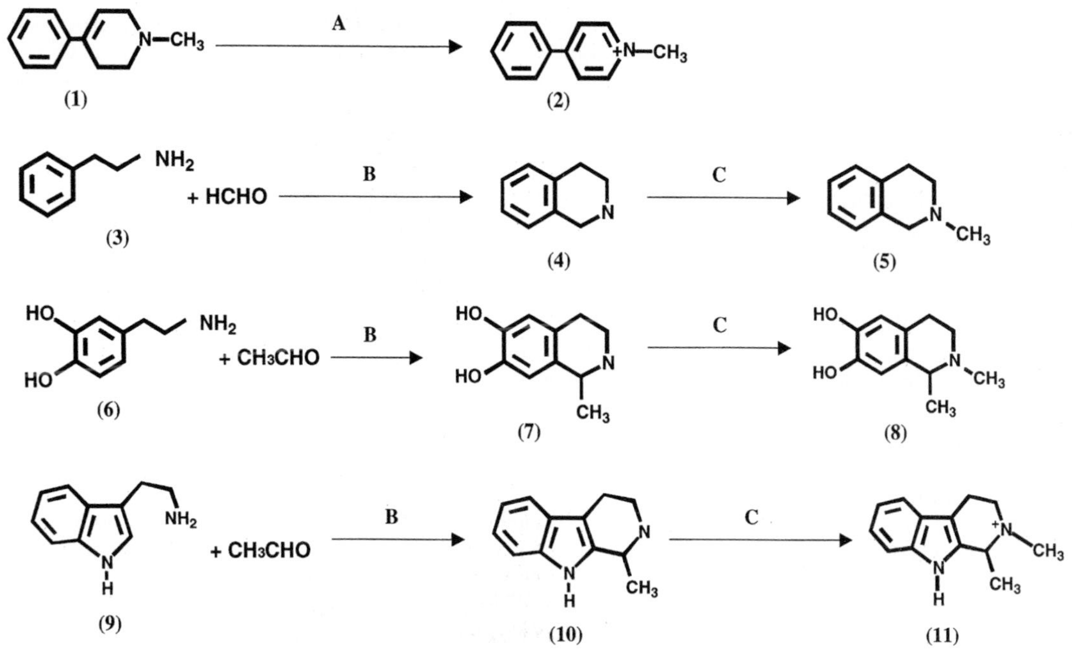

FIGURE 13-2 MPTP and Related Compounds.

1: MPTP, 2: MPP+, 3: Phenylethylamine, 4: Tetrahydroisoquinoline, 5: N-methyl-tetrahydroisoquinoline, 6: Dopamine, 7: Salsolinol, 8: N-methyl-salsolinol, 9: Tryptamine, 10: Beta-carboline, 11: N-methyl-beta-carboline, A: Monoamine oxidase, B: Condensation Reaction, C: N-methyltransferase

reproduced PD-like pathology, including Lewy body-like inclusions, in rats by chronic infusion of rotenone, a complex I inhibitor. In addition, the herbicide paraquat, when given to C57 BL mice, produced a dose-dependent decrease in SN dopaminergic neurons, assessed by a fluorogold prelabeling method, and a decline in striatal dopamine nerve terminal density, assessed by measurement of tyrosine hydroxylase (TH) immunoreactivity.[75]

Pezzoli et al.[76] studied the relationship between hydrocarbon exposure and the age of onset in 188 exposed and 188 nonexposed patients. Hydrocarbon exposure was associated with younger onset (61.0 ± 9.4 versus 64.7 ± 9.4 years, $P = 0.002$) and more severe disease ($r = 0.311$). Tinuvin 123, another industrial chemical, was also found to be a potent nigral neurotoxin, but injection of this compound into the SN causes both TH-positive and glutamic acid decarboxylase-positive neuronal destruction.[77,78]

By reviewing the literature, it is clear that further studies are definitely necessary to make any definite conclusion about the role of environmental neurotoxins in the etiology of PD.

SMOKING

Smoking has been inversely associated with PD.[65,68,69,73,79,80] It has been assumed that the risk of parkinsonism in smokers is reduced by 20–70 percent of that of nonsmokers.[80] Nicotine increases the firing rate of dopaminegic nigrostriatal

neurons,[81,82] and causes increased striatal dopamine release;[83,84] thus nicotine may have a symptomatic effect on parkinsonism.

Regarding the neuroprotective role of cigarette smoking, Calne and Langston[85] postulated that carbon monoxide (CO), which is produced during cigarette smoking, might have a scavenging action on free radicals that are produced in nigral neurons. Inhibition of MAO-B by cigarette smoking[86] may also be a neuroprotective mechanism. Based on an epidemiological study, Hellenbrand et al.[87] also concluded that smoking was neuroprotective. They studied the smoking histories of 380 PD patients, 379 age- and sex-matched control subjects, and 376 controls from the same region. Among parkinsonian patients, 44 percent had ever smoked, compared with 59 percent in both control groups. Among ever-smoking patients, 74 percent quit prior to the date of diagnosis, compared with roughly 45 percent of the ever-smoking control subjects. The odds ratio for ever having smoked was 0.5 (95% confidence interval (CI) 0.3–0.7).

However, there are controversies among the studies on smoking and PD. Some studies show no significant difference in the incidence of previous exposure to smoking between PD patients and control subjects.[67,70,88] It is also a possibility that, because of a premorbid personality change, people who eventually develop PD tend to dislike habitual smoking.

Recently, Elbaz et al.[89] studied interaction of familial history and smoking habit as a risk factor for PD.

When ever-smoking was associated with a history of PD in first-degree relatives, it was a significant risk factor for developing PD.

ENDOGENOUS NEUROTOXINS

The discovery of MPTP stimulated extensive studies on endogenous and exogenous neurotoxins which may accumulate in the SN and cause nigral cell death. Of these, tetrahydroisoquinolines (TIQs) and beta-carbolines have been most extensively studied. TIQs are a group of compounds that are formed by condensation of aldehyde and phenylethylamine or its derivatives. Some representative compounds are shown in Fig. 13-2. Beta-carbolines are derived from indolamines and aldehydes. These substances are structurally similar to MPTP or MPP$^+$.

Isoquinoline derivatives are widely distributed in the environment, being present in many plants and foodstuffs, and readily cross the blood-brain barrier. Some are potent inhibitors of mitochondrial complex I and generate reactive oxygen species when oxidized by MAO.[90]

Monkeys chronically treated with TIQ showed a clinical syndrome similar to parkinsonism,[91] and decreased dopamine, biopterine, and TH activity in the striatum.[92] Exogenously introduced TIQ, the prototype of TIQ compounds, can easily be transported into the brain.[93] The mechanism of toxicity of TIQ on dopaminergic neurons has not yet been well elucidated; however, mitochondrial toxicity appears to be one of the possibilities, as TIQ inhibits complex I[94] and mitochondrial state 3 respiration.[95] In contrast to these findings, 1-methyl-TIQ prevented MPTP-induced parkinsonism in mice,[96] and, interestingly enough, 1-methyl-TIQ was reduced in the striatum of PD.[97] Thus, structurally related less-toxic compounds may prevent nigral lesions being caused by more-toxic substances.

Maruyama et al.[98] studied dopamine-derived endogenous TIQs extensively and extracted N-methyl(R)salsolinol as a candidate PD-inducing substance.[98] N-methyl(R)salsolinol is formed by an endogenous enzyme (N-methyltransferase) from (R)salsolinol, which is formed from dopamine and acetaldehyde. N-methyl(R)salsolinol induces apoptotic cell death in SH-SY5Y cells, and this apoptotic cell death was inhibited by antioxidants[99] or a caspase inhibitor.[100] Cytotoxicity of N-methyl(R)salsolinol was ascribed to its oxidation into 1,2-dimethyl-6,7-dihydroxylisoquinolinium ion with generation of hydroxyl radicals. The isoquinolinium ion, when given locally, caused massive necrosis in the striatum, whereas N-methyl(R)salsolinol depleted dopaminergic neurons in the SN without necrotic tissue reaction.[101] Furthermore, Maruyama et al.[102] found increased N-methyltransferase activity in lymphocytes of patients with PD. In addition, N-methyl(R)salsolinol levels were increased in the cerebrospinal fluid (CSF) of untreated parkinsonian patients.[103] Thus, N-methyl(R)salsolinol appears to be a candidate PD-inducing substance, but what is lacking is the proof of accumulation of this compound in the nigrostriatal

system of PD patients. 1-(3',4'-Dihydroxybenzyl)-1,2,3,4-tetrahydroisoquinoline (a 1-benzyl-TIQ derivative with a dopamine moiety) was also reported to be a potent parkinsonism-inducing agent in rat. This compound is actively taken up into dopaminergic neurons through the dopamine transporter.[104]

Beta-carbolines are other interesting endogenous compounds structurally similar to MPP$^+$.[105–107] Derivatives of beta-carbolines show differential toxicity on PC12 cells.[108] Some inhibit MAO,[109] dopamine uptake,[110] and mitochondrial respiration.[111] Matsubara et al.[112] reported in vivo N-methylation of beta-carbolines and decreased in dopamine of the striatum of C57BL/6 mice. Kuhn et al.[113] measured plasma harman and norharman in 36 patients with PD and found that plasma norharman levels were significantly elevated compared with those of age- and sex-matched control subjects.

By reviewing the literature, it appears to be too early to conclude that any single toxin definitely plays an etiological role in PD.

GENETIC PREDISPOSITION

There is no question about the genetic influence on the development of PD (see Chap. 1). Studies of PD among first-degree relatives of index patients with PD reported a frequency 2–3 times higher than that in the control population.[114–117]

On the other hand, results of twin studies are not so convincing about the role of genetic factors. Concordance rate between monozygotic (MZ) twins was low, and was not much higher than that of dizygotic (DZ) twins (2.3 percent versus 0 percent).[118] A more recent study on a large veterans cohort showed high concordance rate in MZ twins with onset before age 50 (100 percent) and low in those with onset after age 50 years (10.4 percent). In DZ twins, concordance rate was 16.7 percent before age 50 and 10.2 percent after age 50.[119] When positron emission tomography scanning was included in the evaluation of the nigrostriatal involvement, the concordance rate in MZ twins was much higher (55.6 percent) than that in DZ twins (18.8 percent).[120] Thus, genetic factors appear to be important in early-onset PD patients.

GENETIC ASSOCIATION STUDIES

Genetic predisposition may be encoded in a subtle difference in base sequences (polymorphism) of some of the important proteins and enzymes. A single polymorphism may not produce significant disturbance in neuronal metabolism; however, when it is combined with exposure to environmental neurotoxins, or when multiple polymorphic mutations are combined in the same patient, they may become important genetic risk factors of PD. Based on this premise, many candidate genes have been studied. Genetic markers that have been studied in PD are shown in Table 13-1.

TABLE 13-1 Association Studies in PD

Single positive results
  Glutathione S-transferase
  N-Acetyltransferase 2
  Tau
  NDUFV2 (24-kDa subunit of mitochondrial complex I)
  Dihydrolipoamide succinyltransferase
Controversial results
  CYP2D6
  S-Methyltransferase
  Monoamine oxidase A (MAO-A)
  Monoamine oxidase B (MAO-B)
  Catechol O-methyltransferase
  D2 dopamine receptor
  D3 dopamine receptor
  D4 dopamine receptor
  Mn superoxide dismutase (Mn SOD)
  Alpha-synuclein
  Parkin
  Apolipoprotein epsilon4
  Alpha-antichymotrypsin
  Mitochondrial DNA
Negative results
  D5 dopamine receptor
  Dopamine transporter
  Tyrosine hydroxylase (TH)
  Cu-Zn superoxide dismutase (Cu-Zn SOD)
  8-Oxo-dGTPase
  Interleukin (IL)-1beta
  IL-1alpha
  IL-1 receptor antagonist

CYP2D6

The first enzyme studied was debrisoquine hydroxylase. Debrisoquine has a structure similar to that of TIQ, and is metabolized by one of the hepatic cytochrome P450 enzymes, CYP2D6 (debrisoquine hydroxylase). The activity level of debrisoquine hydroxylase is genetically determined by the CYP2D6 gene; thus subjects can be described as extensive or poor debrisoquine metabolizers. Barbeau et al.[121] reported a significant increase in the proportion of poor debrisoquine metabolizers in PD patients compared to the controls; however, this increase was later ascribed to the antihistamine drugs that those patients were taking.[122] Since then many studies have been reported, but controversy exists over the results. Positive results were reported by Benitez et al.,[123] and negative results were reported by Marttila et al.,[124] and Liu et al.[125]

Armstrong et al.[126] and Smith et al.[127] addressed this question by analyzing the gene for CYP2D6. Smith et al.[127] examined the frequency of mutant CYP2D6 alleles in 229 patients with PD and 720 controls. Individuals with a metabolic defect in the CYP2D6 gene with the poor metabolizer phenotype had a 2.54-fold (95% CI 1.51–4.28) increased risk for PD. The frequency of poor metabolizers among PD patients was 11.8 percent.

Since then, a number of studies have been performed. Positive results were reported by Armstrong et al.,[126] Kurth and Kurth,[128] Kondo and Kanazawa,[129] and Tsuneoka et al.,[130] but negative results were reported by Sandy et al.,[131] Diederich et al.,[132] and Joost et al.[133]

Recently, Payami et al.[134] addressed the question as to whether the age of onset was earlier in poor metabolizers (CYP2D6*4). They analyzed 576 PD patients and 247 control subjects. Contrary to expectation, the mean age of onset was significantly later in *4-positive patients. The frequency of *4 was significantly higher in late-onset PD than in early-onset PD. Poor metabolizers may even be protected from the disease.

Christensen et al.[135] made a meta-analysis of case-control studies on CYP2D6. They calculated the odds ratio for the risk of PD among poor metabolizers compared with extensive metabolizers. They identified 21 studies until 1998, from which they excluded 6 because the studies were incomplete. The overall odds ratio was 1.48 (95% CI 1.10–1.99). This difference was caused by a single large study using genotyping. They concluded that there was no convincing evidence of an association between debrisoquine/spartan polymorphism and PD.

S-METHYLTRANSFERASE

S-Methylation is another detoxifying system for exogenous substances. Waring et al.[136] reported reduced activity of erythrocyte S-methyltransferase in PD; however, we could not reproduce this result on Japanese PD patients.[137]

MONOAMINE OXIDASE A (MAO-A)

MAO-A is located in the X chromosome and regulates the metabolism of monoamines, including catecholamines. Hotamisligil et al.[138] examined 91 male patients with PD and 129 male controls for polymorphisms of a $(GT)_n$ repeat in the MAO-A locus. One particular haplotype, marked by restriction fragment length polymorphisms (RFLPs) at MAO-A, was 3 times more frequent in patients with PD than in controls, and the overall distribution of these alleles was significantly different ($P = 0.03$) between the two groups. Nakatome et al.[139] examined the polymorphism in 228 Japanese controls and 68 patients with PD. Although analysis of the MAO-A marker demonstrated no overall association between its alleles and PD, a significant difference in the frequency of one particular MAO-A allele between controls and patients with PD was found.

However, a negative association between MAO-A gene polymorphisms and PD was reported by Nanko et al.,[140] Plante-Bordeneuve et al.,[141] and Costa-Mallen et al.[142]

MONOAMINE OXIDASE B (MAO-B)

The MAO-B gene is located in the X chromosome and has two polymorphisms: $(GT)_n$ repeat length polymorphism in intron 2, and G-T substitution in intron 13.

Kurth et al.[143] examined the single base change (A or G) in intron 13 in 122 controls and 46 PD patients. The frequencies of alleles 1 (A allele) and 2 (G allele) were 0.62 and 0.38 for PD patients and 0.45 and 0.55 for control subjects, respectively. The presence of MAO-B allele 1 was associated with a relative risk of 2.03-fold for PD (95% CI 1.44–2.61; $P < 0.02$).

Costa et al.[144] examined the same polymorphism in 62 Caucasian PD patients and 79 controls. The age-adjusted odds ratio for the G allele in males was 1.87 (95% CI 0.78–4.47). Among females the age-adjusted odds ratios were 5.00 (95% CI 1.13–22.1) for the GA genotype and 5.60 (95% CI 1.01–30.9) for the GG genotype. They suggested that the G allele of this MAO-B polymorphism might relate to PD risk. Wu et al.[145] examined the same polymorphism in 224 Taiwanese PD patients and 197 controls. The MAO-B G genotype (G in men and G/G in women) was associated with a 2.07-fold increased relative risk of PD. When this mutation was combined with the COMT L (low) polymorphism, a significant synergistic enhancement was found. MAO-B G and COMT L alleles were 2.4 times more frequent in patients with PD ($P = 0.023$).

However, Ho et al.,[146] Morimoto et al.,[147] Nanko et al.,[140] Plante-Bordeneuve et al.,[141] and Nakatome et al.[139] found no association with the above genotypes and PD.

Regarding the dinucleotide repeat $(GT)_n$ polymorphism, Hotamisligil et al.[138] examined 91 male patients with PD and 129 male controls. No associations were observed between individual MAO-B alleles and the disease state, but the frequency distribution for all alleles was significantly different in the two populations ($P = 0.046$).

Mellick et al.[148] examined the length of $(GT)_n$ repeat sequence and the G-A genotype of the MAO-B gene polymorphism in 204 Australians with PD and 285 controls. The G-A polymorphism showed no association with PD (odds ratio 0.80; $P = 0.51$; 95% CI 0.42–1.53). There was a significant difference in frequencies of the $(GT)_n$ repeat allelic variation between patients and control subjects ($\chi^2 = 20.09$; $P<0.01$). The $(GT)_n$ repeat alleles ≥ 188 base pairs (bp) were significantly associated with PD (odds ratio 4.60; $P<0.00005$; 95% CI 1.97–10.77). The 186-bp allele was also significantly associated with PD (odds ratio 1.85; $P = 0.048$; 95% CI 1.01–3.42). They concluded that the $(GT)_n$ repeat in intron 2 of the MAO-B gene was a powerful marker for PD in their large Australian cohort. Mellick et al.[149] examined the $(GT)_n$ repeat in 176 Chinese PD patients and 203 controls. There was no significant difference in the frequencies of the $(GT)_n$ repeat allelic variation between patients and controls.

CATECHOL-O-METHYLTRANSFERASE (COMT)

Catechol-O-methyltransferase (COMT) is an enzyme that inactivates catecholamines. An amino acid change at Val108Met determines the high-activity and low-activity forms of the enzyme (Val/Val = high, Met/Met = low).

Kunugi et al.[150] examined this polymorphism in 109 Japanese patients with PD and 153 controls. The frequency of low-activity allele in the controls was 0.29, which was significantly different from that reported in Caucasians (0.50). Homozygosity for the low-activity allele was significantly more common among the patients than the controls (15 percent versus 6 percent; $P = 0.017$; odds ratio 2.8; 95% CI 1.2–6.5).

Yoritaka et al.[151] examined the same polymorphism in 176 Japanese PD patients and 156 controls. Contrary to the report by Kunugi et al.,[150] homozygosity for the high activity was significantly higher in PD patients (56.8 percent versus 44.2 percent).

Hoda et al.,[152] Syvanen et al.,[153] Xie et al.,[154] and Lee et al.[155] did not find any association between the polymorphism and PD. Thus there is no conclusive evidence to indicate that the polymorphism of COMT plays a role in the etiology of PD.

DOPAMINE RECEPTORS (D2, D3, D4, AND D5)

Plante-Bordeneuve et al.[141] examined the polymorphism of the D2 dopamine receptor gene in 100 white PD patients and 100 white controls. The overall allelic distribution was significantly different in sporadic PD ($P < 0.01$). The odds ratios were significant ($P < 0.01$) for allele 3, with respective values of 1.84 (95% CI 1.23-2.74). Individuals who were homozygous for allele 3 were 2.3 times more frequent in the sporadic PD than in controls. Grevle et al.[156] examined a TaqI A RFLP located in the untranslated region, approximately 10 kilobases from the 3' end of the D2 dopamine receptor gene. They examined 72 patients with PD and 81 controls. They found significant differences in allelic distribution between the overall PD group and control groups ($\chi^2 = 5.009$; $P = 0.025$). When only patients with definite PD were considered, an even more significant association was found ($\chi^3 = 8.2121$; $P = 0.004$). Among the overall PD group, the odds ratio for having the variant allele A1 was 2.2 (95% CI 1.1–4.4), whereas it was calculated to be 3.0 (95% CI 1.4–6.4) when only patients with definite PD were considered.

Ricketts et al.[157] examined the polymorphism of the exon 3 variants of the D4 dopamine receptor gene in 95 PD patients and 47 controls. They found a significantly higher frequency of exon 3 alleles with 6 or more repeat units in the PD group ($P = 0.039$).

On the other hand, Nanko et al.,[158] and Higuchi et al.[159] did not find any association between dopamine D2, D3, and D4 receptor gene polymorphisms and PD in 71 Japanese patients. Also, Pastor et al.[160] examined the intronic allele 3 of the D2 dopamine receptor gene and found no association in Spanish PD patients.

Wan et al.[161] did not find association between the dopamine D4 receptor gene polymorphism and PD in Chinese patients in Hong Kong. Wang et al.[162] also examined T978C polymorphism of the D5 dopamine receptor gene in 120 Chinese PD patients and 110 controls. The overall allelic and genotypic frequencies did not differ significantly between the two groups.

DOPAMINE TRANSPORTER

Higuchi et al.[159] examined a dopamine transporter gene polymorphism in 70 Japanese PD patients and 70 controls. No significant difference was noted between the two groups. Plante-Bordeneuve et al.[141] examined the polymorphism of the dopamine transporter gene in 60 white PD patients and 60 white controls. There was no significant difference between the groups.

TYROSINE HYDROXYLASE (TH)

Plante-Bordeneuve et al.[163] examined the highly variable GT repeat polymorphism at the TH locus in 44 patients with sporadic PD, 48 patients with familial PD, and 50 controls. No association or linkage was found between this locus and sporadic or familial PD.

Cu-Zn SUPEROXIDE DISMUTASE (Cu-Zn SOD)

Parboosingh et al.[164] screened for mutations in the Cu-Zn SOD gene by single-strand conformation analysis in unrelated patients with PD from two populations (familial and sporadic). No mutations were identified. Farin et al.[165] studied polymorphisms in the coding region of Cu-Zn SOD and found no difference between PD patients and controls, but the number of subjects studied was small (45 PD patients, and 49 controls).

Mn SUPEROXIDE DISMUTASE (Mn SOD)

Parboosingh et al.[164] screened mutations in the Mn SOD gene by single-strand conformation analysis in unrelated patients with PD from two PD populations (familial and sporadic). No mutations were identified.

Shimoda-Matsubayashi et al.[166] genotyped the −Val9Ala polymorphism in the mitochondrial targeting sequence of the Mn SOD gene. The -9Ala allele was significantly more frequent in PD patients (12.1 percent versus 19.3 percent; $P < 0.05$).

Grasbon-Frodl et al.[167] examined two polymorphisms of the Mn SOD gene (Ile58Thr, and Ala9Val) in 63 German Caucasian PD patients. All 63 PD patients exhibited a T at nucleotide position 5777 in exon 3 of the Mn SOD gene, corresponding to ATA, or Ile at the peptide level; no other sequence variants were found. In addition, both alleles of the −Ala9Val polymorphism in the mitochondrial targeting sequence of Mn SOD were equally distributed between German PD patients and controls, excluding this gene variant as a risk factor for PD in Caucasian subjects.

Farin et al.[165] studied polymorphisms in the coding region of the Mn SOD gene and found no difference between PD patients and the controls. They also studied the polymorphism in the mitochondrial signal peptide (C47T, exon 2), but they found no difference between PD patients ($n = 155$) and the controls ($n = 231$).

CATALASE

Parboosingh et al.[164] screened for mutations in the catalase gene by single-strand conformation analysis in unrelated patients with PD from two populations (familial and sporadic). They identified an amino acid substitution (glycine to aspartic acid) in exon 9 of the catalase gene in one familial patient; decreased red blood cell catalase activity was observed in this patient.

GLUTATHIONE-*S*-TRANSFERASE

Stroombergen et al.[168] examined glutathione-*S*-transferase gene M1 polymorphism in 122 Caucasian PD patients and 84 age- and sex-matched control subjects. Glutathione-*S*-transferase M1 null frequency was significantly higher in PD patients (67 percent versus 51 percent, $P < 0.025$). Glutathione-*S*-transferase itself has an antioxidant property. They postulated that deletion of the glutathione-*S*-transferase gene might be associated with a susceptibility to PD.

8-Oxo-dGTPase, MTH1

8-Oxo-7,8-dihydrodeoxyguanosine triphosphatase (8-oxo-dGTPase, MTH1) is a key enzyme for preventing oxidative stress-induced DNA damage. Satoh and Kuroda[169] recently studied polymorphism of the gene encoding this protein. They studied the Val to Met polymorphism at codon 83 in exon 4 of the MTH1 gene in 73 patients with sporadic PD and 151 age-matched controls. The frequency of either the 83Val or the 83Met allele was not statistically different between PD patients (92.5 percent or 7.5 percent) and the controls (88.7 percent or 11.3 percent) ($\chi^2 = 1.511$; $P = 0.2190$).

N-ACETYLTRANSFERASE 2

Bandmann et al.[170] examined *N*-acetyltransferase 2 gene polymorphism in 100 sporadic parkinsonian brains and 100 control brains. The frequency of the polymorphism, which renders the subjects slow acetylators, was 59 percent in PD patients and 37 percent in the controls. The difference was statistically significant (95% CI 1.37–4.38). They also studied 100 blood samples from familial PD patients. The frequency of slow acetylators was 69 percent (95% CI 2.08–6.90) compared to the controls.

INTERLEUKIN (IL) 1BETA, IL-1ALPHA, AND IL-1 RECEPTOR ANTAGONIST

Nishimura et al.[171] studied genetic polymorphisms of the IL-1beta gene (position -511 in the promoter region, and position +3953 in exon 5), the IL-1alpha, and the IL-1 receptor antagonist genes in 122 Japanese patients with PD and 112 controls. No significant difference was found in these genetic markers between PD patients and controls.

ALPHA-SYNUCLEIN

Kruger et al.[172] studied a polymorphism of the alpha-synuclein gene in 193 German PD patients and 200 healthy control subjects matched for age, sex, and origin. They genotyped a polymorphism in the promoter region of the alpha-synuclein gene, as well as of the closely linked DNA markers D4S1647 and D4S1628. They found significant differences in the allelic distributions between PD patients and the controls. They also analyzed the apolipoprotein (Apo) epsilon4 allele and found that it was significantly more frequent among early-onset PD patients (age at onset <50 years) than in late-onset PD patients. The combination of the Apo epsilon4 allele and allele 1 of the alpha-synuclein promoter polymorphism gave a 12.8-fold increased relative risk for development of PD.

Farrer et al.[173] also found significant association between the dinucleotide repeat polymorphism in the promoter region of the alpha-synuclein gene. Izumi et al.[174] did not find association between the dinucleotide repeat polymorphism in the promoter region of the alpha-synuclein gene in a Japanese population.

PARKIN

Wang et al.[175] examined three polymorphisms of the parkin gene—i.e., G to A transition in exon 4 (S/N167), C to T transition in exon 10 (R/W366), and G to C transition in exon 10 (V/L380)—in 160 Japanese sporadic PD patients and 160 age- and sex-matched control subjects. The C to T transition (R/W366) was significantly lower in PD patients (1.2 percent versus 4.4 percent), suggesting that it might be a protective factor against PD. Hu et al.[176] also studied the same parkin gene polymorphisms (S/N167, R/W366, V/L380) in 92 sporadic PD patients and in 98 controls in Chinese in Taiwan. They found that a polymorphism of R/W366 in the parkin gene was associated with a protective factor for sporadic PD.

Satoh and Kuroda[177] studied a codon 167 serine/asparagine (S/N167) polymorphism located in exon 4 in 71 patients with sporadic PD and 109 age-matched controls. The frequency of either the 167S or the 167N allele was not statistically different between PD patients and controls, but the frequency of 167S/N heterozygotes was significantly higher in PD patients (62.0 percent versus 45.9 percent) compared with that of both 167S/S and 167N/N homozygotes combined ($\chi^2 = 4.467$; $P = 0.0346$; odds ratio 1.92; 95% CI 1.05–3.54). They suggested that the heterozygosity at codon 167 in the parkin gene might represent a genetic risk factor for development of sporadic PD.

TAU

Pastor et al.[178] studied a dinucleotide repeat marker at intron 11 of the tau gene in 152 patients with PD and 150 healthy controls. They detected a significant difference in A0 allelic frequency in the PD group (79.27 percent) compared with the control group (71 percent). Individuals homozygous for the A0 allele were also detected significantly more frequently in the PD group (63.8 percent) compared with the control group (52.66 percent).

APOLIPOPROTEIN EPSILON4

Koller et al.[179] studied the ApoE gene type 4 allele in a cohort of 52 PD patients with dementia, 61 patients without dementia, and 78 nondemented controls. ApoE genotype and allele frequencies did not differ between demented and nondemented PD patients. Neither group's genotype or allele frequencies differed from those of a nondemented population of 78 controls.

ALPHA-ANTICHYMOTRYPSIN (ACT)

Yamamoto et al.[180] analyzed the alpha-antichymotrypsin gene in Japanese patients with PD. The number of individuals with two copies of the ACT-A allele (ACT-AA genotype) was increased significantly in patients with PD compared to that in healthy controls (19.9 percent versus 8.3 percent; $P < 0.02$), and the ACT-A allele frequency in patients with PD was significantly higher than that in healthy controls ($\chi^2 = 5.96$; df = 1; $P < 0.015$). The odds ratio for developing PD in individuals with the ACT-AA genotype was 3.36 compared to individuals with two copies of another allele, the ACT-T allele (ACT-TT genotype).

Grasbon-Frodl et al.[181] studied this allele frequency in 62 German PD patients and in 53 controls without clinical or pathological evidence of neurodegenerative diseases. The A allele frequency was 47 percent in PD patients compared to 54 percent in control cases. The difference was not significant; however, ACT-A allele frequencies were significantly different ($P < 0.001$) between Japanese and German controls.

Munoz et al.[182] genotyped ACT-AA in 71 patients with clinically definite PD and 109 age-matched healthy control subjects. They found no significant difference between the two groups (31 percent in the PD group versus 28.4 percent in the control group).

24-kDa SUBUNIT OF MITOCHONDRIAL COMPLEX I

Hattori et al.[183] genotyped a novel polymorphism (Ala29Val) in the mitochondrial targeting sequence of NDUFV2 (the 24-kDa subunit of mitochondrial complex I) in 126 Japanese patients with PD and 113 controls. The distribution of the three genotypes was significantly different between the two groups ($\chi^2 = 7.53$; df = 2; $P = 0.023$). The frequency of homozygotes for the mutation was significantly higher in PD patients (23.8 percent) than in control subjects (11.5 percent; Fisher's exact test, $P = 0.0099 < 0.01$). The risk of developing Parkinson's disease associated with homozygosity for this mutation was calculated as 2.40 (95% CI 1.18–4.88).

DIHYDROLIPOAMIDE SUCCINYLTRANSFERASE

Kobayashi et al.[184] examined a G to A polymorphism in exon 8 of dihydrolipoamide succinyltransferase (E2 of the alpha-ketoglutarate dehydrogenase complex in mitochondria) in 176 PD patients and 223 controls, and found a higher frequency of the A allele in PD patients compared with the

TABLE 13-2 Familial Forms of PD

Name	Chromosome	Locus	Gene	Inheritance	Reference(s)
PARK1	4	4q21-23	Alpha-synuclein	AD	192, 193
PARK2	6	6q25.2-27	Parkin	AR	194, 195
PARK3	2	2p13	Unknown	AD	196
PARK4 (=PARK1)	4	4p21-23	Alpha-synuclein	AD	197, 197'
PARK5	4	4p14-15.1	UCH-L1	AR	201
PARK6	1	1p35-36	Unknown	AR	198
PARK7	1	1p36	D.T-1	AR	199, 199'
PARK8	12	12	Unknown	AD	200
PARK9	1	1p36	Unknown	AR	
FTDP-17	17	17q21-23	Tau	AD	202–204
Dystonia-parkinsonism	19	19q13	Unknown	AD	205
Lubag dystonia	X	Xq13.1	Unknown	XR	206, 207

AD, autosomal-dominant; AR, autosomal-recessive; XR, X-linked recessive.

controls (41.5 percent versus 28.4 percent). This substitution does not change the amino acid sequence.

MITOCHONDRIAL DNA (mtDNA)

There are reports on mtDNA in PD.[185–191] However, there is no convincing evidence to indicate that mtDNA mutations are etiologically related to PD.

FAMILIAL PD

Recently, there has been a great progress in the investigation of the familial forms of PD. So far, 12 forms have been assigned to different chromosome loci[192–207] (Table 13-2). Among these, alpha-synuclein mutations cause an autosomal-dominant form and parkin mutations cause an autosomal-recessive form of the disease. In addition, tau gene mutations cause familial frontotemporal dementia and parkinsonism. The disease genes for other inherited forms of PD have not yet been identified. As an extensive review of familial forms of PD is beyond the scope of this chapter, only findings that may help understanding of sporadic PD will be discussed briefly.

PARK1

PARK1 is an autosomal-dominant L-dopa-responsive PD. The age of onset is younger than that of sporadic cases.[208] Alpha-synuclein is a neuron-specific protein expressed in the presynaptic terminal region. Two mutations are known (Ala30Pro, and Ala53Thr).[193,209] Mutated alpha-synuclein proteins have an increased tendency to self-aggregation and deposition in the cytoplasm and neuritic processes.[210] This is a very rare familial form of PD, but what is interesting about alpha-synuclein is the observation that the major component of the Lewy body has been found to be alpha-synuclein.[211,212] Alpha-synuclein aggregates are also seen in the SN of sporadic PD cases.

It would be interesting to know whether or not transgenic animals for these mutations might be more or less susceptible to nigral neurotoxins. Rathke-Hartlieb et al.[213] treated alpha-synuclein transgenic mice (Ala30Pro alpha-synuclein under control of neuron-specific Thy-1 or a TH promoter) with MPTP. The number of remaining nigral neurons was the same as in wild-type mice treated with MPTP. There was no increase in sensitivity to this putative environmental neurotoxin. These transgenic mice did not show nigral neuronal death or striatal dopamine loss before treatment with MPTP.

However, an in vitro overexpression study clearly showed neurotoxicity of mutated alpha-synuclein. Zhou et al.[214] overexpressed Ala53Thr alpha-synuclein in rat primary mesencephalic cultures and in N27 cells, a rat dopaminergic cell line. Overexpression of wild-type human alpha-synuclein was not directly neurotoxic but did increase dopamine cell death after 6-hydroxy dopamine. Overexpression of the mutated alpha-synuclein selectively induced apoptotic cell death of primary dopamine neurons as well as N27 cells.

Furthermore, Kanda et al.[215] showed a link between alpha-synuclein mutation and oxidative stress. They constructed SH-SY5Y cells overexpressing alpha-synuclein Ala53Thr and Ala30Pro, and studied the effect of hydrogen peroxide exposure. Cells expressing the 2 point mutant isoforms of alpha-synuclein were significantly more vulnerable to oxidative stress than the cells expressing the wild isoform.

Thus accumulation of normal alpha-synuclein in nigral neurons in PD is believed to play an important role in the neurodegeneration; however, the message of alpha-synuclein was reported to be diminished in PD.[216] This downregulation may be a reflection of neuronal degeneration. The question is whether or not transient overexpression of alpha-synuclein exists in the initial stage of neurodegeneration. In dementia with Lewy bodies, the mRNA level of alpha-synuclein in the cingulated cortical neurons was reported to be unchanged compared with control brains.[217]

PARK2

PARK2 is an autosomal-recessive young-onset familial PD linked to the long arm of chromosome 6.[194] Clinical features were first delineated by Yamamura et al. in 1973.[218] The disease gene was identified and named *parkin*.[195] A wide variety of deletion mutations and point mutations were found in affected patients.[219,220] The parkin protein is expressed in synaptic vesicle membranes and in Golgi bodies,[221] and it was found to be a ubiquitin-protein ligase.[222] Ubiquitin ligase is the third enzyme of the ubiquitin system, which transfers ubiquitin molecules to target proteins. Polyubiquitinated proteins are rapidly destroyed by 26S proteasome.[223] The ubiquitin system is not only important for the quality control of proteins but it also plays important roles in many vital reactions, such as cell cycling, ontogenesis, the immune system, carcinogenesis, and neurodegeneration.

As ubiquitin ligase is an enzyme, there must be specific substrates. Recently, several candidate substrates were reported and some were found in the brains of young-onset PD with parkin mutations. They include CDCrel1,[224] 22-kDa alpha-synuclein,[225] PAEL (parkin-associated endothelin receptor-like) receptor,[226] and synphilin 1.[227] In this form, accumulation of such compounds within nigral neurons may play a role in neurodegeneration. Discovery of parkin and parkin protein opened up a new approach to the etiopathogenesis of PD.

MITOCHONDRIA IN PD

There is ample evidence to indicate that there is a selective loss of complex I of the mitochondrial electron transport system in PD.[228–231] This decrease is specific for SN and is not seen in other brain regions, as well as being specific for PD.[84] A small but significant decrease in the activity of complex I was also reported in platelets, lymphocytes, and skeletal muscle.[232–241] However, results are not consistent among different reports.[242–245] Thus it appears likely that loss of complex I in PD is not a primary event and does not play an etiologic role. Complex I deficiency is likely to be a secondary phenomenon, but it appears to be an important contributing factor to neurodegeneration. The magnitude of loss of complex I in PD is not so marked as to knock out ATP formation, but it may increase the production of reactive oxygen species contributing to oxidative damage.

OXIDATIVE STRESS IN PD

There is ample evidence to indicate the presence of oxidative damage to high molecular weight substances such as proteins, lipids, and nucleic acids in the SN of patients with PD. Generally, free radicals are highly reactive, oxidizing other substances by extracting electrons; they may oxidize various substances nonselectively by cross-linkaging sulfhydryl bonds of proteins, inactivating certain enzymes, and by inducing acquired DNA mutations.[246] Evidence of oxidative damage is summarized in Table 13-3.

TABLE 13-3 Evidence of Oxidative Damage in PD

Increase in iron
Increase in Cu-Zn superoxide dismutase?
Increase in Mn superoxide dismutase?
Increase in malondialdehyde (lipid peroxidation)
Decrease in reduced form of glutathione
Increase in 8-hydroxydeoxyguanine (oxidative damage to DNA)
Increase in hydroxynonenal-modified proteins (oxidative damage to proteins)
Increase in protein carbonyl (oxidative damage to proteins)
Increase in protein nitration (oxidative damage to proteins)

IRON

Among the reactive oxygen species, hydroxyl radicals are most cytotoxic. These radicals are formed by Fenton reaction (Fig. 13-3) in the presence of ferrous iron. Increased iron in the SN of PD patients has been reported by many groups.[247–252] Iron exists in two forms (i.e., Fe^{3+} and Fe^{2+}). Most of the tissue iron is believed to be in the ferric form (Fe^{3+}), although, small amounts of ferrous iron (Fe^{2+}) may exist.[253] In the presence of reducing substance, Fe^{3+} can be reduced to Fe^{2+}; Fe^{2+} is highly reactive and may induce free radical reactions, Fe^{2+} catalyzes the Fenton reaction, and Fe^{3+} mediates iron-catalyzed Haber-Weiss reaction (Fig. 13-3); both reactions produce hydroxyl radicals from hydrogen peroxide. Neuromelanin has high-affinity binding sites for iron,[253,254] and, in the presence of neuromelanin, Fe^{3+} is believed to be reduced to Fe^{2+}.[255] The mechanism of iron accumulation in the SN in PD is not known.

1. $^3O_2 + e^- \longrightarrow O_2^-$

2. $2O_2^- + 2H^+ \longrightarrow H_2O_2 + {}^3O_2$

3. $H_2O_2 + Fe^{2+} \longrightarrow HO\cdot + OH^- + Fe^{3+}$

4. $O_2^- + H_2O_2 \longrightarrow HO\cdot + OH^- + {}^1O_2$

5. $O_2^- + H_2O_2 \xrightarrow{(Fe^{3+})} HO\cdot + OH^- + {}^3O_2$

6. $NO + O_2^- \longrightarrow ONOO^-$

7. $ONOO^- + H^+ \longrightarrow HO\cdot + NO_2\cdot$

8. $R\text{-}CH_2\text{-}NH_2 + O_2 + H_2O \longrightarrow RCHO + NH_3 + H_2O_2$

FIGURE 13-3 Reactive Oxygen Species and their Formation.
1. Formation of superoxide anion, 2. Reaction catalyzed by superoxide dismutase, 3. Fenton reaction, 4. Haber-Weiss reaction, 5. Iron-catalyzed Haber-Weiss reaction, 6. Formation of peroxynitrite, 7. Formation of hydroxyl radical from peroxynitrite, 8. Reaction catalyzed by monoamine oxidase, $^3O_2$: triplet oxygen, O_2^-: superoxide anion, H_2O_2: hydrogen peroxide, HO: hydroxyl radical, $^1O_2$: singlet oxygen, NO: nitric oxide, $ONOO^-$: peroxynitrite, NO_2: nitric dioxide.

In addition to iron, aluminum was reported to be increased in the SN of PD.[251,252] Aluminum may also accelerate membrane lipid peroxidation in the presence of Fe^{2+}.[256]

FREE RADICAL SCAVENGING ENZYMES

There are no consistent changes in the enzymes regulating the metabolism of reactive oxygen species, such as SOD,[257,258] glutathione peroxidase,[259,260] or glutathione reductase,[259] in PD. Recently, Radunovic et al.[261] measured Mn SOD in the frontal cortex of PD patients and found a significant increase compared to controls and patients with amyotrophic lateral sclerosis.

MALONDIALDEHYDE

Dexter et al.[262] reported increased lipid peroxidation, as measured by an increase in malondialdehyde, in the SN of patients with PD.

GLUTATHIONE

Further evidence to suggest oxidative stress is a decrease in the amount of reduced glutathione; 30–60 percent reduction in the reduced form of glutathione has been reported in the SN of PD.[263–266]

In the central nervous system, glutathione is believed to be synthesized mainly in glial cells;[267,268] thus most neuronal glutathione is probably transported from glial cells. A reduced level of glutathione is indirect evidence of oxidative stress.

OXIDATIVE DNA DAMAGE

One of the important aspects of oxidative stress is damage to DNA. Hydroxyl radicals interact with guanine molecules of DNA to yield 8-hydroxydeoxyguanine, which may be read as thymine at the time of DNA duplication; thus a GC to AT pair mutation will be induced.[269]

Interestingly, Sanchez-Ramos et al.[270] recently reported an increase in 8-hydroxydeoxyguanosine in the nigrostriatum of PD brain. This would suggest that acquired mutation of nuclear DNA as well as of mtDNA might occur under oxidative stress.

Alam et al.[271] measured 8-hydroxy-2'-deoxyguanine by gas chromatography-mass spectrometry and found that levels of 8-hydroxyguanine (8-OHG) tended to be elevated and levels of 2,6-diamino-4-hydroxy-5-formamidopyrimidine (FAP guanine) tended to be decreased in PD. The most striking difference was a rise in 8-OHG in PD SN ($P = 0.0002$). They postulated that the rise in 8-OHG could be due to a change in 8-OHG/FAP guanine ratios rather than to an increase in total oxidative guanine damage.

Zhang et al.[272] studied 8-hydroxyguanosine (8OHG) in PD, multisystem atrophy, and in dementia with Lewy bodies. In PD patients, cytoplasmic 8OHG immunoreactivity was intense in neurons of the SN. The proportion of 8OHG-immunoreactive SN neurons was significantly greater in PD patients compared to age-matched controls. Midbrain sections from patients with multi system atrophy-parkinsonian type and dementia with Lewy bodies showed increased cytoplasmic 8OHG immunoreactivity in SN neurons compared to controls; however, the proportion of positive neurons was significantly less than in PD. Nuclear 8OHG immunoreactivity was not observed in any individual.

Shimura et al.[273] studied 8-oxo-dGTPase and 8-oxo-7,8-deoxyguanosine (8-oxo-dG) in 6 autopsied PD brains. 8-Oxo-dGTPase is an enzyme that metabolizes 8-oxo-7,8-deoxyguanosine triphosphate. There was a significant increase in the amount of enzyme and 8-oxo-dG immunoreactivity in the nigral neurons of PD compared with the age-matched control brains. Immunostaining was mainly cytoplasmic, indicating that mtDNA is the target of oxidative DNA damage.

OXIDATIVE PROTEIN DAMAGE

Using an immunohistochemical method, Yoritaka et al.[274] reported an increase in hydroxynonenal-modified proteins in the nigral neurons of 7 patients who died of PD compared to control subjects. 4-Hydroxy-2-nonenal (HNE) is an unsaturated aldehyde released from fatty acids by lipid peroxidation. It reacts with proteins to form stable adducts, which represent a marker of oxidative stress-induced cellular damage. They found that 58 percent of nigral neurons were positively stained for HNE-modified proteins in PD, in contrast to 9 percent in the control subjects ($P < 0.01$).

Protein carbonyl is another indicator of oxidative brain damage. Alam et al.[275] measured protein carbonyl in postmortem brain tissues from patients with PD and age-matched controls. There was a significant increase in carbonyl levels in the SN, putamen, and caudate in PD. However, increased carbonyl levels were also found in areas of the brain not thought to be affected in PD. They suggested that protein carbonyl formation was related to therapy with L-dopa.

Floor and Wetzer[276] measured carbonyl modifications of soluble proteins in postmortem samples of SN, basal ganglia, and prefrontal cortex from neurologically normal subjects by 2,4-dinitrophenylhydrazine assay. They found a 2-fold increase in the protein carbonyl in substantia nigra pars compacta (SNp) than in other regions. They suggested that elevated oxidative damage might contribute to the degeneration of nigral dopaminergic neurons in aging and in PD.

Protein nitration is another way of damaging normal protein functions. Giasson et al.[277] reported nitration of aggregated alpha-synuclein proteins in brains of PD, dementia with Lewy bodies, the Lewy body variant of Alzheimer's disease, and multisystem atrophy brains using antibodies to specific nitrated tyrosine residues in alpha-synuclein.

CYTOKINES

Cytokines are bioactive substances released from cells to the surrounding media (not to the synaptic cleft), acting on

TABLE 13-4 Cytokines in PD

Increased
  Beta2-Microglobulin
  Tumor necrosis factor-alpha (TNF-alpha)
  Interleukin 2 (IL-2)
  Transforming growth factor-beta (TGF-beta)
  Epidermal growth factor (EGF)
Decreased
  Interleukin 1alpha (IL-1alpha)
  Basic fibroblast growth factor (bFGF)
  Glial cell line-derived neurotrophic factor (GDNF)
  Brain-derived neurotrophic factor (BDNF)
  Nerve growth factor (NGF)
  Ciliary neurotrophic factor (CNTF)
No change
  Neurotrophin-3 (NT-3)
  Neurotrophin-4 (NT-4)
Controversial
  Interleukin 1beta (IL-1beta)
  Interleukin 6 (IL-6)

other cells. Levels of many cytokines have been measured in PD (Table 13-4).

BETA2-MICROGLOBULIN

Mogi et al.[278] reported an increase in beta2-microglobulin in the striatum, but not in the cortex, of patients with PD.

TUMOR NECROSIS FACTOR-ALPHA (TNF-ALPHA)

Mogi et al.[278] reported increased TNF-alpha in the striatum, but not in the cortex, of patients with PD. TNF-alpha may induce beta2-microglobulin expression. TNF-alpha receptors in the peripheral lymphocytes were also reported to be increased in PD.[279] Activated T lymphocytes have increased amounts of TNF-alpha receptors, but TNF-alpha production by peripheral mononuclear cells was decreased in PD.[280]

INTERLEUKINS

Blum-Degen et al.[281] measured CSF IL-1beta, IL-2, and IL-6 in 22 de novo PD patients and found increased IL-1beta, and IL-6. They suggested the involvement of immunologic events in the complex process of neurodegeneration in PD. Mogi et al.[282] also reported an increase in IL-2 and IL-2 in ventricular fluid in patients with PD. They also reported significantly elevated IL-2 in the striatum,[283] as well as in the blood of PD patients.[284] On the other hand, Wandinger et al.[285] reported decreased IL-2 and interferon-gamma-forming activity in the peripheral blood of PD patients.[285] Interestingly, this decrease was normalized by treatment with amantadine HCl. Hasegawa et al.[280] also reported decreased IL-1alpha, IL-1beta, and IL-6 formation by peripheral blood mononuclear cells in PD. More recently, Muller et al.[286] found increased IL-6 in the CSF of PD patients, and its level was inversely correlated with the disease severity. IL-6 is a member of the neuropoietic cytokine family and has an essential role in the development, differentiation, regeneration, and degeneration of neurons in the peripheral and central nervous systems. It is expressed in both neurons and glial cells. IL-6 can exert completely opposite actions on neurons, triggering either neuronal survival after injury or causing neuronal degeneration and cell death in disorders such as Alzheimer's disease.[287]

TRANSFORMING GROWTH FACTOR-BETA (TGF-BETA)

Mogi et al.[288] reported increased TGF-beta in the striatum, but not in the cortex, of patients with PD. TGF-beta was also increased in the CSF compared with the controls. Vawter et al.[289] reported increased TGF-beta1 ($P = 0.015$) and TGF-beta2 ($P = 0.012$) in the ventricular CSF of PD patients compared to normal controls. TGF-beta is expressed in both neurons and glial cells from early embryonic stages to adulthood. TGF-beta is a potent antiapoptotic and neuroprotective agent and is significantly upregulated in response to lesions.

BASIC FIBROBLAST GROWTH FACTOR (bFGF)

Tooyama et al.[290] reported decreased bFGF in the SN of PD patients, but there was no decrease in the striatum.[283]

GLIAL CELL LINE-DERIVED NEUROTROPHIC FACTOR (GDNF)

Glial cell line-derived neurotrophic factor (GDNF) is a potent neurotrophic factor for dopaminergic neurons. Hunot et al.[291] examined GDNF gene expression in 8 PD patients and 6 controls by in situ hybridization using riboprobes corresponding to a sequence of the exon 2 human GDNF gene. No labeling was observed in nigral or striatal neurons in either group of patients. The expression level of GDNF in adult brain must be very low.

Mogi et al.[292] reported a significant decrease in GDNF in the nigrostriatal region in PD using highly sensitive sandwich enzyme-linked immunosorbent assays (ELISAs). Chauhan et al.[293] examined GDNF in the substantia nigra by quantitative immunofluorescence histochemistry. Compared to the controls, the intensity of immunostaining for GDNF was decreased by 19.4 percent per neuron ($P<0.0001$) and 20.2 percent per neuropil ($P<0.0001$). Among the 6 neurotrophic factors (GDNF, BDNF, CNTF, NGF, NT-3, NT-4) that they studied, the decrease in GDNF was most prominent.

BRAIN-DERIVED NEUROTROPHIC FACTOR (BDNF)

Parain et al.[294] studied the expression of the BDNF protein at the cellular level in postmortem mesencephalon of control subjects and patients with PD. In control subjects, BDNF was expressed in all mesencephalic regions containing dopaminergic neurons, and, in the SN, 65 percent of the melanized neurons expressed BDNF. In the PD SN, the total number of pigmented neurons containing BDNF was reduced to 9.6 percent of the corresponding control value.

Howells et al.[295] reported a 70 percent decrease in expression of BDNF mRNA in SN in PD. They suggested that neurons expressing particularly low levels of BDNF mRNA might be those at greatest risk of injury in PD. Normally, BDNF promotes survival of damaged mesencephalic dopaminergic neurons. Mogi et al.[292] also reported a significant decrease in BDNF in the nigrostriatal region in PD using highly sensitive sandwich ELISAs. Chauhan et al.[293] examined BDNF in the SN by quantitative immunofluorescence histochemistry. Compared to the controls, the intensity of immunostaining for BDNF was decreased by 8.6 percent per neuron ($P < 0.0001$) and 2.5 percent per neuropil compared to the controls.

NERVE GROWTH FACTOR (NGF)

Mogi et al.[292] reported a significant decrease in NGF in the SN of parkinsonian patients in comparison with that in the controls.

CILIARY NEUROTROPHIC FACTOR (CNTF)

Chauhan et al.[293] examined CNTF in the SN by quantitative immunofluorescence histochemistry. Compared to the controls, the intensity of immunostaining for CNTF was decreased by 11.1 percent per neuron ($P<0.0001$) and 9.4 percent per neuropil ($P<0.0001$).

EPIDERMAL GROWTH FACTOR (EGF)

Villares et al.[296] examined EGF expression in the striatum of PD. They found increased density of ^{125}I-EGF binding at anterior levels in the dorsal striatum, but not in the pallidum. EGF protects and stimulates the activity of dopaminergic neurons.

NEUROTROPHIN-3 (NT-3) AND NEUROTROPHIN-4 (NT-4)

Chauhan et al.[293] examined NT-3 and NT-4 in the SN by quantitative immunofluorescence histochemistry. There was no difference in the intensity of immunostaining in PD compared with the controls.

OTHER FACTORS CONTRIBUTING TO NIGRAL NEURODEGENERATION

Glutamate toxicity has been implicated as a pathogenetic factor contributing to nigral cell death in PD,[297] but it does not appear to be a primary etiologic factor in the disease. Further studies are needed to make any definite conclusion on the role of glutamate in nigral neuronal death in PD.

PD AND APOPTOSIS

In PD, nigral dopaminergic neurons are believed to die of apoptosis. The apoptosis cascade is shown in Fig. 13-4.

TUNEL

Mochizuki et al.[37] first applied the TUNEL method to autopsied brains of PD patients and found positive staining in 4 out of 7 cases. Tompkins et al.[38] also examined the substantia nigra by in situ end-labeling (TUNEL). Neurons demonstrated changes resembling apoptosis (i.e., nuclear condensation, chromatin fragmentation, and formation of apoptotic-like bodies). Ultrastructural analysis confirmed nuclear condensation and the formation of apoptotic-like bodies in PD, and diffuse Lewy body disease. Anglade et al.[39] examined the SN by electron microscopy and found characteristic changes of apoptosis and autophagic degeneration in melanized neurons of the SN in PD.

Kingsbury et al.[298] examined the influence of poor agonal condition on the end-labeling of fragmented DNA. They examined 16 PD brains and 14 controls. In the control group, labeling of neurons and glia was strongly associated with poor agonal status as assessed by tissue pH, a marker for antemortem hypoxia. The mean tissue pH of the control group with neuronal labeling was 6.28 (SEM 0.057), which was significantly different from that of the unlabeled group (6.55, SEM 0.055). There was no association of nigral neuronal labeling with poor agonal status in the PD cases, which showed labeling throughout the range of pH values. Their results suggest apoptotic neuronal death in PD.

Tatton[299] combined TUNEL and YOYO-1 dye binding to demonstrate apoptosis. YOYO-1 binds to DNA, demonstrating chromatin condensation. Tatton found TUNEL- and YOYO-1-positive neurons in the SN of PD patients. He identified increased numbers of apoptotic neuronal nuclei in the PD SN compared with age-matched controls. In addition, caspase 3 and Bax showed increased immunoreactivity in melanized neurons of the PD SN compared with controls. Furthermore, she observed glyceraldehyde-3-phosphate dehydrogenase nuclear accumulation in the PD SN. He suggested apoptotic rather than necrotic cell death in PD.

On the other hand, Kosel et al.[300] did not find TUNEL-positive neurons in the SN of 22 patients with PD. They thought that apoptotic neuronal death was unlikely in PD. Banati et al.[301] also failed to find TUNEL-positive neurons in the SN of 10 PD patients. Wullner et al.[302] also did not find TUNEL-positive neurons in the SN of PD patients.

SOLUBLE Fas

Mogi et al.[303] measured the soluble form of Fas (sFas) in the caudate and putamen of PD patients by a highly sensitive two-site sandwich ELISA. They found a significant increase in sFas in the caudate and putamen compared with the controls. Fas is an apoptosis-signaling receptor molecule on the surface of a number of cell types. Mogi et al. interpreted their results as indicating the presence of apoptotic neuronal death in PD.

NF-KAPPAB

Hunot et al.[304] examined nuclear translocation of NF-kappaB from cytoplasm to the nucleus. NF-kappaB is a transcription

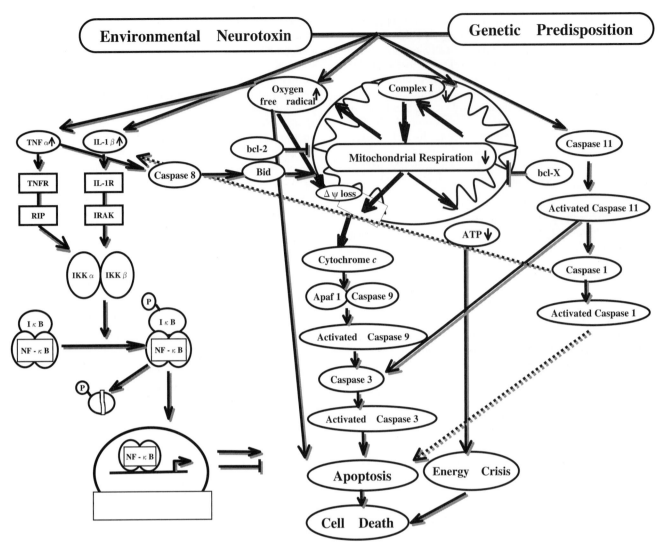

FIGURE 13-4 A schematic representation of apoptosis cascades that may be induced in nigral neurons as a result as a result of interaction of environmental neurotoxins and genetic predisposition.

factor that is activated by oxidative stress-induced apoptosis, and its activation causes it to migrate from the cytoplasm to the nucleus. They examined 5 PD patients and 7 controls. They found that the proportion of dopaminergic neurons with immunoreactive NF-kappaB in their nuclei was more than 70-fold that in control subjects. They interpreted their data as suggesting that the oxidant-mediated apoptogenic transduction pathway might play a role in the mechanism of neuronal death in PD.

Bcl-2 AND BAX
Mogi et al.[305] reported an increase in bcl-2 protein in the caudate and the putamen, but not in the cerebral cortex, of PD patients. Bcl-2 is an antiapoptotic protein located in the mitochondrial membrane, regulating the opening of the

permeability transition pore. Opening of the transition pore is associated with a proapoptotic molecule, cytochrome c. The increase in bcl-2 was interpreted as a neuronal response to counterbalance the reactive oxygen species-mediated apoptotic process. Marshall et al.[306] confirmed the increase in bcl-2 expression in the basal ganglia of PD patients.

On the other hand, Vyas et al.[307] reported a normal amount of bcl-2 mRNA expression in the SN and nucleus basalis of Meynert in PD. Wullner et al.[302] examined Bcl-2, BAX, and BCL-x expression in the SN by immunohistochemistry. They found no difference between PD patients and the controls.

Hartmann et al.[308] examined BAX expression in PD by immunohistochemistry. Bax is a proapoptotic member of the Bcl-2 family of proteins. It is believed to exert its action primarily by facilitating the release of cytochrome c from the mitochondrial intermembrane space into the cytosol, leading to caspase activation and cell death. They found that Bax was expressed ubiquitously by dopaminergic neurons in post-mortem brain of normal and PD subjects. Using an antibody to Bax inserted into the outer mitochondrial membrane as an index of Bax activation, no significant differences were observed between control and PD subjects, regardless of the mesencephalic subregion analyzed.

CASPASES

Hartmann et al.[309] recently examined caspase 3 in PD by immunohistochemistry. Caspase 3 is an effector of apoptosis. They observed a positive correlation between the degree of neuronal loss in dopaminergic cell groups in PD patients and a decrease of caspase 3-positive pigmented neurons in the SN. They interpreted their observation as suggesting that neurons expressing caspase 3 were more sensitive to the pathological process than those that did not express the protein. In addition, the percentage of active caspase 3-positive neurons among dopaminergic neurons was significantly higher in PD patients than in controls. Their results suggest apoptotic neuronal death in PD.

Hartmann et al.[310] examined caspase 8 expression in PD. Caspase 8 is a proximal effector protein of the TNF receptor family death pathway. They observed a significantly higher percentage of dopaminergic neurons displaying caspase 8 activation in PD patients compared with controls. Furthermore, they showed that caspase 8 inhibition did not result in neuroprotection, but triggered a switch from apoptosis to necrosis in a mouse MPTP model.

Summary and Conclusion

Despite our increased knowledge about the biochemical and molecular biological abnormalities in PD, we still do not know the exact etiology of sporadic PD. Many believe that the interaction of environmental factors and genetic predisposition initiates the neurodegenerative process in the nigral neurons, leading to mitochondrial respiratory failure and oxidative stress. The latter two abnormalities are believed to induce apoptotic cell death. However, no single environmental molecule or any genetic polymorphism has been identified at the molecular level. As PD is a very slowly progressing disease and asymmetry of symptoms is the rule, initial insults may be very subtle, such as minor trauma, viral infection, or subclinical intoxication. But once a portion of nigral neurons are destroyed, the expelled content of the dying neurons may be toxic to adjacent nigral neurons. As our molecular understanding of familial PD progresses, we may be able to obtain more fruitful clues to explore sporadic PD in the near future.

Acknowledgments

This study was supported in part by Grant-in-Aid for Priority Areas and Grant-in-Aid for Neuroscience Research from the Ministry of Education and Science, Japan, Grant-in-Aid for Brain Science from the Ministry of Health and Labor, Japan, and a "Center of Excellence" project grant from the National Parkinson Foundation, Miami.

References

1. Parkinson J: *An Essay on the Shaking Palsy.* London: Sherwood, Neely, and Jones, 1817.
2. Von Economo C: Encephalitis lethargica. *Wien Klin Wochenschr* 30:581–585, 1917.
3. Duvoisin RC, Yahr MD: Encephalitis and parkinsonism. *Arch Neurol* 12:227–239, 1965.
4. Holt WL Jr: Epidemic encephalitis. A follow-up study of two hundred and sixty-six cases. *Arch Neurol Psychiatry* 38:1135–1144, 1937.
5. Hallervorden J: Anatomische Untersuchungen zur Pathogenese des postencephalitischen Parkinsonismus. *Dtsch Z Nervenheilk* 136:68–77, 1935.
6. Hirano A, Zimmerman HM: Alzheimer's neurofibrillary changes: A topographic study. *Arch Neurol* 7:227–242, 1962.
7. Duvoisin RC, Yahr MD: Encephalitis and parkinsonism. *Arch Neurol* 12:227–329, 1955.
8. Goto A: A long duration follow-up study of encephalitis japonica. *Folia Psychiatr Neurol Jpn* 17:326–334, 1963.
9. Mulder DW, Parrott M, Thaler M: Sequelae of Western equine encephalitis. *Neurology* 1:318–327, 1951.
10. Schultz DR, Barthal JS, Garrett C: Western equine encephalitis with rapid onset of parkinsonism. *Neurology* 27:1095–1096, 1977.
11. Walters JH: Post-encephalitic Parkinson syndrome after meningoencephalitis due to Coxsackie virus B, type 2. *N Engl J Med* 263:744–747, 1960.
12. Henner K, Hanzal F: Les encéphalitides européennes à tiques. *Rev Neurol* 108:697–752, 1963.
13. Lycke E, Modigh K, Roos BE: The monoamine metabolism in viral encephalitides of the mouse. I. Virological and biochemical results. *Brain Res* 23:235–246, 1970.
14. Knotts FB, Cook ML, Stevens JG: Latent Herpes simplex virus in the central nervous system of rabbits and mice. *J Exp Med* 138:740–744, 1973.
15. Marttila RJ, Arstila P, Nikoskelainen J, et al: Viral antibodies in the sera from patients with Parkinson's disease. *Eur Neurol* 15:25–33, 1977.
16. Marttila RJ, Kalimo KOK, Ziola BR, et al: Herpes simplex virus subunit antibodies in patients with Parkinson's disease. *Arch Neurol* 35:668–671, 1978.
17. Schwartz J, Elizan TS: Search for viral particles and virus-specific products in idiopathic Parkinson disease brain material. *Ann Neurol* 6:261–263, 1979.
18. Wetmur JG, Schwartz J, Elizan TS: Nucleic acid homology studies of viral nucleic acids in idiopathic Parkinson's disease. *Arch Neurol* 36:462–464, 1979.
19. Rinne UK: Recent advances in research on parkinsonism. *Acta Neurol Scand* 57(suppl 67):77–113, 1978.
20. Marttila RJ, Halonen P, Rinne UK: Influenza virus antibodies in parkinsonism. *Arch Neurol* 34:99–100, 1977.
21. Elizan TS, Madden DL, Noble GR, et al: Viral antibodies in serum and CSF of parkinsonian patients and controls. *Arch Neurol* 36:529–534, 1979.

22. Mena I, Marin O, Fuenzalida S, Cotzias GC: Chronic manganese poisoning. Clinical picture and manganese turnover. *Neurology* 17:128–136, 1967.

23. Cotzias GC: Metabolic modification of some neurologic disorders. *JAMA* 210:1255–1262, 1969.

24. Yase Y: The pathogenesis of amyotrophic lateral sclerosis. *Lancet* ii:292–296, 1972.

25. Pentschew A, Ebner FF, Kovatch RM: Experimental manganese encephalopathy in monkeys. A preliminary report. *J Neuropathol Exp Neurol* 22:488–499, 1963.

26. Larsen NA, Pakkenberg H, Damsgaard E, et al: Distribution of arsenic, manganese, and selenium in the human brain in chronic renal insufficiency, Parkinson's disease, and amyotrophic lateral sclerosis. *J Neurol Sci* 51:437–446, 1981.

27. Barbeau A: Parkinson's disease: Etiological considerations. *Res Publ Assoc Res Nerv Ment Dis* 55:281–292, 1976.

28. Nair RMG, Kastin AJ, Schally AV: Isolation and structure of hypothalamic MSH release-inhibiting hormone. *Biochem Biophys Res Commun* 43:1376–1381, 1971.

29. Shuster S, Burton JL, Thody AJ, et al: Melanocyte-stimulating hormone in parkinsonism. *Lancet* i:463–464, 1973.

30. Cotzias GC, Van Woert MH, Schiffer LM: Aromatic amino acids and modification of parkinsonism. *N Engl J Med* 276:374–379, 1967.

31. Kastin AJ, Barbeau A: Preliminary clinical studies with L-prolyl-L-leucyl-glycine amide in Parkinson's disease. *Can Med Assoc J* 107:1079–1081, 1972.

32. Chase TN, Woods AC, Lipton MA, et al: Hypothalamic releasing factors and Parkinson's disease. *Arch Neurol* 31:55–56, 1974.

33. Mizuno Y, Hattori N, Matsumine H: Neurochemical and neurogenetic correlates of Parkinson's disease. *J Neurochem* 71:893–902, 1998.

34. Feldman RG, Ratner MH: The pathogenesis of neurodegenerative disease: neurotoxic mechanisms of action and genetics. *Curr Opin Neurol* 12:725–731, 1999.

35. Olanow CW, Tatton WG: Etiology and pathogenesis of Parkinson's disease. *Annu Rev Neurosci* 22:123–144, 1999.

36. Zhang Y, Dawson VL, Dawson TM: Oxidative stress and genetics in the pathogenesis of Parkinson's disease. *Neurobiol Dis* 7:240–250, 2000.

37. Mochizuki H, Goto G, Mori H, Mizuno Y: Histochemical detection of apoptosis in Parkinson's disease. *J Neurol Sci* 137:120–123, 1996.

38. Tompkins MM, Basgall EJ, Zamrini E, Hill WD: Apoptotic-like changes in Lewy-body-associated disorders and normal aging in substantia nigral neurons. *Am J Pathol* 150:119–131, 1997.

39. Anglade P, Vyas S, Javoy-Agid F, et al: Apoptosis and autophagy in nigral neurons of patients with Parkinson's disease. *Histol Histopathol* 12:25–31, 1997.

40. Davis GC, Williams AC, Markey SP, et al: Chronic parkinsonism secondary to intravenous injection of meperidine analogues. *Psychiatry Res* 1:249–254, 1979.

41. Langston JW, Ballard P, Tetrud JW, Irwin I: Chronic parkinsonism in humans due to a product of meperidine-analog synthesis. *Science* 219:979–980, 1983.

42. Ballard PA, Tetrud JW, Langston JW: Permanent human parkinsonism due to 1-methyl-4-phenyl-1,2,3,6-tetrahydropyridine (MPTP): Seven cases. *Neurology* 35:949–956, 1985.

43. Langston JW, Forno LS, Tetrud J, et al: Evidence of active nerve cell degeneration in the substantia nigra of humans years after 1-methyl-4-phenyl-1,2,3,6-tetrahydropyridine exposure. *Ann Neurol* 46:598–605, 1999.

44. Chiba K, Trevor AJ, Castagnoli N Jr: Metabolism of the neurotoxic tertiary amine, MPTP, by brain monoamine oxidase. *Biochem Biophys Res Commun* 120:574–578, 1984.

45. Javitch JA, D'Amato RJ, Strittmatter SM, Snyder SH: Parkinsonism-inducing neurotoxin, N-methyl-4-phenyl-1,2,3,6-tetrahydropyridine: Uptake of the metabolite N-methyl-4-phenylpyridine by dopamine neurons explains selective toxicity. *Proc Natl Acad Sci U S A* 82:2173–2177, 1985.

46. Ricaurte GA, Langston JW, Delanney LE, et al: Dopamine uptake blockers protect against the dopamine depleting effect of 1-methyl-4-phenyl-1,2,3,6-tetrahydropyridine (MPTP) in the mouse striatum. *Neurosci Lett* 59:259–264, 1985.

47. Irwin I, Langston JW: Selective accumulation of MPP$^+$ in the substantia nigra: A key to neurotoxicity? *Life Sci* 36:207–212, 1985.

48. Ramsay RR, Singer TP: Energy-dependent uptake of N-methyl-4-phenylpyridinium, the neurotoxic metabolite of 1-methyl-4-phenyl-1,2,3,6-tetrahydropyridine, by mitochondria. *J Biol Chem* 261:7585–7587, 1986.

49. Nicklas WJ, Vyas I, Heikkila RE: Inhibition of NADH-linked oxidation in brain mitochondria by 1-methyl-4-phenyl-pyridine, a metabolite of the neurotoxin, 1-methyl-4-phenyl-1,2,5,6-tetrahydropyridine. *Life Sci* 36:2503–2508, 1985.

50. Mizuno Y, Saitoh T, Sone N: Inhibition of mitochondrial NADH-ubiquinone oxidoreductase activity by 1-methyl-4-phenylpyridinium ion. *Biochem Biophys Res Commun* 143:294–299, 1987.

51. Mizuno Y, Suzuki K, Sone N, Saitoh T: Inhibition of ATP synthesis by 1-methyl-4-phenylpyridinium ion (MPP$^+$) in isolated mitochondria from mouse brains. *Neurosci Lett* 81:204–208, 1987.

52. Ramsay RR, McKeown KA, Johnson EA, et al: Inhibition of NADH oxidation by pyridine derivatives. *Biochem Biophys Res Commun* 146:53–60, 1987.

53. Mizuno Y, Saitoh T, Sone N: Inhibition of mitochondrial alpha-ketoglutarate dehydrogenase by 1-methyl-4-phenylpyridinium ion. *Biochem Biophys Res Commun* 143:971–976, 1987.

54. Dipasquale B, Marini M, Youl RJ: Apoptosis and DNA degradation by 1-methyl-4-phenylpyridinium in neurons. *Biochem Biophys Res Commun* 181:1442–1448, 1991.

55. Mochizuki H, Nakamura N, Nishi K, Mizuno Y: Apoptosis is induced by 1-methyl-4-phenylpyridinium ion (MPP$^+$) in a ventral mesencephalic-striatal co-culture. *Neurosci Lett* 170:191–194, 1994.

56. Vila M, Jackson-Lewis V, Vukosavic S, et al: Bax ablation prevents dopaminergic neurodegeneration in the 1-methyl-4-phenyl-1,2,3,6-tetrahydropyridine mouse model of Parkinson's disease. *Proc Natl Acad Sci U S A* 98:2837–2842, 2001.

57. Turmel H, Hartmann A, Parain K, et al: Caspase-3 activation in 1-methyl-4-phenyl-1,2,3,6-tetrahydropyridine (MPTP)-treated mice. *Mov Disord* 16:185–189, 2001.

58. Goodwin BL, Kite GC. Environmental MPTP as a factor in the aetiology of Parkinson's disease? *J Neural Transm* 105:1265–1269, 1998.

59. Rajput AH, Uitti RJ, Stern W, Laverty W: Early onset Parkinson's disease in Saskatchewan: Environmental considerations for etiology. *Can J Neurol Sci* 13:312–316, 1986.

60. Tanner CM, Langston JW: Do environmental toxins cause Parkinson's disease? A critical review. *Neurology* 40(suppl 3): 17–31, 1990.

61. Koller W, Vetere-Overfield B, Gray C, et al: Environmental risk factors in Parkinson's disease. *Neurology* 40:1218–1221, 1991.

62. Wong GF, Gray CS, Hassanein RS, Koller WC: Environmental risk factors in siblings with Parkinson's disease. *Arch Neurol* 48:287–289, 1991.

63. Hubble JP, Cao T, Hassanein RES, et al: Risk factors for Parkinson's disease. *Neurology* 43:1693–1697, 1993.

64. McCann SJ, LeCouteur DG, Green AC, et al: The epidemiology of Parkinson's disease in an Australian population. *Neuroepidemiology* 17:310–317, 1998.

65. De Michele G, Filla A, Volpe G, et al: Environmental and genetic risk factors in Parkinson's disease: A case-control study in southern Italy. *Mov Disord* 11:17–23, 1996.

66. Schoenberg BS: Environmental risk factors for Parkinson's disease: The epidemiologic evidence. *Can J Neurol Sci* 14:407–413, 1987.

67. Semchuck KM, Love EJ, Lee RG: Parkinson's disease: A test of the multifactorial etiologic hypothesis. *Neurology* 43:1173–1180, 1993.

68. Butterfield PG, Valanis BG, Spencer PS, et al: Environmental antecedents of young-onset Parkinson's disease. *Neurology* 43:1150–1158, 1993.

69. Seidler A, Hellenbrand W, Robra BP, et al: Possible environmental, occupational, and other etiologic factors for Parkinson's disease: A case-control study in Germany. *Neurology* 46:1275–1284, 1996.

70. Tanner CM, Chen B, Wang W, et al: Environmental factors and Parkinson's disease: A case-control study in China. *Neurology* 39:660–664, 1989.

71. Taylor CA, Saint-Hilaire MH, Cupples LA, et al: Environmental, medical, and family history risk factors for Parkinson's disease: A New England-based case control study. *Am J Med Genet* 88:742–749, 1999.

72. Rajput AH, Uitti RJ, Stern W, et al: Geography, drinking water chemistry, pesticides and herbicides and the etiology of Parkinson's disease. *Can J Neurol Sci* 14:414–418, 1987.

73. Stern M, Dulaney E, Gruber SB, et al: The epidemiology of Parkinson's disease. A case controlled study of young-onset and old-onset patients. *Arch Neurol* 48:903–907, 1991.

74. Beterbet R, Sherer TB, MacKenzie G, et al: Chronic systemic pesticide exposure reproduces features of disease. *Nat Neurosci* 3:1301–1306, 2000.

75. Brooks AI, Chadwick CA, Gelbard HA, et al: Paraquat elicited neurobehavioral syndrome caused by dopaminergic neuron loss. *Brain Res* 823:1–10, 1999.

76. Pezzoli G, Canesi M, Antonini A, et al: Hydrocarbon exposure and Parkinson's disease. *Neurology* 55:667–673, 2000.

77. Masalha R, Herishaunu Y, Alfahel-Kakunda A, Silverman WF: Selective dopamine neurotoxicity by an industrial chemical: An environmental cause of Parkinson's disease? *Brain Res* 774:260–264, 1997.

78. Jackson-Lewis V, Liberatore G: Effects of a unilateral stereotaxic injection of Tinuvin 123 into the substantia nigra on the nigrostriatal dopaminergic pathway in the rat. *Brain Res* 866:197–210, 2000.

79. Godwin-Austen RB, Lee PN, Marmot MG, Stern GM: Smoking and Parkinson's disease. *J Neurol Neurosurg Psychiatry* 45:577–581, 1982.

80. Baron JA: Cigarette smoking and Parkinson's disease. *Neurology* 36:1490–1496, 1986.

81. Lichtensteiger W, Felix D, Lienhart R, Hefti F: A quantitative correlation between single unit activity and fluorescence intensity of dopamine neurons in zona compacta of substantia nigra, as demonstrated under the influence of nicotine and physostigmine. *Brain Res* 117:85–103, 1976.

82. Anderson K, Fuxe K, Agnati LF: Effects of single injections of nicotine on the ascending dopamine pathways in the rat. *Acta Physiol Scand* 112:345–347, 1981.

83. Arqueros L, Naquira D, Zunino E: Nicotine-induced release of catecholamines from rat hippocampus and striatum. *Biochem Pharmacol* 27:2667–2674, 1978.

84. Giorguieff-Chesselet MF, Kemel ML, Wandscheer D, Glowinski J: Regulation of dopamine release by presynaptic nicotine receptors in rat striatal slices: Effect of nicotine in a low concentration. *Life Sci* 25:1257–1262, 1979.

85. Calne DB, Langston JW: Aetiology of Parkinson's disease. *Lancet* ii:1457–1459, 1983.

86. Oreland L, Fowler CJ, Schalling D: Low platelet monoamine oxidase activity in cigarette smokers. *Life Sci* 29:2511–2518, 1981.

87. Hellenbrand W, Seidler A, Robra BP, et al: Smoking and Parkinson's disease: A case-control study in Germany. *Int J Epidemiol* 26:328–339, 1997.

88. Rajput AH, Offord KP, Beard CM, Kurland LT: A case-control study of smoking habits, dementia, and other illnesses in idiopathic Parkinson's disease. *Neurology* 37:226–232, 1987.

89. Elbaz A, Manubens-Bertran JM, Baldereschi M, et al: Parkinson's disease, smoking, and family history. EUROPARKINSON Study Group. *J Neurol* 247:793–798, 2000.

90. McNaught KS, Carrupt PA, Altomare C, et al: Isoquinoline derivatives as endogenous neurotoxins in the aetiology of Parkinson's disease. *Biochem Pharmacol* 56:921–933, 1998.

91. Yoshida M, Niwa T, Nagatsu T: Parkinsonism in monkeys produced by chronic administration of an endogenous substance of the brain, tetrahydroisoquinoline: The behavioral and biochemical changes. *Neurosci Lett* 119:109–113, 1990.

92. Nagatsu T, Yoshida M: An endogenous substance of the brain, tetrahydroisoquinoline, produces parkinsonism in primates with decreased dopamine, tyrosine hydroxylase and biopterine in the nigrostriatal regions. *Neurosci Lett* 87:178–182, 1988.

93. Niwa T, Takeda N, Tatematsu A, et al: Migration of tetrahydroisoquinoline, a possible parkinsonian neurotoxin, into monkey brain from blood as proved by gas chromatography-mass spectrometry. *J Chromatogr* 452:85–91, 1988.

94. Suzuki K, Mizuno Y, Yoshida M: Inhibition of mitochondrial NADH-ubiquinone oxidoreductase activity and ATP synthesis by tetrahydroisoquinoline. *Neurosci Lett* 86: 105–108, 1988.

95. Suzuki K, Mizuno Y, Yoshida M: Inhibition of mitochondrial respiration by 1,2,3,4-tetrahydroisoquinoline-like endogenous alkaloids in mouse brain. *Neurochem Res* 15: 705–710, 1990.

96. Tasaki Y, Makino Y, Ohta S, Hirobe M: 1-Methyl-1,2,3,4-tetrahydroisoquinoline, decreasing in 1-methyl-4-phenyl-1,2,3,6-terahydropyridine-treated mouse, prevents parkinsonism-like behavior abnormalities. *J Neurochem* 57:1940–1943, 1991.

97. Ohta S, Kohno M, Makino Y, et al: Tetrahydroisoquinoline and 1-methyl-tetrahydroisoquinoline are present in the human brain: relation to Parkinson's disease. *Biomed Res* 8:453–456, 1987.

98. Maruyama W, Nakahara D, Ota M, et al: N-Methylation of dopamine-derived 6,7-dihydroxy-1,2,3,4-tetrahydroisoquinoline, (R)-salsolinol, in rat brains: In vivo microdialysis study. *J Neurochem* 59:395–400, 1992.

99. Maruyama W, Benedetti MS, Takahashi T, Naoi M: A neurotoxin N-methyl(R)salsolinol induces apoptotic cell death in differentiated human dopaminergic neuroblastoma SH-SY5Y cells. *Neurosci Lett* 232:147–150, 1997.

100. Akao Y, Nakagawa Y, Maruyama W, et al: Apoptosis induced by an endogenous neurotoxin, N-methyl(R)salsolinol, is mediated by activation of caspase 3. *Neurosci Lett* 267:153–156, 1999.

101. Naoi M, Maruyama W, Kasamatsu T, Dostert P: Oxidation of N-methyl(R)salsolinol: Involvement to neurotoxicity and neuroprotection by endogenous catechol isoquinolines. *J Neural Transm Suppl* 52:125–138, 1998.

102. Maruyama W, Strolin-Benedetti M, Naoi M: N-Methyl-(R)salsolinol and a neutral N-methyltransferase as pathogenic factors in Parkinson's disease. *Neurobiology* 8:55–68, 2000.

103. Maruyama W, Narabayashi H, Dostert P, Naoi M: Stereospecific occurrence of a parkinsonism-inducing catechol isoquinoline, N-methyl(R)salsolinol, in the human intraventricular fluid. *J Neural Transm* 103:1069–1076, 1996.

104. Kawai H, Makino Y, Hirobe M, Ohta S: Novel endogenous 1,2,3,4-tetrahydroisoquinoline derivatives: Uptake by dopamine transporter and activity to induce parkinsonism. *J Neurochem* 70:745–751, 1998.

105. Collins MA, Neafsey E: β-Carboline analogues of N-methyl-4-phenyl-1,2,5,6-tetrahydropyridine (MPTP): Endogenous factors underlying idiopathic parkinsonism? *Neurosci Lett* 55:179–184, 1985.

106. Collins MA, Neafsey EJ, Matsubara K, et al: Indo-N-methylated β-carbolinium ions as potential brain-bioactivated neurotoxins. *Brain Res* 570:154–160, 1992.

107. Matsubara K, Collins MA, Akane A, et al: Potential bioactivated neurotoxins, N-methylated β-carbolinium ions, are present in human brain. *Brain Res* 610:90–96, 1993.

108. Cobuzzi RJ Jr, Neafsey EJ, Collins MA: Differential cytotoxicities of N-methyl-beta-carbolinium analogues of MPP$^+$ in PC12 cells: Insights into potential neurotoxicants in Parkinson's disease. *J Neurochem* 62:1503–1510, 1994.

109. Kojima T, Naoi M, Wakabayashi K, et al: 3-Amino-1-methyl-5H-pyrido[4,3-b]indole(Trp-P-2) and other heterocyclic amines as inhibitors of mitochondrial monoamine oxidases separated from human brain synaptosomes. *Neurochem Int* 16:51–57, 1990.

110. Drucker G, Raikoff K, Neafsey EJ, Collins MA: Dopamine uptake inhibitory capacities of beta-carboline and 3,4-dihydro-beta-carboline analogs of N-methyl-4-phenyl-1,2,3,6-tetrahydropyridine (MPTP) oxidation products. *Brain Res*, 509:125–133, 1990.

111. Albores R, Heafsey EJ, Drucker G, et al: Mitochondrial respiratory inhibition by N-methylated beta-carboline derivatives structurally resembling N-methyl-4-phenylpyridine. *Proc Natl Acad Sci U S A* 87:9368–9372, 1990.

112. Matsubara K, Gonda T, Sawada H, et al: Endogenously occurring beta-carboline induces parkinsonism in nonprimate animals: A possible causative protoxin in idiopathic Parkinson's disease. *J Neurochem* 70:727–735, 1998.

113. Kuhn W, Muller T, Grosse H, Rommelspacher H: Plasma harman and norharman in Parkinson's disease. *J Neural Transm Suppl* 46:291–295, 1995.

114. Payami H, Bernard S, Larsen K, et al: Genetic anticipation in Parkinson's disease. *Neurology* 45:135–138, 1995.

115. Marder K, Tang M-X, Mejia H, et al: Risk of Parkinson's disease among first-degree relatives: A community-based study. *Neurology* 47:155–160, 1996.

116. Rybicki BA, Johnson CC, Peterson EL, et al: A family history of Parkinson's disease and its effect on other PD risk factors. *Neuroepidemiology* 18:270-278, 1999.

117. Elbaz A, Grigoletto F, Baldereschi M, et al: European Parkinson Study Group: Familial aggregation of Parkinson's disease. A population-based case-control study in Europe. *Neurology* 52:1876–1882, 1999.

118. Ward CD, Duvoisin RC, Ince SE, et al: Parkinson's disease in 65 pairs of twins and in a set of quadruplets. *Neurology* 33:815–824, 1983.

119. Tanner CM, Ottman R, Goldman SM, et al: Parkinson's disease in twins: An etiologic study. *JAMA* 281:341–346, 1999.

120. Piccini P, Burn DJ, Ceravolo R, et al: The role of inheritance in sporadic Parkinson's disease: Evidence from a longitudinal study of dopaminergic function in twins. *Ann Neurol* 45:577–582, 1999.

121. Barbeau A, Cloutier T, Roy M, et al: Ecogenetics of Parkinson's disease: 4-Hydroxylation of debrisoquine. *Lancet* ii:1213–1215, 1985.

122. Poirier J, Roy M, Campanella G, et al: Debrisoquine metabolism in parkinsonian patients treated with antihistamine drugs. *Lancet* ii:386–387, 1987.

123. Benitez J, Ladero JM, Jimenez-Jimenez C, et al: Oxidative polymorphism of debrisoquine in Parkinson's disease. *J Neurol Neurosurg Psychiatry* 53:289–292, 1990.

124. Marttila KJ, Rinne UK, Sonninen V, Syvälahti E: Debrisoquine oxidation in Parkinson's disease. *Acta Neurol Scand* 83:194–197, 1991.

125. Liu TY, Chi CW, Yang JC, et al: Debrisoquine metabolism in Chinese patients with Alzheimer's and Parkinson's diseases. *Mol Chem Neuropathol* 17:31–37, 1992.

126. Armstrong M, Daly AK, Cholerton S, et al: Mutant debrisoquine hydroxylation genes in Parkinson's disease. *Lancet* 339:1017–1018, 1992.

127. Smith CA, Gough AC, Leigh PN, et al: Debrisoquine hydroxylase gene polymorphism and susceptibility to Parkinson's disease. *Lancet* 339:1375–1377, 1992.

128. Kurth MC, Kurth JH: Variant cytochrome P450 CYP2D6 allelic frequencies in Parkinson's disease. *Am J Med Genet* 48:166–168, 1993.

129. Kondo I, Kanazawa I: Debrisoquine hydroxylase and Parkinson's disease. *Adv Neurol* 60:338–342, 1993.

130. Tsuneoka Y, Matsuo Y, Iwahashi K, et al: A novel cytochrome P-450IID6 gene associated with Parkinson's disease. *J Biochem* 114:263–266, 1993.

131. Sandy MS, Armstrong M, Tanner CM, et al: CYP2D6 allelic frequencies in young-onset Parkinson's disease. *Neurology* 47:225–230, 1996.

132. Diederich N, Hilger C, Goetz CG, et al: Genetic variability of the CYP 2D6 gene is not a risk factor for sporadic Parkinson's disease. *Ann Neurol* 40:463–465, 1996.

133. Joost O, Taylor CA, Thomas CA, et al: Absence of effect of seven functional mutations in the CYP2D6 gene in Parkinson's disease. *Mov Disord* 14:590–595, 1999.

134. Payami H, Lee N, Zareparsi S, et al: Parkinson's disease, CYP2D6 polymorphism, and age. *Neurology* 56:1363–1370, 2001.

135. Christensen PM, Gotzsche PC, Brosen K: The sparteine/debrisoquine (CYP2D6) oxidation polymorphism and the risk of Parkinson's disease: A meta-analysis. *Pharmacogenetics* 8:473–479, 1998.

136. Waring RH, Steventon GB, Sturman SG, et al: *S*-Methylation in motoneuron disease and Parkinson's disease. *Lancet* ii: 356–357, 1989.

137. Nakagawa-Hattori Y, Hattori T, Kondo T, Mizuno Y: *S*–Methylation in Parkinson's disease. *Neurology* (in press).

138. Hotamisligil GS, Girmen AS, Fink JS, et al: Hereditary variations in monoamine oxidase as a risk factor for Parkinson's disease. *Mov Disord* 9:305–310, 1994.

139. Nakatome M, Tun Z, Shimada S, Honda K: Detection and analysis of four polymorphic markers at the human monoamine oxidase (MAO) gene in Japanese controls and patients with Parkinson's disease. *Biochem Biophys Res Commun* 247:452–456, 1998.

140. Nanko S, Ueki A, Hattori M: No association between Parkinson's disease and monoamine oxidase A and B gene polymorphisms. *Neurosci Lett* 204:125–127, 1996.

141. Plante-Bordeneuve V, Taussig D, Thomas F, et al: Evaluation of four candidate genes encoding proteins of the dopamine pathway in familial and sporadic Parkinson's disease: Evidence for association of a DRD2 allele. *Neurology* 48:1589–1593, 1997.

142. Costa-Mallen P, Checkoway H, Fishel M, et al: The EcoRV genetic polymorphism of human monoamine oxidase type A is not associated with Parkinson's disease and does not modify the effect of smoking on Parkinson's disease. *Neurosci Lett* 278:33–36, 2000.

143. Kurth JH, Kurth MC, Poduslo SE, Schwankhaus JD: Association of a monoamine oxidase B allele with Parkinson's disease. *Ann Neurol* 33:368–372, 1993.

144. Costa P, Checkoway H, Levy D, et al: Association of a polymorphism in intron 13 of the monoamine oxidase B gene with Parkinson disease. *Am J Med Genet* 74:154–156, 1997.

145. Wu RM, Cheng CW, Chen KH, et al: The COMT L allele modifies the association between MAOB polymorphism and PD in Taiwanese. *Neurology* 56:375–382, 2001.

146. Ho SL, Kapadí AL, Ramsden DB, Williams AC: An allelic association study of monoamine oxidase B in Parkinson's disease. *Ann Neurol* 37:403–405, 1995.

147. Morimoto Y, Murayama N, Kuwano A, et al: Association analysis of a polymorphism of the monoamine oxidase B gene with Parkinson's disease in a Japanese population. *Am J Med Genet* 60:570–572, 1995.

148. Mellick GD, Buchanan DD, McCann SJ, et al: Variations in the monoamine oxidase B (MAOB) gene are associated with Parkinson's disease. *Mov Disord* 14:219–224, 1999.

149. Mellick GD, Buchanan DD, Silburn PA, et al: The monoamine oxidase B gene GT repeat polymorphism and Parkinson's disease in a Chinese population. *J Neurol* 247:52–55, 2000.

150. Kunugi H, Nanko S, Ueki A, et al: High and low activity alleles of catechol-*O*-methyltransferase gene: Ethnic difference and possible association with Parkinson's disease. *Neurosci Lett* 221:202–204, 1997.

151. Yoritaka A, Hattori N, Yoshino H, Mizuno Y: Catechol-*O*-methyltransferase genotype and susceptibility to Parkinson's disease in Japan. *J Neural Transm* 104:1313–1317, 1997.

152. Hoda F, Nicholl D, Bennett P, et al: No association between Parkinson's disease and low-activity alleles of catechol-*O*-methyltransferase. *Biochem Biophys Res Commun* 228:780–784, 1996.

153. Syvanen AC, Tilgmann C, Rinne J, Ulmanen I: Genetic polymorphism of catechol-*O*-methyltransferase (COMT): Correlation of genotype with individual variation of *S*-COMT activity and comparison of the allele frequencies in the normal population and parkinsonian patients in Finland. *Pharmacogenetics* 7:65–71, 1997.

154. Xie T, Ho SL, Li LS, Ma OC: G/A1947 polymorphism in catechol-*O*-methyltransferase (COMT) gene in Parkinson's disease. *Mov Disord* 12:426–427, 1997.

155. Lee MS, Lyoo CH, Ulmanen I, et al: Genotypes of catechol-*O*-methyltransferase and response to levodopa treatment in patients with Parkinson's disease. *Neurosci Lett* 298:131–134, 2001.

156. Grevle L, Guzey C, Hadidi H, et al: Allelic association between the DRD2 *Taq*I A polymorphism and Parkinson's disease. *Mov Disord* 15:1070–1074, 2000.

157. Ricketts MH, Hamer RM, Manowitz P, et al: Association of long variants of the dopamine D4 receptor exon 3 repeat polymorphism with Parkinson's disease. *Clin Genet* 54:33–38, 1998.

158. Nanko S, Ueki A, Hattori M, et al: No allelic association between Parkinson's disease and dopamine D2, D3, and D4 receptor gene polymorphisms. *Am J Med Genet* 54:361–364, 1994.

159. Higuchi S, Muramatsu T, Arai H, et al: Polymorphisms of dopamine receptor and transporter genes and Parkinson's disease. *J Neural Transm* 10:107–113, 1995.

160. Pastor P, Munoz E, Obach V, et al: Dopamine receptor D2 intronic polymorphism in patients with Parkinson's disease. *Neurosci Lett* 273:151–154, 1999.

161. Wan DC, Law LK, Ip DT, et al: Lack of allelic association of dopamine D4 receptor gene polymorphisms with Parkinson's disease in a Chinese population. *Mov Disord* 14:225–229, 1999.

162. Wang J, Liu ZL, Chen B: Dopamine D5 receptor gene polymorphism and the risk of levodopa-induced motor fluctuations in patients with Parkinson's disease. *Neurosci Lett* 308:21–24, 2001.

163. Plante-Bordeneuve V, Davis MB, Maraganore DM, et al: Tyrosine hydroxylase polymorphisms in familial and sporadic Parkinson's disease. *Mov Disord* 9:337–339, 1994.

164. Parboosingh JS, Rousseau M, Rogan F, et al: Absence of mutations in superoxide dismutase and catalase genes in patients with Parkinson's disease. Absence of mutations in superoxide dismutase and catalase genes in patients with Parkinson's disease. *Arch Neurol* 52:1160–1163, 1995.

165. Farin FM, Hitosis Y, Hallagan SE, et al: Genetic polymorphisms of superoxide dismutase in Parkinson's disease. *Mov Disord* 16:705–707, 2001.

166. Shimoda-Matsubayashi S, Hattori T, Matsumine H, et al: Mn SOD activity and protein in a patient with chromosome 6-linked autosomal recessive parkinsonism in comparison with Parkinson's disease and control. *Neurology* 49:1257–1262, 1997.

167. Grasbon-Frodl EM, Kosel S, Riess O, et al: Analysis of mitochondrial targeting sequence and coding region polymorphisms of the manganese superoxide dismutase gene in German Parkinson disease patients. *Biochem Biophys Res Commun* 255:749–752, 1999.

168. Stroombergen MCMJ, Waring RH, Bennett P, Williams AC: Determination of the GSTM1 gene deletion frequency in Parkinson's disease by allele specific PCR. *Parkinsonism Relat Disord* 2:151–154, 1996.

169. Satoh J, Kuroda Y: A valine to methionine polymorphism at codon 83 in the 8-oxo-dGTPase gene MTH1 is not associated with sporadic Parkinson's disease. *Eur J Neurol* 7:673–677, 2000.

170. Bandmann O, Vaughan J, Holmans P, et al: Association of slow acetylator genotype for *N*-acetyltransferase 2 with familial Parkinson's disease. *Lancet* 350:1136–1139, 1997.

171. Nishimura M, Mizuta I, Mizuta E, et al: Influence of interleukin-1beta gene polymorphisms on age-at-onset of sporadic Parkinson's disease. *Neurosci Lett* 284:73–76, 2000.

172. Kruger R, Vieira-Saecker AM, Kuhn W, et al: Increased susceptibility to sporadic Parkinson's disease by a certain combined alpha-synuclein/apolipoprotein E genotype. *Ann Neurol* 45:611–617, 1999.

173. Farrer M, Marananore DM, Lackhart P, et al: Alpha-synuclein gene haplotypes are associated with Parkinson's disease. *Hum Mol Genet* 10:1847–1851, 2001.

174. Izumi Y, Morino H, Oda M, et al: Genetic studies in Parkinson's disease with an alpha-synuclein/NACP gene polymorphism in Japan. *Neurosci Lett* 300:125–127, 2001.

175. Wang M, Hattori N, Matsumine H, et al: Polymorphism in the Parkin gene in sporadic Parkinson's disease. *Ann Neurol* 45:655–658, 1999.

176. Hu CJ, Sung SM, Liu HC, et al: Polymorphisms of the parkin gene in sporadic Parkinson's disease among Chinese in Taiwan. *Eur Neurol* 44:90–93, 2000.

177. Satoh J, Kuroda Y: Association of codon 167 Ser/Asn heterozygosity in the parkin gene with sporadic Parkinson's disease. *Neuroreport* 10:2735–2739, 1999.

178. Pastor P, Ezquerra M, Munoz E, et al: Significant association between the tau gene A0/A0 genotype and Parkinson's disease. *Ann Neurol* 47:242–245, 2000.

179. Koller WC, Glatt SL, Hubble JP, et al: Apolipoprotein E genotypes in Parkinson's disease with and without dementia. *Ann Neurol* 37:242–245, 1995.

180. Yamamoto M, Kondo I, Ogawa N, et al: Genetic association between susceptibility to Parkinson's disease and alpha1-antichymotrypsin polymorphism. *Brain Res* 759:153–155, 1997.

181. Grasbon-Frodl EM, Egensperger R, Kosel S, et al: The alpha1-antichymotrypsin A-allele in German Parkinson disease patients. *J Neural Transm* 106:729–736, 1999.

182. Munoz E, Obach V, Oliva R, et al: Alpha1-antichymotrypsin gene polymorphism and susceptibility to Parkinson's disease. *Neurology* 52:297–301, 1999.

183. Hattori N, Yoshino H, Tanaka M, et al: Genotype in the 24-kDa subunit gene (NDUFV2) of mitochondrial complex I and susceptibility to Parkinson disease. *Genomics* 49:52–58, 1998.

184. Kobayashi T, Matsumine H, Matsubayashi S, et al: Polymorphism of the gene encoding dihydrolipoamide succinyltransferase, a subunit of α-ketoglutarate dehydrogenase complex, is associated with the susceptibility to Parkinson disease: A population based study. *Ann Neurol* 43;120–123, 1998.

185. Ikebe S, Tanaka M, Ohno K, et al: Increase of deleted mitochondrial DNA in the striatum in Parkinson's disease and senescence. *Biochem Biophys Res Commun* 170:1044–1048, 1990.

186. Shoffner JM, Brown MD, Torroni A, et al: Mitochondrial DNA variants observed in Alzheimer disease and Parkinson disease patients. *Genomics* 17:171–184, 1993.

187. Ikebe S, Tanaka M, Ozawa T: Point mutations of mitochondrial genome in Parkinson's disease. *Mol Brain Res* 28:281–295, 1995.

188. Lücking CB, Kösel S, Mehraein P, Graeber MB: Absence of the mitochondrial A7237T mutation in Parkinson's disease. *Biochem Biophys Res Commun* 211:700–704, 1995.

189. Kapsa RM, Jeean-Francois MJ, Lertrit P, et al: Mitochondrial DNA polymorphism in substantia nigra. *J Neurol Sci* 144:204–211, 1996.

190. Schnopp NM, Kösel S, Egensperger R, Graeber MB: Regional heterogeneity of mtDNA heteroplasmy in parkinsonian brain. *Clin Neuropathol* 15:348–352, 1996.

191. Mayr-Wohlfart U, Rodel G, Hennesberg A: Mitochondrial tRNA(Gln) and tRNA(Thr) gene variants in Parkinson's disease. *Eur J Med Res* 2:111–113, 1997.

192. Polymeropoulos MH, Higgins JJ, Golbe LI, et al: Mapping of a gene for Parkinson's disease to chromosome 4q21–q23. *Science* 274:1197–1199, 1996.

193. Polymeropoulos MH, Lavedan C, Leroy E, et al: Mutation in the α-synuclein gene identified in families with Parkinson's disease. *Science* 276:2045–2047, 1997.

194. Matsumine H, Saito M, Shimoda-Matsubayashi S, et al: Localization of a gene for autosomal recessive form of juvenile parkinsonism (AR-JP) to chromosome 6q25.2–27. *Am J Hum Genet* 60:588–596, 1997.

195. Kitada T, Asakawa S, Hattori N, et al: Deletion mutation in a novel protein "Parkin" gene causes autosomal recessive juvenile parkinsonism (AR-JP). *Nature* 392:605–608, 1998.

196. Gasser T, Müller-Myhsok B, Wszolek ZK, et al: A susceptibility locus for Parkinson's disease maps to chromosome 2p13. *Nat Genet* 18:262–265, 1998.

197. Farrer M, Gwinn-Hardy K, Muenter M, et al: A chromosome 4p haplotype segregating with Parkinson's disease and postural tremor. *Hum Mol Genet* 8:81–85, 1999.

197'. Singleton AB, Farrer M, Johston J, et al: α-Synuclein locus triplication causes Parkinson's disease. *Science* 302:841, 2003.

198. Valente EM, Bentivolglio AR, Dixon PH, et al: Localization of a novel locus for autosomal recessive early-onset parkinsonims, PARK6, on human chromosome 1p35–36. *Am J Hum Genet* 68:895–900, 2001.

199. Duijin CMV, Dekker MCJ, Bonifati V, et al: PARK7, a novel locus for autosomal recessive early-onset parkinsonism, on chromosome 1p36. *Am J Hum Genet* 69:629–634, 2001.

199'. Bonifati V, Rizzu P, van Baren MJ, et al: Mutations in the DJ-1 gene associated with autosomal recessive early-onset parkinsonism. *Science* 299:256–259, 2003.

200. Funayama M, Hasegawa K, Kowa H, et al: A new locus for Parkinson's disease (PARK 8) maps to chromosome 12p11.2-q13.1. *Ann Neurol* (in press).

201. Leroy E, Boyer R, Auburger G, et al: The ubiquitin pathway in Parkinson's disease. *Nature* 395:451–452, 1998.

202. Wilhelmsen KC, Lynch T, Pavlou E, et al: Localization of disinhibition-dementia-parkinsonism-amyotrophy complex to 17q21-22. *Am J Hum Genet* 55:1159–1165, 1994.

203. Poorkaj P, Bird TD, Wijsman E, et al: Tau is a candidate gene for chromosome 17 frontotemporal dementia. *Ann Neurol* 43:815–825, 1998.

204. Hutton M, Lendon CL, Rizzu P, et al: Association of missense and 5'-splice-site mutations in *tau* with the inherited dementia FRDP-17. *Nature* 393:702–705, 1998.

205. Kramer PL, Mineta M, Klein C, et al: Rapid-onset dystonia-parkinsonism: Linkage to chromosome 19q13. *Ann Neurol* 46:176–182, 1999.

206. Kupke RG, Lee LV, Müller U: Assignment of the X-linked torsion dystonia gene to Xq21 by linkage analysis. *Neurology* 40:1438–1442, 1990.

207. Wilhelmsen KC, Weeks DE, Nygaard TG, et al: Genetic mapping of "Lubag" (X-linked dystonia-parkinsonism) in a Filipino

kindred to the pericentromeric region of the X chromosome. *Ann Neurol* 29:124–131., 1991.

208. Golbe LI, Di Iorio G, Bonavita V, et al: A large kindred with autosomal dominant Parkinson's disease. *Ann Neurol* 27:276–282, 1990.

209. Krüger R, Kuhn W, Müller T, et al: Ala30Pro mutation in the gene encoding α-synuclein in Parkinson's disease. *Nat Genet* 18:106–108, 1998.

210. El Agnaf OM, Jakes R, Curran MD, Wallace A: Effects of the mutations Ala30 to Pro and Ala53 to Thr on the physical and morphological properties of α-synuclein protein implicated in Parkinson's disease. *FEBS Lett* 440:67–70, 1998.

211. Spillantini MG, Schmidt ML, Lee AMY, et al: α-Synuclein in Lewy bodies. *Nature* 388:839–840, 1997.

212. Wakabayashi K, Matsumoto K, Takayama K, et al: NACP, a presynaptic protein, immunoreactivity in Lewy bodies in Parkinson's disease. *Neurosci Lett* 239:45–48, 1997.

213. Rathke-Hartlieb S, Kahle PJ, Neumann M, et al: Sensitivity to MPTP is not increased in Parkinson's disease-associated mutant alpha-synuclein transgenic mice. *J Neurochem* 77:1181–1124, 2001.

214. Zhou W, Hurlbert MS, Schaack J, et al: Overexpression of human alpha-synuclein causes dopamine neuron death in rat primary culture and immortalized mesencephalon-derived cells. *Brain Res* 866:33–43, 2000.

215. Kanda S, Bishop JF, Eglitis MA, et al: Enhanced vulnerability to oxidative stress by alpha-synuclein mutations and C-terminal truncation. *Neuroscience* 97:279–284, 2000.

216. Neystat M, Lynch T, Przedborski S, et al: Alpha-synuclein expression in substantia nigra and cortex in Parkinson's disease. *Mov Disord* 14:417–422, 1999.

217. Wirdefeldt K, Bogdanovic N, Westerberg L, et al: Expression of alpha-synuclein in the human brain: Relation to Lewy body disease. *Mol Brain Res* 92:58–65, 2001.

218. Yamamura Y, Sobue I, Ando K, et al: Paralysis agitans of early onset with marked diurnal fluctuation of symptoms. *Neurology* 23:239–244, 1973.

219. Hattori N, Matsumine H, Kitada T, et al: Molecular analysis of a novel ubiquitin-like protein (PARKIN) gene in Japanese families with AR-JP: Evidence of homozygous deletions in the PARKIN gene in affected individuals. *Ann Neurol* 44:935–941, 1998.

220. Abbas N, Lücking CB, Ricard S, et al: The French Parkinson's Disease Genetics Study Group and the European Consortium on Genetic Susceptibility in Parkinson's Disease: A wide variety of mutations in the parkin gene are responsible for autosomal recessive parkinsonism in Europe. *Hum Mol Genet* 8:567–574, 1999.

221. Kubo S, Kitami T, Noda S, et al: Parkin is associated with cellular vesicles. *J Neurochem* 78:42–54, 2001.

222. Shimura H, Hattori N, Kubo S, et al: Familial Parkinson's disease gene product, Parkin, is a ubiquitin-protein ligase. *Nature Genet* 25:302–305, 2000.

223. Tanaka K, Suzuki T, Chiba T: The ligation systems for ubiquitin and ubiquitin-like proteins. *Mol Cells* 8:503–512, 1998.

224. Zhang Y, Gao J, Chung KK, et al: Parkin functions as an E2 dependent ubiquitin-protein ligase and promotes the degradation of the synaptic vesicle associated protein, CDCrel-1. *Proc Natl Acad Sci U S A* 21:13354–13359, 2000.

225. Shimura H, Schlossmacher MG, Hattori N, et al: Ubiquitination of a new form of alpha-synuclein by parkin from human brain: Implication for Parkinson's disease. *Science* 293:263–269, 2001.

226. Imai Y, Soda M, Takahashi R: Parkin suppresses unfolded protein stress induced cell death through its E3 ubiquitin-protein ligase activity. *J Biol Chem* 275:35661–35664, 2000.

227. Chung KKK, Zhang Y, Lim KL, et al: Parkin ubiquitinates the alpha-synuclein-interacting protein, synphilin-1: Implications for Lewy-body formation in Parkinson disease. *Nat Med* 7:1144–1150, 2001.

228. Schapira AHV, Cooper JM, Dexter D, et al: Mitochondrial complex I deficiency in Parkinson's disease. *Lancet* i:1269, 1989.

229. Schapira AHV, Cooper JM, Dexter D, et al: Mitochondrial complex I deficiency in Parkinson's disease. *J Neurochem* 54:823–827, 1990.

230. Mizuno Y, Ohta S, Tanaka M, et al: Deficiencies in complex I subunits of the respiratory chain in Parkinson's disease. *Biochem Biophys Res Commun* 163:1450–1455, 1989.

231. Hattori N, Tanaka M, Ozawa T, Mizuno Y: Immunohistochemical studies on complex I, II, III, and IV of mitochondria in Parkinson's disease. *Ann Neurol* 30:563–571, 1991.

232. Parker WD Jr, Boyson SJ, Parks JK: Abnormalities of the electron transport chain in idiopathic Parkinson's disease. *Ann Neurol* 26:719–723, 1989.

233. Kriege D, Carroll MT, Cooper JM, et al: Platelet mitochondrial function in Parkinson's disease. *Ann Neurol* 32:782–788, 1992.

234. Yoshino H, Nakagawa-Hattori Y, Kondo T, Mizuno Y: Mitochondrial complex I and II activities of lymphocytes and platelets in Parkinson's disease. *J Neural Transm* 4:27–34, 1992.

235. Bindoff LA, Birch-Machin M, Cartlidge NEF, et al: Mitochondrial function in Parkinson's disease. *Lancet* ii: 49, 1989.

236. Bindoff LA, Birch-Machin M, Cartlidge NEF, et al: Respiratory chain abnormalities in skeletal muscle from patients with Parkinson's disease. *J Neurol Sci* 104:203–208, 1991.

237. Nakagawa-Hattori Y, Yoshino H, Kondo T, et al: Is Parkinson's disease a mitochondrial disorder? *J Neurol Sci* 107:29–33, 1992.

238. Cardellach F, Martí MJ, Fernández-Solá J, et al: Mitochondrial respiratory chain activity in skeletal muscle from patients with Parkinson's disease. *Neurology* 43:2258–2262, 1993.

239. Blin O, Dsnuelle C, Rascol O, et al: Mitochondrial respiratory failure in skeletal muscle from patients with Parkinson's disease and multiple system atrophy. *J Neurol Sci* 125:95–101, 1994.

240. Shoffner JM, Watts RL, Juncos JL, et al: Mitochondrial oxidative phosphorylation defects in Parkinson's disease. *Ann Neurol* 30:332–339, 1991.

241. Haas RH, Nasirian F, Nakano K, et al: Low platelet mitochondrial complex I and complex II/III activity in early untreated Parkinson's disease. *Ann Neurol* 37:714–722, 1995.

242. Mann VM, Cooper JM, Krige D, et al: Brain, skeletal muscle and platelet homogenate mitochondrial function in Parkinson's disease. *Brain* 115:333–342, 1992.

243. Anderson JJ, Ferrari R, Davis TL, et al: No evidence for altered muscle mitochondrial function in Parkinson's disease. *J Neurol Neurosurg Psychiatry* 56;477–480, 1993.

244. DiDonato S, Zeviani M, Giovannini P, et al: Respiratory chain and mitochondrial DNA in muscle and brain in Parkinson's disease patients. *Neurology* 43:2262–2268, 1993.

245. DiMauro S: Mitochondrial involvement in Parkinson's disease: The controversy continues. *Neurology* 43:2170–2178, 1993.

246. Halliwell B: Oxidants and the central nervous system: Some fundamental questions. *Acta Neurol Scand* 126:23–33, 1989.

247. Riederer P, Sofic E, Rausch WD, et al: Transition metals, ferritin, glutathione, and ascorbic acid in parkinsonian brains. *J Neurochem* 52:515–520, 1989.

248. Youdim MBH, Ben-Shachar D, Riederer P: Is Parkinson's disease a progressive siderosis of substantia nigra resulting in ion and melanin induced neurodegeneration? *Acta Neurol Scand* 126:47–54, 1989.

249. Dexter DT, Wells FR, Lees AJ, et al: Increased nigral iron content and alterations in other metal ions occurring in brain in Parkinson's disease. *J Neurochem* 52:1830–1836, 1989.

250. Jellinger K, Paulus W, Grundke-Iqbal P, et al: Brain iron and ferritin in Parkinson's and Alzheimer's disease. *J Neural Transm* 2:327–340, 1990.

251. Hirsch EC, Brandel JP, Galle P, et al: Iron and aluminum increase in the substantia nigra of patients with Parkinson's disease: An X-ray microanalysis. *J Neurochem* 56:446–451, 1991.

252. Good PF, Olanow CW, Perl DP: Neuromelanin-containing neurons of the substantia nigra accumulate iron and aluminum in Parkinson's disease: a LAMMA study. *Brain Res* 593:343–346, 1992.

253. Gutteridge JNC: Iron and oxygen radicals in brain. *Ann Neurol* 32:S16–S21, 1992.

254. Ben-Shachar D, Riederer P, Youdim MBH: Iron-melanin interaction and lipid peroxidation: Implications for Parkinson's disease. *J Neurochem* 57:1609–1614, 1991.

255. Youdim MBH, Ben-Shachar, Riederer P: The possible role of iron in the etiopathology of Parkinson's disease. *Mov Disord* 8:1–12, 1993.

256. Gutteridge JM, Quinlan GJ, Clark I, Halliwell B: Aluminum salts accelerate peroxidation of membrane lipids stimulated by iron salts. *Biochim Biophys Acta* 835:441–447, 1985.

257. Marttila RJ, Lorentz H, Rinne UK: Oxygen toxicity protecting enzymes in Parkinson's disease: Increase of superoxide dismutase-like activity in the substantia nigra and basal nucleus. *J Neurol Sci* 86:321–331, 1988.

258. Saggu H, Cooksey J, Dexter D, et al: A selective increase in particulate superoxide dismutase activity in parkinsonian substantia nigra. *J Neurochem* 53:692–697, 1989.

259. Sian J, Dexter DT, Lees AJ, et al: Glutathione-related enzymes in brain in Parkinson's disease. *Ann Neurol* 36:356–361, 1994.

260. Kish SJ, Morito C, Hornykiewicz O: Glutathione peroxidase activity in Parkinson's disease. *Neurosci Lett* 58:343–346, 1985.

261. Radunovic A, Porto WG, Zeman S, Leigh PN: Increased mitochondrial superoxide dismutase activity in Parkinson's disease but not amyotrophic lateral sclerosis motor cortex. *Neurosci Lett* 239:105–108, 1997.

262. Dexter DT, Carter CJ, Wells FR, et al: Basal lipid peroxidation in substantia nigra is increased in Parkinson's disease. *J Neurochem* 52:381–389, 1989.

263. Perry TL, Yong VW: Idiopathic Parkinson's disease, progressive supranuclear palsy and glutathione metabolism in the substantia nigra of patients. *Neurosci Lett* 67:269–274, 1986.

264. Sofic E, Lange KW, Jellinger K, Riederer P: Reduced and oxidized glutathione in the substantia nigra of patients with Parkinson's disease. *Neurosci Lett* 142:128–130, 1992.

265. Sian J, Dexter DT, Lees AJ, et al: Alterations in glutathione levels in Parkinson's disease and other neurodegenerative disorders affecting basal ganglia. *Ann Neurol* 36:348–355, 1994.

266. Jenner P, Dexter DT, Sian J, et al: Oxidative stress as a cause of nigral cell death in Parkinson's disease and incidental Lewy body disease. *Ann Neurol* 32:S82–S87, 1992.

267. Slivka A, Mytilineou C, Cohen C: Histochemical evaluation of glutathione in human and monkey brain. *Brain Res* 409:275–284, 1987.

268. Raps SP, Lai JC, Hertz L, Cooper AJ: Glutathione is present in high concentrations in cultured astrocytes but not in cultured neurons. *Brain Res* 493:398–401, 1989.

269. Cheng KC, Cahill DS, Kasai H, et al: 8-Hydroxyguanine, an abundant form of oxidative DNA damage, cause G→T and A→C substitutions. *J Biol Chem* 267:166–172, 1992.

270. Sanchez-Ramos JR, Övervik E, Ames BN: A marker of oxyradical-mediated DNA damage (8-hydroxy-2'-deoxyguanosine) is increased in nigro-striatum of Parkinson's disease brain. *Neurodegeneration* 3:197–204, 1994.

271. Alam ZI, Jenner A, Daniel SE, et al: Oxidative DNA damage in the parkinsonian brain: An apparent selective increase in 8-hydroxyguanine levels in substantia nigra. *J Neurochem* 69:1196–1203, 1997.

272. Zhang J, Perry G, Smith MA, et al: Parkinson's disease is associated with oxidative damage to cytoplasmic DNA and RNA in substantia nigra neurons. *Am J Pathol* 154:1423–1429, 1999.

273. Shimura H, Hattori N, Kang D, et al: Increase of 8-oxo-dGTPase in the mitochondria of substantia nigral neurons in Parkinson's disease. *Ann Neurol* 46:920–924, 1999.

274. Yoritaka A, Hattori N, Uchida K, et al: Immunohistochemical detection of 4-hydroxynonenal protein adducts in Parkinson disease. *Proc Natl Acad Sci U S A* 93:2696–2701, 1996.

275. Alam ZI, Daniel SE, Lees AJ, et al: A generalised increase in protein carbonyls in the brain in Parkinson's but not incidental Lewy body disease. *J Neurochem* 69:1326–1329, 1997.

276. Floor E, Wetzel MG: Increased protein oxidation in human substantia nigra pars compacta in comparison with basal ganglia and prefrontal cortex measured with an improved dinitrophenylhydrazine assay. *J Neurochem* 70:268–275, 1998.

277. Giasson BI, Duda JE, Murray IV, et al: Oxidative damage linked to neurodegeneration by selective alpha-synuclein nitration in synucleinopathy lesions. *Science* 290:985–989, 2000.

278. Mogi M, Harada M, Kondo T, et al: Brain beta 2-microglobulin levels are elevated in the striatum in Parkinson's disease. *J Neural Transm* 9:87–92, 1995.

279. Bongioanni P, Castagna M, Maltinti S, et al: T-lymphocyte tumor necrosis factor-alpha receptor binding in patients with Parkinson's disease. *J Neurol Sci* 149:41–45, 1997.

280. Hasegawa Y, Inagaki T, Sawada M, Suzumura A: Impaired cytokine production by peripheral blood mononuclear cells and monocytes/macrophages in Parkinson's disease. *Acta Neurol Scand* 10:159–164, 2000.

281. Blum-Degen D, Muller T, Kuhn W, et al: Interleukin-1 beta and interleukin-6 are elevated in the cerebrospinal fluid of Alzheimer's and de novo Parkinson's disease patients. *Neurosci Lett* 202:17–20, 1995.

282. Mogi M, Harada M, Narabayashi H, et al: Interleukin (IL)-1beta, IL-2, IL-4, IL-6 and transforming growth factor-alpha levels are elevated in ventricular cerebrospinal fluid in juvenile parkinsonism and Parkinson's disease. *Neurosci Lett* 211:13–16, 1996.

283. Mogi M, Harada M, Kondo T, et al: Interleukin-2 but not basic fibroblast growth factor is elevated in parkinsonian brain. *J Neural Transm* 103:1077–1081, 1996.

284. Stypula G, Kunert-Radek J, Stepien H, et al: Evaluation of interleukins, ACTH, cortisol and prolactin concentrations in the blood of patients with Parkinson's disease. *Neuroimmunomodulation* 3:131–134, 1996.

285. Wandinger KP, Hagenah JM, Kluter H, et al: Effects of amantadine treatment on in vitro production of interleukin-2 in de-novo patients with idiopathic Parkinson's disease. *J Neuroimmunol* 98:214–220, 1999.

286. Muller T, Blum-Degen D, Przuntek H, Kuhn W: Interleukin-6 levels in cerebrospinal fluid inversely correlate to severity of Parkinson's disease. *Acta Neurol Scand* 98:142–144, 1998.

287. Gadient RA, Otten UH: Interleukin-6 (IL-6): A molecule with both beneficial and destructive potentials. *Prog Neurobiol* 52: 379–390, 1997.

288. Mogi M, Harada M, Kondo T, et al: Transforming growth factor-beta 1 levels are elevated in the striatum and in ventricular cerebrospinal fluid in Parkinson's disease. *Neurosci Lett* 193:129–132, 1995.

289. Vawter MP, Dillon-Carter O, Tourtellotte WW, et al: TGFbeta1 and TGFbeta2 concentrations are elevated in Parkinson's disease in ventricular cerebrospinal fluid. *Exp Neurol* 142:313–322, 1996.

290. Tooyama I, Kawamata T, Walker D, et al: Loss of basic fibroblast growth factor in substantia nigra neurons in Parkinson's disease. *Neurology* 43:372–376, 1993.

291. Hunot S, Bernard V, Faucheux B, et al: Glial cell line-derived neurotrophic factor (GDNF) gene expression in the human brain: A post mortem in situ hybridization study with special reference to Parkinson's disease. *J Neural Transm* 103:1043–1052, 1996.

292. Mogi M, Togari A, Kondo T, et al: Brain-derived growth factor and nerve growth factor concentrations are decreased in the substantia nigra in Parkinson's disease. *Neurosci Lett* 270:45–48, 1999.

293. Chauhan NB, Siegel GJ, Lee JM: Depletion of glial cell line-derived neurotrophic factor in substantia nigra neurons of Parkinson's disease brain. *J Chem Neuroanat* 21:277–288, 2001.

294. Parain K, Murer MG, Yan Q, et al: Reduced expression of brain-derived neurotrophic factor protein in Parkinson's disease substantia nigra. *Neuroreport* 10:557–561, 1999.

295. Howells DW, Porritt MJ, Wong JY, et al: Reduced BDNF mRNA expression in the Parkinson's disease substantia nigra. *Exp Neurol* 166:127–135, 2000.

296. Villares J, Faucheux B, Herrero MT, et al: [125I]EGF binding in basal ganglia of patients with Parkinson's disease and progressive supranuclear palsy and in MPTP-treated monkeys. *Exp Neurol* 154:146–156, 1998.

297. Beal MF: Excitotoxicity and nitric oxide in Parkinson's disease pathogenesis. *Ann Neurol* 44(3 suppl 1):S110–114, 1998.

298. Kingsbury AE, Mardsen CD, Foster OJ: DNA fragmentation in human substantia nigra: Apoptosis or perimortem effect? *Mov Disord* 13:877–884, 1998.

299. Tatton NA: Increased caspase 3 and Bax immunoreactivity accompany nuclear GAPDH translocation and neuronal apoptosis in Parkinson's disease. *Exp Neurol* 166:29–43, 2000.

300. Kosel S, Egensperger R, von Eitzen U, et al: On the question of apoptosis in the parkinsonian substantia nigra. *Acta Neuropathol (Berl)* 93:105–108, 1997.

301. Banati RB, Daniel SE, Blunt SB: Glial pathology but absence of apoptotic nigral neurons in long-standing Parkinson's disease. *Mov Disord* 13:221–227, 1998.

302. Wullner U, Kornhuber J, Weller M, et al: Cell death and apoptosis regulating proteins in Parkinson's disease: A cautionary note. *Acta Neuropathol (Berl)* 97:408–412, 1999.

303. Mogi M, Harada M, Kondo T, et al: The soluble form of Fas molecule is elevated in parkinsonian brain tissues. *Neurosci Lett* 220:195–198, 1996.

304. Hunot S, Brugg B, Ricard D, et al: Nuclear translocation of NF-kappaB is increased in dopaminergic neurons of patients with parkinson disease. *Proc Natl Acad Sci U S A* 94:7531–7536, 1997.

305. Mogi M, Harada M, Kondo T, et al: Bcl-2 protein is increased in the brain from parkinsonian patients. *Neurosci Lett* 215:137–139, 1996.

306. Marshall KA, Daniel SE, Cairns N, et al: Upregulation of the anti-apoptotic protein Bcl-2 may be an early event in neurodegeneration: Studies on Parkinson's and incidental Lewy body disease. *Biochem Biophys Res Commun* 240:84–87, 1997.

307. Vyas S, Javoy-Agid F, Herrero MT, et al: Expression of Bcl-2 in adult human brain regions with special reference to neurodegenerative disorders. *J Neurochem* 69:223–231, 1997.

308. Hartmann A, Michel PP, Troadec JD, et al: Is Bax a mitochondrial mediator in apoptotic death of dopaminergic neurons in Parkinson's disease? *J Neurochem* 76:1785–1793, 2001.

309. Hartmann A, Hunot S, Michel PP, et al: Caspase-3: A vulnerability factor and final effector in apoptotic death of dopaminergic neurons in Parkinson's disease. *Proc Natl Acad Sci USA* 97:2875–2880, 2000.

310. Hartmann A, Troadec JD, Hunot S, et al: Caspase-8 is an effector in apoptotic death of dopaminergic neurons in Parkinson's disease, but pathway inhibition results in neuronal necrosis. *J Neurosci* 21:2247–2255, 2001.

Chapter 14

CLINICAL MANIFESTATIONS OF PARKINSON'S DISEASE

HENRY L. PAULSON and MATTHEW B. STERN

DEFINITIONS 233
DISEASE ONSET 234
CARDINAL MANIFESTATIONS 235
    Tremor 235
    Rigidity 235
    Akinesia/Bradykinesia 236
    Postural Instability 236
SECONDARY MANIFESTATIONS 237
    Cognitive Dysfunction 237
    Ocular Dysfunction 237
    Facial and Oropharyngeal Dysfunction 238
    Musculoskeletal Deformities 238
    Pain and Sensory Symptoms 238
    Autonomic Dysfunction 238
    Dermatologic Problems 239
    Sleep Disorders 239
ATYPICAL FEATURES AND DIFFERENTIAL
   DIAGNOSIS 239
    Young-Onset Patient 240
    Absent or Atypical Tremor 240
    Predominant Postural Instability 241
    Early Dementia 241
    Persistent Asymmetry 242
TREATMENT-RELATED MANIFESTATIONS 242
    Dyskinesias 242
    Motor Fluctuations 242
    Cognitive and Behavioral Disturbances 242
    Orthostatic Hypotension 243
CLINICAL RATING SCALES 243

James Parkinson's original 1817 description of the "shaking palsy" remains a remarkably accurate account of the disease now bearing his name.[1] Although the cardinal manifestations of Parkinson's disease (PD) are no different today, our understanding of the full array of parkinsonian signs and symptoms has grown immeasurably. Because of continuing advances in therapy, it is increasingly important that clinicians recognize PD in its earliest stages. Equally critical, PD must be distinguished from less common forms of parkinsonism, because prognosis and treatment may differ. In this chapter we discuss the primary and secondary clinical manifestations of PD,

then address ways in which clinical signs can help distinguish it from other parkinsonian syndromes.

Definitions

Parkinsonism is a clinical syndrome characterized by specific motor deficits: tremor, akinesia (or bradykinesia), rigidity, and postural instability. At least two of these should be present to make the diagnosis. A wide variety of unrelated disease states can result in parkinsonism. The common thread linking these disorders is an underlying disruption of the dopaminergic nigrostriatal pathways which play a central role in controlling voluntary movements. This disruption can take one of many forms. It may be chemical, as is seen with drugs that deplete dopamine from intraneuronal storage sites (reserpine, tetrabenazine), or block striatal dopamine receptors (the phenothiazine and butyrophenone neuroleptics, as well as metoclopramide). Alternatively, it may stem from acute or chronic metabolic insults that cause destruction of neurons within the striatum or substantia nigra. Less commonly, the disruption may be structural, as with hydrocephalus and brain tumors. Finally, many inherited neurodegenerative disorders cause parkinsonism when the degenerative process involves the substantia nigra or striatum (as well as, depending on the particular disease, other brain regions). Causes of parkinsonism can be grouped into primary (or idiopathic), secondary (or symptomatic), the parkinsonism-plus syndromes, and hereditary neurodegenerative diseases (Table 14-1).

In contrast to parkinsonism, *Parkinson's disease* is a distinct clinical and pathological entity. It is the most common form of parkinsonism, accounting for approximately 75 percent of all cases seen in a movement disorders clinic. The pathologic definition of PD includes massive loss of pigmented neurons in the substantia nigra and the presence of Lewy bodies.[2] Although a uniform clinical definition of PD has not been established, most movement disorder specialists consider the presence of two of three cardinal motor signs (tremor, rigidity, bradykinesia) and a consistent response to L-dopa indicative of clinical PD.[3] The fourth clinical feature of parkinsonism, postural instability, is not included in this definition because of its frequent occurrence in other forms of parkinsonism, such as multisystem atrophy (MSA), and progressive supranuclear palsy (PSP) (see Chaps. 21 and 22). Because of the broad phenotypic variability in PD, the lack of a precise and rigid clinical definition may be inevitable and perhaps even appropriate. A definition relying too heavily on any one clinical feature runs the risk of excluding legitimate cases. For example, one could argue that rest tremor should always be present, because this is the single most reliable sign of PD. However, a small percentage of patients without tremor will have a good response to L-dopa and display, at autopsy, the pathological hallmarks of PD. Also, response to L-dopa is not unique to PD, as other forms of parkinsonism

TABLE 14-1 Classification of Parkinsonism

Primary (idiopathic)
    Parkinson's disease
Secondary (symptomatic)
    Drug-induced (phenothiazines, butyrophenones,
        metoclopramide, reserpine, alpha-methyldopa)
    Infectious (postencephalitic, syphilis)
    Metabolic (hepatocerebral degeneration, hypoxia, parathyroid
        dysfunction)
    Structural (brain tumor, hydrocephalus, trauma)
    Toxin (carbon monoxide, carbon disulphide, cyanide, manganese,
        MPTP)
    Vascular
Parkinsonism-plus syndromes
    Corticobasal ganglionic degeneration
    Hemiparkinsonism-hemiatrophy
    Dementia syndromes
        Alzheimer's disease
        Diffuse Lewy body disease
    Multisystem atrophy
        Parkinsonism-amyotrophy
        Shy-Drager syndrome
        Sporadic olivopontocerebellar degeneration
        Striatonigral degeneration
    Parkinsonism-dementia-ALS complex of Guam
    Progressive supranuclear palsy
Hereditary degenerative diseases
    Genetic forms of PD
        Autosomal dominant (including alpha-synuclein mutations)
        Autosomal recessive (including parkin mutations)
    Spinocerebellar ataxias (especially Machado-Joseph disease)
    Hallervorden-Spatz disease/PKAN
    Juvenile Huntington's disease
    Mitochondrial disorders
    Neuroacanthocytosis
    Wilson's disease

MPTP, 1-methyl-4-phenyl-1,2,3,6-tetrahydropyridine; ALS, amyotrophic lateral sclerosis; PKAN, pantothenate kinase-associated neurodegeneration.

may also improve with L-dopa.[4,5] Any clinical definition of PD must be flexible enough to accommodate such exceptions to the general rule.

PD is also defined, in part, by the absence of other causes of parkinsonism. Proposed exclusionary criteria for the diagnosis of PD include more than one affected relative, a remitting course, neuroleptic use within the past year, a history of encephalitis lethargica or repeated head trauma, oculogyric crisis, cerebellar signs, autonomic neuropathy, dementia from the onset of symptoms, pyramidal tract signs not explained by other focal neurological disease, and evidence of cerebrovascular disease. Some of these criteria (the use of neuroleptics, for example) make the diagnosis of PD unlikely. Others, however, do not entirely rule out the possibility of PD. There is, for example, a familial tendency in a subset of PD (including rare inherited forms of PD), and autonomic dysfunction is quite common among PD patients. In such cases, exclusionary criteria should weigh heavily, but not solely, in deciding whether a patient has PD. As a case in point, the patient who initially presents with disabling and overwhelming autonomic dysfunction is unlikely to have PD, but the tremulous and bradykinetic patient with minor autonomic complaints may well have it.

Its wide clinical variability has led some investigators to group PD into several subtypes,[6,7] including *juvenile* and *young-onset* forms, *tremor-predominant* versus *postural instability-dominant* forms, and *benign* versus *malignant* forms of PD. Whether these clinically defined subtypes correspond to differences at the biochemical or pathophysiological levels is unknown. Regardless, making such distinctions seems valid and useful. Studies indicate, for example, that young-onset patients are more likely to display exquisite sensitivity to L-dopa and develop drug-related dyskinesias sooner than older patients do.[8–10] Likewise, tremor-predominant PD tends to follow a slower, more benign course than postural instability-predominant disease.[6,7,11]

Disease Onset

PD is one of the most common causes of neurological disability, affecting 1 percent of the population over age 55. It is typically a disease of the middle to late years, beginning at a mean age of 50–60 years and progressing slowly over a 10–20-year period.[12–14] The age of onset assumes a broad bell-shaped distribution, with roughly 5 percent of cases beginning before age 40 (by definition, young-onset PD).

The underlying pathology of PD, the loss of nigral neurons, is believed to occur slowly in the decades preceding the onset of symptoms. Up to 80 percent of dopaminergic neurons are lost before the cardinal signs and symptoms of PD first appear. It is not surprising, then, that PD usually begins insidiously and is heralded by a prodrome of nonspecific symptoms.[15] Easy fatigability, malaise or personality changes may appear years before the first motor sign. Patients frequently first experience motor signs in subtle ways, such as a feeling of weakness, mild incoordination or difficulty writing. The "sudden weakness" that some patients describe may prove, after questioning, to be sudden awareness of problems in movement (getting out a chair, swinging a golf club). Many will also complain of pain or tension confined to the muscles of one shoulder or arm, prompting a visit to an orthopedist before a neurologist. Asymmetric onset is typical in PD and has even been proposed as a defining criterion.[16]

Diagnosing PD in this earliest stage is difficult. The nonspecific nature of the symptoms and signs suggests a broad differential diagnosis, including myasthenia gravis, cerebrovascular disease, and multiple sclerosis. Mild parkinsonian features on examination—an intermittent rest tremor confined to one or several fingers, subtle cogwheel rigidity—may be the first clue that PD is the underlying problem. In many cases, the diagnosis will only become apparent as motor signs develop in the ensuing years.

Cardinal Manifestations

TREMOR

The rest tremor of PD, the "involuntary tremulous motion" first noted by Parkinson, remains the best-known and most readily identifiable sign of disease (Table 14-2). In about 75 percent of patients it is the first motor manifestation, usually beginning unilaterally in the distal limb, in most cases an arm. In some patients, the tremor may be confined to a single finger before the appearance of other signs. The tremor often involves rhythmic, alternating opposition of the forefinger and thumb in the classic, stereotypic "pill-rolling" tremor. In others, it takes the form of a simple to-and-fro motion of the hand or arm. Occasionally, patients will complain that their tremor is felt internally, with only subtle external signs. In all cases, it oscillates with a characteristic

TABLE 14-2 Manifestations of PD

Cardinal manifestations
  Rest tremor
  Rigidity
  Akinesia/bradykinesia
  Postural instability
Secondary manifestations
  Cognitive/neuropsychiatric
    Anxiety
    Bradyphrenia
    Dementia
    Depression
    Sleep disturbances
  Cranial nerve/facial
    Blurred vision (impaired upgaze, blepharospasm)
    Dysarthria
    Dysphagia
    Glabellar reflex (Myerson's sign)
    Masked facies
    Olfactory dysfunction
    Sialorrhea
  Musculoskeletal
    Compression neuropathies
    Dystonia
    Hand and foot deformities
    Kyphoscoliosis
    Peripheral edema
  Autonomic (including gastrointestinal and genitourinary symptoms)
    Constipation
    Lightheadedness (orthostatic hypotension)
    Increased sweating
    Sexual dysfunction (impotence, loss of libido)
    Urinary dysfunction (frequency, hesitancy or urgency)
  Sensory
    Cramps
    Pain
    Paresthesias
    Restless leg syndrome
  Skin
    Seborrhea

frequency of 3–7 cycles/s (Hz), most commonly 4–5 Hz. Over several years, the tremor may spread proximally in the affected arm before involving the ipsilateral leg, and finally the contralateral limbs. Of the cardinal features of PD, however, tremor progresses at a slower rate than the other three.[17] Although tremor is bilateral in advanced disease, it often maintains some asymmetry throughout the course. In later stages, an accompanying tremor of the face, lips, or chin is not uncommon.

The tremor of PD is termed a rest tremor because it is present at rest and usually abates when the affected limb performs a motor task. Not uncommonly, at the same time that tremor decreases in an affected arm during voluntary movement, it increases asynchronously in the resting contralateral limb. When lower limbs are involved, tremor will be present in the legs when the patient is supine or sitting but disappears when the patient bears weight. Tremor often increases in the arms during walking; hence, the clinician should watch the arms as closely as the legs when examining a patient's gait. In the course of a day, tremor will occur intermittently and vary in intensity. It disappears in sleep and worsens with stress or anxiety. It is important to note that patients often also have a postural or kinetic component to their tremor, as well as an exaggerated physiological tremor. A moderate degree of action tremor is consistent with PD.[18,19] However, a pronounced action tremor at disease onset should suggest other diagnoses.

The pathophysiological basis of the parkinsonian tremor is uncertain.[20] Although several brain regions likely contribute to the tremor, the major source is thought to be a pathological central oscillator of 3–5 Hz. Cells of the ventral intermediate nucleus of the thalamus show oscillatory behavior correlating with the tremor, but it is unclear whether thalamic neurons are true pacemakers or simply oscillating as part of a long-loop reflex arc. Tremor can be affected by emotional state, motor activity, and general health. This suggests that the involved circuitry is linked to, and modulated by, other circuits within the nervous system.

RIGIDITY

The stiffness of PD is caused by an involuntary increase in muscle tone that can affect all muscle groups—axial and limb muscles, flexor as well as extensor muscles. On examination, rigidity is noted as increased resistance to passive movement of a limb segment. The amount of resistance remains fairly constant through the entire range of motion, both flexion and extension, and is not greatly influenced by the speed or force with which the movement is performed. This distinguishes it from spasticity, which displays a velocity-dependent increase in tone and variable resistance through the range of motion (clasp-knife phenomenon). Spasticity is further distinguished from PD by its associated pathological reflexes, weakness, and silent electromyogram (EMG) at rest; in PD, the EMG resembles ordinary tonic voluntary muscle activity.[21] Likewise, rigidity can be distinguished from the Gegenhalten tone seen in a variety of encephalopathic conditions, because Gegenhalten is intermittent and tends to increase in opposition to an applied force.

The rigidity of PD can be either smooth (lead pipe) or rachety (cogwheel). Cogwheeling is thought to reflect the superimposed rest tremor. Both rigidity and cogwheeling can be brought out, or reinforced, by voluntary movement in the contralateral limb. As with tremor, rigidity frequently begins unilaterally, may vary during the course of the day, and is influenced by mood, stress, and medications.

Although the rigidity of PD limits the speed of voluntary movements, it is unclear to what degree it contributes to motor impairment. Some patients with prominent rigidity have relatively unimpeded motor function. Bradykinesia probably plays a greater role than rigidity in determining a patient's degree of disability.

As with tremor, the pathophysiological basis of rigidity is not fully understood.[20] Afferent impulses must play a role, because sectioning of dorsal roots or application of local anesthetic in the epidural or subarachnoid space decreases rigidity. Competing theories explaining rigidity—not necessarily mutually exclusive—have invoked either increased activity in long-loop reflex pathways or abnormalities in spinal interneuron function because of altered input from descending tracts. There may be changes intrinsic to the muscle as well. The rigidity of PD usually responds to dopaminergic therapy.

AKINESIA/BRADYKINESIA

Akinesia means the absence or failure of movement; bradykinesia means slowness of movement. Together they are the terms used to define the difficulty PD patients have in initiating and executing a motor plan. It is often the most disabling sign of PD, experienced by virtually all patients and manifested in a variety of ways (see Table 14-3). As a general rule, the nature and severity of akinesia/bradykinesia worsen over the course of illness. Early on, hypokinesia (falling short of the mark when executing a movement) is nearly always present, later progressing to bradykinesia (slowed movements) and, finally, to akinesia. Early signs may be confined to distal muscles (micrographia, decreased dexterity, impaired sequential finger movements), but, eventually, all muscle groups can be affected. Particularly difficult for patients are sequential motor acts, such as alternating pronation-supination of the hand, and complex motor acts, such as buttoning a shirt. Quick repetitive movements, such as repeated opposition of the forefinger and thumb, will typically show a rapid decrease in amplitude and frequency. In more advanced stages, patients have difficulty rising from a chair and display a generalized slowing of voluntary movements. Facial and vocal manifestations of bradykinesia (hypomimia, hypophonia, dysarthria, and sialorrhea) are often apparent to the clinician before the formal examination has even begun.

The pathophysiology of motor control in PD is a field in itself. Researchers generally agree that patients with PD have

TABLE 14-3 Signs of Akinesia in PD

General
    Delayed motor initiation
    Slowed voluntary movements (bradykinesia)
    Diminution in voluntary movements (hypokinesia)
    Rapid fatigue with repetitive movements
    Difficulty executing sequential actions
    Inability to perform simultaneous actions
    Decreased dexterity
    Freezing
Specific
    Masked facies (hypomimia)
    Decreased blink
    Hypometric saccades
    Hypophonia
    Dysarthria
    Sialorrhea
    Micrographia
    Dysdiadochokinesia
    Difficulty rising from a chair
    Shuffling gait, short steps
    Decreased arm swing

little or no trouble "planning" a motor task. The problem lies in initiating and executing the sequential motor acts that comprise a particular motor program.[20,22,23] When a simple movement at one joint is attempted, the initial burst of agonist activity is inappropriately small; hence, the resulting movement is too slow and falls short of the intended target. The problem is further exacerbated in complex motor acts, as it is particularly difficult for PD patients to execute two motor programs simultaneously. Because these are the kinds of movements necessary for performing normal daily activities, it is understandable why bradykinesia is usually the most disabling sign of PD.

It is increasingly clear that dopamine plays a central role in modulating the striatal pathways that control motor initiation, execution, and adaptation.[24] Fortunately, dopaminergic therapy is often quite effective in treating the varied manifestations of akinesia/bradykinesia.

POSTURAL INSTABILITY

Postural instability with associated gait disorder is usually the last of the four cardinal signs to appear. Yet it often proves to be the most disabling, least treatable manifestation of the disease and represents the major contributing factor in progression from mild bilateral disease (Hoehn and Yahr stage 2) to wheelchair confinement (stage 5).[25] No single factor is alone responsible for postural instability and gait disturbance. Rather, it stems from a combination of deficits, including changes in postural adjustment, the loss of postural reflexes, rigidity, and akinesia.

Loss of postural reflexes often occurs early but is rarely disabling until years later. The patient adopts a stooped posture with flexion of the neck and trunk. The arms are held in an adducted position with elbows flexed. Once a patient starts to lose the ability to make rapid postural corrections, a tendency to fall forward or backward becomes evident. The examiner can elicit this finding with the "pull test," standing behind the patient and pulling backward on the shoulders: patients with decreased righting reflexes will take more than two steps backwards before catching themselves (retropulsion), while others with more advanced disease will fall unless caught.

The earliest sign of gait disturbance is often decreased arm swing, but over time patients also begin to walk with a short, shuffling, uncertain step. Gait initiation and turning become particularly difficult. Once walking has begun, the loss of postural reflexes and stooped posture combine to produce a festinating gait: in an effort to retain balance, the patient walks faster and faster in a shuffling manner, as the legs try to catch up with the body's forward momentum. In many cases, stopping is accomplished only by grabbing onto an object or running into a wall. Although the gait is unsteady, the base is usually minimally or not at all widened, and truncal ataxia is absent. Falls become increasingly common over time, in many cases resulting in hip fracture.

Freezing is a phenomenon distinct from other forms of akinesia. We discuss this poorly understood phenomenon here in relation to the gait disorder, because it is during ambulation that freezing proves most troublesome.[26] Patients freeze especially when starting to walk (start-hesitation), attempting to turn, or approaching a narrow or crowded space (doorways, corners, closets, a sidewalk with heavy traffic). Also called "motor blocks," freezing may occur just before the patient reaches an intended target (e.g., a chair or bed). Sitting "en bloc" represents a special form of freezing in which a patient literally falls into a chair. Freezing more often occurs in advanced disease and after years of dopaminergic therapy.

The opposite of freezing can also occur in PD. *Kinesia paradoxica* is the term used to describe sudden short periods of relatively effortless mobility experienced by a few patients. These episodes are unrelated to medication and should not be confused with the "on-off" phenomenon that occurs in advanced patients on dopaminergic therapy.

The mechanisms that control normal locomotion and postural stability are complex, involving neural structures from cerebral cortex to proprioceptive sensory afferents. The pathophysiological basis of gait and postural abnormalities in PD is not well understood but is almost certainly multifactorial. Its multifactorial origin may help explain why postural instability and gait disturbance are the least treatable signs of PD.

Secondary Manifestations

Many secondary manifestations[27] actually represent special cases of one of the four cardinal signs, yet are common and distinct enough to merit separate discussion (see Table 14-2).

COGNITIVE DYSFUNCTION

Cognitive and behavioral disturbances are common in PD and often are more disabling than the motor manifestations.[28] Although prodromal symptoms of PD can include changes in mood or personality, the mental status remains relatively intact in early PD. Tests of cognitive function demonstrate mild-to-moderate deficits, including visuospatial impairment, attentional set-shifting difficulties, and poor executive function, as demonstrated in the Wisconsin Card Sorting and verbal fluency tests.[29-32] Patients demonstrate slowed thinking and slow responses to questions (bradyphrenia) but usually get the answers right.[33] Bradyphrenia may represent the cognitive analogue of bradykinesia but does not correlate with the degree of motor deficits and may, in part, reflect disruption of nondopaminergic pathways. Signs of dementia, if present at the onset of illness, should suggest diseases other than PD, including Alzheimer's disease (AD), diffuse Lewy body disease, PSP, and Creutzfeldt-Jakob disease (CJD).

Although not an early finding in PD, dementia eventually occurs in 20–30 percent of PD patients, making it the third most common cause of dementia in the elderly.[34,35] Affected patients perform poorly on visuospatial and perceptual motor tests, but language function is typically spared (although grammatic complexity is reduced, aphasia is not present). Delayed recall memory is not impaired to the degree it is in AD.[36] The dementia of PD has been called a "subcortical" dementia, although there is considerable overlap with cortical forms of dementia, such as AD.[29,36] Subcortical features of PD dementia include bradyphrenia, psychomotor retardation and depression, the absence of aphasia, and relatively mild memory impairment. Many patients will nonetheless develop dementia that is not unlike that of AD. Risk factors for dementia include older age and masked facies at onset of PD, depression, L-dopa-induced hallucinations, and akinetic-rigid predominant features.[37,38] In one study, dementia in PD was associated with a 2-fold increase in mortality risk.[39]

As PD progresses, patients often become passive and apathetic, relying on others to make decisions or do their talking. Many will become reclusive, fearful of going outside. Depression is common in PD, affecting up to one-half of patients.[40-44] It is generally mild to moderately severe and can take the form of chronic major depression or fluctuating dysthymia. Serotonin metabolites are reduced in depressed PD patients, suggesting an endogenous form of depression that may be intrinsic to the parkinsonian disease process. However, depression also can occur in reaction to chronic motor disability. Antidepressants prove helpful for both reactive and endogenous depression in PD.

OCULAR DYSFUNCTION

Oculomotor function is generally preserved in PD, in contrast to what is found in many parkinsonism-plus syndromes. Some patients will complain of blurred vision or difficulty reading, which may be a result of weakened convergence. Limited upgaze is common in PD patients but can also be seen in the asymptomatic elderly. Vertical gaze paresis downwards is not seen in PD. If it is present, one should consider the diagnosis of PSP or MSA. Although slow saccades and jerky ocular pursuits are often seen in PD, ophthalmoparesis does not occur, and lid retraction is uncommon.

The frequency of spontaneous eye blinking is reduced. A typical feature of PD is persistent eye blinking when the forehead is repeatedly tapped; this is called the sustained glabellar reflex or Myerson's sign. This primitive reflex is intrinsic to the disease process and does not indicate dementia. Other primitive reflexes can also be seen in PD without associated dementia, most commonly the snout reflex.[45]

FACIAL AND OROPHARYNGEAL DYSFUNCTION

Facial bradykinesia leads to a mask-like, staring expression (masked facies). The speech of PD is a hypokinetic dysarthria, typically monotonal, hypophonic, and muffled. The first syllable may be repeated (pallilalia), and words and phrases may rush together. Excessive saliva with drooling occurs in up to 80 percent of patients and is a consequence of decreased transfer of saliva to the pharynx.[46] Dysphagia, a consequence of pharyngeal bradykinesia, usually occurs later in disease and may prove life-threatening. Early and prominent dysphagia should suggest other forms of parkinsonism (PSP, MSA).

Decreased olfactory function is an early sign in PD.[47,48] Reduced ability to smell is not something patients complain about unless specifically asked; even then, only 25 percent will have noticed a change. However, testing indicates that decreased sense of smell is a significant and widespread manifestation, occurring early in disease and bilaterally. It neither correlates with motor signs nor progresses over the course of illness. Olfactory dysfunction may help distinguish PD from other forms of parkinsonism, because patients with PSP and essential tremor do not show similar changes.

MUSCULOSKELETAL DEFORMITIES

Deformities of the hands and feet are common in PD. The parkinsonian hand displays ulnar deviation, flexion of the metacarpophalangeal and distal interphalangeal joints, and extension of the proximal interphalangeal joints (so-called striatal hand). Likewise, the great toe can be tonically extended, with the remaining toes curled claw-like. Dystonic cramps, particularly of the feet, may be troublesome. These can occur before medication or as a side-effect of dopaminergic therapy.

Coincident with rigidity, changes occur in the curvature of the spine. Early on, mild scoliosis may be seen, concave contralateral to the affected side. As a result the patient may walk tilted away from the affected side. Later, kyphosis becomes prominent and contributes to the disabling postural changes of advanced disease.

Many patients complain of swelling in the extremities. This is probably a consequence of immobility, representing peripheral edema from venous stasis. Measures taken to improve mobility will often reduce the swelling. Rarely, the profoundly immobile patient will develop compression neuropathies.

PAIN AND SENSORY SYMPTOMS

Although peripheral nerve disease is not associated with PD, pain and sensory complaints are surprisingly common. In a random group of parkinsonian patients, approximately 50 percent complained of pain directly related to their parkinsonism.[49,50] Pain is often proportional to the degree of motor dysfunction and may take the form of muscle cramps, stiffness, dystonia, radiculopathy or arthralgias.

Sensory complaints, also very common, are usually not associated with signs of peripheral neuropathy. Numbness, burning, or tingling may occur at any stage of the disease, independent of medications and the degree of motor deficits, and, in some cases, even precedes motor manifestations. Paresthesias were noted in 40 percent of patients in one series, more commonly occurring on the affected side in hemiparkinsonians.[49] The basis of sensory disturbance in PD is unknown, but possibly reflects a role for the basal ganglia in sensory processing. One postulated mechanism is altered striatal input to sensory centers in the thalamus.

In PD, sensory complaints in the legs may be a sign of restless leg syndrome, which occurs more commonly in PD patients than in normal controls.[51,52] Typically, symptoms of restless leg syndrome begin well after PD symptoms and may be associated with lower serum ferritin levels[52] (see Chap. 55). Having restless leg syndrome earlier in life does not appear to be a predisposing factor for later development of PD.

AUTONOMIC DYSFUNCTION

Although autonomic signs are more closely associated with MSA, nearly all PD patients experience some degree of autonomic dysfunction during the course of illness.[53] Careful measurements of autonomic function in PD (pulse variability, orthostatic blood pressure, responses to Valsalva maneuver, and cold pressor stimuli) indicate that the underlying disease does cause mild autonomic insufficiency.[54]

By far the most frequent complaints referrable to autonomic insufficiency are bowel and bladder symptoms. Constipation is an exceedingly common problem that can become serious, occasionally leading to intestinal pseudo-obstruction or megacolon.[46] The basis of constipation is reduced colonic motility, possibly a direct consequence of PD as Lewy body neuropathology has been described within the myenteric plexus. Other factors exacerbate the problem, including poor diet, fluid depletion, reduced physical activity, and antiparkinsonian medications. Urinary difficulties include hesitancy, urgency, and increased frequency. Rarely, catheterization is required for an atonic bladder.

TABLE 14-4 Atypical Features in Parkinsonism

Early or Predominant Feature	Disease
Young-onset	Juvenile PD, WD, HS/PKAN
Minimal or absent tremor	SND, PSP, SDS, vascular parkinsonism, hydrocephalic parkinsonism
Atypical tremor	CBGD, OPCD
Postural instability	PSP, MSA (all forms), vascular parkinsonism, hydrocephalic parkinsonism
Ataxia	MSA (particularly OPCD)
Pyramidal signs	MSA (particularly SND), CBGD, vascular or hydrocephalic parkinsonism
Neuropathy	MSA (particularly parkinsonism-amyotrophy)
Marked motor asymmetry	Hemiparkinsonism-hemiatrophy, CBGD
Symmetric onset	SND, vascular or hydrocephalic parkinsonism
Myoclonus	CBGD, CJD
Dementia	DLBD, AD, CJD, MID, PSP
Focal cortical signs	CBGD
Alien limb sign	CBGD
Oculomotor deficits	PSP, OPCA, CBGD
Dysautonomia	MSA (particularly SDS)

AD, Alzheimer's disease; CBGD, corticobasal ganglionic degeneration; CJD, Creutzfeldt-Jakob disease; DLBD, diffuse Lewy body disease; MID, multi-infarct dementia; MSA, multisystem atrophy; OPCD, olivopontocerebellar degeneration; PSP, progressive supranuclear palsy; SDS, Shy-Drager syndrome; SND, striatonigral degeneration; WD, Wilson's disease; HS/PKAN, pantothenate kinase-associated neurodegeneration, formerly known as Hallervorden-Spatz disease.

Sexual dysfunction is a frequent complaint and may involve both loss of libido and impotence. The cause of sexual problems is likely multifactorial, with possible contributing factors including a depressed mood, chronic motor disability, and partial or complete loss of autonomic innervation. Episodic sweating occurs in some patients. Frank orthostatic hypotension is uncommon in PD and is more likely a result of medications (particularly dopamine agonists) than of the underlying disease.

DERMATOLOGIC PROBLEMS

Chronic seborrhea is a common finding. This leads to greasy skin, particularly on the face, which can be associated with erythema, and scaly patches in skin creases.

SLEEP DISORDERS

Problems with nocturnal sleep and excessive daytime drowsiness are very common in persons with PD[55] (see Chap. 52). Various sleep disorders in PD may be due to parkinsonian symptoms that disrupt sleep, adverse effects of medications, or a direct effect of the pathophysiological processes of PD on central sleep mechanisms. In patients with mild-to-moderate PD and not on medications, sleep efficiency and total sleep time are reduced and periodic leg movements are increased.[56] A significant subset of predominantly male PD patients have rapid eye movement (REM) sleep behavior disorder, in which excessive motor activity occurs during dreaming.[57,58] In many cases, symptoms of REM sleep behavior disorder predate symptoms of PD. Finally, dopaminergic therapy is known to cause daytime sleepiness,

more common with agonists than with L-dopa.[59] Sleep issues often go unrecognized unless the clinician directly asks about them (see Chap. 52).

Atypical Features and Differential Diagnosis

Recognizing classic cases of PD should not be difficult. The 60-year-old person who presents with a unilateral rest tremor and whose examination reveals masked facies, hypophonic dysarthria, generally slowed movements, and cogwheel rigidity almost certainly has PD. A good response to L-dopa will clinch the diagnosis. Yet many cases are not so straightforward. When the history is suggestive but the signs not obvious, every effort should be made to bring out cardinal features; for example, subtle cogwheel rigidity in a limb might only be present with reinforcement, and a hand tremor may appear only when a patient walks. Atypical features, particularly at the onset of symptoms, should raise suspicion of other forms of parkinsonism (see Table 14-4).[60,61]

A complete history remains critical in establishing the correct diagnosis. The physician must inquire thoroughly about medications, possible environmental exposures, and family history of neurological disease, including essential tremor, dominantly inherited spinocerebellar ataxias, and dementia, as well as parkinsonism. Careful attention should be paid to the precise sequence of symptoms experienced by the patient. For example, did tremor or rigidity begin unilaterally, as is typically the case in PD? In the patient on L-dopa, which symptoms improved in response to medications, by how much and for how long? Accurately reconstructing a patient's disease history may be difficult, given the insidious onset of PD, but well worth the effort if atypical features are uncovered.

YOUNG-ONSET PATIENT

Most movement disorder specialists define patients whose symptoms begin before age 40 as "young-onset PD."[62,63] "Juvenile-onset" is a separate term used by many authors to refer to patients whose parkinsonism begins in childhood (before age 20). Disease in the former group resembles older-onset PD in most respects, and probably represents the tail end of the bell-shaped distribution for PD on the younger side. In contrast, juvenile-onset disease, although also resembling adult-onset PD in many ways,[64] differs in some respects. Juvenile-onset patients are more likely to have a family history of PD and to display dystonic features as part of their parkinsonism. It is important not to confuse dystonia in juvenile-onset parkinsonism with dopa-responsive dystonia, another juvenile-onset disease that is successfully and chronically treated with low doses of L-dopa.

Parkinsonism in the adolescent or young adult should never be assumed to be PD until other causes have been ruled out. If the clinical features resemble PD in all respects and there is an affected sibling, then there is a good possibility that the disease is caused by recessive mutations in the parkin gene. If, however, the parkinsonism is accompanied by other features, then other hereditary neurodegenerative diseases should be considered. Wilson's disease must be excluded by a slit-lamp examination and laboratory tests of copper, ceruloplasmin, and hepatocellular enzymes. A family history of neurological disease should raise concern about dynamic repeat expansion disorders, including Huntington's and Machado-Joseph disease (also known as spinocerebellar ataxia type 3), both of which show anticipation in families and can present as juvenile parkinsonism. Signs of spasticity and retinal degeneration suggest Hallervorden-Spatz disease, also now known as pantothenate kinase-associated neurodegeneration (HS/PKAN). The diagnosis of HS/PKAN is further supported by magnetic resonance imaging (MRI) evidence of symmetric signal abnormalities in the globus pallidus ("eye of the tiger" sign).[65]

ABSENT OR ATYPICAL TREMOR

The absence of rest tremor, both by history and examination, makes the diagnosis of PD difficult. If the patient also fails to respond to L-dopa, the diagnosis is in serious doubt. A careful search, once again, for symptomatic causes of parkinsonism must be undertaken. The patient should be re-examined with a close look for down-gaze paresis and facial dystonia (PSP), orthostatic hypotension (Shy-Drager syndrome, SDS), bulbar dysfunction with truncal ataxia (sporadic olivopontocerebellar degeneration and the autosomal-dominant hereditary ataxias), and pyramidal signs (cerebrovascular disease and hydrocephalus, among other disorders).

In the patient without tremor, risk factors for cerebrovascular disease should raise concern of vascular parkinsonism (see Chap. 27). In rare cases, the vascular parkinsonian will fulfill clinical criteria for PD, but most patients will have minimal tremor, poor response to L-dopa and, occasionally, pyramidal signs and a stepwise progression. Brain MRI supports the diagnosis, demonstrating widespread small-vessel ischemic changes. The MRI is frequently helpful in other forms of parkinsonism as well: symmetric abnormal signal in the basal ganglia suggests manganese or iron deposition, and atrophy within the brainstem, cerebellum, or striatum suggests several different parkinsonism-plus conditions.

Parkinsonism-plus syndromes frequently present with minimal or no tremor. Of these, striatonigral degeneration (SND)[66] (see Chap. 22) most closely resembles PD and is often confused with it, especially when patients respond to L-dopa.[67] Like other disorders falling under the heading MSA, SND frequently presents with an early and pronounced gait disorder. Other features helpful in distinguishing it from PD include symmetrical onset, severe dysarthria or dysphonia, respiratory stridor, rapid progression, pyramidal signs, and a poor or transient response to L-dopa.[68]

Essential tremor is often mistaken for the tremor of PD (see Chap. 29). The patient with pronounced kinetic or postural tremor, minimal or no signs of rigidity and bradykinesia, and a strong family history of tremor is much more likely to have essential tremor than PD. However, it is important to remember that many patients with PD have, as part of their disease, a superimposed kinetic tremor that may resemble essential tremor. PD patients rarely display the tremulous voice that is characteristic of familial essential tremor, and this may serve as a clue. It is important to remember that cogwheeling is not pathognomonic for PD; essential tremor can also cause ratcheting during passive movement of the limb, but without rigidity. Because both PD and essential tremor are common disorders, a small number of PD patients will inherit the trait for familial tremor as well.

A coarse kinetic tremor originating proximally in the limb is probably not parkinsonian, because the rest tremor of PD typically originates distally. Degenerative diseases affecting the cerebellum and its outflow tracts can cause a coarse, proximal kinetic tremor (sometimes known as a rubral tremor) associated with other cerebellar signs.

A markedly asymmetric tremor with myoclonic features suggests corticobasal ganglionic degeneration (CBGD) (see Chap. 48). Initially described by Rebeiz et al.,[69] this disorder is characterized by progressive asymmetric motor impairment and both cortical and basal ganglionic dysfunction.[70,71] Typical features include asymmetric parkinsonism with dystonia and myoclonus, apraxia, cortical sensory loss, the alien-limb phenomenon, ocular motility disturbance, and late-onset dementia. The tremor of CBGD often begins as an action tremor in an arm that, over time, becomes increasingly rigid and contracted. By late stages of disease, stimulus-induced myoclonus in the affected arm is often apparent. Although stimulus-induced myoclonus is also seen in CJD disease and occasionally in SND, the combination of focal cortical and extrapyramidal signs usually distinguishes CBGD from these two diseases.

PREDOMINANT POSTURAL INSTABILITY

Although postural instability is one of the cardinal features of PD, it is usually not prominent early in disease. When initial signs include pronounced postural instability out of proportion to other manifestations, the clinician should look hard for other forms of parkinsonism. In particular, several parkinsonism-plus syndromes can present with postural instability and gait disorder, including progressive supranuclear palsy and the various forms of MSA.

PSP[72,73] may be the most common parkinsonism-plus syndrome, accounting for 7.5 percent of cases of parkinsonism in one series[61] (see Chap. 21). In early PSP, pronounced postural instability is a clue to the diagnosis, because the disease otherwise can resemble PD. Instead of the stooped, shuffling gait of PD, patients with PSP may walk stiffly with extended trunk and knees. It is important to note that in early stages of PSP the most characteristic feature—vertical and (later) horizontal ophthalmoparesis—may be absent or manifested only by abnormal vertical optokinetic nystagmus. The vestibulo-ocular reflex remains intact, even in advanced disease, hence the designation supranuclear. Other early clues distinguishing PSP from PD include a less prominent tremor, more prominent cognitive deficits, and a poor or transient response to L-dopa. Additional features include axial and nuchal rigidity with opisthotonic neck posturing, and a fixed facial expression with dystonic features such as blepharospasm. Dementia is more common in PSP than in PD, and the cognitive disturbance of PSP tends to have more frontal lobe features.[74] These differences, however, are not reliable enough to be diagnostic (see Chap. 19).

MSA also frequently presents with marked postural instability. MSA represents a spectrum of related clinical syndromes characterized by deficits in the extrapyramidal and pyramidal systems, cerebellum, and autonomic nervous system (see Chap. 22). Particular forms of MSA are identified by the predominant involvement of one of these neural systems: the cerebellum in sporadic olivopontocerebellar degeneration (OPCD), the autonomic nervous system in SDS, the extrapyramidal and pyramidal systems in SND, and lower motoneurons in parkinsonism-amyotrophy. Still, there is considerable overlap between them, and parkinsonism is common to all. In addition to postural instability, the parkinsonism of MSA typically shows features of an akinetic rigid form of disease. Clues to the diagnosis of OPCD include progressive truncal and gait ataxia, ophthalmoparesis, and bulbar dysfunction. If a strong family history is present, the patient may have dominantly inherited cerebellar ataxia instead of sporadic OPCD. The dominant spinocerebellar ataxias include at least nine expanded repeat diseases for

which genetic testing is readily available.[75] In SDS, the diagnosis is supported by evidence of autonomic dysfunction, including orthostatic hypotension, sexual dysfunction, urinary urgency or frequency, and anhydrosis.[76] Frequent falls in the SDS patient may be the result of orthostatic hypotension rather than postural instability.

Marked postural instability with parkinsonism also occurs in normal pressure hydrocephalus, in which it is usually accompanied by urinary incontinence and dementia. When attempting to walk, patients with normal pressure hydrocephalus may find it difficult to raise their leg from the floor (magnetic gait). The gait is slow, apraxic, and characterized by short mincing, irregular steps ("march à petits pas"). Leg function usually improves markedly in the recumbent position. Hydrocephalic parkinsonism is not limited to normal pressure hydrocephalus, as noncommunicating hydrocephalus has also been reported with parkinsonian features. Clinical features suggesting hydrocephalic parkinsonism include a history of head trauma, subarachnoid hemorrhage, or meningitis, symmetrical onset involving the lower extremities, prominent gait disturbance, early cognitive or urinary symptoms, minimal or absent tremor, position-dependent bradykinesia (less when lying down), and brisk leg reflexes. A similar clinical picture may be seen in multi-infarct dementia. MRI can distinguish between hydrocephalus and multi-infarct dementia, as the former typically shows prominent dilated ventricles and an aqueductal void on MRI.

Finally, it is important to remember that the differential diagnosis of early postural instability includes PD itself. Early postural instability in PD is of prognostic importance, because evidence suggests that postural instability-predominant disease tends to progress more rapidly and show a less effective response to medication than tremor-predominant PD.[6]

EARLY DEMENTIA

Dementia at the onset of illness argues against PD, suggesting instead primary dementia with parkinsonian features. Forms of dementia with parkinsonian features include diffuse Lewy body disease (DLBD), and CJD. Early cognitive changes are also common in PSP, which may be misdiagnosed as AD. Although parkinsonism is not a classic feature of AD, some patients will have subtle bradykinesia and rigidity. DLBD was until recently an underdiagnosed cause of dementia with parkinsonism, accounting for up to 20 percent of all dementia in the elderly.[77] Early psychiatric disturbance is said to be more common in DLBD, but in fact there is no sure way of clinically distinguishing the dementia of AD from that of DLBD, except that the latter often displays parkinsonian features and fluctuating levels of consciousness. CJD typically progresses rapidly, over months instead of years, and usually can be identified by the presence of startle myoclonus and periodic complexes on the electroencephalogram; 5–10 percent of CJD patients will have a long-duration variant in which disease may last for more than 2 years. There is considerable overlap in the clinical and pathological features of the various dementia syndromes, meaning that the diagnosis in some patients cannot be made until autopsy.[78]

It is important to recognize that PD can exist concurrently with depression, masquerading as dementia, so-called pseudodementia. Compared to PD patients who are not depressed, those with depression show greater cognitive deficits and are more likely to show a rapid decline in global function.[37,44,79] Formal neuropsychological testing may distinguish bona fide dementia from PD associated with depression.

PERSISTENT ASYMMETRY

Although usually unilateral in onset, PD typically becomes bilateral within several years. A patient whose disease persists in a markedly asymmetric manner may have CBGD, discussed earlier, or hemiparkinsonism-hemiatrophy (HPHA). The latter is a rare condition characterized by unilateral body atrophy (face, arm, or leg), ipsilateral parkinsonism often accompanied by dystonia, and poor response to L-dopa.[80,81] Parkinsonism in this condition may represent a late manifestation of hypoxic-ischemic injury during brain development. Although imaging studies in CBGD and HPHA may demonstrate similar focal brain metabolic abnormalities, the two are distinguishable by the younger-onset, slower progression and focal body atrophy in HPHA, and by the prominence of cortical signs in CBGD.

Just as persistent asymmetry is unusual, so is symmetrical onset of disease. It is more commonly seen in forms of parkinsonism other than PD, including vascular and hydrocephalic parkinsonism and several parkinsonism-plus syndromes.

Treatment-Related Manifestations

The aim in this section is not to list all the potential side-effects of antiparkinsonian drugs, which many patients will experience, in one form or another, during the course of their illness. Instead, we discuss specific treatment-related manifestations that can be mistaken for, or cloud the interpretation of, motor and cognitive deficits intrinsic to the disease. These include dyskinesias, motor fluctuations, cognitive and behavioral disturbances, and orthostatic hypotension.

DYSKINESIAS

Most parkinsonian patients experience L-dopa- or dopamine agonist-induced dyskinesias at some point in their illness.[82,83] Dyskinesias typically begin later in the course of disease and are greatest on the side most affected with parkinsonism. A variety of dyskinesias can be seen, including chorea, athetosis, ballismus, myoclonus, dystonia, and akathisia. Their relationship to medication dosage is often clear, falling under one of three temporal patterns: peak-dose, biphasic (onset and end-of-dose), and off-period dyskinesias. Peak-dose dyskinesias are usually choreic movements, whereas end-of-dose or off-period dyskinesias are typically dystonic. The severity of peak-dose dyskinesias has been shown to be dose-dependent and correlated with higher plasma levels of L-dopa. Frequently, patients do not notice or are not bothered by choreic movements, even when they are obvious and distressing to other family members. In contrast, off-period dystonia (e.g., early-morning foot dystonia) can be quite painful and disabling. Akathisia is another common form of dyskinesia, occurring in about 40 percent of patients.[84]

MOTOR FLUCTUATIONS

Motor fluctuations, such as kinesia paradoxica and freezing, are an intrinsic feature of PD that can occur prior to any dopaminergic therapy. Yet, fluctuations do not usually become a significant problem until after years of dopaminergic therapy.[85–87] At first, most patients derive sustained and fairly steady benefit from L-dopa and/or dopamine agonists throughout the day. As PD advances, however, the duration of benefit shortens for each dose. For example, L-dopa takes longer to "kick in," and "works" for a shorter length of time. Patients may start to experience extreme fluctuations from an "on" to an "off" state. These can occur suddenly and unpredictably, and the transition from "on" to "off" is often accompanied by a short period of severe dyskinesias. Measures to alleviate fluctuations include using more frequent or higher doses of L-dopa or adding a dopamine agonist or catechol-O-methyl transferase inhibitor. Despite these measures, fluctuations may persist and, for many patients, prove to be one of the most disabling aspects of disease. In advanced disease, drug-resistant off-periods also may occur. Most often a late-afternoon or early-evening phenomenon, these off-periods fail to respond to increasing doses of L-dopa or dopamine agonist. Increasingly surgical approaches have become an integral part of the treatment of advanced PD, particularly for patients experiencing disabling medication-related fluctuations and dyskinesias.

COGNITIVE AND BEHAVIORAL DISTURBANCES

Dopaminergic agents can cause a number of psychiatric side-effects. Although these typically do not occur until after several years of treatment, they may happen sooner in patients with dementia or prior psychiatric history. Early effects include disruption of the sleep cycle, vivid dreams, and nightmares. Over time these may progress to daytime visual hallucinations, a common and disabling side-effect of L-dopa or dopamine agonists. These are typically formed, stereotyped images of people or animals that are not threatening. However, a small percentage of patients will develop a paranoid psychosis. Hallucinations are dose-related; hence efforts should be made to lower dopaminergic stimulation in affected patients. Adding an atypical antipsychotic may control hallucinations while permitting continued dopaminergic therapy.

Panic attacks have also been described in late PD.[88] These tend to occur during off-periods in patients experiencing fluctuations and dyskinesias, and may be relieved by additional dopaminergic therapy.

ORTHOSTATIC HYPOTENSION

Although more characteristic of MSA, autonomic dysfunction can cause postural hypotension in some untreated PD patients. More commonly in PD, however, postural hypotension occurs as a side-effect of dopaminergic therapy, particularly dopamine agonists. In one study of the dopamine agonists pergolide and bromocriptine, one-third of patients had postural hypotension.[89] Measures to treat this drug-related effect are the same as for dysautonomia: increased salt and fluid intake, fitted elastic stockings, fludrocortisone or other drugs to correct orthostatic hypotension, and rising slowly to the standing position.

Clinical Rating Scales

In order to evaluate the efficacy of new pharmacotherapies for PD, it is crucial to have standardized methods to quantify disease severity, motor manifestations, and quality of life. Rating scales serve this purpose. Moreover, they prove useful in evaluating an individual patient's response to medication changes, and in assessing the contribution of treatment-related fluctuations and dyskinesias to a patient's disability. For these reasons, a variety of PD rating scales have been developed, three of which are discussed here. Other ways of assessing manifestations of PD are available, including videotape analysis (routinely used in movement disorders centers), patient diaries to assess on-off status, and simple timed maneuvers such as walking a defined distance. For a more detailed discussion, we refer the reader to Lang's thorough review.[90]

The Hoehn and Yahr Staging Scale[13] is a widely adopted and useful scale designed to give a rough estimate of disease severity. Its developers designed five stages of disease severity:

1. Unilateral disease only.
2. Bilateral mild disease, with or without axial involvement.
3. Mild-to-moderate bilateral disease, with first signs of deteriorating balance.
4. Severe disease requiring considerable assistance.
5. Confinement to wheelchair or bed unless aided.

Stage 3 is distinguished from stage 2 by the appearance of postural instability. The stage 3 patient remains fully independent, whereas the stage 4 patient is unable to live alone without assistance. Interrater correlation with the Hoehn and Yahr Staging Scale is excellent. It was not designed for use in therapeutic trials and is clearly inadequate for such purposes

when used in isolation. However, it has been incorporated into several recent rating scales as one arm in patient assessment, including the Unified Parkinson's Disease Rating Scale (UPDRS). Two additional stages, 1.5 and 2.5, have been added to the Hoehn and Yahr component of the UPDRS.

The Schwab and England Capacity for Daily Living Scale is a widely used scale to assess patient disability in performing activities of daily living. It has a 10-point scoring system, with 100 percent representing completely normal function and 0 percent total helplessness. The UPDRS has incorporated the Schwab and England Capacity for Daily Living Scale as the sixth and final arm of patient assessment. It provides an accurate assessment of disability and has the highest interrater concordance rate of the seven stages in the UPDRS.[91]

Investigators created the Unified Parkinson's Disease Rating Scale in the 1980s, in response to the need for standardized assessment of PD. Now widely used, the UPDRS has undergone several revisions. Its major strength is that it provides a detailed and accurate assessment of PD in a variety of respects. This also may be its greatest weakness, because completing the entire scale can prove somewhat cumbersome in a routine clinic practice. Studies have confirmed the high interrater reliability of the UPDRS and suggest possible ways of further shortening the scale without compromising detail and accuracy.[92–94]

The UPDRS contains six sections. The first is a limited assessment of mood and cognition, which in some patients will need to be supplemented with other tests for depression or cognitive disturbance. The second is an assessment of activities of daily living in both the "on" and "off" state, as determined by history. The third is a detailed motor examination based on the widely used Columbia scale. The fourth is a questionnaire assessing complications of therapy, focusing principally on fluctuations and dyskinesias. The fifth and sixth sections are, respectively, a modified Hoehn and Yahr scale and the Schwab and England scale. Added stages in the Hoehn and Yahr scale take into account axial involvement (stage 1.5) and mild postural instability (stage 2.5). Taken together, the six stages provide a detailed and accurate assessment of a patient's global function, level of disability, mood, and both disease-related and treatment-related manifestations of PD.

References

1. Parkinson J: *An Essay on the Shaking Palsy.* London: Sherwood, Neely, and Jones, 1817.
2. Gibb WR: The neuropathology of Parkinson disorders, in Jankovic J, Tolosa E (eds): *Parkinson's Disease and Movement Disorders.* Baltimore: Williams and Wilkins, 1993, pp 205–233.
3. Stern MB: Parkinson's disease, in Stern MB, Koller WC (eds): *Parkinsonian Syndromes.* New York: Marcel Dekker, 1993.
4. Curran T, Lang AE: Parkinsonian syndromes associated with hydrocephalus: Case reports, a review of the literature, and pathophysiological hypotheses. *Mov Disord* 9:508–520, 1994.

5. Rajput AH, et al: Levodopa efficacy and pathological basis of Parkinson syndrome. *Clin Neuropharmacol* 13:553–558, 1990.

6. Jankovic J, et al: Variable expression of Parkinson's disease: A base-line analysis of the DATATOP cohort. The Parkinson Study Group. *Neurology* 40:1529–1534, 1990.

7. Zetusky WJ, Jankovic J, Pirozzolo FJ: The heterogeneity of Parkinson's disease: Clinical and prognostic implications. *Neurology* 35:522–526, 1985.

8. Gibb WR, Lees AJ: A comparison of clinical and pathological features of young- and old-onset Parkinson's disease. *Neurology* 38:1402–1406, 1988.

9. Goetz CG, et al: Risk factors for progression in Parkinson's disease. *Neurology* 38:1841–1844, 1988.

10. Kostic V, et al: Early development of levodopa-induced dyskinesias and response fluctuations in young-onset Parkinson's disease. *Neurology* 41(2 Pt 1):202–205, 1991.

11. Elbaz A, et al: Survival study of Parkinson disease in Olmsted County, Minnesota. *Arch Neurol* 60:91–96, 2003.

12. Hoehn MM, Yahr MD: Parkinsonism: Onset, progression and mortality. *Neurology* 17:427–442, 1967.

13. Hoehn MM: The natural history of Parkinson's disease in the pre-levodopa and post-levodopa eras. *Neurol Clin* 10:331–339, 1992.

14. Rajput AH, et al: Epidemiology of parkinsonism: Incidence, classification, and mortality. *Ann Neurol* 16:278–282, 1984.

15. Koller WC: When does Parkinson's disease begin? *Neurology* 42(4 suppl 4):27–31, discussion 41–48, 1992.

16. Hughes AJ, et al: What features improve the accuracy of clinical diagnosis in Parkinson's disease: A clinicopathologic study. 1992. *Neurology* 57(10 suppl 3):S34–S38, 2001.

17. Louis ED, et al: Progression of parkinsonian signs in Parkinson disease. *Arch Neurol* 56:334–337, 1999.

18. Lance JW, Schwab RS, Peterson EA: Action tremor and the cogwheel phenomenon in Parkinson's disease. *Brain* 86:95–110, 1963.

19. Louis ED, et al: Clinical correlates of action tremor in Parkinson disease. *Arch Neurol* 58:1630–1634, 2001.

20. Hallett M: Parkinson revisited: Pathophysiology of motor signs. *Adv Neurol* 91:19–28, 2003.

21. Hoefer PF, Putnam TJ: Action potentials of muscles in rigidity and tremor. *Arch Neurol Psychiatry* 43:704–725, 1940.

22. Bloxham CA, Mindel TA, Frith CD: Initiation and execution of predictable and unpredictable movements in Parkinson's disease. *Brain* 107(Pt 2):371–384, 1984.

23. Marsden CD: Defects of movement in Parkinson's disease, in Delwaide PJ, Agnoli A (eds): *Clinical Neurophysiology in Parkinsonism.* Amsterdam: Elsevier, 1985.

24. Graybiel AM, et al: The basal ganglia and adaptive motor control. *Science* 265:1826–1831, 1994.

25. Klawans HL: Individual manifestations of Parkinson's disease after ten or more years of levodopa. *Mov Disord* 1:187–192, 1986.

26. Giladi N, et al: Motor blocks in Parkinson's disease. *Neurology* 42:333–339, 1992.

27. Stern MB: The clinical characteristics of Parkinson's disease and parkinsonian syndromes: Diagnosis and assessment, in Stern MB, Hurtig HI (eds) *The Comprehensive Management of Parkinson's Disease.* New York: PMA Publishing, 1988.

28. Friedman JH: Behavioral dysfunction in Parkinson's disease. *Clin Neurosci* 5:87–93, 1998.

29. Levin BE, Tomer R, Rey GJ: Cognitive impairments in Parkinson's disease. *Neurol Clin* 10:471–485, 1992.

30. Boller F, et al: Visuospatial impairment in Parkinson's disease. Role of perceptual and motor factors. *Arch Neurol* 41:485–490, 1984.

31. Cooper JA, et al: Cognitive impairment in early, untreated Parkinson's disease and its relationship to motor disability. *Brain* 114(Pt 5):2095–2122, 1991.

32. Stam CJ, et al: Disturbed frontal regulation of attention in Parkinson's disease. *Brain* 116(Pt 5):1139–1158, 1993.

33. Pate DS, Margolin DI: Cognitive slowing in Parkinson's and Alzheimer's patients: Distinguishing bradyphrenia from dementia. *Neurology* 44:669–674, 1994.

34. Brown RG, Marsden CD: How common is dementia in Parkinson's disease? *Lancet* ii:1262–1265, 1984.

35. Mayeux R, et al: An estimate of the incidence of dementia in idiopathic Parkinson's disease. *Neurology* 40:1513–1517, 1990.

36. Stern Y, et al: Comparison of cognitive changes in patients with Alzheimer's and Parkinson's disease. *Arch Neurol* 50:1040–1045, 1993.

37. Stern Y, et al: Antecedent clinical features associated with dementia in Parkinson's disease. *Neurology* 43:1690–1692, 1993.

38. Starkstein SE, et al: A prospective longitudinal study of depression, cognitive decline, and physical impairments in patients with Parkinson's disease. *J Neurol Neurosurg Psychiatry* 55:377–382, 1992.

39. Levy G, et al: The association of incident dementia with mortality in PD. *Neurology* 59:1708–1713, 2002.

40. Gotham AM, Brown RG, Marsden CD: Depression in Parkinson's disease: A quantitative and qualitative analysis. *J Neurol Neurosurg Psychiatry* 49:381–389, 1986.

41. Taylor AE, et al: Parkinson's disease and depression. A critical re-evaluation. *Brain* 109(Pt 2):279–292, 1986.

42. Aarsland D, et al: Range of neuropsychiatric disturbances in patients with Parkinson's disease. *J Neurol Neurosurg Psychiatry* 67:492–496, 1999.

43. Poewe W, Luginger E: Depression in Parkinson's disease: Impediments to recognition and treatment options. *Neurology* 52(7 suppl 3):S2–6, 1999.

44. Slaughter JR, et al: Prevalence, clinical manifestations, etiology, and treatment of depression in Parkinson's disease. *J Neuropsychiatry Clin Neurosci* 13:187–196, 2001.

45. Vreeling FW, et al: Primitive reflexes in Parkinson's disease. *J Neurol Neurosurg Psychiatry* 56:1323–1326, 1993.

46. Edwards LL, Quigley EM, Pfeiffer RF: Gastrointestinal dysfunction in Parkinson's disease: Frequency and pathophysiology. *Neurology* 42:726–732, 1992.

47. Doty RL, et al: Olfactory testing differentiates between progressive supranuclear palsy and idiopathic Parkinson's disease. *Neurology* 43:962–965, 1993.

48. Stern MB, et al: Olfactory function in Parkinson's disease subtypes. *Neurology* 44:266–268, 1994.

49. Koller WC: Sensory symptoms in Parkinson's disease. *Neurology* 34:957–959, 1984.

50. Snider SR, et al: Primary sensory symptoms in parkinsonism. *Neurology* 26:423–429, 1976.

51. Krishnan PR, Bhatia M, Behari M: Restless legs syndrome in Parkinson's disease: A case-controlled study. *Mov Disord* 18:181–185, 2003.

52. Ondo WG, Vuong KD, Jankovic J: Exploring the relationship between Parkinson disease and restless legs syndrome. *Arch Neurol* 59:421–424, 2002.

53. Appenzeller O, Goss JE: Autonomic deficits in Parkinson's syndrome. *Arch Neurol* 24:50–57, 1971.

54. Goetz CG, Lutge W, Tanner CM: Autonomic dysfunction in Parkinson's disease. *Neurology* 36:73–75, 1986.

55. Comella CL: Sleep disturbances in Parkinson's disease. *Curr Neurol Neurosci Rep* 3:173–180, 2003.

56. Wetter TC, et al: Sleep and periodic leg movement patterns in drug-free patients with Parkinson's disease and multiple system atrophy. *Sleep* 23:361–367, 2000.

57. Gagnon JF, et al: REM sleep behavior disorder and REM sleep without atonia in Parkinson's disease. *Neurology* 59:585–589, 2002.

58. Olson EJ, Boeve BF, Silber MH: Rapid eye movement sleep behaviour disorder: Demographic, clinical and laboratory findings in 93 cases. *Brain* 123(Pt 2):331–339, 2000.

59. Cantor CR, Stern MB: Dopamine agonists and sleep in Parkinson's disease. *Neurology* 58(4 suppl 1):S71–S78, 2002.

60. Facca AG, Koller WC: Differential diagnosis of parkinsonism. *Adv Neurol* 91:383–396, 2003.

61. Stacy M, Jankovic J: Differential diagnosis of Parkinson's disease and the parkinsonism plus syndromes. *Neurol Clin* 10:341–359, 1992.

62. Giovannini P, et al: Early-onset Parkinson's disease. *Mov Disord* 6:36–42, 1991.

63. Quinn N, Critchley P, Marsden CD: Young onset Parkinson's disease. *Mov Disord* 2:73–91, 1987.

64. Muthane UB, et al: Early onset Parkinson's disease: Are juvenile- and young-onset different? *Mov Disord* 9:539–544, 1994.

65. Hayflick SJ, et al: Genetic, clinical, and radiographic delineation of Hallervorden-Spatz syndrome. *N Engl J Med* 348:33–40, 2003.

66. Adams RD, Victor M: [Hepato-cerebral degeneration, especially of the acquired non-Wilsonian type.] *Rev Med Suisse Romande* 86:655–665, 1966.

67. Fearnley JM, Lees AJ: Striatonigral degeneration. A clinico-pathological study. *Brain* 113(Pt 6):1823–1842,1990.

68. Gouider-Khouja N, et al: "Pure" striatonigral degeneration and Parkinson's disease: A comparative clinical study. *Mov Disord* 10:288–294, 1995.

69. Rebeiz JJ, Kolodny EH, Richardson EP Jr: Corticodentatonigral degeneration with neuronal achromasia. *Arch Neurol* 18:20–33, 1968.

70. Brunt ER, et al: Unique myoclonic pattern in corticobasal degeneration. *Mov Disord* 10:132–142, 1995.

71. Riley DE, et al: Cortical-basal ganglionic degeneration. *Neurology* 40:1203–1212, 1990.

72. Gearing M, et al: Progressive supranuclear palsy: Neuropathologic and clinical heterogeneity. *Neurology* 44:1015–1024, 1994.

73. Steele JC, Richardson JC, Olszewski J: Progressive supranuclear palsy: A heterogeneous degeneration involving the brainstem, basal ganglia and cerebellum with vertical gaze and pseudobulbar palsy, nuchal dystonia and dementia. *Arch Neurol* 10:333–359, 1964.

74. Pillon B, et al: Severity and specificity of cognitive impairment in Alzheimer's, Huntington's, and Parkinson's diseases and progressive supranuclear palsy. *Neurology* 41:634–643, 1991.

75. Paulson H, Ammache Z: Ataxia and hereditary disorders. *Neurol Clin* 19:759–782, 2001.

76. Shy GM, Drager GA: A neurologic syndrome associated with orthostatic hypotension: A clinical-pathologic study. *Arch Neurol* 2:511–527, 1960.

77. McKeith IG: Spectrum of Parkinson's disease, Parkinson's dementia, and Lewy body dementia. *Neurol Clin* 18:865–902, 2000.

78. Wojcieszek J, et al: What is it? Case 1, 1994: Rapidly progressive aphasia, apraxia, dementia, myoclonus, and parkinsonism. *Mov Disord* 9:358–366, 1994.

79. Troster AI, et al: The influence of depression on cognition in Parkinson's disease: A pattern of impairment distinguishable from Alzheimer's disease. *Neurology* 45:672–676, 1995.

80. Giladi N, et al: Hemiparkinsonism-hemiatrophy syndrome: Clinical and neuroradiologic features. *Neurology* 40:1731–1734, 1990.

81. Klawans HL: Hemiparkinsonism as a late complication of hemiatrophy: A new syndrome. *Neurology* 31:625–628, 1981.

82. Nutt JG: Levodopa-induced dyskinesia: Review, observations, and speculations. *Neurology* 40:340–345, 1990.

83. Marconi R, et al: Levodopa-induced dyskinesias in Parkinson's disease phenomenology and pathophysiology. *Mov Disord* 9:2–12, 1994.

84. Comella CL, Goetz CG: Akathisia in Parkinson's disease. *Mov Disord* 9:545–549, 1994.

85. Fahn S: "On-off" phenomenon with levodopa therapy in parkinsonism. Clinical and pharmacologic correlations and the effect of intramuscular pyridoxine. *Neurology* 24:431–441, 1974.

86. Marsden CD, Parkes JP, Quinn N: Fluctuations of disability in Parkinson's disease, in Marsden CD, Fahn S (eds): *Movement Disorders*. London: Butterworth, 1982.

87. Nutt JG, et al: The "on-off" phenomenon in Parkinson's disease. Relation to levodopa absorption and transport. *N Engl J Med* 310:483–488, 1984.

88. Vazquez A, et al: "Panic attacks" in Parkinson's disease. A long-term complication of levodopa therapy. *Acta Neurol Scand* 87:14–18, 1993.

89. LeWitt PA, et al: Comparison of pergolide and bromocriptine therapy in parkinsonism. *Neurology* 33:1009–1014, 1983.

90. Lang AE: Clinical rating scales and videotape analysis, in Paulson GW, Koller WC (eds): *Therapy of Parkinson's Disease*. New York: Marcel Dekker, 1995.

91. Fahn S, Elton RL, M.o.U.D. Committee: Unified Parkinson's disease rating scale, in Fahn S, et al (eds): *Recent Developments in Parkinson's Disease*. New York: Macmillan, 1987.

92. van Hilten JJ, et al: Rating impairment and disability in Parkinson's disease: Evaluation of the Unified Parkinson's Disease Rating Scale. *Mov Disord* 9:84–88, 1994.

93. Martinez-Martin P, et al: Unified Parkinson's Disease Rating Scale characteristics and structure. The Cooperative Multicentric Group. *Mov Disord* 9:76–83, 1994.

94. Richards M, et al: Interrater reliability of the Unified Parkinson's Disease Rating Scale motor examination. *Mov Disord* 9:89–91, 1994.

Chapter 15

PHARMACOLOGIC TREATMENT OF PARKINSON'S DISEASE

W. POEWE, R. GRANATA, and F. GESER

THE MAJOR CLASSES OF ANTIPARKINSONIAN
   DRUGS   247
      Dopaminergic Agents   247
      Nondopaminergic Agents   257
PRACTICAL TREATMENT DECISIONS IN PD   258
      Early Monotherapy   258
      Treatment of Advanced PD   260

The first empirical attempts at a pharmacologic treatment of Parkinson's disease (PD) were made in the 1860s by Ordenstein and Charcot in Paris, using extracts from *Hyscyamus niger, Atropa belladonna,* and *Datura stramonium* containing the anticholinergic compounds hyoscine and scopolamine.[1,2] With the development of synthetic anticholinergic drugs in the 1940s,[3] these agents became the mainstay of antiparkinsonian drug treatment, but, while improving tremor and rigidity, they had little effect on akinesia.[4]

The classical experiments on reserpinized animals by Carlsson in 1957, which showed that the akinesia of catecholamine-depleted animals could be reversed by *dl*-dopa administration,[5] led to the hypothesis of a dopaminergic disorder as the pathophysiological basis of PD. Shortly afterwards, the finding in postmortem studies of dopamine deficiency in the striatum of PD patients, by Ehringer and Hornykiewicz in Vienna in 1960,[6] and the observation of reduced dopamine excretion in the urine of PD patients by Barbeau et al.,[7] marked the beginning of a new "era" in the treatment of PD. In 1961, two groups, in Vienna and in Montreal, independently reported positive results of open-label small-scale clinical trials with L-dopa in parkinsonian patients.[8,9] Five years later, Cotzias et al. demonstrated striking efficacy of high-dose oral L-dopa,[10] the potentiation of its effects and the improvement of side-effects with co-administration of peripheral dopa decarboxylase inhibitors,[11] as well as the long-term side-effects of L-dopa treatment.[12]

Until now, L-dopa substitution has remained the gold standard of antiparkinsonian drug therapy, although important advances have been made, including the introduction of directly acting dopamine agonists, monoamine oxidase B (MAO-B) inhibitors, L-dopa slow-release formulations, or the

experimental use of catechol-*O*-methyltransferase (COMT) inhibitors. In addition, new concepts of "neuroprotection" have led to the search for drugs that may halt or slow down the progression of nigral cell death undergoing PD. So far, however, none of the agents tested have proven to be unequivocally effective. This chapter first reviews the clinical pharmacology of currently available agents for the symptomatic treatment of PD, followed by a brief review of the present status of "neuroprotective" therapies. The final section deals with the clinically most important practical treatment decision in the course of PD.

The Major Classes of Antiparkinsonian Drugs

This section reviews the most commonly used drugs to treat motor symptoms of PD by class of agents. For each drug, a brief synopsis of its clinical pharmacology, current indications in PD, and safety is provided.

DOPAMINERGIC AGENTS

L-DOPA

Basic Pharmacology and Mechanisms of Action

L-Dopa is absorbed in the gastrointestinal tract at the level of the small bowel, utilizing the large neutral amino acid (LNAA) transport system. It is then rapidly distributed into other tissues, mainly muscle, with a half-life of 5–10 minutes. It crosses the blood-brain barrier via LNAA, competing with the normal concentration of plasma amino acids. Peripherally, L-dopa is rapidly catabolized by aromatic amino acid decarboxylase (AADC) and COMT (Fig. 15-1), and eliminated from plasma with a half-life of approximately 60–90 minutes (Table 15-1). The amount of L-dopa that eventually reaches the brain following ingestion of an oral dose is dependent on a number of variables that may interfere with absorption and transport of the drug.[13,14] The speed of gastric emptying is crucial for the time interval to reach plasma levels as absorption sites for L-dopa are in the intestinal wall. Food may delay gastric transit time and, in the case of protein-rich meals, competition between L-dopa and dietary LNAA for transmucosal transport further contributes to erratic intestinal absorption. L-Dopa versus LNAA transport competition may also significantly reduce the amount of plasma L-dopa crossing the endothelial blood-brain barrier.[15,16] The stomach mucosa, as well as the bowel and the liver, are rich in AADC and COMT. Those enzymes convert L-dopa into dopamine and *O*-methyldopa, reducing the bioavailability of L-dopa.[17,18] For this reason, commonly used L-dopa preparations contain inhibitors of peripheral AADC (benserazide or carbidopa; see Table 15-2),[19,20] and, more recently, inhibitors of COMT have been introduced into clinical practice.

Co-administration of peripherally acting AADC inhibitors doubles the bioavailability of L-dopa without significant

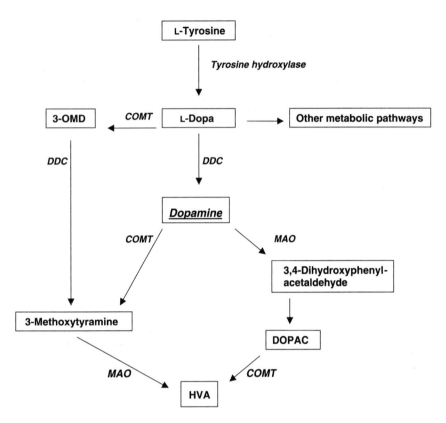

FIGURE 15-1 Metabolic pathways of dopamine and ʟ-dopa in brain and periphery. COMT, catechol-*O*-methyltransferase; DDC, dopa decarboxylase; DOPAC, 3,4-dihydroxyphenylacetic acid; HVA, homovanillic acid; MAO, monoamine oxidase; 3-OMD, 3-*O*-methyldopa.

effects on elimination half-life.[17] Consequently, therapeutically effective ʟ-dopa doses are much lower when administered in combination with a dopa decarboxylase inhibitor, and the incidence of peripheral side-effects such as nausea, vomiting, and hypotension is markedly reduced. Inhibition of COMT is associated with an increase in the plasma half-life of ʟ-dopa and an increase in bioavailability without significant changes in maximal plasma concentrations following a dose (C_{max}) or the time to peak plasma levels (t_{max}).[21,22]

TABLE 15-1 ʟ-Dopa Pharmacokinetic Parameters: Summary of Human Studies

Study	Apparent Volume of Distribution	Plasma Clearance	Half-life (alpha)	Half-life (beta)
Hardie et al., 1986[273]	83.1 L	36.2 L/h	5.5 min	1.6 h
Sasahara et al., 1980[274]	87.8 L	96.6 L/h	—	0.6 h
Fabbrini et al., 1988[275]	0.26 L/kg	0.13 L/h	—	1.4 h
Nutt and Fellman, 1984[13]	0.67 L/kg	0.3 L/h	—	1.4 h
Poewe et al. (unpublished data)	3 L/kg	1.4 L/h	5.4 min	1.5 h

The exact central mechanisms of ʟ-dopa action are disputed. The classical hypothesis assumes that ʟ-dopa is taken up by residual dopaminergic neurons, decarboxylated by AADC in these surviving cells, and finally synaptically released.[23] According to this hypothesis, there should be a continuous loss of ʟ-dopa efficacy with disease duration, which is clearly not observed in some PD patients. This suggests alternative mechanisms of presynaptic handling of ʟ-dopa, and the exact site of decarboxylation of exogenous ʟ-dopa to dopamine remains unknown.[24]

Current Indications

Despite numerous advances in the development of dopaminergic drugs, ʟ-dopa substitution continues to be regarded as the gold standard of antiparkinsonian pharmacotherapy. ʟ-Dopa responsiveness is considered as one of the diagnostic criteria differentiating PD from other parkinsonian syndromes—multiple system atrophy (MSA), progressive supranuclear palsy, or secondary parkinsonism,[25] although some patients with MSA may initially respond to ʟ-dopa.[26] On the other hand, a majority of patients chronically exposed to oral ʟ-dopa therapy will eventually develop motor complications, including response oscillations and drug-induced involuntary movements (see below). Dose and duration of

TABLE 15-2 Commonly Used L-Dopa Preparations

Substance	Commercial Name	Dosage
L-Dopa/carbidopa	Sinemet (tablets)	100/10
		100/25[a]
		250/25
L-Dopa/carbidopa slow-release	Sinemet CR (tablets)	100/25
		200/50
L-Dopa/benserazide[a]	Madopar (capsule)	50/12.5
		100/25
		200/50
	Madopar (tablets)	100/25
		200/50
L-Dopa/benserazide slow-release[a]	Madopar CR (capsule)	100/25
	Madopar HBS (capsule)	100/25
L-Dopa/benserazide dispersible[a]	Madopar LT (tablets)	100/25
L-Dopa/benserazide dual-release[b]	Madopar DR (tablets)	200/50

[a]Not available in the US.
[b]Available only in Switzerland.

L-dopa treatment are the most consistent risk factors.[27] In addition, young age at onset of PD is associated with a striking propensity to develop L-dopa-induced dyskinesias even after a relatively short period of exposure.[28] Several recent randomized prospective controlled trials have compared L-dopa with dopamine agonists as early monotherapy regarding relative risks to develop motor complications.[29–33] These trials have consistently demonstrated significantly reduced incidences of motor complications with early agonist monotherapy over L-dopa even if dopamine agonists are later on supplemented with adjunct L-dopa.

As a consequence, there is growing consensus that dopamine replacement therapy in early PD should be started with a dopamine agonist to be supplemented by adjunct L-dopa when required for sufficient symptomatic control.[34] Elderly patients, particularly those with cerebrovascular comorbidity and/or cognitive decline, may be at greater risk to develop neuropsychiatric side-effects with dopamine agonists and have lesser risk of developing L-dopa-induced dyskinesias. They continue to be candidates for first-line treatment with L-dopa. Moreover, L-dopa treatment is indicated in patients in whom symptoms cause significant disability and/or interfere with performance at work and in whom alternative strategies fail to produce sufficient benefit.

The current available formulations of L-dopa in association with a peripheral AADC inhibitor are shown in Table 15-2.

Side-Effects and Late L-Dopa Failure

Despite coadministration of an AADC inhibitor some patients initially experience nausea and vomiting when L-dopa treatment is started. Most patients, however, develop tolerance to these side-effects within days. In severe cases they may be controlled (outside the US) by coadministration of domperidone (10–20 mg) 1 hour before dosing. The same is

true for postural hypotension induced by L-dopa.[35] In the US, the use of extra carbidopa (25 mg, Lodosyn) or Tigan (trimethobenzamide) 100–200 mg with each L-dopa dosage helps alleviate nausea and vomiting until tolerance develops (weeks or months). Sedation and daytime sleepiness is another common and occasionally dose-limiting side-effect of L-dopa. Although randomized controlled comparative trials of L-dopa versus various dopamine agonists suggest a decreased incidence of this side-effect with L-dopa compared to dopamine agonists, attacks of irresistible sleep following L-dopa have been occasionally described.[36,37] In addition, L-dopa is known to trigger a variety of psychiatric symptoms, particularly in elderly people or in patients with a history of psychiatric disease. Unusually vivid dreams may represent the first signs of L-dopa psychotoxicity, which may progress to visual delusions, hallucinations, and paranoid psychosis.

Although marked clinical responsiveness to oral L-dopa is one of the diagnostic hallmarks of PD, advanced stages of the disease are accompanied by both the development of disease-related motor and nonmotor symptoms, which are largely unresponsive to L-dopa, as well as by L-dopa-related motor complications (see Table 15-3). Up to 50 percent of all patients treated with L-dopa for 5 years or more develop motor response fluctuations.[27,29,38] Initially, these motor response oscillations are related to dose intervals and are characterized by re-emergence of parkinsonian symptoms some 3–4 hours post dosing ("wearing-off phenomenon"). In addition to such "end-of-dose" problems, patients may begin to experience "delayed-on" phenomena consisting of lag times of more than 30 minutes from oral drug intake until onset of clinical effect.[39] While wearing-off fluctuations are related to L-dopa half-life, delayed-on or complete dose failure ("no-on") have been shown to best correlate with erratic gastric emptying.[40]

A minority of patients progress to develop more malignant and unpredictable "on-off" swings, with sudden releases of parkinsonian symptoms without apparent relation to their L-dopa dosing schedule. This latter type of response oscillation has been linked to postsynaptic changes in receptor pharmacodynamics induced by long-term pulsatile stimulation.[41] This pathophysiological classification into presynaptic pharmacokinetic changes giving rise to predictable wearing-off

TABLE 15-3 Complications of Disease Progression in PD

L-Dopa-related motor complications
  Response fluctuations
  Dyskinesias
Disease-related motor complications
  Freezing
  Postural imbalance
  Dysarthria and dysphagia
Nonmotor complications
  Neuropsychiatric morbidity
  Sleep disorders
  Autonomic dysfunction

TABLE 15-4 Classification of L-Dopa-Related Motor Fluctuations in PD

Clinical pattern	Pathophysiology
Wearing-off	Short L-dopa half-life
	Reduced presynaptic storage
Delayed-on	Delayed gastric emptying
	Delayed intestinal absorption
Dose failures (No-on)	Deficient gastric emptying
	Deficient intestinal absorption
	Insufficient blood-brain barrier transport
Complex on-off	Striatal pharmacodynamic changes

TABLE 15-5 Drug-Induced Dyskinesias in PD

On-period dyskinesias (interdose)
Phasic (choreic) limb movements
Dystonic craniocervical movements
More pronounced on side initially affected by PD

Biphasic dyskinesias
At onset or wearing-off of clinical benefit from a dose of L-dopa (or both)
Mix of phasic and dystonic movements (mobile dystonia)

Off-period dystonia
Most often distal limb (feet)
Painful

effects, and postsynaptic pharmacodynamic alterations producing sudden on-off swings may be too simplistic since even the "long-duration" response to L-dopa is likely to involve postsynaptic mechanisms.[42] Table 15-4 summarizes the different types of motor response oscillations by their underlying pathophysiology.

On-off oscillations may be associated with prominent mood swings where depression, anxiety or panic attacks accompany off-states while dysphoria, hypomania or mania may be noted during on-periods. Patients with a fluctuating motor response to L-dopa may be exquisitely responsive to such behavioral stimulatory L-dopa effects, leading to uncontrolled drug intake and severe behavioral disturbances.[43]

The emergence of response oscillations is usually associated with the appearance of L-dopa-induced abnormal involuntary movements. These may occur in 30 percent of patients after 2 years of L-dopa exposure,[32] or even earlier in patients with young-onset PD.[28] According to their relation to L-dopa response cycles they are commonly divided into three main types. (1) "Peak dose" or "interdose" dyskinesias occur at times of a full L-dopa motor response and are characterized by phasic (choreic or ballistic) asymmetric limb movements, but may also involve facial grimacing as well as trunk and neck rotations. (2) "Diphasic" dyskinesias are clinically linked to transition periods (onset or wearing-off of benefit from an individual dose) and frequently contain phasic and dystonic elements causing bizarre twisting movements of the trunk and extremities; again, limb involvement may be asymmetric. (3) "Off-period" dystonia occurs after the motor response has worn off, and may initially be linked to the early morning hours ("early morning dystonia"). It characteristically consists of unilateral distal painful dystonic limb cramps, most often involving one foot[44] (see Table 15-5).

The exact pathophysiology of dyskinesias is not fully understood, but they are probably related to striatal dopamine receptor changes following dopaminergic denervation and chronic exposure to L-dopa. These receptor alterations include changes of sensitivity, relative balance between different dopamine receptor subtypes, and different translational and neuromodulatory system responses.[45,46] The denervation induced imbalance between the D1 and D2

receptor-controlled direct and indirect outflow pathways appears to be sustained by L-dopa, perhaps through its predominant action on the D1 receptor.[47]

Recent studies on 1-methyl-4-phenyl-1,2,3,6-tetrahydropyridine (MPTP)-treated monkeys show that abnormal pulsatile stimulation of denerved striatal dopamine receptor results in molecular modifications in the basal ganglia, such as upregulation of immediate early genes in the Fos family and of preproenkephalin (PPE) mRNA expression, which could be at the origin of L-dopa-induced dyskinesias.[48] The upregulation of Fos protein and PPE induced by short-acting dopaminergic agents such as L-dopa are avoided with longer-acting drugs. Furthermore, in MPTP-treated monkeys it has been shown that, when long-acting dopaminergic agents are introduced, the frequency and severity of dyskinesias are significantly reduced as compared to treatment with short-acting dopamine agonists or standard L-dopa.[49] Based on these observations, it has been proposed that long-acting dopamine agonists and the administration of L-dopa, in combination with COMT to extend its half-life, may avoid or delay the onset of dyskinesias.[50] Further prospective double-blind clinical studies are required to support this hypothesis.

L-Dopa Slow-Release Preparations

L-Dopa slow-release preparations have been introduced in an attempt to produce prolonged clinical effects from each individual dose and thereby smooth out response oscillations. Two formulations are currently available: Sinemet CR and Madopar CR (Madopar HBS). Sinemet CR is a combination of 200 mg of L-dopa and 50 mg of carbidopa, imbedded in a slowly eroding matrix.[51,52] A rate-controlled erosion and dissolution takes place as the preparation passes along the duodenal-jejunal mucosa. Madopar CR contains 100 mg of L-dopa and 25 mg of benserazide which, upon gastric contact, are transformed into a gelatinous diffusion body which floats on the fluid contents of the stomach.[53] Both these controlled-release preparations cause a delayed onset of peak L-dopa concentrations (t_{max}), and a prolonged decline of plasma levels compared to conventional preparations. Further pharmacokinetic features of L-dopa slow-release preparations include reduced peak plasma levels and decreased bioavailability of about 25 percent compared to conventional L-dopa formulations.[54]

These pharmacokinetic characteristics have several clinical consequences. (1) The delay in t_{max} causes delayed "on" effects, particularly after the first morning dose. (2) With multiple daily doses L-dopa, plasma levels during the day are generally more stable compared to standard L-dopa, thereby reducing end-of-dose response swings; however, results of 10 randomized controlled trials comparing L-dopa standard versus slow-release formulations to control motor fluctuations in advanced PD have produced inconsistent results.[55] (3) In patients with mild wearing-off-type motor fluctuations, interdose intervals can be stretched, resulting in a decreased dosing frequency, although this is usually not dramatic. (4) The decreased bioavailability of slow-release L-dopa requires greater total daily doses compared to standard preparations.

The combined use of slow-release plus standard L-dopa formulations may overcome delayed "on" effects and generally increases the predictability of onset of clinical effects for the patients. Not all patients with fluctuating PD, however, are helped by controlled-release preparations.[56,57] The main reason for failure are a lack of predictability of onset of clinical effects and increased peak-dose, or prolonged biphasic, dyskinesias.[58]

Two randomized controlled long-term trials have compared standard versus slow-release L-dopa as initial treatment in de novo patients[38,59,60] with the rate of occurrence of motor fluctuations and dyskinesias after 5 years as their primary endpoint. Both trials failed to detect significant differences in the rate of motor complications observed with either type of initial treatment, thereby failing to show efficacy of slow-release L-dopa regarding prevention of motor complications.

New Pharmacokinetic Formulations of L-Dopa

While L-dopa slow-release preparations and add-on treatment with COMT inhibitors (see below) are aimed at increasing the half-life of L-dopa, a number of strategies have been used to improve gastrointestinal absorption of L-dopa to overcome onset-of-dose difficulties. Such formulations include dispersible L-dopa preparations which have been shown to produce shorter t_{max} and more rapid onset of clinical effects as compared to standard formulations.[61] Dispersible L-dopa is marketed as Madopar LT in several European countries.

Recently a novel dual-release preparation of L-dopa, consisting of a 3-layer tablet combining immediate and slow-release properties, has been developed; small-scale open-label studies have reported significantly shorter times to switch on compared to slow-release formulations and a trend to longer on-duration.[62] This formulation is currently only marketed in Switzerland.

L-Dopa ethyl ester is a highly water-soluble prodrug of L-dopa, which is rapidly hydrolyzed in the stomach to release L-dopa. Phase II clinical trials have shown shortened t_{max} and decreased time-to-on in patients with fluctuating

PD compared to standard L-dopa.[63,64] Two large double-blind randomized controlled trials assessing the efficacy of L-dopa ethyl ester in improving time-to-on and reducing total daily off-time compared to standard L-dopa have just been completed and results will be available soon.

COMT INHIBITORS

Basic Pharmacology and Mechanisms of Action

Following continued administration of L-dopa with AADC inhibitors, the major catabolism of the drug is shifted to conversion to 3-O-methyldopa (3-OMD) by the action of COMT (Fig. 15-1). 3-OMD, because of its long half-life of approximately 15 hours, accumulates during chronic L-dopa treatment and competes with L-dopa for intestinal absorption and active transport through the blood-brain barrier. By inhibiting COMT, it is possible to prolong the pharmacological half-life of L-dopa in plasma and brain. Two COMT inhibitors, tolcapone and entacapone, have been introduced into clinical practice.

Entacapone acts as a reversible inhibitor of peripheral COMT,[65] with a half-life of approximately 1.5 hours;[66] it inhibits erythrocyte COMT activity in a dose-dependent fashion.[67] Clinical pharmacokinetic studies have shown that coadministration of 200 mg of entacapone prolongs the elimination half-life and approximately doubles the bioavailability of L-dopa due to significantly reduced metabolic loss of L-dopa into 3-OMD.[21,22,68–70] Plasma 3-OMD levels from a given dose of L-dopa are reduced by 40–60 percent. ^{18}F-Fluoro-L-dopa positron emission tomography (PET) studies have shown a significant increase in striatal signal following coadministration of entacapone.[71,72] The average L-dopa maximum plasma concentration (C_{max}) and the time to C_{max} (t_{max}) are generally unaffected.

Tolcapone has a very similar pharmacological profile to entacapone. However, high doses of tolcapone may cross the blood-brain barrier in humans and also block central COMT in addition to peripheral blocking effects.

Current Indications

Both tolcapone and entacapone have been shown to reduce off-time and increase on-time in L-dopa-treated patients with motor fluctuations. Randomized placebo-controlled trials in patients with wearing-off type of response oscillations have consistently shown increases in on-time by about 1–2 hours with tolcapone[73–77] and entacapone.[78–81] The clinically effective dose of entacapone is 200 mg, and the drug has to be given with every L-dopa dose for up to a maximum of 10 doses per day. Beneficial effects have been reported with both 100 mg and 200 mg of tolcapone using a three times daily dosing scheme.

Entacapone has also been shown to improve symptomatic control of parkinsonism by enhancing "on" motor functions in patients with fluctuating PD.[79,80] In addition, both COMT inhibitors are able to improve symptomatic control in PD patients with a stable response to L-dopa.[81,82]

When adding COMT inhibitors, the total daily dose of L-dopa can be reduced. The reported dose reductions of L-dopa were generally above 100 mg/day in clinical trials with tolcapone, and somewhat lower in studies with entacapone.

A triple L-dopa tablet containing both the AADC inhibitor carbidopa and the COMT inhibitor entacapone has just been released onto the market in the US and Europe.

Side-Effects

Worsening of pre-existing L-dopa-induced dyskinesias and nausea are the most common dopaminergic adverse reactions when COMT inhibitors are added to L-dopa. They are usually transient and can be relieved by reducing the L-dopa dose. Newly emergent dyskinesias or hallucinations are rare. Diarrhea is the most common nondopaminergic side-effect of both tolcapone and entacapone, but diarrhea-related withdrawal was somewhat rarer in studies with entacapone compared to tolcapone. Urine discoloration in up to 40 percent of patients taking entacapone is a clinically irrelevant side-effect related to the formulation.

Tolcapone exposure has been associated with liver toxicity and after published reports on 3 fetal cases of fulminant liver failure following treatment with tolcapone the drug was withdrawn from the market in the European Union, and labeling was changed in the US, restricting its use to patients for whom there is no alternative treatment and requiring regular monitoring of liver enzymes. The exact mechanism of the liver toxicity of tolcapone is not clear.[83,84] No such monitoring is required for entacapone and there have been no cases of fetal liver injury associated with entacapone in postmarketing surveillance.

MAO-B INHIBITORS

Basic Pharmacology and Mechanisms of Action

MAO-B plays an important role in the biotransformation of dopamine in human brain. Inhibitors of this enzyme block the oxidative deamination of dopamine, and increase its half-life in the brain. The selective and irreversible MAO-B inhibitor *selegiline (deprenyl)* potentiates the efficacy of L-dopa and improves motor fluctuations in one-half to two-thirds of patients.[85–87] At the dose commonly given in PD (10–20 mg/day), selegiline effects a complete and irreversible inhibition of MAO-B, with only minimal effects on MAO-A, an enzyme that oxidatively deaminates serotonin and noradrenaline. Selegiline has a half-life of approximately 40 hours, with cumulative MAO inhibition at repeated doses. It has been shown that a 50 percent restoration of MAO-B activity in rat brain occurs within approximately 10 days after discontinuation of the drug via de novo synthesis of the enzyme.[88] Selegiline is metabolized to metamphetamine, and to a lesser extent to amphetamine,[89] which blocks dopamine reuptake and releases dopamine, and may account for some of the dopaminergic effects. Although a clear antidepressant and amphetamine-like action has not been demonstrated in

man, the partial anti-MAO-A activity, as well as the effects exerted by its amphetamine metabolites, may explain some of the mood brightening and stimulating properties that can be observed in individual patients.

Current Indications

When given as monotherapy to de novo patients with PD, selegiline has a small but definitive symptomatic effect according to several placebo-controlled trials, usually with doses of 10 mg/day.[90–93] Improved symptomatic control and reduced need for L-dopa was also observed in studies where selegiline was given as adjunct therapy in patients with stable PD, but effect sizes were small and results inconsistent between trials.[55]

Some studies have shown that adjunct therapy with selegiline in L-dopa-treated patients with motor fluctuations will induce some increase in daily on-time and decrease in wearing-off symptoms.[94,95]

The majority of randomized controlled trials conducted with selegiline were designed to assess the potential of selegiline to modify PD progression. Some of these demonstrated delayed need for L-dopa,[90,91,96] but such results are insufficient to demonstrate neuroprotective properties because of selegiline's symptomatic efficacy, as evident from "wash-in" effects.[90,93] One study found improved scores after 12 months of selegiline versus placebo treatment added to L-dopa or bromocriptine in de novo patients after an extended 2-month wash-out period, and argued that such effects were more readily explained by neuroprotective than symptomatic properties of selegiline.[97] Overall, the evidence available is insufficient to demonstrate neuroprotection through selegiline.

Side-Effects

Selegiline is generally well tolerated, and many studies failed to detect differences in the incidence of adverse reactions between selegiline and placebo. Increased dyskinesia, nausea, and hypotension are the most commonly observed dopaminergic side-effects when selegiline is added to L-dopa; occasionally, adjunct selegiline may trigger hallucinations. Insomnia, particularly if doses are given late in the day, has been linked to selegiline's metabolism to amphetamine-like compounds. Most studies have failed to detect significant changes in blood pressure and other cardiovascular parameters with selegiline treatment, but one large prospective study in de novo patients reported increased mortality after 2 and 4 years of treatment with L-dopa plus selegiline compared to L-dopa alone.[98] This has not been confirmed through any other trial and is generally regarded as a statistical artefact.[99]

New MAO-B Inhibitors

Rasagiline mesylate is an irreversible inhibitor of MAO-B and more potent than selegiline on a milligram basis; 0.5–1 mg/day completely inhibits platelet MAO-B in humans.[100] Unlike selegiline, the drug does not give rise to amphetamine-like metabolites. One small placebo-controlled short-term trial in

TABLE 15-6 Clinical Pharmacology of Dopamine Agonists

Substance	Dopamine Receptor Interaction*	Interaction with Other Receptors		Half-life (h)	Average Daily Dose (mg)	
		α_1/α_2 adrenergic	5-HT		Monotherapy	Adjunct to L-Dopa
Bromocriptine	D2	+	+	3–6	25–45	15–25
Lisuride	D2	+	+	2–3	0.8–1.6	0.6–1.2
Pergolide	D2>D1	+	+	15	1.5–5.0	0.75–5
Cabergoline	D2	+	+	65	2–6	2–4
Dihydroergocriptine**	D2 (± D1)	+	+	12–16	60–80	40
Apomorphine**	D2/D1	−	−	0.5	−	1.5–6 (s.c. bolus)
Piribedil**	D2	+	−	20	150–250	150–250
Pramipexole	D2	±	−	10	0.375–4.5	0.375–4.5
Ropinirole	D2	−	−	6	6–18	6–12

*Within the D2 family, all agonists have a D3/D2 affinity ratio of >1, except for lisuride, bromocriptine, and dihydroergocryptine.

**NA, Not available in the US; 5-HT, 5-hydroxytryptamine (serotonin).

L-dopa-treated patients demonstrated symptomatic efficacy of rasagiline,[101] and further randomized controlled trials in both de novo patients and patients with motor fluctuations have just been completed.

DOPAMINE AGONISTS

Clinical Pharmacology

Dopamine agonists act directly on postsynaptic dopamine receptors, thereby bypassing the need for metabolic conversion, storage and release in degenerating nigrostriatal nerve terminals as required for the action of L-dopa. Furthermore, dopamine agonists decrease endogenous dopamine turnover, which is even enhanced by L-dopa and may be one source of potentially neurotoxic free radical formation through auto-oxidation of accumulating dopamine. In addition, while they all act on D2-like dopamine receptors, dopamine agonists have selective subspecificities within the D2 family, offering the potential of specific clinical profiles and reduced risks for adverse reactions associated with specific types of receptor stimulation. Finally, a number of in vitro and in vivo studies have produced findings suggestive of potential neuroprotective effects of dopamine agonists related to antioxidative, radical scavenging, and antiapoptotic properties.[102,103]

Despite these considerable theoretical advantages of dopamine agonists over L-dopa, they have so far failed to parallel L-dopa's clinical efficacy or tolerability. When introduced clinically in the 1970s, dopamine agonists were primarily used as add-on treatment to patients with a failing L-dopa response. The current debate on their clinical role, however, is focused on early treatment, alone or combined with L-dopa, in de novo patients. Currently used dopamine agonists include the ergot derivatives bromocriptine, cabergoline, dihydroergocriptine, lisuride and pergolide, as well as nonergot compounds such as apomorphine, piribedil,

pramipexole, and ropinirole. Their clinical pharmacology is summarized in Table 15-6.

Bromocriptine mesylate is a tetracyclic ergoline derivative and was the first dopamine agonist to be marketed for the treatment of PD. Bromocriptine is not completely absorbed via the oral route and is extensively metabolized in the liver. Absolute oral bioavailability is less than 10 percent, maximum plasma levels are reached within 1–2 hours, and plasma half-life is 6–8 hours.[104]

It acts as a D2 agonist with a D1 antagonist activity in nanomolar concentrations, and as a partial D1 agonist in micromolar concentrations.[105]

Like most ergot compounds, bromocriptine also has 5-HT$_2$ receptor antagonistic efficacy, and some adrenergic, efficacy.

The clinical efficacy of bromocriptine as add-on treatment to L-dopa was shown in the 1970s.[106] When added to L-dopa, bromocriptine can reduce "wearing-off" and "on-off" phenomena in patients with fluctuating PD,[107,108] at the same time decreasing L-dopa dose requirements by about 10 percent,[109] which may in turn reduce pre-existing L-dopa-induced dyskinesias. Later, placebo-controlled studies confirmed the efficacy of bromocriptine monotherapy in de novo patients with PD,[110] and L-dopa-controlled trials of early bromocriptine monotherapy in PD consistently found lower incidences of long-term motor complications compared to L-dopa.[111–113] Some of these studies have also found that the overall antiparkinsonian efficacy of bromocriptine monotherapy is less than that of L-dopa, and overall tolerability is also inferior to L-dopa. One study[112] found that only about 30 percent of patients can be satisfactorily controlled by bromocriptine monotherapy for more than 3 years, and virtually all patients eventually require L-dopa by 10 years.[114] The optimal dose of bromocriptine has been a matter of controversy. Some authors have proposed daily doses as low as 7.5–12.5 mg added to L-dopa. The vast majority of clinical trials, however, have come up with considerably higher doses, and the current consensus is that the bromocriptine dose required for effective monotherapy lies between 20 and 40 mg/day,[109] while slightly smaller doses may suffice when given as adjunct to L-dopa.

Dihydroergocriptine is a dihydro derivative of ergocriptine, with a similar pharmacological profile to that of bromocriptine. It is marketed in several European countries but is not available in the US. Efficacy has been established in placebo-controlled studies in de novo patients as well as an adjunct to L-dopa in stable responders;[115,116] there are limited trial data on its use to control motor complications. Therapeutic doses reported in clinical trials range between 30 and 60 mg/day.

Cabergoline is another orally active synthetic tetracyclic ergoline derivative with selective D2 receptor agonist properties, but with no significant affinity for D1 receptors. Its nondopaminergic receptor profile (noradrenergic agonist, serotonergic antagonist) is similar to other ergot dopamine agonists such as bromocriptine. A unique characteristic of cabergoline is its very long elimination half-life of approximately 65 hours, with an associated long duration of clinical effect.[117,118] A single 1-mg oral dose of cabergoline has been shown to suppress prolactin levels for up to 21 days.[119] The pharmacokinetic profile of cabergoline therefore allows for once-daily dosing regimens.[120]

Add-on treatment with cabergoline in patients experiencing motor fluctuations with L-dopa therapy reduces off-time and increases on-time.[121,122] Early monotherapy with cabergoline is superior to L-dopa in delaying the onset of motor complications (fluctuations and dyskinesias) based on one large randomized prospective controlled trial with a follow-up between 3 and 5 years.[123,124]

In most studies, cabergoline was used at daily doses in the range 2–5 mg/day. When given as adjunct to L-dopa to treat motor fluctuations, it is frequently necessary to employ a twice-daily dosing schedule despite the very long half-life of cabergoline.

Lisuride is a semisynthetic alpha-aminoergoline with D2 dopaminergic activity and no apparent D1 receptor agonism. Lisuride has a relatively short half-life of about 2 hours and its absolute oral bioavailability is low due to extensive first-pass metabolism. As with most other ergot agonists, lisuride has also 5-HT$_2$ receptor activity.

Lisuride is effective when given as initial monotherapy in early PD, but symptomatic efficacy is less than seen with L-dopa.[125] One 4-year prospective study in de novo patients has suggested that either lisuride monotherapy or early combined treatment with L-dopa and lisuride will result in significantly fewer motor complications at 4 years compared to L-dopa alone.

When given as adjunct treatment to L-dopa in patients with motor fluctuations, lisuride may reduce motor fluctuations; this effect has been reported to be similar to that seen with bromocriptine.[126]

Unlike the other available ergot dopamine agonists, lisuride is readily water-soluble, which make it a suitable candidate for parenteral administration. Continuous subcutaneous infusions of lisuride via portable minipumps were introduced in the late 1980s by Vaamonde et al. for PD patients with refractory response oscillations, but this approach is associated with an unacceptable incidence of drug-induced psychosis in the long term.[127] Some authors have reported evidence for pharmacodynamic dopamine receptor changes with increases of dyskinetic thresholds following subcutaneous lisuride infusions in patients with late L-dopa failure, arguing for continuous dopaminergic stimulation as the optimal treatment modality in PD.[128] A recent prospective randomized clinical trial comparing standard oral L-dopa-based therapy with subcutaneous lisuride infusions in patients with advanced disease and motor complications has found significantly reduced dyskinesia scores with subcutaneous lisuride infusions.[129]

Pergolide mesylate is a semisynthetic ergot derivative that acts at both D2 and D1 receptors. Pergolide reaches plasma peak concentrations in 1–3 hours; a single dose is completely cleared within 7 days, with a half-life of 15–42 hours.[130] Molecular biological studies have shown that pergolide also has a high affinity for the D3 receptor.[131] Studies using catecholamine synthesis inhibitors have shown that the dopaminergic action of pergolide is much less dependent on intact dopamine stores than that of bromocriptine, and this difference may be related to the mixed D1/D2 agonistic properties of pergolide.[132]

Pergolide has been in general clinical use since 1989; numerous studies in patients with fluctuating PD have shown that it can reduce motor fluctuations by at least 30 percent and that concomitant L-dopa dose requirements go down by more than 25 percent.[133,134] Studies comparing pergolide and bromocriptine as add-on drugs in L-dopa-treated patients with response oscillations and dyskinesias have revealed slight advantages for pergolide in terms of both efficacy and tolerability.[109,135,136]

More recently, efficacy of pergolide monotherapy in de novo patients with PD has been demonstrated in one large randomized double-blind placebo-controlled study at a mean daily dose of 2 mg/day of pergolide; highly significantly more patients experienced 30 percent or greater improvement on the Unified Parkinson's Disease Rating Scale (UPDRS) motor score compared to placebo.[137] A 3-year double-blind prospective L-dopa controlled study of pergolide in de novo patients assessed the relative incidence of motor complications with either treatment as primary endpoint. Results have only been presented in abstract form and show significantly reduced frequencies of motor fluctuations and dyskinesias with pergolide monotherapy compared to L-dopa. Symptomatic efficacy as judged by the UPDRS motor score, however, was also significantly less with pergolide at a mean dose of slightly more than 3 mg/day (compared to 500 mg/day of L-dopa).[31]

Apomorphine was first described in the early 1950s by Schwab as an antiparkinsonian agent, reversing all cardinal features of PD,[138] followed by observations on its antitremor effect by Struppler and von Uexküll.[139] Lack of knowledge about the underlying mechanism of action, the need for parenteral application, and reports of reversible azotemia with high-dose oral apomorphine[140] initially prevented the further pursuit of apomorphine as an antiparkinsonian drug.

Apomorphine is now known to be a potent mixed D1- and D2-type dopamine receptor agonist with powerful antiparkinsonian effects. It has poor bioavailability when administered orally due to extensive first-pass metabolism. It is readily absorbed via sublingual, intranasal, or rectal routes. With subcutaneous or intravenous injections it has a half-life of about 30 minutes,[141] corresponding to a 45–60-minute duration of clinical effect. Following a subcutaneous bolus injection, maximal plasma concentrations are reached in about 8 minutes, and clinical effects have a latency of 10–20 minutes. Latencies are longer for the various transmucosal routes.[142–146]

Apomorphine is currently marketed in several European countries for subcutaneous therapy of L-dopa-treated patients with motor fluctuations. A number of open-label studies have consistently found reliable reversal of the off-period with intermittent subcutaneous apomorphine injections, and marked reductions in daily off-time with continuous subcutaneous apomorphine infusions.[55,147–149] Intermittent subcutaneous apomorphine injections are able to reverse off-periods within 10–15 minutes ("rescue injections") at single doses between 2 mg and 7 mg. These effects have recently been confirmed in a double-blind placebo-controlled trial.[150] Special pen injection systems for subcutaneous apomorphine self-administration are currently marketed in several European countries.

Several groups have advocated the use of continuous subcutaneous apomorphine infusions via portable minipumps in patients suffering from complex unpredictable on-off oscillations refractory to conventional oral treatment.[149] Continuous subcutaneous apomorphine monotherapy may be associated with marked downregulation of pre-existing L-dopa-induced dyskinesias.[151,152]

Piribedil is a non-ergot, mixed D2/D3 agonist with some alpha2-antagonistic effects.[153] After oral administration, t_{max} is reached within 1 hour. Piribedil has a long half-life of about 20 hours.

Although there are no randomized controlled trials available regarding efficacy of piribedil given as monotherapy or adjunct to L-dopa in patients with PD, the drug is currently marketed as an antiparkinsonian agent in several European countries.

Pramipexole is a benzothiazole derivative with full agonism at the D2 receptor family with preferential affinity for the D3 receptor subtype.[154,155] Pramipexole has no D1 affinity and very low affinity for nondopamine receptors. Pramipexole has been shown to improve parkinsonism in the 6-hydroxydopamine rat model, as well as in MPTP-treated primates.[156] Pramipexole is completely absorbed after oral administration with a bioavailability of more than 90 percent. Maximal plasma concentration (t_{max}) is reached within 1–3 hours, and the half-life is 9–12 hours.[157]

Pramipexole monotherapy has been shown to be effective in the treatment of de novo patients with PD in double-blind placebo-controlled short-term trials.[158–160] Daily doses were between 1.5 and 6 mg, but a dose-range trial found no evidence for significant further improvement in total UPDRS scores beyond daily doses of 1.5 mg compared to placebo.[159] Mean effective doses in the largest placebo-controlled de novo study of pramipexole were 3.8 mg/day.[160] An L-dopa controlled randomized double-blind prospective trial found somewhat inferior symptomatic efficacy, as assessed by UPDRS motor scores, of pramipexole compared to L-dopa in de novo PD patients.[32] Early monotherapy with pramipexole, however, was associated with a significantly reduced risk of motor complications both at 2 and at 4 years compared to L-dopa.[32,33] This effect was particularly significant for drug-induced dyskinesias.

Recently, results of a beta-CIT-SPECT progression substudy to the pramipexole versus L-dopa monotherapy 4-year study have become available.[33] Eighty-one patients were randomized to either pramipexole or L-dopa monotherapy, and sequential beta-CIT-SPECT scans were used to monitor progression of dopamine transporter dysfunction over a 4-year follow-up period. Similar to the main study, these patients were given supplementary open-label L-dopa as clinically required. Beta-CIT-SPECT results at 22, 34, and 46 months showed significantly reduced declines in striatal beta-CIT findings in the pramipexole- versus L-dopa-treated patients. The exact interpretation of these results is difficult due to the lack of a placebo arm. Also, there were no clinical differences in UPDRS off-scores at 3 and 4 years between the two patient groups.

Four randomized double-blind placebo-controlled studies have also shown efficacy of pramipexole as adjunct to L-dopa in patients with motor fluctuations.[161–164] One further placebo-controlled randomized double-blind trial has been conducted specifically in patients with insufficient control of tremor using a variety of premedications. Adjunct treatment with pramipexole was superior to placebo in reducing tremor in this cohort.[165]

Adjunct therapy with pramipexole in patients with motor fluctuations is associated with significant reductions in daily "off-time,"[161–164] and daily L-dopa can be reduced by up to 27 percent.[161]

Ropinirole is a selective nonergoline dopamine agonist at D2-like receptors, with greatest affinity for the D3 subtype but no significant D1 activity. There is also no interaction with nondopamine receptors.[166,167] Ropinirole is rapidly absorbed at slightly more than 1 hour after oral administration; its bioavailability is around 15 percent and its half-life around 6 hours.

Ropinirole monotherapy is effective in improving symptomatic control in de novo patients with early PD as assessed in randomized double-blind placebo-controlled trials.[168,169] One trial found a trend towards greater improvement with ropinirole compared to bromocriptine monotherapy,[170] but efficacy is less than that seen with L-dopa.[171] Effective doses for ropinirole monotherapy in early PD are generally above 9 mg/day, and between 12 and 16 mg/day after 2–5 years of therapy.[172,173]

A 5-year L-dopa controlled double-blind randomized prospective trial in de novo patients demonstrated significantly reduced incidences of drug-induced dyskinesias with ropinirole monotherapy compared to L-dopa. Even after open-label L-dopa supplementation to initial ropinirole monotherapy, the reduction of dyskinesia incidence remained significant compared with L-dopa.[29]

A 2-year randomized double-blind prospective trial of ropinirole versus L-dopa used ^{18}F-dopa PET scanning as a surrogate marker to assess differential rates of progression of nigrostriatal dysfunction with either type of treatment in 186 de novo patients not previously exposed to any dopaminergic therapy.[173] Ropinirole-treated patients had a significantly reduced rate of decline of putaminal ^{18}F-dopa uptake compared to L-dopa-treated patients, with a relative difference in favor of ropinirole of around 40 percent. Similarly to the pramipexole versus L-dopa beta-CIT-SPECT study, these results are difficult to interpret in the absence of a placebo control and without a clear clinical correlate.

Adjunct therapy with ropinirole to L-dopa in patients with motor fluctuations reduces daily off-time.[174,175]

Current Indications

Dopamine agonists are first-line therapeutic agents in both early and advanced PD, where they are commonly used as initial monotherapy or adjunct to L-dopa, respectively. In spite of their different pharmacological profiles, there seem to be only minor differences between the various ergot and nonergot compounds regarding efficacy and safety. The robustness of evidence from high-quality controlled clinical trials supporting their use, however, varies between different agents of this class.[55,176]

There is growing consensus that dopamine replacement therapy in early PD should generally be initiated with a dopamine agonist.[177] Bromocriptine, dihydroergocriptine, pergolide, pramipexole, and ropinirole have all been shown to be effective in placebo-controlled double-blind trials, while lisuride and cabergoline have only been compared to L-dopa as initial monotherapy in de novo PD patients. All dopamine agonists that have been tested in randomized controlled studies versus L-dopa (bromocriptine, cabergoline, lisuride, pergolide, pramipexole, ropinirole) have been somewhat less effective based on motor scores of different rating scales (most often UPDRS). Because of this difference in symptomatic efficacy, most patients started on dopamine agonist monotherapy will eventually require adjunct L-dopa. In recent L-dopa controlled clinical trials, this proportion was close to 80 percent of the intent-to-treat population at 5 years,[29] and greater than 90 percent in the 10-year follow-up of the bromocriptine versus L-dopa comparative trial conducted by the UK Parkinson's Disease Research Group.[114]

Initial monotherapy with dopamine agonists is effective in delaying the onset of motor complications, in

particular drug-induced dyskinesias. This has been convincingly demonstrated for bromocriptine, cabergoline, pergolide, pramipexole, and ropinirole.[55] Doses of dopamine agonists required for sufficient symptomatic control in early monotherapy are summarized in Table 15-6.

There is experimental evidence for potential neuroprotective properties of dopamine agonists (see above), and two recent L-dopa controlled trials with pramipexole and ropinirole have used functional neuroimaging surrogate markers (beta-CIT-SPECT, ^{18}F-dopa PET) to assess differential effects of these agonists versus L-dopa on the rate of progression of nigrostriatal terminal dysfunction. Both trials have found similar reductions in the rate of decline of functional markers of nigrostriatal terminal activity in favor of the dopamine agonists.[33,173] These findings do not, however, provide clear evidence for neuroprotective properties since both trials lacked placebo controls and there was no clinical evidence of different effects on progression of motor impairment between the agonists and L-dopa.

Dopamine agonists can effectively be added to L-dopa to enhance symptomatic control, in patients without and with motor fluctuations. This has been convincingly shown in randomized controlled trials of bromocriptine, cabergoline, pergolide, and pramipexole, while there is less robust evidence for apomorphine, lisuride, or ropinirole. Doses required in this indication are generally similar to those required for initial monotherapy (see Table 15-6).

Apomorphine, bromocriptine, cabergoline, pergolide, pramipexole, and ropinirole have all been demonstrated to reduce motor fluctuations with an increase in on-time and reduction in off-time in L-dopa-treated patients with response oscillations,[55] while lisuride and dihydroergocriptine have been insufficiently tested in this regard. Adding dopamine agonists to L-dopa in patients with advanced disease and motor complications generally allows for L-dopa dose reductions, and this may help to reduce the duration and/or intensity of pre-existing L-dopa-induced dyskinesias.

Side-Effects

Currently available dopamine agonists share a wide range of side-effects with L-dopa, due to peripheral and central dopaminergic stimulation. Nausea and vomiting, postural hypotension, dizziness, bradycardia, and other signs of autonomic peripheral stimulation are common peripheral dopaminergic side-effects of all dopamine agonists. In a small number of patients, the first dopamine agonist dose can induce severe hypotensive reactions, so that small starting doses and slow titration schemes are recommended. Outside of the US coadministration of the peripheral dopamine receptor blocker domperidone can be used to counteract these peripherally induced dopaminergic side-effects if necessary. Both ergot and nonergot dopamine agonists have been reported to induce leg edema.[178]

In patients with L-dopa-induced dyskinesias, adjunct therapy with dopamine agonists can exacerbate these motor complications, but these can be counteracted by reducing the dose of L-dopa. In individual patients with disabling L-dopa-induced dyskinesias, switching to high-dose oral dopamine agonist monotherapy may significantly reduce pre-existing dyskinesias.[179] Dopamine agonists appear to have a slightly greater potential than L-dopa to induce central side-effects such as sedation, confusional states, and hallucinosis or paranoid psychosis.[36] Elderly patients over 70, and those with concomitant cerebrovascular disease and cognitive decline or antecedent history of psychiatric complications, are at particular risk.

Some case reports suggested that nonergot dopamine agonists such as pramipexole and ropinirole may induce sleep attacks without warning,[180,181] raising the question of safety of these medications for patients who drive. Subsequent reports described similar side-effects of excessive daytime sleepiness, including sleep episodes at the wheel caused by ergot dopamine agonists, including bromocriptine, pergolide, cabergoline,[182–185] and also by L-dopa monotherapy.[37,186] Daytime sedation, therefore, must be regarded as a side-effect common to all dopaminergic agents, and patients must be warned of this in particular with respect to driving. Ergot-derivative dopamine agonists have been associated with the occurrence of pleuropulmonary and/or peritoneal fibrosis.[187–192] So far, this has not been reported with nonergot agonists such as pramipexole and ropinirole.

Subcutaneous injections frequently cause red itching nodules at injection sites; these are usually well tolerated and transient. Problems of local tolerability with large areas of inflammation or subcutaneous abscesses or necrosis have been recorded, and are often related to noncompliance with hygiene rules for needle use.[152,193] Sexual dysfunction (i.e., frequent erections, and hypersexuality) have also been reported with subcutaneous apomorphine. Apomorphine-induced autoimmune hemolytic anemia is a rare complication, requiring monthly blood counts in patients on continuous subcutaneous infusions.[194]

NONDOPAMINERGIC AGENTS

ANTICHOLINERGICS

Basic Pharmacology and Mechanisms of Action

The interaction of dopaminergic and acetycholine-containing neurons in the striatum has been extensively documented. For example, D2 receptor stimulation inhibits the release of acetylcholine in the striatum,[195,196] whereas D1 receptor stimulation has the opposite effect.[197] In animal experiments, cholinergic muscarinic agonists have been shown to block dopamine reuptake into presynaptic dopaminergic terminals,[198] and also to influence the regulation of striatal neuropeptide expression.[199]

The effect of striatal dopamine deficiency in human PD on these various aspects of dopaminergic/cholinergic interaction are not entirely clear, but it is commonly assumed that there is a relative cholinergic muscarinic overactivity.[200] From the first empirical use of the anticholinergic drug hyoscine in PD by Charcot in the 19th century, it took more

TABLE 15-7 Commonly Available Anticholinergic Drugs

Substance	Recommended Daily Dose
Benzatropine mesylate	3–6 mg
Biperiden HCl/lactate	4–8 mg
Trihexiphenidyl HCl	4–8 mg
Orphenadrine HCl	150–300 mg
Procyclidine HCl	10–15 mg

than 60 years to develop the first synthetic anticholinergic drugs; and Table 15-7 summarizes the most commonly available compounds of this class.

Current Indications

Symptomatic efficacy of the various anticholinergic agents is less than that observed with L-dopa or other dopaminergic compounds, although high-quality comparative trials of anticholinergic monotherapy in de novo patients are lacking.[55] This, and the potential to induce mental side-effects, has largely restricted their use in current clinical practice. Anticholinergics should not be given to patients with cognitive decline or to elderly patients over 65 years of age.[201] Overall, clinical studies suggest that anticholinergic drugs improve rigidity and tremor with little effect on akinesia.[55] Occasionally, anticholinergic monotherapy can be employed in de novo patients when symptoms are still mild and tremor is the predominant complaint.

Side-Effects

Due to their peripheral antimuscarinic action, anticholinergics are contraindicated in narrow-angle glaucoma, tachycardia, prostate hypertrophy, gastrointestinal obstruction, and megacolon. They may cause blurred vision, urinary retention, nausea, and constipation, rarely paralytic ileus. Reduced sweating may interfere with temperature regulation, and central anticholinergic activity may interfere with mental function. Particularly in the elderly, anticholinergics may induce acute confusion and hallucinations. The use of anticholinergics is contraindicated in patients with cognitive decline and dementia. There are some reports suggesting that anticholinergic treatment may induce or exacerbate dyskinesias.

The abrupt withdrawal of anticholinergic drugs may induce marked worsening of parkinsonism, so these agents should be discontinued gradually.

GLUTAMATE ANTAGONISTS

Basic Pharmacology and Mechanisms of Action

According to current models of basal ganglia function, increased glutamatergic neurotransmission contributes to parkinsonian motor dysfunction at multiple levels. Increased glutamatergic drive from the subthalamic nucleus to the internal pallidum contributes to increased inhibitory pallidal input to the motor thalamus and is therefore involved in the pathophysiology of akinesia.[202] Pharmacodynamic changes of striatal *N*-methyl-D-aspartate (NMDA) receptors may be involved in the development of L-dopa-induced dyskinesias.[203] Consistent with these concepts, NMDA receptor antagonists such as MK-801, 3-[(±)-2-carboxypiperazin-4-yl]-propyl-1-phosphonate and ramacemide, can potentiate the ability of L-dopa to reverse akinesia in monoamine-depleted rats.[204,205] Non-NMDA antagonists, such as 2,3-dihydroxy-6-nitro-7-sulfamoyl-benzo-(*f*)quinoxaline, have also been reported to improve parkinsonian symptoms and to potentiate the effect of L-dopa in animal models of parkinsonism.[206] It has also been shown that specific stimulation of either NMDA or non-NMDA glutamate receptors by stereotactic injection in different subcortical targets induces parkinsonian features in rodents in a regionally specific manner.[207] The application of glutamate antagonists in PD may therefore require both receptor specificity plus regional selectivity. In addition to these experimental symptomatic antiparkinsonian effects, glutamate antagonists also have a neuroprotective potential, via blockade of excitatory amino acid receptors, which can mediate excitotoxic neuronal cell death.[208]

Amantadine's antiparkinsonian efficacy was first reported in 1969 by Schwab et al.[209] Its exact mechanism of action remains uncertain. Amantadine has been shown to enhance the release of catecholamines from intact dopaminergic terminals,[210] and also to inhibit catecholamine reuptake; other studies have suggested effects on dopamine receptors as well as anticholinergic activity.[211,212] More recently, amantadine has been shown to block NMDA glutamate receptors.[213,214]

Amantadine hydrochloride produces peak plasma levels 1–4 hours after an oral dose, with a clinical duration of action of up to 8 hours. In most countries, the drug is available as amantadine hydrochloride, 100-mg capsules or coated tablets; in some countries, it is also available as a liquid formulation of 50 mg/mL as well as in a parenteral form for infusions (200 mg/500 mL). The recommended daily oral dose is 200–400 mg.

Current Indications

Oral treatment with amantadine 200–300 mg/day has consistently been shown to produce mild-to-moderate antiparkinsonian effects both as monotherapy or as adjunct to L-dopa.[55] Some studies have suggested that these effects may be short-lived, but others have found continuous benefit over more than 1 year.[215] While virtually all trials studying symptomatic efficacy of amantadine were formed in the 1970s and generally did not meet modern standards of trial methodology, recent PD trials assessing the antidyskinetic potential of amantadine have been high-quality placebo-controlled studies.[216–219] These trials have consistently shown adjunct treatment with oral amantadine at 300–400 mg/day to significantly reduce the intensity of pre-existing L-dopa-induced dyskinesias. Such benefit may be maintained for at least 12 months.[217]

Side-Effects

Amantadine is generally well tolerated. It should be used with caution in patients with azotemia because of its largely renal elimination. The same applies to patients with cognitive dysfunction in whom amantadine may induce confusional states or hallucinosis. Occasionally, amantadine may cause ankle edema and livedo reticularis, for which the underlying mechanism is unclear. Occasional urinary retention and constipation have been related to anticholinergic properties of the drug.

Practical Treatment Decisions in PD

Beyond the presenting motor symptoms, treatment of PD has to take into account a number of additional issues, including age of the patient, employment status, associated nonmotor symptoms, and concomitant nonparkinsonian morbidity. Since treatment options include pharmacological as well as nonpharmacological interventions, treatment decisions in PD are usually highly individualized and can be complex.

The best way to guide clinicians through practical pharmacological treatment decisions is by referral to controlled clinical trials assessing the potential benefit and risk of candidate drugs for the various clinical indications. Unfortunately, the available evidence from clinical trials in PD is insufficient to draw conclusions about effectiveness and clinical usefulness of every type of intervention for every indication.[55] Nevertheless, some generally accepted principles for rational pharmacotherapy of PD at certain clinically relevant stages have emerged; these are summarized below (see Table 15-8).

EARLY MONOTHERAPY

Although medical and psychosocial counseling, together with group support and physiotherapy, may for a limited time in a limited number of patients be sufficient as treatment of early PD, there is generally no advantage in withholding effective pharmacotherapy from an PD patient with subjectively or objectively disabling motor symptoms. The optimal time at which to start effective symptomatic pharmacotherapy, however, not only depends on objective parameters in terms of severity of motor symptoms, but also has to take into account the individual patient's psychological and socioeconomic status. Interference with performance at work is usually a powerful argument for starting rigorous antiparkinsonian drug therapy.

Symptomatic control of motor symptoms is not the only goal when deciding on which strategy to use as initial monotherapy. Prevention of motor complications and potential modification of disease progression are additional important considerations.

NEUROPROTECTION

Neuroprotective intervention in PD has been defined as treatment that will significantly and in a clinically meaningful

TABLE 15-8 Drug Approaches to Early Monotherapy in IPD

	Clinical Indication			
	Neuroprotection*	Symptomatic Efficacy**	Prevention of Motor Complications	Safety Restrictions***
Nondopaminergic				
Anticholinergics	–	+/++ (rigidity, tremor)	–	Avoid in the elderly and in patients with cognitive impairment
Amantadine	–	+/++	–	Avoid in patients with cognitive impairment
Dopaminergic				
L-Dopa	–	+++	–	Enhanced risk of motor complications in young-onset PD
Dopamine agonists	±	++/+++	+	Increased risk of hallucinosis versus L-dopa (caution in patients with cognitive impairment) Monitor daytime somnolence and sudden onset of sleep (caution with driving)
MAO-B inhibitors	±	+	–	Small risk of serotonin syndrome in combination with SSRIs

*Neuroprotection/prevention of motor complications: –, no evidence; ±, equivocal evidence; +, unequivocal positive evidence.
**Symptomatic efficacy: +, mild; ++, moderate; +++, marked.
***For detailed description of side-effects see text.

way modify the underlying neuronal degeneration and thereby forestall the onset of clinical disability or slow its progression.[220] One of the major problems of potentially neuroprotective drugs in PD has been the confounding symptomatic effect of many candidate agents, as well as the difficulty of defining appropriate endpoints.[176] Surrogate markers of functional imaging of nigrostriatal dopaminergic terminal function, as employed in recent trials of dopamine agonists versus L-dopa, are a promising approach, but will not obviate the need for meaningful clinical endpoints. A number of interventions have been tested in clinical neuroprotection studies of PD.

Monotherapy trials of deprenyl (Selegiline), while consistently showing a delayed need for L-dopa versus placebo, have remained inconclusive due to symptomatic efficacy of deprenyl. Comparative trials of dopamine agonists such as pramipexole and ropinirole vs. L-dopa using beta-CIT-SPECT[33] or ^{18}F-dopa PET[173] as surrogate markers to assess progression of nigrostriatal terminal function loss have shown significant differences in favor of either agonist, but results have again remained inconclusive due to the lack of a placebo arm, lack of clinical correlates, and unresolved questions related to mechanisms underlying differential effects on imaging markers between L-dopa and dopamine agonists.[221]

A recent trial of coenzyme Q has suggested possible reductions in the rate of progression of UPDRS scores in patients receiving 1200 mg/day of coenzyme Q in the absence of any known symptomatic efficacy of this agent. Again, numbers are too small and trial duration is too short to allow definitive conclusions.[222]

At present, none of the available agents to treat PD has been proven to exert clinically meaningful disease-modifying effects in terms of neuroprotection, and whether or not to start patients on any of them once clinically diagnosed is a matter of the physician's belief and the patient's perception.

SYMPTOMATIC CONTROL OF MOTOR SYMPTOMS

Virtually all nondopaminergic and dopaminergic agents currently marketed for the treatment of PD have some degree of symptomatic efficacy, and are potential candidates for early monotherapy to control motor symptoms. Major differences exist regarding their potency, safety profiles, costs, and the body of evidence supporting their clinical use (see Table 15-8).

Nondopaminergic Drugs

There is a paucity of controlled clinical trials assessing amantadine monotherapy of PD, but it appears to affect all cardinal symptoms in at least two-thirds of patients.[55] The clinical benefit from amantadine is often transient with about a third of patients showing slight to moderate loss of improvement within the first months of treatment, but some studies have reported sustained benefit for more than a year.[215] Amantadine is therefore best used as short-term monotherapy in early PD with mild functional impairment. Doses of 100 to 300 mg per day, given in two or three divided doses, are usually well tolerated.

Age and cognitive status are important factors for deciding for or against anticholinergic monotherapy in early PD. Generally patients about 60 years of age or those exhibiting clinical signs of cognitive impairment should be excluded from anticholinergic therapy. Since anticholinergic drugs mainly influence tremor and rigidity without much effect on akinesia, tremor-dominant patients with mild to moderate functional impairment are the best candidates for this type of treatment. Clinically there is little difference between the various available anticholinergic agents but trihexyphenidyl and benztropine are the two most widely used candidates worldwide.

Dopaminergic Agents

L-Dopa continues to be the single most effective and best tolerated drug for the treatment of PD. An excellent response to oral L-dopa with motor improvement exceeding 70 percent is one of the diagnostic criteria differentiating PD from other parkinsonian disorders.[223] However, exposure to oral L-dopa will lead to motor complications in 30–40 percent of patients already after 2 years of treatment.[32] This number further increases year by year so that, after 6 or more years of treatment, up to 80 per cent of patients will develop fluctuations in motor response and L-dopa-induced dyskinesias.[114,224]

Patients under the age of 50 are particularly likely to develop disabling motor complications after a few years of L-dopa treatment,[28] so strategies delaying L-dopa exposure are particularly important in this group of patients.

The incidence of motor response oscillations and dyskinesias is correlated with dose and duration of L-dopa therapy,[27,224] so most clinicians will try to obtain sufficient symptomatic relief with the lowest dose of L-dopa possible. For many de novo patients, this means treatment with daily doses of between 300 and 500 mg of L-dopa, plus carbidopa or benserazide. Initiating treatment with sustained-release instead of standard L-dopa does not confer additional benefit regarding prevention of motor complications.[38,59] Starting L-dopa therapy in combination with COMT inhibitors may enhance symptomatic control and reduce dose requirements,[82] but there are no data from controlled trials in de novo patients, and it is unknown if combined L-dopa plus dopa decarboxylase inhibitor, plus COMT inhibitor ("triple combination") will prevent motor complications.

There have been concerns that L-dopa via its oxidative metabolism might further induce oxidative stress in nigral neurons, thereby enhancing neuronal cell death and ultimately progression of PD.[225] However, evidence from in vitro and in vivo studies of potential L-dopa toxicity has been conflicting, showing both neurotoxicity and neuroprotection.[226] Likewise, after more than 30 years of extensive use in PD, there is no clinical indication of deleterious effects of L-dopa treatment on the progression of PD. A recent placebo-controlled 9-month trial of early L-dopa monotherapy, on the other hand, has found sustained beneficial effects on symptomatic scores, even after washout for 2 weeks.[227]

All available dopamine agonists, with the exception of apomorphine, have been shown to improve motor symptoms in early PD. Based on data from L-dopa controlled monotherapy trials in de novo patients (see above), dopamine agonists as a class demonstrate reduced motor complications but are less potent than L-dopa. Differences in improvement of motor scores versus L-dopa that have been reported are in the order of 3–6 points of the UPDRS motor subsection.[31,32,36]

Given that there are no data on the minimal clinically relevant change for the UPDRS, there is ongoing controversy as to whether such differences are clinically meaningful. On the other hand, the majority of patients started on dopamine agonist monotherapy will eventually require add-on L-dopa for sufficient symptomatic control. There are almost no data from controlled trials to guide clinicians regarding potential differences in efficacy and safety between the various dopamine agonists when given as early monotherapy. The only available long-term double-blind prospective trial provides some evidence for slightly superior efficacy of ropinirole over bromocriptine without differences in side-effects.[170,172]

While overall safety is similar for L-dopa and dopamine agonists, specific side-effects are more commonly seen with dopamine agonists than with L-dopa, including hallucinosis and possibly daytime sleepiness.

MAO-B Inhibitors

Selegiline monotherapy is associated with mild but definitive symptomatic improvement of motor symptoms at a dose of 10 mg/day (5 mg twice daily). It is a well-tolerated drug and may be a monotherapy option for the short-term management of patients with mild disease.

PREVENTION OF MOTOR COMPLICATIONS

Dopamine agonists are the only class of antiparkinsonian agents with proven efficacy regarding prevention of motor complications. This has been demonstrated in L-dopa controlled trials for bromocriptine over 5 years,[113] for cabergoline over 3–5 years,[124] pergolide over 3 years,[31] ropinirole over 5 years,[29] and pramipexole over 4 years.[32,33] Even after the addition of L-dopa when eventually required, there is a statistically significant reduction of drug-induced dyskinesias over L-dopa monotherapy. Controlled-release L-dopa is not effective in reducing the rate of long-term motor complications,[38,59] and the combination of L-dopa with COMT inhibitors has not been studied for this indication in PD patients.

TREATMENT OF ADVANCED PD

With advancing disease, pharmacotherapy of PD becomes increasingly more complex and difficult due to motor complications of prolonged L-dopa treatment, progressive gait and balance problems, increasing neuropsychiatric morbidity, and other nonmotor complications.

MANAGEMENT OF MOTOR FLUCTUATIONS

Management of L-dopa-related motor response oscillations is aimed at various aspects of the underlying pathophysiology, and includes measures to enhance absorption and transport of L-dopa, stabilizing L-dopa plasma levels via changes of drug delivery and L-dopa pharmakokinetics, and also through non-L-dopa-related strategies of continuous

TABLE 15-9 Pharmacological Management of Motor Fluctuations

1. Improve L-dopa absorption and transport
   Avoid dosing with protein-rich food
   Enhance gastric motility (avoid anticholinergics or dosing with meals)
   Soluble L-dopa preparations (Madopar dispersible*; L-dopa ethyl ester**)
   Duodenal L-dopa infusions**

2. Stabilize L-dopa plasma levels
   Increase dosing frequency
   Introduce sustained-release formulations
   Add COMT inhibitors

3. Introduce subcutaneous apomorphine "rescue" injections*

4. Provide prolonged striatal dopaminergic stimulation
   Add MAO-B inhibitors
   Add orally active dopamine agonists
   Introduce subcutaneous apomorphine infusions
   Use transdermal dopamine agonist delivery (Rotigotine**)

*Not available in the US.
**Experimental.

dopaminergic receptor stimulation (see Table 15-9). Which of the different options listed in Table 15-9 is used will depend on the type of drug regimen the patient is on when motor fluctuations begin, patient factors such as age and comorbidity, as well as ease of use and complexity of motor response swings.

Patients with beginning and mild wearing-off effects on a three or four times daily L-dopa regimen will profit from the addition of a COMT inhibitor such as entacapone with every L-dopa dose, with or without increases in L-dopa dosing frequency. Occasionally, the addition of L-dopa controlled release preparations may confer some additional benefit, particularly regarding nighttime disabilities. The addition of MAO-B inhibitors such as selegiline may also reduce wearing-off fluctuations to some extent.

Patients with motor fluctuations on L-dopa monotherapy will also benefit from the addition of one of the dopamine agonists, particularly those with longer half-lives of more than 6 hours, such as bromocriptine, pergolide, cabergoline, pramipexole, and ropinirole. All of these compounds have been shown to increase on-time in patients with motor fluctuations. Theoretically, drugs such as pergolide and cabergoline, with half-lives of more than 20 hours, should be superior to those with shorter pharmacokinetics, but control comparative trials showing such a difference are not available. Cabergoline, however, can be given as a once or twice daily dosing regimen while all the other agonists require dosing three times a day.

Intermittent subcutaneous apomorphine rescue injections or continuous subcutaneous infusions of apomorphine have been used in Europe to manage complex on-off swings that are refractory to oral treatment.

MANAGEMENT OF DRUG-INDUCED DYSKINESIAS

L-Dopa-induced dyskinesias most often consist of choreic movements involving the trunk and extremities at times of peak effect (on-period dyskinesia).[228] Some 30 percent of patients additionally suffer from painful dystonic cramps, particularly involving the foot and leg at times of wearing-off of L-dopa effects (off-period dystonia).[35] Still another variety of L-dopa-induced involuntary movements is linked to the phases of onset or waning of a motor response to an individual dose of L-dopa.[229,230] These biphasic dyskinesias also may contain prominent dystonic elements intermingled with jerky and ballastic limb movements (mobile dystonia as opposed to the fixed painful cramps in off-period dystonia) (see Table 15-5).

Adjunct therapy with oral amantadine 300–400 mg/day usually reduces pre-existing on-period dyskinesias by some 40–60 percent. Disabling interdose choreic dyskinesias usually require L-dopa dose reductions, which in turn may require the introduction or increase of a dopamine agonist to prevent motor worsening. Some patients become intolerant even to small L-dopa doses, so agonist monotherapy (usually high-dose) may be tried. Subcutaneous continuous apomorphine infusions with a discontinuation of all oral treatment have been reported to control dyskinesias in individual cases.[152] The addition of atypical neuroleptics such as olanzapine may also lessen dyskinesias, but at some cost regarding motor control.[231] Table 15-10 summarizes the most commonly used drug options to treat L-dopa-induced dyskinesias.

A number of experimental drug approaches have produced promising results in animal models or small clinical series, and include opioid agonists and antagonists, alpha2-adrenergic antagonists, and adenosine antagonists, but these agents are not available in clinical practice.[232]

Off-period dystonia usually responds to measures smoothing out motor fluctuations (see above). Nocturnal or early-morning painful off-period cramps can be treated by bedtime doses of a long-acting dopamine agonist, while controlled release L-dopa is less reliable in this indication.

Disabling dyskinesias can be refractory to drug therapy, and these patients are candidates for deep brain surgery (globus pallidus interna pallidotomy or subthalamic nucleus stimulation; see Chap. 17).

TABLE 15-10 Pharmacological Management of L-Dopa-Induced Dyskinesias

Add amantadine

Reduce L-dopa (increase dopamine agonists if required)

Switch to dopamine agonist monotherapy

Use continuous drug delivery (duodenal L-dopa, subcutaneous apomorphine)

MANAGEMENT OF NONMOTOR COMPLICATIONS
Management of Depression
Depression is a common nonmotor complication, affecting about 40–50 percent of PD patients.[233,234] It can occur before the onset of motor PD symptoms in up to 30 percent of cases,[235] and shows two peaks in prevalence over the various stages of PD, one early and one late.[236] Some authors have suggested that depression may be more frequent in younger patients and in the akinetic-rigid compared to tremor-dominant subtype of PD,[237] and to be a risk factor for more rapid progression of motor and cognitive decline.[238,239] Most studies, however, failed to demonstrate a correlation between depression and individual motor features (bradykinesia, rigidity, tremor) or severity or duration of the illness.[236,240] Depression in PD patients is usually mild-to-moderate, with low major depression and suicide rates despite higher frequency of suicide ideation,[241,242] and it is frequently associated with anxiety and panic attacks.

The pathophysiology of depression in PD is still a matter of debate, and there are many theories regarding the neurobiological substrate of this nonmotor PD complication, including dopaminergic degeneration of pontomesencephalic and forebrain structures projecting to cortical and subcortical areas related to the limbic system (mesocorticolimbic projections),[243,244] noradrenergic deficiency in the locus ceruleus,[245] and reduction of serotonergic neurons within the raphe nucleus.[246] It is possible that a multifactorial etiology including multiple neurotransmitter deficiencies and genetic influences may be involved.[240]

Medical and psychosocial counseling as well as good management of motor PD features through dopaminergic drugs (L-dopa and dopamine agonists), which also have antidepressant properties, may be of some help in some cases of depression in PD. However, since depression has been shown to have a major impact on quality of life, to be a risk factor for insomnia, and to worsen other PD symptoms and therapy compliance, antidepressants should be added to the treatment regimen, including selective serotonin reuptake inhibitors (SSRIs) and tricyclic antidepressants (TCAs). Both classes of antidepressant agents have been shown to be efficacious in the treatment of depression in PD patients, with improvement of parkinsonian motor symptoms once the depression is under control. Most studies, however, have not been well controlled or lack double-blinding.

SSRIs (paroxetine, sertraline, fluoxetine, citalopram, fluvoxamine) in the dose normally used for non-PD depressed patients are commonly prescribed in depressed PD patients. There is anecdotal evidence that SSRIs may worsen parkinsonian motor features—in particular tremor—in individual patients, but this is a very rare cause for discontinuation.[247,248] Some caution should be taken in the case of concomitant therapy with selegiline since a "serotonin syndrome" (delusions, confusion, hypomania stupor, myoclonus, sweating, tremor, diarrhea, shivering, fever) may rarely occur.[249]

Since tricyclic antidepressants (TCAs) have a higher incidence of side-effects, mostly due to their anticholinergic and antiadrenergic properties, they should be avoided in elderly patients and in those with cognitive impairment. In some cases, particularly with high doses, they can worsen drug-induced psychiatric side-effects of dopaminergic stimulation and motor fluctuations by slowing the gastrointestinal absorption of L-dopa. In limited PD patients, TCAs can be of some benefit in sleep disorders due to their sedative effect, and may have some benefit on tremor.

Other antidepressant drugs may be tried, including MAO-A (moclobenide) and MAO-B inhibitors (selegiline), mixed serotonin and nonadrenaline reuptake inhibitors (venlafaxine), pure nonadrenaline reuptake inhibitors (reboxetine), or the presynaptic alpha2-antagonist mirtazapine. For all these drugs, as well as for the SSRIs and TCAs, there are no adequate prospective double-blind placebo-controlled studies specifically assessing their efficacy and safety in depression in PD patients.[55]

Management of Cognitive Dysfunction
Between 20 and 40 percent of patients with PD will develop cognitive decline, leading on to dementia, in the course of their illness.[250–253] While dementia is very rare in patients with young-onset disease,[254] it has been found in up to 70 percent of patients aged above 80 years.[252] Onset of dementia within the first year of motor presentation of parkinsonism is regarded as an exclusion criterion for a diagnosis of PD,[255] and a defining feature of dementia with Lewy bodies (DLB).[256]

Cholinergic deficiency is regarded as the hallmark neurochemical finding underlying cognitive decline in dementia of PD cell loss in the cholinergic nucleus basalis of Meynert, and the degree of cortical cholinergic denervation has been shown to correlate with cognitive dysfunction in PD.[257,258] The pharmacological management of dementia in PD should therefore always include discontinuation of potential aggravators of central cholinergic dysfunctions, such as anticholinergic drugs, amantadine, and TCAs (see Table 15-11). Cholinesterase inhibitors were first shown to improve cognitive dysfunction and particularly behavioral symptoms in a double-blind placebo-controlled prospective study of rivastigmine (6–12 mg/day) in patients with DLB.[259] Similar results have been recently reported with rivastigmine treatment of patients with PD and dementia experiencing recurrent hallucinations. A small randomized placebo-controlled crossover study has also reported beneficial cognitive effects of treatment with donepezil 10 mg/day in 14 PD patients with mild-to-moderate dementia.[260]

PD patients with cognitive dysfunction are at particular risk of becoming demented compared to the general population. These patients are also at particular risk to develop acute toxic confusional states or paranoid hallucinosis in response to L-dopa or dopamine agonists. Confusion is frequently dose-related, and occurs more frequently with agonists than with L-dopa treatment. Although drug-related, the occurrence of confusion and hallucinosis in a patient receiving ongoing

TABLE 15-11 Pharmacological Management of Psychosis in PD

1. Control nondrug triggers and aggravators
   Treat infection
   Rectify fluid/electrolyte balance
   Exclude acute organic brain disease (stroke, encephalitis)
      if reasonable
2. Reduce polypharmacy
   Discontinue tricyclic antidepressants
   Discontinue anticholinergics and/or amantadine
   Reduce/discontinue dopamine agonists before L-dopa
   Discontinue COMT inhibitors before L-dopa
3. Add antipsychotics
   Clozapine (start with 6.25–12.5 mg at bedtime,
      monitor blood counts)
   Quetiapine (start with 12.5–25 mg)

   CAVEAT: olanzapine has failed efficacy in controlled trials of PD
      and may induce motor worsening.
4. Add cholinesterase inhibitors in patients with cognitive
   impairment (donepezil 5–10 mg, rivastigmine 4.5–9 mg)*

*Experimental.

antiparkinsonian medication should initially prompt a search for intercurrent illnesses, particularly infections or metabolic disturbances. Dopaminergic-induced psychosis may be preceded by patients reporting unusually vivid dreaming followed by hallucinations at night, when they may see familiar human-beings or animals without a sense of being threatened. In such situations, as in florid paranoid drug-induced psychosis, the first step is to reduce polypharmacy. In patients on combined regimens containing anticholinergics and/or amantadine in addition to L-dopa or dopamine agonists, the former should be discontinued first. In combined treatment with L-dopa plus a dopamine agonist, the latter should be reduced or discontinued first, before L-dopa is reduced to the minimum effective dose. Those patients continuing to hallucinate despite antiparkinsonian drug reductions have to be treated with atypical antipsychotic agents (see Table 15-11). Clozapine given as a starting bedtime dose of 6.25 mg and an average dose requirement of usually less than 50 mg/day remains the only atypical neuroleptic with proven efficacy based on randomized controlled trials.[261,262] Clozapine does not worsen parkinsonism, as demonstrated in placebo-controlled trials, but has other safety hazards, including a small but definite risk of leukopenia, requiring weekly blood monitoring for the first 6 months of treatment and biweekly thereafter. There have been instances of cardiomyopathy, venous thromboembolism, and interstitial nephritis in young schizophrenic patients receiving higher doses of clozapine than those used in parkinsonian psychosis.[263]

More recently, the atypical neuroleptic quetiapine, which has similar pharmacology to clozapine but without hematological safety risks, has been used in a number of open-label studies in patients with PD and psychosis. Overall, 80 percent of patients have been reported to respond to doses of 25–150 mg/day of quetiapine, so this agent may be a safer option to use than clozapine. There are, however, no placebo-controlled or clozapine-controlled trials of quetiapine in PD. There have been some reports of motor worsening with quetiapine among those open-label studies reported.

Olanzapine, while initially hoped to be a safe alternative to clozapine, has consistently failed to improve parkinsonian psychosis to a greater extent than placebo in several controlled trials.[264,265] At doses between 4 and 11 mg/day olanzapine has consistently been shown to significantly worsen parkinsonism.[264,265,266] Motor worsening has also been a frequent finding with risperidone treatment of drug-induced psychosis in PD at doses between 0.5 and 4 mg/day.[263]

More recently, a number of small open-label studies have reported beneficial effects of adjunct treatment with either rivastigmine or donepezil in PD patients with hallucinations and psychosis.[267–269] One study reported motor worsening in individual patients.[268] Given the low numbers of patients and the open-label design, no definite conclusions on the potential role of cholinesterase inhibitors in the treatment of drug-induced psychosis in PD are currently possible.

Management of Sleep Problems

Sleep disorders are very common in patients with PD, and various series have documented different kinds of sleep problems in 70–98 percent of PD patients (see Chap. 52).[270–272] Subjective complaints about sleep in patients with PD include difficulties falling sleep, frequent awakenings, discomfort and pain in the legs, difficulties turning in bed, nycturia, nocturnal confusion, and hallucinosis, as well as daytime sleepiness. Management has to be based on the type of problem and identifiable underlying causes. These include motor abnormalities such as nocturnal akinesia and/or tremor, nocturnal off-period dystonia, as well as coexistent restless legs syndrome or periodic leg movements in sleep. In addition, patients with PD have the same or even a greater prevalence of sleep-disordered breathing, and a number of disease-specific abnormalities of sleep structure, including fragmentation, reduced sleep efficiency, reduced REM (rapid eye movement) sleep and REM-sleep behavior disorder. Table 15-12 summarizes the principles of managing sleep problems in PD.

Management of Autonomic Dysfunction

Autonomic dysfunction is common in PD. It usually occurs in advanced disease (in contrast to atypical parkinsonism such as multiple system atrophy, where it occurs early). Autonomic features may include orthostatic hypotension, urinary dysfunction (urinary frequency, urgency, and urge incontinence), erectile dysfunction and impotence, gastrointestinal motility problems, and constipation. A number of therapeutic strategies are available for various manifestations of autonomic dysfunction; these are listed in Table 15-13.

TABLE 15-12 Management of Sleep Disorders in PD

Treatment of underlying causes
  Nocturnal motor problems (tremor, nocturnal akinesia, off-period dystonia): bedtime doses of controlled-release L-dopa or dopamine agonists (see Table 15-9)
  RLS/PLMS: bedtime doses of controlled-release L-dopa or dopamine agonists
  Sleep-disordered breathing: CPAP if necessary
  REM sleep behavior disorder: clonazepam 0.5 mg
  Nocturia: consider oxybutynin, tolterodine (see Table 15-13)
  Nocturnal hallucinosis/confusion (see Table 15-11)

Symptomatic treatment
  Sleep hygiene
  Avoid substances that might interfere with sleep (e.g., caffeine, alcohol)
  Short-acting benzodiazepines (e.g., triazolam) or zolpidem
  Low-dose, sedating antidepressants (e.g., trazadone, amitriptylin, reboxetine)

RLS, restless leg syndrome; PLMS, periodic leg movements in sleep; CPAP, continuous positive airway pressure.

TABLE 15-13 Practical Management of Dysautonomia in PD

For orthostatic hypotension
  Head-up tilt of bed at night
  Elastic stockings or tights
  Increased salt intake
  Fludrocortisone 0.1–0.3 mg/day
  Ephedrine 15–45 mg three times a day
  Midodrine 2.5–10 mg three times a day
For postprandial hypotension
  Octreotide 25–50 µg s.c. 30 min before a meal
For bladder symptoms
  Oxybutynin for detrusor hyperreflexia (2.5-5 mg two to three times a day)
  Tolterodine
  Intermittent self-catheterization for retention or residual volume > 100 mL
For erectile failure
  Sidenafil
  Yohimbine
  Intracavernosal injection of papaverine
  Penis implant
For gastrointestinal motility problems
  Domperidone up to 150 mg/day
  Metoclopramide* (10 mg i.m.)
For constipation
  Macrogol-water solution to increase intraluminal fluid
  Stool softeners
  Increase fiber intake

*Caution: may cause worsening of PD symptoms.

References

1. Ordenstein L: *Sur la Paralysie Agitante et la Sclérose en Plaque Généralisée*. Doctoral Thesis. Paris: Martinet, 1867.
2. Charcot J-M: *Leçons sur les Maladies du Système Nerveux*. Paris: A Delahaye, 1872–1873.
3. Schwab RS, Leigh D: Parpanit in the treatment of Parkinson's disease. *JAMA* 139:629–634, 1939.
4. Corbin KB: Trihexyphenidyl (Artane): The evaluation of a new agent in the treatment of parkinsonism. *JAMA* 141:377–382, 1949.
5. Carlsson A, Lindqvist M, Magnusson T: 3,4-Dihydroxyphenyl-alanine and 5-hydroxytryptophan as reserpine antagonists. *Nature* 180:1200–1201, 1957.
6. Ehringer H, Hornykiewicz O: Verteilung von Noradrenalin und Dopamin (3-Hydroxytyramin) im Gehirn des Menschen und ihr Verhalten bei Erkrangungen des extrapyramidalen Systems. *Klin Wochenschr* 38:1236–1239, 1960.
7. Barbeau A, Murphy CF, Sourkes TL: Excretion of dopamine in diseases of basal ganglia. *Science* 133:1706–1707, 1961.
8. Birkmayer W, Hornykiewicz O: Der l-3,4-Dioxyphenylalanin (=DOPA): Effekt bei der Parkinson-Akinese. *Wien Klin Wochenschr* 73:787–788, 1961.
9. Barbeau A, Sourkes TL, Murphy CF: Les catécholamines dans la maladie de Parkinson, in J de Ajuriaguerra (ed): *Monoamines et Système Nerveaux Central*. Geneva: Georg, 1962, pp 247–262.
10. Cotzias GC, Van Woert MH, Schiffer L: Aromatic amino acids and modification of parkinsonism. *N Engl J Med* 276:374–379, 1967.
11. Papavasiliou PS, Cotzias GC, Duby S, et al: Levodopa in parkinsonism: potentiation of central effects with a peripheral inhibitor. *N Engl J Med* 285:814, 1972.
12. Cotzias GC, Papavasiliou PS, Gellene R: Modification of parkinsonism: Chronic treatment with l-DOPA. *N Engl J Med* 280:337–345, 1969.
13. Nutt JG, Fellman JH: Pharmacokinetics of levodopa. *Clin Neuropharmacol* 7:35–49, 1984.
14. Rivera-Calimin L, Duyovne CA, Morgan JP, et al: Absorbtion and metabolism of L-dopa by the human stomach. *Eur J Clin Invest* 1:313–320, 1971.
15. Nutt JG, Woodward WR, Hammerstad JP, et al: The "on-off" phenomenon in Parkinson's disease: Relation to levodopa absorption and transport. *N Engl J Med* 310:483–488, 1984.
16. Leenders KL, Poewe W, Palmer A, et al: Inhibition of L-[18F]fluorodopa uptake into human brain by amino acids demonstrated by positron emission tomography. *Ann Neurol* 20:258–262, 1986.
17. Nutt JG, Woodward WR, Anderson JL: The effect of carbidopa on the pharmacokinetics of intravenously administered levodopa: The mechanism of action in the treatment of Parkinsonism. *Ann Neurol* 18:537–543, 1985.
18. Schultz E: Catechol-*O*-methyltransferase and aromatic l-amino acid decarboxylase activities in human gastrointestinal tissues. *Life Sci* 49:721–725, 1991.
19. Barbeau A, Gillo-Joffroy L, Mars H: Treatment of Parkinson's disease with levodopa and Ro 4-4602. *Clin Pharmacol Ther* 12:353–359, 1971.
20. Calne DB, Reid JL, Vakil SD, et al: Idiopathic parkinsonism treated with an extra-cerebral decarboxylase inhibitor in combination with levodopa. *BMJ* 3:7299–7732, 1971.

21. Merello M, Lees AJ, Webster R, et al: Effect of entacapone, a peripherally acting catechol-*O*-methyltransferase inhibitor, on the motor response to acute treatment with levodopa in patients with Parkinson's disease. *J Neurol Neurosurg Psychiatry* 57:186–189, 1994.

22. Kaakkola S, Teräväinen H, Ahtila S, et al: Effect of entacapone, a COMT inhibitor, on clinical disability and levodopa metabolism in parkinsonian patients. *Neurology* 44:77–80, 1994.

23. Hefti F, Melamed E, Wurtman RJ: The site of dopamine formation in rat striatum after L-dopa administration. *J Pharmacol Exp Ther* 217:189–197, 1980.

24. Poewe W, Wenning G: L-Dopa in Parkinson's disease: Mechanisms of action and pathophysiology of late failure, in Jankovic J, Tolosa E (eds): *Parkinson's Disease and Movement Disorders*, 4th ed. Baltimore: Williams & Wilkins, 2002, pp 104–115.

25. Hughes AJ, Daniel SE, Kilford L, Lees AJ: Accuracy of clinical diagnosis of idiopathic Parkinson's disease: A clinico-pathological study of 100 cases. *J Neurol Neurosurg Psychiatry* 55:181–184, 1992.

26. Wenning GK, Ben Shlomo Y, Magalhães M, et al: Clinical features and natural history of multiple system atrophy. An analysis of 100 cases. *Brain* 117:835–845, 1994.

27. Schrag A, Quinn N: Dyskinesias and motor fluctuations in Parkinson's disease. A community-based study. *Brain* 123:2297–2305, 2000.

28. Schrag A, Ben-Shlomo Y, Brown R, et al: Young-onset Parkinson's disease revisited: Clinical features, natural history and mortality. *Mov Disord* 13:885–894, 1998.

29. Rascol O, Brooks DJ, Korczyn AD, et al: A five-year study of the incidence of dyskinesia in patients with early Parkinson's disease who were treated with ropinirole or levodopa. *N Engl J Med* 342:1484–1491, 2000.

30. Rinne UK, Bracco F, Chouza C, et al: Cabergoline in the treatment of early Parkinson's disease: Results of the first year of treatment in a double-blind comparison of cabergoline and levodopa. *Neurology* 48:363–368, 1997.

31. Oertel WH: Pergolide versus L-dopa (PELMOPET). *Mov Disord* 15(suppl 3):4, 2000.

32. Parkinson Study Group. Pramipexole vs. levodopa as initial treatment for Parkinson's disease. *JAMA* 284:1931–1938, 2000.

33. Marek K, Seibyl J, Shoulson I, et al: Dopamine transporter brain imaging to assess the effect of pramipexole vs levodopa on Parkinson disease progression. *JAMA* 287:1653–1661, 2002.

34. Olanow CW: The role of dopamine agonists in the treatment of early Parkinson's disease. *Neurology* 58(4 suppl 1):S33–41, 2002.

35. Quinn NP: Anti-parkinsonian drugs today. *Drugs* 28:236–262, 1984.

36. Hubble JP: Long-term studies of dopamine agonists. *Neurology* 58(suppl 1):S42–S50, 2002.

37. Högl B, Seppi K, Brandauer E, et al: Irresistible onset of sleep during acute levodopa challenge in a patient with multiple system atrophy (MSA): Placebo-controlled, polysomnographic case report. *Mov Disord* 16:1177–1179, 2001.

38. Koller WC, Hutton JT, Tolosa E, Capildeo R, Carbidopa/Levodopa Study Group. Immediate-release and controlled-release carbidopa/levodopa in PD: A 5-year randomized multicenter study. *Neurology* 53:1012–1019, 1999.

39. Djaldetti R, Achiron A, Ziv I, Melamed E: First emergence of "delayed-on" and "dose failure" phenomena in a patient with Parkinson's disease following vagotomy. *Mov Disord* 9:582–583, 1994.

40. Djaldetti R, Baron J, Ziv I, Melamed E: Gastric emptying in Parkinson's disease: Patients with and without response fluctuations. *Neurology* 46:1051–1054, 1996.

41. Mouradian MM, Juncos JL, Fabbrini G, et al: Motor fluctuations in Parkinson's disease: Central pathophysiological mechanisms, part II. *Ann Neurol* 24:372–378, 1988.

42. Nutt JG, Woodward WR: Levodopa pharmacokinetics and pharmacodynamics in fluctuating parkinsonian patients. *Neurology* 36:739–744, 1986.

43. Giovannoni G, O'Sullivan JD, Turner K, et al: Hedonistic homeostatic dysregulation in patients with Parkinson's disease on dopamine replacement therapies. *J Neurol Neurosurg Psychiatry* 68:423–428, 2000.

44. Poewe W, Lees AJ, Stern GM: Dystonia in Parkinson's disease: Clinical and pharmacological features. *Ann Neurol* 23:73–78, 1988.

45. Savasta M, Dubois A, Feuerstein C, et al: Denervation supersensitivity of striatal D-2 receptors is restricted to the ventro- and dorsolateral regions of the striatum. *Neurosci Lett* 74:180–186, 1987.

46. Chase TN, Engber TM, Mouradian MM: Striatal dopaminoceptive system changes and motor response complications in L-dopa-treated patients with advanced Parkinson's disease. *Adv Neurol* 60:181–185, 1993.

47. Jenner P: The rationale for the use of dopamine agonists in Parkinson's disease. *Neurology* 45(suppl 3):S6–S12, 1995.

48. Brotchie JM: The neural mechanism underlying levodopa-induced dyskinesia in Parkinson's disease. *Ann Neurol* 47(suppl 1):105–114, 2000.

49. Jenner P: Factors influencing the onset and persistence of dyskinesias in the parkinsonian primate. *Ann Neurol* 47:S90–S104, 2000.

50. Obeso JA, Olanow CW, Nutt JG: Levodopa motor complications in parkinson's disease. *Trends Neurosci* 23(suppl):S2–S7, 2000.

51. LeWitt PA, Nelson MV, Berchou RC, et al: Controlled-release carbodopa/levodopa (Sinemet 50/200 CR4): Clinical and pharmacokinetic studies. *Neurology* 39(suppl 2):45–53, 1989.

52. Yeh KC, August TF, Bush DF, et al: Pharmacokinetics and bioavailability of Sinemet CR: A summary of human studies. *Neurology* 39:25–38, 1989.

53. Erni W, Held K: The hydrodynamically balanced system: A novel principle of controlled drug release. *Eur Neurol* 27(suppl 1):21–27, 1987.

54. Koller W, Pahwa R: Treating motor fluctuations with controlled-release levodopa preparations. *Neurology* 44(suppl 6): S23–S28, 1994.

55. Goetz CG, Koller WC, Poewe W, et al: Management of Parkinson's disease: An evidence based review. *Mov Disord* 17(suppl 4), 2002.

56. Poewe WH, Lees AJ, Stern GM: Treatment of motor fluctuations in Parkinson's disease with an oral sustained-release preparation of L-dopa: Clinical and pharmacological observations. *Clin Neuropharmacol* 9:430–439, 1986.

57. Kleedorfer B, Poewe W: Comparative efficacy of two oral sustained-release preparations of L-dopa in fluctuating Parkinson's disease. Preliminary findings in 20 patients. *J Neural Transm* 4:173–178, 1992.

58. Le Witt PA: Clinical studies with and pharmacokinetic considerations of sustained-release levodopa. *Neurology* 42(suppl 1):28–31, 1992.

59. Dupont E, Anderson A, Boqs J, et al: Sustained-release Madopar HBS compared with standard Madopar in the long-term treatment of de novo parkinsonian patients. *Acta Neurol Scand* 93:14–20, 1996.

60. Block G, Liss C, Scott R, et al: Comparison of immediate-release and controlled release carbidopa/levodopa in Parkinson's disease. A multicenter 5-year study. *Eur Neurol* 37:23–27, 1997.

61. Contin M, Riva R, Martinelli P, et al: Concentration-effect relationship of levodopa-benserazide dispersible formulation versus standard form in the treatment of complicated motor response fluctuations in Parkinson's disease. *Clin Neuropharmacol* 22:351–355, 1999.

62. Descombes S, Bonnet AM, Gasser UE, et al: Dual-release formulation, a novel principle in L-dopa treatment of Parkinson's disease. *Neurology* 56:1239–1242, 2001.

63. Djaldetti R, Atlas D, Melamed E: Effect of subcutaneous administration of levodopa ethyl ester, a soluble prodrug of levodopa, on dopamine metabolism in rodent striatum: Implication for treatment of Parkinson's disease. *Clin Neuropharmacol* 19:65–71, 1996.

64. Djaldetti R, Inzelberg R, Giladi N, et al: Oral solution of levodopa ethylester for treatment of response fluctuations in patients with advanced Parkinson's disease. *Mov Disord* 17:297–302, 2002.

65. Kaakkola S, Wurtman RJ: Effects of COMT inhibitors on striatal dopamine metabolism: A microdialysis study. *Brain Res* 587:241–249, 1992.

66. Keränen T, Gordin A, Karlsson M, et al: Inhibition of soluble catechol-*O*-methyltransferase and single-dose pharmacokinetics after oral and intravenous administration of entacapone. *Eur J Clin Pharmacol* 46:151–157, 1994.

67. Nissinen E, Lindén IB, Schultz E, Pohto P: Biochemical and pharmacological properties of a peripherally acting catechol-*O*-methyltransferase inhibitor entacapone. *Naunyn Schmiederbergs Arch Pharmacol* 346:262–266, 1992.

68. Myllyla VV, Sotaniemi KA, Illi A, et al: Effect of entacapone, a COMT inhibitor, on the pharmacokinetics of levodopa and on cardiovascular responses in patients with Parkinson's disease. *Eur J Clin Pharmacol* 45:419–423, 1993.

69. Keränen T, Gordin A, Harjola VP, et al: The effect of catechol-*O*-methyltransferase inhibition by entacapone on the pharmacokinetics and metabolism of levodopa in healthy volunteers. *Clin Neuropharmacol* 16:145–156, 1993.

70. Sawle GV, Burn DJ, Morrish PK, et al: The effect of entacapone (OR-611) on brain [18F]-6-L-fluorodopa metabolism: Implications for levodopa therapy of Parkinson's disease. *Neurology* 44:1292–1297, 1994.

71. Nutt JG, Woodward WR, Beckner RM, et al: Effect of peripheral catechol-*O*-methyltransferase inhibition on the pharmacokinetics and pharmacodynamics of levodopa in parkinsonian patients. *Neurology* 44:913–919, 1994.

72. Limousin P, Pollak P, Gervason-Tournier CL, et al: Ro 40–7592, a COMT inhibitor, plus levodopa in Parkinson's disease. *Lancet* 341:1605, 1993.

73. Rajput AH, Martin W, Saint-Hilaire MH, et al: Tolcapone improves motor function in parkinsonian patients with the "wearing-off" phenomenon: A double-blind, placebo-controlled, multicenter trial. *Neurology* 49:1066–1071, 1997.

74. Kurth MC, Adler CH, Hilaire MS, et al: Tolcapone improves motor function and reduces levodopa requirement in patients with Parkinson's disease experiencing motor fluctuations: A multicenter, double-blind, randomized, placebo-controlled trial. Tolcapone Fluctuator Study Group I. *Neurology* 48:81–87, 1997.

75. Myllyla VV, Jackson M, Larsen JP, Baas H: Efficacy and safety of tolcapone in levodopa-treated Parkinson's disease patients with "wearing off" phenomenon: A multicenter, double blind, randomized, placebo controlled trial. *Eur J Neurol* 4:333–341, 1997.

76. Baas H, Beiske AG, Ghika J, et al: Catechol-*O*-methyltransferase inhibition with tolcapone reduces the "wearing off" phenomenon and levodopa requirements in fluctuating parkinsonian patients. *J Neurol Neurosurg Psychiatry* 63:421–428, 1997.

77. Adler CH, Singer C, O'Brien C, et al: Randomized, placebo-controlled study of tolcapone in patients with fluctuating Parkinson disease treated with levodopa-carbidopa. Tolcapone Fluctuator Study Group III. *Arch Neurol* 55:1089–1095, 1998.

78. Ruottinen HM, Rinne UK: Entacapone prolongs levodopa response in a one month double blind study in parkinsonian patients with levodopa related fluctuations. *J Neurol Neurosurg Psychiatry* 60:36–40, 1996.

79. Parkinson Study Group: Entacapone improves motor fluctuations in levodopa-treated Parkinson's disease patients. *Ann Neurol* 42:747–755, 1997.

80. Rinne UK, Larsen JP, Siden A, Worm-Petersen J: Entacapone enhances the response to levodopa in parkinsonian patients with motor fluctuations. Nomecomt Study Group. *Neurology* 51:1309–1314, 1998.

81. Poewe WH, Deuschl G, Gordin A, et al, the Celomen Study Group: Efficacy and safety of entacapone in Parkinson's disease patients with suboptimal levodopa response: A 6-month randomised placebo-controlled double-blind study in Germany and Austria (Celomen study). *Acta Neurol Scand* 105:245–255, 2002.

82. Waters CH, Kurth M, Bailey P, et al: Tolcapone in stable Parkinson's disease: Efficacy and safety of long-term treatment. The Tolcapone Stable Study Group. *Neurology* 49:665–671, 1997.

83. Assal F, Spahr L, Hadengue A, et al: Tolcapone and fulminant hepatitis. *Lancet* 352:958, 1998.

84. Colosimo C: The rise and fall of tolcapone. *J Neurol* 246:880–882, 1999.

85. Birkmayer W, Riederer P, Youdim MBH, Linauer W: The potentiation of the anti-akinetic effect after levodopa treatment by an inhibitor of MAO-B, deprenyl. *J Neural Transm* 36:303–326, 1975.

86. Rinne UK, Siirtola T, Sonninen V: L-Deprenyl treatment of on-off phenomena in Parkinson's disease. *J Neural Transm* 43:253–262, 1978.

87. Golbe LI, Lieberman AN, Muenter MD, et al: Deprenyl in the treatment of symptom fluctuations in advanced Parkinson's disease. *Clin Neuropharmacol* 11:45–55, 1988.

88. Turkish S, Tu PH, Grenshaw AJ: Monoamine oxidase-B inhibition: A comparison of in vivo and ex vivo measures of reversible effects. *J Neural Transm* 74:141–148, 1988.

89. Reynolds GP, Elsworth JD, Blau K: Deprenyl is metabolized to methamphetamine and amphetamine in man. *Br J Clin Pharmacol* 6:542–544, 1978.

90. Parkinson's Study Group: Effect of deprenyl on the progression of disability in early Parkinson's disease. *N Engl J Med* 321:1364–1371, 1989.

91. Myllyla VV, Sotaniemic KA, Vuorinen JA, Heinonen EA: Selegiline as initial treatment in de novo parkinsonian patients. *Neurology* 42:339–343, 1992.

92. Mally J, Kovacs AB, Slone TW: Delayed development of symptomatic improvement by (−)-deprenyl in Parkinson's disease. *J Neurol Sci* 134:143–145, 1995.

93. Palhagen S, Heinonan EH, Hagglund J, et al: Selegiline delays the onset of disability in de novo parkinsonian patients. Swedish Parkinson Study Group. *Neurology* 51:520–525, 1998.

94. Lees AJ, Shaw KM, Kohout LJ, et al: Deprenyl in Parkinson's disease. *Lancet* ii:791–795, 1977.

95. Golbe LI, Lieberman AN, Muenter MD, et al: Deprenyl in the treatment of symptom fluctuations in advanced Parkinson's disease. *Clin Neuropharmacol* 11:45–55, 1988.

96. Tetrud JW, Langston JW: The effect of deprenyl (selegiline) in the natural history of Parkinson's disease. *Science* 245:519–522, 1989.

97. Olanow CW, Hauser A, Gauger L, et al: The effect of deprenyl and levodopa on the progression of Parkinson's disease. *Ann Neurol* 38:771–777, 1995.

98. Lees A: Comparison of therapeutic effects and mortality data of levodopa and levodopa combined with selegiline in patients with early, mild Parkinson's disease. Parkinson's Disease Research Group of the United Kingdom. *BMJ* 311:1602–1607, 1995.

99. Wheatley K, Stowe RL, Clarke CE, et al: Evaluating drug treatments for Parkinson's disease: How good are the trials? *BMJ* 324:1508–1511, 2002.

100. Sterling J, Veinberg A, Lerner D, et al: R(+)N-propargyl-1-aminoindan (rasagiline) and derivatives: Highly selective and potent inhibitors of monoamine-oxidase B. *J Neural Transm Suppl* 52:301–305, 1998.

101. Rabey JM, Sagi I, Huberman M, et al: Rasagiline mesylate, a new MAO-B inhibitor for the treatment of Parkinson's disease: A double-blind study as adjunctive therapy to levodopa. *Clin Neuropharmacol* 23:324–330, 2000.

102. Olanow CW, Jenner P, Brooks D: Dopamine agonists and neuroprotection in Parkinson's disease. *Ann Neurol* 44(3 suppl 1):S167–174, 1998.

103. Schapira AH: Neuroprotection and dopamine agonists. *Neurology* 58(4 suppl 1):S9–S18, 2002.

104. Lieberman A, Gopinathan G, Neophydites A, et al: Dopamine agonists in Parkinson's disease, in Stern G (ed): *Parkinson's Disease*. London: Chapman & Hall, 1990, pp 509–557.

105. Schachter M, Bedard P, Debona AG, et al: The role of D-1 and D-2 receptors. *Nature* 286:157–159, 1980.

106. Calne DB, Teychenne PF, Claveria LE, et al: Bromocriptine in parkinsonism. *BMJ* 4:442–444, 1974.

107. Olanow CW: Single blind double observer-controlled study of carbidopa/levodopa vs bromocriptine in untreated Parkinson patients. *Arch Neurol* 45:206, 1988.

108. Lieberman A, Gopinathan G, Neophytides A: Management of levodopa failures: The use of dopamine agonists. *Clin Neuropharmacol* 9(suppl 2):S9–S21, 1986.

109. Lieberman AN, Neophytides A, Leibowitz M, et al: Comparative efficacy of pergolide and bromocriptine in patients with advanced Parkinson's disease. *Adv Neurol* 37:95–108, 1983.

110. Staal-Schreinemachers AL, Wesseling H, Kamphuis DJ, et al: Low-dose bromocriptine therapy in Parkinson's disease: Double-blind, placebo-controlled study. *Neurology* 36:291–293, 1986.

111. Lees AJ, Stern GM: Sustained bromocriptine therapy in previously untreated patients with Parkinson's disease. *J Neurol Neurosurg Psychiatry* 44:1020–1023, 1981.

112. Parkinson's Disease Research Group in the United Kingdom: Comparisons of therapeutic effects of levodopa, levodopa and selegiline, and bromocriptine in patients with early, mild Parkinson's disease: Three year interim report. *BMJ* 307:469–472, 1993.

113. Montastruc JL, Rascol O, Senard JM, Rascol A: A randomised controlled study comparing bromocriptine to which levodopa was later added, with levodopa alone in previously untreated patients with Parkinson's disease: A five year follow-up. *J Neurol Neurosurg Psychiatry* 57:1034–1038, 1994.

114. Lees AJ, Katzenschlager R, Head J, Ben-Shlomo Y: Ten-year follow-up of three different initial treatments in de-novo PD: A randomized trial. *Neurology* 57:1687–1694, 2001.

115. Bergamasco B, Frattola L, Muratorio A, et al: Alpha-dihydroergocryptine in the treatment of de novo parkinsonian patients: Results of a multicentre, randomized, double-blind, placebo-controlled study. *Acta Neurol Scand* 101:372–380, 2000.

116. Martignoni E, Pacchetti C, Sibilla L, et al: Dihydroergocryptine in the treatment of Parkinson's disease: A six month's double-blind clinical trial. *Clin Neuropharmacol* 14:78–83, 1991.

117. Obeso JA, Lera G, Vaamonde J, et al: Cabergoline for the treatment of motor complications in PD. *Neurology* 41(suppl 1):172, 1991.

118. Ferrari C, Barbieri C, Caldara R: Long-lasting prolactin lowering effect of cabergoline, a new dopamine agonist, in hyperprolactinemic patients. *J Clin Endocrinol Metab* 63:941–945, 1986.

119. Webster J, Piscitelli G, Polli A, et al: A comparison of cabergoline and bromocriptine in the treatment of hyperprolactinemic amenorrhea. Cabergoline Comparative Study Group. *N Engl J Med* 331:904–909, 1994.

120. Lera G, Vaamonde J, Rodriguez M, Obeso JA: Cabergoline in Parkinson's disease. *Neurology* 43:2587–2590, 1993.

121. Hutton JT, Koller WC, Ahlskog JE, et al: Multicenter, placebo-controlled trial of cabergoline taken once daily in the treatment of Parkinson's disease. *Neurology* 46:1062–1065, 1996.

122. Inzelberg R, Nisipeanu P, Rabey JM, et al: Double-blind comparison of cabergoline and bromocriptine in Parkinson's disease patients with motor fluctuations. *Neurology* 47:785–788, 1996.

123. Rinne UK, Bracco F, Chouza C, et al: Cabergoline in the treatment of early Parkinson's disease: Results of the first year of treatment in a double-blind comparison of cabergoline and levodopa. The PKDS009 Collaborative Study Group. *Neurology* 48:363–368, 1997.

124. Rinne UK, Bracco F, Chouza C, et al: Early treatment of Parkinson's disease with cabergoline delays the onset of motor complications. Results of a double-blind levodopa controlled trial. The PKDS009 Study Group. *Drugs* 55(suppl1):23–30, 1998.

125. Rinne UK: Lisuride, a dopamine agonist in the treatment of early Parkinson's disease. *Neurology* 39:336–339, 1989.

126. Laihinen A, Rinne UK, Suchy I: Comparison of lisuride and bromocriptine in the treatment of advanced Parkinson's disease. *Acta Neurol Scand* 86:593–595, 1992.

127. Vaamonde J, Luquin MR, Obeso JA: Subcutaneous lisuride infusion in Parkinson's disease. Response to chronic administration in 34 patients. *Brain* 114:601–617, 1991.

128. Baronti F, Mouradian M, Davis LT: Continuous lisuride effects on central dopaminergic mechanisms in Parkinson's disease. *Ann Neurol* 32:776–781, 1992.

129. Stocchi F, Ruggieri S, Vacca L, Olanow CW: Prospective randomized trial of lisuride infusion versus oral levodopa in patients with Parkinson's disease. *Brain* 125:2058–2066, 2002.

130. Rubin A, Leneberger L, Dhahir P: Physiologic disposition of pergolide. *Clin Pharmacol Ther* 30:258–265, 1981.

131. Sokoloff P, Giros B, Martres M-P, et al: Molecular cloning and characterization of a novel dopamine receptor (D-3) as a target for neuroleptics. *Nature* 347:146–151, 1990.

132. Duvoisin RC, Hekkila RE: Pergolide-induced circling in rats with 6-hydroxydopamine lesions of the nigro-striatal pathway. *Neurology* 31(suppl 2):133, 1981.

133. Olanow CW, Fahn S, Muenter M, et al: A multicenter double-blind placebo-controlled trial of pergolide as an adjunct to sinemet in Parkinson's disease. *Mov Disord* 9:40–47, 1994.

134. Langtry HD, Clissold SP: Pergolide. A review of its pharmacological properties and therapeutic potential in Parkinson's disease. *Drugs* 39:491–506, 1990.

135. Pezzoli G, Martignoni E, Pacchetti C, et al: A crossover, controlled study comparing pergolide with bromocriptine as an adjunct to levodopa for the treatment of Parkinson's disease. *Neurology* 45(suppl 3):S22–27, 1995.

136. Goetz CG, Tanner CM, Glantz RH, Klawans HL: Chronic agonist therapy for Parkinson's disease: A five year study of bromocriptine and pergolide. *Neurology* 35:749–751, 1985.

137. Barone P, Bravi D, Bermejo-Pareja F, and the Pergolide Monotherapy Study Group: Pergolide monotherapy in the treatment of early PD. A randomized controlled study. *Neurology* 53:573–579, 1999.

138. Schwab RS, Amador LV, Lettvin JY: Apomorphine in Parkinson's disease. *Trans Am Neurol Ass* 76:251–253, 1951.

139. Struppler A, von Uexküll T: Untersuchungen über die Wirkungsweise des Apomorphin auf Parkinsonstremor. *Z Klin M* 152:46–57, 1953.

140. Cotzias GC, Papavasiliou PS, Tolosa ES, et al: Treatment of Parkinson's disease with aporphines. Possible role of growth hormone. *N Engl J Med* 294:567–572, 1976.

141. Gancher ST, Woodward WR, Boucher B, Nutt JG: Peripheral pharmacokinetics of apomorphine in humans. *Ann Neurol* 26:232–238, 1989.

142. Durif F, Deffond D, Tournilhac M, et al: Efficacy of sublingual apomorphine in Parkinson's disease. *J Neurol Neurosurg Psychiatry* 53:1105, 1990.

143. Kapoor R, Turjanski N, Frankel J, et al: Intranasal apomorphine: A new treatment in Parkinson's disease. *J Neurol Neurosurg Psychiatry* 53:1015, 1990.

144. van Laar T, Jansen EN, Neef C, et al: Pharmacokinetics and clinical efficacy of rectal apomorphine in patients with Parkinson's disease: A study of five different suppositories. *Mov Disord* 10:433–439, 1995.

145. van Laar T, Neef C, Danhof M, et al: A new sublingual formulation of apomorphine in the treatment of patients with Parkinson's disease. *Mov Disord* 11:633–638, 1996.

146. van Laar T, Jansen EN, Essink AW, Neef C: Intranasal apomorphine in parkinsonian on-off fluctuations. *Arch Neurol* 49:482–484, 1992.

147. Stibe CM, Lees AJ, Kempster PA, Stern GM: Subcutaneous apomorphine in Parkinsonian on-off oscillations. *Lancet* i:403–406, 1988.

148. Frankel JP, Lees AJ, Kempster PA, Stern GM: Subcutaneous apomorphine in the treatment of Parkinson's disease. *J Neurol Neurosurg Psychiatry* 53:96–101, 1990.

149. Poewe W, Wenning GK: Apomorphine: An underutilized therapy for Parkinson's disease. *Mov Disord* 15:789–794, 2000.

150. Dewey RB Jr, Hutton JT, LeWitt PA, Factor SA: A randomized, double-blind, placebo-controlled trial of subcutaneously injected apomorphine for parkinsonian off-state events. *Arch Neurol* 58:1385–1392, 2001.

151. Colzi A, Turner K, Lees AJ: Continuous subcutaneous waking day apomorphine in the long term treatment of levodopa induced interdose dyskinesias in Parkinson's disease. *J Neurol Neurosurg Psychiatry* 64:573–576, 1998.

152. Poewe W, Kleedorfer B, Wagner M, et al: Continuous subcutaneous apomorphine infusions for fluctuating Parkinson's disease. Long term follow-up in 18 patients. *Adv Neurol* 60:656–659, 1993.

153. Millan MJ, Cussac D, Milligan G, et al: Antiparkinsonian agent piribedil displays antagonist properties at native, rat, and cloned, human alpha(2)-adrenoceptors: Cellular and functional characterization. *J Pharmacol Exp Ther* 297:876–887, 2001.

154. Dooley M, Markham A: Pramipexole. A review of its use in the management of early and advanced Parkinson's disease. *Drugs Aging* 12:495–514, 1998.

155. Piercey MF: Pharmacology of pramipexole, a dopamine D3-preferring agonist useful in treating Parkinson's disease. *Clin Neuropharmacol* 21:141–151, 1998.

156. Mierau J, Schingnitz G: Biochemical and pharamacological studies on pramipexole, a potent selective D2 receptor agonist. *Eur J Pharmacol* 215:161–170, 1992.

157. Wright CE, Sisson TL, Ichhpurani AK, Peters GR: Steady-state pharmacokinetic properties of pramipexole in healthy volunteers. *J Clin Pharmacol* 37:520–525, 1997.

158. Hubble JP, Koller WC, Cutler NR, et al: Pramipexole in patients with early Parkinson's disease. *Clin Neuropharmacol* 18:338–347, 1995.

159. Parkinson Study Group: Safety and efficacy of pramipexole in early Parkinson disease. A randomized dose-ranging study. *JAMA* 278:125–130, 1997.

160. Shannon KM, Bennett JP Jr, Friedman JH: Efficacy of pramipexole, a novel dopamine agonist, as monotherapy in mild to moderate Parkinson's disease. The Pramipexole Study Group. *Neurology* 49:724–728, 1997.

161. Lieberman A, Ranhosky A, Korts D: Clinical evaluation of pramipexole in advanced Parkinson's disease: Results of a double-blind, placebo-controlled, parallel-group study. *Neurology* 49:162–168, 1997.

162. Guttman M, and the International Pramipexole-Bromocriptine Study Group: Double-blind comparison of pramipexole and bromocriptine treatment with placebo in advanced Parkinson's disease. *Neurology* 49:1060–1065, 1997.

163. Wermuth L, and The Danish Pramipexole Study Group: A double-blind, placebo-controlled, randomized, multi-center study of pramipexole in advanced Parkinson's disease. *Eur J Neurol* 5:235–242, 1998.

164. Pinter MM, Pogarell O, Oertel WH: Efficacy, safety, and tolerance of the non-ergoline dopamine agonist pramipexole in

the treatment of advanced Parkinson's disease: A double-blind, placebo controlled, randomised, multicentre study. *J Neurol Neurosurg Psychiatry* 66:436–441, 1999.

165. Pogarell O, Gasser T, van Hilten JJ, et al: Pramipexole in patients with Parkinson's disease and marked drug resistant tremor: A randomised, double blind, placebo controlled multicentre study. *J Neurol Neurosurg Psychiatry* 72:713–720, 2002.

166. Matheson AJ, Spencer CM: Ropinirole: A review of its use in the management of Parkinson's disease. *Drugs* 60:115–137, 2000.

167. Tulloch IF: Pharmacologic profile of ropinirole : A nonergoline dopamine agonist. *Neurology* 49(suppl 1):S58–S62, 1997.

168. Adler CH, Sethi KD, Hauser RA, et al. for the Ropinirole Study Group: Ropinirole for the treatment of early Parkinson's disease. *Neurology* 49:393–399, 1997.

169. Brooks DJ, Abbott RJ, Lees AJ, et al: A placebo-controlled evaluation of ropinirole, a novel D2 agonist, as sole dopaminergic therapy in Parkinson's disease. *Clin Neuropharmacol* 21:101–107, 1998.

170. Korczyn AD, Brooks DJ, Brunt ER, et al. on behalf of the 053 Study Group: Ropinirole versus bromocriptine in the treatment of early Parkinson's disease: A 6-month interim report of a 3-year study. *Mov Disord* 13:46–51, 1998.

171. Rascol O, Brooks DJ, Brunt ER, et al. on behalf of the 056 Study Group: Ropinirole in the treatment of early Parkinson's disease: A 6-month interim report of a 5-year levodopa-controlled study. *Mov Disord* 13:39–45, 1998.

172. Korczyn AD, Brunt ER, Larsen JP, et al. for the 053 Study Group: A 3-year randomized trial of ropinirole and bromocriptine in early Parkinson's disease. *Neurology* 53:364–370, 1999.

173. Whone AL, Watts RL, Stoessl AJ, et al: Slower progression of Parkinson's disease with ropinirole versus levodopa: The REAL-PET study. *Ann Neurol* 54:93–101, 2003.

174. Rascol O, Lees AJ, Senard JM, et al: Ropinirole in the treatment of levodopa-induced motor fluctuations in patients with Parkinson's disease. *Clin Neuropharmacol* 19:234–245, 1996.

175. Lieberman A, Olanow CW, Sethi K, et al., and the Ropinirole Study Group. A multicenter trial of ropinirole as adjunct treatment for Parkinson's disease. *Neurology* 51:1057–1062, 1998.

176. Rascol O, Goetz C, Koller W, et al: Treatment interventions for Parkinson's disease: an evidence based assessment. *Lancet* 359:1589–1598, 2002.

177. Olanow CW: The role of dopamine agonists in the treatment of early Parkinson's disease. *Neurology* 58(4 suppl 1):S33–S41, 2002.

178. Tan EK, Ondo W: Clinical characteristics of pramipexole-induced peripheral edema. *Arch Neurol* 57:729–732, 2000.

179. Facca A, Sanchez-Ramos J: High-dose pergolide monotherapy in the treatment of severe levodopa-induced dyskinesias. *Mov Disord* 11:327–329, 1996.

180. Frucht S, Rogers JD, Greene PE, et al: Falling asleep at the wheel: Motor vehicle mishaps in persons taking pramipexole and ropinirole. *Neurology* 52:1908–1910, 1999.

181. Ryan M, Slevin JT, Wells A: Non-ergot dopamine agonist-induced sleep attacks. *Pharmacotherapy* 20:724–726, 2000.

182. Ferreira JJ, Desboeuf K, Galitzky M, et al: "Sleep attacks" and Parkinson's disease: Results of a questionnaire survey in a movement disorders outpatient clinic. *Mov Disord* 15(suppl 3):187, 2000.

183. Ferreira JJ, Galitzky M, Montastruc JL, Rascol O: Sleep attacks and Parkinson's disease treatment. *Lancet* 355:1333–1334, 2000.

184. Schapira AH: Sleep attack (sleep episodes) with pergolide. *Lancet* 355:1332–1333, 2000.

185. Ebersbach G, Norden J, Tracik F: Sleep attacks in Parkinson's disease: Polysomnographic recordings. *Mov Disord* 15(suppl 3): 89, 2000.

186. Ferreira JJ, Galitzky M, Brefel-Courbon C, et al: "Sleep attacks" as an adverse drug reaction of levodopa monotherapy. *Mov Disord* 15(suppl 3):129, 2000.

187. Ben-Noun L: Drug-induced respiratory disorders: Incidence, prevention and management. *Drug Saf* 23:143–164, 2000.

188. Geminiani G, Fetoni V, Genitrini S, et al: Cabergoline in Parkinson's disease complicated by motor fluctuations. *Mov Disord* 11:495–500, 1996.

189. Ling LH, Ahlskog JE, Munger TM, et al: Constrictive pericarditis and pleuropulmonary disease linked to ergot dopamine agonist therapy (cabergoline) for Parkinson's disease. *Mayo Clin Proc* 74:371–375, 1999.

190. Oechsner M, Groenke L, Mueller D: Pleural fibrosis associated with dihydroergocryptine treatment. *Acta Neurol Scand* 101:283–285, 2000.

191. Bhatt MH, Keenan SP, Fleetham JA, Calne DB: Pleuropulmonary disease associated with dopamine agonist therapy. *Ann Neurol* 30:613–616, 1991.

192. Shaunak S, Wilkins A, Pilling JB, Dick DJ: Pericardial, retroperitoneal, and pleural fibrosis induced by pergolide. *J Neurol Neurosurg Psychiatry* 66:79–81, 1999.

193. Hughes AJ, Bishop S, Kleedorfer B, et al: Subcutaneous apomorphine in Parkinson's disease: Response to chronic administration for up to five years. *Mov Disord* 8:165–170, 1993.

194. Poewe W, Kleedorfer B, Gerstenbrand F, Oertel W: Subcutaneous apomorphine in Parkinson's disease. *Lancet* i:943, 1988.

195. Stoof JC, Kebabian JW: Independent in vitro regulation by the dopamine-stimulated efflux of cyclic AMP and K$^+$-stimulated release of acetylcholine from rat neostriatum. *Brain Res* 250:263–270, 1982.

196. Friedman E, Wang H-Y, Butkerait P: Decreased striatal release of acetylcholine following withdrawal from long-term treatment with haloperidol: Modulation by cholinergic, dopamine D-1, D-2 mechanisms. *Neuropharmacology* 29:537–544, 1990.

197. Damsma G, Tham CS, Robertson GS, Fibiger HC: Dopamine D-1 receptor stimulation increases striatal acetylcholine release in the rat. *Eur J Pharmacol* 186:335–338, 1990.

198. Coyle JT, Snyder SH: Antiparkinsonian drugs: Inhibition of dopamine uptake in the corpus striatum as a possible mechanism of action. *Science* 166:899–901, 1969.

199. Pollack AE, Wooten GF: D2 dopaminergic regulation of striatal preproenkephalin mRNA levels is mediated at least in part through cholinergic interneurons. *Mol Brain Res* 13:35–41, 1992.

200. Duvoisin RC, Cholinergic-anticholinergic antagonism in parkinsonism. *Arch Neurol* 17:124–136, 1967.

201. Olanow CW, Watts RL, Koller WC: An algorithm (decision tree) for the management of Parkinson's disease (2001): Treatment guidelines. *Neurology* 56(11 suppl 5):S1–S88, 2001.

202. Obeso JA, Rodriguez-Oroz MC, Rodriguez M, et al: Pathophysiology of the basal ganglia in Parkinson's disease. *Trends Neurosci* 23(suppl 10):S8–S19, 2000.

203. Chase TN, Oh JD: Striatal dopamine- and glutamate-mediated dysregulation in experimental parkinsonism. *Trends Neurosci* 23(suppl 10):S86–S91, 2000.

204. Klockgether T, Turski L: NMDA antagonists potentiate antiparkinsonian actions of L-dopa in monoamine-depleted rats. *Ann Neurol* 28:539–546, 1990.

205. Greenamyre JT, Eller RV, Zhang Z, et al: Antiparkinsonian effects of ramacemide hydrochloride, a glutamate antagonist, in rodent and primate models of Parkinson's disease. *Ann Neurol* 35:655–661, 1994.

206. Klockgether T, Turski L, Honoré T, et al: The AMPA receptor antagonist NBQX has antiparkinsonian effects in monoamine-depleted rats and MPTP-treated monkeys. *Ann Neurol* 30:717–723, 1991.

207. Klockgether T, Turski L: Toward an understanding of the role of glutamate in experimental parkinsonism: Agonist-sensitive sites in the basal ganglia. *Ann Neurol* 34:585–593, 1993.

208. Albin RL, Greenamyre JT: Alternative excitotoxic hypotheses. *Neurology* 42:733–738, 1992.

209. Schwab RS, England AC Jr, Poskancer DC, Young RR: Amantadine in the treatment of Parkinson's disease. *JAMA* 208:1168–1170, 1969.

210. Von Voigtlander PF, Moore KE: Dopamine: Release from the brain in vivo by amantadine. *Science* 174:408–410, 1971.

211. Gianutsos G, Chute S, Dunn JP: Pharmacological changes in dopaminergic systems induced by long-term administration of amantadine. *Eur J Pharmacol* 110:357–361, 1985.

212. Nastuck WC, Su PC, Doubilet P: Anticholinergic and membrane activities of amantadine in neuromuscular transmission. *Nature* 264:76–79, 1976.

213. Stoof JC, Booij J, Drukarch B: Amantadine as *N*-methyl-D-aspartic acid receptor antagonist. New possibilities for therapeutic application? *Clin Neurol Neurosurg* 94(suppl):S4–S6, 1992.

214. Greenamyre JT, O'Brien CF: *N*-Methyl-D-aspartate antagonists in the treatment of Parkinson's disease. *Arch Neurol* 48:977–981, 1991.

215. Parkes JD, Baxter RC, Curzon G, et al: Treatment of Parkinson's disease with amantadine and levodopa. A one-year study. *Lancet* i:1083–1086, 1971.

216. Verhagen Metman L, Del Dotto P, van den Munckhof P, et al: Amantadine as treatment for dyskinesias and motor fluctuations in Parkinson's disease. *Neurology* 50:1323–1326, 1998.

217. Verhagen Metman LV, Del Dotto P, LePoole K, et al: Amantadine for levodopa-induced dyskinesias. A 1-year follow-up study. *Arch Neurol* 56:1383–1386, 1999.

218. Snow BJ, Macdonald L, Mcauley D, Wallis W: The effect of amantadine on levodopa-induced dyskinesias in Parkinson's disease: A double-blind, placebo-controlled study. *Clin Neuropharmacol* 23:82–85, 2000.

219. Luginger E, Wenning GK, Bosch S, Poewe W: Beneficial effects of amantadine on L-dopa-induced dyskinesias in Parkinson's disease. *Mov Disord* 15:873–878, 2000.

220. Shoulson I: Experimental therapeutics of neurodegenerative disorders: Unmet needs. *Science* 282:1072–1074, 1998.

221. Clarke CE, Guttman M: Dopamine agonist monotherapy in Parkinson's disease. *Lancet* 360:1767–1769, 2002.

222. Shults CW, Oakes D, Kieburtz K, et al: Effects of coenzyme Q10 in early Parkinson disease: Evidence of slowing of the functional decline. *Arch Neurol* 59:1541–1550, 2002.

223. Hughes AJ, Ben-Shlomo Y, Daniel SE, Lees AJ: What features improve the accuracy of clinical diagnosis in Parkinson's disease: A clinicopathologic study. *Neurology* 42:1142–1146, 1992.

224. Poewe WH, Lees AJ, Stern GM: Low-dose L-dopa therapy in Parkinson's disease: A six-year follow-up study. *Neurology* 36:1528–1530, 1986.

225. Fahn S: Is levodopa toxic? *Neurology* 47(6 suppl 3):S184–S195, 1996.

226. Agid Y, Olanow CW, Mizuno Y: Levodopa: Why the controversy? *Lancet* 360:575, 2002.

227. Fahn S, Parkinson's Study Group: Results of the ELLDOPA (Earlier vs. Later Levodopa) study. *Mov Disord* 17(suppl 5):S13–S14, 2002.

228. Nutt GJ: Levodopa-induced dyskinesia: Review, observations and speculations. *Neurology* 40:340–345, 1990.

229. Muenter MD, Sharpless NS, Tyce GM, Darley FL: Patterns of dystonia ("I-D-I" and "D-I-D") in response to L-dopa therapy for Parkinson's disease. *Mayo Clinic Proc* 52:163–174, 1977.

230. Marsden CD, Parkes JD, Quinn N: Fluctuations of disability in Parkinson's disease. Clinical aspects, in Marsden CD, Fahn S (eds): *Movement Disorders*. London: Butterworth Scientific, 1981, pp 96–122.

231. Manson AJ, Schrag A, Lees AJ: Low-dose olanzapine for levodopa induced dyskinesias. *Neurology* 55:795–799, 2000.

232. Brotchie JM: Adjuncts to dopamine replacement: A pragmatic approach to reducing the problem of dyskinesia in Parkinson's disease. *Mov Disord* 13:871–876, 1998.

233. Gotham AM, Brown RG, Marsden CD: Depression in Parkinson's disease: A quantitative and qualitative analysis. *J Neurol Neurosurg Psychiatry* 49:381–389, 1986.

234. Cummings JL: Depression and Parkinson's disease: A review. *Am J Psychiatry* 149:443–454, 1992.

235. Santamaria J, Tolosa E, Valles A: Parkinson's disease: A possible subground of idiopathic parkinsonism. *Neurology* 36:1130–1133, 1986.

236. Brown RG, Jahanshahi M: Depression in Parkinson's disease: A psychosocial viewpoint. *Adv Neurol* 65:61–84, 1995.

237. Starkstein SE, Petracca G, Chemerinski E, et al: Depression in classic versus akinetic-rigid Parkinson's disease. *Mov Disord* 13:29–33, 1998.

238. Brown RG, MacCarthy B, Jahanshahi M, Marsden CD: Accuracy of self-reported disability in patients with parkinsonism. *Arch Neurol* 46:955–959, 1989.

239. Starkstein SE, Preziosi TJ, Bolduc PL, Robinson RG: Depression in Parkinson's disease. *J Ment Dis* 178:27–31, 1990.

240. Burn DJ: Beyond the iron mask: Towards better recognition and treatment of depression associated with Parkinson's disease. *Mov Disord* 17:445–454, 2002.

241. Brown RG, MacCarthy B, Gotham A-M, et al: Depression and disability in Parkinson's disease: A follow-up of 132 cases. *Psychol Med* 18:49–55, 1988.

242. Tandberg E, Larsen JP, Aarsland D, Cumming JI: The occurrence of depression in Parkinson's disease. A community-based study. *Arch Neurol* 53:175–179, 1996.

243. Damier P, Hirsch EC, Agid Y, Graybiel AM: The substantia nigra of the human brain II. Patterns of loss of dopamine-containing neurons in Parkinson's disease. *Brain* 122:1437–1448, 1999.

244. Charlton CG: Depletion of nigrostriatal and forebrain tyrosine hydroxylase by *S*-adenosylmethionine: A model that may explain the occurrence of depression in Parkinson's disease. *Life Sci* 61:495–502, 1997.

245. Chan Palav V, Asan E: Alterations in catecholamine neurons of the locus coeruleus in senile dementia of the Alzheimer type

and in Parkinson's disease with and without dementia and depression. *J Comp Neurol* 287:373–392, 1989.

246. Doder M, Rabiner EA, Turjanski N, et al: Brain serotonin 1A receptors in Parkinson's disease with and without depression measured by positron emission tomography with 11C-WAY 100635. *Mov Disord* 15(suppl 3):213, 2000.

247. Caley CF, Friedman JH: Does fluoxetine exacerbate Parkinson's disease? *J Clin Psychiatry* 53:278–282, 1992.

248. Tesei S, Antonini A, Canesi M, et al: Tolerability of paroxetine in Parkinson's disease: A prospective study. *Mov Disord* 15:986–989, 2000.

249. Richard IH, Kurlan R, Tanner C, et al: Serotonin syndrome and the combined use of deprenyl and an antidepressant in Parkinson's disease. Parkinson Study Group. *Neurology* 48:1070–1077, 1997.

250. Brown RG, Marsden CD: How common is dementia in Parkinson disease. *Lancet* ii:1262–1265, 1984.

251. Mayeux R, Chen J, Mirabello E, et al: An estimate of the incidence of dementia in idiopathic Parkinson's disease. *Neurology* 40:1513–1517, 1990.

252. Mayeux R, Denaro J, Hemenegildo N, et al: A population-based investigation of Parkinson's disease with and without dementia. Relationship to age and gender. *Arch Neurol* 49:492–497, 1992.

253. Aarsland D, Tandberg E, Larsen JP, Cummings JL: Frequency of dementia in Parkinson disease. *Arch Neurol* 53:538–542, 1996.

254. Quinn N, Critchley P, Marsden CD: Young onset Parkinson's disease. *Mov Disord* 2:73–91, 1987.

255. Hughes AJ, Daniel SE, Blankson S, Lees AJ: A clinicopathologic study of 100 cases of Parkinson's disease. *Arch Neurol* 50:140–148, 1993.

256. McKeith IG, Galasko D, Kosaka K, et al: Consensus guidelines for the clinical and pathologic diagnosis of dementia with Lewy bodies (DLB): Report of the consortium on DLB international workshop. *Neurology* 47:1113–1124, 1996.

257. Whitehouse PJ, Hedreen JC, White CL 3rd, Price DL: Basal forebrain neurons in the dementia of Parkinson disease. *Ann Neurol* 13:243–248, 1983.

258. Perry EK, Irving D, Kerwin JM, et al: Cholinergic transmitter and neurotrophic activities in Lewy body dementia: Similarity to Parkinson's and distinction from Alzheimer disease. *Alzheimer Dis Assoc Disord* 7:69–79, 1993.

259. McKeith I, Del Ser T, Spano P, et al: Efficacy of rivastigmine in dementia with Lewy bodies: A randomised, double-blind, placebo-controlled international study. *Lancet* 356:2031–2036, 2000.

260. Aarsland D, Laake K, Larsen JP, Janvin C: Donepezil for cognitive impairment in Parkinson's disease: A randomised

controlled study. *J Neurol Neurosurg Psychiatry* 72:708–712, 2002.

261. The Parkinson Study Group: Low-dose clozapine for the treatment of drug-induced psychosis in Parkinson's disease. *N Engl J Med* 340:757–763, 1999.

262. The French Clozapine Parkinson Study Group: Clozapine in drug-induced psychosis in Parkinson's disease. *Lancet* 353:2041–2042, 1999.

263. Poewe W, Seppi K: Treatment options for depression and psychosis in Parkinson's disease. *J Neurol* 248(suppl 3):12–21, 2001.

264. Ondo WG, Levy JK, Vuong KD, et al: Olanzapine treatment for dopaminergic-induced hallucinations. *Mov Disord* 17:1031–1035, 2002.

265. Breier A, Sutton VK, Feldman PD, et al: Olanzapine in the treatment of dopamimetic-induced psychosis in patients with Parkinson's disease. *Biol Psychiatry* 52:438–445, 2002.

266. Goetz CG, Blasucci LM, Leurgans S, Pappert EJ: Olanzapine and clozapine: Comparative effects on motor function in hallucinating PD patients. *Neurology* 55:789–794, 2000.

267. Reading PJ, Luce AK, McKeith IG: Rivastigmine in the treatment of parkinsonian psychosis and cognitive impairment: Preliminary findings from an open trial. *Mov Disord* 16:1171–1174, 2001.

268. Fabbrini G, Barbanti P, Aurilia C, et al: Donepezil in the treatment of hallucinations and delusions in Parkinson's disease. *Neurol Sci* 23:41–43, 2002.

269. Bergman J, Lerner V: Successful use of donepezil for the treatment of psychotic symptoms in patients with Parkinson's disease. *Clin Neuropharmacol* 25:107–110, 2002.

270. Lees AJ, Blackburn NA, Campbell VL: The nighttime problems of Parkinson's disease. *Clin Neuropharmacol* 11:512–519, 1988.

271. Factor SA, McAlarney T, Sanchez-Ramos JR, Weiner WJ: Sleep disorders and sleep effect in Parkinson's disease. *Mov Disord* 5:280–285, 1990.

272. Tandberg E, Larsen JP, Karlsen K: A community-based study of sleep disorders in patients with Parkinson's disease. *Mov Disord* 13:895–899, 1998.

273. Hardie RJ, Malcom SL, Lees AJ, et al: The pharmacokinetics of intravenous and oral levodopa in patients with Parkinson's disease who exhibit on-off fluctuations. *Br J Pharmacol* 22:429–436, 1986.

274. Sasahara K, Habara T, Morioka T, Nakajima E: Bioavailability of marketed levodopa preparations in dogs and parkinsonian patients. *J Pharm Sci* 69:261–265, 1980.

275. Fabbrini G, Mouradian MM, Juncos JL, et al: Motor fluctuations in Parkinson's disease: Central pathophysiological mechanisms, part I. *Ann Neurol* 24:366–371, 1988.

Chapter 16

TRANSPLANTATION AND RESTORATIVE THERAPIES FOR PARKINSON'S DISEASE

C. WARREN OLANOW, THOMAS B. FREEMAN, and
JEFFREY H. KORDOWER

INTRODUCTION   273
FETAL NIGRAL TRANSPLANTATION IN
   PARKINSON'S DISEASE   274
     Preclinical Issues   274
     Clinical Issues   277
FETAL NIGRAL TRANSPLANTATION: OPEN-LABEL
   CLINICAL TRIALS IN PARKINSON'S DISEASE   279
     Adverse Events and Neuropathologic Results   279
FETAL NIGRAL TRANSPLANTATION:
   DOUBLE-BLIND CONTROLLED STUDIES   280
OTHER DIRECTIONS   281
     Future Directions: Fetal Nigral Transplantation   282
     Future Directions: Stem Cells   282
     Future Directions: Gene Therapy   283
CONCLUSION   283

Since the last writing of this chapter there have been several important developments in the field of transplantation. Double-blind controlled trials of human and porcine fetal nigral transplantation have been completed and results have been somewhat disappointing. Nonetheless, as discussed in this chapter, there are many different ways of performing transplantation and it is possible that better results can be obtained with different transplant variables. More concerning are reports in transplanted patients of off-medication dyskinesias that occur in response even to small doses of L-dopa and may persist for days or even weeks after L-dopa is stopped. In contrast, enthusiasm about the potential of stem cells persists, and preclinical studies provide exciting evidence of benefit associated with trophic factors such as glial cell line-derived neurotrophic factor.

Introduction

Parkinson's disease (PD) is an age-related neurodegenerative disorder characterized by loss of melanin-containing neurons in the substantia nigra pars compacta (SNc) and a reduction in striatal dopamine.[1] Treatment typically consists of dopaminergic agents in the form of a dopamine agonist and/or L-dopa coupled with the peripheral decarboxylase inhibitor carbidopa. Initially, treatment provides substantial antiparkinsonian benefit, but long-term treatment is frequently complicated by debilitating side-effects such as motor fluctuations, dyskinesia, and neuropsychiatric problems.[2] In addition, disease progression is frequently associated with the development of postural instability, freezing episodes, autonomic disturbances, and dementia which are not satisfactorily controlled with dopaminergic or other available therapies. A number of new medical and surgical therapies have been recently developed in an attempt to overcome these problems,[3] and although they offer meaningful advances over treatments of a decade ago, they generally do not provide benefits superior to those obtained with L-dopa. Finally, PD is inexorably progressive, and none of the currently available medications has yet been established to provide neuroprotective or rescue effects. Thus, despite the flurry of activity in this field and the many new therapeutic approaches that have been introduced, PD patients ultimately suffer disability that interferes with their activities of daily living and their quality of life. Accordingly, there is an ongoing search for alternative treatments that can restore function to this population of patients.

Neural transplantation is a rational consideration for the treatment of PD because: (1) PD is associated with a relatively specific dopamine neuronal degeneration; (2) dopaminergic neurons provide tonic innervation to postsynaptic dopamine receptors; (3) dopamine replacement therapies provide dramatic clinical benefits; and (4) there are well-defined target areas for neural transplantation. Based on these considerations, transplantation strategies have been investigated in experimental models and in PD patients.

In the 1970s and 1980s, it was first demonstrated that implanted fetal mesencephalic neurons could survive, manufacture and secrete dopamine, form synaptic connections, and reduce motor abnormalities in 6-hydroxydopamine (6-OHDA)-lesioned rats[4–8] and 1-methyl-4-phenyl-1,2,3,6-tetrahydropyridine (MPTP)-treated primates.[9–14] Fetal dopaminergic allografts have also been shown to form normal appearing graft-host interconnections and to reinnervate the striatum in an organotypic pattern.[15,16] Grafts also exhibit normal electrical firing patterns and spontaneous dopamine synthesis and release.[17,18] Functional benefits can be long-lasting and have been observed to persist in rodents for more than 2 years.[19] Human fetal nigral grafts transplanted into immunocompromised rats also survive and form synaptic connections with host cells.[20–23] They can more completely reinnervate the host striatum, although neuritic outgrowth and functional recovery occur over a protracted period of time. Benefits following fetal nigral transplantation are dependent on the continued presence of donor mesencephalic cells and are lost following their removal or destruction.[24] Behavioral effects are also dependent on the type of tissue transplanted and the site of implantation. Thus, benefits are not seen with intrastriatal grafts of nondopaminergic tissue or when dopaminergic grafts are implanted into nonstriatal regions.[25]

These studies illustrate that grafting of species-specific and human fetal nigral cells can provide functional benefits in rodent and primate models of dopamine deficiency and suggest that this strategy may be beneficial in patients with PD. Alternate sources of dopamine-producing cells have also been studied. Fetal porcine nigral cells, sympathetic ganglia, carotid body glomus cells, PC-12 cells, neuroblastoma cells, and retinal pigmented epithelial cells do not produce behavioral effects in laboratory models that are as prominent or as long-lasting as those observed with embryonic nigral grafts.[26–30] There has also been interest in transplantation using chromaffin cells of the adrenal medulla, which normally produce epinephrine and norepinephrine, but only small amounts of dopamine. However, dopamine levels are increased if medullary cells are separated from the overlying adrenal cortex and the influence of glucocorticoids. Grafts of adrenal medulla placed into the denervated striatum or lateral ventricle of 6-OHDA-lesioned rats or MPTP-treated primates provide some behavioral improvement;[31–34] however, these effects are not as great in magnitude or duration as those observed with fetal nigral implants. Initial trials of cell suspensions of autologous adrenal medullary cells stereotactically implanted into the putamen of PD patients did not provide significant clinical benefit.[35,36] A report from Mexico of "dramatic amelioration" of symptoms in 2 PD patients following transplantation of solid grafts of autologous adrenal medullary tissue into the head of the caudate nucleus sparked renewed interest in this area,[37] but results could not be confirmed in subsequent studies.[38–41]

Further, the procedure was associated with significant morbidity and mortality, reflecting the need for a craniotomy and laparotomy in a patient with advanced PD,[41] and the procedure has largely been abandoned. The lack of a dramatic benefit following adrenal medullary transplantation may reflect the fact that chromaffin cells survive poorly following transplantation and do not send out neurites or form well-defined synaptic contacts with host neurons.[43] Transplantation using fetal nigral cells is thus associated with the best behavioral results in animal models of PD.

Fetal Nigral Transplantation in Parkinson's Disease

PRECLINICAL ISSUES

In considering a fetal nigral transplantation program, it is important to appreciate that many transplant variables can influence the likelihood that implanted cells will survive, innervate the target region, and provide optimal clinical benefits. These include: (1) tissue acquisition; (2) age of donor tissue; (3) tissue storage; (4) type of transplant; (5) site of implant; (6) volume of tissue; and (7) distribution of tissue. Decisions as to which transplant variables to employ are likely to impact upon whether or not implanted cells survive and the clinical results.

TISSUE ACQUISITION

Fetal tissue can be obtained from women undergoing spontaneous or elective abortion. It has been argued that fetal cells for transplantation can be derived from spontaneous abortions[44] based on studies demonstrating that these grafts provide functional benefits in rodent models of parkinsonism.[45] However, most research centers use fetal tissue derived from elective abortions[46] because spontaneously aborted fetal tissue is more likely to (1) contain genetic or central nervous system (CNS) defects, (2) be infected, (3) be disrupted making it difficult to identify critical landmarks, stage tissue, and dissect dopaminergic cells, and (4) provide a nonviable graft. In addition, it is more difficult to obtain donors from spontaneous abortions in such a way as to permit the use of multiple grafts or to schedule the timing of surgery reliably. To ensure that women will not become pregnant solely to provide tissue for transplantation and to comply with all current guidelines, we routinely employ the following guidelines in our program:

1. Consent for use of donor tissue is requested only after consent for the abortion has been signed.
2. There is no monetary or other inducement provided to either the mother or participating physicians.
3. There is no advertising for donors.
4. Patients are not denied medical care for refusal to donate tissue for transplantation.
5. Confidentiality of donor and recipient are maintained.
6. There is no linkage between the donor of the embryonic tissue and the recipient.
7. It is not stipulated that donated tissue will be employed for clinical or animal research.
8. Tissue is acquired in concert with all existing federal, state, and institutional regulations.

It is highly unlikely that the decision to have an abortion will be influenced by the prospects of participating in fetal research. During the 30-year history of fetal tissue research in the US, there is no evidence that research has influenced the demographics of abortion. At the present time, voluntary abortion is permitted under the laws of the United States of America. More than 1 million abortions are performed annually, and it is estimated that tissue from less than 0.01 percent of these is used for research purposes.[47] In addition, there is no alteration in the timing or indication for the abortion, the abortion is performed in a routine manner, and the fetus is pronounced dead by a physician not related to the transplantation process. The research study involves only the use of otherwise discarded fetal tissue. Recipients are informed that they are receiving transplanted fetal tissue derived from an elective abortion. All involved hospital staff are also fully informed as to the nature of the procedure.

DONOR AGE

The optimal donor age for graft survival is between the time dopaminergic cells are first detected in the subventricular zone until they differentiate and extend neuritic processes. Once neuritic processes are formed, cells are less likely to survive transplantation, possibly because they tend to be axotomized during preparation. We performed a study of the ontogeny of human embryonic dopamine-producing cells and found that tyrosine hydroxylase-immunoreactive (TH-IR) dopaminergic neurons were first detected in the subventricular floor at approximately 5–6.5 weeks postconception (PC).[48] Neuritic process were first identified at approximately 8 weeks PC and extended to reach the striatum at 9 weeks PC. By approximately 11 weeks PC, all TH-IR cells had migrated from the subventricular zone towards their adult location in the ventral portion of the mesencephalon. These observations suggest that the ideal donor age for transplantation of human embryonic mesencephalic dopamine cells is between 5.5 and 9 weeks PC (Fig. 16-1). Human-to-rodent nigral xenografts confirm these assumptions, demonstrating that optimal survival is between 5.5 and 8 weeks PC for suspension grafts and between 6.5 and 9 weeks PC for solid grafts.[49]

TISSUE STORAGE

It is necessary to store embryonic tissue in order to permit time for transportation to the medical center, screening for infectious agents, acquisition of multiple donors, and scheduling of surgery. Redmond et al. used cryopreservation to store fetal tissue prior to grafting.[50] However, cryopreservation of cells for 1 year is associated with a significant reduction in cell viability and neuritic outgrowth following transplantation in vivo,[51] even though there is no fall in dopamine levels in vitro.[52] Freed et al. cultured tissue for up to 4 weeks before use, but there is also a concern that there will be a loss of viability in implanted dopaminergic neurons.[53] We employ a chemically defined "hibernation medium" in which tissue is stored at 8°C. Using this cold-storage medium, we have demonstrated robust cell survival without evident degradation in either the viability or number of transplanted neurons following transplantation in animal models after storage for up to 4 days (Fig. 16-1).[54]

TYPE OF TRANSPLANT

Fetal mesencephalic cells can be transplanted as either cell suspension or solid grafts. Suspension grafts provide more homogeneous tissue distribution and have been employed by most transplant groups. However, this necessitates pooling of tissue, and infection or rejection of any one donor could adversely affect all graft deposits. Additionally, cells are more likely to be injured during graft preparation. We routinely employ solid grafts as these have an extended donor window, are easier to prepare, and preserve cytoarchitectural relationships.[55] Comparable survival has been demonstrated following transplantation of solid or suspension grafts of human ventral mesencephalon into immunosuppressed rats.[54]

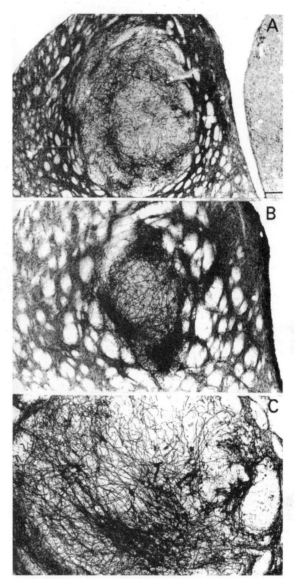

FIGURE 16-1 Low- (A, B) and medium- (C) power photomicrographs of TH-immunostained sections through the striatum of 6-OHDA-lesioned immunosuppressed rats receiving fetal human nigral xenografts from the optimal donor window. Grafted TH-IR neurons survived in an organotypic manner and extensively innervated the surrounding host striatum. Tissue was stored for 4 days in "hibernation" medium prior to transplantation. Scale bars: A, B, 250 μm; C, 100 μm.

SITE OF IMPLANT

Although the striatum is separated anatomically into a distinct putamen and caudate nucleus, functional relationships are not based on these anatomic boundaries (Fig. 16-2). Embryological development of the posterior two-thirds or the postcommissural portion of the putamen differs from that of the anterior putamen, which is more closely linked

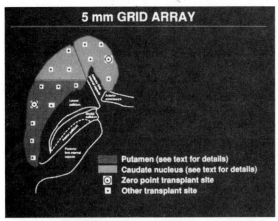

FIGURE 16-2 Schematic representation of putamen and caudate nucleus. While the putamen and caudate nucleus are anatomically distinct, we divide the striatum into the postcommissural putamen (shown in darker gray) and anterior putamen and caudate nucleus (shown in lighter gray), because they are more related functionally and embryologically. The postcommissural putamen is more affected in PD and is the target of our transplant procedure. We implant tissue at 5-mm intervals in three dimensions (as illustrated in this diagram) in order to try and obtain seamless dopaminergic innervation between transplant deposits throughout the entire extent of the target region.

functionally to the caudate nucleus.[56] The postcommissural putamen also differs from the anterior putamen-caudate nucleus complex in its anatomical connections. The postcommissural putamen has reciprocal connections with the precentral motor fields,[57,58] and microstimulation in this area evokes discrete movements of contralateral body parts.[59] In contrast, the caudate nucleus and anterior putamen are less related to primary motor circuitry but rather have extensive neuronal interconnections with the prefrontal cortex, frontal eye fields, and association cortex.[60] Functional recovery is also site-specific in models of parkinsonism. Grafts placed into the dorsal striatum of 6-OHDA-lesioned rats ameliorate drug-induced rotational asymmetries, whereas those placed into the ventrolateral striatum ameliorate sensorimotor attentional deficits.[61,62] Similarly, the pattern of behavioral improvement may differ in MPTP-treated primates following grafting into the caudate and putamen.[63]

There are several reasons to consider the postcommissural putamen as the primary site for neural grafting in PD. Both autopsy and positron emission tomography (PET) scan studies demonstrate greater dopamine depletion in the posterior putamen in PD patients.[64–66] In addition, degeneration of the SNc in PD preferentially occurs in regions that project to the posterior putamen.[67] Indeed, dopamine grafts placed exclusively into the putamen of MPTP-treated primates induce significant improvement in motor function.[12,63] There is, however, also evidence suggesting that the anterior putamen-caudate nucleus may be an important target for transplantation in PD. Hemiparkinsonism can be induced

by injecting MPTP into the caudate nucleus,[68] and fetal nigral grafts placed into the caudate nucleus of MPTP-treated monkeys can produce significant functional recovery with benefits different from those associated with grafting into the posterior putamen.[10,13] Preliminary studies also suggest that grafting into the SNc can provide enhanced benefits in MPTP-treated monkeys.[69] The effect of grafting into other potentially relevant brain regions, such as the nucleus accumbens, remains to be studied. Ultimately, the best clinical results may be associated with grafting into all of these areas.

VOLUME AND DISTRIBUTION OF TISSUE

A determination of the volume of tissue required to provide optimal results following fetal nigral grafting is complicated by the fact that dopaminergic neurons comprise only about 5 of the cells in a mesencephalic graft, and only 5–10 percent of transplanted cells survive the grafting procedure.[70] Behavioral improvement can be observed in rodents following transplantation of a fragment of a single human embryonic ventral mesencephalon.[20] The human striatum is markedly larger, however, and it is therefore likely that transplantation of a substantially greater number of nigral neurons will be required to achieve meaningful clinical benefit. There are approximately 500,000 dopamine neurons in the human SN, of which an estimated 60,000 project to the posterior putamen.[71] Approximately 20,000 dopamine neurons from a single human fetus survive transplantation into immunosuppressed rodents.[20,72] Thus, it may be necessary to transplant mesencephalic tissue from 3 or more donors into each putamen in order to completely restore the normal number of dopaminergic neurons. However, complete replacement of dopamine cells may not be required as clinical features do not emerge in PD until there has been a 50–60 percent reduction in the number of nigral neurons. On the other hand, it is possible that the number of dopaminergic neurons that survive transplantation overestimates the number capable of reinnervating the striatum as these grafts include neurons from the ventral tegmental area which do not normally project to the striatum or provide innervation to the striatum.[73] It may also be that it is necessary to have an excess number of dopaminergic neurons in order to compensate for ongoing neuronal degeneration that occurs as a result of immune rejection or the neurodegenerative process. Preliminary open-label studies in humans suggest that good results with transplantation can be obtained with tissue derived from 3–4 donors per side. Ultimately, a dose-response study will be required to determine the optimal number of donors for fetal nigral grafting in PD.

TISSUE DISTRIBUTION

The human striatum is approximately 500 times larger in volume than the striatum of the rodent. This presents a significant technical challenge for neural transplantation. Even if the correct numbers of donor cells are transplanted, improper distribution may result in a suboptimal clinical response. Based on our preclinical experiments, we estimate that implanted human fetal nigral neurons uniformly innervate a region of the striatum with a radius of approximately 2.5 mm, although more extensive fiber outgrowth may occur in a single direction. Dopamine diffusion from genetically engineered cells or following intracerebral microperfusion also appears to be limited.[74,75] To achieve confluent dopamine innervation of the target region, it may thus be necessary to distribute deposits of embryonic nigral cells at no greater than 5-mm intervals throughout its three-dimensional configuration. This can be accomplished in the postcommissural putamen or in the anterior putamen-caudate complex by placing four deposits in each of 6–8 needle tracts (Fig. 16-2). Utilizing such a protocol, we have observed confluent dopaminergic reinnervation following transplantation on autopsy studies.[55,76]

CLINICAL ISSUES

PATIENT SELECTION

It is not yet known which PD patients are the best candidates for a neural transplantation procedure. At the present time, it is easiest to justify performing an experimental procedure on patients with advanced PD who cannot be satisfactorily controlled with established medical or surgical therapies. However, these patients have greater perioperative risk. In addition, they are more likely to have clinical features that do not respond to L-dopa, and accordingly may not be capable of responding to grafted dopaminergic neurons. These problems may be less significant, and it may be easier to detect transplant benefits in patients with early PD. These patients may also not require drug therapy, thereby avoiding theoretical concerns relating to the potential toxic effects of the oxidative metabolites of L-dopa on graft viability.[77] Double-blind studies described below suggest that younger patients and those with milder disease might be better candidates for a transplantation procedure.

INFECTIOUS DISEASE ISSUES

Recipient

We routinely screen all patients who are candidates for a transplantation procedure for the following laboratory studies: complete blood count (CBC), Chem 18, HIV-1 (Ab, Ag), HIV-2 (Ab), hepatitis B (HBsAg, HBcAb), hepatitis C (HCVAb), cytomegalovirus (CMV IgG), toxoplasma (TOXO IgG), syphilis (VDRL or RPR), and herpes simplex (HSV IgG). Patients are excluded if they test positive for HIV. In the past we restricted participation to patients who were CMV- and TOXO-positive in order to minimize the risk of infection with transplantation of one of these contagious agents into a naive recipient. This may not be necessary in the case of CMV, as exposure in recipients is so common and active infection with this organism has not been detected in any of the donors we have tested to date.

Donor

We meticulously evaluate donors for the possibility of contagious agents in order to reduce the risk of transmitting infection and because infection can stimulate graft rejection. We screen each donor using maternal blood for: CBC, HIV-1 (Ab, Ag), HIV-2 (Ab), HTLV-I (Ab), hepatitis A (HAV IgM), hepatitis B (HBsAg, HBcAb), hepatitis C (HCVAb), CMV (IgM), toxoplasma (IgM), syphilis (VDRL or RPR), and herpes simplex (HSV IgM). In addition, fetal tissue is cultured for aerobic and anaerobic bacteria, and yeast. Donors are excluded if there is evidence of infection with HIV-1, HIV-2, HTLV-I, syphilis, hepatitis B transmissability, or hepatitis C. In addition, donors are not used from mothers who have been the recipient of multiple blood transfusions, have a temperature above 100.5° F, a white blood cell count greater than 15,000, a history of prostitution, or evidence of active genital herpes simplex.

IMMUNOSUPPRESSION

The CNS is an immunologically privileged site and it may be that immunosuppression is not essential for successful nigral grafting. Fetal allografts have been observed to survive for extended periods of time without immunosuppression in rodents and nonhuman primates.[8,78] Further, clinical improvement has been reported in open-label studies in PD patients who received fetal grafts without immunosuppression.[79,80] However, graft rejection in transplanted patients who do not receive immunosuppression might preclude development of a graft-related clinical benefit. Surgical trauma or the graft itself could disrupt the blood-brain barrier and permit the immune system access to graft antigens within the brain.[81] This is particularly relevant to protocols utilizing multiple immunologically unrelated donors. Immunosuppression has been shown to improve survival of xenografts in rodent models of parkinsonism,[70,82] and allograft rejection has been described in immunologically disparate rodents.[83] Indeed, we have seen HLA-DR immunoreactivity as well as T-cells and B-cells in what are otherwise seemingly intact nigral grafts.[84] For these reasons, most transplant groups have employed immunosuppression. In our own studies, we treat patients with cyclosporin A (CsA) 6 mg/kg for approximately 1 month. Thereafter, the dose of CsA is reduced to 2 mg/kg and the drug is discontinued after 6 months, at which time the blood-brain barrier is expected to be closed. Using this treatment protocol, we have noted robust survival of implanted neurons without evidence of immune rejection 18 months after transplantation and 12 months after discontinuation of CsA.[76] This suggests that prolonged treatment with CsA may not be necessary. It remains to be determined if CsA can be withheld entirely or even discontinued from the transplant protocol.

If CsA is to be employed, it is reasonable to consider the possibility that it may also affect PD signs and symptoms and confound interpretation of transplant benefits. CsA induces increased spontaneous and dopamine agonist-induced motor activity in rodents.[84] There is also evidence of inflammation in the SNc of PD patients,[85] raising the possibility that an inflammatory reaction may contribute to the pathogenesis of cell degeneration in PD and be attenuated by CsA administration. Perhaps most importantly, CsA is a potent antiapoptotic agent that binds to cyclophilins, and promotes closure of the mitochondrial permeability transition pore and preservation of the mitochondrial membrane potential.[86] As there is evidence that cell death in PD occurs by way of an apoptotic process, it is possible that CsA might influence the natural progression of PD. These factors must be considered in interpreting study results and comparing the benefit of a transplant procedure to unoperated PD controls.

CLINICAL EVALUATIONS

Clinical evaluations of transplantation typically include motor assessments of parkinsonism, neuropsychologic assessments of cognitive function, and PET scan measures of fluorodopa (FD) uptake as a surrogate marker of the number of surviving dopaminergic neurons.

MOTOR ASSESSMENT

The core assessment protocol for intracerebral transplantation (CAPIT) and its more recent revision have been developed to facilitate comparison of results among different transplant centers.[88,89] Clinical evaluations include measures of disability, motor function, and timed motor tasks during the "practically defined off" state (approximately 12 hours after overnight withdrawal of antiparkinsonian medication) and "best on" state (1–2 hours after usual dose of antiparkinsonian medication). The CAPIT also includes a self-administered home diary determination of the time during the waking day that the patient spends in the "on," "on with dyskinesia," and "off" states. Many centers also perform an L-dopa response test, timed measures of specified motor functions, and standardized videotape evaluations.

COGNITIVE FUNCTION

Changes in cognitive function can frequently be detected even in nondemented PD patients. Specific impairments are most frequently seen in strategic cognitive abilities such as recall of information,[90] dual-process tasks,[91] memory for temporal order,[92] and switching of cognitive sets.[93] These deficits are thought to be due primarily to impairment of the caudate outflow to the frontal lobes. No data have yet been presented on the effect of fetal nigral transplant surgery on cognitive function, but such studies are important both from the standpoint of detecting putative site-specific benefits of transplantation as well as to assess possible adverse effects of the transplant procedure.

PET STUDIES

Striatal fluorodopa (FD) uptake on PET is employed in most clinical trials as a surrogate measure of the number

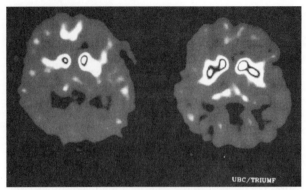

FIGURE 16-3 PET scan showing decreased striatal fluorodopa (FD) uptake preoperatively, particularly in the region of the postcommissural putamen (*left*). Note dramatic increase in striatal FD uptake bilaterally in the target region of transplantation (*right*). This magnitude of improvement has been seen in each of our transplanted patients and may continue to increase over time, but levels continue to remain below the lower limits of normal.

of surviving dopaminergic neurons.[94] FD is decarboxylated to fluorodopamine in the brain and retained in the striatum, probably within nigrostriatal dopaminergic nerve terminals. A steady-state striatal FD uptake rate constant can be calculated by the graphic method of Patlak and Blasberg,[95] and has been shown to correlate with dopamine cell counts and levels.[96] More recent studies utilize striatal/occipital ratio to assess fluorodopa uptake. Three-dimensional PET studies offer an opportunity to assess fluorodopa uptake throughout all brain regions, including the SNc.[97] There are several reports indicating that increased striatal FD uptake on PET can occur following fetal nigral grafting in PD or MPTP-parkinsonism and that changes correlate with clinical benefits [55,98–101] (Fig. 16-3). Following unilateral transplantation, striatal FD uptake has been reported to be increased on the transplanted side, but to be decreased on the contralateral (unoperated) side, possibly due to disease progression.[102] A progressive increase in striatal FD uptake has been observed in a few patients who have undergone sequential postoperative PET studies.[102]

It is likely that increased striatal FD uptake on PET following transplantation reflects graft survival and neuritic outgrowth based on pathological confirmation in 2 cases.[76,103] It is unlikely that increased FD uptake is due to the surgical trauma and/or a trophic effect as PET changes were not seen following adrenal transplantation despite a greater degree of trauma,[104] and host-derived sprouting has not been reported to occur in the putamen where PET changes have been most prominent. There has recently been interest in measuring β-CIT uptake with single photon emission tomography (SPECT) to measure ligands for the dopamine transporter as a marker of dopaminergic terminals. In addition, PET-raclopride binding studies performed before and after a dose of L-dopa permit a measure of dopamine release from grafts and have been used to demonstrate the capacity of implanted neurons to store and secrete dopamine as long as 10 years following transplantation.[105] These techniques offer considerable promise for evaluating transplantation in an objective fashion, as well as for better understanding the nature of the pathophysiologic defect in PD.

DRUG MANAGEMENT

There are several concerns about the use of L-dopa following a transplantation procedure for PD. Break-down of the blood-brain barrier following transplantation could theoretically permit carbidopa administered with L-dopa to inhibit central decarboxylase activity. However, L-dopa has not been shown to be more effective than L-dopa/carbidopa, and carbidopa was not identified in the ventricular cerebrospinal fluid of levodopa/carbidopa-treated PD patients 6 months following adrenal transplantation.[106] L-Dopa undergoes oxidative metabolism and has the potential to generate cytotoxic free radicals;[107] it can induce degeneration of cultured fetal nigral cells.[108] However, the bulk of laboratory and clinical data suggest that L-dopa is not likely to be toxic in PD,[109] and clinical benefits, increased FD uptake on PET, and survival of grafted cells postmortem have all been observed years following transplantation in L-dopa-treated patients.[110] There are also clinical trial issues with regard to the management of L-dopa. Lowering the L-dopa dose can paradoxically lead to symptomatic improvement in some PD patients and confound interpretation of transplant benefits. Accordingly, caution must be exercised in using a decrease in L-dopa dosage as an index of clinical improvement. On the other hand, elimination of the need for L-dopa in a patient with advanced PD would be clear evidence of a transplant effect. While total drug withdrawal is a desirable goal, only a small number of patients have been able to be completely withdrawn from L-dopa following a transplant procedure.[110]

Fetal Nigral Transplantation: Open-Label Clinical Trials in Parkinson's Disease

Several open-label transplant studies have been reported demonstrating the feasibility of performing fetal nigral transplantation in PD patients.[53,55,76,99,100,110–117] However, results have been inconsistent and difficult to compare because of variations in patient selection, transplant variables, rating system employed, level of scrutiny, and clinical expertise.[118] Some trials have reported consistent clinical benefit,[55,110,114–116] but others have had more inconsistent or negative results.[53,111,113] In general, better results correlated with the use of larger numbers of donors, using the correct donor window, and improvement on PET. Benefits typically consisted of improvement in UPDRS (Unified Parkinson's Disease Rating Scale) motor scores during "off" periods, percent "on" time without dyskinesia, and Schwab-England

disability scores when "off." Increased striatal FD uptake on PET has been observed by 6 months following the grafting procedure and has continued to increase to near normal levels in some patients.[98,100,116]

ADVERSE EVENTS AND NEUROPATHOLOGIC RESULTS

For the most part, fetal nigral transplantation has been well tolerated in these open-label studies, and in most studies there were no reports of serious transplant-related morbidity or mortality. There have only been two deaths that are thought to directly relate to the transplant procedure: one from a perioperative complication,[119] and one from obstructive hydrocephalus due to migration of a misplaced graft into the fourth ventricle and subsequent brainstem compression.[120,121] Postmortem study in the latter case revealed that the tissue derived from multiple germ layers and contained bone, cartilage, hair, and squamous epithelium.[121] This case illustrates the dangers that can occur when inexperienced investigators employ improper dissection and transplant techniques, and underscores the importance of adequate training prior to performing a transplant procedure.[122]

Early pathologic studies following transplantation did not show survival of meaningful numbers of implanted neurons,[79,123] probably because of the transplant variables employed in these studies. Indeed, some of the cells contained extraordinarily large amounts of neuromelanin suggestive of pathologic dopamine auto-oxidation.[79] It is noteworthy that poor cell survival in these cases was associated with little, if any, clinical benefit. Subsequently, postmortem studies were performed in 2 patients who died 18 months after transplantation from unrelated causes.[76,103,117,124] Each had experienced clinically meaningful benefit and increased striatal FD uptake on PET. At autopsy, large viable transplants were observed bilaterally in grafted regions (Fig. 16-4) containing approximately 82,000–138,000 dopaminergic neurons per side.[124] Abundant neuritic processes extended from graft deposits into the neighboring striatum where they were seamlessly integrated into the host tissue. Innervation of the striatum was contiguous between graft deposits and organized in a classic patch-matrix fashion. This was in stark contrast to ungrafted regions that demonstrated virtually no TH-immunoreactive staining. Cytochrome oxidase staining, an index of metabolic activity, was markedly increased in transplanted regions. Similarly, there was extensive staining for the dopamine transporter, a marker of dopamine terminals, in grafted regions of the putamen, but not in ungrafted regions of the striatum. In situ hybridization studies demonstrated extensive TH mRNA formation in grafted neurons within the striatum, but not in host neurons in the SNc, suggesting that implanted but not host neurons were functional and had the capacity to manufacture dopamine. Ultrastructural studies demonstrated normal appearing graft-host and host-graft synaptic connections.

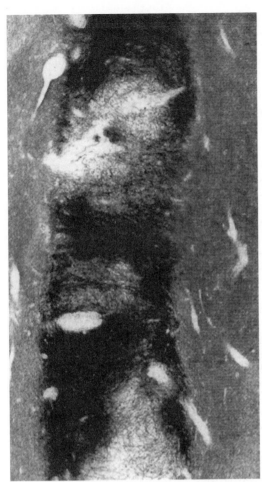

FIGURE 16-4 Low-power photomicrograph showing a TH-immunostained graft deposit in a PD patient. Note the robust survival of implanted neurons, and the extensive and seamless innervation of the surrounding striatum.

No evidence for graft-mediated host sprouting or cellular infiltration was detected. Nonetheless, a few macrophages and T4 and T8 cells were observed, indicating the possibility that some degree of graft rejection might have occurred.[125] The possibility that sprouting of host dopaminergic fibers due to local trauma or implanted trophic factors might account for the clinical benefits and postmortem changes found in transplanted patients has been considered. Host-derived sprouting has been observed in PD patients as well as in rodent and primate models of PD following adrenal medullary transplant procedures.[126,127] In patients transplanted with fetal nigral cells, sprouting of host fibers was carefully sought but not detected. In addition, adrenal transplant did not induce PET changes despite more extensive trauma,[128] and sprouting has not been detected in the putamen in preclinical studies. These findings suggest that the increased FD uptake on PET and striatal innervation observed following fetal nigral grafting procedures represents graft survival.

Fetal Nigral Transplantation: Double-Blind Controlled Studies

While open-label uncontrolled clinical trials suggest that fetal nigral transplantation might be valuable in the treatment of PD, formal confirmation in the form of double-blind, placebo-controlled trials is required to assess the true safety and efficacy of this procedure. While there is controversy regarding the use of surgical placebo controls in evaluating surgical procedures, surgery is well known to be associated with the development of a placebo response that can confound interpretation of any procedure-derived benefit.[129] Furthermore, there is the potential for physician bias in the evaluation of patients. There are numerous examples of surgical procedures that have been employed in routine practice only to be found lacking when held to the light of a controlled trial.[130,131] Accordingly, we have argued for placebo-controlled trials in evaluating cell-based therapies such as transplantation.[132] To date, two NIH-supported, prospective, double-blind, placebo-controlled studies have been performed testing fetal nigral transplantation in patients with advanced PD.

The first study was a 1-year trial in which 40 patients with advanced PD were randomized to receive bilateral transplantation versus an imitation placebo procedure.[133] Those in the transplant group received solid grafts or "noodles" on each side of the brain. Donor tissue was derived from the mesencephalon of 2 embryos aged 7–8 weeks PC. Tissue was implanted using two needle-tracks per side. Prior to transplantation, tissue was stored in tissue culture for 1–4 weeks in order to test for cell viability. Immunosuppression was not employed. Placebo-treated patients received a burr hole, but a needle was not passed into the brain and fetal tissue was not implanted. Change in quality of life between baseline and final visit was selected as the primary endpoint.

With respect to the primary endpoint, patients in the transplant group had a change of 0.0±2.1 compared to −0.4±1.7 in the sham-surgery group. This difference was not significant, and the study must therefore be considered to have failed to establish the benefit of fetal nigral transplantation in PD using the selected parameters. However, transplanted patients under the age of 60 years were significantly improved in comparison to placebo patients with respect to some secondary endpoints, including UPDRS motor score ($P = 0.01$) and Schwab-England disability score ($P = 0.006$) during the "practically defined off" stages. No significant benefits were observed in older patients (> 60 years). Interestingly, PET studies showed a significant increase in striatal FD uptake in both younger patients who had motor improvement as well as in older patients who did not.[134] The procedure was generally well tolerated, but, after a latency of approximately 18 months, 15 percent of transplanted patients developed a dyskinesia/dystonia that persisted for days or even weeks following withdrawal of dopaminergic medication.[135] This off-medication dyskinesia was a source of considerable disability to some individuals and is not seen in patients who did not undergo transplantatation.[136] The authors postulate that these dyskinesias are due to dopamine overproduction and report focal areas of increased striatal uptake on PET.[137]

The second study is also a prospective, randomized, double-blind, placebo-controlled trial of bilateral human fetal nigral transplantation. In this study, a total of 34 patients were enrolled into the study and randomized to one of three treatment groups: (1) bilateral transplantation with 4 donors per side, (2) bilateral transplantation with 1 donor per side, or (3) bilateral sham placebo procedures. Differences from the first study include a restricted target (the postcommissural putamen), distribution of deposits so that they are separated by no more than 5 mm in three dimensions, the use of immunosuppressant agents during the first 6 months following transplantation, a comparison of the effect of implanting relatively large numbers (4 donors per side) versus small numbers (1 donor per side) of donors per side, and 2 years of follow-up. In addition, tissue was stored in fresh hibernation media for no more than 48 hours. The primary endpoint in this study was the change from baseline in UPDRS motor score in the "practically defined off" state. Secondary endpoints included percent of time in the "on" state without dyskinesia, timed motor tasks, neuropsychological measures of cognitive function, and PET measures of FD uptake. The formal results have not been published, but preliminary presentations indicate that transplanted patients were not significantly improved in comparison to placebo patients despite evidence of graft survival on PET and postmortem studies (Olanow et al., personal observations). Further, approximately half of transplanted patients developed off-medication dyskinesia which was sufficiently severe as to necessitate surgical intervention in some individuals, thus confirming the results reported in the first trial.

These two trials leave us with troubling problems that must be resolved before transplantation can be reconsidered as a treatment for PD. Why did patients not experience enhanced benefits despite graft survival on PET and postmortem examinations? And secondly, what are off-medication dyskinesias? The specific answers to these questions are not known. Current information suggests that dyskinesia in PD patients relates to intermittent pulsatile stimulation of striatal dopamine receptors related to disease severity and the use of short-acting dopaminergic agents such as L-dopa.[138] This theory has led to the concept that treatments that provide more "continuous dopaminergic stimulation" might reduce the risk of developing motor complications. Indeed, studies in both MPTP-treated monkeys and PD patients show that long-acting dopamine agonists are much less likely to induce dyskinesia than short-acting dopaminergic agents such as L-dopa. These findings are difficult to reconcile with the observations reported in transplanted patients. Quite the contrary, one might have expected that dyskinesia would be alleviated in transplanted patients who now have an increased number of dopamine terminals in which to store dopamine and buffer fluctuations in the plasma L-dopa concentration. Indeed, Lee et al. have reported that transplantation sufficient

to partially restore dopamine transporter staining (an index of the number of dopamine terminals) alleviates dyskinesia in a rodent model.[139] Precisely what is going on in the double-blind studies, and why some, but not all, patients developed this troublesome side-effect remains to be determined. Unfortunately, preclinical trials did not assess the effects of transplants in L-dopa-treated primates that had been primed to express dyskinesia. It might be that implantation of small numbers of dopaminergic neurons in relatively separated deposits recreates pulsatile stimulation of primed striatal neurons and that more diffuse innervation of the striatum might avoid this problem. Alternatively, it is possible that the answer to both questions relates to incomplete dopamine reinnervation of the striatum. This hypothesis would explain why patients do not have a more profound antiparkinsonian response and would argue that off-medication dyskinesia is a form of diphasic dyskinesia that is related to the effects of suboptimal levels of striatal dopamine. Further experiments to test these hypotheses are required.

Other Directions

Fetal porcine nigral transplantation was introduced in an attempt to avoid the societal and logistical issues associated with the use of human embryonic tissue. Because of the relatively large size of porcine litters, they provide a readily available and controlled source of fetal tissue for transplantation. Issues involved in transplantation are similar to those discussed with human embryonic tissue. However, to avoid the greater risk of rejection associated with xenografts, CsA has to be co-administered. Alternatively, attempts have been made to reduce immunogenicity by pretreating donor cells with antibodies to MHC sites. Preclinical studies demonstrated the capacity of porcine nigral cells to survive transplantation and to reverse motor abnormalities in rodent models of PD, although results were not of the same magnitude as observed with human embryonic nigral cells. Open studies in a small number of PD patients have not been impressive. Clinical improvement has been variable and modest at best. PET studies show no significant improvement in striatal FD uptake, and a single postmortem study showed poor graft survival.[140] Despite these results, a prospective double-blind placebo-controlled study was performed in a small number of advanced PD patients. While the results of the study have not been formally published, preliminary reports indicate that transplantation was not superior to placebo. Interestingly, there was a striking placebo effect that persisted for the entire 18-month duration of the study, illustrating the importance of performing double-blind placebo-controlled trials. It is not clear at this time if further work will continue with porcine fetal nigral transplants based on these results.

There has also been some early work with transplantation of pigmented retinal epithelia cells that manufacture and release L-dopa. They are administered bound to spheroids and degenerate quickly if dissociated. They can be developed in abundant supply, but may have limited potential because they do not extend processes or form connections with host neurons, and it is not certain how far L-dopa can diffuse from the deposit site. Benefits were reported in an open-label unpublished study in a small number of patients (R Watts, unpublished data), and double-blind trials are presently underway.

FUTURE DIRECTIONS: FETAL NIGRAL TRANSPLANTATION

Our finding of robust survival of TH-IR neurons with organotypic striatal reinnervation in PD patients who had undergone a fetal nigral transplant procedure provided essential confirmation of the hypothesis that fetal nigral grafts can survive and mediate clinical recovery as predicted by animal studies. As exciting as these observations are, enthusiasm is tempered by the fact that, despite excellent graft survival and impressive striatal innervation, no patient has yet been cured of parkinsonism, and there is a major concern that transplantation may be complicated by severe dyskinesia. We observed the survival of seemingly supranormal numbers of dopamine-containing neurons within the putamen in both of our transplant cases which came to autopsy, but patients only displayed partial recovery. The most parsimonious explanation is that, despite supranormal numbers of grafted nigral neurons, there was a subnormal pattern of innervation. In our first case, the graft provided dopaminergic innervation to only 53 percent and 28 percent of the right and left putamen, respectively.[124] It is possible that this innervation pattern might have continued to increase over time as progressive increases in FD uptake were seen on PET scan in both of these cases. Furthermore, grafted patients from other centers have continued to show clinical improvement over prolonged periods of time.[112] However, more immediate clinical benefits are required. In this regard, it is noteworthy that, even though we observed an impressive number of surviving dopaminergic neurons following transplant, this still represents only a small fraction (5–10 percent) of the original population of grafted cells. Enhanced survival or larger numbers of donors might provide better clinical results. It is thus possible that there is a window of opportunity to improve upon the transplantation procedure and improve on clinical results by manipulation of transplant variables. Towards that end there is interest in combining transplantation with antioxidants, and antiapoptotic agents.[141,142] It is also possible that transplantation into multiple or different targets such as the SNc might enhance clinical benefit.[69]

Improving neurite outgrowth from the graft might also enhance the magnitude of functional benefit and the speed over which recovery occurs. One method for improving neurite outgrowth from grafted dopaminergic neurons is to expose them in vitro or in vivo to trophic factors. Many different neurotrophic factors support the viability and/or phenotypic expression of dopaminergic neurons,[143] including brain-derived neurotrophic factor (BDNF), basic fibroblast growth factor (bFGF), and glial cell-derived neurotrophic factor (GDNF). BDNF has been demonstrated to enhance neurite outgrowth from BDNF-producing cells in vitro.[144] We have genetically modified oligodendroglia to secrete BDNF and shown that, when these cells are co-cultured with fetal nigral neurons, neurite outgrowth and neuron viability can be enhanced. After grafting fetal nigral tissue to the dopamine-depleted striatum, rats treated with chronic intraventricular infusions or daily intrastriatal injections of BDNF display a significant reduction in ipsiversive rotations following amphetamine administration.[144] However, BDNF has not been shown to have a significant effect upon cell survival, suggesting that BDNF may act as a tropic rather than a trophic factor for implanted fetal nigral neurons. Other trophic factors can also influence the effects of fetal nigral grafting. GDNF has also been shown to promote the survival and phenotypic differentiation of fetal rat midbrain dopaminergic neurons in culture.[145] GDNF has also been shown to enhance the viability and neurite outgrowth of grafted nigral neurons, and to potentiate functional recovery in unilateral 6-OHDA-lesioned rats and MPTP-lesioned primates.[146] Ultimately, the use of these trophic factors, either alone or in combination, may optimize graft viability, neurite outgrowth, and hopefully functional recovery. In addition, there is emerging interest in the direct delivery of trophic factors to the striatum as a treatment for PD. Initial trials failed to benefit PD patients with delivery of GDNF to the lateral ventricle, but this approach may not have resulted in adequate brain penetration.[147] More recently, clinical improvement has been reported in small numbers of patients with direct infusion of GDNF into the striatum.[148] Prospective double-blind trials of this therapy is now being tested.

FUTURE DIRECTIONS: STEM CELLS

Even if the parameters for fetal nigral grafting can be optimized so as to provide greater clinical efficacy and the issue of off-medication dyskinesia can be resolved, difficulties in tissue procurement as well as societal and ethical concerns related to the use of embryonic tissue makes this source of tissue impractical for treating large numbers of PD patients. The future of cell replacement therapy seems to clearly rest with the use of stem cells, a multipotential self-renewing source of neurons and glia. Stem cells can be obtained from embryos, fetuses, bone marrow, and even adult CNS, although presently the embryonic stem cell is the most manipulable in vitro and the best donor source for transplantation. It has now been shown that embryonic stem cells can be induced to differentiate in dopamine cells,[149] and that grafts of mouse embryonic stem cells can survive and reverse motor features of parkinsonism in the 6-OHDA rodent model of parkinsonism.[150,151] However, behavioral results are not as profound as are seen with transplantation of fetal nigral cells. Further, in one study significant numbers of animals developed teratomas.[150] Understanding growth control parameters for stem cell transplants as well as how to enhance upon the benefits found with fetal cells as well as avoid problems such as off-medication dyskinesia are critical to bringing this technology forward for clinical trials in PD patients. Studies are ongoing from multiple groups around the world testing the ability of human stem cells to survive, innervate the striatum and reverse functional deficits in rodent and nonhuman primate models of PD.

FUTURE DIRECTIONS: GENE THERAPY

The entrance of molecular biology into the field of neural transplantation has greatly extended our ability to generate cell lines that may be candidates for transplantation in PD. Ex vivo and in vivo gene therapy approaches have now become commonplace methods for inducing the expression of a particular gene product. In a relatively straightforward manner, genes encoding specific proteins can be transfected into dividing cells using viral vectors and then transplanted into the brain where these proteins will hopefully continue to be expressed. In some circumstances, cells manipulated in this manner have been shown to induce anatomical and/or functional changes following grafting in a manner comparable to that seen following direct infusion of the specific protein. Rosenberg et al.[152] and Wolff et al.,[153] as well as others,[154] initially utilized genetically modified fibroblasts as donor cells for transplantation. Currently, in vivo gene therapy has been used to deliver therapeutic molecules to the brain in rodent and nonhuman primate models of PD. We have used a lentivirus to deliver GDNF to aged and MPTP-treated monkeys based on the beneficial results observed with direct injections in rodent and primate models of parkinsonism. In parkinsonian monkeys, we observed behavioral improvement coupled with complete protection of nigral neurons and striatal dopamine.[155] Gene delivery of GDNF also increases TH mRNA expression in nigral neurons in aged and parkinsonian monkeys. Studies in rodents also demonstrate the ability of gene delivery of GDNF and other proteins to prevent the structural and functional consequences of experimental parkinsonism. These results can be obtained with no evident adverse effects to the animal, although long-term studies, particularly with respect to the risk of inducing dyskinesia, are required. Initial studies in marmosets suggest that gene delivery of GDNF reduces, and does not exacerbate, dyskinesias. Further studies are needed to confirm this observation. Instead of aiming for neuroprotection, Bankiewicz et al. have used gene therapy to deliver amino acid decarboxylase to parkinsonian monkeys. The premise behind this approach is to augment the ability of exogenous L-dopa to provide symptomatic benefit by enhancing its conversion to dopamine. This approach may reduce the likelihood of dyskinesias by permitting dopamine to be delivered to the brain in a more continuous manner. There is also interest in using gene therapy to deliver glutamic acid decarboxylase to the subthalamic nucleus (STN) in an attempt to suppress the overexpression of neuronal firing in this target that is thought to contribute to PD features. However, excessive suppression of STN activity could lead to hemiballismus, and trials in nonhuman primates should be performed prior to entering into clinical trials in PD.

In considering gene therapies for PD, several issues need to be considered, including the specific protein that should be transferred, the target site, the vector, the promoter, and whether or not to include a regulatory system that has the capacity to control excessive growth of the virus or the protein.[156] While there are many issues to resolve, this approach offers the prospect of being able to deliver a desired protein to a specific brain target and accordingly offers hope as a treatment for PD.

Conclusion

In summary, the status of transplantation as a treatment for PD is more confusing than at the time of the last writing. Today, we have demonstrated that large numbers of fetal neurons can survive grafting and reinnervate the striatum. However, transplantation was not demonstrated to provide clinical benefits superior to placebo in double-blind studies, and treatment is complicated by a potentially disabling off-medication dyskinesia. Thus, fetal nigral transplantation cannot be recommended as a therapy for PD today, and further testing in PD patients cannot be performed until we understand why these problems have occurred. The mechanisms responsible for these limitations are not known, but a body of evidence is beginning to suggest that both problems may be related to incomplete striatal reinnervation. It is possible that transplant protocols that permit survival of larger numbers of cells may provide better results. The development of stem cell transplantation, gene therapy, and trophic factors as treatments for PD offer additional opportunities. Current experience, however, indicates that the safety and efficacy of these approaches will have to be well studied in the laboratory before beginning clinical trials and that ultimately success in double-blind controlled studies will be required.

References

1. Olanow CW: Parkinson's disease: Clinical crossroads. *JAMA* 275:716–722, 1996.
2. Fahn S: Adverse effects of levodopa, in Olanow CW, Lieberman AN (eds): *The Scientific Basis for the Treatment of Parkinson's Disease.* Lancaster: Parthenon, 1992, pp 89–112.
3. Olanow CW, Watts RL, Koller WC: An algorithm (decision tree) for the management of Parkinson's disease (2001): Treatment guidelines. *Neurology* 56(suppl 5):1–88, 2001.
4. Bjorklund A, Stenevi U: Reconstruction of the nigrostriatal dopamine pathway by intracerebral nigral transplants. *Brain Res* 177:555–560, 1979.
5. Dunnett SB, Bjorklund A, Stenevi U, Iversen SD: Behavioral recovery following transplantation of substantia nigra in rats

subjected to 6-OHDA lesions of the nigrostriatal pathway. *Brain Res* 215:147–161, 1981.

6. Perlow MJ, Freed WJ, Hoffer BJ, et al: Brain grafts reduce motor abnormalities produced by destruction of nigro-striatal dopamine system. *Science* 204:643–647, 1979.

7. Bjorklund A, Stenevi U, Dunnett SB, et al: Functional reactivation of the deafferented neostriatum by nigral transplants. *Nature* 289:497–499, 1981.

8. Brundin P, Bjorklund A: Survival, growth and function of dopaminergic neurons grafted to the brain. *Prog Brain Res* 71:293–308, 1987.

9. Sladek JR Jr, Collier TC, Haber SN, et al: Survival and growth of fetal catecholamine neurons transplanted into the primate brain. *Brain Res Bull* 17:809–818, 1986.

10. Sladek JR Jr, Redmond DE, Collier TC, et al: Fetal dopamine neural grafts: Extended reversal of methylphenyltetrahydropyridine-induced parkinsonism in primates. *Prog Brain Res* 78:497–506, 1988.

11. Redmond DE, Roth RH, Elsworth JD, et al: Fetal neuronal grafts in monkeys given methyl-phenyl-tetrahydro-pyridine. *Lancet* May:1125–1127, 1986.

12. Bakay RAE, Barrow DL, Fiandaca MS, et al: Biochemical and behavioral correction of MPTP-like syndrome by fetal cell transplantation. *Ann N Y Acad Sci* 495:623–640, 1987.

13. Fine A, Hunt SB, Oertel WH, et al: Transplantation of embryonic dopaminergic neurons to the corpus striatum of marmosets rendered parkinsonian by 1-methyl-4-phenyl-1,2,3,6–tetrahydropyridine. *Prog Brain Res* 78:479–490, 1988.

14. Bankiewicz KS, Plunkett RJ, Jacobawitz DM, et al: The effect of fetal mesencephalon implants on primate MPTP-induced parkinsonism. *J Neurosurg* 72:231–244, 1990.

15. Mahalick TJ, Finger TE, Stromberg I, et al: Substantia nigra transplants into denervated striatum of the rat: Ultrastructure of graft-host interconnections. *J Comp Neurol* 240:60–70, 1985.

16. Bjorklund A, Stenevi U, Schmidt RH, et al: Intracerebral grafting of neuronal cell suspensions. II. Survival and growth of nigral cell suspensions implanted in different brain sites. *Acta Physiol Scand* 522:9–18, 1983.

17. Wuerthele SM, Freed WJ, Olson L, et al: Effects of dopamine agonists and antagonists on the electrical activity of substantia nigra neurons transplanted into the lateral of the rat. *Exp Brain Res* 44:1–10, 1981.

18. Schmidt RH, Ingvar M, Lindvall O, et al: Functional activity of substantia nigra grafts reinnervating the striatum: Neurotransmitter metabolism and (14C)-2-deoxy-D-glucose autoradiography. *J Neurochem* 38:737–748, 1982.

19. Freed WJ, Perlow MJ, Karoum F, et al: Restoration of dopamine brain function by grafting fetal substantia nigra to the caudate nucleus: Long term behavioral, biochemical, and histological studies. *Ann Neurol* 8:510–523, 1980.

20. Brundin P, Strecker RE, Widner H, et al: Human fetal dopamine neurons grafted in a rat model of Parkinson's disease: Immunological aspects, spontaneous and drug-induced behavior, and dopamine release. *Exp Brain Res* 70:192–208, 1988.

21. Stromberg I, Almqvist P, Bygdeman M, et al: Human fetal mesencephalic tissue grafted to dopamine-denervated striatum of athymic rats: Light and electron microscopic histochemical and in vivo chronoamperometric studies. *J Neurosci* 614–624, 1989.

22. van Horne CG, Mahalik T, Hoffer B, et al: Behavioral and electrophysiological correlates of human mesencephalic dopamine

xenograft function in the rat striatum. *Brain Res Bull* 25:325–334, 1990.

23. Clarke DJ, Brundin P, Strecker RE, et al: Human fetal dopamine neurons grafted in a rat model of Parkinson's disease: Ultrastructural evidence for synapse formation using tyrosine hydroxylase immunocytochemistry. *Exp Brain Res* 73:115–126, 1988.

24. Brundin P, Widner H, Nilsson OG, et al: Intracerebral xenografts of dopamine neurons: The role of immunosuppression and the blood-brain barrier. *Exp Brain Res* 75:195–207, 1989.

25. Dunnett SB, Hernandez TD, Summerfield A, et al: Graft-derived recovery from 6-OHDA lesions: Specificity of ventral mesencephalic graft tissues. *Exp Brain Res* 71:411–424, 1988.

26. Itakura T, Kamei I, Nakai K, et al: Autotransplantation of the superior cervical ganglion into the brain. A possible therapy for Parkinson's disease. *J Neurosurg* 68:955–959, 1988.

27. Pasik P, Martinez JF, Yahr MD, et al: Grafting of human sympathetic ganglia into the brain of MPTP-treated monkeys. *Soc Neurosci Abstr* 5–6, 1988.

28. Hefti F, Hartikka J, Schlumpf M: Implantation of PC12 cells into the corpus striatum of rats with lesions of the dopaminergic nigrostriatal neurons. *Brain Res* 348:283–288, 1985.

29. Freed WJ, Patel-Vaidya U, Geller HM: Properties of PC12 pheochromocytoma cells transplanted to the adult rat brain. *Exp Brain Res* 63:557–566, 1986.

30. Jaeger CB: Morphological and immunocytochemical characteristics of PC12 cell grafts in rat brain. *Ann N Y Acad Sci* 495:334–349, 1987.

31. Freed WJ, Morihisa JM, Spoor E, et al: Transplanted adrenal chromaffin cells in rat brain reduce lesion-induced rotational behavior. *Nature* 292:351–352, 1981.

32. Stromberg I, Herrera-Marschitz M, Ungerstedt U, et al: Chronic implants of chromaffin tissue into the dopamine-denervated striatum. Effects of NGF on graft survival, fiber growth and rotational behavior. *Exp Brain Res* 60:335–349, 1985.

33. Freed WJ, Cannon-Spoor HE, Krauthamer E: Intrastriatal adrenal medulla grafts in rats: Long-term survival and behavioral effects. *J Neurosurg* 65:664–670, 1986.

34. Bankiewicz KS, Plunkett RJ, Jacobowitz DM, et al: Fetal non-dopaminergic neural implants in parkinsonian primates. *J Neurosurg* 74:97–104, 1991.

35. Backlund EO, Granberg PO, Hamberger B, et al: Transplantation of adrenal medullary tissue to striatum in parkinsonism. First clinical trials. *J Neurosurg* 62:169–173, 1985.

36. Lindvall O, Backlund EO, Farde L, et al: Transplantation in Parkinson's disease: Two cases of adrenal medullary grafts to the putamen. *Ann Neurol* 22:457–468, 1987.

37. Madrazo I, Drucker-Colin R, Diaz V, et al: Open microsurgical autograft of adrenal medulla to right caudate nucleus in two patients with intractable Parkinson's disease. *N Engl J Med* 316:831–834, 1987.

38. Goetz CG, Olanow CW, Koller WC, et al: Multicenter study of autologous adrenal medullary transplantation to the corpus striatum in patients with advanced Parkinson's disease. *N Engl J Med* 320:337–341, 1989.

39. Olanow CW, Koller W, Goetz CG, et al: Autologous transplantation of adrenal medulla in Parkinson's disease. *Arch Neurol* 47:1286–1289, 1990.

40. Allen GS, Burns RS, Tulipan NB, Parker RA: Adrenal medullary transplantation to the caudate nucleus in Parkinson's disease.

Initial clinical results in 18 patients. *Arch Neurol* 46:487–491, 1989.

41. Jankovic J, Grossman R, Goodman C, et al: Clinical, biochemical, and neuropathologic findings following transplantation of adrenal medulla to the caudate nucleus for treatment of Parkinson's disease. *Neurology* 39:1227–1234, 1989.

42. Goetz CG, Stebbins GT, Klawans HL, et al: United Parkinson Foundation Neurotransplantation Registry on adrenal medullary transplants: Presurgical, and 1- and 2-year followup. *Neurology* 41:1719–1722, 1991.

43. Kordower JH, Cochran E, Penn R, et al: Putative chromaffin cell survival and enhanced host derived TH-fiber innervation following a functional adrenal medulla autograft for Parkinson's disease. *Ann Neurol* 29:405–412, 1991.

44. Branch DW, Ducat L, Fantel A, et al: Suitability of fetal tissue from spontaneous abortions and from ectopic pregnancies for transplantation. *JAMA* 273:64–65, 1995.

45. Kondoh T, Blount JP, Conrad JA, et al: Functional effects of transplanted human fetal ventral mesencephalic brain tissue from spontaneous abortions into a rodent model of Parkinson's disease. *Transplant Proc* 26:335, 1994.

46. Freeman TB, Olanow CW: Fetal homotransplants. *Arch Neurol* 40:1529–1534, 1990.

47. Center for Disease Control: *Abortion Surveillance 1981*. Atlanta: US DHHS Public Health Service, 1985.

48. Freeman TB, Spence MS, Boss BD, et al: Development of dopaminergic neurons in the human substantia nigra. *Exp Neurol* 113:344–353, 1991.

49. Freeman TB, Sanberg PR, Nauert GM, et al: The influence of donor age on the survival of solid and suspension intraparenchymal human embryonic nigral grafts. *Cell Transplant* 4:141–154, 1995.

50. Redmond DE Jr, Naftolin F, Collier TJ, et al: Cryopreservation, culture, and transplantation of human fetal mesencephalic tissue into monkeys. *Science* 242:820–822, 1988.

51. Collier TJ, Gallagher MJ, Sladek CD: Cryopreservation and storage of embryonic rat mesencephalic dopamine neurons for one year: Comparison to fresh tissue in culture and neural grafts. *Brain Res* 623:249–256, 1993.

52. Kontur PJ, Leranth C, Redmond DE Jr, et al: Tyrosine hydroxylase immunoreactivity and monoamine metabolite levels in cryopreserved human fetal ventral mesencephalon. *Exp Neurol* 121:172–180, 1993.

53. Freed CR, Breeze RE, Rosenberg NL, et al: Survival of implanted fetal dopamine cells and neurologic improvement 12 to 46 months after transplantation for Parkinson's disease. *N Engl J Med* 327:1549–1555, 1992.

54. Freeman TB, Kordower JH: Human cadaver embryonic substantia nigra grafts: Effects of ontogeny, pre-operative graft preparation and tissue storage, in Lindvall O, Bjorklund A, Widner H (eds): *Intracerebral Transplantation in Movement Disorders*. New York: Elsevier, 1991, pp 163–184.

55. Freeman TB, Olanow CW, Hauser RA, et al: Bilateral fetal nigral transplantation as a treatment for Parkinson's disease. *Ann Neurol* 38:379–388, 1995.

56. Bayer SA: Neurogenesis in the rat neostriatum. *Int J Dev Neurosci* 2:1163–1175, 1984.

57. Kunzle H: Bilateral projections from precentral motor cortex to the putamen and other parts of the basal ganglia. An autoradiographic study in *Macaca fascicularis*. *Brain Behav Evol* 88:195–209, 1975.

58. Alexander GE, Crutcher MD, DeLong MR: Basal ganglia-thalamocortical circuits: Parallel substrates for motor, oculomotor, 'prefrontal' and 'limbic' functions. *Prog Brain Res* 85:119–146, 1990.

59. Alexander GE, DeLong MR: Microstimulation of the primate neostriatum. II. Somatotopic organization of striatal microexcitable zones and their relation to neuronal response properties. *J Neurophysiol* 53:1417–1430, 1985.

60. Kunzle H: An autoradiographic analysis of the efferent connections from premotor and adjacent prefrontal regions (areas 6 and 9) in *Macaca fascicularis*. *Brain Behav Evol* 15:185–234, 1978.

61. Dunnett SB, Bjorklund A, Stenevi U, Iversen SD: Behavioral recovery following transplantation of substantia nigra in rats subjected to 6-OHDA lesions of the nigrostriatal pathway. *Brain Res* 215:147–161, 1981.

62. Dunnett SB, Bjorklund A, Schmidt RH, et al: Intracerebral grafting of neuronal cell suspensions IV. Behavioral recovery in rats with unilateral 6-OHDA lesions following implantation of nigral cell suspensions in different forebrain sites. *Acta Physiol Scand* 522:29–37, 1983.

63. Dunnett SB, Annett LE: Nigral transplants in primate models of parkinsonism, in Lindvall O, Bjorklund A, Widner H (eds): *Intracerebral Transplantation in Movement Disorders*. New York: Elsevier, 1991, pp 27–50.

64. Kish SJ, Shannak K, Hornykiewica O: Uneven pattern of dopamine loss in the striatum of patients with idiopathic Parkinson's disease. Pathophysiologic and clinical implications. *N Engl J Med* 318:876–880, 1988.

65. Nyberg P, Nordberg A, Webster P: Dopaminergic deficiency is more pronounced in putamen than in nucleus caudatus in Parkinson's disease. *Neurochem Pathol* 1:193–202, 1983.

66. Leenders KL, Salmon EP, Tyrrell P, et al: The nigrostriatal dopaminergic system assessed in vivo by positron emission tomography in healthy volunteer subjects and patients with Parkinson's disease. *Arch Neurol* 47:1290–1297, 1990.

67. Szabo J: Organization of the ascending striatal afferents in monkeys. *J Comp Neurol* 189:307–321, 1980.

68. Imai H, Nakamura T, Endo K, et al: Hemiparkinsonism in monkeys after unilateral caudate nucleus infusion of 1-methyl-4-phenyl-1,2,3,6-tetrahydropyridine (MPTP): Behavior and histology. *Brain Res* 474:327–332, 1988.

69. Mendez I, Dagher A, Hong M, et al: Simultaneous intrastriatal and intranigral fetal dopaminergic grafts in patients with Parkinson disease: A pilot study. Report of three cases. *J Neurosurg* 96:589–596, 2002.

70. Brundin P, Isacson O, Bjorklund A: Monitoring of cell viability in suspensions of embryonic CNS tissue and its use as a criterion for intracerebral graft survival. *Brain Res* 331:251–259, 1985.

71. Pakkenberg B, Moller A, Gunderson HJG, et al: The absolute number of nerve cells in substantia nigra normal subjects and in patients with Parkinson's disease estimated with an unbiased stereological method. *J Neurol Neurosurg Psychiatry* 54:30–33, 1991.

72. Frodl EM, Duan WM, Sauer H, et al: Human embryonic dopamine neurons xenografted to rat: Effect of cryopreservation and varying regional source of donor cells on transplant survival and morphology. *Brain Res* 647:286–298, 1994.

73. Schultzberg M, Dunnett SB, Bjorklund A, et al: Dopamine and cholecystokinin immunoreactive neurones in mesencephalic

grafts reinnervating the neostriatum: Evidence for selective growth regulation. *Neuroscience* 12:17–32, 1984.

74. Horellou P, Brundin P, Kalen P, et al: In vivo release of DOPA and dopamine from genetically engineered cells grafted to the denervated rat striatum. *Neuron* 5:393–402, 1990.

75. Sendeldeck SL, Urquhart J: Spatial distribution of dopamine, methotrexate, and antipyrine during continuous intracerebral microperfusion. *Brain Res* 328:251–258, 1985.

76. Kordower JH, Freeman TB, Snow BJ, et al: Neuropathological evidence of graft survival and striatal reinnervation after the transplantation of fetal mesencephalic tissue in a patient with Parkinson's disease. *N Engl J Med* 332:1118–1124, 1995.

77. Yurek DM, Steece-Collier K, Collier TJ, Sladek JR Jr: Chronic levodopa impairs the recovery of dopamine agonist-induced rotational behavior following neural grafting. *Exp Brain Res* 86:97–107, 1991.

78. Fiandaca MS, Kordower JH, Hansen JT, et al: Adrenal medullary autografts into the basal ganglia of Cebus monkeys: Injury-induced regeneration. *Exp Neurol* 102:76–91, 1988.

79. Hitchcock ER, Clough C, Hughes R, Kenny B: Embryos and Parkinson's disease. *Lancet* i:1274, 1988.

80. Freed CR, Breeze RE, Rosenberg NL, et al: Transplantation of human fetal dopamine cells for Parkinson's disease. Results at one year. *Arch Neurol* 47:505–512, 1990.

81. Wekerle H, Linington C, Lassmann H, Meyerman R: Cellular reactivity within the CNS. *Trends Neurosci* 6:271, 1986.

82. Inoue H, Kohsaka S, Yoshida K, et al: Cyclosporin A enhances the survivability of mouse cerebral cortex grafted into the third ventricle of rat brain. *Neurosci Lett* 54:85, 1985.

83. Nicholas MK, Antel JP, Stefansson K, Arnason BGW: Rejection of fetal neocortical neural transplants by H-2 incompatible mice. *J Immunol* 139:2275–2283, 1987.

84. Kordower JH, Styren S, DeKosky ST, et al: Fetal grafting for Parkinson's disease: Expression of immune markers in two patients with functional fetal nigral implants. *Cell Transplant* 6:213–219, 1997.

85. Borlongan CV, Freeman TB, Sorcia TA, et al: Cyclosporine A increases spontaneous and dopamine agonist-induced locomotor behavior in normal rats. *Cell Transplant* 4:65–73, 1995.

86. McGeer PL, Itagaki S, Boyes BE, McGeer EG: Reactive microglia are positive for HLA-DR in the substantia nigra of Parkinson and Alzheimer's disease brains. *Neurology* 38:1285–1291, 1988.

87. Scorrano L, Nicolli A, Basso E, et al: Two modes of activation of the permeability transition pore: The role of mitochondrial cyclophilin. *Mol Cell Biochem* 174:181–184, 1997.

88. Langston JW, Widner H, Brooks D, et al: Core assessment program for intracerebral transplantations (CAPIT). *Mov Disord* 7:2–13, 1992.

89. Lang AE, Benabid A-I, Koller WC, et al: The core assessment program for cerebral transplantation. *Mov Disord* 10:527–528, 1995.

90. Pirrozzolo FJ, Hansch EC, Mortimer JA, et al: Dementia in Parkinson's disease: A neuropsychological analysis. *Brain Cogn* 1:71–83, 1982.

91. Brown RG, Marsden CD: Dual tasks performance and processing resources in normal subjects and patients with Parkinson's disease. *Brain* 114:1215–1231, 1991.

92. Sagar HJ, Sullivan EV, Gabrieli JDE, et al: Temporal ordering and short-term memory deficits in Parkinson's disease. *Brain* 111:525–539, 1988.

93. Taylor AE, Saint-Cyr JA, Lang AE: Frontal lobe dysfunction in Parkinson's disease. *Brain* 109:845–883, 1986.

94. Martin WRW, Palmer MR, Patlak CS, Calne DB: Nigrostriatal function in man studied with positron emission tomography. *Ann Neurol* 26:535–542, 1989.

95. Patlak CS, Blasberg RG: Graphical evaluation of blood-to-brain transfer constants from multiple-time uptake data. Generalizations. *J Cereb Blood Flow Metab* 5:584–590, 1985.

96. Snow BJ, Tooyama I, McGeer EG, et al: Human positron emission tomographic [18F]-fluorodopa studies correlate with dopamine cell counts and levels. *Ann Neurol* 34:324–330, 1993.

97. de la Fuente-Fernandez R, Stoessl AJ: Parkinson's disease: Imaging update. *Curr Opin Neurol* 15:477–482, 2002.

98. Remy P, Samson Y, Hantraye P, et al: Clinical correlates of [18F] fluorodopa uptake in five grafted Parkinsonian patients. *Ann Neurol* 38:580–588, 1995.

99. Lindvall O, Brundin P, Widner H, et al: Grafts of fetal dopamine neurons survive and improve motor function in Parkinson's disease. *Science* 247:574–577, 1990.

100. Sawle GV, Bloomfield PM, Bjorklund A, et al: Transplantation of fetal dopamine neurons in Parkinson's disease: PET [18F]-6-L-fluorodopa studies in two patients with putaminal implants. *Ann Neurol* 31:166–173, 1992.

101. Widner H, Tetrud JW, Rehncrona S, et al: Bilateral fetal mesencephalic grafting in two patients with MPTP-induced parkinsonism. *N Engl J Med* 327:1556–1563, 1992.

102. Sawle GV, Myers R: The role of positron emission tomography in the assessment of human neurotransplantation. *Trends Neurosci* 16:172–176, 1993.

103. Kordower JH, Freeman TB, Olanow CW: Neuropathology of fetal nigral grafts in patients with Parkinson's disease. *Mov Disord* 13:88–95, 1998.

104. Guttman M, Burns RS, Martin WRW, et al: PET studies of parkinsonian patients treated with autologous adrenal transplants. *Can J Neurol Sci* 16:305–309, 1989.

105. Piccini P, Brooks DJ, Bjorklund A, et al: Dopamine release from nigral transplants visualized in vivo in a parkinsonian patient. *Nat Neurosci* 2:1137–1140, 1999.

106. Olanow CW, Gauger LL, Cedarbaum J: Temporal relationships between plasma and CSF pharmacokinetics of levodopa and clinical effect in Parkinson's disease. *Ann Neurol* 29:556–559, 1991.

107. Olanow CW: Oxidation reactions in Parkinson's disease. *Neurology* 40:32–37, 1990.

108. Mytilineou C, Han S-K, Cohen G: Toxic and protective effects of L-DOPA on mesencephalic cell cultures. *J Neurochem* 61:1470–1478, 1993.

109. Agid Y, Olanow CW, Mizuno Y: Levodopa: Why the controversy? *Lancet* 360:575, 2002.

110. Lindvall O, Sawle G, Widner H, et al: Evidence for long-term survival and function of dopaminergic grafts in progressive Parkinson's disease. *Ann Neurol* 35:1172–1180, 1994.

111. Lindvall O, Rechncrona S, Brundin P, et al: Human fetal dopamine neurons grafted into the striatum in two patients with Parkinson's disease: A detailed account of methodology and 6 month follow-up. *Arch Neurol* 46:615–631, 1989.

112. Lindvall O, Widner H, Rehncrona S, et al: Transplantation of fetal dopamine neurons in Parkinson's disease: One-year clinical and neurophysiological observations in two patients with putaminal implants. *Ann Neurol* 31:155–165, 1992.

113. Spencer DD, Robbins RJ, Naftolin F, et al: Unilateral transplantation of human fetal mesencephalic tissue into the caudate nucleus of patients with Parkinson's disease. *N Engl J Med* 327:1541–1548, 1992.

114. Peschanski M, Defer G, N'Guyen JP, et al: Bilateral motor improvement and alteration of L-dopa effect in 2 patients with Parkinson's disease following intrastriatal transplantation of foetal ventral mesencephalon. *Brain* 117:487–499, 1994.

115. Defer GL, Geny C, Ficolfi F, et al: Long-term outcome of unilaterally transplanted parkinsonian patients. I. Clinical approach. *Brain* 119:41–50, 1996.

116. Hauser RA, Freeman TB, Snow BJ, et al: Long-term evaluation of bilateral fetal nigral transplantation in Parkinson's disease. *Arch Neurol* 56:179–187, 1999.

117. Kordower JH, Freeman TB, Chen E-Y, et al: Fetal nigral grafts survive and mediate clinical benefit in a patient with Parkinson's disease. *Mov Disord* 13:383–393, 1998.

118. Olanow CW, Freeman TB, Kordower JH: Fetal nigral transplantation as a therapy for Parkinson's disease. *Trends Neurosci* 19:102–109, 1996.

119. Hitchcock ER, Clough C, Hughes R, Kenny B: Embryos and Parkinson's disease. *Lancet* i:1274, 1988.

120.

121.

122. Kordower JH, Freeman TB, Bakay RAE, et al: Treatment with fetal allografts. *Neurology* 48:1737–1738, 1997.

123. Redmond DE Jr, Leranth C, Spencer DD, et al: Fetal neural graft survival. *Lancet* 336:820–822, 1990.

124. Kordower JH, Rosenstein JM, Collier TM, et al: Functional fetal nigral grafts in a patient with Parkinson's disease: Chemoanatomic, quantitative, ultrastructural, and metabolic studies. *JCN* 370:203–230, 1996.

125. Kordower JH, Styren S, DeKosky ST, et al: Fetal grafting for Parkinson's disease: Expression of immune markers in two patients with functional fetal nigral implants. *Cell Transplant* 6:213–219, 1997.

126. Bohn MC, Cupit L, Marciano F, et al: Adrenal medulla grafts enhance recovery of striatal dopaminergic fibers. *Science* 237:913–915, 1987.

127. Bohn MC, Cupit L, Marciano F, et al: Adrenal medulla autografts into the basal ganglia of cebus monkeys: Injury-induced regeneration. *Exp Neurol* 102:76–91, 1988.

128. Guttman M, Burns RS, Martin WRW, et al: PET studies of parkinsonian patients treated with autologous adrenal transplants. *Can J Neurol Sci* 16:305–309, 1989.

129. Beecher HK: Surgery as placebo. *JAMA* 176:1102–1107, 1961.

130. The EC/IC Bypass Study Group: Failure of extracranial/intra-cranial arterial bypass to reduce the risk of ischemic stroke. *N Engl J Med* 313:1191–1200, 1985.

131. Orthopedic study.

132. Freeman TB, Vawter DE, Leaverton PE, et al: The use of a surgical placebo-control in evaluating cellular-based therapy for Parkinson's disease. *N Engl J Med* 341:988–992, 1999.

133. Freed CR, Greene PE, Breeze RE, et al: Transplantation of embryonic dopamine neurons for severe Parkinson's disease. *N Engl J Med* 344:710–719, 2001.

134. Dhawan V, Nakamura T, Margouleff C, et al: Double-blind controlled trial of human embryonic dopaminergic tissue transplants in advanced Parkinson's disease: Fluorodopa PET imaging. *Neurology* 52:405, 1999.

135. Greene PE, Fahn S, Tsai WY, et al: Severe spontaneous dyskinesias: A disabling complication of embryonic dopaminergic tissue implants in a subset of transplanted patients with advanced Parkinson's disease. *Mov Disord* 904, 1999.

136. Cubo E, Gracies JM, Benabou R, et al: Early morning off-medication dyskinesias, dystonia, and choreic subtypes. *Arch Neurol* 58:1379–1382, 2001.

137. Ma Y, Feigin A, Dhawan V, et al: Dyskinesia after fetal cell transplantation for parkinsonism: A PET study. *Ann Neurol* 52:628–634, 2002.

138. Obeso JA, Rodriguez-Oroz MC, Rodriguez M, et al: Pathophysiology of levodopa-induced dyskinesias in Parkinson's disease: Problems with current models of the basal ganglia. *Ann Neurol* 47:22–34, 2000.

139. Lee CS, Cenci MA, Schulzer M, Bjorklund A: Embryonic ventral mesencephalic grafts improve levodopa-induced dyskinesia in a rat model of Parkinson's disease. *Brain* 123:1365–1379, 2000.

140. Deacon T, Schumacher J, Dinsmore J, et al: Histological evidence of fetal pig neural cell survival after transplantation into a patient with Parkinson's disease. *Nat Med* 3:350–353, 1997.

141. Brundin P, Pogarell O, Hagell P, et al: Bilateral caudate and putamen grafts of embryonic mesencephalic tissue treated with lazaroids in Parkinson's disease. *Brain* 123:1380–1390, 2000.

142. Hansson O, Castilho RF, Kaminski Schierle GS, et al: Additive effects of caspase inhibitor and lazaroid on the survival of transplanted rat and human embryonic dopamine neurons. *Exp Neurol* 164:102–111, 2000.

143. Lindsay RM, Wiegand SJ, Altar CA, Distephano PS: Neurotrophic factors: From molecule to man. *Trends Neurosci* 17:182–190, 1994.

144. Hyman C, Hofer M, Barde Y-A, et al: BDNF is a neurotrophic factor for dopaminergic neurons of the substantia nigra. *Nature* 350:230–232, 1991.

145. Sauer H, Fischer W, Nikkah G, et al: Brain derived neurotrophic factors enhance function rather than survival of intrastriatal dopamine cell-rich grafts. *Brain Res* 626:37–44, 1993.

146. Lin L-F, Doherty DH, Lile JD, et al: A glial cell line-derived neurotrophic factor for midbrain dopaminergic neurons. *Science* 260:1130–1132, 1993.

147. Gash DM, Zhang Z, Ovadia A, et al: Functional recovery in parkinsonian monkeys treated with GDNF. *Nature* 380:252–255, 1996.

148. Nutt JG, Burchiel KG, Comella CL, et al: Randomized double blind trial of glial cell line derived neurotrophic factor (GDNF) in PD. *Neurology* 14:69–73, 2003.

149. Gill SS, Patel NK, Hotton GR, et al: Direct brain infusion of glial cell line derived neurotrophic factor in Parkinson's disease. *Nat Med* 9:589–595, 2003.

150. Lee SA, Lumelsky N, Studer L, et al: Efficient generation of midbrain and hindbrain neurons from mouse embryonic stem cells. *Nat Biotechnol* 18:675–679, 2000.

151. Bjorklund LM, Sánchez-Pernaute R, Chung S, et al: Embryonic stem cells develop into functional dopaminergic neurons after transplantation in a Parkinson rat model. *Proc Natl Acad Sci U S A* 99:2344–2349, 2000.

152. Kim J-H, Auerbach JM, Rodriguez-Gomez JA, et al: Dopamine neurons derived from embryonic stem cells function in an animal model of Parkinson's disease. *Nature* 418:50–56, 2002.

153. Rosenberg MB, Friedmann T, Robertson RC, et al: Grafting genetically modified cells to the damaged brain: Restorative effects of NGF expression. *Science* 242:157, 1988.

154. Wolff JA, Fisher LJ, Xu L, et al: Grafting fibroblasts genetically modified to produce L-dopa in a rat model of Parkinson's disease. *Proc Natl Acad Sci U S A* 86:9011, 1989.

155. Frim DM, Short MP, Rosenberg UC, et al: Local protective effects of nerve growth factor secreting fibroblasts against excitotoxic lesions in the rat striatum. *J Neurosurg* 78:267, 1993.

156. Kordower JH, Emborg ME, Bloch J, et al: Neurodegeneration prevented by lentiviral vector delivery of GDNF in primate models of Parkinson's disease. *Science* 290:767–773, 2000.

157. Bjorklund A, Kirik D, Rosenblad C, et al: Towards a neuroprotective gene therapy for Parkinson's disease: Use of adenovirus, AAV and lentivirus vectors for gene transfer of GDNF to the nigrostriatal system in the rat Parkinson model. *Brain Res* 886:82–98, 2000.

STEREOTAXIC SURGERY AND DEEP BRAIN STIMULATION FOR PARKINSON'S DISEASE AND MOVEMENT DISORDERS

BENJAMIN L. WALTER and JERROLD L. VITEK

HISTORY OF STEREOTAXIC SURGERY FOR
MOVEMENT DISORDERS   289
PATHOPHYSIOLOGICAL BASIS OF HYPO- AND
HYPERKINETIC MOVEMENT DISORDERS   290
    Organization of Basal Ganglia and
       Thalamocortical Circuits   290
    Pathophysiology Underlying Hypo- and
       Hyperkinetic Movement Disorders   292
    Summary   295
RADIOGRAPHIC AND MICROELECTRODE
MAPPING TECHNIQUES FOR TARGET
LOCALIZATION   295
    Radiographic Techniques   295
    Microelectrode Mapping Technique for
       Physiological Localization of the Target Site   296
    Semimicroelectrode Technique   300
ABLATIVE SURGERY TECHNIQUE   300
DEEP BRAIN STIMULATION SURGICAL
TECHNIQUE   300
SURGICAL APPROACH TO SPECIFIC MOVEMENT
DISORDERS   301
    Parkinson's Disease (PD)   301
    Essential Tremor (ET) and Other Tremors   306
    Dystonia   307
    Hemiballismus   309
POTENTIAL MECHANISM(S) UNDERLYING THE
BENEFICIAL EFFECT OF DBS AND ABLATIVE
THERAPY   309

Functional surgery for movement disorders can significantly alleviate symptoms and improve the quality of life for disabling diseases such as Parkinson's disease (PD), essential tremor (ET) and dystonia in appropriately selected patients. The surgical approach to movement disorders has evolved dramatically from the pre-L-dopa era to the development of modern magnetic resonance imaging (MRI)-based stereotaxic and neurophysiologic guided targeting. New techniques benefited from the concurrent growth in our understanding of the pathophysiological basis of these disorders and physiology of the target structures. Initial experience with ablative therapy has given rise to the advent of deep brain stimulation (DBS). DBS provides more surgical options while allowing for reversibility of side-effects and postoperative modification of stimulation parameters to optimize results. For PD, medical treatment with L-dopa is not the panacea it was initially thought to be, particularly due to the late complications of L-dopa-induced dyskinesias. Even with molecular- and genetic-based therapies on the horizon aimed at slowing the progression of PD, there is and will be for the foreseeable future a large population of patients significantly burdened by these neurodegenerative diseases.

While many patients with essential tremor have mild symptoms that may be controlled with medication, others are refractory to medication, have significant disability, and are unable to perform simple activities of daily living or maintain employment.

Dystonia is a particularly disabling condition and, although many patients with focal dystonias involving small muscle groups may respond to botulinum toxin, others with more diffuse involvement or involvement of larger muscle groups do not. In many cases, other medical therapies available may not provide sufficient relief.

As data from larger controlled trials become available, neurologists and neurosurgeons will be able to tailor therapy for their patient by appropriate choice of target site and mode of treatment (ablative or stimulation), depending on the patient's disease characteristics. Furthermore, we will be better able to stratify the risk of adverse side-effects based on the characteristics of the patient's disease, age, and other risk factors.

History of Stereotaxic Surgery for Movement Disorders

The history of the development of stereotaxic surgery for the treatment of movement disorders is replete with a multitude of approaches to different targets in an attempt to ameliorate a variety of movement disorders. Reports of remarkable successes are mixed with complete failures after the same stereotaxic intervention.[1,2] The earliest approaches were generally not based on sound scientific principles but were empirically driven or based on simplistic rationales that led to what often appears as a desperate search for an effective target. The first known attempts to treat PD surgically were based on the presumed relationship between the motor symptoms and the foci of infection in patients with encephalitis lethargica. These consisted of removing the various organs suspected of harboring the infection evolving to sympathetic ramisectomies and cervical ganglionectomies. In 1930, Pollack and Davis,[3] in a failed attempt to relieve parkinsonian tremor, sectioned the dorsal roots of 1 patient. Although the rigidity was lessened, the tremor remained. Subsequent attempts included antero-lateral cordotomies,[4,5] dentatectomy,[6] and extirpation of the precentral cortex.[7] These were generally unsuccessful and were associated with considerable morbidity. Meyers[2] subsequently reported improvements in some patients in which various parts of the basal ganglia, including the caudate, putamen, and globus pallidus (GP) or its outflow tracts, the ansa lenticularis or fascicularis lenticularis, were removed or sectioned, respectively. However, there remained significant morbidity and mortality associated with these procedures. In 1952, Cooper observed alleviation of parkinsonian motor signs after accidental ligation of the anterior choroidal artery, which led to a number of unpredictable outcomes after subsequent ligations in other PD patients.[8] A variety of approaches were subsequently used to interrupt the pallidofugal pathways, including heating, freezing, and injections of procaine oil into the pallidum. Results, however, were inconsistent. Was it a problem of appropriate target selection, or an inability to consistently reach the chosen target that led to such a wide variation in the results for patients with similar movement disorders? With the development of stereotaxis by Spiegel et al.,[9] there was an opportunity to improve target localization. Yet results, although somewhat improved, were still quite variable. This led to the report by Svennilson et al., who described the effect of pallidotomy on 81 patients operated on by Lars Leksell.[10] Leksell, varying the lesion site within the globus pallidus pars interna (GPi), observed a clear difference in outcome that was correlated with lesion location. In the last 20 patients with lesions placed in the posteroventral portion of GPi, 19 were substantially improved. With the advent of L-dopa, however, surgical treatment of PD became less frequent. Subsequent approaches were focused on thalamotomy for parkinsonian tremor, because most surgeons, at that time, felt that this was a better target for tremor alleviation.[11] Although Svennilson et al. had reported that more than 80 percent of patients experienced complete tremor alleviation after pallidotomy, the target site was moved to the thalamus.

Thalamotomy, although effective for tremor, rigidity, and L-dopa-induced dyskinesia, was ineffective for akinesia, and often it worsened gait or speech disorders. It remained the target of choice, however, until the early 1990s when pallidotomy was favorably re-explored by Laitinen et al.[12] Laitinen's report of significant improvement in parkinsonian motor signs, and drug-induced dyskinesias after posteroventral pallidotomy, together with separate reports of improvement of parkinsonian motor signs after ablation or inactivation of the subthalamic nucleus (STN) and GPi in animal models of PD, led to a resurgence of stereotaxic pallidotomy for PD. Several centers corroborated earlier reports[10,12] of amelioration of parkinsonian motor signs after stereotaxic pallidotomy.[13–17] Results, however, were not uniformly successful across centers, with some reporting minimal improvement,[18] whereas others, such as Svennilson et al. and Laitinen, reported significant improvement across the vast majority of patients.[13–17] Short- and long-term benefit of pallidotomy for PD has now

been confirmed in a blinded randomized trial versus best medical therapy.[19] Inconsistencies in results of earlier studies were likely due to a variety of clinical variables, including lesion location and size, the patient's age and cognitive state, and other, as yet unidentified variables, including the presence of cerebral atrophy, response to medication, associated medical problems, and varied brain pathology. These variables, of which lesion location, age, and etiology of the movement disorder will likely play a central role, may also account, in part, for the variable success rates of stereotaxic intervention in other movement disorders.

DBS evolved from experience with thalamotomies for PD in the 1950s and 1960s. Hassler and others noted that intraoperative high-frequency stimulation (>100 Hz) in Vim temporarily arrested parkinsonian tremor.[20,21] Chronic Vim stimulation was soon employed as an alternative to thalamotomy for parkinsonian and ET.[22–24] As the revival of pallidotomy for parkinsonism was meeting renewed success with modern techniques, investigators started applying chronic stimulation successfully in Vim,[22–27] GPi,[28–30] and STN.[31] It was not long before DBS was applied to these targets for other movement disorders, including hemiballism,[32] and dystonia.[33–35]

Pathophysiological Basis of Hypo- and Hyperkinetic Movement Disorders

ORGANIZATION OF BASAL GANGLIA AND THALAMOCORTICAL CIRCUITS

Based on our understanding of the anatomy and physiology of the basal ganglia and related structures, a scheme for the functional organization of the basal ganglia has been developed. This scheme views the basal ganglia as a family of larger segregated circuits involving specific portions of the thalamus and cerebral cortex. These circuits take origin from different cortical areas, project to separate portions of the basal ganglia, which in turn project to separate portions of the thalamus, returning to the same areas of the frontal cortex from which they took origin. One of these circuits, the "motor" circuit, has been considered most important in the pathogenesis of hypo- and hyperkinetic movement disorders, including PD, dystonia, hemiballismus, and Huntington's chorea.[36] Parkinsonian tremor, although implicated in this circuit, may have a more diverse etiology,[37,38] whereas ET and intention tremor are most likely a result of alterations in cerebellothalamic pathways.[39–41]

The motor circuit takes origin from precentral motor and postcentral somatosensory cortical areas and projects to motor areas of the basal ganglia and thalamus en route to its return to motor and premotor cortical areas (Fig. 17-1). This circuit is somatotopically organized throughout the different cortical and subcortical motor areas. Cortical input to subcortical portions of the motor circuit occurs via their

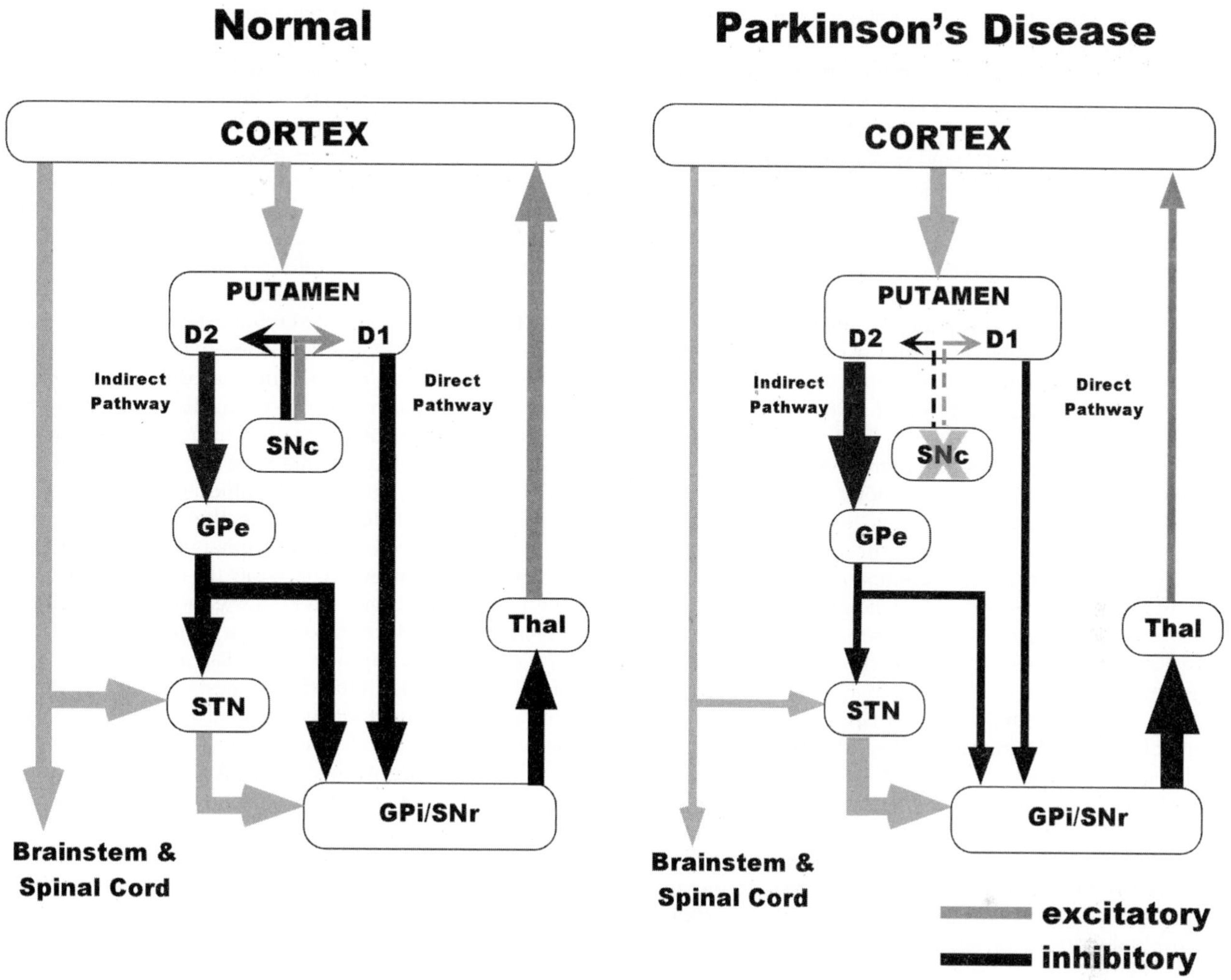

Normal

Parkinson's Disease

FIGURE 17-1 Schematic illustration of the basal ganglia-thalamocortical "motor" circuit and its neurotransmitters in the normal and parkinsonian state. "Indirect" and "direct" pathways from the striatum to basal ganglia output nuclei are shown by the arrows. GPe, globus pallidus par externa; GPi, globus pallidus pars interna; STN, subthalamic nucleus; SNr, substantia nigra pars reticulata; SNc, substantia nigra pars compacta; Thal, thalamus; D1, D2, dopamine receptor subtypes 1 and 2. Wider lines represent an increase in neuronal activity, thinner lines represent a decrease.

projections to the putamen. Putaminal output arrives at the two major output routes from the basal ganglia, the GPi and the substantia nigra pars reticulata (SNr), via two pathways, termed the "direct" and the "indirect" pathways (see Fig. 17-1). The direct pathway takes origin from medium spiny neurons with presumed dopaminergic excitatory responses and monosynaptic projections to GPi and SNr. The indirect pathway takes origin from medium spiny neurons with presumed dopaminergic inhibitory responses that project, via globus pallidus pars externa (GPe) and STN, to the GPi and SNr. In addition, there are return projections from the STN to GPe as well as direct projections from GPe to GPi, SNr, and the reticularis nucleus of the thalamus.[42]

Based on this organizational scheme of the basal ganglia, two putative roles for the pallidothalamocortical motor circuit have been proposed: (1) scaling movement, and (2) focusing motor activity. Basal ganglia output neurons from GPi/SNr may respond to balancing forces from inhibitory direct pathway neurons and excitatory indirect pathway neurons from STN. Thus, movement can be scaled by facilitation of movement through increasing direct pathway activity and inhibition of movement through increased indirect pathway activity converging on these same neurons. Likewise, focusing of movement may occur when neurons controlling agonist activity are facilitated through the direct pathway, while at the same time neurons controlling antagonist activity are inhibited through the indirect pathway.[43]

The primary projection site from GPi is to the "motor" thalamus, ventralis lateralis pars oralis (VLo), and ventralis anterior (VA).[44–48] These areas project predominantly to the supplementary motor area and premotor areas, respectively, but also have projections to the primary motor and arcuate premotor areas.[49–51] The SNr projects predominantly to ventralis anterior magnocellularis (VAmc) which projects to the prefrontal[44] cortex. GPi and SNr also have smaller projections to the midbrain tegmentum and the superior colliculus.[52,53] All intrinsic and output projections from the basal ganglia are GABA-ergic and inhibitory, with the exception of the STN, which is glutaminergic and excitatory. Projections from the cortex to the putamen, and from the thalamus to the cortex are excitatory.

Through the use of retrograde transsynaptic tracers it has been discovered that within the motor circuit there may be a series of segregated subcircuits, each taking origin in different motor and premotor cortical areas (motor cortex, supplementary and arcuate premotor cortex), and involving different portions of the basal ganglia and thalamus.[54,55] The proposal that these subcircuits may differentially affect movement receives some support from the differential role these cortical areas are proposed to play in motor control,[56–59] as well as from observations that neurons in different portions of GPi, electrophysiologically identified to project to different thalamic and cortical motor areas, have characteristic patterns of activity related to different components of the behavioral task.[55] Thus, it appears likely that these subcircuits may indeed be differentially involved in motor control and, when altered in a particular fashion, may lead to the development of specific motor signs (i.e., rigidity, tremor, akinesia, dystonia, and dyskinesias).

PATHOPHYSIOLOGY UNDERLYING HYPO- AND HYPERKINETIC MOVEMENT DISORDERS

PARKINSON'S DISEASE (PD)

The Rate Model

Based on our understanding of the pathophysiological changes that occur in the basal ganglia thalamocortical circuit in the parkinsonian monkey, a rate model for PD was developed (Fig. 17-1). In this model, loss of dopamine in the substantia nigra pars compacta (SNc) is proposed to lead to differential changes in neuronal activity of striatal cells in the direct and indirect pathways. In the direct pathway, loss of dopamine at striatal excitatory D1 receptors leads to a decrease of inhibitory activity from the putamen to GPi. In the indirect pathway, there is loss of dopamine at inhibitory D2 receptors leading to increased activity of inhibitory putaminal neurons projecting to GPe, causing a reduction of GPe activity. The decrease in inhibitory output from GPe to STN leads to excessive excitation from the STN to the GPi. Thus, there is an increase in inhibitory activity from the GPi to the

thalamus and brainstem, which occurs via both the direct and indirect pathways.

In this model, inhibition of thalamocortical and midbrain projections in the motor circuit has been proposed as the primary cause of the development of parkinsonian motor signs and the hypokinetic features associated with PD.[36] Similarly, the model predicts that a loss or lowering of inhibitory input from GPi to the thalamus may result in the hyperkinetic movements associated with drug-induced dyskinesias.[11,60,61] Changes in mean firing rates of neurons in GPe, GPi, STN, and VLo in the 1-methyl-4-phenyl-1,2,3,6-tetrahydropyridine (MPTP) monkey model of PD, and in GPe and GPi in patients with idiopathic PD, are consistent with those predicted by the model; that is, a decrease in mean discharge rates in GPe and VLo and an increase in mean discharge rates in STN and GPi.[36,62–66] Furthermore, positron emission tomography (PET) studies in PD patients have shown increased activity in cortical motor areas after pallidotomy, consistent with disinhibition of thalamocortical pathways.[67]

Patient and experimental animal responses to surgical interventions, however, contradict the expectations based on the rate model. Lesions within the motor thalamus do not exacerbate or induce parkinsonian motor signs but, instead, are reported to improve or abolish parkinsonian tremor, rigidity, and drug-induced dyskinesias.[60,68,69] This suggests that a decrease in activity of thalamic neurons cannot by itself account for the development of parkinsonian motor signs. Furthermore, the rate model would predict that pallidotomy would produce excessive involuntary movements or dyskinesias by disinhibiting the thalamus. It does not, and, in fact, pallidotomy is very effective in alleviating drug-induced dyskinesias. These contradictions of the rate model have led to the development of an alternative, the pattern model.[70–73]

The Pattern Model

Alternatively, parkinsonian motor signs may occur, in part, because of an altered pattern of neuronal activity (see Fig. 17-2). This altered pattern of thalamocortical activity may, in turn, disrupt the normal operation of corticocortical circuits involved in motor control. Our observations of increased bursting and rhythmic oscillatory patterns of activity within the thalamus in parkinsonian monkeys, together with the clear improvement in most parkinsonian motor signs after thalamotomy, lend support to this hypothesis.[66,74,75] Based on this model, pallidotomy or thalamotomy is effective in PD because they remove disorganized output from the basal ganglia that is interrupting the motor circuit.

Additional Pathways

Although altered patterns and rates of neuronal activity within the pallidothalamocortical motor circuit likely provide a significant contribution to the development of the motor signs associated with PD, the contribution of other pathways should not be disregarded, either in terms of their role in the underlying pathophysiology or in our approach

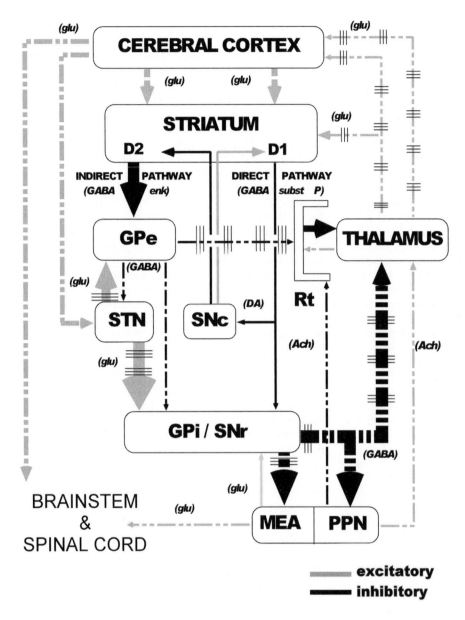

FIGURE 17-2 Schematic illustration of the basal ganglia thalamocortical "motor" circuit incorporating changes in pattern of neuronal activity and alternative pathways from the external segment of the globus pallidus (GPe) and pedunculopontine nucleus (PPN). Interrupted arrows represent an alternation in the pattern of neuronal activity. The grouped lines crossing the projections from the subthalamic nucleus (STN), the internal segment of the globus pallidus (GPi) and thalamus represent the presence of bursting activity. SNc, substantia nigra pars compacta; SNr, substantia nigra pars reticulata; D1, D2, dopamine receptor 1 and 2 subtypes; glu, glutamate; GABA, gamma-aminobutyric acid; enk, enkephalin; DA, dopamine; Rt, nucleus reticularis of the thalamus; Ach, acetylcholine; MEA, midbrain extrapyramidal area; PPN, pedunculopontine nucleus; subst P; substance P.

to treatment. Perhaps the best example of the role of alternative pathways in the development of parkinsonian motor signs is the potential role of the cerebellothalamocortical pathway in the development of parkinsonian tremor. In previous animal models of parkinsonian tremor, in which a portion of the midbrain tegmentum was ablated, it was necessary to include cerebellothalamic projections in order for tremor to develop.[76] Furthermore, whereas lesions in the sensorimotor portion of GPi are effective in improving or ameliorating parkinsonian tremor, lesions within the pallidal receiving area of the thalamus (Vop and Voa) have not generally been reported to be as effective as those within the cerebellar receiving area (Vim).[77–79] Although Hassler et al.

reported that lesions within Vop were effective for parkinsonian tremor, he considered Vop to be a cerebellar receiving area not associated with pallidothalamic input.[11,80] The importance of interrupting the cerebellothalamic pathway in alleviating tremor was emphasized in his report of postmortem material obtained after thalamotomy. In patients with complete tremor arrest, he reported "coagulations either in the Vop or in the dentatothalamic fibers, which end in the Vop." The discrepancy between the observations of Hassler et al. and others concerning the most effective site in the thalamus for alleviation of parkinsonian tremor may be no more than a difference in nomenclature, or may be the result of a difference in interpretation of the cytoarchitectonic boundaries of thalamic subnuclei. Both groups, however, argue that the most effective lesions for relief of parkinsonian tremor lie in the cerebellar receiving area of the motor thalamus.

Additional support for a role of the cerebellothalamic pathway in the pathogenesis of parkinsonian tremor are the observations of rhythmic activity of neurons in Vim strongly correlated with tremor, as well as reports that the optimal location for lesions to alleviate such tremor appears to be within or includes significant portions of this region within Vim.[79,81–84]

Another potentially significant pathway in the development of parkinsonian motor signs is the projection from GPe to the nucleus reticularis of the thalamus (NRT).[42,85] Other than through its effect on the STN, the role of GPe in the development of the motor signs associated with PD has been largely disregarded. Given the significant decrease in mean firing rates in GPe in PD, and the diffuse projections of reticularis neurons within and across thalamic subnuclei, the projection from GPe to NRT may serve an important role in the underlying pathophysiology of PD. Other potentially important pathways in PD involve the role of brainstem regions, including the pedunculopontine nucleus (PPN) and midbrain extrapyramidal area (MEA), which receive input from GPi and SNr and project to the thalamus, as well as the locus ceruleus (LC), which has widespread projections to the thalamus, cerebellum, and brainstem and may suffer significant cellular loss in PD (see Fig. 17-2). The MEA sends projections back to the GPi and SNr, as well as to the brainstem and spinal cord, whereas the PPN has extensive projections to the thalamus.[86–89] Cholinergic projections from the PPN have a differential effect on thalamic relay and reticular neurons, depolarizing relay neurons and hyperpolarizing reticular neurons.[90–93] Thus, cholinergic brainstem projections from the PPN are generally excitatory to thalamic relay neurons and inhibitory to reticular neurons. Therefore, in addition to the direct effect of GPi and PPN projections on thalamic relay cells, there are likely indirect effects on these cells from GPe and PPN projections to the NRT. The extensive projections from NRT and PPN throughout the motor thalamus may explain the observed changes in neuronal activity reported in both pallidal and cerebellar receiving areas in animal models of PD.[66,86–88,94] Such a diffuse change in both the rate and pattern of neuronal activity in the motor thalamus is hard to account for without considering the potential role of GPe and/or brainstem thalamic projections in mediating them (Fig. 17-2).

DYSTONIA

Dystonia is a movement disorder characterized by sustained muscle contractions, leading to twisting, repetitive movements and abnormal postures. Clinicopathological studies in patients with dystonia indicate that the most common site in which a lesion can be identified is in the basal ganglia (i.e., caudate, putamen, or pallidum). Thalamic lesions, although less common, have also been observed in patients with dystonia[95,96] (see also Chap. 33).

In mapping the receptive fields of thalamic neurons in patients with dystonia undergoing microelectrode-guided thalamotomy, an increased area of representation of the affected body part has been reported, compared to that in those patients without dystonia (i.e., patients with ET or intention tremor).[97,98] The incidence of somatosensory responses in Vop and Vim was significantly greater than that in a control group comprising chronic pain or tremor (non-PD) patients.[99,100] In this study, the percentage of sensory cells in the motor thalamus (22 percent) was significantly greater than that observed in control patients (9.5 percent). Notably, the number of sensory cells responding to movement of more than one joint was significantly higher in dystonic patients (23 percent) than in control patients (9 percent), an observation similar to that made in the MPTP monkey model of parkinsonism.[101] In addition, microstimulation in and around Vim produced simultaneous contraction of multiple muscles in the forearm of dystonic patients, with the activity of many neurons in Vop and Vim showing peaks of activity at the frequency of the dystonic movements, which were significantly correlated with electromyogram (EMG) activity in the affected limb segment.[99,100] A small lesion, presumably involving Vop and part of Vim, produced an immediate and dramatic decrease in the involuntary movements of these dystonic patients. These observations provide compelling evidence that pallidal (Vop) and cerebellar (Vim), receiving areas of the motor thalamus, are both involved in the pathogenesis of some types of dystonia.

Pathophysiologically, dystonia may be a presenting symptom in parkinsonian patients who are not taking antiparkinsonian medications, or alternatively may appear as a consequence of L-dopa treatment (peak-dose dystonia). Dystonia can be viewed as either a hypo- or hyperkinetic movement disorder. Whether this reflects etiologically different "types" of dystonia or merely represents a variation along the same general pathophysiological scheme is unclear. Although both types of dystonia likely reflect an alteration in the neural activity in the pallidothalamocortical and, probably, the cerebellothalamocortical circuit, the exact relationship between changes (rate and pattern) in neural activity in these regions and the development of dystonia remains unclear. In addition, pallidal projections to the brainstem are also likely to contribute to the pathogenesis of some "types" of dystonia. As with the pallido- and cerebellothalamic pathways, the particular changes in neural activity in these areas and their relationship to the development of dystonia is unclear.

ESSENTIAL AND ACTION TREMOR

Cerebellothalamic pathways, although likely contributing to the development of parkinsonian tremor, may also play a significant role in the development of ET and intention tremor. In both disorders, tremor-related activity has been identified in Vim, and lesions within this area can significantly reduce or abolish both benign essential and cerebellar outflow tremors.

The physiological basis for the development of these tremors has been a much-debated issue. Neurons in the "cerebellar" thalamus in patients with either ET or cerebellar tremor have rhythmic bursting activity at tremor frequency.[102] Whether this occurs as a result of inherent neuronal rhythmicity expressed secondarily to conditions particular to these disorders and results in tremor, or occurs secondarily to or coincident with the development of these tremors, remains unclear. Thus, although the central mechanisms underlying the development of these tremors is not well defined, they clearly appear to involve thalamic neurons given the resolution of such tremors after thalamotomy.

The contribution of peripheral afferent mechanisms to the development of these tremors is also debated. Some investigators have argued that the contribution of peripheral afferent mechanisms could be assessed by determining the degree of phase resetting of bursting neuronal activity in the thalamus after unexpected perturbations to the tremulous limb, and they termed this the resetting index.[95] An index of 0 suggested that there was no resetting, whereas an index of 1 implied complete resetting. The resetting index for ET was high, suggesting a significant peripheral contribution. It can be argued, however, that the index simply describes the degree to which tremor-related activity may be altered by peripheral input and not necessarily whether it underlies tremor genesis. Support implicating peripheral afferent mechanisms in the genesis of cerebellar tremor was provided by Vilis and Hore, who cooled the deep cerebellar nuclei and examined the change in response of motor cortical neurons, as well as the change in timing and duration of agonist and antagonist EMG responses to torque pulses applied to the upper limb.[41,103,104] They concluded that cerebellar tremor occurred secondary to disordered reflex loops involving the motor cortex, because the delay in the response of motor cortex cells related to agonist-antagonist EMG activity was correlated with the delay observed in these EMG responses to controlled perturbation.[41,103,104] These data, although suggestive of a peripheral contribution to the pathogenesis of cerebellar tremor, however, do not address the role of inherent oscillatory mechanisms in the development of cerebellar tremor. Given the reports of rhythmically bursting neuronal activity in the motor thalamus in patients with cerebellar tremor who undergo thalamotomy, there is likely a significant central component underlying the genesis of this tremor.[68,105] One explanation for the development of cerebellar tremor lies in the inherent tendency for hyperpolarized thalamic neurons to burst after a depolarizing pulse.[93,94,106] Interruption of excitatory cerebellar projections to thalamic neurons could put these neurons into a hyperpolarized "burst-promoting" state. With initiation of movement, depolarizing corticothalamic projections may produce synchronous bursting activity of a population of thalamic neurons. When a critical population of thalamic neurons bursts synchronously, it may lead to the development of rhythmic bursting activity which, when transmitted to a critical number of alpha-motoneurons via the motor cortex induces an action tremor. Thus, although both peripheral and central tremorgenic mechanisms likely contribute to the development of cerebellar tremor, the relative contribution remains unclear.

HEMIBALLISMUS

Hemiballism consists of involuntary, often violent, movements of the contralateral limbs. These movements are most closely associated with inactivation or destruction of the STN or its efferent pathway.[107] Hemiballismus has been observed in humans after vascular lesions restricted to the STN, as well as in monkeys after selective lesioning of the STN with ibotenic acid, and is thought to occur predominantly as a result of disinhibition of the thalamus.[108,109]

This model receives support from both experimental studies in the monkey and studies of patients with intractable hemiballismus,[75,107–111] who undergo microelectrode-guided pallidotomy.[75] In both humans and monkeys, there is a significant reduction in the tonic discharge rate in GPi after an STN lesion and the development of hemiballismus. Consistent with this observation, monkeys with hemiballismus after inactivation of STN show decreased metabolic activity in both GPi and the ventral lateral thalamus.[112] However, the reduced rate in GPi would suggest that thalamotomy and not pallidotomy would effectively treat hemiballism, yet both alleviate hemiballism.[13–16,70,113] This lends further support to the hypothesis that altered patterns of activity in the pallidothalamic motor circuit underlie the abnormal movement found in both hypokinetic and hyperkinetic movement disorders.

SUMMARY

Our understanding of the pathophysiological basis of hypo- and hyperkinetic movement disorders has increased significantly over the last decade. Both rate and pattern are now considered important in the genesis of both hypo- and hyperkinetic movement disorders. The contribution of altered receptive fields and changes in synchrony are just now being appreciated. Additionally, alternative pathways are likely involved with different subcircuits mediating different aspects of involuntary movement.

Radiographic and Microelectrode Mapping Techniques for Target Localization

RADIOGRAPHIC TECHNIQUES

Initial target coordinates are obtained by conventional radiographic techniques using computed tomography (CT), MRI, and/or ventriculography. The location of the anterior (AC) and posterior commissure (PC) relative to fiducial markers on the stereotaxic frame are used to calculate the X, Y, and Z coordinates of the target.

For Vim thalamus, a good starting point is approximately 3 mm anterior to the posterior commissure at 15 mm lateral to the AC-PC line. These coordinates should allow the first pass with the recording electrode to penetrate portions of the sensory thalamus which, combined with determination of the receptive fields of neurons in the adjacent motor thalamus, provides a highly reliable landmark for subsequent penetrations.

For GPi, the coordinates are 21 mm lateral, 3 mm anterior, and 3–6 mm ventral to the midcommissural line. Based on physiological data gathered during microelectrode-guided pallidotomies, these coordinates target the sensorimotor portion of GPi.[62]

For STN, initial targeting coordinates are 2–3 mm posterior to the midcommissural point, 11–13 mm lateral, and 4–6 mm inferior to the AC-PC line.

The final target selection should be based on the type of movement disorder being treated. Other factors that can and should be taken into consideration include the somatotopic organization of the structure, the portion of the body involved, and the relative location of nearby critical structures to be avoided. This information is readily obtained with the use of electrophysiological mapping techniques. Some reports suggest that errors in radiographic targeting are greater than 3 mm in 43 percent of GPi cases and 45 percent of STN cases. Assuming a 3–4-mm diameter spread of current with DBS, with a 3-mm inaccuracy, there would be significantly less than an optimal amount of target effected by the DBS lead in these cases.[114]

Because of individual variation in the length of the AC-PC line, size of the third ventricle, and radiographic distortion inherent in these techniques, these coordinates should serve only as a starting point. MRI is prone to error due to magnetic susceptibility artifact in the direction of frequency encoding (usually the anterior-posterior direction),[115] whereas CT does not provide sufficient contrast of subcortical structures. Some advocate use of combined techniques fusing MRI and CT images to minimize these errors while still providing high resolution.[116–118] There is also a significant degree of anatomical variation from patient to patient. Some of this variation may be accounted for by variation in the width of the third ventricle and one approach advocated is to normalize the lateral coordinate to the width of the third ventricle.[119,120] Another approach is to use direct targeting based on the boundaries of the target.[120] This approach has been shown to be more accurate than reliance on coordinates based on AC-PC dimensions. Microelectrode mapping has an accuracy of approximately 0.1 mm. Thus, despite improvements in MRI- and CT-based targeting techniques, electrophysiological mapping provides information for target verification not available by other means.

MICROELECTRODE MAPPING TECHNIQUE FOR PHYSIOLOGICAL LOCALIZATION OF THE TARGET SITE

Microelectrode recording techniques used in conjunction with radiographic methods and macrostimualtion techniques facilitate identification and localization of the target structure. This approach enhances the ability of the surgeon to locate and place the stimulator or lesion within the identified target or sculpting the lesion to involve as much or as little of the target as deemed necessary to provide the optimal outcome, while avoiding adjacent structures.

TECHNICAL COMMENTS AND ELECTROPHYSIOLOGICAL EQUIPMENT

A variety of electrodes can be used for electrophysiologic recording; however, platinum-iridium glass-coated microelectrodes with a tip diameter of 2–4 µm and an impedance of 0.5–2.0 Mohms (at 1000 Hz) provide excellent recording characteristics that do not deteriorate after microstimulation. The electrode is protected in a stainless steel "carrier" tube attached to a microdrive assembly, which is adapted to fit onto the stereotaxic frame and manually zeroed so that the tip of the electrode is even with the end of the carrier tube when the microdrive is at zero. The microelectrode is then withdrawn by several millimeters to protect it during placement into the outer guide cannula. The microelectrode is then lowered into a protective guide tube and comes to rest at the level of the tip of the guide tube. The recording electrode is connected to standard electrophysiological equipment for amplification, filtering, and discrimination of electrophysiological signals.

Vim ELECTROPHYSIOLOGY

The thalamus contains 50–60 different subnuclei. The targeted subnuclei lie adjacent to regions which, when interrupted, may lead to significant cognitive, language, or sensory impairment. It is important, therefore, to map precisely the boundaries of the region(s) to be included within the target area to obtain the maximal benefit while minimizing potential complications as a result of encroachment on adjacent subnuclei.

The thalamus is approached parasagitally at an angle of approximately 30–35 degrees from the vertical, except for cases in which one wants to include Vop or portions of Voa, in which case one may choose an angle of 45 degrees. A sharper angle allows one microelectrode penetration to cross a greater portion of adjacent thalamic subnuclei and provides a better approximation of the borders between thalamic subnuclei.

Just before the microelectrode enters the thalamus it penetrates neurons with broad receptive fields responding to passive or active movement, confrontational hand gestures, or changes in attention. These types of responses are typical of neurons in the NRT. This nucleus is only a few hundred micrometers thick and is followed by a thin lamina of similar diameter before the characteristic rhythmic discharge of thalamic neurons is encountered. At this point single units are discriminated throughout the track. In patients with tremor, "tremor cells" may be identified in pallidal and cerebellar receiving areas (Vim, Voa, or Vop), where neurons have bursting discharges synchronous with the patient's tremor.

Neuronal responses to passive and active movement of individual body parts are sought, and microstimulation is carried out at 5–50 μA, with trains of symmetric biphasic pulse pairs at a frequency of 300–400 Hz. The patient is instructed to report any change in sensation that occurs with microstimulation, describing its location, quality, and intensity. At each stimulation site, when changes in sensation occur with stimulation, sensory thresholds are determined by decreasing the current intensity progressively, until the stimulus no longer elicits a sensory response. For each microelectrode penetration, response to microstimulation, sensory thresholds, spontaneous activity patterns, and the response of each isolated cell to sensorimotor examination are plotted on plastic overlays, then fitted to computer-generated maps of the human thalamus taken from the Schaltenbrand and Bailey Atlas[121] and scaled to the patient's AC-PC coordinates.

Lateral, anterior, and ventral boundaries of the motor (Voa, Vop, and Vim) and sensory (Vc) thalamus are determined based on microstimulation effects, the presence or absence of neuronal activity, and neuronal response properties to sensorimotor examination. The lateral border of the thalamus is bounded by the internal capsule where microstimulation results in evoked movements, allowing this region to be easily identified. Along the anterior border of the sensory thalamus is the ventrocaudal nucleus (Vc). It is identified by the presence of neurons with small, well-defined fields receptive to tactile sensation in a body region in which low-threshold (5–10 μA) stimulation-induced paresthesias occur. The relative distance of the recording electrode from the anterior border of Vc can be approximated by the sensory

threshold at which microstimulation induces paresthesias. Sites sufficiently anterior to Vc are characterized by a lack of microstimulation-induced paresthesias, even at current intensities of 40–50 μA or greater. The sensorimotor thalamus is somatotopically organized with areas representing leg, arm, jaw, and face, arrayed in a lateral-to-medial direction in onion skin-like lamellae. Thus, penetrations near the lateral border of the sensory thalamus are characterized by microstimulation-induced paresthesias of somatosensory responses predominantly restricted to the leg. Penetrations made progressively more medially will have responses largely restricted to the arm and face, respectively. As one moves rostrally from Vc to Vim, Vop, and Voa, there is a gradation of cell responses to sensorimotor examination: cells in Vc predominantly respond to tactile stimuli, while the most rostral portion of Vc has some proprioceptive responses. Cells in Vim, Vop, and Voa do not respond to tactile stimulation; however, cells in Vim readily respond to passive manipulations of the limbs and orofacial structures. Cells in Vop and Voa tend to respond more selectively to voluntary movement and less to passive manipulations, which is similar to the case described in the monkey for homologous subnuclei.[122,123]

GPi ELECTROPHYSIOLOGY

Microelectrode penetrations are made in the parasagittal plane, proceeding from the anterodorsal to posteroventral direction at an angle of approximately 30–35 degrees from vertical. As the microelectrode is advanced, patterns of neural activity are noted throughout the track. The major structures that are identified using this plane of approach are striatum (caudate and putamen), followed by GPe, GPi, and lastly internal capsule and/or optic tract. The nucleus basalis may be encountered with anteriorly placed penetrations.

Each cellular region has a characteristic pattern of neural activity similar to that described in the monkey[124] (Fig. 17-3).

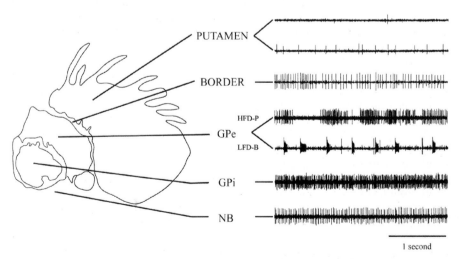

FIGURE 17-3 Microelectrode physiology encountered when targeting GPi. Typical neural activity is shown for striatum (putamen and caudate), GPe (globus pallidus externa), GPi (globus pallidus interna), and NB (nucleus basalis). Populations of high-frequency discharge pausing cells (HFD-P) and low-frequency discharge bursting cells (LFD-B) are found in GPe. The line drawing shows a parasaggital representation of these structures from the Schaltenbrand and Bailey Atlas.[121]

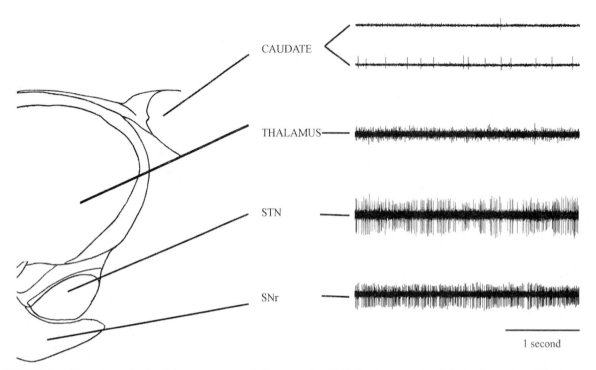

FIGURE 17-4 Microelectrode physiology encountered when targeting STN. Typical neural activity is shown for striatum (putamen and caudate), thalamus, subthalamic nucleus (STN), and substantia nigra pars reticulata (SNr). The line drawing shows a parasaggital representation of these structures from the Schaltenbrand and Bailey Atlas.[121]

Low spontaneous discharge rates (< 1 Hz) that increase transiently up to 4–6 Hz as the electrode is advanced typify neural activity from the striatum. As the electrode enters GPe, two distinct cell types can be identified: (1) units with high-frequency discharges (50±21 Hz) separated by pauses (HFD-P), and (2) units that are active in bursts separated by periods of single-spike discharges at low frequency at 18±12 Hz (LFD-B). Next, in GPi, high-frequency (82±24 Hz) tonic activity characterizes the majority of neural activity, although a variety of other patterns may be present, including bursts with little pause between them, emitting a "chugging" sound, or lower-frequency bursting in the range of 4–6 Hz that may correspond to the patient's tremor frequency ("tremor cells"). Within the laminae of the pallidum (i.e., between the GPe and GPi, as well as laminae within GPi), neurons with slower rates of tonic neural activity ("border" cells) may be encountered. These cells help identify border regions of the pallidal segments.[62]

Once through the pallidum, the optic tract or the internal capsule can be identified by microstimulation. In the optic tract, microstimulation at 5–40 μA typically results in brief flashes of light (phosphenes). In the internal capsule, microstimulation induces movement of the limbs or orofacial structures. The relative proximity of these structures (i.e., optic tract and internal capsule) can be ascertained by the stimulation threshold at which these phosphenes are noted or muscle contraction occurs. The optic tract can also be identified by flashing a light in the patient's eyes and listening for high-frequency modulation of the background audio signal coincident with the light stimulus.

The target region within GPi is determined by identifying neurons with responses to passive manipulations and active movement of the extremities and orofacial structures of the patient. The presence of bursting activity and its relationship to tremor, if present, is noted, along with each type of neural activity. The presence and somatotopic location of neuronal responses in the GPi to passive or active movement, as well as the relative location of the optic tract and internal capsule (noting the thresholds), are used to generate a topographic map of this subcortical region. This topographic map is, in turn, used to determine the location within GPi and guide stimulator or lesion placement.

There is somatotopic organization within the sensorimotor region of GPi, with a preponderance of leg cells found medially, arm cells laterally, and face ventrally (see Fig. 17-5).[122] Neurons in this area are characterized by increased activity to deep-muscle palpation, passive joint movement, or active movement of the somatotopically related body parts. These responses are predominantly contralateral and specific to a single joint, although neurons with responses to multiple

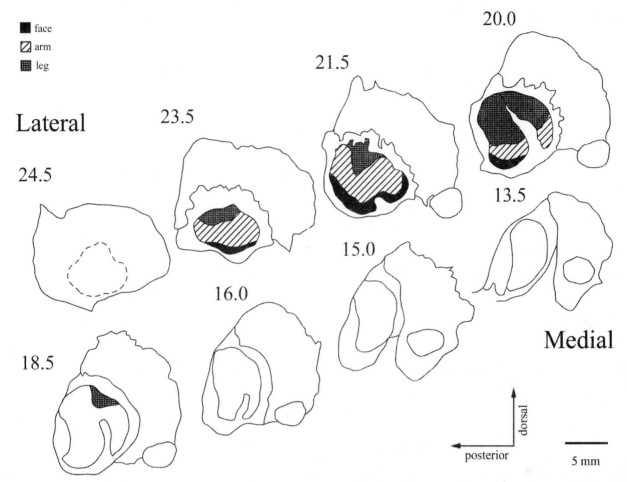

FIGURE 17-5 Somatotopic organization of GPi. Drawing representing a composite of 10 patients showing the somatotopic organization of receptive fields in GPi. The numbers represent the distance in millimeters from the midline of each parasagittal plane.

joints or limbs or even the ipsilateral limb are commonly encountered in patients with PD and dystonia may be encountered.[62,70,125]

Sensorimotor responses are found predominantly in the posterolateral portions of GPi, whereas neurons in regions more anterior and medial are not as likely to respond to active or passive manipulations of the limbs or orofacial structures. Based on anatomical studies these neurons are likely related to nonmotor "associative" functions.[126] Stimulation or lesions in this region alone will likely result in no or partial improvement in the motor symptoms of PD. Targeting this region of GPi is likely to produce similar results for dystonia and hemiballismus.[13,127]

STN ELECTROPHYSIOLOGY

When targeting STN, the microelectrode may pass through the striatum (usually caudate) before coursing through the anterior thalamus. Here the reticular thalamus may be identified with its characteristic units that respond to broad receptive field with active and passive movement.[128] Fig. 17-4 shows examples of characteristic electrophysiological recordings in structures encountered when targeting STN. Anterior thalamic nuclei may be identified by units with a characteristic bursting pattern at about 15 Hz.[128] If the electrode is more anteriorly located, it may pass through the internal capsule with low background noise and a paucity of cellular activity. Just below the thalamus there is a quiet region, likely the thalamic fasciculus (H1 fields of Forel), followed by a narrow strip of cells with large-amplitude neurons or bursting neurons at 25–45 Hz characteristic of zona incerta.[129] Below this, another quiet region is encountered corresponding to the lenticular fasciculus (H2 fields of Forel). As STN is approached further inferiorly, there is a striking increase in background activity, reflecting increased cellular density. STN neurons are then found with a discharge rate of about 37 Hz; however, they may range from 20 to 70 Hz.[129] Two patterns of units can be discerned: (1) a mixed pattern with

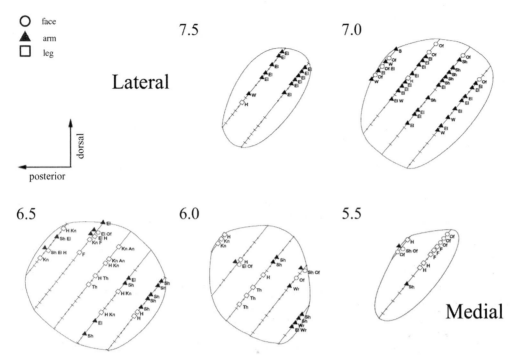

FIGURE 17-6 Somatotopic organization of STN. Monkey data showing distribution of cells responding to somatosensory input in subthalamic nucleus (STN). The numbers represent the distance in millimeters from the midline of each parasagittal plane. (*Modified from Wichmann T, Bergman H, DeLong MR. 1994,*[131] *with Permission.*)

tonic activity, irregular discharges, and occasional bursts, and (2) a burst pattern with periodic oscillating bursts that may or may not be synchronous with the patient's tremor.[129,130] Below the inferior border of STN, there is another short quit area followed by the SNr, which has units with a regular firing pattern at 71±23.2 Hz, similar to those present in GPi.[129]

Careful somatotopic mapping of the subthalamic nucleus in the African green monkey shows that the dorsorostral subthalamic nucleus contains most of the cells responding to somatosensory input, with the face represented dorsomedially, the leg ventrolateral to this and the arm at the most lateral extent of the nucleus (see Fig. 17-6).[131] Our knowledge of the somatotopic organization in the human is incomplete, but existing studies seem to correlate roughly with the monkey data.[132,133]

Micro- and macro-stimulation in STN can be used to help identify its borders and proximity to adjacent structures. Stimulation lateral to STN causes muscle contractions identifying its proximity to the internal capsule. Medially, stimulation may cause ipsilateral adduction of the eye from stimulation of the oculomotor nerve. Caudal stimulation may cause paresthesias from current spread to medial lemniscus.

SEMIMICROELECTRODE TECHNIQUE

An alternative recording technique for physiological localization of target sites involves the use of a bipolar concentric semimicroelectrode with a tip diameter of approximately 0.6 mm and an interpole distance of 0.3–0.6 mm. Although the basic technique is the same as that used for the microelectrode, the type of information provided differs significantly. The semimicroelectrode gives a broader, more integrated sampling of multicellular activity, whereas the microelectrode allows characterization of the response properties of single units. Basically, the semimicroelectrode is better suited to locate and differentiate individual subnuclei, or to identify the borders of the targeted nucleus, whereas the microelectrode is more precise, allowing for the determination of spontaneous activity patterns and sensorimotor response properties of single units.

Ablative Surgery Technique

Ablation for pallidotomy or thalamotomy is commonly performed with a radiofrequency lesioning electrode. Once the target is determined by imaging and electrophysiological mapping the lesioning electrode is advanced into the target. The lesioning electrode should be used for macrostimulation confirmation of the location and to assess side-effects. We have previously determined that, when making 75°C lesions, thresholds of > 0.5 mA at 300 Hz are safe for avoiding encroachment into the internal capsule, while thresholds of > 1.0 mA are safe for avoiding the optic tract. It should be noted that these thresholds may vary depending on the equipment and how it is configured. During macrostimulation and lesioning, the patient is serially examined for side-effects. We generally make our initial lesions at 60°C for 60 seconds. Subsequent lesions can be made at temperatures up to 80–90°C. There is a linear relationship between temperature and lesion diameter; while 60°C lesions are approximately 1 mm in diameter, 90°C lesions are roughly 5 mm.[62]

Deep Brain Stimulation Surgical Technique

After the target nucleus is identified by preoperative radiologic techniques and intraoperative electrophysiology, the stimulator lead is implanted in the chosen target. The FDA-approved Medtronic system has two lead configurations that are commonly used. Both are platinum-iridium quadripolar leads approximately 1.3 mm in diameter. The 3387 lead has four 1.5-mm contacts separated by 1.5-mm, and the 3389 has 1.5-mm contacts separated by 0.5 mm. The device is capable of bipolar stimulation between any of the four contacts or monopolar stimulation using the pulse generator casing as the anode. Before leaving the lead in place, an external pulse generator can be used to try various stimulation settings while examining the patient to assess for improvement or side-effects. Once satisfactory placement is achieved the lead is secured and connected to a programmable pulse generator located in the subclavicular region. This can be done during the same procedure or at a later date once the patient has recovered from the initial surgery.

Surgical Approach to Specific Movement Disorders

PARKINSON'S DISEASE (PD)

PATIENT SELECTION
Patients with medically intractable idiopathic PD with at least two of the four cardinal motor symptoms—i.e., tremor, rigidity, bradykinesia/akinesia, or difficulty with gait and postural instability (freezing, festination)—are considered candidates for surgery. Motor fluctuations, on-off phenomenon, dystonia (off or on) and drug-induced dyskinesia also respond to surgical intervention and may be the predominant feature in some patients for which they are undergoing surgery. Patients should have demonstrated a clear and long-lasting benefit from antiparkinsonian medication, in particular L-dopa preparations and dopamine agonists. Patients with multiple-system atrophy, striatonigral degeneration, progressive supranuclear palsy, or olivopontocerebellar atrophy are not candidates. Medical management of patients with idiopathic PD should be optimized before surgery, depression should be treated, and the cognitive state of patients should be thoroughly assessed. Patients with significant cognitive impairment are less likely to have long-lasting improvement and may be unable to cooperate with motor and visual field testing during the procedure.[14,62]

ABLATIVE THERAPY
Thalamotomy
The thalamus has been targeted predominantly for its benefit on tremor. Lesions within Vim are highly effective in alleviating parkinsonian tremor in more than 85 percent of patients,[77,134] and if extended anteriorly to include Vop, and possibly portions of Voa, they also improve rigidity and dopa-induced dyskinesia.[60] Thalamic lesions generally have not been reported to improve bradykinesia or akinesia and have been reported to exacerbate speech and gait disorders in some patients.[135,136] Studies showing exception to this are sparse; Hassler reported that bradykinesia did improve following lesions that included more anterior portions of the motor thalamus (i.e., Voa).[11] While thalamotomy has similar benefit on parkinsonian tremor as pallidotomy (see below), its efficacy on other symptoms is more limited. As PD progresses, akinesia, rigidity and gait problems invariably become problematic. Given the success of other procedures in improving all of these symptoms, thalamotomy is usually not recommended.

Pallidotomy
Based on the hypokinetic rate model, lesions in either the sensorimotor portion of the GPi or the STN should be effective in reducing or alleviating the motor signs associated with PD. Lesions that lie outside or involve only a portion of this circuit are likely to result in no or only a partial benefit.[137] Optimal benefit is most likely to occur with lesions that most completely interrupt the motor circuit.[10,137] The optimal location and size of the lesion within the GPi, although not yet fully defined, should involve as much of the sensorimotor portion of GPi as possible without infringing on nearby critical structures (i.e., GPe, nucleus basalis, internal capsule, and the optic tract). Modern techniques using MRI-guided stereotaxic targeting, electrophysiological mapping techniques to identify the target structure together with an improved understanding of the pathophysiological basis underlying the development of parkinsonian motor signs have lead to improved and more reliable outcomes.

A prospective single-blind trial randomizing 36 patients to unilateral pallidotomy or best medical therapy was conducted at our center. Results at 6 months showed unilateral pallidotomy improved the total UPDRS (Unified Parkinson's Disease Rating Scale) score by 32 percent over the presurgical baseline while, at the same time, patients with medical therapy alone worsened by 5 percent. The UPDRS "off" motor subscore in the surgical arm improved by 33 percent; there was no significant improvement in the "on"-period motor subscore. There was significant improvement in contralateral tremor, rigidity, bradykinesia, and dyskinesias. Gait and "off"-period freezing were also significantly improved.[19] Significant improvement in ipsilateral rigidity, bradykinesia, and drug-induced dyskinesia was also observed.

After meeting the primary outcome criteria at 6 months, control patients were offered pallidotomy and a total of 20 patients were followed for 2 years. Over this time, the patients continued to have a significant (25 percent) benefit in their off-medicine motor UPDRS subscore. Dyskinesias, rigidity, and bradykinesia continued to show bilateral improvement, and tremor maintained contralateral improvement. However, there was loss of benefit in midline symptoms, including postural stability, gait, and freezing.[19] Although the patients did worsen with time, some of this may have been due to progression of the underlying disease, particularly in the contralateral side where no surgery was performed.

One other randomized study showed similar results with the UPDRS "off" motor score improving 31 percent from baseline in the surgical arm at 6 months.[138] On average, other nonrandomized series showed similar benefit with a roughly 30 percent improvement in the motor "off" score at 6 months postoperatively.[14,15,139–148]

Results of long-term studies are more divergent. Most studies show loss of gait and postural benefit beyond 1 year;[19,149–153] however, a few show persistent benefit beyond 2 years.[10,12,154]

Improvement of ipsilateral "off" rigidity often does not last beyond 1 year,[149,150,152,153,155] although our recent randomized single-blinded study showed a persistent 55 percent reduction at 2 years. Improvement of ipsilateral bradykinesia[19] and dyskinesia[19,150,153,155] is usually more robust than other ipsilateral symptomatology and have been shown to persist for as long as 2 years in several studies. Studies of patients followed for up to 4 years showed significant reductions of contralateral tremor and dyskinesia and a milder reduction of contralateral rigidity and bradykinesia that was not always significant.[150,156]

Current use of pallidotomy for PD is mostly restricted to unilateral procedures due to the finding of significant hypophonia, dysarthria and worsening cognitive and neuropsychiatric function with bilateral pallidotomy.[157–160] With unilateral pallidotomy, cognitive side-effects are mild and often transient. Detailed neuropsychological evaluation of patients randomized to unilateral pallidotomy or medical management found a mild defect in phonemic fluency, with left pallidotomy surgeries producing a slightly higher risk. There was no overall change in mood; however, patients with a history of depression were at risk for recurrence.[161] A detailed analysis of lesion location and outcome showed that anteromedially placed lesions lead to impairment in memory and cognitive impairment, whereas posteriolateral lesions improved cognition as well as motor performance.[162]

Weight gain is common after pallidotomy.[163] More serious but rare complications of pallidotomy include delayed infarction of the internal capsule causing hemiparesis or dysarthria,[14,146,149,164] and compromise of the optic tract from a poorly placed lesion causing visual field defects.[165] Delayed infarctions, although rare, may occur in patients 2 weeks to 3–4 months after surgery. Patients with delayed infarctions often have a history of prior stroke, suggesting that patients with cerebrovascular disease may be at risk for this complication.[164] Most complications of pallidotomy are avoidable by appropriate screening and patient selection, and precise targeting. With careful targeting, lesions can be limited to motor territory and should spare more anterior areas that may be associated with cognitive and neuropsychological changes.

Subthalamotomy

The STN is another potential target in the treatment of parkinsonian motor signs. Although STN lesions in monkeys have been highly successful in ameliorating parkinsonian motor signs,[166–168] there has been reluctance to use this technique in humans because of the association of such lesions with the development of hemiballismus.[67,107–111] Although transient in most cases, intractable hemiballismus may occur after subcortical lesions involving the STN.[169] In addition, although the intensity of hemiballism has been reported to decrease over time, in animal experiments it has been reported to persist to some degree for the duration of the experiments (8 months) and may become intensified after administration of dopaminergic drugs.[166–168] Monkeys in which these observations were made, however, had not been on chronic L-dopa therapy, and the effect of subthalamotomy on dopa-induced dyskinesia in patients with long-term dopaminergic drug use is unclear. These observations, the location of the STN near the internal capsule, together with its rich blood supply, have made this a less popular target for an ablative lesion in the treatment of PD.

With modern neurosurgical techniques, including the use of MRI and neurophysiology for target localization, some groups have re-explored the use of subthalamic lesions for control of parkinsonian symptoms.[170–173] Alvarez et al. performed unilateral subthalamotomies in 10 patients, resulting in a 50 percent decrease in the off-medicine UPDRS motor score, and stable benefit in contralateral symptoms in patients followed up to 2 years. There was a less robust ipsilateral benefit that disappeared at 1 year. "On" time was improved from 53 percent at baseline to 94 percent at 12 months. Hemichorea was common but usually transient, occurring in 6 of 11 patients, and lasted from a few hours to 5 days. One additional patient had a thalamic infarct and developed disabling hemichorea at 7 days, which continued until an ipsilateral pallidotomy was performed.[172] Su et al. performed unilateral subthalamotomy in 13 patients with a 30 percent and 32 percent improvement in off-medicine UPDRS scores at 6 months and 1 year, respectively.[174] Three patients (23 percent) developed hemichorea, two of which resolved spontaneously without treatment. The third patient developed intractable chorea at 1 month postoperatively and died at 5 months from aspiration pneumonia.

Alvarez's group performed bilateral subthalamotomy in 18 patients. One patient dropped out due to ataxia and cognitive decline; the remaining 17 patients were followed for 2 years. Three patients had postoperative chorea and dysarthria. They had a 58 percent reduction in the "off" UPDRS motor subscore. There was also a significant improvement in the "on" subscore of 63 percent. There was an average decrease of L-dopa by 72 percent with five patients stopping L-dopa therapy altogether. At the same time, dopamine dyskinesias were reduced by 50 percent.[175]

These promising results show that subthalamotomy can be performed safely and with efficacy comparable to pallidotomy and that the risk of hemichorea may not be as high as previously thought. Like pallidotomy, this approach is particularly attractive when stimulation therapy is considered too costly or when the associated need for close follow-up, and periodic surgery for battery changes and follow-up visits for programming adjustments are not acceptable or feasible.

DEEP BRAIN STIMULATION (DBS)
Vim DBS
The Vim nucleus of the thalamus, although initially pursued aggressively as a target for stimulation therapy for parkinsonian tremor, has fallen out of favor due to its lack of efficacy on akinesia, rigidity, and L-dopa-induced dyskinesias. Early reports from the Grenoble group showed that, of 80 parkinsonian patients undergoing Vim DBS, 88 percent showed improvement in their tremor;[176] several smaller series from other groups showed similar results ranging from 64 percent to 100 percent of patients having improvement of their contralateral tremor.[24,28,177,178] However, 65 percent of the Grenoble patients eventually required further surgery due to progression of akinetic-rigid symptoms or dyskinesias for which the Vim DBS was ineffective.[130] Although most studies of Vim DBS have not found improvement of dyskinesia or rigidity, one group has shown some improvement in dyskinesia with a more anterior electrode placement.[23,24] At 8 mm anterior to the posterior commissure, they were likely affecting Voa and Vop. Consistent with these observations, others have targeted more anterior portions of the motor thalamus for relief of L-dopa-induced dyskinesias,[60] and rigidity.[11,179,180]

The most common complication of Vim stimulation for PD tremor is worsening dysarthria, which has been reported to occur in approximately 20 percent of patients. It is more common with bilateral stimulation and can often be reduced with reduction of the amplitude of stimulation.[25] In patients who have a contralateral thalamotomy, the incidence of dysarthria following Vim DBS on the intact side is higher, at approximately 27–30 percent.[28,176] This compares to a higher (30–50 percent) incidence of speech difficulties in patients with bilateral thalamotomies. The major advantage

to Vim stimulation over lesioning is that the side-effects associated with stimulation are reversible, whereas those that occur as a result of lesioning are not.[181,182]

Although very effective for tremor, the lack of reliable efficacy on the other cardinal parkinsonian symptoms has limited the use of Vim DBS for PD.[130] Even in patients with tremor predominant disease, other features manifest with time that would have potentially been controlled if another target had been selected.[183] Perhaps, with stimulation of Vim and Voa/Vop tremor, rigidity, and dyskinesia could be controlled, however, this has not been possible with stimulation, as current spread is not sufficient to cover such a broad territory with a single DBS lead.

GPi DBS
After initial successes with modern pallidotomy for PD and Vim stimulation to relieve parkinsonian and essential tremor, GPi DBS has appeared an attractive intervention, which may match the efficacy of pallidotomy with less risk of irreversible disability. Furthermore, bilateral GPi DBS does not have the risk of speech disturbances seen with anteriorly placed bilateral pallidotomy and can therefore be used more safely to obtain better bilateral benefit.

In the largest prospective double-blind multicenter study to date, bilateral GPi DBS showed 37 percent improvement in the off-medicine UPDRS motor subscore in 38 patients at 3 months.[184] Results from other studies have been consistently positive, and long-term studies of bilateral GPi DBS up to 2 years have shown stable benefit (Table 17-1). Two series of 6 patients showed 53 percent and 36 percent improvement at 6 months, and 50 percent and 38 percent at 2 years.[185,186] "On" time is substantially increased; the 38 patients in the DBS for Parkinson's Study improved their percent of "on" time in the day from 28 percent to 64 percent.[184]

Unlike thalamotomy or Vim DBS, GPi DBS has reliably alleviated not only tremor but all the cardinal motor symptoms of PD including akinesia/bradykinesia, rigidity, and gait.[184–194] "Off" dystonia is improved,[195,196] and, like pallidotomy, GPi DBS has a potent direct suppressing effect on L-dopa-induced dyskinesias.[29,185,186,189,197,198]

In gait kinematic studies, GPi DBS has been shown to improve both postural instability and gait, albeit less so than L-dopa. Defebvre et al. found that gait velocity increased with GPi DBS. This was considered to occur as a result of an increased stride length along with a compensatory increase in cadence.[199] Other studies have shown similar improvement along with an approximately 50 percent improvement in the UPDRS gait subscore.[30,187,188,190,200] These changes tended to be more dramatic in patients with bilateral rather than unilateral stimulation.

Complications directly due to GPi DBS are minimal and are usually eliminated with adjustment of the stimulation parameters. There are fewer reports of adverse effects on speech, mood, and cognition reported with GPi DBS than have been reported for stimulation in STN (see below).[201]

TABLE 17-1 Comparison of Results from Studies with Bilateral STN or GPi DBS

Study	3 Months	6 Months	9 Months	12 Months	24 Months	36 Months
Bilateral STN DBS						
Krack 1998[190]		71 (8)				
Burchiel 1999[189]				44 (5)		
Scotto di Luzio 2001[191]	44 (9)	54 (9)		57 (9)		
DBS Study Group 2001[184]	49 (96)					
Volkmann 2001[192]		67 (16)		60 (16)		
Limousin 1998[190]				60 (20)		
Brown 1999[301]	57 (6)					
Moro 1999[302]	34 (7)	36 (6)		41 (5)		
Pinter 1999[303]	54 (9)			55 (8)		
Bejjani 2000[305]		62 (10)				
Fraix 2000[306]	17 (24)			9 (24)		
Molinuevo 2000[307]		66 (15)				
Alegret 2001[308]	57 (15)					
Capus 2001[309]		56 (7)				
Lopiano 2001[310]	57 (16)					
Figueiras-Mendez 2002[208]				63 (22)	49 (9)	
Iansek 2002[311]						
Ostergaard 2002[312]	57 (26)			64 (26)		
Romito 2002[206]					49 (10)	49 (7)
Simuni 2002[313]				47 (12)		
Thobois 2002[227]		55 (18)		62 (14)		
Vingerhoets 2002[207]	46 (19)	49 (19)		49 (19)	63 (10)	
Average	47 (227)	58 (108)		49 (180)	50 (29)	49 (7)
Bilateral GPI DBS						
Krack 1998[190]		39 (5)				
Burchiel 1999[189]				39 (4)		
Scotto di Luzio 2001[191]	49 (5)	44 (5)		42 (5)		
DBS Study Group 2001[184]	37 (38)					
Volkmann 2001[192]		56 (11)		51 (11)		
Ghika 1998[185]		53 (6)	52 (6)	55 (6)		
Volkmann 1998[187]	44 (9)					
Kumar 2000[193]		31 (17)				
Durif 2002[304]		36 (6)		26 (6)		
Loher 2002[195]	36 (10)			41 (10)		
Average	39 (62)	42 (50)	52 (6)	43 (42)		

Data are presented as percent improvement from preoperative off-medication UPDRS motor score, by postoperative months. Number of patients are given in parentheses.

There are, however, case reports of mania,[202] apathy,[203] and mild decline in lexical verbal memory with GPi DBS.[185] Of the studies that have performed detailed neuropsychological testing, most have shown minimal subclinical changes in some patients, and overall no significant change.[204,205]

STN DBS

Like GPi stimulation, bilateral STN stimulation has been shown to improve all of the cardinal motor symptoms of PD. A multicenter double-blinded crossover study showed 49 percent improvement in the off-medicine UPDRS motor subscore in 96 patients after bilateral STN stimulation.[184]

These results and those of other studies have been consistently robust, with most studies showing 45–55 percent improvement and some showing as high as 60–70 percent improvement in the off-medicine motor subscore (Table 17-1). Like GPi DBS, improvement appears to be relatively stable to at least 24–36 months,[206,207] with only one study showing any decline[208] (see Table 17-1). "On" time is also increased: the 96 patients in the DBS for Parkinson's Study improved from spending 27 percent at baseline to 74 percent at 3 months of the day in an "on" state.[184]

Bilateral STN stimulation may produce dramatic beneficial effects on midline symptoms such as gait, posture, and balance.[190,209] Unlike GPi DBS, it has been reported to increase walking velocity to a degree that is comparable to that of L-dopa.[210,211] Most studies of patients with bilateral STN DBS attribute this increase in velocity to an increase in stride length and thus more closely approximating normal gait.[210,212–214]

STN DBS has an additive effect to L-dopa on dyskinesias and, if stimulation parameters are titrated too quickly, the patient can have distressing choreic dyskinesias.[215] As stimulation is also very effective on all the cardinal motor signs of PD, postoperative dopamine and dopamine-agonist therapy can (and usually must) be decreased.[31,216,217] If done properly, patients tolerate this well, and postoperative UPDRS scores in most studies demonstrate significant benefit despite lower doses of dopaminergic therapy.[31] In turn, by treating patients with less L-dopa, particularly if done early in their disease course, the long-term side-effect of inducing motor fluctuations and dyskinesia may be minimized.

In addition to stimulation-induced dyskinesias, there are more reports of mood, behavioral, and cognitive side-effects associated with STN than with GPi stimulation. This may be due to the fact that more centers perform STN stimulation and therefore there are more reports of side-effects; however, the STN also has unique anatomical characteristics that may make stimulation in this site more likely to be associated with such side-effects. These include (1) its small size, requiring implantation of the DBS lead in regions near nonmotor portions of the STN, and (2) its close proximity to important neighboring structures such as the median forebrain bundle and lateral hypothalamus. Because of its small size and location to nonmotor structures, inadvertent current spread into nonmotor STN or adjacent structures may affect cognition and behavior by modulating frontal and limbic function.

Worsening cognitive function has been reported in some patients with subthalamic stimulation, more commonly in older patients[218] and patients who demonstrate preoperative cognitive decline.[219] In contrast, as a whole, young and nondemented patients show no significant cognitive change.[220] Several reports show worsening of frontal lobe function as demonstrated on the Stroop test.[221,222] PET studies done during evaluation of patients taking the Stroop test implicate changes in striatoanterior cingulate cortex circuits as potentially having a role in this disturbance.[222] Whereas such findings are subclinical to routine examination, modulation of these important frontal circuits may become more important in older or demented patients with less cognitive reserve.

Limbic circuits have strong connections with medial STN and not surprisingly STN stimulation has been reported to cause apathy, depression, or mania.[192,218,223–227] Depression and apathy may also occur in part due to a reduction or sudden withdrawal of L-dopa, as such patients may show improvement with increasing dopaminergic treatment.[228] Depression has also been reported to occur in some patients, particularly with left STN stimulation.[223,229] Right-sided STN DBS may produce laughter.[230] We observed a patient who appeared to have a pseudobulbar depression with uncontrollable crying associated only with left STN stimulation, while

having no change in the Geriatric Depression Scale. She also had an exaggerated gag reflex that was present only when stimulation was turned on (unpublished observations).

Whereas speech can improve with STN stimulation, current spread in the neighboring corticobulbar fibers may cause poorer speech production.[228] Subthalamic stimulation can also induce conjugate horizontal or vertical eye deviation that is usually contraversive to the stimulation side. This is most common with a laterally placed lead and may involve the oculomotor loop.[228] Ipsilateral deviation of the homolateral eye, on the other hand, is common with medially placed leads and is likely due to direct stimulation of the oculomotor nerve.[228] Many of the side-effects of STN stimulation are limited to when stimulation is on and can often be ameliorated by changing the stimulation contact or parameter; however, mood and cognitive changes can be more occult, and may not be noticed immediately.

In addition to its size and location, the rapid medication adjustments necessitated by the prodyskinetic effect may also lead to induction of side-effects associated with too rapid a reduction in dopaminergic medications. STN stimulation also provides for more difficult postoperative management of dopamine agonist therapy in patients with dyskinesias; however, the benefits are very rewarding in properly selected patients when managed closely in the postoperative period.

Target/Procedure Selection

STN and GPi DBS are the most common neurosurgical procedures performed today for PD. Although most studies of STN stimulation have shown greater improvement in off-medicine motor subscores than those of GPi stimulation (Table 17-1), large randomized comparisons of these two targets have not been completed. One small study of 10 patients randomized to GPi or STN showed no significant difference between the two targets, with STN showing a slightly higher improvement of 44 percent as compared to 39 percent with GPi stimulation.[189] The errors in taking these data at face value without proper comparison are numerous. Average improvement is inextricably linked to targeting accuracy. There is a great degree of center-to-center variability in targeting techniques used, ranging from combined stereotaxic MRI-guided initial targeting with microelectrode and macroelectrode neurophysiologic characterization of the target structure to just CT-guided targeting with minimal or no neurophysiology. If there is a difference in targeting accuracy between these structures when targeting techniques are limited (as may be suggested by their differing size and proximity to neighboring structures with adverse stimulatory effects), then a bias can be predicted. We must also be reminded that different centers target different areas within these structures and there is not a clear consensus on the site of optimal lead placement, nor has the relationship between lead location and clinical outcome been defined. Furthermore, most STN leads are placed bilaterally whereas more GPi leads are unilateral, thus these patients cannot be directly compared. The side-effect profile differs between the two targets with, STN stimulation having more reports of mood, cognitive, and speech effects[201] and may be more difficult to manage postoperatively.[228] As more data are collected directly comparing these procedures, it may be determined that there is a select patient population better suited for each procedure. At present, however, the data by which we could make these decisions do not exist.

In PD, bilateral pallidotomies are now generally felt to have unjustifiable side-effects of hypophonia and dysarthria. Unilateral pallidotomy, however, is safe, has proven efficacy, and still exists as a good alternative to DBS for some patients. It has clear advantages when cost is an issue, when patients do not want repeated procedures for battery replacement, or programming along with the risk of infection of the implanted hardware. If the patient has bilateral disease, a different procedure may eventually be necessary for the unoperated side. Subthalamotomy, although studied less, may provide a safe alternative. More studies regarding the use of this approach for the treatment of PD are clearly needed.

ESSENTIAL TREMOR (ET) AND OTHER TREMORS

PATIENT SELECTION

ET is the most common movement disorder. It is often mild and controlled symptomatically with oral medications. However, approximately 10 percent of patients have severe disabling tremor that is refractory to medical therapy.[231] Patients with medically intractable ET who are functionally compromised in performing activities of daily living are considered candidates for surgical intervention. Maximal doses of propranolol and primidone alone and in combination should be tried before recommending surgical intervention. Deuschl and Bain also recommend a trial of gabapentin and a test dose of 12.5 mg of clozapine (if significant hand and head tremor is present) or a trial of botulinum toxin (if significant head and voice tremor is present) before declaring patients medically refractory.[231]

Patients with predominantly distal limb postural tremor are most likely to benefit from surgery. There may be a physiological explanation for this observation. The thalamus has a somatotopic lamellar organization with leg, trunk, proximal arm, distal arm, and face arranged in sequential lamellae towards the center of the nuclei.[122] Due to this somatotopic organization, proximal tremors are more difficult to treat surgically and require a larger lesion or larger area of current spread to affect more proximal limb segments. Improvement following surgery is contralateral to the side of the lesion, with little or no improvement in the ipsilateral side. Those patients with bilateral tremor should have the side operated on which, in the patient's and surgeon's view, will give the most functional benefit.

Midline symptoms such as head and voice tremor have generally been felt to require bilateral procedures. When bilateral procedures are needed, DBS is the method of choice over thalamotomy for at least one side due to the significantly high risk of dysarthria after bilateral thalamotomy.

Patients with other non-Parkinson tremor etiologies can sometime benefit from surgery as well. Patients with cerebellar outflow tremors, multiple sclerosis, or posttraumatic brain injury, may be considered for surgery as these tremors rarely respond well to medical therapy. However, success among this group of patients has been highly variable, with many undergoing several procedures, only to have their tremor return. Larger lesions or areas of current spread are required for these tremors and should involve as much of the affected limb region within Vim, and possibly Vop, as possible. These patients usually have extensive and diffuse brain pathology and thus may have less functional reserve, raising the risk of adverse outcomes with surgery. Thus, the risk versus benefit ratio must be carefully weighed for these patients before recommending surgical intervention.

RESULTS: THALAMOTOMY VERSUS Vim DBS

Both thalamic stimulation and thalamotomy have been shown to be effective in the relief of postural tremor in patients with ET. Most studies show approximately 90 percent of patients having marked improvement or complete elimination of tremor with either thalamotomy[232–241] or Vim stimulation.[176,239,240,242–247] Long-term follow-up of patients with thalamotomies shows that nearly 80 percent of patients continue to have significant improvement.[234–236]

Voice tremor is less responsive to unilateral thalamotomy but has been reported to improve in some series.[241] Several studies have noted improvement of voice and head tremors with thalamic DBS most consistently when performed bilaterally.[245,248–252] However, there is some evidence that unilateral stimulation can be efficacious in treating voice and head tremor. Koller et al. reported that 71 percent of patients had improvement in head tremor with unilateral Vim DBS and maintained this benefit when re-examined 1 year later.[244] There was also improvement in voice tremor in 57 percent of patients with voice involvement. Others have also seen similar improvement in both head[253] and voice tremor[250] with unilateral stimulation.

Complications of unilateral thalamotomy are often mild and transient, lasting only a few days to weeks postoperatively. Two to 9 percent of patients may experience some permanent neurological deficit. These deficits include numbness, weakness, dysarthria, ataxia, and cognitive problems.[233–237] There are few data on adverse outcome with bilateral thalamotomy in ET patients in the modern era. Many do not suggest bilateral thalamotomy, based on the high incidence of speech and cognitive dysfunction found in patients operated for parkinsonian tremor.[231,238,239] No recent study operated more than 3 patients bilaterally for ET.[233,234,236,237] One such study showed that 2 of 3 patients with ET had dysarthria after bilateral thalamotomy.[237] Vim DBS has a comparatively lower incidence of permanent neurological complications but does carry all the common risks of implantation of stimulation hardware, including infection and device failure, which may necessitate repeated surgical procedures. One major advantage to Vim DBS over thalamotomy is the ability to perform bilateral surgeries without the side-effects associated with bilateral thalamotomy. Alternatively, unilateral thalamotomy can be combined with contralateral Vim stimulation safely and at the same time reduce the number of battery replacements.

DYSTONIA

PATIENT SELECTION

Patients with generalized or focal dystonia, either primary or secondary, have been considered candidates for stereotaxic functional surgery. Although all groups of patients have been reported to benefit from ablative and stimulation procedures in both the thalamus and pallidum, results vary considerable across studies. No randomized trials comparing either the site (pallidum or thalamus) or technique (ablation versus stimulation) have been conducted.

Interpretation of results is also difficult due to the fact that dystonia is not a single disease, but rather a syndrome that has been traditionally divided into subcategories based on etiologic and phenomenologic criteria. Some processes that cause dystonia also cause more diffuse brain pathology and may lead to a higher risk of neuropsychological or other complications. It is also important to consider whether the disease process is progressive, raising the risk of early recurrence due to progression of the underlying disease. As our understanding of the molecular and genetic basis of these diseases and the circuitry involved improves, we will be better able to categorize patients so that subsequent studies of surgical therapy will be able to provide the necessary information to better predict which patients are most likely to respond to surgery.

Such studies will be critically dependent on the use of validated, standardized rating scales to allow comparisons across studies. In contemporary studies, patients are usually assessed by one of three commonly used scales: the Burke-Fahn-Marsden Dystonia Rating Scale (BFMDRS), the Unified Dystonia Rating Scale (UDRS) and the Physicians Global Dystonia Rating Scale (PGDS). All three have been compared in a multicenter trial and show excellent internal consistency, interrater reliability and high correlation ($r = 0.977$–0.983).[254] Additionally, the Toronto Western Spasmodic Torticollis Rating Scale (TWSTRS) has been used in several studies for cervical dystonia.[255–257]

ABLATIVE THERAPY
Thalamotomy

The thalamus was initially the preferred target for surgical therapy for dystonia. In 1976, Cooper published long-term follow-up results on 226 dystonia patients (followed on average for 7.9 years) showing that, overall, 70 percent of patients had mild-to-marked improvement with thalamotomy.[258]

Cardoso et al. showed that 47 percent of patients improved in his series.[261] Other major studies also reported positive results, which varied depending on the disease characteristics.[259,260]

Andrew et al. found that 64 percent of patients with generalized dystonia improved with thalamotomy (most of which were bilateral);[259] however, 1 year after surgery, only 35 percent retained benefit and by 3 years only 19 percent were still improved. In contrast, Cardoso found in his series that 80 percent of patients with generalized dystonia had moderate-to-marked improvement, and did better than other subgroups.[261]

Patients with hemidystonia had dramatic initial postoperative improvement in Andrew's series, with 100 percent showing improvement—91 percent were rated as good to excellent and 9 percent as fair.[259] However, after 3 years, the benefit was greatly diminished with only 17 percent continuing to show improvement. In contrast, Cardoso found that only 33 percent of patients with hemidystonia had a moderate or better response to thalamotomy.[261] He also found that 1 of 3 patients with segmental dystonia improved.

For spasmodic torticollis four major studies of thalamotomy showed that, on average, 63 percent of patients had good-to-excellent improvement. Lathien's series had only poor-to-fair improvement in all patients with significant (63 percent) major complications. The three other studies had fewer complications, with 54–82 percent of patients demonstrating good results.

Forty-five percent of patients with primary dystonia had greater than 25 percent improvement in Tasker et al.'s series.[260] Cooper also found significant improvement, and noted that Jewish patients with a significant family history of dystonia did better than others, with 85 percent improving significantly.[258] Although this series preceded the discovery of the DYT1 gene, it is likely that many of these patients may have been DYT1-positive. In contrast, non-Jewish patients with familial dystonia only improved in 56 percent of cases.

Broggi's group performed thalamic lesions in patients with cerebral palsy and dystonia and achieved a good benefit in 46 percent of patients, and a fair benefit in 18 percent.[262] Others have reported only transient benefit, not lasting longer than a year.[263,264]

Lesion location and size vary dramatically from study to study making direct comparisons difficult. Having performed a large number of thalamotomies in varied locations, Cooper suggested that the best target for dystonia is the posterior half of the ventrolateral thalamus extending into VPL, VPM, and centromedian thalamus. Targets chosen by others vary greatly, and include Vim, Voa, Vop, Vce, Vci, CeM, and pulvinar.

Complications varied significantly by series. Cooper reported a 0.7 percent mortality rate per operation and 2 percent per patient.[258] Similarly, Tasker had a 1.8 percent mortality rate per patient.[260] Dysarthria or dysphonia occurs in 18–25 percent of all dystonia patients after thalamotomy.[258,260] There is a greater incidence of dysarthria, ranging from

56 percent to 73 percent after bilateral thalamotomies compared with only 8–11 percent of patients after unilateral thalamotomy.[259,260] Additionally, Tasker reported that 6 percent of patients undergoing thalamotomy for secondary dystonia developed permanent dysphagia. Overall, Tasker noted a 21 percent incidence of major complications in patients with secondary dystonia and 25 percent in primary dystonia patients undergoing surgery.[260]

In summary, thalamotomy can have dramatic benefit in carefully selected patients. Side-effects are not trivial, particularly when bilateral procedures are required, as is the case with axial-predominant symptoms. In these instances, one must consider whether the underlying disability is significant enough to warrant the risk of surgery.

Pallidotomy

Early surgeries for dystonia were principally thalamotomies. After witnessing the beneficial effect of pallidotomy on dystonia in patients undergoing surgery for PD, several groups pursued the use of pallidotomy for other dystonic syndromes. Our group, as well as Iacono and Lozano, reported individual cases of primary generalized dystonia with dramatic improvement,[265–268] which was soon followed by several case series.[72,269–271]

In all of the series reported to date, the vast majority of idiopathic generalized dystonia patients have improved following pallidotomy. Although many of the secondary dystonia patients have improved as well, their response has generally been less dramatic and less consistent.[269–271] In primary dystonia, the BFMDRS has been reported to improve 67–80 percent,[72,270,271] whereas improvement in secondary dystonia is approximately 18 percent. This has ranged from transient benefit that was lost by 3 months in a patient reported by Teive et al.,[269] to 13 percent benefit found in 18 patients reported by Lin et al.,[270] to 59 percent average improvement in 4 patients reported by Ondo et al.[271] Even in Ondo's series, in which the results in secondary dystonia were comparatively better than others, primary dystonia still had a better response. All case series reported have been retrospective and many consist of patients who have had unilateral or bilateral pallidotomies with variable length of follow-up. In most cases, improvement is gradual, and patients continue to improve for 3–6 months or more after surgery.

Most complications reported in unilateral or bilateral pallidotomy for dystonia are mild and transient, ranging from 0 percent to 38 percent of patients.[72,268–272] Of note, unlike cases with PD, dystonia patients have not been reported to develop incapacitating hypophonia with bilateral pallidotomy.[269–271]

To date, there has been no randomized prospective trial comparing surgical targets for dystonia. One group has retrospectively compared thalamotomy and pallidotomy and suggests that pallidotomy is more effective in primary dystonia, whereas thalamotomy may be better in focal secondary dystonia.[272] However, this study was limited not only because it was retrospective but also because unilateral or bilateral surgeries were performed and some patients underwent both pallidotomy and thalamotomy. Future studies are also needed with careful characterization of patients into focal, segmental, hemi- and generalized dystonia to document carefully which patient populations respond best to the various therapies.

DEEP BRAIN STIMULATION (DBS)

Thalamic DBS

Given the data from pallidotomy and thalamotomy studies suggesting that pallidotomy may be more effective and safer and allows for bilateral procedures in patients without the high incidence of side-effects seen with bilateral thalamotomy, most studies of DBS for dystonia have chosen GPi as the target. Nevertheless, some studies have investigated thalamic stimulation in patients with primary and secondary dystonia.

Vercueil has the largest series of thalamic stimulation patients, and implanted 12 patients (4 primary, 8 secondary) in VLp thalamus.[273] Five of these patients had moderate to marked improvement of their dystonia and 3 of the remaining 7 were reimplanted in GPi with good benefit in 2. Three of the 4 primary dystonia patients had good improvement with VLp stimulation and the fourth patient had benefit in her dystonic tremor but not other dystonic movements until her thalamic leads were removed and GPi was implanted. This study shows one group's clinical experience with DBS for dystonia suggesting that GPi may be a superior target; however, it is limited by its retrospective design, variable follow-up, and study of a mixed population of primary and secondary dystonia. There is also limited support from individual case reports also suggesting that thalamic stimulation is not as good as GPi.

Trottenburg et al. implanted bilateral leads each with contacts in Vim and GPi in a single patient with tardive dystonia.[274] There was no benefit with Vim stimulation but 73 percent improvement in the BMFDS with bilateral GPi stimulation. They reported 1 other patient with dystonia-myoclonus with Vim stimulation who had improvement of the myoclonus but not dystonia.[275] In contrast, Ghika reported a case of postanoxic dystonia who failed to improve from bilateral pallidal DBS but subsequently improved after explanting and reimplanting in bilateral Voa thalamus.[276] This is an interesting finding. The patient had MRI evidence of bilateral pallidal anoxic damage possibly rendering it a poor target due to lack of functional brain to stimulate. However, by stimulating Voa thalamus, a pallidal receiving area, they may have disrupted abnormal pallidal output responsible for the patient's symptoms. Thus, theoretically the motor thalamus is a sound target for the treatment of dystonia. Experimentally it has been demonstrated that lesions or stimulation in Voa and Vop can be effective in treating the symptoms of dystonia. Lest we make the mistakes of the past, we should not dismiss the motor thalamus as a viable target for the treatment of dystonia.

GPi DBS

Pallidal stimulation has also been successful for the treatment of primary dystonia. Similar to the experience with pallidotomy, the experience with GPi DBS is predominately in patients with primary dystonia in particular, DYT1 dystonia. Coubes et al. reported seven patients with DYT1-positive dystonia, with all patients having a dramatic response to bilateral pallidal stimulation with an average improvement in the BFMDRS of 90.3 percent (range 60–100 percent) with stable results for over 1 year.[34,35] They also reported a larger series including the seven DYT1 patients as well as 9 DYT1-negative primary generalized dystonia patients with an average improvement in the BFMDRS of 80.3 percent.[35] Vercueil's series included 1 patient with DYT1-positive generalized dystonia with 86 percent improvement in the BMFDRS and 3 patients with DYT1-negative primary generalized or multifocal dystonia with an average improvement of 59 percent. Additionally, 1 secondary posttraumatic patient with hemidystonia had 72 percent improvement. Others have also showed significant improvement in patients with segmental and cervical dystonia.[277–280] It is important to note that the literature has a selective bias against reporting negative results and there have been a few DYT1-positive patients with reportedly good placement and poor outcome that have been described in unpublished abstracts.[281] The reasons for this while unclear remain important and require further study. It is also important to note that there have been no randomized trials comparing pallidal DBS to other therapies, either medical or surgical. It is important to keep in mind that the recommendations we make today are based on nonrandomized series with little documentation of the location of the lesion or lead within the targeted structure.

TARGET/PROCEDURE SELECTION

Despite the lack of careful controlled prospective trials, given the dramatic benefit, relative safety, and reversibility of GPi DBS most physicians consider GPi DBS the preferred surgical approach to dystonia.[273,281,282] Thalamic DBS may still have a role, and has not been thoroughly evaluated. Some have suggested that Vim thalamic DBS may be particularly beneficial in patients with secondary dystonia or in patients with dystonia and tremor or other hyperkinetic movements.[273,281,283] Others have suggested that Vim is the wrong thalamic target for dystonia and instead the pallidal receiving areas Voa and Vop should be targeted. Just as we should not dismiss the thalamus as a potential target for dystonia, we should not disregard pallidotomy for the treatment of dystonia. Although there has been no randomized evaluation of pallidotomy versus GPi DBS they appear to have roughly similar efficacy in improving the symptoms of primary dystonia as measured by the BFMRS.[34,35,62,267,269,271,274,281,284] Unlike patients with PD, patients with dystonia appear to tolerate bilateral pallidotomy and do not appear to develop hypophonia.[269–271] Pallidotomy may also have some advantages over pallidal DBS for dystonia since many dystonia patients require high voltages with DBS thus leading to frequent battery changes. The associated risks of surgery for battery replacements, although small, are ever present and should not be dismissed, particularly in young patients in whom battery replacements could be required every couple of years. Given the associated issues of safety and efficacy it will be important that these techniques are compared in a randomized clinical study to assess their relative efficacy, complications, and economic implications.

HEMIBALLISMUS

PATIENT SELECTION

Hemiballism is most often secondary to acute stroke but may also be due to trauma or other insult involving the subthalamic region. Medical therapies include haloperidol, diazepam, and clozapine. Many patients (56 percent) fully recover spontaneously or with medical therapy alone within 15 days of the event.[285] There is a high rate of death after poststroke hemiballism, but the vast majority of deaths are due to cerebrovascular, or cardiac etiologies. A small percentage of patients have such severe hemiballism that physical exhaustion eventually leads to death.

Patients in whom medical therapy has been unsuccessful and/or whose health is at risk secondary to continuous excessive hemiballistic movements should be considered candidates for surgery.

TARGET/PROCEDURE SELECTION

Both thalamotomy and pallidotomy have been reported to be effective in the surgical treatment of intractable hemiballismus.[75,107,113,261,286] Although there are few cases with histological confirmation of lesion location, the effective lesions in GPi are reported to lie in the posterior pallidum.[75] Those in the thalamus are placed in the ventrolateral thalamus and would appear to include portions of what is now termed Vop and Vim. These lesions, however, likely involve surrounding subnuclei and, in some histologically verified cases, involve portions of the zona incerta and reticular nucleus of the thalamus.[258,287] DBS in Vim thalamus has also been reported to be successful in isolated cases of hemiballism.[32]

Potential Mechanism(s) Underlying the Beneficial Effect of DBS and Ablative Therapy

As the surgical treatment of PD and other movement disorders has evolved from ablative techniques such as pallidotomy and thalamotomy to DBS, the traditional models of hypo- and hyperkinetic movement disorders have been challenged and revised. Alternative models of basal ganglia function were developed that focused attention on the pattern of neural discharges and the content of information that it represents.[43,70,288] Subsequent studies of DBS supported and reinforced these alternative models. This transition from the rate model to models focusing on altered patterns and uncontrolled synchrony of neuronal activity remains in a dynamic state with modifications occurring with each new piece of data supplied through experimental studies.

Based on the rate model, one might assume that pallidal or subthalamic stimulation must be inhibitory, thus explaining the similar effect of stimulation to ablation on tremor and PD motor signs. However, there is an evolving consensus based on neurophysiologic data from primate animal models and functional imaging of patients that DBS is likely *excitatory* and causes an increased output from its target nuclei.

The mechanisms proposed by which DBS may paradoxically ameliorate symptoms of PD with comparable efficacy to ablation at the same sites are numerous, and include: (1) activation of inhibitory presynaptic axons terminating in the target structure, (2) depolarization blockade, (3) block of ion channels, (4) synaptic exhaustion, or (5) jamming.[289–291] Theories (1)–(4) would require stimulation to have an inhibitory effect on target nucleus activity, which is not supported by the majority of data available to us today. Our group and others are now proposing that DBS causes an alteration of the pattern of neural activity possibly by "jamming" or interrupting abnormal neural signals responsible for many of the symptoms of PD.[292–295]

Hashimoto et al. showed that chronic stimulation of the STN in parkinsonian monkeys causes an increased mean discharge of neurons in GPi during stimulation, suggesting activation of glutamatergic subthalamic neuron projecting to GPi.[297] There appeared to be a dose-response relationship between STN stimulation and GPi activity: with subtherapeutic stimulation parameters, there were nearly equal numbers of neurons with increased, decreased or unchanged activity. At stimulation parameters that improved bradykinesia and rigidity (i.e., therapeutic stimulation), there was a dramatic shift in the percentage of neurons with increased mean discharge rates in GPi.[293] Furthermore, the pattern of neural activity was stimulus locked with an increased regularity. As mean discharge rate increased, parkinsonian symptoms paradoxically improved. Thus, a rate model does not explain the mechanism by which pallidal DBS is improving PD while a normalization of pattern further supports the role of hypo- and hyperkinetic movement disorders focusing on patterns of neuronal activity.

Support for activation of the output from the site of stimulation was also supported by studies in normal monkeys. Anderson et al. demonstrated that GPi stimulation inhibited thalamic neuronal activity consistent with activation of GABAergic GPi projections.[292] In further support of these data, microdialysis performed in GPi and SNr during STN stimulation in the rat showed increased extracellular levels of glutamate, consistent with increased activity of STN efferent projections during STN stimulation.[295]

Functional MRI (fMRI) studies of patients with deep brain stimulators implanted in STN are also consistent with stimulation-induced neuronal activation. In a study by Jech et al., increased BOLD (blood oxygenation level-dependent) signal changes were seen in ipsilateral GPi in 2 of 3 patients, and in ipsilateral thalamus in all 3 patients with STN stimulation.[294] Interestingly, the only patient that did not have GPi activation lost benefit of stimulation within 4 weeks of surgery and required reimplantation inferiorly before gaining benefit. In a recent report, these authors extended the work to 8 patients with STN DBS, all of which had ipsilateral GPi and thalamic BOLD signal changes with stimulation parameters giving the patient clinical benefit.[297] A PET study of 6 patients with GPi stimulation showed increased cerebral blood flow in ipsilateral thalamus.[298] With Vim thalamic stimulation both PET and fMRI studies have shown ipsilateral thalamic activation and ipsilateral supplementary motor area activation—an efferent target of Vim.[294,297,299] Further clues to our understanding of how DBS works may be gained from functional imaging during motor tasks. Parkinson patients have abnormal hyperactivation of SM1 and SMA. With STN or Vim stimulation, Jech et al. found that contralateral hand movement caused less activity in these areas when stimulation was turned on. Thus, there seems to be a normalization of cortical activity with stimulation.[298]

Although experimental support for activation of the site of stimulation is substantial, there remains disagreement as to whether DBS activates or inhibits neurons. Early reports that STN stimulation caused a subsequent decreased activity of neurons in SNr and the enteropeduncular nucleus (analogous to GPi) as well as VL thalamus in the anesthetized rat, led many to believe that stimulation may have a net inhibitory effect.[290,291] However, this conflicts with primate studies mentioned above.[292,296] One major difference in these studies is that in both primate studies data were collected during the stimulus train by using a spike sorter, whereas in the rat experiments data were collected after the stimulus and may not reflect the true concurrent effects of the electrical stimulation. Additionally, the anesthesia used in the rat model could have affected firing rates. Dostrovsky et al. used low current stimulation in GPi in order to record close to the stimulating electrode and found inhibition, they suggested that pallidal DBS causes excitation of inhibitory subthalamic axon terminals synapsing in GPi.[300] However, their stimulation was at a much lower intensity and frequency than that of DBS, and may not be comparable. In evidence of this, our data did not show net stimulation of GPi until stimulation reached therapeutic parameters.[293]

In summary, there is substantial evidence that DBS causes activation of fibers exiting the targeted structures (GPi, STN, or thalamus). More importantly, however, is that the pattern of activity in these pathways has been changed, replacing what may have been abnormal feedback loops with a less-disruptive more regular pattern of activation. Therefore, the clinical effect of DBS may be similar to ablative therapy in that an abnormal pattern of activity is removed, allowing the cortex to process information in a more normal manner.

References

1. Cooper IS: A review of surgical approaches to the treatment of parkinsonism, in Cooper IS (ed): *Parkinsonism: Its Medical and Surgical Therapy.* Springfield, IL: Charles C Thomas, 1960, pp 14–128.

2. Meyers R: Surgical interruption of pallidofugal fibres: Its effect on the syndrome paralysis agitans and technical considerations in its application. *N Y State J Med* 42:317–325, 1942.

3. Pollack LT, Davis L: Muscle tone in parkinsonian states. *Arch Neurol Psychiatry* 23:303–319, 1930.

4. Putnam TJ: Treatment of unilateral paralysis agitans by section of the lateral pyramidal tract. *Arch Neurol Psychiatry* 44:950–976, 1940.

5. Foerster O, Gagel O: Die Vorderseitenstrangdurchschneidung beim Menschen. *Z Neurol Psychiatr* 138:1, 1932.

6. Delmas-Marsalat P, Van Bogaert L: Sur un cas de myoclonies rhythmique continues par une intervention chirurgicale sur le tronc cerebral. *Rev Neurol* 64:728–740, 1935.

7. Bucy JC: Cortical extirpation in the treatment of involuntary movement. *Arch Neurol Psychiatry* 21, 1942.

8. Cooper IS: Ligation of the anterior choroidal artery for involuntary movements of parkinsonism. *Arch Neurol* 75:36–48, 1952.

9. Spiegel EA, Wycis HT, Marks M, Lee AJ: Stereotaxic apparatus for operations on the human brain. *Science* 106:349–350, 1946.

10. Svennilson E, Torvik A, Lowe R, Leksell L: Treatment of parkinsonism by stereotactic thermolesions in the pallidal region: A clinical evaluation of 81 cases. *Acta Psychiatr Neurol Scand* 35:358–377, 1960.

11. Hassler R, Mundinger F, Reichert T: *Stereotaxis in Parkinsonian Syndromes.* Berlin: Springer-Verlag, 1979.

12. Laitinen LV, Bergenheim AT, Hariz MI: Leksell's posteroventral pallidotomy in the treatment of Parkinson's disease. *J Neurosurg* 76:53–61, 1992.

13. Vitek JL, Bakay RA, DeLong MR: Microelectrode-guided pallidotomy for medically intractable Parkinson's disease. *Adv Neurol* 74:183–198, 1997.

14. Baron MS, Vitek JL, Bakay RA, et al: Treatment of advanced Parkinson's disease by posterior GPi pallidotomy: 1-year results of a pilot study. *Ann Neurol* 40:355–366, 1996.

15. Dogali M, Fazzini E, Kolodny E, et al: Stereotactic ventral pallidotomy for Parkinson's disease. *Neurology* 45:753–761, 1995.

16. Lozano AM, Lang AE, Galvez-Jimenez N, et al: Effect of GPi pallidotomy on motor function in Parkinson's disease. *Lancet* 346:1383–1387, 1995.

17. Vitek JL, Baron M, Kaneoke Y: Microelectrode-guided pallidotomy is an effective treatment for medically intractable Parkinson's disease. *Neurology* 44:P703, 1994.

18. Sutton JP, Couldwell W, Lew MF, et al: Ventroposterior medial pallidotomy in patients with advanced Parkinson's disease. *Neurosurgery* 36:1112–1116, 1995; discussion 1116–1117.

19. Vitek JL, Bakay RA, Freeman A, et al: Randomized trial of pallidotomy versus medical therapy for Parkinson's disease. *Ann Neurol* 53:558–569, 2003.

20. Hassler R, Reichert T, Mundinger F: Physiological observations in stereotaxic operations in extrapyramidal motor disturbances. *Brain* 83:337–350, 1960.

21. Ohye C, Kubota K, Hooper HE: Ventrolateral and subventrolateral thalamic stimulation. *Arch Neurol* 11:427–434, 1964.

22. Benabid AL, Pollak P, Seigneuret E, et al: Chronic VIM thalamic stimulation in Parkinson's disease, essential tremor and extra-pyramidal dyskinesias. *Acta Neurochir Suppl (Wien)* 58:39–44, 1993.

23. Caparros-Lefebvre D, Blond S, Vermersch P, et al: Chronic thalamic stimulation improves tremor and levodopa induced dyskinesias in Parkinson's disease. *J Neurol Neurosurg Psychiatry* 56:268–273, 1993.

24. Blond S, Caparros-Lefebvre D, Parker F, et al: Control of tremor and involuntary movement disorders by chronic stereotactic stimulation of the ventral intermediate thalamic nucleus. *J Neurosurg* 77:62–68, 1992.

25. Benabid AL, Pollak P, Gervason C, et al: Long-term suppression of tremor by chronic stimulation of the ventral intermediate thalamic nucleus. *Lancet* 337:403–406, 1991.

26. Blond S, Siegfried J: Thalamic stimulation for the treatment of tremor and other movement disorders. *Acta Neurochir Suppl (Wien)* 52:109–111, 1991.

27. Benabid AL, Pollak P, Louveau A, et al: Combined (thalamotomy and stimulation) stereotactic surgery of the VIM thalamic nucleus for bilateral Parkinson disease. *Appl Neurophysiol* 50:344-346, 1987.

28. Siegfried J, Lippitz B: Chronic electrical stimulation of the VL-VPL complex and of the pallidum in the treatment of movement disorders: Personal experience since 1982. *Stereotact Funct Neurosurg* 62:71–75, 1994.

29. Gross C, Rougier A, Guehl D, et al: High-frequency stimulation of the globus pallidus internalis in Parkinson's disease: A study of seven cases. *J Neurosurg* 87:491–498, 1997.

30. Pahwa R, Wilkinson S, Smith D, et al: High-frequency stimulation of the globus pallidus for the treatment of Parkinson's disease. *Neurology* 49:249–253, 1997.

31. Limousin P, Krack P, Pollak P, et al: Electrical stimulation of the subthalamic nucleus in advanced Parkinson's disease. *N Engl J Med* 339:1105–1111, 1998.

32. Tsubokawa T, Katayama Y, Yamamoto T: Control of persistent hemiballismus by chronic thalamic stimulation. Report of two cases. *J Neurosurg* 82:501–505, 1995.

33. Islekel S, Zileli M, Zileli B: Unilateral pallidal stimulation in cervical dystonia. *Stereotact Funct Neurosurg* 72:248–252, 1999.

34. Coubes P, Roubertie A, Vayssiere N, et al: Treatment of DYT1-generalised dystonia by stimulation of the internal globus pallidus. *Lancet* 355:2220–2221, 2000.

35. Coubes P, Roubertie A, Vayssiere N, et al: Early onset generalised dystonia: Neurosurgical treatment by continuous bilateral stimulation of the internal globus pallidus in sixteen patients. *Mov Disord* 15:S154, 2000.

36. DeLong MR: Primate models of movement disorders of basal ganglia origin. *Trends Neurosci* 13:281–285, 1990.

37. Vitek JL, Wichmann T, Delong MR: Current concepts of basal ganglia neurophysiology with respect to tremorgenesis, in Findley LJ, Koller W (eds): *Handbook of Tremor Disorders.* New York: Marcel Dekker, 1994, pp 37–50.

38. Lamarre Y, Joffroy AJ: Experimental tremor in monkey: Activity of thalamic and precentral cortical neurons in the absence of peripheral feedback. *Adv Neurol* 24:109–122, 1979.

39. Lamarre Y: Tremorgenic mechanisms in primates. *Adv Neurol* 10:23–34, 1975.

40. Llinas RR: Rebound excitation as the physiological basis for tremor: A biophysical study of the oscillatory properties of mamalian central neurones in vitro, in Findley LJ, Capildeo R (eds): *Movement Disorders: Tremor.* New York: Oxford University Press, 1984.

41. Vilis T, Hore J: Central neural mechanisms contributing to cerebellar tremor produced by limb perturbations. *J Neurophysiol* 43:279–291, 1980.

42. Hazrati LN, Parent A: Projection from the external pallidum to the reticular thalamic nucleus in the squirrel monkey. *Brain Res* 550:142–146, 1991.

43. Vitek JL, Giroux M: Physiology of hypokinetic and hyperkinetic movement disorders: Model for dyskinesia. *Ann Neurol* 47:S131–140, 2000.

44. Ilinsky IA, Jouandet ML, Goldman-Rakic PS: Organization of the nigrothalamocortical system in the rhesus monkey. *J Comp Neurol* 236:315–330, 1985.

45. Asanuma C, Thach WT, Jones EG: Distribution of cerebellar terminations and their relation to other afferent terminations in the ventral lateral thalamic region of the monkey. *Brain Res* 286:237–265, 1983.

46. Asanuma C, Thach WR, Jones EG: Anatomical evidence for segregated focal groupings of efferent cells and their terminal ramifications in the cerebellothalamic pathway of the monkey. *Brain Res* 286:267–297, 1983.

47. Asanuma C, Thach WT, Jones EG: Cytoarchitectonic delineation of the ventral lateral thalamic region in the monkey. *Brain Res* 286:219–235, 1983.

48. DeVito JL, Anderson ME: An autoradiographic study of efferent connections of the globus pallidus in *Macaca mulatta*. *Exp Brain Res* 46:107–117, 1982.

49. Schell GR, Strick PL: The origin of thalamic inputs to the arcuate premotor and supplementary motor areas. *J Neurosci* 4:539–560, 1984.

50. Jones EG, Coulter JD, Burton H, Porter R: Cells of origin and terminal distribution of corticostriatal fibers arising in the sensory-motor cortex of monkeys. *J Comp Neurol* 173:53–80, 1977.

51. Darian-Smith C, Darian-Smith I, Cheema SS: Thalamic projections to sensorimotor cortex in the macaque monkey: Use of multiple retrograde fluorescent tracers. *J Comp Neurol* 299:17–46, 1990.

52. Hamois C, Filion M: Pallidofugal projections to thalamus and midbrain: A quantitative antidromic activation study in monkeys and cats. *Exp Brain Res* 47:277–285, 1982.

53. Parent A, De Bellefeuille L: Organization of efferent projections from the internal segment of globus pallidus in primate as revealed by fluorescence retrograde labeling method. *Brain Res* 245:201–213, 1982.

54. Hoover JE, Strick PL: Multiple output channels in the basal ganglia. *Science* 259:819–821, 1993.

55. Jinnai K, Nambu A, Yoshida S, Tanibuchi I: The two separate neuron circuits through the basal ganglia concerning the preparatory or execution processes of motor control, in Mano N, Hamada I, DeLong MR (eds): *Role of the Cerebellum and Basal Ganglia in Voluntary Movement*. New York: Elsevier, 1985, pp 153–161.

56. Tanji J: Comparison of neuronal activities in the monkey supplementary and precentral motor areas. *Behav Brain Res* 18:137–142, 1985.

57. Tanji J, Kurata K: Contrasting neuronal activity in supplementary and precentral motor cortex of monkeys. I. Responses to instructions determining motor responses to forthcoming signals of different modalities. *J Neurophysiol* 53:129–141, 1985.

58. Tanji J, Okano K, Sato KC: Relation of neurons in the nonprimary motor cortex to bilateral hand movement. *Nature* 327:618–620, 1987.

59. Wise SP, Godschalk M: Functional fractionation of frontal fields. *Trends Neurosci* 10:449–450, 1987.

60. Narabayashi H, Yokochi F, Nakajima Y: Levodopa-induced dyskinesia and thalamotomy. *J Neurol Neurosurg Psychiatry* 47:831–839, 1984.

61. Ohye C: Depth microelectrode studies, in Walker AE (ed): *Stereotaxy of the Human Brain*. New York, 1982, pp 372–389.

62. Vitek JL, Bakay RA, Hashimoto T, et al: Microelectrode-guided pallidotomy: Technical approach and its application in medically intractable Parkinson's disease. *J Neurosurg* 88:1027–1043, 1998.

63. Miller WC, DeLong MR: Altered tonic activity of neurons in the globus pallidus and subthalamic nucleus in the porimate MPTP model of parkinsonism, in Carpenter MB, Jayaraman A (eds): *The Basal Ganglia II*. New York: Plenum Press, 1987, pp 415–427.

64. Filion M, Tremblay L: Abnormal spontaneous activity of globus pallidus neurons in monkeys with MPTP-induced parkinsonism. *Brain Res* 547:142–151, 1991.

65. Vitek JL, Kaneoke Y, Turner R: Neuronal activity in the internal (GPi) and external (GPe) segments of the globus pallidus (GP) of parkinsonian patients is similar to that in the MPTP-treated primate model of parkinsonism. *Soc Neurosci* 19:561, 1993.

66. Vitek JL, Ashe J, Kaneoke Y: Spontaneous neuronal activity in the motor thalamus: Alternation in pattern and rate in parkinsonism. *Soc Neurosci* 20:561, 1994.

67. Ceballos-Baumann AO, Obeso JA, Vitek JL, et al: Restoration of thalamocortical activity after posteroventral pallidotomy in Parkinson's disease. *Lancet* 344:814, 1994.

68. Narabayashi H: Tremor mechanisms, in Schaltenbrand G, Walker AE (eds): *Stereotaxy of the Human Brain*. Stuttgart: Thieme, 1982.

69. Hassler R, Dieckmann G: Stereotactic treatment of different kinds of spasmodic torticollis. *Confin Neurol* 32:135–143, 1970.

70. Vitek JL, Chockkan V, Zhang JY, et al: Neuronal activity in the basal ganglia in patients with generalized dystonia and hemiballismus. *Ann Neurol* 46:22–35, 1999.

71. Vitek JL, Ashe J, Kaneoke Y: Spontaneous neuronal activity in the motor thalamus: Alteration in pattern and rate in parkinsonism. *Neuroscience* 20(Pt 1):561, 1994.

72. Vitek JL, Zhang J, Evatt M, et al: GPi pallidotomy for dystonia: Clinical outcome and neuronal activity. *Adv Neurol* 78:211–219, 1998.

73. Wichmann T, DeLong M: Functional and pathophysiological models of the basal ganglia. *Curr Opin Neurobiol* 6:751–758, 1996.

74. Tasker RR, Yamashiro K, Lenz F, Dostrovsky JO: Thalamotomy in Parkinson's disease: Microelectrode techniques, in Lundsford D (ed): *Modern Stereotactic Surgery*. Norwell, MA: Academic Press, 1988, pp 297–313.

75. Kaneoke Y, Vitek JL: The motor thalamus in the parkinsonian primate: Enhanced burst and oscillatory activities. *Soc Neurosci* 21:1428, 1995.

76. Nakaoka T: Experimental tremor produced by ventromedial tegmental lesion in monkeys. Neuroanatomical study. *Appl Neurophysiol* 46:92–106, 1983.

77. Narabayashi H: Surgical approach to tremor, in Marsden CD (ed): *Neurology 2: Movement Disorders*. London: Butterworth, 1982.

78. Ohye C, Nakamura R, Fukamachi A, Narabayashi H: Recording and stimulation of the ventralis intermedius nucleus of the human thalamus. *Confin Neurol* 37:258, 1975.

79. Ohye C, Narabayashi H: Physiological study of presumed ventralis intermedius neurons in the human thalamus. *J Neurosurg* 50:290–297, 1979.

80. Hassler R, Mundinger F, Riechert T: Correlations between clinical and autoptic findings in stereotaxic operations of parkinsonism. *Confin Neurol* 26:282–290, 1965.

81. Hirai T, Miyazaki M, Nakajima H, et al: The correlation between tremor characteristics and the predicted volume of effective lesions in stereotaxic nucleus ventralis intermedius thalamotomy. *Brain* 106(Pt 4):1001–1018, 1983.

82. Lenz FA, Schnider S, Tasker RR, et al: The role of feedback in the tremor frequency activity of tremor cells in the ventral nuclear group of human thalamus. *Acta Neurochir Suppl (Wien)* 39:54–56, 1987.

83. Narabayashi H: Tremor: Its generation mechanism and treatment. *Handb Clin Neurol* 5:597–607, 1986.

84. Lenz FA, Kwan HC, Martin RL, et al: Single unit analysis of the human ventral thalamic nuclear group. Tremor-related activity in functionally identified cells. *Brain* 117(Pt 3):531–543, 1994.

85. Asanuma C: Organization of the external pallidal projection upon the thalamic reticular nucleus in squirrel monkeys. *Soc Neurosci* 20:332, 1994.

86. Hallanger AE, Levey AI, Lee HJ, et al: The origins of cholinergic and other subcortical afferents to the thalamus in the rat. *J Comp Neurol* 262:105–124, 1987.

87. Levey AI, Hallanger AE, Wainer BH: Cholinergic nucleus basalis neurons may influence the cortex via the thalamus. *Neurosci Lett* 74:7–13, 1987.

88. Pare D, Smith Y, Parent A, Steriade M: Projections of brainstem core cholinergic and non-cholinergic neurons of cat to intralaminar and reticular thalamic nuclei. *Neuroscience* 25:69–86, 1988.

89. Steriade M, Pare D, Parent A, Smith Y: Projections of cholinergic and non-cholinergic neurons of the brainstem core to relay and associational thalamic nuclei in the cat and macaque monkey. *Neuroscience* 25:47–67, 1988.

90. McCormick DA, Prince DA: Acetylcholine induces burst firing in thalamic reticular neurones by activating a potassium conductance. *Nature* 319:402–405, 1986.

91. McCormick DA, Prince DA: Actions of acetylcholine in the guinea-pig and cat medial and lateral geniculate nuclei, in vitro. *J Physiol* 392:147–165, 1987.

92. McCormick DA, Pape HC: Acetylcholine inhibits identified interneurons in the cat lateral geniculate nucleus. *Nature* 334:246–248, 1988.

93. McCormick DA: Cholinergic and noradrenergic modulation of thalamocortical processing. *Trends Neurosci* 12:215–221, 1989.

94. Steriade M, Jones EG, Llinas RR: *Thalamic Oscillations and Signaling.* New York: Wiley-Interscience, 1990.

95. Lee MS, Marsden CD: Movement disorders following lesions of the thalamus or subthalamic region. *Mov Disord* 9:493–507, 1994.

96. Marsden CD, Obeso JA, Zarranz JJ, Lang AE: The anatomical basis of symptomatic hemidystonia. *Brain* 108(Pt 2):463–483, 1985.

97. Lenz F, Byl N, Garonzik I, et al: Microelectrode studies of basal ganglia and VA, VL and VP thalamus in patients with dystonia: dystonia-related activity and sensory reorganization, in Kultas-Ilinsky K, Ilinsky I (eds): *Basal Ganglia and Thalamus in Health and Movement Disorders.* New York: Kluwer Academic/Plenum Publishers, 2001, pp 225–237.

98. Lenz FA, Seike MS, Jaeger CJ, et al: Thalamic single neuron activity in patients with dystonia: Dystonia-related activity and somatic sensory reorganization. *J Neurophysiology* 82:2372–2392, 1999.

99. Lenz FA, Tasker RR, Kwan HC, et al: Cross-correlation analysis of thalamic neurons and EMG activity in parkinsonian tremor. *Appl Neurophysiol* 48:305–308, 1985.

100. Lenz FA, Jaeger CJ, Seike MS, et al: Single-neuron analysis of human thalamus in patients with intention tremor and other clinical signs of cerebellar disease. *J Neurophysiol* 87:2084–2094, 2002.

101. Vitek JL, Ashe J, DeLong MR, Alexander GE: Altered somatosensory response properties of neurons in the "motor" thalamus of MPTP treated parkinsonian monkeys. *Soc Neurosci* 16:425, 1989.

102. Narabayashi H, Ohye C: Importance of microstereoencephalotomy for tremor alleviation. *Appl Neurophysiol* 43:222–227, 1980.

103. Vilis T, Hore J: Effects of changes in mechanical state of limb on cerebellar intention tremor. *J Neurophysiol* 40:1214–1224, 1977.

104. Hore J, Flament D: Changes in motor cortex neural discharge associated with the development of cerebellar limb ataxia. *J Neurophysiol* 60:1285–1302, 1988.

105. Narabayashi H: A consideration of intention tremor, in Ito M (ed): *Integrative Control Function of the Brain.* Tokyo: Kodansha, 1979, vol 2, 185–187.

106. Llinas RR: The intrinsic electrophysiological properties of mammalian neurons: Insights into central nervous system function. *Science* 242:1654–1664, 1988.

107. Carpenter MB, Whittier JR, Mettler FA: Analysis of choroid hyperkinesia in the rhesus monkey: Surgical and pharmacological analysis of hyperkinesia resulting from lesions in the subthalamic nucleus of Luys. *J Comp Neurol* 92:293–332, 1950.

108. Hamada I, DeLong MR: Excitotoxic acid lesions of the primate subthalamic nucleus result in reduced pallidal neuronal activity during active holding. *J Neurophysiol* 68:1859–1866, 1992.

109. Hamada I, DeLong MR: Excitotoxic acid lesions of the primate subthalamic nucleus result in transient dyskinesias of the contralateral limbs. *J Neurophysiol* 68:1850–1858, 1992.

110. Whittier JR, Mettler FA: Studies of subthalamus of the rhesus monkey. II. Hyperkinesia and other physiologic effects of subthalamic lesions with special reference to the subthalamic nucleus of Luys. *J Comp Neurol* 90:319–372, 1949.

111. Martin JP: Hemichorea (hemiballismus) without lesions in the corpus luysii. *Brain* 80:1–10, 1957.

112. Crossman AR, Mitchell IJ, Sambrook MA: Regional brain uptake of 2-deoxyglucose in *N*-methyl-4-phenyl-1,2,3,6-tetrahydropyridine (MPTP)-induced parkinsonism in the macaque monkey. *Neuropharmacology* 24:587–591, 1985.

113. Suarez JI, Metman LV, Reich SG, et al: Pallidotomy for hemiballismus: Efficacy and characteristics of neuronal activity. *Ann Neurol* 42:807–811, 1997.

114. Guridi J, Rodriguez-Oroz MC, Lozano AM, et al: Targeting the basal ganglia for deep brain stimulation in Parkinson's disease. *Neurology* 55:S21–28, 2000.

115. Burchiel KJ, Nguyen TT, Coombs BD, Szumoski J: MRI distortion and stereotactic neurosurgery using the Cosman-Roberts-Wells and Leksell frames. *Stereotact Funct Neurosurg* 66:123–136, 1996.

116. Liu X, Rowe J, Nandi D, et al: Localisation of the subthalamic nucleus using Radionics Image Fusion and Stereoplan combined with field potential recording. A technical note. *Stereotact Funct Neurosurg* 76:63–73, 2001.

117. Duffner F, Schiffbauer H, Breit S, et al: Relevance of image fusion for target point determination in functional neurosurgery. *Acta Neurochir* 144:445–451, 2002.

118. Egidi M, Rampini P, Locatelli M, et al: Visualisation of the subthalamic nucleus: A multiple sequential image fusion (MuSIF) technique for direct stereotaxic localisation and postoperative control. *Neurol Sci* 23:S71–72, 2002.

119. Kelly PJ, Derome P, Guiot G: Thalamic spatial variability and the surgical end results of lesions placed with neurophysiologic control. *Surg Neurol* 9:307–315, 1978.

120. Starr PA, Vitek JL, DeLong M, Bakay RA: Magnetic resonance imaging-based stereotactic localization of the globus pallidus and subthalamic nucleus. *Neurosurgery* 44:303–313, 1999; discussion 313–304.

121. Schaltenbrand G, Bailey P: *Introduction to Stereotaxis with an Atlas of the Human Brain*, II. New York: Grune & Stratton, 1959.

122. Vitek JL, Ashe J, DeLong MR, Alexander GE: Physiologic properties and somatotopic organization of the primate motor thalamus. *J Neurophysiol* 71:1498–1513, 1994.

123. Hirai T, Jones EG: A new parcellation of the human thalamus on the basis of histochemical staining. *Brain Res Brain Res Rev* 14:1–34, 1989.

124. DeLong MR: Activity of pallidal neurons during movement. *J Neurophysiol* 34:414–427, 1971.

125. Vitek JL, Bakay RAE, Hashimoto T, et al: Microelectrode-guided pallidotomy: Technical approach and application for treatment of medically intractable Parkinson's disease. *J Neurosurg* 88:1027–1043, 1998.

126. DeLong MR, Alexander GE, Miller WC, Crutcher MD: Anatomical and functional aspects of basal ganglia-thalamocortical circuits, in Winslow W (ed): *Studies in Neuroscience*. Manchester: Manchester University Press, 1989.

127. Bronte-Stewart H, Hill B, Molander M, et al: Lesion location predicts clinical outcome of pallidotomy. *Mov Disord* 13:300, 1998.

128. Hutchison WD, Allan RJ, Opitz H, et al: Neurophysiological identification of the subthalamic nucleus in surgery for Parkinson's disease. *Ann Neurol* 44:622–628, 1998.

129. Sterio D, Zonenshayn M, Mogilner AY, et al: Neurophysiological refinement of subthalamic nucleus targeting. *Neurosurgery* 50:58–67, 2002; discussion 67–59.

130. Benazzouz A, Breit S, Koudsie A, et al: Intraoperative microrecordings of the subthalamic nucleus in Parkinson's disease. *Mov Disord* 17(suppl 3):S145–149, 2002.

131. Wichmann T, Bergman H, DeLong MR: The primate subthalamic nucleus. I. Functional properties in intact animals. *J Neurophysiol* 72:494–506, 1994.

132. Abosch A, Hutchison WD, Saint-Cyr JA, et al: Movement-related neurons of the subthalamic nucleus in patients with Parkinson disease. *J Neurosurg* 97:1167–1172, 2002.

133. Rodriguez-Oroz MC, Rodriguez M, Guridi J, et al: The subthalamic nucleus in Parkinson's disease: Somatotopic organization and physiological characteristics. *Brain* 124:1777–1790, 2001.

134. Kelly PJ, Ahlskog JE, Goerss SJ, et al: Computer-assisted stereotactic ventralis lateralis thalamotomy with microelectrode recording control in patients with Parkinson's disease. *Mayo Clin Proc* 62:655–664, 1987.

135. Selby G: Stereotactic surgery for the relief of Parkinson's disease. 1. A critical review. *J Neurol Sci* 5:315–342, 1967.

136. Speelman JD: *Parkinson's Disease and Stereotaxic Surgery*. Amsterdam: Elsevier, 1991.

137. Vitek JL, Hashimoto T, Baron M: Lesion location related to outcome in microelectrode-guided pallidotomy. *Ann Neurol* 36:279, 1994.

138. de Bie RM, de Haan RJ, Nijssen PC, et al: Unilateral pallidotomy in Parkinson's disease: A randomised, single-blind, multicentre trial. *Lancet* 354:1665–1669, 1999.

139. Uitti RJ, Wharen RE, Jr, Turk MF, et al: Unilateral pallidotomy for Parkinson's disease: Comparison of outcome in younger versus elderly patients. *Neurology* 49:1072–1077, 1997.

140. Shannon KM, Penn RD, Kroin JS, et al: Stereotactic pallidotomy for the treatment of Parkinson's disease. Efficacy and adverse effects at 6 months in 26 patients. *Neurology* 50:434–438, 1998.

141. Scott R, Gregory R, Hines N, et al: Neuropsychological, neurological and functional outcome following pallidotomy for Parkinson's disease. A consecutive series of eight simultaneous bilateral and twelve unilateral procedures. *Brain* 121(Pt 4):659–675, 1998.

142. Samuel M, Caputo E, Brooks DJ, et al: A study of medial pallidotomy for Parkinson's disease: Clinical outcome, MRI location and complications. *Brain* 121(Pt 1):59–75, 1998.

143. Ondo WG, Jankovic J, Lai EC, et al: Assessment of motor function after stereotactic pallidotomy. *Neurology* 50:266–270, 1998.

144. Lang AE: Pallidal surgery. Pallidotomy vs. pallidal stimulation: Which to choose? Teaching Courses of the American Academy Meeting 1999. Saint Paul, MN: American Academy of Neurology, 1999, pp 1–7.

145. Kopyov O, Jacques D, Duma C, et al: Microelectrode-guided posteroventral medial radiofrequency pallidotomy for Parkinson's disease. *J Neurosurg* 87:52–59, 1997.

146. Giller CA, Dewey RB, Ginsburg MI, et al: Stereotactic pallidotomy and thalamotomy using individual variations of anatomic landmarks for localization. *Neurosurgery* 42:56–62, 1998; discussion 62–55.

147. Kishore A, Turnbull IM, Snow BJ, et al: Efficacy, stability and predictors of outcome of pallidotomy for Parkinson's disease. Six-month follow-up with additional 1-year observations. *Brain* 120(Pt 5):729–737, 1997.

148. Krack P, Poepping M, Weinert D, et al: Thalamic, pallidal, or subthalamic surgery for Parkinson's disease? *J Neurol* 247:II122–134, 2000.

149. Lang AE, Lozano AM, Montgomery E, et al: Posteroventral medial pallidotomy in advanced Parkinson's disease. *N Engl J Med* 337:1036–1042, 1997.

150. Baron MS, Vitek JL, Bakay RA, et al: Treatment of advanced Parkinson's disease by unilateral posterior GPi pallidotomy: 4-year results of a pilot study. *Mov Disord* 15:230–237, 2000.

151. Pal PK, Samii A, Kishore A, et al: Long term outcome of unilateral pallidotomy: Follow up of 15 patients for 3 years. *J Neurol Neurosurg Psychiatry* 69:337–344, 2000.

152. Lai EC, Jankovic J, Krauss JK, et al: Long-term efficacy of posteroventral pallidotomy in the treatment of Parkinson's disease. *Neurology* 55:1218–1222, 2000.

153. Kondziolka D, Bonaroti E, Baser S, et al: Outcomes after stereotactically guided pallidotomy for advanced Parkinson's disease. *J Neurosurg* 90:197–202, 1999.

154. Fazzini E, Dogali M, Sterio D, et al: Stereotactic pallidotomy for Parkinson's disease: A long-term follow-up of unilateral pallidotomy. *Neurology* 48:1273–1277, 1997.

155. Samii A, Turnbull IM, Kishore A, et al: Reassessment of unilateral pallidotomy in Parkinson's disease. A 2-year follow-up study. *Brain* 122(Pt 3):417–425, 1999.

156. Fine J, Duff J, Chen R, et al: Long-term follow-up of unilateral pallidotomy in advanced Parkinson's disease. *N Engl J Med* 342:1708–1714, 2000.

157. De Bie RM, Schuurman PR, Esselink RA, et al: Bilateral pallidotomy in Parkinson's disease: A retrospective study. *Mov Disord* 17:533–538, 2002.

158. Favre J, Burchiel KJ, Taha JM, Hammerstad J: Outcome of unilateral and bilateral pallidotomy for Parkinson's disease: Patient assessment. *Neurosurgery* 46:344–353, 2000; discussion 353–345.

159. Intemann PM, Masterman D, Subramanian I, et al: Staged bilateral pallidotomy for treatment of Parkinson disease. *J Neurosurg* 94:437–444, 2001.

160. Merello M, Starkstein S, Nouzeilles MI, et al: Bilateral pallidotomy for treatment of Parkinson's disease induced corticobulbar syndrome and psychic akinesia avoidable by globus pallidus lesion combined with contralateral stimulation. *J Neurol Neurosurg Psychiatry* 71:611–614, 2001.

161. Green J, McDonald WM, Vitek JL, et al: Neuropsychological and psychiatric sequelae of pallidotomy for PD: Clinical trial findings. *Neurology* 58:858–865, 2002.

162. Lombardi WJ, Gross RE, Trepanier LL, et al: Relationship of lesion location to cognitive outcome following microelectrode-guided pallidotomy for Parkinson's disease: Support for the existence of cognitive circuits in the human pallidum. *Brain* 123(Pt 4):746–758, 2000.

163. Lang AE, Lozano A, Tasker R, et al: Neuropsychological and behavioral changes and weight gain after medial pallidotomy. *Ann Neurol* 41:834–836, 1997.

164. Lim JY, De Salles AA, Bronstein J, et al: Delayed internal capsule infarctions following radiofrequency pallidotomy. Report of three cases. *J Neurosurg* 87:955–960, 1997.

165. Biousse V, Newman NJ, Carroll C, et al: Visual fields in patients with posterior GPi pallidotomy. *Neurology* 50:258–265, 1998.

166. Bergman H, Wichmann T, DeLong MR: Reversal of experimental parkinsonism by lesions of the subthalamic nucleus. *Science* 249:1436–1438, 1990.

167. Guridi J, Luquin MR, Herrero MT, Obeso JA: The subthalamic nucleus: A possible target for stereotaxic surgery in Parkinson's disease. *Mov Disord* 8:421–429, 1993.

168. Aziz TZ, Peggs D, Sambrook MA, Crossman AR: Lesion of the subthalamic nucleus for the alleviation of 1-methyl-4-phenyl-1,2,3,6-tetrahydropyridine (MPTP)-induced parkinsonism in the primate. *Mov Disord* 6:288–292, 1991.

169. Lang AE: Persistent hemiballismus with lesions outside the subthalamic nucleus. *Can J Neurol Sci* 12:125–128, 1985.

170. Su PC, Tseng HM: Subthalamotomy for end-stage severe Parkinson's disease. *Mov Disord* 17:625–627, 2002; author reply 627.

171. Su PC, Tseng HM, Liu HM, et al: Subthalamotomy for advanced Parkinson disease. *J Neurosurg* 97:598–606, 2002.

172. Alvarez L, Macias R, Guridi J, et al: Dorsal subthalamotomy for Parkinson's disease. *Mov Disord* 16:72–78, 2001.

173. Gill SS, Heywood P: Bilateral dorsolateral subthalamotomy for advanced Parkinson's disease. *Lancet* 350:1224, 1997.

174. Su PC, Tseng HM, Liu HM, et al: Treatment of advanced Parkinson's disease by subthalamotomy: One-year results. *Mov Disord* 18:531–538, 2003.

175. Alvarez L, Macias R, Lopez G, et al: Bilateral dorsal subthalamotomy in Parkinson's disease (PD): Initial response and evolution after 2 years. *Mov Disord* 17:S95, 2002.

176. Benabid AL, Pollak P, Gao D, et al: Chronic electrical stimulation of the ventralis intermedius nucleus of the thalamus as a treatment of movement disorders. *J Neurosurg* 84:203–214, 1996.

177. Hubble JP, Busenbark KL, Wilkinson S, et al: Effects of thalamic deep brain stimulation based on tremor type and diagnosis. *Mov Disord* 12:337–341, 1997.

178. Alesch F, Pinter MM, Helscher RJ, et al: Stimulation of the ventral intermediate thalamic nucleus in tremor dominated Parkinson's disease and essential tremor. *Acta Neurochir (Wien)* 136:75–81, 1995.

179. Smith MC: Location of stereotactic lesions confirmed at necropsy. *Br Med J* 1962:900–906.

180. Ohye C. Functional organization of the human thalamus: Stereotactic interventions, in Steriade M, Jones EG, McCormick DA (eds): *Thalamus.* Amsterdam: Elsevier, 1997, vol 2, pp 517–542.

181. Wester K, Hauglie-Hanssen E: Stereotaxic thalamotomy: Experiences from the levodopa era. *J Neurol Neurosurg Psychiatry* 53:427–430, 1990.

182. Matsumoto K, Shichijo F, Fukami T: Long-term follow-up review of cases of Parkinson's disease after unilateral or bilateral thalamotomy. *J Neurosurg* 60:1033–1044, 1984.

183. Krack P, Pollak P, Limousin P, et al: Stimulation of subthalamic nucleus alleviates tremor in Parkinson's disease. *Lancet* 350: 1675, 1997.

184. The Deep-Brain Stimulation for Parkinson's Disease Study Group: Deep-brain stimulation of the subthalamic nucleus or the pars interna of the globus pallidus in Parkinson's disease. *N Engl J Med* 345:956–963, 2001.

185. Ghika J, Villemure JG, Fankhauser H, et al: Efficiency and safety of bilateral contemporaneous pallidal stimulation (deep brain stimulation) in levodopa-responsive patients with Parkinson's disease with severe motor fluctuations: A 2-year follow-up review. *J Neurosurg* 89:713–718, 1998.

186. Durif F, Lemaire JJ, Debilly B, Dordain G: Long-term follow-up of globus pallidus chronic stimulation in advanced Parkinson's disease. *Mov Disord* 17:803–807, 2002.

187. Volkmann J, Sturm V, Weiss P, et al: Bilateral high-frequency stimulation of the internal globus pallidus in advanced Parkinson's disease. *Ann Neurol* 44:953–961, 1998.

188. Krack P, Pollak P, Limousin P, et al: Opposite motor effects of pallidal stimulation in Parkinson's disease. *Ann Neurol* 43:180–192, 1998.

189. Burchiel KJ, Anderson VC, Favre J, Hammerstad JP: Comparison of pallidal and subthalamic nucleus deep brain stimulation for advanced Parkinson's disease: Results of a randomized, blinded pilot study. *Neurosurgery* 45:1375–1382, 1999; discussion 1382–1374.

190. Krack P, Pollak P, Limousin P, et al: Subthalamic nucleus or internal pallidal stimulation in young onset Parkinson's disease. *Brain* 121:451–457, 1998.

191. Scotto di Luzio AE, Ammannati F, Marini P, et al: Which target for DBS in Parkinson's disease? Subthalamic nucleus versus globus pallidus internus. *Neurol Sci* 22:87–88, 2001.

192. Volkmann J, Allert N, Voges J, et al: Safety and efficacy of pallidal or subthalamic nucleus stimulation in advanced PD. *Neurology* 56:548–551, 2001.

193. Kumar R, Lang AE, Rodriguez-Oroz MC, et al: Deep brain stimulation of the globus pallidus pars interna in advanced Parkinson's disease. *Neurology* 55:S34–39, 2000.

194. Loher TJ, Burgunder JM, Pohle T, et al: Long-term pallidal deep brain stimulation in patients with advanced Parkinson disease: 1-year follow-up study. *J Neurosurg* 96:844–853, 2002.

195. Loher TJ, Burgunder JM, Weber S, et al: Effect of chronic pallidal deep brain stimulation on off period dystonia and sensory symptoms in advanced Parkinson's disease. *J Neurol Neurosurg Psychiatry* 73:395–399, 2002.

196. Sugiyama K, Yokoyama T, Namba H: Neurosurgical treatment for dopamine-induced dyskinesias in Parkinson's disease patients. *Nippon Rinsho* 58:2115–2119, 2000.

197. Nutt JG, Rufener SL, Carter JH, et al: Interactions between deep brain stimulation and levodopa in Parkinson's disease. *Neurology* 57:1835–1842, 2001.

198. Katayama Y: Deep brain stimulation (DBS) therapy for Parkinson's disease. *Nippon Rinsho* 58:2078–2083, 2000.

199. Defebvre LJ, Krystkowiak P, Blatt JL, et al: Influence of pallidal stimulation and levodopa on gait and preparatory postural adjustments in Parkinson's disease. *Mov Disord* 17:76–83, 2002.

200. Krystkowiak P, Blatt JL, Bourriez JL, et al: Chronic bilateral pallidal stimulation and levodopa do not improve gait in the same way in Parkinson's disease: A study using a video motion analysis system. *J Neurol* 248:944–949, 2001.

201. Vitek JL: Deep brain stimulation for Parkinson's disease. A critical re-evaluation of STN versus GPi DBS. *Stereotact Funct Neurosurg* 78:119–131, 2002.

202. Miyawaki E, Perlmutter JS, Troster AI, et al: The behavioral complications of pallidal stimulation: A case report. *Brain Cogn* 42:417–434, 2000.

203. Dujardin K, Krystkowiak P, Defebvre L, et al: A case of severe dysexecutive syndrome consecutive to chronic bilateral pallidal stimulation. *Neuropsychologia* 38:1305–1315, 2000.

204. Troster AI, Fields JA, Wilkinson SB, et al: Unilateral pallidal stimulation for Parkinson's disease: Neurobehavioral functioning before and 3 months after electrode implantation. *Neurology* 49:1078–1083, 1997.

205. Vingerhoets G, van der Linden C, Lannoo E, et al: Cognitive outcome after unilateral pallidal stimulation in Parkinson's disease. *J Neurol Neurosurg Psychiatry* 66:297–304, 1999.

206. Romito LM, Scerrati M, Contarino MF, et al: Long-term follow up of subthalamic nucleus stimulation in Parkinson's disease. *Neurology* 58:1546–1550, 2002.

207. Vingerhoets FJ, Villemure JG, Temperli P, et al: Subthalamic DBS replaces levodopa in Parkinson's disease: Two-year follow-up. *Neurology* 58:396–401, 2002.

208. Figueiras-Mendez R, Regidor I, Riva-Meana C, Magarinos-Ascone CM: Further supporting evidence of beneficial subthalamic stimulation in Parkinson's patients. *Neurology* 58:469–470, 2002.

209. Limousin P, Pollak P, Benazzouz A, et al: Effect of parkinsonian signs and symptoms of bilateral subthalamic nucleus stimulation. *Lancet* 345:91–95, 1995.

210. Faist M, Xie J, Kurz D, et al: Effect of bilateral subthalamic nucleus stimulation on gait in Parkinson's disease. *Brain* 124:1590–1600, 2001.

211. Yokoyama T, Sugiyama K, Nishizawa S, et al: Subthalamic nucleus stimulation for gait disturbance in Parkinson's disease. *Neurosurgery* 45:41–47, 1999; discussion 47–49.

212. Rizzone M, Ferrarin M, Pedotti A, et al: High-frequency electrical stimulation of the subthalamic nucleus in Parkinson's disease: Kinetic and kinematic gait analysis. *Neurol Sci* 23(suppl 2):S103–104, 2002.

213. Allert N, Volkmann J, Sturm V, et al: Improvement of gait in Parkinson patients treated by bilateral stimulation of subthalamic nucleus or internal pallidum. *Mov Disord* 15:51, 2000.

214. Krystkowiak P, Defebvre L, Blatt JL, et al: Influence of subthalamic nucleus stimulation on gait in Parkinson's disease: A study using the optoelectronic VICON system. *Mov Disord* 15:48, 2000 (abstract).

215. Benabid AL, Benazzouz A, Limousin P, et al: Dyskinesias and the subthalamic nucleus. *Ann Neurol* 47:S189–192, 2000.

216. Vingerhoets FJ, Villemure JG, Temperli P, et al: Subthalamic DBS replaces levodopa in Parkinson's disease: Two-year follow-up. *Neurology* 58:396–401, 2002.

217. Albanese A, Nordera GP, Caraceni T, Moro E: Long-term ventralis intermedius thalamic stimulation for parkinsonian tremor. Italian Registry for Neuromodulation in Movement Disorders. *Adv Neurol* 80:631–634, 1999.

218. Saint-Cyr JA, Trepanier LL: Neuropsychologic assessment of patients for movement disorder surgery. *Mov Disord* 15:771–783, 2000.

219. Hariz MI, Johansson F, Shamsgovara P, et al: Bilateral subthalamic nucleus stimulation in a parkinsonian patient with preoperative deficits in speech and cognition: persistent improvement in mobility but increased dependency: A case study. *Mov Disord* 15:136–139, 2000.

220. Ardouin C, Pillon B, Peiffer E, et al: Bilateral subthalamic or pallidal stimulation for Parkinson's disease affects neither memory nor executive functions: A consecutive series of 62 patients. *Ann Neurol* 46:217–223, 1999.

221. Pillon B, Ardouin C, Damier P, et al: Neuropsychological changes between "off" and "on" STN or GPi stimulation in Parkinson's disease. *Neurology* 55:411–418, 2000.

222. Schroeder U, Kuehler A, Haslinger B, et al: Subthalamic nucleus stimulation affects striato-anterior cingulate cortex circuit in a response conflict task: A PET study. *Brain* 125:1995–2004, 2002.

223. Bejjani BP, Damier P, Arnulf I, et al: Transient acute depression induced by high-frequency deep-brain stimulation. *N Engl J Med* 340:1476–1480, 1999.

224. Dujardin K, Defebvre L, Krystkowiak P, et al: Influence of chronic bilateral stimulation of the subthalamic nucleus on cognitive function in Parkinson's disease. *J Neurol* 248:603–611, 2001.

225. Kulisevsky J, Berthier ML, Gironell A, et al: Mania following deep brain stimulation for Parkinson's disease. *Neurology* 59:1421–1424, 2002.

226. Berney A, Vingerhoets F, Perrin A, et al: Effect on mood of subthalamic DBS for Parkinson's disease: A consecutive series of 24 patients. *Neurology* 59:1427–1429, 2002.

227. Thobois S, Mertens P, Guenot M, et al: Subthalamic nucleus stimulation in Parkinson's disease: Clinical evaluation of 18 patients. *J Neurol* 249:529–534, 2002.

228. Krack P, Fraix V, Mendes A, et al: Postoperative management of subthalamic nucleus stimulation for Parkinson's disease. *Mov Disord* 17:S188–197, 2002.

229. Kumar R, Krack P, Pollak P: Transient acute depression induced by high-frequency deep-brain stimulation. *N Engl J Med* 341:1003–1004, 1999; author reply 1004.

230. Krack P, Kumar R, Ardouin C, et al: Mirthful laughter induced by subthalamic nucleus stimulation. *Mov Disord* 16:867–875, 2001.

231. Deuschl G, Bain P: Deep brain stimulation for tremor: Patient selection and evaluation. *Mov Disord* 17:S102–111, 2002.

232. Riechert T, Richter D: [Surgical treatment of multiple sclerosis tremor and essential tremor]. *Muench Med Wochenschr* 114:2025–2028, 1972.

233. Ohye C, Hirai T, Miyazaki M, et al: Vim thalamotomy for the treatment of various kinds of tremor. *Appl Neurophysiol* 45:275–280, 1982.

234. Nagaseki Y, Shibazaki T, Hirai T, et al: Long-term follow-up results of selective VIM-thalamotomy. *J Neurosurg* 65:296–302, 1986.

235. Mohadjer M, Goerke H, Milios E, et al: Long-term results of stereotaxy in the treatment of essential tremor. *Stereotact Funct Neurosurg* 54/55:125–129, 1990.

236. Shahzadi S, Tasker RR, Lozano A: Thalamotomy for essential and cerebellar tremor. *Stereotact Funct Neurosurg* 65:11–17, 1995.

237. Zirh A, Reich SG, Dougherty PM, Lenz FA: Stereotactic thalamotomy in the treatment of essential tremor of the upper extremity: Reassessment including a blinded measure of outcome. *J Neurol Neurosurg Psychiatry* 66:772–775, 1999.

238. Pahwa R, Lyons K, Koller WC: Surgical treatment of essential tremor. *Neurology* 54:S39–44, 2000.

239. Schuurman PR, Bosch DA, Bossuyt PM, et al: A comparison of continuous thalamic stimulation and thalamotomy for suppression of severe tremor. *N Engl J Med* 342:461–468, 2000.

240. Pahwa R, Lyons KE, Wilkinson SB, et al: Comparison of thalamotomy to deep brain stimulation of the thalamus in essential tremor. *Mov Disord* 16:140–143, 2001.

241. Goldman MS, Ahlskog JE, Kelly PJ: The symptomatic and functional outcome of stereotactic thalamotomy for medically intractable essential tremor. *J Neurosurg* 76:924–928, 1992.

242. Pahwa R, Lyons KL, Wilkinson SB, et al: Bilateral thalamic stimulation for the treatment of essential tremor. *Neurology* 53:1447–1450, 1999.

243. Limousin P, Speelman JD, Gielen F, Janssens M: Multicentre European study of thalamic stimulation in parkinsonian and essential tremor. *J Neurol Neurosurg Psychiatry* 66:289–296, 1999.

244. Koller WC, Lyons KE, Wilkinson SB, et al: Long-term safety and efficacy of unilateral deep brain stimulation of the thalamus in essential tremor. *Mov Disord* 16:464–468, 2001.

245. Koller WC, Lyons KE, Wilkinson SB, Pahwa R: Efficacy of unilateral deep brain stimulation of the VIM nucleus of the thalamus for essential head tremor. *Mov Disord* 14:847–850, 1999.

246. Obwegeser AA, Uitti RJ, Turk MF, et al: Thalamic stimulation for the treatment of midline tremors in essential tremor patients. *Neurology* 54:2342–2344, 2000.

247. Hariz MI, Shamsgovara P, Johansson F, et al: Tolerance and tremor rebound following long-term chronic thalamic stimulation for Parkinsonian and essential tremor. *Stereotact Funct Neurosurg* 72:208–218, 1999.

248. Taha JM, Janszen MA, Favre J: Thalamic deep brain stimulation for the treatment of head, voice, and bilateral limb tremor. *J Neurosurg* 91:68–72, 1999.

249. Yoon MS, Munz M, Sataloff RT, et al: Vocal tremor reduction with deep brain stimulation. *Stereotact Funct Neurosurg* 72:241–244, 1999.

250. Carpenter MA, Pahwa R, Miyawaki KL, et al: Reduction in voice tremor under thalamic stimulation. *Neurology* 50:796–798, 1998.

251. Berk C, Honey CR: Bilateral thalamic deep brain stimulation for the treatment of head tremor. Report of two cases. *J Neurosurg* 96:615–618, 2002.

252. Ondo W, Almaguer M, Jankovic J, Simpson RK: Thalamic deep brain stimulation: Comparison between unilateral and bilateral placement. *Arch Neurol* 58:218–222, 2001.

253. Ondo W, Jankovic J, Schwartz K, et al: Unilateral thalamic deep brain stimulation for refractory essential tremor and Parkinson's disease tremor. *Neurology* 51:1063–1069, 1998.

254. Comella CL, Leurgans S, Wuu J, et al: Rating scales for dystonia: A multicenter assessment. *Mov Disord* 18:303–312, 2003.

255. Lindeboom R, Brans JW, Aramideh M, et al: Treatment of cervical dystonia: A comparison of measures for outcome assessment. *Mov Disord* 13:706–712, 1998.

256. Comella CL, Stebbins GT, Goetz CG, et al: Teaching tape for the motor section of the Toronto Western Spasmodic Torticollis Scale. *Mov Disord* 12:570–575, 1997.

257. Tarsy D: Comparison of clinical rating scales in treatment of cervical dystonia with botulinum toxin. *Mov Disord* 12:100–102, 1997.

258. Cooper IS: 20-year follow up study of the neurosurgical treatment of dystonia musculorum deformans. *Adv Neurol* 14:423–452, 1976.

259. Andrew J, Fowler CJ, Harrison MJ: Stereotaxic thalamotomy in 55 cases of dystonia. *Brain* 106(Pt 4):981–1000, 1983.

260. Tasker RR, Doorly T, Yamashiro K: Thalamotomy in generalized dystonia. *Adv Neurol* 50:615–631, 1988.

261. Cardoso F, Jankovic J, Grossman RG, Hamilton WJ: Outcome after stereotactic thalamotomy for dystonia and hemiballismus. *Neurosurgery* 36:501–507, 1995; discussion 507–508.

262. Broggi G, Angelini L, Bono R, et al: Long term results of stereotactic thalamotomy for cerebral palsy. *Neurosurgery* 12:195–202, 1983.

263. Speigel E, Wycis H, Freed H: Stereoencephalotomy: Thalamotomy and related procedures. *JAMA* 148:446–451, 1952.

264. Gros C, Frerebeau P, Perez-Dominguez E, et al: Long term results of stereotaxic surgery for infantile dystonia and dyskinesia. *Neurochirurgie* 19:171–178, 1976.

265. Vitek J, Evatt M, Zhang J, et al: Pallidotomy as a treatment for medically intractable dystonia. *Ann Neurol* 42:409, 1997.

266. Vitek JL, Evatt ML, Zhang J, et al: Pallidotomy is an effective treatment for patients with medically intractable dystonia. *Mov Disord* 12:31, 1996.

267. Lozano AM, Kumar R, Gross RE, et al: Globus pallidus internus pallidotomy for generalized dystonia. *Mov Disord* 12:865–870, 1997.

268. Iacono RP, Kuniyoshi SM, Lonser RR, et al: Simultaneous bilateral pallidoansotomy for idiopathic dystonia musculorum deformans. *Pediatr Neurol* 14:145–148, 1996.

269. Teive HA, Sa DS, Grande CV, et al: Bilateral pallidotomy for generalized dystonia. *Arq Neuropsiquiatr* 59:353–357, 2001.

270. Lin JJ, Lin SZ, Lin GY, et al: Treatment of intractable generalized dystonia by bilateral posteroventral pallidotomy: One-year results. *Zhonghua Yi Xue Za Zhi (Taipei)* 64:231–238, 2001.

271. Ondo WG, Desaloms JM, Jankovic J, Grossman RG: Pallidotomy for generalized dystonia. *Mov Disord* 13:693–698, 1998.

272. Yoshor D, Hamilton WJ, Ondo W, et al: Comparison of thalamotomy and pallidotomy for the treatment of dystonia. *Neurosurgery* 48:818–824, 2001; discussion 814–816.

273. Vercueil L, Pollak P, Fraix V, et al: Deep brain stimulation in the treatment of severe dystonia. *J Neurol* 248:695–700, 2001.

274. Trottenberg T, Paul G, Meissner W, et al: Pallidal and thalamic neurostimulation in severe tardive dystonia. *J Neurol Neurosurg Psychiatry* 70:557–559, 2001.

275. Trottenberg T, Meissner W, Kabus C, et al: Neurostimulation of the ventral intermediate thalamic nucleus in inherited myoclonus-dystonia syndrome. *Mov Disord* 16:769–771, 2001.

276. Ghika J, Villemure JC, Miklossy J, et al. Postanoxic generalized dystonia improved by bilateral Voa thalamic deep brain stimulation. *Neural* 58(2):311–313, 2002.

277. Bereznai B, Steude U, Seelos K, Botzel K: Chronic high-frequency globus pallidus internus stimulation in different types of dystonia: A clinical, video, and MRI report of six patients presenting with segmental, cervical, and generalized dystonia. *Mov Disord* 17:138–144, 2002.

278. Chang JW, Choi JY, Lee BW, et al: Unilateral globus pallidus internus stimulation improves delayed onset post-traumatic cervical dystonia with an ipsilateral focal basal ganglia lesion. *J Neurol Neurosurg Psychiatry* 73:588–590, 2002.

279. Krauss JK, Loher TJ, Pohle T, et al: Pallidal deep brain stimulation in patients with cervical dystonia and severe cervical dyskinesias with cervical myelopathy. *J Neurol Neurosurg Psychiatry* 72:249–256, 2002.

280. Andaluz N, Taha JM, Dalvi A: Bilateral pallidal deep brain stimulation for cervical and truncal dystonia. *Neurology* 57:557–558, 2001.

281. Vercueil L, Krack P, Pollak P: Results of deep brain stimulation for dystonia: A critical reappraisal. *Mov Disord* 17(suppl 3):S89–93, 2002.

282. Volkmann J, Benecke R: Deep brain stimulation for dystonia: Patient selection and evaluation. *Mov Disord* 17(suppl 3):S112–115, 2002.

283. Thompson TP, Kondziolka D, Albright AL: Thalamic stimulation for choreiform movement disorders in children. Report of two cases. *J Neurosurg* 92:718–721, 2000.

284. Tronnier VM, Fogel W: Pallidal stimulation for generalized dystonia. Report of three cases. *J Neurosurg* 92:453–456, 2000.

285. Ristic A, Marinkovic J, Dragasevic N, et al: Long-term prognosis of vascular hemiballismus. *Stroke* 33:2109–2111, 2002.

286. Jallo GI, Dogali M: Ventral intermediate thalamotomy for hemiballismus. *Stereotact Funct Neurosurg* 65:23–25, 1995.

287. Gioino GG, Dierssen G, Cooper IS: The effect of subcortical lesions on production and alleviation of hemiballic or hemichoreic movements. *J Neurol Sci* 3:10–36, 1966.

288. Nini A, Feingold A, Slovin H, Bergman H: Neurons in the globus pallidus do not show correlated activity in the normal monkey, but phase-locked oscillations appear in the MPTP model of parkinsonism. *J Neurophysiol* 74:1800–1805, 1995.

289. Benabid AL, Benazzous A, Pollak P: Mechanisms of deep brain stimulation. *Mov Disord* 17(suppl 3):S73–74, 2002.

290. Benazzouz A, Gao DM, Ni ZG, et al: Effect of high-frequency stimulation of the subthalamic nucleus on the neuronal activities of the substantia nigra pars reticulata and ventrolateral nucleus of the thalamus in the rat. *Neuroscience* 99:289–295, 2000.

291. Benazzouz A, Piallat B, Pollak P, Benabid AL: Responses of substantia nigra pars reticulata and globus pallidus complex to high frequency stimulation of the subthalamic nucleus in rats: Electrophysiological data. *Neurosci Lett* 189:77–80, 1995.

292. Anderson ME, Postupna N, Ruffo M: Effects of high-frequency stimulation in the internal globus pallidus on the activity of thalamic neurons in the awake monkey. *J Neurophysiol* 89:1150–1160, 2003.

293. Vitek JL: Mechanisms of deep brain stimulation: Excitation or inhibition. *Mov Disord* 17(suppl 3):S69–72, 2002.

294. Jech R, Urgosik D, Tintera J, et al: Functional magnetic resonance imaging during deep brain stimulation: A pilot study in four patients with Parkinson's disease. *Mov Disord* 16:1126–1132, 2001.

295. Windels F, Bruet N, Poupard A, et al: Effects of high frequency stimulation of subthalamic nucleus on extracellular glutamate and GABA in substantia nigra and globus pallidus in the normal rat. *Eur J Neurosci* 12:4141–4146, 2000.

296. Hashimoto T, Elder CM, Okun MS, et al: Stimulation of the subthalamic nucleus changes the firing pattern of pallidal neurons. *J Neurosci* 23:1916–1923, 2003.

297. Jech R: Effects of deep brain stimulation of the STN and Vim nuclei in the resting state and during simple movement task. A functional MRI study at 1.5 Tesla. *Mov Disord* 17:S173, 2002.

298. Fukuda M, Mentis M, Ghilardi MF, et al: Functional correlates of pallidal stimulation for Parkinson's disease. *Ann Neurol* 49:155–164, 2001.

299. Perlmutter JS, Mink JW, Bastian AJ, et al: Blood flow responses to deep brain stimulation of thalamus. *Neurology* 58:1388–1394, 2002.

300. Dostrovsky JO, Levy R, Wu JP, et al: Microstimulation-induced inhibition of neuronal firing in human globus pallidus. *J Neurophysiol* 84:570–574, 2000.

301. Brown RG, Dowsey PL, Brown P, et al: Impact of deep brain stimulation on upper limb akinesia in Parkinson's disease. *Ann Neurol* 45:473–488, 1999.

302. Moro E, Scerrati M, Romito LM, et al: Chronic subthalamic nucleus stimulation reduces medication requirements in Parkinson's disease. *Neurology* 53:85–90, 1999.

303. Pinter MM, Alesch F, Murg M, et al: Deep brain stimulation of the subthalamic nucleus for control of extrapyramidal features in advanced idiopathic Parkinson's disease: One year follow-up. *J Neural Transm* 106:693–709, 1999.

304. Durif F, Lemaire JJ, Debilly B, Dordain G: Acute and chronic effects of anteromedial globus pallidus stimulation in Parkinson's disease. *J Neurol Neurosurg Psychiatry* 67:315–322, 1999.

305. Bejjani BP, Gervais D, Arnulf I, et al: Axial parkinsonian symptoms can be improved: The role of levodopa and bilateral subthalamic stimulation. *J Neurol Neurosurg Psychiatry* 68:595–600, 2000.

306. Fraix V, Pollak P, Van Blercom N, et al: Effect of subthalamic nucleus stimulation on levodopa-induced dyskinesia in Parkinson's disease. *Neurology* 55:1921–1923, 2000.

307. Molinuevo JL, Valldeoriola F, Tolosa E, et al: Levodopa withdrawal after bilateral subthalamic nucleus stimulation in advanced Parkinson disease. *Arch Neurol* 57:983–988, 2000.

308. Alegret M, Junque C, Valldeoriola F, et al: Effects of bilateral subthalamic stimulation on cognitive function in Parkinson disease. *Arch Neurol* 58:1223–1227, 2001.

309. Capus L, Melatini A, Zorzon M, et al: Chronic bilateral electrical stimulation of the subthalamic nucleus for the treatment of advanced Parkinson's disease. *Neurol Sci* 22:57–58, 2001.

310. Lopiano L, Rizzone M, Bergamasco B, et al: Deep brain stimulation of the subthalamic nucleus: Clinical effectiveness and safety. *Neurology* 56:552–554, 2001.

311. Iansek R, Rosenfeld JV, Huxham FE: Deep brain stimulation of the subthalamic nucleus in Parkinson's disease. *Med J Aust* 177:142–146, 2002.

312. Ostergaard K, Sunde N, Dupont E: Effects of bilateral stimulation of the subthalamic nucleus in patients with severe Parkinson's disease and motor fluctuations. *Mov Disord* 17:693–700, 2002.

313. Simuni T, Jaggi JL, Mulholland H, et al: Bilateral stimulation of the subthalamic nucleus in patients with Parkinson disease: A study of efficacy and safety. *J Neurosurg* 96:666–672, 2002.

Chapter 18

NEUROBEHAVIORAL ABNORMALITIES IN PARKINSON'S DISEASE

RUTH DJALDETTI and ELDAD MELAMED

IS THERE A SPECIFIC PARKINSONIAN
PERSONALITY TRAIT?   319
DEPRESSION   319
ANXIETY DISORDERS   320
SLEEP DISORDERS   321
PSYCHOSIS   321

Although Parkinson's disease (PD) is best known as a movement disorder, dysfunction is by no means limited to the motor domain. In addition to nonmotor autonomic and cognitive impairments, such as dementia (see Chap. 2), there are also important neurobehavioral abnormalities that affect, and are in turn affected, by the illness (see Table 18-1). These include mainly personality changes, depression, anxiety and panic attacks, sleep alterations (including vivid dreams), and psychosis. The problems may be related to the basic pathology of PD, the effect of antiparkinsonian drugs, or both. Sometimes, the neurobehavioral impairments become dominant and functional disability, influence motor function, cognition, and the response to L-dopa and other medications.

Is There a Specific Parkinsonian Personality Trait?

There have been many attempts to define a characteristic premorbid personality type in PD.[1–3] Although findings are inconclusive, it seems that individuals who are passive, anxious, moody, insecure, punctual, cautious, and morally rigid have a greater tendency to develop the disease. For instance,

TABLE 18-1 Neurobehavioral Abnormalities in PD

Personality changes
Depression
Anxiety and panic attacks
Sleep disorders
Psychosis

a cessation or reduction in smoking, which is common in PD, may simply be related to a premorbid personality trait and not to an antiparkinsonian protective effect of cigarette smoke. The personality type is apparently not dopamine-dependent.[4]

Depression

Depression is by far the most common psychiatric or neurobehavioral problem in PD.[5–10] Its prevalence varies in the different series, but is generally estimated within the range of 25–40 percent.[5–11] It is not unlikely that part of the depression may be reactive to the presence of a chronic progressive illness, particularly the incapacitating movement abnormalities.[10–13] However, researchers now accept that most of the depression in PD is endogenous and constitutes an important and common component of the disease symptomatology. This view is supported by several observations: (1) in 15–25 percent of patients, depression precedes the emergence of the motor signs and symptoms,[5–10] often by a year to even several years; (2) depression is relatively more prevalent in patients with PD than in patients with chronic disorders involving similar disability;[10] (3) depression is not necessarily correlated directly with the severity of the disease.[13] Risk factors for depression in PD are akinesia and increased severity of disability, anxiety, and psychosis. The role of female gender, onset of parkinsonism at a younger age, and use of L-dopa is still debatable.[14,15] Moreover, depression itself has a strong positive association with subsequent risk of PD.[16]

In general, parkinsonian depression is mild to moderate, and in some cases it is revealed only by direct questioning or the use of various neuropsychological tests and scales. Only in a small percentage of patients is it severe, and only rarely associated with suicidal attempts.[10–12] The depression may be permanent and chronic in some patients and relapsing-remitting in others. There seems to be no direct association with the type of depression and sex, age, duration of disease, and antiparkinsonian drugs.

The presence and severity of depression may have an impact on several aspects of the disease. It can adversely affect the basic parkinsonian symptomatology and even the response to drugs. Treating neurologists should be alerted to the possible presence of depression in patients with a good objective motor improvement in response to onset of L-dopa treatment, but no concomitant satisfaction, and in optimally managed patients with more advanced illness who show a sudden deterioration in motor ability without an obvious cause (such as infection, physical trauma, stroke, noncompliance, or inappropriate medication). Depression may affect sleep and contribute to insomnia. Prognostically, it is considered a risk factor for cognitive decline, particularly in memory and selective attention.[17–20] These comorbidities are due to the common involvement of anterior cingulate regions. Accordingly, depressed patients with cognitive decline are predisposed to even deeper depression. Depression may amplify the basic fatigue and lack of energy that are quite common in PD[21] and reduce the patient's general drive and desire to engage in physical activities. It commonly leads to loss of appetite and reduced caloric intake. Hence, depression-associated anorexia is an important cause of loss of weight, even leading to emaciation, particularly in patients in the more advanced stages.

The pathogenic mechanisms responsible for the occurrence of depression in PD are unknown. One possibility is the loss of dopaminergic innervation in specific parts of the basal ganglia or, more likely, the limbic system. There is evidence of a major degeneration of the nigromesolimbic dopaminergic neurons emanating from the A10 region within the midbrain in parkinsonism. Indeed, the most common adverse reactions to reserpine, a drug that depletes dopamine in vesicular sites, are parkinsonism and depression. Furthermore, in patients with response fluctuations due to chronic L-dopa administration, "off" periods are commonly associated with severe depression but rapidly disappear when a dose of L-dopa successfully turns them "on."[15,22,23] At the same time, the role of dopamine depletion in parkinsonian depression is negated by studies showing that, although the administration of L-dopa and other antiparkinsonian drugs increases dopamine concentrations and restores dopaminergic transmission in the striatum (caudate and putamen nuclei) and in the limbic system (e.g., nucleus accumbens, and hippocampus), it significantly improved only the motor functioning, but not the depression. Others have suggested that serotonergic mechanisms may be important.[24] Serotonergic projections originating from the raphe nuclei in the brainstem are variably involved in the degenerating process of PD. Generally, in depression, and also in parkinsonian depression, there is a reduction in the major metabolite of serotonin, 5-hydroxyindoleacetic acid (5-HIAA), in the cerebrospinal fluid, indicating reduced central serotonergic neurotransmission.[10] This is supported by findings of polymorphism of the serotonin transporter expression in patients with PD.[25] Autopsy studies have also revealed that brains of PD patients have not only reduced levels of serotonin and dopamine, but also reduced levels of norepinephrine.

Neurologists usually fail to identify the presence of depression and fatigue during routine office visits. Yet, it is mandatory that depression be sought and diagnosed, and, when present, brought to the attention of the patients and their families and properly treated. Sometimes reassurance alone, without supplementary psychotherapy, is sufficient. More often than not, however, patients require antidepressant medications. Amazingly, there are almost no randomized controlled clinical studies on the effect of antidepressants in patients with PD. Tricyclics are the only group of medications tested so far and found to be effective.[26] Serotonin uptake inhibitors, and more recently, combined serotonin-norepinephrine reuptake inhibitors are promising but still unproven.[27–29] Apparently, these drugs rarely induce parkinsonism, aggravate existing PD, or block the antiparkinsonian efficacy of L-dopa.[28] Electroconvulsive therapy is not contraindicated and may be used successfully in selected, severely depressed patients or in those who do not respond well to pharmacotherapy.[30,31]

Anxiety Disorders

Anxiety is extremely common in PD. It may adversely affect the basic parkinsonian symptomatology, and it is correlated with a greater level of disability.[21,32] A sudden unexplained deterioration in a well-balanced patient receiving optimal medication should alert the treating neurologist to the possibility of new-onset or exacerbation of anxiety. Anxiety particularly increases the parkinsonian tremor, and the severity of the tremor may often serve as an index for anxiety rather than the basic PD. Many affected patients claim their tremor is aggravated even when they just think that others are looking at their hands. An increase in anxiety can also dramatically enhance the frequency and severity of freezing gait, and amplify L-dopa-induced dyskinesias. Anxiety adversely affects sleep, appetite, and general functioning. Recurrent or persistent side-effects of various antiparkinsonian drugs (e.g., nausea) may originate psychogenically from anxiety. Patients with anxiety may develop various phobic disorders, including fear of gait, fear of falling, fear of being alone, and fear of open places or crowds,[10] leading to a reluctance to leave the home and even severe social withdrawal. Anxiety and depression are commonly interrelated.[6,32]

Most devastating within the scope of anxiety disorders are panic attacks.[33,34] These are manifested by a sudden extreme enhancement of anxiety and unexplained fear in association with sympathetic overactivity, including palpitations, sweating, heat waves, and dry mouth. Panic attacks may occur rarely or several times a day. In patients with response fluctuations, panic attacks commonly coincide with "off" phases, particularly those linked to "wearing-off" or "on-off" phenomena, and they subside when an "on" period is achieved by a successful dose of L-dopa. Panic attacks can be totally dissociated from the motor fluctuations, even appearing abruptly, without any obvious cause, at the peak of a good motor response to L-dopa. In a fluctuating patient, a panic attack can often prematurely terminate an "on" period.

Anxiety can cause certain patients to take an excessive amount of L-dopa and thus aggravate dyskinesias and induce hallucinosis. In others, it may lead to inadvertent cessation of medications, resulting in a parkinsonian crisis. Therefore, anxiety needs to be vigorously treated by reassurance, psychotherapy, and drugs (including benzodiazepines such as alprazolam). The latter rarely exacerbate parkinsonian symptoms or reduce the efficacy of L-dopa. The new generation of serotonin reuptake inhibitors is generally recommended, with only a few case reports of their aggravation of motor symptoms.

Sleep Disorders

The spectrum of sleep disorders in PD is wide and includes excessive daytime sleepiness (19.25 percent), sleep fragmentation, insomnia, and parasomnias[35–38] (see Chap. 55). Rapid eye movement (REM) sleep behavior disorder (RBD) is the most common disorder, occurring in 15–47 percent of patients. Vivid dreams and night terrors are also common.

Many patients suffer from "paradoxical sleep"; that is, they do not sleep well or remain awake at nights and are hypersomnolent during the day. The presence of anxiety, depression, or psychosis (particularly if associated with agitation) may aggravate the insomnia.[39] Nocturnal akinesia and rigidity, and the resultant discomfort in bed, which are linked to inadequate dopaminergic coverage at night, may be important factors contributing to sleep difficulties.

Tremors and dyskinesia usually disappear during sleep. Nocturnal foot dystonia and leg cramps may occur, and the associated pain and discomfort can cause premature awakening. Paradoxically, there may be an increase in nocturnal myoclonic phenomena and periodic sleep movements. Patients sometimes toss and turn excessively in bed, particularly during REM sleep, and have violent thrashing movements. They may unknowingly beat or kick their bed partners, forcing them to seek other sleeping quarters.

Many patients, particularly those being treated with L-dopa, have vivid dreams, which are sometimes colorful, friendly, and pleasant but, more often, frightening, menacing, and associated with past unpleasant and threatening experiences. Patients frequently report dreaming about long-deceased family members (particularly parents) or friends, and they may exhibit nocturnal vocalizations and talking in their sleep. Vivid dreams may cause excessive body movements and they can become so frightening that they take the form of night terrors (pavor nocturnus). Patients may shout, cry, and show signs of intense fear during these episodes, sometimes waking themselves up. It is commonly believed that vivid dreams, particularly the night-terror type, herald the development of parkinsonian psychosis, and that the psychosis reflects a narcolepsy-like REM sleep disorder.[39] Sleep attacks have recently drawn attention owing to several reports of motor vehicle accidents involving participants in clinical trials of ropinirole and pramipexole,[40] as well with pergolide and L-dopa preparations. Overall, however, sleep attacks are rare, and it is not entirely clear if they are a consequence of the medication or the disease or both. Patients should be made aware of this danger, and those with troublesome daytime sleepiness might be advised to give up driving.

Treatment of sleep disorders is complicated and should be tailored to the problems and requirements of the individual patient (see Chap. 52). Nocturnal akinesia responds favorably to the addition of a slow-release L-dopa preparation, taken immediately before sleep. It may sometimes be necessary to administer a regular, immediate-release L-dopa preparation at bedtime so the patient can get into bed and fall asleep.

Nocturnal insomnia, excessive periodic sleep movements, and vivid dreams may improve after the administration of benzodiazepines or alprazolam. RBD is quite efficiently alleviated with clonazepam. Caution is necessary, however, because these drugs may sometimes cause or increase awakening, confusion, and instability and lead to the loss of balance and falling, particularly in males who need to urinate frequently during the night. Selegiline (L-deprenyl) may cause sleep difficulties in some patients, and, if necessary, should be discontinued or taken only in the morning. Reduction of the L-dopa dosage and intake of the last dose in the early evening can prevent or reduce vivid dreams and night terrors, but it may be intolerable because of the resultant increase in nocturnal akinesia and rigidity. Excessive daytime somnolence is one of the reasons for insomnia, and it should be treated mainly by instructing patients in sleep hygiene, increasing their physical and mental activity, and, rarely, with the use of mild psychostimulants such as methylphenidate.

In a small percentage of patients, particularly those in the advanced stage of disease who already have motor response fluctuations, individual L-dopa doses (particularly the first morning dose) may cause narcolepsy-like irresistible somnolence. Episodes of L-dopa-induced sleep may last for 30–60 minutes, and they represent an additional disabling side-effect of chronic L-dopa therapy. It is noteworthy that in certain patients, an "on" response to a single dose of L-dopa is heralded by grotesque involuntary yawning. This phenomenon is more commonly seen after apomorphine injections, used as rescue from "off" situations. The mechanisms responsible for L-dopa-induced somnolence and yawning are unknown and may involve serotonergic or cholinergic abnormalities within the reticular activating system.

Psychosis

Psychosis affects one-third of patients with PD, and is one of its most disabling complications.[10,41–44] It is actually a spectrum of disorders, consisting of illusions and hallucinosis, predominantly the visual type, paranoid delusions, agitation, aggression, confusion, and delirium. The presence of vivid dreams and night terrors may herald a transition to psychosis. Psychosis occurs more frequently in elderly patients with signs of impaired cognition and a longer duration of illness and L-dopa treatment.[45] It usually, but not always, emerges after an attempt to increase the L-dopa dose or to initiate or add other antiparkinsonian drugs. Sometimes it is triggered by a very small increase in drug dose, although its development and severity are usually dose-dependent. Although associated mainly with chronic L-dopa administration, the psychosis in some cases may be initially caused or aggravated by other antiparkinsonian drugs, namely selegiline (L-deprenyl), anticholinergics, and dopamine agonists. Use of a combination of several antiparkinsonian drugs increases susceptibility. It rarely occurs after abrupt discontinuation of

L-dopa owing, for instance, to patient's noncompliance or a planned L-dopa "holiday". In an optimally managed patient, psychosis may suddenly appear after infection, physical or mental trauma, or surgery, particularly surgery with general anesthesia.

Very seldom are there de novo patients with PD who, for unknown reasons, are extremely sensitive and develop psychosis in response to the initiation of even a small L-dopa dose. In some of these patients, this early and usually unexpected adverse reaction is transitory and does not recur when L-dopa is reinitiated after a brief interval. In others, it may indicate the presence of dementia (e.g., Lewy body dementia).

The development of psychosis in the later stages of the disease is a grave milestone indicating further deterioration and bad prognosis. It is the most common reason for transferring patients to a nursing home.[46] Family members who, despite great difficulties, continue to cope with the many incapacitating aspects of this chronic disease, including decline in L-dopa efficacy, response fluctuations, dyskinesias, and postural instability, may become helpless and discouraged when psychosis emerges. More importantly, parkinsonian psychosis is the predominant limiting factor to the optimal antiparkinsonian drug therapy. Its presence prevents an increase in L-dopa dosage or the addition of other drugs to improve motor function, particularly in advanced stages of illness, which are almost invariably associated with intolerable worsening of the psychotic phenomena. When L-dopa is discontinued or reduced, the psychosis may improve or even subside, but the parkinsonian motor signs and symptoms, and especially bradykinesia and rigidity, soon worsen, and the patient may develop a catastrophic and life-threatening parkinsonian crisis.

The clinical features of parkinsonian psychosis are varied and complex, yet quite stereotypical. The central symptom is hallucinosis, mainly of visual type (see Table 18-2). Occasionally, there are hallucinations of "presence"; that is, a physical sensation that someone or something is standing at the side or behind the patient. Auditory hallucinations are rare. When they predominate, other types of psychosis should be considered. Visual hallucinations usually involve human images: single or many, males or females, adults or children, whole or partial, colorless, dressed or naked, normal-appearing or distorted (sometimes, faceless or demoniacal), usually, but not always, unfamiliar to the patient, located in various parts of the house. They may be threatening, indifferent, or even invited and welcome.

TABLE 18-2 Manifestations of Psychosis in PD

Vivid dreams/illusions
Benign visual hallucinosis
Visual, auditory or tactile hallucinations that are threatening or disturbing
Paranoid delusions
Agitated delirium

Hallucinations may also take the form of such nonhuman images as dogs, cats, rodents, lizards, snakes, worms, and insects (e.g., ants, scorpions, cockroaches). Patients may even stop eating and lose weight, imagining that insects or worms are in their food, making it repulsive and inedible. Less often, patients report plant-like images (trees, flowers), colorful tapestry, or monstrous mythological apparitions. The hallucinations may occur only at night (e.g., when waking up, during the lingering of a dream into a state of wakefulness, when turning on the light, etc.), or during the whole 24-hour day. They may occur only rarely or become established as a common regular daily phenomenon. The frequency and intensity of the hallucinosis may increase or decrease in a given subject. Sometimes, the hallucinations are of a "benign" nature, occurring only sporadically and nonthreatening. Patients with this type tend to have partial or complete insight. If the visual hallucinations seem very real, patients find it difficult to believe otherwise, though they can often be convinced. Most people learn "how to live" with the hallucinations, mainly by developing a type of tolerance or to disregard them. Some deny their existence, even though they continue to appear, because they are ashamed to admit having them. When the hallucinations are frequent and frightening and when paranoid delusions emerge, the psychosis is considered malignant and incapacitating. It may then be associated with persecutory thoughts, suspiciousness, negativism, agitation, aggression, hypersexuality, or abnormal sexual behavior and confusion (with disorientation in time and place). Patients feel threatened. They accuse family members and other individuals of cheating, stealing, adultery, or other aggressive motives. They sometimes do not recognize their spouses and invent imaginary ones. They become fearful and restless, have no insight, and cannot be convinced of the illusory nature of the images. They wake up in the middle of the night, and, in confusion, partially dress themselves and try to go out. Nightmares may become frequent. It is at this stage that the situation at home may become intolerable.

The mechanisms responsible for the development of psychosis in PD are not yet completely understood. One major theory attributes the psychosis to an impairment in central dopaminergic neurotransmission.[47] PD is characterized by a progressive degeneration not only of the nigrostriatal dopaminergic neurons but also of the nigromesolimbic and nigrocortical projections.[48] Such denervation may render the postsynaptic dopaminergic receptors in the limbic system and cortex supersensitive. Treatment with exogenous L-dopa increases dopamine formation in both the striatum and the limbic and cortical regions. This theory is supported by the fact that the psychosis may be attenuated by a reduction or withdrawal of L-dopa or the addition of typical (phenothiazines or butyrophenones) or atypical (clozapine) dopamine receptor-blocking neuroleptics.

Another emerging hypothesis is that the psychosis is due to abnormalities in central serotonergic (5-hydroxytryptamine, 5-HT) neurotransmission.[48–50] The 5-HT raphe nuclei in the brainstem may be involved in the degenerative process of PD.[50] Exogenous L-dopa enters the brain and can be taken up by 5-HT nerve terminals, where it is inadvertently metabolized to dopamine by the enzyme dopa decarboxylase (aromatic amino acid decarboxylase).[51,52] This enzyme normally catalyzes the conversion of L-dopa to dopamine in dopaminergic nerve terminals, and L-5-hydroxytryptophan to 5-HT in serotonergic nerve endings.[51] Acute and chronic treatment with L-dopa decreases 5-HT levels and increases 5-HIAA concentrations in various brain regions, indicating increased 5-HT turnover.[50] There is evidence of both 5-HT and dopaminergic innervation within the mammalian visual cortex. Therefore, visual hallucinations in parkinsonian psychosis may be a result of nonphysiological serotonin release or displacement of serotonin from its nerve terminals in the cortex and limbic systems due to the dopamine generated from the exogenous L-dopa. These serotonin molecules may reach and activate 5-HT receptors, which are supersensitive because of previous raphe degeneration. It should also be noted that dopamine agonists and dopamine-blocking neuroleptics (including clozapine) are not entirely selective and may interact with 5-HT receptors in the brain.

Treatment of parkinsonian psychosis is both difficult and frustrating.[53,54] Sporadic, benign hallucinations usually require no treatment, although antiparkinsonian medication should not be increased because of the potential of malignant transformation. In more severe cases, the first step should be correction of possible triggering factors (see Table 18-3), followed by a reduction and possible discontinuation of non-L-dopa antiparkinsonian medications, including

anticholinergics, amantadine, selegiline, and dopamine agonists. At this stage, these drugs may not be particularly useful for the motor signs and may aggravate the psychosis. When this is not helpful, the total L-dopa daily dose and the number of doses should be reduced to a tolerable minimum. This may lead to worsening of the parkinsonism. If such worsening is disabling, L-dopa should again be slowly increased. It may be necessary to avoid alleviating the psychosis completely in order to keep the patient partially mobile. As mentioned above, the addition of classical dopamine receptor-blocking neuroleptics of the phenothiazine (e.g., chlorpromazine) or butyrophenone (e.g., haloperidol) subtypes may attenuate the psychosis, but they also aggravate parkinsonian signs and inhibit the efficacy of L-dopa.

Currently, treatment of psychosis that cannot be alleviated by lowering of dopaminergic medications is best achieved with the newer, selective ("atypical") neuroleptics. A few randomized controlled clinical studies have proven the efficacy of clozapine in the treatment of drug-induced psychosis.[55–57] Clozapine is an atypical neuroleptic agent in that it is a D4 dopamine receptor antagonist and has little effect on the D2 receptor, which is crucial in motor control. It exerts its inhibitory activity principally within the limbic system, where the D4 receptors are abundant. Studies in patients with schizophrenia have shown that, because the striatum lacks D4 receptors, clozapine may induce an antipsychotic effect without causing drug-induced parkinsonism; the dose required in these cases is in the range of hundreds of milligrams daily. Apparently, small doses of clozapine (e.g., 10–50 mg daily) in one to three divided doses can also satisfactorily attenuate parkinsonian psychosis without exacerbating motor disability or blocking L-dopa efficacy.[56–58] However, 1–2 percent of patients may develop drug-induced neutropenia, which necessitates weekly white blood counts during treatment. Other side-effects are hypersomnolence, orthostatic hypotension, sialorrhea, and paradoxical worsening of confusion in moderately to severely demented patients.

Another promising atypical neuroleptic agent is quetiapine, an atypical benzothiazepine with a low D2 receptor antagonism and a high affinity for 5-HT$_2$ receptors, which acts selectively in the mesolimbic system. These characteristics allow good control of psychotic symptoms, apparently with almost no harmful effect on parkinsonian motor symptoms.[59–61] The key is to start with a low dose at bedtime (e.g., 12.5 mg) and titrate the dose upwards in a gradual manner until the hallucinations are controlled and sleep has been consolidated (usually 25–75 mg at bedtime, but sometimes more is required) (see Table 18-3). Olanzapine is also effective, although less than clozapine, in reducing hallucinations, but it aggravates the motor symptoms.[62] There are as yet no solid data regarding other atypical neuroleptic agents (risperidone, zotepine, mianserin) for the treatment of L-dopa-induced psychosis. Cholinergic neurotransmission appears also to be involved in cognitive, behavioral and psychic symptoms in PD patients. Preliminary studies with

TABLE 18-3 Treatment Approach for Psychosis in PD

1. Correction of triggering factors (infections, dehydration, change of medication)
2. Reduction of antiparkinsonian drugs (aim: minimal effective monotherapy)
   - Reduction/discontinuation of anticholinergics or amantadine
   - Reduction of selegiline
   - In case of combined L-dopa/dopamine agonists the latter should be reduced first
   - Reduction of L-dopa at the minimal effective dose
3. Administration of antipsychotics
   - Clozapine:12.5–25 mg in the evening in case of mild psychosis, up to 100–200 mg in 2–4 dosages/day in severe psychosis
   - Quetiapine: 25–75 mg in the evening (higher bedtime doses and 1 or 2 daytime doses of 12.5–25 mg may be required in more serious cases)
   - Classic neuroleptics (i.e., haloperidol) only in case of florid paranoid psychosis for a very brief period when parenteral administration is necessary
   - Ondansetron or other 5-HT receptor antagonists
   - Cholinesterase inhibitors (donepezil, rivastigmine) in mild cases of cognitive changes and mild hallucinations

Adapted from Table 15-11.

cholinesterase inhibitors (donepezil, rivastigmine) reported a reduced severity of the psychotic symptoms and improved social behavior.[63,64]

Because serotonergic overactivity may be partially responsible for the parkinsonian psychosis, Zoldan et al.[65] recently tried treating affected patients with ondansetron, a selective 5-HT$_3$ receptor antagonist. This drug is used as an antiemetic treatment in cancer patients receiving chemotherapy. In an open protocol, ondansetron at an average daily dose of 18 mg proved effective against the visual hallucinosis and paranoid delusions without causing any worsening in the parkinsonian motor signs or suppression of the efficacy of L-dopa. The drug was well tolerated with only minimal side-effects. If the results are borne out in the controlled trial, it may become possible to treat parkinsonian psychosis with these new pharmacological strategies. This may permit increases in the daily L-dopa dosage without risking psychotic relapses, thereby improving patients' quality of life and enabling them to remain at home with their families.

Special attention should be focused on the effect of surgery (pallidotomy, deep brain stimulation) on depression, anxiety and psychosis in PD. First, researchers need to determine if the outcome presents an improvement or is mainly an epiphenomenon of motor symptom amelioration. The findings are still inconclusive, with some studies reporting marked improvement in mood, decreased anxiety, and decreased perceived stigma,[66,67] and others reporting no improvement in psychic function or even a deterioration.[68-70] In some cases, a brief euphoria caused by the improvement in motor symptoms was followed by anxiety: fear of withdrawing to the preoperative condition, psychological dependence on caregivers and medical staff, etc., which led to a vicious cycle of increased anxiety. There are a few anecdotal reports of transient increased hypersexuality and mania following deep brain stimulation.[71-73] Better understanding of the mechanisms underlying deep brain stimulation will shed light on the mechanisms responsible for psychosis.

References

1. Menza M: The personality associated with Parkinson's disease. *Curr Psychiatry Rep* 2:421–426, 2000.
2. Poewe W, Gerstenbrand F, Ransmyr G, Plorer S: Premorbid personality in Parkinson patients. *J Neurol Transm* 19:215–224, 1983.
3. Todes CJ, Lees AJ: The premorbid personality of patients with Parkinson's disease. *J Neurol Neurosurg Psychiatry* 48:97–100, 1983.
4. Kaasinen V, Nurmi E, Bergman J, et al: Personality trait and brain dopaminergic function in Parkinson's disease. *Proc Natl Acad Sci U S A* 98:13272–13277, 2001.
5. Cummings JL: Depression and Parkinson's disease: A review. *Am J Psychiatry* 149:443–454, 1992.
6. Doonreief G, Mirabello E, Bell K, et al: An estimate of the incidence of depression in idiopathic Parkinson's disease. *Arch Neurol* 49:305–307, 1992.
7. Starkstein SE, Preziosi TJ, Berthier ML, et al: Depression and cognitive impairment in Parkinson's disease. *Brain* 112:1141–1153, 1983.
8. Yamamoto M: Depression in Parkinson's disease: Its prevalence, diagnosis, and neurochemical background. *J Neurol* 248(suppl 3):5–11, 2001.
9. Brown R, Jahanshan M: Depression in Parkinson's disease: A psychological viewpoint, in Weiner WJ, Lang AE (eds): *Advances in Neurology.* New York: Raven Press, 1995, pp 61–68.
10. Mayeux R: Mental state, in Koller WC (ed): *Handbook of Parkinson's Disease.* New York: Marcel Dekker, 1987, pp 127–143.
11. Santamaria J, Tolosa E, Valles A: Parkinson's disease with depression: A possible subgroup of idiopathic parkinsonism. *Neurology* 36:1130–1133, 1986.
12. Mindham RHS, Marsden CD, Parkes JD: Psychiatric symptoms during L-dopa therapy for Parkinson's disease and their relationship to physical disability. *Psychiatr Med* 6:23–33, 1976.
13. Huber SJ, Paulson GW, Shuttleworth EC: Relationship of motor symptoms, intellectual impairment and depression in Parkinson's disease. *J Neurol Neurosurg Psychiatry* 51:855–858, 1988.
14. Schuurman AG, van den Akker M, Ensinck KTJL, et al: Increased risk of Parkinson's disease after depression: A retrospective cohort study. *Neurology* 58:1501–1504, 2002.
15. Maricle RA, Nutt JG, Valentine RJ, Carter JH: Dose response relationship of levodopa with mood and anxiety in fluctuating Parkinson's disease: A double blind, placebo-controlled study. *Neurology* 45:1757–1760, 1995.
16. Shiba M, Bower JH, Maraganore DM, et al: Anxiety disorders and depressive disorders preceding Parkinson's disease: A case-control study. *Mov Disord* 15:669–677, 2000.
17. Mayeux R, Stern Y, Rosen J, Leventhal J: Depression, intellectual impairment and Parkinson's disease. *Neurology* 31:645–650, 1981.
18. Starkstein SE, Bolduc PL, Mayberg HS, et al: Cognitive impairments and depression in Parkinson's disease: A follow-up study. *J Neurol Neurosurg Psychiatry* 53:594–602, 1990.
19. Wertman E, Speedie L, Shemesh Z, et al: Cognitive disturbances in parkinsonian patients with depression. *Neuropsychiatry Neuropsychol Behav Neurol* 6:31–37, 1993.
20. Troster AI, Paolo AM, Lyons KE, et al: The influence of depression on cognition in Parkinson's disease: A pattern of impairment distinguishable from Alzheimer's disease. *Neurology* 45:672–676, 1995.
21. Witjas T, Kaphan E, Azulay JP, et al: Nonmotor fluctuations in Parkinson's disease: Frequent and disabling. *Neurology* 59:408–413, 2002.
22. Menza MA, Sage J, Marshall E, et al: Mood changes and "on-off" phenomena in Parkinson's disease. *Mov Disord* 5:148–151, 1990.
23. Nissenbaum H, Quinn NP, Brown RG, et al: Mood swings associated with the "on-off" phenomenon in Parkinson's disease. *Psychol Med* 17:899–904, 1987.
24. Mayeux R: The serotonin hypothesis for depression in Parkinson's disease. *Adv Neurol* 53:163–166, 1990.
25. Mossner R, Hennenerg A, Schmitt A, et al: Allelic variation of serotonin transporter expression is associated with depression in Parkinson's disease. *Mol Psychiatry* 6:350–352, 2001.
26. Strang RR: Imipramine in treatment of Parkinson's disease: A double-blind placebo study. *BMJ* 2:33–34, 1965.
27. Anderson J, Aabro E, Gulman N, et al: Antidepressant treatment of Parkinson's disease. *Acta Neurol Scand* 62:210–219, 1980.

28. Montastruc JL, Fabre N, Blin O, et al: Does fluoxetine aggravate Parkinson's disease? A pilot prospective study. *Mov Disord* 10:355–357, 1995.

29. Kent JM: SNaRIs, NaSSAs and NaRIs: New agents for the treatment of depression. *Lancet* 355:911–918, 2000.

30. Douyon R, Serby M, Klutchko B, Rotrosen J: ECT and Parkinson's disease revisited: A "naturalistic" study. *Am J Psychiatry* 146:1451–1455, 1989.

31. Moellentine C, Rummans T, Ahlskog JE, et al: Effectiveness of ECT in patients with parkinsonism. *J Neuropsychiatry Clin Neurosci* 10:187–193, 1998.

32. Henderson R, Kurlan R, Kersun JM, Como P: Preliminary examination of the co-morbidity of anxiety and depression in Parkinson's disease. *J Neuropsychiatry Clin Neurosci* 4:257–264, 1992.

33. Vasquez A, Jimenez-Jimenez FJ, Garcia-Ruiz P, Garcia-Urra D: "Panic attacks" in Parkinson's disease: A long-term complication of L-dopa therapy. *Acta Neurol Scand* 87:14–18, 1993.

34. Maricle RA, Nutt JG, Carter JH: Mood and anxiety fluctuation in Parkinson's disease associated with L-dopa infusion. Preliminary findings. *Mov Disord* 10:329–332, 1995.

35. Nausieda PA: Sleep disorders, in Koller WC (ed): *Handbook of Parkinson's Disease*. New York: Marcel Dekker, 1987, pp 371–380.

36. Arnulf I, Konofal E, Merino-Andren M, et al: Parkinson's disease and sleepiness: An integral part of PD. *Neurology* 58:1019–1024, 2002.

37. Larsen JP, Tandberg E: Sleep disorders in patients with Parkinson's disease: Epidemiology and management. *CNS Drugs* 15:267–275, 2001.

38. Hobson DE, Lang AE, Martin WRW, et al: Excessive daytime sleepiness and sudden-onset sleep in Parkinson's disease: A survey by the Canadian Movement Disorders Group. *JAMA* 287:455–463, 2002.

39. Arnulf I, Bonnet AM, Damier P, et al: Hallucinations, REM sleep, and Parkinson's disease: A medical hypothesis. *Neurology* 55:281–288, 2000.

40. Frucht S, Rogers JD, Greene PE, et al: Falling asleep at the wheel: Motor vehicle mishaps in person taking pramipexole and ropinirole. *Neurology* 52:1908–1910, 1999.

41. Celesia GC, Barr AN: Psychosis and other psychiatric manifestations of L-dopa therapy. *Arch Neurol* 23:193–200, 1970.

42. Tanner CM, Vogel C, Goetz CG, Klawans HL: Hallucinations in Parkinson's disease: A population study. *Ann Neurol* 14:136–139, 1983.

43. Klawans HL: Psychiatric side effects during treatment of Parkinson's disease. *J Neurol Transm* 27(suppl):117–122, 1988.

44. Nausieda PA, Glantz R, Weber S, et al: Psychiatric complications of L-dopa therapy of Parkinson's disease. *Adv Neurol* 40:271–277, 1984.

45. Fahn S: Adverse effects of L-dopa, in Olanow CW, Lieberman AN (eds): *The Scientific Basis of the Treatment of Parkinson's Disease*. New York: Parthenon, 1992, pp 89–112.

46. Goetz CG, Stebbins GT: Risk factors for nursing home placement in advanced Parkinson's disease. *Neurology* 43:2227–2229, 1993.

47. Goetz CG, Tanner CM, Klawans HL: Pharmacology of hallucinations induced by long-term drug therapy. *Am J Psychiatry* 139:494–497, 1982.

48. Agid Y, Javoy-Agid F, Ruberge M: Biochemistry of neurotransmitters in Parkinson's disease, in Marsden CD, Fahn S (eds): *Movement Disorders*. London: Butterworth, 1987, pp 166–230.

49. Nausieda PA, Tanner CW, Klawans HL: Serotonergically active agents in L-dopa-induced psychiatric toxicity reactions. *Adv Neurol* 37:23–32, 1983.

50. Melamed E, Zoldan J, Friedberg G, Weizmann A: Involvement of serotonin in clinical features of Parkinson's disease and complications of L-dopa therapy. *Adv Neurol* 69:545–550, 1996.

51. Melamed E, Hefti F, Wurtman RJ: L-3,4-Dihydroxyphenylalanine and L-5-hydroxytryptophan decarboxylase activities in rat striatum: Effect of selective destruction of dopaminergic and serotonergic inputs. *J Neurochem* 34:1753–1756, 1980.

52. Melamed E, Hefti F, Wurtman RJ: Non-aminergic striatal neurons convert exogenous L-dopa to dopamine in parkinsonism. *Ann Neurol* 8:558–563, 1980.

53. Friedman JH: The management of L-dopa psychosis. *Clin Neuropharmacol* 14:283–295, 1991.

54. Juncos JL: Management of psychotic aspects of Parkinson's disease. *J Clin Psychiatry* 60:842–853, 1999.

55. Kahn N, Freeman A, Juncos JL, et al: Clozapine is beneficial for psychosis in Parkinson's disease. *Neurology* 41:1699–1700, 1991.

56. Parkinson Study Group. Low-dose clozapine for the treatment of drug-induced psychosis in idiopathic Parkinson's disease: Results of the double-blind, placebo controlled PSYCLOPS trial. *N Engl J Med* 340:757–763, 1999.

57. The French Clozapine Parkinson Study Group: Clozapine in drug-induced psychosis in Parkinson's disease. *Lancet* 353:2041–2042, 1999.

58. Factor SA, Brown D, Molho ES, Podskalny GD: Clozapine: A 2-year open trial in Parkinson's disease patients with psychosis. *Neurology* 44:544–546, 1994.

59. Fernandez HH: Quetiapine for the treatment of drug-induced psychosis in Parkinson's disease. *Mov Disord* 14:484–487, 1999.

60. Fernandez HH: Quetiapine for L-dopa-induced psychosis in Parkinson's disease. *Neurology* 55:899, 2000.

61. Dewey RB, O'Suileabhain PE: Treatment of drug-induced psychosis with quetiapine and clozapine in Parkinson's disease. *Neurology* 55:1753–1754, 2000.

62. Goetz CG, Blasucci LM, Leurgans S, Pappert EJ: Olanzapine and clozapine. Comparative effects on motor function in hallucinating PD patients. *Neurology* 55:748–749, 2000.

63. Bergman J, Lerner V: Successful use of donepezil for the treatment of psychotic symptoms in patients with Parkinson's disease. *Clin Neuropharmacol* 25:107–110, 2002.

64. Fabbrini G, Barbanti P, Aurilia C, et al: Donepezil in the treatment of hallucinations and delusions in Parkinson's disease. *Neurol Sci* 23:41–43, 2002.

65. Zoldan J, Friedberg G, Livneh M, Melamed E: Psychosis in advanced Parkinson's disease: Treatment with ondansetron, a 5-HT3 receptor antagonist. *Neurology* 45:1305–1308, 1995.

66. Straits Troster K, Fields JA, Wilkinson SB, et al: Health-related quality of life in Parkinson's disease after pallidotomy and deep brain stimulation. *Brain Cogn* 42:399–416, 2000.

67. Higginson CI, Fields JA, Troster AI: Which symptoms of anxiety diminish after surgical interventions of Parkinson's disease? *Neuropsychiatry Neuropsychol Behav Neurol* 14:117–121, 2001.

68. Ardouin C, Pillon B, Peiffer E, et al: Bilateral subthalamic or pallidal stimulation for Parkinson's disease affects neither memory or executive function: A consecutive series of 62 patients. *Ann Neurol* 46:217–223, 1999.

69. Trepanier LL, Saint Cyr JA, Lozano AM, Lang AE: Neuropsychological consequences of posteroventral pallidotomy for the treatment of Parkinson's disease. *Neurology* 51:207–215, 1998.

70. Houeto JL, Mesnage V, Mallet L, et al: Behavioral disorders, Parkinson's disease and subthalamic stimulation. *J Neurol Neurosurg Psychiatry* 72:701–707, 2002.

71. Romito LMA, Scerrati M, Contarino MF, et al: Long-term follow-up of subthalamic stimulation in Parkinson's disease. *Neurology* 58:1546–1550, 2002.

72. Kulisevsky J, Berthier ML, Gironell A, et al: Mania following deep brain stimulation for Parkinson's disease. *Neurology* 59:1421–1424, 2002.

73. Berney A, Vingerhoets F, Perrin A, et al: Effect on mood of subthalamic DBS for Parkinson's disease: A consecutive series of 24 patients. *Neurology* 59:1427–1428, 2002.

Chapter 19

PARKINSON'S DISEASE: NEUROPATHOLOGY

BRUCE H. WAINER and NATIVIDAD P. STOVER

GROSS PATHOLOGY   327
MICROSCOPIC PATHOLOGY   327
PATHOGENESIS   330
GENETICS, ANIMAL MODELS, AND RISK FACTORS   331

The past decade has witnessed dramatic advances in understanding the pathogenesis of neurodegenerative diseases. These advances should lead to novel therapeutic approaches, which will delay the onset, improve the rationality for symptomatic treatment, or slow down the progression of many of these diseases. The most striking discovery is that a final common pathway for many of these diseases involves the abnormal aggregation of proteins that are ultimately toxic to cellular function.[1–5] This mechanism has been implicated in trinucleotide repeat diseases, tauopathies, Alzheimer's disease (AD), multiple-system atrophy (MSA), and, as discussed in this chapter, Parkinson's disease (PD). Some of these entities exhibit Mendelian patterns of inheritance (e.g., trinucleotide repeat diseases), but the more common age-associated diseases such as PD and AD are for the most part sporadic. However, the small percentage (10 percent or less) of familial cases of PD and AD share the same pathogenic pathway as the sporadic forms. Therefore, the mutated genes have been invaluable for defining disease genotypes and their corresponding phenotypes, for generating animal models to study pathogenic mechanisms, and for the identification of logical targets for eventual therapeutic intervention. A major challenge for the future will be to identify both the genetic and environmental risk factors that trigger the development of disease. It is highly likely that preventive measures will be as important for controlling PD and AD as they are today for cardiovascular diseases and many forms of cancer.

The purpose of this chapter is to review the neuropathology of PD in the context of what is now known concerning its pathogenesis and the criteria for pathologic diagnosis. The pathological features of other diseases that have parkinsonian features are discussed elsewhere in this volume. For a comprehensive discussion of comparative pathology see the review by Dickson[6] and respective chapters in Greenfield.[7,8] Currently, the diagnosis of possible or probable idiopathic PD is a clinical exercise, and the accuracy is quite high, as confirmed by autopsy.[9] The clinical history of the typical syndrome of asymmetric resting tremor, bradykinesia-akinesia, rigidity, postural instability, and response to dopaminergic medication supports a diagnosis of PD. In contrast, other signs such as gaze palsies, dystonia, ataxia, and poor response to dopaminergic treatment, suggest an alternative diagnosis such as progressive supranuclear palsy (PSP) or MSA. Nonetheless, the final diagnosis requires careful neuropathologic evaluation and correlation with the clinical history.

Gross Pathology

The salient gross feature of a brain with PD is pallor of the substantia nigra (SN), which is seen on inspection of the cut surface of the midbrain (Fig. 19-1). The SN may also exhibit a reddish-brown discoloration, in association with pallor, and indicative of iron deposition. When there is some pigmentation remaining, it frequently has a "smeared" appearance, in contrast to the relatively sharp margins of the pigmented bands in a normal midbrain (Fig. 19-1). In many cases there is relative sparing of pigmentation in the medial quadrants where the ventral tegmental area is located. The locus ceruleus (LC) in the upper pons may also exhibit pallor, although changes appreciated on visual inspection can be quite variable. In contrast, it is common to observe significant pallor of the LC and normal pigmentation of the SN in AD cases.

While there is significant pathology in numerous other brainstem nuclei in PD (Table 19-1), very little is usually evident on gross inspection. Similarly, the forebrain, including the cortex and major basal ganglia structures, is usually unremarkable. There may be evidence of frontal cortical atrophy, but these changes are not of diagnostic significance in PD, since they may be age-related or a result of concominant Alzheimer's pathology.

Microscopic Pathology

On microscopic examination, the major diagnostic features consist of dopaminergic cell loss in the SN (Fig. 19-2A,B), and the presence of Lewy bodies (Fig. 19-2D). The cell loss is usually associated with release of neuromelanin pigment from dying neurons, and subsequent phagocytosis (melanophagia) (Fig. 19-2C). There is usually astrogliosis and microgliosis but the severity is quite variable. More detailed studies have reported increased vulnerability of the ventrolateral tier cell group of the pars compacta of the SN in PD,[10] but this may not be readily apparent without detailed morphometric analysis. The physiological basis for this selective vulnerability is not understood.

Lewy bodies (LB) were originally described by the German pathologist Lewy and then given their eponymous title by Tretiakoff.[11,12] They are round eosinophilic cytoplasmic inclusions that frequently have a pale peripheral rim, particularly in the brainstem. It is important to distinguish

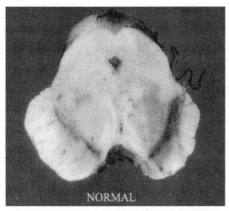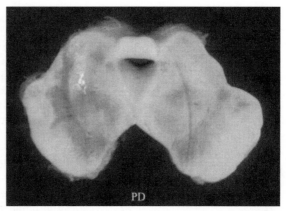

FIGURE 19-1 Gross photograph of a coronal section through the midbrain from a normal brain (*left*) and from a case of PD (*right*). Note the normal pigmentation pattern of the substantia nigra in the normal specimen, and the loss of pigmentation in the case of PD. See Color Plate Section.

LB from "Marinesco bodies," which are intranuclear hyaline inclusions, increased in toxic encephalopathies, but of no pathologic significance in neurodegenerative diseases.[13] Although the presence of LB has long constituted the

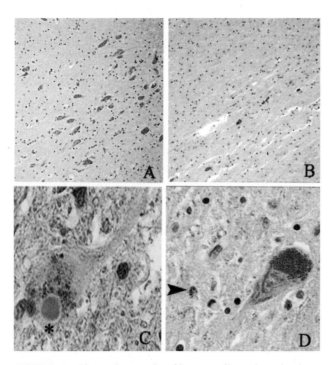

FIGURE 19-2 Photomicrographs of hematoxylin eosin-stained sections of the midbrain from a normal brain (A), and from a case of PD (B–D). In the low-power images (A, B), note the normal complement of pigmented dopamine neurons in the substantia nigra (A), and the marked loss of dopamine neurons (B) in the case of PD. In higher-power photomicrographs (C, D), note the presence of a Lewy body (C, asterisk), and phagocytosis of melanin pigment (melanophagia) (D, arrowhead). A normal remaining dopamine neuron is also present (D). See Color Plate Section.

basis for pathologic diagnosis of PD, the principal protein aggregate responsible for its formation was only recently identified. It is now known that the vesicle-associated protein, alpha-synuclein, is the key constituent of the LB.[14–19] Other filamentous proteins are associated with LB,[20–23] but alpha-synuclein is considered to play a central role in the pathogenesis of PD. Prior to the identification of alpha-synuclein in LB, ubiquitin immunocytochemistry was commonly employed, indicating the presence of proteins targeted for degradation through the ubiquitin ATP-dependent nonlysosomal proteolysis system.[21,24,25] One problem with ubiquitin is that it will also stain abnormal protein deposits present in AD, so that the latter structures, particularly globoid-shaped neurofibrillary tangles (NFT), have to be differentiated from LB. Immunohistochemistry for alpha-synuclein provides the most sensitive indicator for PD pathology,[18] and has provided evidence of pathological changes that are far more extensive, particularly in the brainstem, than previously appreciated.

LBs are usually present throughout the brainstem axis, with particular frequency in the SN, LC, and dorsal motor vagus nuclei (Table 19-1). LB can also be widely distributed in sites ranging from the cerebral cortex to the myenteric plexus of the intestine. In the dorsal motor vagus nucleus, hypothalamus, and sympathetic ganglia, LBs can be multiple and merge to form elongated serpiginous inclusions. It is not unusual to find LB in the limbic cortices, including hippocampus-amygdala, entorhinal-perirhinal cingulate, and insular areas. In the cortex, LB do not usually exhibit the sharp laminated profiles seen in the brainstem (Fig. 19-3A,B), and they tend to be present in the deeper cortical layers (V–VI) which may be difficult to identify on hematoxylin-eosin preparations. In instances where there are high densities of LB in limbic as well as neocortical structures, a diagnosis of dementia with Lewy bodies (DLB) needs to be considered, and appropriate clinico-pathologic correlations performed.[26–31] McKeith et al. have provided a semiquantitative approach to assess cortical

TABLE 19-1 Distribution of Lewy Bodies in Idiopathic PD

Telencephalon	
Limbic/neocortex	
Nucleus basalis of Meynert	
Diencephalon	
Hypothalamus	
Thalamus	Subthalamic nucleus
Nucleus mammilloinfundibularis	Olfactory bulb
Midbrain	
Substantia nigra	Ventral tegmental area
Oculomotor nucleus	Edinger-Wesphal nucleus
Periaqueductal gray	Pedunculopontine nucleus
Nucleus of Darkschewitsch	Dorsal tegmental nucleus
Pons	
Locus ceruleus	Nucleus pontis centralis
Nucleus subceruleus	Central superior raphe nucleus
Pontine nucleus	Central pontine gray
Medulla	
Dorsal motor vagal nucleus	Perihypoglossal nucleus
Inferior olive	
Spinal cord	
Intermediolateral column	
Vertebral sympathetic ganglia	
Gastrointestinal tract	
Esophagus	Colon and rectum

LB involvement.[26] Although less sensitive stains such as hematoxylin-eosin or ubiquitin immunocytochemistry were used, similar approaches can be employed using immunocytochemistry for alpha-synuclein. The technique employed by our laboratory (B Wainer and M Gearing) is to score at least 5 separate 10× objective fields as either: no LB identified; sparse, 0–2; moderate, 2–5; or frequent, >5. This approach is analogous to the scoring of neuritic plaque density in

AD using CERAD criteria.[32] Another classification scheme, proposed by Braak and Braak,[33] involves the assessment of LB frequency at different levels of the brainstem-forebrain axis. This scheme makes some assumptions about pathogenesis and is analogous to the Braak staging scheme for AD, which focuses on the progression of NFT involvement in the forebrain.[34] Finally, the immunologic stain allows one to identify more loosely organized aggregates of cytoplasmic alpha-synuclein, which are difficult to characterize as LBs with hematoxylin-eosin stains, and were formally described as "pale bodies."[6]

LBs have been reported in a number of disparate conditions, including Hallervorden-Spatz disease,[35] ataxia telangiectasia,[36–38] and subacute sclerosing panencephalitis.[39] Some of these descriptions have been questioned.[28] There are also instances where LB pathology may coexist with other disease conditions such as AD. In the latter instance, there may be important factors linking disease mechanisms (see Chap. 46 and the discussion by Dickson[28]). Previous descriptions of LB in MSA[40] are now explained by the fact that both PD and MSA involve abnormal aggregates of alpha-synuclein, as discussed below.[41–45] LBs are also a frequent finding in the elderly, and most likely represent presymptomatic PD. It is not unusual to find LB and mild SN cell loss in cases where there is no documented history of a movement disorder, since the onset of parkinsonian symptoms requires loss of 50 percent or more of the dopaminergic cell population.[46,47] In our laboratory, such changes are reported as Parkinson-related pathology (BH Wainer and M Gearing).

It is now appreciated that there is extensive alpha-synuclein neuritic pathology in PD.[6,18] One interesting finding, albeit unexplained, is the presence of dystrophic neurites in the hippocampus at the CA2/CA3 pyramidal cell field junction (Fig. 19-4A,B).[48] This finding is present even when significant LB pathology is not identified in the hippocampus.

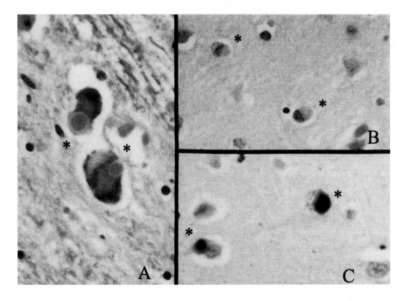

FIGURE 19-3 Photomicrographs of Lewy bodies stained with hematoxylin eosin (A, B), and with antibodies against alpha-synuclein (C). In (A), the typical appearance of Lewy bodies in the brainstem is illustrated (asterisks) as cytoplasmic inclusions with a compact eosinophilic center and a pale peripheral rim. In (B), cortical Lewy bodies are illustrated (asterisks) in small neurons and lacking the sharp laminated structure of the brainstem inclusions. Alpha-synuclein staining of the cortex (D, asterisks) clearly identifies the abnormal deposits. See Color Plate Section.

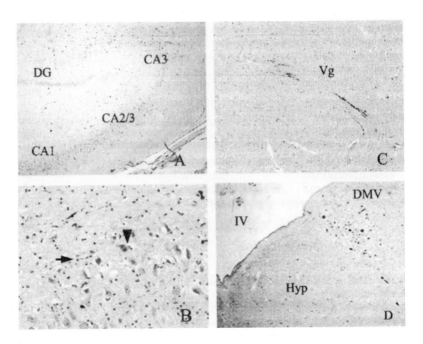

FIGURE 19-4 Immunostaining of neuritic deposits of alpha-synuclein. In (A), staining of the CA2-3 field of the hippocampus is illustrated at low power. In (B), a higher-power magnification from (A) is illustrated, showing alpha-synuclein-positive neurites (arrow) and a Lewy body (arrowhead). In (C), a low-power magnification of the medulla illustrates alpha-synuclein-positive neurites within the vagus nerve (Vg). In (D), low-power magnification of the medullary tegmentum shows Lewy bodies and dystrophic neurites in the dorsal motor vagus nucleus (DMV) and sparing of the hypoglossal nucleus (Hyp). The ventricle is at the top (IV). The section has been counterstained with hematoxylin. See Color Plate Section.

Dystrophic neurites are seen in all areas with LB-containing cells, and also within white matter axon fascicles. For example, the dorsal motor vagus nucleus and adjacent medullary tegmentum show much more extensive pathology using alpha-synuclein immunocytochemical preparations than appreciated with silver stains or with ubiquitin antibodies (Fig. 19-4C,D). It is not uncommon to observe axon fascicles within the vagus nerve stuffed with alpha-synuclein-positive immunoreactivity as it courses through the ventrolateral medullary tegmentum, and which can sometimes be appreciated by holding the slide up to the naked eye. These findings provide clear pathologic evidence for the sleep and autonomic symptomatology frequently seen in PD.[49,50]

Various other inclusions have been described in PD, and most have been found not to be specific for PD. Pale bodies, as discussed above, represent loosely organized aggregations of alpha-synuclein,[6] and probably represent an evolution step in the formation of LB. "Spheroids" are swellings of dystrophic axons, which can be seen in a variety of neurodegenerative conditions as well as in normal aging.[13]

Pathogenesis

The discovery of alpha-synuclein as a central component of LBs has contributed to a better understanding of the pathogenesis of PD, and has revealed a spectrum of possibilities for therapeutic interventions.[14,15,17–19,51] It has also revolutionized the classification of neurodegenerative disorders, which are now based on more precise pathophysiological mechanisms.[28,41,42,52,53]

Alpha-synuclein was first cloned by Maroteaux et al. from torpedo electroplax.[54] Initial reports demonstrated alpha-synuclein localization in the nucleus and synaptic vesicles; however, nuclear localization was not later confirmed. Subsequent studies of alpha-synuclein processing demonstrated that a cleaved fragment was associated with neuritic plaques of AD, and was termed the nonamyloid component (NAC) of plaques.[55] Follow-up studies, however, demonstrated that NAC does not localize within the amyloid cores of neuritic plaques but can be found in occasional dystrophic neurites associated with plaques.[56] Therefore, a role for NAC in the development of AD pathology has not been confirmed.[28] Alpha-synuclein was also found to strongly localize to the ubiquitin-positive glial inclusions described in MSA, and the dystrophic neurites seen in both PD and MSA.[16,43–45,57] It is now proposed that PD and MSA are different phenotypes of a general disease family, the synucleinopathies.[28,41,52,53] Thus the reported instances of LB in MSA are not surprising given common disease mechanisms.[28] In fact, the presence of glial pathology has been reported in both sporadic and familial PD.[58–60]

We have studied the case of a patient presenting initially as probable PD who was L-dopa-responsive, but progressed to L-dopa resistance, dystonia, bulbar signs, autonomic insufficiency, and ataxia.[61] Following death, the neuropathologic examination showed clear evidence of LB pathology and cell loss in the substantia nigra, as well as extensive glial inclusion pathology throughout the brainstem and deep cerebellar nuclei. The case was signed out as a synucleinopathy with overlapping features of PD and MSA. Previous reports of overlap were common for Pick's disease, corticobasal ganglionic degeneration, and PSP, particularly prior to the recognition that these diseases all arise from abnormalities of tau.[62,63]

Alpha-synuclein is a member of a family of proteins that are conserved throughout evolution.[64,65] The other family members include beta- and gamma-synuclein. The synucleins are expressed in a variety of tissues and all three are expressed in the brain. The function of synucleins is not known but some studies suggest an interaction of alpha- and beta-synucleins with phospholipase D_2, and involvement in directed movement of vesicles as well as signal-induced cytoskeletal regulation.[66] The mechanism of alpha-synuclein-mediated toxicity is not understood, but it is known that NAC exhibits the capacity for self-aggregation and the formation of amyloid fibrils.[55,67–69] It is suggested that either mutations of the alpha-synuclein gene or damage to the protein from oxidative stress or other insults may induce conformational changes that render the protein toxic and resistant to normal degradation by the ubiquitin proteasome system.[25,64,70–76] Detailed ultrastructural and biophysical studies of alpha-synuclein fibrils have provided several interesting observations and speculations.[76] First, both wild-type and mutant forms of alpha-synuclein can form the typical beta-pleated sheet conformation of amyloid. This structure is in beta-amyloid deposits of AD, NFT of AD and tauopathy, and prion disease. These findings suggest that AD, tauopathies, prion diseases and now PD may share a final common pathway of amyloid-mediated cellular toxicity. A second finding is that mutant alpha-synuclein and smaller fragments, such as NAC, more readily form protease-resistant amyloid fibrils than the whole length molecule. In fact, some investigators have suggested that small soluble protofibrils may be of more significance for cellular toxicity than the large complexes.[28,70,76] It has even been suggested that LBs may represent an adaptive response on the part of the cell to sequester small toxic aggregates into large insoluble and less harmful complexes. LBs in the SN are invariably accompanied by neuronal loss, and in other brain regions the presence of LBs is believed usually to indicate associated neuronal damage. However, LBs are frequently observed in cells that appear otherwise healthy. For example, no significant neuronal loss has been found in the hypothalamus of 7 cases with PD, despite the presence of LBs.[77] A logical extension of this hypothesis is that attempts to prevent LB formation could result in more severe cell toxicity and death. It is clear that there is still much to learn about the cellular and molecular pathology of PD.

Genetics, Animal Models, and Risk Factors

Several major areas of research have provided fundamental insights into the pathogenesis of PD. These areas include the identification of genetic loci for familial forms of PD, the generation of transgenic models of PD, insights into the role of abnormalities of protein processing in PD, and further insights into the role of environmental factors, particularly injury to bioenergetic mechanisms. These advances are briefly summarized here, and the reader is referred to other chapters of this volume and several excellent reviews for a more detailed consideration.[70,71,78–80]

Several animal models of PD have been available for a number of years and have employed toxins that elicit selective injury to dopamine neurons.[78] In addition, the development of stable gene-delivery systems has also made possible the generation of animal models by overexpressing the alpha-synuclein gene.[81] Perhaps the best studied have been 6-hydroxydopamine and 1-methyl-4-phenyl-1,2,3,6-tetra-hydropyridine (MPTP). These toxins have been valuable for assessing therapeutic modalities, particularly transplantation, in PD as well as focusing attention on the role of oxidative stress as a risk factor.[82] It is now appreciated that various neuronal systems are vulnerable to this kind of injury because of the biosynthetic and degradative pathways that are active within these cells, and even by the presence of the neurotransmitter dopamine which has the capacity by itself to enhance alpha-synuclein-mediated neurotoxicity.[83,84] More recently, attention has focused on the possible role of environmental toxins, such as the pesticides paraquat, rotenone, and maneb, as contributors to dopamine cell toxicity.[85–88] The basic model is that such agents interfere with mitochondrial function by inhibiting complex I, the first step in the respiratory chain, which results in elevated levels of reactive oxygen species (ROS) (Fig. 19-5).[71,72,82] Elevated levels of ROS can have several deleterious effects. First, the direct action of these molecules can injure cellular constituents leading to necrosis. Second, elevated ROS within the mitochondria can trigger signaling pathways, leading to programmed cell death or apoptosis. Finally, recent studies have indicated that ROS can also influence the normal processing of protein species such as alpha-synuclein and induce the formation of toxic aggregates.[70,76] Some investigators have suggested a role for inflammatory mediators in this scheme,[89,90] but other studies suggest that such mechanisms may be more evident in AD compared to PD.[28,91–93] As more is learned about these cellular pathways of injury, it is likely that a growing number of environmental risk factors as well as genetic polymorphisms associated with risk will be identified. For example, the apolipoprotein E4 allele, a known risk factor for AD and cardiovascular disease, can also increase the risk for developing PD when expressed with certain polymorphisms of the alpha-synuclein promotor region.[94]

The identification of genetic loci responsible for familial forms of PD has contributed to our understanding of the role of the synucleins in PD, as well as for the development of transgenetic animal models.[78–80] The following genetic loci have been identified as responsible for either autosomal-dominant or autosomal-recessive forms of familial PD (Table 19-2). PARK1 has been mapped to chromosome 4, and the gene of interest codes for alpha-synuclein. The mutations identified include an alanine-to-threonine

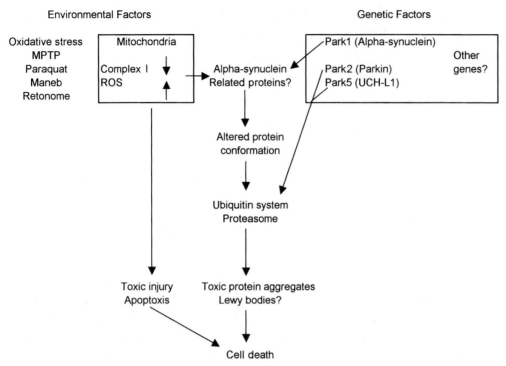

Environmental Factors   Genetic Factors

FIGURE 19-5 Hypothetical pathways to neurodegeneration in PD. A schematic illustrating the interplay of environmental and genetic factors impinging on dopamine neurons. Various environmental factors such as the illicit drug impurities (MPTP), pesticides (paraquat, maneb, rotenone) or other causes of oxidative stress lead to inhibition of complex I and the elevation of reactive oxygen species (ROS). ROS can directly injure cells or alternately facilitate aggregation of alpha-synuclein or related protein. Mitochondrial dysfunction can also trigger programmed cell death (apoptosis). Aggregation of alpha-synuclein can also be facilitated through direct genetic mutations (Park1), or through mutations that affect the ubiquitination system (Park2, parkin, an E3 ligase; or Park5, UCH-L1, an E1 ligase). Abnormal processing through the ubiquitin-proteasome system fails to remove toxic aggregates leading to cell injury and death. The significance of Lewy bodies is questioned (?) given the uncertainty of whether they signify cell injury or an adaptive response as discussed in the text. The figure is modified from Refs 71, 72 and 82.

substitution at position 53 (A53T) in 13 families of Italian/Greek descent,[95] and an alanine-to-proline substitution at position 30 (A30P) in a single German kindred.[96] These mutations lead to early onset PD (mean age of onset 46) with typical LB-neuritic pathology. In contrast, the PARK2 locus codes for the protein parkin: parkin mutations are responsible for autosomal-recessive juvenile PD (AR-JP).[97] Parkin has been identified as an E3 ubiquitin

TABLE 19-2 Familial PD*

Locus	Chromosome	Inheritance	Phenotype	Lewy Bodies
PARK1 (alpha-synuclein)	4q21.3	AD	Slightly early-onset	+
PARK2 (parkin)	6q25.2-27	AR	Juvenile-onset	−/+
PARK3	2p13	AD	Typical PD	+
PARK4	4p15	AD	PD/essential tremor	+
PARK5 (UCH-L1)	4p14	AD	Typical PD	?
PARK6	1p35-p36	AR	Early-onset	?
PARK7 (DJ-1)	1p36	AR	Early-onset	?
PARK8	12p11.2-q13.1	AD	Partial penetration	
PARK9	1p36	AR (Kufor-Rakeb syndrome)		
PARK10	1p32	Late-onset Susceptibility gene		
SCA3	14q32.1	Apparent AD	Apparent typical PD	?
SCA2	12q23-q24.1	Apparent AD	PD/ataxia/supranuclear gene palsy	?

*Modified from Refs 71–72.
AD, autosomal-dominant; AR, autosomal-recessive.

ligase.[98–100] Several substrates for parkin have been identified, including CDRrel-1,[101] a novel glycolated form of alpha-synuclein,[102] the pael receptor,[103] and synphilin-1.[104] Interestingly, CDRrel is a vesicle-associated protein like alpha-synuclein, and is also present in LB.[105,106] Although LBs were not reported initially in AR-JP, subsequent studies have identified cases where LB are present and where the mutations are present in the heterozygous state.[107] More detailed analyses have revealed additional intronic mutations as well as promoter variations.[108] These findings suggest that parkin haploinsufficiency may also be sufficient to induce sporadic disease in some instances. Another genetic locus on chromosome 4, UCH-L1, also involves the ubiquitin system, with a mutation of an E1 ligase.[109] As more of these loci are better understood, it is anticipated that a complex interplay of mutations in either alpha-synuclein or related vesicle-associated proteins, abnormalities of ubiquitination and proteasome processing, and perhaps others sites of protein trafficking, will be identified as sites of vulnerability predisposing to PD (Fig. 19-5). While LBs and neuritic aggregates of alpha-synuclein are considered to be the hallmark of idiopathic PD and in some of the familial forms, it is possible that abnormal aggregates of other related proteins will be identified in the future.

The identification of these several genetic loci has prompted the development of transgenetic animal models that have ranged from *Drosophila*[110,111] to mice.[112–117] These models have demonstrated alpha-synuclein neuronal and neuritic deposits in conjunction with motor abnormalities. While the motor abnormalities appear to be most selective in the *Drosophila* model for dopamine cells and basal ganglia-like functional impairment, the mouse models generated to date are not highly specific for dopamine systems.[28] Clearly, more work is needed to be done to reproduce the functional impairment typical of PD in these models. In summary, the pathologic diagnosis of PD is now understood more clearly from the perspective of the disease spectrum of synucleinopathy. Future prospects are to understand better the complex interactions of environmental factors leading to bioenergetic stress, as well as genetic factors that alter the processing of synucleins and associated proteins, and result in the generation of toxic oligomers or fibrils. Insights gained from these studies will clearly point to rational avenues of therapeutic intervention.

References

1. Hardy J: Pathways to primary neurodegenerative disease. *Mayo Clin Proc* 74:835–837, 1999.
2. Martin JB: Molecular basis of the neurodegenerative disorders. *N Engl J Med* 340:1970–1980, 1999 [erratum appears in *N Engl J Med* 341:1407, 1999].
3. Schulz JB, Dichgans J: Molecular pathogenesis of movement disorders: Are protein aggregates a common link in neuronal degeneration? *Curr Opin Neurol* 12:433–439, 1999.
4. Kaytor MD, Warren ST: Aberrant protein deposition and neurological disease. *J Biol Chem* 274:37507–37510, 1999.
5. Taylor JP, Hardy J, Fischbeck KH: Toxic proteins in neurodegenerative disease. *Science* 296:1991–1995, 2002.
6. Dickson DW: Neuropathology of parkinsonism, in Pahwa R, Lyons KE, Koller WC (eds): *Handbook of Parkinson's Disease*. New York: Marcel Dekker, 2003, pp 203–220.
7. Mirra SS, Hyman B: Ageing and dementia, in Graham D, Lantos P (eds): *Greenfield's Neuropathology*. New York: Gray Publishing, 2002, pp 195–271.
8. Lowe J, Leigh N: Disorders of movement and system degenerations, in Graham D, Lantos P (eds): *Greenfield's Neuropathology*. New York: Gray Publishing, 2002, pp 325–430.
9. Hughes A, Daniel S, Lees A: Improved accuracy of clinical diagnosis of Lewy body Parkinson's disease. *Neurology* 57:1497–1499, 2001.
10. Gibb W, Lees A: Anatomy, pigmentation, ventral and dorsal subpopulations of the substantia nigra, and differential cell death in Parkinson's disease. *J Neurol Neurosurg Psychiatry* 54:388–396, 1991.
11. Lewy F: Zur pathologischen Anatomie der Paralysis Agitans. *Dtsch Z Nervenheilkd* 50:50–55, 1914.
12. Tretiakoff C: *Contribution a l'étude de l'anatomie pathologique du locus niger de Soemmering avec quelques déductions relatives à la pathogénie des troubles du tonus musculaire et de la maladie de Parkinson.* University of Paris, Paris: 1919.
13. Hirano A, Llena J: Structures of neurons in the aging nervous system, in Calne D (ed): *Neurodegenerative Diseases*. Vancouver: W B Saunders, 1994, pp 3–14.
14. Spillantini M, Schmidt M, VM-Y, L, et al: Alpha-synuclein in Lewy bodies. *Nature* 388:839–840, 1997.
15. Wakabayashi K, Matsumoto K, Takayama K, et al: NACP, a presynaptic protein, immunoreactivity in Lewy bodies in Parkinson's disease. *Neurosci Lett* 239:45–48, 1997.
16. Wakabayashi K, Hayashi S, Kakita A, et al: Accumulation of alpha-synuclein/NACP is a cytopathological feature common to Lewy body disease and multiple system atrophy. *Acta Neuropathol* 96:445–452, 1998.
17. Takeda A, Mallory M, Sundsmo M, et al: Abnormal accumulation of NACP/alpha-synuclein in neurodegenerative disorders. *Am J Pathol* 152:367–372, 1998.
18. Spillantini MG, Crowther RA, Jakes R, et al: Alpha-synuclein in filamentous inclusions of Lewy bodies from Parkinson's disease and dementia with Lewy bodies. *Proc Natl Acad Sci U S A* 95:6469–6473, 1998.
19. Irizarry MC, Growdon W, Gomez-Isla T, et al: Nigral and cortical Lewy bodies and dystrophic nigral neurites in Parkinson's disease and cortical Lewy body disease contain alpha-synuclein immunoreactivity. *J Neuropath Exp Neurol* 57:334–337, 1998.
20. Goldman J, Yen SH, Chiu F-C, NS P: Lewy bodies of Parkinson's disease contain neurofilament antigens. *Science* 221:1082–1084, 1983.
21. Kuzuhara S, Mori H, N I, et al: Lewy bodies are ubiquitinated: A light and electron microscopy study. *Acta Neuropath* 75:345–352, 1988.
22. Pollanen M, Bergeron C, L W: Detergent-insoluble Lewy body fibrils share epitopes with neurofilament and tau. *J Neurochem* 58:1953–1956, 1992.
23. Iwatsubo T, H Y, M F, et al: Purification and characterization of Lewy bodies from the brains of patients with diffuse Lewy body disease. *Am J Pathol* 148:1517–1529, 1996.

24. Mayer J, Rezvani K, Layfield R, Dawson S: The ubiquitin pathway, neurodegeneration and brain function, in Dickson DW (ed): *Neurodegeneration: The Molecular Pathology of Dementia and Movement Disorders*. ISN Neuropath Press, 2003, pp 14–16.

25. Bennett MC, Bishop JF, Leng Y, et al: Degradation of alpha-synuclein by proteasome. *J Biol Chem* 274:33855–33858, 1999.

26. McKeith IG, Galasko D, Kosaka K, et al: Consensus guidelines for the clinical and pathologic diagnosis of dementia with Lewy bodies (DLB): Report of the consortium on DLB international workshop. *Neurology* 47:1113–1124, 1996.

27. McKeith IG, Ballard CG, Perry RH, et al: Prospective validation of consensus criteria for the diagnosis of dementia with Lewy bodies. *Neurology* 54:1050–1058, 2000.

28. Dickson DW: Alpha-synuclein and the Lewy body disorders. *Curr Opin Neurol* 14:423–432, 2001.

29. Campbell BC, Li QX, Culvenor JG, et al: Accumulation of insoluble alpha-synuclein in dementia with Lewy bodies. *Neurobiol Dis* 7:192–200, 2000.

30. Mattila PM, Rinne JO, Helenius H, et al: Alpha-synuclein-immunoreactive cortical Lewy bodies are associated with cognitive impairment in Parkinson's disease. *Acta Neuropath* 100:285–290, 2000.

31. Haroutunian V, Serby M, Purohit DP, et al: Contribution of Lewy body inclusions to dementia in patients with and without Alzheimer disease neuropathological conditions. *Arch Neurol* 57:1145–1150, 2000.

32. Mirra SS, Heyman A, McKeel D, et al: The Consortium to Establish a Registry for Alzheimer's Disease (CERAD). Part II. Standardization of the neuropathologic assessment of Alzheimer's disease. *Neurology* 41:479–486, 1991.

33. Braak H, Del Tredici K, Rub U, et al: Staging of brain pathology related to sporadic Parkinson's disease. *Neurobiol Aging* 24:197–211, 2003.

34. Braak H, Braak E: Neuropathological staging of Alzheimer-related changes. *Acta Neuropathol* 82:239–259, 1991.

35. Gibb WR: Neuropathology in movement disorders. *J Neurol Neurosurg Psychiatry* suppl:55–67, 1989.

36. De Leon GA, Grover WD, Huff DS: Neuropathologic changes in ataxia-telangiectasia. *Neurology* 26:947–951, 1976.

37. Agamanolis DP, Greenstein JI: Ataxia-telangiectasia. Report of a case with Lewy bodies and vascular abnormalities within cerebral tissue. *J Neuropathol Exp Neurol* 38:475–489, 1979.

38. Monaco S, Nardelli E, Moretto G, et al: Cytoskeletal pathology in ataxia-telangiectasia. *Clin Neuropath* 7:44–46, 1988.

39. Gibb WR, Scaravilli F, Michund J: Lewy bodies and subacute sclerosing panencephalitis. *J Neurol Neurosurg Psychiatry* 53:710–711, 1990.

40. Gibb WR: The Lewy body in autonomic failure, in Bannister R (ed): *Autonomic Failure*. Oxford: Oxford University Press, 1988, pp 484–497.

41. Galvin JE, Lee VM, Trojanowski JQ: Synucleinopathies: Clinical and pathological implications. *Arch Neurol* 58:186–190, 2001.

42. Goedert M: Alpha-synuclein and neurodegenerative diseases. *Nat Neurosci* 2:492–501, 2001.

43. Dickson DW, Lin W, Liu WK, Yen SH: Multiple system atrophy: A sporadic synucleinopathy. *Brain Pathol* 9:721–732, 1999.

44. Dickson DW, Liu W, Hardy J, et al: Widespread alterations of alpha-synuclein in multiple system atrophy. *Am J Pathol* 155:1241–1251, 1999.

45. Duda JE, Giasson BI, Gur TL, et al: Immunohistochemical and biochemical studies demonstrate a distinct profile of alpha-synuclein permutations in multiple system atrophy. *J Neuropathol Exp Neurol* 59:830–841, 2000.

46. Fearnley JM, Lees AJ: Ageing and Parkinson's disease: Substantia nigra regional selectivity. *Brain* 114:2283–2301, 1991.

47. Bernheimer H, Birkmayer W, Hornykiewicz O, et al: Brain dopamine and the syndromes of Parkinson and Huntington. Clinical, morphological and neurochemical correlations. *J Neurol Sci* 20:415–455, 1973.

48. Dickson DW, Ruan D, H C, et al: Hippocampal degeneration differentiates diffuse Lewy body disease (DLBD) from Alzheimer's disease: Light and electron microscopic immunocytochemistry of CA2-3 neurites specific to DLBD. *Neurology* 41:1402–1409, 1991.

49. Poewe W, Hogl B: Parkinson's disease and sleep. *Curr Opin Neurol* 13:423–426, 2000.

50. Chaudhuri KR: Autonomic dysfunction in movement disorders. *Curr Opin Neurol* 14:505–511, 2001.

51. Beites CL, Xie H, Bowser R, Trimble WS: The septin CDCrel-1 binds syntaxin and inhibits exocytosis. *Nat Neurosci* 2:434–439, 1999.

52. Hashimoto M, Masliah E: Alpha-synuclein in Lewy body disease and Alzheimer's disease. *Brain Pathol* 9:707–720, 1999.

53. Lucking CB, Brice A: Alpha-synuclein and Parkinson's disease. *Cell Mol Life Sci* 57:1894–1908, 2000.

54. Maroteaux L, Campanelli JT, Scheller RH: Synuclein: A neuron-specific protein localized to the nucleus and presynaptic nerve terminal. *J Neurosci* 8:2804–2815, 1988.

55. Iwai A, Masliah E, Yoshimoto M, et al: The precursor protein of non-A beta component of Alzheimer's disease amyloid is a presynaptic protein of the central nervous system. *Neuron* 14:467–475, 1995.

56. Culvenor JG, McLean CA, Cutt S, et al: Non-abeta component of Alzheimer's disease amyloid (NAC) revisited. NAC and alpha-synuclein are not associated with abeta amyloid. *Am J Pathol* 155:1173–1181, 1999.

57. Wakabayashi K, Yoshimoto M, Tsuji S, Takahashi H: Alpha-synuclein immunoreactivity in glial cytoplasmic inclusions in multiple system atrophy. *Neurosci Lett* 249:180–182, 1998.

58. Gwinn-Hardy K, Mehta ND, Farrer M, et al: Distinctive neuropathology revealed by alpha-synuclein antibodies in hereditary parkinsonism and dementia linked to chromosome 4p. *Acta Neuropathol* 99:663–672, 2000.

59. Arai T, Ueda K, Ikeda K, et al: Argyrophilic glial inclusions in the midbrain of patients with Parkinson's disease and diffuse Lewy body disease are immunopositive for NACP/alpha-synuclein. *Neurosci Lett* 259:83–86, 1999.

60. Wakabayashi K, Hayashi S, Yoshimoto M, et al: NACP/alpha-synuclein-positive filamentous inclusions in astrocytes and oligodendrocytes of Parkinson's disease brains. *Acta Neuropathol* 99:14–20, 2000.

61. Gearing M, Juncos J, Farrer M, et al: Multiple system atrophy (MSA) and Parkinson's disease (PD) pathology with diffuse cortical Lewy bodies in a patient evidencing multiple clinical phenotypes. *J Neuropathol Exp Neurol* 60:548, 2001.

62. Buee L, Delacourte A: Comparative biochemistry of tau in progressive supranuclear palsy, corticobasal degeneration, FTDP-17 and Pick's disease. *Brain Pathol* 9:681–693, 1999.

63. Arvanitakis Z, Wszolek ZK: Recent advances in the understanding of tau protein and movement disorders. *Curr Opin Neurol* 14:491-497, 2001.

64. Clayton DF, George JM: The synucleins: A family of proteins involved in synaptic function, plasticity, neurodegeneration and disease. *Trends Neurosci* 21:249–254, 1998.

65. Lavedan C: The synuclein family. *Genome Res* 8:871–880, 1998.

66. Jenco JM, Rawlingson A, Daniels B, Morris AJ: Regulation of phospholipase D2: Selective inhibition of mammalian phospholipase D isoenzymes by alpha- and beta-synucleins. *Biochemistry* 37:4901–4909, 1998.

67. Jensen PH, Hojrup P, Hager H, et al: Binding of Abeta to alpha- and beta-synucleins: Identification of segments in alpha-synuclein/NAC precursor that bind Abeta and NAC. *Biochem J* 323(Pt 2):539–546, 1997.

68. Hashimoto M, Hsu LJ, Sisk A, et al: Human recombinant NACP/alpha-synuclein is aggregated and fibrillated in vitro: Relevance for Lewy body disease. *Brain Res* 799:301–306, 1998.

69. Paik SR, Lee JH, Kim DH, et al: Self-oligomerization of NACP, the precursor protein of the non-amyloid beta/A4 protein (A beta) component of Alzheimer's disease amyloid, observed in the presence of a C-terminal A beta fragment (residues 25–35). *FEBS Lett* 421:73–76, 1998.

70. Lansbury PT Jr, Brice A: Genetics of Parkinson's disease and biochemical studies of implicated gene products. *Curr Opin Genet Dev* 12:299–306, 2002.

71. Mouradian MM: Recent advances in the genetics and pathogenesis of Parkinson disease. *Neurology* 58:179–185, 2002.

72. Dawson TM, Dawson VL: Rare genetic mutations shed light on the pathogenesis of Parkinson disease. *J Clin Invest* 111:145–151, 2003.

73. Wickner S, Maurizi M, Gottesman S: Posttranslational quality control: Folding, refolding, and degrading proteins. *Science* 286:1888–1893, 1999.

74. Ancolio K, Alves da Costa C, Ueda K, Checler F: Alpha-synuclein and the Parkinson's disease-related mutant Ala53Thr-alpha-synuclein do not undergo proteasomal degradation in HEK293 and neuronal cells. *Neurosci Lett* 285:79–82, 2000.

75. McNaught KS, Jenner P: Proteasomal function is impaired in substantia nigra in Parkinson's disease. *Neurosci Lett* 297:191–194, 2001.

76. Conway KA, Harper JD, Lansbury PT Jr: Fibrils formed in vitro from alpha-synuclein and two mutant forms linked to Parkinson's disease are typical amyloid. *Biochemistry* 39:2552–2563, 2000.

77. Kremer HP, Bots GT: Lewy bodies in the lateral hypothalamus: Do they imply neuronal loss? *Mov Disord* 8:315–320, 1993.

78. Beal MF: Experimental models of Parkinson's disease. *Nat Neurosci* 2:325–334, 2001.

79. Lee M, Price DL: Advances in genetic models of Parkinson's disease. *Clin Neurosci Res* 1:456–466, 2001.

80. Dawson T, Mandir A, Lee M: Animal models of PD: Pieces of the same puzzle? *Neuron* 35:219–222, 2002.

81. Kirik D, Rosenblad C, Burger C, et al: Parkinson-like neurodegeneration induced by targeted overexpression of alpha-synuclein in the nigrostriatal system. *J Neurosci* 22:2780–2791, 2002.

82. Ischiropoulos H, Beckman JS: Oxidative stress and nitration in neurodegeneration: Cause, effect, or association? *J Clin Invest* 111:163–169, 2003.

83. Tabrizi SJ, Orth M, Wilkinson JM, et al: Expression of mutant alpha-synuclein causes increased susceptibility to dopamine toxicity. *Hum Mol Genet* 9:2683–2689, 2000.

84. Xu J, Kao SY, Lee FJ, et al: Dopamine-dependent neurotoxicity of alpha-synuclein: A mechanism for selective neurodegeneration in Parkinson disease. *Nat Med* 8:600–606, 2002.

85. Lockwood AH: Pesticides and parkinsonism: Is there an etiological link? *Curr Opin Neurol* 13:687-690, 2000.

86. Thiruchelvam M, Richfield EK, Baggs RB, et al: The nigrostriatal dopaminergic system as a preferential target of repeated exposures to combined paraquat and maneb: Implications for Parkinson's disease. *J Neurosci* 20:9207–9214, 2000.

87. Betarbet R, Sherer TB, MacKenzie G, et al: Chronic systemic pesticide exposure reproduces features of Parkinson's disease. *Nat Neurosci* 3:1301–1306, 2000.

88. Manning-Bog AB, McCormack AL, Li J, et al: The herbicide paraquat causes up-regulation and aggregation of alpha-synuclein in mice: Paraquat and alpha-synuclein. *J Biol Chem* 277:1641–1644, 2002.

89. Hunot S, Hirsch EC: Neuroinflammatory processes in Parkinson's disease. *Ann Neurol* 53(suppl 3):S49–S60, 2003.

90. Orr CF, Rowe DB, Halliday GM: An inflammatory review of Parkinson's disease. *Prog Neurobiol* 68:325–340, 2002.

91. Mackenzie IR: Activated microglia in dementia with Lewy bodies. *Neurology* 55:132–134, 2000.

92. Rozemuller AJ, Eikelenboom P, Theeuwes JW, et al: Activated microglial cells and complement factors are unrelated to cortical Lewy bodies. *Acta Neuropathol* 100:701–708, 2000.

93. Shepherd CE, Thiel E, McCann H, et al: Cortical inflammation in Alzheimer disease but not dementia with Lewy bodies. *Arch Neurol* 57:817–822, 2000.

94. Kruger R, Vieira-Saecker AM, Kuhn W, et al: Increased susceptibility to sporadic Parkinson's disease by a certain combined alpha-synuclein/apolipoprotein E genotype. *Ann Neurol* 45:611–617, 1999.

95. Polymeropoulos M, C L, E L, et al: Mutation in the alpha-synuclein gene identified in families with Parkinson's disease. *Science* 276:2045–2047, 1997.

96. Kruger R, Kuhn W, Muller T, et al: Ala30Pro mutation in the gene encoding alpha-synuclein in Parkinson's disease. *Nat Genet* 18:106–108, 1998.

97. Kitada T, Asakawa S, Hattori N, et al: Mutations in the parkin gene cause autosomal recessive juvenile parkinsonism. *Nature* 392:605-608, 1998.

98. Shimura H, Hattori N, Kubo S, et al: Familial Parkinson disease gene product, parkin, is a ubiquitin-protein ligase. *Nat Genet* 25:302–305, 2000.

99. Imai Y, Soda M, Takahashi R: Parkin suppresses unfolded protein stress-induced cell death through its E3 ubiquitin-protein ligase activity. *J Biol Chem* 275:35661–35664, 2000.

100. Mizuno Y, Hattori N, Mori H, et al: Parkin and Parkinson's disease. *Curr Opin Neurol* 14:477–482, 2001.

101. Zhang Y, Gao J, Chung KK, et al: Parkin functions as an E2-dependent ubiquitin-protein ligase and promotes the degradation of the synaptic vesicle-associated protein, CDCrel-1. *Proc Nat Acad Sci U S A* 97:13354–13359, 2000.

102. Shimura H, Schlossmacher MG, Hattori N, et al: Ubiquitination of a new form of alpha-synuclein by parkin from human brain: Implications for Parkinson's disease. *Science* 293:263–269, 2001.

103. Imai Y, Soda M, Inoue H, et al: An unfolded putative transmembrane polypeptide, which can lead to endoplasmic reticulum stress, is a substrate of parkin. *Cell* 105:891–902, 2001.

104. Chung KK, Zhang Y, Lim KL, et al: Parkin ubiquitinates the alpha-synuclein-interacting protein, synphilin-1: Implications

for Lewy-body formation in Parkinson disease. *Nat Med* 7:1144–1150, 2001.

105. Engelender S, Kaminsky Z, Guo, X, et al: Synphilin-1 associates with alpha-synuclein and promotes the formation of cytosolic inclusions. *Nat Genet* 22:110–114, 1999.

106. Wakabayashi K, Engelender S, Yoshimoto M, et al: Synphilin-1 is present in Lewy bodies in Parkinson's disease. *Ann Neurol* 47:521–523, 2000.

107. Farrer M, Chan P, R C, et al: Lewy bodies and parkinsonism in families with parkin mutations. *Ann Neurol* 50:293–300, 2001.

108. West A, Periquet M, Lincoln S, et al: French Parkinson's Disease Genetics Study, and the European Consortium on Genetic Susceptibility on Parkinson's Disease: Complex relationship between Parkin mutations and Parkinson disease. *Am J Med Genet* 114:584–591, 2002.

109. Maraganore DM, Farrer MJ, Hardy JA, et al: Case-control study of the ubiquitin carboxy-terminal hydrolase L1 gene in Parkinson's disease. *Neurology* 53:1858–1860, 1999.

110. Feany MB, Bender WW: A *Drosophila* model of Parkinson's disease. *Nature* 404:394–398, 2000.

111. Auluck PK, Chan HY, Trojanowski JQ, et al: Chaperone suppression of alpha-synuclein toxicity in a *Drosophila* model for Parkinson's disease. *Science* 295:865–868, 2002.

112. Lee MK, Stirling W, Xu Y, et al: Human alpha-synuclein-harboring familial Parkinson's disease-linked Ala-53→Thr mutation causes neurodegenerative disease with alpha-synuclein aggregation in transgenic mice. *Proc Natl Acad Sci U S A* 99:8968–8973, 2002.

113. Giasson BI, Duda JE, Quinn SM, et al: Neuronal alpha-synucleinopathy with severe movement disorder in mice expressing A53T human alpha-synuclein. *Neuron* 34:521–533, 2002.

114. Richfield EK, Thiruchelvam MJ, Cory-Slechta DA, et al: Behavioral and neurochemical effects of wild-type and mutated human alpha-synuclein in transgenic mice. *Exp Neurol* 175:35–48, 2002.

115. Masliah E, Rockenstein E, Veinbergs I, et al: Dopaminergic loss and inclusion body formation in alpha-synuclein mice: Implications for neurodegenerative disorders. *Science* 287:1265–1269, 2000.

116. van der Putten H, Wiederhold KH, Probst A, et al: Neuropathology in mice expressing human alpha-synuclein. *J Neurosci* 20:6021–6029, 2000.

117. Kahle PJ, Neumann M, Ozmen L, et al: Subcellular localization of wild-type and Parkinson's disease-associated mutant alpha-synuclein in human and transgenic mouse brain. *J Neurosci* 20:6365–6373, 2000.

I. PARKINSONIAN STATES
AKINETIC-RIGID SYNDROMES

Chapter 20

PROGRESSIVE SUPRANUCLEAR PALSY (RICHARDSON'S DISEASE)

LAWRENCE I. GOLBE

CLINICAL SUMMARY   339
    Presenting Features and Clinical Course   339
    PSP versus PD   340
    Atypical Features   340
DIAGNOSTIC CRITERIA   340
    Differential Diagnosis   341
    Clinical Evaluation   341
    Radiologic Evaluation   341
    Cerebrospinal Fluid (CSF) Studies   342
NEUROPATHOLOGY, NEUROCHEMISTRY, AND
    THEIR CLINICAL CORRELATES   342
    Overview   342
    Neurofibrillary Tangles (NFTs)   342
    Tau Protein   342
    Other Changes   343
ANATOMIC DISTRIBUTION OF DEGENERATION   343
    Cerebral Cortex   343
    Hippocampus   344
    Nigrostriatal System   344
    Other Basal Ganglia   345
    Mesencephalic and Pontine Ocular Motor Areas   345
    Brainstem Centers Controlling Sleep and Arousal   346
    Brainstem Centers Controlling Speech and
        Swallowing   347
    Spinal and Autonomic Centers   347
EPIDEMIOLOGY AND ETIOLOGY   347
    Descriptive Epidemiology   347
    Analytic Epidemiology   348
    An Hereditary Component?   348
    Geographic Clusters   349
    A Mitochondrial or Oxidative Mechanism?   349
    A Nuclear Genetic Mechanism?   349
TREATMENT   350
    Pharmacotherapy   350
    Nonpharmacologic Therapy   351
PATIENT RESOURCES   351

The first clinicopathologic descriptions of progressive supranuclear palsy (PSP) to draw widespread attention were published in 1963 and 1964.[1-3] The full-blown, typical case is at once unusually complex in its combination of motor and behavioral features and so distinctive that the diagnosis is unmistakable at a glance. While lack of objective diagnostic markers and poor response to treatment make PSP a challenge for the clinician, recent progress in understanding its genetic, molecular, and cellular pathology offer hope that PSP will become more easily diagnosed and treated in the near future.

Clinical Summary

PRESENTING FEATURES AND CLINICAL COURSE

Two retrospective studies found gait disturbance, often unheralded falls, to be a presenting feature in 90 percent and 62 percent, respectively.[4,5] In contrast, Parkinson's disease (PD) presents with gait disturbance in only 11 percent of cases.[6] The falls may prompt a workup for vestibulopathy, myelopathy, basilar artery ischemia, cardiac syncope or epilepsy. However, in most cases, the gait disturbance is accompanied by enough bradykinesia and/or rigidity to prompt an initial diagnosis of PD.

The next most common presenting feature is a nonspecific mental and physical slowness, irritability, social withdrawal or fatigability[7] that is usually interpreted by the patient as normal aging. If medical attention is sought at this point, a diagnosis of primary depression or Alzheimer's disease (AD) is common.

In the minority of cases that present with gaze palsy, dysarthria or dysphagia, the initial workup may embark on a search for myasthenia gravis, progressive bulbar palsy or local causes of esophageal dysmotility. Cataract extraction may be performed in a futile effort to correct the nonrefractible visual deficit of early, unrecognized supranuclear gaze fixation instability. Gaze palsy is often absent until the middle of the illness and is only rarely the presenting symptom (Table 20-1). In one series of autopsy-confirmed patients, gaze palsy failed to appear during life in half of cases.[8] Yet many physicians fail to consider the diagnosis of PSP until vertical gaze restriction occurs.

In its full-blown clinical state, PSP will not be confused with other illnesses. There can be little diagnostic doubt in a patient with a progressive syndrome of gait instability with early falls, predominantly proximal rigidity and bradykinesia (recently found to be localized to the neck, with no

TABLE 20-1 Median Actuarially Adjusted Interval from Initial Symptom to Onset of Disease Milestones for PSP

	Years
Initial gait difficulty	0.3
Cane or helper needed to walk	3.1
Dysarthria	3.4
Visual symptoms	3.9
Dysphagia	4.4
Confined to bed or wheelchair	8.2
Death	9.7

Data obtained by retrospective interview of patient and family.[4]

more trunkal rigidity than in PD),[9] predominantly vertical supranuclear gaze abnormality, spastic dysarthria, dangerous dysphagia, and behavioral abnormalities referrable disproportionately to frontal lobe dysfunction. The illness progresses to an immobile state over less than a decade in most cases.[4,5]

A clinical disability rating scale, the PSP Rating Scale, has been devised.[10,11] It requires about 10 minutes to administer and can be performed by a neurologist with no specialized familiarity with PSP. The scores span 0 (normal) to 100 and progress an average of 10–12 points per year.

PSP VERSUS PD

The most important competing diagnostic consideration, PD, may often be discarded by a glance at the patient's tonically contracted facial muscles, unmoving gaze with coarse square-wave jerks and unexpectedly erect posture for the degree of bradykinesia. More careful clinical inquiry and examination are likely to reveal a history of poor response to dopaminergic treatment (a common reason for the patient's referral), pseudobulbar affect, slow or hypometric saccades in the upward or downward directions, dysarthria that is too spastic or cerebellar in quality for PD, unexpected mildness of rigidity in the wrists and elbows, and postural instability as the most disabling feature of all.

One pathologically based series using logistic regression analysis found gait instability, paucity of tremor and poor L-dopa response to be the features that best differentiated PSP from PD.[12] The same series found that falls in the first year of illness had high sensitivity and positive predictive value in distinguishing PSP from PD, multiple-system atrophy (MSA), dementia with Lewy bodies and corticobasal degeneration.[13] While PD may display restrictions of vertical gaze and early PSP may not, a sign that is highly sensitive and specific for PSP is slowing of downward saccades.[14] Another that is quite sensitive for PSP but shared with other conditions involving the cerebellum is square-wave jerks.[15]

ATYPICAL FEATURES

Cases departing from this typical picture are common. Some patients with PSP have prominent dementia suggestive of AD.[16] Others have asymmetric apraxia or dystonia suggestive of corticobasal degeneration,[1] and others resemble PD or MSA of the parkinsonian type (formerly called striatonigral degeneration) until late in the illness, when marked vertical supranuclear gaze abnormalities finally appear. Even such findings as moderate asymmetry and mild rest tremor,[17,18] claimed by earlier authors to virtually exclude PSP, occurred in 2 of 12 pathologically confirmed cases in a recent series.[19] Another autopsy series[20] found asymmetric onset in 3 of 16 cases.

Atypical clinical features tend to cluster in patients with atypical pathological and molecular features that occur in AD.[21] This suggests that there may be two or more disease entities presently lumped as "PSP."

Diagnostic Criteria

A set of diagnostic criteria formulated by Golbe et al.[4] for use in settings that permit detailed examination of patients are shown in Table 20-2. This set is suitable for drug trials or for small epidemiologic studies in which an experienced neurologist examines each patient. Under such conditions, its specificity is 98 percent and its positive predictive value 92 percent.[23] It would not be suitable when only retrospective examination data by nonneurologists are available. Likewise, its sensitivity, 50 percent, is insufficient for prevalence or incidence surveys.

Litvan et al.[23] formulated a now widely accepted set of "probable" clinical criteria (Table 20-3) that achieves 100 percent specificity and positive predictive value while sacrificing sensitivity (50 percent). They reviewed clinical records of 24 patients with autopsy-proven PSP and approximately three times that number with other conditions in the differential diagnosis of PSP. The same project also formulated a set of "possible" criteria with the higher sensitivity, 83 percent, necessary to a prevalence or incidence study. The "possible" criteria sacrifice only little specificity (93 percent) and positive predictive value (83 percent) in achieving this goal. These criteria have been named the National Institute of Neurological Disorders and Stroke/Society for Progressive

TABLE 20-2 Diagnostic Criteria for PSP (proposed by Golbe et al.[4])

All 4 of these:
  Onset at age 40 or later
  Progressive course
  Bradykinesia
  Supranuclear gaze palsy, per criteria below
Plus any 3 of these:
  Dysarthria or dysphagia
  Neck rigidity (to flexion/extension) greater than limb rigidity
  Neck in a posture of extension
  Minimal or absent tremor
  Frequent falls or gait disturbance early in course
Without any of these:
  Early or prominent cerebellar signs
  Unexplained polyneuropathy
  Prominent noniatrogenic dysautonomia other than isolated postural hypotension
  Criteria for supranuclear gaze palsy
EITHER both of these:
  Voluntary downgaze less than 15 degrees (tested by instructing patient to "look down" without presenting a specific target; accept the best result after several attempts)
  Preserved horizontal oculocephalic reflexes (except in very advanced stages)
OR all 3 of these:
  Slowed downward saccades (defined as slow enough for the examiner to perceive the movement itself)
  Impaired opticokinetic nystagmus with the stimulus moving downward
  Poor voluntary suppression of vertical vestibulo-ocular reflex

TABLE 20-3 NINDS-SPSP Criteria for the Diagnosis of PSP (proposed by Litvan et al.[23])

"Possible" PSP
All 3 of these:
1. Gradually progressive disorder
2. Onset at age 40 or later
3. No evidence for competing diagnostic possibilities
Plus either of these:
4. Vertical gaze palsy
   or
5. Slowing of vertical saccades *and* prominent postural instability with falls in the first year

"Probable" PSP
All 5 of these:
1. Gradually progressive disorder
2. Onset at age 40 or later
3. No evidence for competing diagnostic possibilities
4. Vertical gaze palsy
5. Slowing of vertical saccades *and* prominent postural instability with falls in the first year

Criteria that would exclude PSP from consideration
1. Recent encephalitis
2. Alien limb syndrome, cortical sensory defects or temporoparietal atrophy
3. Psychosis unrelated to dopaminergic treatment
4. Important cerebellar signs
5. Important unexplained dysautonomia
6. Severe, asymmetric parkinsonian signs
7. Relevant structural abnormality of basal ganglia on neuroimaging
8. Whipple's disease on CSF PCR, if indicated

PCR, polymerase chain reaction.

Supranuclear Palsy (NINDS-SPSP) Criteria in honor of the co-sponsors of the project.

DIFFERENTIAL DIAGNOSIS

For a neuropathologist with access to the full range of modern, but routine, histopathologic techniques, the principal entities competing with PSP are only corticobasal degeneration (CBD), postencephalitic parkinsonism (PEP) and the Parkinson-dementia complex of Guam (PDC) (Table 20-4). The clinician must contend with a longer list that includes some cases of PD, CBD, MSA (principally striatonigral degeneration but also olivopontocerebellar atrophy),[24] progressive subcortical gliosis,[25] Creutzfeldt-Jakob disease,[26] AD with parkinsonism, diffuse Lewy body disease,[27] Pick's disease and the primary pallidal atrophies, including dentatorubropallidoluysian atrophy.[28] The mitochondrial encephalomyopathies, which are protean in their presentations, can rarely resemble PSP.[29]

Some clinical points by which PSP can be differentiated from some of the most common of these entities are listed in Table 20-4. Perhaps the most difficult differentiation of PSP is from MSA. One recent study[20] found that certain clinical features could distinguish MSA from PD with acceptable certainty, but that they could not distinguish MSA from PSP

TABLE 20-4 Clinical Points Differentiating PSP from Some Other Parkinsonian Disorders

	PSP	PD	MSA (SND)	CBD
Symmetry of deficit	+++	+	+++	−
Axial rigidity	+++	++	++	++
Limb dystonia	+	+	+	+++
Postural instability	+++	++	++	+
Vertical supranuclear gaze restriction	+++	+	++	++
Frontal behavior	+++	+	+	++
Dysautonomia	−	+	++	−
L-Dopa response early in course	+	+++	+	−
L-Dopa response late in course	−	++	+	−
Asymmetric cortical atrophy on MRI	−	−	−	++

SND, striatonigral degeneration.

in the absence of specific signs such as downgaze palsy or extensor axial dystonia.

CLINICAL EVALUATION

A thorough clinical examination and history will generally reveal PEP, PDC, myasthenia gravis (as a cause of gaze palsy, dysarthria, and dysphagia), mitochondrial myopathy (as a cause of gaze palsy), and bulbar amyotrophic lateral sclerosis. Magnetic resonance imaging (MRI) or X-ray computed tomography (CT) will reveal, although not necessarily incriminate, mimics such as hydrocephalus,[30] midbrain tumors, and a multi-infarct state. The last is the most common nondegenerative PSP mimic. In fact, lacunar state can reproduce virtually the full range of clinical features of PSP, as it can the features of AD and PD.[31−33] It may be suspected in the patient with stepwise progression, marked pyramidal signs, focal weakness, and, as mentioned, ischemic changes on MRI or CT.

RADIOLOGIC EVALUATION

Positron emission tomography using ^{18}F-dopa distinguished 90 percent of patients with clinically diagnosed PSP from a group with PD.[34] Similar results are produced by use of ^{18}F-glucose as a marker of cortical and subcortical metabolic rate,[34−37] and by calculating the relative deficiencies of caudate and putamen with regard to uptake of a dopamine transporter marker.[38]

Although ^{18}F-dopa and ^{18}FDG (fluorodeoxyglucose) positron emission tomography (PET) can identify presymptomatic members of families with PSP,[39] the sensitivity and specificity of PET in distinguishing patients with clinically equivocal or early PSP from other conditions has not been assessed. For this reason, PET is not yet considered a standard diagnostic tool in PSP. The cost of that technology is a separate problem that would limit the use of PET in PSP to research settings for the foreseeable future.

MRI and CT imaging are nonspecific in most cases of PSP (Table 20-5). In the moderate to advanced stages, they

TABLE 20-5 MRI Features of PSP and Some Other Conditions

	PSP	PD	MSA (OPCA)	MSA (SND)	CBD	AD
Cortical atrophy	++	+	+/−	+	++/−	++
Putamenal atrophy	−	−	−	++	−	−
Pontine atrophy	+	−	+++	−	+/−	−
Midbrain atrophy	++	−	+	−	+/−	−
Cerebellar atrophy	−	−	++/−	−	−	−
High putamenal iron	−	−	+/−	+/−	−	−

− absent or rare; +, occasional, mild or late; ++, usual, moderate; +++, usual, severe or early; OPCA, olivopontocerebellar atrophy; SND, striatonigral degeneration.

may reveal thinning of the anteroposterior diameter of the midbrain tectum and tegmentum with atrophy of the colliculi and disproportionate enlargement of the sylvian fissures and posterior third ventricle.[40−45] MRI may show high signal in the periaqueductal gray compatible with gliotic change, a nonspecific finding in the parkinsonisms. The MRI features that are most likely to permit a differentiation of PSP from MSA are the absence (in PSP) of abnormal signal and/or atrophy in the cerebellum, middle cerebellar peduncle, pons and inferior olive, and of the hyperintense putaminal rim caused by iron deposition.[45] The MRI features most helpful in distinguishing PSP from CBD are the absence of asymmetric frontal atrophy and the presence of midbrain atrophy.

As is the case with PET imaging, the value of MRI and CT in the early, diagnostically doubtful case is not established, except to rule out nondegenerative pathology or to rule out cerebellar atrophy that would direct suspicion toward olivopontocerebellar atrophy as the diagnosis.

A similar challenge faces the use of single photon emission computed tomography (SPECT) using markers of cerebral blood flow and/or metabolism. Such studies show bifrontal hypometabolism in established PSP[48−50] and have yet to be evaluated in equivocal cases. However, SPECT imaging of D2 receptor sites using ^{123}I-iodobenzamide is promising as a means of differentiating PSP, where there is often detectable striatal D2 loss, from PD, where there is not.[51,52]

Magnetic resonance spectroscopy is starting to show promise as a means of differentiating PSP from PD or other states.[53−55] The diagnostic finding is a reduction in the ratio of *N*-acetylaspartate to creatine in the region of the putamen and/or pallidum. However, as for PET, the ability of this modality to distinguish the conditions during their early, clinically equivocal phases is unproven.

CEREBROSPINAL FLUID (CSF) STUDIES

CSF tau levels are elevated in CBD but not in PSP[56,57] or AD.[57] The CSF level of neurofilament protein has been found to distinguish PSP from PD and controls but not from MSA.[58] Oligoclonal bands occurred in 1 of 2 patients with PSP in whom they were sought.[59] Protein, glucose, and cell counts are uniformly normal in PSP.

Neuropathology, Neurochemistry, and their Clinical Correlates

OVERVIEW

PSP is one of the neurofibrillary tangle (NFT) diseases. This group also includes: AD, corticobasal degeneration, dementia pugilistica, Down's syndrome, frontotemporal dementia, Guadelouopean tauopathy, PDC, Pick's disease, postencephalitic parkinsonism.

Dopaminergic damage in the nigrostriatal pathway and cholinergic damage in many areas are the most consistent, severe neurotransmitter-related changes in PSP.[60−63] GABAergic function of the basal ganglia (in striatum, globus pallidus interna, GPi, and globus pallidus externa, GPe) is moderately but widely impaired.[64] Unlike the case in PD, the peptidergic systems and the mesolimbic and mesocortical dopaminergic systems are intact. Serotonergic receptor sites are reduced in the cortex, but unlike in PD, are normal in basal ganglia.[65] The loss of adrenoceptors is widespread,[66] reflecting the wide projections of the severely damaged locus ceruleus.

NEUROFIBRILLARY TANGLES (NFTs)

While neuronal loss and gliosis are the most prominent microanatomic features of PSP[67] and their characteristic anatomic distribution can produce suspicion of PSP, that diagnosis cannot be made in the absence of NFTs. While most of the NFTs of most brains with PSP have a rounded ("globose") shape, a few are "flame-shaped". This situation is reversed in AD and seems to relate more closely to the structure of the neuron containing the tangle than to the disease producing the damage.[68]

The filaments composing the NFTs of PSP are unpaired straight filaments 15–18 nm in diameter, comprising at least 6 protofilaments 2–5 nm in diameter.[69−72] Filaments of AD, by contrast, are mostly paired helical filaments 22 nm in diameter with a minor component of straight filaments similar to those of PSP.[73] A few cortical areas in PSP, or even subcortical nuclei, may display paired helical filaments of the Alzheimer type.[74−75] Paired straight filaments and unpaired twisted filaments, which may be a more advanced stage of filament formation, also occur occasionally in PSP.[75]

The immunostaining and ultrastructural properties of the filaments of PSP tangles are nearly identical to those of CBD.[75,76] However, the white matter tangles of CBD occur in oligodendroglia rather than in astrocytes, as in most[77] but not all[78] cases of PSP. Furthermore, "pretangles" are far more frequent in CBD than in PSP.[79]

TAU PROTEIN

Cortical NFTs of PSP appear to be antigenically identical to those of AD, most notably with regard to the presence of abnormally phosphorylated tau protein.[80–84] Tau is a low molecular weight component of microtubule-associated protein. The latter is involved in axonal transport of vesicles. PSP tau exhibits bands of 64 and 69 kDa on Western blot, while AD and Down's syndrome tau has those two bands plus one of 55 kDa.[85,86]

Staining with anti-tau antibody greatly aids the identification of NFTs in PSP and has largely replaced silver stains and hematoxylin and eosin for this purpose, at least in the research setting. Anti-tau staining has revealed the existence of neuropil threads, also known as curly fibers, in the same neurons that include NFTs and in oligodendroglia of white matter tracts connecting affected areas of subcortical gray matter.[87–89] Most neuropil threads of AD, on the other hand, occur in neurons, sparing glia. Staining for ubiquitin, a peptide involved in proteolysis and occurring in NFTs of AD and Lewy bodies of PD, is weak or variable in the NFTs of PSP.[90]

A mouse model of PSP has recently been described.[91] It expresses one of the mutant forms of tau that causes frontotemporal dementia, but the distribution of lesions is closely analogous to that of human PSP. *Drosophila* models of a generic tauopathy have also been reported.[92,93] In one of these, intriguingly, adult-onset, selective neurodegeneration with accumulation of abnormal tau occurred without formation of NFTs.[92] This and other experimental evidence from many sources suggests that the toxic species is tau in an early stage of aggregation, not mature NFTs.

The molecular biology of tau abnormalities in PSP is discussed in more detail in the section on genetics below.

OTHER CHANGES

Grumose degeneration, in which eosinophilic material surrounds degenerating neurons, accompanied by spherical argentophilic components, occurs in a significant minority of cases with PSP, particularly in the cerebellar dentate nucleus.[2,94] It appears to comprise abnormally regenerated synaptic terminal material of Purkinje cells. Grumose degeneration of the dentate occurs also in dentatorubropallidoluysian atrophy, a condition with more obvious ataxia than occurs in PSP.

While amyloid or senile plaques do not occur in PSP, another hallmark of AD, granulovacuolar degeneration, does occur to a mild extent. In addition, swollen, achromatic neurons characteristic of CBD or Pick's disease occur in a few cases of otherwise typical PSP, generally in tegmental and inferior temporal areas.[95]

The overlap of PSP with AD is illustrated by a recent series of 13 autopsies with the full pathologic picture of PSP.[96] Four of the 13 also exhibited pathologic changes of "definite AD" and two had "probable AD." A primary clinical diagnosis of AD with memory loss as the first neurologic symptom was present in 2 of these 6 and in 3 of the 7 without AD pathology.

Microglial activation, another pathologic change that occurs in some neurodegenerative disorders, has recently been found to be common in PSP.[97] In the brainstem in PSP, microglial activation does not correlate well with the presence of NFTs. This suggests that neither is the direct cause of the other and that microglia may help produce the neuronal loss of PSP.

Anatomic Distribution of Degeneration

The major areas of primary involvement in PSP, together with an oversimplified but convenient scheme of their clinical correlates are: the cerebral cortex, producing cognitive and behavioral changes; the nigrostriatalpallidal area, producing rigidity, bradykinesia, and postural instability; the cholinergic pontomesencephalic nuclei area, producing gaze palsies, sleep disturbances, and axial motor abnormalities; and the hindbrain area, producing dysarthria, and dysphagia. The daunting complexity of this syndrome, the interactions of its parts, and its tremendous interpatient variability may be the principal reason for the continuing resistance of PSP to pathophysiologic understanding and pharmacologic intervention.

CEREBRAL CORTEX

PATHOANATOMY
The marked central and cortical atrophy of cerebrum seen on gross postmortem examination in AD is only mild in PSP.[98] Early studies of PSP found little microscopical pathology in cerebral cortex, but the advent of tau immunostaining has permitted identification of the motor strip (area 4) and a partly ocular motor association area (area 39) as the most important sites of pathology.[99–101] Many other cortical areas are affected, but much less severely. The least affected area appears to be the primary visual cortex (area 17), as is the case in AD.[102] The affection of the motor area of cortex may be secondary to the severe degeneration of subcortical areas, such as the subthalamic nucleus, that have projections to cortex.[103] Overlap with the topography of the pathology of corticobasal degeneration can produce in some cases of PSP cortical signs such as apraxia.[104]

PSP affects the large pyramidal and small neurons of layers V and VI, while AD affects the medium-sized neurons of layers III and V.[104]

Cortical involvement in PSP therefore differs importantly from that in AD at the gyral, laminar, cytologic, ultrastructural, and biochemical levels.

FRONTAL LOBES
Behavioral changes were the initial symptom of PSP in 22 percent of patients in one series[4] that used family interview data, and in 2 of 24 (8 percent) in a series with autopsy confirmation and good clinical records (I Litvan, personal communication). Disabling mental changes eventually occur in 80 percent or more of cases.[5,105]

ANATOMIC AND NEUROCHEMICAL CHANGES

The prefrontal areas, which are the most obviously affected by behavioral testing and by measures of cerebral blood flow,[48–50,106–109] display relatively little neurofibrillary pathology or neuronal loss in PSP.[99,102] This suggests that, in PSP, secondary cortical dysfunction is caused by subcortical pathology, as in the cholinergic nucleus basalis of Meynert and the cholinergic pedunculopontine nucleus, both important and relatively constant sites of involvement.[110–112] The situation is not so simple, however, because, in PSP, unlike in PD, dementia does not correlate with the degree of reduction in choline acetyltransferase activity.[61,113] Frontal cortical degeneration in PSP correlates well with the atrophy of the anterior corpus callosum, which presumably is its result[114] and with disproportionate slowing of the EEG frontally.[115]

Damage to the striatopallidal complex may also contribute to dementia via reduction of its output to the frontal lobes.[103,116] However, in PSP, unlike in PD, damage to noncholinergic subcorticocortical projections via dopaminergic, noradrenergic, and serotonergic pathways is minimal.

CLINICAL CORRELATES

Clinically, the frontal lobe dysfunction in PSP is often striking and rapidly progressing.[117] Apathy, intellectual slowing and impairment of "executive" functions are the consistent findings. These are partly related to slowed central sensory processing.[118,119] Tests of reaction time that control for motor slowing show that the cognitive component of such tasks is greatly prolonged in PSP, approximately 50 percent longer than in PD.[120] It is a common clinical observation that the patient with PSP can supply correct answers to complex questions after a delay of several minutes.

The executive dysfunction[121] is illustrated by difficulty in shifting mental set, as between following a numerical trail and an alphabetical trail with a pencil.[122] Other defects are poor performance of sorting, problem-solving, abstract thinking, and lexical fluency (as when given 1 minute to name as many items as possible from a given category such as words starting with "m").[123,124] Other examining room tasks that can reveal a frontal defect are the ability to perform task A (e.g., tapping once) when the examiner performs task B (e.g., tapping twice) and vice versa, and the ability, when confronted by the examiner's widely separated hands, to direct horizontal gaze toward the hand that does not wave, the "antisaccade task." Disinhibition in other forms occurs in a significant minority.

Prominent frontal deficits of this sort with little agitation, irritability or abnormal motor behaviors helps distinguish the dementia of PSP from that of AD.[125]

Spontaneous frontal motor behaviors can also be dramatic in some patients with PSP.[122,126] Most obvious are forced grasping (either with the hand or with the gaze), imitative behavior (such as mimicking the examiner's hand movements), and motor perseveration (as when unable to cease clapping after being asked to imitate the examiner's three handclaps—the "applause sign"). These signs in the presence of parkinsonism are a useful alert to the possibility of PSP, but the combination also occurs in PD and SND.[24] Arm levitation[127] and other forms of apraxia[128] have been described. Palilalia is a common and, at times, disabling problem in PSP.[123]

HIPPOCAMPUS

The hippocampus, a primary site of pathology in AD, is involved in only half of cases of PSP.[129] This probably explains the relative preservation of memory in PSP, at least until late in the course.[16] The qualitative pattern of involvement of the hippocampus in PSP, however, is similar to that in AD and PD.[101] Memory tasks that require goal-directed searching of memory are, as one would expect given the frontal lobe function, an early area of impairment in PSP.[130] The pattern of memory impairment is similar to that of PD and Huntington's disease and different from that in AD, where forgetting is more rapid.[131]

NIGROSTRIATAL SYSTEM

DISTRIBUTION OF PATHOLOGY

Damage to the pigmented neurons of the zona compacta of the substantia nigra, the most consistent abnormality in PSP, occurs in a different distribution than in PD.[132] In PSP, the damage is relatively uniform except for relative sparing of a small, extreme lateral portion, while, in PD, both the dorsal and extreme lateral portions are relatively spared. A similar pattern occurs in striatonigral degeneration.[132] The dorsal portion projects principally to the caudate, the ventral to the putamen. This probably explains the relative sparing of presynaptic caudate dopamine reuptake in PD and its involvement in PSP, as measured by ^{18}F-fluorodopa PET.[34,133]

In the striatum, there is also severe loss of acetylcholinergic activity,[62] although the majority of affected striatal cells appear to be astrocytes rather than neurons ("tufted" astrocytes).[83] They include tau-positive, argyrophilic tangles and neuropil threads similar to those in affected neurons. Such astrocytic pathology may be unique to PSP. Most of the few affected striatal neurons are probably cholinergic interneurons.[63,134,135]

It is unclear whether the poor response of the parkinsonian components of PSP to dopamine replacement therapy and the relative resistance of PSP to the hyperkinetic side-effects of such therapy are the result of pathology in the striatum or further downstream in the striatal system. It is also unclear whether the loss of the cholinergic striatal interneurons explains the failure of anticholinergic treatment (relative to its success in PD) and the hints of improvement from cholinergic treatment.[136]

As predicted from the paucity of striatal neuronal damage, there is no loss of postsynaptic dopamine D1 receptors, as measured by binding studies, and by D1 receptor mRNA levels.[65] Density of D2 receptors is probably normal or only slightly decreased.[65,137,138]

CLINICAL COURSE

Postural instability is the initial symptom in approximately two-thirds of patients with PSP.[4,5] Frank falls start a median of 1.8 years into the illness.[104] The falls are often unheralded in that the patient had had no concomitant gait difficulty and typically complains of having "tripped over nothing." This has prompted the term "paroxysmal dysequilibrium." Patients often have a normal neurological examination at this point and are investigated for vestibulopathy, syncope, epilepsy, or myelopathy. The initial or only gait abnormality occasionally takes the form of severe gait "freezing" or "apraxia"[139–142] with no rigidity. In PD, by contrast, gait difficulty or postural instability is a presenting feature in only 11 percent.[6]

The postural instability is usually the most disabling feature of later PSP. The median intervals from initial symptom, corrected by the Kaplan-Meier lifetable method, are 3.1 years until assistance is required, and 8.2 years until wheelchair confinement.[4]

Contrary to widespread impression, rest tremor is not unknown in PSP, occurring in about 5–10 percent of patients, usually early in the course.[143,144] Action or postural tremor occurs in about 25 percent. The limb rigidity and distal bradykinesia are mild relative to axial rigidity and bradykinesia. The rigidity tends to increase from wrist to elbow to shoulder.

OTHER BASAL GANGLIA

SUBTHALAMIC NUCLEUS

Damage to the subthalamic nucleus ranks beside that of the substantia nigra as a constant in PSP and is far more specific to PSP. Subthalamic neuronal depletion is so severe that the posteroinferior portion of the third ventricle may be disproportionately dilated on CT or magnetic resonance MRI.[40] This can give the third ventricle the shape of a bowling pin on axial imaging, contrasting with the cigar shape characteristic of AD.

GLOBUS PALLIDUS INTERNA (GPi)

The basal ganglia damage that is furthest "downstream" and therefore perhaps the most relevant with regard to therapeutic intervention in PSP is in the GPi. This structure acts as the common outflow pathway from the basal ganglia to the thalamus. This lesion is not quite as constant as that of the substantia nigra (SN) or subthalamic nucleus, but it probably explains the failure of stereotactic GPi lesions to ameliorate PSP despite their efficacy against PD. Similarly, the outflow function of the GPi probably explains the therapeutic failure of fetal mesencephalic implants into the striatum in PSP.

GLOBUS PALLIDUS EXTERNA (GPe)

A careful comparison of PSP with PD and controls with regard to neuronal counts in the GPe showed an important loss in PSP but not in PD.[145] This offers the possibility that GPe dysfunction provides the most direct source of the hypokinesis of PSP by increasing thalamic inhibition, particularly in patients lacking the excitatory input from the subthalamic nucleus.

PEDUNCULOPONTINE NUCLEUS

Despite the status of the GABAergic GPi (and the partly GABAergic substantia nigra reticulata, SNr) as the final outflow from the basal ganglia, and despite low GABAergic activity in many parts of the basal ganglia, efforts to treat PSP with the GABAergic drug valproic acid have failed, at least on informal assessment at the symptomatic level.[146] Part of the explanation may be that the GPi projects not only to the thalamus, which is nearly intact in PSP, but also to the cholinergic pedunculopontine nucleus (PPN), which is severely affected.[111,112,147] There is evidence that lesions of the PPN alone can cause severe postural instability.[148] Nevertheless, GABA agonists more selective for basal ganglia function should be tested in PSP.

THALAMUS

Although the thalamus is not classically considered a major center of pathology in PSP, Steele et al.[1–3] did mention the presence of tangles in the glutamatergic caudal intralaminar nuclei, which regulate caudate and putamen, and recent studies have confirmed this quantitatively.[149] PET using a cholinergic marker has documented loss of those thalamic neurons, producing a picture different from that of the cholinergic loss in PD.[150]

OTHERS

The GPe, ventral tegmental area, red nucleus, intralaminar nuclei of the thalamus, and locus ceruleus are also involved in PSP, although not as constantly or as severely as the foregoing areas. The reported[151] slight therapeutic benefit of a noradrenergic drug, idazoxan, suggests that the locus ceruleus pathology may play a pivotal role.

Experimental lesions of the interstitial nucleus of Cajal in monkeys produce extensor rigidity at the neck and postural instability,[152] and this nucleus is characteristically affected in PSP.[153] However, the severe damage in the striatopallidal pathway could also help explain the unusual extensor tone of PSP.[154]

MESENCEPHALIC AND PONTINE OCULAR MOTOR AREAS

PATHOANATOMY

The supranuclear, predominantly vertical, eye movement abnormality for which PSP was named presumably originates in the rostral midbrain, where there is variable involvement of the interstitial nucleus of Cajal, the nucleus of Darkschewitsch, the rostral interstitial nucleus of the

TABLE 20-6 Components of Dysarthria in PSP and Some Related Conditions (from Hardman and Halliday[145])

	Hypokinesia	Ataxia	Spasticity
PSP	++	+	+++
PD	+++	−	−
MSA (striatonigral degeneration)	+++	++	+
MSA (olivopontocerebellar atrophy)	+	+++	++

medial longitudinal fasciculus, and the mesencephalic reticular formation.[103,111,153,155] The relative contributions of these nuclei have not been sorted out.

There have been cases of damage to some of these areas in patients without clinical supranuclear gaze abnormality.[156–159] Conversely, there is one report of idiopathic calcification of basal ganglia sparing dorsal midbrain with PSP-like gaze palsy.[160] One quantitative study of neuronal loss in the SNr[161] found a correlation of damage there with gaze palsy in patients with PSP. This may be explained by the projection of the SNr to the superior colliculus.

Some of the vertical paresis may result from subselective involvement of these nuclei themselves, followed by nuclear ocular paresis at the endstage of PSP in some cases. The horizontal gaze palsy that appears eventually in most cases is attributable to degeneration of nuclei of the pontine base.[162] The ocular motor cranial nerve nuclei are perhaps the sole example of cholinergic nuclei to escape important involvement in PSP.

CLINICAL PHENOMENOLOGY

Symptomatic eye movement difficulty does not begin until a median of 3.9 years after disease onset, nearly half the clinical course.[4] Before that time, however, most patients with otherwise diagnosable PSP will exhibit slowing of vertical saccades, saccadic pursuit, breakdown of opticokinetic nystagmus in the vertical plane, disordered Bell's phenomenon, poor convergence, and subtle square-wave jerks.[163–165] The last finding has perhaps the greatest sensitivity for PSP, occurring in all or nearly all patients with PSP.[165,166] Square-wave jerks occur in very few patients with PD, but are sufficiently common in MSA and other conditions that they cannot be used to differentiate them from PSP.[166] Of great specificity for PSP is a delay in saccade initiation, at times so prolonged as to give the appearance of the patient's not having heard or attended to the examiner's command. Such delays may constitute visual prehension, also called perseveration of gaze, a result of frontal lobe damage.[167]

The frontal dysfunction is also expressed via such ocular motor phenomena as poor performance on the antisaccade task. Here, the patient quickly directs the gaze to the examiner's hand that does *not* move. An altitudinal visual attentional deficit[168] arising from damaged tectal centers may contribute to overloading the fork, poor aim of the urinary stream, and poor attention to dress out of proportion to

dementia. In addition, patients with PSP seem less aware of their postural instability than do patients with other causes of the same degree of instability.

Later in the course, the patient loses range of vertical gaze, with downgaze usually, but far from always, worse than upgaze. Voluntary gaze without a specific target (i.e., "look down") is usually worse than command gaze to a target, which is worse than pursuit, and reflex gaze is by far the least affected. Some patients with autopsy-confirmed PSP never display gaze paresis during life, even on careful prospective examination.[8]

REFLEX GAZE

From the earliest stages, most patients also suffer loss of the ability to voluntarily suppress the vestibulo-ocular reflex.[169] This may be tested by seating the patient in a swivel chair or wheelchair and asking him to extend the arms at the level of the eyes, clasp his hands and fixate on one thumbnail as the examiner slowly rotates the chair and patient en bloc. Patients with PSP (and many other basal ganglia disorders) are unable to suppress the opticokinetic nystagmus produced by relative movement of the environment. Performing this maneuver in the vertical plane, if the patient's axial rigidity permits, reveals an abnormality which, when out of proportion to concomitant poor horizontal vestibulo-ocular reflex suppression, may be a valuable clue to the presence of very early PSP.

EYELID MOVEMENT

Eyelid movement abnormalities, particularly apraxia of eyelid opening (perhaps better termed "lid levator inhibition"[170]), and blepharospasm, occur in about one-third of patients and can cause functional blindness.[171–173] Apraxia of lid closing and the very slow blink rate of PSP, often less than 5/minute, can allow conjunctival drying with annoying reactive inflammation and lacrimation. The electrical blink reflex is severely impaired, unlike in PD, CBD or MSA,[174] testament to the profound brainstem pathology in PSP.

BRAINSTEM CENTERS CONTROLLING SLEEP AND AROUSAL

Sleep disturbance is a prominent abnormality in PSP. It is presumably related principally to damage to the (serotonergic) raphe nuclei, the (cholinergic) pedunculopontine nucleus and others, the (noradrenergic) locus ceruleus, and the periaqueductal gray. The most important clinical component is a severe reduction in rapid eye movement (REM) sleep.[175] There is a loss of sleep spindles and K-complexes. During what REM sleep remains, there are abnormal slow waves and absence of normal sawtooth waves.[176] The diagnostic value of the REM abnormalities prompted Agid et al.[129] to advocate polysomnography in all patients with a suspicion of PSP.

Daytime hypersomnolence, probably related to damage of dopaminergic systems that maintain wakefulness, is a disabling problem in PSP. There is a fragmentation of sleep-wake

TABLE 20-7 Drugs Most Likely to Relieve Symptoms in PSP

Drug	Starting dosage	Maximum dosage in PSP
L-Dopa (with carbidopa)	100 mg per day	2000 mg per day
Amantadine	100 mg once daily	100 mg twice daily
Amitriptyline	10 mg at bedtime	20 mg in the morning, 20 mg at bedtime

Note: L-Dopa as a rule will only relieve.

periods that culminates, at the endstage of PSP, in a constant sleep-like or stuporous state from which the patient can be roused but briefly.

The auditory startle and auditory blink reflexes are absent or severely impaired in PSP[177] despite normal auditory evoked potentials.[178] Startle is mediated via the lower pontine reticular formation, in particular the nucleus reticularis pontis caudalis, which degenerates in PSP.

BRAINSTEM CENTERS CONTROLLING SPEECH AND SWALLOWING

DYSARTHRIA

Steele et al.[3] were referring to the lower brainstem functions as much as to the eye movements in applying the term "supranuclear palsy." Indeed, degeneration of the cranial nerve nuclei in PSP is mild except in the oculomotor nucleus.[179] Likewise, the dysarthria of PSP reveals no lower motoneuron features. Rather, it is a variable combination of, in descending order of importance, spasticity, hypophonia, and ataxia.[180] The combination is unique among the competing diagnostic considerations, at least from a statistical standpoint (Table 20-7). The slow rate of speech with a strained and strangled quality and some hyperkinetic, ataxic components is highly specific for PSP.

Dysarthria can be an early symptom that often brings the patient to a physician.[5] Within 2 years after disease onset, 41 percent of patients or their families have detected dysarthria. By the fifth year, the figure is 68 percent.[4]

DYSPHAGIA

Relative to the morbidity it causes, the dysphagia of PSP has received only little and belated research attention. Aspiration pneumonia is a major risk in advanced PSP, but only 18 percent of patients report symptomatic dysphagia within 2 years after PSP onset and 46 percent do so by 5 years.[4] Dysphagia occurred in 26 of 27 patients in one study in which their mean disease duration was 52 months.[181,182] The median latency to onset of dysarthria was 48 months in one study,[4] and 42 in another.[183]

In a study[184] that performed videofluoroscopy in 22 patients with mild to moderate PSP with symptomatic dysphagia, at least 80 percent of patients exhibited abnormalities attributable to parkinsonian rigidity of the oral and pharyngeal muscles. Esophageal problems occurred in fewer than half of patients and nasal reflux occurred in none. Only 1 patient (4.5%) aspirated contrast material, but 27 percent coughed or choked. The dysphagia of PSP, while arising from many levels of the oropharyngeal axis,[182] emphasizes oral rather than pharyngeal abnormalities, distinguishing it from the dysphagia of PD.[185]

It is common for patients with PSP, but not with PD, to exacerbate the effects of dysphagia by overloading the fork, probably through a combination of poor downgaze, frontal disinhibition, and vertical visual inattention.[186] The neck hyperextension that occurs eventually in some patients with PSP may decrease the ability of the epiglottis to protect the airway. However, relative to patients with PD, those with PSP appear more aware of their dysphagia and have less rigidity and tremor of the tongue, major causes of dysphagia in PD.[184]

SPINAL AND AUTONOMIC CENTERS

PSP includes less dysautonomia than PD,[187,188] a point useful in its clinical differentiation from MSA. Nevertheless, there can be disabling bladder dysfunction,[189] which is probably the result of the severe degeneration of brainstem autonomic nuclei,[190] and of some white matter tracts in the spinal cord.[191] The latter occurs mainly in the motor area (lamina IX) and the intermediolateral column. There is also mild gray matter tract degeneration in the spinal cord.[103] In one series,[80] urinary incontinence occurred in 42 percent of patients, beginning a mean of 3.5 years into the disease course.

Epidemiology and Etiology

DESCRIPTIVE EPIDEMIOLOGY

ONSET AGE

In most series, PSP begins, on average, in the late fifties to mid-sixties, as is the case for PD. Approximately a third of cases begin before age 60.[4] The standard deviation of the onset age is typically between 6 and 7 years,[4] far less than the 11 years typical for PD. For a late-life-onset condition, such raw onset age data are less useful to the epidemiologist than age-specific incidence figures, which do not exist for PSP. That is, we do not know whether there is an age of maximal risk for PSP or whether the incidence of new cases in a given age group relative to the number of people alive in that age group declines after a certain age. This would have implications for etiology and pathogenesis.

SURVIVAL

Death occurred at an actuarially corrected median of 9.7, 7.0 and 5.9 years in three studies.[4,5,192] Ten-year survival is typically approximately 30 percent.[192] In a study based on complete ascertainment of a well-documented community

(Olmsted County, Minnesota), median survival was only 5.3 years.[193] The onset age distribution was older in that study than in many others that were based on referred cases. Therefore, the median survival in that study may be a more valid measure of the natural history of PSP in general.

Death is usually related to pneumonia and other inevitable complications of immobility, but frank aspiration, head trauma due to falls, and complications of hip fracture are important preventable causes of death in PSP.

PREVALENCE

The prevalence ratio of previously diagnosed PSP was found by one study in three counties in central New Jersey[4] to be 1.4 per 100,000, and by another in the UK[194] to be 1.0 per 100,000. This figure would be useful in determining the demand for PSP-specific services or treatment.

Two studies, one in London[195] and the other in the north of England,[194] examined patients in defined geographical areas whose medical records suggested any sort of parkinsonism. Most of the patients thereby identified as having PSP had not previously received that diagnosis. The age-adjusted prevalence ratios were 6.4[195] and 5.0[194] per 100,000. These figures would be useful in determining the actual burden of PSP in the population for purposes of public policymaking or research administration. The 4–5-fold difference between these prevalence ratios and those based only on previously diagnosed cases is a measure of the difficulty in accurately diagnosing PSP when the index of suspicion is low.

INCIDENCE

For a chronic disease, incidence (the number of new cases in a defined population per year) gives a more valid measure than prevalence of the intensity of the etiologic agent in the population or environment. The incidence of PSP has been measured directly in Rochester, Minnesota (population 50,000) by two separate studies. The first used patients previously diagnosed over the interval 1967–1979, giving an incidence of 0.3 per 100,000 per year.[196] The second, which covered the years 1976–1990 and used a more thorough method that captured patients with inobvious clinical presentations, gave an annual incidence of 1.1 per 100,000 per year.[193] This compares with approximately 20 per 100,000 per year for PD.[197]

SEX RATIO

Published cases of PSP reveal a sex ratio (M/F) of approximately 2:1.[15] The absence of so asymmetric a ratio in other highly referred neurodegenerative disorders is a point against gender-related referral bias as the explanation in PSP and points to an occupational toxin as an etiologic factor.

ANALYTIC EPIDEMIOLOGY

In one case-control study of risk factors in PSP, an 85-item questionnaire administered to 50 patients and 100 matched controls in New Jersey,[198] patients were 3.1 times more likely than controls to have completed high school, and 2.9 times as likely to have completed college. Patients were also 2.4 times more likely to have lived as an adult over age 40 in a locality of population less than 10,000. These both reached statistical significance, but were interpreted by the authors as probable effects of ascertainment bias or referral bias. Items that gave statistically nonsignificant results concerned living overseas, occupations implicated in other neurologic illnesses, potential exposure to occupational toxins, smoking, alcohol, caffeine, contact sports, head trauma, type A personality, early menopause, estrogen supplementation, multiparity, various medical conditions, surgical history, psychiatric history, animal exposure, maternal age, birth order, and family neurologic history.

Anecdotal reports from one investigator in Canada suggest greater than expected exposure to hydrocarbons in a small series of patients with PSP.[199,200] This may help explain the asymmetric sex ratio, but has not yet been specifically examined in a controlled study. Smoking, which is negatively correlated with PD and MSA, has no relation to PSP.[201]

A TRANSMISSIBLE AGENT?

The pathologic and clinical similarity between PSP and PDC aroused suspicion that a slow virus may be their cause, as it is in Kuru, another neurodegenerative disease of the western Pacific. However, after a mean of 9.1 (range 3–24) years' observation of 29 chimpanzees receiving intracerebral inoculation of brain tissue from 10 patients with PSP, results are negative.[202] A search for prion protein in PSP and other parkinsonian disorders, despite the pathologic similarities between PSP and Creutzfeldt-Jakob disease, was also negative.[203]

In PD and AD, but not in PSP,[22,204] there is a deficit in the sense of smell, the function of which involves dopaminergic transmission. This is evidence against the hypothesis that, at least in PSP, an etiologic agent gains entry to the CNS via the olfactory epithelium. An alternative explanation is simply that for unknown reasons the dopaminergic involvement in PSP spares the olfactory pathway, just as it does many other areas involved by PD.

AN HEREDITARY COMPONENT?

In reviewing the records of 104 patients with PSP, Jankovic et al.[205] found no allegations of secondary cases of PSP among their 409 relatives, and the frequency of PD, tremor and dementia among the relatives was only that expected in the population. A retrospectively controlled survey from the same clinic[206] found a family history of tremor in relatives of patients with (nonfamilial) PSP (2.6 percent) to be similar to that among relatives of controls (2.2 percent). However, in a formal case-control study,[198] the question inquiring into the presence of "Parkinson's disease" among parents, siblings, grandparents, aunts, uncles, and first cousins elicited a positive answer 5.0 times as frequently in those with PSP as in controls. For "Alzheimer's or dementia," the ratio was 3.6.

Recent reports of families with more than one member with PSP give additional reason to reconsider the issue of a genetic factor in the cause of PSP. Eight such reports with autopsy confirmation in at least one member have appeared, all most compatible with autosomal-dominant transmission.[209–215] Paternal transmission was a component of the mechanism in most of these families, a strong point against a mitochondrial gene as the sole culprit. It is intriguing that some of these families, including a Spanish family that is by far the largest, include additional members with reports of typical PD or essential tremor.[216] Some asymptomatic members of such families show caudate and putaminal abnormalities in ^{18}F-fluorodopa uptake on PET.[217]

GEOGRAPHIC CLUSTERS

Two geographic clusters of PSP-like tauopathies are known. Lytigo-bodig, or the amyotrophic lateral sclerosis-parkinsonism-dementia complex of Guam (PDC), has resisted multiple careful etiologic investigations, but its markedly declining incidence since the westernization of Guam after World War II suggests an environmental cause.[218] The anatomic pathology of PDC has been called both easily distinguishable[79] and indistinguishable[219] from PSP. At the biochemical level, however, the predominance of 4-repeat tau in PSP tangles is absent in PDC, where the ratio is unity, as in controls and AD.[79]

An unusual concentration of a PSP-like tauopathy on the Caribbean island of Guadeloupe was described in 1999 by Caparros-Lefebvre et al.[220] Their case-control survey found that illness to be associated with dietary or medicinal use of two indigenous plants, soursop and sweetsop (*Annona muricata* and *A. squamosa*). These species contain reticuline and corexime, which are dopaminergic toxins.[221] Discontinuing the use of these products resulted in marked and prolonged clinical improvement in some of the younger patients on Guadeloupe. The use of these compounds to produce an animal model and to understand tauopathies in general is starting to be explored.[218]

A MITOCHONDRIAL OR OXIDATIVE MECHANISM?

Molecular genetic study of PSP has been advancing in recent years. One candidate locus, the apolipoprotein E (ApoE) locus, which exhibits a disproportionate prevalence of the ε4 allele in AD, exhibits only the normal distribution of alleles in PSP.[222,223] Other candidate genes could be subjected to similar allelic association studies in PSP, but there are as yet too few multiplex families or affected sibling pairs to perform linkage analysis.

A more promising lead arises from the finding[225] that skeletal muscle mitochondrial respiratory function, assessed at the biochemical level, is reduced by about 30 percent in PSP.

In brain tissue, activity levels of superoxide dismutase 1 and/or 2,[226] malondialdehyde,[227] and lipid peroxidation products[228] are markedly increased specifically in areas that degenerate in PSP as a result of oxidative stress.

Evidence that deficiency of complex I of mitochondrial genetic origin contributes to the cause of typical PSP is provided by the observation of low complex I activity and mitochondrial dysfunction in cultured neuronal cells in which native mitochondria were replaced by mitochondria from patients with PSP.[229,230]

An area of recent inquiry is the role of transglutaminases in PSP.[231] Enzymes normally important in stabilizing protein structure, they are aberrantly activated in PSP and other neurodegenerative disorders by oxidative stress. The resulting crosslinking of tau protein could help explain the formation of NFTs or the dysfunction of other proteins. This observation offers a promising site of action for neuroprotective therapy.

A NUCLEAR GENETIC MECHANISM?

TAU ISOFORMS

In normal human brain, tau occurs in approximately equal proportions of two isoforms: with either 3 or 4 repeats of the microtubule-binding peptide domain.[232] The isoform is determined by whether the transcript of the tau gene's exon 10 is spliced in or out of the final tau protein product. In PSP, the ratio is at least 3:1 in favor of 4-repeat tau.[85] In some other tauopathies such as Pick's disease, 3-repeat tau predominates; in others, such as AD, the normal 1:1 ratio occurs. Disordered regulation of exon 10 splicing may therefore explain tau aggregation into NFTs in PSP and other tauopathies.

The PSP-like illness highly prevalent on Guadeloupe, at least in the three cases autopsied so far,[233] is biochemically identical to PSP itself. That is, the NFTs in both conditions present a major doublet at 64 and 69 kDa and a minor 74 kDa band, and the tau is predominantly 4-repeat.[233] This contrasts with the Guamanian disease, where there is a triplet at 60, 64 and 69 kDa, and the tau occurs equally in 3-repeat and 4-repeat forms.[234] The Guamanian biochemical signature is therefore closer to that of AD than PSP.[218]

A CLUE FROM FTD

A valuable clue to PSP, a sporadically occurring tauopathy, arises from frontotemporal dementia (FTD), a dominantly inherited tauopathy.[235] Several mutations in and near the 5′ splice site downstream of exon 10 have been described in FTD families. Here, the 3-repeat 4-repeat skew is similar to that of PSP.[236] The pathogenic mechanism of these mutations is probably disruption of a stem-loop structure in the RNA transcribed at the downstream end of exon 10. This stem-loop regulates splicing of the exon 10 transcript. Its dysfunction in FTD produces predominantly 4-repeat tau. The cause, then, of PSP and other sporadic tauopathies may be dysfunction of the same RNA stem-loop, but of nongenetic or nonmendelian genetic cause. This prospect has been strengthened by the description[237] of a family with inherited, autopsy-typical PSP and a mutation at the downstream end of exon 10 close to those described in FTD. This single nucleotide substitution does not alter the tau amino acid sequence but would disrupt the RNA stem-loop.

A TAU ALLELIC VARIANT

Following the lead of the FTD story, Conrad et al.[238] found an association between sporadic PSP and a genetic marker, the A0 allele, located in the intron upstream of exon 10. This has been amply confirmed, and patients with PSP who lack the A0/A0 genotype experience later disease onset.[239] Subsequently, two haplotypes delineating the same chromosome consisting of markers spanning most of the tau gene have been associated with PSP more strongly than the A0 allele alone.[240,241] Each haplotype is present in nearly all patients with PSP but also in a significant minority of controls. This suggests that a genetic variation necessary but not sufficient to cause PSP is located in or near the tau gene at chromosome 17q21. The precise mutation is not known, but mutations in the tau promoter region that are in linkage disequilibrium with these haplotypes have been described and may explain the dysfunction of that version of tau.[242,243]

The occurrence of PSP in sporadic rather than familial fashion must then require an additional exogenous or genetic factor. It is sobering in this regard to note that corticobasal degeneration shares the haplotype that characterizes PSP,[244–246] as does PD to a lesser degree.[247] It is equally sobering that the presence or absence of this H1 haplotype or the H1/H1 genotype has no effect on the age of onset, clinical progression,[248,249] the anatomical distribution of degeneration, or on the biochemical features of the abnormal tau protein.[250]

Variants in apoE that are associated with AD and variants in α-synuclein and synphilin that are associated with PD are absent in PSP.[251]

Treatment

PHARMACOTHERAPY

As is the case for most other degenerative disorders, neurotransmitter replacement or receptor stimulation in PSP encounters little or none of the success it has with PD.[146,252]

DOPAMINERGICS

The extent and nature of the benefit of L-dopa in PSP has not been adequately studied in double-blind fashion, but any benefit is nearly always mild and/or brief. In two retrospective, uncontrolled studies, 51 percent[253] and 38 percent[146] of patients responded, most of them minimally. (The placebo response rate in PD drug trials is generally about 30 percent.)

Only the rigidity and bradykinesia, including those components of dysarthria and dysphagia attributable to them, may respond more than would be expected from placebo. Therefore, there is no reason to prescribe dopaminergic treatment for patients whose activities are not impaired by those specific abnormalities.

While hyperkinetic side-effects and response fluctuations of L-dopa are very rare in PSP (0 of 82 patients in one survey[146]), agitation, confusion, and/or hallucinations are less rare (5 of 82, 6 percent). Still, it is the author's practice to prescribe for PSP approximately twice the L-dopa/carbidopa dosages used for PD with the equivalent degree of parkinsonism. Dopamine receptor agonists give similar benefit with additional risks.[146,254] This impression has recently been confirmed by a multicenter double-blind trial of pramipexole as well as anecdotal experience with that drug.[255]

CHOLINERGICS AND ANTICHOLINERGICS

It is perhaps symptomatic of our state of knowledge of PSP therapy that opposite directions in cholinergic intervention have been advocated. Anticholinergics have been used by analogy with PD, but are far less efficacious than L-dopa.[146,253,256] An exception may be amantadine, which has dopaminergic and antiglutamatergic properties as well, and is a close second to L-dopa in risk/benefit ratio.[146] A trial of amantadine starting at 100 mg daily and increasing to a maximum of 100 mg twice daily is worthwhile for most patients with PSP. It should be tapered and discontinued if symptomatic benefit is not apparent within a month.

Trials of cholinergics have been inspired by the severe and widespread degeneration of acetylcholinergic systems in PSP. The cholinesterase inhibitor physostigmine was reported to improve PET evidence of prefrontal dysfunction, longterm verbal memory, and visuospatial attention, all very slightly,[119,136] but a subsequent trial by one of these groups gave negative results, with worsening of gait.[258] Donepezil, a commercially available cholinesterase inhibitor minimally effective in AD, has no benefit against PSP.[257] The benefits of RS-86, another cholinergic agent, were limited to some aspects of sleep.[259]

ANTIDEPRESSANTS AND ANTISEROTONERGICS

In a double-blind trial,[261] amitriptyline improved gait and rigidity in 3 of 4 patients, and desipramine improved "apraxia" of eyelid opening in both of 2 patients. In a retrospective series,[146] amitriptyline gave a risk/benefit ratio that was slightly less favorable than those of L-dopa and amantadine. Amitriptyline is generally safest started at 10 mg at bedtime, increasing by that amount each week, given in two divided doses. If 20 mg twice daily proves ineffective, higher dosages are unlikely do otherwise. Amitriptyline may paradoxically worsen postural instability in PSP and its anticholinergic effect may the worsen the cognitive impairment of the illness. Imipramine confers a slightly less favorable risk/benefit ratio than amitriptyline,[115] and desipramine a quite unfavorable ratio. There is also a case report of benefit from trazodone.[260]

The antiserotonergic drug methysergide was found moderately efficacious in a controlled trial published in 1981,[186] but subsequent informal experience has not confirmed this benefit.[146,262]

GABAergics

Zolpidem, a commonly prescribed bedtime sedative, has been reported to ameliorate overall parkinsonian scores and some eye movement problems in PSP,[263] but the benefit lasts only a few hours at best and has not been confirmed. Sedation is common.

BOTULINUM TOXIN

Blepharospasm in PSP responds well to botulinum A injections.[264] Even "apraxia" of lid opening may respond to botulinum A.[265] Torticollis or retrocollis in PSP may also respond, but the occasional occurrence of mild dysphagia after botulinum injection for idiopathic spasmodic torticollis dictates caution in the case of PSP, where slight exacerbation of dysphagia could allow aspiration. Botulinum toxin may also be useful in focal dystonia of PSP.[266]

NONPHARMACOLOGIC THERAPY

GAZE AND LID PARESES

Blepharospasm or lid levator inhibition may be overcome if a family member presents a finger-counting task. Some patients can overcome the voluntary downgaze palsy that impairs eating by using their remaining pursuit downgaze ability to follow the fork down to the plate. If downgaze palsy or inattention to the lower half of space is present, low-lying objects such as children's toys, loose rugs, and coffee tables should be removed from the patient's path. While prisms are not usually useful in correcting the patient's inability to attend to the lower half of space, they may help diplopia related to dysconjugate gaze.

The chronic conjunctivitis and reactive lacrimation caused by the low blink rate may be treated by instillation of methylcellulose or polyvinyl alcohol drops when awake, and a petrolatum-based ointment or mineral oil at bedtime.

PHYSICAL, SPEECH, AND SWALLOWING THERAPY

Physical therapy seems to be of little or no benefit against the postural instability of PSP, but instruction for the family in the physical care of the poorly ambulatory patient may be useful, and regular exercise has a clear psychological benefit.[267] Similarly, speech therapy has proved of little benefit in most patients, but the speech pathologist may be able to arrange adjunctive means of communication such as electronic typing devices or simple pointing boards.

Dysphagia in PSP is also unlikely to respond to therapy. However, the family may be instructed in the preparation of foods of proper consistency, using a blender or cornstarch-based thickeners as necessary. A barium swallow radiograph using boluses of varying consistency will guide this advice. The speech pathologist can teach the patient safer swallowing techniques and can monitor the patient for the need for a feeding gastrostomy. The high morbidity and mortality related to aspiration in advanced PSP has led the author to recommend endoscopic placement of a feeding gastrostomy after the first episode of aspiration pneumonitis, if the patient requires more time to finish a meal than the family can practically provide, if there is significant weight loss because of reduced intake, or if a minor degree of aspiration occurs with every mouthful (K Kluin, personal communication).

SURGICAL IMPLANTS

Fetal or porcine nigral cell striatal allografts have not been attempted in PSP, but the advanced state of degeneration of centers downstream from the striatum, contrasting with the situation in PD, suggests that such procedure is unlikely to be of benefit. This prediction is supported by the unfavorable results of a trial of adrenal medullary tissue autografts to striatum.[268]

A similar rationale predicts that deep brain stimulation would not help PSP. Stimulation of the subthalamic nucleus or GPi in PD, in which those nuclei do not degenerate, ameliorates the symptoms, presumably by mitigating the disinhibited activity in those areas. In PSP, however, both areas are among the most severely affected by the degenerative process, and reduction in activity there could be expected only to exacerbate the functional abnormality.

ELECTROCONVULSIVE THERAPY (ECT)

Two personal cases and one from the literature[269] have markedly worsened with ECT with regard to both motor and cognitive functioning. All 3 patients improved nearly to baseline over subsequent weeks. This contrasts with the benefit of ECT in PD.[270]

Patient Resources

The Society for Progressive Supranuclear Palsy is headquartered in Baltimore and serves North America. The Progressive Supranuclear Palsy Association is based in the UK and serves all of Europe. Smaller organizations have recently been founded in other countries. These patient service and advocacy organizations offer support meetings and lay-language literature. The two listed below also offer research funding to scientists in all countries. Just as important as these formal activities is these organizations' message to patients that having an "orphan disease" does not mean neglect by the medical world.

The Society for Progressive
   Supranuclear Palsy, Inc.
Woodholme Medical Building
1838 Greene Tree Rd, Suite 515
Baltimore, MD 21208
USA
Phone 1-800-457-4777
Fax 410-486-4283
spsp@psp.org
http://www.psp.org

The Progressive
   Supranuclear Palsy
   Association (Europe)
The Old Rectory
Wappenham
Towcester NN12 8SQ
UK
Phone +44 1327 860299
Fax +44 1327 861007
psp.eur@virgin.net
http://www.pspeur.org

References

1. Richardson JC, Steele J, Olszewski J: Supranuclear ophthalmoplegia, pseudobulbar palsy, nuchal dystonia and dementia: A clinical report on eight cases of "heterogeneous system degeneration." *Trans Am Neurol Assoc* 88:25–29, 1963.

2. Olszewski J, Steele J, Richardson JC: Pathological report on six cases of heterogeneous system degeneration. *J Neuropathol Exp Neurol* 23:187–188, 1963.

3. Steele JC, Richardson JC, Olszewski J: PSP: A heterogeneous degeneration involving the brain stem, basal ganglia and cerebellum, with vertical gaze and pseudobulbar palsy, nuchal dystonia and dementia. *Arch Neurol* 10:333-359, 1964.

4. Golbe LI, Davis PH, Schoenberg BS, Duvoisin RC: Prevalence and natural history of PSP. *Neurology* 38:1031–1034, 1988.

5. Maher ER, Lees AJ: The clinical features and natural history of the Steele-Richardson-Olszewski syndrome (PSP). *Neurology* 36:1005–1008, 1986.

6. Hoehn MM, Yahr MD: Parkinsonism: Onset, progression, and mortality. *Neurology* 17:427–442, 1967.

7. Duvoisin RC: Clinical diagnosis, in Litvan I, Agid Y (eds): *PSP: Clinical and Research Approaches.* New York: Oxford University Press, 1992, pp 15–33.

8. Birdi S, Rajput AH, Fenton M, et al: PSP diagnosis and confounding features: Report on 16 autopsied cases. *Mov Disord* 17:1255–1267, 2002.

9. Tanigawa A, Komiyama A, Hasegawa O: Truncal muscle tonus in PSP. *J Neurol Neurosurg Psychiatry* 64:190–196, 1998.

10. Golbe LI and the Medical Advisory Board of the Society for Progressive Supranuclear Palsy: A clinical rating scale and staging system for PSP. *Neurology* 48(suppl):A326, 1997.

11. Golbe LI, Lepore FE, Johnson WG, et al: Inter-rater reliability of the PSP rating scale. *Neurology* 52(suppl):A227, 1999.

12. Litvan I, Campbell G, Mangone CA, et al: Which clinical features differentiate PSP from related disorders? A clinicopathological study. *Brain* 120:65–74, 1997.

13. Wenning GK, Ebersbach G, Verny M, et al: Progression of falls in postmortem-confirmed parkinsonian disorders. *Mov Disord* 14:947–950, 1999.

14. Leigh RJ, Riley DE: Eye movements in parkinsonism: It's saccadic speed that counts. *Neurology* 54:1018–1019, 2000.

15. Rivaud-Péchoux S, Vidailhet M, Gallouedec G, et al: Longitudinal ocular motor study in corticobasal degeneration and PSP. *Neurology* 54:1029–1032, 2000.

16. Milberg W, Albert M: Cognitive differences between patients with PSP and Alzheimer's disease. *J Clin Exp Neuropsychol* 11:605–611, 1989.

17. Rivest J, Quinn N, Marsden CD: Dystonia in Parkinson's disease, multiple system atrophy, and PSP. *Neurology* 40:1571–1578, 1990.

18. Gibb WRG, Luthert PJ, Marsden CD: Corticobasal degeneration. *Brain* 112:1171–1192, 1989.

19. Collins SJ, Ahlskog JE, Parisi JE, Maraganore DM: PSP: Neuropathologically based diagnostic clinical criteria. *J Neurol Neurosurg Psychiatry* 58:167–173, 1995.

20. Colosimo C, Albanese A, Hughes AJ, et al: Some specific clinical features differentiate multiple system atrophy (striatonigral variety) from Parkinson's disease. *Arch Neurol* 52:294–298, 1995.

21. Morris HR, Gibb G, Katzenschlager R, et al: Pathological, clinical and genetic heterogeneity in PSP. *Brain* 125:969–975, 2002.

22. Müller A, Müngersdorf M, Reichmann H, et al: Olfactory function in parkinsonian syndromes. *J Clin Neurosci* 9:521–524, 2002.

23. Litvan I, Agid Y, Calne D, et al: Clinical research criteria for the diagnosis of PSP: Report of the NINDS-SPSP International Workshop. *Neurology* 47:1–9, 1996.

24. Robbins TW, James M, Owen AM, et al: Cognitive deficits in PSP, Parkinson's disease, and multiple system atrophy in tests sensitive to frontal lobe dysfunction. *J Neurol Neurosurg Psychiatry* 57:79–88, 1994.

25. Will RG, Lees AJ, Gibb W, Barnard RO: A case of progressive subcortical gliosis presenting clinically as Steele-Richardson-Olszewski syndrome. *J Neurol Neurosurg Psychiatry* 51:1224–1227, 1988.

26. Bertoni JN, Label LS, Sackellares C, Hicks SP: Supranuclear gaze palsy in familial Creutzfeldt-Jakob disease. *Arch Neurol* 40:618–622, 1983.

27. Fearnley JM, Revesz T, Brooks DJ, et al: Diffuse Lewy body disease presenting with a supranuclear gaze palsy. *J Neurol Neurosurg Psychiatry* 54:159–161, 1991.

28. Pahwa R, Koller WC, Stern MB: Primary pallidal atrophy, in Stern MB, Koller WC (eds): *Parkinsonian Syndromes.* New York: Marcel Dekker, 1993, pp 433–440.

29. Truong DD, Harding AE, Scaravilli F, et al: Movement disorders in mitochondrial myopathies: A study of nine cases with two autopsy studies. *Mov Disord* 5:109–117, 1990.

30. Curran T, Lang AE: Parkinsonian syndromes associated with hydrocephalus: Case reports, a review of the literature, and pathophysiological hypotheses. *Mov Disord* 9:508–520, 1994.

31. Tanner CM, Goetz CG, Klawans HL: Multi-infarct PSP. *Neurology* 37:1819, 1987.

32. Winikates J, Jankovic J: Vascular PSP. *J Neural Transm Suppl* 42:189–201, 1994.

33. Dubinsky RM, Jankovic J: PSP and a multi-infarct state. *Neurology* 37:570–576, 1987.

34. Burn DJ, Sawle GV, Brooks DJ: Differential diagnosis of Parkinson's disease, multiple system atrophy, and Steele-Richardson-Olszewski syndrome: Discriminant analysis of striatal ^{18}F-dopa PET data. *J Neurol Neurosurg Psychiatry* 57:278–284, 1994.

35. Foster NL, Gilman S, Berent S, et al: Cerebral hypometabolism in PSP studied with PET. *Ann Neurol* 24:399–406, 1988.

36. D'Antona R, Baron JC, Samson Y, et al: Subcortical dementia: Frontal cortex hypometabolism detected by PET in patients with PSP. *Brain* 108:785–799, 1985.

37. Nagahama Y, Fukuyama H, Turjanski N, et al: Cerebral glucose metabolism in corticobasal degeneration: Comparison with PSP and normal controls. *Mov Disord* 12:691–696, 1997.

38. Ilgin N, Zubieta J, Reich SG, et al: PET imaging of the dopamine transporter in PSP and PD. *Neurology* 52:1221–1226, 1999.

39. Piccini P, Lees AJ, de Yébenes JG, et al: ^{18}F-dopa and [18]FDG studies in 3 kindreds with familial PSP. *Neurology* 50:A429, 1998.

40. Schonfeld SM, Golbe LI, Safer J, et al: Computed tomographic findings in PSP: Correlation with clinical grade. *Mov Disord* 2:263–278, 1987.

41. Drayer BP, Olanow W, Burger P, et al: Parkinson plus syndrome: Diagnosis using high field MR imaging of brain iron. *Radiology* 159:493–498, 1986.

42. Savoiardo M, Strada L, Girotti F, et al: MR imaging in PSP and Shy-Drager syndrome. *J Comput Assist Tomogr* 13:555–560, 1989.

43. Saitoh H, Yoshii F, Shinohara Y: Computed tomographic findings in PSP. *Neuroradiology* 29:168–171, 1987.

44. Yuki N, Sato S, Yuasa T, et al: Computed tomographic findings of PSP compared with Parkinson's disease. *Jpn J Med* 29:506–511, 1990.

45. Stern MB, Braffman BH, Skolnick BE, et al: Magnetic resonance imaging in Parkinson's disease and parkinsonian syndromes. *Neurology* 39:1524–1526, 1989.

46. Schrag A, Good CD, Miszkiel K, et al: Differentiation of atypical parkinsonian syndromes with routine MRI. *Neurology* 54:697–702, 2000.

47. Wenning GK, Ebersbach G, Verny M, et al: Progression of falls in postmortem-confirmed parkinsonian disorders. *Mov Disord* 14:947–950, 1999.

48. Timmons JH, Bonikowski FW, Harshorne MF: Iodoamphetamine-123 brain imaging demonstrating cortical deactivation in a patient with PSP. *Clin Nucl Med* 14:841–842, 1989.

49. Habert MO, Spampinato U, Mas JL, et al: A comparative technetium 99m hexamethylpropylene amine oxime SPECT study in different types of dementia. *Eur J Nucl Med* 18:3–11, 1991.

50. Neary D, Snowdon JS, Shields RA, et al: Single photon emission tomography using [99]mTc-HM-PAO in the investigation of dementia. *J Neurol Neurosurg Psychiatry* 50:1101–1109, 1987.

51. van Royen E, Verhoeff NF, Speelman JD, et al: Multiple system atrophy and PSP: Diminished striatal D2 dopamine receptor activity demonstrated by ^{123}I-IBZM single photon emission computed tomography. *Arch Neurol* 50:513–516, 1993.

52. Schwarz J, Tatsch K, Arnold G, et al: ^{123}I-Iodobenzamide-SPECT predicts dopaminergic responsiveness in patients with de novo parkinsonism. *Neurology* 42:556–561, 1992.

53. Davie CA, Barker GJ, Machado C, et al: Proton magnetic resonance spectroscopy in Steele-Richardson-Olszewski syndrome. *Mov Disord* 12:767–771, 1997.

54. Abe K, Terakawa H, Takanashi M, et al: Proton magnetic resonance spectroscopy of patients with parkinsonism. *Brain Res Bull* 52:589–595, 2000.

55. Clarke CE, Lowry M: Systematic review of proton magnetic resonance spectroscopy of the striatum in parkinsonian syndromes. *Eur J Neurol* 8:573–577, 2001.

56. Urakami K, Mori M, Wada K, et al: A comparison of tau protein in CSF between CBD and PSP. *Neurosci Lett* 259:127–129, 1999.

57. Arai H, Morikawa Y, Higuchi M, et al: Cerebrospinal fluid tau levels in neurodegenerative diseases with distinct tau-related pathology. *Biochem Biophys Res Commun* 236:262–264, 1997.

58. Bolmberg B, Rosengren L, Karlsson J-E, Johnels B: Increased cerebrospinal fluid levels of neurofilament protein in PSP and MSA compared with PD. *Mov Disord* 13:70–77, 1998.

59. Miller JR, Burke AM, Bever CT: Occurrence of oligoclonal bands in multiple sclerosis and other CNS diseases. *Ann Neurol* 13:53–58, 1983.

60. Jellinger K, Riederer P, Tomonaga M: PSP: Clinicopathological and biochemical studies. *J Neural Transm Suppl* 16:111–128, 1980.

61. Kish SJ, Chang LJ, Mirchandani L, et al: PSP: Relationship between extrapyramidal disturbances, dementia and brain neurotransmitter markers. *Ann Neurol* 18:530–536, 1985.

62. Ruberg M, Javoy-Agid F, Hirsch E, et al: Dopaminergic and cholinergic lesions in PSP. *Ann Neurol* 18:523–529, 1985.

63. Young AB: PSP: Postmortem chemical analysis. *Neurology* 18:521–522, 1985.

64. Levy R, Ruberg M, Herrero MT, et al: Alterations of GABAergic neurons in the basal ganglia of patients with PSP: An in situ hybridization study of GAD_{67} messenger RNA. *Neurology* 45:127–134, 1995.

65. Landwehrmeyer B, Palacios JM: Neurotransmitter receptors in PSP. *J Neural Transm Suppl* 42:229–246, 1994.

66. Pascual J, Berciano J, Gonzalez AM, et al: Autoradiographic demonstration of loss of alpha-2-adrenoceptors in PSP: Preliminary report. *J Neurol Sci* 114:165–169, 1993.

67. Hauw J-J, Daniel SE, Dickson D, et al: Preliminary NINDS neuropathologic criteria for Steele-Richardson-Olszewski syndrome (PSP). *Neurology* 44:2015–2019, 1994.

68. Ishino H, Otsuki S: Frequency of Alzheimer's neurofibrillary tangles in the cerebral cortex in PSP. *J Neurol Sci* 28:309–316, 1976.

69. Powell HC, London GW, Lampert PW: Neurofibrillary tangles in PSP. *J Neuropathol Exp Neurol* 33:98–106, 1974.

70. Tellez-Nagel I, Wisniewski HM: Ultrastructure of neurofibrillary tangles in Steele-Richardson-Olszewski syndrome. *Arch Neurol* 29:324–327, 1973.

71. Tomonaga M: Ultrastructure of neurofibrillary tangles in PSP. *Acta Neuropathol (Berl)* 37:1771–1781, 1977.

72. Montpetit V, Clapin DR, Guberman A: Substructure of 20 nm filaments of PSP. *Acta Neuropathol* 68:311–318, 1985.

73. Dickson DW, Kress Y, Crowe A, Yen S-H: Monoclonal antibodies to Alzheimer neurofibrillary tangles (ANT): 2. Demonstration of a common antigenic determinant between ANT and neurofibrillary degeneration in PSP. *Am J Pathol* 120:292–303, 1985.

74. Ghatak NR, Nochlin D, Hadfield MG: Neurofibrillary pathology in PSP. *Acta Neuropathol (Berl)* 52:73–76, 1980.

75. Ikeda K, Akiyama H, Haga C, et al: Argyrophilic thread-like structure in corticobasal degeneration and supranuclear palsy. *Neurosci Lett* 174:157–159, 1994.

76. Mori H, Nishimura M, Namba Y, Oda M: Corticobasal degeneration: A disease with widespread appearance of abnormal tau and neurofibrillary tangles, and its relation to PSP. *Acta Neuropathol* 88:113–121, 1994.

77. Wakabayashi K, Oyanagi K, Makifuchi T, et al: Corticobasal degeneration: Etiopathological significance of the cytoskeletal alterations. *Acta Neuropathol* 87:545–553, 1994.

78. Inagaki T, Ishino H, Seno H, et al: An autopsy case of PSP with astrocytic inclusions. *Jpn J Psychiatry Neurol* 48:85–89, 1994.

79. Oyanagi K, Tsuchiya K, Yamazaki M, Ikeda K: Substantia nigra in PSP, corticobasal degeneration and parkinsonism-dementia

complex of Guam: Specific pathological features. *J Neuropathol Exp Neurol* 60:393–402, 2001.

80. Pollock NJ, Mirra SS, Binder LI, et al: Filamentous aggregates in Pick's disease, PSP, and Alzheimer's disease share antigenic determinants with microtubule-associated protein, tau. *Lancet* ii: 1211, 1986.

81. Love S, Saitoh T, Quijada S, et al: Alz-50, ubiquitin and tau immunoreactivity of neurofibrillary tangles, Pick bodies and Lewy bodies. *J Neuropathol Exp Neurol* 47:393–405, 1988.

82. Tabaton M, Whitehouse PJ, Perry G, et al: Alz 50 recognized abnormal filaments in Alzheimer's disease and PSP. *Ann Neurol* 24:407–413, 1988.

83. Yamada T, Calne DB, Akiyama H, et al: Further observations on tau-positive glia in the brains with PSP. *Acta Neuropathol* 85:308–315, 1993.

84. Schmidt ML, Huang R, Martin JA, et al: Neurofibrillary tangles in PSP contain the same tau epitopes identified in Alzheimer's disease PHFtau. *J Neuropathol Exp Neurol* 55:534–539, 1996.

85. Flament S, Delacourte A, Verny M, et al: Abnormal tau proteins in PSP. *Acta Neuropathol (Berl)* 81:591–596, 1991.

86. Vermersch P, Robitaille Y, Bernier L, et al: Biochemical mapping of neurofibrillary degeneration in a case of PSP: Evidence for general cortical involvement. *Acta Neuropathol* 87:572–577, 1994.

87. Probst A, Langui D, Lautenschlager C, et al: PSP: Extensive neuropil threads in addition to neurofibrillary tangles. *Acta Neuropathol (Berl)* 77:61–68, 1988.

88. Nelson SJ, Yen S-H, Davies P, Dickson DW: Basal ganglia neuropil threads in PSP. *J Neuropathol Exp Neurol* 48:324, 1989.

89. Iwatsubo T, Hasegawa M, Ihara Y: Neuronal and glial tau-positive inclusions in diverse neurologic diseases share common phosphorylation characteristics. *Acta Neuropathol (Berl)* 88:129–136, 1994.

90. Lennox G, Lowe J, Morrell K, et al: Ubiquitin is a component of neurofibrillary tangles in a variety of neurodegenerative diseases. *Neurosci Lett* 94:211–217, 1988.

91. Lewis J, McGowan E, Rockwood J, et al: Neurofibrillary tangles, amyotrophy and progressive motor disturbance in mice expressing mutant (P301L) tau protein. *Nat Genet* 25:402–405, 2000.

92. Wittmann CW, Wszolek MF, Shulman JM, et al: Tauopathy in *Drosophila*: Neurodegeneration without neurofibrillary tangles. *Science* 293:711–714, 2001.

93. Lewis J, Dickson KW, Lin W-L, et al: Enhanced neurofibrillary degeneration in transgenic mice expressing mutant tau and APP. *Science* 293:1487–1491, 2001.

94. Arai N: "Grumose degeneration" of the dentate nucleus: A light and electron microscopic study in PSP and dentatorubropallidoluysian atrophy. *J Neurol Sci* 90:131–145, 1987.

95. Giaccone G, Tagliavini F, Street JS, et al: PSP with hypertrophy of the olives: An immunohistochemical study of artyrophilic neurons. *Acta Neuropathol (Berl)* 77:14–20, 1988.

96. Gearing M, Olson DA, Watts RL, Mirra SS: PSP: Neuropathologic and clinical heterogeneity. *Neurology* 44:1015–1024, 1994.

97. Ishizawa K, Dickson DW: Microglial activation parallels system degeneration in PSP and corticobasal degeneration. *J Neuropathol Exp Neurol* 60:647–657, 2001.

98. Cordato NJ, Halliday GM, Harding AJ, et al: Regional brain atrophy in PSP and Lewy body disease. *Ann Neurol* 47:718–728, 2000.

99. Hauw J-J, Verny M, Delaere P, et al: Constant neurofibrillary changes in the neocortex in PSP. Basic differences with Alzheimer's disease and aging. *Neurosci Lett* 119:182–186, 1990.

100. Hof PR, Delacourte A, Bouras C: Distribution of cortical neurofibrillary tangles in PSP: A quantitative analysis of six cases. *Acta Neuropathol (Berl)* 84:45–51, 1992.

101. Braak H, Jellinger K, Braak E, Bohl J: Allocortical neurofibrillary changes in PSP. *Acta Neuropathol* 84:478–483, 1992.

102. Verny M, Duyckaerts C, Delaére P, et al: Cortical tangles in PSP. *J Neural Transm Suppl* 42:179–188, 1994.

103. Jellinger KA, Bancher C: Neuropathology, in Litvan I, Agid Y (eds): *PSP: Clinical and Research Approaches.* New York: Oxford University Press, 1992, pp 44–88.

104. Bergeron C, Pollanen MS, Weyer L, Lang AE: Cortical degeneration in PSP: A comparison with cortical-basal ganglionic degeneration. *J Neuropathol Exp Neurol* 56:726–734, 1997.

105. Jankovic J, Van der Linden C: PSP, in Chokroverty S (ed): *Movement Disorders.* New York: PMA Publishing, 1990, pp 267–286.

106. D'Antona R, Baron JC, Sanson Y, et al: Subcortical dementia: Frontal cortex hypometabolism detected by positron tomography in patients with PSP. *Brain* 108:785–799, 1985.

107. Foster NL, Gilman S, Berent S, et al: Cerebral hypometabolism in PSP studied with positron emission tomography. *Ann Neurol* 24:399–406, 1988.

108. Leenders KL, Frackowiak RSJ, Lees AJ: Steele-Richardson-Olszewski syndrome: Brain energy metabolism, blood flow and fluorodopa uptake measured by positron emission tomography. *Brain* 111:615–630, 1988.

109. Goffinet AM, De Volder AG, Guillain C, et al: Positron tomography demonstrates frontal lobe hypometabolism in PSP. *Ann Neurol* 25:131–139, 1989.

110. Tagliavini F, Pilleri G, Bouras C, Constantinidis J: The basal nucleus of Meynert in patients with PSP. *Neurosci Lett* 44:37–42, 1984.

111. Zweig RM, Whitehouse PJ, Casanova MF, et al: Loss of pedunculopontine neurons in PSP. *Ann Neurol* 22:18–25, 1987.

112. Jellinger K: The pedunculopontine nucleus in Parkinson's disease, PSP and Alzheimer's disease. *J Neurol Neurosurg Psychiatry* 52:540–543, 1988.

113. Perry RH, Tomlinson BE, Candy JM, et al: Cortical cholinergic deficit in mentally impaired parkinsonian patients. *Lancet* ii:789–790, 1983.

114. Yamauchi H, Fukuyama H, Nagahama Y, et al: Atrophy of the corpus callosum, cognitive impairment, and cortical hypometabolism in PSP. *Ann Neurol* 41:606–614, 1997.

115. Montplaisir J, Petit D, Decary A, et al: Sleep and quantitative EEG in patients with PSP. *Neurology* 49:999–1003, 1997.

116. Agid Y, Graybiel AM, Ruberg M, et al: The efficacy of levodopa treatment declines in the course of Parkinson disease: Do nondopaminergic lesions play a role? *Adv Neurol* 53:83–100, 1990.

117. Soliveri P, Monza D, Paridi D, et al: Neuropsychological follow up in patients with PD, SND-type MSA, and PSP. *J Neurol Neurosurg Psychiatry* 69:313–318, 2000.

118. Johnson R, Litvan I, Grafman J: PSP: Altered sensory processing leads to degraded cognition. *Neurology* 41:1257–1262, 1991.

119. Kertzman C, Robinson DL, Litvan I: Effects of physostigmine on spatial attention in patients with PSP. *Arch Neurol* 47:1346–1350, 1990.

120. Dubois B, Pillon B, Legault F, et al: Slowing of cognitive processing in PSP. *Arch Neurol* 45:1194–1199, 1988.

121. Pillon B, Gouider-Khouja N, Deweer B, et al: Neuropsychological pattern of striatonigral degeneration: Comparison with Parkinson's disease and PSP. *J Neurol Neurosurg Psychiatry* 58:174–179, 1995.

122. Grafman J, Litvan I, Gomez C, Chase TN: Frontal lobe function in PSP. *Arch Neurol* 47:553–558, 1990.

123. Podoll K, Schwarz M, Noth J: Language functions in PSP. *Brain* 114:1457–1472, 1991.

124. Rosser A, Hodges JR: Initial letter and semantic category fluency in Alzheimer's disease, Huntington's disease, and PSP. *J Neurol Neurosurg Psychiatry* 57:1389–1394, 1994.

125. Litvan I, Mega MS, Cummings JL, Fairbanks L: Neuropsychiatric aspects of PSP. *Neurology* 47:1184–1189, 1996.

126. Cambier J, Masson M, Viader F, et al: Le syndrome frontal de paralysie supranucleaire progressive. *Rev Neurol (Paris)* 141:528–536, 1985.

127. Barclay CL, Bergeron C, Lang AE: Arm levitation in PSP. *Neurology* 52:879–882, 1999.

128. Leiguarda RC, Pramstaller PP, Merello M, et al: Apraxia in PD, PSP, MSA and neuroleptic-induced parkinsonism. *Brain* 120:75–90, 1997.

129. Agid Y, Javoy-Agid F, Ruberg M, et al: PSP: Anatomo-clinical and biochemical considerations. *Adv Neurol* 45:191–206, 1987.

130. Pillon B, Dubois B: Cognitive and behavioral impairments, in Litvan I, Agid Y (eds): *PSP: Clinical and Research Approaches*. New York: Oxford University Press, 1992, pp 223–239.

131. Pillon B, Deweer B, Michon A, et al: Are explicit memory disorders of PSP related to damage to striatofrontal circuits? Comparison with Alzheimer's, Parkinson's and Huntington's diseases. *Neurology* 44:1264–1270, 1994.

132. Fearnley JM, Lees AJ: Ageing and Parkinson's disease: Substantia nigra regional selectivity. *Brain* 114:2283–2301, 1991.

133. Brooks DJ, Ibanez V, Sawle GV, et al: Differing patterns of striatal ^{18}F-dopa uptake in Parkinson's disease, multiple system atrophy, and PSP. *Ann Neurol* 28:547–555, 1990.

134. Villares J, Strada O, Faucheux B, et al: Loss of striatal high affinity NGF binding sites in PSP but not in Parkinson's disease. *Neurosci Lett* 182:59–62, 1994.

135. Oyanaki K, Takahashi H, Wakabayashi K, Ikuta F: Large neurons in the neostriatum in Alzheimer's disease and PSP: A topographic, histologic and ultrastructural investigation. *Brain Res* 544:221–226, 1991.

136. Litvan I, Gomez C, Atack JR, et al: Physostigmine treatment of PSP. *Ann Neurol* 26:404–407, 1989.

137. Baron JC, Mazière B, Loc'h C, et al: Loss of striatal [^{76}Br] bromospiperone binding sites demonstrated by positron emission tomography in PSP. *J Cereb Blood Flow Metab* 6:131–136, 1986.

138. Brooks DJ, Ibanez V, Sawle GV, et al: Striatal D_2 receptor status in patients with Parkinson's disease, striatonigral degeneration, and PSP, measured with ^{11}C-raclopride and positron emission tomography. *Ann Neurol* 31:184–192, 1992.

139. Matsuo H, Takashima H, Kishikawa M, et al: Pure akinesia: An atypical manifestation of PSP. *J Neurol Neurosurg Psychiatry* 54:397, 1991.

140. Imai H, Nakamura T, Kondo T, Narabayashi H: Dopa-unresponsive pure akinesia or freezing: A condition with a wide spectrum of PSP? *Adv Neurol* 60:622–625, 1993.

141. Mizusawa H, Mochizuki A, Ohkoshi N, et al: PSP presenting with pure akinesia. *Adv Neurol* 60:618–621, 1993.

142. Riley DE, Fogt N, Leigh RJ: The syndrome of "pure akinesia" and its relationship to PSP. *Neurology* 44:1025–1029, 1994.

143. Masucci EF, Kurtzke JF: Tremor in PSP. *Acta Neurol Scand* 80:296–300, 1989.

144. Jankovic J, Van der Linden C: PSP (Steele-Richardson-Olszewski syndrome), in Chokroverty S (ed): *Movement Disorders*. New York: PMA Publishing, 1990, pp 267–286.

145. Hardman CD, Halliday GM: The external globus pallidus in patients with PD and PSP. *Mov Disord* 14:626–633, 1999.

146. Nieforth KA, Golbe LI: Retrospective study of drug response in 87 patients with PSP. *Clin Neuropharmacol* 16:338–346, 1993.

147. Moriizumi T, Hattori T: Separate neuronal populations of the rat globus pallidus projecting to the subthalamic nucleus, auditory cortex and pedunculopontine tegmental area. *Neuroscience* 46:701–710, 1992.

148. Masdeu JC, Alampur U, Cavaliere R, Tavoulareas G: Astasia and gait failure with damage of the pontomesencephalic locomotor region. *Ann Neurol* 35:619–621, 1994.

149. Henderson JM, Carpenter K, Cartwright H, Halliday GM: Loss of thalamic intralaminar nuclei in PSP and PD: Clinical and therapeutic implications. *Brain* 123:1410–1421, 2000.

150. Shinotoh H, Namba H, Yamaguchi M, et al: PET measurement of acetylcholinesterase activity reveals differential loss of ascending cholinergic systems in PD and PSP. *Ann Neurol* 46:62–69, 1999.

151. Ghika J, Tennis M, Hoffman E, et al: Idazoxan treatment in PSP. *Neurology* 41:986–991, 1991.

152. Carpenter MB, Harbison JW, Peter P: Accessory oculomotor nuclei in the monkey: Projections and effects of discrete lesions. *J Comp Neurol* 140:131–147, 1970.

153. Fukushima-Kudo J, Fukushima K, Tahiro K: Rigidity and dorsiflexion of the neck in PSP and the interstitial nucleus of Cajal. *J Neurol Neurosurg Psychiatry* 50:1197–1203, 1987.

154. Lees AJ: The Steele-Richardson-Olszewski syndrome (PSP). *Mov Disord* 2:272–287, 1987.

155. Juncos JL, Hirsch EC, Malessa S, et al: Mesencephalic cholinergic nuclei in PSP. *Neurology* 41:25–30, 1991.

156. Davis PH, Bergeron C, McLachlan DR: Atypical presentation of PSP. *Ann Neurol* 17:337–343, 1985.

157. Dubas F, Gray F, Escourolle R: Maladie de steele-Richardson-Olszewski sans ophthalmoplégie: 6 cas anatomo-cliniques. *Rev Neurol (Paris)* 139:407–416, 1992.

158. Nuwer MR: PSP despite normal eye movements. *Arch Neurol* 38:784, 1981.

159. Kida E, Barcikowska M, Niemszewska M: Immunohistochemical study of a case with PSP without ophthalmoplegia. *Acta Neuropathol* 83:328–332, 1992.

160. Saver, Liu GT, Charness ME: Idiopathic striopallidodentate calcification with prominent supranuclear abnormality of eye movement. *J Neuroophthalmol* 14:29–33, 1994.

161. Halliday GM, Hardman CD, Cordato NJ, et al: A role for the substantia nigra pars reticulata in the gaze palsy of PSP. *Brain* 123:724–732, 2000.

162. Malessa S, Gaymard B, Rivaud S, et al: Role of pontine nuclei damage in smooth pursuit impairment of PSP: A clinical-pathologic study. *Neurology* 44:716–721, 1994.

163. Pfaffenbach DD, Layton DD, Kearns TP: Ocular manifestations in PSP. *Am J Ophthalmol* 74:1179–1184, 1972.

164. Chu FC, Reingold DB, Cogan DG, Williams AC: The eye movement disorders of PSP. *Ophthalmology* 86:422–428, 1979.

165. Troost BT, Daroff RB: The ocular motor defects in PSP. *Ann Neurol* 2:397–403, 1977.

166. Rascol O, Sabatini U, Simonetta-Moreau M, et al: Square wave jerks in parkinsonian syndromes. *J Neurol Neurosurg Psychiatry* 54:599–602, 1991.

167. Pierrot-Deseilligny C, Rivaud S, Pillon B, et al: Lateral visually-guided saccades in PSP. *Brain* 112:471–487, 1989.

168. Rafal RD, Posner MI, Friedman JH, et al: Orienting of visual attention in PSP. *Brain* 111:267–280, 1988.

169. Rascol OJ, Clanet M, Senard JM, et al: Vestibulo-ocular reflex in Parkinson's disease and multiple system atrophy. *Adv Neurol* 60:395–397, 1993.

170. Lepore FE, Duvoisin RC: "Apraxia" of eyelid opening: An involuntary levator inhibition. *Neurology* 35:423–427, 1985.

171. Dehaene I: Apraxia of eyelid opening in PSP. *Neurology* 15:115–116, 1984.

172. Jankovic J: Apraxia of eyelid opening in PSP: Reply. *Neurology* 15:116, 1984.

173. Golbe LI, Davis PH, Lepore FE: Eyelid movement abnormalities in PSP. *Mov Disord* 4:297–302, 1989.

174. Valls-Solé J, Valldeoriola F, Tolosa E, Marti MJ: Distinctive abnormalities of facial reflexes in patients with PSP. *Brain* 120:1877–1883, 1997.

175. Aldrich MS, Foster NL, White RF, et al: Sleep abnormalities in PSP. *Ann Neurol* 25:577–581, 1989.

176. Leygonie F, Thomas J, Degos JD, et al: Troubles du sommeil dans la maladie de Steele-Richardson: Étude polygraphique de 3 cas. *Rev Neurol (Paris)* 132:125–136, 1976.

177. Vidailhet M, Rothwell JC, Thompson PD, et al: The auditory startle response in the Steele-Richardson-Olszewski syndrome and Parkinson's disease. *Brain* 115:1181–1192, 1992.

178. Tolosa ES, Zeese JA: Brainstem auditory evoked responses in PSP. *Ann Neurol* 6:369, 1979.

179. De Bruin VMS, Lees AJ: Subcortical neurofibrillary degeneration presenting as Steele-Richardson-Olszewski and other related syndromes: A review of 90 pathologically verified cases. *Mov Disord* 9:381–389, 1994.

180. Kluin KJ, Foster NL, Berent S, Gilman S: Perceptual analysis of speech disorders in PSP. *Neurology* 43:563–566, 1993.

181. Litvan I, Sastry N, Sonies BC: Characterizing swallowing abnormalities in PSP. *Neurology* 48:1654–1662, 1997.

182. Leopold NA, Kagel MC: Dysphagia in PSP: Radiologic features. *Dysphagia* 12:140–143, 1997.

183. Muller J, Wenning GK, Verny M, et al: Progression of dysarthria and dysphagia in postmortem-confirmed parkinsonian disorders. *Arch Neurol* 58:259–264, 2001.

184. Sonies BC: Swallowing and speech disturbances, in Litvan I, Agid Y (eds): *PSP: Clinical and Research Approaches.* New York: Oxford University Press, 1992, pp 240–254.

185. Johnston BT, Castell JA, Stumacher S, et al: Comparison of swallowing function in PD and PSP. *Mov Disord* 12:322–327, 1997.

186. Rafal RD, Grimm RJ: PSP: Functional analysis of the response to methysergide and antiparkinsonian agents. *Neurology* 31:1507–1518, 1981.

187. Gert van Dijk J, Haan J, Koenderink M, Roos RAC: Autonomic nervous function of PSP. *Arch Neurol* 48:1083–1084, 1991.

188. Kimber J, Mathias CJ, Lees AJ, et al: Physiological, pharmacological and neurohormonal assessment of autonomic function in PSP. *Brain* 123:1422–1430, 2000.

189. Sakakibara R, Hattori T, Tojo M, et al: Micturitional disturbance in PSP. *J Auton Nerv Syst* 45:101–106, 1993.

190. Rub U, Del Tredici K, Schultz C, et al: PSP: Neuronal and glial cytoskeletal pathology in the higher order processing autonomic nuclei of the lower brainstem. *Neuropathol Appl Neurobiol* 28:12–22, 2002.

191. Vitaliani R, Scaravilli T, Egarter-Vigl E, et al: The pathology of the spinal cord in PSP. *J Neuropathol Appl Neurol* 61:268–274, 2002.

192. Testa D, Monza D, Ferrarini M, et al: Comparison of natural histories of PSP and multiple system atrophy. *Neurol Sci* 22:247–251, 2001.

193. Bower JH, Maraganore DM, McDonnell SK, Rossa WA: Incidence of PSP and multiple system atrophy in Olmsted County, Minnesota, 1976 to 1990. *Neurology* 49:1284–1288, 1997.

194. Nath U, Ben-Shlomo Y, Thomson RG, et al: The prevalence of PSP (Steele-Richardson-Olszewski syndrome) in the UK. *Brain* 124:1438–1449, 2001.

195. Schrag A, Ben-Shlomo Y, Quinn N: Prevalence of PSP and MSA: A cross-sectional study. *Lancet* 354:1771–1772, 1999.

196. Rajput AH, Offord KP, Beard CM, Kurland LT: Epidemiology of parkinsonism: Incidence, classification, and mortality. *Ann Neurol* 16:278–282, 1984.

197. Kurtzke JF, Kurland LT: Neuroepidemiology: A Summation, in Kurland LT, Kurtzke JF, Goldberg ID (eds): *Epidemiology of Neurologic and Sense Organ Disorders.* Cambridge: Harvard University Press, 1973, pp 305–332.

198. Davis PH, Golbe LI, Duvoisin RC, Schoenberg BS: Risk factors for PSP. *Neurology* 38:1546–1552, 1988.

199. McCrank E: PSP risk factors. *Neurology* 40:1637, 1990.

200. McCrank E, Rabheru K: Four cases of PSP in patients exposed to organic solvents. *Can J Psychiatry* 34:934–935, 1989.

201. Vanacore N, Bonifati V, Fabbrini G, et al: Smoking habits in multiple system atrophy and PSP. *Neurology* 54:114–119, 2000.

202. Doty RL, Golbe LI, McKeown DA, et al: Olfactory testing differentiates between PSP and Parkinson's disease. *Neurology* 43:962–965, 1993.

203. Jendroska K, Hoffmann O, Schelosky L, et al: Absence of disease related prion protein in neurodegenerative disorders presenting with Parkinson's syndrome. *J Neurol Neurosurg Psychiatry* 57:1249–1251, 1994.

204. Brown P, Gibbs CJ, Rodgers-Johnson P, et al: Human spongiform encephalopathy: The National Institutes of Health series of 300 cases of experimentally transmitted disease. *Ann Neurol* 35:513–529, 1994.

205. Jankovic J, Friedman DI, Pirozzolo FJ, McCrary JA: PSP: Motor, neurobehavioral, and neuro-ophthalmic findings. *Adv Neurol* 53:293–304, 1990.

206. Jankovic J, Beach J, Schwartz K, Contant C: Tremor and longevity in relatives of patients with Parkinson's disease, essential tremor, and control subjects. *Neurology* 45:645–648, 1995.

207. Elipe JG, Sanchez Pernaute R, Sandiumenge A, de Yebenes JG: Clinical symptoms in relatives of probands with PSP. *Neurology* 46:A386–A387, 1996.

208. Golbe LI: The epidemiology of PSP. *Adv Neurol* 69:25–31, 1996.

209. Brown J, Lantos P, Stratton M, et al: Familial PSP. *J Neurol Neurosurg Psychiatry* 56:473–476, 1993.

210. Ohara S, Kondo K, Morita H, et al: PSP-like syndrome in two siblings of a consanguineous marriage. *Neurology* 42:1009–1014, 1992.

211. Golbe LI, Dickson DW: Familial autopsy-proven PSP. *Neurology* 45(suppl 4):A255, 1995.

212. Tetrud JW, Golbe LI, Farmer PM, Forno LS: Autopsy-proven PSP in two siblings. *Neurology* 46:931–934, 1996
213. Gazely S, Maguire J: Familial PSP. *Brain Pathol* 4:534, 1994.
214. García de Yébenes J, Sarasa JL, Daniel SE, Lees AJ: Autosomal dominant PSP. *Eur Neurol* (in press).
215. Uitti R, Evidente VGH, Dickson DW, Graff-Radford N: A kindred with familial PSP. *Neurology* 52:A227, 1999.
216. Rojo A, Pernaute S, Fontán A, et al: Clinical genetics of familial PSP. *Brain* 122:1233–1245, 1999.
217. Piccini P, de Yebenes, Lees AJ, et al: Familial PSP: Detection of subclinical cases using 18F-dopa and 18-fluorodeoxyglucose positron emission tomography. *Arch Neurol* 58:1846–1851, 2001.
218. Steele JC, Caparros-Lefebvre D, Lees AJ, Sacks OW: PSP and its relation to Pacific foci of the Parkinson-dementia complex and Guadeloupean parkinsonism. *Parkinsonism Rel Dis* 9:39–54, 2002.
219. Geddes JF, Hughes AJ, Lees AJ, Daniel SE: Pathological overlap in cases of parkinsonism associated with neurofibrillary tangles: A study of recent cases of postencephalitic parkinsonism and comparison with PSP and Guamanian parkinsonism-dementia complex. *Brain* 116:281–302, 1993.
220. Caparros-Lefebvre D, Elbaz A and the Caribbean Parkinsonism Study Group: Possible relation of atypical parkinsonism in the French West Indies with consumption of tropical plants: A case-control study. *Lancet* 354:281–286, 1999.
221. Lannuzel A, Michel PP, Caparros-Lefebvre D, et al: Toxicity of Annonaceae for dopaminergic neurons: Potential role in atypical parkinsonism in Guadeloupe. *Mov Disord* 17:84–90, 2002.
222. Anouti A, Schmidt K, Lyons KE, et al: Normal distribution of apolipoprotein E alleles in progressive supranuclear palsy. *Neurology* 46:1156–1157, 1996.
223. Morris HR, Schrag A, Nath U, et al. Effect of ApoE and tau on age of onset of progressive supranuclear palsy and multiple system atrophy. *Neurosci Lett* 312:118–120, 2001.
224. Schneider JA, Gearing M, Robbins RS, et al: Apolipoprotein E genotype in diverse neurodegenerative disorders. *Ann Neurol* 38:131–135, 1995.
225. Di Monte CA, Harati Y, Jankovic J, et al: Muscle mitochondrial ATP production in PSP. *J Neurochem* 62:1631–1634, 1994.
226. Cantuti-Castelvetri I, Standaert DG, Albers DS, et al: Antioxidant enzymes in the PSP brain. *Mov Disord* 15:1045, 2000.
227. Albers DS, Augood SJ, Martin DM, et al: Evidence for oxidative stress in the subthalamic nucleus in PSP. *J Neurochem* 73:881–884, 1999.
228. Odetti P, Garibaldi S, Norese R, et al: Lipoperoxidation is selectively involved in PSP. *J Neuropathol Exp Neurol* 59:393–397, 2000.
229. Swerdlow RH, Golbe LI, Parks JK, et al: Mitochondrial dysfunction in cybrid lines expressing mitochondrial genes from patients with PSP. *J Neurochem* 75:1681–1684, 2000.
230. Chirichigno J, Manfredi G, Beal M, Albers D: Stress-induced mitochondrial depolarization and oxidative damage in PSP cybrids. *Brain Res* 95:31–35, 2002.
231. Kim SY, Jeiter TM, Steinert PM: Transglutaminases in disease. *Neurochem Int* 40:85–103, 2002.
232. Dickson DW: Neurodegenerative diseases with cytoskeletal pathology: A biochemical classification. *Ann Neurol* 42:541–544, 1997.
233. Caparros-Lefebvre D, Sergeant N, Lees A, et al: Guadeloupean parkinsonism: A cluster of PSP-like tauopathy. *Brain* 125:801–811, 2002.

234. Bueé-Scherrer V, Bueé L, Hof PR, et al: Neurofibrillary degeneration in amyotrophic lateral sclerosis/parkinsonism-dementia complex of Guam. Immunochemical characterisation of tau proteins. *Am J Pathol* 146:924–932, 1995.
235. Hutton M, Lendon CL, Rizzu P, et al: Association of missense and 5′-splice-site mutation in tau with the inherited dementia FTDP-17. *Nature* 393:702–705, 1998.
236. Spillantini MG, Murrell JR, Goedert M, et al: Mutation in the tau gene in familial multiple system tauopathy with presenile dementia. *Proc Natl Acad Sci U S A* 95:7737–7741, 1998.
237. Stanford PM, Halliday GM, Brooks WS, et al: PSP pathology caused by a novel silent mutation in exon 10 of the tau gene. *Brain* 123:880–893, 2000.
238. Conrad C, Andreadis A, Trojanowski JQ, et al: Genetic evidence for the involvement of tau in PSP. *Ann Neurol* 41:277–281, 1997.
239. Molinuevo JL, Valldeoriola F, Alegret M, et al: Earlier age of onset in patients with the tau protein A0/A0 genotype. *J Neurol* 247:206–208, 2000.
240. Baker M, Litvan I, Houlden H, et al: Association of an extended haplotype in the tau gene with PSP. *Hum Mol Genet* 8:711–715, 1999.
241. Higgins JJ, Adler RL, Loveless JM: Mutational analysis of the tau gene in PSP. *Neurology* 53:1421–1424, 1999.
242. Ezquerra M, Pastor P, Valldeoriola F, et al: Identification of a novel polymorphism in the promoter region of the tau gene highly associated to PSP in humans. *Neurosci Lett* 275:183–186, 1999.
243. de Silva R, Weiler M, Morris HR, et al: Strong association of a novel tau promoter haplotype in PSP. *Neurosci Lett* 311:145–148, 2001.
244. Pastor P, Ezquerra M, Tolosa E, et al: Further extension of the H1 haplotype associated with PSP. *Mov Disord* 17:550–556, 2002.
245. Di Maria E, Tabaton M, Vigo T, et al: Corticobasal degeneration shares a common genetic background with PSP. *Ann Neurol* 47:374–377, 2000.
246. Houlden H, Baker M, Morris HR, et al: Corticobasal degeneration and PSP share a common tau haplotype. *Neurology* 56:1702–1706, 2001.
247. Golbe LI, Lazzarini AM, Spychala JR, et al: The *tau* A0 allele in Parkinson's disease. *Mov Disord* 16:442–447, 2001.
248. Morris HR, Schrag A, Nath U, et al: Effect of ApoE and tau on age of onset of PSP and multiple system atrophy. *Neurosci Lett* 312:118–120, 2001.
249. Litvan I, Baker M, Hutton M: Tau genotype: No effect on onset, symptom severity, or survival in PSP. *Neurology* 57:138–140, 2001.
250. Liu WK, Le TV, Adamson J, et al: Relationship of the extended tau haplotype to tau biochemistry and neuropathology in PSP. *Ann Neurol* 50:494–502, 2001.
251. Morris HR, Vaughan JR, Datta SR, et al: Multiple system atrophy/PSP: α-Synuclein, synphilin, tau, and APOE. *Neurology* 55:1918–1920, 2000.
252. Kompoliti K, Goetz CG, Litvan I, et al: Pharmacological therapy in PSP. *Arch Neurol* 55:1099–1102, 1998.
253. Jankovic J: PSP: Clinical and pharmacologic update. *Neurol Clin* 2:473–486, 1984.
254. Jankovic J: Controlled trial of pergolide mesylate in Parkinson's disease and PSP. *Neurology* 33:505–507, 1983.
255. Weiner WJ, Minagar A, Shulman LM: Pramipexole in PSP. *Neurology* 52:873–874, 1999.

256. Jackson JA, Jankovic J, Ford J: PSP: Clinical features and response to treatment in 16 patients. *Ann Neurol* 13:273–278, 1983.

257. Litvan I, Phipps M, Pharr VL, et al: Randomized placebo-controlled trial of donepezil in patients with PSP. *Neurology* 57:467–473, 2001.

258. Litvan I, Blesa R, Clark K, et al: Pharmacological evaluation of the cholinergic system in PSP. *Ann Neurol* 36:55–61, 1994.

259. Foster NL, Aldrich MS, Bluemlein L, et al: Failure of cholinergic agonist RS-86 to improve cognition and movement in PSP despite effects on sleep. *Neurology* 39:257–261, 1989.

260. Kato E, Takahashi S, Abe T, et al: A case of PSP showing improvement of rigidity, nuchal dystonia and autonomic failure with trazodone. *Rinsho Shinkeigaku* 34:1013–1017, 1994.

261. Newman GC: Treatment of PSP with tricyclic antidepressants. *Neurology* 35:1189–1193, 1985.

262. Gaudet RJ, Kessler II: Transparently blinded trials of methysergide. *N Engl J Med* 316:279–280, 1987.

263. Daniele A, Moro E, Bentivoglio AR: Zolpidem in PSP. *N Engl J Med* 341:543–544, 1999.

264. Lepore FE: PSP, in Tusa RJ, Newman SA (eds): *Neuro-Ophthalmological Disorders: Diagnostic Workup and Management.* New York: Marcel Dekker (in press).

265. Piccione F, Mancini E, Tonin P, Bizzarini M: Botulinum toxin treatment of apraxia of eyelid opening in PSP: Report of two cases. *Arch Phys Med Rehab* 78:525–529, 1997.

266. Polo KB, Jabbari B: Botulinum toxin-A improves the rigidity of progressive supranculear palsy. *Ann Neurol* 35:237–239, 1994.

267. Sosner J, Wall GC, Sznajder J: PSP: Clinical presentation and rehabilitation of two patients. *Arch Phys Med Rehab* 74:537–539, 1993.

268. Koller WC, Morantz R, Vetere-Overfield B, Waxman M: Autologous adrenal medullary transplant in PSP. *Neurology* 39:1066–1068, 1989.

269. Hauser RA, Trehan R: Initial experience with electroconvulsive therapy for PSP. *Mov Disord* 9:466–468, 1994.

270. Rasmussen K, Abrams R: Treatment of Parkinson's disease with electroconvulsive therapy. *Psychiatr Clin North Am* 14:925–933, 1991.

Chapter 21 _____

MULTIPLE-SYSTEM ATROPHY

LISA M. SHULMAN, ALIREZA MINAGAR, and
WILLIAM J. WEINER

HISTORICAL BACKGROUND AND NOSOLOGY   359
EPIDEMIOLOGY   360
CLINICAL DIAGNOSIS   360
    Extrapyramidal Features   361
    Autonomic Failure   362
    Cerebellar Dysfunction   363
    Pyramidal Signs   363
    Cognitive Function and Behavior   363
DIAGNOSTIC INVESTIGATIONS   363
NEUROPATHOLOGY   365
DIFFERENTIAL DIAGNOSIS   365
TREATMENT   367

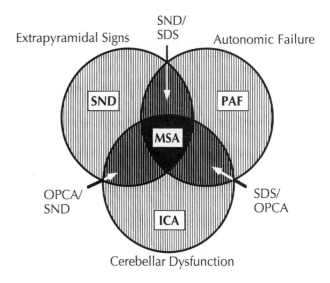

ICA: idiopathic cerebellar ataxia	PAF: pure autonomic failure
MSA: multiple-system atrophy	SDS: Shy-Drager syndrome
OPCA: olivopontocerebellar atrophy	SND: striatonigral degeneration

FIGURE 21-1 Cardinal features of MSA. Diagnostic representation of the overlapping combination of signs and symptoms in MSA.

The topic multiple-system atrophy (MSA) alerts the reader that a description of a subset of neurodegenerative disorders characterized by predominant involvement of the extrapyramidal, cerebellar, and autonomic pathways (Fig. 21-1) follows. The uninitiated may be understandably misled by the broad inference of the term MSA. We later describe the historical derivation of this appellation, although perhaps we should not dismiss the impulse to reexamine the congruity of this diagnostic subset with the range of patients seen in the clinical setting. The sharp distinction of MSA from the other neurodegenerative processes, as depicted in discrete chapters of this book, belies the challenge facing the clinician when diagnosing the individual patient. Despite the prodigious advances in medicine, MSA and the neurodegenerative disorders as a group remain clinical diagnoses, and the heterogeneity of our patients defies simple classification.

Historical Background and Nosology

The conceptualization of the diagnosis MSA emerged from a series of publications that each described fragments of a larger picture. Dejerine and Thomas[1] first coined the term olivopontocerebellar atrophy (OPCA) in 1900 to describe two sporadic cases of progressive cerebellar degeneration with parkinsonism. Sixty years later, Shy and Drager[2] published the first clinicopathological study of a patient with idiopathic orthostatic hypotension. They recognized the association of orthostatic hypotension with a primary

degenerative disorder of the nervous system involving the intermediolateral cell column of the spinal cord, medulla, pons, midbrain, cerebellum, and basal ganglia. The full clinical syndrome comprised "orthostatic hypotension, urinary and rectal incontinence, loss of sweating, iris atrophy, external ocular palsies, rigidity, tremor, loss of associated movement, impotence, the findings of an atonic bladder and loss of the rectal sphincter tone, fasciculations, wasting of distal muscles, and evidence of a neuropathic lesion."[2]

Also in 1960, van der Eecken et al.[3] described a unique pathological subgroup among a large number of patients with paralysis agitans. Striatopallidonigral degeneration was identified with "virtual disappearance of the small cells of the caudate nucleus and putamen" in a few patients with extrapyramidal rigidity but minimal tremor. The full clinicopathological study was published the following year.[4] In addition to parkinsonism, the diagnostic signs of brisk reflexes, extensor plantar responses, ataxia, dysarthria, syncope, incontinence, and impotence were described among the three patients reported. Neurodegeneration was also identified in the cerebellum, olivary nuclei, and pons.

The conceptual threads of the three disorders, OPCA, Shy-Drager syndrome (SDS), and striatonigral degeneration (SND), were tied together in a seminal paper by Graham and Oppenheimer[5] in 1969:

> What is needed is a general term to cover this collection of overlapping progressive presenile multisystem degenerations. As the causes of this group of conditions are still unknown,

such a general term would merely be a temporary practical convenience... What we wish to avoid is the multiplication of names for 'disease entities' which in fact are merely the expressions of neuronal atrophy in a variety of overlapping combinations. We therefore propose to use the term multiple system atrophy to cover the whole group.

Graham and Oppenheimer also identified two subgroups of patients with idiopathic orthostatic hypotension: those with Lewy body pathology and those without. This latter group comprised the patients with MSA. Bannister and Oppenheimer[6] again highlighted this distinction in their clinicopathological review of 16 patients in 1972. Although parkinsonian features and lesions of the pigmented nuclei were common to both groups, MSA was distinguished by an earlier mean age of onset than idiopathic paralysis agitans (49 years, as compared to 65), and a worsened prognosis.

Although the existence of MSA as a unique pathological disorder remains unproven, we believe that the term retains clinical usefulness. The usage of the terms SND, OPCA, or SDS confers additional information about the predominant clinical presentation. Nevertheless, the close relationship between these three subgroups is implicit. Although either parkinsonism, autonomic failure, or cerebellar dysfunction may mark the beginning of the disease, the emergence of the other two syndromes can be predicted when the patient survives long enough.

Familial associations of SND or SDS are rarely observed; however, OPCA is distinguished in this regard. Although nonfamilial idiopathic cerebellar degeneration is more common, much of the medical literature regarding OPCA has focused on the hereditary, autosomal-dominant cerebellar ataxias (see Chap. 45). In fact, familial cerebellar ataxia was initially described by Menzel[7] in 1891, before the introduction of the term OPCA by Dejerine and Thomas. Greenfield[8] initially subdivided OPCA into the familial Menzel-type and the sporadic Dejerine and Thomas-type. It is unclear whether or not both types are properly classified as MSA. Penney pointed out that there is a growing body of evidence from positron emission tomography (PET) studies and pathology to indicate that sporadic OPCA of the Dejerine and Thomas-type is MSA and is distinct from the dominantly inherited cerebellar degenerations.[9] In a further comparison of the clinical features of sporadic and familial OPCA by Harding,[10] retinal degeneration was confined to the familial cases. Also, both optic atrophy and ophthalmoplegia occurred with far greater frequency in the familial cases. Patients with familial history developed their initial symptoms at a younger age.

We use the term MSA to refer to a gradually progressive, idiopathic neurodegenerative process of adult onset characterized by varying proportions of cerebellar dysfunction, autonomic failure, and parkinsonism that is poorly responsive to L-dopa therapy. The clinical syndrome is dominated but not confined to these features. Familial presentations will heretofore be excluded from the discussion (see Chap. 45). It is understood that these lines are currently drawn more to conform with precedent and practicality than to reflect genuine and fundamental attributes of pathophysiology.

Epidemiology

MSA affects both sexes equally. The exact prevalence of MSA due to limited epidemiologic data is unknown. However, one cross-sectional study in a primary care service reported a prevalence of 4.4 per 100,000 in the UK.[11] Vanacore et al.[12] reported the annual incidence of new cases as about 0.6 per 100,000 population. Ben-Shlomo et al., in a meta-analysis of published cases of pathologically proven MSA, calculated a mean age at onset of 54.2 years and a median survival of 6.2 years.[13] MSA usually begins in middle age and advances over a period of 1–18 years.[14,15]

Clinical Diagnosis

The initial evaluation of a patient with MSA is simply a "snapshot" of the evolving neurodegenerative process. Although the initial presentation may suggest the diagnosis, often the full picture will remain obscured for some time. In fact, the akinetic-rigid patient who is poorly responsive to L-dopa therapy has a broad differential diagnosis. The impression will be later refined by the emerging signs: a vertical supranuclear ophthalmoparesis suggests progressive supranuclear palsy, whereas prominent orthostatic hypotension suggests MSA. Ironically, an initial evaluation of a patient with an advanced neurodegenerative disorder may also be difficult to sort out, particularly when historical data regarding the order and time frame of the symptoms are lacking. For example, cerebellar signs may be difficult to appreciate in the wheelchair-bound patient with profound rigidity and bradykinesia. Therefore, diagnostic accuracy requires either long-term follow-up of the individual patient or the good fortune to be confronted by the patient when all the diagnostic pieces of the puzzle are in place. Even then, confidence in our diagnostic impression is tempered by the inability to confirm our clinical intuition.

Although MSA patients can manifest any combination of extrapyramidal, autonomic, and cerebellar features, extrapyramidal signs are the most common. Quinn[16] reported that parkinsonism was present in 89 percent of MSA case reports at some point in the course of their illness. Autonomic failure occurred in 78 percent and cerebellar signs in 55 percent. Pyramidal involvement is also very common, occurring in 61 percent. Twenty-eight percent of MSA patients developed the full clinical spectrum (i.e., parkinsonism, autonomic failure, cerebellar signs, pyramidal signs) before death.

Quinn[17] proposed a set of clinical diagnostic criteria for MSA. Definite MSA is restricted to patients with postmortem pathological confirmation. A possible diagnosis may be conferred in patients with either parkinsonism with poor L-dopa responsiveness or cerebellar parkinsonism. Lastly, a probable diagnosis of MSA applies to patients presenting with the many possible permutations of the designated clinical syndromes (i.e., extrapyramidal, pyramidal, cerebellar, and autonomic). Exclusionary criteria include age less than 30 years, a family history, or the presence of another identifiable cause.

A consensus conference on diagnosis of MSA was convened in 1998 and a statement on the diagnosis of MSA was published.[18] The guidelines for inclusion and exclusion criteria for MSA are presented in Tables 21-1–21-3. Application of either Quinn or consensus criteria is far superior to actual clinical diagnosis made early in the disease.[19]

TABLE 21-1 Clinical Domains, Features, and Criteria Used in the Diagnosis of MSA

I. Autonomatic and urinary dysfunction
  (A) Autonomic and urinary features
    1. Orthostatic hypotension (by 20 mmHg systolic or 10 mmHg diastolic)
    2. Urinary incontinence or incomplete bladder emptying
  (B) Criterion for autonomic failure or urinary dysfunction in MSA Orthostatic fall in blood pressure (by 30 mmHg systolic or 15 mmHg diastolic) or urinary incontinence (persistent, involuntary partial or total bladder emptying, accompanied by erectile dysfunction in men) or both
II. Parkinsonism
  (A) Parkinsonian features
    1. Bradykinesia (slowness of voluntary movement progressive reduction in speed and amplitude during repetitive actions)
    2. Rigidity
    3. Postural instability (not caused by primary visual, vestibular, cerebellar, or proprioceptive dysfunction)
    4. Tremor (postural, resting, or both)
  (B) Criterion for parkinsonism in MSA Bradykinesia plus at least one of items 2–4
III. Cerebellar dysfunction
  (A) Cerebellar features
    1. Gait ataxia (wide-based stance with steps of irregular length and direction)
    2. Ataxic dysarthria
    3. Limb ataxia
    4. Sustained gaze-evoked nystagmus
  (B) Criterion for cerebellar dysfunction in MSA Gait ataxia plus at least one of parkinsonism items 2–4
IV. Corticospinal tract dysfunction
  (A) Corticospinal tract features
    1. Extensor plantar responses with hyperreflexia
  (B) Corticospinal tract dysfunction in MSA: no corticospinal tract features are used in defining the diagnosis of MSA

Feature (A) is a characteristic of the disease and a criterion; Feature (B) is a defining feature or composite of features required for diagnosis.
Source: Gilman S, Low P, Quinn N, et al: Consensus statement on the diagnosis of multiple system atrophy. American Autonomic Society and American Academy of Neurology. *Clin Auton Res* 8:359–362, 1998. *Used with permission.*

EXTRAPYRAMIDAL FEATURES

Progressive akinesia, rigidity, and postural instability are common features of MSA. Tremor may occur, although it is less frequent than in idiopathic Parkinson's disease (PD). Bilateral onset of symptoms favors MSA over PD, although unilateral presentations do occur.[20] Diminished facial expressivity, micrographia, and a narrowly based shuffling gait with flexion posture appear. The primary distinguishing factors between PD and MSA presenting with isolated extrapyramidal signs are early postural instability, rapid progression, and a poor or atypical response to dopaminergic therapy.[21]

TABLE 21-2 Diagnostic Categories of MSA

I. Possible MSA: one criterion plus two features from separate domains. When the criterion is parkinsonism, a poor L-dopa response qualifies as one feature (hence only one additional feature is required)
II. Probable MSA: criterion for autonomic failure/urinary dysfunction plus poor L-dopa-responsive parkinsonism or cerebellar dysfunction
III. Definite MSA: pathologically confirmed by the presence of a high density of glial cytoplasmic inclusions in association with a combination of degenerative changes in the nigrostriatal and olivopontocerebellar pathways

The features and criteria for each clinical domain are shown in the diagnosis, but are less important than abnormalities.
Source: Gilman S, Low P, Quinn N, et al: Consensus statement on the diagnosis of multiple system atrophy. American Autonomic Society and American Academy of Neurology. *Clin Auton Res* 8:359–362, 1998. *Used with permission.*

TABLE 21-3 Exclusion Criteria for the Diagnosis of MSA

I. History
  Symptomatic onset under 30 years of age
  Family history of a similar disorder
  Systemic diseases or other identifiable causes for features listed in Table 21-1
  Hallucinations unrelated to medication
II. Physical examination
  DSM criteria for dementia
  Prominent slowing of vertical saccades or vertical supranuclear gaze palsy
  Evidence of focal cortical dysfunction such as aphasia, alien hand syndrome, and parietal dysfunction
III. Laboratory investigation
  Metabolic, molecular genetic, and imaging evidence of an alternative cause of features listed in Table 21-1

In practice, MSA is most frequently confused with PD or progressive supranuclear palsy (PSP). Mild limitation of upward gaze alone is nonspecific, whereas a prominent (>50 percent) limitation of upward gaze or any limitation of downward gaze suggests PSP. Before the onset of vertical gaze limitation, a clinically obvious slowing of voluntary vertical saccades is usually easily detectable in PSP and assists in the easy differentiation of these two disorders.
Source: Gilman S, Low P, Quinn N, et al: Consensus statement on the diagnosis of multiple system atrophy. American Autonomic Society and American Academy of Neurology. *Clin Auton Res* 8:359–362, 1998. *Used with permission.*

An adequate trial of L-dopa assumes a central role in identifying patients with MSA, although one can be misled. One-third of early MSA patients reported by Rajput et al.[22] experienced a moderate-to-marked improvement with L-dopa therapy, and Quinn[16] similarly observed a moderate-to-good response in one-third. Hughes et al.[23] reported that 65 percent of pathologically confirmed MSA patients had an initial response to L-dopa, and 35 percent remained partially responsive until death. The benefits are generally less impressive than that observed in PD and tend to decline over 1–2 years of treatment. L-Dopa-induced dyskinesias occur in MSA. They may appear unusually early and with an atypical predilection for the face and neck. Dyskinesias may be observed without concomitant symptomatic improvement. It is uncommon to obtain symptomatic relief from other antiparkinsonian agents in the absence of a response to L-dopa. Although the benefits are less gratifying than in PD, this should not discourage the clinician from attempting an adequate trial of high-dose L-dopa (1500 mg/day) in MSA patients with parkinsonism. We also try to treat these patients with dopamine agonists (e.g., bromocriptine, pergolide, pramipexole, or ropinirole).

AUTONOMIC FAILURE

Practically all patients with MSA develop some degree of clinically apparent autonomic failure. For example, postural hypotension ranging from mild postural dizziness to frequent black-outs, manifests in 88 percent of patients.[2,24,25] From the perspective of a neurological clinic, where the neurological history and examination are more intensive than the autonomic evaluation, the prevalence, severity, and time frame of the dysautonomia is often underestimated. Although orthostasis and genitourinary difficulties are most likely to be brought to the attention of the physician, problems of thermoregulation and gastrointestinal and respiratory function are not uncommon.

Autonomic dysfunction may also occur in idiopathic PD and, therefore, this array of symptoms and signs in a patient with an akinetic-rigid syndrome does not immediately imply a diagnosis of MSA. Magalhaes et al.,[24] in a retrospective review of autonomic dysfunction in pathologically confirmed cases of MSA and PD, identified certain distinctions regarding prevalence and severity that may prove useful in differentiating MSA and PD when autonomic signs and symptoms are present. All patients with MSA had some autonomic involvement, whereas 24 percent of PD had none. Autonomic dysfunction in MSA involved more autonomic functions and was more severe than that seen in PD, particularly with regard to inspiratory stridor. Although this investigation concluded that autonomic disturbance alone does not distinguish among MSA and PD in individual patients, the presence of severe autonomic dysfunction, autonomic dysfunction that precedes parkinsonism, or inspiratory stridor are all suggestive of MSA.

On initial evaluation of the patient with autonomic signs, the distinction between the primary autonomic failure of MSA and secondary autonomic dysfunction should be considered. Common medical disorders, including diabetes mellitus, autoimmune disease, neoplasia, and renal failure, may give rise to autonomic dysfunction. A variety of medications, including antihypertensives, cardiovascular agents, diuretics, tricyclic antidepressants, and antiparkinsonian drugs, may contribute to postural hypotension.

Orthostatic hypotension (OH) is the most commonly recognized symptom of autonomic dysfunction and develops in nearly all patients with autonomic failure. OH is generally defined as a fall of more than 20 mmHg systolic blood pressure when the patient stands from a seated position. Not infrequently, significant orthostasis is documented in asymptomatic patients, as gradually progressive and chronic autonomic failure promotes compensatory adjustments of cerebral autoregulation. The symptoms related to postural hypotension are variable, ranging from vague descriptions of lethargy or weakness to full syncope. Other complaints include dizziness, visual disturbances, and craniocervical discomfort, although patients rarely relate their symptoms to changes of position without direct questioning.

Postural hypotension is exacerbated after prolonged recumbency, mealtime, and physical exertion. Other contributory factors are heat, alcohol, coughing, and defecation.[26,27] Management of OH involves a number of prophylactic measures. As nocturnal diuresis in the elderly contributes to inadequate blood volume and OH upon arising, recommendations are designed to improve intravascular volume and diminish peripheral edema. Liberalizing salt and water intake, the application of elastic stockings before arising, elevation of the legs periodically during the day, and elevation of the head at night may be helpful (Table 21-1). Physical exertion should be delayed until the afternoon and should not closely follow mealtime. Pharmacotherapy of OH may include the use of fludrocortisone, midodrine, recombinant human erythropoietin, phenylpropanolamine, indomethacin, dihydroxyphenylserine, caffeine, and ergots.[28]

Genitourinary dysfunction in MSA is very common. Beck et al.[29] studied neurourological features of 62 patients clinically diagnosed with MSA. All patients had abnormal urethral or anal sphincter electromyograms, a finding the authors considered diagnostic in the appropriate clinical setting. Impotence was the presenting symptom in 37 percent of men and occurred in 96 percent with progression of the illness. Frequent spontaneous penile erections may antedate erectile failure. The absence of penile erection upon awakening in the morning favors a neurogenic rather than a functional etiology for impotence. Urinary symptoms resulted from a combination of detrusor hyperreflexia, urethral sphincter weakness and, finally, failure of detrusor contraction. The urinary symptoms simulated outflow obstruction in men, and 43 percent underwent prostatic or bladder neck surgery. Fifty-seven percent of the women had stress incontinence, and one-half had undergone surgical bladder repair.

The results of operative procedures in both sexes were poor. Nonsurgical treatment with intermittent catheterization, anticholinergic medication, and desmopressin spray improved continence in over one-half of the patients. Anticholinergic medication may result in urinary retention, and intermittent catheterization may result in recurrent infection.

Sakakibara et al. also studied micturitional disturbance in 86 patients with clinically diagnosed MSA.[30] The authors subdivided their MSA patients into those with SDS, SND, and OPCA to further classify urinary dysfunction. Micturitional symptoms were found in more than 90 percent of patients, regardless of MSA subdivision. Urinary symptoms appeared earlier and were more severe in SDS than in SND or OPCA. Urinary symptoms progressed with disease progression.

Constipation is the most common gastrointestinal symptom and affects 57 percent of patients.[31] Straining during evacuation or micturition elevates intrathoracic pressure and may result in symptomatic hypotension. Daily use of dietary fiber, adequate liquid intake, and laxatives is helpful. Fecal incontinence occasionally occurs, although it is less common than urinary incontinence. Dysphagia is not uncommon in more advanced stages of the disorder. Laryngeal stridor is another serious manifestation of MSA, which may be due to the loss of motor neurons of the nucleus ambiguus innervating the laryngeal abductor muscles.[32] However, a recent study of the number of cholinergic neurons in the nucleus ambiguus of patients with MSA and PD failed to confirm neuronal loss as the sole cause of stridor in patients with MSA.[33] Bilateral abductor vocal fold paresis, a life-threatening condition, has also been reported in patients with MSA.[34] The advisability of either gastrostomy or tracheostomy should be approached on an individual basis with a realistic appraisal of the patient's general quality of life.

There is often a mild, normocytic-normochromic anemia that may be caused by loss of sympathetic stimulation of renal erythropoietin production.[35]

CEREBELLAR DYSFUNCTION

Whereas the majority of MSA patients present with bradykinetic parkinsonian signs, in others a cerebellar syndrome heralds the development of multisystem involvement. The initial manifestation is frequently gait ataxia with eventual involvement of the upper limbs.[36] Dysarthria is nearly universal, although its nature may vary. Speech may be scanning, bulbar, pseudobulbar, monotone, slow, or hypophonic. Kinetic tremor with dysmetria may occur. Other cerebellar features include hypotonia and exaggerated rebound with loss of checking response. Myoclonus is less common. Ocular motor signs frequently emerge, although they are more common in the familial form of OPCA than in the sporadic form. Supranuclear ophthalmoplegia occurs primarily in familial OPCA[36] or, of course, progressive supranuclear palsy (PSP), whereas nystagmus, jerky pursuit, ocular dysmetria, fixation instability, and slowing of saccades are common in MSA patients.[37] Mild limitations of gaze are also common.

However, Quinn believes that a prominent downgaze palsy is an exclusion criterion for a clinical diagnosis of MSA.[16]

Therapeutics for cerebellar signs remains a disappointing and frustrating area for the clinician. When tremor or myoclonus are prominent, trials of clonazepam or valproate may prove worthwhile. Patients with isolated cerebellar dysfunction are frequently diagnosed with cerebellar degeneration. The later emergence of autonomic, extrapyramidal, and pyramidal signs is often overlooked for some time, delaying both appropriate diagnosis as well as therapeutic opportunities for parkinsonian or autonomic symptoms. A clinicopathological study of 35 patients with MSA revealed that 88 percent had evidence of OPCA, with the cerebellar vermis usually more involved than the cerebellar hemispheres. Surprisingly, the presence of cerebellar pathology was unrelated to the presence of cerebellar signs in life.[38]

PYRAMIDAL SIGNS

Exaggerated deep tendon reflexes, extensor plantar responses, pseudobulbar palsy, and spasticity are present in the majority of MSA patients, often early in the disorder. The presence of prominent extrapyramidal rigidity and bradykinesia often masks both pyramidal spasticity and cerebellar incoordination.

COGNITIVE FUNCTION AND BEHAVIOR

Although progressive dementia is not a feature of MSA, cognitive deficits and alterations of personality and mood are common. When the cognitive performance of 16 patients with probable MSA of the striatonigral type (mean Hoehn and Yahr stage 3.7) was studied and compared to that of normal controls, the MSA group showed significant deficits on tests of frontal lobe function.[39] Specifically, attentional set shifting and speed of thinking were impaired, although there was no consistent evidence of intellectual deterioration, as measured by the Wechsler Adult Intelligence Scale. Cognitive deficits were not correlated with either the duration or severity of disease. The pattern of deficits was distinctive, markedly in contrast to Alzheimer's dementia, less in contrast to PD. Personality alterations include apathy, passivity, emotional lability, and depression. This confluence of impaired executive functions, apathy, and impulsivity is characteristic of frontal subcortical circuit dysfunction.[40] Treatment of associated psychotic disturbances is often complicated and unsuccessful. A single patient with OPCA and neuroleptic-resistant depression was treated successfully with clozapine without compromise of neurological function.[41]

Diagnostic Investigations

Neuroradiological evaluation is routinely performed in the investigation of a patient with progressive neurological deficits. Cranial computed tomography (CT) may reveal

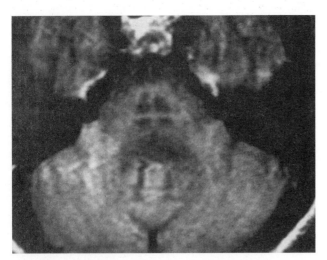

FIGURE 21-2 MRI proton density image demonstrating increased signal in the brainstem involving the midline raphe and transverse pontine fibers and sparing the tegmentum, pyramidal tracts, and superior cerebellar peduncles. (*Courtesy of Dr. Brian Bowen.*)

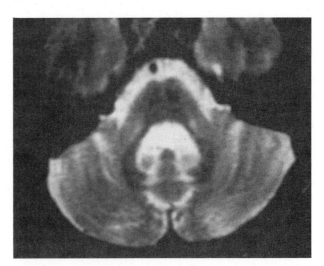

FIGURE 21-3 OPCA. Increased signal on MRI in the middle cerebellar peduncles. (*Courtesy of Dr. Brian Bowen.*)

infratentorial atrophy. When CT images of 33 MSA patients and 40 age-matched controls were blindly analyzed by neuroradiologists, atrophy of the cerebellar hemispheres, vermis, pons, midbrain, and cerebral hemispheres, as well as enlargement of the basilar cisterns and fourth ventricle, were differentially discriminated between the two groups.[42] However, in no case did CT imaging confirm cerebellar or brainstem involvement that was not clinically evident. Wenning et al.[42] concluded that CT is of limited diagnostic use in MSA.

Magnetic resonance imaging (MRI) of the brain can differentiate MSA from multi-infarct conditions or normal pressure hydrocephalus as a cause of dopa-unresponsive parkinsonism. MRI also shows cerebellar and brainstem atrophy in patients with MSA, olivopontocerebellar atrophy type.

In more than half of patients with MSA and in a higher proportion of patients with SND, iron deposition manifesting as hypointense signals on T_2-weighted images as well as gliosis presenting as slit-like hyperintense signals on T_2-weighted images at the posterolateral border of the putamen occur.[43,44] However, the diagnostic significance of these findings has not been established, but may be sensitive and specific findings in patients who are already clinically diagnosed.[11,45] Infratentorial atrophy may be seen more readily with MRI than with CT and may assist in differentiating idiopathic PD from MSA/OPCA before the full clinical picture is apparent (Figs. 21-2–21-5).

PET studies have been performed with ^{18}F-6-fluorodopa (FD), ^{11}C-raclopride (RAC), and ^{11}C-diprenorphine in order to examine both the pre- and postsynaptic segments of the

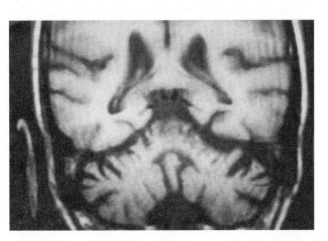

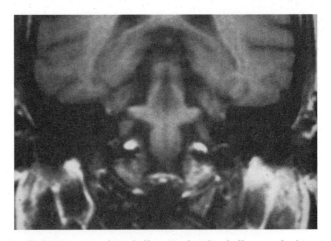

FIGURES 21-4 and 21-5 OPCA. MRI T_1-weighted coronal images showing the brainstem and cerebellar atrophy. Cerebellar atrophy is often worse for the hemispheres than the vermis. Atrophy of the middle cerebellar peduncles results in a "cross" or "t" appearance on the coronal image. (*Courtesy of Dr. Brian Bowen.*)

dopaminergic pathway. Reduced putaminal uptake of FD has been reported in MSA, as well as reduced striatal binding of diprenorphine and RAC.[46–48] Abnormalities of striatal glucose metabolism have also been demonstrated with ^{18}F-fluorodeoxyglucose PET studies.[49–51] These results suggest that selective metabolic reduction in the putamen and cerebellum may be a marker for MSA. In addition, PET studies have contributed to the evidence that sporadic OPCA is MSA, whereas dominantly inherited OPCA is a separate entity. ^{123}I-Iodobenzamide single-photon emission computed tomography scanning may be useful in assessing the integrity of striatal dopamine receptors in early parkinsonians.[52] Proton magnetic resonance spectroscopy (MRS) has been reported to differentiate MSA from PD.[43–54] In patients with the SND form of MSA the N-acetylaspartate/creatine ratio and the choline/creatine ratio were significantly reduced in the putamen and globus pallidus, compared to the preserved ratio in patients with PD. OPCA patients showed a significant but less marked reduction in these ratios. The reduced ratio probably reflects neuronal loss occurring predominantly in the putamen. It is suggested that proton MRS may prove to be a useful noninvasive technique to diagnose MSA. However, whether or not this technique can differentiate MSA from PSP or other akinetic-rigid syndromes is unknown. Experience is currently insufficient to state whether any of these studies will reliably distinguish MSA from the spectrum of neurological disorders. Recently, brain parenchyma sonography (BPS) has been used to differentiate idiopathic PD from atypical parkinsonian syndromes including MSA. BPS is a novel and noninvasive method that may differentiate between idiopathic PD and atypical parkinsonism.[53]

Nerve conduction and electromyographic (EMG) studies may reveal subclinical polyneuropathy in MSA. EMG of external urethral sphincter demonstrates denervation in almost all patients with MSA.[54] However, the capability of this test to differentiate patients with MSA from those with PD has been challenged.[55] Electroencephalographic studies are normal in MSA, and evoked responses yield widely varying results.

Although autonomic failure is commonly diagnosed in the setting of the appropriate history and the demonstration of a significant drop in blood pressure upon arising, there are a number of sophisticated investigations of autonomic function available.[27] Postural hypotension is best evaluated with the use of a tilt table. Plasma norepinephrine responses to postural change may provide a quantitative biochemical assessment of the sympathetic nervous system. In individual patients, barium swallowing studies for dysphagia, urodynamic studies for urinary difficulties, and laryngoscopy or sleep studies for respiratory stridor may be useful for both diagnosis and management.

In summary, although diagnostic investigations are routinely pursued, their major contribution is in the exclusion of diagnoses that are more amenable to therapy than MSA. The accumulated data may add to the clinical impression; however, no diagnostic study can reliably distinguish the autonomic failure, electrophysiology, or neuroradiology of MSA from the other possible etiologies in this setting.

Neuropathology

Postmortem brains of MSA patients demonstrate selective neuronal loss and gliosis in an assortment of the following regions: striatum, substantia nigra, locus ceruleus, Edinger-Westphal nucleus, dorsal motor nucleus of the vagus, middle cerebellar peduncles, cerebellar Purkinje cells, inferior olives, intermediolateral cell columns, and Onuf's nucleus (Figs. 21-6–21-8).[16,56] Characteristic neuropathological features of MSA include glial cytoplasmic inclusions (GCIs), neuronal cytoplasmic inclusions, neuronal nuclear inclusions, glial nuclear inclusions, and neuropil threads. However, the clinicopathological correlation of MSA is not high, particularly in the early stages of the disorder. GCIs (also known as Papp-Lantos inclusions) are the most significant neuropathological feature of MSA[57,58] (Fig. 21-9). GCIs surround the nuclei of oligodendroglia with a crescent- or flame-shaped morphology. They are found in large numbers in many regions of the central nervous system, with a particular predilection for the white matter tracts. The mechanism(s) of cell loss in MSA remains unknown; however, the oligodendroglia GCIs stain heavily for alpha-synuclein.[59–61] The GCIs also demonstrate variable immunoreactivity for tau protein,[62] ubiquitin, tubulin, microtubule-binding protein, and alphaB-crystallin. Ultrastructural examination of GCIs has shown inclusions composed of randomly arranged tubules or filaments with a diameter alternating with a diameter of 20–40 nm associated with granular material.[58] Another more recent study using sarcosyl-extracted material, showed two forms of filaments: twisted and straight filaments.[63] Neuronal cytoplasmic inclusions may be located in neurons of pontine nuclei, putamen, subthalamic nucleus, arcuate nucleus, subiculum, amygdala, inferior olivary nucleus, and the reticular formation of brainstem. These neuronal inclusions are argentophilic and show immunoreactivity with anti-alpha-synuclein. Argentophilic inclusions are both alpha-synuclein- and ubiquitin-positive, and may be observed in both neuronal and glial nuclei.

Differential Diagnosis

The most instrumental tool currently available to the clinician to make the diagnosis of MSA is the passage of time. Indeed, we all have congratulated ourselves for diagnosing MSA in patients with previous misdiagnoses of idiopathic PD or cerebellar ataxia, when we simply have been the beneficiary of information unavailable to our predecessors. There is considerable similarity between the neurological signs

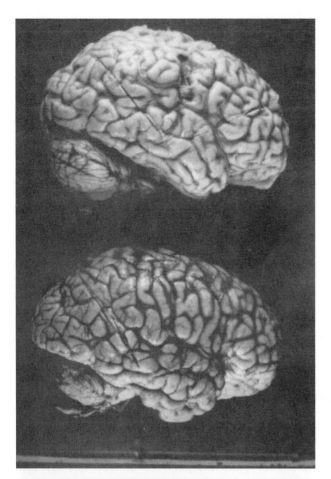

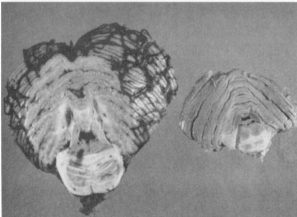

FIGURE 21-6 *Top:* OPCA *below* with the control brain *above.* *(Courtesy of Dr. Michael Norenberg.) Bottom:* OPCA on *right,* control on *left.* *(Courtesy of Dr. Michael Norenberg.)*

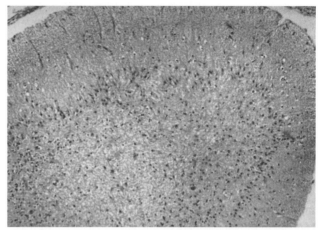

FIGURE 21-7 OPCA with loss of Purkinje and granule cells associated with Bergmann gliosis. *(Courtesy of Dr. Michael Norenberg.)*

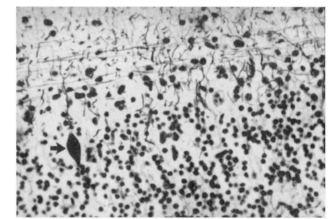

FIGURE 21-8 OPCA. Biotin stain showing loss of Purkinje cells. A torpedo is indicated by the arrow. *(Courtesy of Dr. Michael Norenberg.)*

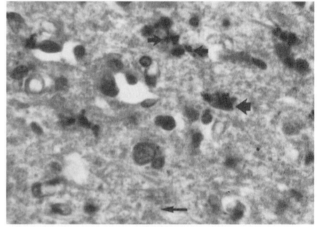

FIGURE 21-9 The arrows indicate pigmented inclusions in glial cells within the striatum in a patient with nigrostriatal degeneration. Hematoxylin-eosin stain. *(Courtesy of Dr. Michael Norenberg.)*

TABLE 21-4 Neurological Signs in the Neurodegenerative Disorders

	MSA			PSP	PD	DLBD	CBD	AD
	SND	SDS	OPCA					
Parkinsonism	++++	+++	++	++++	++++	++++	++++	++
Cerebellar signs	++	+	++++	+	0	0	+	+
Autonomic failure	++	++++	++	+	++	++	+	+
Pyramidal signs	++	+	++	++	0	+	++	++++
Cognitive dysfunction	++	+	++	+++	++	++++	++	++++
Oculomotor impairment	+	+	+++	++++	++	++	++	+
Dysarthria	+++	+	+++	+++	++	++	+++	++
Dysphagia	++	+	++	+++	++	++	+	++
Peripheral neuropathy	+	+	++	+	0	0	++	+
Involuntary movements	+	+	++	+	+++	+++	++	+

0, none; +, uncommon or unusual; ++, common or moderate; +++, frequent or marked; ++++, present in nearly all cases or severe. DLBD, diffuse Lewy body disease; CBD, corticobasal degeneration; AD, Alzheimer's disease.

that appear in the various neurodegenerative disorders (Table 21-4). The particular vulnerability of the substantia nigra and striatum to neuronal injury is borne out by the presence of moderate-to-severe parkinsonism in the full range of disorders. Autonomic failure, cognitive dysfunction, oculomotor impairment, dysarthria, dysphagia, and involuntary movements are also pervasive. The clinical impression is formed by the relative proportions of a similar array of neurological signs, tempered by knowledge of the natural history of the individual disorders. Nonetheless, the astute clinician can be sensitized to clues or idiosyncrasies that suggest the presence of one disorder over another.

MSA is most commonly confused with PD, although PSP often bears the greatest similarity (see Chaps. 15 and 21). Corticobasal degeneration (CBD) also deserves consideration in the differential diagnosis of atypical parkinsonism, especially in the early years before the fully developed clinical picture emerges (see Chap. 46). In a prospective clinical pathological study of diagnostic accuracy in parkinsonism, the initial diagnosis of idiopathic PD was correct in 65 percent of cases, and improved to 76 percent with follow-up.[22] The diagnostic accuracy for MSA with at least 5 years of follow-up was 69 percent. SND and SND/SDS were misdiagnosed as idiopathic PD in 31 percent, whereas OPCA was accurately identified in this study.

The major clinical features that raises suspicion about a diagnosis of idiopathic PD are: a poor response to L-dopa; the presence of pyramidal, cerebellar, or autonomic signs; early postural instability; and rapid clinical deterioration. Questions are also raised by the absence of rest tremor, the presence of a symmetrical onset of signs, a severe dysarthria, disproportionate antecollis, and respiratory stridor. PSP is most frequently distinguished from MSA by the appearance of a prominent supranuclear vertical ophthalmoparesis with associated visual impairment (see Chap. 21). Hyperextension of the head or unusually erect posture, lid retraction associated with a surprised facial expression, disproportionate nuchal and axial rigidity, and apraxia of eyelid opening also

suggest the presence of PSP. CBD is most frequently distinguished from MSA by the presence of early signs of cortical dysfunction (especially apraxia, and cortical sensory loss), prominent myoclonus, and asymmetric perirolandic frontoparietal cortical atrophy on CT or MRI (see Chap. 46). Vascular parkinsonism may be confused with MSA; however, a good history, the association of hypertension or other stroke risk factors, and modern neuroimaging help the clinician distinguish between them (see Chap. 26).

Our current knowledge of MSA and other neurodegenerative disorders that have similar presentations is fragmentary, and the conundrum of where to draw the lines that define and compartmentalize "unique" disorders remains an ongoing challenge. Clinical description, diagnostic investigations, and neuropathology are insufficient. Advances in cellular biochemistry and molecular biology will ultimately identify the fundamental distinguishing attributes of these disorders.

Treatment

There is great variability of therapeutic results from L-dopa in patients win MSA. L-Dopa may improve rigidity, bradykinesia, and postural instability in possible and probable MSA patients.[64,65] L-Dopa therapy can be started with (carbidopa/L-dopa 25/100 0.5–1 tablet twice daily). The dosage can then be increased until patients show toxicity or response. Compared with patients with PD, MSA patients may need far larger doses of L-dopa.

Dopamine agonists have been used in treatment of MSA with variable results. Generally, these agents are not as effective of L-dopa. Bromocriptine (10–80 mg daily) and lisuride (up to 2.4 mg daily) have been used. No formal efficacy trials of pramipexole or ropinirole are available. Hallucinations caused by use of dopamine agonists in this situation usually resolve in response to clozapine 6.25–50 mg or quetiapine 25–75 mg at bedtime.

Apomorphine, a powerful dopamine agonist, has been used in a clinical trial involving 28 patients with MSA. This trial demonstrated that apomorphine had some positive effects on these patients with an average improvement in motor scores of 11.9, 14.3, and 13.3 percent at doses of 1.5, 3, and 4.5 mg daily.[66]

Symptomatic orthostatic hypotension can be managed with sodium and volume replacement, unless there are contraindications such as congestive heart failure or renal failure. The mineralocorticoid fludrocortisone may be initiated at 0.1 mg daily and escalated to a maximum of four tablets per day in two divided doses, given with fluid replacement. Midodrine, an alpha-adrenergic agonist, is a suitable alternative. Treatment starts with 2.5 mg three times a day, increasing to 10 mg three times a day.

In patients with MSA, urinary symptoms such as frequency or incontinence may result from a combination of detrusor hyperreflexia and urethral sphincter weakness. Urinary frequency may be managed with anticholinergic agents such as oxybutynin 5–10 mg or tolterodine 2 mg at bedtime or propantheline 15–30 mg at bedtime. Recently, sildenafil citrate has been used for treatment of erectile dysfunction in patients with MSA. Despite its efficacy, sildenafil often worsens the orthostatic hypotension.[67]

References

1. Dejerine J, Thomas A: L'atrophie olivo-ponto-cerebelleuse. *Nouv Iconogr Salpet* 13:330–370, 1900.
2. Shy GM, Drager GA: A neurological syndrome associated with orthostatic hypotension. *Arch Neurol* 2:511–527, 1960.
3. van der Eecken H, Adams RD, van Bogaert L: Striopallidal-nigral degeneration: A hitherto undescribed lesion in paralysis agitans. *J Neuropathol Exp Neurol* 19:159–161, 1960.
4. Adams RD, vonBogaert L, van der Eecken H: Degeneres cences nigro-striees et cerebello-nigro-striees. *Psychiatr Neurol* 142:219–259, 1961.
5. Graham JG, Oppenheimer DR: Orthostatic hypotension and nicotine sensitivity in a case of multiple system atrophy. *J Neurol Neurosurg Psychiatry* 32:28–34, 1969.
6. Bannister R, Oppenheimer DR: Degenerative diseases of the nervous system associated with autonomic failure. *Brain* 95:457–474, 1972.
7. Menzel P: Beitrag zur Kenntniss der hereditaren Ataxie und Kleinhirnatrophie. *Arch Psychiatr Nervenkr* 22:160–190, 1891.
8. Greenfield JG: *The Spino-Cerebellar Degenerations.* Springfield, IL: Charles C Thomas, 1954.
9. Penney JB: Multiple systems atrophy and nonfamilial olivopontocerebellar atrophy are the same disease. *Ann Neurol* 37:553–554, 1995.
10. Harding AE: 'Idiopathic' late onset cerebellar ataxia, in Harding AE (ed): *The Hereditary Ataxias and Related Disorders.* New York: Churchill Livingstone, 1984, pp 166–173.
11. Schrag A, Ben-Shlomo Y, Quinn NP: Prevalence of progressive supranuclear palsy and multiple system atrophy: A cross-sectional study. *Lancet* 354:1771–1775, 1999.
12. Vanacore N, Bonifati V, Colosimo C, et al: Epidemiology of progressive supranuclear palsy. ESGAP Consortium. European Study Group on Atypical Parkinsonisms. *Neurol Sci* 22:101–103, 2001.
13. Ben-Shlomo Y, Wenning GK, Tison F, Quinn NP: Survival of patients with pathologically proven multiple system atrophy: A meta-analysis. *Neurology* 48:384–393, 1997.
14. Wenning GK, Ben Shlomo Y, Magalhaes M, et al: Clinical features and natural history of multiple system atrophy: An analysis of 100 cases. *Brain* 117:835–845, 1994.
15. Klockgether T, Ludtke R, Kramer B, et al: The natural history of degenerative ataxia: A retrospective study in 466 patients. *Brain* 121:589–600, 1998.
16. Quinn NP: Multiple system atrophy, in Marsden CD, Fahn S (eds): *Movement Disorders 3.* Oxford: Butterworth-Heinemann, 1994, pp 262–281.
17. Quinn N: Multiple system atrophy: The nature of the beast. *J Neurol Neurosurg Psychiatry* (suppl):1989, 78–89.
18. Gilman S, Low P, Quinn N, et al: Consensus statement on the diagnosis of multiple system atrophy. American Autonomic Society and American Academy of Neurology. *Clin Auton Res* 8:359–362, 1998.
19. Osaki Y, Wenning GK, Daniel SE, et al: Do published criteria improve clinical diagnostic accuracy in multiple system atrophy? *Neurology* 59:1486–1491, 2002.
20. Adams RD, Salam-Adams M: Striatonigral degeneration, in Vinken PJ, Bruyn GW, Klawans HL (eds): *Extrapyramidal Disorders.* Amsterdam: Elsevier Science Publishers, 1986, pp 205–212.
21. Gouider-Khouja N, Vidailhef M, Bonnef AM, et al: "Pure" striatonigral degeneration and Parkinson's disease: A comparative clinical study. *Mov Disord* 10:288–294, 1995.
22. Rajput AH, Rodzilsky B, Rajput A: Accuracy of clinical diagnosis in parkinsonism: A prospective study. *Can J Neurol Sci* 18:275–278, 1991.
23. Hughes AJ, Colosimo C, Kleedorfen B, et al: The dopaminergic response in multiple system atrophy. *J Neurol Neurosurg Psychiatry* 55:1009–1013, 1992.
24. Magalhaes M, Wenning GK, Daniel SE, Quinn NP: Autonomic dysfunction in pathologically confirmed multiple system atrophy and idiopathic Parkinson's disease: A retrospective comparison. *Acta Neurol Scand* 91:98–102, 1995.
25. Mathias CJ: Autonomic disorders and their recognition. *N Engl J Med* 336:721–724, 1997.
26. Mathias CJ: Orthostatic hypotension: Causes, mechanisms and influencing factors. *Neurology* 45:S6–S11, 1995.
27. Robertson D, Davis TL: Recent advances in the treatment of orthostatic hypotension. *Neurology* 45:S26–S32, 1995.
28. Mathias CJ, Williams AC: The Shy-Drager syndrome and multiple system atrophy, in Calne DB (ed): *Neurodegenerative Diseases.* Philadelphia: WB Saunders, 1994, pp 743–767.
29. Beck RO, Betts CD, Fowler CJ: Genitourinary dysfunction in multiple system atrophy: Clinical features and treatment in 62 cases. *J Urol* 151:1336–1341, 1994.
30. Sakakibara R, Hattori T, Tojo M, et al: Micturitional disturbance in multiple system atrophy. *Jpn J Psychiatry Neurol* 47:591–598, 1993.
31. Stocchi F, Badiali D, Vacca L, et al: Anorectal function in multiple system atrophy and Parkinson's disease. *Mov Disord* 15:71-76, 2000.
32. Isozaki E, Matsubara S, Hayashida T, et al: Morphometric study of nucleus ambiguus in multiple system atrophy presenting with vocal cord abductor paralysis. *Clin Neuropathol* 19:213–220, 2000.

33. Benarroch EE, Schmeichel AM, Parisi JE: Preservation of branchi-motor neurons of the nucleus ambiguus in multiple system atrophy. *Neurology* 60:115–117, 2003.

34. Blumin JH, Berke GS: Bilateral vocal fold paresis and multiple system atrophy. *Arch Otolaryngol Head Neck Surg* 128:1404–1407, 2002.

35. Winkler AS, Marsden J, Parton M, et al: Erythropoietin deficiency and anaemia in multiple system atrophy. *Mov Disord* 16:233–239, 2001.

36. Berciano J: Olivopontocerebellar atrophy, in Jankovic J, Tolosa E (eds): *Parkinson's Disease and Movement Disorders*. Baltimore: Williams & Wilkins, 1993, pp 163–189.

37. Duvoisin RC: The olivopontocerebellar atrophies, in Marsden CD, Fahn S (eds): *Movement Disorders 2*. London: Butterworth, 1987, pp 249–271.

38. Wenning GK, Ben-Shlomo Y, Magalhaes M, et al: Clinicopatho-logical study of 35 cases of multiple system atrophy. *J Neurol Neurosurg Psychiatry* 58:160–166, 1995.

39. Robbins TW, James M, Lange KW, et al: Cognitive performance in multiple system atrophy. *Brain* 115:271–291, 1992.

40. Cummings JL: Frontal-subcortical circuits and human behavior. *Arch Neurol* 50:873–880, 1993.

41. Parsa MA, Simon M, Dubrow C, et al: Psychiatric manifestations of olivopontocerebellar atrophy and treatment with clozapine. *Int J Psychiatry Med* 23:149–156, 1993.

42. Wenning GK, Jager K, Kendall B, et al: Is cranial computerized tomography useful in the diagnosis of multiple system atrophy? *Mov Disord* 9:333–336, 1994.

43. Konagaya M, Konagaya Y, Iida M: Clinical and magnetic resonance imaging study of extrapyramidal symptoms in multi-ple system atrophy. *J Neurol Neurosurg Psychiatry* 57:1528–1531, 1994.

44. Macia F, Yekhlef F, Ballan G, et al: T2-hyperintense lateral rim and hypointense putamen are typical but not exclusive of multiple system atrophy. *Arch Neurol* 58:1024–1026, 2001.

45. Kraft E, Schwarz J, Trenkwalder C, et al: The combination of hypointense and hyperintense signal changes on T2-weighted magnetic resonance imaging sequences: A specific marker of multiple system atrophy? *Arch Neurol* 56:225-228, 1999.

46. Brooks DJ, Ibanez V, Sawle GV, et al: Differing patterns of stri-atal 18F-dopa uptake in Parkinson's disease, multiple system atrophy, and progressive supranuclear palsy. *Ann Neurol* 28: 547–555, 1990.

47. Sawle GV, Playford ED, Brooks DJ, et al: Asymmetrical pre-synaptic and post-synaptic changes to the striatal dopamine projection in dopa naive parkinsonism: Diagnostic implications of the D2 receptor status. *Brain* 116:853–867, 1993.

48. Rinne JO, Burn DJ, Mathias CJ, et al: Positron emission tomog-raphy studies on the dopaminergic system and striatal opioid binding in the olivopontocerebellar atrophy variant of multiple system atrophy. *Ann Neurol* 37:568–573, 1995.

49. Eidelberg D, Takikawa S, Moeller JR, et al: Striatal hypometabolism distinguishes striatonigral degeneration from Parkinson's disease. *Ann Neurol* 33:518–527, 1993.

50. Perani D, Bressi S, Testa D, et al: Clinical/metabolic correlations in multiple system atrophy: A fluorodeoxyglucose F18 positron emission tomographic study. *Arch Neurol* 52:179–185, 1995.

51. Gilman S, Koeppe RA, Junck L, et al: Patterns of cerebral glucose metabolism detected with positron emission tomography differ in multiple system atrophy and olivopontocerebellar atrophy. *Ann Neurol* 36:166–175, 1994.

52. Schwarz J, Taksen K, Arnold G, et al: 123I-iodobenzamide SPECT predicts dopaminergic responsiveness in patients with de novo parkinsonism. *Neurology* 42:556–561, 1992.

53. Walter U, Niehaus L, Probst T, et al: Brain parenchyma sonogra-phy discriminates Parkinson's disease and atypical parkinsonian syndromes. *Neurology* 60:74-77, 2003.

54. Wenning GK, Kraft E, Beck R, et al: Cerebellar presentation of multiple system atrophy. *Mov Disord* 12:115-117, 1997.

55. Giladi N, Simon ES, Korczyn AD, et al: Anal sphincter EMG does not distinguish between multiple system atrophy and Parkinson's disease. *Muscle Nerve* 23:731-734, 2000.

56. Wenning GK, Ebersbach G, Verny M, et al: Progression of falls in postmortem-confirmed parkinsonism disorders. *Mov Disord* 14:947–950, 1999.

57. Papp MI, Kahn JE, Lantos PL: Glial cytoplasmic inclusions in the CNS of patients with multiple system atrophy (striatonigral degeneration, olivopontocerebellar atrophy and Shy-Drager syn-drome). *J Neurol Sci* 94:79–100, 1989.

58. Papp MI, Lantos PL: Accumulation of tubular structures in oligo-dendroglial and neuronal cells as the basic alteration in multiple system atrophy. *J Neurol Sci* 107:172–182, 1992.

59. Arima K, Ueda K, Sunohara N, et al: NACP/alpha-synuclein immunoreactivity in fibrillary components of neuronal and oligo-dendroglial cytoplasmic inclusions in the pontine nuclei in multiple system atrophy. *Acta Neuropathol (Berl)* 96:439–444, 1998.

60. Gai WP, Power JH, Blumbergs PC, Blessing WW: Multiple-system atrophy: a new alpha-synuclein disease? *Lancet* 352:547–548, 1998.

61. Duda JE, Giasson BI, Gur TL, et al: Immunohistochemical and biochemical studies demonstrate a distinct profile of alpha-synuclein permutations in multiple system atrophy. *J Neuropathol Exp Neurol* 59:830–841, 2000.

62. Piao YS, Hayashi S, Hasegawa M, et al: Co-localization of alpha-synuclein and phosphorylated tau in neuronal and glial cytoplas-mic inclusions in a patient with multiple system atrophy of long duration. *Acta Neuropathol (Berl)* 101:285–293, 2001.

63. Spillantini MG, Crowther RA, Jakes R, et al: Filamentous alpha-synuclein inclusions link multiple system atrophy with Parkin-son's disease and dementia with Lewy bodies. *Neurosci Lett* 251:205–208, 1998.

64. Hughes AJ, Colosimo C, Kleedorfer B, et al: The dopaminergic response in multiple system atrophy. *J Neurol Neurosurg Psychiatry* 55:1009–1013, 1992.

65. Parati EA, Fetoni V, Geminiani GC, et al: Response to L-DOPA in multiple system atrophy. *Clin Neuropharmacol* 16:139-144, 1993.

66. Rossi P, Colosimo C, Moro E, et al: Acute challenge with apo-morphine and levodopa in Parkinsonism. *Eur Neurol* 43:95–101, 2000.

67. Hussain IF, Brady CM, Swinn MJ, et al: Treatment of erectile dys-function with sildenafil citrate (Viagra) in parkinsonism due to Parkinson's disease or multiple system atrophy with observa-tions on orthostatic hypotension. *J Neurol Neurosurg Psychiatry* 71:371–374, 2001.

I. PARKINSONIAN STATES

OTHER PARKINSONIAN SYNDROMES

Chapter 22 _____

INFECTIOUS AND POSTINFECTIOUS PARKINSONISM

PUIU NISIPEANU, DIANA PALEACU, and AMOS D. KORCZYN

CLINICAL FEATURES OF ENCEPHALITIS
  LETHARGICA   373
POSTENCEPHALITIC PARKINSONISM   374
  Clinical Features   374
  Pathophysiology   375
  Pathology   375
  Treatment   376
PARKINSONISM RESULTING FROM OTHER
  INFECTIOUS CAUSES   376
  Acquired Immune Deficiency Syndrome (AIDS)   377
  Nonviral Infections   378
  Syphilis   378
  Fungal and Parasitic Infections   378
  Creutzfeldt-Jakob Disease (CJD)   378
  Whipple's Disease   379

Parkinsonian features can develop during or after various infectious diseases. A major cause of parkinsonism in earlier decades of the 20th century, fortunately of historical interest at the present time, was encephalitis lethargica (EL). This disease, also called von Economo's disease, appeared as an epidemic during World War I, and many new cases were reported for more than 10 years. In Austria and France, EL was first described in 1917 by von Economo[1] and Cruchet et al.[2]

By 1918 the disease had spread throughout Europe to England and Germany, and later it spread to North America and China. By 1919 it had overrun Europe and disseminated to Central America, India, and, later, to Japan, Africa, and Australia.[3,4] However, after 1935, the number of new cases was negligible and the disease essentially disappeared from public health reports and mortality data in 1940, when the term EL was replaced by the more inclusive "infectious encephalitides" on the international list of the causes of death.[5]

Postencephalitic parkinsonism (PEP) was a frequently seen variant of parkinsonism in the 1920s; probably the best estimates were provided by Dimsdale's review of the patients seen in London clinics between 1900 and 1942.[6] Her data indicate that EL accounted for two-thirds of the cases of parkinsonism seen in the period 1920–1930, and for one-half of the cases seen during the following decade.[6]

In a later retrospective study, conducted in 1959 and 1960, a history suggesting EL was obtained from 13 percent of 107 consecutive patients with parkinsonism and a history of other encephalitides from a further 16 percent.[4] A progressive decline of PEP was seen over time: whereas, in 1955, 20 percent of the parkinsonian population was diagnosed as suffering from PEP, 10 years later PEP contributed only 6.6 percent of patients. In 1968, Duvoisin[7] noted that PEP represented less than 1 percent of patients. Nevertheless, considering the prior high frequency of PEP, it was suggested that many cases of "idiopathic" Parkinson's disease (PD) were actually caused by the EL pandemic during the 1920s, in which these subjects had been affected, even if subclinically. It was further suggested that, as the cohort of patients who had undergone subclinical infection died, the frequency of PD would decrease dramatically, so that PD would cease to exist as a major entity.[8] This theory, known as the cohort theory, was supported by observations that the mean age at onset of parkinsonism rose progressively during subsequent calendar years from 1920 to 1955. However, an alternative interpretation may be more valid, namely that the increasing age of onset of PD could be a result of the increasing number of elderly people, and increased attention to their medical disorders. Today, several decades later, the cohort theory is obsolete. There is no trend towards a decrease in PD prevalence, although PEP has all but disappeared.

Clinical Features of Encephalitis Lethargica

The initial clinical features of EL were of a nonspecific viral infection. Von Economo's description of EL was as follows: "The patients all showed a slight influenza-like prodromal condition with pharyngeal symptoms, a slight rise of temperature which was soon followed by a variety of nervous system symptoms of which generally one or another pointed to the midbrain as the source."[9]

Most patients exhibited a persistent pathological somnolence, or sleep lasting for days to weeks (a feature giving the disease its name), from which they could be aroused briefly by vigorous stimulation. Another prominent feature was ophthalmoplegia, usually in combination with somnolence (the "somnolent ophthalmoplegic" form). Wilson, one of the leading neurologists of the period, remarked that every type of internal or external ophthalmoplegia could be found.[10] This common somnolent ophthalmoplegic form suggested to von Economo an inflammatory involvement of the upper midbrain. Signs of cortical dysfunction, such as aphasia, convulsions, psychosis, and sensory impairment, including disorders of hearing and vision, were notably rare. A small percentage of patients were overactive, rather than somnolent, and an even smaller fraction exhibited movement disorders such as chorea or myoclonus on a cataplectic background. Bradykinesia and mutism were predominant in yet another small group. As in other viral encephalitides, fever was a constant feature, whereas elevated cerebrospinal fluid (CSF) protein level with lymphocytic pleocytosis was seen in about one-half of patients.

The clinical, laboratory, and pathological features of EL were highly suggestive of a viral infection. Von Economo even reported successful transmission to nonhuman primates.[9] However, no virus was ever convincingly identified and the disease was not contagious. Attempts to establish a link between EL/PEP and a number of viruses, notably influenza strains A and B and herpes viruses, were unsuccessful.[11–13] The role of retroviruses was discussed by Elizan and Casals,[14] who found white matter astrogliosis in EL and PEP brains, similar to the astrogliosis seen in human immunodeficiency virus-1 (HIV-1) encephalopathy. The addition of polymerase chain reaction techniques that may be applied to detect viral genomes in paraffin-embedded tissues provided new impetus to continue the search for a viral etiology of EL.[15] The hypothesis that an influenza virus strain was the responsible agent is more attractive than that of a one-time unidentified virus, particularly because sporadic cases have appeared in which a relationship to influenza has been suggested.[16] However, as stressed by Casals et al.,[17] the pandemic of EL began in January 1917 (or perhaps earlier in 1915, in Romania), whereas the influenza epidemic started later (1918–19). More recent epidemiological studies[18] have found that earlier outbreaks of influenza actually occurred during the winter in the years 1915–1917. Nevertheless, McCall et al.[19] did not detect influenza viral RNA in brains from patients with acute EL and with PEP, including in some from substantia nigra.

The onset of EL was acute or subacute. The disease lasted for several weeks, and the mortality in some areas was as high as 40 percent. Many of those who survived the acute phase of the illness were left with a wide variety of symptoms, including: mental impairment, difficulty in re-establishing a normal sleep-wake cycle, myoclonus, dystonia, tics and other bizarre movements, postures, or gait; bulimia and obesity; sociopathic behavior in adults; and personality changes in children with compulsive behavior.[20,21] However, three very specific delayed features became evident: (1) oculogyric crises (OGC); (2) central respiratory irregularities, including increased respiratory rate, apneic episodes, myoclonic jerks of the diaphragm, and cluster breathing resulting in hypoxia; and (3) parkinsonism.

OGC apparently were not seen, or at least not reported, during the epidemic of EL, and were first reported by Oeckinghaus[22] in 1921, consisting of forceful deviation of the eyes, almost always upwards or upwards and laterally, seldom in a horizontal or downward direction, and, rarely, convergence. Most attacks were of a sustained tonic nature (usually continuing for minutes or hours and disappearing during sleep), but instances of repeated clonic spasms of ocular deviation also occurred. Almost always OGC appeared in patients who had already developed parkinsonism, although rarely they preceded it by a short period. Their prevalence was probably close to 20 percent of PEP patients.[23]

Once present, OGC tended to persist, possibly later decreasing in intensity.

In some patients with OGC, deviation of the head, blepharospasm, contractions of muscles of the tongue and jaws evoking cranial dystonia similar to that in Meige's syndrome, or dystonia of limbs also occurred. Remarkably, patients frequently complained of fear, anxiety, depression, or suicidal ideation which preceded or accompanied OGC.

The only other encephalitic patient with OGC unrelated to epidemic EL who developed parkinsonism (after acute Western equine encephalitis) was followed by Mulder et al.[24] They only mentioned two short episodes of upward deviation of the eyes in a 6-month period. More recently, few patients were reported with OGC during acute encephalitis considered to represent sporadic EL.[25]

The pathophysiology of OGC and of thought changes was discussed by Leigh et al.[26] Because OGC was well controlled by anticholinergic medication, they may be caused by a transient disequilibrium between increased cholinergic and low dopaminergic activity in supranuclear areas affecting ocular movements. In contrast to postencephalitic OGC, the acute drug-induced OGC is not usually associated with parkinsonism.[27]

Postencephalitic Parkinsonism

CLINICAL FEATURES

Given the clinical features described below, and a history of encephalitis, the diagnosis of PEP is straightforward.[28] Dating the onset of PEP is more difficult because of the insidious development of symptomatology. A few of the survivors of acute EL probably went on to develop parkinsonism immediately. Reviewing the data, Duvoisin and Yahr[5] found that, in about one-half of the patients who developed parkinsonism, this feature was present 5 years after EL, in 80 percent or more at 10 years, and that by 1950 most of the long-term survivors had already developed parkinsonism. As some patients never reported a clear-cut episode of EL but exhibited features typical of PEP, it was accepted that PEP may occur without overt infection and that its occurrence is not related to the severity of EL. The symptom-free period may have had variable lengths, presumably depending on the extent of cell destruction, compensatory hyperactivity of those neurons that survived, and supersensitivity of postsynaptic dopamine receptors to dopamine.

It seems, however, that some EL epidemics were "bad for parkinsonism," according to Wilson.[10] Von Economo stated that he knew of only 2 patients in whom parkinsonism had occurred who suffered from EL in 1916 and 1917, but that many of those who were acutely ill in 1920 and 1921 developed PEP.[9]

The extrapyramidal features, which appeared after a variable latent "parkinsonism-free" period, included rigidity, mask face, bradykinesia, impaired gait, and dysarthria, but clinicians were impressed by differences between PEP and "cryptogenic" parkinsonism. Wilson noted not only that PEP patients were usually much younger but also that they had many features unseen in idiopathic parkinsonism, such as myoclonus, chorea, tics or spasms, OGC, respiratory disturbances, pupillary dysfunction, ocular palsies, and behavioral disorders.[10] Interestingly, the study of PEP patients contributed to the delineation of "bradyphrenia," as Naville[29] termed the slowing of cognitive processing in these patients.

When present, the resting "coarse," or typical pill-rolling, tremor was less prominent than rigidity ("paralysis agitans without agitation"); sometimes, a disabling rigidity of neck extension was encountered. Many patients manifested catatonic akinesia, whereas others were embarrassed by akathisia. Another notable feature was that some PEP patients demonstrated a striking fluctuation of their rigidity and motor impairment.

It should be recalled that vertical gaze paresis and eyelid opening apraxia may occur in PEP, making the distinction from progressive supranuclear palsy important.[30] Two reports have appeared which portray the photographic and cinematographic features of PEP.[31,32]

The evolution of PEP is still debatable. Wilson expressed the view that "the course of residua and sequelae is difficult to foretell" and that "among the sequelae parkinsonism seems least likely to alter," whereas Duncan[33] mentioned the worsening of parkinsonian symptomatology. This view was confirmed by Duvoisin and Yahr who, in a retrospective study in the early 1960s, observed that, on the whole, the encephalitic sequelae had been rather mild and remarkably stable but also that in the previous 10 years there had been a definite slow and insidious progression in about one-half of the patients.[5] Two more recent studies[34,35] have shown late progression of PEP patients, most of whom were in their seventies. Motor deterioration exceeded changes naturally seen in normal elderly populations. In a clinicopathological study of 8 long survivors of PEP, Geddes et al.[35] found that 7 had a slowly progressive disease. This progression manifested, as was noted also by Calne and Lees,[34] by increased bradykinesia, rigidity, and postural instability. In a brief reference, however, Agid[36] considered motor decline in PEP patients to be related to aging and not to progression of the disease.

Vierrege et al.[37] studied retrospectively 10 autopsied PEP cases and found that 4 of them had motor worsening before death but no intellectual decline. It is of interest to emphasize that dementia was rare among PEP patients, in contrast to its relatively high prevalence in PD.[38]

PATHOPHYSIOLOGY

The issue of whether PEP patients manifest delayed exacerbation of the parkinsonism may be important, because it may provide clues to the hypothesis of interaction between acute environmental damage and age-related neuronal attrition.[38,39] When this late progression exists, is it phenomenologically different from the initial development of parkinsonism after years of "PEP-free" period? How consistent is this difference with the hypothesis that a one-time exposure to a very aggressive agent will be followed by a short presymptomatic period, as happened in 1-methyl-4-phenyl-1,2,3,6-tetrahydropyridine (MPTP)-induced acute parkinsonism? Or is the long presymptomatic phase the expression of a continuous or intermittent but mildly potent inducer of dopaminergic neuronal death, by different mechanisms, possibly autoimmune, because there is some experimental evidence suggesting that autoimmunity may be relevant to the pathogenesis of parkinsonism?[40] Unfortunately, most EL survivors have now died, so that more answers as to the progression of PEP are unlikely to be forthcoming. The demonstration of immunoglobulin G oligoclonal bands in the cerebrospinal fluid (CSF) of PEP patients[41] may provide additional evidence of an intrathecal immune response. The nature of the antigen provoking the response, or even whether the response is directly triggered by a virus, is not known, and the persistence of oligoclonal bands does not necessarily signify a response to an active infection.

There are contradictory data concerning the role of genetic factors in the development of PEP, as in the report of Elizan et al.,[42] which found an increased frequency of HLA-B4 in PEP patients compared with that of matched controls, and which was not replicated.[43]

PATHOLOGY

Brain weight and macroscopic cortical atrophy were similar in long-standing PEP and an age-matched control group.[44] The earlier studies concentrated on basal ganglia and brainstem pathology, with less emphasis on other brain structures.[45,46] The characteristic macroscopic change is depigmentation of the substantia nigra and, to a lesser degree, of the locus ceruleus.

The microscopic examination was typical for severe and diffuse neuronal loss and gliosis in the substantia nigra, and inflammatory perivascular lymphocytic cuffing, such as was seen in EL, was present also in PEP brains examined a long time after EL. Gibb and Lees[44] found that the loss of pigmented nigral cells was significantly higher than that in PD, exceeding 90 percent. The locus ceruleus was also affected, as well as raphe nuclei. Even more widespread astrocytic changes were found by Haraguchi et al.[47]

The hallmark of PD is eosinophilic inclusions in certain neurons in the brain, the so-called Lewy bodies. These are conspicuously absent in PEP. The important pathological feature of PEP is the presence of neurofibrillary tangles (NFTs).[48] The NFTs consist of straight filaments 15 mμ in width. Notably, NFTs are not found in PD. NFTs are widely distributed and are usually present not only in the substantia nigra and locus ceruleus, but also in the nuclei of the reticular formation, hippocampus, nucleus basalis of Meynert, and variably in other structures, including neocortex and spinal cord. A detailed analysis of NFTs allowed Geddes et al.[35] to suggest that PEP is an active degenerative process, rather than the expression of delayed cell decompensation and aging after an initial acute illness. They found that the few surviving neurons in which NFTs were already present showed granular cytoplasmic staining. The NFTs of the substantia nigra in PEP reacted positively with anti-tau antibodies, and with antisera raised against a purified human brain microtubule fraction.[48] The accumulation of abnormal tau protein starts in neuronal soma, and the gradual formation of mature NFTs is followed after neuronal death by extracellular NFT "ghosts."

Buee-Scherrer et al. stressed the widespread distribution of NFTs in hippocampus entorhinal cortex, areas 4, 9, and 20, globus pallidum, and putamen. Biochemically, NFT were composed of a triplet made of tau 55, 64, and 69, similar to the tau triplet seen in Alzheimer's disease but different from the tau doublet (tau 55 and 64) described in progressive supranuclear palsy (PSP) and corticobasal degeneration.[49]

The presence of granular cytoplasmic staining for tau protein was believed then to represent an early stage in NFT formation, which would be unexpected after many years during which the disease process was apparently inactive. Furthermore, relatively few extracellular "ghosts" were seen, again in contrast to the expected total extracellular occurrence after a very long disease duration.

In addition to the neuronal changes, PEP brains were found to contain tau-immunoreactive astrocytes (glial fibrillary tangles).[46]

NFTs are found in a diversity of genetic and acquired conditions, such as Alzheimer's disease, PSP, parkinsonism-dementia complex of Guam (PDC), subacute sclerosing panencephalitis, and myotonic dystrophy, and thus may constitute a final common pathway for different types of cellular injury. Moreover, the NFT distribution, morphology, and antigenic profile are essentially the same in PEP and PDC, suggesting a common pathogenesis, if not etiology, in these disorders. PDC is a disease that affects the Chamorro population and its etiology is still elusive; an environmental risk factor is highly suspected.[50] As happened in some PEP patients, PDC was reported to be present or to progress decades after withdrawal from the exposure to the presumed environmental risk factor, and this disease is also disappearing.

It must be emphasized that Geddes et al.[35] in contrast to Viarregi et al.,[37] failed to find inflammatory changes of nigral dopaminergic cells, accepted markers of an active pathological process.[51]

There was no correlation between the clinical symptomatology and the above-mentioned pathological findings (neuronal loss, gliosis, or NFT load and distribution).[35]

TREATMENT

Amphetamines were widely used to treat patients with PEP. Initially recommended for their alerting effect, amphetamines were found not only to produce subjective improvement but also to reduce motor disability slightly.[52,53]

Before the introduction of L-dopa, the belladonna alkaloids proved to be most effective.[54] Anticholinergic drugs continued to be used extensively for decades, because their long-term tolerance was better than that of L-dopa (see below). Tics, OGC and, sometimes, behavioral disturbances were influenced in addition to objective improvement of extrapyramidal symptomatology. Surprisingly, in the long-term use of anticholinergics dystonia has been reported as the most prominent adverse effect.

The introduction of L-dopa as therapy for idiopathic parkinsonism was extended to PEP, and it was proven to be of some benefit. The first double-blind controlled trial of L-dopa in PEP was conducted by Calne et al.[55] They administered maximally tolerated doses of L-dopa for more than 6 weeks to a group of 20 institutionalized PEP "active" patients. The maximum tolerated dose was 2.5 g daily (without decarboxylase inhibitors), considerably lower than the doses used in the same period for idiopathic parkinsonism. Ten patients improved, 5 did not, and 5 were withdrawn because of side-effects. The main improvement occurred in walking, but OGC crises and drooling were also alleviated. Side-effects included disturbing dyskinesias and pathological restlessness.

An open trial was reported by Hunter et al.[56] Of 50 patients, 16 had maintained benefit, 16 showed no change, and 18 were unable to tolerate L-dopa. The conclusion of this study was that the majority of PEP patients do not benefit or tolerate L-dopa for extended periods of time. The observation of limited tolerance of L-dopa was confirmed by Krasner and Cornelius,[57] by Sacks et al.,[58] and by Duvoisin et al.,[59] who were also concerned about the high incidence of side-effects, especially respiratory crises, respiratory or phonatory tics, and exacerbation of OGC.

Parkinsonism Resulting from Other Infectious Causes

Although EL ceased to occur, at least in an epidemic form, in the 1930s, parkinsonian syndromes were infrequently described in association with acute encephalitic illness, sometimes supposed to represent sporadic cases of EL. More often they appeared during or following an episode of poorly documented febrile illness or after an encephalitis not resembling EL.

Duvoisin and Yahr[5] concluded that "the rare association of a progressive parkinsonian syndrome such as is understood by the term PD with any known type of viral encephalitis (except for EL) had not been shown to be more than coincidental." A similar approach was expressed by Schwab and England.[60] Extrapyramidal features such as hypomimia, rigidity, tremor, impaired posture, and gait that are somewhat similar to those seen in PD may occur during the acute phase of various encephalitides, notably Japanese encephalitis and Western equine encephalitis.

Parkinsonian symptomatology in such cases was most often transient, and nonprogressive, and the free period after the infection, characteristic for EL and PEP, was not seen.

Single-patient reports or small series of patients have been described.[60–70] Both Rail et al.[63] and Howard and Lees[64] were concerned with a strict definition of EL, consisting of an episode of acute or subacute encephalitis, presence of extrapyramidal signs, ocular palsies, oculogyric crises, and behavioral disturbances. Undoubtedly, in the absence of a specific diagnostic test for EL, and because of the variability of the clinical manifestations, many of the reported cases remain questionable.

An extended list of viral infections, other than Japanese and Western equine encephalitis, reported to be associated with parkinsonism generally compliant to the conclusions expressed by Duvoisin and Yahr,[5] includes coxsackie B types 2 and 4, measles, post-measles encephalitis, poliomyelitis, and possibly herpes simplex, Epstein-Barr virus, and West Nile virus.[71–79] A particularly interesting patient was reported by Lin et al.[80] This young patient developed a pure extrapyramidal syndrome after 1 week of headache and intermittent fever, attributed to a probable viral (herpes simplex type 1) infection. Magnetic resonance imaging (MRI) showed hyperintense (T_2-weighted) signals bilaterally within the substantia nigra which almost disappeared 2 months later. Clinical improvement occurred and, when asymptomatic after 8 months, positron emission tomography scanning with fluorodopa and raclopride revealed a pattern similar to that seen in idiopathic parkinsonism. This may represent the first in vivo demonstration of isolated involvement of the substantia nigra by means of an external agent also inducing a reduction of fluorodopa uptake more marked in the putamen than in the caudate. Other reports showing substantia nigra lesions by MRI were published in patients with Japanese encephalitis, St Louis encephalitis, and other acute encephalitides.[81–85] Rarely, the substantia nigra lesions were associated with persistent parkinsonism after Japanese encephalitis.[86]

L-Dopa therapy was found to help in some patients.[66,68]

ACQUIRED IMMUNE DEFICIENCY SYNDROME (AIDS)

Neurological complications occur in about 70 percent of AIDS patients, and in more than 90 percent of autopsied cases pathologic examination disclosed brain abnormalities.[87] Clinically, the primary HIV-related neurological syndromes are HIV-1 encephalopathy (HIV-1-associated cognitive/motor abnormalities), neuropathy, and myelopathy. Movement disorders including parkinsonism, are as a rule seen in patients with HIV encephalopathy, those exposed to neuroleptics or as a consequence of opportunistic infections.

When exposed to neuroleptic drugs, many patients with HIV encephalopathy showed an unusual sensitivity, dopamine receptor blockade resulting in overt parkinsonism.[88] About 80 percent of patients younger than 50 years who received more than 4 mg/kg per day of chlorpromazine equivalents developed parkinsonism.[89] This suggested the vulnerability of their striatal dopaminergic system, possibly resulting from subclinical neuronal loss in the pars compacta of the substantia nigra,[90] and neuronal loss in the globus pallidum.[91] Pathological studies of the substantia nigra have found substantial neuronal degeneration, possibly related to the toxicity of some viral proteins (gp120 and Tat, proteins known to inhibit tyrosine hydroxylase expression).[92–94]

HIV-1 DNA was recently detected in macrophages and microglia, as well as in basal ganglia astrocytes and neurons.[95] HIV infection greatly increases apoptosis of basal ganglia astrocytes which, together with activation of astrocytes, produces dysfunction of the astrocyte-neuron network.[96,97]

CSF dopamine seems to be reduced, especially in neurologically impaired patients with lower CD4 lymphocyte counts.[98]

Additionally, spectroscopic abnormalities were found, even in neurologically intact HIV patients,[99] and PET showed hypermetabolism of basal ganglia in HIV-positive patients, which changed to hypometabolism as they developed extrapyramidal symptomatology.[100] Motor abnormalities can be identified in nonimpaired HIV-infected persons by quantifying rapid alternating finger movements and reaction time.[101] Nevertheless, parkinsonian features such as bradykinesia, rigidity, slow gait, postural instability, hypomimia, and hypophonia occur in a minority. Mattos et al.[102,103] detected neurological manifestations in 42.8 percent of 2460 HIV-positive patients. Movement disorders were present in 2.7 percent of them, while parkinsonism was seen in 14 patients (0.56 percent). The mean time after HIV diagnosis to the appearance of parkinsonism was 5 months. A much higher prevalence was reported by Mirsattari et al.,[104] who found 6 parkinsonians and another 10 patients with parkinsonian features among 115 consecutive HIV patients. Predictably the patients were young, suggesting that HIV should be investigated in young-onset nonfamilial PD patients.

It must be remembered that hyperkinesias (chorea, postural tremor) are the most commonly observed movement disorders in AIDS patients.[105]

In a few, parkinsonism was related to focal lesions of basal ganglia by opportunistic infections, toxoplasmosis, tuberculosi revealed by brain imaging and CSF data.[106–108] Exceptionally, parkinsonism was the presenting manifestation of HIV infection. Hersh et al.[109] reported a 37-year-old man with rapidly evolving atypical parkinsonism in the absence of neuroleptic exposure.

Koutsilieri et al.[93] have shown in monkeys infected with simian immunodeficiency virus a reduction in striatal dopamine as early as 2 months without a similar reduction in nigral dopamine, which may indicate initial involvement of dopaminergic terminals.

TREATMENT

L-Dopa use was followed by mild or no improvement.[103,107] However, Mintz et al.[110] followed a small group of children with severe parkinsonian-like dysfunction and found a relatively sustained benefit of L-dopa therapy. Nevertheless, the use of L-dopa may be deleterious. Czub et al.[111] have shown that L-dopa and selegiline may accelerate the infection in macaques infected with simian immunodeficiency virus. In psychotic patients who developed neuroleptic-induced parkinsonism, clozapine provided, in a pilot study, an important reduction in both psychopathology and parkinsonism.[112] Etiologic treatment of opportunistic infections also improved parkinsonism.[107,108]

The advent of highly active antiretroviral therapy was expected to reduce or to change the patterns of HIV-associated encephalopathy, and some data supported this hope.[113-115] However, the virus may persist in the central nervous system (CNS)[116] and an increasing resistance of HIV strains was noted. This contrasts with the reduction in prevalence of CNS opportunistic infections and of primary CNS lymphoma. Prolonged survival, older patients, longer duration of antiretroviral complex therapy with possible interactions of drugs with cerebral endothelium and brain white matter may contribute to a future increase of HIV encephalopathy.[117]

NONVIRAL INFECTIONS

Nonviral infections were also found to induce acute parkinsonism. Several children developed extrapyramidal features associated with proven or probable *Mycoplasma pneumoniae*.[119-121] The symptomatology included bradykinesia, rigidity, dystonia, and choreic movements and was reversible. In 1 patient, brain MRI showed bilateral lesions in the basal ganglia with hemiparkinsonism that later disappeared in parallel with resolution of midbrain MRI enhancement.[121]

SYPHILIS

Because meningovascular syphilis involves the midbrain, it is conceivable that parkinsonian features may be induced or precipitated. However, most cases that were reported when neurosyphilis was a more common disease probably reflected the coincidence of two independent diseases.[121]

A more stringent link can be made to a 43-year-old patient with active neurosyphilis, who developed typical parkinsonism insidiously.[122] Penicillin treatment was followed by definite improvement in the parkinsonism. Another report mentioned a 66-year-old male with general paresis who developed bradykinesia and rigidity much later and in whom autopsy findings were similar to those found in PEP.[123]

FUNGAL AND PARASITIC INFECTIONS

Cryptococcal infection in the mesencephalon and specifically in the substantia nigra was sometimes demonstrated on autopsy.[124] Bilateral, small, hyperintense signals in basal ganglia were shown on MRI (on long T$_2$ weighted images) in a patient with AIDS and cryptococcal meningitis.[125] However, the development of subacute parkinsonism in patients with cryptococcal meningoencephalitis or cryptococcal granulomata is probably exceedingly rare.

The permanent parkinsonian syndrome that appeared in a young patient with cryptococcal meningitis after intraventricular administration of amphotericin B was considered to be a result of amphotericin B rather than the infection.[126]

Another patient developed parkinsonian features before the onset of meningoencephalitic symptoms, but they worsened dramatically thereafter and improved following anticryptococcal therapy. No basal ganglia lesions were seen on cranial computed tomography.[127] The role of cryptococcal infection remained unclear, as the period of observation was too short before the patient's death, and no autopsy was performed.

A more impressive correlation between parkinsonism and fungal infection was shown in a patient reported by Adler et al.[128] The patient, a young intravenous-drug user, developed subacute, asymmetric, severe parkinsonism, including pharyngeal akinesia. MRI revealed bilateral striatal abscesses which, at biopsy, showed the presence of hyphae, consistent with either aspergillus or mucor. After systemic amphotericin B therapy, the parkinsonism improved, together with shrinkage of the striatal lesions.

Interestingly, in an experimental model, mice injected with *Nocardia asteroides* developed L-dopa-responsive extrapyramidal disorder, associated with hyaline inclusion bodies that resembled Lewy bodies, suggesting that *Nocardia* may localize and grow within the brain.[129]

Neurocysticercosis as a cause of acute-onset parkinsonism was reported in a single case. During an abrupt aggravation of known neurocysticercosis treated with praziquantel, this patient developed asymmetric parkinsonism that was attributed to cysticercus cysts located by MRI within the midbrain. The extrapyramidal symptoms were entirely reversible.[130]

CREUTZFELDT-JAKOB DISEASE (CJD)

Although CJD is not strictly an infectious disease, it is potentially transmissible.[131,132] The symptomatology is diverse and, even in one subtype, the genetic form related to the codon 200 mutation in the prion protein gene, there is phenotypic variability.[133,134] The main features are mental deterioration, cerebellar ataxia, and involuntary movements. The characteristic pathology, spongiform changes, predominates within the cortex and basal ganglia. Rigidity very rarely occurs at onset but later is quite common. Brown et al.[134] have found that 56 percent of patients with sporadic CJD developed extrapyramidal symptomatology during the course of the disease, as compared with 9 percent on their first examination.

In new-variant CJD, which is a definitely transmitted disease, parkinsonism has not been described. However, these patients are younger than sporadic CJD cases, and this might explain their resistance.

WHIPPLE'S DISEASE

The pathognomonic movement disorder in Whipple's disease is oculomasticatory myorhythmia. A unique patient who developed bilateral rigidity and bradykinesia was reported by Uldry and Bogousslavsky.[123a,135] MRI showed lesions in basal ganglia. Treatment with trimethoprim-sulfamethoxazole partially reversed the extrapyramidal features.

References

1. von Economo C: Encephalitis lethargica. *Wien Klin Wochnschr* 30:581–585, 1917.

2. Cruchet JR, Moutier J, Calmettes: A quarante cas d'encephalomyelite subaigue. *Bull Soc Med Hop Paris* 41: 614–646, 1917.

3. Anonymous: Encephalitis lethargica. *Lancet* 19:1396–1397, 1981.

4. Eadie MJ, Sutherland JM, Doherty RL: Encephalitis in the etiology of parkinsonism in Australia. *Arch Neurol* 12:240–245, 1965.

5. Duvoisin RC, Yahr MD: Encephalitis and parkinsonism. *Arch Neurol* 12:227–239, 1965.

6. Dimsdale H: Changes in Parkinson syndrome in the 20th century. *Q J Med* 15:155–170, 1946.

7. Duvoisin RC: Genetics of Parkinson's disease. *Adv Neurol* 45:447–480, 1986.

8. Poskanzer DC, Schwab RS: Studies in the epidemiology of Parkinson's disease predicting its disappearance as a major clinical entity by 1980. *Trans Am Neurol Assoc* 86:234–245, 1961.

9. von Economo C: *Encephalitis Lethargica: Its Sequelae and Treatment.* New York: Oxford University Press, 1931.

10. Wilson SAK: Epidemic encephalitis, in AN Bruce (ed): *Neurology.* London: Arnold, 1940, vol I, pp 99–144.

11. Martilla RJ, Halonen P, Rinne UK: Influenza virus antibodies in parkinsonism: Comparison of postencephalitic and idiopathic Parkinson patients and matched controls. *Arch Neurol* 34:99–100, 1977.

12. Esiri MK, Swash M: Absence of herpes simplex virus antigen in brain in encephalitis lethargica. *J Neurol Neurosurg Psychiatry* 47:1049–1050, 1984.

13. Elizan TS, Madden DL, Noble GR, et al: Viral antibodies in serum and CSF of parkinsonian patients and controls. *Arch Neurol* 36:529–534, 1979.

14. Elizan TS, Casals J: Astrogliosis in von Economi's and postencephalitic Parkinson's disease supports probable viral etiology. *J Neurol Sci* 105:131–134, 1991.

15. Reid AH, McCall S, Henry JM, Taubenberger JK: Experimenting on the past: The enigma of von Economo's encephalitis lethargica. *J Neuropathol Exp Neurol* 60:663–670, 2001.

16. Ravenholt RT, Foege WH: 1918 influenza, encephalitis lethargica, parkinsonism. *Lancet* 2:860–4, 1982.

17. Casals J, Elizan TS, Yahr MD: Postencephalitic parkinsonism: A review. *J Neural Transm* 105:645–676, 1998.

18. Oxford JS: Influenza A pandemics of the 20th century with special reference to 1918: Virology, pathology and epidemiology. *Rev Med Virol* 10:119–133, 2000.

19. McCall S, Henry JM, Reid AH, Taubenberger JK: Influenza RNA not detected in archival brain tissues from acute encephalitis lethargica cases or in postencephalitic Parkinson cases. *J Neuropathol Exp Neurol* 60:696–704, 2001.

20. Grinker RR, Bucy PC: *Epidemic Encephalitis in Neurology*, 4th edn. Oxford: Blackwell Scientific 1949, pp 651–663.

21. Krusz JC, Koller WC, Ziegler DK: Historical review: Abnormal movements associated with epidemic encephalitis lethargica. *Mov Disord* 2:137–141, 1987.

22. Oeckinghaus W: Encephalitis epidemica und Wilsonsches Krankleithbild. *Dtsch Z Nervenkr* 72:294–309, 1921.

23. McCowan PK, Cook LC: Oculogyric crises in chronic epidemic encephalitis. *Brain* 51:285–309, 1928.

24. Mulder DW, Parrott M, Thaler M: Sequelae of western equine encephalitis. *Neurology* 1:318–327, 1950.

25. Clough CG, Plaitakis A, Yahr MD: Oculogyric crises and parkinsonism. *Arch Neurol* 40:36–37, 1983.

26. Leigh RJ, Foley JM, Remler BF, Civil RH: Oculogyric crisis: A syndrome of thought disorder and ocular deviation. *Ann Neurol* 22:13–17, 1987.

27. Korczyn AD, Goldberg GJ: Extrapyramidal effects of neuroleptics. *J Neurol Neurosurg Psychiatry* 39:866–869, 1976.

28. Litvan II, Jankovic J, Goetz CG, et al: Accuracy of the clinical diagnosis of postencephalitic parkinsonism: A clinicopathologic study. *Eur J Neurol* 5:451–457, 1998.

29. Naville F: Etudes sur les complications et les sequelles mentales de l'encephalite epidemique: La bradyphrenie. *Encephale* 17:423–436, 1922.

30. Wenning GK, Jellinger K, Litvan I: Supranuclear gaze palsy and eyelid apraxia in postencephalitic parkinsonism. *J Neural Transm* 104:845–865, 1997.

31. Evidente VG, Gwinn KA: Post-encephalitic parkinsonism. *J Neurol Neurosurg Psychiatry* 5:64, 1998.

32. Evidente VG, Gwinn KA, Caviness JN, et al: Early cinematographic cases of postencephalitic parkinsonism and other movement disorders. *Mov Disord* 13:167–169, 1998.

33. Duncan AG: The sequelae of encephalitis lethargica. *Brain* 47:76–95, 1924.

34. Calne DB, Lees AJ: Late progression of postencephalitic Parkinson's syndrome. *Can J Neurol Sci* 15:135–138, 1988.

35. Geddes JF, Hughes A, Lees AJ, Daniel SE: Pathological overlap in cases of parkinsonism associated with neurofibrillary tangles: A study of recent cases of postencephalitic parkinsonism and comparison with supranuclear palsy and Guamanian Parkinson dementia complex. *Brain* 116:281–302, 1993.

36. Agid Y: Parkinson's disease. Pathophysiology. *Lancet* 337:1321–1324, 1991.

37. Vierrege P, Reinhardt V, Houauft B: Is progression in postencephalitic Parkinson's disease late and age-related? *J Neurol* 238:299–303, 1991.

38. Korczyn AD: Dementia in Parkinson's disease. *J Neurol* 248(suppl 3):1–4, 2001.

39. Calne DB: Is idiopathic parkinsonism the consequence of an event or a process? *Neurology* 44:5–10, 1994.

40. Appel SH, Le WD, Taijti J, et al: Nigral damage and dopaminergic hypofunction in mesencephalon-immunized guinea pigs. *Ann Neurol* 32:494–501, 1992.

41. Williams A, Houff S, Lees A, Calne DB: Oligoclonal banding in the cerebrospinal fluid of patients with postencephalitic parkinsonism. *J Neurol Neurosurg Psychiatry* 42:790–792, 1979.

42. Elizan TS, Terasky PL, Yahr MD: HLA-B14 antigen and postencephalic Parkinson's disease, their association in an American Jewish ethnic group. *Arch Neurol* 37:542–544, 1980.

43. Lees AJ, Stern GM, Compston DAS: Histocompatibility antigens and postencephalitic parkinsonism. *J Neurol Neurosurg Psychiatry* 45:1060–1061, 1982.

44. Gibb WR, Lees AJ: The progression of idiopathic Parkinson's disease is not explained by age-related changes: Clinical and pathological comparisons with postencephalitic parkinsonian syndrome. *Acta Neuropathol* 73:195–201, 1987.

45. Greenfield JG, Bosanquet FD. The brain stem lesions in parkinsonism. *J Neurochem* 16:213–226, 1953.

46. Forno LS: Pathology of parkinsonism. A preliminary report of 24 cases. *J Neurosurg* 1:266–271, 1966.

47. Haraguchi T, Ishizu H, Terada S, et al: An autopsy case of postencephalitic parkinsonism of von Economo type: Some new observations concerning neurofibrillary tangles and astrocytic tangles. *Neuropathology* 20:143–148, 2000.

48. Yen SH, Houroupian DS, Terry RD: Immunocytochemical comparison of neurofibrillary tangles in Alzheimer type dementia, progressive supranuclear palsy and postencephalitic parkinsonism. *Ann Neurol* 13:172–175, 1982.

49. Buee-Scherrer V, Buee L, Leveugle B, et al: Pathological tau proteins in postencephalitic parkinsonism: Comparison with Alzheimer's disease and other neurodegenerative disorders. *Ann Neurol* 42:356–359, 1997.

50. Hudson AY, Rice GPA: Similarities of Guamanian ALS/PD to postencephalitic parkinsonism/ALS: Possible viral cause. *Can J Neurol Sci* 17:427–433, 1990.

51. McGeer PL, Itagaki S, Akiyama H, McGeer EG: Rate of cell death in parkinsonism indicates active neuropathological process. *Ann Neurol* 24:574–576, 1988.

52. Solomon P, Mitchell RS, Prinzmetal M: The use of benzedrine sulfate in postencephalitic Parkinson's disease. *J Am Med Assoc* 108:1765–1770, 1937.

53. Parkes JD, Tarsy D, Marsden CD, et al: Amphetamines in the treatment of Parkinson's disease. *J Neurol Neurosurg Psychiatry* 38:232–237, 1937.

54. Mark MH, Duvoisin RC: The history of the medical therapy of Parkinson's disease, in Koller WC, Paulson G (eds): *Therapy of Parkinson's Disease*, 2nd edn. New York: Marcel Dekker, 1995, pp 1–20.

55. Calne DB, Stern GM, Laurence DR, et al: L-Dopa in postencephalitic parkinsonism. *Lancet* 12:744–747, 1969.

56. Hunter KR, Stern GM, Sharkey J: L-Dopa in postencephalitic parkinsonisms. *Lancet* ii:1366–1367, 1970.

57. Krasner N, Cornelius JM: L-Dopa for postencephalitic parkinsonism. *Br Med J* 4:496, 1970.

58. Sacks OW, Kohl M, Schwartz W, Messeloff C: Side effects of L-dopa in postencephalitic parkinsonism. *Lancet* i:1006, 1970.

59. Duvoisin RC, Antunes JL, Yahr MD: Response of patients with postencephalitic parkinsonism to L-dopa. *J Neurol Neurosurg Psychiatry* 35:487–495, 1977.

60. Schwab RS, England AC: Parkinsonian syndrome due to various specific causes, in Vinken PY, Bruyn GW (eds): *Handbook of Clinical Neurology*. Amsterdam: North-Holland, vol. 6, 1968, pp 227–245,

61. Bojinov S: Encephalitis with acute parkinsonism syndrome and bilateral inflammatory necrosis of substantia nigra. *J Neurol Sci* 12:383–415, 1971.

62. Herishanu Y, Noah Z: On acute encephalitic parkinsonism syndrome. *Eur Neurol* 10:117–124, 1973.

63. Rail D, Scholtz C, Swash M: Postencephalitic parkinsonism: Current experience. *J Neurol Neurosurg Psychiatry* 44:670–676, 1981.

64. Howard RS, Lees AJ: Encephalitis lethargica: A report of four recent cases. *Brain* 110:19–33, 1987.

65. Blunt SB, Lane RJM, Perkin GD: Encephalitis lethargica: Clinical features and management. *Mov Disord* 9:73, 1994.

66. Blunt SB, Lane RJ, Turjanski N, Perkin GD: Clinical features and management of two cases of encephalitis lethargica. *Mov Disord* 12:354–359, 1997.

67. Shen WC, Ho YJ, Lee SK, Lee KR: MRI of transient postencephalitic parkinsonism. *J Comput Assist Tomogr* 18:155–156, 1994.

68. McAuley J, Shahmanesh M, Swash M: Dopaminergic therapy in acute encephalitis lethargica. *Eur J Neurol* 6:235–237, 1999.

69. Kiley M, Esiri MM: A contemporary case of encephalitis lethargica. *Clin Neuropathol* 20:2–7, 2001.

70. Ghaemi M, Rudolf J, Schmulling S, et al: FDG- and Dopa-PET in postencephalitic parkinsonism. *J Neural Transm* 107:1289–1295, 2000.

71. Poser CM, Huntley CJ, Poland JD: Paraencephalitic parkinsonism: Report of an acute case due to coxsackie virus type B and re-examination of the aetiologic concepts of post-encephalitic parkinsonism. *Acta Neurol Scand* 45:199–215, 1969.

72. Walters JH: Postencephalitic parkinsonism syndrome after meningoencephalitis due to coxsackie virus group B, type 2. *N Engl J Med* 263:744–747, 1960.

73. Cree BC, Bernardini GL, Hays AD, Lowe G: A fatal case of coxsackievirus 4 meningo-encephalitis. *Arch Neurol* 60:107–112, 2003.

74. Yazaki M, Yamazaki M, Urasawa N, et al: Successful treatment with alpha-interferon of a patient with chronic measles infection of the brain and parkinsonism. *Eur Neurol* 44:184–186, 2000.

74a. Bennett N McK: Murray Valley Encephalitis, 1947: Clinical features. *Med J Aus* 2:746–750, 1976.

75. Alves RSC, Barbosa ER, Scaff M: Postvaccinal parkinsonism. *Mov Disord* 7:178–180, 1992.

76. Thieffry S: Enterovirus (poliomyelite, coxsackie, ECHO) et maladies du systeme nerveux: Revision critique et experience personnelle. *Rev Neurol* 105:753–776, 1963.

77. Solbrig M, Nashuf L: Acute parkinsonism in suspected herpes simplex encephalitis. *Mov Disord* 8:233–234, 1993.

78. Hsieh JC, Lue KH, Lee YL: Parkinson-like syndrome as the major presenting symptoms of Epstein-Barr virus encephalitis. *Arch Dis Child* 87:358, 2002.

79. Solomon T, Ooi MH, Beasley DWC, Mallewa M: West Nile encephalitis. *BMJ* 26:865–869, 2003.

80. Lin SK, Lu CS, Vingerhoets F, et al: Isolated involvement of substantia nigra in acute transient parkinsonism: MRI and PET observations. *Parkinsonism Relat Disord* 1:367–372, 1995.

81. Cerna F, Mehrad B, Luby JP, et al: St Louis encephalitis and the substantia nigra: MR imaging evaluation. *AJNR Am J Neuroradiol* 20:1281–1283, 1999.

82. Savant CS, Singhal BS, Jankovic J, et al: Substantia nigra lesions in viral encephalitis. *Mov Disord* 2:213–217, 2003.

83. Kun LN, Yian SY, Haur LS, Tjia H: Bilateral substantia nigra changes on MRI in a patient with encephalitis lethargica. *Neurology* 53:1860–1862, 1999.

84. Pradhan S, Pandey N, Shashank S, et al: Parkinsonism due to predominant involvement of substantia nigra in Japanese encephalitis. *Neurology* 53:1781–1786, 1999.

85. Verschuren H, Crols R: Bilateral substantia nigra lesions on magnetic resonance imaging in a patient with encephalitis lethargica. *J Neurol Neurosurg Psychiatry* 271:75, 2001.

86. Murgod UA, Muthane UB, Ravi V, et al: Persistent movement disorder following Japanese encephalitis. *Neurology* 57:2313–2335, 2001.

87. Holloway RG, Kieburtz KD: Neurologic manifestations of human immunodeficiency virus infection, in Mandell GL, Bennett JE, Polin R (eds): *Mandell, Douglas and Bennett's Principles and Practice of Infectious Diseases*, 5 edn. Philadelphia: Churchill-Livingstone, 2000, pp 1432–1439.

88. Berger JR, Arendt G: HIV dementia: The role of the basal ganglia and dopaminergic systems. *J Psychopharmacol* 14:214–221, 2000.

89. Hriso E, Kuhn T, Masdeu JC, Grundman M: Extrapyramidal symptoms due to dopamine-blocking agents in patients with AIDS encephalopathy. *Am J Psychiatry* 148:1558–1561, 1991.

90. Reyes MG, Faraldi A, Senseng CS, et al: Nigral degeneration in acquired immune deficiency syndrome (AIDS). *Acta Neuropathol* 82:39–44, 1991.

91. Factor SA, Podskalny GD, Barron KD: Persistent neuroleptic-induced rigidity and dystonia in AIDS dementia complex: A clinicopathological case report. *J Neurol Sci* 127:114-120, 1994.

92. Nath A, Anderson C, Jones M, et al: Neurotoxicity and dysfunction of dopaminergic systems associated with AIDS dementia. *J Psychopharmacol* 14:222–227, 2000.

93. Koutsilieri E, Sopper S, Scheller C, et al: Parkinsonism in HIV dementia. *J Neural Transm* 109:767–775, 2002.

94. Itoh K, Mehrain P, Weis S: Neuronal damage of the substantia nigra in HIV-1 infected brains. *Acta Neuropathol (Berl)* 99:376–384, 2000.

95. Trillo-Pazos G, Diamanturos A, Rislove L, et al: Detection of HIV-1 DNA in microglia/macrophages, astrocytes and neurons isolated from brain tissue with HIV-1 encephalitis by laser capture microdissection. *Brain Pathol* 13:144–154, 2003.

96. Thompson KA, McArthur JC, Wesselingh SL: Correlation between neurological progression and astrocyte apoptosis in HIV-associated dementia. *Ann Neurol* 49:745–752, 2001.

97. Sabri F, Titanji K, De Milito A, Chiodi F: Astrocyte activation and apoptosis: Their roles in the neuropathology of HIV infection. *Brain Pathol* 13:84–94, 2003.

98. Berger JR, Kumar K, Kumar A, et al: Cerebral fluid dopamine in HIV-1 infection. *AIDS* 8:67–71, 1994.

99. Moller HE, Vermathen P, Lentschig MG, et al: Metabolic characterization of AIDS dementia complex by spectroscopic imaging. *J Magn Reson Imaging* 9:10–18, 1999.

100. von Giesen HJ, Antke C, Hefter H, et al: Potential time course of human immunodeficiency virus type 1-associated minor motor deficits: Electrophysiologic and positron emission tomography findings. *Arch Neurol* 57:160–167, 2000.

101. Arendt G, von Giesen HJ: Human immunodeficiency virus dementia: Evidence of a subcortical process from studies of fine finger movements. *J Neurovirol* 8(suppl 2):27–32, 2002.

102. De Mattos JP, Rosso AL, Correa RB, Novis S: Involuntary movements and AIDS. Report of seven cases and review of the literature. *Arq Neuropsiquiatr* 51:4917, 1993.

103. De Mattos JP, Rosso AL, Correa RB, Novis SA: Movement disorders in 28 HIV-infected patients. *Arq Neuropsiquiatr* 60:525–530, 2002.

104. Mirsattari SM, Power C, Nath A: Parkinsonism with HIV infection. *Mov Disord* 13:684–689, 1998.

105. Cardoso F: HIV-related movement disorders. *CNS Drugs* 16:663–668, 2002.

106. De la Fuente-Aguado J, Bordon J, Moreno JA, et al: Parkinsonism in an HIV-infected patient with hypodense cerebral lesion. *Tuber Lung Dis* 77:191–192, 1996.

107. Maggi P, Mari M, Moramarco A, et al: Parkinsonism in a patient with AIDS and cerebral opportunistic granulomatous lesions. *Neurol Sci* 21:173–176, 2000.

108. Murakami T, Nakajima M, Nakamura T, et al: Parkinsonian symptoms as an initial manifestation in a Japanese patient with acquired immunodeficiency syndrome and *Toxoplasma* infection. *Int Med* 39:1111–1114, 2000.

109. Hersh BP, Rajendran PR, Battinelli D: Parkinsonism as the presenting manifestation of HIV infection: Improvement on HAART. *Neurology* 56:278–279, 2001.

110. Mintz M, Tardieu M, Hoyt L, et al: Levodopa therapy improves motor function in HIV-children with extrapyramidal syndromes. *Neurology* 47:1583–1585, 1995.

111. Czub S, Koutsilieri E, Sopper S, et al: Enhancement of CNS pathology in early simian immunodeficiency virus infection by dopaminergic drugs. *Acta Neuropathol* 101:85–91, 2001.

112. Lera G, Zirulnik J. Pilot study with clozapine in patients with HIV-associated psychosis and drug-induced parkinsonism. *Mov Disord* 14:128–131, 1999.

113. Sacktor N: The epidemiology of human immunodeficiency virus-associated neurological disease in the era of highly active antiretroviral therapy. *J Neurovirol* 8:115–121, 2002.

114. Langford TD, Letendre SL, Larrea GJ, Masliach E: Changing patterns in the neuropathogenesis of HIV during the HAART era. *Brain Pathol* 13:195–210, 2003.

115. Kandanearatchi A, Williams B, Everall IP: Assessing the efficacy of highly active antiretroviral therapy in the brain. *Brain Pathol* 13:104–110, 2003.

116. Lambotte O, Deiva K, Tardieu M: HIV-1 persistence viral reservoir and the central nervous system in the HAART era. *Brain Pathol* 13:95–103, 2003.

117. Neuenburg JK, Brodt HR, Herndier BG, et al: HIV-related neuropathology, 1985 to 1999: Rising prevalence of HIV encephalopathy in the era of highly active antiretroviral therapy. *J Acquir Immune Defic Syndr* 31:171–177, 2002.

118. Al Mateen M, Gibbs M, Dietrich R, et al: Encephalitis lethargica-like illness in a girl with mycoplasma infection. *Neurology* 38:1155–1158, 1988.

119. Saitoh S, Wada T, Narita M, et al: *Mycoplasma pneumoniae* infection may cause striatal lesions leading to acute neurologic dysfunction. *Neurology* 43:2150–2151, 1993.

120. Kim JS, Choi IS, Lee MC: Reversible parkinsonism and dystonia following probable *Mycoplasma pneumoniae* infection. *Mov Disord* 10:510–512, 1995.

121. Denny-Brown D: Syphilitic parkinsonism, in *Diseases of the Basal Ganglia and Subthalamic Nucleus*. New York: Oxford University Press, 1945, p 299.

122. Neill KJ: An unusual case of syphilitic parkinsonism. *Br Med J* 2:320–322, 1953.

123. Matsuyama Y, Fukunaga H, Takayama S: Parkinson's disease of postencephalitic type following general paresis: An autopsied case. *Folia Psychiatr Neurol Jpn* 37:85–93, 1983.

124. Weenink HR, Bruyn GW: Cryptococcosis of the nervous system, in Vinken PJ, Bruyn GW, Klawans HL (eds): *Handbook of Clinical*

Neurology. Amsterdam: Elsevier/North-Holland, 1978, vol 35, pp 459–502.

125. Balakrishnau J, Becker PS, Jumar AY, et al: Acquired immune deficiency syndrome: Correlation of radiologic and pathologic findings in the brain. *Radiographics* 10:201–216, 1990.

126. Fisher JF, Dewald J: Parkinsonism associated with intraventricular amphotericin B. *J Antimicrob Chemother* 12:97–99, 1983.

127. Wszolek Z, Monsour H, Smith P, Pfeiffer R: Cryptococcal meningoencephalitis with Parkinsonian features. *Mov Disord* 3:271–273, 1988.

128. Adler CH, Stern MB, Brooks ML: Parkinsonism secondary to bilateral striatal fungal abscesses. *Mov Disord* 4:333–337, 1989.

129. Kohbata S, Beaman BL: L–Dopa-responsive movement disorder caused by *Nocardia asteroides* localized in the brains of mice. *Infect Immun* 59:181–191, 1991.

130. Verma A, Berger JR, Bower BC, Sanchez-Ramos J: Reversible parkinsonism syndrome complicating cysticercus midbrain encephalitis. *Mov Disord* 10:215–219, 1995.

131. Brown P, Gibbs CY, Rodgers-Johnson P, et al: Human spongiform encephalopathy: The NIH series of 300 cases of experimentally transmitted disease. *Ann Neurol* 35:513–529, 1994.

132. Chapman J, Brown P, Rabey JM, et al: Transmission of spongiform encephalopathy from a familial Creutzfeldt-Jakob disease patient of Jewish Libyan origin carrying the PRNP codon 200 mutation. *Neurology* 42:1249–1250, 1992.

133. Korczyn AD: Creutzfeldt-Jakob disease among Libyan Jews. *Eur J Epidemiol* 7:490–493, 1991.

134. Chapman J, Korczyn AD: Genetic and environmental factors determining the development of Creutzfeld-Jakob disease in Libyan Jews. *Neuroepidemiology* 10:228–231, 1991.

135. Uldry PA, Bogousslavsky J: Partially reversible parkinsonism in Whipple's disease with antibiotherapy. *Eur Neurol* 32:151–153, 1992.

Chapter 23

TOXIN-INDUCED PARKINSONIAN SYNDROMES

RAJESH PAHWA

MPTP-INDUCED PARKINSONISM   383
    Clinical Features   383
    Pathology   384
    Mechanism of Toxicity   384
    Treatment   384
MANGANESE   385
    Clinical Features   385
    Pathology   385
    Mechanism of Toxicity   386
    Treatment   386
CARBON MONOXIDE   386
    Clinical Features   386
    Pathology   387
    Mechanism of Toxicity   387
    Treatment   387
CARBON DISULFIDE   387
    Clinical Features   387
    Pathology   387
    Mechanism of Toxicity   388
    Treatment   388
CYANIDE   388
    Clinical Features   388
    Pathology   388
    Mechanism of Toxicity   388
    Treatment   388
METHANOL   388
    Clinical Features   388
    Pathology   388
    Mechanism of Toxicity   389
    Treatment   389
OTHER SOLVENTS   389
SUMMARY   389

A variety of toxins can induce parkinsonian syndrome, characterized by tremor, bradykinesia, rigidity, and postural instability. Manganese was the first toxin reported to cause parkinsonism in 1837.[1] The discovery of the neurotoxin MPTP (1-methyl-4-phenyl-1,2,3,6-tetrahydropyridine) as a cause of parkinsonism has benefited almost every aspect of Parkinson's disease (PD) research.[2] MPTP-induced parkinsonism in laboratory animals has become a standard and powerful tool in the laboratory investigation of parkinsonism.[2] In this chapter, we discuss the various toxins that can induce parkinsonism (Table 23-1).

TABLE 23-1 Various Toxins that Can Induce Parkinsonism

1-Methyl-4-phenyl-1,2,3,6-tetrahydropyridine (MPTP)
Manganese
Carbon monoxide
Carbon disulfide
Cyanide
Methanol

MPTP-Induced Parkinsonism

In 1947, Ziering et al.[3] synthesized the compound 1-methyl-4-phenyl-4-propionoxypiperdine (MPPP). This compound underwent testing as a possible antiparkinsonian drug.[4] Primates who received this compound became rigid and unable to move, and two humans died during or shortly after the study; this agent was therefore abandoned as a possible therapeutic agent.[4]

In 1979, Davis et al.[5] reported a 23-year-old college student who became parkinsonian after injecting a compound that he had synthesized. It is believed that the offending agent was a mixture of MPPP and MPTP.[6] The parkinsonian symptoms responded to L-dopa and bromocriptine and at autopsy there was neuronal loss in the substantia nigra.[5]

In 1982, an illicit chemist in northern California synthesized and distributed MPPP as a heroin substitute.[7] Due to shortcuts in the synthesis, he produced a mixture of MPPP and MPTP that resulted in a number of young addicts being admitted with acute parkinsonism. Samples of the substance used by the addicts were analyzed and MPPP and MPTP were identified in the samples, and in one batch MPTP was the only compound identified.[8] Subsequent animal studies confirmed that MPTP was the neurotoxin that caused selective and irreversible damage to the substantia nigra and produced clinical characteristics similar to those of PD.[9]

CLINICAL FEATURES

Although the majority of the 400 intravenous-drug users estimated to be exposed to MPTP[10] have remained asymptomatic, there are reports of addicts who developed mild-to-severe parkinsonism.[11-13] In the 7 patients reported to have developed moderate-to-severe parkinsonism, the acute reactions associated with intravenous use of MPTP included a burning sensation at the site of the injection followed by a high sensation and visual changes with hallucinations.[11] The majority of these patients experienced generalized jerking movements and 1 patient reported twisting postures of arms, legs, and neck. Within a few days, patients developed drooling, oily face, slow generalized movements, low-volume speech, and tremor.

All 7 of these patients developed rapidly progressive parkinsonian features within 2 weeks. The patients had the cardinal signs of PD, namely resting tremor, bradykinesia, rigidity, and postural instability. Other features of PD, including flexed posture, shuffling gait, micrographia, loss of associated movements, masked facies, freezing, and akinesia paradoxica, were also present. None of the patients had dementia[14] or associated corticospinal tract, cerebellar, or sensory findings.[11] These patients had a dramatic response to L-dopa and long-term complications of L-dopa therapy, namely dyskinesias, motor fluctuations, and psychiatric disturbances, occurred within weeks to months.[15] This is in contrast to PD, where it usually takes years for these adverse effects to occur. All these side-effects related to L-dopa therapy worsened over time.[2]

Tetrud and Langston[2] reported a series of 22 individuals who developed mild parkinsonism after exposure to MPTP. These individuals demonstrated parkinsonian features similar to early PD patients and the symptoms got progressively worse. Some of the asymptomatic individuals develop features of early PD over time. Two surveys carried out in a group of MPTP-exposed individuals have supported the findings of symptom progression.[10,16] One of the surveys was a retrospective chart review of individuals who complained of typical PD symptoms,[16] the second was a survey of 83 individuals exposed to MPTP who developed parkinsonian symptoms about 1 year after exposure.[10] Although these surveys suggest symptom progression, they cannot be considered definite as they relied on patient reports.

Snow et al.[17] used positron emission tomography (PET) scans to examine the distribution of striatal dopaminergic function in MPTP-induced parkinsonian patients. They scanned 9 patients with MPTP-induced parkinsonism and compared them to 10 patients with PD and 6 normal subjects. In the MPTP group there was an equal reduction of dopaminergic function in the caudate and putamen, in contrast to PD where there was a greater putaminal than caudate loss.

PATHOLOGY

Brains of 3 subjects with MPTP-induced parkinsonism have undergone detailed neuropathological evaluations.[5,18] Gross examination of the brain shows pale to almost completely depigmented substantia nigra. Microscopically there is moderate to severe depletion of pigmented nerve cells of the substantia nigra, along with gliosis and clustering of microglia around nerve cells. Lewy bodies or other inclusions are not present. One of the cases had large amounts of extraneuronal melanin.

In nonhuman primates, MPTP also causes selective pathologic changes. There is extensive damage to the tyrosine hydrolase-positive dopamine cells of the substantia nigra.[19–21] The cells in the centrolateral area of the zona compacta are more extensively damaged than the cells in the medial portion of the substantia nigra,[22] similar to the findings in PD.

MECHANISM OF TOXICITY

MPTP is the protoxin and is converted to MPP^+, which is the toxin responsible for cell damage in the substantia nigra.[23,24] MPTP is metabolized by extraneuronal monoamine oxidase B (MAO-B), located in the glial cells,[25] to 1-methyl-4-phenyl-2,3-dihydropyridinium ($MPDP^+$), which is converted to MPP^+.[26] Pretreatment of animals with MAO-B inhibitor blocks the toxicity of MPTP.[27,28]

MPP^+ enters the neurons through the dopamine uptake systems.[29] It is not exactly known why the toxicity is limited to the dopaminergic neurons in the substantia nigra. However, Langston and Irwin[30] proposed the following hypothesis. If the presence of a dopamine uptake system is a prerequisite for MPTP toxicity, there are three primary dopaminergic projection systems in the brain: hypothalamic dopaminergic system, ventral tegmental system, and the nigrostriatal system. The hypothalamic dopaminergic system is less avid[31] and hence would be more resistant to the toxicity of MPTP. The glia surrounding the substantia nigra but not the ventral tegmental area is rich in MAO-B,[30] and, hence, only the substantia nigra has all the requirements for the generation of toxic MPP^+.

Once MPP^+ enters the neuron, it was believed that it might kill cells through a process of free radical generation. The reason for this speculation was that MPP^+ has structural similarities to paraquat, which is a herbicide. Paraquat generates highly reactive oxygen species by a process called redox cycling.[32] However, with the use of isolated hepatocyte preparations, investigators have shown that MPP^+ alone does not undergo redox cycling and does not produce free radicals.[33,34]

Once within the cell, MPP^+ is accumulated by the mitochondria.[35] This process is dependent on the mitochondrial membrane gradient and appears to be driven by the mitochondrial membrane potential. In the mitochondria, MPP^+ appears to act by interfering with the mitochondrial energy metabolism, inhibiting nicotinamide adenine dinucleotide (NAD^+)-linked oxidation in complex J,[36–38] thereby interrupting the process of cellular energy production. In spite of lack of definitive evidence, most investigators believe that this energy depletion is the ultimate cause of cell death.[35]

TREATMENT

Patients with MPTP-induced parkinsonism have a dramatic and unequivocal response to L-dopa and dopamine agonists.[8,11,15] Unfortunately, they develop the long-term complications of L-dopa therapy, such as end-of-dose "wearing-off," peak-dose dyskinesias, on-off phenomenon, and psychiatric complications, including hallucinations and agitation.[15] However, these L-dopa complications occur much more rapidly than seen with PD.

In 1992, Widner et al.[39] reported the outcome of grafting human fetal tissue bilaterally to the caudate and putamen in

2 immunosuppressed patients with MPTP-induced parkinsonism. The patients were assessed 18 months preoperatively and 22–24 months after the surgery. Both patients had substantial, sustained improvement in motor function. Striatal uptake of fluorodopa as measured by PET scans showed marked increase in uptake on both sides, paralleling the patients' clinical improvement. However, this surgical technique is investigational and not widely used.

Manganese

Manganese is the twelfth most common element in the earth's crust and the fourth most widely used metal in the world.[40] Its main application is in the manufacture of steel. Manganese dioxide is used in the manufacture of dry batteries; methylcyclopentadienyl manganese tricarbonyl is used as an antiknock agent in gasoline. Potassium permanganate is used industrially for bleaching resins and fabrics, in printing fabrics, dyeing wood, tanning leather and for water purification, and these can also be sources of manganese intoxication.[41,42] Maneb, a fungicide, also contains manganese. Manganese plays an important role as a cofactor in many enzymatic reactions in humans, but excess amounts can cause irreversible damage to the central nervous system (CNS).

CLINICAL FEATURES

Couper[43] was the first to describe the effects of chronic manganese intoxication in 1837. He described 5 patients who worked in a manganese ore-crushing plant and developed clinical features similar to those of PD. The clinical syndrome has since been reported in miners, smelters, industrial and agricultural workers, in patients on long-term parenteral nutrition, and after ingestion of Chinese herbal pills.[44–49] The clinical syndrome of manganese intoxication can be divided into three stages: behavioral and psychiatric manifestations, parkinsonian features, and dystonia with severe gait disturbances.[42] The initial symptoms are nonspecific, such as fatigue, headache, muscle cramps, anorexia, insomnia, memory problems, and impotence. The miners usually have the psychiatric and behavioral manifestations ("manganese madness" or "locura manganesa") which are not present in industrial workers.[50,51] Psychiatric disturbances include nervousness, irritability, emotional instability, illusions, and hallucinations.[50,51] These usually last for 1–3 months. Parkinsonian features are similar to those of PD, and include seborrhea, increased sweating, soft speech, clumsiness with impaired dexterity, dystonic reactions, balance difficulties, and gait problems.[52] Bradykinesia and rigidity are the predominant signs. Tremor is infrequently observed and is usually upper extremity postural tremor. In the later stages of the disease, parkinsonian features are accompanied by severe dystonia of the trunk and extremities. The patients often have a peculiar gait ("cock walk"), in which the trunk is extended, arms are flexed and patients swagger on their toes. Limb and truncal dystonia is often present, resulting in painful cramps.[53,54] Other neurologic signs include corticospinal signs, dementia, cranial nerve palsies, sensory deficits, muscle weakness, and cerebellar dysfunction.[42] There may be progression of signs and symptoms even after withdrawal from the exposure.[52]

Manganese-induced parkinsonism should be suspected in patients with dystonic parkinsonism. Tremor is usually absent, and dystonia along with postural impairment occur early in the course of the illness. In addition, there is failure to have a sustained response to dopaminomimetic agents.[40] A history of occupational exposure to manganese is helpful. The value of testing biological specimens (blood, hair) for diagnosing manganese-induced parkinsonism is controversial. Blood manganese levels have been reported to be higher in healthy individuals exposed to manganese and lower in manganese-induced parkinsonian patients if they have been removed from exposure.[50] Manganese can be estimated in hair but the concentrations increase with the degree of pigmentation.[42] Electroencephalography, cerebrospinal fluid, and evoked potentials are generally normal.[52,55] Magnetic-resonance imaging (MRI) of the brain usually shows high signal intensity on T_1-weighted images in the globus pallidus.[56] These hyperintense signals on T_1-weighted images gradually disappear after cessation of exposure.[48,56] In patients with manganese-induced parkinsonism, PET studies with ^{18}F-6-fluoro-L-dopa are normal, and ^{11}C-raclopride (RAC) studies show that RAC binding is mildly reduced in the caudate and normal in the putamen; cerebral glucose metabolism studies show widespread decline in cortical glucose metabolism.[57,58]

PATHOLOGY

Pathological changes with manganesium intoxication result in neuronal loss and gliosis in the globus pallidus.[59,60] The changes are more extensive in the medial segment of the globus pallidus compared with the lateral segment. There is also some degeneration of the caudate nucleus and the substantia nigra reticulata. The areas of the brain that are affected inconsistently include the substantia nigra compacta, the pons, cerebral cortex, the thalamus, the hypothalamus, the red nucleus, and the cerebellum. Histologically, there is a prominent reduction of the myelinated fibers and astrocyte proliferation.[60,61] Bernheimer et al.[62] reported a case of depigmentation and cell damage in the substantia nigra with Lewy bodies; however, the case is atypical and the patient may have had PD.[40]

In primates exposed to manganese, postmortem studies have shown widespread lesions in the caudate and putamen,[63] as well as no significant atrophy in the pallidum or striatum.[64] There is a report of degeneration and depigmentation of the substantia nigra in primates after 18 months of exposure to manganese.[65]

MECHANISM OF TOXICITY

Normally, manganese functions in carbohydrate metabolism and gluconeogenesis. However, overexposure to manganese will result in neurotoxicity, possibly due to increased auto-oxidation of dopamine by a higher valence manganese (Mn^{3+}) ion causing increased generation of free radicals.[66,67] However, manganese in its Mn^{2+} form or in complexes such as superoxide dismutase is normally a scavenger of free radicals.[68,69] Barbeau[54] proposed that brain regions with high concentrations of oxidative enzymes, such as nuclei of the basal ganglia, promote the oxidation of Mn^{2+} to Mn^{3+}, which causes increased auto-oxidation of dopamine to toxic quinones and hydroxyl radicals. However, manganese toxicity also results in degeneration of nondopaminergic neurons in the pallidum, caudate, and putamen. It is postulated that the rich dopaminergic innervation of the striatum results in high extracellular concentrations of dopamine, which in the presence of Mn^{3+} are sufficient to injure the adjacent neurons.[51,70] Other possible theories include mitochondrial damage, leading to excitotoxic cell death, and enhanced iron and aluminum in the brain.[42] Manganese accumulates within the mitochondria[71] and can inhibit both the sodium-dependent and sodium-independent calcium efflux in the brain.[72] It can produce a bioenergetic defect by impairing oxidative phosphorylation and reducing ATP synthesis.[73] This can lead to calcium-dependent enzyme activation and cell death.

TREATMENT

Administration of the chelating agent ethylenediaminetetraacetic acid (EDTA) has not resulted in significant clinical improvement.[74] Open-label studies with L-dopa have reported some response to L-dopa.[53,75] Mena et al.[53] reported dramatic improvement with L-dopa of rigidity, hypokinesia, postural reflexes, and balance in 5 patients, and dystonia in 2 patients. One of the patients had L-dopa aggravation of weakness, postural impairment, tremor, hypokinesia, and hypotonia which improved with 5-hydroxytryptophan. There is another L-dopa report of cognitive improvement along with bradykinesia but not dystonia in 1 patient.[75] Cook et al.[74] and Greenhouse[76] reported patients that had none to some benefit with L-dopa. However, in a placebo-controlled study with L-dopa there was no change in motor scores, finger tapping, gait or dystonia in 6 patients.[77] There is one report of para-aminosalicylic acid improving two patients with chronic manganese poisoning.[78]

Carbon Monoxide

Carbon monoxide is a colorless, odorless, nonirritating gas that can cause CNS damage. Approximately 2–26 percent of affected individuals die due to acute intoxication with carbon monoxide,[79–83] and 2–49 percent of the survivors develop sequelae.[79,83–86] The recovery in patients with sequelae is 53–75 percent; the morbidity is 17–21 percent, and mortality is 8–25 percent.[79,85]

CLINICAL FEATURES

The sequelae due to carbon monoxide intoxication are divided into progressive and delayed relapsing.[87] In the progressive-type, acute encephalopathy due to carbon monoxide intoxication progresses directly into the vegetative state, whereas, in the delayed relapsing-type, neurological deficits develop after a period of recovery from the acute poisoning. Lee and Marsden[87] described 8 patients with progressive-type sequelae. The patients opened their eyes spontaneously 2–15 days after recovery from coma, but remained in a mute vegetative state. The patients were nonresponsive, rigid, spastic, bed-bound, and exhibited little or no spontaneous movement. In patients with delayed relapsing-type carbon monoxide intoxication, after the initial coma they recovered completely after a period of days to weeks.[85,88] The delayed symptoms may be parkinsonian or akinetic-mute. The parkinsonian patients have slow shuffling gait, loss of armswing, retropulsion, bradykinesia, rigidity, masked face, and occasionally resting tremor.[89] There may be fixed dystonia of the hands and feet.[87] Emotional change, confusion, memory disturbances, anxiety, and depression may occur.[79,85,87,90] In the akinetic-mute patients, initial mental changes progress to apathy and mutism along with motor deterioration. Incontinence, rigidity and primitive responses to painful stimuli may be present.[87] The delayed deterioration may progress, stop at any time during the progression or may improve subsequently.[87,91]

In a series of 156 patients evaluated 33 years after carbon monoxide poisoning, neurological symptoms were reported in approximately 49 percent of the patients.[92] These included sensory disturbances (26 percent), peripheral nerve symptoms (16 percent), pyramidal symptoms (14 percent), ataxia and cranial nerve abnormalities (7 percent), paroxysmal symptoms (6 percent), focal symptoms (5 percent), extrapyramidal symptoms (22 percent), and vegetative symptoms (37 percent).

Rare patients with tremor,[87,93] chorea,[94,95] myoclonus,[86,96] and Tourette syndrome[97] have also been described as sequelae of carbon monoxide intoxication. Choi and Cheon[98] examined 242 patients with carbon monoxide poisoning and reported movement disorders in 32 (13.2 percent). These included parkinsonism in 23 patients, dystonia in 5 patients, chorea in 3 patients, and myoclonus in 1 patient. Median latency for onset of these disorders included parkinsonism and chorea 4 weeks after exposure, dystonia 51 weeks after exposure, and myoclonus 8 weeks after exposure.

Patients with carbon monoxide intoxication may have a normal CT scan, white matter low-density lesions, bilateral globus pallidus lesions, or both white matter and globus pallidus lesions.[87,99–101] Mimura et al.[92] performed MRI in 129 of their 156 patients. They reported abnormal findings of cerebral atrophy (72 percent), pallidum lesions (38 percent), lacunar and cerebral infarctions (53 percent), and hippocampal atrophy (19 percent). Among the patients with extrapyramidal symptoms, pallidum lesions occurred in 59 percent of the cases. Follow-up computed tomography (CT) scans may show new lesions or progression of white matter and globus pallidus lesions.[87,102–104] Sohn et al.[105] reported a couple who were exposed to carbon monoxide and underwent MRI of the brain, proton magnetic resonance spectroscopy (MRS) and [123]I-*N*-(3-iodoprophene-2-yl)-2β-carbomethoxy-3β-(4-chlorophenyl)tropane dopamine transporter brain single-photon emission computed tomography (SPECT). MRI findings were compatible with other cases of carbon monoxide poisoning, and included white matter hyperintensities and hemorrhagic necrosis of the pallidum. SPECT scan showed a significant dopamine neuronal loss. MRS showed significant increase in Cho/Cr (Choline containing compounds/creatine) ratio and decreased NAA/Cr (*N*-acetyl-aspartate/creatine) ratio in the white matter, but not in the cortex. These results indicate severe white matter damage, including demyelination, axonal damage, and gliosis. Follow-up neurological examinations revealed complete recovery, including improvement in the high signals on the MRI, and improvements in the MRS in the white matter.

PATHOLOGY

The most prominent pathological changes with carbon monoxide poisoning are white matter changes and necrosis of the globus pallidus.[106–108] If death occurs a few hours after acute intoxication the pathological changes are similar to those seen with asphyxia. The brain appears swollen, with congestion of the capillaries and veins, along with petechial hemorrhages.[109] Three types of white matter damage have been reported: small multifocal necrotic lesions with fragmentation of axis cylinders, extensive diffuse necrotic lesions with severe axis cylinder damage, and diffuse demyelination with sparing of axis cylinders.[108,110] These changes may be due to differences in the severity of poisoning.[111]

Unilateral or bilateral necrosis of the globus pallidus is the most striking finding.[109,112] The hemorrhage or necrosis of the globus pallidus is limited to the anterior and superior part of the inner pallidum.[106,108,109] Rarely, the pallidum may be spared in cases of carbon monoxide encephalopathy, where the predominant finding is white matter lesions.[109,113]

MECHANISM OF TOXICITY

Carbon monoxide is an asphyxiant that has a much greater affinity for hemoglobin oxygen-binding sites compared to oxygen. It enters the blood, where it binds with the ferrous ion complex of protoporphyrin IX in hemoglobin and hence blocks the binding of oxygen.[41] This results in anoxia, leading to tissue damage. The globus pallidus is vulnerable to anoxic injury, which could be due to intrinsic metabolic

susceptibility[114] such as high oxygen consumption[115] and high iron content.[116] Carbon monoxide also blocks ATP production by binding to the cytochrome oxidase of the mitochondrial chain[41] and potentiates the injury due to anoxia.

TREATMENT

There have been some reports that L-dopa and anticholinergics have been helpful in a few patients.[117,118] Lee and Marsden[87] used anticholinergic drugs and carbidopa/L-dopa (375–750 mg/day) in 23 patients. Due to spontaneous improvement of the symptoms, they found it difficult to evaluate the benefits of these medications. None of their patients had a dramatic response, nor was there any deterioration after the medications were discontinued. Hyperbaric oxygen therapy is the fastest method of reversing the effects of acute carbon monoxide and prevents the development of delayed neurological sequelae.

Carbon Disulfide

Carbon disulfide is a clear, colorless and highly volatile liquid used in various industries, such as: the production of cellophane and viscose rayon; as a solvent for resins, fats, and rubber; the manufacture of carbon tetrachloride. It is also used as a fumigant, in combination with carbon tetrachloride, to treat corn, wheat, rye, and other grains.

CLINICAL FEATURES

There are three principal manifestations of carbon disulfide neurotoxicity: acute and chronic encephalopathy, peripheral and cranial neuropathies, and movement disorders. Nervousness, irritability, confusion, disorientation, insomnia, memory problems, and hallucinations are mental changes that can be seen with carbon disulfide intoxication.[119] Neurological findings associated with carbon disulfide exposure include peripheral sensorimotor neuropathy, cranial nerve and brainstem abnormalities, pyramidal and extrapyramidal dysfunction, cerebellar dysfunction, and rarely dystonia and choreoathetosis.[119–122] Resting tremor, gait abnormalities, decreased associated movements, and rigidity are the common parkinsonian features.[123,124] MRI may be normal or show a pattern consistent with central demyelination or lesions of the basal ganglia and corona radiata.[120,125]

PATHOLOGY

There have been very few reports of pathological findings after chronic carbon disulfide intoxication. The pathological changes in the brain show diffuse neuronal degeneration over the cerebral cortex, globus pallidus and putamen, and a decrease in Purkinje cells in the cerebellar cortex.[126,127]

In a rhesus monkey, following chronic exposure to carbon disulfide, bilateral necrosis of the globus pallidus and zona reticulata of the substantia nigra has been reported.[128]

MECHANISM OF TOXICITY

Carbon disulfide may induce neurotoxicity by the formation of dithiocarbamate metabolites.[129] Dithiocarbamate complexes are capable of chelating metal ions such as copper and zinc, which are of physiological importance.[130] It is also possible that carbon disulfide inhibits cytochrome oxidase and brain tissue respiration,[131] which induces lesions of the striatopallidum.

TREATMENT

There are no reports of dramatic improvement in parkinsonian features with L-dopa.

Cyanide

CLINICAL FEATURES

Cyanide poisoning may result from accidental or suicidal exposure through ingestion, injection, or asphyxiation with hydrocyanic fumes. A dose of 50 mg[132] or 0.5 mg per kg of body weight[133] has been estimated as the minimum lethal dose. Acute intoxication results in dizziness, headaches, confusion, restlessness, coma, and convulsions; death usually occurs within seconds to minutes.[51,134] The clinical picture also includes cardiac arrhythmias, and hypotension.[134] The mortality rate with acute cyanide poisoning is 95 percent.[135] Although survival following acute intoxication is rare, in those who recover consciousness parkinsonian features develop over a period of days.[135–137] Gait abnormalities, masked facies, infrequent blinking, rigidity, and weak hypophonic voice are the common parkinsonian features.[135–137] Mild postural and resting tremor has been reported.[135,136] Dystonia and dementia are other features that may occur.[135,137,138]

Immediately following acute intoxication, neuroimaging studies are unremarkable; however, after 3–6 months, bilateral symmetric lesions in the globus pallidus and posterior putamen are reported.[136–138] 6-Fluorodopa PET scan has revealed diffuse decreased activity in the posterior regions of the basal ganglia, similar to that in patients with PD.[136]

PATHOLOGY

Pathologic changes after acute cyanide intoxication have demonstrated selective destruction of the striatum, especially the globus pallidus.[139,140] Pathological findings in a patient with cyanide-induced parkinsonism demonstrated destruction of the putamen and globus pallidus.[135] There was also atrophy of the cerebellum, subthalamic nucleus and complete nerve cell loss, along with marked fibrous gliosis in the zona reticularis of the substantia nigra.[135] In experimental animals, multifocal lesions in the basal ganglia, cerebral cortex, cerebellum, and white matter are reported following a single large dose,[141–143] or many small doses, of cyanide.[143]

MECHANISM OF TOXICITY

Similar to the other neurotoxins discussed in this chapter, cyanide radicals inactivate cytochrome oxidase and other oxidative enzymes, leading to cell death due to tissue anoxia.[143]

TREATMENT

Amantadine, anticholinergics and carbidopa/L-dopa have been used in patients with cyanide-induced parkinsonism.[135–137] None of the patients had a dramatic response to these medications.

Methanol

Methanol is a common industrial solvent. It is a colorless, clear, volatile liquid with a weak odor and is slightly sweeter than ethanol.[144] Methanol poisoning commonly occurs from illegal adulteration of ethanol with methanol.[145,146] Suicidal or accidental poisoning can also occur from ingestion of industrial or household products that contain methanol (e.g., windshield wiper fluid).[147,148]

CLINICAL FEATURES

Acute intoxication with methanol results in severe acidosis, confusion, and coma.[149] Blindness due to retinal degeneration and subsequent optic atrophy is the most common deficit in patients who survive the acute intoxication.[149,150] There are multiple reports of parkinsonism developing a few days after acute intoxication with methanol.[149–153] Soft voice, masked facies, drooling, tremulousness, rigidity, bradykinesia, and slow shuffling gait are the common parkinsonian features reported. Limb and foot dystonia has also been reported.[153] CT and MRI scans demonstrate bilateral putaminal abnormalities, localized areas of cerebral edema, with necrosis and hemorrhage in the cortex, subcortical white matter, cerebellum, brainstem, and optic nerve.[149,151,153]

PATHOLOGY

Bilateral necrosis of the putamen along with optic atrophy and widespread lesions in the cerebral cortex, anterior horn and other gray matter nuclei are lesions often induced by methanol intoxication.[109,149,151] Although the duration of

TABLE 23-2 Clinical Features that are Common to MPTP-Induced Parkinsonism and PD

Resting tremor
Bradykinesia
Rigidity
Dramatic response of motor disabilities to L-dopa
Development of motor fluctuations, and dyskinesias
Progression of symptoms over time

survival after methanol ingestion determines the severity of the lesions, bilateral putaminal necrosis has been reported after survival of at least 24 hours.[152]

MECHANISM OF TOXICITY

The exact pathogenesis of methanol intoxication is controversial. Methanol is metabolized to formaldehyde and formic acid by liver alcohol dehydrogenase.[154] Formic acid is believed to be largely responsible for the severe systemic acidosis.[155,156] Since formaldehyde and formic acid achieve high concentrations within the putamen,[157] it is believed to have selective toxicity to the putamen. Toxicity of methanol is delayed in monkeys who receive 4-methylpyrazole, an inhibitor of liver alcohol dehydrogenase as formic acid is not produced.[156]

TREATMENT

There are reports of L-dopa and bromocriptine having dramatic improvement in rigidity, tremor, and hypokinesia in patients with methanol-induced parkinsonism;[150,153] however, other reports have not confirmed this finding.[149]

Other Solvents

Various other solvents have also been reported to cause parkinsonism. Uitti et al.[158] described a case of parkinsonism after the patient was sniffing lacquer thinner daily for 9 months. The constituents of lacquer thinner are toluene, methanol, ethyl acetate, xylene, n-hexane, isopropyl alcohol, isobutyl acetate, and isobutyl isobutyrate. Although methanol and n-hexane[159] have been reported to cause parkinsonism, the authors believed that toluene was the most likely toxin that produced parkinsonism in their patient. Hageman et al.[160] described 3 patients who developed a

TABLE 23-3 Clinical Features in MPTP-Induced Parkinsonism that Differentiate it and PD

Young age of onset (less than 40 years)
History of intravenous drug abuse
Rapidly progressive symptoms and complications of L-dopa therapy

variety of neurological features, including parkinsonism, after exposure to a variety of organic solvents, including toluene, xylene, methyl ethyl ketone, and resins. It is possible that mixtures of organic solvents may have a synergistic effect or an antagonistic effect, depending on the solvents in the mixture. Studies of long-term exposure to solvents may lead to identification of other specific neurotoxins that can cause parkinsonism.

Summary

Parkinsonism (especially rigidity and bradykinesia) following exposure to toxins is rare but can be present. MPTP-induced parkinsonism has clinical characteristics similar to those of PD (Tables 23-2 and 23-3). Unlike parkinsonism induced by MPTP, the other toxins usually cause rigidity and bradykinesia and usually do not respond to L-dopa (Table 23-4). These cases have lesions primarily in the pallidostriatum. Better understanding of toxin-induced parkinsonism may help find the cause of PD.

TABLE 23-4 Clinical Features Associated with PD and Toxin-Induced Parkinsonism

Clinical Features	PD	MPTP	Mn	CO	CS	CN	Methanol
Tremor	++	++	±	±	+	±	+
Bradykinesia	++	++	++	++	++	++	++
Rigidity	++	++	++	++	++	++	++
Gait abnormality	++	++	++	++	++	++	++
Dystonia	±	±	++	+	±	±	±
Mental changes	+	±	++	+	−	+	−
L-Dopa response	++	++	±	±	−	±	+
Motor fluctuations	++	++	−	−	−	−	−

PD, Parkinson's disease; MPTP, 1-methyl-4-phenyl-1,2,3,6-tetrahydropyridine-induced parkinsonism; MN, manganese-induced parkinsonism; CO, carbon monoxide-induced parkinsonism; CS, carbon disulfide-induced parkinsonism; CN, cyanide-induced parkinsonism; methanol, methanol-induced parkinsonism.
−, not present; ±, may be present; +, rarely present; ++, commonly present.

References

1. Crouper J: Sur les effets du peroxide de managanese. *J Chim Med Pharm Toxicol* 3:223–225, 1837.
2. Tetrud JW: Langston JW: MPTP and Parkinson's disease: One decade later, in Stern MB, Koller WC (eds): *Parkinsonian Syndromes*. New York: Marcel Dekker, 1993, pp 173–193.
3. Ziering A, Berger L, Heineman SD, Lee J: Piperidine derivatives. Part III. 4-Arylpiperidines. *J Org Chem* 12:911–914, 1947.
4. Langston JW, Langston EB, Irwin I: MPTP-induced parkinsonism in human and non-human primates: Clinical and experimental aspects. *Acta Neurol Scand* 70:49–54, 1984.
5. Davis GC, Williams AC, Markey SP, et al: Chronic parkinsonism secondary to intravenous injection of meperidine analogues. *Psychiatry Res* 1:249–254, 1979.

6. Markey SP: MPTP: A new tool to understand Parkinson's disease. *Discuss Neurosci* 3:11–51, 1986.

7. Langston JW: MPTP: The promise of a new neurotoxin, in Marsden CD, Fahn S (eds): *Movement Disorders 2*. London: Butterworths, 1987, pp 73–90.

8. Langston JW, Ballard P, Tetrud J, Irwin I: Chronic parkinsonism in humans due to a product of meperidine-analog synthesis. *Science* 219:979–980, 1983.

9. Langston JW, Forno LS, Rebert CS, Irwin I. Selective nigral toxicity after systemic administration of 1-methyl-4-phenyl-1,2,5,6-tetrahydropyridine (MPTP) in the squirrel monkey. *Brain Res* 292:390–394, 1984.

10. Ruttenber AJ, Garbe PL, Kalter HD, et al: Meperidine analog exposure in California narcotics abusers: Initial epidemiologic findings, in Markey SP, Castagnoli N Jr, Trevor AJ, Kopin IJ (eds): *MPTP: A Neurotoxin Producing a Parkinsonian Syndrome*. New York: Academic Press, 1986, pp 339–353.

11. Ballard PA, Tetrud JW, Langston JW: Permanent parkinsonism in humans due to 1-methyl-4-phenyl-1,2,3,6-tetrahydropyridine (MPTP): Seven cases. *Neurology* 35:949–956, 1985.

12. Tetrud JW, Langston JW, Redmond DE Jr, et al: MPTP-induced tremor in human and non-human primates. *Neurology* 36:308, 1986.

13. Tetrud JW, Langston JW, Garbe PL, Ruttenber JA: Early parkinsonism in persons exposed to 1-methyl-4-phenyl-1,2,3,6-tetrahydropyridine (MPTP). *Neurology* 39:1483–1487, 1989.

14. Stern Y, Langston JW: Intellectual changes in patients with MPTP-induced parkinsonism. *Neurology* 35:1506–1509, 1985.

15. Langston JW, Ballard PA: Parkinsonism induced by 1-methyl-4-phenyl-1,2,3,6-tetrahydropyridine (MPTP): Implications for treatment and the pathogenesis of Parkinson's disease. *Can J Neurol Sci* 11:160–165, 1984.

16. Langston JW: MPTP-induced parkinsonism: How good a model is it? in Fahn S, Marsden CD, Teychenne P, Jenner P (eds): *Recent Advances in Parkinson's Disease*. New York: Raven Press, 1986, pp 119–126.

17. Snow BJ, Vingerhoets FJG, Langston JW, et al: Pattern of dopaminergic loss in the striatum of humans with MPTP induced parkinsonism. *J Neurol Neurosurg Psychiatry* 68:313–316, 2000.

18. Langston JW, Forno LS, Tetrud J, et al: Evidence of active nerve cell degeneration in the substantia nigra of humans years after 1-methyl-4-phenyl-1,2,3,6-tetrahydropyridine exposure. *Ann Neurol* 46:598–605, 1999.

19. Burns RS, Chiueh CC, Markey SP, Ebert MN, et al: A primate model of parkinsonism: Selective destruction of dopaminergic neurones in the pars compacta of the substantia nigra by N-methyl-4-phenyl-1,2,3,6-tetrahydropyridine. *Proc Natl Acad Sci U S A* 80:4546–4550, 1983.

20. Langston JW, Forno LS, Rebert SC, Irwin I. Selective nigral toxicity after systemic administration of 1-methyl-4-phenyl-1,2,3,6-tetrahydropyridine (MPTP) in the squirrel monkey. *Brain Res* 292:390–394, 1984.

21. Waters CM, Hunt SP, Bond AB, et al: Neuropathological, immunohistochemical and receptor changes seen in marmosets treated with MPTP, in Markey SP, Castagnoli N Jr, Trevor AJ, Kopin IJ (eds): *MPTP: A Neurotoxin Producing a Parkinsonian Syndrome*. New York: Academic Press, 1986, pp 637–642.

22. Gibb WRG, Lees AJ, Jenner P, Marsden CD: Effects of MPTP in the mid-brain of the marmoset, in Markey SP, Castagnoli N Jr, Trevor AJ, Kopin I (eds): *MPTP: A Neurotoxin Producing a Parkinsonian Syndrome*. New York: Academic Press, 1986, pp 607–614.

23. Langston JW, Irwin I, Langston EB, Forno LS: 1-Methyl-4-phenyl-pyridinium ion (MPP$^+$): Identification of a metabolite of MPTP, a toxin selective to the substantia nigra. *Neurosci Lett* 48:87–92, 1984.

24. Sanchez-Ramos JR, Barrett JN, Goldstein M, et al: 1-Methyl-4-phenylpyridinium (MPP$^+$) but not 1-methyl-4-phenyl-1,2,3,6-tetrahydropyridine (MPTP) selectively destroys dopaminergic neurons in cultures of dissociated rat mesencephalic neurons. *Neurosci Lett* 72:215–220, 1986.

25. Uhl GR, Javitch JA, Snyder SH: Normal MPTP binding in parkinsonian substantia nigra: Evidence for extraneuronal toxin conversion in human brain. *Lancet* i:956–957, 1985.

26. Chiba K, Trevor AJ, Castagnoli N Jr: Metabolism of the neurotoxic tertiary amine, MPTP, by brain monoamine oxidase. *Biochem Biophys Res Commun* 120:574–578, 1984.

27. Langston JW, Irwin I, Langston EB, Forno LS: Pargyline prevents MPTP-induced parkinsonism in primates. *Science* 225:1480–1482, 1984.

28. Cohen G, Pasik P, Cohen B, et al: Pargyline and deprenyl prevent the neurotoxicity of 1-methyl-4-phenyl-1,2,3,6-tetrahydropyridine (MPTP) in monkeys. *Eur J Pharmacol* 106:209–210, 1985.

29. Javitch DA, D'Amato RJ, Strittmatter SM, Snyder SH: Parkinsonism-inducing neurotoxin, N-methyl-4-phenyl-1,2,3,6-tetrahydropyridine: Uptake of the metabolite N-methyl-4-phenylpyridine by dopamine neurones explains selective toxicity. *Proc Natl Acad Sci U S A* 82:2173–2177, 1985.

30. Langston JW, Irwin I: MPTP: Current concepts and controversies. *Clin Neuropharmacol* 9:485–507, 1986.

31. Demarest KT, Moore KE: Lack of high affinity transport system for dopamine in the median eminence and posterior pituitary. *Brain Res* 171:545–551, 1979.

32. Bus JS, Aust SD, Gibson JE: Paraquat: Model for oxidant-initiated toxicity. *Environ Health Perspect* 55:37–46, 1984.

33. Di Monte D, Jewell SA, Ekstrom G, et al: 1-Methyl-4-phenyl-1,2,3,6-tetrahydropyridine (MPTP) and 1-methyl-4-phenylpyridine (MPP$^+$) cause rapid ATP depletion in isolation hepatocytes. *Biochem Biophys Res Commun* 137:310–315, 1986.

34. Smith MT, Ekstrom G, Sandy MS, Di Monte D: Studies on the mechanism of 1-methyl-4-phenyl-1,2,3,6-tetrahydropyridine cytotoxicity in isolated hepatocytes. *Life Sci* 40:747–748, 1987.

35. Di Monte DA: Mitochondrial DNA and Parkinson's disease. *Neurology* 4(suppl 2):38–42, 1991.

36. Nicklas WJ, Vyas I, Heikkila RE: Inhibition of NADH-linked oxidation in brain mitochondria by 1-methyl-4-phenyl-1,2,3,6-tetrahydropyridine. *Life Sci* 36:2503–2508, 1985.

37. Poirier J, Barbeau A: 1-Methyl-4-phenyl-pyridinium-induced inhibition of nicotinamide adenosine dinucleotide cytochrome c reductase. *Neurosci Lett* 62:7–11, 1985.

38. Mizuno Y, Suzuki K, Sone N, Saitoh T: Inhibition of ATP synthesis by 1-methyl-4-phenylpyridinium ion (MPP$^+$) in isolated mitochondria from mouse brains. *Neurosci Lett* 81:204–208, 1987.

39. Widner H, Tetrud J, Rehncrona S, et al: Bilateral fetal mesencephalic grafting in two patients with parkinsonism induced by 1-methyl-4-phenyl-1,2,3,6-tetrahydropyridine (MPTP). *N Engl J Med* 327:1556–1563, 1992.

40. Calne DB, Chu NS, Huang CC, et al: Manganism and idiopathic parkinsonism: Similarities and differences. *Neurology* 44:1583–1586, 1994.

41. Spencer PS, Butterfield PG: Environmental agents and Parkinson's disease, in Ellenberg JH, Koller WC, Langston JW (eds): *Etiology of Parkinson's Disease.* New York: Marcel Dekker, 1995, pp 319–365.

42. Pal PK, Samii A, Calne DB: Manganese neurotoxicity: A review of clinical features, imaging and pathology. *Neurotoxicology* 20:227–238, 1999.

43. Couper J: On the effects of black oxide of manganese when inhaled into the lungs. *Br Ann Med Pharm* 1:41–42, 1987.

44. Canavan MM, Cobb S, Drinker CK: Chronic manganese poisoning. *Arch Neurol Psychiatry* 32:501–512, 1934.

45. Flinn RH, Neal PA, Fulton WB: Industrial manganese poisoning. *J Ind Hyg Toxicol* 23:374–387, 1941.

46. Rodier J: Manganese poisoning in Moroccan miners. *Br J Ind Med* 12:21–35, 1955.

47. Emara AM, El-Shawabi SH, Madkour OI, El-Samra GH: Chronic manganese poisoning in the dry battery industry. *Br J Ind Med* 28:78–82, 1971.

48. Ejima A, Imamura T, Nakamura S, et al: Manganese intoxication during total parenteral nutrition. *Lancet* 426:339, 1992.

49. De Krom MC, Boreas AM, Hardy EL: Manganese poisoning due to use of Chien Pu Wan tablets. *Ned Tijdschr Geneesk* 138:2010–2012, 1994.

50. Mena I, Marin O, Fuenzalida S, Cotzias GC: Chronic manganese poisoning: Clinical picture and manganese turnover. *Neurology* 17:128–136, 1967.

51. Sanchez-Ramos JR: Toxin-induced parkinsonism, in Stern MB, Koller WC (eds): *Parkinsonian Syndromes.* New York: Marcel Dekker, 1993, pp 155–172.

52. Huang CC, Chu NS, Song C, Wang JD: Chronic manganese intoxication. *Arch Neurol* 46:1104–1112, 1989.

53. Mena I, Court J, Fuenzalida S, et al: Modification of chronic manganese poisoning-treatment with L-dopa or 5-OH tryptophane. *N Engl J Med* 282:5–10, 1970.

54. Barbeau A: Manganese and extrapyramidal disorders. *Neurotoxicology* 5:13–36, 1984.

55. Mena I: Manganese poisoning, in Vinken PJ, Bruyn EW, Cohen MM, Klawans HL (eds): *Intoxications of the Nervous System, Part I. Handbook of Clinical Neurology.* Amsterdam: North-Holland, 1979, vol 36, pp 217–237.

56. Nelson K, Golnick J, Korn T, Angle C: Manganese encephalopathy: Utility of early magnetic resonance imaging. *Br J Ind Med* 50:510–513, 1993.

57. Wolters EC, Huang CC, Clark C, et al: Positron emission tomography in manganese intoxication. *Ann Neurol* 26:647–651, 1989.

58. Shinotoh H, Snow BJ, Chu NS, et al: Presynaptic and postsynaptic striatal dopaminergic function in patients with manganese intoxication: A positron emission tomography study. *Neurology* 48:1053–1056, 1997.

59. Canavan M, Cobb S, Drinker CK: Chronic manganese poisoning: Report of a case with autopsy. *Arch Neurol Psychiatry* 32:500–505, 1934.

60. Yamada M, Ohno S, Okayasu I, et al: Chronic manganese poisoning: A neuropathological study with determination of manganese distribution. *Acta Neuropathol* 70:173–178, 1986.

61. Banta RG, Markesbery WR: Elevated manganese levels associated with dementia and extrapyramidal signs. *Neurology* 27:213–216, 1977.

62. Bernheimer H, Birkmayer W, Hornykiewicz O, et al: Brain dopamine and the syndromes of Parkinson and Huntington: Clinical, morphological and neurochemical correlations. *J Neurol Sci* 20:415–425, 1973.

63. Mella H: The experimental production of basal ganglia symptomatology in macaque rhesus. *Arch Neurol Psychiatry* 11:405–417, 1923.

64. Van Bogaert L, Dallemagne MJ: Approaches expérimentales des troubles nerveux du manganisme. *Monatsschr Psychiatr Neurol* II: 60–89, 1943.

65. Gupta SK, Murthy RC, Chandra SV: Neuromelanin in manganese-exposed primates. *Toxicol Lett* 6:17–20, 1980.

66. Donaldson J, Labaella FS, Gesser D: Enhanced autoxidation of dopamine as a possible basis of manganese neurotoxicity. *Neurotoxicity* 2:53–64, 1981.

67. Donaldson J: The pathophysiology of trace metal: Neurotransmitter interaction in the CNS. *Trends Pharmacol Sci* 1:75–77, 1981.

68. Kono Y, Takahashi M, Asada K: Oxidation of manganous pyrophosphate by superoxide radicals and illuminated spinach chloroplasts. *Arch Biochem Biophys* 174:454–461, 1976.

69. Archibald FS, Fridovich I: Manganese, superoxide dismutase and oxygen tolerance in some lactic acid bacteria. *J Bacteriol* 146:928–936, 1981.

70. Graham DG: Catecholamine toxicity: A proposal for the molecular pathogenesis of manganese neurotoxicity and Parkinson's disease. *Neurotoxicology* 5:83–96, 1984.

71. Maynard LS, Cotzias GC: The partition of manganese among organs and intracellular organelles of the rat. *J Biol Chem* 214:489–495, 1955.

72. Gavin CE, Gunter KK, Gunter TE: Manganese and calcium efflux kinetics in brain mitochondria. Relevance to manganese toxicity. *Biochem J* 266:329–334, 1990.

73. Brouillet EP, Shinobu L, McGarvey U, et al: Manganese injection into the rat striatum produces excitotoxic lesions by impairing energy metabolism. *Exp Neurol* 120:89–94, 1993.

74. Cook DG, Fahn S, Brait KA: Chronic manganese intoxication. *Arch Neurol* 30:59–64, 1974.

75. Rosenstock HA, Simons DG, Meyer JS: Chronic manganism: neurologic and laboratory studies during treatment with levodopa. *JAMA* 217:1354–1358, 1971.

76. Greenhouse AH: Manganese intoxication in the United States. *Trans Am Neurol Assoc* 96:248–249, 1971.

77. Lu CS, Huang CC, Chu NS, Calne DB: Levodopa failure in chronic manganism. *Neurology* 44:1600–1602, 1994.

78. Ky S, Deng H, Xie P, Hu W: A report of two cases of chronic serious manganese poisoning treated with sodium paraaminosalicylic acid. *Br J Ind Med* 49:66–69, 1992.

79. Shillito JH, Drinker CK, Sahgnessy TJ: The problem of nervous and mental sequelae in carbon monoxide poisoning. *JAMA* 106:669–674, 1936.

80. Meigs JW, Hughes JPW: Acute carbon monoxide poisoning. *Arch Ind Hyg Occup Med* 6:344–356, 1952.

81. Richarson JC, Chambers RA, Heywood PM: Encephalopathies of anoxia and hypoglycemia. *Arch Neurol* 1:178–182, 1959.

82. Bour H, Tutin M, Pasquier P: The central nervous system and carbon monoxide poisoning. I. Clinical data with reference to 20 fatal cases. *Prog Brain Res* 24:1–30, 1967.

83. Smith J, Brandon S: Morbidity from acute carbon monoxide poisoning at three year follow up. *Br Med J* 1:318–320, 1970.

84. Norkool DM, Kirkpatrick JN: Treatment of acute carbon monoxide poisoning with hyperbaric oxygen: A review of 115 cases. *Ann Emerg Med* 14:1168–1171, 1985.

85. Choi IS: Delayed neurological sequelae in carbon monoxide intoxication. *Arch Neurol* 40:433–435, 1983.

86. Mathieu D, Nolf M, Durocher A, et al: Acute carbon monoxide poisoning. Risk of late sequelae and treatment by hyperbaric oxygen. *Clin Toxicol* 23:315–324, 1985.

87. Lee MS, Marsden CD: Neurological sequelae following carbon monoxide poisoning. Clinical course and outcome according to the clinical types and brain computed tomography scan findings. *Mov Disord* 9:550–558, 1994.

88. Siesjö BK: Carbon monoxide poisoning: Mechanism of damage, late sequelae and therapy. *Clin Toxicol* 23:247–248, 1985.

89. Min SK: A brain syndrome associated with delayed neuropsychiatric sequelae following acute carbon monoxide intoxication. *Acta Psychiatr Scand* 73:80–86, 1986.

90. Lacey DJ: Neurological sequelae of acute carbon monoxide intoxication. *Am J Dis Child* 135:145–147, 1981.

91. Ginsberg MD: Delayed neurological deterioration following hypoxia. *Adv Neurol* 26:21–43, 1979.

92. Mimura K, Harada M, Sumiyoshi S, et al: Long-term follow-up study on sequelae of carbon monoxide poisoning: Serial investigation 33 years after poisoning. *Seishin Shinkeigaku Zasshi* 101:592–618, 1999.

93. Raskin N, Mullaney OC: The mental and neurological sequelae of carbon monoxide asphyxia in a case observed for fifteen years. *J Nerv Ment Dis* 92:640–659, 1940.

94. Schwarz A, Hennerici M, Wegener OH: Delayed choreoathetosis following carbon monoxide poisoning. *Neurology* 35:98–99, 1985.

95. Davous P, Rondot P, Marion MH, Guerguen B: Severe chorea after carbon monoxide poisoning. *J Neurol Neurosurg Psychiatry* 49:206–208, 1986.

96. Kim JS, Lee SA, Kim JS: Myoclonus, delayed sequelae of carbon monoxide poisoning. Piracetam trial. *Yonsei Med J* 28:231–233, 1987.

97. Pulst SM, Walshe TM, Rovero JA: Carbon monoxide poisoning with features of Gilles de la Tourette's syndrome. *Arch Neurol* 40:443–444, 1983.

98. Choi IS, Cheon HY: Delayed movement disorders after carbon monoxide poisoning. *Eur Neurol* 42:141–144, 1999.

99. Sawada Y, Takahashi M, Ohashi N, et al: Computed tomography as an indication of long-term outcome after acute carbon monoxide poisoning. *Lancet* i:783–784, 1980.

100. Miura T, Mitomo M, Kawai R, Harada M: CT of the brain in acute carbon monoxide intoxication: Characteristic features and prognosis. *Am J Neuroradiol* 6:739–742, 1985.

101. Hayashi R, Hayashi K, Inoue K, Yanagiasawa N: A serial computerized tomographic study of the interval form of CO poisoning. *Eur Neurol* 33:27–29, 1993.

102. Destee A, Courteville V, Devos PH, et al: Computed tomography and acute carbon monoxide poisoning. *J Neurol Neurosurg Psychiatry* 48:281–282, 1985.

103. Jaeckle RS, Nasrallah HA: Major depression and carbon monoxide-induced parkinsonism: Diagnosis, computerized axial tomography, and response to L-dopa. *J Nerv Ment Dis* 173:503–508, 1985.

104. Vieregge P, Klostermann W, Blümm RG, Borgis KJ: Carbon monoxide poisoning: Clinical, neurophysiological, and brain imaging observations in acute disease and follow-up. *J Neurol* 236:478–481, 1989.

105. Sohn YH, Jeong Y, Kim HS, et al: The brain lesion responsible for parkinsonism after carbon monoxide poisoning. *Arch Neurol* 57:1214–1218, 2000.

106. Garland H, Pearce J: Neurological complication of carbon monoxide poisoning. *Q J Med* 36:445–475, 1967.

107. Gordon EB: Carbon monoxide encephalopathy. *Br Med J* 1:1232, 1965.

108. Lapresle J, Fardeau M: The central nervous system and carbon monoxide poisoning. II. Anatomical study of brain lesion following intoxication with carbon monoxide, in Bour H, Ledingham IM (eds): *Progress in Brain Research*. Amsterdam: Elsevier, 1967, pp 31–74.

109. Jellinger K: Exogenous lesions of the pallidum, in Vincken PJ, Bruyn GW (eds): *Handbook of Clinical Neurology*. New York: Elsevier, 1986, pp 465–491.

110. Kobayashi K, Isaki K, Fukutani Y, et al: CT findings of the interval form of carbon monoxide poisoning compared with neuropathological findings. *Eur Neurol* 23:34–43, 1984.

111. Jefferson JW: Subtle neuropsychiatric sequelae of carbon monoxide intoxication: Two case reports. *Am J Psychiatry* 133:961–964, 1976.

112. Shiraki H: The neuropathology of carbon monoxide poisoning in humans with special reference to the change of globus pallidus. *Adv Neurol Sci* 13:25–32, 1969.

113. Ginsberg MD, Hedley-White ET, Richardson EP Jr: Hypoxic-ischemic leukoencephalopathy in man. *Arch Neurol* 33:5–14, 1976.

114. Vogt C, Vogt O: Erkrandungen der Grosshirnrunde im Lichte der Topistik, Pathoklise und Pathoarchitektonik. *J Psychol Neurol* 28:1–171, 1922.

115. Friede RL: Chemoarchitecture and neuropathology. *Proceedings of the 4th International Congress on Neuropathology*. Stuttgart: G Thieme, 1962, pp 70–75.

116. Dexter DT, Wells FR, Lees AJ, et al: Increased nigral iron content in post-mortem parkinsonian brain. *Lancet* ii:1219–1220, 1967.

117. Ringel RW, Klawans HL: Carbon monoxide induced parkinsonism. *J Neurol Sci* 16:245–251, 1972.

118. Klawans HL, Stein RW, Tanner CM, Goetz CG: A pure parkinsonian syndrome following acute carbon monoxide poisoning. *Arch Neurol* 39:302–304, 1982.

119. Lewey FH: Neurological, medical and biochemical signs and symptoms indicating chronic industrial carbon disulfide absorption. *Ann Intern Med* 15:869–883, 1941.

120. Peters HA, Levine RL, Matthews CG, Chapman LJ: Extrapyramidal and other neurological manifestations associated with carbon disulfide fumigant exposure. *Arch Neurol* 45:537–540, 1988.

121. Pentschew A: Intoxications, in Menckler J (ed): *Pathology of the Nervous System*. New York: McGraw-Hill, 1971, pp 1618–1650.

122. Frumkin H: Multiple system atrophy following chronic carbon disulfide exposure. *Environ Health Perspect* 106:611–613, 1998.

123. Peters HA, Levine RL, Mattews CG, et al: Carbon disulfide-induced neuropsychiatric changes in grain storage workers. *Am J Ind Med* 3:373–391, 1982.

124. Peters HA, Levine RL, Mattews CG, et al: Synergistic neurotoxicity of carbon tetrachloride/carbon disulfide (80/20 fumigants) and other pesticides in grain storage workers: *Acta Pharmacol Toxicol* 59(suppl 7):535–546, 1986.

125. Huang CC, Chu CC, Chen RS, et al: Chronic carbon disulfide encephalopathy. *Eur Neurol* 36:364–368, 1996.

126. Alpers BJ, Lewy FH: Changes in the nervous system following carbon disulfide poisoning in animals and in man. *Arch Neurol Psychiatry* 44:725–726, 1940.

127. Ferraro A, Jervis GA, Flicker DJ: Neuropathologic changes in experimental carbon disulfide poisoning in cats. *Arch Pathol* 32:723–738, 1941.
128. Richter R: Degeneration of the basal ganglia in monkeys from chronic carbon disulfide poisoning. *J Neuropathol Exp Neurol* 4:324–353, 1945.
129. Bus JS: The relationship of carbon disulfide metabolism to development of toxicity. *Neurotoxicology* 4:73–80, 1985.
130. Barbeau A, Pourcher E: New data on the genetics of Parkinson's disease. *Can J Neurol Sci* 9:53–60, 1982.
131. Seppalainen AKM, Haltia M: Carbon disulfide, in Spencer RS, Schaumburg HM (eds): *Experimental Clinical Neurotoxicology.* Baltimore: Williams & Wilkins, 1980, pp 356–373.
132. Naughton M: Acute cyanide poisoning. *Anaesth Intensive Care* 2:351–356, 1974.
133. Dreisbach RH: *Handbook of Poisoning Prevention, Diagnosis and Treatment,* 11th edn. Los Altos, CA: Lange Med, 1993.
134. Pentore R, Venneri A, Nichelli P: Accidental choke cherry poisoning: Early symptoms and neurological sequelae of an unusual case of cyanide intoxication. *Ital J Neurol Sci* 17:233–235, 1996.
135. Uitti RJ, Rajput AH, Ashenhurst EM, Rozkilsky B: Cyanide-induced parkinsonism: A clinicopathologic report. *Neurology* 35:921–925, 1985.
136. Rosenberg NL, Myers JA, Wayne WR: Cyanide-induced parkinsonism: Clinical, MRI, and 6-fluorodopa PET studies. *Neurology* 39:142–144, 1989.
137. Feldman JL, Feldman MD: Sequelae of attempted suicide by cyanide ingestion: A case report. *Int J Psychiatry Med* 20:173–179, 1990.
138. Grandas F, Artieda J, Obesco JA: Clinical and CT scan findings in a case of cyanide intoxication. *Mov Disord* 4:188–193, 1989.
139. Edelman F: Ein Beitrag zur Vergiftung mit gasformiger Blausäure insbesondere zu den dabei auftretenden Geheinveränderungen. *Dtsch Z Nervenheilkd* 72:259–287, 1921.
140. Schmorl G: Demonstrationen 3. Gehirn bei Blausäurevergiftung. *Muench Med Wochenschr* 67:913, 1920.
141. Meyer A: Experimentelle Vergiftungsstudien. III. Über Gehirnveränderungen bei experimenteller Blausäurevergiftung. *Z Gesamte Neurol Psychiatr* 143:333–348, 1933.
142. Hurst EW: Experimental demyelination of the central nervous system. I. The encephalopathy produced by potassium cyanide. *Aust J Exp Biol Med Sci* 18:210–223, 1940.
143. Haymaker W, Ginzler AM, Ferguson RL: Residual neuropathological effects of cyanide poisoning: A study of the central nervous system of 23 dogs exposed to cyanide compounds. *Mil Surg* 111:231–246, 1952.
144. Von Burg R: Methanol toxicology update. *J Appl Toxicol* 14:309–313, 1994.
145. Bennett IL, Cary FH, Mitchell GL, Cooper MN: Acute methyl-alcohol poisoning: A review based on experiences in an outbreak of 323 cases. *Medicine* 32:431–463, 1953.
146. Mittal BV, Desai AP, Khade KR: Methyl alcohol poisoning: An autopsy study of 28 cases. *J Postgrad Med* 37:9–13, 1990.
147. Gonda A, Gault H, Churchill D, Hollomby D: Hemodialysis for methanol intoxication. *Am J Med* 64:749–758, 1978.
148. Glazer M, Dross P: Necrosis of the putamen caused by methanol intoxication: MR findings. *Am J Roentgenol* 160:1105–1106, 1993.
149. Mclean DR, Jacobs H, Mielke BW: Methanol poisoning: A clinical and pathological study. *Ann Neurol* 8:161–167, 1980.
150. Guggenheim MA, Couch JR, Weinberg W: Motor dysfunction as a permanent complication of methanol ingestion. *Arch Neurol* 24:550–554, 1971.
151. Potts AM, Praglin J, Farkas J, et al: Studies on the visual toxicity of methanol. *Am J Ophthalmol* 40:76–83, 1955.
152. Erlanson P, Frisz H, Hagstram K: Severe methanol intoxication. *Acta Med Scand* 117:393–408, 1965.
153. Davis LE, Adair JC: Parkinsonism from methanol poisoning: Benefit from treatment with anti-parkinsonian drugs. *Mov Disord* 14:520–522, 1999.
154. Ritchie JM: The aliphatic alcohols, in Goodman LS, Gilman A (eds): *The Pharmacological Basis of Therapeutics.* London: Macmillan, 1970, pp 135–150.
155. Clay KL, Murphy RC, Watkins WD: Experimental methanol toxicity in the primates: Analysis of metabolic acidosis. *Toxicol Appl Pharmacol* 34:49–61, 1975.
156. McMartin KE, Makar AB, Martin A, et al: Methanol poisoning. I. The role of formic acid in the development of metabolic acidosis of the monkey and the reversal by 4-methylpyrazole. *Biochem Med* 13:319–333, 1975.
157. Symon L, Pasztor E, Dorsch NWC: Physiological responses of local areas of the cerebral circulation in experimental primates determined by the method of hydrogen clearance. *Stroke* 4:632–634, 1973.
158. Uitti RJ, Snow BJ, Shinotoh H, et al: Parkinsonism induced by solvent abuse. *Ann Neurol* 35:616–619, 1994.
159. Tanner CM: Occupational and environmental causes of parkinsonism. *Occup Med* 7:503–513, 1992.
160. Hageman G, Van der Hoek J, Van Hout M, et al: Parkinsonism, pyramidal signs, polyneuropathy, and cognitive decline after long-term occupational solvent exposure. *J Neurol* 246:198–206, 199.

DRUG-INDUCED PARKINSONISM

JEAN P. HUBBLE

SPECIFIC NEUROLEPTIC AGENTS 395
CLINICAL FEATURES 396
PATHOGENESIS 397
TREATMENT OF NEUROLEPTIC-INDUCED
   PARKINSONISM 398
   Dopamine Storage and Transport Inhibitors 398
   Calcium-Channel Blockers 399
   Other Medications 399
SUMMARY 400

Many drugs can produce parkinsonism. The antipsychotic drugs or neuroleptics are well recognized in this regard. In the early 1950s, after its introduction for the treatment of psychiatric illness, reports were issued linking the neuroleptic chlorpromazine with various neurological side-effects, including parkinsonism.[1,2] In these early series, the incidence of drug-induced parkinsonism (DIP) varied from 4 percent to 40 percent.[3–5] Whereas investigators agreed on the clinical manifestations of the syndrome, they varied in their opinions regarding causative mechanism and identification of at-risk individuals. A clear dose-response was lacking: that is, there was no correlation between occurrence of parkinsonian signs and the amount of chlorpromazine administered.[5] It was initially hypothesized that DIP may be related to chlorpromazine-induced liver damage. In their study of DIP, Hall et al. found no relationship between liver function tests and the occurrence of this syndrome.[5] Similarly, these investigators were unable to corroborate the claim, made by others, that patients with the most pronounced antipsychotic drug benefit were most apt to develop DIP.

In subsequent years, additional neuroleptic compounds were developed and marketed. As the number of individuals exposed to this class of drugs grew, several distinct adverse reactions involving abnormalities in movement and tone were described. In 1961, Ayd reported extrapyramidal reactions, including DIP, dyskinesia, and akathisia in 39 percent of 3775 neuroleptic-treated patients.[6] In searching for clues to the cause of DIP, Ayd found that the syndrome developed over a shorter time period in individuals treated with the piperazine and fluorinated phenothiazine compounds.

Specific Neuroleptic Agents

It is now recognized that parkinsonism can result from the use of numerous drugs among the various types of neuroleptics (Table 24-1). Certain neuroleptics, such as thioridazine and molindone, have fewer reported extrapyramidal side-effects; thus, the risk of DIP may be less with their use. However, well-controlled comparison studies substantiating this notion are lacking. In one series, thioridazine was the third most common offending drug, after haloperidol and amitriptyline-perphenazine, among 125 patients followed for drug-induced movement disorders at a referral specialty clinic.[7]

The atypical neuroleptic, clozapine, has a low incidence of extrapyramidal side-effects, including parkinsonism.[8] This is attributed to the relative specificity of clozapine's dopamine receptor blockade. The introduction of clozapine offered particular promise for the treatment of psychosis in patients with Parkinson's disease (PD).[9] Confusion, agitation, and hallucinations can occur in PD as a result of dopaminergic

TABLE 24-1 Neuroleptics and Related Agents

Trade Name	Generic Name
Phenothiazines	
Compazine	Prochlorperazine
Etrafon (Triavil)	Perphenazine and amitripyline
Levoprome	Methotrimeprazine
Mellaril	Thioridazine
Phenergen	Promethazine
Prolixin	Fluphenazine
Norzine	Thiethylperazine
Serentil	Mesoridazine
Sparine	Promaxine
Stelazine	Trifluoperazine
Thorazine	Chlorpromazine
Torecan	Thiethylperazine
Trilafon	Perphenazine
Butyrophenones	
Haldol	Haloperidol
Fentanyl	Droperidol
Thioxanthenes	
Navane	Thiothixene
Taractran	Chlorprothixene
Benzamides	
Reglan	Metoclopramide
Dihydroindolone	
Moban	Molindone
Dibenzoxazepine	
Loxitane	Loxapine
Dibenzodiazepine	
Clozaril	Clozapine
Seroquel	Quetiapine
Others	
Zofran	Ondansetron
Geodon	Ziprasidone

drug therapy, the primary disease process or unrelated psychiatric disorders. Conventional antipsychotics are poorly tolerated in the PD patient because of the propensity of these drugs to exacerbate parkinsonian symptoms. In addition to its reported efficacy in the control of psychosis, clozapine may reduce tremor and motor fluctuations in PD.[10,11] However, clozapine at higher doses (75–250 mg/day) in PD patients has been associated with sedation and delirium.[12] In a placebo-controlled study, clozapine has shown to be a relatively safe and effective remedy for drug-induced psychosis in PD.[13] In this study, relatively small doses of clozapine (25–75 mg at bedtime) suppressed hallucinations and other psychotic features in the majority of subjects. In an open-label study, the effects of clozapine was studied in 6 patients with HIV-associated psychosis who had developed DIP in the past when taking typical neuroleptic drugs.[14] Significant improvement in psychotic symptoms were achieved in all subjects with an average drug dose of 27 mg/day. Parkinsonian features were reported to improve by an average of 76 percent by the end of this 3-month study. The association of this drug with hematologic abnormalities, including fatal agranulocytosis, necessitates frequent blood count monitoring in all treated individuals. The concern over the potential for neutropenia, coupled with the cost and inconvenience of frequent blood tests, has limited the use of this agent.

Other atypical antipsychotic drugs have been developed and released subsequent to clozapine. Included among these medications are risperidone, olanzapine, and quetiapine. The effects of olanzapine in the treatment of drug-induced psychosis in PD has been studied.[15] In this report, Goetz et al. found olanzapine to be effective in reducing hallucinations and other psychotic symptoms in this PD patient population, but the drug appeared to worsen the primary motor manifestations of the disease. The atypical neuroleptic agent quetiapine has also been studied as a potentially safe antipsychotic agent for PD patients.[16,17] Based on these open-label reports, quetiapine may effectively reduce psychotic symptoms (particularly visual hallucinations) in PD patients without worsening the primary motor manifestations of the disease. Doses of quetiapine used in these studies varied from 25 to 300 mg/day.

Although neuroleptics are used primarily as antipsychotic agents, it is important to recognize their other nonpsychiatric uses. These drugs are sometimes prescribed for depression, anxiety, and insomnia. Typically used to control nausea and vomiting, prochlorperazine and related agents belong to the neuroleptic class of drugs and can produce DIP.[18] Metoclopramide, an atypical neuroleptic belonging to the benzamide class, is used to ameliorate gastric stasis and is used as an antiemetic; various extrapyramidal reactions, including parkinsonism, have been associated with its use.[19–21] In one series, 5 of 2557 metoclopramide-treated patients developed parkinsonism; all affected individuals were over 40 years of age.[22] In countries outside the US, other benzamide derivatives are available. This includes sulpiride, tiapride, metoclopramide, and cisapride, which were all associated

with drug-induced parkinsonism in a review by Kuzuhara in Japan.[23]

Clinical Features

Clinical descriptions of neuroleptic-induced parkinsonism date back to the original reports in the 1960s. In 1961, Ayd reported on DIP's responsiveness to anticholinergic medications, noted its usual abatement with the discontinuation of the offending drug and distinguished it clinically from PD.[6] Ayd also reported it to be more common in women and in the elderly. It was initially suggested that neuroleptic-induced parkinsonism resembled postencephalitic parkinsonism, rather than PD.[24] However, subsequent work suggests that the clinical manifestation of this syndrome is quite similar to that of PD.[25] Bradykinesia, rigidity, postural abnormalities, and tremor may occur. Bradykinesia is the earliest, most common and, frequently, the only manifestation of DIP, accounting for the expressionless face, loss of associated movements, slow initiation of motor activity, and disturbed speech. Rigidity of the extremities, neck, or trunk, usually without a "cogwheel" phenomenon, may occur after the onset of bradykinesia. Although the characteristic parkinsonian "pill-rolling" tremor at rest may be present, postural tremor resembling essential tremor may also be seen.[26,27] Gait difficulties and falling have also been reported as common features in DIP.[28]

Although DIP may be clinically indistinguishable from PD, some differentiating characteristics may occur[29] (Table 24-2). The signs and symptoms of PD usually begin insidiously on one side of the body; with time, the opposite side is also affected but to a lesser degree. The manifestations of neuroleptic-induced parkinsonism are frequently bilateral and symmetric, and often develop acutely or subacutely. In one series, the signs of parkinsonism emerged within a few days of neuroleptic treatment with a gradual increase in incidence, so that 50–70 percent of cases appeared by 1 month

TABLE 24-2 Clinical Features that May Distinguish Drug-Induced Parkinsonism from Idiopathic PD

	Drug-Induced Parkinsonism	PD
Symptom at onset	Bilateral and symmetric	Unilateral or asymmetrical
Course	Acute or subacute	Insidious, chronic
Tremor type	Bilateral or symmetric postural or rest tremor	Unilateral or asymmetric rest tremor
Anticholinergic drug response	May be pronounced	Usually mild-to-moderate
Withdrawal of suspected offending drug	Remittance typically within weeks to months	Symptoms and signs slowly progress

and 90 percent of cases within 3 months.[25] It is often stated that tolerance develops to neuroleptic-induced parkinsonism. However, prospective studies to verify this phenomenon are lacking. The only clinical basis for this assumption is the observation that withdrawal of anticholinergic drugs, co-administered for several months with neuroleptics, is followed by the appearance of relatively few cases of DIP.

After discontinuation of neuroleptics, the majority of patients are free of parkinsonian signs within a few weeks. However, the effects may last longer, in some cases for up to several years.[29] Metoclopramide-induced parkinsonism has been reported to take several months to resolve completely.[30,31] The potentially long duration of neuroleptic-induced parkinsonism is important to appreciate so that one can avoid diagnostic error. DIP will usually improve slowly over time with reduction or discontinuation of the drug, whereas the signs and symptoms of PD will progressively worsen.

Neuroleptic-induced movement disorders, including DIP, frequently go unrecognized.[31] This lack of recognition on the part of treating physicians is suggested by Miller and Jankovic in their review of metoclopramide-induced movement disorders; they found that the offending drug was continued for an average of 6 months after the onset of extrapyramidal symptoms.[21] Hansen et al. found that resident psychiatry physicians diagnosed DIP in 11 percent of neuroleptic-treated patients, whereas researchers determined the prevalence to be 26 percent in this study population.[32] The work of Albanese et al. further emphasizes that the proper diagnosis of DIP depends on a high index of suspicion.[33] These authors detail 3 cases in which individuals developed parkinsonism while unwittingly ingesting neuroleptics being surreptitiously administered to them by their consorts.

Pathogenesis

The primary neurochemical of PD is striatal dopamine depletion.[34] Because neuroleptic drugs function as dopamine receptor blockers, it is not surprising that clinical features of parkinsonism can result from their use. It is not plausible that DIP is simply the result of dopamine receptor blockade. If this were true, then the incidence and severity of DIP should correlate with drug dosage, but this type of clear dose-effect relationship has never been established;[5] furthermore, plasma neuroleptic drug levels do not usually correlate with the severity of DIP.[35] Spina et al. reported a correlation between plasma levels of risperidone and its active metabolite and the occurrence of DIP; however, the drug dose (ranging from 4 to 9 mg/day) did not predict the occurrence or severity of parkinsonism in this study.[36] Parkinsonism appearing within several days of treatment with relatively small drug doses is a common clinical experience; yet, other patients are successfully maintained on relatively high doses for several years without developing parkinsonism. It had been suggested that DIP is simply idiopathic PD occurring

by chance in neuroleptic-treated individuals, as in the general population. The reported prevalence of neuroleptic-induced parkinsonism varies, but clinically significant parkinsonism reportedly occurs in 10–15 percent of treated individuals.[37,38] These rates of DIP are probably underestimates;[39] thus, coincidental idiopathic PD could not account for all cases of DIP, because the occurrence rate of parkinsonism in neuroleptic-treated individuals is much greater than estimates of PD in the general populace.

The mechanisms determining individual susceptibility to DIP remain unclear. Some studies suggest that women are at an increased risk for the development of neuroleptic-induced movement disorders, including tardive dyskinesia[40,41] and DIP.[6,37] Estrogen-related dopamine receptor blockade has been offered as the explanation for this female preponderance.[42] Others have not substantiated a gender influence.[43,44] These discrepancies could be explained by disparities in case ascertainment and by differences in medication prescription and usage based on sex. In one report, low urinary levels of free dopamine were associated with the subsequent development of phenothiazine-induced parkinsonism, suggesting that an inherent metabolic defect may be causative.[45] Human leukocyte antigen B44 (HLA-B44) is reported to be common in DIP, suggesting a genetic influence.[46] In one series, 5 of 16 patients with metoclopramide-induced movement disorders had family members with reported parkinsonism, tremor, or chorea.[21] However, the precise role of genetics in DIP remains uncertain.

The possibility that increased susceptibility to DIP might be related to subclinical PD has also been considered.[47,48] In some instances, it appears that PD becomes clinically overt during neuroleptic therapy and then subsides when the drug is discontinued, only to reappear years later.[49–51] In addition, Rajput et al. described 2 patients with drug-induced parkinsonism that completely remitted upon drug withdrawal; postmortem examination ultimately revealed pathological changes consistent with PD.[52] Brooks reported reduced putamen ^{22}F-dopa uptake on positron emission tomography (PET) in 2 of 7 individuals with DIP;[53] 4 of the 5 patients with normal PET scans recovered fully with cessation of drug therapy. Two patients with abnormal scans had persistent evidence of parkinsonism requiring L-dopa therapy, suggesting underlying PD. Chabolla et al. reported on DIP as a risk factor for the development of PD utilizing a large medical record database in Olmstead County, Minnesota.[54] These authors reported that 2 of 24 DIP patients went on to be characterized as having typical PD. This is a greater number than expected based on the observed number of cases in the general population. In a separate study, 140 middle-aged and elderly psychiatric outpatients who had a history of neuroleptic drug exposure, but were now on no drug therapy, were assessed for the presence of parkinsonian features.[55] Thirty-one of the 140 subjects were characterized as having persistent parkinsonism. Patients who were older and who had lower Mini-Mental State Examination scores were more likely to be characterized as having persistent parkinsonian features. The occurrence of parkinsonism in this psychiatric drug-exposed patient group did not differ from findings in the age-matched normal control population. These findings would suggest that neuroleptic drugs do not cause longlasting pharmacological or pathological changes resulting in persistent parkinsonism but, instead, uncover parkinsonian features in a population at risk for PD.

The relationship of DIP to other neuroleptic-induced extrapyramidal syndromes is intriguing. Like DIP, tardive dyskinesia is reported to occur more frequently in the elderly.[56–58] Saltz et al. followed 215 patients over 55 years of age after the initiation of neuroleptic therapy.[59] Evidence of parkinsonism was found in 103 patients by week 43; tardive dyskinesia developed in 40 percent of the parkinsonian patients, compared to 12 percent of the nonparkinsonian subjects. The coexistence of DIP and tardive dyskinesia has been reported by others.[60–62] The occurrence of both hypokinetic and hyperkinetic drug-induced side-effects in a common patient population is difficult to explain. In reviewing the effects of neuroleptics, Seeman et al. postulated action at the presynaptic site as causative in both DIP and tardive dyskinesia.[63] This may reflect the differential effects of neuroleptics on dopamine receptor subtypes; the geriatric patient population may be especially vulnerable to such effects because of diminished drug metabolism, dopaminergic neuron loss, or alterations in dopamine receptors.[42,64,65] Advancing age has often been cited as the chief risk factor for DIP. Baldereschi et al. reported that DIP was the second most common form of parkinsonism following PD in a population-based prospective study of the incidence of parkinsonism in individuals over the age of 65 years in Italy.[66] Caligiuri et al. determined the incidence of neuroleptic-induced parkinsonism in 56 elderly, newly medicated, psychiatric patients.[67] Predictors of neuroleptic-induced parkinsonism in this study included older age, presence of tremor, the presence of extrapyramidal signs prior to drug exposure, and underlying dementia. In this project, low doses of risperidone appear to be better tolerated than the other more potent conventional neuroleptics. Controlled comparison studies of conventional versus atypical neuroleptics in the elderly have not been conducted. Nevertheless, it is probably prudent to use low doses of atypical neuroleptics judiciously in this age group. It has been suggested that antioxidant drugs (e.g., vitamin E) may prevent or lessen the risk of neuroleptic-induced movement disorders including tardive dyskinesia.[68] There is no evidence substantiating the benefit of vitamin E or other antioxidants in the prevention or treatment of DIP.

Treatment of Neuroleptic-Induced Parkinsonism

Withdrawal of the offending drug when possible is the obvious treatment choice. This, however, is done at the risk of exacerbating the underlying condition for which the drug was initially prescribed. This is a particular difficulty in the instance of psychosis associated with schizophrenia. It is prudent to weigh the benefits that the patient derives from the drug against the severity and disability of DIP. Mild nondisabling DIP occurring in individuals who have achieved good control of psychotic symptoms on a stable dose of neuroleptic may require only observation and no intervention. Alternatively, the patient can be switched to a neuroleptic with fewer potential side-effects (e.g., quetiapine or clozapine). As described above, the atypical antipsychotic clozapine is an effective antipsychotic, having virtually no parkinsonian side-effects, but requiring weekly blood tests and close follow-up. In lieu of the antiemetics metoclopramide and chlorpromazine, the peripherally acting dopamine antagonist, domperidone, is sometimes used.[69] Domperidone is not commercially available within the US. Despite its reportedly low central nervous system (CNS) penetration, drug-induced movement disorders have occasionally been associated with the use of domperidone.[70] Antiemetics that do not act via dopamine blockade, such as ondansetron and benzquinamide hydrochloride, can be used in some instances.

Standard antiparkinsonian drugs can be used to treat DIP. Anticholinergic compounds are frequently used in this regard. Anticholinergic drugs reportedly decrease the signs and symptoms of neuroleptic-induced parkinsonism to a greater degree than in PD. This drug response is touted to be of use as a means of distinguishing between DIP and PD, but this has not been explored in a rigorous fashion.[71] Dopaminergic drugs, including L-dopa, can ameliorate DIP but may provoke the very symptoms for which the neuroleptic drug was prescribed, such as nausea and hallucinations.[72] In a single case report, pyridoxine was reported to ameliorate DIP and tardive dyskinesia in an individual with neuroleptic-treated schizophrenia.[73]

DOPAMINE STORAGE AND TRANSPORT INHIBITORS

Reserpine, an antihypertensive, depletes brain dopamine and other biogenic amines by interfering with presynaptic vesicular storage mechanisms. It can produce both clinical and experimental parkinsonism.[74] With numerous other antihypertensives now available, reserpine is rarely used to control blood pressure but is sometimes prescribed to treat tardive dyskinesia.[75,76] Because individuals with tardive dyskinesia may be at increased risk for DIP, close monitoring of these patients is warranted if treatment with reserpine is used. Tetrabenazine, a synthetic analogue of reserpine, also depletes amines and may also block postsynaptic dopamine receptors.[77] Not currently marketed in the US, tetrabenazine, like reserpine, may be useful in the treatment of hyperkinetic disorders.[78,79] Jankovic and Orman reported parkinsonism as the most common side-effect of tetrabenazine exposure, affecting 53 of 217 patients receiving the drug for hyperkinesia.[79]

Two cases of PD exacerbated by alpha-methylodopa have been observed, as well as several cases of parkinsonism reported to be induced by the drug.[80,81] Theorized as acting as a "false" neurotransmitter, alpha-methyldopa has been used in the treatment of PD.[82] Therefore, the significance of the few reported cases of alpha-methyldopa-induced parkinsonism is unclear.

CALCIUM-CHANNEL BLOCKERS

Available in Europe and Latin America, the piperazine derivatives, flunarizine and cinnarizine, act as calcium-entry blockers and have been prescribed for various disorders, including vertigo, migraine, and tinnitus.[83,84] Extrapyramidal reactions, including DIP and exacerbation of PD, have been associated with their use.[85,86] A primate model of cinnarizine-induced parkinsonism has also been described.[87] Parkinsonism is thought to be a result of the antidopaminergic effects of these compounds which may be pre- or postsynaptic.[88,89] Based on laboratory model data, it is theorized that cinnarizine and flunarizine inhibit the energy-dependent vesicular uptake of dopamine (a presynaptic event).[90] Other postulated mechanisms for DIP with this class of calcium-channel blockers include dopaminergic D2 receptor blockade,[91] mitochondrial damage,[92] and inhibition of catecholamine transport.[93] Garcia-Ruiz et al. reported persistence of parkinsonian signs, particularly in the aged, many months after the cessation of the offending drug.[94] Negrotti et al. suggested that DIP resulting from calcium-channel blockers may have a genetic component, because they found a relatively higher occurrence of other movement disorders among relatives of affected individuals.[95] Marti-Masso and Poza reported their experience in a 15-year follow-up of individuals with cinnarizine-induced parkinsonism.[96] They followed a total of 74 cases of cinnarizine-induced parkinsonism. They found this to be more common among women. The majority of patients recovered after the offending drug was withdrawn within a 16-month period. However, 11 of the 74 patients later went on to develop more typical PD. In addition, 5 patients had persistent features of tardive dyskinesia. Calcium-channel blockers, widely available in the US, are rarely associated with parkinsonism,[97] although the antidopaminergic effect of one such agent, nimodipine, has been demonstrated experimentally.[98]

OTHER MEDICATIONS

Drugs of various other types have occasionally been associated with parkinsonism (Table 24-3). The cardiac antiarrhythmic agent, amiodarone, may cause sundry neurological side-effects, including tremor. Amiodarone-induced tremor is typically of the postural type, resembling essential tremor; however, parkinsonian signs and symptoms have also been described with this drug.[99–101]

TABLE 24-3 Miscellaneous Drugs Associated with Parkinsonism

Reserpine
Tetrabenazine
Alpha-methyldopa
Calcium-channel blockers (cinnarizine, flunarizine)
Amiodarone
Bethanechol
Pyridostigmine
Lithium
Diazepam
Fluoxetine
Phenelzine
Procaine
Meperidine
Amphotericin B
Cephaloridine
5-Fluorouracil
Doxorubicin hydrochloride

In single case reports, parkinsonism has been ascribed to cholinergic drugs, including bethanechol and the cholinesterase inhibitor pyridostigmine.[102,103] This side-effect is theorized to be a result of drug-induced cholinergic overactivity, that is an imbalance of striatal acetylcholine-dopamine activity. In one instance of bethanechol-induced parkinsonism, postmortem analysis demonstrated pathological changes consistent with PD, suggesting that the drug may clinically manifest the underlying nigrostriatal pathology.[102] However, it is more difficult to explain parkinsonism secondary to pyridostigmine, because this drug appears to penetrate the blood-brain barrier poorly, and CNS effects would not be anticipated.

Lithium commonly produces a postural tremor, but whether it can induce parkinsonism is not firmly established. Cogwheel rigidity has been found on examination in a small percentage of patients taking lithium.[104] Two patients were reported to develop parkinsonian symptoms after lithium therapy but both had prior exposure to neuroleptics.[105] Lutz described transient parkinsonism in an individual with elevated lithium blood levels who had been taking a liquid protein diet.[106] Pentoxifylline is a synthetic derivative of xanthine which stimulates adenosine receptors which inhibit phosphodiesterase and increases cyclic monophosphate adenosine. Serrano-Duenas described 4 cases of pentoxifylline-induced parkinsonism following therapy with an average dose of 1100 mg/day.[107]

DIP was reported in 4 patients on high dose ($\geq$100 mg/day) diazepam in the treatment of schizophrenia.[108] Fluoxetine, alone and in conjunction with neuroleptics or carbamazapine, has been associated with parkinsonism.[109–111] Isolated instances of parkinsonism have been ascribed to sundry other agents, including phenelzine,[112] procaine,[113] meperidine,[114] amphotericin B,[115] cephaloridine,[116] 5-fluorouracil,[117] and vincristine combined with doxorubicin hydrochloride.[118]

Summary

In summary, parkinsonism secondary to drug ingestion is common, particularly in the elderly. Dopamine receptor blockers, used primarily as antipsychotics and antiemetics, are the most frequent offending agents. Other pharmacological classes of medications have also been impugned, although the mechanism of DIP in such instances is less certain. The susceptibility of the individual to developing DIP has not been established, but may represent latent PD or a heritable trait, in some instances. Further scrutiny of the occurrence and characteristics of DIP would yield a better understanding of this phenomenon and may also provide greater insight into the cause and pathogenesis of PD.

References

1. Anton-Stephens D: Preliminary observations on the psychiatric uses of chlorpromazine (Largactil). *J Ment Sci* 100:543–545, 1954.
2. Lehmann HE, Hanrahan GE: Chlorpromazine: New inhibiting agent for psychomotor excitement and manic states. *Arch Neurol Psychiatry* 71:227, 1954.
3. Kinross-Wright V: Chlorpromazine: A major advance in psychiatric treatment. *Postgrad Med* 16:297, 1954.
4. Goldman D: Treatment of psychotic states with chlorpromazine. *J Am Med Assoc* 157:1274–1277, 1955.
5. Hall RA, Jackson RB, Swain JM: Neurotoxic reactions resulting from chlorpromazine administration. *J Am Med Assoc* 161:214–218, 1956.
6. Ayd FJ Jr: A survey of drug-induced extrapyramidal reactions. *J Am Med Assoc* 175:1054–1060, 1961.
7. Miller LG, Jankovic J: Neurologic approach to drug-induced movement disorders: A study of 125 patients. *South Med J* 83:525–532, 1990.
8. Baldessarini RJ, Frankenburg FR: Clozapine: A novel antipsychotic agent. *N Engl J Med* 324:746–754, 1991.
9. Friedman JH, Lannon MC: Clozapine in the treatment of psychosis in Parkinson's disease. *Neurology* 39:1219–1221, 1989.
10. Bennet JP, Landow ER, Schuh LA: Suppression of dyskinesias in advanced Parkinson's disease. II. Increasing daily clozapine doses suppress dyskinesias and improve parkinsonian symptoms. *Neurology* 43:1551–1555, 1993.
11. Friedman JH, Lannon MC: Clozapine treatment of tremor in Parkinson's disease. *Mov Disord* 5(suppl 1):50, 1990.
12. Wolters EC, Hurwitz TA, Mak E, et al: Clozapine in the treatment of parkinsonian patients with dopaminometic psychosis. *Neurology* 40:832–834, 1990.
13. The Parkinson Study Group: Low-dose clozapine for the treatment of drug-induced psychosis in Parkinson's disease. *N Engl J Med* 340:757–763, 1999.
14. Lera G, Zirulnik J: Pilot study in patients with HIV-associated psychosis and drug-induced parkinsonism. *Mov Disord* 14:128–131, 1999.
15. Goetz CG, Blasucci LM, Leurgans S, Pappert EJ: Olanzapine and clozapine: Comparative effects on motor function in hallucinating PD patients. *Neurology* 55:789–794, 2000.
16. Juncos JL: Management of psychotic aspects of Parkinson's disease. *J Clin Psychiatry* 60(suppl 8):42–53, 1999.
17. Targum SD, Abbot JL: Efficacy of quetiapine in Parkinson's patients with psychosis. *J Clin Psychopharmacol* 20:54–60, 2000.
18. Bateman DN, Rawlins MC, Simpson JM: Extrapyramidal reactions to prochlorperazine and haloperidol in the United Kingdom. *Q J Med* 59:549–556, 1986.
19. Grimes D, Hassan MN, Preston DN: Adverse neurologic effects of metoclopramide. *Can Med Assoc J* 126:23–25, 1982.
20. Sethi KD, Patel B, Meador KJ: Metoclopramide-induced parkinsonism. *South Med J* 82:1581–1582, 1989.
21. Miller LG, Jankovic J: Metoclopramide-induced movement disorders. *Arch Intern Med* 149:2486–2492, 1989.
22. Bateman DN, Darling WM, Boys R, Rawlins MD: Extrapyramidal reactions to metoclopramide and prochlorperazine. *Q J Med* 71:307–311, 1989.
23. Kuzuhara S: Essential points to differentiate various diseases causing parkinsonism. *Nippon Rinsho* 58:2049–2053, 2000.
24. Steck H: Le syndrome extra-pyramidal et diencephalique au cours des traitements au forgacril au Serpasil. *Ann Med Psychol* 1/2:737–743, 1954.
25. Marsden CD, Tarsy D, Bladessarini RH: Spontaneous and drug-induced movement disorders, in Benson DF, Blumer D (eds): *Psychiatric Aspects of Neurologic Disease*. New York: Grune & Stratton, 1975.
26. Indo T, Ando K: Metoclopramide induced parkinsonism: Clinical characteristics of ten cases. *Arch Neurol* 39:494–496, 1982.
27. Hershey LA, Gift T, Rivera-Calminlin L: Not Parkinson's disease. *Lancet* ii:49, 1982.
28. Akbostanci MC, Atbasoglu EC, Balaban H: Tardive dyskinesia, mild drug-induced dyskinesia, and drug-induced parkinsonism: risk factors and topographic distribution. *Acta Neurol Belg* 3:176–181, 1999.
29. Klawans HL, Bergen D, Bruyn GW: Prolonged drug-induced parkinsonism. *Confin Neurol* 35:368–377, 1973.
30. Yamamoto M, Ujike H, Ogawa N: Metoclopramide-induced parkinsonism. *Clin Neuropharmacol* 10:287–289, 1987.
31. Weiden PJ, Mann JJ, Haas G, et al: Clinical nonrecognition of neuroleptic-induced movement disorders: A cautionary study. *Am J Psychiatry* 144:1148–1153, 1987.
32. Hansen TE, Brown WL, Weigel RM, Casey DE: Underrecognition of tardive dyskinesia and drug-induced parkinsonism by psychiatric residents. *Gen Hosp Psychiatry* 14:340–344, 1992.
33. Albanese A, Colosimo C, Bentivoglio AR, Bergonzi P: Unsuspected, surreptitious drug-induced parkinsonism. *Neurology* 42:459, 1992.
34. Ehringer H, Hornykiewicz O: Verteilung von Noradrenalin und Dopamin (3-Hydroxytyramin) im Gehirn des Menshen und ihr Verhalften bei Erkrankungen des extrapyramidalen Systems. *Klin Wochenschr* 38:1236–1260, 1960.
35. Crowley TJ, Hoehn MM, Rutledge CD, et al: Dopamine excretion and vulnerability to drug-induced parkinsonism. *Arch Gen Psychiatry* 35:97–401, 1978.
36. Spina E, Avenoso A, Facciolà G, et al: Relationship between plasma risperidone and 9-hydroxyrisperdone concentrations and clinical response in patients with schizophrenia. *Psychopharmacology* 153:238–243, 2001.
37. Koczyn AD, Goldberg GJ: Extrapyramidal effects of neuroleptics. *J Neurol Neurosurg Psychiatry* 39:866–869, 1976.
38. Moleman P, Janzen G, von Bargen BA, et al: Relationship between age and incidence of parkinsonism in psychiatric

patients treated with haloperidol. *Am J Psychiatry* 143:232–234, 1986.

39. McClelland HA: Discussion on assessment of drug-induced extrapyramidal reactions. *Br J Clin Pharmacol* 3:401–403, 1976.

40. Kane JM, Smith JM: Tardive dyskinesia: Prevalence and risk factors, 1959–1979. *Arch Gen Psychiatry* 39:473–481, 1982.

41. Jus A, Pineau R, Lachance R, et al: Epidemiology of tardive dyskinesia. Part I. *Dis Nerv Syst* 37:210–214, 1976.

42. Glazer WM, Naftolin F, Moore DL, et al: The relationship of circulating estradiol to tardive dyskinesia in men and postmenopausal women. *Psychoneuroendocrinology* 8:429–434, 1983.

43. Moleman P, Schmitz PJM, Ladee GA: Extrapyramidal side effects and oral haloperidol: An analysis of explanatory patient and treatment characteristics. *J Clin Psychiatry* 43:492–496, 1982.

44. Kennedy PF, Hershon HI, McGuire RJ: Extrapyramidal disorders after prolonged phenothiazine therapy. *Br J Psychiatry* 118:509–518, 1971.

45. Crowley TJ, Rutledge CO, Hoehn MM, et al: Low urinary dopamine and prediction of phenothiazine induced parkinsonism: A preliminary report. *Am J Psychiatry* 133:703–706, 1976.

46. Metzer WS, Newton JEO, Steele RW, et al: HLA antigens in drug-induced parkinsonism. *Mov Disord* 4:121–128, 1989.

47. Gelay J, Deniker P: Drug-induced extrapyramidal syndromes, in Vinken PJ, Bruyn GW (eds): *Handbook of Clinical Neurology: Diseases of the Basal Ganglia.* Amsterdam: North-Holland, 1968, vol 6.

48. Duvoisin RC: Problems in the treatment of parkinsonism. *Adv Exp Med Biol* 90:131–155, 1977.

49. Goetz CG: Drug-induced parkinsonism and idiopathic Parkinson's disease. *Arch Neurol* 40:325–326, 1983.

50. Stephen PJ, Williamson J: Drug-induced parkinsonism in the elderly. *Lancet* ii:1082–1083, 1984.

51. Hardie RJ, Lees AJ: Neuroleptic-induced Parkinson's syndrome: Clinical features and results of treatment with levodopa. *J Neurol Neurosurg Psychiatry* 8:850–854, 1988.

52. Rajput AH, Rozdilsky B, Hornykiewicz O, et al: Reversible drug-induced parkinsonism: Clinicopathologic study of two cases. *Arch Neurol* 39:644–646, 1982.

53. Brooks DJ: Detection of preclinical Parkinson's disease with PET. *Neurology* 41(5, suppl 2):24–27, 1991.

54. Chabolla DR, Maraganore DM, Ahlskog JE, et al: Drug-induced parkinsonism as a risk factor for Parkinson's disease: A historical cohort study in Olmstead County, Minnesota. *Mayo Clin Proc* 8:724–727, 1998.

55. Jeste DV, Lohr JB, Eastham JH, et al: Adverse neurobiological effects of long-term use of neuroleptics: Human and animal studies. *J Psychiatr Res* 32:201–214, 1998.

56. Jeste DV, Wyatt RJ: *Understanding and Treating Tardive Dyskinesia.* New York: Guilford Press, 1982.

57. Crane GE, Smeets RA: Tardive dyskinesia and drug therapy in geriatric patients. *Arch Gen Psychiatry* 30:314–343, 1974.

58. Woerner MG, Kane JM, Lieberman JA, et al: The prevalence of tardive dyskinesia. *J Clin Psychopharmacol* 11:34–42, 1991.

59. Saltz BL, Woerner MG, Kane JM, et al: Prospective study of tardive dyskinesia incidence in the elderly. *JAMA* 266:2402–2406, 1991.

60. DeFraited EG, Davis KL, Berger PA: Coexisting tardive dyskinesia and parkinsonsim: A case report. *Biol Psychiatry* 12:267–272, 1977.

61. Fahn WE, Lake CR: On the co-existence of parkinsonism and tardive dyskinesia. *Dis Nerv Syst* 35:325–326, 1974.

62. Rao JM, Cowie VA, Mathew B: Tardive dyskinesia in neuroleptic medicated mentally handicapped subjects. *Acta Psychiatr Scand* 76:507–513, 1987.

63. Seeman P, Staiman A, Lee T, et al: The membrane action of tranquilizers in relation to neuroleptic-induced parkinsonism and tardive dyskinesia, in Forrest IS, Carr CJ, Usdin E (eds): *The Phenothiazine and Structurally Related Drugs.* New York: Raven Press, 1974.

64. Finch CE: Catecholamine metabolism in the brains of aging male mice. *Brain Res* 52:261–276, 1973.

65. Goetz CG, Weiner WJ, Nausieda PA, Klawans HL: Tardive dyskinesia: Pharmacology and clinical implications. *Clin Neuropharmacol* 5:3–22, 1983.

66. Baldereschi M, DiCarlo A, Rocca WA, et al: Parkinson's disease and parkinsonism in a longitudinal study: Two-fold higher incidence in men. *Neurology* 55:1358–1363, 2000.

67. Caligiuri MP, Lacro JP, Jeste DV: Incidence and predictors of drug-induced parkinsonism in older psychiatric patients treated with very low doses of neuroleptics. *J Clin Psychopharmacol* 4:322–328, 1999.

68. Caligiuri MR, Jeste DV, Lacro JP: Antipsychotic-induced movement disorders in the elderly: Epidemiology and treatment recommendations. *Drugs Aging* 5:363–384, 2000.

69. Parkes JD: Domperidone and Parkinson's disease. *Clin Neuropharmacol* 9:517–532, 1986.

70. Debontridder O: Dystonic reactions after domperidone. *Lancet* ii:1259, 1980.

71. Hornykiewicz O: Parkinsonism induced by dopaminergic antagonists. *Adv Neurol* 9:155–164, 1975.

72. Hausner RS: Amantadine-associated recurrence of psychosis. *Am J Psychiatry* 137:240–242, 1980.

73. Sandyk R, Pardeshi R: Pyridoxine improves drug-induced parkinsonism and psychosis in a schizophrenic patient. *Int J Neurosci* 52:225–232, 1990.

74. Carlsson A, Londquist M, Magnusson T: 3,4-Dihydroxytryptophan as reserpine antagonist. *Nature* 180:1200–1201, 1957.

75. Fahn S: Treatment of tardive dyskinesia: Use of dopamine-depleting agents. *Clin Neuropharmacol* 6:151–157, 1983.

76. Klawans HL, Tanner CM: The reversibility of permanent tardive dyskinesia. *Neurology* 33(suppl 2):163, 1983.

77. Reches A, Burke RE, Kahn C, Fahn S: Tetrabenazine, an amine depleting agent, also blocks dopamine receptors in rat brain. *J Pharmacol Exp Ther* 225:515–521, 1983.

78. Jankovic J: Tetrabenazine in the treatment of hyperkinetic movement disorders. *Adv Neurol* 37:227–289, 1983.

79. Jankovic J, Orman J: Tetrabenazine therapy of dystonia, chorea, tics, and other dyskinesias. *Neurology* 38:391–394, 1988.

80. Rosenblum AM, Montgomery EB: Exacerbation of parkinsonism by methyldopa. *JAMA* 244:2727–2728, 1980.

81. Gillman MA, Sandyk R: Parkinsonism inducing by methyldopa. *S Afr Med J* 65:194, 1984.

82. Fermaglich J, Chase TN: Methyldopa or methyldopahydrazine as levodopa synergists. *Lancet* i:1261–1262, 1973.

83. Godfrain T, Towse G, VanNueten JM: Cinnarizine: A selective calcium entry blocker. *Drugs Today* 18:27–42, 1982.

84. Holmes B, Brogden RN, Heel RC, et al: Flunarizine: A review of its pharmacodynamic and pharmacokinetic properties and therapeutic use. *Drugs* 27:6–44, 1984.

85. Micheli F, Pardal MF, Gatto M, et al: Flunarizine- and cinnarizine-induced extrapyramidal reactions. *Neurology* 37:881–884, 1987.

86. Micheli FE, Pardal MF, Giannaula R, et al: Movement disorders and depression due to flunarizine and cinnarizine. *Mov Disord* 4:139–146, 1989.

87. Martin Masso JF, Obeso JA, Carrera N, Martinez-Lage JM: Aggravation of Parkinson's disease by cinnarizine. *J Neurol Neurosurg Psychiatry* 50:804–805, 1987.

88. Fadda F, Gessa GL, Mosca E, Stefanini E: Different effects of the calcium antagonists nimodipine and flunarizine on dopamine metabolism in the rat brain. *J Neural Transm* 75:195–200, 1989.

89. DeVries DJ, Beart PM: Competitive inhibition of [^{3}H] spiperone binding to D_2 dopamine receptors in striatal homogenates by organic calcium-channel antagonists and polyvalent cations. *Eur J Pharmacol* 106:133–139, 1985.

90. Terland O, Flatmark T: Drug-induced parkinsonism: cinnarizine and flunarizine are potent uncouplers of the vacuolar H^+-ATPase in catecholamine storage vesicles. *Neuropharmacology* 38:879–882, 1999.

91. Brücke T, Wöber C, Podreka I, et al: D_2 receptor blockade by flunarizine and cinnarizine explains extrapyramidal side-effects. A SPECT study. *J Cereb Blood Flow Metab* 15:513–518, 1995.

92. Veitch K, Hue L: Flunarizine and cinnarizine inhibit mitochondrial complexes I and II: Possible implication for parkinsonism. *Mol Pharmacol* 45:158–163, 1994.

93. Vaccari A, Saba PL, Gessa GL: Potent, extra-channel influence of several calcium channel modulators on striatal binding of [^{3}H] tyramine. *Neurochem Res* 18:1125–1130, 1993.

94. Garcia-Ruiz PJ, de Yebenes JG, Jimenez-Jimenez FJ, et al: Parkinsonism associated with calcium channel blockers: A prospective follow-up study. *Clin Neuropharmacol* 15:19–26, 1992.

95. Negrotti A, Calzetti S, Sasso E: Calcium-entry blockers-induced parkinsonism: Possible role of inherited susceptibility. *Neurotoxicology* 13:261–264, 1992.

96. Marti-Masso JF, Poza JJ: Cinnarizine-induced parkinsonsim: ten years later. *Mov Disord* 3:453–456, 1998.

97. Dick RS, Barold SS: Diltiazem-induced parkinsonism. *Am J Med* 87:95–96, 1989.

98. Pileblad E, Carlsson A: In vivo effects of the Ca^{++} antagonist nimodipine on dopamine metabolism in mouse brain. *J Neural Transm* 66:171–187, 1986.

99. LeMaire JF, Autret A, Biziere K, et al: Amiodarone neuropathy: Further arguments for human drug-induced neurolipidosis. *Eur Neurol* 21:65–68, 1982.

100. Palakurthy PR, Iyer V, Meckler RJ: Unusual neurotoxicity associated with amiodarone therapy. *Arch Intern Med* 147:881–884, 1987.

101. Werner EG, Olanow CW: Parkinsonism and amiodarone therapy. *Ann Neurol* 25:630–632, 1989.

102. Fox JH, Bennett DA, Goetz CG, et al: Induction of parkinsonism by intraventricular bethanechol in a patient with Alzheimer's disease. *Neurology* 39:1265, 1989.

103. Iwasaki Y, Wakata N, Kinoshita M: Parkinsonism induced by pyridostigmine. *Acta Neurol Scand* 78:236, 1988.

104. Kane J, Rifkin A, Quitkin F, Klein D: Extrapyramidal side effects with lithium treatment. *Am J Psychiatry* 135:851–853, 1978.

105. Tyrer P, Alexander MS, Regan A, Lee I: An extrapyramidal syndrome after lithium therapy. *Br J Psychiatry* 136:191–194, 1980.

106. Lutz EG: Acute lithium-induced parkinsonism precipitated by liquid protein diet. *J Med Soc N J* 75:165–166, 1978.

107. Serrano-Duenas M: Parkinsonisma o enfermedad de Parkinson desedmascarada por pentoxifilina? *Neurologia* 1:39–42, 2001.

108. Suranyi-Cadotte BE, Nestoros JN, Nair NPV, et al: Parkinsonism induced by high doses of diazepam. *Biol Psychiatry* 20:451–460, 1985.

109. Bouchard RH, Pourcher E, Vincent P: Fluoxetine and extrapyramidal side effects. *Am J Psychiatry* 146:1352–1353, 1989.

110. Tate JL: Extrapyramidal symptoms in a patient taking haloperidol and fluoxetine. *Am J Psychiatry* 146:339–340, 1989.

111. Gernaat HBPE, Van de Woude J, Touw DJ: Fluoxetine and parkinsonism in patients taking carbamazepine. *Am J Psychiatry* 148:1604–1605, 1991.

112. Teusink JP, Alexopoulos GS, Shamoian CA: Parkinsonian side effects induced by a monoamine oxidase inhibitor. *Am J Psychiatry* 141:118–119, 1984.

113. Gjerris F: Transitory procaine-induced parkinsonism. *J Neurol Neurosurg Psychiatry* 34:20–22, 1971.

114. Lieberman AN, Goldstein M: Reversible parkinsonism related to meperidine. *N Engl J Med* 8:509, 1985.

115. Fisher JF, Dewald J: Parkinsonism associated with intraventricular amphotericin B. *J Antimicrob Ther* 12:97–99, 1983.

116. Mintz U, Lieberman UA, Vries A: Parkinsonism syndrome due to cephaloridine. *J Am Med Assoc* 216:1200, 1971.

117. Bergevin PR, Patwardhan VC, Weissman J, et al: Neurotoxicity of 5-fluorouracil. *Lancet* i:410, 1975.

118. Boranic M, Raci F: A Parkinson-like syndrome as a side effect of chemotherapy with vincristine and Adriamycin in a child with acute leukemia. *Biomedicine* 31:124–125, 1979.

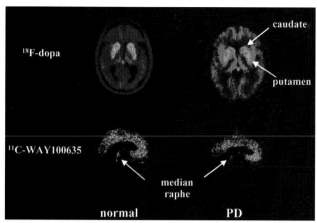

FIGURE 3-2 Dopamine terminal and serotonin HT$_{1A}$ function in PD. ^{18}F-dopa and ^{11}C-WAY100635 PET images for a normal subject and a PD patient. There is a selective loss of putamen dopamine storage and median raphe HT$_{1A}$ binding in PD. (Courtesy of M. Doder.)

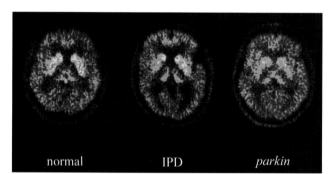

FIGURE 3-3 F-dopa uptake in PD. ^{18}F-dopa PET in idiopathic (IPD) and *parkin*-associated PD. There is a selective loss of putamen dopamine storage in IPD but uniform striatal involvement in *parkin* disease. (Courtesy of N. Khan.)

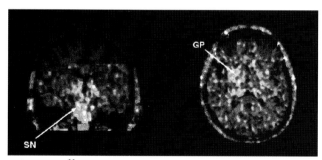

FIGURE 3-4 ^{11}C-PK11195 PET images for a PD patient showing microglial activation in the midbrain and pallidum. SN, Substantia Nigra; GP, Globus Pallidus. (Courtesy of A. Gerhard.)

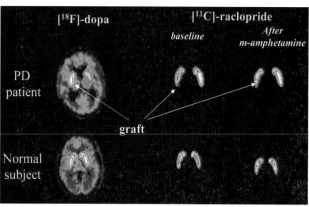

FIGURE 3-5 Dopamine release from nigral transplants visualized *in vivo* in Parkinson's Disease. ^{18}F-dopa and ^{11}C-raclopride PET images before and after amphetamine for a normal subject and a PD patient. It can be seen that the PD patient takes up normal levels of striatal ^{18}F-dopa on the unilaterally grafted side and that striatal ^{11}C-raclopride falls normally after amphetamine. (Courtesy of P. Piccini.)

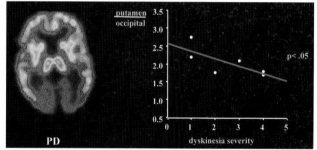

FIGURE 3-6 ^{11}C-Diprenorphine binding in PD, showing an inverse correlation between levels of putamen uptake and dyskinesia severity. (Courtesy of P. Piccini.)

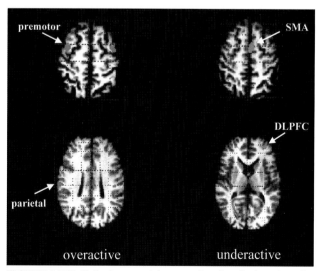

FIGURE 3-7 Statistical parametric maps showing the location of reduced and increased activation during sequential finger movements in PD. SMA, supplementary motor area; DLPFC, dorsolateral prefrontal cortex. (Courtesy of M. Samuel.)

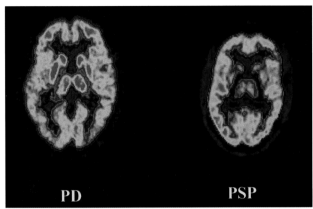

FIGURE 3-8 ^{18}FDG PET showing reduced resting basal ganglia glucose metabolism in PSP. (Courtesy of P. Piccini.)

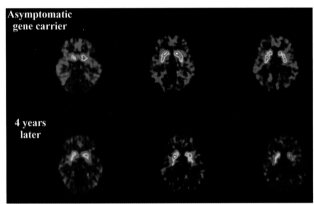

FIGURE 3-9 Dopamine D1 binding in HD. Serial ^{11}C-SCH23390 PET scans in a HD gene carrier, showing loss of striatal binding over 4 years. (Courtesy of T. Andrews.)

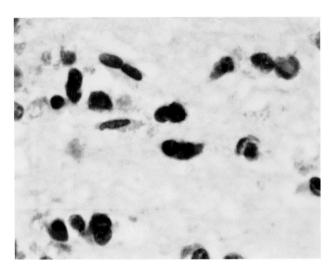

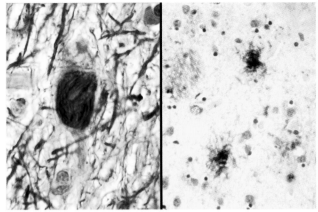

FIGURE 9-9 Progressive supranuclear palsy. A neuron in the globus pallidus contains a characteristic globose neurofibrillary tangle (*left*, Bielschowsky silver preparation). Tau immunohistochemistry reveals tufted astrocytes in the putamen (*right*).

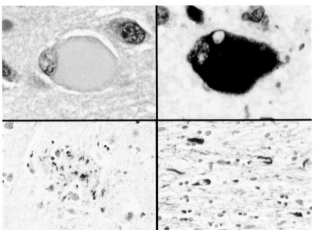

FIGURE 9-10 Corticobasal degeneration. Ballooned neurons are present in multiple regions of neocortex (*top left*, hematoxylin-eosin stain; *top right*, alpha-B-crystallin immunohistochemistry). Tau immunohistochemistry reveals astrocytic plaques in neocortical gray matter (*bottom left*), and coiled bodies and threads in the white matter (*bottom right*).

FIGURE 9-7 Alpha-synuclein immunohistochemistry reveals glial cytoplasmic inclusions in the putamen in a case of multisystem atrophy.

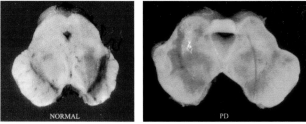

FIGURE 19-1 Gross photograph of a coronal section through the midbrain from a normal brain (*left*) and from a case of PD (*right*). Note the normal pigmentation pattern of the substantia nigra in the normal specimen, and the loss of pigmentation in the case of PD.

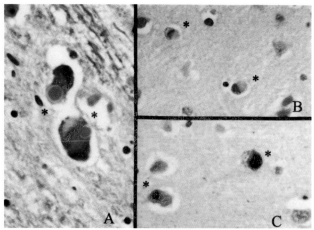

FIGURE 19-3 Photomicrographs of Lewy bodies stained with hematoxylin eosin (A, B), and with antibodies against alpha-synuclein (C). In (A), the typical appearance of Lewy bodies in the brainstem is illustrated (asterisks) as cytoplasmic inclusions with a compact eosinophilic center and a pale peripheral rim. In (B), cortical Lewy bodies are illustrated (asterisks) in small neurons and lacking the sharp laminated structure of the brainstem inclusions. Alpha-synuclein staining of the cortex (D, asterisks) clearly identifies the abnormal deposits.

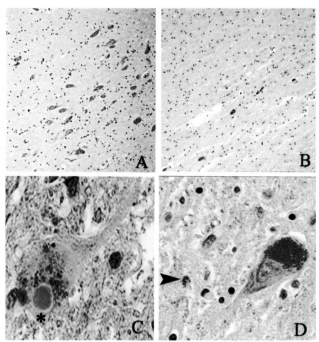

FIGURE 19-2 Photomicrographs of hematoxylin eosin-stained sections of the midbrain from a normal brain (A), and from a case of PD (B–D). In the low-power images (A, B), note the normal complement of pigmented dopamine neurons in the substantia nigra (A), and the marked loss of dopamine neurons (B) in the case of PD. In higher-power photomicrographs (C, D), note the presence of a Lewy body (C, asterisk), and phagocytosis of melanin pigment (melanophagia) (D, arrowhead). A normal remaining dopamine neuron is also present (D).

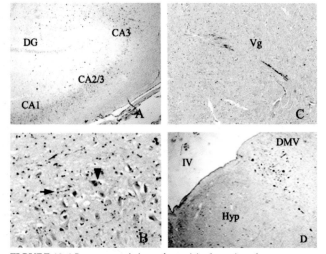

FIGURE 19-4 Immunostaining of neuritic deposits of alpha-synuclein. In (A), staining of the CA2-3 field of the hippocampus is illustrated at low power. In (B), a higher-power magnification from (A) is illustrated, showing alpha-synuclein-positive neurites (arrow) and a Lewy body (arrowhead). In (C), a low-power magnification of the medulla illustrates alpha-synuclein-positive neurites within the vagus nerve (Vg). In (D), low-power magnification of the medullary tegmentum shows Lewy bodies and dystrophic neurites in the dorsal motor vagus nucleus (DMV) and sparing of the hypoglossal nucleus (Hyp). The ventricle is at the top (IV). The section has been counterstained with hematoxylin.

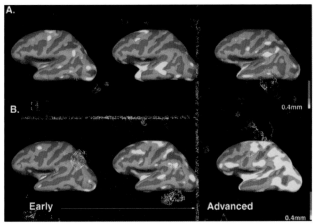

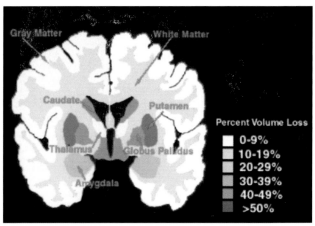

FIGURE 36-12 Cortical thinning in vivo in patients with HD determined in the left hemisphere by MRI. *A* demonstrates heterogeneity of regional involvement. All three individual subjects were in similar stages of disease. The left and middle mean thickness maps are from a set of twins. *B* demonstrates the progression of cortical thinning with advancing disease. Full yellow corresponds to >0.4 mm of cortical thinning. The mean thickness of the cortex normally varies from 2.5 to 4 mm.

FIGURE 36-13 MRI brain segmentation. Composite representation of volume loss occurring in the brains of 18 individuals in the early stages of HD. In addition to the expected marked atrophy of the striatum, significant volume loss is also evident in the globus pallidus, amygdala, hypothalamus, and cortical white and gray matters.

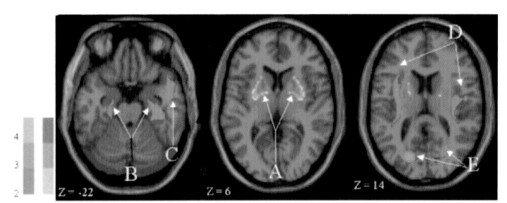

FIGURE 36-15 Voxel-based network analysis utilizing a principal component analysis applied to flourodeoxyglucose/PET scans from a group of 12 presymptomatic HD gene carriers and 11 age-matched controls. The first principal component discriminated the HD gene carriers from controls ($P < 0.005$), and was characterized by hypometabolism in bilateral striatum (A), covarying with hypermetabolism in bilateral hippocampi (B), right superior temporal gyrus (C), bilateral insula (D), and cuneus (E). *Courtesy of Andy Feigin.*

RARE DEGENERATIVE SYNDROMES ASSOCIATED WITH PARKINSONISM

WOLFGANG H. OERTEL and J. CARSTEN MÖLLER

FRONTOTEMPORAL DEMENTIA AND
  PARKINSONISM LINKED TO CHROMOSOME 17
  (FTDP-17)   404
    Clinical Definition   404
    Epidemiology   404
    Neurogenetics   404
    Pathogenesis   404
    Neuropathology   404
    Clinical Manifestations   404
    Central Nervous System (CNS) Manifestations   404
    Cardinal Neurological Symptoms   404
    Psychiatric Symptoms   404
    Diagnosis/Differential Diagnosis   405
    Biochemical Criteria   405
    Neuroimaging   405
    Therapy   405
PANTOTHENATE KINASE-ASSOCIATED
  NEURODEGENERATION (HALLERVORDEN-SPATZ
  SYNDROME)   405
    Clinical Definition   405
    Epidemiology   405
    Neurogenetics   405
    Pathogenesis   405
    Neuropathology   405
    Clinical Manifestations   406
    CNS Manifestations   406
    Cardinal Neurological Symptoms   406
    Psychiatric Symptoms   406
    Diagnosis/Differential Diagnosis   406
    Biochemical Criteria   406
    Neuroimaging   406
    Therapy   406
HEMIPARKINSON-HEMIATROPHY SYNDROME
  (HPHA)   407
    Clinical Definition   407
    Epidemiology   407
    Neurogenetics   407
    Pathogenesis   407
    Neuropathology   407
    Clinical Manifestations   407
    CNS Manifestations   407
    Cardinal Neurological Symptoms   407
    Psychiatric Symptoms   407
    Diagnosis/Differential Diagnosis   407
    Biochemical Criteria   408

    Neuroimaging   408
    Therapy   408
DEMENTIA WITH LEWY BODIES   408
    Clinical Definition   408
    Epidemiology   408
    Neurogenetics   408
    Pathogenesis   408
    Neuropathology   408
    Clinical Manifestations   408
    CNS Manifestations   408
    Cardinal Neurological Symptoms   408
    Psychiatric Symptoms   409
    Diagnosis/Differential Diagnosis   409
    Biochemical Criteria   409
    Neuroimaging   409
    Therapy   409
X-LINKED DYSTONIA-PARKINSONISM SYNDROME
  (LUBAG)   409
    Clinical Definition   409
    Epidemiology   409
    Neurogenetics   409
    Pathogenesis   409
    Neuropathology   410
    Clinical Manifestations   410
    CNS Manifestations   410
    Cardinal Neurological Symptoms   410
    Psychiatric Symptoms   410
    Diagnosis/Differential Diagnosis   410
    Biochemical Criteria   410
    Neuroimaging   410
    Therapy   410
CHOREA-ACANTHOCYTOSIS (CHAC)   410
    Clinical Definition   410
    Epidemiology   411
    Neurogenetics   411
    Pathogenesis   411
    Neuropathology   411
    Clinical Manifestations   411
    Neurological Manifestations   411
    Cardinal Neurological Symptoms   411
    Psychiatric Symptoms   411
    Diagnosis/Differential Diagnosis   411
    Biochemical Criteria   412
    Neuroimaging   412
    Therapy   412
PALLIDONIGROLUYSIAN DEGENERATION (PNLD)   412
    Clinical Definition   412
    Epidemiology   412
    Neurogenetics   412
    Pathogenesis   412
    Neuropathology   412
    Clinical Manifestations   413
    CNS Manifestations   413
    Cardinal Neurological Symptoms   413
    Psychiatric Symptoms   413
    Diagnosis/Differential Diagnosis   413
    Biochemical Criteria   413
    Neuroimaging   413
    Therapy   413
PALLIDOPYRAMIDAL DISEASE   413
    Clinical Definition   413

Epidemiology 414
Neurogenetics 414
Pathogenesis 414
Neuropathology 414
Clinical Manifestations 414
CNS Manifestations 414
Cardinal Neurological Symptoms 414
Psychiatric Symptoms 414
Diagnosis/Differential Diagnosis 414
Biochemical Criteria 414
Neuroimaging 414
Therapy 414
RETT SYNDROME 414
Clinical Definition 414
Epidemiology 415
Neurogenetics 415
Pathogenesis 415
Neuropathology 415
Clinical Manifestations 415
CNS Manifestations 415
Cardinal Neurological Symptoms 415
Psychiatric Symptoms 415
Diagnosis/Differential Diagnosis 416
Biochemical Criteria 416
Neuroimaging 416
Therapy 416

Frontotemporal Dementia and Parkinsonism Linked to Chromosome 17 (FTDP-17)

CLINICAL DEFINITION

In the previous edition of this textbook, disinhibition-dementia-parkinsonism-amyotrophy complex (DDPAC) was described as one example of familial parkinsonism-dementia syndromes.[1] Today, DDPAC and other familial parkinsonism-dementia syndromes such as autosomal-dominant parkinsonism and dementia with pallidoponto-nigral degeneration have been summarized and termed FTDP-17.[2,3] Since this disorder is presented elsewhere in more detail, only a brief overview is provided in this chapter.

EPIDEMIOLOGY

The estimated total number of affected patients from 62 known families is 470.[4]

NEUROGENETICS

In 1998, mutations in the tau gene were found to be associated with FTDP-17 in several affected families.[5] So far, 26 different mutations have been reported, with the exon-10 P301L missense mutation being most prevalent.[4]

PATHOGENESIS

Tau is an intracellular protein that promotes assembly and stabilization of microtubules. Mutations in the tau gene can be distinguished into two types.[6] The first type of (missense) mutations reduces the ability of the tau protein to bind to microtubuli. The second type of mutation results in a change in the ratio (and subsequent accumulation) of tau isoforms with 3 amino acid repeats to those with 4 amino acid repeats.

NEUROPATHOLOGY

Macroscopically, frontotemporal and basal ganglia atrophy and substantia nigra (SN) depigmentation are usually found. Microscopic examination reveals neuronal loss and gliosis of variable intensity, tau-positive intraneuronal (and glial) inclusions without the characteristics of Pick bodies, and ballooned neurons.[2]

CLINICAL MANIFESTATIONS

Manifestations other than neurological and psychiatric symptoms do not usually occur.

CENTRAL NERVOUS SYSTEM (CNS) MANIFESTATIONS

The mean age at disease onset is 49 years, and the average disease duration is 8.5 years.[4] The principal CNS manifestations consist of behavioral, cognitive, and motor disturbances.[2] The behavioral symptoms include impaired social conduct, hyperorality, hyperphagia, obsessive stereotyped behavior, and psychosis. The cognitive disturbances consist of impaired executive functions with visuospatial, orientation, and common memory functions being relatively preserved until later stages of the disease. The motor symptoms include akinetic-rigid parkinsonian features without resting tremor, dystonia, spasticity, supranuclear gaze palsy, and occasionally amyotrophy. Most patients harboring exon-10 missense and intronic mutations in the tau gene develop a parkinsonism-predominant phenotype.[4] FTDP-17 features a wide range of phenotypic variations between kindreds with different tau mutations but also among family members from the same kindred.

CARDINAL NEUROLOGICAL SYMPTOMS

The cardinal neurological symptoms are the simultaneous occurrence of parkinsonism and dementia.

PSYCHIATRIC SYMPTOMS

The psychiatric symptoms are described above.

DIAGNOSIS / DIFFERENTIAL DIAGNOSIS

Useful diagnostic criteria are age at disease onset between the third and the fifth decade, rapid disease progression, personality and behavioral abnormalities, frontotemporal dementia (see above), and parkinsonism-plus symptoms (i.e., akinetic-rigid features associated with early falls, supranuclear gaze palsy, apraxia, dystonia, and lateralization).[4] The diagnosis can be confirmed by genetic testing, if available.

There is a wide range of possible differential diagnoses, including sporadic tauopathies such as progressive supranuclear palsy, corticobasal ganglionic degeneration (CBDG), and Pick's disease. Besides FTDP-17 there are also other types of familial frontotemporal dementia (FTD)—i.e., familial ubiquitin-positive FTD and dementia lacking distinctive histology.[7] Parkinson's disease (PD) with dementia, dementia with lewy bodies (DLB), and Alzheimer's disease represent further differential diagnoses of FTDP-17.

BIOCHEMICAL CRITERIA

No biochemical criteria exist.

NEUROIMAGING

Systematic studies have not yet been performed. Structural and functional imaging may reveal frontotemporal atrophy and/or hypometabolism.

THERAPY

A specific therapy is not known. The patients usually show poor response to L-dopa. Psychiatric treatment may be necessary.

Pantothenate Kinase-Associated Neurodegeneration (Hallervorden-Spatz Syndrome)

CLINICAL DEFINITION

In 1922, Hallervorden and Spatz reported a sibship affected by a new disease characterized by gait impairment resulting from rigidity of legs and feet deformity and mental deterioration with juvenile onset.[8] Recently, it has been shown that this disease is due to mutations in the gene for pantothenate kinase 2 (PANK2).[9] In response to the unethical activities of Hallervorden and Spatz during World War II, it has been suggested to replace the name "Hallervorden-Spatz syndrome" by the term "panthothenate kinase-associated neurodegeneration" (PKAN).

EPIDEMIOLOGY

The disease is rare. No sufficient epidemiological data are available.

NEUROGENETICS

PKAN is usually an autosomal-recessive disorder. The disease locus was localized to chromosome 20p13.[10] Recently, mutations in the PANK2 gene have been shown to cause PKAN.[9] In some cases, the PANK2 mutation was suggested to be semidominant. Mutations were found in all patients with classic Hallervorden-Spatz syndrome and in one-third of those with so-called atypical disease.[11] In these publications classic Hallervorden-Spatz syndrome was diagnosed in patients with disease onset during the first two decades, dystonia, and high globus pallidus (GP) iron with characteristic radiographic appearance. The term "atypical disease" was applied to individuals not fitting the above criteria but with radiographic evidence of increased basal ganglia iron.[9] Patients with the classic variant of the disease turned out usually to have mutations resulting in predicted protein truncation.[11]

PATHOGENESIS

The precise pathophysiology of PKAN is unknown. It has been suggested that the PANK2 mutations lead to coenzyme A depletion associated with defective membrane biosynthesis.[9] Furthermore, accumulated cysteine, which would normally condense with phosphopantothenate, may form complexes with iron and cause oxidative damage in the brain.[11]

NEUROPATHOLOGY

Macroscopically, the most striking neuropathologic feature is the rust-brown pigmentation of GP and pars reticulata of substantia nigra (SNr). On the microscopic level, iron granules were found in neurons, microglial cells, and astrocytes. Some iron was also localized extracellularly. Furthermore, "mulberry" concretions were observed in tissue and regarded as so-called pseudocalcium. A further prominent finding of the disease is a widely distributed distal axonal swelling. These swellings may be surrounded by glial cells and contain pigment granules, particularly when located in GP or SNr. These structures are known as spheroid bodies[8,12] and resemble those found in neuroaxonal dystrophy,[13] but in the latter the spheroids in the pallidum store fatty material and not pigments. These neuropathological alterations are accompanied by some loss of neurons and myelinated fibers as well as by gliosis. In analogy to PD, Lewy body-like intraneuronal inclusions containing alpha-synuclein were also observed in PKAN.[14]

CLINICAL MANIFESTATIONS

Apart from CNS manifestations, foot deformities were frequently observed, and skin pigmentation was noted in some cases.[15] As mentioned below, abnormal cytosomes in circulating lymphocytes and sea-blue histiocytes in the bone marrow were reported.

CNS MANIFESTATIONS

Dooling et al.[16] examined 42 patients who fulfilled both clinical and neuropathological criteria for PKAN. Onset of disease occurred in 24 patients before the age of 10 years, and 39 patients were ill before age 22. The mean duration of disease was 11 years. Gait difficulty and postural impairment were noted as initial symptoms in 37 patients. This may have been the result of spasticity, since symptoms of extrapyramidal dysfunction could be delayed by one to several years. However, the usual course included progression of rigidity and the presence of posture abnormalities. Other basal ganglia signs were observed, including dystonia in 23 patients, choreoathethosis in 19 patients, and tremor without any distinctive character in 15 patients. Additionally, mental impairment was common, and seizures occurred in 9 out of 42 patients. Generally, there was a wide spectrum of variation in the clinical manifestations of PKAN. It is noteworthy that one case of late-onset PKAN presenting as familial parkinsonism was reported.[17] A more detailed summary of the CNS manifestations based on a genotype-phenotype analysis is presented below.

CARDINAL NEUROLOGICAL SYMPTOMS

The cardinal neurological symptoms consist of an extrapyramidal movement disorder, intellectual impairment, and pyramidal tract signs with onset usually after early childhood.

PSYCHIATRIC SYMPTOMS

Apart from mental deterioration, personality changes such as impulsivity and violent outbursts, depression, and emotional lability were observed in patients with atypical disease and PANK2 mutations (see below).[11]

DIAGNOSIS/DIFFERENTIAL DIAGNOSIS

Several obligatory and corroborative symptoms for the diagnosis of PKAN were defined in 1991.[12] The obligatory symptoms were onset during the first two decades of life, a progressive course, and evidence of extrapyramidal dysfunction. The corroborative symptoms included pyramidal tract signs, progressive mental deterioration, hypodensities in basal ganglia on magnetic resonance imaging (MRI), occurrence of seizures, ophthalmological symptoms such as retinitis pigmentosa or optic atrophy, positive family history, and abnormal cytosomes in circulating lymphocytes and sea-blue histiocytes in bone marrow.

A recent genotype-phenotype analysis provided a novel concept of the clinical presentation of PKAN. (1) Patients with classic Hallervorden-Spatz syndrome had a mean age of onset of 3.4 years; usually presented with gait or postural symptoms; featured dystonia, dysarthria, rigidity, and choreoathetosis; and frequently developed spasticity and cognitive decline. (2) Atypical patients with PANK2 mutations had a mean age of onset of 13.7 years and featured less severe and more slowly progressive extrapyramidal symptoms. Furthermore, patients with classic disease more often suffered from retinopathy. Conversely, atypical patients more frequently presented with speech problems as part of the early disease.

It should be noted that two-thirds of the so-called atypical patients do not feature PANK2 mutations and are thus not covered by this description. Possible differential diagnoses of PKAN include Wilson's disease, Huntington's disease, chorea-acanthocytosis, neurometabolic disorders, and other diseases with brain iron accumulation such as neuroferritinopathy and aceruloplasminemia.[18,19] Clinical diagnosis of PKAN can be confirmed by MRI and genetic testing, if available.

BIOCHEMICAL CRITERIA

Laboratory investigations do not reveal any distinctive abnormalities. Hematologic studies have shown vacuolated circulating lymphocytes containing abnormal cytosomes, and the occurrence of sea-blue histiocytes in bone marrow in some patients.[20] HARP syndrome (hypoprebetalipoproteinemia, acanthocytosis, retinitis pigmentosa, pallidal degeneration) has been shown to be allelic with PKAN.[21]

NEUROIMAGING

Computed tomography (CT) in patients with PKAN has been reported to show atrophy and low-density lesions in basal ganglia.[22] MRI using a high field-strength unit (1.5 Tesla) showed decreased signal intensity in GP and SNr in T_2-weighted images, which is compatible with heavy metal (iron) deposits, and a small area of hyperintensity in the internal segment of pallidum, constituting the so-called "eye of the tiger" sign.[23,24] In all (homozygous and heterozygous) PKAN patients, whether classic or atypical, MRI showed the "eye of the tiger" sign, whereas this pattern was not seen in atypical patients without PANK2 mutations.[11]

THERAPY

There is no specific therapy for PKAN. Symptomatic management, such as L-dopa and dopamine agonists, may be beneficial to patients.[12] Hypothetically, supplementation of panthothenate could ameliorate the symptoms.[11] Simple case reports described a dramatic improvement with pantothenate, but no studies yet have been performed.

Hemiparkinson-Hemiatrophy Syndrome (HPHA)

CLINICAL DEFINITION

The HPHA syndrome is defined by the occurrence of a body hemiatrophy with features of a highly asymmetric, often L-dopa-responsive, parkinsonism more prominent on the side of the hemiatrophy.[25,26] Other characteristics are an early age of onset, ipsilateral dystonia, and a slowly progressive course. An association with contralateral brain atrophy was also shown.[27]

EPIDEMIOLOGY

There are no epidemiologic data available. So far a total of 40 patients has been published.

NEUROGENETICS

Parkin mutations have been found in 1 patient with HPHA.[28] Other neurogenetic studies have not been performed.

PATHOGENESIS

So far, no brains have been subjected to a postmortem examination. It has been reported that lesions of the postcentral gyrus before the age of 3 are associated with a relative smallness of the contralateral parts of the body.[29] Accordingly, it was suggested that the occurrence of parkinsonism in HPHA patients is related to an additional subcortical lesion.[25] In support of this point of view, Giladi et al. presented neuroradiological evidence of a contralateral brain hemiatrophy in 64 percent of their patients.[27] Since an association between perinatal asphyxia, brain hemiatrophy, and delayed-onset hemidystonia has been shown, HPHA could represent an example of a movement disorder with delayed onset as a consequence of neonatal brain injury.[27]

Recently, other authors reported 4 patients with dopa-responsive dystonia and hemiatrophy.[30] Since dopa-responsive dystonia results from a purely biochemical deficit in the brain, these authors suggested that a deficiency of the nigrostriatal dopamine system may by itself be sufficient to cause body hemiatrophy. However, neonatal ablation of the nigrostriatal pathway did not influence limb development in rats.[31] The variable response to L-dopa and the striatal hypometabolism as shown by ^{18}F-fluorodeoxyglucose and positron emission tomography (PET) suggest that both presynaptic and postsynaptic mechanisms contribute to HPHA.

NEUROPATHOLOGY

No postmortem analysis has been performed.

CLINICAL MANIFESTATIONS

In addition to the CNS manifestations, patients suffer from a body hemiatrophy with small and narrow extremities on one side. There is a wide variation in the degree of hemiatrophy: in some patients the face, arm, and a leg are affected, whereas in other patients only the hand seems to be affected. The most likely part of the hand to demonstrate hemiatrophy is the thumb. It has to be kept in mind that there is "normal" asymmetry of the two halves of the human body. The term "normal" asymmetry can be applied only to differences in opposite limb length that are not visually apparent in the absence of measurements.[32] Interestingly, one patient showed no hemiatrophy, but an enlarged lateral ventricle was the sign of brain hemiatrophy.[27]

CNS MANIFESTATIONS

With respect to the CNS manifestations, Buchman et al. reported that the mean age of onset of parkinsonism was 43.7 years.[26] The course of the disease is slowly progressive (the mean duration of disease until initiation of L-dopa therapy was 14.2 years). In contrast, in patients suffering from idiopathic PD, L-dopa treatment was started after 4.1 years.[26] Furthermore, no progression to Hoehn and Yahr stage IV or V was observed. Eight out of 15 patients remained asymmetric after the development of bilateral disease. Giladi et al. found a more variable clinical course; for instance, one patient progressed from Hoehn and Yahr stage I to stage V during "off" within 2.5 years.[27] Ipsilateral dystonic movements, sometimes presenting as the first symptom, often occur early in the course of the disease before exposure to L-dopa. Ten of 15 patients showed tremor as their initial symptom. Apart from the parkinsonian features, pyramidal tract dysfunction ipsilateral to the side of HPHA was present in 8 of 15 patients.[26]

CARDINAL NEUROLOGICAL SYMPTOMS

The cardinal neurological symptoms include early age of onset of unilateral parkinsonism, as well as ipsilateral dystonia occurring prior to L-dopa therapy.

PSYCHIATRIC SYMPTOMS

Psychiatric symptoms are not a major feature of this syndrome.

DIAGNOSIS/DIFFERENTIAL DIAGNOSIS

In the differential diagnosis a benign, early-onset parkinsonism has to be considered. Common features are early age of onset and unilateral symptoms with mild progression. The main differences are the evidence of ipsilateral hemiatrophy and the prominence of early dystonia in HPHA patients.

Therefore, the diagnosis depends on a thorough physical examination. Neuroradiological methods might be helpful: 64 percent of the patients examined by Giladi et al. showed a brain asymmetry on CT or MRI. Furthermore, ^{18}F-fluorodeoxyglucose and PET may be helpful in differentiating HPHA from typical asymmetric PD. Moreover, early on, the differential diagnosis may include CBGD, since HPHA may mimic its early stage.[33]

BIOCHEMICAL CRITERIA

Due to the involvement of the nigrostriatal dopaminergic system, the level of homovanillic acid in the cerebrospinal fluid can be reduced.[27]

NEUROIMAGING

CT and MRI showed contralateral brain asymmetry in 64 percent of investigated patients.[27] However, Buchman et al. found no evidence of cerebral hemiatrophy (cortical or ventricular asymmetry) in 11 of 12 patients.[26] Studies using ^{18}F-fluorodeoxyglucose and PET showed a focal hypometabolism in the basal ganglia and the medial frontal cortex of the contralateral side, whereas ^{18}F-fluorodopa and PET revealed a reduction in striatal ^{18}F-fluorodopa uptake. Hence, the former examination might be useful to distinguish HPHA from typical unilateral idiopathic PD.[34,35] This observation was not confirmed by other authors.[28]

THERAPY

Seven of 9 investigated patients showed a good response to L-dopa therapy, and 7 of 8 patients responded well to a combination of amantadine and anticholinergics.[26] Other investigators found a good response to L-dopa treatment in 7 of 11 patients.[27] One patient showed dramatic improvement after subthalamic nucleus stimulation.[36]

Dementia with Lewy Bodies

CLINICAL DEFINITION

In the previous edition of this textbook it was still controversial whether diffuse Lewy body disease (DLBD) is a variant form of PD or a disease entity. Although this issue is far from being definitely resolved, many authors now agree that DLBD represents a clinical entity. Usually the term dementia with Lewy bodies (DLB) is used for this disorder. Since DLB is described elsewhere in more detail, only a brief overview is provided in this chapter.

EPIDEMIOLOGY

In 1990, 90 autopsy cases were reviewed for the first time by Kosaka.[37] Subsequent autopsy studies estimated a prevalence of DLB in demented patients of 15–25 percent.[38]

NEUROGENETICS

DLB is usually sporadic. Because of the close relationship to PD, the same considerations regarding possible neurogenetic mechanisms might hold true for both conditions. So far it has been shown that the apolipoprotein ε4 allele is overrepresented in DLB cases with concomitant Alzheimer pathology, and that the CYP2D6B allele is overrepresented in both PD and DLB.[39,40]

PATHOGENESIS

The common pathological hallmark of PD and DLB, the Lewy body, suggests a closely related pathogenesis of these two conditions. Since alpha-synuclein, and parkin, were found in cortical Lewy bodies of DLB patients, this condition also belongs to the recently established group of synucleinopathies.[41] The overlap between PD and DLB is further emphasized by the cognitive impairment with cortical Lewy bodies in patients with familial parkinsonism linked to chromosome 4p15.[42]

NEUROPATHOLOGY

The following neuropathological features associated with DLB were defined at the first Consensus meeting in 1996. (1) Brainstem and cortical Lewy bodies. Usually more than 5 Lewy bodies per area are to be found by hematoxylin-eosin or ubiquitin staining in the neocortex, the cingulate cortex, and the transentorhinal cortex. Tau immunostaining may be used to distinguish cortical Lewy bodies from small tangles. (2) Lewy-body neurites. (3) Plaques. (4) Neurofibrillary tangles. (5) Regional neuronal loss. (6) Microvacuolation and synapse loss. (7) Neurochemical abnormalities and neurotransmitter deficits.[38] Lewy bodies represent the only essential feature for the diagnosis of DLB. Alzheimer pathology was found to be a concomitant feature in most DLB cases. The precise nosological relationship between DLB and Alzheimer's disease is therefore still uncertain.

CLINICAL MANIFESTATIONS

Manifestations other than the neurological and psychiatric symptoms usually do not occur.

CNS MANIFESTATIONS

The CNS manifestations are described below.

CARDINAL NEUROLOGICAL SYMPTOMS

DLB presents with dementia often associated with parkinsonian features.

PSYCHIATRIC SYMPTOMS

The psychiatric symptoms are described below.

DIAGNOSIS/DIFFERENTIAL DIAGNOSIS

The central feature required for the diagnosis of DLB is progressive cognitive decline.[38] Additional core features of DLB are fluctuating cognition with pronounced variations in attention, recurrent visual hallucinations, and parkinsonian motor symptoms. Two of these additional core features are essential for the diagnosis of probable DLB, and one is essential for possible DLB. Features supportive of the diagnosis are repeated falls, syncope, and transient loss of consciousness, neuroleptic sensitivity, and systematized delusion and hallucinations in other modalities. In 1999, REM (rapid eye movement) sleep behavior disorder and depression were added to the list of supportive features.[43] These consensus criteria were found to have a sensitivity of 0.83 and a specificity of 0.95 in predicting neuropathologically proven DLB in one study.[44] The phenomenon of neuroleptic sensitivity deserves particular attention. A severe sensitivity reaction, including the new appearance or worsening of parkinsonism, an irreversible cognitive decline, delirium, and features of neuroleptic malignant syndrome, was observed in 29 percent of DLB patients within 2 weeks of a neuroleptic prescription or a dose change.[45] These sensitivity reactions can occur despite low dosing and the use of atypical neuroleptics. Quetiapine has been suggested to represent a relatively safe option for the treatment of psychosis in DLB.[46]

Due to the assumed overlap between DLB and PD with dementia, it has been suggested to use DLB as a diagnosis if dementia occurs within 12 months of the onset of parkinsonian motor symptoms.[38] If history of parkinsonism is longer than 12 months, PD with dementia should be used as diagnostic label. However, since a recent study failed to find a significant difference in the neuropsychological assessment of DLB versus PD patients with dementia, it has been proposed to drop definitional distinctions between these two conditions.[47]

Despite the apparently high specificity of the above diagnostic criteria it might be difficult to distinguish safely DLB or PD with dementia from advanced AD with parkinsonian features on the one hand, or other syndromes associated with parkinsonism and dementia on the other hand. Therefore, the correct diagnosis should be confirmed by postmortem analysis.

BIOCHEMICAL CRITERIA

There are no known biochemical criteria.

NEUROIMAGING

CT or MRI may show generalized cortical atrophy. Medial temporal lobe atrophy on MRI is significantly less pronounced in DLB than in Alzheimer's disease, and reduced striatal dopamine transporter activity may be found by SPECT (single-photon emission computed tomography) imaging in DLB but hardly in Alzheimer's disease.[48,49]

THERAPY

A smaller proportion of DLB than PD patients showed motor improvement in response to treatment with L-dopa.[38] Cholinesterase inhibitors, as shown for rivastigmine in a double-blind placebo-controlled randomized trial, produced significant and clinically relevant behavioral effects in DLB.[50] Donepezil and tacrine have also been found useful in several smaller studies or case series.

X-Linked Dystonia-Parkinsonism Syndrome (Lubag)

CLINICAL DEFINITION

Lubag is an X-linked recessive form of movement disorder, prevalent among Filipino men born on Panay island. This entity was first reported by Lee et al.[51] Onset occurs at 30–45 years of age with focal dystonia, subsequently generalizing within approximately 5 years. Parkinsonism develops usually after the onset of dystonia and becomes the predominant symptom beyond the tenth year of illness.[52]

EPIDEMIOLOGY

Lubag occurs endemically in the Philippines. As of June 2001, 376 lubag cases have been registered.[52] The prevalence of lubag on the island of Panay is 5.24 per 100,000.[52] Presumably, the disease originated from a common ancestor on the island, suggesting a single gene mutation. The neuropathological similarity between a patient with lubag and a non-Filipino patient with dystonia suggests that this mutation may not be restricted to the Filipino population.[53]

NEUROGENETICS

An X-linked recessive mode of inheritance has been suggested. Linkage between the phenotype lubag and the DXS7117-DXS559 region on chromosome Xq13.1 has recently been established.[54] However, the affected gene, which was named DYT3, has not yet been identified. It should be mentioned that women can also be affected, leading to the hypothesis that lubag may be a codominant disorder.[55]

PATHOGENESIS

The pathogenesis of this disease is unknown.

NEUROPATHOLOGY

A subtle astrocytosis in a mosaic pattern was found in the caudate and putamen in 1 case.[53] The lateral part of the putamen was the most severely gliotic. Gliotic areas also exhibited neuronal loss. Postmortem examinations were subsequently performed in 5 additional patients.[52] Overall, varying degrees of neuronal loss and astrogliosis involving the caudate and putamen were observed. Other brain areas such as the cerebral cortices and SN were unremarkable.

CLINICAL MANIFESTATIONS

There are no other clinical manifestations beyond the CNS symptoms.

CNS MANIFESTATIONS

Three hundred and seventy-six lubag patients were clinically assessed.[52] The mean age of onset was 39.5 years. Ninety-four percent presented with focal dystonia (33 percent dystonia involving the lower extremities; 27 percent blepharospasm, jaw opening and closing, or tongue protrusion; 25 percent torticollis, retrocollis, anterocollis, neck stiffness, tremors, or shoulder dystonia; 14 percent tremors, and cramps of the upper extremities). The symptoms usually progressed to involve other body parts leading to generalized dystonia within 5 years in 84 percent.

Six percent presented with initial parkinsonian symptoms, (i.e., predominantly hand or foot tremor).[52] In most patients, dystonia becomes less intense as the tenth year of illness is approached. Then bradykinesia sets in, and a festinating gait, freezing, and masked facies can be observed. Rigidity and cogwheeling, however, are rare. The mean duration of illness until parkinsonism has become predominant is 13.4 years. Other symptoms that have been observed in lubag include myorhythmia and myoclonus.[56]

Recently, 3 patients with predominant parkinsonism with late-onset or no dystonia were reported.[57] Pure or predominant parkinsonism may be a phenotypic variation of lubag with a more benign course. It remains uncertain whether dystonia will universally develop over time in such patients.

CARDINAL NEUROLOGICAL SYMPTOMS

The cardinal neurological symptoms are focal, multifocal, or generalized dystonia, as well as parkinsonism.

PSYCHIATRIC SYMPTOMS

Primary psychiatric symptoms have not been reported.

DIAGNOSIS/DIFFERENTIAL DIAGNOSIS

Lubag can be diagnosed by its typical clinical features. In the differential diagnosis, any of the dystonias associated with parkinsonism should be considered, such as Wilson's disease, PKAN, chorea-acanthocytosis (CHAC), and dopa-responsive dystonia. Significant differences between the latter and lubag are age of onset, the sex predominance, and the distinct response to L-dopa therapy. In the future, routine diagnosis of lubag will be possible by neurogenetic methods.

BIOCHEMICAL CRITERIA

With the exception of an elevated manganese value obtained in the serum of affected Filipino men, laboratory studies showed no abnormalities.[51]

NEUROIMAGING

CT may reveal mild cerebral atrophy. Sixteen patients were analysed by MRI.[52] At an early disease stage the outer rim of the putamen may feature an increased signal intensity in T_2-weighted images. Later on the atrophy of the caudate and putamen becomes visible. Using ^{18}F-fluorodeoxyglucose and PET, a selective reduction of striatal glucose metabolism was determined, whereas the ^{18}F-fluorodopa uptake was found to be in the normal range.[58]

THERAPY

Patients were treated with trihexyphenidyl, L-dopa, lorazepam, diazepam, or diphenhydramine, either alone or in combination, with no or only moderate improvement of symptoms.[59] Surgical treatment provided no lasting relief.[52] Patients may benefit from the local administration of botulinum toxin. Furthermore treatment with zolpidem, which selectively binds to the alpha1- subunit of the $GABA_A$ receptor, improved dystonia and, less perceptibly, parkinsonism in three lubag patients.[60] Patients with parkinsonism as only or predominant manifestation may benefit from L-dopa therapy.[57]

Chorea-Acanthocytosis (CHAC)

CLINICAL DEFINITION

Acanthocytes are erythrocytes with changed morphology bearing spicules of variable length and breadth.[61] If they occur in association with neurological symptoms, the term neuroacanthocytosis is used. Four different types of neuroacanthocytosis are known. Acanthocytes are observed in abetalipoproteinemia, the so-called Bassen-Kornzweig syndrome,[62] and in familial hypobetalipoproteinemia.[63] Furthermore, they are detectable in CHAC.[64,65] Finally, the McLeod syndrome represents a further entity with the occurrence of acanthocytes and neurological symptoms.[66-68] There are also some other conditions in which a sporadic association with acanthocytes has been described (i.e., PKAN and mitochondrial encephalomyopathies).[69]

Here, the focus will be on CHAC. This is a disorder characterized by chorea, oromandibular dyskinesias, dementia, seizures, and peripheral neuropathy. Additionally, parkinsonism may occur either with chorea or as a subsequent feature when the hyperkinetic movement disorder subsides.[70,71] In contrast to the Bassen-Kornzweig syndrome and to familial hypobetalipoproteinemia, decreased serum lipid levels are not found in CHAC. Therefore, and due to its distinct neurological manifestations, it represents an independent entity presenting primarily as a movement disorder.

EPIDEMIOLOGY

Sufficient epidemiological data are not available.

NEUROGENETICS

CHAC is an autosomal-recessive disorder. The disease gene has recently been identified and named chorein.[72,73] The gene is localized to chromosome 9q21 and flanked by the markers GATA89A11 and D9S1843. In 43 CHAC patients, 57 different chorein mutations were found, indicating a strong allelic heterogeneity with no single mutation causing the majority of cases.[74] Most mutations, however, lead to premature termination codons and therefore predict absence or marked reduction of the chorein gene product.

PATHOGENESIS

The function of chorein is not known. Based on homology studies, it has been hypothesized that the gene product could be involved in intracellular protein cycling. Absence of the functional gene product may therefore lead to destabilization of the plasma membrane structure, and hence acanthocytosis.[73] The suggested occurrence of CHAC without acanthocytes may indicate that the gene can be variably expressed in different tissues and may cause neurological abnormalities alone. In a family with CHAC featuring an autosomal-dominant transmission and polyglutamine-containing neuronal inclusions, abnormalities of the membrane protein band 3 were demonstrated by gel electrophoresis of red blood cell membranes.[75]

NEUROPATHOLOGY

Macroscopically the brains showed enlargement of the ventricles, particularly of the frontal horns. Caudate and putamen were the most severely affected brain areas showing atrophy, neuronal loss, and gliosis. Depletion of small- and medium-sized striatal neurons was most apparent. Involvement of GP was also present, and in some cases thalamus and the anterior horns of spinal cord showed neuronal loss and mild gliosis.[76] The SN of 3 CHAC patients was investigated in more detail.[77] In CHAC with parkinsonism, a reduced neuronal density (particularly in the ventrolateral region) of the

SN was determined, whereas in 1 CHAC patient without parkinsonian features the number of neurons was at the lower limit of the control range.

CLINICAL MANIFESTATIONS

The salient clinical features are mainly characterized by the neurological symptoms.

NEUROLOGICAL MANIFESTATIONS

The mean age of onset was 32 years, ranging from 8 to 62 years. The most striking symptoms were involuntary movements affecting the orofacial region, and the limbs presenting as orofacial dyskinesias and limb chorea.[78] The former can cause tongue and lip biting and very often interferes with speech and swallowing. Accordingly, involuntary vocalizations were frequently observed. In some cases, the predominant manifestation was dystonia, rather than chorea, and tics were noticed. Additionally, hypo- or areflexia was repeatedly found. In many cases muscle wasting occurred, and an axonal neuropathy was demonstrated.[79] Moreover, one-third of patients suffered from seizures, and in more than half of the cases cognitive impairment, psychiatric features, and personality change were seen.[69,80] Spitz et al. reported two CHAC cases presenting as tics, but these were subsequently and progressively replaced or masked by progressive parkinsonism.[71] Furthermore, Yamamoto et al.[70] and Hardie et al.[80] described the occurrence of akinetic-rigid features simultaneously with the appearance of hyperkinetic disorders in 2 of 2 and in 5 of 19 cases, respectively. However, in 2 of 19 patients, no movement disorder could be established, indicating that this might not be a necessary condition.[80]

CARDINAL NEUROLOGICAL SYMPTOMS

A movement disorder presenting with orofacial dyskinesias and as limb chorea is most frequently observed.

PSYCHIATRIC SYMPTOMS

Eleven of 19 examined patients showed psychiatric symptoms.[80] The most consistent symptom was personality change, with impulsive and distractable behavior, apathy, and loss of insight. Additionally, depression, anxiety, paranoid delusions, and obsessive-compulsive features were seen.

DIAGNOSIS/DIFFERENTIAL DIAGNOSIS

The correct diagnosis depends on the combination of significant acanthocytosis with normal plasma lipoproteins and neurological abnormalities. In this context the clinical picture of CHAC with a predominantly hyperkinetic movement disorder, personality change, and cognitive impairment may resemble that of Huntington's disease. Therefore, in any suspected case of Huntington's disease, acanthocytosis should be excluded. Usually diagnosis of Huntington's disease will be confirmed by neurogenetic methods. This will likely be the case for CHAC in the near future as well.

Significant acanthocytosis is defined by the presence of >3 percent acanthocytes in dried blood smears. Acanthocytes have to be thoroughly distinguished from echinocytes. Scanning electron microscopy may be helpful in measuring the extent of the erythrocyte morphological abnormalities when in doubt.[80]

BIOCHEMICAL CRITERIA

Apart from acanthocytosis, only modestly elevated creatine kinase levels have been reported.[78] Other laboratory parameters, especially plasma lipoproteins, show no abnormalities.

NEUROIMAGING

CT revealed cortical or occasional caudate atrophy as significant features.[79,80] MRI showed focal and symmetric signal abnormalities in the caudate and lentiform nuclei in 3 out of 4 cases.[80] In another study, increased signal intensity accompanied by scattered bright spots in the striatum in T_2-weighted images was observed.[81] PET revealed the following alterations: mean posterior putamen ^{18}F-fluorodopa uptake was reduced to 42 percent of normal; depressed frontal and striatal blood flow was seen; and a loss of caudate and putamen D2 receptors was observed.[81,82]

THERAPY

Because there is no specific treatment known, therapy remains symptomatic. However, parkinsonian symptoms did not respond to high dosages of L-dopa,[71] and the response of the involuntary movements to drug treatment was generally poor.[69] Severe trunk spasms were improved by bilateral thalamic stimulation in one case.[83]

Pallidonigroluysian Degeneration (PNLD)

CLINICAL DEFINITION

The pallidal, pallidonigral, pallidoluysian, and pallidonigroluysian degenerations include a number of familial or sporadically occurring movement disorders clinically defined by a slowly progressive course and a wide variety of extrapyramidal symptoms. Morphologically, a degeneration of the pallidum alone or in association with the substantia nigra and/or the nucleus subthalamicus (of Luys) is found. The first 4 sporadic cases were described by Hunt.[84] This category of disorders with predominant affection of the pallidonigroluysian system has previously been classified

into four distinct groups: (1) pure pallidal atrophy, (2) pure pallidoluysian atrophy, (3) extended forms of pallidal degeneration (i.e., pallidonigral and the pallidoluysionigral atrophy), and (4) variable forms of these subtypes with other cerebrospinal degenerations.[85] For instance, the separately described pallidopyramidal disease (see below) could be considered a member of this group.[85] Furthermore, the relation of the familial pallidonigral system degeneration with cystic damage reported by McCormick and Lemmi[86] to the diseases discussed here is not known. Finally, in a small number of cases there is evidence of a possibly different movement disorder, characterized by the isolated degeneration of the external pallidum or status marmoratus of the basal ganglia in association with the occurrence of intraneuronal polyglucosan (Bielschowsky) bodies.[87] In this section we will focus on PNLD.

EPIDEMIOLOGY

No epidemiological data are available due to the small number of investigated cases.

NEUROGENETICS

In most of the reported families the condition appears to be of autosomal-recessive inheritance.[85] Recently, a mutation in the microtubule-associated protein tau has been found in a PNLD case.[88] This mutation, a substitution at codon 279, had previously been reported in a family with pallidopontonigral degeneration and in a family with dementia and supranuclear palsy.[89]

PATHOGENESIS

The pathogenesis of this (these) disorder(s) is not exactly known. The recent discovery of a mutation in the tau gene and the histopathological demonstration of hyperphosphorylated tau in one PLND case each suggest that this disorder is a tauopathy.[88,90] It can therefore be speculated that PNLD is related to FTDP-17 (see above). It is not clear whether pallidal, pallidoluysian, and pallidonigral degeneration are tauopathies as well.

NEUROPATHOLOGY

A progressive loss of nerve cells and fibers accompanied by proportional gliosis, particularly in the GP and the subthalamic nucleus, has been found.[85] The changes may vary in their extent. In rare instances they might be associated with further degenerative lesions in other extrapyramidal, motor neuron, or spinocerebellar systems. A pure pallidal atrophy with gliosis and locally differing neuronal loss was reported by Lange et al.[91] In another case of pure pallidal atrophy,[92] morphometric analysis revealed a shrinkage of the globus pallidus externus (GPe) to 59 percent of normal and of the globus pallidus internus (GPi) to 37 percent of normal, but the neuron density seemed not to be affected. Bilateral symmetrical loss of neurons and myelin with gliosis mainly in the outer pallidum was combined with pallor of the ansa lenticularis and atrophy of subthalamic nucleus in a case of pallidoluysian degeneration.[93] These changes are consistent with the findings observed in the various (extended) forms of this group of neurodegenerative disorders. Other observations include the occurrence of corpora amylacea throughout the CNS and brown granular deposits showing a positive reaction to iron in the degenerated nuclei and the striatum in PNLD.[94,95] Only recently, hyperphosphorylated tau was observed in a patient with PNLD.[90]

CLINICAL MANIFESTATIONS

Except for the CNS and psychiatric symptoms (see below), no other clinical manifestations are known.

CNS MANIFESTATIONS

The disorders demonstrate an insidious onset and a slowly progressive course. Onset of illness in familial cases was between ages 5 and 40, and in sporadic cases between ages 30 and 64. Depending on the variable pattern of morphological alterations, there may be distinct predominant symptoms. In pure pallidal degeneration the clinical picture is characterized by the development of progressive choreoathetotic hyperkinesias with axial dystonia, followed by the appearance of progressive rigidity. Finally, the involuntary movements are overcome by permanent rigidity, and the patients become bedridden.[85] In contrast, Aizawa et al. reported a case of pallidal degeneration with an extreme slowness of movements without rigidity as the main symptom.[92] In pallidoluysian degeneration, additional symptoms are torticollis, head tremor, and distal movements with or without a ballistic component.[85] Another case of pallidoluysian degeneration presented with 20 years of progressive generalized dystonia, dysarthria, gait disorder, vertical gaze palsy, and bradykinesia.[96] In PNLD the most apparent symptoms are progressive akinesia and rigidity with little or no tremor.[85] Additionally, upward gaze palsy or Parinaud's syndrome have been observed. Recently, a PNLD case with rapidly progressive hemidystonia was reported.[97] In conclusion, a wide spectrum of different clinical manifestations exists, depending on the spatial and temporal pattern of affection of the distinct brain areas. Consequently, because of their rarity, the clinical correlates of the distinct forms are still not well described.

CARDINAL NEUROLOGICAL SYMPTOMS

Familial occurrence of the combination of progressive rigidity and choreoathethosis or torsion dystonia with an early onset may suggest one of these disorders.

PSYCHIATRIC SYMPTOMS

The disorders may be accompanied by mental deterioration, but intellectual impairment may be absent, even in advanced disease stages.[85] A history of psychosis was reported in several cases.[94,95] The PNLD patient with the mutation in the tau gene featured dementia, whereas no dementia was observed in the case with the accumulation of hyperphosphorylated tau.[88,90]

DIAGNOSIS/DIFFERENTIAL DIAGNOSIS

The diagnosis of these rare conditions can only be proven by means of postmortem examination. Possible differential diagnoses include juvenile parkinsonism, idiopathic torsion dystonia, PKAN, dentatorubropallidoluysian atrophy, progressive supranuclear palsy, striatonigral degeneration, corticobasal degeneration, and others. Sequencing of the tau gene, if available, should be performed.

BIOCHEMICAL CRITERIA

Routine laboratory date are unremarkable.

NEUROIMAGING

CT in younger patients was normal;[85] minimal atrophy of the brainstem and dilation of the brainstem and of the sylvian fissure were seen in a single case.[92] MRI of the brain in a patient with pallidoluysian degeneration showed no abnormalities.[96] T_2-weighted MRI demonstrated increased signal intensity in pallidum and SN in a PNLD patient with hemidystonia.[97] Furthermore, contralateral cortical hyperperfusion was observed in this patient.

THERAPY

Treatment with L-dopa has produced only equivocal improvement of the movement disorder.[92,98] However, 1 patient with dystonic symptoms was reported to benefit from baclofen.[96]

Pallidopyramidal Disease

CLINICAL DEFINITION

Pallidopyramidal disease is thought to be an autosomal-recessive disorder with onset in the second or early third decade, with a clinical picture consisting of parkinsonism and pyramidal tract signs.[99–102] Furthermore, a syndrome was reported that is closely related but not identical to pallidopyramidal disease. It is called Kufor-Rakeb syndrome and additionally characterized by supranuclear upgaze paresis and dementia.[103]

EPIDEMIOLOGY

Until now 11 familial and 4 nonfamilial cases have been described.

NEUROGENETICS

It has been suggested that pallidopyramidal disease is recessively inherited.[102] The disease locus for Kufor-Rakeb syndrome has been mapped to chromosome 1p36.[104]

PATHOGENESIS

The pathogenesis of pallidopyramidal disease is unknown.

NEUROPATHOLOGY

Until now only one autopsy in a nonfamilial patient 50 years after onset has been performed.[99] A pallor of the pallidal segments, slight shrinkage and cellular change of the substantia nigra, a thinning of the ansa lenticularis, and early demyelination of the pyramids and crossed pyramidal tracts were observed. The latter extended from the lower parts of the medulla oblongata into the spinal cord.

CLINICAL MANIFESTATIONS

Pallidopyramidal disease is characterized by its CNS symptoms.

CNS MANIFESTATIONS

In general, disease onset occurred during the second or the early third decade. The 2 siblings reported by Horowitz and Greenberg[100] developed their first symptoms in the first decade of life. The classical parkinsonian features were observed in all cases. Pyramidal tract signs, consisting of hyperreflexia, spastic muscle tone, and bilateral extensor plantar responses, were also found. In the patients described by Nisipeanu et al. the occurrence of pyramidal tract signs preceded the appearance of extrapyramidal symptoms.[102] Only a slow progression of the disorder was noted. The two patients investigated by Horowitz et al.[100] were still ambulatory after 10–13 years of disease. No diurnal variation was observed. Some patients examined by Davison showed additional symptoms such as horizontal nystagmus, intention tremor, poor memory, and impaired intelligence.[99]

CARDINAL NEUROLOGICAL SYMPTOMS

The cardinal neurological symptoms are featured by the co-occurrence of young-onset parkinsonism and pyramidal tract signs.

PSYCHIATRIC SYMPTOMS

Psychiatric symptoms have not been observed in this syndrome. However, 1 patient reported by Davison had impaired intelligence. Furthermore, 3 out of the 5 patients with Kufor-Rakeb syndrome were demented.[103]

DIAGNOSIS/DIFFERENTIAL DIAGNOSIS

The diagnostic possibilities are limited. Evidence of isolated extrapyramidal and pyramidal signs and normal laboratory and neuroradiologic investigations in a young adult are suggestive of pallidopyramidal disease. Possible differential diagnoses are juvenile parkinsonism and L-dopa-responsive dystonia.

BIOCHEMICAL CRITERIA

No biochemical criteria for diagnosis are known.

NEUROIMAGING

Three out of the 4 patients examined by Nisipeanu et al. were subjected to cranial CT and MRI. No abnormalities were found. Patients suffering from Kufor-Rakeb syndrome showed, in contrast, generalized atrophy on MRI with pronounced atrophy of the lentiform nuclei and the pyramids.[103] PET with ^{18}F-fluorodopa was performed in 2 patients with pallidopyramidal disease and showed marked dopaminergic denervation of the striatum.[105] PET with ^{11}C-flumazenil demonstrated a marked decrease in benzodiazepine receptor density in the precentral gyrus and the mesial frontal cortex.[106]

THERAPY

Extrapyramidal symptoms improved with L-dopa therapy. Typically, the pyramidal symptoms were not influenced by this treatment. However, Tranchant et al. reported a worsening of pyramidal tract signs due to the medication regimen.[101] Response to L-dopa was somewhat variable; most patients responded rapidly to low doses with improvement persisting for a long period. After many years of treatment, "wearing-off" phenomena occurred. The daily dose of L-dopa used in the patients reported by Nisipeanu et al. was 500–1000 mg.[102]

Rett Syndrome

CLINICAL DEFINITION

Rett syndrome is a progressive neurodegenerative disorder, which is reported almost exclusively in females and characterized by a wide spectrum of motor and behavioral abnormalities. It was first described by Rett in 1966,[107,108] and subsequently investigated by other authors.[109,110]

The most typical symptoms are stereotyped movements and gait disturbance. Furthermore, parkinsonism and hyperkinetic disorders can be associated with Rett syndrome.

EPIDEMIOLOGY

The prevalence of Rett syndrome is estimated to be about 0.44/10,000.[111]

NEUROGENETICS

It has been proposed that Rett syndrome is the result of an X-linked-dominant mutation with mortality for hemizygous males with each case representing a new mutation.[112] Previous studies mapped the disease locus to Xq28.[113] Recently, de novo mutations in the gene encoding X-linked methyl-CpG-binding protein 2 (MeCP2) have been identified as a cause of Rett syndrome.[114] Methylation of CpG dinucleotides in genomic DNA represents a fundamental epigenetic mechanism of gene expression control. MeCP2 likely causes transcriptional repression through an interaction with core histones since the MeCP2 binding domain was shown to associate with histone deacetylases. Mutations in the MECP2 gene have been identified in 75–90 percent of sporadic cases, and approximately 50 percent of the rare familial cases.[115] However, MECP2 mutations can also be found in individuals lacking the clinical features of Rett syndrome.[116]

PATHOGENESIS

Rett syndrome is likely due to a loss of function of MeCP2. Genotype-phenotype studies suggest that the pattern of X-chromosome inactivation has a more prominent effect on clinical severity than the type of mutation.[115] It still remains to be determined why mutations of the widely expressed MECP2 gene give rise to a predominantly neuronal phenotype. So far it is not known what subset of genes is regulated by MeCP2.

NEUROPATHOLOGY

Autopsy studies showed diffuse cerebral atrophy with a decrease in brain weight of 14–34 percent compared to that of age-matched controls, with increased amounts of lipofuscin and, occasionally, mild astrocytosis seen microscopically. Moreover, mild but inconsistent spongy changes of white matter were found. Most apparent was a low level of pigmentation of the substantia nigra, whereas the number of nigral neurons was normal.[117] In addition, selective dendritic alterations in the cortex of patients with Rett syndrome were reported.[118]

CLINICAL MANIFESTATIONS

Rett syndrome leads not only to neurological abnormalities, but also to dysfunction of other organs.[119]

Gastrointestinal complaints include constipation and weight loss. Swallowing difficulties are also common. Furthermore, an unusual breathing pattern with central apnea intermixed with hyperventilation is frequently observed. Scoliosis occurs often. Patients with Rett syndrome have significantly longer corrected QT intervals and T-wave abnormalities on electrocardiograms, which might explain sudden death in Rett syndrome.[120]

CNS MANIFESTATIONS

A 4-stage model for the description of Rett syndrome was proposed.[110] Stage 1 is defined by developmental stagnation, hypotonia, and deceleration of head growth (onset 6 months to 1.5 years). Stage 2 is characterized by loss of functional hand use, stereotypic hand-wringing, loss of expressive language, rapid developmental regression, and occasional seizures (onset 1–3 or 4 years). Stage 3 is termed a pseudostationary period because of some restitution of communication, but increasing ataxia, hyperreflexia, and rigidity, as well as breathing dysfunction and bruxism, are observed. After several years stage 4 develops with the so-called late motor deterioration and growth retardation.

With respect to extrapyramidal dysfunction, bruxism (97 percent), oculogyric crises (63 percent), and parkinsonism and dystonia (59 percent) are common features.[121] Myoclonus and choreoatheosis were seen only infrequently. In younger patients (<4 years) hyperkinetic disorders were more evident, whereas in older patients (>8 years) the bradykinetic syndrome tended to predominate. Drooling (75 percent), rigidity (44 percent), and bradykinesia (41 percent) were the most often observed parkinsonian symptoms. Parkinsonism has so far not been included among the diagnostic criteria of Rett syndrome or variant Rett syndrome (see below).[116,122]

CARDINAL NEUROLOGICAL SYMPTOMS

The cardinal neurological symptoms are developmental stagnation followed by dementia, autism, loss of purposeful hand movements, and jerky truncal ataxia in a stage-dependent manner.[109] It has been suggested that the jerky truncal ataxia represents a combination of cerebellar ataxia and myoclonus.[121]

PSYCHIATRIC SYMPTOMS

Sleep disturbances, mainly in the early stages, are frequently present in Rett syndrome. They are characterized by an overall increase in daytime sleep and a delayed onset of sleep at night. Despite their mental retardation and their loss of expressive language, these patients tend to appear happy and enjoy close physical contact.

DIAGNOSIS/DIFFERENTIAL DIAGNOSIS

Criteria for the diagnosis of Rett syndrome were initially developed by The Rett Syndrome Diagnostic Criteria Work Group in 1988.[122] These criteria have been revised in the light of the recent advances in the understanding of the molecular biology of Rett syndrome.[116] Necessary criteria for the diagnosis of Rett syndrome are apparently normal prenatal and perinatal history; a largely normal (or delayed) psychomotor development through the first 6 months; normal head circumference at birth; postnatal deceleration of head growth in the majority; loss of purposeful hand skills at the age of 0.5–2.5 years; stereotypic hand movements; emerging social withdrawal, communication dysfunction, loss of learned words, and cognitive impairment; and impaired or failing locomotion. Supportive criteria include awake disturbances of breathing; bruxism; impaired sleep pattern from early infancy; abnormal muscle tone; peripheral vasomotor disturbances; scoliosis/kyphosis progressing through childhood; growth retardation; and small hands and feet. Diagnostic criteria for variant Rett syndrome have also been developed.[123]

Infantile autism is one of the most important differential diagnoses. Further differential diagnoses include other neurodevelopmental disorders with mental retardation and motor impairment. Sequencing of the MECP2 gene, if available, is advisable.

BIOCHEMICAL CRITERIA

It was proposed that hyperammonemia could be an essential sign of this condition,[107,108] but further investigations did not reproduce the findings of hyperammonemia in most patients.[109] Significant reductions in the metabolites of norepinephrine, dopamine, and serotonin, as well as an elevation of biopterin in the cerebrospinal fluid, constituted the first detected biochemical alterations.[124] Additionally, there is evidence of elevation of lactate, pyruvate, alpha-ketoglutarate, malate, and glutamate in the cerebrospinal fluid.[125,126]

NEUROIMAGING

MRI indicated a global hypoplasia of brain and progressive cerebellar atrophy increasing with age.[127] An increased density of D2 receptors in the striatum of patients suffering from Rett syndrome using SPECT imaging was found.[128] ^{18}F-fluorodeoxyglucose PET showed several areas of hypometabolism with markedly lower metabolism in the occipital lobes.[129] Furthermore, a mild presynaptic deficit of nigrostriatal activity was demonstrated by ^{18}F-fluorodopa and PET.[130]

THERAPY

There is no specific treatment. Naltrexone appears to provide clinical benefit in the treatment of breathing dysfunction and cognitive impairment.[131] Furthermore, bromocriptine, L-carnitine, and lamotrigine can be tried to improve certain disease symptoms.[132–134] Symptomatic therapeutic approaches also include physio- and music therapy.[118]

References

1. Lynch T, Sano M, Marder KS, et al: Clinical characteristics of a family with chromosome 17-linked disinhibition-dementia-parkinsonism-amyotrophy complex. *Neurology* 44:1878–1884, 1994.
2. Foster NL, Wilhelmsen K, Sima AA, et al: Frontotemporal dementia and parkinsonism linked to chromosome 17: A consensus conference. *Ann Neurol* 41:706–715, 1997.
3. Wszolek ZK, Pfeiffer RF, Bhatt MH, et al: Rapidly progressive autosomal dominant parkinsonism and dementia with pallido-ponto-nigral degeneration. *Ann Neurol* 32:312–320, 1992.
4. Wszolek ZK, Tsuboi Y, Farrer M, et al: Hereditary tauopathies and parkinsonism. *Adv Neurol* 91:153–163, 2003.
5. Hutton M, Lendon CL, Rizzu P, et al: Association of missense and 5′-splice-site mutations in tau with the inherited dementia FTDP-17. *Nature* 393:702–705, 1998.
6. Rosso SM, van Swieten JC: New developments in frontotemporal dementia and parkinsonism linked to chromosome 17. *Curr Opin Neurol* 15:423–428, 2002.
7. Morris HR, Kanh MN, Janssen JC, et al: The genetic and pathological classification of familial frontotemporal dementia. *Arch Neurol* 58:1813–1816, 2001.
8. Hallervorden J, Spatz H: Eigenartige Erkrankung im extrapyramidalen System mit besonderer Beteiligung des Globus Pallidus und der Substantia Nigra. *Z Gesamte Neurol Psychiatr* 79:254–302, 1922.
9. Zhou B, Westaway SK, Levinson B, et al: A novel pantothenate kinase gene (PANK2) is defective in Hallervorden-Spatz syndrome. *Nat Genet* 28:345–349, 2001.
10. Taylor TD, Litt M, Kramer P, et al: Homozygosity mapping of Hallervorden-Spatz syndrome to chromosome 20p12.3-p13. *Nat Genet* 14:479–481, 1996.
11. Hayflick SJ, Westaway SK, Levinson B, et al: Genetic, clinical, and radiographic delineation of Hallervorden-Spatz syndrome. *N Engl J Med* 348:33–40, 2003.
12. Swaiman KF: Hallervorden-Spatz syndrome and brain iron metabolism. *Arch Neurol* 48:1285–1293, 1991.
13. Seitelberger F: Zur Morphologie und Histochemie der degenerativen Axonveränderungen vom Zentralnervensystem, in: *Proceedings of the 3rd International Congress of Neuropathology* 1957, pp 127–147.
14. Galvin JE, Giasson B, Hurtig HI, et al: Neurodegeneration with brain iron accumulation, type 1 is characterized by alpha-, beta-, and gamma-synuclein neuropathology. *Am J Pathol* 157:361–368, 2000.
15. Wigboldus JM, Bruyn GW: Hallervorden-Spatz disease, in Vinken PJ, Bruyn GW (eds): *Handbook of Clinical Neurology: Diseases of the Basal Ganglia.* Amsterdam: Elsevier, 1968, pp 604–631.
16. Dooling EC, Schoene WC, Richardson EP Jr: Hallervorden-Spatz syndrome. *Arch Neurol* 30:70–83, 1974.

17. Jankovic J, Kirkpatrick JB, Blomquist KA, et al: Late-onset Hallervorden-Spatz disease presenting as familial parkinsonism. *Neurology* 35:227–234, 1985.

18. Curtis AR, Fey C, Morris CM, et al: Mutation in the gene encoding ferritin light polypeptide causes dominant adult-onset basal ganglia disease. *Nat Genet* 28:350–354, 2001.

19. Gitlin JD: Aceruloplasminemia. *Pediatr Res* 44:271–276, 1998.

20. Swaiman KF, Smith KA, Trock GL, et al: Sea-blue histiocytes, lymphocytic cytosomes and 59Fe-studies in Hallervorden-Spatz syndrome. *Neurology* 33:301–305, 1983.

21. Ching KH, Westaway SK, Gitschier J, et al: HARP syndrome is allelic with pantothenate kinase-associated neurodegeneration. *Neurology* 58:1673–1674, 2002.

22. Dooling EC, Richardson EP Jr, Davis KR: Computed tomography in Hallervorden-Spatz disease. *Neurology* 30:1128–1130, 1980.

23. Rutledge JN, Hilal SK, Silver AJ, et al: Study of movement disorders and brain iron by MR. *Am J Roentgenol* 149:365–379, 1987.

24. Sethi KD, Adams RJ, Loring DW, et al: Hallervorden-Spatz syndrome: Clinical and magnetic resonance imaging correlations. *Ann Neurol* 24:692–694, 1988.

25. Klawans HL: Hemiparkinsonism as a late complication of hemiatrophy: A new syndrome. *Neurology* 31:625–628, 1981.

26. Buchman AS, Goetz CG, Klawans HL: Hemiparkinsonism with hemiatrophy. *Neurology* 38:527–530, 1988.

27. Giladi N, Burke RE, Kostic V, et al: Hemiparkinsonism-hemiatrophy syndrome: Clinical and neuroradiologic features. *Neurology* 40:1731–1734, 1990.

28. Pramstaller PP, Kunig G, Leenders K, et al: Parkin mutations in a patient with hemiparkinsonism-hemiatrophy: A clinical-genetic and PET study. *Neurology* 58:808–810, 2002.

29. Penfield W, Robertson JSM: Growth asymmetry due to lesions of the post central cortex. *Arch Neurol Psychiatry* 50:405–430, 1943.

30. Greene PE, Bressman SB, Ford B, et al: Parkinsonism, dystonia, and hemiatrophy. *Mov Disord* 15:537–541, 2000.

31. Hebb MO, Lang AE, Fletcher PJ, et al: Neonatal ablation of the nigrostriatal dopamine pathway does not influence limb developments in rats. *Exp Neurol* 177: 547–556, 2002.

32. Halperin G: Normal asymmetry and unilateral hypertrophy. *Arch Intern Med* 48:676–684, 1931.

33. Giladi N, Fahn S: Hemiparkinsonism-hemiatrophy syndrome may mimic early-stage cortical-basal ganglionic degeneration. *Mov Disord* 7:384–385, 1992.

34. Przedborski S, Goldman S, Levivier M, et al: Brain glucose metabolism and dopamine D2 receptor analysis in a patient with hemiparkinsonism-hemiatrophy syndrome. *Mov Disord* 8:391–395, 1993.

35. Przedborski S, Giladi N, Takikawa S, et al: Metabolic topography of the hemiparkinsonism-hemiatrophy syndrome. *Neurology* 44:1622–1628, 1994.

36. Jenkins M, Mendonca D, Parrent A, et al: Hemiparkinsonism-somatic hemiatrophy syndrome. *Can J Neurol Sci* 29:184–187, 2002.

37. Kosaka K: Diffuse Lewy body disease in Japan. *J Neurol* 237:197–204, 1990.

38. McKeith IG, Galasko D, Kosaka K, et al: Consensus guidelines for the clinical and pathologic diagnosis of dementia with Lewy bodies (DLB): Report of the consortium on DLB international workshop. *Neurology* 47:1113–1124, 1996.

39. Olichney JM, Hansen LA, Galasko D, et al: The apolipoprotein E epsilon 4 allele is associated with increased neuritic plaques and cerebral amyloid angiopathy in Alzheimers's disease and Lewy body variant. *Neurology* 47:190–196, 1996.

40. Tanaka S, Chen X, Xia Y, et al: Association of CYP2D microsatellite polymorphism with Lewy body variant of Alzheimer's disease. *Neurology* 50:1556–1562, 1993.

41. Schlossmacher MG, Frosch MP, Gai WP, et al: Parkin localizes to the Lewy bodies of Parkinson disease and dementia with Lewy body. *Am J Pathol* 160:1655–1667, 2002.

42. Gwinn-Hardy K, Mehta ND, Farrer M, et al: Distinctive neuropathology revealed by alpha-synuclein antibodies in hereditary parkinsonism and dementia linked to chromosome 4p. *Acta Neuropathol (Berl)* 99:663–672, 2000.

43. McKeith IG, Perry EK, Perry RH: Diagnosis and treatment of dementia with Lewy bodies (DLB): Report on the second DLB International Workshop. *Neurology* 53:902–905, 1999.

44. McKeith IG, Ballard CG, Perry RH, et al: Prospective validation of consensus criteria for the diagnosis of dementia with Lewy bodies. *Neurology* 54:1050–1058, 2000.

45. Ballard C, Grace J, McKeith I, et al: Neuroleptic sensitivity in dementia with Lewy bodies and Alzheimer's disease. *Lancet* 351:1032–1033, 1998.

46. Fernandez HH, Trieschmann ME, Burke MA, et al: Quetiapine for psychosis in Parkinson's disease versus dementia with Lewy bodies. *J Clin Psychiatry* 63:513–515, 2002.

47. Ballard CG, Aarsland D, McKeith I, et al: Fluctuations in attention: PD dementia vs DLB with parkinsonism. *Neurology* 59:1714–1720, 2002.

48. Barber R, Gholkar A, Scheltens P, et al: Medial temporal lobe atrophy on MRI in dementia with Lewy bodies. *Neurology* 52:1153–1158, 1999.

49. Walker Z, Costa DC, Ince P, et al: In-vivo demonstration of dopaminergic degeneration in dementia with Lewy bodies. *Lancet* 354:646–647, 1999.

50. McKeith I, Del Ser, Spano P, et al: Efficacy of rivastigmine in dementia with Lewy bodies: A randomised, double-blind, placebo-controlled international study. *Lancet* 356:2024–2025, 2000.

51. Lee LV, Pascasio FM, Fuentes FD, et al: Torsion dystonia in Panay, Philippines. *Adv Neurol* 14:137–151, 1976.

52. Lee LV, Maranon E, Demaisip C, et al: The natural history of sex-linked recessive dystonia parkinsonism of Panay, Philippines (XDP). *Parkinsonism Relat Disord* 9:29–38, 2002.

53. Waters CH, Faust PL, Powers J, et al: Neuropathology of lubag (X-linked dystonia parkinsonism). *Mov Disord* 8:387–390, 1993.

54. Nemeth AH, Nolte D, Dunne E, et al: Refined linkage disequilibrium and physical mapping of the gene locus for X-linked dystonia-parkinsonism (DYT3). *Genomics* 60:320–329, 1999.

55. Waters CH, Takahashi H, Wilhelmsen KC, et al: Phenotypic expression of X-linked dystonia-parkinsonism (lubag) in two women. *Neurology* 43:1555–1558, 1993.

56. Evidente VG, Advincula J, Esteban R, et al: Phenomenology of lubag or X-linked dystonia-parkinsonism. *Mov Disord* 17:1271–1277, 2002.

57. Evidente VG, Gwinn-Hardy K, Hardy J, et al: X-linked dystonia (lubag) presenting predominantly with parkinsonism: A more benign phenotype? *Mov Disord* 17:200–202, 2002.

58. Eidelberg D, Takikawa S, Wilhelmsen K, et al: Positron emission tomographic findings in Filipino X-linked dystonia-parkinsonism. *Ann Neurol* 34:185–191, 1993.

59. Lee LV, Kupke KG, Caballar-Gonzaga F, et al: The phenotype of the X-linked dystonia-parkinsonism syndrome. An assessment of 42 cases in the Philippines. *Medicine* 70:179–187, 1991.

60. Evidente VG: Zolpidem improves dystonia in lubag or X-linked dystonia-parkinsonism syndrome. *Neurology* 58:662–663, 2002.

61. Brecher G, Bessis M: Present status of spiculed red cells and their relationship to the discocyte-echinocyte transformation: A critical review. *Blood* 40:333–344, 1972.

62. Kornzweig AL, Bassen FA: Retinitis pigmentosa, acanthocytosis and hererodegenerative neuromuscular disease. *Arch Ophthalmol* 58:183–187, 1957.

63. Young SG, Bertics SJ, Curtiss LK, et al: Genetic analysis of a kindred with familial hypobetalipoproteinemia. Evidence for two separate gene defects: One associated with an abnormal apolipoprotein B species, apolipoprotein B-37; and a second associated with low plasma concentrations of apolipoprotein B-100. *J Clin Invest* 79:1842–1851, 1987.

64. Levine IM, Estes JW, Looney JM: Hereditary neurological disease with acanthocytosis. *Arch Neurol* 19:403–409, 1968.

65. Critchley EM, Clark DB, Wikler A: Acanthocytosis and neurological disorder without betalipoproteinemia. *Arch Neurol* 18:134–140, 1968.

66. Allen FH, Krabbe FMR, Corcoran PA: A new phenotype (McLeod) in the Kell blood group system. *Vox Sang* 6:555–560, 1961.

67. Danek A, Rubio JP, Rampoldi L, et al: McLeod neuroacanthocytosis: Genotype and phenotype. *Ann Neurol* 50:755–764, 2001.

68. Swash M, Schwartz MS, Carter ND, et al: Benign X-linked myopathy with acanthocytes (McLeod syndrome). Its relationship to X-linked muscular dystrophy. *Brain* 106:717–733, 1983.

69. Hardie RJ: Acanthocytosis and neurological impairment: A review. *Q J Med* 71:291–306, 1989.

70. Yamamoto T, Hirose G, Shimazaki K, et al: Movement disorders of familial neuroacanthocytosis syndrome. *Arch Neurol* 39:298–301, 1982.

71. Spitz MC, Jankovic J, Killian JM: Familial tic disorder, parkinsonism, motor neuron disease and acanthocytosis: A new syndrome. *Neurology* 35:366–370, 1985.

72. Ueno S, Maruki Y, Nakamura M, et al: The gene encoding a newly discovered protein, chorein, is mutated in chorea-acanthocytosis. *Nat Genet* 28:121–122, 2001.

73. Rampoldi L, Dobson-Stone C, Rubio JP, et al: A conserved sorting-associated protein is mutant in chorea-acanthocytosis. *Nat Genet* 28:119–120, 2001.

74. Dobson-Stone C, Danek A, Rampoldi L, et al: Mutational spectrum of the CHAC gene in patients with chorea-acanthocytosis. *Eur J Hum Genet* 10:773–781, 2002.

75. Walker RH, Morgello S, Davidoff-Feldman B, et al: Autosomal dominant chorea-acanthocytosis with polyglutamine-containing neuronal inclusions. *Neurology* 58:1031–1037, 2002.

76. Rinne JO, Daniel SE, Scaravilli F, et al: The neuropathological features of neuroacanthocytosis. *Mov Disord* 9:297–304, 1994.

77. Rinne JO, Daniel SE, Scaravilli F, et al: Nigral degeneration in neuroacanthocytosis. *Neurology* 44:1629–1632, 1994.

78. Sakai T, Mawatari S, Iwashita H, et al: Choreoacanthocytosis. Clues to clinical diagnosis. *Arch Neurol* 38:335–338, 1981.

79. Serra S, Xerra A, Scribano E, et al: Computerized tomography in amyotrophic choreo-acanthocytosis. *Neuroradiology* 29:480–482, 1987.

80. Hardie RJ, Pullon HW, Harding AE, et al: Neuroacanthocytosis. A clinical, haematological and pathological study of 19 cases. *Brain* 114:13–49, 1991.

81. Tanaka M, Hirai S, Kondo S, et al: Cerebral hypoperfusion and hypometabolism with altered striatal signal intensity in chorea-acanthocytosis: A combined PET and MRI study. *Mov Disord* 13:100–107, 1998.

82. Brooks DJ, Ibanez V, Playford ED, et al: Presynaptic and postsynaptic striatal dopaminergic function in neuroacanthocytosis: A positron emission tomographic study. *Ann Neurol* 30:166–171, 1991.

83. Burbaud P, Rougier A, Ferrer X, et al: Improvement of severe trunk spasms by bilateral high-frequency stimulation of the motor thalamus in a patient with chorea-acanthocytosis. *Mov Disord* 17:204–207, 2002.

84. Hunt JR: Progressive atrophy of the globus pallidus (primary atrophy of the pallidal system): A system disease of the paralysis agitans type, characterized by atrophy of the motor cells of the corpus striatum. A contribution to the functions of the corpus striatum. *Brain* 40:58–148, 1917.

85. Jellinger K: Pallidal, pallidonigral, and pallidoluysionigral degenerations including association with thalamic and dentate degenerations, in Vinken PJ, Bruyn GW (eds): *Handbook of Clinical Neurology*. Amsterdam: Elsevier, 1986, pp 445–463.

86. McCormick WF, Lemmi H: Familial degeneration of the pallidonigral system. *Neurology* 15:141–153, 1965.

87. Yagishita S, Itoh Y, Nakano T, et al: Pleomorphic intra-neuronal polyglucosan bodies mainly restricted to the pallidium. A case report. *Acta Neuropathol* 62:159–163, 1983.

88. Yasuda M, Kawamata T, Komure O, et al: A mutation in the microtubule-associated protein tau in pallido-nigro-luysian degeneration. *Neurology* 53:864–868, 1999.

89. Wszolek ZK, Uitti RJ, Hutton M: A mutation in the microtubule-associated protein tau in pallido-nigro-luysian degeneration. *Neurology* 54:2028–2030, 2000.

90. Mori H, Motoi Y, Kobayashi T, et al: Tau accumulation in a patient with pallidonigroluysian atrophy. *Neurosci Lett* 309:89–92, 2001.

91. Lange E, Poppe W, Scholtze P: Familial progressive pallidum atrophy. *Eur Neurol* 3:265–267, 1970.

92. Aizawa H, Kwak S, Shimizu T, et al: A case of adult onset pure pallidal degeneration. I. Clinical manifestations and neuropathological observations. *J Neurol Sci* 102:76–82, 1991.

93. van Bogaert L: Aspects cliniques et pathologiques des atrophies pallidales et pallido-luysiennes progressives. *J Belge Neurol Psychiatr* 47:268–286, 1947.

94. Kosaka K, Matsushita M, Oyanagi S, et al: Pallido-nigro-luysial atrophy with massive appearance of corpora amylacea in the CNS. *Acta Neuropathol* 53:169–172, 1981.

95. Kawai J, Sasahara M, Hazama F, et al: Pallidonigroluysian degeneration with iron deposition: A study of three autopsy cases. *Acta Neuropathol* 86:609–616, 1993.

96. Wooten GF, Lopes MB, Harris WO, et al: Pallidoluysian atrophy: Dystonia and basal ganglia functional anatomy. *Neurology* 43:1764–1768, 1993.

97. Vercueil L, Hammouti A, Andriantseheno ML, et al: Pallido-luysio-nigral atrophy revealed by rapidly progressive hemidystonia: A clinical, radiologic, functional, and neuropathologic study. *Mov Disord* 15:947–953, 2000.

98. Yamamoto T, Kawamura J, Hashimoto S, et al: Pallido-nigro-luysian atrophy, progressive supranuclear palsy and adult onset Hallervorden-Spatz disease: A case of akinesia as a predominant feature of parkinsonism. *J Neurol Sci* 101:98–106, 1991.

99. Davison C: Pallido-pyramidal disease. *J Neuropathol Exp Neurol* 13:50–59, 1954.

100. Horowitz G, Greenberg J: Pallido-pyramidal syndrome treated with levodopa. *J Neurol Neurosurg Psychiatry* 38:238–240, 1975.

101. Tranchant C, Boulay C, Warter JM: [Pallido-pyramidal syndrome: An unrecognized entity]. *Rev Neurol (Paris)* 147:308–310, 1991.

102. Nisipeanu P, Kuritzky A, Korczyn AD: Familial levodopa-responsive parkinsonian-pyramidal syndrome. *Mov Disord* 9:673–675, 1994.

103. Najim al-Din AS, Wriekat A, Mubaidin A, et al: Pallido-pyramidal degeneration, supranuclear upgaze paresis and dementia: Kufor-Rakeb syndrome. *Acta Neurol Scand* 89:347–352, 1994.

104. Hampshire DJ, Roberts E, Crow Y, et al: Kufor-Rakeb syndrome, pallido-pyramidal degeneration with supranuclear upgaze paresis and dementia, maps to 1p36. *J Med Genet* 38:680–682, 2001.

105. Remy P, Hosseini H, Degos JD, et al: Striatal dopaminergic denervation in pallidopyramidal disease demonstrated by positron emission tomography. *Ann Neurol* 38:954–956, 1995.

106. Pradat PF, Dupel-Pottier C, Lacomblez L, et al: Case report of pallido-pyramidal disease with supplementary motor area involvement. *Mov Disord* 16:762–764, 2001.

107. Rett A: [On an until now unknown disease of a congenital metabolic disorder]. *Krankenschwester* 19:121–122, 1966.

108. Rett A: Cerebral atrophy with hyperammonaemia, in Vinken PJ, Bruyn GW (eds): *Handbook of Clinical Neurology*. Amsterdam: Elsevier, 1977, pp 305–329.

109. Hagberg B, Aicardi J, Dias K, et al: A progressive syndrome of autism, dementia, ataxia, and loss of purposeful hand use in girls: Rett's syndrome: Report of 35 cases. *Ann Neurol* 14:471–479, 1983.

110. Hagberg B, Witt-Engerstrom I: Rett syndrome: A suggested staging system for describing impairment profile with increasing age towards adolescence. *Am J Med Genet Suppl* 1:47–59, 1986.

111. Kozinetz CA, Skender ML, MacNaughton N, et al: Epidemiology of Rett syndrome: A population-based registry. *Pediatrics* 91:445–450, 1993.

112. Comings DE: The genetics of Rett syndrome: The consequences of a disorder where every case is a new mutation. *Am J Med Genet Suppl* 1:383–388, 1986.

113. Sirianni N, Naidu S, Pereira J, et al: Rett syndrome: Confirmation of X-linked dominant inheritance, and localization of the gene to Xq28. *Am J Hum Genet* 63:1781–1785, 1998.

114. Amir RE, Van den Veyver IB, Wan M, et al: Rett syndrome is caused by mutations in X-linked MECP2, encoding methyl-CpG-binding protein 2. *Nat Genet* 23:185–188, 1999.

115. Shahbazian MD, Zoghbi HY: Molecular genetics of Rett syndrome and clinical spectrum of MECP2 mutations. *Curr Opin Neurol* 14:171–176, 2001.

116. Hagberg B, Hanefeld F, Percy A, et al: An update on clinically applicable diagnostic criteria in Rett syndrome. Comments to Rett Syndrome Clinical Criteria Consensus Panel Satellite to European Paediatric Neurology Society Meeting. *Eur J Paediatr Neurol* 6:293–297, 2002.

117. Jellinger K, Seitelberger F: Neuropathology of Rett syndrome. *Am J Med Genet Suppl* 1:259–288, 1986.

118. Armstrong D, Dunn JK, Antalffy B, et al: Selective dendritic alterations in the cortex of Rett syndrome. *J Neuropathol Exp Neurol* 54:195–201, 1995.

119. Braddock SR, Braddock BA, Graham JM Jr: Rett syndrome. An update and review for the primary pediatrician. *Clin Pediatr (Phila)* 32:613–626, 1993.

120. Sekul EA, Moak JP, Schultz RJ, et al: Electrocardiographic findings in Rett syndrome: An explanation for sudden death? *J Pediatr* 125:80–82, 1994.

121. FitzGerald PM, Jankovic J, Percy AK: Rett syndrome and associated movement disorders. *Mov Disord* 5:195–202, 1990.

122. The Rett Syndrome Diagnostic Criteria Work Group: Criteria for Rett syndrome. *Ann Neurol* 23:425–428, 1988.

123. Hagberg BA, Skjeldal OH: Rett variants: A suggested model for inclusion criteria. *Pediatr Neurol* 11:5–11, 1994.

124. Zoghbi HY, Milstien S, Butler IJ, et al: Cerebrospinal fluid biogenic amines and biopterin in Rett syndrome. *Ann Neurol* 25:56–60, 1989.

125. Hamberger A, Gillberg C, Palm A, et al: Elevated CSF glutamate in Rett syndrome. *Neuropediatrics* 23:212–213, 1992.

126. Matsuishi T, Urabe F, Percy AK, et al: Abnormal carbohydrate metabolism in cerebrospinal fluid in Rett syndrome. *J Child Neurol* 9:26–30, 1994.

127. Murakami JW, Courchesne E, Haas RH, et al: Cerebellar and cerebral abnormalities in Rett syndrome: A quantitative MR analysis. *Am J Roentgenol* 159:177–183, 1992.

128. Chiron C, Bulteau B, Loch C, et al: Dopaminergic D2 receptor SPECT imaging in Rett syndrome: Increase of specific binding in striatum. *J Nucl Med* 34:1717–1721, 1993.

129. Naidu S, Wong DF, Kitt C, et al: Positron emission tomography in the Rett syndrome: Clinical, biochemical and pathological correlates. *Brain Dev* 14:S75–79, 1992.

130. Dunn HG, Stoessl AJ, Ho HH, et al: Rett syndrome: Investigation of nine patients, including PET scan. *Can J Neurol Sci* 29:345–357, 2002.

131. Percy AK, Glaze DG, Schultz RJ, et al: Rett syndrome: Controlled study of an oral opiate antagonist, naltrexone. *Ann Neurol* 35:464–470, 1994.

132. Kumandas S, Caksen H, Ciftci A, et al: Lamotrigine in two cases of Rett syndrome. *Brain Dev* 23:240–242, 2001.

133. Plioplys AV, Kasnicka I: L-Carnitine as a treatment for Rett syndrome. *South Med J* 86:1411–1412, 1993.

134. Zappella M, Genazzani A, Facchinetti F, et al: Bromocriptine in the Rett syndrome. *Brain Dev* 12:221–225, 1990.

Chapter 26

OTHER CENTRAL NERVOUS SYSTEM CONDITIONS

JACOB I. SAGE

VASCULAR PARKINSONISM   421
TRAUMA AS A CAUSE OF PARKINSONISM   422
PARKINSONISM AND HYDROCEPHALUS   423
STRUCTURAL LESIONS PRODUCING
    PARKINSONISM   424
CALCIFICATION OF THE BASAL GANGLIA,
    DISORDERS OF CALCIUM METABOLISM AND
    PARKINSONISM   424
NEUROLEPTIC-MALIGNANT SYNDROME
    (PARKINSONISM-HYPERPYREXIA SYNDROME)   424

This chapter will cover parkinsonian syndromes caused by the following: vascular disease, trauma, hydrocephalus, structural lesions, disorders of calcium metabolism, and the neuroleptic-malignant syndrome. For the most part, these entities present with atypical findings in the sense that the complete clinical syndrome associated with most cases of Lewy body Parkinson's disease (PD) (resting tremor, rigidity, bradykinesia, and postural instability) is not present. Generally, but not always, resting tremor and L-dopa responsiveness are not features of these forms of parkinsonism. More importantly, however, it is the historical setting, associated clinical and laboratory findings, and disease course that lead to a diagnosis of one of these conditions rather than PD.

Vascular Parkinsonism

Vascular parkinsonism is a condition whose nosology is still under debate. Our concept of its contribution in terms of numbers to the parkinsonian disorders, even its distinctness as a separate entity, has changed over the past 100 years and continues to change. One recent analysis suggests that as many as 6 percent of all cases of parkinsonism have a vascular cause.[1] It is therefore useful to review briefly the history of this syndrome.[2]

Near the end of the nineteenth century, an arteriosclerotic disorder was delineated that resembled the disease described by James Parkinson most prominently as a disorder of gait in the elderly. To this short-stepped gait, which came to be known as "marche à petit pas," were added the additional characteristics of dementia, pyramidal signs, and symptoms, including mild hemiparesis, urinary and emotional incontinence, and dysarthria. This clinical syndrome was correlated to multiple basal ganglia cavitations (etat crible) and infarcts (etat lacunaris). By the 1920s parkinsonism was defined by the anatomic site of the lesion in the basal ganglia for which could be found a number of causes, one of which was vascular.

Despite the lack of a clear pathological substrate defining PD in the late 1920s, there was a feeling that PD was a separate entity from other possible causes of parkinsonism. In 1929, this underlying sense that PD was different from vascular parkinsonism lead to Critchley's monograph on arteriosclerotic parkinsonism.[3] Despite nearly 70 years of technological advances and debate, this paper remains the single most useful contribution delineating vascular parkinsonism from PD. To the features of vascular parkinsonism described in the previous paragraph, he adds Gegenhalten, pseudobulbar palsy, a shuffling gait with persistent freezing but *without* festination, diminished armswing, tremor or associated seborrhea. Signs are usually symmetrical in vascular parkinsonism. Cerebellar system involvement is seen in some cases. There is a history of hypertension and stepwise progression with distinct plateaus in the clinical course. In contrast, patients with PD tend to be younger at disease onset, have cogwheel rigidity, asymmetrical findings, festination but only transient freezing, diminished armswing, and a resting tremor. Today, we must add that a good response to L-dopa strongly favors a diagnosis of PD.[4]

Since Critchley's paper, attempts to redefine the limits of vascular parkinsonism have lead to the concept of "lower body parkinsonism."[5,6] Such refinement occurred partly because substantia nigra degeneration with Lewy bodies was now accepted as the pathological substrate of PD,[7] and L-dopa responsiveness was taken as convincing evidence in favor of that diagnosis during life. This knowledge eliminated some of the confusion facing neurologists and pathologists prior to the 1960s and 1970s in that it largely separated PD from other forms of parkinsonism. A lower body gait disorder, different but not entirely distinct from senile gait[8,9] without apparent cause, came to be associated with vascular brain pathology and not with Lewy body disease.

The evolving definition of vascular parkinsonism also came about because the advent of computed tomography (CT) during the 1970s revealed changes suggesting deep white matter vasculopathy in a group of patients presenting predominantly with disorders of gait.[10] White matter periventricular low-density changes correlated with gait apraxia and poor balance. These patients exhibited a wide-based ataxic gait, presumably similar to the cerebellar gait alluded to in Critchley's description. This gait was dissimilar to the narrow-based gait seen in patients with PD. The periventricular location of these radiographic abnormalities presumably accounted for lower body parkinsonism by disrupting pathways to the legs in preference to those to the upper body. Subsequent studies in the magnetic resonance imaging (MRI) era support but by no means prove these speculations.[11]

The idea that lower body parkinsonism is primarily due to arteriosclerotic cerebral vascular disease has been extended to include clinical syndromes suggesting postencephalitic parkinsonism with oculogyric-like crises,[12] basal ganglia infarction due to cocaine and heroin[13] or secondary to hemodynamic changes from large vessel disease,[14] and progressive supranuclear palsy (PSP).[6,10] In one study, 19 of 58 patients with a clinical diagnosis of PSP had radiographic evidence of multiple small infarcts in the brainstem and deep white matter.[10] These patients were more likely to be hypertensive than those with PD. As with many diagnoses relying on imaging studies in elderly patients, it remains to be seen whether the white matter changes and small infarcts are truly indicative of the underlying pathology or simply a finding seen with increasing frequency in the aged.[11] White matter changes in older patients may turn out to be unrelated to the cause of their parkinsonism.

In a number of patients, however, it is impossible not to relate widespread abnormalities in the deep cerebral white matter to neurologic deterioration. This subcortical arteriosclerotic encephalopathy (Binswanger's disease) is usually characterized by a gradually worsening dementia in the setting of vascular risk factors.[15] Atypical gait, often having elements of both parkinsonism and ataxia, may be the initial symptom. Criteria to aid in the diagnosis of Binswanger's disease have recently been proposed.[16] They include dementia, abnormalities on imaging studies suggestive of rarefaction bilaterally in the deep white matter, and any two of the following findings: vascular risk factor, focal cerebral vascular disease or subcortical cerebral dysfunction (parkinsonism). Some patients may present with a PSP-like syndrome. Although most patients are L-dopa-unresponsive, cases have been reported that did improve with L-dopa.[17] Furthermore, at least one pathologically documented case did not have dementia during life.[18] Binswanger's disease remains difficult to diagnose with certainty before death.

Hurtig outlined a set of criteria for the diagnosis for vascular parkinsonism which it seems prudent to follow.[2] They include the acute or subacute (preferably stepwise) evolution of an akinetic rigid syndrome in the setting of documented vascular risk factors (hypertension, previous strokes, lipid abnormalities including anticardiolipin antibodies,[17] systemic arteriosclerotic vascular disease). Imaging studies should show at least two infarcts in the basal ganglia. To this may be added widespread and severe white matter disease on MRI consistent with Binswanger's pathology. There should be improvement in clinical signs without the use of L-dopa therapy or after it has been withdrawn, if given acutely. Adherence to these criteria may miss some cases of bona fide vascular parkinsonism but will minimize confusion among the various forms of parkinsonism not attributable to Lewy body disease. Treatment is directed at control of underlying risk factors, as with other forms of cerebral vascular disease. One recent study suggests that cerebrospinal fluid (CSF) drainage to improve gait disturbances in patients with subcortical white matter ischemic changes merits further study.[19]

Trauma as a Cause of Parkinsonism

The exact relationship between trauma and parkinsonism has been a subject of debate[20] since James Parkinson first speculated that it might be responsible for the syndrome he described in 1817. By the late nineteenth century, traumatic parkinsonism due to everything from emotional stress to moral lapses became a fashionable diagnosis with no solid clinical or pathological basis.[21] In particular, peripheral limb trauma was thought to be causative if parkinsonism subsequently developed in the same extremity. In retrospect, many cases were clearly misdiagnosed and in others evidence for the relation between the trauma and parkinsonism was weak.[22] By the early decades of the twentieth century, only concussion remained as a significant cause of posttraumatic parkinsonism. Experience during the great war made many neurologists sceptical even of this relation, since parkinsonism was not a noticeable sequela of hundreds and thousands of concussions from combat wounds.

In the years after the war, however, as neurologists sought to delineate postencephalitic from other types of parkinsonism, cases of posttraumatic parkinsonism with more specific clinical and pathologic characteristics began to accumulate.[23] With these cases in mind, neurologists developed specific criteria for the diagnosis of posttraumatic parkinsonism that are still relevant today. They include the onset of a bradykinetic, rigid syndrome (often unilateral with variable degree of tremor) which slowly becomes generalized. Postural instability, gait disorders, headache, psychiatric and cognitive dysfunction, and pyramidal signs are often present. More recently, posttraumatic parkinsonism resembling PSP[24] and the hemiparkinsonism-hemiatrophy syndrome[25] also have been described. The latter disorder includes such features as slow progression, dystonia, and pyramidal dysfunction.

Diagnostic criteria to justify a diagnosis of posttraumatic parkinsonism include a short duration of time from the trauma to the onset of clinical symptoms, and a sufficiently violent blow to cause a concussion. Pathologic evidence for necrosis or hemorrhage in the basal ganglia or midbrain should be found at autopsy. At present, in the absence of postmortem examinations, imaging studies showing structural damage in the basal ganglia or midbrain following concussion may be taken as evidence in favor of a diagnosis of traumatic parkinsonism.[26] Midbrain injury occurs either by direct damage from basilar skull fractures, hemorrhage, and infarction, or indirectly by the effects of herniation from supratentorial or infratentorial mass lesions. Shearing injury with axonal damage may occur in the midbrain as it rotates from the impact of a blow to the head.[27] A diagnosis of posttraumatic parkinsonism should not be made in the absence of evidence for structural damage to basal ganglia or midbrain.

Dementia pugilistica represents a somewhat different form of posttraumatic parkinsonism.[28] It usually results from a long career of blows to the head and is insidious in onset. Ataxia, dysarthria, personality changes, psychosis, and resting tremor frequently accompany the cognitive decline and other features of parkinsonism.[29,30] Imaging studies show generalized brain atrophy and frequently a cavum septum pellucidum.[31,32] Pathologic studies correlate well to the clinical syndrome, showing loss of cells in the substantia nigra, hippocampal gyrus, and amygdala. Neurofibrillary tangles are seen. Cerebellar infarctions and loss of Purkinje cells have been noted.[33] L-Dopa may be of benefit and should be tried in most patients with traumatic parkinsonism.

Although head trauma does not cause PD, there is some controversy about the effect of head trauma on the onset and progression of Lewy body PD. A number of retrospective studies support the notion that head trauma is a risk factor for the subsequent development of PD;[34,35] others do not.[36] A single prospective study of 821 patients did not a show a relationship between previous head trauma and PD, suggesting that other studies supporting the opposite position may suffer from recall bias.[37] What is clear from a prospective study of patients with already diagnosed PD is that trauma may worsen existing symptoms.[38] This worsening, however, is generally reversible by 3 months after the injury. It is therefore possible that head trauma may precipitate symptoms of PD in patients with nigral loss just below the threshold for symptoms to appear. In this sense, PD may appear after head injury, the assumption being that it would have occurred anyway, just a little later.

Parkinsonism and Hydrocephalus

Although hydrocephalus from any cause may include parkinsonian symptoms and signs, normal-pressure hydrocephalus (NPH) has received the most attention since described in 1965.[39] The clinical picture of the complete syndrome includes the gradual onset of dementia, gait ataxia, and urinary incontinence, although all three components of this picture are not always present. The description of the gait disorder has variously been described as magnetic, apraxic or ataxic. More often it appears to include elements of all three gait types with a tendency to lurch and fall. All the typical features of parkinsonism have been described in one or another patient, including resting tremor, hypophonia, hypomimia, bradykinesia, and rigidity.[40] Occasionally, altered levels of consciousness, oculomotor dysfunction or headache may be present. Corticospinal signs, nystagmus, and even seizures have been reported.

The pathophysiology of NPH is still obscure. The initial event may be a deficiency of CSF absorption at the arachnoid villi, making this entity one of the types of extraventricular obstructive hydrocephalus, a term preferred by some authors.[40] This obstruction to CSF flow results in transient high-pressure hydrocephalus with subsequent ventricular enlargement. As the ventricles enlarge, the intraventricular pressure may return to normal but the force generated at the ventricular surface may increase (Pascal's law), leading to further increases in ventricular size.[41] This enlargement of the ventricles compromises corticospinal pathways, especially those to the legs, leading to the characteristic gait abnormalities. Parkinsonism from basal ganglia compromise, and dementia and incontinence from frontal lobe dysfunction may also be explained in part from this mechanism.

Although some patients with parkinsonian features have responded to L-dopa,[42] surgical shunting remains the main mode of therapy.[43] A major unresolved issue is that of predicting which patients will respond favorably to shunting. Imaging studies reveal enlargement of the ventricular system without significant cortical atrophy. In the appropriate clinical setting described above, this radiographic picture is sufficient to suggest the diagnosis of NPH. All other radiologic signs and clinical tests must be considered as possibly helpful but not clearly diagnostic. These include a CSF flow void in the aqueduct of Sylvius.[44] The absence of this finding may be suggestive of hydrocephalus not associated with NPH. Isotope cisternography with reversal of CSF flow into the lateral ventricles and delayed clearance from the subarachnoid space has not proven a reliable indicator of success following shunting procedures. Removal of 50 mL of CSF from lumbar puncture, with subsequent clinical improvement over the next few hours or days or with increases in cerebral blood flow, may be more helpful.[45] Removal of lumbar CSF temporarily abolishes bladder hyperactivity in some patients with NPH and may predict good outcome from shunting.[46] Continuous external lumbar drainage of CSF has reportedly produced amelioration of symptoms and may give some indication as to the effect of a more permanent shunting procedure.[47] In one study, a ratio of cerebral blood flow from anterior to posterior of greater than 1.05 correctly predicted surgical outcome.[48]

Making the correct diagnosis and predicting outcome is of paramount importance because the results of shunting procedures are not stunning and the complications are frequent. Early reports of universal success, usually from neurosurgical centers, were clearly unreliable, but lead to surgery for many patients with various forms of dementia. In fact, it may be precisely this lack of an exact diagnosis that is responsible for the low percentage of patients who improved following shunt. In a recent retrospective, but reliable, multicenter study, marked improvement was seen in only 21 percent of patients.[49] The complication rate was nearly 30 percent. Thus it seems prudent to resort to shunting only in patients with a relatively complete clinical picture compatible with NPH and one or more imaging and other studies consistent with that diagnosis. Some patients can be treated with repeated lumbar puncture without resorting to the use of intracranial shunting procedures.

As reviewed by Shannon, features of more or less typical parkinsonism are seen with intraventricular obstructive hydrocephalus as well.[40] Most prominent are parkinsonian gait disorders with small shuffling steps. Rigidity and bradykinesia are not infrequent and resting tremor is present in as many as half the reported cases. It must be kept in mind, however, that all cases also have signs to suggest dysfunction of brain areas other than the basal ganglia, most frequently pyramidal and cerebellar systems. Etiology of the hydrocephalus includes aqueductal stenosis, posterior fossa tumors, Paget's disease, head trauma, and encephalitis.

Parkinsonism due to extraventricular hydrocephalus related to specific causes other than NPH has been reported. The clinical syndromes are similar to that described above for intraventricular hydrocephalus, again with the emphasis that signs suggesting involvement of other systems than the basal ganglia are almost always present.[40] Head trauma, subarachnoid hemorrhage, and subdural hematoma have all been implicated in small numbers of patients. A few patients responded to L-dopa, suggesting that two disease processes (PD, and hydrocephalus) were involved.[42] While this may be possible, it need not be the case, since L-dopa could benefit parkinsonian symptoms related to midbrain dysfunction caused by entities other than PD.

Structural Lesions Producing Parkinsonism

Structural lesions associated with cases of parkinsonism in which at least two of the four cardinal signs and symptoms were present have been catalogued by Waters in a recent review.[50] Tumors comprise most of the documented cases. Somewhat surprisingly, tumors of the striatum presenting with parkinsonian features are rare. Tumors in other brain areas (frontal, parietal, temporal, thalamus, midbrain, and third ventricle) presumably are responsible for parkinsonian features due to compression of the basal ganglia, or by compression or direct involvement of the midbrain. As expected, gliomas and menigiomas are the most frequently noted tumors. The few additional cases are of metastatic tumor, lymphoma, and fibrosarcoma.

Subdural hematoma may also cause parkinsonism, presumably by compression of basal ganglia or midbrain depending on location and type of herniation. These symptoms have generally been reversible with evacuation. It should be remembered that in most cases additional clues were present that lead to the correct diagnosis, most prominently headache, decreased level of consciousness, and confusion.

Striatal abscess, midbrain tuberculoma, vascular malformations, and posterior fossa cysts have all been reported to include features of parkinsonism in the clinical picture.

Calcification of the Basal Ganglia, Disorders of Calcium Metabolism and Parkinsonism

Since the advent of CT, it has been possible to ascertain the prevalence of basal ganglia calcification (sometimes called Fahr's disease) in large, if selected, groups of patients undergoing imaging studies for various reasons. In these studies, basal ganglia calcification is noted in less than 0.7 percent of patients, in whom less than 7 percent had a clinical disorder related to the basal ganglia.[51–53] Even fewer of these patients had parkinsonism. From these studies and from reports of families with familial basal ganglia calcification, it is clear that calcification of the basal ganglia (from whatever cause) is not sufficient in itself to cause symptoms of parkinsonism.[54]

Although case reports of basal ganglia calcification have been described in numerous diseases, it is most frequently associated with hypoparathyroidism. Basal ganglia calcification is reported in over 70 percent of patients with idiopathic hypoparathyroidism,[55] and in nearly all patients with pseudohypoparathyroidism.[56] Most descriptions of parkinsonism with hypoparathyroidism have been anecdotal, although one study notes that nearly one-quarter of patients with hypoparathyroidism may have some features of parkinsonism along with a picture of more diffuse neurologic involvement.[55] Secondary hypoparathyroidism is much less likely to be associated with calcification, presumably due to the shorter duration of disease before treatment begins in this disorder. Symptoms of parkinsonism generally improve following treatment of hypocalcemia, but this favorable outcome is not universal.[57] L-Dopa is of little benefit.[58] Other neurologic abnormalities seen in all three major types of hypoparathyroidism include tetany, chorea, psychiatric symptoms, and seizures, all of which may in fact be more common than parkinsonism in these disorders.

Neuroleptic-Malignant Syndrome (Parkinsonism-Hyperpyrexia Syndrome)

Neuroleptic-malignant syndrome (NMS) is a rare condition that occurs in the setting of either withdrawal of dopaminergic drugs in patients with Parkinson's disease or in patients receiving central dopamine-blocking agents. It can be considered, therefore, a state of acute dopamine deficiency. Parkinson patients with a prior episode of NMS, for example, have lower CSF levels of homovanillic acid than those with no such history.[59] In a single patient with NMS, there was no binding of iodobenzamide to D2 receptors 6 days into the illness, a finding that demonstrates complete receptor occupancy during the acute phase.[60] It has been argued that the obligate clinical characteristics of NMS are hyperpyrexia and a parkinsonian picture consisting most prominently of severe rigidity, hence the term parkinsonism-hyperpyrexia syndrome.[61] Other clinical features include autonomic dysfunction (diaphoresis, incontinence, tachycardia, blood pressure changes), tremor, akinesia, and an altered level of consciousness.[62] Leukocytosis may occur. The clinical course usually begins with rigidity and autonomic changes followed by fever within several hours of onset. Medical complications of NMS include aspiration pneumonia, myocardial infarction, rhabdomyolysis, and subsequent renal failure. Hemodialysis may be required. The duration of NMS is typically between 1 and 2 weeks. Much has been made of concomitant elevations in creatine kinase, although this finding may be present in only about half the cases.[63]

Although the incidence of NMS in patients taking neuroleptics is probably less than 1 in 1000,[64] a number of factors that increase risk emerge from epidemiologic and case studies. Men are more commonly affected than women.[65] Dehydration, exposure to heat, and organic brain disease seem to put patients at increased risk for NMS.[66] Multiple neuroleptics, depot forms of neuroleptics, and the additional use of lithium confer particular risk.[63,67] Lithium may even adversely affect outcome.[68] All types of dopamine-blocking agents have been associated with NMS, including resperidone,[69–72] tetrabenazine,[73] droperidol,[74] clozapine,[75] olanzapine,[72,76] compazine, and metoclopramide.[77,78]

There are a number of other medical and psychiatric conditions that may mimic NMS and must be excluded. Lethal catatonia usually begins with agitation and fever, followed shortly by catatonia.[79] Muscle rigidity may be difficult to distinguish from catatonia. A prior history of catatonia in the absence of neuroleptic treatment favors this diagnosis rather than NMS. When there is doubt, it is probably prudent to treat for NMS (see below).[61] Both systemic and central nervous system infections must be considered early in the differential diagnosis; evaluations by lumbar puncture and cultures are mandatory. Syndromes of serotonin excess are associated with confusion and autonomic changes, and must therefore be considered in the differential diagnosis of NMS in psychiatric and parkinson patients.[80,81] Drug-withdrawal syndromes may cause fever, altered consciousness, and autonomic instability, which might be confused with NMS. In Parkinson patients, withdrawal of amantadine,[82] tolcapone,[83] L-dopa,[84] and even rapid switching from one dopamine receptor agonist to another[85] have been reported to cause NMS. There is a single reported case of baclofen withdrawal causing an NMS-like syndrome.[86] Rigidity can occur in alcohol- and benzodiazepine-withdrawal states but are not likely to cause full-blown parkinsonism. An accurate history should clarify the situation. Heat stroke (fever and altered consciousness) also is generally obvious from the setting. Neuroleptic drugs, however, by altering sweating, may contribute to the risk of hot humid conditions and may confuse the diagnosis. The same is true of malignant hyperthermia (fever and rigidity) in which a genetic risk factor predisposes some patients to this condition which occurs shortly after exposure to inhalation anesthetics.[87] Despite reports that tricyclic antidepressants, phenytoin, and cocaine may cause NMS, it is unlikely that these agents by themselves are responsible for more than drug-induced fever associated with other nonspecific neurologic signs and symptoms.[61] Ecstacy (3,4-methylenedioxymethamphetamine) seems to produce an overlapping NMS and serotonin syndrome.[88] There are single case reports of thrombocytopenia,[89] hypernatremia,[90] and hyponatremia[91] precipitating NMS-like syndromes.

Treatment of NMS depends on recognition and immediate stopping of neuroleptic drugs. Patients should be hydrated, fever reduced, and medical support instituted. Hemodialysis should be started in those in acute renal failure. Therapy with bromocriptine (2.5–10 mg three times a day) is aimed at reducing parkinsonism.[92] It may be used alone or in combination with dantrolene (up to 3 mg/kg/day), which acts directly at the sarcoplasmic reticulum to reduce muscle rigidity.[93] Fever also responds to dantrolene, presumably by decreasing that component of fever caused by peripheral heat production. There is some evidence suggesting that combination therapy (bromocriptine and dantrolene) shortens the course of illness,[94] although either therapy alone has been shown to be effective. Other antiparkinsonian therapy, particularly L-dopa, would be expected to work, although the number of patients treated with this approach has been far fewer than with either bromocriptine or dantrolene. There is a single report of successful treatment of NMS with apomorphine.[95] Electroconvulsive therapy may be effective in some cases,[96] but should not be used as primary treatment for NMS. Clonidine has been effective in the management of autonomic overactivity in NMS.[97] Once an episode of NMS is over, only patients absolutely requiring neuroleptics should be restarted on these drugs. Waiting 2 weeks before rechallenge is a prudent absolute minimum, and close monitoring is necessary to look for recurrence of symptoms.[98]

References

1. Foltynie T, Barker R, Brayne C: Vascular parkinsonism: A review of the precision and frequency of diagnosis. *Neuroepidemiology* 21:1–7, 2002.
2. Hurtig HI: Vascular parkinsonism, in Stern MB, Koller WC (eds): *Parkinsonian Syndromes*. New York: Marcel Dekker, 1993, pp 81–93.
3. Critchley M: Arteriosclerotic parkinsonism. *Brain* 52:23–83, 1929.
4. Parkes JD, Marsden CD, Rees JE, et al: Parkinson's disease, cerebral arteriosclerosis and senile dementia. *Q J Med* 43:49–61, 1974.
5. Thompson PD, Marsden CD: Gait disorder of subcortical arteriosclerotic encephalopathy: Binswanger's disease. *Mov Disord* 2:1–8, 1987.
6. Fitzgerald PM, Jancovic J: Lower body parkinsonism: Evidence for a vascular etiology. *Mov Disord* 4:249–260, 1989.
7. Greenfield JG, Bosanquet FD: Brainstem lesions in parkinsonism. *J Neurol Neurosurg Psychiatry* 16:213–226, 1953.

8. Critchley M: On senile disorders of gait including the so-called senile paraplegia. *Geriatrics* 3:364–370, 1948.

9. Sudarsky L: Gait disorders in the elderly. *N Engl J Med* 322:1441, 1990.

10. Dubinsky RM, Jankovic J: Progressive supranuclear palsy and a multi-infarct state. *Neurology* 37:570–576, 1987.

11. Fazekas F, Niederkorn K, Schmidt R, et al: White matter signal abnormalities in normal individuals: Correlation with carotid ultrasound, cerebral blood flow measurements, and cerebrovascular disease risk factors. *Stroke* 19:1285–1288, 1988.

12. Scarmeas N, Eidelberg D, Frucht SJ, Scarmato N: Oculogyric-like crises in a 92-year old woman with vascular parkinsonism. *Mov Disord* 17:353–355, 2002.

13. Daras MD, Orrego JJ, Akfirat GL, et al: Bilateral symmetrical basal ganglia infarction after intravenous use of cocaine and heroin. *Clin Imaging* 25:1–4, 2001.

14. Yamauchi H, Fukuyama H, Nagahama Y, et al: Brain arteriosclerosis and hemodynamic disturbance may induce leukoaraiosis. *Neurology* 53:1833–1838, 1999.

15. Pellissier JF, Poncet M: Binswanger's encephalopathy, in Toole JF (ed): *Vascular Diseases 2. Handbook of Clinical Neurology.* Amsterdam: Elsevier, 1989, vol 54, pp 221–233.

16. Bennett DA, Wilson RS, Gilley DW, Fox JH: Clinical diagnosis of Binswanger's disease. *J Neurol Neurosurg Psychiatry* 53:961–965, 1990.

17. Huang Z, Jacewicz M, Pfeiffer RF: Anticardiolopin antibody in vascuolar parkinsonism. *Mov Disord* 17:992–997, 2002.

18. Mark MH, Sage JI, Walters AS, et al: Binswanger's disease presenting as levodopa-responsive parkinsonism: Clinicopathologic study of three cases. *Mov Disord* 10:450–454, 1995.

19. Ondo WG, Chan LL, Levy JK: Vascular parkinsonism: Clinical correlates predicting motor improvement after lumbar puncture. *Mov Disord* 17:91–97, 2002.

20. Factor SA: Posttraumatic parkinsonism, in Stern MB, Koller WC (eds): *Parkinsonian Syndromes.* New York: Marcel Dekker, 1993, pp 95–110.

21. Factor SA, Sanchez-Ramos J, Weiner WJ: Trauma as an etiology of parkinsonism: A historical review of the concept. *Mov Disord* 3:30–36, 1988.

22. Grimberg L: Paralysis agitans and trauma. *J Nerv Ment Dis* 79:14–42, 1934.

23. Crouzan O, Justin-Besancon L: Le parkinsonisms traumatique. *Presse Med* 37:1325–1327, 1929.

24. Koller WC, Wong GF, Lang A: Posttraumatic movement disorders: A review. *Mov Disord* 4:20–36, 1989.

25. Giladi N, Burke RE, Kostic V, et al: Hemiparkinsonism-hemiatrophy syndrome: Clinical and neuroradiologic features. *Neurology* 40:1731–1734, 1990.

26. Nayernouri T: Posttraumatic parkinsonism. *Surg Neurol* 24:263–264, 1985.

27. Peerless SJ, Rewcastle NB: Shear injuries of the brain. *Can Med Assoc J* 96:577–582, 1967.

28. Martland HS: Punch drunk. *J Am Med Assoc* 91:1103–1107, 1928.

29. Critchley M: Medical aspects of boxing, particularly from a neurological standpoint. *Br Med J* 1:357–362, 1957.

30. Johnson J: Organic psychosyndromes due to boxing. *Br J Psychiatry* 115:45–53, 1969.

31. Casson IR: Neurologic syndromes in boxers. *Neuroview* 1:1–3, 1985.

32. Jordan BD: Neurologic aspects of boxing. *Arch Neurol* 44:453–459, 1987.

33. Lampert PW, Hardman JM: Morphological changes in brains of boxers. *JAMA* 251:2676–2679, 1984.

34. Factor SA, Weiner WJ: Prior history of head trauma in Parkinson's disease. *Mov Disord* 6:225–229, 1991.

35. Stern M, Dulaney E, Gruber SB, et al: The epidemiology of Parkinson's disease: A case-control study of young onset and old onset patients. *Arch Neurol* 48:903–907, 1991.

36. Ward CD, Duvoisin RC, Ince RE, et al: Parkinson's disease in 65 pairs of twins and in a set of quadruplets. *Neurology* 33:815–824, 1983.

37. Williams DB, Anneyers JF, Kohmen E, et al: Brain injury and neurologic sequelae: A cohort study of dementia, parkinsonism and amyotrophic lateral sclerosis. *Neurology* 41:1554–1557, 1991.

38. Goetz CG, Stebbins GT: Effects of head trauma from motor vehicle accidents on Parkinson's disease. *Ann Neurol* 29:191–193, 1991.

39. Hakim S, Adams RD: The special clinical problem of symptomatic hydrocephalus with normal cerebrospinal fluid pressure: Observations on cerebrospinal fluid hydrodynamics. *J Neurol Sci* 2:307–327, 1965.

40. Shannon KM: Hydrocephalus and parkinsonism, in Stern MB, Koller WC (eds): *Parkinsonian Syndromes.* New York: Marcel Dekker, 1993, pp 123–136.

41. Prockop LD: Hydrocephalus, in Rowland LP (ed): *Merritt's Textbook of Neurology.* Baltimore: Williams & Wilkins, 1995, pp 294–302.

42. Jacobs L, Conti D, Kinkel WR, Manning EG: "Normal pressure" hydrocephalus. Relationship of clinical and radiographic findings to improvement following shunt surgery. *JAMA* 235:510–512, 1976.

43. Sage JI, Duvoisin RC: The Parkinson plus syndromes. *Curr Opin Neurol Neurosurg* 2:314–318, 1989.

44. Jack CR Jr, Mokri B, Laws ER Jr, et al: MR findings in normal-pressure hydrocephalus: Significance and comparison with other forms of dementia. *J Comput Assist Tomogr* 11:923–931, 1987.

45. Mamo HL, Meric PC, Ponsin JC, et al: Cerebral blood flow in normal pressure hydrocephalus. *Stroke* 18:1074–1080, 1987.

46. Ahlberg J, Norlen L, Blomstrand C, Wikkelso C: Outcome of shunt operation on urinary incontinence in normal pressure hydrocephalus predicted by lumbar puncture. *J Neurol Neurosurg Psychiatry* 51:105–108, 1988.

47. Haan J, Thomeer RTWM: Predictive value of temporary external lumbar drainage in normal pressure hydrocephalus. *Neurosurgery* 22:388–391, 1988.

48. Graff-Radford NR, Rezai K, Godersky JC, et al: Regional cerebral blood flow in normal pressure hydrocephalus. *J Neurol Neurosurg Psychiatry* 50:1589–1596, 1987.

49. Vanneste J, Augustijn P, Dirven C, et al: Shunting normal-pressure hydrocephalus: Do the benefits outweigh the risks? A multicenter study and literature review. *Neurology* 42:54–59, 1992.

50. Waters CH: Structural lesions and parkinsonism, in Stern MB, Koller WC (eds): *Parkinsonian Syndromes.* New York: Marcel Dekker, 1993, pp 137–144.

51. Comella CL: Bilateral striopallidodentate calcinosis, in Stern MB, Koller WC (eds): *Parkinsonian Syndromes.* New York: Marcel Dekker, 1993, pp 483–501.

52. Murphy MJ: Clinical correlations of CT scan-detected calcifications of the basal ganglia. *Ann Neurol* 6:507–511, 1979.

53. Brannan TS, Burger AA, Chaudhary MY: Bilateral basal ganglia calcification visualized on CT scan. *J Neurol Neurosurg Psychiatry* 40:403–406, 1980.

54. Okada J, Takeuchi K, Ohkado M, Hoshina K: Familial basal ganglia calcifications visualized by computed tomography. *Acta Neurol Scand* 64:273–279, 1981.

55. Sachs C, Sjoberg HE, Ericson K: Basal ganglia calcification on CT: Relation to hypoparathyroidism. *Neurology* 32:779–782, 1982.

56. Illum F, Dupont E: Prevalence of CT-detected calcification in the basal ganglia in idiopathic hypoparathyroidism and pseudohypoparathyroidism. *Neuroradiology* 27:32–37, 1985.

57. Muenter MD, Whisnant JP: Basal ganglia calcification, hypoparathyroidism, and extrapyramidal motor manifestations. *Neurology* 18:1075–1082, 1968.

58. Klawans HL, Lupton M, Simon L: Calcification of the basal ganglia as a cause of levodopa-resistant parkinsonism. *Neurology* 26:221–225, 1976.

59. Ueda M, Hamamoto M, Nagayama H, et al: Susceptibility to neuroleptic malignant syndrome in Parkinson's disease. *Neurology* 52:777–781, 1999.

60. Jauss M, Krack P, Franz M, et al: Imaging of dopamine receptors with (123I)iodobenzamide single-photon emission-computed tomography in neuroleptic malignant syndrome. *Mov Disord* 11:726–728, 1996.

61. Granner MA, Wooten GF: Neuroleptic maligant syndrome or parkinsonism hyperpyrexia syndrome. *Semin Neurol* 11:228–234, 1991.

62. Buckley PF, Hutchinson M: Neuroleptic malignant syndrome. *J Neurol Neurosurg Psychiatry* 59:271–273, 1995.

63. Kurlan R, Hamill R, Shoulson I: Neuroleptic malignant syndrome. *Clin Neuropharmacol* 7:109–120, 1984.

64. Keck PE, Pope HG, McElroy SL: Declining frequency of neuroleptic malignant syndrome in a hospital population. *Am J Psychiatry* 148:880–882, 1991.

65. Caroff SN: The neuroleptic malignant syndrome. *J Clin Psychiatry* 41:79–83, 1980.

66. Guze BH, Baxter LR: Current concepts: Neuroleptic malignant syndrome. *N Engl J Med* 313:163–166, 1985.

67. Kirkpatrick B, Edelsohn GA: Risk factors for the neuroleptic malignant syndrome. *Psychiatr Med* 2:371–381, 1985.

68. Cohen WJ, Cohen NH: Lithium carbonate, haloperidol, and irreversible brain damage. *JAMA* 230:1283–1287, 1974.

69. Tarsy D: Risperidone and neuroleptic malignant syndrome. *JAMA* 275:446, 1996.

70. Sechi G, Agnetti V, Masuri R, et al: Risperidone, neuroleptic malignant syndrome and probably dementia with Lewy bodies. *Prog Neuropsychopharmacol Biol Psychiatry* 24:1043–1051, 2000.

71. Robb AS, Chang W, Lee HK, Cook MS: Case study. Risperidone-induced neuroleptic malignant syndrome in an adolescent. *J Child Adolesc Psychopharmacol* 10:327–330, 2000.

72. Aboraya A, Schumacher J, Abdalla E, et al: Neuroleptic malignant syndrome associated with risperidone and olanzapine in first-episode schizophrenia. *W V Medi J* 98:63–65, 2002.

73. Petzinger GM, Bressman SB: A case of tetrabenazine-induced neuroleptic malignant syndrome after prolonged treatment. *Mov Disord* 12:246–248, 1997.

74. So PC: Neuroleptic malignant syndrome induced by droperidol. *Hong Kong Med J* 7:101–103, 2001.

75. Blttlender R, Jager M, Hofschuster E, et al: Neuroleptic malignant syndrome due to atypical neuroleptics: Three episodes in one patient. *Pharmacopsychiatry* 35:119–121, 2002.

76. Kontaxakis VP, Havaki-Kontaxaki BJ, Christodoulou NG, Paplos KG: Olanzapine-associated neuroleptic malignant syndrome. *Prog Neuropsychopharmacol Biol Psychiatry* 26:897–902, 2002.

77. Nonino F, Campomori A: Neuroleptic malignant syndrome associated with metoclopramide. *Ann Pharmacother* 33:644–645, 1999.

78. Friedman LS, Weinrauch LA, D'Elia JA: Metoclopramide-induced neuroleptic malignant syndrome. *Arch Intern Med* 147:1495–1497, 1987.

79. Mann SC, Caroff SN, Bleier HR, et al: Lethal catatonia. *Am J Psychiatry* 143:1374–1381, 1986.

80. Martin TG: Serotonin syndrome. *Ann Emerg Med* 28:520–526, 1996.

81. Fink M: Toxic serotonin syndrome or neuroleptic malignant syndrome. *Pharmacopsychiatry* 29:159–161, 1996.

82. Ito T, Shibata K, Watanabe A, Akabane J: Neuroleptic malignant syndrome following withdrawal of amantadine in a patient with influenza A encephalopathy. *Eur J Pediatr* 160:401, 2001.

83. Iwuagwu CU, Riley D, Bonoma RA: Neuroleptic malignant-like syndrome in an elderly patient caused by abrupt withdrawal of tolcapone, a catechol-*O*-methyl transferase inhibitor. *Am J Med* 108:517–518, 2000.

84. Gordon PH, Frucht SJ: Neuroleptic malignant syndrome in advanced Parkinson's disease. *Mov Disord* 16:960–962, 2001.

85. Reimer J, Kuhlmann A, Muller T: Neuroleptic malignant-like syndrome after rapid switch from bromocriptine to pergolide. *Parkinsonism Relat Disord* 9:115–116, 2002.

86. Turner MR, Bainsborough N: Neuroleptic malignant-like syndrome after abrupt withdrawal of baclofen. *J Psychopharmacol* 15:61–63, 2001.

87. Heiman-Patterson TD: Neuroleptic malignant syndrome and malignant hyperthermia. *Med Clin North Am* 71:477–492, 1993.

88. Demirkiran M, Jankovic J, Dean JM: Ecstasy intoxication: An overlap between serotonin syndrome and neuroleptic malignant syndrome. *Clin Neuropharmacol* 19:157–164, 1996.

89. Ray JG: Neuroleptic malignant syndrome associated with severe thrombocytopenia. *J Intern Med* 241:245–247, 1997.

90. Cao L, Katz RH: Acute hypernatremia and neuroleptic malignant syndrome in Parkinson's disease. *Am J Med Sci* 318:67–68, 1999.

91. Elizalde-Sciavolino C, Racco A, Proscia-Lieto T, Kleiner M: Severe hyponatremia, neuroleptic malignant syndrome, rhabdomyolysis and acute renal failure: A case report. *Mt Sinai J Med* 65:284–288, 1998.

92. Sakkas P, Davis JM, Jancak PG, Wang Z: Drug treatment of the neuroleptic malignant syndrome. *Psychopharmacol Bull* 27:381–384, 1991.

93. Nisijima K, Ishiguro I: Does dantrolene influence central dopamine and serotonin metabolism in the neuroleptic malignant syndrome? A retrospective study. *Biol Psychiatry* 33:45–48, 1993.

94. Rosenberg MR, Green M: Neuroleptic malignant syndrome: Review of response to therapy. *Arch Intern Med* 149:1927–1931, 1989.

95. Wang HC, Hsieh Y: Treatment of neuroleptic malignant syndrome with subcutaneous apomorphine monotherapy. *Mov Disord* 16:765–767, 2001.

96. Davis JM, Janicak PG, Sakkas P, et al: Electroconvulsive therapy in the treatment of neuroleptic malignant syndrome. *Convulsive Ther* 7:111–120, 1991.

97. Gregorakos L, Thomaides T, Stratouli S, Sakayanni E: The use of clinidine in the management of autonomic overactivity in neuroleptic malignant syndrome. *Clin Auton Res* 10:193–196, 2000.

98. Wells AJ, Sommi RW, Crismon ML: Neuroleptic rechallenge after neuroleptic malignant syndrome: Case report and literature review. *Drug Intelligence Clin Pharm* 22:475–480, 1988.

II. TREMOR DISORDERS

ESSENTIAL TREMOR

MARIA GRACIELA CERSOSIMO and WILLIAM C. KOLLER

HISTORY   431
EPIDEMIOLOGY OF ESSENTIAL TREMOR   432
GENETICS   433
CLINICAL MANIFESTATIONS   434
    Neuropsychological Deficits   435
    Classification   435
    Body Region Affected by ET   436
    Disease Onset and Progression   436
    Factors Influencing ET   436
    Disability   436
    Diagnostic Pitfalls   437
    Clinical Variants   438
ASSOCIATED CONDITIONS   439
PATHOPHYSIOLOGY   441
ASSESSMENT OF TREMOR   442
    Tremor   442
    Speaking Phonation   442
    Feeding (Other Than Liquids)   442
    Bringing Liquids to Mouth (Drinking)   442
    Hygiene   443
    Dressing   443
    Writing   443
    Working   443
    Fine Movements   443
    Embarrassment   443
    Handwriting   443
    Drawing   443
    Pouring   444
TREATMENT   444
    Alcohol   444
    Beta-Adrenergic Blockers   445
    Primidone   446
    Phenobarbital   446
    Benzodiazepines   446
    Carbonic Anhydrase Inhibitors   447
    Gabapentin   447
    Other Drugs   447
    Botulinum Toxin Injection   449
    Thalamotomy   449
    Thalamic Stimulation   449
    Behavioral Therapy   450
    Drugs of Choice   451
SUMMARY   451

Essential tremor (ET) is most likely the most common movement disorder. We will review the history, epidemiology, genetics, clinical features, pathophysiology, and therapy of ET and expand on previous reviews of ET.[1–7]

History

Historically, tremor as an affliction of the elderly has long been noted; however, tremor as an isolated symptom commencing before old age and occurring within families has been clearly described only within the past two centuries. Critchley[8] provided a detailed chronological review of the history of ET. He cites one of the earlier references to tremor: "The keepers of the house shall tremble" (Ecclesiastes XII.3). Galen in the second century described tremor as "an involuntary alternating up-and-down motion" differentiating it from other movements in his treatise on tremor, palpitation, spasm, and rigor.[9] In 1817 James Parkinson,[10] in his landmark monograph, *An Essay on the Shaking Palsy*, distinguished senile tremor as a separate entity from the tremor of paralysis agitans. In the late nineteenth century, Charcot[11] commented on the salient clinical features of familial and senile tremor. In addition, the variability of clinical expression in ET was recognized by Charcot;[12] he described head tremor in two elderly female patients: "The head participates in the shaking, on its own account; the movements which are both vertical and horizontal succeed each other with regularity, and in these the patient seems, by her gesture, to say yes or no."

Credit for first noting the familial form of tremor is usually given to Most who, in 1836, reported briefly on several cases of tremor in a single family.[8,13,14] However, in 1887, Dana[14] wrote the first thorough account of familial tremor; he described three families with tremor, detailing 45 patients with tremor within a single pedigree. In addition to the excellent family history, Dana provided a thorough clinical description of ET. He noted the body parts affected, variability in severity and age of onset, remission during sleep, and lack of increased mortality. Regarding familial and senile tremor as two distinct entities, Dana wrote that senile tremor "generally affects first and entirely the head and neck." In addition, he considered ET to be associated with neuroses, psychoses, epilepsy, unique talents, and high intellect. He reported that ET "illustrates the fact that a neuropathic taint in a family may develop as a disease, or as some brilliant mental endowment."

The notion of the ET patient as having unique characteristics was shared by others. Critchley[8] reviewed the work of the Russian neurologist, Minor, who in the early 1920s proposed the concept of status macrobioticus multiparus: the trial of familial tremor, longevity, and fecundity. This association of tremor with long life and profligacy has not been corroborated by others when examining families with ET.[15,16] Other traits have also been ascribed to ET patients over the years. Inebriety, nervousness, emotivity, and anxiety have been reported in association with ET.[17] Raymond[18] considered "neuropathic shock" to be the precipitant of ET. From the contrary viewpoint, Katzenstein[19] considered families affected with tremor to be unusually accomplished and highly intelligent. Critchley[8] observed that ET has been noted among individuals of great intelligence giving, as an example, Joseph Babinski. These divergent views of the ET patient have not been addressed in recent times. Detailed epidemiological and genetic studies performed within the past 25 years offer no substantiation of these notions.[16,20]

Epidemiology of Essential Tremor

The epidemiology of ET is only partly understood. ET has been described as "common," "not uncommon," and "rare."[8,21,22] Reports of ET have been issued from around the world, indicating a global occurrence.[23–28] Depending on the study methods,[23,25,28] prevalence estimates vary widely (0.0005–5.55 percent). As part of a door-to-door neuroepidemiological survey, Salemi et al.[29] investigated the frequency and distribution of ET in a Sicilian municipality. They administered a screening instrument for tremor to 7653 persons residing in Terrasini (Palermo province). Neurologists evaluated those subjects who had screened positively. They found 31 subjects affected by ET (17 men, 14 women); 11 patients (35.5 percent) reported a familial aggregation. The prevalence of ET was for the total population, and 1074.9 per 100,000 for those 40 years old or older. The prevalence increased with advancing age for both sexes and was slightly but consistently higher in men.[29] Epidemiological surveys are complicated by less-than-ideal case ascertainment. As ET is usually monosymptomatic and often minimally disabling, it is likely to be underrepresented in surveys of neurological disorders.[16] Only a small percentage of individuals with ET comes to medical attention; in the series of Rautakorpi et al.[25] only 10 percent of identified ET patients had sought treatment. Even if the patient seeks medical advice, the disorder

may not be properly recognized. Mild forms of ET may be dismissed as incidental, particularly in the elderly; Critchley[8] noted that tremor is not simply a characteristic of aging when he cited Charcot's report of tremor in only 1–2 percent of the aged inmates of the Salpetaire. The symptom of ET may also be ascribed incorrectly to other medical conditions, with severe tremor commonly misdiagnosed as Parkinson's disease (PD).[30] For these reasons, medical registries cannot be relied on in studying the epidemiology of ET. Instead, a population-based approach is suggested,[31] in which an entire community is surveyed for features of ET.

Several epidemiological surveys for ET have been undertaken (Table 27-1). Larsson and Sjögren[16] conducted a comprehensive epidemiological survey in an isolated region of northern Sweden (population, 7451) in which a high frequency of ET had been previously noted. The prevalence of the condition was 1.4 percent for the general population and rose to 3.7 percent in the over-40-year-old age group. Similarly, Hornabrook and Nagurney[26] examined a region in New Guinea in which a propensity for tremor had been described. When five language groups in this area are considered, prevalence rates were reported of 0.35 percent in the general population and 1.64 percent in the over-40-year-old age group. However, in other nearby communities with distinct linguistic and ethnic features, ET was remarkably uncommon. The New Guinea study was distinctive in that over-40-year-old subjects comprised only 21 percent of the study population; in addition, a significantly greater prevalence of ET among females was found. The investigators speculated that tremor might be more frequently detected in females because of the heavy manual labor performed by the

TABLE 27-1 Epidemiological Studies of Essential Tremor

Methodology	Reference	Prevalence (percent)	
		Total Population	Over-40-Year-Old Population
Population survey	Larsson and Sjögren (1960)[16]	1.7	3.73
Population survey	Hornabrook and Nagurney (1976) [26]	0.35	1.64
			2.12 females
			1.03 males
Population survey	Rautakorpi (1978)[20]		5.55
			4.73 females
			6.62 males
Population survey	Haerer et al. (1982)[4]		0.45 white females
			0.41 white males
			0.41 black females
			0.33 black males
Medical record review	Rajput et al. (1982)[33]	0.31	
Medical record review	Aiyesiloju et al. (1984)[8]	0.0005	
Population survey	Bharucha et al. (1988)[32]	1.59	2.76
			2.81 females
			2.71 males

women of this society. Because of their restricted geographic, ethnic, and cultural features, the findings of the Swedish and New Guinea studies cannot easily be generalized to other more diversified populations.

Rautakorpi et al.,[25] in a two-phase population-based study, examined the occurrence of ET in over-40-year-old patients in two rural communities in Finland. In the first phase, community members with tremor were identified by questionnaire. Clinical examinations were performed in phase two. Based on their findings, a minimal prevalence rate of 5.55 percent for ET in the over-40-year-old age group was reported. The authors suggested that the actual prevalence of ET among over-40-year-old patients may be close to 10 percent, as their data did not consider cases lost as a result of nonparticipation or incorrect reporting. A male preponderance was seen, and ET occurred more frequently with advancing age; the peak prevalence (12.6 percent) was in the 70–79-year-old age group. In the US, Haerer et al.[24] reported on the prevalence of ET derived from a survey of major neurological disorders in a biracial Mississippi county. A screening questionnaire was administered to Copiah County residents. Based on questionnaire responses, individuals suspected of having ET were examined. The minimal prevalence rate of ET in this population was 0.41 percent, with the condition more common in whites than in blacks, for either sex; it was more common in women than men, for either race. The occurrence of ET was approximately 10-fold greater in the 70–79-year-old age group, as compared to the 40–69-year-old group (1.18 versus 0.12 percent). The lower prevalence rates obtained in this study may, at least in part, be attributed to more stringent diagnostic criteria. Only tremor that significantly interfered with activities of daily living was considered; in addition, a 10-year or more history of tremor or a positive family history was required. A similar population-based study was conducted in the Parsi community of Bombay, India.[32] The prevalence of ET in this group was 1.52 percent. Age-adjusted prevalence rates were similar for men and women. A second epidemiological study of ET in the US was reported by Rajput et al.[23,33] Their findings were based on the retrospective review of medical records from a 45-year period in Rochester, Minnesota. The estimated prevalence rate was 0.31 percent. The incidence of ET rose sharply after age 49 years. No difference in the incidence rates between males and females was found. Survival of patients diagnosed as having ET was comparable to that of the sex- and age-matched control population. Interestingly, when the data were considered in 15-year intervals a progressive increase in the incidence rate of ET was noted; that is, the diagnosis of ET was being made more frequently with the passage of time. The authors attributed this rise to the greater availability of health care and increased physician awareness of ET in recent years.

A similar retrospective review of hospital records was conducted by Aiyesiloju et al. in Nigeria.[28] A strikingly low prevalence rate of 0.0005 percent for ET was found. Other inheritable neurodegenerative disorders were also noted to be quite rare in this population. Genetic, environmental, and cultural features unique to this populace may explain these findings. In addition, ET as a sole medical condition would be expected to result rarely in hospital admission, making case ascertainment quite limited in this survey. In a report from a Chinese clinic, 146 of 258 tremor patients were thought to have ET.[34] There were 96 males and 50 females, ranging from 14 to 89 years of age. The hands were affected in all cases. A familial tendency was obvious in 32 percent. Epidemiological studies reveal that ET is more common than PD. The marked difference in prevalence ratios for PD and ET is attributed to: (1) higher incidence of ET in the general population; (2) a greater possibility that most, if not all, ET patients would reside in the community, whereas a sizable proportion of elderly PD patients may be institutionalized, and (3) shortened survival in PD but a normal life-expectancy in ET.[35] Louis et al.[36] found that relatives of ET patients were 5 times more likely to develop ET than members of the normal population and 10 times more likely if the proband's tremor started at an early age. These investigators[37] found in cases of normal relatives over the age of 60 an increased prevalence of tremor and they suggested that, in this age group, ET may be present and that penetrance may be incomplete.

Age appears to be a risk factor for ET. Data from the Mayo Clinic show a dramatic increase in the prevalence of ET with aging.[23] Anecdotal experience in the clinic also indicates that postural tremors are common in the aging population. Therefore, ET can be viewed as a disorder that is closely linked to the aging nervous system. A better understanding of ET will undoubtedly increase our knowledge of nervous system changes that occur with aging.

In summary, despite the variability in data, epidemiological studies illustrate ET to be a frequently encountered disorder, especially among the elderly. Applying the prevalence rate of ET derived from the Finnish study to US Census Bureau population statistics, one can estimate that more than 5 million individuals over 40 years of age in the US are affected. ET would, therefore, appear to be the most common movement disorder.[1,13,23]

Genetics

The tendency of ET to run in families has been recognized for many years. In the American medical literature Dana[14] reported on 3 families with tremor in 1887. In the intervening years authors reviewing ET have reaffirmed its heritable nature.[8,13,16,18] Family history positivity varies by report from 17 percent to 70 percent.[20,23,25,28,38] Pedigree charts have been published, providing details on families with ET. Although Critchley cautioned that "more than one type of inheritance may be concerned," the genealogical reports published to date support the assumption that familial ET is inherited in an autosomal-dominant manner.[8,14,39–41]

A comprehensive genetic population study was conducted in a region of northern Sweden by Larsson and Sjögren.[16]

In this study, 210 cases of ET were traced to 9 ancestral families in this geographically and ethnically restricted area. The pattern of occurrence of ET in this study was consistent with autosomal-dominant transmittance. Despite reports by others to the contrary,[8,20] Larsson and Sjögren[16] reported no instance of familial ET skipping generations. In 10 families both parents were affected with ET; estimating that approximately one-third of the affected offspring could be expected to be homozygotes, the investigators could identify no clinical features distinguishing homozygotes from heterozygotes. The disease manifested itself by age 70 in virtually all patients; that is complete penetrance by 70 years of age. Rautakorpi[10] reported a similar age of onset of familial ET, with virtually all patients becoming symptomatic by age 65 and more than 50 percent of patients having tremor by age 40. This relatively early age of onset may distinguish familial ET from sporadic cases in which the peak age of onset is later.[20] Critchley[8] remarked on the occurrence of "anticipation;" that is, younger age of onset of tremor in each succeeding generation within a given family. This phenomenon was not observed by Larsson and Sjögren.[16] In keeping with the observations of others, our experience with familial ET indicates that remarkable variability in age of onset and clinical expression may occur within a given family.[16,40] The cause of sporadic ET is unclear. Many of these cases may, indeed, have a familial basis, as family history can be unreliable or unattainable.

It should be noted that for most studies the presence or absence of a family history of ET was ascertained simply by inquiring from the patient. Therefore, there is the strong possibility of underreporting. For instance, a mild postural tremor could be present in a family member, or an individual who has a tremor may deny its existence to others. Acknowledgment of a familial disease may even be socially unacceptable.[28] It is possible that all cases of ET have a genetic basis and that the existence of sporadic cases is an artifact related to the method of data collection. Indeed, one study suggests that most reported negative family histories are positive when more thoroughly investigated.[42]

Another problem related to the issue of heredity and ET is how to define the presence of familial occurrence. If ET does occur sporadically and ET is a very common condition, then how does one define familiar occurrence? Criteria need to be developed that clearly separate familial from sporadic cases. Also, investigation of possible clinical and pharmacological differences between hereditary and sporadic ET (if it exists) needs to be performed. There is a report of an association of ET and CAG repeats in the androgen receptor gene;[43] however, this needs to be confirmed. A tremor indistinguishable from ET may be observed in patients with autosomal-dominant idiopathic torsion dystonia (ITD), in which the disease locus has been mapped to 9q32-34 in some kindreds, tightly linked to the argininosuccinate synthetase (ASS) locus. Conway et al.[44] performed linkage analysis in 15 families with ET containing 60 definitely affected individuals, using dinucleotide repeat polymorphisms at the ASS locus and the Abelson locus (ABL). Cumulative LOD

TABLE 27-2 Genetic Linkage Studies in Essential Tremors

Study	Population	Locus	LOD Scores
Gulcher et al. (1997)[45]	16 Icelandic families with 75 affected	3q13	3.71
Higgins et al. (1997)[46]	1 family	2p22-25	5.92
Farrer et al. (1999)[47]	1 family	4p	>3.0

LOD, logarithm of the odds.

(logarithm of the odds) scores were −19.5 for ASS and −10.8 for ABL at a recombination fraction of 0.01, and tight linkage to ASS was excluded individually in 11 of the families. These data indicate that the ET gene is not allelic to that causing ITD.

Several genetic linkage studies have identified gene loci[45–47] (Table 27-2). Gulcher et al.[45] studied 16 Icelandic families and reported linkage to 3q13. Higgins et al.[46] evaluated 1 large family and reported a LOD score of almost 6 with linkage to 2p22-25. Farrer et al.[47] investigated a large family with L-dopa-responsive parkinsonism that appeared to aggregate as an autosomal-dominant trait. Chromosome 4p haplotype segregated not only for the parkinsonism but also for patients with a postural tremor which they thought was consistent with the diagnosis of ET. However, the responsible gene and the function of these potential genes has not been identified. Hopefully, further studies will provide more information about the dysfunction due to genetic abnormalities and this potentially can result in novel forms of treatment strategies.

It is clear that genetic heterogeneity does exist in ET. For instance, Kovach et al.[48] did a genetic linkage study in a family of 68 members. Linkage to loci ETM-1 and ETM-2 as well as chromosome 4 did not occur, suggesting that other gene loci exist for ET. Tan et al.[49] found certain alleles were higher in PD and ET patients. They suggested a possible association of the alleles 263bp with PD and ET.

Tanner et al.[50] attempted to assess the relative contribution of genetics and environment in 16 ET twin pairs. They found that concordance ratio in monozygotic twins was approximately 2 times that in dizygotic twins. These findings are consistent with the genetic cause of ET. However, the concordance of monozygotic twins was not 100 percent, suggesting that other factors, perhaps environmental, may also play a role in the cause of ET.[50]

Clinical Manifestations

ET has as its sole clinical manifestation tremor. The diagnosis is made either incidentally or when the patient presents because of the functional or social disability resulting from the tremor. Other neurological signs or symptoms are typically absent.[6,13,40,51] Mild abnormalities of tone or gait are occasionally reported.[13,16] Singer et al.[52] found that 50 percent of

ET patients exhibited tandem gait abnormalities, as compared to 28 percent of age-matched controls. Stolze et al.[53] investigated the gait disorder of advanced ET quantitatively. ET patients exhibited abnormalities in tandem gait with increased number of missteps and a broad-based ataxia and dysmetric gait indistinguishable from the findings of patients with primary cerebellar-disease. The gait disorder was more severe in ET patients who had intention tremor. The authors concluded that this finding provided evidence for a cerebellar-like disturbance in ET.[53] Tremor, indistinguishable in appearance from ET, can be seen in association with other neurological disorders (see section on associated conditions below).[8,13,54] Clinical findings of a group of largely untreated, unselected cases of ET that would not otherwise come to neurologic assessment revealed that intention tremor was mild, often asymmetrical and not uniformly present throughout the examination.[55]

It has been suggested that social phobia is common among patients with ET. However, Schneier et al.[56] studied 94 patients with ET with mild-to-moderate tremor and found that only a minority had social phobia features that were associated with disability. They noted that the social phobia with ET appears to be different from persons with anxiety, phobia disorder.[56]

In general, tremor is rarely confused with other involuntary movements.[57] Its rhythmic, oscillating nature allows relatively easy recognition.[30,58] Physiologically, tremor has been defined as an "involuntary oscillation of a body part produced by alternating or synchronous contractions of reciprocally innervated antagonistic muscles."[58] Essential tremor is typically of the postural type; that is, the tremor is best seen with maintenance of a fixed posture.[13,30] It may be accentuated with goal-directed movement of the limbs (kinetic tremor), and, in some instances, may be present at rest.[8,13,59] The tremor may also occur only during the maintenance of a specific position. Changing the angle of the position may significantly alter the severity of the tremor. Sanes and Hallett[60] examined the influence of limb positioning in ET and other pathological tremors and found that different postures of the arm affected the magnitude of the tremor. This phenomenon was more evident in instances of postural tremor other than in ET.

A clinical and polyelectromyographic study in patients with essential head tremor, tremendous cervical dystonia, and dystonic head tremor found that sensory tricks (geste antagonistique) were helpful in reducing dystonic head tremors but not essential head tremor.[61] The authors conclude that the effect of sensory tricks is helpful in the differential diagnosis of head tremor.

NEUROPSYCHOLOGICAL DEFICITS

Patients with ET may have deficits on neuropsychological functioning, particularly those involving prefrontal and frontal cortex. Gasparini et al.[62] found that 27 ET patients showed significant impairments both in intentional and conceptual thinking tasks similar to those observed in a PD group. Similarly, Lombardi et al.[63] studied cognitive performance and mood in 18 ET patients and reported deficits on tests of verbal fluency, mainly mental set shifting, verbal memory and working memory, as well as higher levels of depression. Patients with PD had deficits on the same tests and on tests of visuospatial processes. Troster et al.[64] also found neuropsychological deficits in a subgroup of ET patients, documenting problems with visuoperceptual function, verbal fluency, and encoding. These studies suggest possible dysfunction in the cerebellothalamocerebral circuitry.

CLASSIFICATION

Critchley[8] noted that ET may occur in a wide range of frequencies (4–12 cycles/second) with an inverse relationship between amplitude size and tremor rate. It has been suggested that ET is simply exaggerated physiological tremor, following the same frequency pattern.[38] More recent electrophysiological data do not support this assumption.[65,66] With the recognition that ET is a heterogeneous condition, various classification schemes have been proposed. Findley and Gretsy[65] separated two types of ET on the basis of frequency analysis: those with frequencies between 7 and 11 Hz, having features of enhanced physiological tremor, and those with frequencies below 6.5 Hz. Categorizing ET on the basis of frequency alone, however, is not optimal, as it may vary within a single family or even in a given individual.[59] Marsden et al.[54] proposed a classification into four types, based on the presence or absence of a family history, response to alcohol, and response to beta-adrenergic-blocking drugs. Responsiveness to primidone was not addressed. Only types 2 and 3 of this classification should be considered ET. Currently, there are no data to support this classification, but this proposal does form the basis for future investigation. Deuschl et al.[67] have proposed another classification, based on pharmacological and electrophysiological properties. They tested 25 patients and found one group had normal long latency and synchronous tremor burst in antagonists or activity of antigravity muscles alone. The second group was characterized by abnormal long-latency reflexes and reciprocal electromyographic (EMG) activity in antagonists. It was further suggested that patients of the first group respond to propranolol, whereas those of the second group do not. However, pharmacological responsiveness was tested in only some subjects, and no objective measure of drug response was performed. Koller et al.[68] attempted to classify ET, using tremor frequency, tremor duration, family history of tremor, responsiveness to alcohol, propranolol, and primidone, muscle contraction pattern, and by using long-latency reflexes. They collected information from 61 patterns and found few correlations. It was concluded that ET could not be divided into subtypes using these characteristics. More investigation is needed to clarify the proper classification of ET.

BODY REGION AFFECTED BY ET

ET appears most frequently in the hands.[7,69–71] An adduction-abduction movement of the fingers and a flexion-extension movement of the hand is typical; less often, a pronation-supination movement (similar to the tremor of PD) is seen. Frequently, the tremor is unilateral at the onset, but, with time, both sides become involved.[8,16,54] With hand tremor, handwriting may become tremulous, and rounded letters take on a sharp angularity. Critchley[8] provided a handwriting example of both clinical and historical note when he reproduced the normal and tremor-affected signatures of Oliver Cromwell. The handwriting in ET does not become micrographic, distinguishing it from the script in PD.

The next most frequently affected body area is cranial musculature.[7,70] Although the tongue, head, or voice may be affected in isolation (see section on clinical variants below), it is most common for tremor in these regions to occur in association with hand tremor.[16,72,73] In advanced cases, tremor of the palate, voice, and tongue may result in dysarthric speech, but this infrequently occurs before 65 years of age.[16] The legs and trunk become affected infrequently and usually in the later stages of the illness.[30]

DISEASE ONSET AND PROGRESSION

ET may commence at any age, but its incidence rises with advancing years (see section on epidemiology). The onset of ET may be earlier in the familial form, as compared to the sporadic form.[16,20] It is rarely reported in infancy and childhood.[74] Categorizing ET by age of onset has not proved useful, as it does not assist in predicting clinical outcome or therapeutic response.[8,13,18] In the nineteenth century, Dana[14] distinguished between senile tremor and hereditary tremor, but this differentiation was soon recognized as arbitrary, and both entities are now considered to be manifestations of the same disease.[18,75]

ET is generally considered to be a slowly progressive disorder, but variability in its clinical course has been noted. The progression of this disease can be defined as an increase in tremor amplitude or extension of tremor to previously unaffected body parts. It is the former that impairs the patient's voluntary movements and results in disability. Critchley[8] characterized the illness as occurring in stages: in the initial 1–2 years a slow deterioration occurs, then little or no change in the tremor may be noted for several years, and then in later life the tremor may suddenly worsen. Larsson and Sjögren[16] in their study of familial ET suggest that the disease typically appears before age 50 with a fine rapid hand tremor of little consequence, by age 65 years the tremor is moderate, and at 70 years it is quite pronounced (increased in amplitude and diminished in frequency). We have observed patients who present in later life who have a very rapid progression of their tremors but otherwise appear to have typical ET. Despite its progressive nature, it has long been recognized that the diagnosis of ET is not associated with increased mortality.[14]

FACTORS INFLUENCING ET

Tremor can be affected by a host of factors. Overall, it tends to progress with age, so that, with advancing years, tremor frequency declines and amplitude increases.[38,40] Handedness may play a role in the expression and severity of ET. Biary and Koller[76] found a higher incidence of left-handedness among ET patients than controls; in addition, a direct relationship was found between hand dominance and tremor severity. It is not unusual for patients to associate the onset of tremor with a specific incident or circumstance; however, establishing causal relationship is difficult. Tremor, resembling ET, has been reported following head trauma;[77] it is unlikely that this phenomenon represents a form of ET, given the abruptness of onset, temporal link to the trauma, and refractoriness to therapy.

A number of things can affect tremor in the short term. In 1887, Dana[14] remarked that "everything that produces excitement or nervousness" may increase ET. In the intervening years a number of specific factors that may exacerbate ET have been suggested: fatigue, extremes of temperature, emotional upset, sexual arousal, central nervous system (CNS) stimulants, and diurnal fluctuations in catecholamine levels.[8,13,78] Alcohol may produce a remarkable ameliorative effect on ET. In many patients, tremor is lessened by ingesting even a small amount of alcoholic beverage. Intravenous alcohol infusion, but not local intra-arterial injection, decreases ET[79] and suggests that the effect of alcohol is centrally mediated. Indeed, alcohol is able to reverse the increase in cerebral regional blood flow seen in ET.[80] Although the therapeutic effect of alcohol is most typical of ET, it has been reported to occur rarely in other forms of tremor.[81] Caffeine is commonly considered to be a precipitant of tremor; however, in a formal study evaluating 20 ET patients, caffeine produced no discernible effect.[82] As is the case with most involuntary movements, ET typically remits during sleep; there are, however, rare reports of its persistence during slumber.[8,51]

In summary, the appearance of tremor in a given patient may vary, not only with the passage of years but even over the course of a single day.

DISABILITY

The patient with ET may be handicapped by the physical limitations that the tremor may create (e.g., writing, drinking liquids, etc.) or by the social embarrassment that it may cause. The physical disability is directly related to tremor amplitude; with aging or disease progression, amplitude increases, and the ability to execute fine, discrete movements may be impaired. Compromise of occupational skills may occur; approximately 15 percent of ET patients referred to a university clinic were pensioned as a result of tremor. Cooper noted that, in 1962, in rare cases, tremor is so severe as to warrant surgical intervention.[83] One cannot estimate to what extent ET alters quality of life, given the variability in social limitations that patients may impose on themselves because of embarrassment resulting from tremor. Although ET is sometimes preceded by the prefix "benign," the condition is clearly very disabling in some individuals. Busenbark et al.[84] analyzed the results of the Sickness Impact Profile, a standardized assessment tool that measures illness-related dysfunction, in 753 ET patients, 145 parkinsonians, and 87 controls. ET patients had greater dysfunction than the controls but less than the parkinsonians. Communication, work, emotional behavior, home management, and reactions and pastimes were particularly impaired in ET. The investigators concluded that significant disability can occur in ET and, compared to PD, ET tends to be less severe but causes relatively greater psychosocial dysfunction. Social phobia-like symptoms can occur in ET,[85] and several surveys[7,70] have documented the high prevalence of disability in ET. Depression, anxiety, and age, independent of the severity of tremor, were associated with greater functional disability in ET. It has therefore been suggested that these factors should be considered when assessing the impact of treatments in ET.[86]

DIAGNOSTIC PITFALLS

ET can be misdiagnosed, being most commonly mislabeled as incipient PD.[30] The correct diagnosis of ET can also be clouded by the consideration of other neurological illnesses that may have tremor as a clinical manifestation. This would include multiple sclerosis, Wilson's disease, Huntington's disease, and cerebellar degenerative diseases. In addition, tremor can be precipitated by drugs and toxins (e.g., lithium and valproic acid), and by systemic illness (e.g., thyrotoxicosis).[30] Laboratory studies are not considered helpful in diagnosing ET. However, in one study there was substantial agreement between clinical and electrophysiological definitions of ET.[87] In an effort to minimize diagnostic errors, we have adopted the use of diagnostic criteria for ET. Such guidelines not only assist in individual case assessment but also are crucial to ensure validity in the clinical investigation of ET. The Tremor Research Investigation Group, a committee of scientists studying ET, recently proposed a working definition of ET for research studies.[88]

DEFINITE ESSENTIAL TREMOR

1. Presence of postural tremor in the arms that worsens with action, in the absence of any condition or drug known to cause enhanced physiological tremor (listed below), in the absence of cerebellar symptoms and signs, and in the absence of PD dystonia, hyperthyroidism, chronic alcoholism, peripheral neuropathy, and an anxiety state. Medications known to be tremorgenic, such as (1) beta-agonists, (e.g., terbutaline), (2) lithium, (3) neuroleptics, (4) valproate, (5) tricyclic antidepressants, (6) antihistamines, (7) anticholinergics, (8) corticosteroids, and (9) dopamine agonists.

OR

2. Postural tremor of arms without action tremor of arms, plus head (neck) tremor, in the absence of any condition or drug known to cause enhanced physiological tremor, in the absence of cerebellar symptoms and signs, and in the absence of PD and dystonia.

PROBABLE ESSENTIAL TREMOR

1. Presence of both postural tremor and action tremor of arms, without an increase during action, in the absence of any condition or drug known to cause enhanced physiological tremor, in the absence of cerebellar symptoms and signs, and in the absence of PD and dystonia.

OR

2. Presence of action tremor alone, in the absence of any condition or drug known to cause enhanced physiological tremor, in the absence of cerebellar symptoms and signs, and in the absence of PD and dystonia.

OR

3. Postural tremor of arms that gets better with action, in the absence of any condition or drug known to cause enhanced physiological tremor, in the absence of cerebellar symptoms and signs, and in the absence of PD and dystonia.

OR

4. Postural tremor of arms and vocal tremor, in the absence of any condition or drug known to cause enhanced physiological tremor, in the absence of cerebellar symptoms and signs, and in the absence of PD and dystonia.

OR

5. Vocal and head or neck tremor without other known causes present, in the absence of any condition or drug known to cause enhanced physiological tremor, in the absence of cerebellar symptoms and signs, and in the absence of PD and dystonia.

POSSIBLE ESSENTIAL TREMOR

1. Postural tremor of arms and action tremor of arms, in the absence of any condition or drug known to cause enhanced physiological tremor, and in the absence of cerebellar symptoms and signs, but in the presence of PD or dystonia affecting those limbs.

OR

2. Postural tremor that goes away with action or remains unchanged with action, in the absence of any condition or drug known to cause enhanced physiological tremor, and in the absence of cerebellar symptoms and signs, but in the presence of PD or dystonia affecting those limbs.

OR

3. Leg or head or neck or lingual tremor alone, in the absence of any condition or drug known to cause enhanced physiological tremor, and in the absence of cerebellar symptoms and signs, but in the presence of PD or dystonia affecting those limbs.

CLINICAL VARIANTS

A variety of atypical tremor disorders exists that appear to be related to ET.[89] An association of these conditions with ET is suggested by a high occurrence of a family history of ET, frequent presence of a mild postural tremor, and tremor reduction with alcohol ingestion. In most patients with ET, varying degrees of postural and kinetic tremor are observed; however, in kinetic predominant tremor a marked dissociation occurs, with the postural component minimal or absent.[90] Cerebellar signs are absent. Disability may be severe in these patients. A resting tremor is not a defined component of ET, although it has been observed in severely affected or elderly patients. Koller and Rubino[91] reported a group of patients with a combined resting and postural tremor with minimal kinetic tremor. A postural tremor often occurs in PD, but the patients reported by Koller and Rubino[91] had no other parkinsonian features, despite a long duration of tremor. Tremor reduction did not occur with antiparkinsonian drugs in these patients. Several case reports of familial paroxysmal tremor with clinical features similar to ET exist.[92,93]

A task-specific or selective action tremor affecting the hands is primary writing tremor, in which pronation of the forearm elicits a pronation-supination tremor that is not seen during other movements of the arm.[94–96] Other activities involving pronation may also result in tremor; however, the major disability is impaired handwriting, which may be the patient's sole complaint. Tremor is present for the duration of writing, often making the task impossible. Postural and kinetic tremors, when present, are usually mild. EMG findings show an alteration of antagonist muscles, and there is no significant increase of reflex excitability or evidence of cortical hyperexcitability.[96] Primary writing tremor needs to be distinguished from a segmental dystonia of the hands, or writer's cramp.[97] Dystonic spasms are observed in writer's cramp, rather than in tremor. However, tremor may occur secondary to trying to control the dystonia, and some families have been reported as having different members who exhibit writer's cramp, ET, and primary writing tremor.[98] Elble et al.[99] studied 5 patients who had severe 5–7-Hz tremor when attempting to write or draw. They noted abnormal coactivation of the antagonistic muscles, which produced subtle dystonic posturing of the affected limb that was overshadowed by the tremor. The authors suggested that the nonspecificity of dystonia and postural tremor should be considered when discussing the pathophysiology of primary writing tremor.

ET can affect solely or predominantly one body part. Therefore, isolated tremors of the tongue, chin, and voice may occur. Tongue tremor is commonly found when the patient

is tested for it in the postural position, although the patient is often unaware of any difficulty with the tongue. However, a tongue tremor can be a patient's chief complaint. Tongue shaking may interfere both with speaking and eating. An isolated chin tremor (geniospasm) not involving the lips may also occur. Isolated trembling of the chin may also occur in families, transmitted as an autosomal-dominant gene.[100,101] This hereditary condition is stimulus-sensitive, may begin at birth, and may improve with age. Quavering of the lower lip can occur in PD but is almost always associated with other parkinsonian signs. Speech involvement in ET is not uncommon and, occasionally, may be the predominant or sole symptom.[102,103] Riveat and Marsden[104] suggested that some of these tremors may be associated with dystonia. They studied 5 patients who had an isolated tremor of the trunk or neck and found that their clinical characteristics were similar to those of other patients who presented with tremors and eventually developed torticollis or arm dystonia. They concluded that isolated tremors of the trunk and head, especially when of slow frequency (e.g., 2–3 Hz), may be the initial manifestation of a focal dystonia.

Truncal tremor is occasionally observed in ET patients with a long history of severe hand and head tremors. Truncal tremor occurring as a presenting symptom is rare. Heilman[105] first reported 3 patients with the sole symptom of orthostatic tremor of the trunk and the proximal legs. Wee et al.[106] described a family that had both typical ET of the hands and orthostatic trunk tremor. Pape and Gershanik[107] reported patients similar to those of Heilman. Tremor was present after standing for several seconds, increased with time, and could lead to falling. There was no tremor during sitting, walking, or leaning against a firm support. Gabellini et al.[108] described 8 cases of orthostatic tremor: 6 were thought to be idiopathic; 1 was said to be a result of hydrocephalus; and 1 was a result of chronic relapsing polyradiculoneuropathy. They suggested a relationship between orthostatic tremor and ET. Pape and Gershanik[107] reported EMG findings in orthostatic tremor that were similar to those of ET in the upper and lower limbs. However, standing or sustaining certain positions with the arms and legs would bring about dramatic changes in the pattern of rhythmic discharges, with a high-frequency activity of 15–16 Hz.[106,109] They thought that the clinical manifestations could be a result of instability caused by stiffness of the legs, depending on the high-frequency tremor, which is not clearly visible. Thompson et al.[110] described electrophysiological findings in 1 patient with orthostatic tremor. In this patient the tremor affected primarily the legs and was alternating between antagonist muscle groups and had a high frequency of 16 Hz. The tremor was present only during certain postures. A tremor of the same frequency was also recorded in the arms during particular movements. It was suggested that orthostatic tremor is generated by spontaneous oscillations responsible for organizing the motor programs for standing.

An orthostatic tremor patient was described by Walker et al.[111] in which EMG revealed tremor burst of 15 Hz in the lower extremities while standing and with isometric activation of the muscles, but the bursts disappeared with isotonic activation of muscles. Uncini et al.[112] reported 2 patients with orthostatic tremor with 10–12- and 16-Hz EMG bursts in antagonistic muscles. EMG activity was synchronous in corresponding muscles of both legs. They suggested that orthostatic tremor may be an exaggeration of physiological tremor resulting from synchronization of motor units by spontaneous oscillations in central structures. Lewitt[113] hypothesized that orthostatic tremor shares a similar mechanism with the entity of "paradoxical clonus" or shorting reaction. Drugs that may be useful for orthostatic tremor include clonazepam, gabapentin, and mysoline.

Associated Conditions

ET has been described in association with various disorders and conditions. The chance of simultaneous occurrence of such a common disorder with other diseases must be considered when one is reviewing the long list of "associated conditions." In an epidemiological study in Finland by Rautakorpi,[20] there was a significantly higher incidence of cardiovascular disorders, including arterial hypertension, coronary heart disease, and cerebrovascular disease, in ET patients than in controls. He proposed that this association may depend on the occurrence of a selection bias in the control group or a genetic linkage between ET and certain risk factors of cardiovascular disease. Other studies have not substantiated this link between cardiovascular disorders and ET. In a 45-year retrospective study based on original medical records, Rajput et al.[23] reported that diagnosis of hypertension was made at some time or another in 30 percent of the cases. There was no significant difference between patients and controls for risk of hypertension subsequent to the diagnosis of ET. In their study of ET in Papua, New Guinea, Hornabrook and Nagurney[26] found that blood pressures and electrocardiographs of their ET population were comparable with those of a control series.

The incidence of nonspecific neurological abnormalities in ET patients has been studied with various conclusions. Larsson and Sjögren[16] described stiff gait, slight rigidity, or other nonspecific neurological abnormalities in 17 of the 81 cases. Hornabrook and Nagurney[26] also noted a certain stiffness in some patients, stating that it is "perhaps better described as a tenseness of the general musculature. This was qualitatively distinct from the akinetic rigidity so familiar in paralysis agitans. Patients appeared to hold themselves stiffly, perhaps in order to give themselves less opportunity for the involuntary tremors to become manifest." A study of 200 ET patients observed mild reduction of upper limb synkinetic movements during gait in 4 patients (2 percent), and hypomimic facies in 2 patients (1 percent).[114] The authors speculated that extrapyramidal impairment may be common in the normal aging population as a result of progressive loss

of nigrostriatal neurons and brain dopamine.[115,116] Therefore, they concluded, it was not surprising to find similar signs in elderly ET patients. In a study of 247 ET patients in London and Chicago, mild extrapyramidal signs occurred in only 4.5 percent of ET patients and did not differ significantly from the findings in age-matched controls.[117]

The relationship of ET and PD has been controversial since James Parkinson (1817) first commented on the distinction between paralysis agitans and senile (essential) tremor in 1817.[10] Gowers[118] in 1888 did not make this distinction, but rather, he stated that "it is doubtful whether this senile tremor is essentially different from paralysis agitans. Some cases are met with a character intermediate between the two affections." He also described "simple" tremor and stated that "in spite of the occasional collateral relation to paralysis agitans, it seems to have little tendency to develop into the latter disease, and certainly is less closely connected with it than is senile tremor."[118] In 1949, Critchley[8] stressed that, because both disorders are relatively common, chance may account for the presence of ET or PD in family members and cases of concurrent ET-PD. In a clinical series, Duvoisin et al.[21] noted that the incidence of ET among the 85 index PD patients' siblings and spouses was the same.

In their study in New Guinea, Hornabrook and Nagurney[26] reported that there "is slight evidence from this series that the two conditions are in some way linked." In another epidemiological study, Marttilla and Rinne[119] found no association, reporting that 5.8 percent of PD patients and 8.1 percent of control subjects had relatives with probable ET. More recent epidemiological studies have also concluded that ET and PD are genetically independent diseases.[23,120]

Barbeau and Pourcher[121] reported a strong family history of ET in early-onset PD. In a clinical series of 50 cases of familial PD, Roy et al.[122] proposed two main patterns of genetic transmission within parkinsonian patients, with one a parkinsonism related to hereditary ET. They reported a high prevalence of ET in families of PD patients who had tremor as their initial symptom. Geraghty et al.,[123] in a clinical series of 130 ET patients, concluded that the risk of PD is 24 times greater than in an age-matched, randomly selected population. In a report from the same clinic, the clinical correlates of 350 ET patients were reported.[124] Twenty percent of patients were thought to have parkinsonism. However, this conclusion has been challenged because of methodological flaws of the study, which include the problem of dual reporting and unclear definition of postural tremors and ET.[125] Lang et al.[126] also found a higher incidence of familial tremor in PD patients than in controls but not the striking association reported by Geraghty et al.[123] Cleeves et al.[117] found no association or genetic link between ET and PD in their clinical series of 237 ET patients, 100 PD patients, and 100 normal controls. Frequency of family history of ET was higher among PD patients than controls but was not statistically significant. The authors propose that, although there is no overall relationship, there may be an association between ET and a distinct subgroup of PD patients, as suggested earlier by

Barbeau and Pourcher.[121] In a clinical series examining the occurrence of PD and ET in parents and siblings of early-onset parkinsonian patients, the incidence of PD or ET did not differ significantly from the relevant expected incidence in any group.[127] In a study of several kindreds of ET, Bain et al.[5] found no association with PD, and in an investigation of over 800 ET patients, only 7 percent were thought to have concomitant PD.[70] Montgomery et al.[128] found that both ET and PD had longer reaction times and slower movements velocities as compared to controls. They suggested that a similar pathogenetic motor mechanism may occur in both diseases. Also visuomotor impairment has been found in a minority of ET patients, which is similar to that seen in early PD.[129]

The controversy over the relationship of PD and ET continues and is compounded by the frequent inability to distinguish the two disorders.[30] Parkinsonian signs, such as cogwheeling and tremor at rest, may be seen in ET,[130] and postural tremor is not uncommon in PD. However, recent observations have further suggested that ET is unrelated to PD.[131,132] Rajput et al.[133] reported the postmortem results of 6 patients with ET. There was no neuronal loss in the substantia nigra, and Lewy bodies were not observed. Positron emission tomography (PET) scanning indicates that striatal fluorodopa uptake is normal in ET.[134] Olfaction function, measured by the University of Pennsylvania Smell Identification Test, was found to be normal in ET, whereas dysfunction in olfaction is a common and early sign in PD.[135]

The presence of a postural tremor in patients with focal or generalized dystonia is not uncommon. Whether this can truly be labeled "ET" is debatable. Yanagisawa et al.[136] described 6 generations of a Japanese family with 149 members, 5 of whom had dystonia musculorum deformans, another 12 of whom had a forme fruste of this disease, and all 17 of whom had a postural tremor. In their study of patients with torsion dystonia, Johnson et al.[137] found a large number of family members with tremor. In reviewing the records of 100 patients with the diagnosis of ET, familial, or senile tremor, Baxter and Lal[138] found dystonic symptoms in 12 cases. Other studies have reported a 1–3 percent incidence of dystonia in their ET populations.[16,114] In 1949, Critchley[8] summarized the European literature on ET and reported individual cases of torticollis and ET. A strong association between spasmodic torticollis and ET was reported by Couch.[139] Of 30 patients with idiopathic spasmodic torticollis, 26 demonstrated tremor, "usually rhythmic" and resembling ET. A family history of tremor was present in 16 of the patients who had tremor with dystonia. Couch[139] proposed that ET is a forme fruste of dystonia but acknowledged the association of postural tremor with a wide variety of basal ganglia disorders. Duane[140] noted that, although idiopathic spasmodic torticollis and essential head tremor may coexist, patients who have essential head tremor commonly tilt their head to one side in an effort to suppress the tremor. In the database of the Dystonia Clinic at the University of Kansas Medical Center for patients with dystonia and tremor,

Dubinsky et al.[141] found that, of 296 patients with idiopathic dystonia, 24 had dystonic tremor, 20 with cervical dystonia had an isolated head-nodding tremor, 2 with writer's cramp had ipsilateral hand tremor, and 2 with generalized dystonia had arm tremor. Eight patients, all with cervical dystonia, had essential tremor that preceded the onset of their dystonia.

Using surface EMG, Yanagisawa and Goto[142] showed that an irregular 1–6.5-Hz grouping of motor unit discharges is often associated with the involuntary dystonic contractions, but a more rhythmic 5–11-Hz grouping is seen during voluntary contraction. The rhythmic motor unit grouping is indistinguishable from that of ET, but the irregular 1–6.5-Hz tremor bears very little resemblance to ET, making a proposed relationship questionable.

The presence of tremor in writer's cramp has been recognized, but the specific relationship is unclear.[96,97] Ravits et al.[96] described 4 patients with tremor upon writing that they consider to have a form of focal dystonia with tremor, noting similar physiological findings in a patient with myoclonic writer's cramp and in tremor patients. Klawans et al.[94] described 6 patients who had a tremor upon writing, 5 of whom responded to anticholinergic therapy and none of whom responded to propranolol. Sheehy and Marsden[97] proposed that patients who present clinically with primary writing tremor may have a variant of ET that is responsive to alcohol and propranolol, or a tremulous form of dystonia, as described by Ravits et al.[96] and Klawans et al.[94] Rosenbaum and Jankovic[143] studied focal task-specific tremor and dystonia and noted that the two disorders shared many clinical, genetic, physiological, and pharmacological features with the more common generalized movement disorders, and suggested interrelationships between the focal and the generalized forms of tremor and dystonia. In one report, 47 percent of ET patients were said to have some form of dystonia.[124] This observation is contrary to most clinicians' experience, and the findings may represent a referral bias to a specialty clinic.

Tremor may occur in familial and acquired peripheral neuropathies.[144–147] Roussy and Lévy[144] provided the classic description of a hereditary neuropathy patient who had tremor as a clinical manifestation. In more recent years, it has been suggested that the Roussy-Lévy syndrome does not represent a distinct entity but that tremor may be seen in hereditary motor-sensory neuropathies of both the hypertrophic and nonhypertrophic types.[148–150] This association of tremor with familial neuropathies has led to consideration as to whether this represents the expression of linked genetic material ("Charcot-Marie-Tooth gene" linked to the "ET gene" in a given family), the expression of a single genetic aberration (independent of Charcot-Marie-Tooth disease and ET), or that tremor may simply occur in hereditary neuropathies owing to pathophysiological circumstances within the peripheral nervous system.[150] The heterogeneous nature of such tremors is illustrated by the diversity of genetic, clinical, physiological, and pharmacological features in the reported cases.[150,151] Similarly, tremors of sundry natures have been associated with acquired peripheral neuropathies, including neuropathies of the chronic relapsing type and those attributed to dysgammaglobulinemia, diabetes, uremia, and amyloidosis.[145,147,152] It has been suggested that such tremor represents physiological tremor, enhanced by weakness or impaired stretch reflexes.[145,153] In summary, although neuropathic tremor remains an obscure entity in terms of its pathogenesis and nosological significance, it should be considered distinct from ET.

Baughman[154] and Pittman et al.[155] described several patients with concurrent Klinefelter's syndrome and ET. Baughman[154] studied 13 males in a private neurology practice and 11 institutionalized male retardates, all with known sex chromosome abnormalities. ET was present in 5 from each group, 10 of 24 total. They concluded that "ET is a common and significant component of the male supernumerary X syndromes and probably supernumerary Y syndromes."

In summary, postural and kinetic tremors are a common accompaniment of many illnesses, both systemic and neurological. Characteristics of these tremors are so nonspecific as to preclude firm conclusions regarding a pathophysiological relationship. Consequently, reported associations with other medical conditions must be interpreted with caution.

Pathophysiology

Unfortunately, our knowledge regarding the anatomic localization of possible neural abnormalities in ET is minimal, and, likewise, there is almost no understanding of possible pathophysiological mechanisms. Is the pathogenesis of ET related to dysfunction of the peripheral or central nervous system? The anatomic basis of tremor could be a result of oscillation in the stretch reflex or in a centrally located network of neurons. It is clear that tremor can be modified by various maneuvers that perturb both the stretch reflex and cortical mechanisms, such as transcranial magnetic stimulation.[156–159] However, when ET is produced by a central oscillator, the tremor must be expressed through the neuromuscular machinery of the stretch reflex and limb mechanisms. Several observations suggest that ET does not result solely from peripheral mechanisms. There is no correlation between tremor frequency and nerve conduction velocities,[145] and the frequency of ET has no relationship to the reflex loop time. Furthermore, there is a lack of tremor entrainment produced by peripheral rhythmic inputs.[54] It is interesting to note that tremor frequency tends to be lower in older patients. As there is a linear relationship between age and tremor frequency the decrease in ET frequency might reflect age-related changes in cerebellum or other parts of the nervous system.[160]

A central site for the abnormality in ET is supported by the beneficial effect of thalamotomy and by drugs that

appear to act centrally.[30,79] ET has been reported to be alleviated unilaterally in 2 patients with strokes that involved the pyramidal tracts[161,162] and in patients with homolateral cerebellar infarction.[163] Several brain areas are candidates for the exaggerated oscillations responsible for ET. Areas with inherent rhythmicity in the frequency range of ET included the inferior olivary and thalamic nuclei.[164–166] Hypermetabolism of the inferior olive can be observed on PET during tremor activation.[167] Colebatch et al.[168] also studied cerebral blood flow, using ^{15}C-labeled carbon dioxide with PET technology in 4 ET patients and 4 controls. They found that the cerebellum was selectively activated in ET and suggested that the increased blood flow in the cerebellum represented neural activity involved in tremor generation. These investigators concluded that ET is the result of oscillation within the cerebello-olivary pathways that is relayed by way of the thalamus and motor cortex to the spinal cord. Increased activity of the cerebellum in ET, both at rest and when the tremor is advanced, has been observed in other PET studies.[169] A tremor disorder that resembles ET can be caused by vascular or traumatic insults to the brainstem, particularly around the area of the red nucleus.[170] Because of the lack of human data, animal models of ET would be important. Tremors can be induced by drugs such as harmaline and oxotremorine and by anatomic lesions.[171,172] However, the relevance of these conditions to ET is uncertain.

The cerebellum appears to be a prime candidate for the site of dysfunction in ET. Animal models of tremor can involve cerebellar dysfunction or pathology.[173] Furthermore, both qualitative and quantitative studies of advanced ET show similarities of gait disturbances and intention tremor to patients with cerebellar disease.[174] Postmortem anatomical studies of the cerebellum need to be performed in ET.

Thus, it appears that ET may be a result of an abnormal oscillation of a CNS "pacemaker," the location of which is currently unknown. The proposed circuitry for the genesis of ET is shown in Fig. 27-1. There have been only approximately 20 reported postmortem examinations of patients with ET.[3,175–179] These investigations have reported nonspecific changes, and it would appear that gross anatomic change may not occur in ET. Studies of possible neurochemical changes in ET brains have not to date been performed. Drug trials with gamma-aminobutyric acid (GABA, progabide) and serotonergic (trazodone) agonists, using these drugs as pharmacological probes, have not indicated a role for these neurotransmitters in ET.[180,181] Using simultaneously EEG-EMG correlates Heilwig et al.[182] found significant correlations between the sensorimotor cortex and ET tremor frequency and suggested that the sensorimotor cortex was involved in the generation of ET. However, their conclusion has been criticized by McAuley[183] for methodological and other reasons.

It can be concluded that ET is probably produced by a central oscillator that can be enhanced or suppressed by reflex pathways. Analysis of postmortem material from

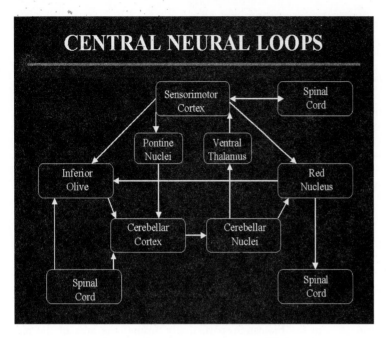

CENTRAL NEURAL LOOPS

FIGURE 27-1 Proposed circuitry underlying the pathophysiology of essential tremor.

ET brains is needed if we are to further understand the pathophysiology of ET.

Assessment of Tremor

A variety of means have been used in the assessment of ET.[5,184,185] One major difficulty with attempts to quantify ET is that the severity of tremor can fluctuate significantly over short periods of time. The changing intensity of tremor relates probably both to an inherent rhythm of ET and to the influence of external factors. Assessment of tremor severity has been reported using a modified Klove-Matthews-Motor-Steadiness Battery.[186] Also a tremor scale (the Columbia University Disability Questionnaire for essential tremor) was reported to be reliable and to correlate with measures of tremor severity.[187] A teaching videotape for this tremor rating scale has also been published.[188]

Clinical rating scales have been used to assess tremor. One such scale that is currently in use is shown below.

TREMOR

0—No tremor perceived.
1—Slight (barely noticeable).
2—Moderate, noticeable, probably not disabling, less than 2-cm excursions of affected part.
3—Marked, probably partially disabling (2–4-cm excursions).
4—Severe, disabling (more than 4-cm excursion).

Tremor can be rated for the resting, postural, and kinetic positions and for the affected body part.

Self-assessment scales have also been developed to quantify the functional disability associated with ET.

SPEAKING PHONATION

0—Normal.
1—Mild speech difficulty and/or voice tremulousness when "nervous" only.
2—Mild speech difficulty and/or voice tremor, most of the time.
3—Moderate speech difficulty and/or voice tremor constant.
4—Severe speech difficulty and/or voice tremor. Most words or phrases difficult to understand.

FEEDING (OTHER THAN LIQUIDS)

0—Normal.
1—Mildly abnormal. Can bring all solids to mouth, spilling only rarely.
2—Moderately abnormal. Frequently spills peas and similar foods. May bring head at least halfway to meet food.
3—Markedly abnormal. Unable to cut or uses both hands to feed.
4—Severely abnormal. Needs help to feed.

BRINGING LIQUIDS TO MOUTH (DRINKING)

0—Normal.
1—Mildly abnormal. Can still use a spoon but spills if completely full.

2—Moderately abnormal. Unable to use a spoon. Still uses cup or glass but spills more frequently if more than half full.

3—Markedly abnormal. Can drink from cup or glass but needs both hands.

4—Severely abnormal. Must use a straw.

HYGIENE

0—Normal.

1—Mildly abnormal. Able to do everything but is more careful than average person.

2—Moderately abnormal. Able to do everything but with errors; for example, uses an electric shaver because of tremor.

3—Markedly abnormal. Unable to do most fine tasks, such as putting on lipstick or shaving (even with electric shaver), unless using both hands.

4—Severely abnormal. Unable to do any fine movement tasks.

DRESSING

0—Normal.

1—Mildly abnormal. Able to do everything but is clumsier than average person.

2—Moderately abnormal. Able to do everything but with difficulty.

3—Markedly abnormal. Needs some assistance with buttoning or tying shoelaces.

4—Severely abnormal. Requires assistance with most dressing activities.

WRITING

0—Normal.

1—Mildly abnormal. Legible. Continues to write letters.

2—Moderately abnormal. Legible but no longer writes letters.

3—Markedly abnormal. Illegible.

4—Severely abnormal. Unable to sign checks or other documents requiring signature.

WORKING

0—Tremor does not interfere with primary occupation.

1—Able to perform primary occupation but requires more effort than the average person.

2—Able to do everything but with errors. Poorer than usual performance because of tremor.

3—Unable to do primary occupation. Many have changed to a different job because of tremor. Tremor limits housework, such as ironing.

4—Unable to do outside job. Housework very limited.

FINE MOVEMENTS

0—Normal.

1—Minimal impairment. Difficulty threading needles.

2—Moderate impairment. Difficulty buttoning shirt buttons.

3—Marked impairment. Difficulty placing a key in a lock.

4—Severe impairment. Requires both hands to put on glasses.

EMBARRASSMENT

0—None.

1—Minimal change in social activities, still socializes.

2—Moderate change in social activities, avoids encounters with strangers.

3—Marked change in social activities, avoids encounters with friends.

4—Severe change in social activities, avoiding public encounters.

Functional disability can also be assessed by scales when a rater scores the patient's ability to perform motor tasks.

HANDWRITING

Have the subject write the standard sentence "Today is a nice day" with dominant hand.

WITH STRATEGY (COMPENSATORY MANEUVERS)
Describe strategy.

0—Normal.

1—Mildly abnormal. Slightly untidy, tremulous.

2—Moderately abnormal. Legible but with considerable tremor.

3—Markedly abnormal. Illegible.

4—Severely abnormal. Unable to keep pencil or pen on paper without holding down with the other hand.

WITHOUT STRATEGY
0—Normal.

1—Mildly abnormal. Slightly untidy, tremulous.

2—Moderately abnormal. Legible but with considerable tremor.

3—Markedly abnormal. Illegible.

4—Severely abnormal. Unable to keep pencil or pen on paper without holding down with the other hand.

DRAWING

Ask the subject to draw the requested figures. Test each hand without leaning the hand or arm on the table. Use a ballpoint pen only.

SPIRAL
0—Normal.
1—Slightly tremulous.
2—Moderately tremulous.
3—Accomplishes the task with great difficulty. Figure still recognizable.
4—Unable to complete drawing. Figure not recognizable.

DRAW A STRAIGHT LINE BETWEEN LINES (PATIENT WORKSHEET ATTACHED)
0—Normal.
1—Slightly tremulous.
2—Moderately tremulous.
3—Accomplishes the task with great difficulty. Figure still recognizable.
4—Unable to complete drawing. Figure not recognizable.

DRAW SINE WAVE BETWEEN LINES
0—Normal.
1—Slightly tremulous.
2—Moderately tremulous.
3—Accomplishes the task with great difficulty. Many errors.
4—Unable to complete drawing. Figure not recognizable.

POURING

Use firm plastic cups (8 cm tall, without handles) filled with water 1 cm from the top. Ask patient to pour water from one cup to another.

0—Normal.
1—More careful than a person without tremor, but no water is spilled.
2—Spills a small amount of water (up to 10 percent of the total amount).
3—Spills a considerable amount of water (>10–50 percent).
4—Unable to pour without spilling most of the water.

The rhythmic, oscillatory kinetics of tremor make it suitable for quantification by objective means. Both acute and chronic recordings have been performed.[3,189] A variety of recording systems have been used. An accelerometer (velocity transducer), which is sensitive to movement (displacement), is attached to the hand or another body part. The signal is then amplified, and a summating technique such as spectral analysis is applied to an epoch of tremor (e.g., 60 s). An amplitude measurement is then generated at a peak frequency. Attempts have been made to develop an ambulatory tremor-recording device the size of a wrist watch which can be worn for a prolonged period of time, such as days or weeks.[189] To date, none of these devices has been perfected. One difficulty is separating normal rhythmic movements from tremor. However, with new developments in technology, it is likely that such

an ambulatory recording device will become commercially available in the near future.

Matsumoto et al.[190] reported a mechanical linkage device that they used to measure the three-dimensional position of the fingertip during a postural task. They found the device superior to uniaxial accelerometry. Elble et al.[191] evaluated another device for quantifying ET. They used a digitizing tablet to record oscillations during writing and drawing.

Treatment

Magee[192] stated in 1965 that there was no effective therapy for ET. Recent advances have now resulted in successful treatment for ET. A variety of pharmacological approaches to ET is available, and new strategies are being studied. However, tremor of different body parts and various tremor variants may have different pharmacological responsiveness and some patients still cannot be effectively treated.[5,69]

ALCOHOL

Alcohol will temporarily cause a dramatic reduction of tremor in the majority of patients.[79,193] Clinical observations suggest that, with time, larger amounts of alcohol may be needed to cause tremor reduction. It is generally recommended that the judicious use of small amounts of alcoholic beverages before meals or other events to reduce tremor is reasonable. Alcohol's mechanism of action is unknown; however, PET studies have shown that alcohol decreases the increase in regional cerebellar blood flow in ET.[80] A better understanding of its action could lead to the development of other pharmacological agents for ET. Teravainen et al.[194] investigated the alcohol derivative, methylpentynol, a 6-carbon alcohol, in ET and found its effect was not different from placebo. Critchley[8] warned that alcohol, when used in ET, "appeared only too often to have served as an excuse for habits of intemperance." The risk of addiction was considered a contraindication to the use of alcohol. However, the rate of chronic alcoholism in ET has only recently been defined. Schroeder and Nasrallah,[195] in a retrospective chart survey, found a 60 percent alcoholic rate in ET and concluded that ET is an important cause of alcoholism. However, Koller,[196] in a prospective study, found that the prevalence of pathological drinking in ET did not differ from other tremor disorders or chronic neurological disease without tremor. Likewise, similar surveys in Finland and Sweden found that ET patients neither used more alcohol nor had a higher prevalence of alcoholism than the general population.[197,198] Moreover, it has been found that chronic alcoholism may itself result in a persistent postural tremor, lasting up to 1 year after complete abstinence.[199] It can be concluded that the occasional use of alcohol in ET is not contraindicated and that the risk of alcoholism is low.

BETA-ADRENERGIC BLOCKERS

Marshall,[200] in 1968, suggested that beta-adrenergic blockers may be useful in the treatment of ET. Winkler and Young[201] and Sevitt[202] both reported that propranolol decreased ET. Several subsequent studies reported a lack of effect of propranolol.[202,203] However, this may have been a result of inadequate doses, small sample size, or lack of objective measurements. Most investigations have confirmed the efficacy of propranolol in reducing postural hand tremor, using both subjective and objective (accelerometer recordings) evaluation.[204–210] Tremor amplitude is decreased, but tremor frequency is unchanged. Propranolol became the drug of choice for ET; however, the clinical response to propranolol is variable and often incomplete.[13,30] It is generally estimated that 50–70 percent of patients will have symptomatic relief. Dramatic improvement occurs in a much smaller percentage, and some patients will have no response. Average tremor reduction of 50–60 percent is suggested by some studies, but the number of patients investigated has been small. There are no well-defined factors that predict therapeutic responsiveness. Dupuis et al.[163] and Murray[206] found that the effect of chronic propranolol treatment was better in younger patients and in those with a shorter duration of disease. However, Teravainen et al.[208] and Larsen et al.[209] found propranolol treatment more effective in older patients and in those with lower frequency of tremor. Calzetti et al.[210] found a better response to a single oral dose of propranolol in patients with a larger tremor amplitude and a lower frequency. With chronic administration, they found no correlation with disease duration, patient's age, or degree of cardiac beta-blockage.[210] The number of patients in the above studies has been small, which may account for the variable findings. In a dose-response study of propranolol, 240–320 mg/day was found to be the optimal dose range.[211] Doses above 320 mg/day conferred no additional benefit. A sustained-release preparation of propranolol (propranolol long-acting) designed for once daily dosage has been reported to provide similar, or, in some cases, greater tremor reduction than divided doses.[212,213] Many patients preferred propranolol long-acting for ease of administration.

Propranolol therapy is usually well tolerated.[214–217] Relative contraindications for propranolol use are (1) heart failure, especially if poorly controlled, (2) second- or third-degree atrioventricular block, (3) asthma or other bronchospastic disease, and (4) insulin-dependent diabetes, in which propranolol may block the adrenergic manifestations of hypoglycemia. Most side-effects of propranolol are related to beta-blockage. The pulse rate will be lowered in most patients. A pulse of 60 beats/minute is usually well tolerated. Other less common adverse reactions include fatigue, weight gain, nausea, diarrhea, rash, impotency, and mental status alterations (e.g., depression). It has been suggested that tolerance may develop to propranolol's effect; however, several studies have found that the majority of patients do not lose any effect of propranolol after 1 year

of therapy, although the dose had to be increased in some patients to maintain the same degree of efficacy.[215,216]

The mechanism of action of propranolol in ET is unknown. Young[217] proposed a central site of action, because he noted no effect of intravenous or intra-arterial propranolol and a delay in the effect of chronic oral therapy. However, several controlled studies have shown that propranolol causes an immediate and sustained reduction in tremor.[218,219] Jefferson et al.[220] have proposed a peripheral site of action. Beta-blockers that enter the CNS with difficulty can reduce ET. Specific beta2-antagonists (ICI 118551, and LI 32-468), which act predominantly peripherally, are effective in decreasing tremor, further supporting a peripheral beta2 mechanism of action.[220,221]

Other orally active beta-adrenergic blocking drugs are available, such as metoprolol, nadolol, atenolol, timolol, and pindolol. The beta-blockers are classified according to the presence or absence of beta1-adrenergic selectivity, intrinsic sympathomimetic activity (partial agonists), and membrane-stabilizing properties. Differences in potency, metabolism, half-life, protein binding, and excretion are recognized. Despite the therapeutic similarity of beta-blocking drugs, differences in their pharmacodynamic properties may be clinically important. The effectiveness of metoprolol in ET has been demonstrated in multiple case reports and a controlled study.[222–227] Metoprolol differs from propranolol in preferentially antagonizing beta1-adrenergic receptors. The selectivity for beta1 receptors is, however, only relative. With higher dosages beta2-adrenergic receptors are also blocked. Some degree of beta2-blockage appears in patients at daily doses above 100 mg. Metoprolol is beneficial in ET at divided doses of 100–200 mg/day. Patients who failed to respond to propranolol also did not respond to metoprolol.[227] It has been suggested that metoprolol is the preferred drug for use in patients with bronchospastic disease. Because of its relative lack of beta2-blocking properties, metoprolol should theoretically be better tolerated than propranolol, a nonspecific blocker. Several asthmatic patients with ET have been reported who could tolerate metoprolol but not propranolol. Metoprolol is, however, capable of causing respiratory distress and should be used with caution in bronchospastic disease. Nadolol, when administered once daily, at doses of 120 and 240 mg/day, was found in a controlled study to significantly decrease ET in patients who also responded to propranolol.[228] Nadolol has a 24-hour half-life and can be taken once daily, avoiding inconveniences and compliance problems of multiple daily drug administration. Atenolol was reported to have no effect on tremor and to cause slight tremor reduction.[229,230] Timolol was found to decrease tremor,[229] and pindolol was found to be ineffective.[211] Pindolol, because of its partial agonist activity, may actually produce tremors.[230] Kuroda et al.[231] reported that arotinolol (30 mg/day), a peripherally acting beta-adrenergic blocker, significantly reduced ET in 15 patients.

The usefulness of other beta-adrenergic blockers is not much different from propranolol. Selective beta-blockers, like metoprolol, can be used at low doses in bronchospastic disease. When a side-effect such as impotence occurs with propranolol, changing to a different beta-blocker may result in disappearance of the adverse affect without loss of beneficial action.

PRIMIDONE

O'Brien et al.[232] noted that primidone given to a patient with epilepsy and ET reduced tremor; they gave the drug to 20 other patients, starting with 125 mg and increasing to 750 mg/day. Six patients, including 4 at the 125-mg dose, could not tolerate the drug because of vertigo, unsteadiness, and nausea. Twelve patients had a good clinical response. Addition of propranolol resulted in further improvement. It was concluded that primidone was more effective than propranolol, but ET patients did not tolerate primidone as well as seizure patients did. However, epileptic patients are often taking other drugs that cause hepatic enzyme induction, which may explain these perceived differences in toxicity. Chakrabarti and Pearce[233] gave primidone to 5 patients, starting at 125 mg for several days with a gradual increase of 750–1000 mg/day. Improvement was evident within a few days with increased functional capabilities. Findley et al.[234] studied 11 patients using objective recording techniques, starting primidone at 62.5 mg and increasing the dose to 750 mg/day. Side-effects occurred in 6 patients, and only 7 patients achieved the maximum dose. Tremor was decreased by an average of 66 percent (mean dose 590 mg/day) and by more than 90 percent in 2 patients. Koller and Royse,[235] in a placebo-controlled study using objective recording techniques, found that primidone (50–1000 mg/day) significantly reduced the amplitude of essential hand tremor in both untreated and propranolol-treated patients. Low doses (i.e., 250 mg/day) were as effective as high doses. Primidone decreased tremor more than propranolol did. There was no correlation between therapeutic response and serum levels. Acute reactions to the initial dose and side-effects of higher dose caused drug intolerance. A single oral dose of 250 mg/day of primidone decreased tremor by 60 percent 1–7 hours after ingestion with stable serum primidone levels but no detectable phenobarbital. Tremor control was lost when primidone was replaced by phenobarbital.[235] Gorman et al.[236] compared primidone, propranolol, and placebo in 14 patients. Both propranolol and primidone significantly reduced tremor, but there was no significant difference in improvement between the drugs. It has been suggested that tolerance to primidone may develop;[237,238] however, two studies that investigated the long-term effects of primidone have found that its antitremor effect was maintained for a 1-year period.[235,239]

The mechanism of action of primidone's antitremor effect is unknown. Primidone is converted to two active metabolites: phenylethylmalonamide (PEMA) with a half-life of approximately 30 hours, and phenobarbital with a half-life of approximately 10 days. The administration of high doses of PEMA had no effect on tremor.[240] Findley and Calzetti[241] suggested that the beneficial effect was mediated by both primidone and phenobarbital. However, primidone decreased tremor when there was no detectable serum phenobarbital, and phenobarbital may have only minimal antitremor action. Primidone itself or an unrecognized metabolite appears to be the responsible agent. It is noted that with primidone monotherapy the ratio of primidone to phenobarbital in the serum is 1:2.

PHENOBARBITAL

Phenobarbital has been used in ET for many years, and generally its effect has been thought to be minimal. However, several studies have demonstrated a beneficial effect of phenobarbital. Procaccianti et al.[242] found that phenobarbital caused a significant reduction in tremor, compared to that in placebo. The effect in 12 patients was comparable to that of propranolol. In a double-blind controlled study, Baruzzi et al.[243] found that both phenobarbital and propranolol were more effective than placebo with objective measures and patient self-assessment. However, clinical evaluation showed no difference between phenobarbital and placebo. Findley and Cleeves[244] gave phenobarbital (120 mg/day) to 12 patients and also found that the drug was better than placebo. They suggested that phenobarbital may be an alternate drug for the treatment of ET. It is possible, however, that the tremolytic effect of phenobarbital might be directly related to the degree of central sedation. Koller and Royse,[235] using objective measures, found no effect of phenobarbital (90 mg/day) in essential hand tremor in 12 patients. In a double-blind comparison of primidone and phenobarbital, Sasso et al.[245] found primidone superior to both placebo and phenobarbital in reducing tremor in 13 patients. Phenobarbital, at a dosage yielding levels greater than those seen with primidone, was not better than placebo. The effectiveness and role of phenobarbital in ET is controversial; however, the drug may be used in patients who do not respond well to propranolol or primidone. Cabrera-Valdivia et al.[246] reported that phenobarbital was a successful treatment in 2 patients with orthostatic truncal tremor.

BENZODIAZEPINES

Benzodiazepines and other sedative-hypnotic drugs have, for a long time, been used in the treatment of ET, perhaps in the mistaken belief that tremor was due to anxiety. Interestingly, there has been no investigation of the most commonly used drug, diazepam, in the treatment of ET. It is generally thought that these medications possess only limited efficacy, which is probably related to a reduction in tension and anxiety that can cause tremor enhancement.

Several compounds have been investigated. The effect of clonazepam in ET was studied by Thompson et al.,[247] who found that the drug had no effect. Sedation was a frequent side-effect. Clonazepam (1–3 mg/day) is, however, very effective in treating kinetic predominant tremor[90] and orthostatic truncal tremor.[105,107] Huber and Paulson[248] studied alprazolam, a triazole analog of the benzodiazepines, in ET in a double-blind, placebo-controlled study of 24 patients. Significant improvement occurred, but transient mild fatigue or sedation occurred in one-half of patients. The contribution of the sedative or anxiolytic effect of alprazolam to tremor reduction is unknown but may be substantial. Gunal et al.[249] found in a double-blind crossover placebo-controlled study that alprazolam was as effective as propranolol in the treatment of ET. The mean daily dose of alprazolam was 0.75 mg and no troublesome side-effects were reported. They suggested that alprazolam may be an alternative drug in advanced ET patients who do not tolerate primidone or propranolol.[249]

CARBONIC ANHYDRASE INHIBITORS

Muenter et al., in 1991,[250] reported that the carbonic anhydrase inhibitor, methazolamide, was highly effective in ET. They administered methazolamide to 28 ET patients in an open trial. Marked improvement was reported in 12 patients, moderate improvement in 4, mild improvement in 4, and no effect in 8 patients. It was noted that head and voice tremor were particularly improved. The mean maximum daily dose was 203 mg. Adverse reactions, including sedation, nausea, epigastric distress, anorexia, and numbness and paresthesias, were common. The authors suggest that perhaps the doses used were too high and that doses were increased too rapidly. Only 10 patients continued on the drug. Busenbark et al.[251] found that acetazolamide, another carbonic anhydrase, significantly decreased tremor on clinical rating scales, and a higher mean dose appeared to have more of an effect. However, no major change was reported by the patients on their assessment of functional disability, and ratings of motor function showed only modest improvement. Therefore, these investigations did not find the dramatic improvement reported with methazolamide. Head and voice tremor did not appear to be particularly sensitive to acetazolamide. A double-blind placebo-controlled study by Busenbark et al.[252] evaluated the effect of methazolamide in 25 patients with ET. Tremor assessment included patient self-reporting of functional disability, clinical rating of motor tasks and tremor severity, and accelerometric measurements. There was no significant difference between methazolamide and placebo in any of the assessments. Side-effects, paresthesias, sedation, headaches, and gastrointestinal symptoms were common. Only 2 patients elected to remain on the drug after the study. It was concluded that methazolamide has only limited efficacy in the treatment of ET.[252]

GABAPENTIN

Gabapentin is an antiepileptic drug which has been used for the treatment of ET. In an open-label study, gabapentin reduced tremor in 5 patients.[253] Three of the 5 patients chose to remain on gabapentin rather than their previous medication. In another open-label study with 5 patients, an excellent response was reported with gabapentin (mean dose 1020 mg/day).[254] However, Pahwa et al.[255] performed a double-blind, placebo-controlled study of gabapentin and found that it was no more effective than placebo. The authors concluded that gabapentin has limited benefit in ET. However, Gironell et al.[256] performed a randomized, blinded, placebo-controlled comparative trial of gabapentin and propranolol in 16 patients with ET. Gabapentin was given at 400 mg three times a day and propranolol at 40 mg three times a day. Tremor was evaluated with a tremor clinical rating scale, accelerometry, and a self-reported disability scale. At day 15 of treatment, both drugs showed significant and comparable efficacy in reducing tremor from baseline in all outcome measures. The authors concluded that gabapentin may be useful for the treatment of ET. Ondo et al.[257] studied gabapentin in a multiple-dose, double-blind, placebo-controlled trial in 25 ET patients. Two doses were evaluated: 1800 mg/day and 3600 mg/day. Patient global assessments, observed tremor, water pouring, and activities of daily living significantly improved. Accelerometry, spirographs, and investigator global impression did not improve. The results were similar for high and low doses. The authors concluded that gabapentin may be effective in some cases of ET. However, we currently do not use this drug to treat ET in our practice.

OTHER DRUGS

Topiramate is a recently released anticonvulsant drug, which enhances GABA activity and inhibits carbonic anhydrase. Also, topiramate appears to act on voltage-gated sodium and calcium channels. Conner[258] reported that 11 ET patients treated with topiramate in an open-label trial had reduction of both hand and head tremor. A large multicenter industry-sponsored clinical trial is being planned for topiramate.

Mirtazapine is a novel antidepressant that disinhibits serotonergic and noradrenergic neurons by its alpha2-antagonist properties. Pact and Giduz[259] reported 5 patients with PD in which tremor was reduced with mirtazapine in an open-label trial. It was also suggested that this drug might be helpful for ET. However, no blinded clinical trials have yet to be reported.

ET patients are sometimes given antiparkinsonian drugs that are usually discontinued because they are ineffective. Therefore, clinical experience indicates that these drugs have no benefit, although there has been no formal study of L-dopa or anticholinergic treatment in ET. It has been suggested that L-dopa therapy may worsen ET.[260] Amantadine, which possesses both dopaminergic and anticholinergic properties, was reported by Critchley[261] to improve tremor in 26 patients. However, this conclusion was based solely on clinical observations. Manyam,[262] using clinical scoring, found that amantadine (100 mg twice per day) caused improvement in 5 patients, had no effect in 1, and worsened tremor in 2 others. Obeso et al.[263] observed 1 patient who had a dramatic response to amantadine therapy. Koller[264] evaluated 6 patients, using objective techniques, and found that amantadine exacerbated tremor in 3 patients and had no effect in the other 3. It would appear that amantadine is not generally useful in ET, but an occasional patient may respond to the drug.

Caccia and Mangoni,[265] in an open trial study, suggested that clonidine might cause improvement of ET. Clonidine's ability to stimulate central alpha-adrenergic receptors was the proposed mechanism of action. Koller et al.[266] studied the effect of clonidine treatment (average dose 0.4 mg/day) in 10 patients in a double-blind placebo-controlled investigation. Tremor amplitude was quantified by an accelerometer. Tremor was not significantly changed by clonidine therapy. Side-effects (dry mouth, decreased urination, tiredness, and lightheadedness) were common and often dose-limiting. It was concluded that clonidine is not effective treatment for ET. Mai and Olsen[267] reported that the alpha-adrenergic-blocking drug, thymoxamine, given intravenously, significantly suppressed ET in 9 patients. However, when Koller[268] studied in a controlled manner the alpha-adrenergic blocker, phenoxybenzamine, no effect on ET could be demonstrated. There is no evidence that alpha-adrenergic mechanisms are involved in the pathogenesis of ET, and alpha-adrenergic drugs, agonists or antagonists, appear to have no role in the treatment of ET. Morris et al.[269] found the serotonergic precursor tryptophan, given with pyridoxine, was ineffective in ET patients. However, McLeod and White[270] observed "significant improvement" of ET in 2 patients with trazodone (150 mg/day), a serotonin agonist. Improvement was observed only after 3 weeks of treatment. No objective measures were made in these open-label observations. Discontinuation of trazodone in 1 patient was said to be associated with an increase in tremor. The authors suggested that serotonergic neurotransmission may be important in ET, because trazodone stimulates serotonin receptors and blocks reuptake mechanisms. Koller[181] performed a double-blind placebo-controlled investigation of trazodone in 24 patients and found that the drug was ineffective. Likewise, Cleeves and Findley[271] found trazodone ineffective in ET. The selective serotonin receptor type 2 antagonist, ritanserin, was found to reduce parkinsonian tremor but to have no effect in ET.[272] Caccia et al.[273] found that the venous infusion of propranolol and clonidine, but not of urapidil or trazodone, reduced ET in 25 patients whose tremor was recorded by accelerometry. Pharmacological studies suggest no role for serotonergic neurotransmission, even though the inferior olivary nucleus, which may be an important structure in the genesis of ET, receives serotonergic input.

Several of the drugs effective in ET affect central GABA neurotransmission, suggesting a possible involvement of this neurotransmitter. However, Koller and Gupta[180] gave progabide, a GABA agonist (30 mg/kg/day) to 10 patients in a double-blind crossover study and found no effect of the drug on tremor.

Mephenesin, a centrally acting muscle relaxant, was touted to have a limited effect in reducing ET; however, the drug never gained widespread use. Topakias et al.[274] studied the acute effects of two calcium-channel blockers, nifedipine and verapamil, in ET. Nifedipine (10 mg) increased tremor intensity, and verapamil (80 mg) had no effect. However, in 14 patients with ET in a crossover study with nicardipine (1 mg/kg/day) and propranolol (160 mg/day), both drugs improved ET, with a nonsignificantly higher efficacy of propranolol.[275] These results suggest that nicardipine might be efficacious for ET. Curran and Lang[276] studied the effects of flunarizine in 10 patients with moderate-to-severe essential tremor. Tremor was evaluated after 6 weeks of treatment, using patient and physician assessment, as well as blinded video analysis. Only 1 patient had mild subjective transient improvement, and 3 experienced worsening of tremor. No patient elected to remain on treatment. They concluded that flumarizine is ineffective for moderate-to-severe ET and may actually worsen the symptoms in some patients. Biary et al.[277] investigated the effect of flunarizine (10 mg/day) in 17 ET patients in a double-blind placebo-controlled trial. Of patients who completed the study, 13 of 15 showed improvement in both subjective and objective measures. The authors concluded that flunarizine is effective treatment for ET. This drug is, however, not available in North America at this time. Pakkenberg and Pakkenberg[278] found, in an open trial, that the atypical neuroleptic, clozapine, decreased ET in 9 of 12 patients. Tremor reduction may be related to sedation, which was a major side-effect. McCarthy[279] also reported some efficacy of clozapine in ET. In another study[280] the effects of a single dose of 12.5 mg of clozapine and placebo were reported in a randomized double-blind, crossover study in 15 drug-resistant patients with ET. Tremor was effectively reduced in 13 of 15 patients. Sedation was the only side-effect reported which disappeared after 6–7 weeks of treatment, whereas the reduction of tremor persisted. However, this drug is associated with the rare occurrence of agranulocytosis which may be associated with fetal infections. Therefore, weekly blood counts are mandatory during the use of clozapine, which represents a major limitation in its use. McDowell[281] reported 2 patients who had suppression of their tremor with glutethimide at doses of 1000–4000 mg/day; 1 patient had taken the drug for 14 years without side-effects. Because of its abuse potential this drug is not in the market in the US.

Xanthine derivatives, such as theophylline, can induce tremor or appear to worsen ET in some patients. However, Mally and Stone[282] administered theophylline to 20 ET patients in a double-blind crossover study. Tremor was said to improve after 4 weeks of treatment. It was suggested that enhancement of GABA sensitivity may be responsible for the therapeutic effect.

BOTULINUM TOXIN INJECTION

Recently, a novel therapeutic approach to the treatment of ET has been reported, using botulinum toxin A intramuscular injections.[283] Botulinum toxin causes some degree of muscle paresis by acting at peripheral nerve endings to block the release of acetylcholine. This agent has been shown to be effective in a variety of focal dystonias and has been suggested as the treatment of choice in these disorders.[283] Jankovic and Schwartz[284] found that injection of this chemical successfully reduced tremor in 67 percent of patients in an open-label trial of botulinum toxin in various tremor disorders. The duration of maximum response was 10.5 weeks. Hand weakness was the most common adverse reaction. In another open-label study, Trosch and Pullman[285] found botulinum toxin subjectively but not objectively improved ET in 14 patients. These initial encouraging results were assessed with a double-blind placebo-controlled study. Brin et al.[286] evaluated 133 ET patients randomized to low-dose (50 U) or high-dose (100 U) botulinum toxin type A or vehicle placebo treatment. Injections were made into the wrist flexors and extensors. Adverse reactions consisted mainly of dose-dependent hand weakness. The authors concluded that botulinum toxin type A injections for ET of the hands resulted in significant improvement of postural, but not kinetic, hand tremors resulting in limited functional efficacy, and that hand weakness was a significant side-effect of treatment at the doses employed. We currently do not use neurotoxin injections for ET of the hand.

Pharmacological treatment of essential head and voice tremor is usually unsuccessful. However, botulinum toxin injection has some efficacy for both head and voice tremor.[287–291] It is estimated that approximately 50 percent of patients with head tremor will respond favorably.[287] Dysphagia and respiratory symptoms can occur as troublesome adverse reactions. The rare conditions of palatal tremor and hereditary chin tremor also respond to botulinum toxin treatment.[292,293] Toxin therapy appears to be the treatment of choice for essential head and voice tremor.

THALAMOTOMY

Stereotaxic thalamotomy is an effective procedure in the treatment of parkinsonian, cerebellar, and essential tremors.[294–300] The technical aspects of the procedure have improved greatly in the last decade. Advances in the neurophysiological confirmation of the site of the lesion now allow for accurate placement. The site of the lesion selected is the ventral anterior or the ventral intermediate (Vim) nucleus of the thalamus. Stereotaxic thalamotomy can be performed with the use of mild sedation and local anesthesia. The neurological status of the patients can, therefore, be monitored.

Stereotaxic coordinates are generated by use of CT head-scanning and computerized programs. A microelectrode with a recording tip is lowered into the brain, and the neuronal response further defines the anatomic site for the lesion. Heating of the electrode tip creates a small lesion. The reported results of thalamotomy in ET have been favorable. Bertrand[294] stated that "the results are most satisfactory and one may expect a marked relief of tremor in 90 percent of cases, with a total relief in a high percentage of these." Ohye et al.[296] reported 15 patients successfully treated with small lesions in the Vim nucleus. No late relapse was noted. Andrew[297] treated 10 patients with thalamotomy. In 3 cases the tremor was improved, and in 5 patients there was almost total suppression of tremor. Functional abilities were said to be markedly improved in these patients. One patient had no change after the operation, and another patient suffered hemiplegia as a complication of the procedure. Stereotaxic thalamotomy currently has a mortality rate of less than 0.3 percent, mostly related to postoperative complications. Temporary intellectual deficits and transitory hemiparesis may occur. A lasting weakness is unusual. Other uncommon adverse reactions include seizures, involuntary movements, and cerebellar signs. A transient deterioration of speech may be seen occasionally after unilateral thalamotomy that will return to normal after several weeks. Bilateral thalamotomy is associated with much more serious complications. In particular, a severe persistent dysarthria occurs. Permanent mental changes may also occur. Therefore, bilateral operations can be recommended only with reservation.

There is only minimal information regarding the long-term effects of thalamotomy for the treatment of ET. Mohadjer et al.[34] reported follow-up from a group of 104 ET patients who were operated on between 1964 and 1984. Sixty-five patients were re-examined who had an average follow-up period of 8.6 years. Eighty percent were found to have evidence of a successful operation, with 69 percent having complete or substantial reduction of tremor, and 11.9 percent having moderate improvement. Also, 11.9 percent of patients showed deterioration on the operated side, compared to 34 percent who showed deterioration on the unoperated side.

Thalamotomy appears in the past to have been a neglected therapeutic option. It should be reserved for those with (1) severe unilateral or asymmetrical tremor, (2) marked functional disability, and (3) a tremor that is unresponsive to maximally tolerated doses of propranolol, primidone, and clonazepam.

THALAMIC STIMULATION

DEEP BRAIN STIMULATION (DBS)

DBS of the thalamus was initially pursued by Benabid et al. colleagues in France because of the high incidence of dysarthia associated with bilateral thalamotomies.[299,301–302] This approach consists of an implanted electrode in the brain connected to a battery source, an implantable pulse generator. A destructive lesion is not made and the amount of stimulus (strength, pulse width, and frequency) can be programmed to increase efficacy or reduce adverse reactions. DBS of the thalamus for the treatment of ET is effective, with over 90 percent of patients having a satisfactory result (Table 27-2).[303–312] The benefit occurs exclusively on the side of the body contralateral to the stimulation, and the effect against tremor in the leg, which is rarely symptomatic, may not be significant. It has been estimated that as many as 50 percent of patients have total abolition of tremor and a highly significant improvement on quality of life scales.[313] This effect clearly cannot be achieved with current pharmacologic therapy. Head tremors also respond to unilateral thalamic DBS.[314] An analysis of 38 patients with head tremor followed for 12 months postoperatively with double-blind evaluation of the effect of stimulation at 3 months in 24 patients showed that stimulation induced a significant reduction in head tremor scores. Voice tremor can also be improved by thalamic DBS but by itself is not considered an indication for surgery.[315,316] Most patients with ET experience a dramatic improvement in their functional disabilities with DBS. Activities such as handwriting, drinking liquids, and eating often return to almost normal function. Many patients return to enjoying activities they had previously abandoned, such as playing golf or other sports. Therefore, there is a high degree of patient satisfaction.

Several studies have demonstrated the long-term efficacy of thalamic DBS in ET. One study showed that there was no loss of effect after 1 year.[311] Similarly, the experience in a European multicenter study found that the effectiveness was maintained over the first several years.[312] A study with follow-up of 40 months showed continued efficacy.[317] However, the long-term (5–10 years) efficacy of thalamic DBS is not well established.

In a small number of patients in a large study,[311] intraoperative suppression of tremor could not be achieved even though it was believed that the electrode was in the Vim nucleus. Therefore, implantation of the permanent stimulation electrodes was not performed. One explanation is that perhaps, in a small minority of patients, the Vim nucleus is not involved in tremor genesis or, more likely, that the recognition of Vim was erroneous. For stereotaxic Vim thalamotomy and thalamic stimulation, it is estimated that there is a 1–2 percent chance of cerebral hemorrhage at the time of operation. In a multicenter study,[312] which included 59 patients with both PD and ET, 1 patient suffered a subdural hematoma and another a cerebral hemorrhage. It appears that the electrode even when implanted for a long time is not associated with any abnormal histologic reaction at the site of the implant.[317]

Adverse reactions related to stimulation are mild and are easily altered by adjusting stimulus parameters. The majority of patients experience a transient paresthesia of the hand that lasts for several seconds when the device is turned on.[311] Other more persistent side-effects are uncommon and include headache disequilibrium, mild paresis, gait disturbances, and dysarthria. These side-effects can usually be treated by adjusting stimulus parameters. However, some patients must make a choice between better control of the tremor or reduction in the side-effects. Many patients prefer to have good control of their tremor and elect to tolerate mild adverse reactions.

Device complications are not uncommon and may necessitate additional surgical operations. Koller et al.[318] reported that device complications were common in 25 ET patients followed for 40 months. These complications frequently required repeated surgical procedures. Improvement in methodology of surgery and devices could reduce these troublesome complications. Also patients should be warned of the possibility of additional surgery procedures before DBS is initiated.

Schuurman et al.[319] compared the effect of DBS of the thalamus to thalamotomy for patients with severe tremor, including 13 patients with ET. They found that functional status improved more in the DBS-treated group, although both therapies were equally effective. Thalamotomies are now only rarely performed, as we prefer DBS as the surgical treatment of choice.

It is concluded that DBS of the Vim nucleus of the thalamus is a safe and effective means of treating disabling ET that is not responsive to medications. However, patients must understand and be willing to accept a 1–2 percent risk of cerebral bleeding at the time of surgery.

GAMMA-KNIFE THALAMOTOMY

The gamma-knife or linear accelerator procedure allows for radiosurgery to be performed noninvasively and does not require general anesthesia.[320] There are few preoperative issues and patients have minimal immediate postoperative problems. However, the effect of surgery is delayed weeks to months as the gamma-knife included lesions develop. This technique has been criticized as the lesion cannot be reliably placed and large lesions lead to severe adverse reactions.[321] However, gamma-knife surgery is sometimes recommended to those patients who are too ill to undergo conventional neurosurgical procedures. Several reports suggest that gamma-knife surgery has efficacy for ET. Niranjan et al.[322] note that 6 of 8 patients had complete relief of their tremors. No persistent adverse reactions were reported. Similarly, Young[323] reported the effects of gamma-knife thalamotomy in 52 ET patients and found that 92 percent of patients were fully or nearly free from tremor after the procedure. Complications were reported as minimal. Nonetheless, we cannot, at this time, recommend gamma-knife Vim thalamotomy for ET because of the lack of precise lesion placement and the possibility of long-term complications.

BEHAVIORAL THERAPY

A variety of behavioral techniques, including psychotherapy, biofeedback, and hypnosis, have been used in the treatment of movement disorders. Any benefit from these procedures has been minimal and short-lived. There is one report of the beneficial effect of psychotherapy in ET.[324] The reported improvement of symptoms was thought to be a result of "mental stabilization" and relaxation of muscle tension.

DRUGS OF CHOICE

Propranolol and other beta-adrenergic blockers and primidone are currently the only drugs that have been clearly shown to be effective in suppressing ET. It is unclear which should be the drug of first choice. As many as 20 percent of patients will suffer side-effects for several days after the first dose of primidone. When the patient is warned of these potential adverse reactions and encouraged to continue to take the drug, only a minority will discontinue primidone. Side-effects with chronic therapy are uncommon with primidone but are much more of a concern with propranolol. Many elderly patients cannot take beta-adrenergic blockers. It appears that marked tremor reduction is more often achieved with primidone than with propranolol. Some patients may require both propranolol and primidone therapy.

We recommend the following treatment schedule:

1. Start with primidone, 50 mg at nighttime. (Warn patient of possible side-effects but recommend continuation of drug even when side-effects occur.)
2. Increase primidone to 125 mg at nighttime when necessary.
3. Increase primidone to 250 mg at nighttime when necessary.
4. Add or switch to propranolol-LA, 80 mg, in the morning.
5. Increase propranolol-LA to 160 mg in the morning, when necessary.
6. Increase propranolol-LA to 240 mg when necessary.
7. Increase propranolol-LA to 320 mg in the morning when necessary.
8. When the patient has no response to either primidone or propranolol, alprazolam or clonazepam should be tried.
9. Lastly, if the patient has severe tremor and is willing to undertake the surgical risk, DBS of the thalamus should be performed.

Hopefully, future research will find new therapeutic agents for those patients not responding to currently used drugs.

Summary

ET is the most common movement disorder, occurring most frequently in individuals over 40 years of age. A positive family history for tremor is obtained in many cases. The affliction usually begins as a postural tremor in the hands, but may later involve the head and other body parts. Typically, tremor amplitude increases, and frequency decreases with age. Disability results from impairment of fine motor skills or social withdrawal. The occurrence of tremor resembling ET in other neurological disorders may lead to misdiagnosis and clouding of nosological classification. The pathophysiological basis of ET is uncertain but is thought to be central in origin. Abnormal oscillation of a CNS pacemaker (presumably within the cerebellar-brainstem circuitry) has been hypothesized. Beta-adrenergic blocking agents and primidone are medications with proven efficacy for the treatment of ET. DBS of the thalamus is highly effective in controlling ET.

References

1. Findley LJ, Koller WC: Essential tremor: A review. *Neurology* 37:1194–1197, 1987.
2. Hubble JP, Busenbark KL, Koller WC: Essential tremor. *Clin Neuropharmacol* 12:453–482, 1989.
3. Elble R, Koller WC: *Tremor.* Baltimore: Johns Hopkins University Press, 1990.
4. Koller WC, Hubble J, Busenbark K: Essential tremor, in Calne DB (ed): *Neurodegenerative Disease.* Philadelphia: WB Saunders, 1994, pp 717–742.
5. Bain PG, Findley LJ, Thompson PD, et al: A study of hereditary essential tremor. *Brain* 117:805–824, 1994.
6. Koller WC, Deuschl G: Essential tremor. *Neurology* 54(suppl 4): S1–S45, 2000.
7. Tremor: Basic mechanism and clinical aspects. *Mov Disord* 13(suppl 3):1–149.
8. Critchley M: Observations on essential (heredofamilial) tremor. *Brain* 72:113–139, 1949.
9. Sider D, McVaugh M: Galen on tremor, palpitation, spasm, and rigor. *Trans Stud Coll Physicians Phila* 1:183–210, 1979.
10. Parkinson J: *An Essay on the Shaking Palsy.* London: Whittingham & Rowland, 1817.
11. Charcot JM: *Policlinique du Mardi: Lecons de Mardi.* Paris: 24 Juillet, 1888, pp 448–451.
12. Charcot JM: Clinical lectures on disease of the nervous system, vol III, lecture XV, translated by Thomas Savill. *The New Sydenham Society (Lond)* 128:183–197, 1889.
13. Larsen TA, Calne DB: Essential tremor. *Clin Neuropharmacol* 6:185–206, 1983.
14. Dana CL: Hereditary tremor, a hitherto undescribed form of motor neurosis. *Am J Med Sci* 94:386–393, 1887.
15. Pintus G: Sul tippo "macrobioticus multiparus" del tremor essenziale. *Riv Patol Nerv Ment* 51:114–124, 1938.
16. Larsson T, Sjögren T: Essential tremor. A clinical and genetic population study. *Acta Psychiatr Neurol Scand* 36(suppl 144): 1–176, 1960.
17. Flatau J: Le tremblement essentiel héréditaire. *Rev Neurol* 17:417, 1909 (abstract).
18. Raymond F: Le tremblement essentiel héréditaire. *Rev Neurol* 17:416–417, 1909 (abstract).
19. Katzenstein E: Uber familiaren Tremor. *Arch Suisses Neurol Psychiatry* 61:380–381, 1948.
20. Rautakorpi I: Essential Tremor: An Epidemiological, Clinical, and Genetic Study. Dissertation, Turku, Finland, 1978.
21. Duvoisin RC, Gearing FR, Schweitzer MD, Yahr MD: A family study of parkinsonism, in Barbeau A, Brunette JR (eds): *Progress in Neurogenetics.* Amsterdam: Excerpta Medica, 1969, pp 492–496.

22. McDowell FH, Lee JE, Sweet RD: Extrapyramidal disease, in Baker AB, Baker LH (eds): *Clinical Neurology*. Philadelphia: Harper & Row, 1938, pp 53–54.

23. Rajput AH, Offord KP, Beard CM, Kurland LT: Essential tremor in Rochester, Minnesota: A 45-year study. *J Neurol Neurosurg Psychiatry* 47:466–470, 1984.

24. Haerer AF, Anderson DW, Schoenberg BS: Prevalence of essential tremor: Results from the Copiah County study. *Arch Neurol* 39:750–751, 1982.

25. Rautakorpi I, Takala J, Marttila RJ, et al: Essential tremor in a Finnish population. *Acta Neurol Scand* 66:58–67, 1982.

26. Hornabrook RW, Nagurney JT: Essential tremor in Papua New Guinea. *Brain* 99:659–672, 1976.

27. Moretti G, Calzetti S, Quartucci G, et al: Epidemiological study on tremor in the aged. *Minerva Med* 74:1701–1705, 1983.

28. Aiyesiloju AB, Osuntodum BO, Bademosi O, Adeuja AO: Hereditary neurodegenerative disorders in Nigerian Africans. *Neurology* 34:361–362, 1984.

29. Salemi G, Savettieri G, Rocca WA, et al: Prevalence of essential tremor: A door-to-door survey in Terrasini, Sicily. Sicilian Neuro-Epidemiologic Study Group. *Neurology* 44:61–64, 1994.

30. Koller WC: Diagnosis and treatment of tremor. *Neurol Clin* 2:499–514, 1984.

31. Rautakorpi I, Marttilla RJ, Rinne UK: Epidemiology of essential tremor, in Findley LJ, Capildeo R (eds): *Movement Disorders: Tremor*. London: Macmillan, 1984, pp 211–218.

32. Bharucha NE, Bharucha EP, Bharuch AE, et al: Prevalence of essential tremor in the Parsi community of Bombay, India. *Arch Neurol* 45:907–908, 1988.

33. Rajput AH, Offord KP, Kurland LT: Epidemiologic survey of essential tremor in Rochester, MN. *Neurology* 32:A128, 1982.

34. Mohadjer M, Goerke H, Milios E, et al: Long-term results of stereotaxy in the treatment of essential tremor. *Stereotact Funct Neurosurg* 54/55:125–129, 1990.

35. Moghal S, Rajput AH, D'Arcy C, Rajput R: Prevalence of movement disorders in elderly community residents. *Neuroepidemiology* 13:175–178, 1994.

36. Louis ED, Ford B, Frucht S, et al: Risk of tremor and impairment from tremor in relatives of patients with essential tremor: A community based family study. *Ann Neurol* 49:761–769, 2001.

37. Louis ED, Ford B, Frucht S, Ottman R: *Arch Neurol* 58:1584–1589, 2001.

38. Marshall J: Observations on essential tremor. *J Neurol Neurosurg Psychiatry* 25:122–125, 1962.

39. Jager BV, King T: Hereditary tremor. *Arch Intern Med* 95:788–793, 1955.

40. Herskovits E, Figueroa E, Mangone C: Hereditary essential tremor in Buenos Aires (Argentina). *Arq Neuropsiquiatr* 46:238–247, 1988.

41. Buckley P: Familial tremor. *Proc R Soc Med* 31:297, 1938.

42. Busenbark K, Barnes P, Lyons K, et al: Accuracy of reported family history of essential tremor. *Neurology* (in press).

43. Kaneko K, Igarashi S, Miyatake T, Tsuiji S: "Essential tremor" and CAG repeats in the androgen receptor gene. *Neurology* 43:1618–1619, 1993.

44. Conway D, Bain PG, Warner TT, et al: Linkage analysis with chromosome 9 markers in hereditary essential tremor. *Mov Disord* 8:374–376, 1993.

45. Gulcher JR, Johnson P, Kong A, et al: Mapping of a family with essential tremor gene, FET1, to chromosome 3q13. *Nat Genet* 17:84–87, 1997.

46. Higgins JJ, Pho LT, Nee LE: A gene (ETM) for essential tremor maps to chromosome 2p22-p25. *Mov Disord* 12:859–869, 1997.

47. Farrer M, Gwinn-Hardy K, Muenter M, et al: A chromosome 4p haplotype segregating with Parkinson's disease and postural tremor. *Hum Mol Genet* 8:81–85, 1999.

48. Kovach MJ, Ruiz J, Kimonis K, et al: Genetic heterogeneity in autosomal dominant essential tremor. *Genet Med* 3:197–199, 2001.

49. Tan EK, Matsurra T, Nagamitsu S, et al: *Neurology* 54:1195–1198, 2000.

50. Tanner CM, Goldman SM, Lyons, KE, et al: Essential tremor in twins. An assessment of genetic vs. environmental determinants of etiology. *Neurology* 57:1389–1391, 2001.

51. Davis CH, Kunkle EC: Benign essential (heredofamilial) tremor. *Arch Intern Med* 87:808–816, 1951.

52. Singer C, Sanchez-Ramos J, Weiner WJ: Gait abnormality in essential tremor. *Mov Disord* 9:193–196, 1994.

53. Stolze H, Petersen G, Raethjen J, et al: The gait disorder of advanced essential tremor. *Brain* 124:2278–2286, 2001.

54. Marsden CD, Obeso J, Rothwell JC: Benign essential tremor is not a single entity, in Yahr MD (ed): *Current Concepts in Parkinson's Disease*. Amsterdam: Excerpta Medica, 1983, pp 31–46.

55. Louis ED, Ford B, Wendt KJ, Cameron G: Clinical characteristics of essential tremor: Data from a community-based study. *Mov Disord* 13:803–808, 1998.

56. Schneier FR, Barnes LF, Albert SM, Louis ED: Characteristics of social phobia among persons with essential tremor. *J Clin Psychiatry* 62:367–372, 2001.

57. Hallett M: Differential diagnosis of tremor, in Vinken PJ, Bruyn GW, Klawans HL (eds): *Handbook of Clinical Neurology*. Amsterdam: Elsevier, 1989, pp 583–595.

58. Jankovic J, Fahn S: Physiologic and pathologic tremors: Diagnosis, mechanism and management. *Ann Intern Med* 93:460–465, 1980.

59. Elble RJ: Physiologic and essential tremor. *Neurology* 36:225–231, 1986.

60. Sanes JN, Hallet M: Limb positioning and magnitude of essential tremor and other pathological tremors. *Mov Disord* 5:304–309, 1990.

61. Masuhr F, Wissel J, Muller J, et al: Quantification of sensory trick impact on tremor amplitude and frequency in 60 patients with head tremor. *Mov Disord* 15:960–964, 2000.

62. Gasparini M, Bonifati V, Fabrizio E, et al: Frontal lobe dysfunction in essential tremor. *J Neurol* 248:399–402, 2001.

63. Lombardi WJ, Woolston DJ, Toberts JW, Gross RE: Cognitive deficits in patients with essential tremor. *Neurology* 57:785–790, 2001.

64. Troster AI, Woods SP, Fields JA, et al: Neuropsychological deficits in essential tremor: An expression of cerebello-thalamo-cortical pathophysiology. *Eur J Neurol* (in press).

65. Findley LF, Gresty MA: Tremor. *Br J Hosp Med* 26:16–32, 1981.

66. Wade P, Gresty MA, Findley LJ: A normative study of postural tremor of the hand. *Arch Neurol* 39:358–362, 1982.

67. Deuschl G, Laucking CH, Schenk E: Essential tremor: Electrophysiological and pharmacological evidence for a subdivision. *J Neurol Neurosurg Psychiatry* 50:1435–1441, 1987.

68. Koller WC, Busenbark KL, Dubinsky R, Hubble J: Classification of essential tremor. *Clin Neuropharmacol* 15:81–88, 1992.

69. Wasielewski PG, Burns JM, Koller WC: Pharmacologic treatment of tremor. *Mov Disord* 13(suppl 3):90–100, 1998.

70. Koller WC, Busenbark K, Miner K: The relationship of essential tremor to other movement disorders: Report on 678 patients. Essential Tremor Study Group. *Ann Neurol* 35:717–723, 1994.

71. Borges V, Ferraz HB, de Andrade LA: Essential tremor: Clinical characterization in a sample of 176 patients. *Arq Neuropsiquiatr* 52:161–165, 1994.

72. Longe AC: Essential tremor in Nigerians: A prospective study of 35 cases. *East Afr Med J* 62:672–676, 1985.

73. Massey EW, Paulson GW: Essential vocal tremor: Clinical characteristics and response to therapy. *South Med J* 78:316–317, 1985.

74. Vanesse M, Bedard P, Andermann F: Shuddering attacks in children: An early clinical manifestation of essential tremor. *Neurology* 26:1027–1030, 1976.

75. Sutherland JM, Edwards VE, Eadie MJ: Essential (hereditary or senile) tremor. *Med J Aust* 2:44–47, 1975.

76. Biary N, Koller W: Handedness and essential tremor. *Arch Neurol* 42:1082–1083, 1985.

77. Biary N, Cleeves L, Findley L, Koller W: Post-traumatic tremor. *Neurology* 39:103–106, 1989.

78. Wake A, Takahashi Y, Onishi T, et al: Treatment of essential tremor through behaviour therapy: Use of Jacobson's progressive relaxation method. *Jpn J Psychiatry Neurol* 76:509–517, 1974.

79. Growdon JH, Shahani BT, Young RR: The effect of alcohol on essential tremor. *Neurology* 28:259–262, 1975.

80. Boecker H, Wills AJ, Ceballos-Baumann A, et al: The effect of ethanol on alcohol-responsive essential tremor: A positron emission tomography study. *Ann Neurol* 39:650–658, 1996.

81. Rajput AH, Jamieson H, Hirsh S, Quraishi A: Relative efficacy of alcohol and propranolol in action tremor. *Can J Neurol Sci* 2:31–35, 1975.

82. Koller W, Cone S, Herbster G: Caffeine and tremor. *Neurology* 37:169–172, 1987.

83. Cooper IS: Heredofamilial tremor abolition by chemothalamectomy. *Arch Neurol* 7:129–131, 1962.

84. Busenbark KL, Nash J, Nash S, et al: Is essential tremor benign? *Neurology* 41:1982–1983, 1991.

85. George MS, Lydiard RB: Social phobia secondary to physical disability: A review of benign essential tremor (BET) and stuttering. *Psychosomatics* 35:520–523, 1994.

86. Louis ED, Barnes L, Albert SM, et al: Correlates of functional disability in essential tremor. *Mov Disord* 16:914–920, 2001.

87. Louis ED, Pullman SL: Comparison of clinical vs. electrophysiological methods of diagnosing of essential tremor. *Mov Disord* 16:668–673, 2001.

88. Findley LJ, Koller WC, De Witt P, et al: Classification and definition of tremor. Cited by Findley LJ, in Lord Walton of Detchant (ed): *Indications for and Clinical Implications of Botulinum Toxin Therapy.* London: Royal Society of Medicine, 1993, pp 22–23.

89. Koller WC, Glatt S, Biary N, Rubino FA: Essential tremor variants: Effect of treatment. *Clin Neuropharmacol* 10:342–350, 1987.

90. Biary N, Koller WC: Kinetic predominant tremor: Effect of clonazepam. *Neurology* 37:471–474, 1987.

91. Koller WC, Rubino FA: Combined resting-postural tremor. *Arch Neurol* 42:683–684, 1985.

92. Bain PG, Findley LJ: Familial paroxysmal tremor: An essential tremor variant [letter]. *J Neurol Neurosurg Psychiatry* 57:1019, 1994.

93. Garcia-Albea E, Jimenez-Jimenez FJ, Ayuso-Peralta L, et al: "Familial paroxysmal tremor": An essential tremor variant? [letter]. *J Neurol Neurosurg Psychiatry* 56:1329, 1993.

94. Klawans HL, Glantz R, Tanner CM, Goetz CG: Primary writing tremor: Selective action tremor. *Neurology* 32:203–206, 1982.

95. Rothwell JC, Traub MM, Marsden CD: Primary writing tremor. *J Neurol Neurosurg Psychiatry* 42:1106–1114, 1979.

96. Ravits J, Hallet M, Baker M, Wilkins D: Primary writing tremor and myoclonic writer's cramp. *Neurology* 35:1387–1391, 1985.

97. Sheehy MP, Marsden CD: Writers' cramp: A focal dystonia. *Brain* 105:461–480, 1982.

98. Cohen LG, Hallett M, Sudarsky L: A single family with writer's cramp, essential tremor, and primary writing tremor. *Mov Disord* 2:109–116, 1987.

99. Elble RJ, Moody C, Higgins C: Primary writing tremor: A form of focal dystonia. *Mov Disord* 5:118–126, 1990.

100. Grossman BJ: Trembling of the chin: An inheritable dominant character. *Pediatrics* 19:453–455, 1957.

101. Lawrence BM, Matthews W, Diggle JA: Hereditary quivering of the chin. *Arch Dis Child* 43:249–254, 1968.

102. Brown JR, Simonson J: Organic voice tremor. *Neurology* 17:520–527, 1967.

103. Hachinski VC, Thomsen IV, Buch NH: The nature of primary vocal tremor. *Can J Neurol Sci* 2:195–197, 1975.

104. Riveat J, Marsden CD: Trunk and head tremor as isolated manifestations of dystonia. *Mov Disord* 5:60–65, 1990.

105. Heilman KM: Orthostatic tremor. *Arch Neurol* 4:880–881, 1984.

106. Wee AS, Subramony SH, Currier RD: Orthostatic tremor: A variant of essential tremor. *Neurology* 36:1241–1245, 1986.

107. Pape SM, Gershanik OS: Orthostatic tremor: An essential tremor variant. *Mov Disord* 3:97–108, 1988.

108. Gabellini AS, Martinelli P, Gulli MR, et al: Orthostatic tremor: Essential and symptomatic cases. *Acta Neurol Scand* 81:111–112, 1990.

109. McManis PG, Sharbrough FW: Orthostatic tremor: Clinical and electrophysiologic characteristics. *Muscle Nerve* 16:1254–1260, 1993.

110. Thompson RD, Rothwell JC, Day BL, et al: The physiology of orthostatic truncal tremor. *Arch Neurol* 43:584–587, 1986.

111. Walker FO, McCormick CM, Hunt VP: Isometric features of orthostatic tremor: An electromyographic analysis. *Muscle Nerve* 13:918–922, 1990.

112. Uncini A, Onofrj M, Basciani M, et al: Orthostatic tremor: Report of 2 cases and an electrophysiological study. *Acta Neurol Scand* 79:119–122, 1989.

113. Lewitt P: Orthostatic tremor: The phenomenon of "paradoxical clonus". *Arch Neurol* 47:501, 1990.

114. Martinelli P, Gabellini AS, Gulli MR, Lugaresi E: Different clinical features of essential tremor: A 200 patient study. *Acta Neurol Scand* 75:106–111, 1987.

115. Newman RP, Lewitt PA, Jaffe M, et al: Motor function in the normal aging population: Treatment with l-dopa. *Neurology* 35:571–573, 1985.

116. McGeer PL, McGeer EG, Siyuki JS: Aging and extrapyramidal function. *Arch Neurol* 34:33–35, 1977.

117. Cleeves L, Findley L, Koller WC: Lack of association between essential tremor and Parkinson's disease. *Ann Neurol* 24:23–26, 1988.

118. Gowers WR: *A Manual of Diseases of the Nervous System.* Philadelphia: P Blakiston, 1888, pp 995–1013.

119. Marttilla RJ, Rinne UK: Arteriosclerosis, heredity and some previous infections in the etiology of Parkinson's disease: A case control study. *Clin Neurol Neurosurg* 79:45–56, 1976.

120. Marttilla RJ, Rautakorpi I, Rinne UK: The relation of essential tremor to Parkinson's disease. *J Neurol Neurosurg Psychiatry* 47:734–735, 1984.

121. Barbeau A, Pourcher E: New data on the genetics of Parkinson's disease. *Can J Neurol Sci* 9:53–60, 1982.

122. Roy M, Boyer L, Barbeau A: A prospective study of 50 cases of familial Parkinson's disease. *Can J Neurol Sci* 10:34–42, 1983.

123. Geraghty JJ, Jankovic J, Zetusky WJ: Association between essential tremor and Parkinson's disease. *Ann Neurol* 17:329–333, 1985.

124. Lou JS, Jankovic J: Essential tremor: Clinical correlates in 350 patients. *Neurology* 41:234–238, 1991.

125. Lang AE, Marsden CD, Findley LJ, et al: Clinical correlates of essential tremor. *Neurology* (in press).

126. Lang AE, Kierans C, Blair RDG: Family history of tremor in Parkinson's disease compared with those of controls and patients with idiopathic dystonia. *Adv Neurol* 45:313–316, 1986.

127. Marttilla RJ, Rinne UK: Parkinson's disease and essential tremor in families of patients with early-onset Parkinson's disease. *J Neurol Neurosurg Psychiatry* 51:429–431, 1988.

128. Montgomery EB, Baker KB, Lyons KE, Koller WC: Motor initiation and execution in essential tremor and Parkinson's disease. *Mov Disord* 15:511–515, 2000.

129. Schwartz M, Badarny S, Gofman S, Hocherman S: Visuomotor performance in patients with essential tremor. *Mov Disord* 14:988–993, 1999.

130. Salisachs P, Findley LJ: Problems in the differential diagnosis of essential tremor, in Findley LJ, Capildeo R (eds): *Movement Disorders: Tremor*. London: Macmillan, 1984, pp 219–224.

131. Rajput AH, Rozdilsky B, Ang L, Rajput A: Significance of parkinsonian manifestations in essential tremor. *Can J Neurol Sci* 20:114–117, 1993.

132. Pahwa R, Koller WC: Is there a relationship between Parkinson's disease and essential tremor? *Clin Neuropharmacol* 16:30–35, 1993.

133. Rajput AH, Rozdilsky B, Ang L, Rajput A: Clinicopathological observations in essential tremor: Report of 6 cases. *Neurology* 41:1422–1424, 1991.

134. Brooks DJ: Detection of preclinical Parkinson's disease with PET. *Neurology* 41(suppl 2):24–28, 1991.

135. Busenbark K, Huber SJ, Greer G, et al: Olfactory function in essential tremor. *Neurology* 42:1631–1632, 1992.

136. Yanagisawa N, Goto A, Narabagashi H: Familial dystonia musculorum deformans and tremor. *J Neurol Sci* 16:125–136, 1971.

137. Johnson W, Schwartz G, Barbeau A: Studies on dystonia musculorum deformans. *Arch Neurol* 7:301–313, 1962.

138. Baxter DW, Lal S: Essential tremor and dystonia syndromes. *Adv Neurol* 24:373–377, 1979.

139. Couch JR: Dystonia and tremor in spasmodic torticollis. *Adv Neurol* 14:245–258, 1976.

140. Duane DD: Spasmodic torticollis. *Adv Neurol* 49:135–150, 1988.

141. Dubinsky RM, Gray CS, Koller WC: Essential tremor and dystonia. *Neurology* 43:2382–2384, 1993.

142. Yanagisawa N, Goto A: Dystonia musculoram deformans: Analysis with electromyography. *J Neurol Sci* 13:39–65, 1971.

143. Rosenbaum F, Jankovic J: Focal task-specific tremor and dystonia: Categorization of occupational movement disorders. *Neurology* 38:522–527, 1988.

144. Roussy G, Lévy G: Sept cas d'une maladie familiale particuliere: Troubles de la march, pieds bots et areflexie tendineuse generalisée avec acessoirement maladresse des mains. *Rev Neurol (Paris)* 2:427–450, 1926.

145. Said G, Bathien N, Cesar P: Peripheral neuropathies and tremor. *Neurology* 32:480–485, 1982.

146. Thomas PK, Lascelles RG, Hallpike JF, Hewer RL: Recurrent and chronic relapsing Guillain-Barré polyneuritis. *Brain* 92:589–606, 1969.

147. Dalakas MC, Teravainen H, Engel WK: Tremor as a feature of chronic relapsing and dysgammaglobulinemic polyneuropathies: Incidence and management. *Arch Neurol* 41:711–714, 1984.

148. Delwaide PJ, Schoenen J: Non-hypertrophic familial neuropathy associated with intention tremor: A variety of Charcot-Marie-Tooth disease? *J Neurol Sci* 27:59–69, 1976.

149. Barbieri F, Filla A, Ragno M, et al: Evidence that Charcot-Marie-Tooth disease with tremor coincides with the Roussy-Lévy syndrome. *Can J Neurol Sci* 11:534–540, 1984.

150. Salisachs P: Charcot-Marie-Tooth disease associated with "essential tremor": Report of 7 cases and a review of the literature. *J Neurol Sci* 28:17–40, 1976.

151. Shahani BT, Young RR, Adams RD: Neuropathic tremor. *Electroencephalogr Clin Neurophysiol* 34:800, 1973.

152. Mendell JR, Sahenk Z, Whitaker JN, et al: Polyneuropathy and IgM monoclonal gammopathy: Studies on the pathogenic role of anti-myelin-associated glycoprotein antibody. *Ann Neurol* 17:243–254, 1985.

153. Adams RD, Shahani BT, Young RR: Tremor in association with polyneuropathy. *Trans Am Neurol Assoc* 97:44–48, 1972.

154. Baughman FA: Klinefelter's syndrome and essential tremor. *Lancet* ii:545, 1969.

155. Pittman CS, Finley WH, Finley SC: Klinefelter's syndrome and essential tremor. *Lancet* ii:749, 1969.

156. Lee RG, Stein RB: Resetting of tremor by mechanical perturbations: A comparison of essential tremor and parkinsonian tremor. *Ann Neurol* 10:523–531, 1981.

157. Elble RJ, Higgens C, Moody CJ: Stretch reflex oscillations and essential tremor. *J Neurol Neurosurg Psychiatry* 50:691–698, 1987.

158. Britton TC, Thompson PD, Day BL, et al: "Resetting" of postural tremors at the wrist with mechanical stretches in Parkinson's disease, essential tremor and normal subjects mimicking tremor. *Ann Neurol* 31:507–514, 1992.

159. Pascual-Leone A, Valls-Sole J, Toro C, et al: Resetting of essential tremor and postural tremor in Parkinson's disease with transcranial magnetic stimulation. *Muscle Nerve* 17:800–807, 1994.

160. Elble R: Essential tremor frequency decreased with time. *Neurology* 55:1547–1551, 2000.

161. Mylle G, Van Bogaert L: Etudes anatomo-cliques de syndromes hypercinétiques complexes. I. Sur le tremblement familial. *Monatsschr Psychiatr Neurol* 103:28–43, 1940.

162. Laitinan F: Stereotaxic treatment of hereditary tremor. *Acta Neurol Scand* 41:74–79, 1965.

163. Dupuis MJM, Delwaide PJ, Boucqucy D, Gonsette RE: Homolateral disappearance of essential tremor after cerebellar stroke. *Mov Disord* 4:180–187, 1989.

164. Jahnsen H, Clinas R: Ionic basis for the electroresponsiveness and oscillatory properties of guinea pig thalamic neurons in vitro. *J Physiol* 349:227–247, 1986.

165. Deschenas M, Paradis M, Roy JP, Steriade N: Electrophysiology of neurons of lateral thalamic nucleus in cat: Resting properties and burst discharges. *J Neurophysiol* 51:1196–1219, 1984.

166. Armstrong DM, Harvey RJ: Responses in the inferior olive to stimulation of the cerebellum and cerebral cortex in the cat. *J Physiol* 187:553–574, 1966.

167. Dubinsky R, Hallet M: Glucose hypermetabolism of the inferior olive in patients with essential tremor. *Ann Neurol* 22:118, 1987.

168. Colebatch JG, Findley LJ, Frackowiak RSJ, et al: Preliminary report: Activation of the cerebellum in essential tremor. *Lancet* 336:1028–1030, 1990.

169. Jenkins IH, Bain PG, Colebatch JG, et al: A positron emission tomography study of essential tremor: Evidence for overactivity of cerebellar connections. *Ann Neurol* 34:82–90, 1993.

170. Samie MR, Selhorst JB, Koller WC: Post-traumatic midbrain tremors. *Neurology* 40:62–66, 1990.

171. Llinas R, Varon Y: Oscillatory properties of guinea pig inferior olivary neurones and their pharmacological modulation: An in vitro study. *J Physiol* 376:163–182, 1986.

172. Gunther H, Brunner R, Klussmann FN: Spectral analysis of tremorine and cold tremor electromyograms in animal species of different size. *Pflugers Arch* 399:180–185, 1983.

173. Wilms H, Sievers J, Deuschl G: Animal models of tremor. *Mov Disord* 14:557–571, 1999.

174. Deuschl G, Wenzelburger R, Loffler K, et al: Essential tremor and cerebellar dysfunction clinical and kinetic analysis of intention tremor. *Brain* 123:1568–1580, 2000.

175. Frankl-Hochwart: *La Degenerescence Hepato-Lenticulaire (Maladies de Wilson, Pseudo-Sclerose)*. Paris: Masson et Cie, 1903.

176. Hassler R: Zur pathologischen Anatomie des Senilen und des parkinsonistischen Tremor. *J Psychol Neurol* 49:193–230, 1939.

177. Mylle G, Van Bogaert L: Du tremblement essential non familial. *Monatsschr Psychiatr Neurol* 115:80–90, 1948.

178. Herskovits E, Blackwood W: Essential (familial, hereditary) tremor: A case report. *J Neurol Neurosurg Psychiatry* 32:509–511, 1969.

179. Lapresle J, Rondot P, Said G: Tremblement idiopathique de repos, d'attitude et d'action. *Rev Neurol (Paris)* 130:343–348, 1974.

180. Koller WC, Gupta S: Pharmacologic probe with progabide of GABA mechanism in essential tremor. *Arch Neurol* 44:905–907, 1987.

181. Koller WC: Trazodone in essential tremor: Probe of serotoninergic mechanisms. *Clin Neuropharmacol* 12:134–137, 1987.

182. Hellwig B, Haubler S, Schelter B, et al: Tremor-correlated cortical activity in essential tremor. *Lancet* 357:519–523, 2001.

183. McAuley S: Does essential tremor originate in the cerebral cortex? *Lancet* 357:492–494, 2001.

184. Fahn S, Tolosa E, Marin C: Clinical rating scale for tremor, in Jankovic J, Tolosa E (eds): *Parkinson's Disease and Movement Disorders*. Baltimore: Urban & Schwarzenberg, 1988.

185. Bain PG, Findley LJ, Atchison P, et al: Assessing tremor severity. *J Neurol Neurosurg Psychiatry* 56:868–873, 1993.

186. Louis ED, Barnes LF, Wendt KJ, et al: Validity and test-retest reliability of a disability questionnaire for essential tremor. *Mov Disord* 15:516–523, 2000.

187. Louis ED, Yousefzadeh E, Barnes LF, et al: Validation of a portable instrument for assessing tremor severity in epidemiological field studies. *Mov Disord* 15:95–102, 2000.

188. Louis ED, Barnes L, Wendt KJ, et al: A teaching videotape for the assessment of essential tremor. *Mov Disord* 16:89–93, 2001.

189. Bacher M, Scholz E, Diener AC: 24-hour continuous tremor quantification based on EMG recordings. *Electroencephalogr Clin Neurophysiol* 72:176–183, 1989.

190. Matsumoto JY, Dodick DW, Stevens LN, et al: Three-dimensional measurement of essential tremor. *Mov Disord* 14:288–294, 1999.

191. Elble RJ, Brilliant M, Leffler K, Higgins C: Quantification of essential tremor in writing and drawing. *Mov Disord* 11:70–78, 1996.

192. Magee KR: Essential tremor: Diagnosis and treatment. *Clin Med* 72:33–41, 1965.

193. Koller WC, Biary N: Effect of alcohol on tremor: Comparison to propranolol. *Neurology* 34:221–222, 1984.

194. Teravainen H, Huttunen J, Lewitt P: Ineffective treatment of essential tremor with an alcohol, methylpentynol. *J Neurol Neurosurg Psychiatry* 49:198–199, 1986.

195. Schroeder D, Nasrallah HA: High alcoholism rate in essential tremor patients. *Am J Psychiatry* 139:1471–1473, 1982.

196. Koller WC: Alcoholism in essential tremor. *Neurology* 33:1074–1076, 1983.

197. Rautakorpi I, Marttila RJ, Rinne UK: Alcohol consumption of patients with essential tremor. *Acta Neurol Scand* 68:177–179, 1983.

198. Martinella P, Gabellini AS, Gulli MR: Different clinical features of essential tremor: A 200-patient study. *Acta Neurol Scand* 75:106–111, 1987.

199. Koller WC, O'Hara R, Dorus W, Bauer J: Tremor in chronic alcoholism. *Neurology* 35:1660–1662, 1985.

200. Marshall J: Tremor, in Vinken PJ, Bruyn GW (eds): *Handbook of Clinical Neurology*. Amsterdam: North-Holland, 1968, vol 6, pp 809–825.

201. Winkler GF, Young RR: Efficacy of chronic propranolol therapy in action tremors of the familial, senile or essential varieties. *N Engl J Med* 290:984–988, 1974.

202. Sevitt I: The effect of adrenergic beta-receptor blocking drugs on tremor. *Practitioner* 207:677–678, 1971.

203. Foster JB, Longley BP, Stewart-Wynne EG: Propranolol in essential tremor. *Lancet* i:1455, 1973.

204. Sweet RD, Blumberg J, Lee JE, McDowell FH: Propranolol treatment of essential tremor. *Neurology* 24:64–67, 1974.

205. Tolosa ES, Loewenson RB: Essential tremor: Treatment with propranolol. *Neurology* 25:1041–1044, 1975.

206. Murray TJ: Treatment of essential tremor with propranolol. *Can Med Assoc J* 107:984–986, 1972.

207. Barbeau A: Traitment du tremblement essentiel familal par le propranolol. *Union Med Can* 102:899–902, 1962.

208. Teravainen H, Fogelholm R, Larsen A: Effect of propranolol on essential tremor. *Neurology* 26:27–30, 1976.

209. Larsen TA, Teravainen H, Calne DB: Atenolol vs propranolol in essential tremor: A controlled, quantitative study. *Acta Neurol Scand* 66:547–554, 1982.

210. Calzetti S, Findley LJ, Gresty MA, et al: Effect of a single dose of propranolol on essential tremor: A double-blind controlled study. *Ann Neurol* 13:165–171, 1983.

211. Koller WC: Dose-response relationship of propranolol in essential tremor. *Arch Neurol* 35:42–43, 1986.

212. Koller WC: Long-acting propranolol in essential tremor. *Neurology* 36:106–108, 1985.

213. Cleeves L, Findley LJ, Koller W: Lack of association between essential tremor and Parkinson's disease. *Ann Neurol* 24:23–26, 1988.

214. Findley LJ, Cleeves L: Beta-adrenoreceptor antagonists in essential tremor. *Lancet* 29:856–857, 1984.

215. Koller WC, Vetere-Overfield B: Acute and chronic affects of propranolol and primidone in essential tremor. *Neurology* 39:1587–1588, 1989.

216. Calzetti S, Sasso E, Baratti M, Faua R: Clinical and computer-based assessment of long-term therapeutic efficacy of propranolol in essential tremor. *Acta Neurol Scand* 81:392–396, 1990.

217. Young RR: Essential-familial tremor and other action tremors. *Semin Neurol* 2:386–391, 1982.

218. Calzettii S, Findley LJ, Perucca E, Richens A: The response of essential tremor to propranolol: Evaluation of clinical variables governing the efficacy on prolonged administration. *J Neurol Neurosurg Psychiatry* 46:393–398, 1983.

219. Koller WC, Royse V: Time course of a single oral dose of propranolol in essential tremor. *Neurology* 35:1494–1499, 1985.

220. Jefferson D, Jenner P, Marsden CD: Beta-adrenoreceptor antagonists in essential tremor. *J Neurol Neurosurg Psychiatry* 42:904–909, 1979.

221. Huttunen J, Teravainen H, Larsen A: Beta-adrenoreceptor antagonist in essential tremor. *Lancet* ii:857, 1984.

222. Britt CR, Peters BH: Metoprolol for essential tremor. *N Engl J Med* 301:31, 1979.

223. Ljung O: Treatment of essential tremor with metoprolol. *N Engl J Med* 301:1005, 1979.

224. Newman RP, Jacobs L: Metoprolol in essential tremor. *Arch Neurol* 37:596–597, 1980.

225. Riley T, Pleet AB: Metoprolol tartrate for essential tremor. *N Engl J Med* 301:663, 1979.

226. Turnbull DM, Shaw DA: Metoprolol in essential tremor. *Lancet* i:95, 1980.

227. Koller WC, Biary N: Metoprolol compared to propranolol in the treatment of essential tremor. *Arch Neurol* 41:171–172, 1984.

228. Koller WC: Nadolol in the treatment of essential tremor. *Neurology* 33:1074–1075, 1983.

229. Dietrichson P, Espen E: Effects of timolol and atenolol on benign essential tremor: Placebo-controlled studies based on quantitative tremor recordings. *J Neurol Neurosurg Psychiatry* 44:677–683, 1981.

230. Koller WC, Larsen L, Potempa K: Pindolol-induced tremor. *Clin Neuropharmacol* 10:449–460, 1987.

231. Kuroda Y, Kakigi R, Shilasaki H: Treatment of essential tremor with arotinolol. *Neurology* 38:650–651, 1988.

232. O'Brien MD, Upton AR, Toseland PA: Benign familial tremor treated with primidone. *Br Med J* 282:178–180, 1981.

233. Chakrabarti A, Pearce JMS: Essential tremor: Response to primidone. *J Neurol Neurosurg Psychiatry* 44:650, 1981.

234. Findley LJ, Cleeves L, Calzetti S: Primidone in essential tremor of the hands and head: A double-blind controlled clinical study. *J Neurol Neurosurg Psychiatry* 481:911–915, 1985.

235. Koller WC, Royse V: Efficacy of primidone in essential tremor. *Neurology* 36:121–124, 1986.

236. Gorman WP, Cooper R, Pocock P, Campbell MJ: A comparison of primidone, propranolol, and placebo in essential tremor using quantitative analysis. *J Neurol Neurosurg Psychiatry* 491:64–68, 1986.

237. Crystal HR: Duration of effectiveness of primidone in essential tremor. *Neurology* 36:1543, 1986.

238. Shale H, Fahn S: Response to essential tremor to treatment with primidone. *Neurology* 37:123, 1987 (abstract).

239. Sasso E, Perucca E, Fava N, Calzetti S: Primidone in the long-term treatment of essential tremor: A prospective study with computerized quantitative analysis. *Clin Neuropharmacol* 13:67–76, 1990.

240. Calzetti S, Findley L, Risani F, Richens A: Phenylethylmalonamide in essential tremor. *J Neurol Neurosurg Psychiatry* 44:932–934, 1981.

241. Findley LJ, Calzetti S: Double-blind controlled study of primidone in essential tremor: Preliminary results. *Br Med J* 285:608, 1982.

242. Procaccianti G, Baruzzi A, Martinelli P, et al: Benign familial tremor treated with primidone. *Br Med J* 283:558, 1981.

243. Baruzzi A, Procaceranti G, Martinelle P: Phenobarbital and propranolol in essential tremor: A double-blind controlled clinical trial. *Neurology* 33:296–300, 1983.

244. Findley LJ, Cleeves L: Phenobarbital in essential tremor. *Neurology* 35:1784–1787, 1985.

245. Sasso E, Perucca E, Calzetti S: Double-blind comparison of primidone and phenobarbital in essential tremor. *Neurology* 38:808–810, 1988.

246. Cabrera-Valdivia F, Jimenez-Jimenez J, Albea EG, et al: Orthostatic tremor: Successful treatment with phenobarbital. *Clin Neuropharmacol* 14:438–441, 1991.

247. Thompson C, Lang A, Parkes JD, Marsden CD: A double-blind trial of clonazepam in benign essential tremor. *Clin Neuropharmacol* 7:83–88, 1984.

248. Huber SJ, Paulson GW: Efficacy of alprazolam for essential tremor. *Neurology* 38:241–243, 1988.

249. Gunal D, Afsar N, Bekiroglu N, Aktan S: New alternative agents in essential tremor therapy: Double-blind placebo-controlled study of alprazolam and acetazolamide. *Neurol Sci* 21:315–317, 2000.

250. Muenter MD, Daube JR, Caviness JN, Miller PN: Treatment of essential tremor with methazolamide. *Mayo Clin Proc* 66:991–997, 1991.

251. Busenbark K, Hubble J, Pahwa P, Koller WC: The effect of acetazolamide on essential tremor. *Neurology* 42:1631–1632, 1992.

252. Busenbark K, Pahwa R, Hubble J, et al: Double-blind controlled study of methazolamide in the treatment of essential tremor. *Neurology* 43:1045–1047, 1993.

253. Burrows GT, King RB: Gapapentin in essential tremor. *Neurology* 38:241–243, 1988 (abstract).

254. Adler CH: Effectiveness of gabapentin in various movement disorders. *Mov Disord* 11(suppl 1):251, 1996 (abstract).

255. Pahwa R, Lyons KE, Hubble JP, et al: Double-blind controlled trial of gabapentin in essential tremor. *Mov Disord* 13:165–167, 1998.

256. Gironell A, Kulisevsky J, Barbanoj M, et al: A randomized placebo-controlled comparative trial of gabapentin and propranolol in essential tremor. *Arch Neurol* 56:475–480, 1999.

257. Ondo W, Hunter C, Vuong KD, et al: Gabapentin for essential tremor: A multiple-dose, double-blind, placebo-controlled trial. *Mov Disord* 15:6787–6782, 2000.

258. Connor GS: Topiramate as a novel treatment for essential tremor. *Mov Disord* 14:908, 1999.

259. Pact V, Giduz T: Mirtazapine treats resting tremor, essential tremor and levodopa-induced dyskinesias. *Neurology* 53:1154, 1999.

260. Barbeau A: L-Dopa therapy in Parkinson's disease: A critical review of nine years' experience. *Can Med Assoc J* 101:791–800, 1969.

261. Critchley E: Clinical manifestation of essential tremor. *J Neurol Neurosurg Psychiatry* 35:365–372, 1972.

262. Manyam BV: Amantadine in essential tremor. *Ann Neurol* 9: 198–199, 1981.

263. Obeso JA, Luguin MR, Artieda J, Martinez-Lage JM: Amantadine may be useful in essential tremor. *Ann Neurol* 19:99–100, 1986.

264. Koller WC: Amantadine in essential tremor. *Ann Neurol* 15:508–509, 1984.

265. Caccia MR, Mangoni A: Clonidine in essential tremor: Preliminary observations from an open trial. *J Neurol* 232:55–57, 1985.

266. Koller WC, Herbster G, Cone S: Clonidine in the treatment of essential tremor. *Mov Disord* 1:235–237, 1986.

267. Mai J, Olsen RB: Depression of essential tremor by alpha-adrenergic blockade. *J Neurol Neurosurg Psychiatry* 44:1171, 1981.

268. Koller WC: Ineffectiveness of phenoxybenzamide in essential tremor. *J Neurol Neurosurg Psychiatry* 49:222, 1986.

269. Morris CE, Prange AJ, Hall CD, Weiss EA: Inefficacy of trypto-phan/pyridoxine in essential tremor. *Lancet* ii:165–166, 1971.

270. McLeod NA, White LE: Trazodone in essential tremor. *JAMA* 256:2675–2676, 1986.

271. Cleeves L, Findley LJ: Trazodone is ineffective in essential tremor. *J Neurol Neurosurg Psychiatry* 53:268–269, 1990.

272. Meert TF, De Beukelaar F, Geldera YG: Ritanserin, a thymos-thenic drug in parkinsonism tremor and drug-induced EPS: A review of existing data. *Tremor 88*. Caesarea, Israel: 1988, p 38.

273. Caccia ML, Oslo M, Galimberti V, et al: Propranolol, clonidine, urapidil, and trazodone in essential tremor. *Acta Neurol Scand* 79:379–383, 1989.

274. Topakias S, Onur R, Dalkara S: Calcium channel blockers and essential tremor. *Eur Neurol* 27:114–119, 1987.

275. Jimenez-Jimenez FJ, Garcia Ruiz PJ, Cabrera-Valdivia F: Nicardipine versus propranolol in essential tremor. *Acta Neurol Napoli* 16:184–188, 1994.

276. Curran T, Lang AE: Flunarizine in essential tremor. *Clin Neuro-pharmacol* 16:460–463, 1993.

277. Biary N, Saleh M, Deeb A, Langenberg P: The effect of flunar-izine on essential tremor. *Neurology* 41:311–312, 1991.

278. Pakkenberg H, Pakkenberg B: Clozapine in the treatment of tremor. *Acta Neurol Scand* 73:295–297, 1986.

279. McCarthy RH: Clozapine reduces essential tremor indepen-dent of its antipsychotic effect: A case report [letter]. *J Clin Psychopharmacol* 14:212–213, 1994.

280. Ceravolo R, Salvetti S, Piccini P, et al: Acute and chronic effects of clozapine in essential tremor. *Mov Disord* 14:468–472, 1999.

281. McDowell FH: The use of glutethimide for treatment of essential tremor. *Mov Disord* 4:75–80, 1989.

282. Mally J, Stone TW: The effect of theophylline on essential tremor: The possible role of GABA. *Pharmacol Biochem Behav* 39:345–349, 1991.

283. American Academy of Neurology Therapeutics and Tech-nology Subcommittee: Assessment: The clinical usefulness of botulinum toxin-A in treating neurologic disorders. Special article. *Neurology* 40:1332–1336, 1990.

284. Jankovic J, Schwartz K: Botulinum toxin treatment of tremors. *Neurology* 41:1185–1188, 1991.

285. Trosch RM, Pullman SL: Botulinum toxin A injections for the treatment of hand tremors. *Mov Disord* 9:601–609, 1994.

286. Brin MF, Lyons KE, Doucette J, et al: A randomized, double masked, controlled trial of botulinum toxin type A in essential hand tremor. *Neurology* 56:1523–1528, 2001.

287. Pahwa R, Busenbark K, Swanson-Hyland EF, et al: Botulinum toxin treatment of essential head tremor. *Neurology* 45:822–824, 1995.

288. Wissel J, Masuhr F, Schelosky L, et al: Quantitative assessment of botulinum toxin treatment in 43 patients with head tremor. *Mov Disord* 12:722–726, 1997.

289. Hertegard S, Granqvist S, Lindestad PA: Botulinum toxin injec-tions for essential voice tremor. *Ann Otol Rhinol Laryngol* 109:204–209, 2000.

290. Warrick P, Dromey C, Irish JC, et al: Botulinum toxin for essen-tial tremor of the voice with multiple anatomical sites of tremor: A crossover design study of unilateral versus bilateral injection. *Laryngoscope* 110:1366–1374, 2000.

291. Stager SV, Ludlow CL: Responses of stutterers and vocal tremor patients to treatment with botulinum toxin, in Jankovic J, Hallett M (eds): *Therapy with Botulinum Toxin*. New York: Marcel Dekker, 1994, pp 481–490.

292. Deuschl G, Lohle E, Heinen F, et al: Ear click in palatal tremor: It's origin and treatment with botulinum toxin. *Neurology* 41:1677–1679, 1991.

293. Gordon K, Cadera W, Hinton G: Successful treatment of hered-itary trembling chin with botulinum toxin. *J Child Neurol* 8:154–156, 1993.

294. Bertrand C: Stereotactic and peripheral surgery for the control of movement disorders, in Barbeau A (ed): *Disorders of Movement*. Lancaster: MTP Press, 1981, pp 191–208.

295. Blocher HM, Bertrand C, Martinez N, et al: Hypotonia accom-panying the neurosurgical relief of essential tremor. *J Nerv Ment Dis* 147:49–55, 1968.

296. Ohye E, Hirai T, Miyazaki M, Shibazaki N: VIM thalamotomy for the treatment of various kinds of tremor. *Appl Neurophysiol* 451:275–280, 1981.

297. Andrew J: Surgical treatment of tremor, in Findley LJ, Capildeo R (eds): *Movement Disorders: Tremor*. London: Macmillan, 1984, pp 339–350.

298. Kelly PJ, Ahlekog JE, Goeres SJ, et al: Computer-assisted stereotactic ventralis lateralis thalamotomy with microelectrode recording in patients with Parkinson's disease. *Mayo Clin Proc* 62:655–664, 1987.

299. Selby G: Stereotaxic surgery, in WC Koller (ed): *Handbook of Parkinson's Disease*. New York: Marcel Dekker, 1987, pp 421–436.

300. Goldman MS, Kelly PJ: Stereotactic thalamotomy for medically intractable essential tremor. *Stereotact Funct Neurosurg* 58:22–25, 1992.

301. Niclot P, Pollin B, N'Guyen J, et al: Treatment of tremor by stereotactic surgery. *Rev Neurol (Paris)* 149:755–763, 1993.

302. Goldman MS, Ahlskog JE, Kelly PJ: The symptomatic and functional outcome of stereotactic thalamotomy for medically intractable essential tremor. *J Neurosurg* 76:924–928, 1992.

303. Benabid AL, Pollak P, Gervason L, et al: Long-term suppres-sion of tremor by chronic stimulation of the ventral intermediate thalamic nucleus. *Lancet* 337:403–406, 1991.

304. Benabid AL, Pollak P, Louveau A, et al: Combined (thalamotomy and stimulation) stereotactic surgery of the Vim thalamic nucleus for bilateral Parkinson's disease. *Appl Neurophysiol* 50:344–346, 1987.

305. Benabid AL, Pollak P, Gao DM, et al: Long-term suppression of tremor by chronic electrical stimulation of the ventralis intermedius nucleus of the thalamus as a treatment of movement disorders. *J Neurosurg* 84:203–214, 1996.

306. Blond S, Caparros-Lefebvre D, Parker F, et al: Control of tremor and involuntary movement disorders by chronic stereotactic stimulation of the ventral intermediate thalamic nucleus. *J Neurosurg* 77:62–68, 1992.

307. Speelman JO, Bosch DA: Continuous electric thalamus stimulation for the treatment of tremor resistant to pharmacotherapy. *Ned Tijdschr Geneeskd* 139:926–930, 1995.

308. Alesch F, Pinter MM, Helscher RJ, et al: Stimulation of the ventral intermediate thalamic nucleus in tremor dominated Parkinson's disease and essential tremor. *Acta Neurochir* 136:75–81, 1995.

309. Benabid AL, Pollak P, Gao DM, et al: Chronic electrical stimulation of the ventralis intermedius nucleus of the thalamus as a treatment of movement disorders. *J Neurosurg* 84:203–214, 1996.

310. Ondo W, Jankovic J, Schwartz K, et al: Unilateral thalamic deep brain stimulation for refractory essential tremor and Parkinson's disease tremor. *Neurology* 51:1063–1069, 1998.

311. Koller W, Pahwa R, Busenbark K, et al: High-frequency unilateral thalamic stimulation in the treatment of essential and parkinsonian tremor. *Ann Neurol* 42:292–299, 1997.

312. Limousin P, Speelman JD, Gielen F, Janssens M: Multicenter European study of thalamic stimulation in parkinsonian and essential tremor. *J Neurol Neurosurg Psychiatry* 66:289–296, 1999.

313. Troster KA, Fields JA, Pahwa R, et al: Neuropsychological and quality of life outcome after thalamic stimulation for essential tremor. *Neurology* 53:1774–1780, 1999.

314. Koller WC, Lyons KE, Wilkinson SB, Pahwa R: Efficacy of unilateral deep brain stimulation of the Vim nucleus of the thalamus for essential head tremor. *Mov Disord* 14:847–850, 1999.

315. Obweggeser AA, Uitti RJ, Turk MF, et al: Thalamic stimulation for the treatment of midline tremors in essential tremor patients. *Neurology* 54:2342–2344, 2000.

316. Taha JM, Janszen Ma, Favre J: Thalamic deep brain stimulation for the treatment of head, voice and bilateral limb tremor. *J Neurosurg* 91:68–72, 1999.

317. Boockvar JA, Telfeian A, Baltuch GH, et al: Long-term deep brain stimulation in a patient with essential tremor: clinical response and postmortem correlation with stimulation termination sites in ventral thalamus. Case report. *J Neurosurg* 93:140–144, 2000.

318. Koller WC, Lyons KE, Wilkinson SB, et al: Long-term safety and efficacy of unilateral deep brain stimulation of the thalamus in essential tremor. *Mov Disord* 16:464–468, 2001.

319. Schuurman PR, Bosch DA, Bossuyt PMM, et al: A comparison of continuous thalamic stimulation and thalamotomy for suppression of severe tremor. *N Engl J Med* 342:462–468, 2000.

320. Young RF, Jacques S, Mark R, et al: Gamma knife thalamotomy for treatment of tremor: Long-term results. *J Neurosurg* 93(suppl 3):128–135, 2000.

321. Okun MS, Natividad P, Stover, et al: Complications of gamma knife surgery for Parkinson's disease. *Arch Neurol* 58:1995–2002, 2001.

322. Niranjan A, Kondziolka D, Baser S, et al: Functional outcomes after gamma knife thalamotomy for essential tremor and MS-related tremor. *Neurology* 55:443–446, 2000.

323. Young R: Functional neurosurgery with the Leksell gamma knife. *Stereotact Funct Neurosurg* 66:19–23, 1996.

324. Wake A, Takahashi Y, Onishi T, et al: Treatment of essential tremor by behavior therapy: Use of Jacobsen's progressive relaxation method. *Psychiatr Neurol Jpn* 76:509–517, 1974.

Chapter 28

UNCOMMON FORMS OF TREMOR

BALA V. MANYAM

PHYSIOLOGICAL TREMOR 459
CORTICAL TREMOR 461
CEREBELLAR TREMOR 461
DYSTONIC TREMOR 462
FOOD-INDUCED TREMOR 462
DRUG-INDUCED TREMOR 463
    Antidepressants 463
    Antiepileptic Drugs 463
    Cardiac Drugs 463
    Dopamine Receptor-Blocking Drugs 464
    Immunosuppressants 464
    Stimulants 464
    Tranquilizers 464
TOXIN-INDUCED TREMOR 465
    Heavy Metals 465
    Insecticides and Herbicides 466
    Solvents 466
HOLMES' (MIDBRAIN) TREMOR 466
PRIMARY ORTHOSTATIC TREMOR 467
PALATAL TREMOR 468
PERIPHERAL NEUROPATHY-ASSOCIATED
   TREMOR 469
PSYCHOGENIC TREMORS 469
REST TREMOR 470
STROKE-ASSOCIATED TREMOR 471
TREMOR IN SYSTEMIC DISORDERS AND
   DISEASES 472
    AIDS 472
    Hereditary Hemochromatosis 472
    Hypoxia/Hypotension 472
    Porphyria 472
    Thyroid Disorders 472
    Wilson's Disease 472
TASK-SPECIFIC TREMOR 472
POSTTRAUMATIC TREMOR 473
VOCAL TREMOR 474

Tremor remains the most common of all movement disorders. The most accepted and simple definition is as follows: "rhythmical involuntary oscillatory movement of a body part."[1] The amplitude of tremor is not critical to the definition. Thus, in any part of the body where agonistic and antagonistic muscles function, tremor could occur. Tremor is most commonly seen in the upper extremities, but tremor of the lower extremities, head, trunk, lips, chin, tongue, and vocal cords could also occur. Functionally, rest tremor is present when the affected part of the body is in repose and is fully supported against gravity, requiring no active muscle contraction.[2] Tremor seen in parkinsonism is typically rest tremor. This tremor typically disappears with onset of movement but, once partial stability is attained in the new position, the tremor returns. When tremor occurs with maintained posture such as holding arms perpendicular to the body, it is called postural tremor. Postural tremor is possibly the most common form of tremor and can be seen in physiological tremor, essential tremor, cerebellar postural tremor, and others. This tremor is often the most functionally disabling. When tremor occurs with movement from one point to another, it is referred to as kinetic or intentional tremor. Kinetic tremor that appears near termination of movement is known as terminal tremor. Kinetic tremor present during specific tasks but absent with other activities involving the same limb is referred to as task-specific tremor. Examples include primary writing tremor, vocal tremor, and orthostatic tremor. Tremor may arise from several anatomic locations within the central nervous system or peripheral nervous system, including the cerebral cortex, white matter, basal ganglia, thalamus, midbrain, cerebellum, and peripheral nerves. In physiological tremor, no known lesion is present. Alterations in neurotransmitters such as dopamine deficiency (as seen in Parkinson's disease), excess epinephrine as seen in anxiety, decreased level of substrate such as glucose (hypoglycemia), reduced level of electrolyte (hyponatremia), and excess level of a hormone such as thyroxin (thyrotoxicosis) can induce tremor leading to biochemical nonspecificity. A simple diagnostic approach is listed in Table 28-1, combining tremor with one other condition.

Frequency of tremor has often been given much importance and is used in classification. Vocal tremor frequency has a narrow range and is generally not altered by treatment. The amplitude of the tremor in patients with the same disease may vary and can be exaggerated by physical and emotional stress. Amplitude of tremor is easily quantifiable and is classified as mild, moderate, or severe on various rating scales. Treatment for tremor disorders is aimed at reducing tremor amplitude, which is responsible for functional disability.

In this chapter, tremor other than that strictly defined as essential tremor will be discussed. However, there may be some degree of overlap of what may be considered "essential tremor variant and tremor other than essential tremor."

Physiological Tremor

Physiological tremor, the invisible mechanical vibration of body parts, is present in all normal people. However, it is barely visible to the naked eye and is symptomatic only during activities that require extreme precision. Physiological tremor has two distinct oscillations. The 8–12-Hz level[5] is very resistant to frequency change. Internal loads,[3,4] elastic

TABLE 28-1 Tremor Differential diagnosis triad

AIDS, Pneumocystis carinii pneumonia and tremor	? Trimethoprim/sulfamethoxazole induced
Bradykinesia, rigidity, and tremor	? Parkinsonism
Weight loss, increased appetite, and tremor	? Hyperthyroidism
Weight gain, decreased appetite, and tremor	? Hypothyroidism
Mania, depression, and tremor	? Lithium induced
Positive Family history, monosymptomatic, and tremor	? Essential tremor
Euphoria, ataxia, and tremor	? Multiple sclerosis
	? Chronic alcoholism
Sweating, Diabetes, and tremor	? Hypoglycemia
Dyspneic, wheezing, and tremor	? Adrenergic drug induced
Urinary frequency, and tremor	? Caffeine induced
Epilepsy and tremor	? Valproic acid induced
Cardiac arrhythmia, ataxia, and tremor	? Amiodarone induced

loads,[5] limb cooling,[6] and torque loads[7] produce less than a 1–2-Hz frequency change. This frequency invariability and the intense synchronous motor unit modulation suggests that the neuronal oscillator is responsible for the 8–12-Hz tremor.[6] It occurs during the maintenance of study limb postures and has a low amplitude. The functional significance of this tremor is not known. The mechanical reflex component is the larger of the two distinct oscillations of physiological tremor and is a result of the internal viscous and elastic properties of the limb or some other body part. The two oscillations are superimposed upon a background of irregular fluctuations in muscle force and limb displacement. The frequency of this mechanical reflex oscillation is determined largely by inertia and stiffness of the body part. Consequently, normal elbow tremors have a frequency of 3–5 Hz, wrist tremors 8–12 Hz, and metacarpophalangeal joint tremors 17–30 Hz. Mechanical reflex tremor is a passive oscillation that occurs in response to broad-frequency, irregular forces that are produced by asynchronous subtetanic motor unit firing. It has been considered that the component of lower frequency originated from the central nervous system as a long loop, and that of higher frequency originated from the muscle-spindle loop system as a short loop.[8] Although both oscillations should be considered together, from a practical standpoint the 8–12-Hz seem to have more practical implications. It has been considered that physiological tremor may be a protective measure against unusual limb posture.[9] Because the physiological tremor has 8–12-Hz, and alpha rhythm in electroencephalogram (EEG) has a similar frequency (7–13), a common central origin was considered. No evidence for such an hypothesis

has been found.[10] Tremor recording with an accelerometer in 1079 healthy subjects showed frequency peaks between 5.85 and 8.80 Hz with spectral analysis. Chronic cigarette smoking and coffee drinking did not modify the tremor. Relaxation sessions decreased tremor significantly.[11]

The frequency of physiological tremor is not influenced by age. Enhanced physiological tremor can occur under various conditions, including emotional stress, fatigue, exercise, hypoglycemia, thyrotoxicosis, pheochromocytoma, hypothermia, alcohol withdrawal, and by means of drugs such as valproic acid, lithium, neuroleptics, and tricyclic antidepressants. Ethanol can also cause a decrease in the amplitude of physiological tremor.[12] In enhanced physiological tremor there is no evidence of an underlying neurologic disease. It has been considered that the stretch-reflex response to oscillation increases during fatigue and in anxiety and response to the several medications named above and to hormones that produce a modulation of motor unit activity. This is what results in an increase in amplitude, being referred to as "enhanced physiological tremor."[13,14] Physiological tremor was not altered by caffeine in controlled studies.[15] Studies with tremorolytic action of beta-adrenoceptor blockers in physiological and isoprenaline-induced tremor suggested that the tremor activity is exerted via the same beta2-adrenoceptors located in a deep peripheral compartment that is thought to be in the muscle spindles.[16] Intravenous propranolol produces a 34–60 percent decrease in the amplitude of physiological tremor. There was a delay of about 10 minutes, suggesting that this was the result of formation of a highly specific, centrally acting metabolite of propranolol.[17]

Postanesthetic tremor may manifest as shivering. Electromyograph (EMG) studies revealed postanesthetic tremor to be consistent with exacerbated physiological tremor and is considered to be secondary to high levels of circulating catecholamines,[18] seldom requiring any treatment. It is not uncommon for nursing staff to cover the patient with an extra blanket.

Physiological tremor can interfere with fine coordinative movements, such as those required for performing microsurgery, watch repair, or diamond cutting. Although knowledge of factors that aggravate physiological tremor should be addressed (e.g., lack of sleep, fatigue, anxiety, etc.), use of a single 40-mg dose of propranolol has been found to be effective. Surgeons who perform microsurgery are known to take such a drug before the start of a procedure.

Cortical Tremor

Cortical tremor is a rare disorder with the electrophysiological characteristics of cortical myoclonus. Most cases are idiopathic or secondary to diffuse brain pathology and lesion localization is generally difficult. The term "cortical tremor" was coined by Ikeda et al.,[19] who described 2 patients with action and postural 9-Hz tremor with electrophysiological evidence of cortical myoclonus, were refractory to beta-blocker therapy but responded to a combination of valproic acid and clonazepam. The authors concluded that this tremor disorder represented a variant of action-induced myoclonus in the setting of cortical myoclonus. Subsequently, Toro et al.[20] described 10 additional cases. Both males and females, with an age range of 16–75 years, shared the common features of these 12 cases equally. The presenting symptom was often tremor or action myoclonus. The etiology was idiopathic in 5, balletic myoclonus in 3, and 1 each of Lafora body disease, postanoxic myoclonus, progressive myoclonic epilepsy of unknown etiology, and opsoclonus myoclonus syndrome. The features common to all patients were abnormal rhythmic bursts on the EMG during voluntary isometric contraction with synchronous activation of agonist and antagonist muscles, alternating periods of near silence, a peak burst frequency of 9–18 Hz with low levels of isometric activation, and an associated cortical potential on EEG back-averaging. In the 10 cases described by Toro et al.,[20] the rhythmic disturbance produced by isometric muscle activation was a source of disabling deception of skill in motor task, such as holding a pen for writing or holding a cup.

Cerebellar Tremor

The main anomaly of cerebellar movement is its discontinuity. When discontinuity in movement becomes rhythmic, the definition of tremor can be applied. Kinetic tremor could occur as the target is reached (as, for example, in the finger-to-nose test). This is referred to as terminal tremor. In the early part of the cerebellar disease (or if the cerebellar damage is minimal), a mild degree of terminal tremor may be the only sign. As the disease advances, the tremor may be present during the entire course of finger-to-nose test. In the early phases, tremor can be present in the extremities, but, as the disease advances, it can involve axial structures. Occasionally, tremor may start as head tremor, although this is less common. The frequency and amplitude of cerebellar tremor are usually irregular. The frequency of cerebellar kinetic tremor is commonly described as being 3–5 Hz, but studies have shown that the frequency of cerebellar tremor is inversely proportional to limb inertia, resulting in the frequency being dependent on the part of the body affected. In the upper extremities, kinetic tremor has a frequency of 3–8 Hz, whereas in the lower extremities it is usually around 3 Hz. The truncal tremor, which is a rhythmic partial sway, usually has a frequency of 2–4 Hz.[21] At times, cerebellar tremor is so irregular it may appear proximal. In cerebellar kinetic tremor the oscillations are of variable amplitude and are perpendicular to the direction of movement. Postural tremor of the head may be the first manifestation of cerebellar disease. Postural tremor of the limb can also occur. Cerebellar tremor is classically elicited by finger-to-nose and heel-to-shin tests. However, the tremor can also be recognized in a patient's handwriting. Each waveform in the helices drawn by a patient with tremor represents upward and downward deflection of a tremor. With this background, the following conditions have to be fulfilled for the diagnosis of cerebellar tremor: pure or dominant intention tremor, uni- or bilateral with a frequency below 5 Hz. There could be presence of postural tremor, but not rest tremor.[1]

Attempts to correlate tremor to cerebellar lesions often results in incomplete results. What is known is that, in humans, lesions in the posterior funiculus aggravate cerebellar tremor, whereas stimulation of Ia fibers by application of vibrations to the tendon diminishes the tremor.[22] In experimental monkeys, damage to dentate, globase, and emboliform nuclei in the cerebellum or to the superior cerebellar peduncles produces tremor.[23] It is also known that, in humans, damage to the superior cerebellar peduncles or to the dentate nucleus is defined as the most common site of focal pathology that leads to severe intention tremor. Head tremor following bilateral cerebellar infarction[24] and cerebellar hemorrhage is reported.[25] Cerebellar axial tremor without apparent palatal tremor with a varied frequency of 3–10 Hz is reported.[26]

The underlying complexity of the transcortical and transcerebellar loops is probably the principal reason why effective pharmacotherapy is not available for cerebellar tremors or, for that matter, cerebellar dysfunction.[21] Nevertheless, several drugs have been tried.[21,27,28] Reports emerging in the literature include either single case reports or open trials in a small number of patients. However, sustained benefit or double-blind studies are few and often do not confirm the initial results. Stereotactic thalamotomy or stimulation in the contralateral ventralis intermedius nucleus is often effective in reducing the amplitude of the tremor but may result in deterioration of other aspects of motor function.[29–31]

Mechanical therapy, such as strapping lead weights to the wrist, has been used and was found to reduce kinetic tremor.[32] Use of weighted instruments during eating and other activities may be helpful,[21] but the mechanical load must be tailored to the need of each patient. Devices for reducing tremor are often cumbersome and may not necessarily improve a patient's functional ability. Thalamic stimulation in 13 patients with cerebellar tremor secondary to multiple sclerosis revealed an improvement of the tremor in 69.2 percent of patients. Functional improvement was more varied and depended on the severity of tremor and coexistence of other neurological symptoms. Of the 8 most severely affected patients, 7 recovered the possibility to easily catch an object and use it.[33] Carbamazepine (400 and 600 mg/day) in 10 patients with cerebellar tremors (7 patients with multiple sclerosis, and 3 with cerebrovascular disease) in a single-blind manner improved tremor on a clinical rating scale and by accelerometric recording. There was no improvement with placebo. This has not been confirmed on a double-blind trial with a larger number of patients.[34] Overall treatment for cerebellar tremor remains unsatisfactory.

Dystonic Tremor

A clear definition of dystonic tremor is still under debate. The Consensus Statement of the Movement Disorder Society on Tremor[1] proposed the following definition: "Tremor in an extremity or body part that is affected by dystonia. Focal tremors, usually have irregular amplitude and variable frequency (mainly less than 7 Hz). Tremor is mainly postural/kinetic and usually not seen during complete rest." A typical example of dystonic tremor is tremulous spasmodic torticollis or dystonic head tremor. On the other hand, tremor can be associated with dystonia, in which case the tremor occurs in a body part not affected by dystonia. An example is the presence of upper limb postural tremor in a patient with cervical dystonia. In this section, both will be discussed together. Oppenheim[35] described presence of tremor associated with dystonic movements. In a review of 42 patients with idiopathic torsion dystonia, tremor was found in 14 percent,[36] but occurrence of tremor before manifestation of dystonia is not uncommon.[37,38] In a series of 271 patients with cervical dystonia, 71 percent had associated tremor.[39] In another series of 308 patients, 10 percent of the patients with varieties of dystonia had tremor.[40] In an accidental toxic exposure to 2,3,7,8-tetrachlorodibenzo-p-dioxin, focal hand dystonia, and intention tremor were present in 22 of the 45 patients.[41] Dystonic tremor is also described as postural, localized, and irregular in amplitude, with periodicity absent during muscle relaxation, exacerbated by smooth muscle contraction, and associated frequently with myoclonus. It is considered a distinct entity from essential tremor, as it is irregular, has a broad range of frequencies, and remains localized.[42] Thus, there is considerable confusion on the very nomenclature. Occurrence of dystonia associated with postural tremor of upper extremity secondary to contralateral anterior thalamic infarct is reported.[43] Head tremor is common in cervical dystonia and is more commonly associated with hand tremor and family history of tremor or other movement disorders.[44] Treatment of dystonia with botulinum often results in significant improvement of tremor as seen in cases of cervical dystonia. Deep brain stimulation of subthalamic area was beneficial in a patient with tremor and dystonia.[45]

Food-Induced Tremor

A tremor is considered to be food- or beverage-induced if it occurs in a reasonable timeframe following ingestion of that particular food or beverage. Tremor secondary to food or beverages can take many forms, including enhanced physiological tremor, precipitated essential tremor, tremor of cerebellar syndrome, or can be associated with peripheral neuropathy. On the other hand, alcohol can suppress essential and certain other forms of tremor.[46]

Coffee, tea, cocoa, and caffeinated soda are sources of caffeine, a stimulant. It is believed that caffeine can induce new onset of tremor or may exacerbate previously existing tremor.[47,48] In a survey of 4558 healthy individuals, 16 percent reported tremor that was sometimes associated with coffee intake.[49] Although a double-blind study has not been done, measurement of tremor using an accelerometer after oral dose of 325 mg of caffeine did not increase physiological, essential tremor, or parkinsonian tremor at 1, 2, or 3 hours after ingestion.[15] Individual sensitivity to caffeine may vary. Under experimental conditions, caffeine at 3 mg/kg, but not at 1 mg/kg body weight, significantly increased whole-arm physiological tremor in young adult males with no effect by time of the day.[50] There appears to be significant variation in drinking caffeinated beverages and in the symptoms attributed to caffeine. Some individuals drink up to 15 cups of coffee per day and still do not have any symptoms attributable to caffeine, whereas others may complain after a single cup. The psychological overlay could also be a factor not only in tremor but also to other symptoms attributed to caffeine, such as insomnia. Decaffeinated beverages may not be totally free of caffeine, and whether other noncaffeine compounds exist in coffee, tea, and cocoa that are tremorogenic has not been proven.

Alcohol, known to suppress essential tremor and a few other forms of tremor,[46] can itself induce tremor through different mechanisms upon withdrawal following chronic ingestion. The most common tremulousness of hepatic encephalopathy, referred to as metabolic tremor, may simply be a less pronounced manifestation.[51] Alcohol withdrawal tremor might be a variant of enhanced physiological tremor, most often caused by anxiety or emotional stress. In 40 patients who had alcohol withdrawal tremor, EMG examination performed 1–10 days following alcohol withdrawal to evaluate the pattern, frequency and amplitude of tremor revealed 8–12 Hz low-amplitude postural tremor with synchronous activity in antagonist muscles. Patients with alcohol withdrawal tremor had significantly higher amplitude tremor compared to patients with anxiety and emotional stress.[52] Alcohol withdrawal tremor is a postural tremor of the upper extremity which, when severe, may spread to other parts of the body (face, tongue, larynx, muscles, and head).[53,54] The tremor from alcohol withdrawal may persist for more than 1 year in the absence of alcohol intake, even though amplitude may diminish.[54] Chronic alcoholism results in cerebellar degeneration, in which case a 3-Hz leg tremor and upper extremity tremor have been demonstrated.[55,56] A variety of movement disorders associated with cirrhosis of the liver occurs in chronic alcoholics and is complicated by portosystemic shunts, resulting in acquired hepatocerebral degeneration. The symptoms include various forms of tremor.[57]

The Chamorro population of the western Pacific islands of Guam and Rota consume palm (*Cycas circinalis*) flour as a staple diet and are known to develop parkinsonism-dementia-amyotrophic lateral sclerosis complex that includes rest tremor. The active compound, beta-*N*-methylamino-L-alanine, is considered the underlying cause,[58] but the exact cause is not fully established.

Tobacco is consumed by chewing, smoking, or sniffing. Nicotine affects both the peripheral and central nervous systems. Nicotine causes tremor in animals[59,60] and is reported to produce tremor in normal individuals.[61,62] However, a controlled study failed to elicit any significant influence of nicotine on either physiological or pathological tremor.[63]

Drug-Induced Tremor

A tremor is considered to be drug-induced if it occurs in a reasonable time frame following drug ingestion. It can have the whole range of clinical presentation of tremor and there could be presence of additional signs depending upon the nature of the drug and individual disposition of the patient. Tremor secondary to drugs and toxins can take many forms, including enhanced physiological tremor, precipitated essential tremor, rest tremor secondary to parkinsonism, tremor of cerebellar syndrome, or can be associated with peripheral neuropathy. The following broad groups of drugs have common features.

ANTIDEPRESSANTS

Tremor is a relatively frequent side-effect of lithium and of antidepressants with serotonergic properties. The risk is greater if the above are combined.[64] Lithium is widely accepted as a prophylactic therapy in recurrent affective disorders and is known to produce enhancement of physiological tremor. The incidence is considered to range from 33 percent to 65 percent,[65] and the occurrence rate increases with increasing serum lithium levels and manifests almost 100 percent in lithium toxicity. Centrally acting beta-blockers, such as propranolol, are effective when tremor occurs, even when lithium is maintained at therapeutic range.

Tricyclic antidepressants are known to produce high-frequency, low-amplitude postural tremor and are considered to represent enhanced physiological tremor.[66] Although specific treatment may not be required, reduction in the dose may be all that is required, as the tremors seem to correlate with the plasma levels of the drug.[67] However, in an occasional case, use of a beta-blocker such as propranolol may be necessary,[68] especially if the tremor is causing social or functional disability.

Monoamine oxide inhibitors are known to cause tremor. The incidence of tremor was 15 percent in a prospective study of phenelzine for depression.[69]

ANTIEPILEPTIC DRUGS

Valproic acid is the most common tremorogenic drug among antiepileptic drugs. In chronic valproic acid therapy, tremor incidence is considered to occur in about one-fourth of patients.[70] Tremor is generally postural, and the frequency may range from 6 to 15 Hz.[70] Tremor may occur even when the dose of valproic acid is within the therapeutic range. Onset of tremor could occur within a few weeks after treatment but generally begins anywhere between 3 and 14 months after the therapy is started.[71,72] Although no correlation between the severity of tremor and serum levels of valproic acid is found, patients may note reduction in the amplitude of tremor when the drug is withheld or after a change in the bioavailability of the drug.[56] Most valproic acid-associated tremor may not require treatment unless the serum level of the drug is at a toxic level. When tremor is persistent, despite serum level of the drug being at a therapeutic level, use of beta-blocking agents such as propranolol may be needed.[56] Lamotrigine is reported to cause tremor, more so when administered in combination with other antiepileptic drugs than as monotherapy.[73,74] Occasional tremor has been reported with phenytoin,[75] carbamazepine,[76] and tiagabine.[77]

CARDIAC DRUGS

Amiodarone, a cardiac antiarrhythmic, in a study involving 70 consecutive patients showed tremor, along with ataxia, in 52 (74 percent) patients on a daily maintenance dose of 600 mg/day.[78] Procainamide, another antiarrhythmic drug, is also known to produce tremor, but this is rare.[79]

Calcium-channel blockers are reported to possess mild D2 receptor-blocking effects.[80,81] As a result, both parkinsonism and rabbit syndrome have been reported to be caused by cinnarizine and flunarizine associated with tremor.[56] Cinnarizine and flunarizine are known to cause isolated tremor.[80] Nifedipine, another calcium-channel blocking agent, is reported to enhance physiological tremor.[81]

Centrally acting beta-blockers such as propranolol are widely used in the treatment of essential tremor and other forms of tremor. Pindolol, a beta-blocker, possesses partial agonist activity. Beta-blockers with partial agonist activity in high doses may stimulate beta-2 musculoskeletal receptors. Development of pindolol-induced tremor during a double-blind, randomized, clinical trial is reported.[82] Cardio-selective beta-blocker, metoprolol, which has been used in the treatment of tremor, is itself reported to cause tremor.[83]

DOPAMINE RECEPTOR-BLOCKING DRUGS

Neurological sequelae resulting from dopamine receptor-blocking medications (neuroleptics) are well recognized. Tremor as a complication of dopamine receptor-blocking therapy could manifest in the form of resting tremor in drug-induced parkinsonism, rabbit syndrome when there is tremor involving mainly the lips, and tremor associated with tardive dyskinesia or tardive tremor. A study of 14 patients clinically diagnosed to have developed dopamine receptor-blocking drug-induced tremor showed both rest and postural tremor with a frequency of 4–7 Hz. The tremor was rhythmic, regular, and sinusoidal. It did not interfere generally with the activities of daily living.[84]

Tremor is often the major concern in patients with drug-induced parkinsonism.[85] Tremor as a result of drug-induced parkinsonism could occur because of either blockage of dopamine receptors[86] or depletion of dopamine stores in the nerve terminal.[87] Tremor is mainly manifested as resting tremor, but it is not uncommon to see partial tremor as well. Although tremor may be more predominant in the upper extremities, it is not uncommon to see head or even lower-extremity tremor. In a detailed study, the incidence of parkinsonian tremor was found to be greater than 13 percent with thioridazine, whereas the incidence with chlorpromazine was less than half of that.[88] However, in this study, about 5 percent of the patients treated with placebo also exhibited tremor. Metoclopramide, a drug used in the treatment of gastroparesis, symptomatic gastroesophageal reflux is known to produce parkinsonism with rest tremor.[89] On discontinuing treatment, the parkinsonism is generally fully reversible. Catecholamine-depleting agents such as reserpine or tetrabenazine (which is less potent than reserpine) may also be capable of producing tremor as part of drug-induced parkinsonism. (Treatment of drug-induced parkinsonism is discussed in detail in Chap. 24.)

In rabbit syndrome—rest tremor affecting the periorbicularis oris muscle of the lips is similar to the movements seen in rabbit's mouth originally described by Villeneuve[90]—there is often a popping-like sound produced as the lips rapidly separate. The frequency is 4–6 Hz. There may be tremor of chin and extremities. Anticholinergics are considered effective in this disorder.

Tardive tremor is predominantly partial and kinetic tremor that interferes with writing, eating, and other activities of daily living. Little or no parkinsonian features were described in patients who were exposed to neuroleptic therapy. The tremor persisted even after 6 years of cessation of neuroleptic therapy. The tremor persisted at rest. Tardive tremor is a rare disorder in patients exposed to neuroleptics, as only 5 patients of 243 patients with drug-induced movement disorders were seen.[91] The mechanism of tardive tremor is not known and may not respond to conventional antitremor therapy. Tetrabenazine and clozapine are reported to be effective.[91,92]

IMMUNOSUPPRESSANTS

Cyclosporin A, an important immunosuppressive agent used in organ transplantation and a variety of other immunological diseases, is known to produce tremor of low amplitude and high frequency.[93] Abnormally increased ^{18}F-fluorodeoxyglucose (^{18}F-FDG) uptake in the basal ganglia was noted by positron emission tomography (PET) in a 37-year-old bone marrow transplant patient who had severe intention tremors of his hands.[94]

Treatment of *Pneumocystis carinii* pneumonia seen in patients with AIDS with trimethoprim/sulfamethoxazole carries a high risk of tremor. Withdrawal of the drug resulted in complete resolution.[95]

STIMULANTS

The enhancement of physiological tremor is often considered to be related to sympathomimetic effects of stimulants via stimulation of peripheral adrenergic receptors. Severe tremor has been reported with intravenous amphetamine abuse.[96] Stimulants may also be associated with increased postural tremor in the upper extremities.[56]

Drugs used in the treatment of asthma can often produce tremor as a common side-effect. These include isoproterenol, terbutaline, aminophylline, and others.[97] Isotributyline produced occasional tremor in 31 percent of patients.[98] Theophylline has a narrow therapeutic margin, and, when the serum level exceeds 15 mg/L, onset of tremor is not uncommon.[99]

TRANQUILIZERS

Tranquilizers, including the benzodiazepine group, are often used in treatment of tremor, because the calming effect on the central nervous system is considered to have therapeutic benefit on tremors. However, occurrence of tremor during diazepam withdrawal in patients who consumed 60–120 mg/day for 3–14 years is reported.[100]

Toxin-Induced Tremor

Toxic tremor occurs after intoxication either acutely or chronically. There may be other clinical signs of central nervous system intoxication such as gait disturbance or eye movement abnormalities. The association of toxins causing tremor has long been known. Jean Fernel, in 1557, linked mercury poisoning to tremor.[101] There are more than 850 neurotoxic chemicals found in the workplace, of which 65 are the most common ones.[102] A conservative estimate of the number of full-time workers exposed to one or more of these neurotoxins is considered to be 7.7 million.[103] Toxins such as harmaline and oxotremorine produce tremor, which has lead to the development of animal models of tremor.[104] Naturally occurring tremorogenic mycotoxins are synthesized by *Aspergillus*, *Penicillium*, and *Claviceps* species. Onset of tremor in cattle and other animals is known. No convincing neurotoxic effects in humans are documented from the above tremorogens.[105]

HEAVY METALS

Neurotoxic effects from ingestion of metals such as mercury, lead, copper, arsenic, and aluminum are well known. However, few of these are known to cause tremor.

Mercury can cause toxic effects in three forms: inorganic mercury salts, organic mercury compounds, and metallic mercury. Inorganic mercury salts are water-soluble, irritate the gut, and cause severe kidney damage. Organic mercury compounds are fat-soluble, can cross the blood-brain barrier, and cause neurological damage. Mercury metal poses two dangers. It can be vaporized: the vapor pressure at room temperature is about 100 times the safe amount, so poisoning can occur if mercury metal is spilled into crevices or cracks in the floorboards. Dentists are occasionally poisoned this way. Mercury easily crosses into the brain, and causes tremor, depression, and behavioral disturbances. A second danger from metallic mercury is that it is biotransformed into organic mercury, by bacteria at the bottom of lakes. This can be passed along through seafood and eventually to man. Mercury was found useful in the treatment of syphilis in the sixteenth century, leading to increased demands for the mineral and, therefore, to heightened mining activities. Miners were said to remain at work rarely for more than a few years because they developed tremor and vertigo. This was considered possibly a result of the toxicity of mercury.[106] Epidemics of inorganic mercury poisoning have occurred, usually manifested by the appearance of tremor. Chronic inorganic exposure to mercury may lead to fine rapid tremor that affects extremities, head, tongue, eyelids, and voice. The incidence of tremor in felt hat makers was found to be 20 percent when exposed for more than 20 years. However, in industrial accidents, the incidence has been 50–90 percent.[106] Organic mercury poisoning was rare before 1953. Industrial pollution in Minamata Bay, Japan, caused an epidemic of mercury poisoning. Ataxic tremor was one of the components. At autopsy, cerebellar atrophy, along with cerebral edema,

was seen.[107] A similar syndrome in a single family from Alamagordo, New Mexico, who consumed meat from hogs that were accidentally fed with grain treated with methyl mercury fungicide, has been reported.[108] Onset of intention tremor along with cerebellar signs has been reported in an agricultural worker after the worker consumed cereal seeds treated with mercury derivative.[109] Accidental acute mercury vapor poisoning with high mercury levels in blood and urine in 3 patients, resulting in tremor, severe pulmonary edema, and coma leading to death, has been reported.[110] Exposure to mercury vapor or mercury-gold amalgam resulted in tremor. Treatment of mercury intoxication is with chelating agent British anti-Lewisite (BAL). Use of *N*-acetyl-DL-penicillamine has been used.[111] Whether BAL alone is effective or penicillamine alone or in combination has not been established. Avoidance of further exposure is equally important.

Chronic exposure to manganese, usually among manganese miners or in an industry where manganese is processed, leads to rest tremor as part of parkinsonism. Manganese is absorbed through the lung and gastrointestinal tract.[106] Experimental animals treated with manganese developed tremor, rigidity, and incoordination. Depletion of dopamine from the basal ganglia is considered to be the underlying cause. In Chilean manganese miners, the incidence of extrapyramidal disease is considered to be 65 percent. In addition, a small number of patients may manifest cerebellar findings. Total parenteral nutritional feeding in a child resulted in tremors and seizures with elevated serum manganese levels. Withdrawal of manganese in the nutritional supplement resulted in full recovery.[112] Chelation is considered not to help in manganese intoxication.[113] L-Dopa showed a varied response.

Tremor is considered a clinical sign of chronic lead exposure. However, the type of tremor and its pathophysiological mechanisms are controversial. Lead neurotoxicity manifests mainly as encephalopathy with irritability, insomnia, memory loss, restlessness, confusion, and hallucinations. Leaded gasoline sniffing leading to lead toxicity in Navajo adolescents resulted in 31 percent having tremor and ataxia. In addition, their blood lead levels were elevated.[114] Twenty-three men with history of chronic lead exposure showed postural and kinetic tremor. EMG examination showed the frequency to be 12 Hz with characteristics of enhanced physiological tremor.[115] The treatment of choice in lead poisoning is chelation with calcium ethylenediaminetetraacetic acid (EDTA). Another single case of postural tremor is reported in a 15-year-old boy who inhaled gasoline for its euphoric effects.[116] Forty-eight of 50 (96 percent) children and adolescents who chronically sniffed leaded gasoline showed exaggerated deep reflexes, postural tremor, and evidence of cerebellar dysfunction. Forty-nine (98 percent) had blood lead levels greater than or equal to 40 µg/dL. The mean blood lead levels were significantly higher in those with abnormally brisk deep reflexes and with evidence of cerebellar dysfunction. Thirty-nine patients received chelation therapy. The neurological abnormalities resolved within 8 weeks in all but 1 patient.[117] When compared with nonsniffers, current sniffers of gasoline showed higher rates of abnormal tandem gait, rapid alternating hand movements, finger-to-nose movements, postural tremor, and brisk deep reflexes. Cognitive deficits occurred in the areas of visual attention, visual recognition memory and visual paired associate learning. Ex-sniffers showed higher rates of abnormal tandem gait and cognitive deficits in the areas of visual recognition memory, and pattern-location paired associate learning. Blood lead levels and length of time of gasoline sniffing correlated significantly with the magnitude of neurological and cognitive deficits. Blood hydrocarbon levels were not related to neurocognitive deficits, although this may have been due to methodological difficulties in obtaining hydrocarbon levels.[118]

INSECTICIDES AND HERBICIDES

Chlordecone (kepone), an organochlorine pesticide, is used as an ant and roach pesticide. Exposure to this pesticide in industrial workers resulted in occurrence of tremor. In the severely affected workers, tremor was present, even at rest, whereas, in those patients moderately affected, tremor was described as irregular and nonpurposive with a frequency of 12 Hz.[119] In addition, workers exhibited ataxia, weight loss, opsoclonus, pleuritic and joint pains, and abnormalities on liver function tests.[120] The tremors were reproducible in mice,[121] and rats.[122] Studies showed that norepinephrine may be involved in the expression of tremor induced by chlordecone.[123] Treatment consists of use of cholestyramine, an anion-exchange resin that would facilitate fecal excretion.[124]

Dichlorodiphenyltrichloroethane (DDT), a residual insecticide, was used worldwide to control mosquitoes, especially in endemic areas where malaria is prevalent, and banned in most places because of its carcinogenicity. DDT is known to produce tremor in experimental animals.[125,126] Inhaling the toxic fumigant, phosphine, 31 crew members aboard a grain freighter exhibited intention tremor, ataxia, diplopia, and other neurological manifestations.[127] Methylbromide is widely used as a fumigant and is known to produce tremor, ataxia, and myoclonus.[128] Dioxin (referred to as agent orange) exposure resulted in postural and intention tremor in 35 of 47 railroad workers during a chemical spillage after damage to a tank car filled with this herbicide.[41] Carbon disulfide, along with carbon tetrachloride, is used as a fumigant. Exposure in 21 grain workers resulted in about half of them developing parkinsonian features, along with resting tremor; the other half developed cerebellar syndrome associated with intention tremor.[129]

Poisoning from herbicides containing glufosinate ammonium used in Japan caused generalized tremor, and dysarthria.[130]

SOLVENTS

Exposure to solvents that contained toluene and methyl ethyl ketone during spray painting in a closed garage resulted in development of intention tremor and other cerebellar signs.[131] Toluene abuse in the form of lacquer sniffing in a 24-year-old man for 5 years resulted in development of tremor with cerebellar signs, with evidence of severe atrophy of cerebellar hemispheres, vermis, and brainstem, as well as mild atrophy of cerebral hemispheres on computed tomography (CT) scan.[132] Irreversible cholinesterase inhibitor soman, used as a nerve gas, is known to produce tremor.[133] In ship painters who were chronically exposed to high concentrations of solvents showed a syndrome of acquired blue-yellow color vision deficits, coarse tremor, impaired vibration sensation in the legs, and cognitive impairment.[134] A 30-year-old man with chronic toluene exposure developed visual impairment, horizontal nystagmus, pyramidal tract signs, postural tremor, and sensory disturbance below the level of T_2 dermatome. T_2-weighted images on magnetic resonance imaging (MRI) of the brain had a marked high-intensity appearance in the posterior limbs of the internal capsule, and in the posterior columns and lateral tracts from the cervical through the upper thoracic cord. The lesions probably reflect demyelination and axonal degeneration produced by chronic toluene abuse.[135]

Holmes' (Midbrain) Tremor

(Synonyms: midbrain tremor, rubral tremor, thalamic tremor, myorhythmia, and Benedikt's syndrome.)

The term "rubral" tremor has been used since 1904, when Holmes described a tremor of the fingers with rotation at wrist and elbow, as he believed that the rubrospinal tract was involved in production of this tremor based on observation of a patient with involvement of the rubrospinal tract in the pons.[136] Subsequent observation showed that the superior cerebellar tract or another cerebellar outflow system may be involved.[137] Studies in experimental animals have demonstrated that this tremor is caused by combined lesion of the red nucleus and neighboring structures.[138,139] However, the red nucleus itself has not been shown to be the source of abnormal oscillation; concomitant damage to the cerebellothalamic fibers and nigrostriatal dopaminergic fibers may be necessary.[21] Most clinical pathological correlations of midbrain tremor have described lesions in the upper brainstem. For this reason, the term midbrain tremor was proposed[140] and accepted by most authors, even though, for want of a better description, the tremor is named on the anatomic site of the lesion.[21,141] It is now believed that this tremor most likely is a result of interruptions of a combination of pathways in the midbrain tegmentum, namely rubro-olivocerebellorubral loop, rubrospinal fibers, dopaminergic nigrostriatal fibers, and the serotonergic brainstem telencephalic fibers.[141] For all these reasons, the tremor has been renamed Holmes' tremor as Holmes gave one of the first concise descriptions and the lesion may be present outside the midbrain.[1] The criteria for Holmes' tremor include rest and intention tremor with

TABLE 28-2 Causes of Holmes' (Midbrain) Tremor

Etiology	Location	Reference
Vascular	Occlusion of post communicating artery	141
	Embolic infarction of right thalamus and left cerebellum (vertebral/basilar artery distribution)	149
	Midbrain region ischemic infarct	150
	Bilateral thalamic infarction	151
	SCP, thalamus (hemorrhage)	142
	SCP (hemorrhage)	142
	SCP, thalamus (hemorrhage AVM)	142
	Subthalamus (hemorrhage)	152
Trauma	Midbrain	153
	SCP (gunshot injury)	142
	SCP and subthalamic region (hemorrhage)	142
	Midbrain	154
	Midbrain	153
	Multiple (punch-drunk syndrome)	141
	SCP, midbrain	146
	Closed head injury nonlocalized (tremor precipitated by neuroleptic)	85
Infection	Midbrain (tuberculoma)	155
	Midbrain (toxoplasma abscess)	137
Multiple sclerosis	Midbrain (demyelination)	156
Neoplastic	Midbrain	156
Radiation	Irradiation of pineal region vascular hamartoma	157

SCP, superior cerebellar peduncle.

a slow frequency of less than 4.5 Hz. The tremor is sometimes irregular in presentation and is often not rhythmic. In many patients postural tremor is also present.

While resting, the amplitude may be small, but, on attempting posture, it becomes uncontrollable, and, on attempting movement (kinetic), the amplitude may be at the peak degree. Occasionally, the tremor at rest can be quite large and irregular and may increase during certain sustained posture. During active movement there may be further terminal acceleration.[141] The proximal muscles may be affected more than the distal muscle, unlike in most other forms of tremor. In addition, there are usually other signs of midbrain damage, such as hemiparesis and cranial nerve palsy. PET and pathoanatomic studies have suggested involvement of the dopaminergic system, and the cerebellothalamic system must be involved for Holmes' tremor to occur.[1] Table 28-2 lists various causes that produce midbrain tremor.

Treatment of Holmes' tremor is generally considered difficult, and spontaneous improvement may occur. Of the various drug treatments tested, response to L-dopa, as reported by Findley and Gresty[142] and, more recently, by Ramy et al.,[143] found that L-dopa with dopa decarboxylase inhibitor showed fair-to-significant improvement. Others found L-dopa disappointing.[144] Clonazepam,[145] a combination of valproic acid and propranolol,[140] anticholinergics,[85,146] and bromocriptine,[85] are reported to be effective. Unfortunately, these are all single case reports or open trials done on a small number of patients, and no controlled studies have been done due to rarity of the disorder. Because of the nature of the underlying pathology, patients with Holmes' tremor

frequently have a shortened life-expectancy.[21] Patients with a long-standing tremor and stable medical illness may be considered for stereotactic thalamotomy or thalamic stimulation in nucleus ventralis intermedius, as significant reduction of tremor has been reported as a result of this procedure.[29,147,148]

Primary Orthostatic Tremor

In orthostatic tremor, also referred to as "shaky leg syndrome," first described by Heilman,[165] there is a subjective feeling of unsteadiness during standing, usually for over 10 seconds. Only in severe cases may fall occur rarely during walking. Standing may induce visible or palpable fine-amplitude ripping in the leg muscles (gastrocnemius or quadriceps). The diagnosis can be confirmed by a surface EMG recording of the above muscles with the patient standing with a typical 13–18-Hz pattern. Similar tremor can be recorded in all leg and trunk muscles, with the tremor disappearing when patient sits or lies down.[1] Walking, sitting, and lying were unaffected. Standing involved a wide base, but gait was normal. There are no other abnormal neurological signs or symptoms. Patients find it harder to stand still, and are forced to take a step to regain balance. Falls and injuries are uncommon, as patients start moving as soon as the sense of imbalance occurs. Within any individual patient the frequency of tremor remains unchanged in all of the muscles examined. The age of onset may vary from the third through

TABLE 28-3 Differences between Orthostatic Tremor and Essential Tremor

	Orthostatic Tremor	Essential Tremor
Age of onset	Late	Early (adult)
Family history of tremor	Rare	Common
Occurrence	Standing	Postural
Legs affected	Always	Rarely
Tremor frequency	14–16 Hz	6–8 Hz
Paraspinal muscle effected	Always	Rarely
Response to		
Alcohol	0	+++
Propranolol	0	+++
Clonazepam	++	+
Phenobarbital	++	++
Primidone	++	++
L-Dopa	++	0
Pramipexole	++	0
Gabapentin	+++	+

0, absent; +, fair response; ++, good response; + + +, excellent response.
SOURCE: Refs. 158–164.

seventh decades of life, with the majority of the patients developing the symptoms in the sixth or seventh decades of life. Men and women seem to be affected equally. Family history of tremor is present only in a small number of patients.[166] The condition is rare. The etiology of this condition is unknown, and the question has been raised as to whether orthostatic tremor is a variant of essential tremor.[159,167] However, there is a considerable difference between the two forms of tremor (Table 28-3), and the general consensus is that the two are separate entities. Symptomatic orthostatic tremor in pontine lesions is reported.[168] Case reports of successful response to clozapine, phenobarbital, primidone, L-dopa, pramipexole,

and valproic acid have been reported, whereas response to propranolol and ethanol remain unsatisfactory.[169] In a placebo-controlled, double-blind, crossover trial, 3 of 4 patients had complete suppression, and the remaining 1 had significant reduction, of orthostatic tremor on gabapentin (dose range 300–2400 mg/day).[160]

Palatal Tremor

What was formerly called palatal myoclonus (synonyms: rhythmic palatal myoclonus, oculopalatal myoclonus, palatal nystagmus, brainstem myorhythmia, and palatal myorhythmia) has been renamed palatal tremor. This reclassification more accurately describes the condition.[171] Palatal tremor is divided into two distinct clinical entities: symptomatic palatal tremor, in which rhythmic movements of the soft palate (levator veli palatini) and often other brainstem-innervated or extremity muscles. Symptoms are preceded by brainstem/cerebellar lesion with subsequent hypertrophic degeneration of inferior olive. In essential palatal tremor, patients often complain of a rhythmic ear click. The rhythmic movements of the soft palate mainly involve the tensor veli palatini. No involvement of extremity or eye muscles occurs. No lesions of brainstem, cerebellum, and olive are known. Table 28-4 gives the criteria for symptomatic and essential forms of palatal tremor. Here, only the symptomatic form will be discussed.

Symptomatic palatal tremor often is a result of an underlying neurological abnormality, such as a previous brainstem stroke, multiple sclerosis, trauma, or degenerative disease. Thus, it is not surprising that the most consistent clinical finding in these patients is a unilateral or bilateral

TABLE 28-4 Criteria for Symptomatic and Essential Forms of Palatal Tremor

Criteria	Symptomatic Palatal Tremor	Essential Palatal Tremor
Cause	Cerebrovascular disease, degenerative disease, encephalitis, multiple sclerosis, trauma	Unknown
Anamnestic or clinical evidence of brainstem or cerebellar disease	Present	Absent
Presenting symptoms	Oscillopsia and others related to brainstem or cerebellar disease	Ear clicks
Involvement of muscle groups other than soft palate	Frequently	Rarely
Involvement of eyes	Frequently	Never
Involvement of extremities	Rarely	Never
Involvement of soft palatal muscles	Levator veli palatini	Tensor veli palatini
Activation of brainstem motor nuclei	Ambiguous nucleus or facial nucleus	Trigeminal nucleus
Cessation of symptoms during sleep	No	Yes
Remote effects of palatal tremor on tonic EMG activity	Unilateral or bilateral	None
Brainstem reflexes	Often abnormal, indicating focal brainstem disease	Normal or nonspecific abnormalities
MRI	Inferior olive abnormality	Normal

From Ref. 170 with permission.

cerebellar syndrome. On MRI scan (provided it is done with a high-field scanner with specific proton density and a T_2-weighted series), unilateral or bilateral hyperintense signals in the upper medulla, consistent with the gliosis representing olivary pseudohypertrophy,[170] which is considered the hallmark for symptomatic palatal tremor, are seen. When unilateral olivary abnormality is seen, palatal tremor and cerebellar signs are present contralateral to the side of olivary hypertrophy. Sleep does not abolish symptomatic palatal tremor. Symptomatic palatal tremor results from activation of levator veli palatini muscle, which is innervated by the seventh or ninth cranial nerves. Frequency of palatal tremor is 2 Hz, which is the range of normal firing frequency of inferior olive cells.[172] The tremor rhythm in symptomatic palatal tremor is highly resistant to both external and internal inferences.[173,174] Improvement of palatal tremor following administration of a calcium entry blocking agent, flunarizine, is reported.[175] Botulinum toxin A injected into each tensor veli palatini is reported to be of benefit.[176]

Peripheral Neuropathy-Associated Tremor

Tremors develop in patients with some forms of peripheral neuropathy more often than others. A variety of tremors has been described in patients with peripheral neuropathy. These include rest tremors, postural tremors, and intention tremors.[177–179] The tremor seen in peripheral neuropathy has been described as irregular, rhythmic, proximal, or distal, with a frequency ranging from 3–10 Hz.[21] Peripheral neuropathies cause slowing of the nerve conduction. No relationship between the degree of conduction velocity and sensory loss has been found.[178,180] Slowing of nerve conduction would increase the delay in stretch reflex, and this may lead to enhancement of tremor.[181] It was suggested that tremor associated with peripheral neuropathy may be an enhancement of physiological tremor secondary to weakness.[180] This hypothesis has been disputed.[182] It was hypothesized that generation of tremor in peripheral neuropathy may be the result of an abnormality in the central nervous system. However, most patients with peripheral neuropathy show normal CT/MRI scans and routine cerebrospinal fluid examination. In dogs (Scottish terriers) with whole-body tremor and ataxia, widespread axonal changes, vacuolation, and gliosis in the white matter of central nervous system were seen at autopsy.[183] Such changes in humans with varieties of peripheral neuropathy have not been reported.

Table 28-5 lists tremor occurring in various peripheral neuropathies. Presence of tremor in Charcot-Marie-Tooth disease was named Roussy-Lévy syndrome. Currently, it is classified as hereditary motor sensory neuropathy (HMSN) type I. Marie observed presence of tremor in HMSN.[184] A detailed evaluation in HMSN type I revealed that tremor was present in 40 percent of patients. The time from appearance of tremor until onset of disease was 16 years, and the tremor involved

TABLE 28-5 Tremor in Peripheral Neuropathy

Hereditary motor and sensory neuropathy type I (HMSN type I)
Chronic inflammatory demyelinating polyneuropathy (CIDP)
Immunoglobulin M (IgM) chronic paraproteinemic demyelinating polyneuropathy
Guillain-Barré syndrome (recovery stage)
Diabetic neuropathy
Uremic neuropathy
Neuropathy associated with porphyria
Amiodarone can cause both tremor and peripheral neuropathy
Neuropathy associated with alcoholism

From Ref. 181 with permission.

mostly hand, followed by arms, legs, and head. Tremor was mostly postural, with rest components but no parkinsonian features. Some patients reported improvement of tremor with alcohol, and some indicated improvement with propranolol. The authors considered that the pattern of tremor seen in HMSN type I resembles essential tremor. Perhaps HMSN type I and essential tremor are related by linkage of a common gene.[185]

In chronic demyelinating polyneuropathy with IgM paraproteinemia, the incidence of tremor is considered to be 47 percent.[181] Tremor is often mild, postural, and seen in the hands. When the amplitude is prominent, tremor may be more disabling than weakness. Treatment with gabapentin is reported to be effective.[186] A range of incidence (3–84 percent) of tremor in chronic sensorimotor neuropathy (CIDP) has been reported. Tremor may appear during relapse and disappear during remission. Tremor subsides with treatment of CIDP with corticosteroid therapy, either alone or in combination with cytotoxic drug, or plasma exchange.[181] In other conditions of peripheral neuropathy associated with tremor, symptomatic treatment with beta-blockers and other drugs used in essential tremor can be tried. When peripheral neuropathy and essential tremor coexist, it may be difficult to establish the etiology unless essential tremor was clearly present prior to development of symptoms and signs of peripheral neuropathy. Tremor can also be seen in peripheral neuropathy associated with diabetes mellitus, uremia, and during the recovery phase of Guillain-Barré syndrome and treatment with amiodarone. Symptomatic treatment with drugs used in the treatment of essential tremor may be attempted in tremor associated with peripheral neuropathy.

Psychogenic Tremors

Occurrence of tremor as a manifestation of hysteria has been known for over a century.[187] Koller et al.[188] reported a more detailed study and established diagnostic criteria (Table 28-6). As with all the psychogenic disorders, psychogenic tremor has higher incidence in females than males, and, while any age is susceptible, it is seldom reported in children.

TABLE 28-6 Clinical Features of Psychogenic Tremor

Abrupt onset
Static course
Spontaneous remissions
Unclassifiable tremors (complex tremors)
Clinical inconsistencies (selective disabilities)
Changing tremor characteristics
Unresponsiveness to antitremor drugs
Tremor increases with attention
Tremor lessens with distractibility
Responsiveness to placebo
Absence of other neurologic signs
Remission with psychotherapy
Multiple somatizations
Multiple undiagnosed conditions
Spontaneous remissions or cures of symptoms
Presence of unphysiologic weakness or sensory complaints
No evidence of disease by laboratory or radiographic procedures
Presence of unwitnessed paroxysmal disorders
Employed in allied health professions
Litigation or compensation pending
Presence of secondary gain
Presence of psychiatric disease
Documented functional disturbances in the past

From Ref. 188 with permission.

The onset is often abrupt with fluctuating severity and is nonprogressive. Tremor is generally bilateral with a mixture of frequencies and patterns. Activities of daily living are not impaired; patients will appear well-groomed, but when asked to demonstrate, significant changes in handwriting and other tasks can be seen. Symptoms present usually when attention is given to the patient, either during clinical examination or by family members, and disappears when attention is drawn to some other task or when the patient is alone. Tremor can be kinetic, postural, or resting but lacks the physiological pattern; for example, postural tremor may be of higher amplitude than the kinetic tremor. The direction of tremor may change from supination-pronation orientation to one of flexion-extension.[188] On the other hand, the amplitude may be strikingly consistent in all positions, a pattern rarely encountered in tremor of organic origin. Often, there is a history of symptoms for a year or longer before the patient seeks medical attention. Details in the history are vague and the patient may become hostile when details are inquired into. Location of the tremor and the pattern may vary from one visit to another. Additional nonphysiological neurological findings may or may not be present, such as split tuning-fork test, clearly detectable physiological weakness, or other sensory changes.

In one large series of 70 patients the incidence of psychogenic tremors usually started abruptly in 73 percent, with the maximal disability at onset in 46 percent that had static course in 46 percent and fluctuating course in 17 percent.[189] Tremorgram recording may reveal marked fluctuation in amplitude and frequency during the same run, a feature

not seen in organic tremors. EMG recordings are of limited diagnostic utility as, for example, when tremor is voluntarily produced an alternating pattern of antagonist muscle interaction can be produced. Pharmacological therapy in organic tremor may reduce amplitude, seldom by 100 percent, but does not alter tremor frequency.[48,190] The effect of therapy in psychogenic tremor may be varied from total suppression of tremor (by placebo effect), especially when associated with the suggestion of a "cure," to no benefit. Some patients may refuse to take medication or, after a short trial, stop the medication with a complaint of side-effects or ineffectiveness. Psychogenic tremor is generally not a diagnosis of exclusion. The presence of characteristic features on history and especially clinical examination can permit an accurate diagnosis and avoid unnecessary investigations. Some patients respond to psychotherapeutic suggestion or placebo treatment. In a small number of patients, psychogenic tremor may be superimposed on other conditions with a preexisting disorder in which tremor is part of the disease, such as Parkinson's disease, and a clear distinction between the psychogenic segment and underlying disease segment may not always be easy to make. It is equally important to realize that all tremors can be exaggerated by anxiety.

Rest Tremor

Rest tremor occurs in a body part that is not voluntarily activated and is completely supported against gravity. Although rest tremor is a descriptive term, it is included in this section because, in addition to parkinsonism, rest tremor can occur in several other conditions (Table 28-7). The most common anatomic site for rest tremor is the distal parts of the upper limbs. It can also be seen in lower extremities and, less commonly, in lips, tongue, and jaw.[191] The characteristic upper limb rest tremor includes pronation-supination of the forearm, flexion-extension of the wrist, or "pill-rolling" movement of the thumb, producing a gliding movement across the first two or three fingers.[192] The rest tremor amplitude increases when movement of another body part is performed, such as walking or under mental stress. Frequency of rest tremor is 4–5.3 Hz, varying only by 0.2–0.3 Hz from person to person.[193] Rest tremor is produced by the alternate contraction of antagonistic muscles.[194] Experimental studies in lesioned monkeys suggest that, for parkinsonism, rest tremor involves ascending nigrostriatal dopaminergic pathway, rubrotegmentospinal fibers, and rubro-olivodentatorubral loop that normally modifies the input into the ventrolateral nucleus of the thalamus.[195] It is a physiologically and clinically separate entity, probably generated by mechanisms unique to this symptom. Studies have shown that rest tremors are a social handicap but do not correlate with the disability or performance items when the tremor is mild-to-moderate; rather, when the tremor is severe, it can interfere with these items. Monosymptomatic rest tremor is a rare condition

TABLE 28-7 Conditions that Cause Rest Tremor

	Number of Patients Studied*	Percent with Rest Tremor	Reference
Idiopathic Parkinson's disease	81	83	
Infarct with striatum			
Thalamic infarct			
Progressive supranuclear palsy	Literature review + author's 5 patients	12–16	
Postencephalopathic			
Multiple system atrophy	100	29	
Olivopontocerebellar atrophy			
Diffuse Lewy body disease	8	29	
Chronic demyelinating polyneuropathy with benign IgM paraproteinemia			
Chronic inflammatory demyelinating neuropathy			
Psychogenic			
Brainstem infarction with palatal tremor	5	80	
Midbrain hemorrhage	1		
Orofacial dystonia	1		
Large subdural hematoma	1		**
Large frontotemporal meningioma	1		

*Blanks indicate that the number of patients was not stated.
**Author's unpublished observation.

where isolated rest tremor is present without other parkinsonian signs such as bradykinesia, rigidity, gait disturbance that is sufficient to diagnose parkinsonism. Despite this isolated finding, PET revealed dopaminergic deficiency.[196]

Parkinson rest tremor may be difficult to control. Controlled-release propranolol hydrochloride (160 mg) reduced the amplitude of rest tremor by 70 percent,[208] anticholinergics and carbidopa/L-dopa by 50 percent, and amantadine by 25 percent.[209] Subcutaneous apomorphine is found to be effective in reducing amplitude by more than 50 percent.[210] Thalamotomy produces a sustained reduction in contralateral rest tremor in at least 85 percent of patients. The optimal site for lesioning is the vastus anterior medialis of the thalamus. Deep brain stimulation may be the treatment of choice when the tremor is severe and pharmacotherapy is not effective or not tolerated and the tremor is disabling.

Stroke-Associated Tremor

The development of tremor subsequent to a thalamic stroke has been known since the time of Dejerine and Roussy.[211] Isolated tremor as a result of stroke is rare. In a review of 62 cases of movement disorders associated with focal lesion in the thalamus and subthalamus, no case of isolated tremor was found.[212] In lesions confined to thalamus, 6 cases of tremor with a postural and kinetic component have been described.[150,213–216] Moroo et al.[217] described 3 patients with postural and kinetic tremor with a frequency of 3–4 Hz whose brain MRI scans showed an ischemic lesion in the midthalamus. Ferbert and Gerwig[218] described 4 patients

with tremor, among whom 3 had associated dystonia and 1 hemiparesis. Dethy et al.[198] reported a patient with pure motor stroke associated with hemibody tremor involving right upper and lower extremities. Tremor frequency was 5–6 Hz. MRI scan showed ischemic lesion in the left centrum semiovale and the left caudate nucleus. PET scan showed glucose hypermetabolism in the ipsilateral sensory motor cortex. Thalamic ataxia syndrome, in which there are significant cerebellar signs, may be associated with intention tremor. Kim,[219] in a prospective study of 35 patients with delayed onset of movement disorder following thalamic infarct, found that action tremor was not an isolated phenomenon but was often accompanied by dystonia-athetosis-chorea. A case of spontaneous tremor following thalamic/subthalamic infarct that subsided in 24 hours is reported.[220] On occasion, acute poststroke movement disorder including tremor may last only a few hours (author's unreported observation). Holmes' (midbrain) tremor, with its classical appearance secondary to stroke, is included in Table 28-2.

Tremor occurring immediately after a stroke seems to have a better prognosis than tremor with delayed onset.[218] Because tremor is not usually an isolated phenomenon and there are associated neurological deficits, treatment needs to address all segments of a patient's disability. A case of "yes-yes" head tremor following right occipital and bilateral cerebellar infarction that responded to botulinum toxin A is reported.[24] However, in general when there is an associated cerebellar component with the tremor, pharmacotherapy is disappointing. In the absence of a cerebellar component, attempts at treatment may be made by using drugs that are used in the treatment of essential tremor. No controlled studies have been done, so the only approach is to use one drug at a time, reaching the maximum dose and trying another when the previous one is proven to be ineffective.

Tremor in Systemic Disorders and Diseases

AIDS

Unilateral postural and action tremor resulting from thalamic toxoplasmosis in a patient with AIDS is reported.[221] There appears to be a high incidence of tremor when patients with AIDS are treated with trimethoprim-sulfamethoxazole.[222]

HEREDITARY HEMOCHROMATOSIS

Neurologic manifestations are rarely described in hereditary hemochromatosis. The putative role of abnormal iron load remains to be ascertained. Arm and head tremor are reported to occur. Phlebotomies and symptomatic treatments may not change the course of the disease.[223]

HYPOXIA/HYPOTENSION

Tremor seen in acute hypoxia is activated physiologic tremor (8–12 Hz). The amplitude of tremor may be higher in hypocapnic hypoxia than during eucapnic hypoxia.[224] Prolonged hypotension may induce localized delayed anoxic lesions in basal ganglia resulting in postural tremor along with bradykinesia, and gait disturbance. MRI showed low signal intensities in the bilateral caudate nuclei and putamen on the T_1-weighted image and high signal intensities on the T_2-weighted images. PET scan with ^{18}F-FDG revealed a severe decrease in glucose metabolism in bilateral basal ganglia.[225]

PORPHYRIA

Presence of tremor is reported in variegate porphyria.[226] Plasma exchange or erythrocytapheresis may not show any beneficial effects on the clinical or laboratory abnormalities.

THYROID DISORDERS

Tremor is a well-known symptom of thyrotoxicosis. Tremor in thyrotoxicosis is an enhanced physiological tremor that cannot be separated clinically or by an EMG examination. Both types of tremor have similar mechanisms and can be distinguished only by the circumstances responsible for their occurrence and presence of other signs and symptoms related to that particular disorder. Only a moderate correlation between tremor intensity and thyroid hormone level is known.[227] Successful treatment of thyrotoxicosis results in

dramatic improvement of tremor. Tremor can also occur in hypothyroidism that often is associated with other cerebellar signs.

WILSON'S DISEASE

Tremor as an initial manifestation of Wilson's disease occurred in 13–32 percent of patients.[228,229] Because of its relative rarity, the initial manifestation may be hepatic or neurological and the diagnosis may be easily missed. With chelation therapy, dramatic improvement of tremor is reported.[230] One patient presented with dystonic tremor.[231]

Task-Specific Tremor

Task-specific tremors are a rare form of tremor that involves skilled, highly learned motor acts. The tremor occurs only when performing a specific repetitive task unique to each individual. Examples include hair-cutting, shaving, putting on make-up, combing hair, use of tools, sewing, use of scissors, golf club swinging, playing a musical instrument, and other activities. Goal-directed movement or certain posture does not often reduce tremor. Generally, no other associated neurological signs and symptoms are present with the exception of focal dystonia. The frequency of tremor is 5–7 Hz.[232] EMG has shown both an alternating and roughly synchronous pattern in the antagonistic muscles, but the alternating pattern appears to be more common.[232]

Primary writing tremor is the most common form of task-specific tremor that occurs predominantly during writing but not during other hand tasks. Primary writing tremor was first described by Rothwell et al. in a 20-year-old man who presented with tremor while writing.[233] Active pronation of his hand produced several beats of pronation-supination tremor. A burst of tremor could also be elicited by tendon taps to the volar surface of the wrist, to the finger extensors, to pectoralis major, and by means of forcible supination of the wrist delivered by torte motor. The subject's writing difficulty and tremor were temporarily abolished by partial motor point anesthesia of pronator teres. The frequency of this tremor was 4 Hz, and EMG revealed tremor in the muscle toward the forearm and arm. Primary writing tremor is considered a form of focal dystonia.[232,234,235] The clinical characteristics of primary writing tremor and focal dystonia of hand (writer's cramp and other occupational cramps) are similar in several respects, as both conditions are more or less task-specific and are not inherited. Patients with primary writing tremor often do not exhibit dystonia. On the other hand, tremor is known to occur in focal dystonia.[236] PET studies of regional cerebral blood flow on voluntary wrist oscillations of control subjects produced ipsilateral cerebellar activation. Patients with primary writing tremor displayed bilateral cerebellar activation only, whereas those with essential tremor displayed bilateral cerebellar activation and activation in red nucleus and thalamus.[237] Two forms of primary writing tremor have been described. Task-induced tremor is characterized by tremor appearing during writing only (type A, task-specific tremor). If it occurs when the hand adopts a writing position, the terms position-specific or position-sensitive tremor (type B) have been used. [238]

Several authors have argued that task-specific tremor is a variant of essential tremor.[234,239,240] However, although essential tremor is generally inherited in an autosomal-dominant fashion, task-specific tremor is most often sporadic. Clinical and neurophysiological characteristics of task-specific tremor compared to essential tremor are too varied. Essential tremor often responds to ethanol, propranolol, and others but not to anticholinergics, whereas these drugs are not as effective in task-specific tremor.

Oral pharmacological treatment for task-specific tremor is disappointing. Botulinum toxin injections have been used with success.[241] Stereotactic selective thalamotomy centered mainly on the nucleus ventralis intermedius has also been successfully used in treatment of this condition.[242] More recently, thalamic stimulation with the electrode lead implanted in the nucleus ventralis intermedius resulted in nearly complete control of primary writing tremor.[243]

Posttraumatic Tremor

In recent times, the definition of trauma has been broadened to include conditions other than those resulting from extrinsic physical injury. Thus, terms such as emotional trauma, metabolic trauma, psychic trauma, and intrinsic trauma (i.e., rupture of an aneurysm, ischemic infarct, etc.) are being used. In this section, trauma will refer to physical trauma, such as injury to a structure that was previously intact. An artificial separation of central versus peripheral injury will also be made, even as we remain fully aware of the intimate relationship between the central and peripheral nervous systems. When tremor is noted with a past history of injury, there is always an interval of days to years before onset of the tremor. Additionally, there are often associated neurological findings, such as rigidity, hemiparesis, reflex sympathetic dystrophy, etc., so tremor generally does not occur in isolation. Tremor does not have a specific anatomic location in the nervous system, because it can occur from lesions of the cerebral cortex, basal ganglia, thalamus, midbrain, cerebellum, and peripheral nerves. Widespread possibilities exist. CT or MRI scan may not show lesions that are tiny and at a cellular or subcellular level. In light of these factors and limitations, one can still find evidence in the literature of tremor being precipitated or caused by various injuries. For an excellent review the reader is referred to Curren and Lang.[244]

Most cases of tremor resulting from severe head injury are believed to result from damage to the midbrain. However, in addition to the typical midbrain tremor discussed above, other forms of tremor are well recognized. The association of head trauma with parkinsonism was made in 1929.[245] A year earlier, parkinsonian symptoms, including rest tremor associated with "punch drunk" syndrome caused by multiple head injuries in boxers, were studied.[246] Subsequently, more clear cases of parkinsonism with known head injury were studied.[247–249] Tremor developing after minor head injury with no loss of consciousness or other neurological deficits was investigated.[145] Tremor was asymmetric with postural and kinetic components. Tremor occurred after sudden twisting of the neck that resulted in an intimal tear of the carotid artery, leading to an embolic infarct.[250] An 18-year-old girl, in a diving accident at a swimming pool, developed ipsilateral tremor in the right upper and lower extremities. The tremor had a kinetic component. The MRI scan showed a lesion in the left ventral lateral thalamus.[251]

Tremor resulting from peripheral nerve injury is rare. There are often other associated neurological abnormalities, such as dystonia or reflex sympathetic dystrophy. In one study of 43 patients with movement disorders associated with reflex sympathetic dystrophy described by Schwartzman and Kerrigan,[252] only 38 demonstrated a history of injury. Deuschl et al.[253] found that 12 of their 21 patients showed a distal tremor with a mean frequency of 7.2 Hz, and those researchers considered it as enhanced physiological tremor. On treatment of reflex sympathetic dystrophy, the tremor completely disappeared. Only 4 of the 23 patients who had tremor did not have reflex sympathetic dystrophy, and 1 of 5 patients with reflex sympathetic dystrophy had tremor in a series reported by Jankovic and Van der Linden.[254] Entrapment of the ulnar nerve in Guyon's canal resulted in development of a tremor in the 4th and 5th fingers with disappearance of tremor after surgery in a secretary/typist subjected to repeated hand movement.[255] This has illustrated the possibility that peripheral trauma could induce tremor. Pathophysiological mechanisms underlying these phenomena are not entirely known, but functional changes in afferent neuronal input to the spinal cord and secondary affection of higher brainstem and subcortical centers are probably involved.[256]

As far as treatment for tremor from central or peripheral trauma is concerned, treating the cause is the key. When the cause can be identified, treatment is often beneficial. Such is the case for compression neuropathy or reflex sympathetic dystrophy. However, where a cause cannot be found or where other associated conditions are present, such as lesion of the midbrain, conventional (pharmacological) therapies have been less than satisfactory. Stereotactic thalamotomy has been tried with success.[147,250] In one long-term follow-up study of patients who developed tremor secondary to trauma, 88 percent showed spontaneous improvement over a period of time with no intervention, and the authors suggested that the surgery be restricted to select cases of disabling tremor.[148] Numerous medications have been studied in the treatment of posttraumatic tremor with variable results. Posttraumatic tremor may respond to clonazepam,[257] propranolol[145,258] alone, or in combination with valproic acid.[259]

Vocal Tremor

Vocal tremor (synonyms: voice, tremulous voice, wavy voice, or tremulous, quivering speech) is defined as involuntary, rhythmic, oscillatory movements that affect the vocal musculature in patients with tremulous diseases. The muscles of the sound production mechanism may also be affected, and rhythm alterations in pitch and loudness may be generated.[260] The "prime generator" of vocal tremor is central nervous system disturbance; the phonatory reflection is typically multifactorial, involving a combination of the extrinsic and intrinsic laryngeal muscles, pharyngeal muscles (including that of the supraglottic structure), and auxiliary respiratory muscles, including the intercostal abdominal muscles and the diaphragm.[260] The frequency of vocal tremor may range from 4 to 8 Hz, with amplitudes of oscillation ranging widely.[261–265] Acoustic analysis has been the primary noninvasive method for quantification of vocal tremor, with most acoustic data obtained by visual inspection of oscillographic displays of the waveform data or graphic record displays of amplitude contours of sustained oral phonation. As a result, the bulk of acoustic data on vocal tremor includes visual quantifiable amplitude oscillations without frequency modulation components.[260,261,264,266,267] Vocal tremor occurs in Parkinson's disease[268] at an incidence rate of 30.5 percent.[269] The tremor frequency is reported to range from 5 to 7 Hz.[247] Despite the recognition of vocal tremor in Parkinson's disease, hypophonia is often the major problem. Vocal tremor is characterized by rhythmic alterations of pitch and loudness of vowels and in some cases with voice arrests, especially during vowel prolongation.[261,264,271]

Mild vocal tremor may be masked during contextual speech[271] and is referred to as essential vocal tremor. Eleven percent of patients with essential tremor are known to suffer from vocal tremor.[272] In a double-blind study, clonazepam, propranolol, and diazepam treatments were effective for vocal and hand tremor, based on clinical and electrophysiological examinations, although hand tremor was more responsive to these drugs.[273] Koller et al. did not find propranolol beneficial in seven patients, compared to placebo in vocal tremor.[274] Koda and Ludlow[273] found that the thyroarytenoid muscle was affected in vocal tremor and suggested that botulinum toxin injections may be beneficial in treating this disorder.

In cerebellar diseases, dysarthria and vocal tremor occur simultaneously.[261,275] Vocal tremor frequency in cerebellar diseases is reported to be 3 Hz, which is similar to that reported for cerebellar and kinetic postural tremor.[276]

In isolated vocal tremor, vocalization is tremulous but no other parts of the body show tremor. It occurs in two variants. The first form is often considered as a form of focal dystonia of the vocal cords, the second form a variant of essential tremor.[1] In the differential diagnoses of vocal tremor, idiopathic spasmodic dysphonia should be considered. In abductor spasmodic dysphonia caused by intermittent abduction of the vocal folds, patients exhibit a breathy effortful voice quality with abrupt termination of voicing, resulting in aphonic, whispered segments of speech. In adductor spasmodic dysphonia caused by irregular hyperabduction of the vocal folds, patients exhibit a choked, strained-strangled vocal quality, with abrupt initiation and termination of voicing, resulting in short breaks in phonation. Some patients can have a combination of the two. Because many patients with spasmodic dysphonia present with a tremulous voice, differential diagnosis between isolated vocal tremor and spasmodic dysphonia may be difficult. Both respond to botulinum treatment. Following bilateral deep brain stimulation of the thalamus, the vocal tremor significantly improved in a single patient.[254]

Acknowledgment

Manuscript preparation help of Angie McReynolds Hitt and Glen Cryer is greatly appreciated.

References

1. Deuschl G, Bain P, Brin M: Consensus Statement of the Movement Disorder Society on Tremor. Ad Hoc Scientific Committee. *Mov Disord* 13(suppl 3):2 1998.
2. Fahn S: Cerebellar tremor: Clinical aspects, in Findley LJ, Capildeo R (eds): *Movement Disorders: Tremor.* London: Macmillan, 1984, pp 355–363.
3. Fox JR, Randall JE: Relationship between forearm tremor and the biceps electromyogram. *J Appl Physiol* 29:103, 1970.
4. Elble RJ, Randall JE: Mechanistic components of normal hand tremor. *Electroencephalogr Clin Neurophysiol* 44:72, 1978.
5. Matthews PBC, Muir RB: Comparison of electromyogram spectra with force spectra during human elbow tremor. *J Physiol (Lond)* 302:427, 1980.
6. Elble RJ, Randall JE: Motor-unit activity responsible for 8- to 12-Hz component of human physiological finger tremor. *J Neurophysiol* 39:370, 1976.
7. Sutton GG, Sykes K: The variation of hand tremor with force in healthy subjects. *J Physiol (Lond)* 191:699, 1967.
8. Sakamoto K, Nishida K, Zhou L, et al: Characteristics of physiological tremor in five fingers and evaluations of fatigue of fingers in typing. *Ann Physiol Anthropol* 11:61, 1992.
9. Elke-Okoro ST: Explanation of physiological muscle tremor. *Electromyogr Clin Neurophysiol* 34:341, 1994.
10. Pizzuti GP, Byford GH, Cifaldi S, et al: Finger tremor and the central nervous system. *J Biomed Eng* 14:356, 1992.
11. Comby B, Chevalier G, Bouchoucha M: A new method for the measurement of tremor at rest. *Arch Int Physiol Biochim Biophys* 100:73, 1992.
12. Lakie M, Frymann K, Villagra F, Jakeman P: The effect of alcohol on physiological tremor. *Exp Physiol* 79:273, 1994.
13. Hagbarth K-E, Young RR: Participation of the stretch reflex in human physiological tremor. *Brain* 102:509, 1979.
14. Young RR, Hagbarth K-E: Physiological tremor enhanced by maneuvers affecting the segmental stretch reflex. *J Neurol Neurosurg Psychiatry* 43:248, 1980.

15. Koller W, Cone S, Herbster G: Caffeine and tremor. *Neurology* 37:169, 1987.

16. Abila B, Wilson JF, Marshall RW, Richens A: The tremorolytic action of beta-adrenoceptor blockers in essential, physiological and isoprenaline-induced tremor is mediated by beta-adrenoceptors located in a deep peripheral compartment. *Br J Clin Pharmacol* 20:369, 1985.

17. Zilm DH: The effect of propranolol on normal physiologic tremor. *Electroencephalogr Clin Neurophysiol* 41:310, 1976.

18. Monso A, Barbal F, Riudeubas J, et al: Electromyographic characteristics of postanesthetic tremor. *Esp Anestesiol Reanim* 324, 1997.

19. Ikeda A, Kakigi A, Funai N, et al: Cortical tremor: A variant of cortical reflex myoclonus. *Neurology* 40:1561, 1990.

20. Toro C, Pascual-Leone A, Deuschl G, et al: Cortical tremor: A common manifestation of cortical myoclonus. *Neurology* 43:2346, 1993.

21. Elble RJ, Koller WC: *Tremor*. Baltimore: The Johns Hopkins University Press, 1990.

22. Rondot P, Bathein N: Motor control in cerebellar tremor, in Findley LJ, Capideo R (eds): *Movement Disorders: Tremor*. London: Macmillan, 1984, pp 366–376.

23. Thach WT, Goodkin HP, Keating JG: The cerebellum and the adaptive coordination of movement. *Annu Rev Neurosci* 15:403, 1992.

24. Finsterer J, Muellbacher W, Mamoli B: Yes/yes head tremor without appendicular tremor after bilateral cerebellar infarction. *J Neurol Sci* 139:242, 1996.

25. Lin JJ, Chang DC: Delayed onset of hand tremor related to cerebellar hemorrhage. *Mov Disord* 14:189, 1999.

26. Brown P, Rothwell JC, Stevens JM, et al: Cerebellar axial postural tremor. *Mov Disord* 12:977, 1997.

27. Manyam BV: Recent advances in the treatment of ataxia. *J Clin Neuropharmacol* 9:508, 1986.

28. Manyam BV: Ataxia, in Klawans HL, Goetz C, Tanner C (eds): *Textbook of Clinical Neuropharmacology*. New York: Raven Press, 1992, pp 297–306.

29. Goldman MS, Kelly PJ: Symptomatic and functional outcome of stereotactic ventralis lateralis thalamotomy for intention tremor. *J Neurosurg* 77:223, 1992.

30. Wester K, Hauglie-Hanssen E: Stereotaxic thalamotomy: Experiences from the levodopa era. *J Neurol Neurosurg Psychiatry* 53:427, 1990.

31. Nguyen JP, Degos JD: Thalamic stimulation and proximal tremor. *Arch Neurol* 50:498, 1993.

32. Hewer RL, Cooper R, Morgan MH: An investigation into the value of treating intention tremor by weighting the affected limb. *Brain* 95:570, 1972.

33. Geny C, Nguyen JP, Pollin B, et al: Improvement of severe postural cerebellar tremor in multiple sclerosis by chronic thalamic stimulation. *Mov Disord* 11:489, 1996.

34. Sechi GP, Zuddas M, Piredda M, et al: Treatment of cerebellar tremors with carbamazepine: A controlled trial with long-term follow-up. *Neurology* 39:1113, 1989.

35. Oppenheim H: Uber eine eigenartige Kramfkrankheit des kindlichen und jungedichen Alters (Dybasia lordotica progressiva, dystonia musculorum deformans): *Neurol Centralbl* 30:1090, 1911.

36. Marsden CE, Harrison MJG: Idiopathic torsion dystonia (dystonia musculorum deformans): A review of forty-two patients. *Brain* 97:793, 1974.

37. Rivest J, Marsden CD: Trunk and head tremor as isolated manifestations of dystonia. *Mov Disord* 5:60, 1990.

38. Hughes AJ, Lees AJ, Marsden CE: Paroxysmal dystonia head tremor. *Mov Disord* 6:85, 1991.

39. Jankovic J, Leder S, Warner D, Schwartz K: Cervical dystonia: clinical findings and associated movement disorders. *Neurology* 41:1088, 1991.

40. Dubinsky RM: Tremor and dystonia, in Findley LJ, Koller WC (eds): *Handbook of Tremor Disorders*. New York: Marcel Dekker, 1995, pp 405–410.

41. Klawans HL: Dystonia and tremor following exposure to 2,3,7,8-tetrachlorodibenzo-*p*-dioxin. *Mov Disord* 2:255, 1987.

42. Jedynak CP, Bonnet AM, Agid Y: Tremor and idiopathic dystonia. *Mov Disord* 6:230, 1991.

43. Cho C, Samkoff LM: A lesion of the anterior thalamus producing dystonic tremor of the head. *Arch Neurol* 57:1353, 2000.

44. Pal PK, Samii A, Schulzer M: Head tremor in cervical dystonia. *Can J Neurol Sci* 27:137, 2000.

45. Kitagawa M, Murata J, Kikuchi S, et al: Deep brain stimulation of subthalamic area for severe proximal tremor. *Neurology* 55:114, 2000.

46. Rajput AH, Jamison H, Hirsh S, Quraishi A: Relative efficacy of alcohol and propranolol in action tremor. *Can J Neurol Sci* 2:31, 1975.

47. Jankovic J, Fahn S: Physiologic and pathologic tremors. *Ann Intern Med* 73:460, 1980.

48. Larsen TA, Calne DB: Essential tremor. *Clin Neuropharmacol* 6:185, 1983.

49. Shirlow MJ, Matheers CS: A study of caffeine consumption and symptoms: Indigestion, palpitations, tremor, headache, and insomnia. *Int J Epidemiol* 14:239, 1985.

50. Miller LS, Lombardo TW, Fowler SC: Caffeine, but not time of day, increases whole-arm physiological tremor in non-smoking moderate users. *Clin Exp Pharmacol Physiol* 25:131, 1998.

51. Leavitt S, Tyler HR: Studies in asterixis. *Arch Neurol* 10:360, 1964.

52. Milanov I, Toteva S, Georgiev D: Alcohol withdrawal tremor. *Electromyogr Clin Neurophysiol* 36:15, 1996.

53. Rondot P, Jedynak CP, Ferrey G: Pathological tremors: Nosological correlates. *Prog Clin Neurophysiol* 5:95, 1978.

54. Koller W, O'Hara R, Durus W, Bauer J: Tremor in chronic alcoholism. *Neurology* 35:1660, 1985.

55. Silverskoid BP: Romberg's test in the cerebellar syndrome occurring in chronic alcoholism. *Acta Neurol Scand* 45:292, 1969.

56. Lang AE: Miscellaneous drug-induced movement disorders, in Lang AE, Weiner WJ (eds): *Drug-Induced Movement Disorders*. Mt Kisco, NY: Futura Publishing, 1992, pp 339–381.

57. Victor M, Adams RD, Cole lM: The acquired (non-Wilsonian) type of chronic hepatocerebral degeneration. *Medicine (Baltimore)* 44:345, 1965.

58. Spencer PS, Nunn PB, Hu J, et al: Guam amyotrophic lateral sclerosis-parkinsonism-dementia linked to a plant excitant. *Science* 237:517, 1987.

59. Bovet D, Longo VG: The action of nicotine-induced tremors of substances effective in parkinsonism. *J Pharmacol Exp Ther* 102:22, 1951.

60. Cahen RL, Thomas JM, Tvede KM: Nicotinolytic drugs. II: Action of adrenergic blocking agents on nicotine-induced tremors. *J Pharmacol Exp Ther* 107:424, 1953.

61. Stiffmaln SM, Fritz ER, Maltese J, et al: Effects of cigarette smoking and oral nicotine on hand tremor. *Clin Pharmacol Ther* 33:800, 1983.

62. Lippold OC, Williams EJ, Wilson CG: Finger tremor and cigarette smoking. *Br J Clin Pharmacol* 10:83, 1980.

63. Zdonczyk D, Royse V, Koller WC: Nicotine and tremor. *Clin Neuropharmacol* 11:282, 1988.

64. Zaninelli R, Bauer M, Jobert M, et al: Changes in quantitatively assessed tremor during treatment of major depression with lithium augmented by paroxetine or amitriptyline. *J Clin Psychopharmacol* 21:190, 2001.

65. Vestergaard P: Clinically important side effects of long-term lithium treatment: A review. *Acta Psychiatr Scand* 67(suppl):11, 1983.

66. Young RR: Physiological and enhanced physiological tremor, in Findley LJ, Capildeo R (eds): *Movement Disorders: Tremor.* New York: Oxford University Press, 1984, pp 127–135.

67. Nelson JC, Jatlow PI, Quinlan DM: Subjective complaints during desipramine treatment. *Arch Gen Psychiatry* 41:55, 1984.

68. Kronfol Z, Greden JF, Zis AP: Imipramine-induced tremor: Effects of a beta-adrenergic blocking agent. *J Clin Psychopharmacol* 44:225, 1983.

69. Evans DL, Davidson J, Raft D: Early and late side effects of phenelzine. *J Clin Psychopharmacol* 2:208, 1982.

70. Karas BJ, Wilder BJ, Hammond EJ, Bauman AW: Valproate tremors. *Neurology* 32:428, 1982.

71. Price DJI: The advantages of sodium valproate in the neurosurgical practice, in Legg NJ (ed): *Clinical and Pharmacological Aspects of Sodium Valproate (Epilim) in the Treatment of Epilepsy.* Tunbridge Wells: MCS Consultants, 1976, pp 44–50.

72. Hyman NM, Dennis PD, Sinclair KGA: Tremor due to sodium valproate. *Neurology* 19:1177, 1979.

73. Duchowny M, Pellock JM, Graf WD, et al: A placebo-controlled trial of lamotrigine add-on therapy for partial seizures in children. Lamictal Pediatric Partial Seizure Study Group. *Neurology* 53:1724, 1999.

74. Messenheimer JA, Giorgi L, Risner ME: The tolerability of lamotrigine in children. *Drug Saf* 22:303, 2000.

75. Prensky AL, DeVivo DC, Palkes H: Severe bradykinesia as a manifestation of toxicity to anti-epileptic medications. *J Pediatr* 78:700, 1974.

76. Hajnsek F, Sartorius N: A case of intoxication with Tegretol. *Epilepsia* 5:371, 1964.

77. Uthman BM, Rowan AJ, Ahmann PA, et al: Tiagabine for complex partial seizures: A randomized, add-on, dose-response trial. *Arch Neurol* 55:56–62, 1998.

78. Greene HL, Graham EL, Werner JA, et al: Toxic and therapeutic effects of amiodarone in the treatment of cardiac arrhythmias. *J Am Coll Cardiol* 2:1114, 1983.

79. Rubinstein A, Cabili S: Tremor induced by procainamide. *Am J Cardiol* 57:340, 1986.

80. Capella D, Laporte JR, Castel JM: Parkinsonism, tremor, and depression induced by cinnarizine and flunarizine. *Br Med J* 297:722, 1988.

81. Amery WK, Heykants J: Essential tremor and flunarizine. *Cephalalgia* 8:227, 1988.

82. Koller W, Orebaugh C, Lawson L, Potempa K: Pindolol-induced tremor. *Clin Neuropharmacol* 5:449, 1987.

83. Zachariah PK, Bonnet G, Chrysant SG, et al: Evaluation of antihypertensive efficacy of lisinopril compared to metoprolol in moderate to severe hypertension. *J Cardiovasc Pharmacol* 9(suppl 3):S53, 1987.

84. Rapoport A, Stein D, Shamir E, et al: Clinico-tremorgraphic features of neuroleptic-induced tremor. *Int Clin Psychopharmacol* 13:115, 1998.

85. Friedman JH: "Rubral" tremor induced by a neuroleptic drug. *Mov Disord* 7:281, 1992.

86. Hornykiewicz O: Parkinsonism induced by dopaminergic antagonists. *Adv Neurol* 9:155, 1975.

87. Freyhan FA: Psychomotility and parkinsonism in treatment with neuroleptic drugs. *Arch Neurol Psychiatry* 78:465, 1957.

88. National Institute of Mental Health Psychopharmacology Service Center Collaborative Study Group: Phenothiazine treatment in acute schizophrenia. *Arch Gen Psychiatry* 10:246, 1964.

89. Indo T, Ando K: Metoclopramide-induced parkinsonism: Clinical characteristics of ten cases. *Arch Neurol* 39:494, 1982.

90. Villeneuve A: The rabbit syndrome: A peculiar extrapyramidal reaction. *Can Psychiatr Assoc J Suppl* 2:SS69, 1972.

91. Stacy M, Jankovic J: Tardive tremor. *Mov Disord* 7:53, 1992.

92. Delecluse F, Elosegi JA, Gerard JM: A case of tardive tremor successfully treated with clozapine. *Mov Disord* 13:846, 1998.

93. Palmer BF, Toto RD: Severe neurologic toxicity induced by cyclosporine A in three renal transplant patients. *Am J Kidney Dis* 18:116, 1991.

94. Meyer MA: Elevated basal ganglia glucose metabolism in cyclosporine neurotoxicity: A positron emission tomography imaging study. *J Neuroimaging* 12:92, 2002.

95. Slavik RS, Rybak MJ, Lerner SA: Trimethoprim/sulfamethoxazole-induced tremor in a patient with AIDS. *Ann Pharmacother* 32:189, 1998.

96. Kramer JC, Fischman VS, Littlefield DC: Amphetamine abuse: Patterns and effects of high doses taken intravenously. *J Am Med Assoc* 201:305, 1967.

97. LeWitt PA: Tremor induced or enhanced by pharmacological means, in Findley LJ.

98. Formgren H: The therapeutic value of oral long-term treatment with terbutaline (Bricanyl) in asthma: A follow-up study of its efficacy and side effects. *Scand J Respir Dis* 56:321, 1975.

99. Heath A, Knudsen K: Role of extracorporeal drug removal in acute theophylline poisoning: A review. *Med Toxicol Adver Drug Exp* 2:294, 1987.

100. Mellor CS, Jain VK: Diazepam withdrawal syndrome: Its prolonged and changing nature. *Can Med Assoc J* 127:1093, 1982.

101. Chang LW: Mercury, in Spencer PS, Schaumburg HH (eds): *Experimental and Clinical Neurotoxicology.* Baltimore: Williams & Wilkins, 1980, pp 508–526.

102. National Institute for Occupational Safety and Health: Leading work-related diseases and injuries: United States. *J Am Med Assoc* 255:1552, 1986.

103. National Institute for Occupational Safety and Health: *National Occupational Hazard Survey, 1972–74.* National Institute for Occupational Safety and Health, Cincinnati, DHEW (NOISH) publication no. 78–114, 1977.

104. Iwata S, Nomoto M, Fukuda T: Effects of beta-adrenergic blockers on drug-induced tremors. *Pharmacol Biochem Behav* 44:611, 1993.

105. Ludolph AC, Spencer PS: Mycotoxins and tremorogens, in Chang LW, Dyer RS (eds): *Handbook of Neurotoxicology.* New York: Marcel Dekker, 1995, pp 601–603.

106. Greenhouse AH: Heavy metals and the nervous system. *Clin Neuropharmacol* 5:45, 1982.

107. Kurland L, Faro S, Siedler H: Minamata disease: The outbreak of a neurologic disorder in Minamata, Japan and its relationship to the ingestion of seafood contaminated by mercuric compounds. *World Neurol* 1:370, 1960.

108. Nelson N, Byerly TC, Kolbye AC, et al: Hazards of mercury: Special report to the secretary's pesticide advisory committee, Department of Health, Education and Welfare. *Environ Res* 4:1, 1971.

109. Lefevre JP, Gil R: Encephalopathy due to organomercuric compounds (translated title). *Sem Hop* 53:165, 1977.

110. Jaeger A, Tempe JD, Haegy JM, et al: Accidental acute mercury vapor poisoning. *Vet Hum Toxicol* 21(suppl):62, 1979.

111. Kark RA, Poskanzer D, Bullock J, Boylen G: Mercury poisoning and its treatment with N-acetyl-D,L-penicillamine. *N Engl J Med* 185:10, 1971.

112. Komaki H, Maisawa S, Sugai K, et al: Tremor and seizures associated with chronic manganese intoxication. *Brain Dev* 21:122, 1999.

113. Mena I, Marin O, Fuenzalida S, Cotzias G: Chronic manganese poisoning: Clinical picture and manganese turnover. *Neurology* 17:128, 1967.

114. Coulehan JL, Hirsch W, Brillman J, et al: Gasoline sniffing and lead toxicity in Navajo adolescents. *Pediatrics* 71:113, 1983.

115. Milanov I, Kolev P: Clinical and electromyographic examinations of patients with tremor after chronic occupational lead exposure. *Occup Med* 51:157, 2001.

116. Goldings AS, Stewart RM: Organic lead encephalopathy: Behavioral change and movement disorder following gasoline inhalation. *J Clin Psychol* 43:70, 1982.

117. Seshia SS, Rjani KR, Boeckx RL, et al: The neurological manifestations of chronic inhalation of leaded gasoline. *Dev Med Child Neurol* 20:323, 1978.

118. Maruff P, Burns CB, Tyler P, et al: Neurological and cognitive abnormalities associated with chronic petrol sniffing. *Brain* 121: 1903, 1998.

119. Gerhart JM, Hong JS, Uphouse LL, Tilson HA: Chlordecone-induced tremor: Quantification and pharmacological analysis. *Toxicol Appl Pharmacol* 66:234, 1982.

120. Taylor JR, Selhorst JB, Houff SA, Martinez AJ: Chlordecone intoxication of man. I: Clinical observations. *Neurology* 28:626, 1978.

121. Huang TP, Ho IK, Mehendale HM: Assessment of neurotoxicity induced by oral administration of chlordecone (Kepone) in the mouse. *Neurotoxicology* 2:113, 1981.

122. Reiter LW, Kidd K, Ledbetter G, et al: Comparative behavioral toxicology of mirex and kepone in the rat. *Toxicol Appl Pharmacol* 41:143, 1977.

123. Chen PH, Tilson HA, Marbury GD, et al: Effect of chlordecone (Kepone) on the rat brain concentration of 3-methoxy-4-hydroxyphenlglycol: Evidence for a possible involvement of the norepinephrine system in chlordecone-induced tremor. *Toxicol Appl Pharmacol* 77:158, 1985.

124. Cohn WJ, Boylan JJ, Blanke RV, et al: Treatment of chlordecone (Kepone) toxicity with cholestyramine. *N Engl J Med* 198:243, 1978.

125. Hietanen E, Vainio H: Effect of administration route on DDT on acute toxicity and on drug biotransformation in various rodents. *Arch Environ Contam Toxicol* 4:201, 1976.

126. Kashyap SK, Nigam SK, Karnik AB, et al: Carcinogenicity of DDT (dichlorodiphenyltrichloroethane) in pure inbred Swiss mice. *Int J Cancer* 19:725, 1977.

127. Wilson R, Lovejoy FH, Jaeger RJ, Landrigan PL: Acute phosphine poisoning aboard a grain freighter: Epidemiologic, clinical, and pathological findings. *J Am Med Assoc* 244:148, 1980.

128. Zatuchni J, Hong K: Methyl bromide poisoning seen initially as psychosis. *Arch Neurol* 38:529, 1981.

129. Peters HA, Levine RL, Matthews CG, Chapman LJ: Extrapyramidal and other neurologic manifestations associated with carbon disulfide fumigant exposure. *Arch Neurol* 45:537, 1988.

130. Hirose Y, Kobayashi M, Koyama K, et al: A toxicokinetic analysis in a patient with acute glufosinate poisoning. *Hum Exp Toxicol* 18:305, 1999.

131. Welch L, Kirschner H, Heath A, et al: Chronic neuropsychological and neurological impairment following acute exposure to a solvent mixture of toluene and methyl ethyl ketone (MEK). *J Toxicol Clin Toxicol* 29:435, 1991.

132. Poungvarin N: Multifocal brain damage due to lacquer sniffing: The first case report of Thailand. *J Med Assoc Thailand* 74:296, 1991.

133. Buccafusco JJ, Heithold DL, Chon SH: Long-term behavioral and learning abnormalities produced by the irreversible cholinesterase inhibitor soman: Effect of a standard pretreatment regimen and clonidine. *Toxicol Lett* 52:319, 1990.

134. Dick F, Semple S, Chen R, et al: Neurological deficits in solvent-exposed painters: A syndrome including impaired colour vision, cognitive defects, tremor and loss of vibration sensation. *Q J Med* 93:655, 2000.

135. Sakai T, Honda S, Kuzuhara S: Encephalomyelopathy demonstrated on MRI in a case of chronic toluene intoxication. *Rinsho Shinkeigaku* 40:571, 2000.

136. Holmes G: On certain tremors in organic cerebral lesions. *Brain* 27:327, 1904.

137. Koppel BS, Daras M: "Rubral" tremor due to midbrain toxoplasma abscess. *Mov Disord* 5:154, 1990.

138. Carpenter MB: A study of the red nucleus in the rhesus monkey. *J Comp Neurol* 105:195, 1956.

139. Ohye C, Shibazaki T, Hirai T, et al: Special role of the parvocellular red nucleus in lesion-induced spontaneous tremor in monkeys. *Behav Brain Res* 28:241, 1988.

140. Samie MR, Selhorst JB, Koller WC: Post-traumatic midbrain tremors. *Neurology* 40:62, 1990.

141. Hopfensperger KJ, Busenbark K, Koller WC: Midbrain tremor, in Findley LJ, Koller WC (eds): *Handbook of Tremor Disorders* New York: Marcel Dekker, 1995, pp 455–459.

142. Findley LF, Gresty MA: Suppression of "rubral" tremor with levodopa. *Br Med J* 28:1043, 1980.

143. Remy P, de Recondo A, Defer G, et al: Peduncular "rubral" tremor and dopaminergic denervation: A PET study. *Neurology* 45:472, 1995.

144. Yuill GM: Suppression of "rubral" tremor with levodopa: Personal observation. *Br Med J* 281:1428, 1980.

145. Biary N, Cleeves L, Findley L, Koller W: Post-traumatic tremor. *Neurology* 39:103, 1989.

146. Krack P, Deuschl G, Kaps M, et al: Delayed onset of "rubral tremor" 23 years after brainstem trauma [letter]. *Mov Disord* 9:240, 1994.

147. Andrew J, Fowler CJ, Harrison MJ: Tremor after head injury and its treatment by sterotaxic surgery. *J Neurol Neurosurg Psychiatry* 45:815, 1982.

148. Krauss JK, Mohadjer M, Nobbe F, Mundinger F: The treatment of posttraumatic tremor by stereotactic surgery: Symptomatic and functional outcome in a series of 35 patients. *J Neurosurg* 80:810, 1994.

149. Yamamoto M, Wakayama Y, Kawasaki H, et al: Symptomatological rubral tremor caused by vertebral-basilar artery embolism. *Rinsho Shinkeigaku* 3l:1110, 1991.

150. Berkovic SF, Bladin PF: Rubral tremor: Clinical features and treatment of three cases. *Clin Exp Neurol* 20:119, 1984.

151. Tan H, Turanli G, Ay H, Saatci I: Rubral tremor after thalamic infarction in childhood. *Pediatr Neurol* 25:409, 2001.

152. Mossuto-Agatiello L, Puccetti G, Castellano AE: "Rubral" tremor after thalamic haemorrhage. *J Neurol* 241:27, 1993.

153. Kremer M, Ritchie Russell W, Smyth GE: A midbrain syndrome following head injury. *J Neurol Neurosurg Psychiatry* 10:49, 1947.

154. De Recondo A, Rondot P, Loc'h C, et al: [Positron-emission tomographic study of the dopaminergic system in a case of secondary unilateral tremor after mesencephalic hematoma]. *Rev Neurol (Paris)* 149:46, 1993.

155. Benedikt M: in Wolf JK (ed): *The Classical Brain Stem Syndromes.* Springfield, IL: Charles C Thomas, 1991, pp 103–109.

156. Deuschl G: Tremor-syndrome, in Hopf HC, Poeck K, Schliak H (eds): *Neurologie in Clinik und Praxis*, 2nd ed. Stuttgart: Thieme, 1992, vol II, pp 53–61.

157. Pomeranz S, Shalit M, Sherman Y: "Rubral" tremor following radiation of a pineal region vascular hamartoma. *Acta Neurochir (Wien)* 103:79, 1990.

158. Thompson PD, Rothwell JC, Day BL, et al: The physiology of orthostatic tremor. *Arch Neurol* 43:584, 1986.

159. FitzGerald PM, Jankovic J: Orthostatic tremor: An association with essential tremor. *Mov Disord* 6:60, 1991.

160. Onofrj M, Thomas A, Paci C, et al: Gabapentin in orthostatic tremor: results of a double-blind crossover with placebo in four patients. *Neurology* 51:880, 1998.

161. Ondo W, Hunter C, Vuong KD, et al: Gabapentin for essential tremor: A multiple-dose, double-blind, placebo-controlled trial. *Mov Disord* 15:678, 2000.

162. Gironell A, Kulisevsky J, Barbanoj M, et al: A randomized placebo-controlled comparative trial of gabapentin and propranolol in essential tremor. *Arch Neurol* 56:475, 1999.

163. Pahwa R, Lyons K, Hubble JP, et al: Double-blind controlled trial of gabapentin in essential tremor. *Mov Disord* 13:465, 1998.

164. McManus PG, Sharbrough FW: Orthostatic tremor: Clinical and electrophysiologic characteristics. *Muscle Nerve* 16:1254, 1993.

165. Heilman KM: Orthostatic tremor. *Arch Neurol* 41:880, 1984.

166. Thompson PD: Primary orthostatic tremor, in Findley LJ, Koller WC (eds): *Handbook of Tremor Disorders.* New York: Marcel Dekker, 1995, pp 387–399.

167. Papa SM, Gershanik OS: Orthostatic tremor: An essential tremor variant? *Mov Disord* 3:97, 1988.

168. Benito-Leon J, Rodriguez J, Orti-Pareja M, et al: Symptomatic orthostatic tremor in pontine lesions. *Neurology* 49:1439, 1997.

169. Cabrera-Valdiva F, Jimenez-Jimenez FJ, Albea EG, et al: Orthostatic tremor: Successful treatment with phenobarbital. *Clin Neuropharmacol* 14:438, 1991.

170. Deuschl G, Toro C, Valls-Sole J, et al: Symptomatic and essential palatal tremor. *Brain* 117:775, 1994.

171. Hallett M, Shibasaki H, Obeso J: Criteria for the visual identification of myoclonus. *Mov Disord* 9:1994.

172. Thack WT: Discharge of cerebellar neurons related to two maintained postures and two prompt movements. I. Nuclear cell output. *J Neurophysiol* 33:527, 1970.

173. Schenck E: *Die Hirnnervenmyorhythmie, ihre Pathogenese und ihre Stellung im myoklonischen Syndrom.* Berlin: Springer Verlag, 1965.

174. Laprsle J: Palatal myoclonus. *Adv Neurol* 43:265, 1986.

175. Cakmur R, Idiman E, Idiman F, et al: Essential palatal tremor successfully treated with flunarizine. *Eur Neurol* 38:133, 1997.

176. Cho JW, Chu K, Jeon BS: Case of essential palatal tremor: atypical features and remarkable benefit from botulinum toxin injection. *Mov Disord* 16:779, 2001.

177. Matthews WB, Howell DA, Hughes RC: Relapsing corticosteroid-dependent polyneuritis. *J Neurol Neurosurg Psychiatry* 33:330, 1970.

178. Smith IS, Furness P, Thomas PK: Tremor in peripheral neuropathy, in Findley LF, Capildeo R (eds): *Movement Disorders: Tremor.* London: Macmillan, 1984, pp 399–406.

179. Thomas PK: Clinical features and differential diagnosis, in Dyck PJ, Thomas PK, Lambert EH, Bunge R (eds): *Peripheral Neuropathy*, 2nd ed. Philadelphia: WB Saunders, 1984, pp

180. Said G, Bathien N, Cesaro P: Peripheral neuropathies and tremor. *Neurology* 32:480, 1982.

181. Smith IS: Tremor in peripheral neuropathy, in Findley LJ, Koller WC (eds): *Handbook of Tremor Disorders.* New York: Marcel Dekker, 1995, pp 443–454.

182. Elble RJ: Peripheral neuropathies and tremor. *Neurology* 33:1389, 1983.

183. Van Ham L, Vandevelde M, Desmidt M, et al: A tremor syndrome with a central axonopathy in Scottish terriers. *J Vet Intern Med* 8:290, 1994.

184. Marie MP: Forme speciale de nevrite interstitielle hypergrophique progressive de l'enfance. *Rev Neurol (Paris)* 14:557, 1906.

185. Cardoso, FEC, Jankovic J: Hereditary motor-sensory neuropathy and movement disorders. *Muscle Nerve* 16:904, 1993.

186. Saverino A, Solaro C, Capello E, et al: Tremor associated with benign IgM paraproteinaemic neuropathy successfully treated with gabapentin. *Mov Disord* 16:967, 2001.

187. Gowers WR: *Disease of the Nervous System.* Philadelphia: Blakiston, 1888.

188. Koller W, Lang A, Vetere-Overfield B, et al: Psychogenic tremors. *Neurology* 39:1094, 1989.

189. Kim YJ, Pakiam AS, Lang AE: Historical and clinical features of psychogenic tremor: A review of 70 cases. *Can J Neurol Sci* 26:190, 1999.

190. Koller WC: Diagnosis and treatment of tremors. *Neurol Clin* 2:499, 1984.

191. Hunker CJ, Abbs JH: Uniform frequency of parkinsonian resting tremor in the lips, jaw, tongue and index finger. *Mov Disord* 5:71, 1990.

192. Rajput AH: Clinical features of tremor in extrapyramidal syndromes, in Findley LJ, Koller WC (eds): *Handbook of Tremor Disorders.* New York: Marcel Dekker, 1995, pp 275–291.

193. Findley LJ, Gresty MA, Halmagi GM: Tremor, the cogwheel phenomenon and clonus in Parkinson's disease. *J Neurol Neurosurg Psychiatry* 44:534, 1981.

194. Shahani BT, Young RR: Physiological and pharmacological aids in the differential diagnosis of tremor. *J Neurol Neurosurg Psychiatry* 39:772, 1976.

195. Pechadre JC, Larochelle L, Poirier LJ: Parkinsonian akinesia, rigidity and tremor in the monkey. *J Neurol Sci* 28:147, 1976.

196. Brooks DJ, Playford ED, Ibanez V, et al: Isolated tremor and disruption of the nigrostriatal dopaminergic system: An 18F-dopa PET study. *Neurology* 42:1554, 1992.

197. Zimmerman R, Deuschl G, Hornig A, et al: Tremors in Parkinson's disease: Symptom analysis and rating. *Clin Neuropharmacol* 17:303, 1994.

198. Dethy S, Luxen A, Bidaut LM, Goldman S: Hemibody tremor related to stroke. *Stroke* 24:2094, 1993.

199. Masucci EF, Kurtzke JF: Tremor in progressive supranuclear palsy. *Acta Neurol Scand* 80:296, 1989.
200. Rail D, Schlotz C, Swash M: Post-encephalitic parkinsonism: Current experience. *J Neurol Neurosurg Psychiatry* 44:670, 1981.
201. Wenning GK, Ben Shlomo Y, Magalhaes M, et al: Clinical features and natural history of multiple system atrophy: An analysis of 100 cases. *Brain* 117:835, 1994.
202. Louis ED, Goldman JE, Powers JM, Fahn S: Parkinsonian features of eight pathologically diagnosed cases of diffuse Lewy body diseases. *Mov Disord* 10:188, 1995.
203. Moon SL, Koller WC: Psychogenic tremor, in Findley LJ, Koller WC (eds): *Handbook of Tremor Disorders.* New York: Marcel Dekker, 1995, pp 491–494.
204. Masucci E, Kurtzke J: Palatal myoclonus associated with extremity tremor. *J Neurol* 236:474, 1989.
205. Defer GL, Remy P, Malapert D, et al: Rest tremor and extrapyramidal symptoms after midbrain haemorrhage: Clinical and 18F-dopa PET evaluation. *J Neurol Neurosurg Psychiatry* 57:987, 1994.
206. Bhatia K, Daniel SE, Marsden CD: Orofacial dystonia and rest tremor in a patient with normal brain pathology. *Mov Disord* 8:361, 1993.
207. Barbosa ER, Teixira MJ, Chaves CJ, Scaff M: Parkinson disease associated to a brain tumor: A case report. *Arq Neuropsiquiatr* 49:338, 1991.
208. Koller WC, Herbster G: Adjuvant therapy of parkinsonian tremor. *Arch Neurol* 44:921, 1987.
209. Koller WC: Pharmacologic treatment of parkinsonian tremor. *Arch Neurol* 43:126, 1986.
210. Hughes AJ, Lees AJ, Stern GM: Apomorphine in the diagnosis and treatment of parkinsonian tremor. *Clin Neuropharmacol* 13:312, 1990.
211. Dejerine J, Roussy G: Le syndrome thalamique. *Rev Neurol* 12:521, 1906.
212. Lee MS, Marsden CD: Movement disorders following lesions of the thalamus or subthalamic region. *Mov Disord* 9:493, 1994.
213. Marsden CD, Obeso JA, Zarranz JJ, Lang AE: The anatomical basis of symptomatic dystonia. *Brain* 108:463, 1985.
214. Pettigrew LC, Jankovic J: Hemidystonia: A report of 22 patients and a review of the literature. *J Neurol Neurosurg Psychiatry* 48:650, 1985.
215. Schlitt M, Brown JW, Zeiger HE, Galbraith JG: Appendicular tremor as a late complication of intracerebral hemorrhage. *Surg Neurol* 25:181, 1986.
216. Kim JS: Delayed onset of hand tremor caused by cerebral infarction. *Stroke* 23:292, 1992.
217. Moroo I, Hirayama K, Kohima S: Involuntary movements caused by thalamic lesion. *Rinsho Shinkeigaku* 34:805, 1994.
218. Ferbert, Gerwig M: Tremor due to stroke. *Mov Disord* 8:179, 1993.
219. Kim JS: Delayed onset mixed involuntary movements after thalamic stroke: Clinical, radiological and pathophysiological findings. *Brain* 124:299, 2001.
220. Kao YF, Shih PY, Chen WH: An unusual concomitant tremor and myoclonus after a contralateral infarct at thalamus and subthalamic nucleus. *Kaohsiung J Med Sci* 15:562, 1999.
221. Micheli F, Granana N, Scorticati MC, et al: Unilateral postural and action tremor resulting from thalamic toxoplasmosis in a patient with acquired immunodeficiency syndrome. *Mov Disord* 12:1096, 1997.
222. Aboulafia DM: Tremors associated with trimethoprim-sulfamethoxazole therapy in a patient with AIDS: Case report and review. *Clin Infect Dis* 22:598, 1996.
223. Demarquay G, Setiey A, Morel Y, et al: Clinical report of three patients with hereditary hemochromatosis and movement disorders. *Mov Disord* 15:1204, 2000.
224. Krause WL, Leiter JC, Marsh Tenney S, et al: Acute hypoxia activates human 8–12 Hz physiological tremor. *Respir Physiol* 123:131, 2000.
225. Takahashi W, Ohnuki Y, Takizawa S, et al: Neuroimaging on delayed postanoxic encephalopathy with lesions localized in basal ganglia. *Clin Imaging* 22:188, 1998.
226. Aizawa T, Hiramatsu K, Ohtsuka H, et al: Defective hepatic anion transport in variegate porphyria. *Am J Gastroenterol* 82:1180, 1987.
227. Milanov I, Sheinkova G: Clinical and electromyographic examination of tremor in patients with thyrotoxicosis. *Int J Clin Pract* 54:364, 2000.
228. Saito T: Presenting symptoms and natural history of Wilson disease. *Eur J Pediatr* 146:261, 1987.
229. Brewer GJ, Yuzbasiyan-Gurkan V: Wilson's disease. *Medicine* 71:139, 1992.
230. Frucht S, Sun D, Schiff N, et al: Arm tremor secondary to Wilson's disease. *Mov Disord* 13:351, 1998.
231. Nicholl DJ, Ferenci P, Polli C, et al: Wilson's disease presenting in a family with an apparent dominant history of tremor. *J Neurol Neurosurg Psychiatry* 70:514, 2001.
232. Elble RJ, Moody C, Higgins C: Primary writing tremor. *Mov Disord* 5:118, 1990.
233. Rothwell JC, Traub MM, Marsden CD: Primary writing tremor. *J Neurol Neurosurg Psychiatry* 42:1106, 1979.
234. Rosenbaum F, Jankovic J: Focal task-specific tremor and dystonia: Categorization of occupational movement disorders. *Neurology* 38:522, 1988.
235. Lang AE: Writing tremor and writing dystonia. *Mov Disord* 5:354, 1990.
236. Sheehy MP, Marsden CD: Writer's cramp: A focal dystonia. *Brain* 105:461, 1982.
237. Wills AJ, Jenkins IH, Thompson PD, et al: A positron emission tomography study of cerebral activation associated with essential and writing tremor. *Arch Neurol* 52:299, 1995.
238. Bain PG, Findley LJ, Britton TC, et al: Primary writing tremor. *Brain* 118:1461, 1995.
239. Kachi T, Rothwell JC, Cowan JMA, Marsden CD: Writing tremor: Its relationship to benign essential tremor. *J Neurol Neurosurg Psychiatry* 48:545, 1985.
240. Koller WC, Martyn B: Writing tremor: Its relationship to essential tremor. *J Neurol Neurosurg Psychiatry* 49:220, 1986.
241. Bain P: Task specific tremor. *ITF Newsletter* 5:3, 1993.
242. Ohye C, Miyazaki M, Hirai T, et al: Primary writing tremor treated by stereotactic selective thalamotomy. *J Neurol Neurosurg Psychiatry* 45:988, 1982.
243. Racette BA, Dowling J, Randle J, et al: Thalamic stimulation for primary writing tremor. *J Neurol* 248:380, 2001.
244. Curren TG, Lang AE: Trauma and tremor, in Findley LJ, Koller WC (eds): *Handbook of Tremor Disorders.* New York: Marcel Dekker, 1995.
245. Crouzon O, Justin-Besancon L: Le parkinsonisme traumatique. *Presse Med* 37:1325, 1929.
246. Martland HS: Punch drunk. *J Am Med Assoc* 91:1103, 1928.

247. Lindenberg R: Die Schadigungmechanismen der Substantia Nigra bei Hirntraumen und das Problem des posttraumatischen Parkinsonismus. *Dtsch Z Nervenheilkd* 185:637, 1964.

248. Nayermouri T: Postraumatic parkinsonism. *Surg Neurol* 24:263, 1985.

249. Bruetsch WL, DeArmond M: The parkinsonian syndrome due to trauma. A clinico-anatomical study of a case. *J Nerv Ment Dis* 81:531, 1935.

250. Andrew J, Fowler CJ, Harrison MJG, Kendall BE: Post-traumatic tremor due to vascular injury and its treatment by stereotactic thalamotomy. *J Neurol Neurosurg Psychiatry* 45:560, 1982.

251. Qureshi F, Morales A, Elble RJ: Tremor due to infarction in the ventrolateral thalamus. *Mov Disord* 11:440, 1996.

252. Schwartzman RJ, Kerrigan J: The movement disorder of reflex sympathetic dystrophy. *Neurology* 40:57, 1990.

253. Deuschl G, Blumberg H, Lucking CH: Tremor in reflex sympathetic dystrophy. *Arch Neurol* 48:1247, 1991.

254. Jankovic J, Van der Linden C: Dystonia and tremor induced by peripheral trauma: Predisposing factors. *J Neurol Neurosurg Psychiatry* 5:1512, 1988.

255. Streib EW: Distal ulnar neuropathy as a cause of finger tremor: A case report. *Neurology* 40:153, 1990.

256. Nobrega JC, Campos CR, Limongi JC, et al: Movement disorders induced by peripheral trauma. *Arq Neuropsiquiatr* 60:17, 2002.

257. Biary N, Koller WC: Kinetic predominant essential tremor: Successful treatment with clonazepam. *Neurology* 37:471, 1988.

258. Ellison PH: Propranolol for severe post-head injury action tremor. *Neurology* 28:197, 1978.

259. Obeso JA, Narbona J: Post-traumatic tremor and myoclonic jerking. *J Neurol Neurosurg Psychiatry* 46:788, 1983.

260. Brin MF, Bilitzer A: Vocal tremor, in Findley LJ, Koller WC (eds): *Handbook of Tremor Disorders*. New York: Marcel Dekker, 1995, pp 495–520.

261. Brown JR, Simonson J: Organic voice tremor: A tremor of phonation. *Neurology* 13:520, 1963.

262. Lebrun Y, Devreux F, Rousseau JJ, Darimont P: Tremulous speech. *Folia Phoniatr* 34:134, 1982.

263. Ludlow C, Bassich C, Connor N, Coulter D: Phonatory characteristics of vocal fold tremor. *J Phonet* 14:509, 1986.

264. Hachinski VC, Thomsen IV, Buch NH: The nature of primary vocal tremor. *Can J Neurol Sci* 2:195, 1975.

265. Ramig LA, Shipp T: Comparative measures of vocal tremor and vocal vibrato. *J Voice* 2:162, 1987.

266. Hartman DE, Overholt SL, Vishwanat B: A case of vocal cord nodules masking essential (voice) tremor. *Arch Otolaryngol* 108:52, 1982.

267. Massey EW, Paulson G: Essential vocal tremor: Response to therapy. *Neurology* 32:A113, 1982.

268. Seguier N, Spira A, Dordain M, et al: Relationship between speech disorders and other clinical manifestations of Parkinson's disease (translated title). *Folia Phoniatr* 16:108, 1974.

269. Logemann J, Fisher H, Boshes B, Blonsky E: Frequency and cooccurrence of vocal tract dysfunctions in the speech of a large sample of Parkinson patients. *J Speech Hear Disord* 43:47, 1978.

270. Ramig LA, Scherer RC, Titze IR, Ringel SP: Acoustic analysis of voices of patients with neurologic disease: Rationale and preliminary data. *Ann Otol Rhinol Laryngol* 97:164, 1988.

271. Aronson AE: Organic (essential) voice tremor, in Aronson AE (ed): *Clinical Voice Disorders*. New York: Thieme-Stratton, 1980, pp 108–111.

272. Findley LJ, Gresty MA: Head, facial, and voice tremor. *Adv Neurol* 239, 1988.

273. Koda J, Ludlow CL: An evaluation of laryngeal muscle activation in patients with voice tremor. *Otolaryngol Head Neck Surg* 107:684, 1992.

274. Koller W, Graner D, Mlcoch A: Essential voice tremor: Treatment with propranol. *Neurology* 35:106, 1985.

275. Ackerman H, Ziegler W: Cerebellar voice tremor: An acoustic analysis. *J Neurol Neurosurg Psychiatry* 54:74, 1991.

276. Silfverskiold BP: A 3 c/sec leg tremor in a "cerebellar" syndrome. *Acta Neurol Scand* 55:385, 1977.

277. Yoon MS, Munz M, Sataloff RT, et al: Vocal tremor reduction with deep brain stimulation. *Stereotact Funct Neurosurg* 72:241, 1999.

Chapter 29

THE PATHOPHYSIOLOGY OF TREMOR

RODGER J. ELBLE

PHYSIOLOGIC TREMOR   481
GENERAL PROPERTIES OF PATHOLOGIC
   TREMORS   482
ESSENTIAL TREMOR   483
PARKINSONIAN TREMOR   485
CEREBELLAR INTENTION TREMOR   485
RUBRAL (HOLMES') TREMOR   486
PALATAL MYOCLONUS   487
STROKE-INDUCED TREMOR   487
TREMOR DUE TO PERIPHERAL NERVE
   PATHOLOGY   488
TASK-SPECIFIC, FOCAL AND DYSTONIC
   TREMORS   488
ORTHOSTATIC TREMOR   488
CORTICAL TREMOR   488
DRUG-INDUCED TREMOR   489
SUMMARY   489

Tremor is an approximately rhythmic, roughly sinusoidal involuntary movement. Despite nearly a century of modern clinical and laboratory investigations, no tremor is understood completely. The more common forms of tremor are reviewed in this chapter, and two basic questions are addressed for each form: what is the source of oscillation and why does the oscillation occur?

Physiologic Tremor

Physiologic tremor is barely visible to the unaided eye and is symptomatic only during activities that require extreme precision. Physiologic tremor consists of two distinct oscillations, mechanical-reflex and 8–12 Hz, which are superimposed upon a background of irregular fluctuations in muscle force and limb displacement.[1,2] These background irregularities have a frequency of 0–15 Hz and are produced by motor units that fire near their threshold.[3] The low-pass filtering property of skeletal muscle attenuates the amplitude of these irregularities at frequencies above 3–5 Hz.[4]

The mechanical-reflex component of physiologic tremor is much larger than the 8–12-Hz component and is exhibited by everyone. The mechanical-reflex component is a passive mechanical oscillation that is produced by the underdamped inertial, viscous and elastic properties of the limbs and other body parts. Participation of the stretch reflex is evident only when physiologic tremor is enhanced by fatigue, anxiety or drugs.[5,6] The mechanical attributes of most body parts are such that damped oscillations occur in response to pulsatile perturbations. The frequency of these mechanical-reflex oscillations (ω) is determined largely by the inertia (I) and stiffness (K) of the body part, according to the formula $\omega \approx \sqrt{K/I}$. Consequently, normal elbow tremor has a frequency, 3–5 Hz, that is lower than the 8–12 Hz frequency of wrist tremor because the forearm has much greater inertia than the hand.[7] Similarly, the finger has even less inertia, so the frequency of metacarpophalangeal joint tremor is 17–30 Hz.[8] Voluntary co-contraction of the muscles about a joint produces a slight increase in tremor frequency due to the increased joint stiffness. Conversely, gradual relaxation of the joint causes the frequency of mechanical-reflex tremor to fall.

The mechanical properties of the body are not sufficient to cause tremor. One or more sources of mechanical energy are required to force or perturb a limb into oscillation at a frequency determined by limb inertia and stiffness. Voluntary muscle contraction contains irregularities in subtetanic motor unit firing that perturb the limb continuously and randomly. The ejection of blood at cardiac systole provides additional perturbations to the limbs. Such cardioballistics account for nearly all of physiologic tremor at rest but only a fraction of physiologic postural and kinetic tremor.[2,9]

Under normal circumstances, somatosensory receptors (e.g., muscle spindles) respond to the mechanical oscillations of physiologic tremor, but the response is usually too weak to entrain motoneurons at the frequency of tremor. Consequently, the power spectrum of the rectified-filtered electromyogram (EMG) is essentially flat during normal steady muscle contraction (Fig. 29-1). The stretch-reflex response to oscillation increases during fatigue and anxiety and in response to some medications, producing a modulation of motor unit activity and so-called enhanced physiologic tremor (Fig. 29-1).[5,6,10] This involvement of the stretch reflex can increase tremor or suppress it, depending upon the dynamics of the reflex loop and limb mechanics.[11] Thus, mechanical-reflex oscillation is minimized when the natural frequency of the mechanical system is far removed from the natural frequencies of associated stretch reflex pathways.

In contrast to the mechanical-reflex oscillation, the 8–12-Hz component of physiologic tremor is always associated with modulation of motor unit activity, even when the 8–12-Hz tremor is much smaller than the mechanical-reflex oscillation (Fig. 29-1). Participating motor units are entrained at 8–12 Hz, regardless of their mean frequency of discharge.[1,12] The 8–12-Hz and mechanical-reflex oscillations are easily distinguished by their response to inertial and elastic loads. The frequency of 8–12-Hz tremor exhibits little or no change when inertial or elastic loads are attached to the limb. By contrast, the frequency of mechanical-reflex oscillation is proportional to $\sqrt{K/I}$, where K is the added stiffness and I is the added inertia.[8,13] Furthermore, the frequency of 8–12-Hz

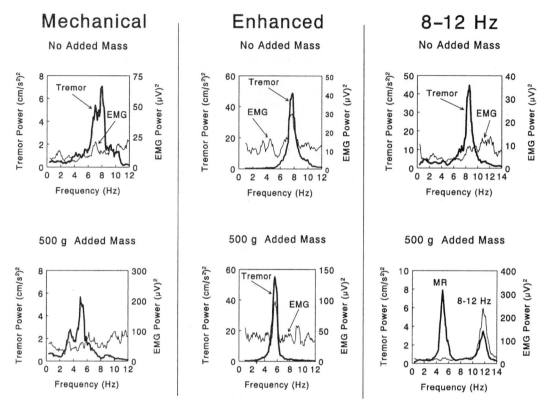

FIGURE 29-1 Fourier power spectra of normal mechanical-reflex tremor (Mechanical), enhanced physiologic tremor due to thyrotoxicosis (Enhanced) and physiologic tremor with a prominent 8–12-Hz component (8–12-Hz). Postural hand tremor was recorded a miniature accelerometer (thick lines), and rectified-filtered EMG of the extensor carpi radialis brevis was recorded with skin electrodes (thin lines). Note how a 500-g load on the hand reduced normal and enhanced mechanical-reflex (MR) tremor. By contrast, the 8–12-Hz tremor increased in amplitude, but its frequency did not change.

tremor is independent of stretch reflex loop time and muscle twitch properties.[12,14,15] For these reasons, the 8–12-Hz tremor probably originates from an unidentified oscillating neuronal network within the central nervous system. The spinal cord, inferior olive, thalamus, and cerebral cortex are only a few of the possible sources of 8–12-Hz tremor.[16]

General Properties of Pathologic Tremors

The segmental stretch reflex and limb mechanics comprise the final common pathway for all forms of tremor (Fig. 29-2). Therefore, the stretch reflex and limb mechanics can influence the frequency or amplitude of a tremor, depending upon its origin. The frequency of normal mechanical-reflex tremor is largely a function of limb inertia and stiffness and is easily changed by added inertia or stiffness because there is little involvement of segmental and long-loop reflexes. However, tremors with greater involvement of segmental and long-loop (e.g., transcortical) sensorimotor pathways have frequencies that are less dependent upon limb mechanics

and more dependent upon reflex loop dynamics (e.g., loop time).[17,18] Consequently, the frequencies of enhanced physiologic tremor and cerebellar tremor are altered less by mechanical loads than the frequency of normal mechanical-reflex tremor.[10,19] Tremors originating from central oscillators have frequencies that are independent of limb mechanics and reflex arc length, except in the hypothetical situation when the stretch reflex is so strong relative to the central oscillator that the central oscillator becomes entrained by stretch-reflex oscillation.[18] Nevertheless, if tremor frequency is independent of limb inertia *and* reflex-arc length, the source of tremor is a central oscillator. Parkinsonian tremor, essential tremor, primary writing tremor, and orthostatic tremor are examples of central oscillation.[16]

Motor pathways are sufficiently integrated that no source of tremor can be isolated completely from the effects of sensory feedback. Consequently, peripheral stretch-reflex manipulations can reset the phase and entrain the frequency of tremors, even when they emerge from central sources of oscillation.[20–24] Similarly, a central oscillator can resonate with the mechanical-reflex system, if their natural frequencies are similar.[22] For example, parkinsonian and essential hand

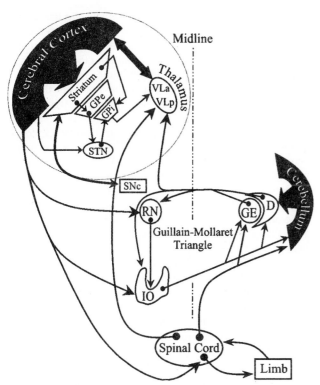

FIGURE 29-2 This simplified schematic diagram illustrates some of the pathways that have been implicated in the various tremors discussed in this chapter. D, dentate nucleus; GE, globose and emboliform nuclei; GPe and GPi, globus pallidus externa and interna; RN, red nucleus; RetN, reticular nuclei; SNc, substantia nigra pars compacta; STN, subthalamic nucleus; IO, inferior olive; VLa and VLp, anterior and posterior ventrolateral thalamic nuclei.

tremors have frequencies that are similar to the mechanical-reflex frequency of the wrist, so there is less mechanical limitation of the tremor than would occur if these tremors had much higher frequencies. The 14–18-Hz frequency of orthostatic tremor is much higher than the natural mechanical-reflex frequency of the lower limbs, so this tremor may not be visible to the examiner until the tremor frequency undergoes subharmonic reduction to 7–9 Hz. Similar dynamical interactions undoubtedly occur between the central oscillators of pathologic tremors and the central neural pathways to which the oscillators are connected. Resonance between a tremor oscillator and other parts of the central nervous system may be as important as the strength of oscillation in determining the amplitude of pathologic tremors.[16]

Magnetic stimulation of the contralateral motor cortex can reset the phase of essential tremor, parkinsonian tremor and normal rapid alternating wrist movements.[25,26] These observations prove that the motor cortex can influence essential tremor (ET) and parkinsonian tremor but do not reveal the anatomic origin of tremor.

Positron emission tomography (PET) has revealed increased cerebellar blood flow in patients with many forms

of tremor, including parkinsonian tremor, writing tremor, orthostatic tremor, and ET.[27] The cerebellum receives all forms of sensory feedback and projects directly or indirectly to all parts of the motor system except the basal ganglia. Thus, cerebellar hyperactivity is a nonspecific abnormality and could be a consequence of tremor rather than its cause.

Nucleus ventralis intermedius of the ventrolateral thalamus is the most effective stereotactic surgical site for treating essential, parkinsonian, cerebellar, rubral, and task-specific tremors,[28–31] even though Vim receives inputs from cerebellum and ascending spinal sensory tracts and only sparse input from the internal pallidum.[32–35] It is unclear whether ventralis intermedius is the primary source of oscillation for any of these tremor disorders. Nevertheless, the oscillatory properties and anatomical connections of ventralis intermedius could facilitate the development of pathologic oscillation originating from virtually any location in the motor system. This may explain why ventralis intermedius is a nonspecific Achilles heel for many forms of pathologic tremor.

Essential Tremor

ET is the most common form of pathologic tremor (see Chap. 27). ET begins at any age but is most common in older people, having a prevalence of at least 1–5 percent in people over the age of 65.[36–38] Thirty to fifty percent of all cases are dominantly inherited, and most patients with ET have no other abnormal neurological signs. ET most commonly affects the hands, but also occurs in the head, voice, face, trunk, and lower extremities.[39] ET is a postural tremor with a variable kinetic component. Tremor in repose is uncommon and is observed only in the most advanced patients, who are typically older. The complex pill-rolling hand movements of parkinsonian tremor are not seen in ET.[39]

Tremor resembling ET is seen in many other neurological disorders, including parkinsonian disease and dystonia, and pathophysiologic relationships between ET and these disorders are frequently debated. These debates will not be resolved until specific diagnostic tests for ET are found. ET in the upper extremities does not have unique diagnostic features, and tremors resembling ET are seen in many neurological disorders, particularly those that produce parkinsonism and dystonia.[40] There is evidence that at least three different genes may be responsible for ET, so ET may not be a single entity.[41–44]

The sine qua non of ET is a rhythmic 4–12-Hz entrainment of motor unit discharge that forces the affected body part into oscillation. The neurophysiologic properties of ET are consistent with a central source of oscillation that is influenced by somatosensory reflex pathways. Mechanical loads have little effect on the frequency of ET (Fig. 29-3), thereby distinguishing this tremor from enhanced physiologic tremor.[40] Cooling the upper extremity reduces tremor amplitude but does not change tremor frequency.[45] Patients with ET exhibit normal mechanical-reflex properties and mechanical-reflex

No Added Mass

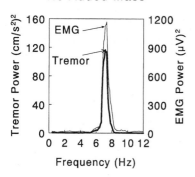

500 g Added Mass

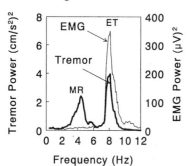

FIGURE 29-3 Fourier power spectra of postural hand tremor recorded from a 57-year-old woman with mild familial tremor. Hand tremor was recorded with a miniature accelerometer (thick lines), and extensor digitorum brevis EMG was recorded with skin electrodes (thin lines). Note the single large spectral peak in tremor and EMG (no added mass). Mass loading reduced the frequency of the mechanical-reflex (MR) oscillation to 4 Hz, leaving the essential tremor (ET) at 8 Hz. This precluded any resonance between the two oscillations. Consequently, the overall amplitude of tremor was reduced (500 g Added Mass).

oscillation, and ET can exhibit mutual frequency entrainment and resonance if their frequencies are similar (Fig. 29-3).[46] When a mechanical load separates the mechanical-reflex and essential tremors, resonance and entrainment are abolished, resulting in reduced tremor amplitude and a more clear demonstration of the frequency of ET (best measured in the rectified-filtered EMG spectrum; Fig. 29-3).

Tremor amplitude bears a logarithmic relationship with the intensity and frequency of motor unit entrainment, according to the equation: $\log(\text{amplitude}) = -2.3\log(\text{frequency}) + 2.3\log(\text{intensity}) + 10$.[47] The frequency-amplitude relationship (slope approximately -2) of ET is predicted by the second-order low-pass filtering properties of skeletal muscle.[4] This relationship also predicts that tremor amplitude could be significantly reduced by increasing tremor frequency. Thus far, no drug or surgical intervention has altered the frequency of ET.[48]

Mild high-frequency ET is qualitatively similar to the 8–12-Hz physiologic tremor, so these tremors could emerge from the same central oscillator.[49] However, oscillators in the frequency range of ET are found throughout the nervous system, and the similarities between ET and physiologic tremor could be fortuitous. Nevertheless, patients within the same family commonly exhibit tremors with different frequencies, ranging from 4 to 12 Hz, and tremor frequency is strongly correlated with the patient's age (in years), according to the equation: frequency $\approx 0.07\text{age} + 10$.[50] The tremor frequency decreases at a rate of approximately 0.07 Hz per year, in the average patient.[50] This drop in tremor frequency presumably is related to age-related changes in the nervous system or to progression of the underlying pathophysiology.[50,51]

The origin of ET is unknown. Routine postmortem examinations have revealed no abnormalities.[52] The inferior olive, thalamus, and cerebral cortex comprise an abbreviated list of plausible candidates.[53] The inferior olive is incriminated by the most experimental data, but the evidence is far from conclusive. Inferior olivary neurons have rhythmic properties and strong interconnectivity that are conducive to the production of tremor, and the enhancement of olivary rhythmicity with harmaline or serotonergic drugs produces an action tremor that is similar to ET.[53,54] Lesions in the cerebellum[55] and thalamus[56] reduce ET, suggesting that abnormal oscillation is transmitted to motor cortex via the cerebellum and its projection to the ventrolateral thalamus (ventralis intermedius, ventralis lateralis posterior). PET studies have revealed bilaterally increased olivary glucose utilization and bilaterally increased blood flow in the cerebellum, red nucleus, and thalamus of patients with ET.[27] The electroencephalogram (EEG) contains cortical rhythmicity that is correlated with essential tremor.[57] Functional magnetic resonance imaging (fMRI) studies have disclosed increased blood flow bilaterally in the cerebellar hemispheres, dentate nucleus, and red nucleus and contralaterally in the globus pallidus, thalamus, and primary sensorimotor cortex.[27]

According to the olivary hypothesis, patients with ET have enhanced synchronization and 4–12-Hz neuronal rhythmicity in their olives. This could result from altered olivary network properties (e.g., enhanced dendrodendritic electrotonic connections), altered neuromodulation of the olivary network (e.g., *N*-methyl-D-aspartate, serotonin, or gamma-aminobutyric acid), abnormal enhancement of the membrane conductances that underlie the neuronal oscillations, or a combination of these mechanisms.[53,58] Olivary oscillation is transmitted and possibly amplified through the cerebellum, producing entrainment of the thalamus, motor cortex and brainstem nuclei.[59] This might explain why patients with advanced ET exhibit intention tremor and subtle signs of ataxia.[60] Widespread entrainment of the motor system by olivary oscillation could explain why lesions in so many areas of the motor system suppress ET.[16]

The mechanism by which stereotactic thalamotomy and deep brain stimulation (DBS) suppress tremor is unclear. One possibility is that tremor is reduced by interrupting resonant oscillation in the thalamocortical loop. This might occur regardless of the primary site of tremorogenic oscillation. An alternative possibility is that the tremorogenic oscillation emerges from the ventralis intermedius, motor cortex or thalamocortical loop.

Noteworthy is a recent report by Kitagawa et al., describing the successful treatment of severe proximal ET with subthalamic nucleus (STN) deep brain stimulation (DBS).[61] The distal postural tremor responded to Vim thalamotomy, but the proximal intention tremor did not. A subsequent STN DBS procedure greatly suppressed the proximal tremor. This observation suggests that the effect of STN DBS is not specific for parkinsonian tremor and that ET may involve tremorogenic reverberation in the basal ganglia.

Ethanol, primidone, and beta-adrenergic blockers suppress ET by mechanisms that are poorly understood.[62] Based on the harmaline model, ethanol and primidone could have direct actions on the neuronal oscillator or could uncouple the oscillation from segmental spinal pathways. Beta-blockers act peripherally, possibly by reducing the sensitivity of sensory receptors (e.g., muscle spindles) and by increasing the low-pass filtering properties of skeletal muscle. A central mode of action is also possible. None of these treatments is specific for ET.

Parkinsonian Tremor

Rest tremor in the upper or lower extremities is the most specific feature of Parkinson's disease (see Chap. 15). Action tremor (i.e., postural tremor or kinetic tremor) is also common and may result from a re-emergent rest tremor or may exist independently of rest tremor.[63] There is no compelling reason to hypothesize different sources of oscillation for parkinsonian action tremor and rest tremor. Both forms of tremor occur in monkeys after destruction of the substantia nigra pars compacta (SNc) with intracarotid injections of MTPT (1-methyl-4-phenyl-1,2,3,6-tetrahydropyridine).[64]

The principal pathology of Parkinson's disease is a loss of dopaminergic cells in the SNc; this deficit is probably sufficient to produce parkinsonian tremor.[65] Neurons in the motor cortex,[66] ventrolateral thalamus,[67,68] globus pallidus,[69] and STN[70–73] oscillate intermittently in correlation with tremor, and a stereotactic lesion or high-frequency stimulation in any of these locations suppresses tremor (Fig. 29-2). The cerebellum is active in patients with parkinsonian tremor, but the cerebellum is not necessary for the production of rest tremor.[74] Thus, many parts of the motor system are clearly involved, and the principal source of oscillation is unclear. Their collective oscillation, rather than individual oscillation, may be necessary for parkinsonian rest tremor.[75,76]

Ventralis intermedius is the most effective stereotactic surgical site for treating parkinsonian tremor, even though Vim receives inputs from cerebellum and ascending spinal sensory tracts and only sparse input from the internal pallidum.[33–35] Stereotactic destruction and DBS of the posteroventrolateral internal pallidum and the subthalamus are effective treatments for tremor,[77] but the thalamic receiving nucleus of the internal pallidum, ventralis oralis posterior (Vop, ventralis lateralis anterior), is not an effective target.[78] How can these paradoxical surgical and anatomical data be reconciled? Of note is recent evidence that the inputs to Vop and Vim (both part of the ventrolateral thalamus) are not completely segregated, and both nuclei project to and receive considerable input from supplementary and primary motor cortices.[35,79] These overlapping corticothalamocortical projections might mediate the entrainment of the pallidothalamic and cerebellothalamic pathways through reverberation within the thalamocortical loops.[72]

Cerebellar Intention Tremor

Holmes used the terms "static tremor" and "intention tremor" to describe the tremors that he observed in patients with cerebellar lesions[80] (see Chap. 30). The following discussion is devoted to kinetic (intention) tremor, which is the most common.

The rhythm and amplitude of cerebellar tremor are usually irregular, and proximal limb muscles are often involved more than distal ones. The frequency of cerebellar tremor is commonly cited as 3–5 Hz, but animal and human studies have shown that tremor frequency is influenced by reflex arc length, and by the inertia and stiffness of the body part.[19,81] These observations are consistent with the mechanistic involvement of somatosensory feedback loops. However, instability in these loops is probably not the sole source of tremor because upper extremity deafferentation in decerebellate monkeys does not eliminate the 2–4-Hz intention tremor that occurs with cerebellar ablation alone.[82] The preservation of tremor following somatosensory deafferentation is probably due to the participation of visual feedback in tremorogenesis,[83] but an additional contribution from a central source of oscillation cannot be excluded.[53]

Classic intention tremor occurs in humans with lesions in the cerebellum or in the brachium conjunctivum pathway from the deep cerebellar nuclei to the contralateral ventrolateral thalamus (Fig. 29-2).[84,85] Small lesions in the vicinity of the ventrolateral thalamus may produce intention tremor with no other signs of ataxia.[84,85] An 8-year-old girl with a ventrolateral infarct and contralateral intention tremor was reported by Qureshi et al.,[85] and this tremor exhibited the properties of a mechanical-reflex oscillation (Fig. 29-4).

A dramatic 3–5-Hz kinetic tremor in the ipsilateral extremities occurs in laboratory primates with lesions in the deep cerebellar nuclei (dentate, globose, and emboliform) or in the outflow tracts of these nuclei (superior cerebellar peduncle). The critical nuclear lesion is still debated, but damage to globose and emboliform (interpositus in monkeys) seems most likely. Tremulous modulation of neuronal activity occurs in the motor cortex, somatosensory cortex, interpositus nucleus,

Hand Tremor (acceleration)

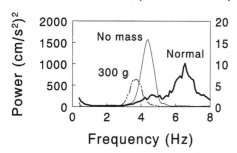

Ext. Carpi Radialis Brevis EMG

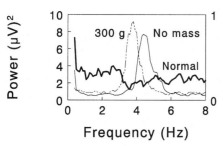

FIGURE 29-4 Fourier power spectra of hand tremor and rectified-filtered forearm EMG that were recorded from an 8-year-old girl who suffered a small infarct in the contralateral ventrolateral thalamus. With horizontal posture, she exhibited normal physiologic tremor (Normal; right vertical axis) with no entrainment of motor units in the extensor carpi radialis brevis (statistically flat spectrum). However, her tremor increased substantially when she pointed at a fixed target without moving her hand, and prominent tremor-related bursts of EMG occurred in the forearm muscles, producing an EMG spectral peak at the frequency of tremor. This abnormal tremor occurred at a lower frequency (No mass), and the frequency of this abnormal tremor decreased further with mass loading (300 g). However, the change in frequency with mass loading was not as great as seen in normal people (Fig. 29-1). Similar abnormal tremor was evident when writing, drawing, and performing finger-to-nose testing.

and somatosensory afferents of monkeys but does not occur in the dentate nucleus, which receives no somatosensory feedback.[19,86] These observations are consistent with the hypothesis that cerebellar tremor is produced by abnormal oscillation in transcortical and transcerebellar sensorimotor feedback loops. Changes in stiffness and inertia influence the frequency of cerebellar tremor less than the frequency of physiologic tremor (mechanical-reflex component) because transcortical and transcerebellar sensorimotor loops are heavily involved in cerebellar tremor but not in physiologic tremor.

Normal rapid limb movements toward a target are decelerated with a burst of antagonist muscle contraction. Target overshoot and limb oscillation occur when this antagonist

activity is delayed or inappropriately sized. Patients with cerebellar damage exhibit delayed antagonist muscle activation and terminal oscillation.[86,87] Cerebellar damage impairs the feedforward control of movement, so that available sensory information and prior experience are not used effectively in the formulation of antagonist muscle activity before the target is reached. Instead, limb movement is guided more by sensory feedback control.[86] Sensory feedback control is too slow and imprecise to prevent ataxia and tremor. Feedforward control (i.e., anticipatory deceleration) of movement is necessary, and the cerebellum plays a critical role in this regard.

Elble et al. found that tremor-related interpositus bursts in a rhesus monkey occurred an average 12.5 ms after the agonist EMG bursts.[19] Murphy et al. found that motor cortex and interpositus were activated nearly simultaneously by agonist muscle stretch.[88] Therefore, the interpositus bursts occurred too late to drive the agonist muscle. Instead, interpositus could be involved in limiting agonist activity through an inhibitory pathway, or it could drive the subsequent burst of antagonist EMG. Li Volsi et al. found that agonist pyramidal tract neurons in the cat were inhibited by the interpositus-thalamocortical pathway, but the antagonist pyramidal tract neurons were either excited or excited and then inhibited.[89] These observations support the notion that the cerebellum plays a critical role in the feedforward control of antagonist activation, which decelerates the limb in a smooth and accurate approach to the intended destination. The participation of these transcortical pathways explains why repetitive transcranial magnetic stimulation of motor cortex produces a cerebellar-like tremor in normal people.[90]

Classic cerebellar intention tremor exhibits a crescendo increase in amplitude as the limb approaches its target. The mechanism of this dramatic terminal accentuation of tremor is unknown. A contribution from a central source of oscillation is likely (e.g., the inferior olive, thalamus, or brainstem reticular formation). The Guillain-Mollaret triangle and other brainstem-cerebellar loops are prone to physiological reverberation and could contribute to the crescendo, nearly paroxysmal features of cerebellar intention tremor.[91,92] Reverberating thalamocortical loops could also contribute in this manner, and this would explain why Vim (ventralis intermedius) thalamotomy is an effective treatment for tremor but not the other manifestations of ataxia.

Rubral (Holmes') Tremor

Rubral tremor is a striking combination of 2–5-Hz rest, postural and kinetic tremor of an upper extremity (see Chap. 30). Frequencies as high as 7 Hz have been reported, and the frequency may vary with posture and movement.[93,94] This unusual tremor is caused by lesions in the vicinity of the red nucleus (Fig. 29-2). Many clinicians prefer the term midbrain tremor because isolated lesions in the red nucleus are not tremorogenic. The participants of the 1997 Tremor Symposium in Kiel, Germany, preferred the term Holmes' tremor.[95] A combination of damage to the neighboring cerebellothalamic, cerebello-olivary and nigrostriatal fiber tracts is required and explains the peculiar rest, postural and kinetic features.[53,96,97]

Rubral tremor usually begins weeks to months after brainstem trauma or stroke, so secondary or compensatory changes in nervous system function participate in tremorogenesis. Additional studies are needed to determine if this tremor is merely a combination of parkinsonian and cerebellar tremors or if a unique source of oscillation emerges from the underlying pathology. Remy et al. demonstrated reduced striatal ^{18}F-fluorodopa uptake in 6 patients with rubral tremor.[94] This finding explains why L-dopa and dopaminergic agonists occasionally are beneficial in these patients. Rubral tremor responds to stereotactic thalamotomy and DBS in ventralis intermedius.[28,98]

Palatal Myoclonus

Palatal myoclonus (or palatal tremor) consists of vertical oscillations of the soft palate at 1–3 Hz (see Chap. 30). Higher frequencies are rarely encountered. There are two forms of palatal myoclonus, symptomatic and essential, which differ clinically and pathophysiologically. Symptomatic palatal myoclonus is produced by damage in the dentato-olivary pathway (Fig. 29-2), which causes secondary hypertrophic olivary degeneration.[99] This anatomical abnormality is often visible with magnetic resonance imaging.[100,101] The palatal movements of symptomatic palatal myoclonus are usually asymptomatic but occasionally cause an ear click by moving the eustachian tube. Symptomatic palatal myoclonus is nearly always associated with other brainstem and cerebellar signs, depending upon the nature and extent of underlying pathology.[99] Synchronous movements of the tongue, floor of the mouth, larynx, face, diaphragm, intercostal muscles, eyes, extremities, and trunk may also occur. By contrast, essential palatal myoclonus causes an annoying ear click but no other neurological signs or symptoms, and the pathophysiology of essential palatal tremor is a complete mystery.[99] The ear click of essential palatal myoclonus is produced by movements of the eustachian tube that are caused by contraction of the tensor veli palatini, which can be suppressed with botulinum toxin injection. The levator veli palatini muscle is rhythmically active in symptomatic palatal myoclonus, and its contraction usually does not cause an ear click.[102,103]

Clinicopathological studies have repeatedly found dentato-olivary pathway damage in patients with symptomatic palatal myoclonus. This leads to secondary hypertrophic olivary degeneration and palatal myoclonus weeks to months after the initial ictus.[100,101,104] Many investigators believe that the hypertrophied olives might oscillate at 1–3 Hz, producing abnormal movements at the same frequency. However, the data supporting this hypothesis are largely inferential and inconclusive. Electrophysiologic studies of olivary hypertrophy in a laboratory animal with palatal myoclonus have not been done.[92]

Symptomatic palatal myoclonus is associated with at least three forms of extremity tremor. An asymptomatic tremor is produced by periodic inhibition of limb muscles at 1–3-Hz, time-locked to the palatal movements.[105] These brief periods of inhibition cause irregularities in muscle force that perturb the limb, producing an enhanced mechanical-reflex tremor. The other two forms of tremor are associated with palatal myoclonus, but it is not clear that these tremors emerge from the same source of oscillation. Masucci and Kurtzke described 5 patients with symptomatic palatal myoclonus and a 2–4-Hz rest tremor of the limbs that persisted during posture and movement.[106] All of their patients had signs of extensive brainstem damage, and only 1 of the 5 patients had tremor that was synchronous with the palatal movements. Masucci et al. also described a 1–3-Hz mixed rest and action tremor, called myorhythmia, that can involve various combinations of one or more extremities, the trunk, head, face, pharynx, jaw, tongue, and eyes.[107] With this tremor, the affected body parts may oscillate synchronously or asynchronously. The distribution of pathology is very similar to that seen in patients with palatal myoclonus, but some patients do not have palatal myoclonus and olivary hypertrophy.

Noteworthy is a recent report of a 49-year-old man who developed disabling right upper-extremity action tremor and palatal myoclonus 4 months after a hemorrhage in the left pontine tegmentum.[108] The distal postural tremor responded to Vim stimulation, but the proximal intention tremor did not. A subsequent left posteroventral pallidotomy greatly suppressed this tremor. This observation suggests that the effect of pallidotomy is not specific for parkinsonian tremor and that lesions in the dentato-olivary pathway can lead to tremorogenic participation of the basal ganglia.

Stroke-Induced Tremor

Tremor frequently follows strokes in the midbrain, superior cerebellar peduncle, and cerebellum, but tremor is a surprisingly uncommon complication of strokes elsewhere in the nervous system. Tremor in the absence of other neurological signs is a very rare. Tremor usually begins weeks to months after the ictus, so secondary neuronal changes are probably involved.[85,109,110]

A review of 240 published cases of focal lesions in the basal ganglia revealed only three cases of tremor, one of which resembled parkinsonian rest tremor. Strokes in the ventrolateral thalamus have produced contralateral action tremor,[110] parkinsonian rest tremor,[109] and intention tremor,[84,85] but in most cases the tremor following ventrolateral thalamic strokes is associated with dystonia.[111]

Tremor due to Peripheral Nerve Pathology

Patients with acquired and hereditary peripheral neuropathies frequently exhibit symptomatic 3–10-Hz action tremors (see Chap. 30). These tremors are usually less rhythmic than ET although some patients with hereditary neuropathy have tremor that is indistinguishable from 6–8-Hz ET.[112] The action tremor in many patients behaves like an abnormal mechanical-reflex oscillation, resembling enhanced physiologic tremor or cerebellar tremor.[113]

The frequency and amplitude of most neuropathic tremors bear no relationship to the degree of sensory loss or velocity of nerve conduction, and the underlying illnesses in most patients do not cause damage to the central nervous system (CNS).[113–115] Compensatory changes in CNS function probably cause abnormal oscillation to emerge from otherwise normal sensorimotor pathways, resulting in symptomatic tremor. The cerebellum has been implicated, but the details are far from clear.[116] Central reorganization in response to altered peripheral sensorimotor function is also hypothesized to cause the rare heterogeneous tremors that occur weeks to months after peripheral nerve trauma.[117]

Task-Specific, Focal and Dystonic Tremors

Patients with primary writing tremor exhibit severe tremor during the act of writing but experience little or no tremor during other activities (see Chap. 33). The frequency of primary writing tremor is not altered by mechanical loads, suggesting a central source of oscillation.[118] It is unclear whether primary writing tremor is a variant of focal dystonia, a variant of ET, or a separate disease entity.[118–121] Dystonic muscle contractions are commonly tremulous, and writer's cramp is no exception.[122–124] Furthermore, the dystonia in patients with isolated writing tremor can be very subtle and difficult or impossible to distinguish from compensatory posturing aimed at stabilizing the hand.[118] Thus, some cases of isolated writing tremor may be a variant of focal dystonia. ET can be relatively task-specific and frequently is most symptomatic during the act of writing. The relationship between primary writing tremor and ET will not be resolved until specific markers for ET and primary writing tremor are found. Both conditions are associated with bilaterally increased cerebellar activity, as measured with $H_2^{15}O$ PET.[125]

Isolated tremors of the voice, chin, tongue, and smile have been described, but these conditions are sufficiently rare that their proper nosology is unclear.[95] Like primary writing tremor, these less common task-specific and focal tremor may be a variant of dystonia, a variant of ET or some other entity.[39] Isolated tremor of the head is commonly due to cervical dystonia, but it may also be a manifestation of ET.[95,124,126]

Orthostatic Tremor

Orthostatic tremor is an unusual postural tremor that develops in the lower extremities and torso within seconds or more of assuming quiet erect stance[127–131] (see Chap. 30). This tremor was initially believed to be restricted to the lower limbs and torso, but it is now clear that the tremor is generalized and nearly synchronous throughout the body.[131] EMG reveals rhythmic bursts of motor unit activity at 14–18 Hz. This activity is usually symptomatic to the patient but barely visible to the examiner. Within seconds to minutes of continued standing, the frequency of body tremor may change to a 7–9-Hz subharmonic oscillation that is more symptomatic and visible. The tremor can reach violent proportions before relief is obtained by walking, sitting or lying down.

The 14–18-Hz frequency of orthostatic tremor is too high to originate in a lower extremity reflex loop, and a central source of oscillation is necessary to produce the dramatic rhythmicity and synchrony of this tremor in muscles of the limbs, torso, and cranium. Involvement of cranial muscles suggests an oscillator above the spinal cord.[131] However, the precise location of the central oscillator is unknown. Wu et al. found that orthostatic tremor is reset by electrical stimulation over the posterior fossa at intensities below the threshold for a motor evoked potential.[132] Like many other tremors, orthostatic tremor is associated with increased cerebellar blood flow, as measured with $H_2^{15}O$ PET.[133] The results of transcranial magnetic stimulation over the motor cortex have been variable.[132,134] Thus, an oscillator within the posterior fossa seems likely.

Although ET affects the lower extremities in 30–45 percent of patients,[135] the unusually high frequency of orthostatic tremor (14–18 Hz) and the marked synchrony among ipsilateral and contralateral muscles are never seen in ET. Therefore, most experts agree that orthostatic tremor is a distinct entity and not a variant of ET.[40,95]

Cortical Tremor

An irregular 7–14-Hz action tremor, resembling ET, occurs in patients with cortical reflex myoclonus and is called cortical tremor. Major motor seizures, myoclonus and a positive family history are characteristic of cortical tremor.[136–138] Cortical tremor is usually suppressed by clonazepam. The enhanced C-reflex and giant sensory evoked potentials in many of these patients are consistent with the presence of enhanced cortical irritability and transcortical reflexes. Like ET and parkinsonian tremor, cortical tremor can be reset by transcranial magnetic stimulation but is relatively refractory to peripheral electrical and mechanical stimuli. An EEG transient preceding the EMG bursts of cortical tremor has been demonstrated with EEG back-averaging.[137,139,140] Thus, the 7–14-Hz oscillation of cortical tremor probably emerges from abnormal cortical oscillation.

Drug-Induced Tremor

Many drugs produce parkinsonian rest tremor (neuroleptics), postural tremor (beta-adrenergic agonists, valproic acid, thyroxine, tricyclic antidepressants and methylxanthines), kinetic tremor (lithium), and combinations thereof (lithium, amiodarone, and valproic acid) (see Chap. 30). Little is known about the mechanisms of these tremors. Amiodarone- and lithium-induced tremors are particularly noteworthy because they are occasionally irreversible.[141–145] Persistent lithium-induced tremor and ataxia are caused by neuronal loss and gliosis of the cerebellar cortex and dentate nuclei.[146] It has long been suspected but never proven that people with subclinical ET and subclinical parkinsonian disease are more susceptible to tremorogenic drugs.[147]

Summary

The motor system contains a vast array of central and peripheral feedback loops, oscillating neuronal networks, and underdamped body mechanics. The complex integration of these sources of oscillation has made the elucidation of all tremors exceedingly difficult. Some tremors may emerge from the interaction of two or more anatomical structures, such that the identification of a single anatomical source of tremor is not possible. Nevertheless, considerable progress has been made, and many patients with disabling tremors are now the beneficiaries of a large and rapidly growing research effort.

Acknowledgments

Supported by NS20973 from the National Institute of Neurological Disorders and Stroke and by the Spastic Paralysis Research Foundation of Kiwanis International, Illinois-Eastern Iowa District.

References

1. Elble RJ, Randall JE: Motor-unit activity responsible for 8- to 12-Hz component of human physiological finger tremor. *J Neurophysiol* 39:370–383, 1976.
2. Elble RJ, Randall JE: Mechanistic components of normal hand tremor. *Electroencephalog Clin Neurophysiol* 44:72–82, 1978.
3. Freund HJ: Motor unit and muscle activity in voluntary motor control. *Physiol Rev* 63:387–436, 1983.
4. Milner-Brown HS, Stein RB, Yemm R: The contractile properties of human motor units during voluntary isometric contractions. *J Physiol (Lond)* 228:285–306, 1973.
5. Hagbarth K-E, Young RR: Participation of the stretch reflex in human physiological tremor. *Brain* 102:509–526, 1979.
6. Young RR, Hagbarth K-E: Physiological tremor enhanced by maneuvers affecting the segmental stretch reflex. *J Neurol Neurosurg Psychiatry* 43:248–256, 1980.
7. Fox JR, Randall JE: Relationship between forearm tremor and the biceps electromyogram. *J Appl Physiol* 29:103–108, 1970.
8. Stiles RN, Randall JE: Mechanical factors in human tremor frequency. *J Appl Physiol* 23:324–330, 1967.
9. Brumlik J, Yap C-B: *Normal Tremor: A Comparative Study.* Springfield, IL: Charles C Thomas, 1970.
10. Stiles RN: Mechanical and neural feedback factors in postural hand tremor of normal subjects. *J Neurophysiol* 44:40–59, 1980.
11. Rack PMH: Limitations of somatosensory feedback in control of posture and movement, in Brooks VB (ed): *Handbook of Physiology: The Nervous System, Motor Control.* Baltimore: Williams & Wilkins, 1981, pp 229–256.
12. Kakuda N, Nagaoka M, Wessberg J: Common modulation of motor unit pairs during slow wrist movement in man. *J Physiol (Lond)* 520:929–940, 1999.
13. Lakie M, Walsh EG, Wright GW: Passive mechanical properties of the wrist and physiological tremor. *J Neurol Neurosurg Psychiatry* 49:669–676, 1986.
14. Brown TI, Rack PM, Ross HF: Different types of tremor in the human thumb. *J Physiol (Lond)* 332:113–123, 1982.
15. Wessberg J, Vallbo ÅB: Pulsatile motor output in human finger movements is not dependent on the stretch reflex. *J Physiol (Lond)* 493:895–908, 1996.
16. Elble RJ: Central mechanisms of tremor. *J Clin Neurophysiol* 13:133–144, 1996.
17. Stein RB, Oguztöreli MN: Tremor and other oscillations in neuromuscular systems. *Biol Cybern* 22:147–157, 1976.
18. Wenderoth N, Bock O: Load dependence of simulated central tremor. *Biol Cybern* 80:285–290, 1999.
19. Elble RJ, Schieber MH, Thach WT Jr: Activity of muscle spindles, motor cortex and cerebellar nuclei during action tremor. *Brain Res* 323:330–334, 1984.
20. Rack PMH, Ross HF: The role of reflexes in the resting tremor of Parkinson's disease. *Brain* 109:115–141, 1986.
21. Britton TC, Thompson PD, Day BL, et al: 'Resetting' of postural tremors at the wrist with mechanical stretches in Parkinson's disease, essential tremor, and normal subjects mimicking tremor. *Ann Neurol* 31:507–514, 1992.
22. Elble RJ, Higgins C, Hughes L: Phase resetting and frequency entrainment of essential tremor. *Exp Neurol* 116:355–361, 1992.
23. Britton TC, Thompson PD, Day BL, et al: Modulation of postural tremors at the wrist by supramaximal electrical median nerve shocks in essential tremor, Parkinson's disease and normal subjects mimicking tremor. *J Neurol Neurosurg Psychiatry* 56:1085–1089, 1993.
24. Bock O, Wenderoth N: Dependence of peripheral tremor on mechanical perturbations: Modeling study. *Biol Cybern* 80:103–108, 1999.
25. Britton TC, Thompson PD, Day BL, et al: Modulation of postural wrist tremors by magnetic stimulation of the motor cortex in patients with PD and essential tremor and in normal subjects mimicking tremor. *Ann Neurol* 33:473–479, 1993.
26. Pascual-Leone A, Valls-Solé J, Toro C, et al: Resetting of essential tremor and postural tremor in Parkinson's disease with transcranial magnetic stimulation. *Muscle Nerve* 17:800–807, 1994.
27. Boecker H, Brooks DJ: Functional imaging of tremor. *Mov Disord* 13(suppl 3):64–72, 1998.
28. Andrew J, Fowler CJ, Harrison MJ: Tremor after head injury and its treatment by stereotaxic surgery. *J Neurol Neurosurg Psychiatry* 45:815–819, 1982.

29. Ohye C, Miyazaki M, Hirai T, et al: Primary writing tremor treated by stereotactic selective thalamotomy. *J Neurol Neurosurg Psychiatry* 45:988–997, 1982.

30. Schuurman PR, Bosch DA, Bossuyt PM, et al: A comparison of continuous thalamic stimulation and thalamotomy for suppression of severe tremor. *N Engl J Med* 342:461–468, 2000.

31. Krauss JK, Simpson RK Jr, Ondo WG, et al: Concepts and methods in chronic thalamic stimulation for treatment of tremor: Technique and application. *Neurosurgery* 48:535–541, 2001, discussion 535–541.

32. Hirai T, Jones EG: A new parcellation of the human thalamus on the basis of histochemical staining. *Brain Res Brain Res Rev* 14:1–34, 1989.

33. Ohye C, Shibazaki T, Hirai T, et al: Further physiological observations on the ventralis intermedius neurons in the human thalamus. *J Neurophysiol* 61:488–500, 1989.

34. Inase M, Tanji J: Thalamic distribution of projection neurons to the primary motor cortex relative to afferent terminal fields from the globus pallidus in the macaque monkey. *J Comp Neurol* 353:415–426, 1995.

35. Sakai ST, Inase M, Tanji J: Comparison of cerebellothalamic and pallidothalamic projections in the monkey (*Macaca fuscata*): A double anterograde labeling study. *J Comp Neurol* 368:215–228, 1996.

36. Elble RJ: Tremor in ostensibly normal elderly people. *Mov Disord* 13:457–464, 1998.

37. Louis ED, Ottman R, Hauser WA: How common is the most common adult movement disorder? Estimates of the prevalence of essential tremor throughout the world. *Mov Disord* 13:5–10, 1998.

38. Louis ED, Wendt KJ, Ford B: Senile tremor: What is the prevalence and severity of tremor in older adults? *Gerontology* 46:12–16, 2000.

39. Elble RJ: Diagnostic criteria for essential tremor and differential diagnosis. *Neurology* 54:S2–6, 2000.

40. Deuschl G, Elble RJ: The pathophysiology of essential tremor. *Neurology* 54:S14–20, 2000.

41. Higgins JJ, Pho LT, Nee LE: A gene (ETM) for essential tremor maps to chromosome 2p22-p25. *Mov Disord* 12:859–864, 1997.

42. Gulcher JR, Jonsson P, Kong A, et al: Mapping of a familial essential tremor gene, FET1, to chromosome 3q13. *Nat Gene* 17:84–87, 1997.

43. Higgins JJ, Loveless JM, Jankovic J, Patel PI: Evidence that a gene for essential tremor maps to chromosome 2p in four families. *Mov Disord* 13:972–977, 1998; erratum appears in *Mov Disord* 14:200, 1999.

44. Kovach MJ, Ruiz J, Kimonis K, et al: Genetic heterogeneity in autosomal dominant essential tremor. *Genet Med* 3:197–199, 2001.

45. Lakie M, Walsh EG, Arblaster LA, et al: Limb temperature and human tremors. *J Neurol Neurosurg Psychiatry* 57:35–42, 1994.

46. Elble RJ, Higgins C, Moody CJ: Stretch reflex oscillations and essential tremor. *J Neurol Neurosurg Psychiatry* 50:691–698, 1987.

47. Elble RJ, Higgins C, Leffler K, Hughes L: Factors influencing the amplitude and frequency of essential tremor. *Mov Disord* 9:589–596, 1994; erratum appears in *Mov Disord* 10:411, 1995.

48. Lakie M, Arblaster LA, Roberts RC, Varma TR: Effect of stereotactic thalamic lesion on essential tremor. *Lancet* 340:206–207, 1992.

49. Elble RJ: Physiologic and essential tremor. *Neurology* 36:225–231, 1986.

50. Elble RJ: Essential tremor frequency decreases with time. *Neurology* 55:1547–1551, 2000.

51. Elble RJ: The role of aging in the clinical expression of essential tremor. *Exp Gerontol* 30:337–347, 1995.

52. Rajput AH, Rozdilsky B, Ang L, Rajput A: Clinicopathologic observations in essential tremor: Report of six cases. *Neurology* 41:1422–1424, 1991.

53. Elble RJ: Animal models of action tremor. *Mov Disord* 13(suppl 3):35–39, 1998.

54. Llinás R, Yarom Y: Oscillatory properties of guinea-pig inferior olivary neurones and their pharmacological modulation: An in vitro study. *J Physiol (Lond)* 376:163–182, 1986.

55. Dupuis MJ, Delwaide PJ, Boucquey D, Gonsette RE: Homolateral disappearance of essential tremor after cerebellar stroke. *Mov Disord* 4:183–187, 1989.

56. Speelman JD, Schuurman PR, de Bie RMA, Bosch DA: Thalamic surgery and tremor. *Mov Disord* 13(suppl 3):103–106, 1998.

57. Hellwig B, Häussler S, Schelter B, et al: Tremor-correlated cortical activity in essential tremor. *Lancet* 357:519–523, 2001.

58. Sugihara I, Lang EJ, Llinas R: Serotonin modulation of inferior olivary oscillations and synchronicity: A multiple-electrode study in the rat cerebellum. *Eur J Neurosci* 7:521–534, 1995.

59. Lamarre Y, Joffroy AJ, Dumont M, et al: Central mechanisms of tremor in some feline and primate models. *Can J Neurol Sci* 2:227–233, 1975.

60. Deuschl G, Wenzelburger R, Loffler K, et al: Essential tremor and cerebellar dysfunction clinical and kinematic analysis of intention tremor. *Brain* 123:1568–1580, 2000.

61. Kitagawa M, Murata J, Kikuchi S, et al: Deep brain stimulation of subthalamic area for severe proximal tremor. *Neurology* 55:114–116, 2000.

62. Koller WC, Hristova A, Brin M: Pharmacologic treatment of essential tremor. *Neurology* 54:S30–38, 2000.

63. Jankovic J, Schwartz KS, Ondo W: Re-emergent tremor of Parkinson's disease. *J Neurol Neurosurg Psychiatry* 67:646–650, 1999.

64. Bergman H, Raz A, Feingold A, et al: Physiology of MPTP tremor. *Mov Disord* 13(suppl 3):29–34, 1998.

65. Tetrud JW, Langston JW: MPTP-induced parkinsonism and tremor, in Findley LJ, Koller WC (eds): *Handbook of Tremor Disorders*. New York: Marcel Dekker, 1995, pp 319–350.

66. Volkmann J, Joliot M, Mogilner A, et al: Central motor loop oscillations in parkinsonian resting tremor revealed by magnetoencephalography. *Neurology* 46:1359–1370, 1996.

67. Lenz FA, Kwan HC, Martin RL, et al: Single unit analysis of the human ventral thalamic nuclear group. Tremor-related activity in functionally identified cells. *Brain* 117:531–543, 1994.

68. Hua S, Reich SG, Zirh AT, et al: The role of the thalamus and basal ganglia in parkinsonian tremor. *Mov Disord* 13(suppl 3):40–42, 1998.

69. Hurtado JM, Gray CM, Tamas LB, Sigvardt KA: Dynamics of tremor-related oscillations in the human globus pallidus: A single case study. *Proc Nat Acad Sci U S A* 96:1674–1679, 1999.

70. Hutchison WD, Allan RJ, Opitz H, et al: Neurophysiological identification of the subthalamic nucleus in surgery for Parkinson's disease. *Ann Neurol* 44:622–628, 1998.

71. Levy R, Hutchison WD, Lozano AM, Dostrovsky JO: High-frequency synchronization of neuronal activity in the

subthalamic nucleus of parkinsonian patients with limb tremor. *J Neurosci* 20:7766–7775, 2000.

72. Magnin M, Morel A, Jeanmonod D: Single-unit analysis of the pallidum, thalamus and subthalamic nucleus in parkinsonian patients. *Neuroscience* 96:549–564, 2000.

73. Magarinos-Ascone CM, Figueiras-Mendez R, Riva-Meana C, Cordoba-Fernandez A: Subthalamic neuron activity related to tremor and movement in Parkinson's disease. *Eur J Neurosci* 12:2597–2607, 2000.

74. Deuschl G, Wilms H, Krack P, et al: Function of the cerebellum in Parkinsonian rest tremor and Holmes' tremor. *Ann Neurol* 46:126–128, 1999.

75. Wichmann T, Bergman H, DeLong MR: The primate subthalamic nucleus. III. Changes in motor behavior and neuronal activity in the internal pallidum induced by subthalamic inactivation in the MPTP model of parkinsonism. *J Neurophysiol* 72:521–530,1994.

76. Elble RJ. Origins of tremor. *Lancet* 355:1113–1114, 2000.

77. Krack P, Poepping M, Weinert D, et al: Thalamic, pallidal, or subthalamic surgery for Parkinson's disease? *J Neurol* 247(suppl 2):II122–134, 2000.

78. Bakay RAE, Vitek JL, DeLong MR: Thalamotomy for tremor. *Neurosurgical Operative Atlas* 2:299–312, 1992.

79. Stepniewska I, Preuss TM, Kaas JH: Thalamic connections of the primary motor cortex (M1) of owl monkeys. *J Comp Neurol* 349:558–582, 1994.

80. Holmes G: The symptoms of acute cerebellar injuries due to gunshot injuries. *Brain* 40:461–535, 1917.

81. Vilis T, Hore J: Effects of changes in mechanical state of limb on cerebellar intention tremor. *J Neurophysiol* 40:1214–1224, 1977.

82. Gilman S, Carr D, Hollenberg J: Kinematic effects of deafferentation and cerebellar ablation. *Brain* 99:311–330, 1976.

83. Sanes JN, LeWitt PA, Mauritz K-H: Visual and mechanical control of postural and kinetic tremor in cerebellar system disorders. *J Neurol Neurosurg Psychiatry* 51:934–943, 1988.

84. Bastian AJ, Thach WT: Cerebellar outflow lesions: A comparison of movement deficits resulting from lesions at the levels of the cerebellum and thalamus. *Ann Neurol* 38:881–892, 1995.

85. Qureshi F, Morales A, Elble RJ: Tremor due to infarction in the ventrolateral thalamus. *Mov Disord* 11:440–444, 1996.

86. Hore J, Vilis T: A cerebellar-dependent efference copy mechanism for generating appropriate muscle responses to limb perturbations, in Bloedel JR, Dichgans J, Precht W (eds): *Cerebellar Functions*. Berlin: Springer-Verlag, 1984, pp 24–35.

87. Diener H-C, Dichgans J: Pathophysiology of cerebellar ataxia. *Mov Disord* 7:95–109, 1992.

88. Murphy JT, Kwan HC, MacKay WA, Wong YC: Physiological basis of cerebellar dysmetria. *Can J Neurol Sci* 2:279–284, 1975.

89. Li Volsi G, Pacitti C, Perciavalle V, et al: Interpositus nucleus influences on pyramidal tract neurons in the cat. *Neuroscience* 7:1929–1936, 1982.

90. Topka H, Mescheriakov S, Boose A, et al: A cerebellar-like terminal and postural tremor induced in normal man by transcranial magnetic stimulation. *Brain* 122:1551–1562, 1999.

91. Houk JC, Keifer J, Barto AG: Distributed motor commands in the limb premotor network. *Trends Neurosci* 16:27–33, 1993.

92. De Zeeuw CI, Simpson JI, Hoogenraad CC, et al: Microcircuitry and function of the inferior olive. *Trends Neurosci* 21:391–400, 1998.

93. Nakamura R, Kamakura K, Tadano Y, et al: MR imaging findings of tremors associated with lesions in cerebellar outflow tracts: Report of two cases. *Mov Disord* 8:209–212, 1993.

94. Remy P, de Recondo A, Defer G, et al: Peduncular "rubral" tremor and dopaminergic denervation: A PET study. *Neurology* 45:472–477, 1995.

95. Deuschl G, Bain P, Brin M: Consensus Statement of the Movement Disorder Society on Tremor. Ad Hoc Scientific Committee. *Mov Disord* 13(suppl 3):2–23, 1998.

96. Holmes G. On certain tremors in organic cerebral lesions. *Brain* 27:327–375, 1904.

97. Ohye C, Shibazaki T, Hirai T, et al: A special role of the parvocellular red nucleus in lesion-induced spontaneous tremor in monkeys. *Behav Brain Res* 28:241–243, 1988.

98. Goldman MS, Kelly PJ: The surgical treatment of tremor, in Findley LJ, Koller WC (eds): *Handbook of Tremor Disorders*. New York: Marcel Dekker, 1995, pp 521–562.

99. Deuschl G, Mischke G, Schenck E, et al: Symptomatic and essential rhythmic palatal myoclonus. *Brain* 113:1645–1672, 1990.

100. Birbamer G, Buchberger W, Kampfl A, Aichner F: Early detection of post-traumatic olivary hypertrophy by MRI. *J Neurol* 240:407–409, 1993.

101. Uchino A, Hasuo K, Uchida K, et al: Olivary degeneration after cerebellar or brain stem haemorrhage: MRI. *Neuroradiology* 35:335–338, 1993.

102. Deuschl G, Toro C, Hallett M: Symptomatic and essential palatal tremor. 2. Differences of palatal movements. *Mov Disord* 9:676–678, 1994.

103. Deuschl G, Toro C, Valls-Sole J, et al: Symptomatic and essential palatal tremor. 1. Clinical, physiological and MRI analysis. *Brain* 117:775–788, 1994.

104. Birbamer G, Gerstenbrand F, Kofler M, et al: Post-traumatic segmental myoclonus associated with bilateral olivary hypertrophy. *Acta Neurol Scand* 87:505–509, 1993.

105. Elble RJ: Inhibition of forearm EMG by palatal myoclonus. *Mov Disord* 6:324–329, 1991.

106. Masucci E, Kurtzke J: Palatal myoclonus associated with extremity tremor. *J Neurol* 236:474–477, 1989.

107. Masucci EF, Kurtzke JF, Saini N: Myorhythmia: A widespread movement disorder. Clinicopathological correlations. *Brain* 107:53–79, 1984.

108. Miyagi Y, Shima F, Ishido K, et al: Posteroventral pallidotomy for midbrain tremor after a pontine hemorrhage. *J Neurosurg* 91:885–888, 1999.

109. Kim JS: Delayed onset hand tremor caused by cerebral infarction. *Stroke* 23:292–294, 1992.

110. Ferbert A, Gerwig M: Tremor due to stroke. *Mov Disord* 8:179–182, 1993.

111. Lee MS, Marsden CD: Movement disorders following lesions of the thalamus or subthalamic region. *Mov Disord* 9:493–507, 1994.

112. Shahani BT: Tremor associated with peripheral neuropathy, in Findley LJ, Capildeo R (eds): *Movement Disorders: Tremor*. London: Macmillan, 1984, pp 389–398.

113. Smith IS, Kahn SN, Lacey BW, et al: Chronic demyelinating neuropathy associated with benign IgM paraproteinaemia. *Brain* 106:169–195, 1983.

114. Said G, Bathien N, Cesaro P: Peripheral neuropathies and tremor. *Neurology* 32:480–485, 1982.

115. Dalakas MC, Teravainen H, Engel WK: Tremor as a feature of chronic relapsing and dysgammaglobulinemic

polyneuropathies. Incidence and management. *Arch Neurol* 41:711–714, 1984.

116. Bain PG, Britton TC, Jenkins IH, et al: Tremor associated with benign IgM paraproteinaemic neuropathy. *Brain* 119:789–799, 1996.

117. Cardoso F, Jankovic J: Peripherally induced tremor and parkinsonism. *Arch Neurol* 52:263–270, 1995.

118. Elble RJ, Moody C, Higgins C: Primary writing tremor. A form of focal dystonia? *Mov Disord* 5:118–126, 1990.

119. Rothwell JC, Traub MM, Marsden CD: Primary writing tremor. *J Neurol Neurosurg Psychiatry* 42:1106–1114, 1979.

120. Ravits J, Hallett M, Baker M, Wilkins D: Primary writing tremor and myoclonic writer's cramp. *Neurology* 35:1387–1391, 1985.

121. Rosenbaum F, Jankovic J: Focal task-specific tremor and dystonia: Categorization of occupational movement disorders. *Neurology* 38:522–527, 1988.

122. Yanagisawa N, Goto A, Narabayashi H: Familial dystonia musculorum deformans and tremor. *J Neurol Sci* 16:125–136, 1972.

123. Sheehy MP, Marsden CD: Writers' cramp: A focal dystonia. *Brain* 105:461–480, 1982.

124. Deuschl G, Heinen F, Kleedorfer B, et al: Clinical and polymyographic investigation of spasmodic torticollis. *J Neurol* 239:9–15, 1992.

125. Wills AJ, Jenkins IH, Thompson PD, et al: A positron emission tomography study of cerebral activation associated with essential and writing tremor. *Arch Neurol* 52:299–305, 1995.

126. Rivest J, Marsden CD: Trunk and head tremor as isolated manifestations of dystonia. *Mov Disord* 5:60–65, 1990.

127. Heilman KM. Orthostatic tremor. *Arch Neurol* 41:880–881, 1984.

128. Thompson PD, Rothwell JC, Day BL, et al: The physiology of orthostatic tremor. *Arch Neurol* 43:584–587, 1986.

129. Kelly JJ, Sharbrough FW: EMG in orthostatic tremor. *Neurology* 37:1434, 1987.

130. McManis PG, Sharbrough FW: Orthostatic tremor: Clinical and electrophysiologic characteristics. *Muscle Nerve* 16:1254–1260, 1993.

131. Köster B, Lauk M, Timmer J, Poersch M, et al: Involvement of cranial muscles and high intermuscular coherence in orthostatic tremor. *Ann Neurol* 45:384–388, 1999.

132. Wu YR, Ashby P, Lang AE: Orthostatic tremor arises from an oscillator in the posterior fossa. *Mov Disord* 16:272–279, 2001.

133. Wills AJ, Thompson PD, Findley LJ, Brooks DJ: A positron emission tomography study of primary orthostatic tremor. *Neurology* 43:747–752, 1996.

134. Tsai CH, Semmler JG, Kimber TE, et al: Modulation of primary orthostatic tremor by magnetic stimulation over the motor cortex. *J Neurol Neurosurg Psychiatry* 64:33–36, 1998.

135. Bain PG, Findley LJ, Thompson PD, et al: A study of hereditary essential tremor. *Brain* 117:805–824, 1994.

136. Ikeda A, Kakigi R, Funai N, et al: Cortical tremor: A variant of cortical reflex myoclonus. *Neurology* 40:1561–1565, 1990.

137. Toro C, Pascual-Leone A, Deuschl G, et al: Cortical tremor. A common manifestation of cortical myoclonus. *Neurology* 43:2346–2353, 1993.

138. Oguni E, Hayashi A, Ishii A, et al: A case of cortical tremor as a variant of cortical reflex myoclonus. *Eur Neurol* 35:63–64, 1995.

139. Terada K, Ikeda A, Mima T, et al: Familial cortical myoclonic tremor as a unique form of cortical reflex myoclonus. *Mov Disord* 12:370–377, 1997.

140. Okuma Y, Shimo Y, Shimura H, et al: Familial cortical tremor with epilepsy: An under-recognized familial tremor. *Clin Neurol Neurosurg* 100:75–78, 1998.

141. Prien RF, Caffey EM Jr, Klett CJ: Lithium carbonate. A survey of the history and current status of lithium in treating mood disorders. *Dis Nerv Syst* 32:521–531, 1971.

142. Donaldson IM, Cuningham J: Persisting neurologic sequelae of lithium carbonate therapy. *Arch Neurol* 40:747–751, 1983.

143. Charness ME, Morady F, Scheinman MM: Frequent neurologic toxicity associated with amiodarone therapy. *Neurology* 34:669–671, 1984.

144. Palakurthy PR, Iyer V, Meckler RJ: Unusual neurotoxicity associated with amiodarone therapy. *Arch Intern Med* 147:881–884, 1987.

145. Werner EG, Olanow CW: Parkinsonism and amiodarone therapy. *Ann Neurol* 25:630–632, 1989.

146. Schneider JA, Mirra SS: Neuropathologic correlates of persistent neurologic deficit in lithium intoxication. *Ann Neurol* 36:928–931, 1994.

147. Burn DJ, Brooks DJ: Nigral dysfunction in drug-induced parkinsonism: An 18F-dopa PET study. *Neurology* 43:552–556, 1993.

III. DYSTONIC DISORDERS

IDIOPATHIC TORSION DYSTONIA

Chapter 30

CHILDHOOD DYSTONIA

MICHELE TAGLIATI, ALANA GOLDEN, and
SUSAN B. BRESSMAN

EPIDEMIOLOGY 496
GENETICS 496
    Inheritance Pattern of Early-Onset Dystonia 496
    Genetic Linkage Studies and Linkage
        Disequilibrium: The DYT1 Story 497
    Gene Identification 498
    Normal Gene and Protein Function 498
    Abnormal Gene and Protein Function 498
PATHOLOGY 499
PATHOPHYSIOLOGY 499
CLINICAL FEATURES 500
    Early-Onset PTD 500
    The Influence of Genetic Phenotype 501
    Clinical Features of PTD 501
DIAGNOSTIC EVALUATION 502
    Genetic Testing 502
    Other Diagnostic Tests 503
TREATMENT 504
DOPA-RESPONSIVE DYSTONIA 504

Dystonia is a movement disorder characterized by involuntary twisting and repetitive movements or abnormal postures resulting from the co-contraction of agonist and antagonist muscles.[1] Different muscle groups can be involved with variable extent and severity, ranging from intermittent contractions limited to a single body region (focal dystonia) to generalized dystonia involving the axial and limb muscles (Table 30-1).

Although a reference to spasmodic torticollis can be found in the notes of the Dutch physician Tulpius as early as 1652,[2] it was Oppenheim who first used the term dystonia in 1911.[3] He described a childhood-onset syndrome characterized by twisted postures, muscle spasms, bizarre walking with bending and twisting of the torso, rapid sometimes rhythmic jerking movements, and progression of symptoms eventually leading to sustained fixed postural deformities that was known for decades as "dystonia musculorum deformans."[4] Many of the early reports of children with dystonia also included descriptions of other affected family members, raising the suspicion that the condition might be inherited.[5–8] Only studies over the past 15 years, however, have elucidated the genetic basis of childhood and adolescent-onset idiopathic dystonia.[9–11]

Three categories are used to classify dystonia: age of onset (early versus late), distribution (focal, segmental, multifocal, and generalized), and etiology.[12] Many different causes of dystonia have been recognized and two large etiologic categories are defined: primary, or idiopathic; and secondary, or symptomatic. Abnormal postures and movements are the only neurological abnormality in primary torsion dystonia (PTD), where no consistent pathologic changes are found and diagnostic studies are unrevealing (Table 30-2). PTD may be inherited, and a gene and several gene loci have been identified. Many adult-onset cases, however, are sporadic, and the genetic contribution remains to be clarified.

Secondary forms of dystonia can result from a variety of lesions, mostly involving the basal ganglia and/or dopamine synthesis, that are either inherited (e.g., dopa-responsive dystonia, Wilson's disease, gangliosidosis), or due to exogenous factors (e.g., perinatal injury, infections, neuroleptic medications). Clinical abnormalities other than dystonia (e.g., parkinsonism, dementia, ataxia, optic atrophy) are frequently present in symptomatic dystonias. Imaging studies often reveal changes involving the basal ganglia and other laboratory findings usually help in diagnosis. Another major distinction between primary and symptomatic dystonias is that a higher proportion of patients with symptomatic dystonia develop hemidystonia.[13]

The vast majority of cases of generalized dystonia begin in childhood or adolescence, with characteristic clinical and epidemiological features. Early-onset PTD has a typical onset around age 9[14] and has a genetic background in the great

TABLE 30-1 Classification of Dystonia According to Distribution of Affected Body Region

Focal: A single area is involved. Typical examples include involvement of:
    Upper face muscles (blepharospasm)
    Lower face muscles (oromandibular dystonia)
    Vocal cords (spasmodic dysphonia)
    Neck muscles (spasmodic torticollis)
    Arm muscles (writer's cramp)

Segmental: Two or more contiguous areas are affected. Examples include involvement of:
    Cranial muscles (face + jaw + tongue + vocal cords)
    Cranial, cervical and brachial muscles
    Bilateral brachial muscles (bibrachial dystonia)
    Axial muscles (neck and trunk)

Multifocal: Two or more noncontiguous body regions are involved. Examples include:
    Involvement of one or both arms plus one leg
    Cranial muscle involvement (e.g., blepharospasm) plus leg dystonia
    Hemidystonia is a type of multifocal dystonia

Generalized: Multiple areas including the legs are involved. Examples include involvement of:
    Both legs with or without the trunk and at least one other region
    One leg and the trunk plus at least one other region.

TABLE 30-2 Etiologic Classification of Dystonia

Primary: Dystonia is the only neurological sign and evaluation does not reveal an identifiable exogenous cause or other inherited or degenerative disease

Childhood- and adolescent-onset
- DYT1: Autosomal-dominant with reduced penetrance (approx. 30 percent), early limb-onset with predominant family phenotype
- Other genes to be identified

Adult onset
- DYT7: Autosomal-dominant, cervical onset in adult life
- Other genes to be identified

Mixed phenotype
- DYT6, DYT13: Autosomal-dominant, early- and late-onset, with possible cranial, cervical and sometimes limb-onset and variable spread
- Other genes to be identified

Secondary: Variety of lesions, mostly involving the basal ganglia and/or dopamine synthesis

Inherited non-degenerative (dystonia plus)
- Dopa-responsive dystonia (DRD): due to DYT5 and other genetic defects
- Myoclonus dystonia: due to DYT11 and possibly other genetic defects
- Rapid-onset dystonia-parkinsonism due to DYT12

Inherited degenerative
- Autosomal-dominant, autosomal-recessive, X-linked (DYT3), mitochondrial

Degenerative disorders of unknown etiology
- Parkinson's disease
- Progressive supranuclear palsy
- Corticobasal ganglionic degeneration

Acquired
- Drugs (dopamine receptor blockers), other toxins
- Head trauma
- Stroke, hypoxia
- Encephalitis, infectious, and postinfectious
- Tumors
- Peripheral injuries

Other movement disorders with dystonic phenomenology
- Tics, paroxysmal dyskinesias (DYT8, 9, 10)

Psychogenic dystonia

majority of cases. Perhaps 80–90 percent of Ashkenazi Jewish children and 50 percent of non-Jewish children who develop PTD test positive for the DYT1 gene defect. The remaining cases are either nongenetic or belong to less common (e.g., DYT6, DYT13) or still unknown genetic causes of dystonia. In this chapter we review the epidemiology, genetics, pathophysiology, clinical features, and treatment of PTD in children and adolescents. A separate section will be dedicated to dopa-responsive dystonia (DRD), a "dystonia-plus" syndrome with typical onset during childhood.

Epidemiology

The prevalence of PTD is difficult to estimate because of the variable expression and tendency for mild cases to go undiagnosed. Family studies have shown that at least one-half of cases of PTD are either not medically diagnosed or are misdiagnosed.[14,15] Using medical records, a study from Rochester, Minnesota calculated the prevalence to be 3.4 per 100,000 for generalized dystonia and 29.5 per 100,000 for focal dystonia.[16] There are also ethnic differences in frequency; childhood and adolescent-onset PTD appears to be more common in Jews of Eastern European or Ashkenazi ancestry. Based on cases reported in the literature, Zeman and Dyken estimated a disease frequency in American Jews (mostly of European ancestry) of 2.7 per 100,000, which is about 5 times the frequency of 0.5 per 100,000 they estimated for the general population.[17] A study of Israeli patients with generalized and segmental PTD found an 8-fold higher frequency among Jews of Eastern European ancestry (6.7 per 100,000) compared to African and Asian Jews (0.85 per 100,000).[18] More recently, a European collaborative study found a crude annual prevalence of 15.2 per 100,000, with most cases (11.7 per 100,000) being focal dystonia.[19] However, this study was based on ascertainment from adult neurology and botulinum toxin clinics and may have significantly underestimated the true prevalence of PTD.

No studies have assessed the frequency of PTD due to DYT1 based on molecular diagnosis. However, using an associated haplotype of alleles surrounding DYT1 in Ashkenazi Jews, the disease frequency in this population is estimated to be between 11/100,000 and 33/100,000,[15] somewhat higher than estimated for generalized and segmental dystonia in Israeli Ashkenazi Jews. Based on previous[17,18] and unpublished (Risch, personal communication) studies, PTD due to DYT1 in the non-Ashkenazi Jewish population and the non-Jewish population is estimated to be about one-third to one-fifth as common.

Genetics

INHERITANCE PATTERN OF EARLY-ONSET DYSTONIA

After the initial work of Oppenheim,[3] early reports of PTD described families with affected siblings, parents, second- and third-degree relatives.[5–8,20–22] Most families had early-onset dystonia and many were of Eastern European Jewish ancestry. However, due to the lack of clear diagnostic criteria,[9] secondary dystonias arising from environmental insults or neurodegenerative disorders were often mixed with PTD, causing Mendel, who coined the term "torsion dystonia" in 1919, to downgrade the disease to a "well-defined syndrome" less than 20 years later.[23,24] In 1944, Herz revived dystonia as a distinct disease entity, but, given the political atmosphere of the time, he chose to overlook a fundamental feature of the disease that would have strengthened his argument: early-onset PTD has increased prevalence among Ashkenazi Jews.[25] Herz also chose to ignore numerous reports of familial clustering, regarding them as exceptional and proclaiming, "hereditary factors are not traceable in the majority of cases of dystonia."[25] Although this notion was challenged in the 1960s, it was not until the end of the 20th century that the true heritable nature of early-onset PTD was conclusively discerned.

In the early 1960s, separate pedigrees with apparent autosomal-dominant transmission were reported.[9] In 1967, Zeman and Dyken reviewed the clinical, pathologic, and genetic aspects of 253 cases of dystonia musculorum deformans.[17] One hundred and forty-eight patients from 31 families (19 Jewish and 12 non-Jewish) were categorized as familial and the remaining 105 (50 Jewish and 55 non-Jewish) were considered sporadic. The median age at onset of the affected individuals was 10 years and over 90 percent were affected by age 21 years. The authors concluded that PTD is inherited in both Jewish and non-Jewish populations as an autosomal-dominant trait with a reduced penetrance of 52 percent. They estimated a higher gene frequency in American Jews, but they did not propose different inheritance patterns, or the presence of two or more genes, based on this difference in disease frequency.

Three years later Eldridge presented a detailed report of 156 cases representing 96 families (41 families were Ashkenazi Jewish) and came to different conclusions.[26] He proposed that PTD is inherited in an autosomal-recessive fashion in Jews and in an autosomal-dominant fashion in most non-Jewish families. He based his hypothesis on three findings: (1) the analysis of sibling risk was consistent with recessive inheritance; (2) the frequency of PTD in Jews is increased over non-Jews, and other disorders that are similarly increased in Jews, such as Tay-Sachs, are autosomal recessive; (3) clinical differences between Jews and non-Jews were noted. Jews were more likely to have progressive childhood-onset disease with first symptoms in a limb compared to non-Jews who had somewhat later onset, less clinical progression, and greater likelihood of initial axial involvement.

A nationwide Israeli study in 1984 rejected autosomal-recessive transmission in favor of autosomal-dominant with reduced penetrance of 51 percent.[18] Yet, despite this finding and numerous criticisms of Eldridge's study, including its lack of quantitative genetic analysis,[27] its failure to examine numerous living parents in affected pedigrees,[9] its erroneous conclusion that there is a significant difference in age and site of onset between Jews and non-Jews,[28] textbooks in the late 1980s still described early-onset PTD as autosomal-recessive in Ashkenazi Jews.[29]

At this time, Bressman and colleagues undertook the first study to include systematic blinded examinations of family members to definitively answer the question of Ashkenazi inheritance.[9,14,30] They studied 39 pedigrees with 43 independently ascertained probands and found an approximately equal frequency of dystonia among parents, siblings, and offspring, a finding consistent with autosomal-dominant inheritance. Moreover, they calculated age-adjusted lifetime risk for first-degree relatives (15.5 percent) to be approximately twice that for second-degree relatives (6.5 percent), consistent with a single locus model of inheritance with reduced penetrance of approximately 30 percent. There was no evidence for sporadic cases or new mutations in these families and the higher frequency of the disorder in Ashkenazim was postulated to be due to founder mutation and genetic drift.[30] An interesting finding in this study was the range of clinical features observed in affected relatives. Although relatives had milder disease (only half were aware they had dystonia), most were affected by age 30. There were no relatives with onset of symptoms >44 years, although over 60 percent of the examined relatives were at least age 45 years. Also none had onset in cranial muscles. These findings are consistent with the hypothesis that early- and late-onset dystonia have different causes, a theory that was subsequently confirmed with the identification of DYT1 (see below).

A subsequent complex segregation analysis on Eldridge's previously reported Ashkenazi families demonstrated that the trait is inherited in an autosomal-dominant fashion with reduced penetrance.[31] In almost all studies of early-onset non-Jewish families with dystonia, the disorder is also found to be inherited as an autosomal-dominant trait[17,21,22,32] with a wide range of penetrance. A systematic analysis[33] of 96 non-Jewish British probands with generalized, multifocal and segmental involvement concluded that approximately 85 percent of cases are inherited as an autosomal-dominant trait with reduced penetrance of 40 percent; the remaining 15 percent are likely to be nongenetic phenocopies. Increased paternal age of singleton cases was found and about 14 percent of genetic cases are thought to be new mutations. As in the study of Ashkenazi families, there was variable and often milder expression in affected relatives although, unlike that population, a larger proportion (10–15 percent) of non-Jewish affected family members had late onset (>44 years). This clinical heterogeneity is a result of the greater genetic heterogeneity in this population where only approximately 50 percent of non-Jewish early limb onset PTD cases harbor the DYT1 GAG deletion mutation.[34–38]

GENETIC LINKAGE STUDIES AND LINKAGE DISEQUILIBRIUM: THE DYT1 STORY

The DYT1 gene was initially mapped to a 30 cM (approximately 30 million base pairs, bp) region on chromosome 9q32-q34 in a single large North American non-Jewish family of French-Canadian ancestry.[10] Shortly thereafter, the same region was linked to 12 Ashkenazi Jewish families,[39] non-Jewish North American families,[40] and some, but not all, European non-Jewish families.[41]

Additional study led to the discovery of linkage disequilibrium in some of the Jewish families, further localizing DYT1 on chromosome 9q34 and suggesting that a single mutational event is responsible for most cases of early-onset PTD in Ashkenazi Jews.[15,42] Using the haplotype data, Risch et al. calculated that the DYT1 founder mutation originated in the Lithuanian or Byelorussian Ashkenazi population 350 years ago.[15] They also reasoned that the current high prevalence of the disease among Ashkenazim is due to the rapid expansion of a small founder group during the 18th century.

Further haplotype analysis within a genomic contig composed of yeast artificial chromosomes and cosmids and spanning 600 kilobase (kb) of chromosome 9q34 refined the localization of the DYT1 gene to a 150-kb region.[11] A cosmid contig was then constructed across the 150-kb target region and screened for transcripts via exon amplification.[43] Five transcripts were identified and inspected for mutation by single-strand conformational polymorphism analysis.

GENE IDENTIFICATION

A trinucleotide GAG deletion in the coding region of one transcript was found in 261 affected and unaffected obligate gene carriers from 64 Ashkenazi families and four non-Jewish families linked to chromosome 9. The GAG deletion results in the loss of one of a pair of glutamic acid residues near the C-terminus of a novel protein termed torsin A.[11]

The deletion, which appears to have arisen multiple times in different ethnic groups, was always heterozygous and never seen in over 500 controls.[11] The finding of de novo GAG deletions in patients of Russian and Mennonite origin added definitive proof that this change causes early-onset dystonia.[44] Subsequently, the GAG deletion has been found in non-Jewish individuals and families of diverse ethnic background.[34,37,45–47] Further, although the GAG deletion in the great majority of Ashkenazim derives from the same founder mutation, a small number of Ashkenazi harbor GAG deletions arising from different mutation events.[46,48] The increased frequency of this mutation is possibly due to genetic instability in an imperfect tandem 24-bp repeat in the region of the deletion.[44] Several studies have been undertaken to determine if other mutations in the DYT1 gene can cause early limb-onset dystonia.[38,49,50] Extensive screening has revealed only a single family with another mutation in the DYT1 gene: an in-frame deletion (18 bp) in the C-terminal region of the protein.[50] However, this family also harbors a mutation in the epsilon-sarcoglycan gene and that co-inherits with a phenotype of early-onset myoclonus and dystonia.[51]

NORMAL GENE AND PROTEIN FUNCTION

DYT1 (also known as TOR1A) is a member of a gene family consisting of three other highly homologous genes in the human genome. TOR1B is adjacent to DYT1 on chromosome 9q34 and is 70 percent identical at both the nucleotide and amino acid levels.[49] These two genes are in opposite orientations in the genome (tail-to-tail) and are assumed to have arisen from a tandem duplication of an evolutionary precursor gene. TOR1B is also ubiquitously expressed. The other

two members of the family, TOR2A and TOR3A, share about 50 percent homology at the amino acid level with DYT1.[49,52] TOR2A resides on chromosome 9q34 and TOR3A is located on chromosome 1q24 and has been independently cloned.[52] Genomic database searches have revealed torsin-like genes, all of unknown function, in mouse, rat, nematode, fruit fly, pig, cow, zebrafish, chicken, hamster, and *Xenopus*.[49]

The DYT1 gene encodes a protein, torsin A, that is 332 amino acids long (approx. 38 kDa), with potential sites for glycosylation and phosphorylation, as well as an N-terminal hydrophobic leader sequence consistent with membrane translocation/targeting.[43] Torsin A shares a similar ATP-binding domain and a predicted secondary structure with the heat-shock protein/Clp ATPase family within the AAA+ (ATPase associated with a variety of cellular activities) superfamily.[49] Members of this family exhibit chaperone activity and, in general, form 6-member, homo-oligomeric ring structures that interact with one or more other proteins.[49] They are associated with a number of functions, including protein folding and degradation, cytoskeletal dynamics, membrane trafficking and vesicle fusion, and response to stress.[53] However, the functions are so diverse that they provide little clue as to how torsin A might act.

In normal adult brain, torsin A is widely distributed, with intense expression in substantia nigra compacta (SNc) dopamine neurons, cerebellar dentate nucleus, Purkinje cells, basis pontis, locus ceruleus (LC), numerous thalamic nuclei, the pedunculopontine nucleus (PPN), the oculomotor nuclei, hippocampal formation, and frontal cortex.[54–57] Both the mRNA and protein were localized to neurons and not to glia, while the protein studies also showed torsin A in neuronal processes. Labeling was predominantly present in cytoplasm with some perinuclear staining.[56,57] A similar widespread pattern of expression was seen in both rat[56,58] and mouse[59] brains. The intense expression in nigral neurons suggests there may be dysfunction in dopamine transmission,[55] while strong labeling of neuronal processes points to a potential role for torsin in synaptic functioning. Two studies have further implicated torsin A in dopamine transmission with the finding of torsin A and alpha-synuclein immunoreactivity colocalized in Lewy bodies.[60,61]

Participation in membrane fusion, vesicle trafficking, and/or chaperoning the proper folding of proteins in the endoplasmic reticulum (ER) are suggested roles for torsin A.[62] Overexpressed wild-type torsin A highly colocalizes with the ER marker PDI, and partially colocalizes with vesicular markers such as VAMP-2 (synaptobrevin). Overexpressed mutant (DYT1 GAG deletion) torsin A accumulated in cytoplasm as ER-derived multilayered, concentric whorls and was frequently accompanied by cell body flattening and neurite retraction.

ABNORMAL GENE AND PROTEIN FUNCTION

Although the exact function of torsin A remains elusive, speculation on the mechanism(s) by which mutant torsin A may compromise neuronal function includes disrupted processing of normal torsin A or other proteins, interference of membrane trafficking, and neurotoxicity due to cytoplasmic inclusions. However, these theories are based upon results of studies based on overexpression of torsin A. So far, no inclusions or neuronal degeneration have been identified in DYT1 dystonia patients, and torsin in DYT1 brains appears normal.[63] Animal models of DYT1 are being developed and will hopefully help to shed light on the function of normal and mutated torsin A.[64]

Pathology

There are no consistent morphological abnormalities in PTD. A review of early pathologic studies on PTD patients showed that, whereas environmental and inherited etiologies of symptomatic dystonia leave their mark on the basal ganglia, the hereditary forms of PTD have no tangible pathologic abnormalities detectable by light microscopy.[65]

Histological analysis of the brainstem in 4 PTD patients (2 with early-onset and 2 with late-onset) yielded inconsistent results.[66] Two cases (1 with early-onset and 1 with adult-onset dystonia) did not show any abnormality. In the other 2 cases, neurofibrillary tangles in the LC and, less numerous, in the SNc, pedunculopontine nucleus, dorsal raphe nucleus and nucleus basalis were described, as well as neuronal loss in the SNc, dorsal raphe, PPN, and LC. The pigmented nuclei had extracellular pigment. The heterogeneity of the clinical presentation and the lack of genetic data make the interpretation of the results of this study very difficult.

The discovery of the DYT1 gene has allowed researchers to study brains with more homogeneous disease. The pathologic study of a single brain found normal nigral cellularity and striatal dopamine and homovanillic acid (HVA) levels, measured by high-performance liquid chromatography, within normal limits except for those in the rostral portions of the putamen and caudate nucleus, which were slightly decreased compared to controls.[67] Another study, again examining a single DYT1-positive dystonia brain, observed no differences in immunoreactivity of torsin A compared to non-DYT1 brains.[63] In addition, the authors found no evidence of intracellular aggregations, or specific colocalization with markers for ER, both of which have been reported in cell culture studies.[63]

Increased 3,4-dihydroxyphenylacetic acid/dopamine and HVA/dopamine ratios, suggestive of increased dopamine turnover, were found in the striatum of 4 DYT1 dystonia brains.[68] Prior to the discovery of the DYT1 gene, changes in norepinephrine, serotonin, and dopamine levels in various regions of brain were described in 2 patients with childhood-onset generalized dystonia[69] and in a single case of adult-onset primary cranial segmental dystonia.[70] Although it is not clear which, if any, of these alterations is related to the pathophysiology of dystonia, large increases in norepinephrine in the caudate nucleus, putamen, globus pallidus, and dentate

nucleus were also described in a patient with dystonia secondary to neuroacanthocytosis.[71] Finally, a significant decrease of complex I activity of platelet mitochondria was observed in several patients with idiopathic dystonia.[72] The severity of the complex I defect was more pronounced in patients with segmental or generalized disease than in those with focal dystonia. Whether abnormalities of complex I activity play a role in the pathogenesis of idiopathic dystonia remains to be determined.

Pathophysiology

Neurophysiological studies show a variety of motor and sensory abnormalities. EMG studies typically show prolonged co-contracting bursts of activity in agonist and antagonist muscles,[73] and a frequent spread of activity to distant muscles not normally used in a particular movement (overflow). These abnormalities can be explained by a loss of inhibitory control at the segmental (spinal cord, brainstem) or cortical level. There is convincing evidence that both spinal cord reciprocal inhibition and brainstem blink reflexes are abnormal in patients with dystonia.[74] However, further studies show that the basic disorder is most likely to be found in supraspinal command signal.[75] Results obtained with several experimental modalities have demonstrated that patients with dystonia have less efficient cortical inhibition than normal subjects.[74,75] A lack of inhibition would lead to excessive cortical activity and abnormal movements. Finally, there is also evidence of abnormal sensory processing in dystonia, and the sensory system may play a crucial role in the development of dystonic movements and postures.[76]

In an attempt to organize these findings, current models of basal ganglia circuitry, based primarily on the study of Parkinson's disease (PD), have been adapted to dystonia. In a very simplified model, the striatum receives glutamatergic input from several areas of the cerebral cortex and dopaminergic input from the SNc. The cortical and nigral inputs are received by the spiny projection neurons, which are pharmacologically and functionally subdivided into two types: those that project directly, and those that project indirectly to the internal segment of the globus pallidus, the major output site of the basal ganglia. The complementary activity of "direct" and "indirect" pathways regulates the function of the output neurons of the globus pallidus pars interna (GPi), which provides tonic inhibitory (GABAergic) input to the thalamic nuclei that project to the frontal cortical and other CNS areas. The "direct" pathway inhibits the substantia nigra pars reticularis (SNr) and the GPi, which results in a net disinhibition and facilitation of the thalamocortical connections. On the other hand, the "indirect" pathway—through serial connections with the globus pallidus pars externa (GPe) and the subthalamic nucleus (STN)—provides excitatory input to the GPi, resulting in further inhibitory action on the thalamocortical pathways. According to these models, the mean discharge rate of the GPi is the key factor associated with hypokinetic and hyperkinetic movements disorders. Increased inhibitory influence of the GPi on the thalamocortical pathway will lead to hypokinetic disorders such as PD, while decreased GPi activity will cause hyperkinetic disorders such as hemiballismus and dystonia. Reduced mean discharge rates in the GPi of patients with dystonia have been documented during surgical procedures using microelectrode guidance.[77]

A basal ganglia dysfunction with imbalance between normal modulation of the direct and indirect pathways is generally considered the basis for cortical disinhibition and abnormal motor output in dystonia. According to this model, both the "direct" and "indirect" pathways are overactive.[77] Overactivity of the "direct" pathway is supported by positron emission tomography (PET) studies showing dissociation of lentiform and thalamic metabolism in dystonia.[78] Overactivity of the "indirect" pathway was suggested by the finding of decreased binding of a D2 receptor ligand (spiperone) in the putamen.[79] However, the improvement in dystonia following pallidotomy (see later) is difficult to reconcile with the simple "rate" hypothesis for hypokinetic and hyperkinetic movement disorders and has led to the development of alternative models that also incorporate abnormalities of pattern, somatosensory responsiveness and degree of synchronization of neuronal activity.[80]

Using ^{18}F-fluorodeoxyglucose (FDG) and network analysis, Eidelberg et al. specifically studied DYT1 GAG deletion mutation carriers, both affected individuals and their asymptomatic gene carrier relatives, and as controls assessed noncarrier family members. They identified two independent abnormal regional metabolic covariance patterns: movement-free (MF) and movement-related (MR).[81] The MR pattern was identified in gene carriers affected with signs of dystonia. It showed increased metabolic activity in the midbrain, cerebellum, and thalamus. The MF pattern was characterized by increased metabolic activity in the lentiform nuclei, cerebellum, and supplementary motor areas, and was seen in both affected and nonmanifesting carriers.[81] More recent PET studies using psychomotor testing show subtle abnormalities in sequence learning both in the motor performance and in recruitment of brain networks.[82] These studies strongly support the presence of abnormal brain processing in gene carriers regardless of overt motor signs of dystonia, expanding the notion of penetrance and phenotype.

Clinical Features

Several features distinguish dystonia from other hyperkinetic movement disorders: the peak of movement is sustained regardless of contraction speed, contractions generally adopt a consistent direction or posture, and particular muscle groups are predictably involved. Additionally, dystonic contractions are often provoked by voluntary movements and can sometimes be alleviated by specific actions providing tactile feedback.[13] We will discuss the main clinical features of

TABLE 30-3 Distribution (percent) of PTD as a Function of Age at Onset

Age at Onset (years)	Generalized	Segmental and Multifocal	Focal	Hemidystonia
< 13	47.5	32.3	18.9	1
13–20	13.5	34.5	50.3	2
> 20	1.9	31.7	53.1	0.5

dystonia, with particular attention to the influence of age of onset and genetic phenotype.

EARLY-ONSET PTD

Clinical studies of dystonia have long noted a relationship between the age at onset of symptoms, the body region first affected, and the progression of disease. There is a well-described bimodal distribution in the age at onset with modes at ages 9 (early-onset) and 45 (late-onset) years, and a nadir at 27 years.[14] Early-onset dystonia usually first involves a leg or arm, and less commonly starts in the neck or vocal cords.[83,84] The majority of early-onset patients progress to involve more than one limb and about 50 percent eventually generalize to involve the legs and arms (Table 30-3). Patients with leg-onset have a somewhat earlier age at onset (8–9 years) compared to those with initial involvement of arm muscles (12–14 years); moreover, those with leg-onset are more likely to evolve into generalized dystonia compared to those patients with dystonia starting in an arm. The rate of progression to generalized dystonia is faster in those with onset in a leg (mean 4.7 years) compared to arm-onset cases (mean 11.4 years).[84] In contrast to early-onset, adult-onset dystonia usually starts in the arm, neck or cranial muscles; onset in a leg is very rare. Adult-onset dystonia tends to remain localized as focal or segmental dystonia and only rarely spreads to involve the legs. In a large series of 1741 patients with PTD, 24 percent had onset before age 21 years and only 9.5 percent had generalized dystonia. Among those with generalized dystonia, 46.5 percent of patients had childhood-onset, 11.8 percent had adolescent-onset and only 1.7 percent had adult-onset of symptoms.

The relationship between age-onset and signs of dystonia is somewhat different for the symptomatic dystonias (Table 30-4). A higher percentage of patients with symptomatic dystonia have early-onset (56 percent) or generalized

TABLE 30-4 Distribution (percent) of Symptomatic Dystonia as a Function of Age at Onset

Age at Onset (years)	Generalized	Segmental and Multifocal	Focal	Hemidystonia
< 13	52.7	23.4	11.3	12.6
13–20	29.9	34.5	25.3	10.3
> 20	13.5	40.6	40.6	5.3

TABLE 30-5 Classification of Genetic Loci Associated with Dystonia

Gene	Location	Inheritance	Phenotype	Gene Product
DYT1	9q34	AD	Early limb-onset PTD	Torsin A
DYT2	Not mapped	AR	Early-onset	
DYT3	Xq13.1	XR	Lubag dystonia/parkinsonism	Not identified
DYT4	Not mapped	AD	Whispering dysphonia	
DYT5	14q22.1	AD	DRD/ parkinsonism	GCH1
DYT6	8p21-p22	AD	"Mixed" cranial/cervical/limb onset	Not identified
DYT7	18p	AD	Adult cervical	Not identified
DYT8	2q33-25	AD	PDC/PNKD	Not identified
DYT9	1p21	AD	Episodic choreoathetosis/ataxia with spasticity	Not identified
DYT10	16	AD	PKC/PKD (EKD1 & 2)	Not identified
DYT11	7q21	AD	Myoclonus dystonia	Epsilon-sarcoglycan
DYT12	19q	AD	Rapid-onset dystonia-parkinsonism	Not identified
DYT13	1p36	AD	Cervical/cranial/brachial	Not identified
DYT14	14q13	AD	DRD	Not identified

Abbreviations: AD: autosomal dominant; AR: autosomal recessive; XR: X-linked recessive; PTD: primary torsion dystonia; DRD: DOPA-responsive dystonia; PDC: paroxysmal dystonic non-kinesigenic choreoathetosis; PNKD: paroxysmal non-kinesigenic dystonia; PKC: paroxysmal kinesigenic choreoathetosis; PKD: paroxysmal kinesigenic dyskinesia; GHC1: GTP Cyclohydrolase 1.

dystonia (27.5 percent); moreover, unlike what is observed in PTD, adult-onset symptomatic dystonia is more likely to generalize (8.3 percent). Another major distinction between idiopathic and symptomatic dystonias is that a much higher proportion of patients with symptomatic dystonia develop hemidystonia (11.4 percent versus 0.5 percent).

THE INFLUENCE OF GENETIC PHENOTYPE

Many genetic defects are associated with the clinical manifestation of dystonia (Table 30-5), and their identification has allowed the direct study of specific phenotypic expressions in affected families. The classic example is DYT1 dystonia, which has no consistent associated pathological abnormality or evidence of neuronal degeneration, and is associated with a GAG deletion mutation in the DYT1 gene on chromosome 9.

Investigators in the US, Europe and Asia have found that clinical expression of the DYT1 GAG deletion is generally similar across ethnic groups.[34,47,48,85,86] In a US study assessing 176 DYT1 mutation carriers, non-Jewish individuals had slightly more progressive disease with more leg-onset compared to Ashkenazi cases,[48] while other authors have noted mild or localized phenotypes in select non-Jewish DYT1 families.[87] No other large-scale systematic studies have further evaluated ethnic differences. One interesting and still unanswered question is whether the DYT1 phenotype or risk for developing dystonia (penetrance) differs between men and women. One study found that, at least among non-Jews, men were somewhat more likely than women to have a DYT1 mutation and developed a more severe disease.[48] However, other studies have not noted gender differences in either risk of developing dystonia due to DYT1 or disease expression.

The great majority of people with the DYT1 GAG deletion have early-onset (before 26 years), with an average age of onset of 14 years.[48] However, later-onset, up to age 64

years, has been described in affected relatives.[88] Disease severity can vary considerably among and within families. Usually dystonia progresses in both its temporal frequency and extent of muscle involvement. Progressively more actions are able to induce the movements and they may eventually occur at rest. Dystonic contractions often spread beyond the muscles first affected. About 65 percent of cases progress to a generalized or multifocal distribution, involving the legs and at least one arm.[48,83] When viewed in terms of body regions ultimately involved, one or more limbs will almost always be affected (over 95 percent have an affected arm). The trunk and neck are affected in about 25–35 percent; the cranial muscles are less likely to be involved (< 15 percent). For the rest, contractions remain more localized as either segmental or focal dystonia. Writer's cramp and bibrachial dystonia are the most common forms of focal and segmental dystonia respectively, and they may be the sole manifestation within a family.[87]

Most patients with adult-onset focal and segmental dystonia are not DYT1 deletion carriers.[48] Two studies looking specifically at adult-onset writer's cramp or musician's dystonia found no DYT1 gene mutations in these patients.[89,90]

CLINICAL FEATURES OF PTD

PTD commonly affects a limb at onset and usually begins with a specific action dystonia; in this case, the abnormal movements are triggered by a particular action and are not present at rest. For example, when idiopathic dystonia begins in a leg, abnormal contraction may be observed only with walking and be distinctively absent with running or walking backwards. As dystonia progresses, less specific actions of the affected leg may activate dystonia (e.g., tapping the floor). Moreover, actions in other parts of the body can induce involuntary movements of the involved leg, configuring the so-called "overflow dystonia." With further worsening, the affected limb can develop dystonic movements while at rest and eventually the leg will progress to sustained posturing. Similarly, arm dystonia typically starts while the individual is performing a specific task, such as writing or playing a musical instrument. Over time, the dystonia may be apparent when another part of the body is engaged in voluntary activity or with less-specific activities of the limb; finally, it may be present at rest. Thus, dystonia at rest is usually a more severe form than pure action dystonia.

Progression proceeds not only in terms of the severity of dystonic contractions in the limb first affected, but also in terms of the spread of dystonia to involve other parts of the body. Usually, dystonia first spreads to adjacent segments of the body and then more distally. Although the ipsilateral limb may be initially affected, producing a hemidystonia, more than 90 percent of the time, hemidystonia indicates that the dystonia is symptomatic rather than idiopathic.[91,92]

Dystonic movements tend to increase with fatigue, stress, and emotional states, and they tend to be suppressed with relaxation, hypnosis, and sleep.[93] One of the characteristic features of dystonic movements is that they can be diminished by tactile or proprioceptive "sensory tricks" (geste antagoniste), usually involving simply touching the involved or adjacent body part. The most common type of dystonia to benefit from sensory tricks is cervical dystonia, where placing a hand on the chin, side of the face, or back of the head reduces, sometime dramatically, neck muscle contractions. The efficacy of the geste antagoniste and the considerable variety in performance, duration, and EMG pattern of these maneuvers[94] warrant further investigation of the therapeutic use of sensorimotor stimulation. Patients with generalized dystonia may also respond to analogous sensory tricks. Not uncommonly, the severe flexed trunk on walking can be overcome by the patient placing one hand on the back of the head.

Usually dystonia is present continually throughout the day, whenever the affected body part is in use, or, in more severe cases, at rest; it disappears with deep sleep. In contrast to DRD, marked diurnal patterns are not common in PTD, although mild variations may occur. Remissions are rare and usually partial in early-onset dystonia,[95] and we have never encountered a patient with generalized dystonia who underwent complete remission of dystonic signs. Complete remissions have been described in patients with cervical dystonia.[96,97]

Pain is uncommon in PTD, with the exception of the involvement of cervical muscles; in fact, 75 percent of patients with cervical dystonia (spasmodic torticollis) have pain.[98] The high incidence of pain in cervical dystonia appears to be due to muscle contractions, because this pain is usually relieved by injections of botulinum toxin.[99] It is believed that the posterior cervical muscles are rich in pain fibers, and that continual contraction of these muscles results in pain. Another potential reason for pain in the cervical area is that dystonia there would increase the likelihood of patients developing cervical osteoarthritis, which would also produce radicular pain.

Because the legs and trunk are so often affected in early-onset dystonia, most children and adolescents with PTD have an abnormal gait. The leg commonly swings abnormally when it is carried forward. There may be abduction at hip and often the foot will swing medially, almost striking the other leg. The knee tends to be abnormally elevated with the foot in an equinovarus posture, but other postures, such as knee extension and foot eversion, are not uncommon. When the trunk is affected, there is commonly a bent-over posture, so called dromedary gait, with the neck extended while there is flexion at the hips. This contrasts to the opisthotonic gait which occurs fairly commonly in patients with tardive dystonia. Some patients with generalized dystonia cannot walk, or can walk only for a few steps before the dystonia overwhelms them. In the early stages of the disease, the trunk may not be dystonic when the patient is sitting or lying down. But with time, there is a tendency for the trunk to become involved in these positions as well.

Patients with PTD sometimes have rhythmic movements manifest as a tremor.[100,101] There are basically two types of tremor seen in dystonic patients: an accompanying tremor that resembles ET, and a tremor that is a rhythmic expression of rapid dystonic movements.[102] The latter can usually be distinguished from the former by showing that the tremor appears only when the affected body part is placed in a position of opposition to the major direction of pulling by the abnormal dystonic contractions. Dystonic tremor appears to be less regular than ET.[103] Sometimes it is very difficult to distinguish between the two types. In a review of 296 patients with primary dystonia, 24 had dystonic tremor, which in the great majority of cases was an isolated head-nodding tremor in the context of focal cervical dystonia. Only 2 patients with generalized dystonia had tremor; both were in the arm.[104]

In PTD, the only neurologic abnormality is dystonic postures and movements, except possibly for tremor.[105] There is no associated loss of postural reflexes, amyotrophy, weakness, spasticity, ataxia, reflex change, abnormality of eye movements, disorder of the retina, dementia, or seizures, except where they may be the result of a concomitant problem such as a complication from a neurosurgical procedure undertaken to correct the dystonia, or the presence of some other incidental neurologic disease. Since many of the symptomatic dystonias are associated with these neurological findings, the presence of any of these abnormalities in a patient with dystonia immediately suggests that one is dealing with symptomatic dystonia (see below). However, the absence of such neurological findings does not necessarily exclude the possibility of a symptomatic dystonia, which may present as a pure dystonia.

Diagnostic Evaluation

GENETIC TESTING

Until recently, no diagnostic test was available to positively identify PTD; the diagnosis depended on excluding secondary causes. With the successful cloning of the DYT1 gene,[43] it is now possible to diagnose one of the leading causes of generalized PTD. The DYT1 GAG deletion accounts for about 90 percent of early limb-onset cases in the Ashkenazi population and about 50–70 percent of non-Jewish early limb-onset PTD.[48] As virtually all cases of DYT1 dystonia are due to the same GAG deletion, screening is relatively easy and commercially available.[106] The test should be considered the first diagnostic test to apply to all PTD patients, whether Ashkenazi or non-Jewish, with onset by age 26, as these criteria result in 100 percent sensitivity with acceptable specificities ranging from 43 percent (in non-Jews) to 63 percent (in Ashkenazi Jews). If criteria are set more narrowly to include only those with early limb-onset, specificity improves (70–80 percent), and sensitivity drops (94–96 percent).[48] It may also be advisable to test individuals with later-onset who have an early-onset blood relative, as genetic studies have revealed that late-onset cases (most with writer's cramp) are found in the families of early-onset patients. It is recommended that, when DYT1 diagnostic and carrier testing are employed, genetic counseling also be provided. The psychological and social implications of a disorder with autosomal-dominant inheritance that has markedly reduced penetrance and very variable expression are complex. For example, even if the test is negative, a genetic etiology is not excluded and this needs to be discussed. If the test is positive, a diagnosis is secured, but this diagnosis impacts on other at-risk family members. Therefore, the need for counseling is particularly important for asymptomatic at-risk family members who wish carrier testing and in cases of prenatal testing.

OTHER DIAGNOSTIC TESTS

For most non-Jewish and the great majority of late-onset Jewish PTD patients, the diagnosis remains one of exclusion. To arrive at the clinical diagnosis of PTD, the examination should be normal, except for dystonia, and the history should not suggest another etiology. Diagnostic tests should be performed only if DYT1 testing is negative (Table 30-6). Diagnostic clues that dystonia is secondary are listed in Table 30-7. The investigation of all children and adolescents with uncomplicated "pure" dystonia must include exclusion of Wilson's disease by measurement of serum ceruloplasmin, slit lamp examination for Kayser-Fleischer rings, and magnetic resonance imaging (MRI). If the history and examination suggest dystonia is symptomatic, a more extensive work-up is indicated (see Table 30-6).

Routine computed tomography (CT) and MRI scans are normal in DYT1 dystonia.[107] FDG PET studies have revealed regional hypometabolism in the frontal cortex[108] and lenticular nucleus hypermetabolism,[109] with dissociation of lentiform and thalamic metabolism.[78] PET scans using a ligand to bind to striatal dopamine D2 receptors showed a trend to higher uptake in the contralateral striatum in subjects showing lateralization of clinical signs,[110] and decreased binding in the putamen.[79]

TABLE 30-6 Diagnostic Evaluation of Dystonia

Examination shows only typical dystonia (primary dystonia)

A. Onset <26 years or older if there is a relative with early onset:
a. DYT1 test with genetic counseling
   If negative
b. L-Dopa trial to rule out DRD
   If negative
c. Ceruloplasmin levels, slit lamp to rule out Wilson's disease

B. Onset >26 years:
a. Ceruloplasmin levels
b. Brain MRI

Examination shows dystonia with other signs and/or history suggests exogenous factor (secondary dystonia)

A. If history suggests tardive dystonia:
Ceruloplasmin levels, slit lamp to rule out Wilson's disease

B. If history and exam suggest structural lesion:
Imaging studies and other appropriate laboratory studies (e.g., CSF)

C. If history and exam suggest metabolic or other inherited disease:
L-Dopa trial
Ceruloplasmin, slit lamp
Brain MRI
And, as per diagnostic likelihood:
- Antiphospholipid antibodies
- Genetic testing (HD, SCA3, mitochondrial)
- Lysosomal analysis
- Alpha-fetoprotein
- Blood smear for acanthocytes
- Lactate/pyruvate
- Amino acids in serum and urine
- Urine organic acids
- Skin, muscle, nerve, bone marrow biopsy
- CSF analysis
- EMG/NCV, EEG

Legend: DRD: DOPA-responsive dystonia; MRI: magnetic resonance imaging; CSF: cerebrospinal fluid; HD: Huntington's disease; SCA: spino-cerebellar atrophy; EMG: electromyography; NCV: nerve conduction velocity; EEG: electroencephalogram.

TABLE 30-7 Clues that Dystonia is Symptomatic

History of possible etiologic factor (e.g., head trauma, peripheral injury, encephalitis, drug or toxin exposure, perinatal anoxia)
Presence of neurological abnormality other than dystonia (e.g., dementia, seizures, ataxia, weakness, spasticity, amiotrophy, ocular abnormalities)
Presence of false weakness or nonphysiological sensory examination, or other clues pointing to psychogenic etiology
Onset at rest instead of action dystonia
Early onset of speech involvement
Hemidystonia
Abnormal brain imaging
Abnormal laboratory workup

Treatment

Treatment for most dystonias, including DYT1, is mainly symptomatic. For patients with childhood- and adolescent-onset dystonia, most of whom have segmental or generalized signs, oral medications are mostly used, although there is increasing evidence that pallidal stimulation may provide dramatic improvement, especially for those with disabling primary dystonia due to the DYT1 GAG deletion. For those with adult-onset focal dystonias, botulinum toxin injections are generally the treatment of choice.

Because of the dramatic response to L-dopa in patients with DRD, most therapeutic recommendations advise trying L-dopa to at least 300 mg combined with carbidopa.[111] However, DYT1 genetic testing is now readily available with a fairly quick turnaround time. Thus, the rational for starting L-dopa in patients suspected clinically to be DYT1 is less compelling as DYT1 rarely substantively improves with low-dose L-dopa, and may actually worsen. Nevertheless, because there often is an urgency to treat, L-dopa with carbidopa frequently is the first drug tried in childhood-onset dystonia. Anticholinergics remain the drugs with the greatest clinical benefit in PTD, with about 40–50 percent of patients responding moderately.[112,113] The dose is slowly titrated up to a maximum tolerated; central side-effects such as memory impairment, confusion, and hallucinations usually limit dose, especially in older individuals. Peripheral side-effects may be controlled with pyridostigmine.

If anticholinergics are not tolerated or not helpful, the next drug tried is usually baclofen.[113,114] Although it appears to be less helpful than anticholinergics in most cases, fairly dramatic response may occur in some children. Other drugs are then usually tried either in combination or alone, and include clonazepam and other benzodiazepines, carbamazepine, mexiletine,[115,116] intravenous methylprednisolone,[117] and tetrabenazine.[113] The latter may be used in primary dystonia in a "cocktail" that includes a dopamine blocker and an anticholinergic.[118] In general, dopamine-blocking agents are not recommended because of acute and tardive side-effects, although risperidone has been reported to be useful in a short trial.[119] In some patients with generalized and segmental dystonia, botulinum toxin A to the most disabling or painful muscles may be given in conjunction with the above therapies.

When oral medications fail to provide symptomatic relief, intrathecal baclofen (ITB) and surgical therapy should be considered. ITB infusions have been shown to be an effective therapy for spasticity[120] and dystonia.[121,122] Both primary and secondary types of dystonia may benefit from this procedure, but it is unclear if the etiology of dystonia and the DYT1 status predict clinical response.[122] ITB may benefit more leg and trunk involvement than arm, neck, or cranial dystonia.[13] However, the proportion of patients showing sustained improvement is not large. Only 2 of 14 patients with primary or secondary dystonia showed unequivocal clinical benefit in a recent series.[122]

Moreover, equipment-related complications are fairly common and potentially serious.[122,123]

Pallidotomy and pallidal stimulation are other options in patients with generalized dystonia unresponsive to other therapies.[124] The more promising of these two surgical approaches appears to be deep brain stimulation (DBS) of the GPi. DBS was first used in the 1970s for the treatment of chronic pain, but over the last 15 years it has been progressively applied to the surgical approach of parkinsonism and other movement disorders. There are significant theoretical advantages of DBS over neuroablative techniques. The effects of DBS are reversible and patients remain eligible for future therapies. Because the DBS lead is left in place, physicians have on-going access to the site, allowing them to adjust stimulation parameters in response to changes in the patient's illness. DBS also allows surgeons to intervene at targets that cannot, or should not, be lesioned. High cost and need for maintenance of the device are the main disadvantages of DBS.

Initial reports describing the use of pallidal DBS in dystonia have been positive.[125–127] The largest experience to date comes from a group in Montpellier (France), which recently reported on 65 patients with different types of dystonia, including 19 with the DYT1 mutation, 26 with primary idiopathic dystonia, and 17 with secondary dystonia, with follow-up from 6 months to 5 years.[128] After 1 year, clinical score of patients with DYT1 dystonia improved on average by 71 percent. A similar improvement (74 percent) was observed in primary non-DYT1 cases, while secondary dystonia showed an average improvement of 44 percent. Stimulation efficiency did not decrease with time, with maximal reported follow-up of 58 months. The clinical improvement for several patients was completed. Side-effects were limited to delayed infection in 3 cases and 1 lead fracture, indicating that electrical stimulation of the GPi may prove to be a safe and effective treatment for advanced primary generalized dystonia with a remarkable tolerance in the pediatric population.

Dopa-Responsive Dystonia

DRD is a "variant" form of childhood-onset dystonia, initially described by Segawa et al.[129] It is a disease characterized by the onset of progressive dystonia, initially and most severely affecting the lower limbs, often marked by diurnal variations, features of parkinsonism, hyperreflexia, and a dramatic and sustained response to low-dose L-dopa therapy. DRD displays genetic and phenotypic heterogeneity and is inherited as an incompletely penetrant autosomal-dominant trait in the majority of cases.[130,131] Segregation analysis suggests a higher penetrance in women as compared to men (2:1–3:1), although it is unclear whether the severity of the disorder differs between the sexes.[131,132] There is no known ethnic predilection, with the prevalence in both England and Japan estimated at 0.5 per million,[130] and it is thought to comprise approximately 5 percent of all childhood dystonias not associated with an obvious etiology.

Since its earliest description, the pathogenesis of DRD was believed to involve a defect in the dopamine synthetic pathway, with evidence from genetic, biochemical, imaging, and pathologic studies. Over the last decade, the cause for most DRD cases has been elucidated and is constituted by a number of heterozygous mutations in the GTP cyclohydrolase I (GCHI) gene located on chromosome 14 (DYT5).[130,133–136] New mutations appear to occur commonly.[137] GCHI is the rate-limiting enzyme in the synthesis of tetrahydrobiopterin, which is an essential cofactor for tyrosine (as well as phenylalanine and tryptophan) hydroxylase (TH), and thus dopamine synthesis.[133,134] It is presumed, then, that DRD is caused by insufficient levels of dopamine as a result of low levels of the converting enzyme in heterozygous carriers. Moreover, homozygous mutations in other enzymes involved in dopamine synthesis, including TH[138–140] and 6-pyruvoyltetrahydropterin synthase (6-PTS), can cause a more severe form of DRD,[141] with associated hypotonia, severe bradykinesia, drooling, and ptosis.

Decreased levels of tetrahydrobiopterin and HVA (a major metabolite of dopamine) in the cerebrospinal fluid (CSF) were historically the first clue to a defect in dopamine synthesis,[142–144] and decreased CSF levels of neopterin may be the most specific biochemical marker for DRD.[145] Fluorodopa-uptake PET scans are virtually normal, indicating intact nigrostriatal pathway and dopamine storage.[146] On the other hand, results obtained with ^{11}C-raclopride PET showed elevated dopamine D2 receptor binding in the striatum of DRD patients, presumably caused by dopaminergic deficiency.[147,148] Confirming the PET studies, which indicate limited structural damage to the nigrostriatal pathway, a single detailed postmortem study described a normal number of dopamine neurons with normal TH activity and protein in the substantia nigra. There were no inclusion bodies or gliosis, and there was no degeneration in the striatum. The nigra dopamine cells, however, were hypopigmented; there was decreased dopamine in the nigra and striatum, and TH protein and activity was diminished in the striatum.[149]

Typically, DRD presents in mid-childhood (5–6 years), and an infantile onset with a picture mimicking cerebral palsy has been reported.[150] In children, the history is usually one of an abnormal gait that worsens as the day progresses and improves with sleep. The gait is frequently stiff-legged and there may be plantar flexion or eversion. Dystonia may also involve the trunk, arms and, less commonly, the neck. Parkinsonian features include postural instability, hypomimia, and bradykinesia, with progressive slowing, decrementing amplitude, and rigidity as rapid successive or alternating movements are attempted.[150,151] In about 25 percent of cases, there is also hyperreflexia, particularly in the legs, and plantar extensor signs; because of the hyperreflexia and also the stiff-legged scissoring gait, children with

DRD are not uncommonly misdiagnosed as having spastic diplegic cerebral palsy.[150] Over the past decade, the clinical spectrum of this disorder has broadened to include focal cervical dystonia,[152] adult-onset parkinsonism,[153,154] adult-onset oromandibular dystonia,[155] spontaneously remitting dystonia,[156] developmental delay and spasticity mimicking cerebral palsy,[157] postural tremor,[152] and limb dystonia that is not only diurnal but clearly related to exercise.[158]

The diagnosis of DRD depends on both the examination findings and a dramatic response to low-dose L-dopa therapy. Total daily dosages of as little as 50–200 mg of L-dopa (together with a dopa decarboxylase inhibitor) usually result in complete or near complete reversal of all signs and symptoms, which is maintained without fluctuations. DRD needs to be distinguished from DYT1 dystonia and juvenile parkinsonism due to homozygous or compound heterozygous parkin gene mutations.[152] Generally, the occurrence of early and prominent parkinsonism and severe dyskinesias with L-dopa treatment indicates a diagnosis of parkinsonism. Fluorodopa PET, which is normal in DRD, can be used to distinguish DRD from juvenile parkinsonism. Single-photon emission tomography using ^{123}I-beta-CIT, a sensitive marker of dopamine uptake sites, is also normal in DRD.[159]

Genetic analysis, although potentially resolutive, is complex. Multiple mutations have been discovered, and this heterogeneity presents a challenge for genetic screening. Moreover, a proportion of cases has no identified mutation[133,160] and may represent mutations of regulatory genes. One test for both affected and nonmanifesting GCHI gene carriers is phenylalanine loading.[161] As DRD patients have normal baseline levels of phenylalanine and tyrosine, a phenylalanine challenge results in abnormal elevations of serum phenylalanine, decreased tyrosine, and elevated phenylalanine/tyrosine ratios at 1, 2, and 4 hours post load. Phenylalanine loading, however, does not distinguish DRD from phenylketoneuria carriers. In this case, either measurement of biopterin (which is decreased in DRD) or repeating the challenge after giving biopterin (which corrects the defect in DRD) will define the diagnosis. In clinical practice, however, the typical phenotype and response to L-dopa are sufficient for the diagnosis.

A remarkable and sustained response to low-dosage L-dopa is the characteristic feature of DRD. Rarely, response may be less dramatic[152] and higher doses may be needed, especially for those patients with compound heterozygous mutations.[137,155] Response to L-dopa occurs within hours to days, and maximal benefit is usually achieved within weeks to months.[134,150,162–164] Even patients who remain untreated for years may show a striking response to L-dopa therapy.[150] It is unclear whether other agents, including anticholinergics and dopamine agonists, should be used instead or more likely in addition to L-dopa. Anticholinergics can be very effective in DRD,[165] as well as carbamazepine.[150] In our experience, dopaminergic agonists can provide further benefit as add-on therapy.

References

1. Fahn S: Concept and classification of dystonia. *Adv Neurol* 50: 1–8, 1988.

2. Redard P: *Le Torticollis et Son Traitement*. Paris: Carre & Naud, 1898.

3. Oppenheim H: Uber eine eigenartige Krampfkrankheit des kindlichen und jugendlichen Alters (Dysbasia lordotica progressiva, Dystonia musculorum deformans). *Neurol Centrabl* 30:1090–1107, 1911.

4. Fahn S: The varied clinical expressions of dystonia. *Neurol Clin* 2:541–554, 1984.

5. Schwalbe W: *Eine eigentumliche tonische Krampfform mit hysterischen Symptomen. Medicin und Chirugie.* Berlin: Universitats-Buchdrukerei von Gustav Schade, 1908.

6. Bernstein S: Ein Fall von Torsionkrampf. *Wien Klin Wochenschr* 25:1567–1571, 1912.

7. Abrahamson I: Presentation of cases of familial dystonia musculorum of Oppenheim. *J Nerv Ment Dis* 51:451–454, 1920.

8. Mankowsky BN, Czerny LI: Zur Frage uber die Heredität der Torsiodystonie. *Monatsschr Psychiatr Neurol* 72:165–179, 1929.

9. Bressman SB, de Leon D, Brin M, et al: Inheritance of idiopathic torsion dystonia among Ashkenazi Jews. *Adv Neurol* 50:45–56, 1988.

10. Ozelius L, Kramer PL, Moskowitz CB, et al: Human gene for torsion dystonia located on chromosome 9q32-9q34. *Neuron* 2:1427–1434, 1989.

11. Ozelius LJ, Hewett J, Kramer P, et al: Fine localization of the torsion dystonia gene (DYT1) on human chromosome 9q34: YAC map and linkage disequilibrium. *Genome Res* 7:483–494, 1997.

12. Fahn S, Bressman SB, Marsden CD: Classification of dystonia. *Adv Neurol* 78:1–10, 1998.

13. Bressman SB, Fahn S: Childhood dystonia, in Watts RL, Koller WC (eds): *Movement Disorders: Neurologic Principles and Practice.* New York: McGraw-Hill, 1997, pp 419–428.

14. Bressman SB, de Leon D, Brin MF, et al: Idiopathic torsion dystonia among Ashkenazi Jews: Evidence for autosomal dominant inheritance. *Ann Neurol* 26:612–620, 1989.

15. Risch N, deLeon D, Ozelius L, et al: Genetic analysis of idiopathic torsion dystonia in Ashkenazi Jews and their recent descent from a small founder population. *Nat Genet* 9:152–159, 1995.

16. Nutt JG, Muenter MD, Aronson A, et al: Epidemiology of focal and generalized dystonia in Rochester, Minnesota. *Mov Disord* 3:188–194, 1988.

17. Zeman W, Dyken P: Dystonia musculorum deformans: Clinical, genetic and pathoanatomical studies. *Psychiatr Neurol Neurochir* 70:77–121, 1967.

18. Zilber N, Korczyn AD, Kahana E, et al: Inheritance of idiopathic torsion dystonia among Jews. *J Med Genet* 21:13–20, 1984.

19. ESDE (Epidemiology Study of Dystonia in Europe Collaborative Group): A prevalence study of primary dystonia in eight European countries. *J Neurol* 247:787–792, 2000.

20. Regensburg J: Zur Klinik des hereditaren torsiondystonischen Symptomen komplexen. *Monatssch Psychiatr Neurol* 75:323–345, 1930.

21. Zeman W, Kaelbling R, Pasamanick B: Idiopathic dystonia musculorum deformans. I. The hereditary pattern. *Am J Hum Genet* 2:188–202, 1959.

22. Johnson W, Schwartz G, Barbeau A: Studies on dystonia musculorum deformans. *Arch Neurol* 7:301–313, 1962.

23. Mendel K: Torsionsdystonie. *Monatsschr Psychiat Neurol* 46: 309–361, 1919.

24. Mendel K: Torsionsdystonie, in Bumke O, Foester O (eds): *Handbuch der Neurologie (Angeborene fruherworbene, heredofamiliare Erkrankungen).* Berlin: Springer-Verlag, 1936, vol 16, pp 848–873.

25. Herz E: Dystonia, Part 2 (clinical classification). *Arch Neurol Psychiatry* 51:319–355, 1944.

26. Eldridge R: The torsion dystonias: Literature review and genetic and clinical studies. *Neurology* 20:1–78, 1970.

27. Korczyn AD, Zilber N, Kahana E, et al: Inheritance of torsion dystonia: Reply. *Ann Neurol* 10:204–205, 1981.

28. Burke RE, Brin MF, Fahn S, et al: Analysis of the clinical course of non-Jewish, autosomal dominant torsion dystonia. *Mov Disord* 1:163–178, 1986.

29. McKusick V: *Mendelian Inheritance in Man,* 7th ed. Baltimore: Johns Hopkins University Press, 1988.

30. Risch NJ, Bressman SB, de Leon D, et al: Segregation analysis of idiopathic torsion dystonia in Ashkenazi Jews suggests autosomal dominant inheritance. *Am J Hum Genet* 46:533–538, 1990.

31. Pauls DL, Korczyn AD: Complex segregation analysis of dystonia pedigrees suggests autosomal dominant inheritance. *Neurology* 40:1107–1110, 1990.

32. Larsson T, Sjögren T: Dystonia musculorum deformans: A genetic and clinical population study of 121 cases. *Acta Neurol Scand Suppl* 17:1–232, 1966.

33. Fletcher NA, Harding AE, Marsden CD: A genetic study of idiopathic torsion dystonia in the United Kingdom. *Brain* 113: 379–395, 1990.

34. Valente EM, Warner TT, Jarman PR, et al: The role of primary torsion dystonia in Europe. *Brain* 121:2335–2339, 1998.

35. Kamm C, Castelon-Konkiewitz E, Naumann M, et al: GAG deletion in the DYT1 gene in early limb-onset idiopathic torsion dystonia in Germany. *Mov Disord* 14:681–683, 1999.

36. Brassat D, Camuzat A, Vidailhet M, et al: Frequency of the DYT1 mutation in primary torsion dystonia without family history. *Arch Neurol* 57:333–335, 2000.

37. Major T, Svetel M, Romac S, et al: DYT1 mutation in primary torsion dystonia in a Serbian population. *J Neurol* 248:940–943, 2001.

38. Tuffery-Giraud S, Cavalier L, Roubertie A, et al: No evidence of allelic heterogeneity in the DYT1 gene of European patients with early onset torsion dystonia. *J Med Genet* 38:E35, 2001.

39. Kramer LP, de Leon D, Ozelius L, et al: Dystonia gene in Ashkenazi Jewish population is located in chromosome 9q32-34. *Ann Neurol* 27:114–120, 1990.

40. Kramer PL, Heiman G, Gasser T, et al: The DYT1 gene on 9q34 is responsible for most cases of early-onset idiopathic torsion dystonia in non-Jews. *Am J Hum Genet* 55:468–475, 1994.

41. Warner T, Fletcher NA, Davis MB, et al: Linkage analysis in British families with idiopathic torsion dystonia. *Brain* 116:739–744, 1993.

42. Ozelius LJ, Kramer PL, de Leon D, et al: Strong allelic association between the torsion dystonia gene (DYT1) and loci on chromosome 9q34 in Ashkenazi Jews. *Am J Hum Genet* 50:619–628, 1992.

43. Ozelius LJ, Hewett JW, Page CE, et al: The early-onset torsion dystonia gene (DYT1) encodes and ATP-binding protein. *Nat Genet* 17:40–48, 1997.

44. Klein C, Brin MF, de Leon D, et al: De novo mutations (GAG deletion) in the DYT1 gene in two non-Jewish patients with early-onset dystonia. *Hum Mol Genet* 7:1133–1136, 1998.

45. Ikeuchi T, Shimohata T, Nakano R, et al: A case of primary torsion dystonia in Japan with the 3-bp (GAG) deletion in the DYT1 gene with a unique clinical presentation. *Neurogenetics* 2:189–190, 1999.

46. Lebre AS, Durr A, Jedtnak P, et al: DYT1 Mutation in French families with idiopathic torsion dystonia. *Brain* 122:41–45, 1999.

47. Slominski PA, Markova ED, Shadrina MI, et al: A common 3-bp deletion in the DYT1 gene in Russian families with early-onset torsion dystonia. *Hum Mutat* 14:269, 1999.

48. Bressman SB, Sabatti C, Raymond D, et al: The DYT1 phenotype and guidelines for diagnostic testing. *Neurology* 54:1746–1752, 2000.

49. Ozelius LJ, Page CE, Klein C, et al: The TOR1A (DYT1) gene family and its role in early onset torsion dystonia. *Genomics* 62:377–384, 1999.

50. Leung J, Klein C, Friedman J, et al: Novel mutation in the TOR1A (DYT1) gene in atypical, early onset dystonia and polymorphisms in dystonia and early onset parkinsonism. *Neurogenetics* 3:133–143, 2001.

51. Klein C, Liu L, Doheny D, et al: Epsilon-sarcoglycan mutations found in combination with other dystonia gene mutations. *Ann Neurol* 52:675–679, 2002.

52. Dron M, Meritet JF, Dandoy-Dron F, et al: Molecular cloning of ADIR, a novel interferon responsive gene encoding a protein related to the torsins. *Genomics* 79:315–325, 2002.

53. Vale RD: AAA proteins: Lords of the ring. *J Cell Biol* 150:F13–F19, 2000.

54. Augood SJ, Penney JB, Friberg I, et al: Expression of the early-onset torsion dystonia gene (DYT1) in human brain. *Ann Neurol* 43:669–673, 1998.

55. Augood SJ, Martin DM, Ozelius LJ, et al: Distribution of the mRNAs encoding torsinA and torsinB in the adult human brain. *Ann Neurol* 46:761–769, 1999.

56. Shashidharan P, Kramer C, Walker R, et al: Immunohistochemical localization and distribution of torsinA in normal human and rat brain. *Brain Res* 853:197–206, 2000.

57. Konakova M, Huynh DP, Yong W, et al: Cellular distribution of torsin A and torsin B in normal human brain. *Arch Neurol* 58:921–927, 2001.

58. Walker RH, Brin MF, Sandu D, et al: Distribution and immunohistochemical characterization of torsinA immunoreactivity in rat brain. *Brain Res* 900:348–354, 2001.

59. Konakova M, Pulst SM: Immunocytochemical characterization of torsin proteins in mouse brain. *Brain Res* 922:1–8, 2001.

60. Shashidharan P, Good PF, Hsu A, et al: TorsinA accumulation in Lewy bodies in sporadic Parkinson's disease. *Brain Res* 877:379–381, 2000.

61. Sharma N, Hewett J, Ozelius LJ, et al: A close association of torsinA and alpha-synuclein in Lewy bodies: A fluorescence resonance energy transfer study. *Am J Pathol* 159:339–344, 2001.

62. Hewett J, Gonzalez-Agosti C, Slater D, et al: Mutant torsinA, responsible for early onset torsion dystonia, forms membrane inclusions in cultured neural cells. *Hum Mol Genet* 22:1403–1413, 2000.

63. Walker RH, Brin MF, Sandu D, et al: TorsinA immunoreactivity in brains of patients with DYT1 and non-DYT1 dystonia. *Neurology* 58:120–124, 2002.

64. Ziefer P, Leung J, Razzano T, et al: Molecular cloning and expression of rat torsinA in the normal and genetically dystonic (dt) rat. *Mol Brain Res* 101:131–135, 2002.

65. Zeman W: Pathology of the torsion dystonias (dystonia musculorum deformans). *Neurology* 20:79–88, 1970.

66. Zweig RM, Hedreen JC, Jankel WR, et al: Pathology in brainstem regions of individuals with primary dystonia. *Neurology* 38:702–706, 1988.

67. Furukawa Y, Hornykiewicz O, Fahn S, et al: Striatal dopamine in early-onset primary torsion dystonia with the DYT1 mutation. *Neurology* 54:1193–1195, 2000.

68. Augood SJ, Hollingsworth Z, Albers DS, et al: Dopamine transmission in DYT1 dystonia: A biochemical and autoradiographical study. *Neurology* 59:445–448, 2002.

69. Hornykiewicz O, Kish SJ, Becker LE, et al: Brain neurotransmitters in dystonia musculorum deformans. *N Engl J Med* 315:347–353, 1986.

70. Jankovic J, Svendsen CN, Bird ED: Brain neurotransmitters in dystonia. *N Engl J Med* 316:278–279, 1987.

71. de Yebenes JG, Brin M, Mena MA, et al: Neurochemical findings in neuroacanthocytosis. *Mov Disord* 3:300–312, 1988.

72. Benecke R, Strumper P, Weiss H: Electron transfer complex I defect in idiopathic dystonia. *Ann Neurol* 32:683–686, 1992.

73. Rothwell JC, Obeso JA: The anatomical and physiological basis of torsion dystonia, in Marsden CD, Fahn S (eds): *Movement Disorders 2*. London: Butterworth, 1987, pp 313–331.

74. Berardelli A, Rothwell JC, Hallett M, et al: The pathophysiology of primary dystonia. *Brain* 121:1195–1212, 1998.

75. Hallett M: The neurophysiology of dystonia. *Arch Neurol* 55:601–603, 1998.

76. Hallett M: Is dystonia a sensory disorder? *Ann Neurol* 38:139–140, 1995.

77. Vitek JL, Chockkan V, Zhang JY, et al: Neuronal activity in the basal ganglia in patients with generalized dystonia and hemiballismus. *Ann Neurol* 46:22–35, 1999.

78. Eidelberg D, Moeller JR, Ishikawa T, et al: The metabolic topography of idiopathic torsion dystonia. *Brain* 118:1473–1484, 1995.

79. Perlmutter J, Stambuk M, Markham J, et al: Decreased [18F] spiperone binding in putamen in idiopathic focal dystonia. *J Neurosci* 17:843–850, 1997.

80. Vitek JL: Pathophysiology of dystonia: A neuronal model. *Mov Disord* 17(suppl 3):S49–62, 2002.

81. Eidelberg D, Moeller JR, Antonini A, et al: Functional brain networks in DYT1 dystonia. *Ann Neurol* 44:303–312, 1998.

82. Carbon M, Ghilardi MF, Dhawan V, et al: Brain networks subserving motor sequence learning in DYT1 gene carriers. *Neurology* 58(suppl 3):A203, 2002.

83. Bressman SB, de Leon D, Kramer PL, et al: Dystonia in Ashkenazi Jews: Clinical characterization of a founder mutation. *Ann Neurol* 35:771, 1994.

84. Greene P, Kang UJ, Fahn S: Spread of symptoms in idiopathic torsion dystonia. *Mov Disord* 10:143–152, 1995.

85. Leube B, Kessler KR, Ferbert A, et al: Phenotypic variability of the DYT1 mutation in German dystonia patients. *Acta Neurol Scand* 99:248–251, 1999.

86. Matsumoto S, Nishimura M, Kaji R, et al: DYT1 mutation in Japanese patients with primary torsion dystonia. *Neuroreport* 12:793–795, 2001.

87. Gasser T, Windgassen K, Bereznai B, et al: Phenotypic expression of the DYT1 mutation: A family with writer's cramp of juvenile onset. *Ann Neurol* 44:126–128, 1998.

88. Opal P, Tintner R, Jankovic J, et al: Intrafamilial phenotypic variability of the DYT1 dystonia: From asymptomatic TOR1A gene carrier status to dystonic storm. *Mov Disord* 17:339–345, 2002.

89. Kamm C, Naumann M, Mueller J, et al: The DYT1 GAG deletion is infrequent in sporadic and familial writer's cramp. *Mov Disord* 15:1238–1241, 2000.

90. Friedman JR, Klein C, Leung J, et al: The GAG deletion of the DYT1 gene is infrequent in musicians with focal dystonia. *Neurology* 55:1417–1418, 2000.

91. Pettigrew LC, Jankovic J, Hemidystonia: A report of 22 patients and a review of the literature. *J Neurol Neurosurg Psychiatry* 48:650–657, 1985.

92. Marsden CD, Obeso JA, Zarranz JJ, Lang AE: The anatomical basis of symptomatic hemidystonia. *Brain* 108:463–483, 1985.

93. Fish DR, Sawyers D, Allen PJ, et al: The effect of sleep on the dyskinetic movements of Parkinson's disease, Gilles de La Tourette syndrome, Huntington's disease, and torsion dystonia. *Arch Neurol* 48:210–214, 1991.

94. Muller J, Wissel J, Masuhr F, et al: Clinical characteristics of the geste antagoniste in cervical dystonia. *J Neurol* 248:478–482, 2001.

95. Eldridge R, Ince SE, Chernow B, et al: Dystonia in 61-year-old identical twins: Observations over 45 years. *Ann Neurol* 16:356–358, 1984.

96. Jayne D, Lees AJ, Stern GM: Remission in spasmodic torticollis. *J Neurol Neurosurg Psychiatry* 47:1236–1237, 1984.

97. Friedman A, Fahn S: Spontaneous remissions in spasmodic torticollis. *Neurology* 36:398–400, 1986.

98. Chan J, Brin MF, Fahn S: Idiopathic cervical dystonia: Clinical characteristics. *Mov Disord* 6:119–126, 1991.

99. Greene P, Kang U, Fahn S, et al: Double-blind, placebo-controlled trial of botulinum toxin injections for the treatment of spasmodic torticollis. *Neurology* 40:1213–1218, 1990.

100. Yanagisawa N, Goto A, Narabayashi H: Familial dystonia musculorum deformans and tremor. *J Neurol Sci* 16:125–136, 1972.

101. Jankovic J, Fahn S: Physiologic and pathologic tremors. Diagnosis, mechanism, and management. *Ann Intern Med* 93:460–465, 1980.

102. Yanagisawa N, Goto A: Dystonia musculorum deformans: Analysis with electromyography. *J Neurol Sci* 13:39–65, 1971.

103. Jedynak CP, Bonnet AM, Agid Y: Tremor and idiopathic dystonia. *Mov Disord* 6:230–236, 1991.

104. Dubinsky RM, Gray CS, Koller WC: Essential tremor and dystonia. *Neurology* 43:2382–2384, 1993.

105. Lou JS, Jankovic J: Essential tremor: Clinical correlates in 350 patients. *Neurology* 41:234–238, 1991.

106. Klein C, Friedman J, Bressman S, et al: Genetic testing for early-onset torsion dystonia (DYT1): Introduction of a simple screening method, experiences from testing of a large patient cohort, and ethical aspects. *Genet Test* 3:323–328, 1999.

107. Rutledge JN, Hilal SK, Silver AJ, et al: Study of movement disorders and brain iron by MR. *Am J Roentgenol* 149:365–379, 1987.

108. Karbe H, Holthoff VA, Rudolf J, et al: Positron emission tomography demonstrates frontal cortex and basal ganglia hypometabolism in dystonia. *Neurology* 42:1540–1544, 1992.

109. Eidelberg D, Dhawan V, Takikawa S, et al: Regional metabolic covariation in idiopathic torsion dystonia: [18F]Fluorodeoxy-glucose PET studies. *Mov Disord* 7:297, 1992.

110. Leenders K, Hartvig P, Forsgren L, et al: Striatal [11-C]-N-methyl-siperone binding in patients with focal dystonia (torticollis) using positron emission tomography. *J Neural Transm* 5:79–87, 1993.

111. Bressman SB, Greene PE: Dystonia. *Curr Treat Options Neurol* 2:275–285, 2000.

112. Burke RE, Fahn S, Marsden CD: Torsion dystonia: A double blind, prospective trial of high dosage trihexyphenidyl. *Neurology* 36:160–164, 1986.

113. Greene PE, Shale H, Fahn S: Analysis of open-label trials in torsion dystonia using high dosages of anticholinergics and other drugs. *Mov Disord* 3:46–60, 1988.

114. Greene PE, Fahn S: Baclofen in the treatment of idiopathic dystonia in children. *Mov Disord* 7:48–52, 1992.

115. Ohara S, Hayashi R, Momoi H, et al: Mexilitine in the treatment of spasmodic torticollis. *Mov Disord* 13:934–940, 1998.

116. Lucetti C, Nuti A, Gambacinni G, et al: Mexiletine in the treatment of torticollis and generalized dystonia. *Clin Neuropharmacol* 23:186–189, 2000.

117. Kumar R, Maraganore DM, Ahlskog JE, et al: Treatment of putative immune-mediated and idiopathic cervical dystonia with intravenous methylprednisolone. *Neurology* 48:732–735, 1997.

118. Marsden CD, Marion MH, Quinn N: The treatment of severe dystonia in children and adults. *J Neurol Neurosurg Psychiatry* 36:160–164, 1984.

119. Zudas A, Cianchetti C: Efficacy of risperidone in idiopathic segmental dystonia. *Lancet* 347:127–128, 1996.

120. Penn RD, Savoy SM, Corcos D, et al: Intrathecal baclofen for severe spinal spasticity. *N Engl J Med* 320:1517–1521, 1989.

121. Ford B, Greene PE, Louis ED, et al: Intrathecal baclofen in the treatment of dystonia. *Adv Neurol* 78:199–210, 1998.

122. Walker RH, Danisi FO, Swope DM, et al: Intrathecal baclofen for dystonia: Benefits and complications during six years of experience. *Mov Disord* 15:1242–1247, 2000.

123. Teddy P, Jamous A, Gardner B, et al: Complications of intrathecal baclofen delivery. *Br J Neurosurg* 6:115–118, 1992.

124. Krack P, Vercueil L: Review of the functional surgical treatment of dystonia. *Eur J Neurol* 8:389–399, 2001.

125. Kumar R, Dagher A, Hutchison WD, et al: Globus pallidus deep brain stimulation for generalized dystonia: Clinical and PET investigation. *Neurology* 11:871–874, 1999.

126. Tronnier VM, Fogel W: Pallidal stimulation for generalized dystonia. Report of three cases. *J Neurosurg* 92:453–456, 2000.

127. Coubes P, Roubertie A, Vayssiere N, et al: Treatment of DYT1: Generalized dystonia by stimulation of the internal globus pallidus. *Lancet* 355:2220–2221, 2000.

128. Coubes P, Echenne B, Cif L, et al: Electrical stimulation of the internal globus pallidus in generalized dystonia. *Mov Disord* 17(suppl 5):S6, 2002.

129. Segawa M, Hosaka A, Miyagawa F, et al: Hereditary progressive dystonia with marked diurnal fluctuation. *Adv Neurol* 14:215–233, 1976.

130. Nygaard TG, Wilhelmsen KC, Risch NJ, et al: Linkage mapping of dopa-responsive dystonia (DRD) to chromosome 14q. *Nat Genet* 5:386–391, 1993.

131. Nygaard TG: An analysis of North American families with dopa-responsive dystonia, in Segawa M (ed):

Hereditary Progressive Dystonia with Marked Diurnal Fluctuation. Carnforth: Parthenon Publishing, 1993, pp 97–104.

132. Louis E, Lynch T, Bressman SB, et al: Gender differences in dopa-responsive dystonia. *Neurology* 44:A368–369, 1994.

133. Ichinose H, Ohye T, Takahashi E, et al: Hereditary progressive dystonia with marked diurnal fluctuations caused by mutations in the GTP cyclohydrolase 1 gene. *Nat Genet* 8:236–242, 1994.

134. Furukawa Y, Shimadzu M, Rajput AH, et al: GTP-cyclohydrolase I gene mutations in hereditary progressive amd dopa-responsive dystonia. *Ann Neurol* 39:609-617, 1996.

135. Ichinose H, Suzuki T, Inagaki H, et al: Molecular genetics of dopa-responsive dystonia. *Biol Chem* 380:1355–1364, 1999.

136. Ichinose H, Inagaki H, Suzuki T, et al: Molecular mechanisms of hereditary progressive dystonia with marked diurnal fluctuation, Segawa's disease. *Brain Dev* 22(suppl 1):S107–110, 2000.

137. Furukawa Y, Kish SJ, Bebin EM, et al: Dystonia with motor delay in compound heterozygotes for GTP-cyclohydrolase I gene mutations. *Ann Neurol* 44:10–16, 1998.

138. Knappskog PM, Flatmark T, Mallet J, et al: Recessively inherited L-DOPA-responsive dystonia caused by a point mutation (Q381K) in the tyrosine hydroxylase gene. *Hum Mol Genet* 4:1209–1212, 1995.

139. Ludecke B, Dworniczak B, Bartholome K: A point mutation in the tyrosine hydroxylase gene associated with Segawa's syndrome. *Hum Genet* 95:123–125, 1995.

140. van den Heuvel LP, Luiten B, Smeitink JA, et al: A common point mutation in the tyrosine hydroxylase gene in autosomal recessive L-DOPA-responsive dystonia in the Dutch population. *Hum Genet* 102:644–646, 1998.

141. Hanihara T, Inoue K, Kawanishi C, et al: 6-Pyruvoyl-tetrahydropterin synthase deficiency with generalized dystonia and diurnal fluctuation of symptoms: A clinical and molecular study. *Mov Disord* 12:408–411, 1997.

142. Williams A, Eldridge R, Levine R, et al: Low CSF hydroxylase cofactor (tetrahydrobiopterin) levels in inherited dystonia. *Lancet* ii:410–411, 1979.

143. LeWitt PA, Miller LP, Levine RA, et al: Tetrahydrobiopterin in dystonia: Identification of abnormal metabolism and therapeutic trials. *Neurology* 36:760–764, 1986.

144. Furukawa Y, Nishi K, Kondo T, et al: CSF biopterin levels and clinical features of patients with juvenile parkinsonism. *Adv Neurol* 60:562–567, 1993.

145. Blau N, Bonafe L, Thony B: Tetrahydrobiopterin deficiencies without hyperphenylalaninemia: Diagnosis and genetics of dopa-responsive dystonia and sepiapterin reductase deficiency. *Mol Genet Metab* 74:172–185, 2001.

146. Snow BJ, Nygaard TG, Takahashi H, et al: Positron emission tomographic studies of dopa-responsive dystonia and early-onset idiopathic parkinsonism. *Ann Neurol* 34:733–738, 1993.

147. Kishore A, Nygaard TG, de la Fuente-Fernandez R, et al: Striatal D2 receptors in symptomatic and asymptomatic carriers of dopa-responsive dystonia measured with [11C]-raclopride and positron-emission tomography. *Neurology* 50:1028–1032, 1998.

148. Kunig G, Leenders KL, Antonini A, et al: D2 receptor binding in dopa-responsive dystonia. *Ann Neurol* 44:758–762, 1998.

149. Rajput AH, Gibb WRG, Zhong XH, et al: Dopa-responsive dystonia: Pathologic and biochemical observations in a case. *Ann Neurol* 35:396–462, 1994.

150. Nygaard TG, Marsden CD, Fahn S: Dopa-responsive dystonia: Long-term treatment response and prognosis. *Neurology* 41:174–181, 1991.

151. Nygaard TG, Marsden CD, Duvoisin RC: Dopa-responsive dystonia. *Adv Neurol* 50:377–384, 1988.

152. Tassin J, Durr A, Bonnet AM, et al: Levodopa-responsive dystonia. GTP cyclohydrolase I or parkin mutations? *Brain* 123:1112–1121, 2000.

153. Nygaard TG, Takahashi H, Heiman GA, et al: Long-term treatment response and fluorodopa positron emission tomographic scanning of parkinsonism in a family with dopa-responsive dystonia. *Ann Neurol* 32:603–608, 1992.

154. Harwood G, Hierons R, Fletcher NA, et al: Lessons from a remarkable family with dopa-responsive dystonia. *J Neurol Neurosurg Psychiatry* 57:460–463, 1994.

155. Steinberger D, Topka H, Fischer D, Muller U: GCH1 mutation in a patient with adult-onset oromandibular dystonia. *Neurology* 52:877–879, 1999.

156. Di Capua M, Bertini E: Remission in dihydroxyphenylalanine-responsive dystonia. *Mov Disord* 10:223, 1995.

157. Nygaard TG, Waran SP, Levine RA, et al: Dopa-responsive dystonia simulating cerebral palsy. *Pediatr Neurol* 11:236–240, 1994.

158. Deonna T, Roulet E, Ghika J, et al: Dopa-responsive childhood dystonia: A forme fruste with writer's cramp, triggered by exercise. *Dev Med Child Neurol* 39:49–53, 1997.

159. Naumann M, Pirker W, Reiners K, et al: [123I]Beta-CIT single-photon emission tomography in DOPA-responsive dystonia. *Mov Disord* 12:448–451, 1997.

160. Bandmann O, Nygaard TG, Surtees R, et al: Dopa-responsive dystonia in British patients: New mutations of the GTP-cyclohydrolase I gene and evidence for genetic heterogeneity. *Hum Mol Genet* 5:403–406, 1996.

161. Hyland K, Fryburg JS, Wilson WG, et al: Oral phenylalanine loading in dopa-responsive dystonia: A possible diagnostic test. *Neurology* 48:1290–1297, 1997.

162. Deonna T: DOPA-sensitive progressive dystonia of childhood with fluctuations of symptoms: Segawa's syndrome and possible variants. *Neuropediatrics* 17:81–85, 1986.

163. Rondot P, Ziegler M: Dystonia: L-Dopa responsive or juvenile parkinsonism? *J Neural Transm Suppl* 19:273–281, 1983.

164. Allen N, Knopp W: Hereditary parkinsonism-dystonia with sustained control by L-dopa and anticholinergic medication. *Adv Neurol* 14:201–213, 1976.

165. Jarman PR, Bandmann O, Marsden CD, et al: GTP cyclohydrolase I mutations in patients with dystonia responsive to anticholinergic drugs. *J Neurol Neurosurg Psychiatry* 63:304–308, 1997.

Chapter 31

ADULT-ONSET IDIOPATHIC TORSION DYSTONIAS

EDUARDO S. TOLOSA and M. J. MARTÍ

CLINICAL FEATURES OF THE IDIOPATHIC
  ADULT-ONSET FOCAL DYSTONIAS 512
    Features Common to the Various IAOFD 512
    Blepharospasm (BSP) 513
    Oromandibular Dystonia (OMD) 513
    Laryngeal Dystonia (Spasmodic Dysphonia) 514
    Cervical Dystonia 514
    Limb Dystonia (LD) 515
    Other Task-Specific Dystonias (TSD) 516
    Other Focal Dystonias 516
ETIOLOGY 516
ANATOMIC SUBSTRATE AND PATHOPHYSIOLOGY
  OF THE FOCAL DYSTONIAS 518
DIFFERENTIAL DIAGNOSIS AND INVESTIGATIONS
  IN PATIENTS WITH FOCAL DYSTONIAS 520

Dystonia is characterized by involuntary muscular contractions causing twisting movements and abnormal postures. Etiologically, dystonia can be classified into primary or idiopathic and secondary or symptomatic. Idiopathic torsion dystonia (ITD) is of unknown cause and is characterized by the development of dystonic movements and postures in the absence of other neurological deficits. Childhood-onset ITD usually involves one lower limb first, with later spread of the dystonia to involve the trunk or other body parts. It is often familial and usually is inherited in an autosomal-dominant pattern with a reduced penetrance (see Chap. 32).[1] The clinical spectrum of idiopathic dystonia in adults is considerably different from the one in childood (Table 31-1). It generally involves the upper body, either the cranial musculature, neck, or arm, and the spasms tend to remain focal or spread only to the adjacent musculature. Idiopathic adult-onset focal dystonias (IAOFD) are sporadic, although, on occasion, more than one member in a family may have a focal dystonia. Table 31-2 lists the various IAOFD.

Rarely, AOFD are a manifestation of unusual forms of hereditary ITD (Table 31-3), including DYT1 dystonia usually starting in childhood. These instances of AOFD include: (1) those occurring in families with DYT1 mutations on chromosome 9q34;[2,3] (2) the AOFD described in a Swedish family (DYT1-negative), starting in adulthood and involving four generations;[4] (3) those that are part of the spectrum of

TABLE 31-1 Early-Onset versus Late-Onset ITD

Early-Onset
  Onset <age 15
  Frequently starts in one leg
  Commonly becomes generalized with involvement of the trunk
  Usually hereditary
Adult-Onset
  Onset >20
  Focal onset
  Tends to remain focal
  Spreads to neighboring regions (segmental dystonia) in
    20 percent of cases
  Usually sporadic

X-linked autosomal-recessive dystonia known to occur on the island of Panay in the Philippines;[5,6] (4) those exceptional cases occurring as a manifestation of the syndrome "rapid-onset dystonia-parkinsonism" linked to chromosome 19q13.[7]

In other chapters in this book, childhood-onset ITD (Chap. 32) and the symptomatic dystonias (Chap. 35) are covered in detail. In this chapter we cover ITD of adult-onset, discussing the clinical manifestations of the various focal dystonias and current thoughts on the underlying pathophysiology. The IAOFD are much more common than previously recognized. Their prevalence has been estimated by Nutt et al.,[8] in the population living in Rochester, Minnesota, at 30 per 100,000, compared to generalized ITD at 3.4 per 100,000. A study in the western area of Tottori Prefecture in

TABLE 31-2 IAOFD Syndromes

Muscle Groups Involved	Terminology
A. Orbicularis oculi and neighboring facial muscles	Essential BSP, dystonic BSP
B. Peribuccal muscles and platysma	Lower facial dystonia
C. Lower facial, masticatory, pharyngeal, and lingual muscles	OMD syndrome
D. A plus B or A plus C	Meige's syndrome, BSP-OMD syndrome
E. Laryngeal muscles	Laryngeal dystonia, spasmodic dysphonia
F. Cervical muscles	Cervical dystonia, ST
G. Hand, forearm, and arm muscles	Upper LD, WC, TSD, musician's dystonia, athlete's TSD

BSP, blepharospasm; OMD, oromandibular dystonia; ST, spasmodic torticollis; LD, limb dystonia; WC, writer's cramp; TSD, task-specific dystonia.

TABLE 31-3 Clinical Variants of ITD that Can Have their Onset in Early Adulthood

1. Adult-onset ITD; autosomal-dominant Swedish family (see Ref. 4)
2. X-linked dystonia-parkinsonism (see Ref. 5)
3. Rapid-onset dystonia-parkinsonism syndrome (see Ref. 5)

Japan encountered a lower prevalence (6.2 per 100,000) for focal dystonias than in western countries.[9] A recent study of primary dystonia in several European countries showed a prevalence rate of 152 per million, being the prevalence rate for focal dystonia of 117 per million.[10] The reasons for these differences in prevalence are unclear. In any case, these figures are probably underestimates, because patients with focal dystonias may go undiagnosed, and others do not seek medical help. Although the prevalence of generalized ITD is higher among the Ashkenazi Jewish population, this is not the case for IAOFD.[11]

Clinical Features of the Idiopathic Adult-Onset Focal Dystonias

FEATURES COMMON TO THE VARIOUS IAOFD

Prolonged muscle contractions producing sustained abnormal movements or postures are the clinical hallmark of dystonia. In the IAOFD, such spasms are limited to a single body region, with clinical symptoms depending primarily on the group of muscles involved.[12–14]

Characteristics common to the various focal dystonias of adulthood are shown in Table 31-4. IAOFD typically have their onset in the 4th or 5th decades but can also begin much earlier, and they typically affect women more than men (3:1). The onset is generally insidious, with symptoms varying depending on the body region involved and degree of spasm intensity. Dystonias occurring in adult life usually progress during the first few years after the initial manifestations. The time from onset to maximal disability, though, can vary considerably from patient to patient; in some patients, intense disabling spasms develop in just a few days or weeks, whereas in others the disorder continues to spread slowly 10–15 years after onset. Symptoms at onset can be intermittent, appearing only during times of emotional stress or without any apparent reason, but eventually they become steadily present. In about 20–30 percent of patients, dystonia extends to neighboring areas where the spasms are generally mild but can be prominent, with the patient then exhibiting signs

TABLE 31-4 Clinical Features Common to the Various Adult-Onset Focal Dystonias

---

Onset generally in 4th to 6th decades
Female predominance
Insidious onset, gradual progression during the first few years
Spread to neighboring regions not uncommon but almost never
    generalizes
Remissions infrequent but can occur in the early years
Worsened by emotional stress and fatigue
Improved by relaxation and rest
Sensory "tricks" transiently improve dystonic spasms
Tremor is common: focal "dystonic" tremor or essential-like tremor

---

of segmental dystonia. Occasionally, progression may skip an adjacent region to involve a more distant one; for example, a patient with blepharospasm (BSP) may later develop writer's cramp (WC) without signs of oromandibular dystonia (OMD) or laryngeal dystonia. In most cases, dystonia stabilizes after a few years and, eventually, may improve slightly with the passage of time.

Remissions, either partial or complete, can occur in all of the IAOFD, almost always during the first 2–3 years from onset, and are always transient, lasting for days to months. At times, symptoms can recur in a different area of the body than was affected originally. Remissions are more common in patients with spasmodic torticollis (ST) than with other types of IAOFD, and they occur more often in those patients with an earlier age of onset.[12–15]

Similar to generalized ITD of childhood, in IAOFD symptoms at onset usually appear during movement (action dystonia) and disappear when the affected body part is at rest. With the passage of time, dystonic movements may involve muscles not normally used in a task or movement. In WC, for example, this phenomenon, which is called "overflow," produces the characteristic posture of elevation of the elbow and abduction of the shoulder. In some patients, dystonia is triggered by actions in other parts of the body, as excessive unwanted movements to attempts at voluntary movements (e.g., dystonic movements appearing in the affected arm in a patient with WC when the patient is attempting to write with the healthy hand). Primary idiopathic dystonia often starts as a task-specific dystonia (TSD). With progression, however, the dystonic movements may appear with other activities. As an example, in patients with limb dystonia, dystonic cramps may occur initially only when writing but later also when using the hands for other tasks such as eating or sawing. In some patients with spasmodic dysphonia, laryngeal spasms occur initially only when the patient is speaking but not when singing or whispering; however, eventually they may be triggered by these actions as well. As the disease progresses, dystonia also may appear even at rest and, if left untreated, may evolve into fixed postures that eventually cause permanent contractures, as can be seen in long-standing untreated cervical dystonia. Although dystonic spasms are usually continuous, the timing and intensity of the movements can be influenced by various factors. Emotional stress and fatigue typically worsen dystonia, whereas rest and relaxation improve the spasms and they disappear during sleep. Some patients notice that certain "sensory tricks" can transiently reduce their dystonia. This reduction in dystonia by tactile or proprioceptive stimuli is a feature almost unique to dystonic movements.[16] Touching the back of the head or chin with one or more fingers, for example, allows some patients with torticollis to straighten their head, and gently leaning on the wall when standing may eliminate truncal dystonia transiently.

In addition to prolonged dystonic spasms, patients with IAOFD, like those with generalized dystonias, can exhibit other types of involuntary movements. In some patients, rapid movements resembling myoclonus occur. Obeso et al.[17] have described myoclonus occurring in patients with idiopathic dystonia that occurs irregularly, is seen mostly on voluntary muscle activation, and is superimposed on dystonic muscle spasms. These rapid movements can cause diagnostic confusion in some cases. Rhythmic, tremor-like movements are not uncommon in patients with dystonia, especially when the patient attempts to actively resist the involuntary movements. This focal, action-type tremor is generally irregular and slow, and is called dystonic tremor.[18] Occasionally, it may precede the onset of dystonia, as described by Rivest and Marsden,[19] or it may be the only manifestation of the dystonic disorder. Another type of tremor encountered in the idiopathic dystonias, in up to 20 percent of patients in some series, is one that resembles essential tremor and is frequently observed in both hands, even though they may not be affected by dystonic spasms, or in the head. It is a regular tremor, generally of modest amplitude, and has been reported in torticollis, WC, Meige's syndrome, and other focal dystonias.[18,20,21] True essential tremor has been said to occur commonly in patients with idiopathic dystonias, but it is not clear whether this type of postural tremor is a form of essential tremor, or whether it is an expression of some dystonia-related physiological abnormality. The finding that families with essential tremor do not have the DYT1 gene, as determined by means of linkage analysis, indicates that the two disorders are not genetically identical.[22] Mild parkinsonism has been described in some of the IAOFD, such as Meige's syndrome 22, and WC.[21]

BLEPHAROSPASM (BSP)

Patients with BSP have intermittent or sustained bilateral eyelid closure as a result of involuntary contractions of the orbicularis oculi muscles. Mild spasms of the frontalis and the middle and lower facial muscles also occur frequently. When the spasms are limited to the orbital or periorbital muscles, it is frequently called essential or dystonic BSP. The association of BSP with OMD is called cranial dystonia, or Meige's syndrome, because it was the French neurologist Henri Meige who, in 1910, first described in detail this syndrome, calling it "spasm facial median."[23,24] BSP affects women more than men and has its onset in about the 6th decade of life.

Patients with BSP, which may begin in one eye only, complain of eye discomfort, involuntary eye closure, eye narrowing or inability to open the eyes. Common complaints at onset are excessive blinking, eye irritation, burning, and photophobia, similar to symptoms of ocular surface, lid margin, and tear film disorders. BSP patients have variable degrees of difficulty with tasks such as reading, watching television, or driving, and they are frequently disabled, both occupationally and socially, by the spasms and the resulting functional blindness.[23-27]

Spasms of eye closure are generally aggravated by stress and disappear during sleep. BSP also is worsened by exposure to bright light, and for this reason most patients with BSP wear dark glasses. Other actions that frequently worsen the spasms are looking upward, walking, and reading and, less commonly driving, watching television, or looking downward. Maneuvers or tricks that alleviate some patients include talking, lying down, humming or singing, yawning, laughing, pressure on the eyebrows or the temple, chewing, and opening the mouth.

There are several clinical presentations of BSP[28] (Table 31-5). In the dystonic variety, the more common type, the spasms are prolonged, lasting for several seconds or even minutes, and the eyebrows are displaced downward, below the superior orbital rim (Charcot's sign). In the clonic form, the repetitive spasms of eye closure (blepharoclonus) are fast and resemble normal blinking. In some patients, as a result of contractions of the pretarsal part of the orbicularis, BSP mimics apraxia of lid opening.[28-31] In these patients, the eyes are closed in the absence of overt spasm, and the patient can not initiate or sustain eye opening. Elevation of the eyebrows, as a result of contraction of the frontalis muscles in an effort by the patient to open the eyelids, is common in this form of BSP (Fig. 31-1). Patients with this type of spasm frequently try to open the eyes with their fingers, pulling the lids apart. At times, reflex BSP is also present, and such attempts to open the eyes manually are met with increasing resistance by stronger spasms of the orbicularis oculi.[32] Yet, in other patients, a persistent narrowing of the palpebral fissure without complete eye closure is observed. The different types of spasms described here can be seen in a given BSP patient but sometimes can occur in isolation.

In most patients, dystonia spreads during the initial 5 years of onset of BSP. Previous head or face trauma with loss of consciousness, age at the onset of BSP, and female sex have been independently associated with an increased risk of spread.[33]

OROMANDIBULAR DYSTONIA (OMD)

In patients with OMD, spasms occur in the region of the jaw, lower face, and mouth.[34-36] Involvement of the masticatory muscles frequently produces spasms of jaw closure or opening, jaw protrusion, or lateral deviation. Spasms of jaw closure associated with involuntary contractions of the temporalis muscle and the masseters can produce trismus and bruxism.

TABLE 31-5 Eyelid Dysfunction in 17 Patients with Dystonic BSP

Eyelid Dysfunction	No. of Patients*
Clonic spasms	17 (3)
Dystonic spasms	9 (6)
"Apraxia" of lid opening	11 (3)
Tonic orbicularis contractions	8 (3)
Reflex BSP	6 (2)

*In parentheses is the number of patients in whom the specific type of eyelid dysfunction is the only or the predominant one.
SOURCE: *Modified from Tolosa and Marti.*[28]

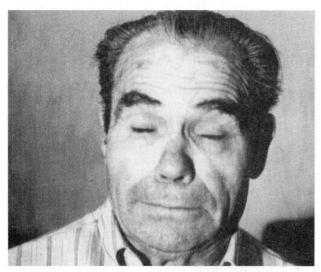

FIGURE 31-1 "Apraxia" of lid opening in patient with BSP. Oribucularis oculi spasms are not clearly evident. The patient tries to open the eyes with vigorous frontalis contraction.

Involuntary contractions of the lower facial muscles result in spasms of lip tightening, involuntary retraction of the corners of the mouth, and lip pursing. Platysmal contractions are also common. Lingual dystonia is manifested by lateral or upper deviation of the tongue, as well as by tongue protrusion. OMD in isolation is a relatively uncommon form of dystonia, but it is usually very disabling, causing jaw pain, dysarthria, and difficulty chewing and eating. Sensory tricks in OMD include touching the chin, chewing gum, biting on a toothpick, talking, and applying pressure in the submental area. In some patients, OMD is triggered by actions such as biting, chewing, or speaking.

In patients with OMD, spasms frequently occur in adjacent regions, and anterocollis, dysphonia, contraction of the nasalis muscles, and BSP are commonly present.

LARYNGEAL DYSTONIA (SPASMODIC DYSPHONIA)

Spasmodic dysphonia (SD) occurs between 30 and 50 years of age and, like other IAOFD, affects women more than men. It was originally described, by Traube in 1871,[37] as "a spastic form of nervous hoarseness" and was wrongly considered to be a psychogenic disorder until recently. Even today, many patients are referred to psychiatrists because the correct diagnosis is not made when the patient presents for treatment. Dystonic spasms in SD occur during speech (action-specific dystonia, and TSD), whereas the muscles and anatomic structures of the larynx are normal during rest. There are two types of SD:[38–42] adductor SD, which is caused by irregular hyperadduction of the vocal cords, and abductor SD, which is characterized by contraction of the posterior cricoarytenoid muscles during the action of speaking, resulting in inappropriate abduction of the vocal cords.

Patients with adductor SD exhibit a choked, strained, staccato, strangled voice quality with abrupt initiation and termination of vocalization, resulting in short breaks in phonation. There is decreased smoothness of speech, which becomes less intelligible. Usually, singing is less affected than speaking, except in severe cases.

Abductor SD is much less frequent. Patients exhibit a breathy, effortful voice, resulting in aphonic whispered segments of speech.[43] The voice is reduced in loudness, and speech is difficult to understand.

Onset of symptoms in SD is usually gradual, at times following an upper respiratory infection and during either occupational or emotional stress.[44] The initial complaints are increased effort and loss of voice and pitch control, at times only during stress. After 1–2 years of progression, the disease tends to stabilize and become chronic. Maneuvers or tricks that ameliorate SD are usually not as obvious as in other focal dystonias, but some patients report improving transiently when they press their hand on the back of their head,[45] or press their hand on their abdomen. Also, speech can improve briefly after a yawn or a sneeze. Laughing, coughing, or crying do not become affected, but, in 20–30 percent of patients, dystonia occurs elsewhere, usually in the cranial or cervical region. About 20 percent of patients have an irregular, audible dystonic voice tremor which can, at times, precede the appearance of the dystonic laryngeal spasms.

CERVICAL DYSTONIA

Dystonia of the neck muscles results in a condition characterized by abnormal head and neck posture called cervical dystonia, commonly referred to as spasmodic torticollis (ST). Patients with ST experience jerky movements of the head and intermittent or constant head deviation at rest. Deviation of the head can take any combination of directions: lateral rotation of the head (torticollis), frequently associated with a head tilt, is the most common,[46–48] but there can be lateral torticollis alone, anterocollis, and retrocollis. Frequently, the shoulder is elevated on the side toward which the chin is pointing, and a mild degree of dystonia can be detected commonly in the proximal muscles of the limbs on the same side. Unlike other focal dystonias, the incidence of pain in ST is remarkably high (over two-thirds of the patients) and contributes to disability.[46–48] Pain is most frequent in patients with constant head deviation, and, although it is usually localized in the neck, patients can develop secondary cervical radiculopathy (over 30 percent of patients in some series) and experience pain radiating into the arm. Head tremor, considered of a dystonic tremor, and/or hand tremor (essential tremor), occur in about one-third of ST patients.[46,49,50]

Sensory tricks used by torticollis patients to reduce the intensity of spasms include touching of the chin, face, or occiput. One such trick, called "geste antagonistique," consists of correction of head position when a very light touch or pressure is applied to the chin, cheek, or elsewhere in the head contralateral to the direction of the head turn. This trick was used in the past to support a psychogenic basis for ST. Symptoms frequently lessen when the patient lies down in bed, and they worsen when the patient walks and/or is under stress. In addition to cervical dystonia, about 20 percent of ST patients exhibit cranial (e.g., BSP) or arm-hand dystonia, which is usually mild.

Reported female to male ratios for idiopathic ST are approximately 2:1. Mean age at onset is between 38 and 42 years, with most cases clustering in the 4th through the 6th decades.[51] Severity of dystonia tends to progress during the first months or years of the illness, and the dystonic spasms can later spread to the oromandibular region or arm and, exceptionally, the leg. Even though ST is mild in some patients, it is usually disabling, interfering with the patient's daily activities and causing frequent pain. In patients with long-standing cervical dystonia, contractures may develop and fixed deformities may occur.

Cervical dystonia has been described after neck trauma. Some of these posttraumatic cases differ clinically from the more typical cases of idiopathic cervical dystonia because of the presence of marked limitation of range of motion, absence of geste antagonistique, and lack of improvement after sleep.[52,53]

About 10 percent of patients experience brief spontaneous remission of symptoms, and another 10 percent, mostly with an earlier age at onset, experience a longer period of remission (2–3 years) that occurs usually during the first 5 years of the illness.[54–56]

LIMB DYSTONIA (LD)

LD is characterized by involuntary contractions of limb musculature that result in twisting and repetitive movements or abnormal postures in the extremities. LD can affect the leg or the arm and can be focal, as in WC, or segmental, as when involving the arm and the neck (brachial) or leg and trunk (crural). It is always present in patients with generalized dystonia and in hemidystonia, when the upper and the lower extremities on one side are affected.[57,58]

Idiopathic LDs are frequently action dystonias, superimposed on voluntary movements such as writing, using eating utensils, or walking. As the disease progresses, the dystonic postures become more sustained and fixed, even more so when they occur in the legs. When occurring in the arm, distal involvement is more common in the form of wrist flexion, ulnar deviation, and supination. However, elevation, internal rotation, and abduction of the arm can occur also. In some patients the arm pulls behind the patient's back spontaneously.[13]

Many upper LDs are task-specific: that is, they occur exclusively or primarily when the patient performs a specific task. The most frequent TSD of the arm is WC but, in addition to writing, a large number of dystonia-inducing tasks have been reported in musicians[59,60] (e.g., guitarists, trumpet players), or sportsmen (e.g., golfers, snooker players, dart throwers).[57,61]

Symptoms of WC appear as soon as the pen is picked up or after a few words of writing. It usually presents as a forceful exaggeration of the usual grip of the pen, but in other instances hyperextension of the fingers may prevent the pen from being held in the hand. The wrist can show hyperextension or flexion, or forced supination or pronation. Arm and shoulder involvement can also occur. Writing is jerky, shaky, and laborious, and it may be accompanied by a sensation of tension and discomfort in the forearm. At times, frank pain is associated with writing. Frequently, writing becomes impossible after a few words. Classically, patients with WC can manage to write on a wallboard. Some patients find relief by stabilizing the writing hand by holding it with the contralateral one or by using thicker writing devices.[62–65]

WC is classified as "simple" when dystonia occurs only when writing, and as "dystonic" when the spasms appear with other hand tasks, such as using a screwdriver or shaving. WC may evolve from simple to dystonic in about one-third of cases but, generally, the severity of the condition remains relatively unchanged. Extension of dystonia to other adjacent or more distant body regions can occur over months to years after onset of symptoms. In about 25 percent of patients who try to write with the noninvolved hand, bilateral WC develops.[56] As with other dystonias, tremor occurs in about one-third of the cases. It can be a postural symmetrical hand tremor or a tremor triggered by writing. In such cases the differentiation with primary writing tremor, a form of task-specific tremor, can be quite difficult.[66,67]

It is not clear whether extensive writing can cause WC. It is likely that patients who write frequently will recognize their symptoms earlier and will seek early medical attention.[55] WC can be the earliest manifestation of idiopathic generalized torsion dystonia, but it can also represent the presenting complaint of neurological disorders, such as Parkinson's disease or progressive supranuclear palsy.[68–71]

In patients with WC, several electrophysiologic abnormalities have been found, and these are shared with other TSD (see Ref. 72 for review). Co-contraction of antagonist muscles occurs, such that movement can be undertaken only with the greatest of effort. There is lack of selectivity in attempts to perform independent finger movements, and neural activation may spread ("overflow") to involve muscles not normally used in the task of writing (e.g., abduction of the shoulder). Failure to activate the appropriate muscles may also occur. These findings highlight the fact that patients have more problems with voluntary actions than with involuntary muscle spasm.

Dystonia occurring in the lower extremities usually affects distal joints, principally the ankle, with plantar flexion and inversion of the foot. The sole of the foot can also cup and the toes can flex. Initially, foot dystonia occurs only when one is walking, being absent with the limb at rest. Frequently, running, walking in tandem, or walking backwards fails to trigger the abnormal posture. The initial equinovarus posture that occurs when the patient is walking may evolve into a fixed dystonic posture, commonly causing plantar flexion, extension of the knee, and extension, internal rotation, and abduction of the hip.

When lower LD occurs in childhood, it usually heralds the onset of early generalized dystonia.[73] When lower LD occurs after the age of 20, it suggests the possibility of focal central nervous system structural disease. Also, when dystonia affects the foot in an adult, the possibility of Parkinson's disease or another parkinsonian syndrome should be considered, because kinesigenic foot dystonia is an early sign of young-onset Parkinson's disease.[69]

OTHER TASK-SPECIFIC DYSTONIAS (TSD)

In addition to WC, other TSD have been described in milkers, seamstresses, cobblers, shoemakers, musicians, and others whose work involves frequent repetitive movements.[57,74] This population of individuals who repeatedly overuse their limbs is also more predisposed to nerve entrapments and muscle and joint disorders. This may lead to some clinical confusion. Tasks capable of inducing action dystonia almost always require either highly repetitive movements or extreme motor precision. The majority of TSD involve the upper limb and, rarely, the leg, probably because the use of the lower limb for precise repetitive tasks is unusual. They have been described in knife sharpeners, dancers, tradesmen, cyclists, sewing machine workers, and cello players.

WC is the most common TSD. Telegraphist cramp, found in one study to affect 14 percent of 516 telegraphists,[75] has been progressively disappearing since the introduction of the modern telephone. It is likely that typist's cramp will become more prevalent with the expansion of keyboard-dependent telecommunication. Musicians, with the years of practice and repetition of precise and complicated movements required to achieve professional status, are prone to overuse syndromes, and as many as 15 percent of professional musicians may be suffering from overuse syndromes.[59] These focal dystonias are particularly devastating. They can occur in musicians using almost any kind of instrument, but are more common in piano players. Newmark and Hochberg,[60] evaluated the focal motor syndromes in 57 instrumental musicians and noted three stereotyped afflictions: (1) flexion of 4th and 5th fingers in pianists, (2) flexion of the 3rd finger in guitarists, and (3) extension of the 3rd finger in clarinetists. The disabilities in these patients were not progressive. In brass instrumentalists, as well as in double-reed players, musician's dystonia may involve the peribuccal and cervical muscles. Frucht et al. have recently reported the clinical observations in 26 brass and woodwind players affected with embouchure dystonia (the pattern of lip, jaw and tongue muscles used to control the flow of air into a mouthpiece). Initial symptoms were limited to one range of notes or style of playing, eventually progressing without remission, although a percentage of patients reported fluctuations in their symptoms.[76]

Musician's cramps are usually refractory to medical treatment, rest, or physical therapy. Alteration of playing technique may help some patients. The response to botulinum toxin injections is generally insufficient, because, for professional musicians, even a marked response to treatment is of no benefit when the abilities needed to play professionally are not maintained.

Athlete's TSD can occur in golfers and other sportsmen, such as tennis players, snooker players, or dart throwers. Golfer's TSD (the "yips") may affect as many as 28 percent of golfers, more commonly afflicting those who have more cumulative years of golfing.[61] Involuntary movements emerge particularly during putting, but are much less evident during chipping or driving.[77] As in patients with other TSD, golfers with the yips use complementary strategies, such as changing hand preference. About one-fourth of them report that other activities can be similarly affected.

OTHER FOCAL DYSTONIAS

Rarely, isolated dystonia of the pharyngeal muscles occurs causing dysphagia (dystonic dysphagia). Disability in these patients may be severe, and surgical section of the crycopharyngeus muscle may be needed to improve swallowing.[78–80] Patients with dystonic dysphagia frequently have OMD or neck dystonia as well. Isolated lingual dystonia is very rare,[81] but lingual dystonia can certainly be the most prominent manifestation of OMD. Another AOFD occasionally encountered is truncal dystonia. In these patients, continuous or repetitive spasms cause flexion, extension, scoliosis, or torsion of the trunk.[78] As with other focal dystonias, spasms at onset may occur only when walking or standing but, eventually, they can be present even when the patient is lying down. In some patients, spasms are rapid enough to resemble myoclonus, and this has been referred to as "woodpecker dystonia." Extension to adjacent regions can occur, such as retrocollis, involvement of proximal limb muscles, or pelvic involvement (so-called copulatory dystonia). Sensory tricks that improve truncal dystonia include gently leaning against the wall when standing, pressing in the back of the neck, or pressing on the hips.

Abdominal wall dystonia (belly dancer's dyskinesia) has recently been described,[82] and Caviness et al.[83] have reported a group of patients with focal or segmental dyskinesias affecting the ears, back, shoulder girdle, abdomen, and pelvic girdle that closely resemble focal dystonias. In these patients the movements were slow, sinuous, semirhythmic, and associated with long-duration bursts of electromyogram (EMG) activity in neurophysiologic studies. Peripheral trauma may have played a role in the pathogenesis of the movements in some patients.

Etiology

The cause of AOFD remains unknown in the majority of cases. Unlike childhood-onset classic ITD, in which current evidence indicates that the mode of inheritance is autosomal-dominant with reduced penetrance in both Jews and non-Jews,[84] the role of heredity in adult-onset cases is not well understood. It is not clear to what extent the clinical distinction between early- and late-onset ITD reflects underlying genetic distinctions. A genetic study, performed prior to the availability of DYT1 testing, of ITD in the UK[85] suggests that in the non-Jewish population a proportion of late-onset cases may be because of the same genetic factors that underlie early onset ITD. On the other hand, findings by Bressman et al.[86] and by Risch et al.[87] suggest that most late-onset ITD in the Ashkenazi Jewish population is etiologically distinct from early-onset ITD. The systematic study of the DYT1 gene in many patients with familial focal dystonia, or generalized dystonia beginning as focal cervical dystonia, have given only positive results in a family recently described by Gasser et al.[88] In this family of German origin, 4 out of 5 members affected had only a WC after many years of disease. Although DYT1 dystonia, in general, responds to a determined phenotypic pattern, some recently published cases have indicated that intrafamilial variability of the disease phenotype can exist, regarding both distribution and age of onset of dystonia.[2,3]

A role for heredity in adult-onset dystonias is suggested by the observed familial cases of orofacial dystonia, WC, and ST,[89,90] and the reports of Meige's syndrome and cervical dystonia in apparently identical twins.[91] Furthermore, several large studies of focal dystonias have reported positive family histories, ranging from 2 to 15 percent of patients.[92] Affected relatives displayed focal and segmental signs but not generalized dystonia. Waddy et al.[93] found that 25 percent of 40 non-Jewish patients with focal dystonia had relatives in whom dystonia could be identified. Most of the secondary cases were not aware of any dystonia. It was concluded, on the basis of segregation analysis, that focal dystonia is commonly transmitted by an autosomal-dominant gene with reduced penetrance and variable expressivity, and they suggested that a single gene may account for inherited dystonias, regardless of whether they are generalized or focal. Defazio et al. made similar observations in a family study of 29 patients with BSP and craniocervical dystonia.[94] Familial patients were clinically indistinguishable from sporadic ones. Besides these studies suggesting that focal dystonia has a genetic basis, several autosomal-dominant families with adult onset focal and/or segmental dystonia have been reported in the last years. To date, only one locus for pure focal dystonia, DYT7, and two loci for the mixed dystonias (generalized and focal dystonia in the same family), DYT6 and DYT13, have been found, but no gene mutation has been identified. The fact that many other families do not show linkage to these loci indicates probable genetic heterogeneity. DYT7 has been described in a large German family with autosomal-dominant focal dystonia with incomplete penetrance.[95] The more common phenotype presented was ST, but one had laryngeal dystonia and several had postural hand tremor. In this family, dystonia began in adulthood, ranging between 28 and 78 years. The gene candidate was localized in the short arm of chromosome 18p.

Almasy et al. reported, in 1997, the clinical and genetic analysis performed in two Mennonite families that presented with autosomal-dominant ITD with an incomplete penetrance pattern.[96] The phenotype was the same as that observed in the DYT1 gene mutation, but in most of the patients dystonia started on the craniocervical region and mean age of disease onset was later. In 2 of the cases, the dystonia remained focal. Linkage studies allowed the gene (DYT6) to be localized on chromosome 8p21-8q22. Finally, an Italian family with focal or segmental dystonia, usually of early adult-onset, has been reported. In general, the patients presented symptoms involving the craniocervical region or the upper limb, but some of them developed generalized dystonia or had an early-onset dystonia.[97] Recently, a genome-wide analysis performed in this family identified the locus gene, DYT13, on the short arm of chromosome 1.[98] A patient suffering from a sporadic oromandibular dystonia who presented a mutation of the DYT5 gene, which is the gene responsible for dopa-responsive dystonia, has been reported.[99] Until now, more than 28 mutations of this gene have been described.

Recently, two controlled allelic association studies with polymorphism in dopamine receptors and transported genes has been reported in a cohort of patient with primary cervical dystonia[100] and BSP.[101] In both, the authors found significant associations for allele 2 of the dinucleotide repeat in the D5 receptor gene on chromosome 4. They suggested that this association could confer susceptibility to develop focal dystonias.

Autoimmune disorders, such as thyroid disease, systemic lupus erythematosus, rheumatoid arthritis, or myasthenia gravis, have been associated with primary dystonia.[27,102] Nivaler et al.,[103] however, could not find anti-central nervous system antibodies in the serum of 11 patients with cranial dystonia, using the direct immunoperoxidase technique. More recently, a study directed to detect basal ganglia-specific antibodies in serum of 7 patients with primary BSP also failed to find them.[104] Use of sympathicomimetic drugs, eye color, and focal brainstem and diencephalic lesions have been associated with the focal dystonias only in occasional patients. Therefore, they are not widely accepted as risk factors.

Several studies have indicated that dystonia may be precipitated by peripheral factors such as overuse, misuse, or trauma.[105] Fletcher et al.[106] showed that peripheral trauma may trigger dystonia in carriers of the ITD gene. A similar phenomenon in isolated BSP is suggested by the finding that up to 12 percent of patients report the occurrence of ocular trauma or lesion before the onset of the movement disorder.[107] Peripheral trauma has also been reported in 5–12 percent of patients with cervical dystonia,[108,109] occurring 3–6 months before the onset of symptoms. Similarly, cases of OMD have occurred soon after facial lacerations and dental work.[110] Laryngitis can precede spasmodic dysphonia.[111] Occasionally, focal LD may be associated with extremity injury, such as electrical injury,[112] or with reflex sympathetic dystrophy. Tremor and dystonia are the movement disorders most often associated with reflex sympathetic dystrophy ("causalgia-dystonia syndrome"),[113,114] and it almost always develops after peripheral trauma. In these cases the development of pain may be of importance.

Peripheral factors are also generally accepted to play a role in a variety of occupational or TSD, such as WC, typist's cramp, or the focal dystonias occurring in musicians or sportsmen. A recently described case of OMD occurring in an auctioneer is another example of a focal dystonia that was possibly related to muscle overuse.[115] Inzelberg et al.[116] found a highly significant relationship between motor dominance and the laterality of limb onset in ITD patients, which suggests that the preferred use of a limb may trigger the onset of dystonia.

The exact role of muscle overuse or trauma in the genesis of dystonia remains to be clarified. A study by Fletcher et al.[117] did not support the notion that trauma is important in idiopathic dystonia. In their study of 71 patients with ITD and 71 matched controls investigating the role of environmental factors in the development of the disorder, trauma was no more frequent among patients than among control subjects, either in the year preceding the onset of dystonia in the index patients or at any other time. It is unlikely that trauma alone is sufficient for dystonia to develop, because, if this were the case, dystonia would be much more common. It has been postulated that trauma may trigger the expression of a previously subclinical or very mild dystonia or trigger dystonia only in patients with pre-existing susceptibility, perhaps on a genetic basis.[12,105,118] A recently developed rat model has supported these concepts. A combination of partial dopaminergic cell destruction in the substantia nigra and a lesion on the zygomatic branch of the facial nerve lead the animal to present spontaneous spasms of eyelid closure. Individually, both of these lesions produced a hyperexcitability of the blink reflex, but BSP was only observed when they were performed on the same animal. This model suggested that a subclinical loss of striatal dopamine confers a susceptibility to developing dystonia, which can be apparent when an external insult occurs.[119]

It has been suggested that complex movement disorders like dystonia, occurring after a peripheral nerve or spinal nerve root lesion, are generated by reorganization of spinal motor circuitry or by changes in supraspinal somatosensory integration that result in altered basal ganglia function.[119] Some authors believe that there may be a psychogenic basis for many cases of posttraumatic dystonia.[120]

Anatomic Substrate and Pathophysiology of the Focal Dystonias

Autopsy studies have been performed in 10 patients with presumed idiopathic cranial dystonia. No significant abnormalities were found in 4; 1 had an "incidental" small angioma

of the pons, and the other patients had relatively nonspecific abnormalities.[121,122] Mosaic neuronal cell loss and gliosis have been seen in 2 patients,[123] and 3 patients have been reported as having cell loss and gliosis of the substantia nigra pars compacta and other brainstem nuclei.[124,125] In 2 of these patients, abundant Lewy bodies were present. Lesions in the basal ganglia, thalamus, cerebral cortex, diencephalon, and brainstem have been reported to be associated with some of the focal dystonias.[126,127]

Mostly based on the correlations that exist between the secondary dystonias and lesions of the putamen and thalamus, it is currently believed that the focal dystonias result from an abnormality in the basal ganglia. Static imaging studies have not identified any definite abnormalities in the idiopathic focal dystonias. Dynamic imaging studies, using positron emission tomography (PET), showed hypometabolism in the caudate and lentiform nucleus, and in the frontal projection fields of the mediodorsal thalamic nucleus.[128] Hence, functional disturbance in the basal ganglia and their frontal connections is thought to be the underlying cause of the dystonias. In Meige's syndrome, relative glucose hypermetabolism of the putamen was detected.[129] In addition, bilateral relative increments in glucose utilization for the thalamus and primary sensorimotor cortices has been observed. When the subjects are studied during sleep, the same pattern of hypermetabolism is present, even though no dystonic spasms are occurring.[130] Recently, some PET studies using ^{18}F-fluorodeoxyglucose (FDG) or regional cerebral blood flow (rCBF) measuring methods have shown abnormalities in the activation pattern of cortical structures. In a recent study, CBF was measured using $H_2^{15}O$ and PET, at rest and during movement, in a group of 6 patients with ITD, 1 of whom had isolated WC. Results demonstrated overactivity of the striatum and its frontal association projection areas. Reduced activity in motor executive areas was also detected.[131] Using rCBF PET, Ibañez et al.[132] studied 7 patients with WC during rest and performing different tasks with the right hand. Patients showed a deficient activation of the sensorimotor and premotor cortex and decreased correlation between premotor cortical regions and putamen, suggesting a dysfunction of the premotor cortical network. Similar results, with decreased activation of the primary sensory motor area, were observed in patients with BSP in response to vibration.[133] Hutchinson et al.[134] used FDG PET to investigate the metabolic topography of BSP in 6 patients. During wakefulness, patients showed hypermetabolism of the cerebellum and pons compared with controls. While a sleep, the BSP group exhibited superomediofrontal hypometabolism, in a region associated with cortical control of eyelid movements.

Measures of the index binding in putamen of the dopaminergic radioligand ^{18}F-spiperone in patients with facial dystonia and WC were 29 percent lower in patients than in controls, suggesting abnormality of dopaminergic receptors in primary dystonia.[135]

Recently, studies with proton magnetic resonance spectroscopy in patients with BSP[136] and torticollis[137] showed

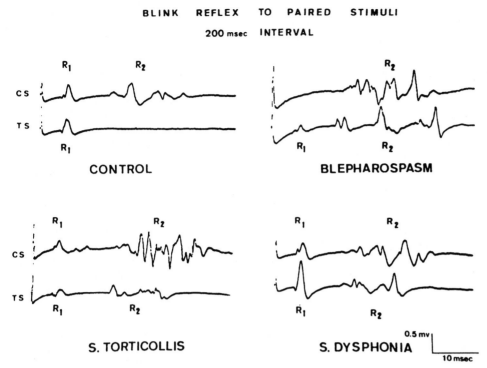

FIGURE 31-2 Blink reflexes to pairs of stimuli given at an interstimulus interval of 200 ms in a normal control subject and in patients with focal dystonia. In the normal control subject the conditioning stimulus (CS) completely inhibits the R_2 of the test stimulus (TS). In the patients, on the other hand, a clear R_2 follows the TS already at this short interstimuli interval. Stimuli were delivered at the supraorbital nerve, and the reflex responses (R_1 and R_2) were recorded with surface electrodes from the ipsilateral orbicularis oculi. *(From Tolosa et al.[144] Used with permission.)*

a reduction in N-acetylaspartate(NAA)/choline and NAA/creatine ratios in the lentiform nucleus, indicating neuronal dysfunction in this region. By contrast, no differences in metabolite levels were seen in another study comparing normal subjects and patients with primary focal hand dystonia.[138]

How dysfunction of the basal ganglia results in dystonia is unclear. In dystonia, basal ganglia dysfunction may result in an inability to target inhibition to opposite sets of neurons in the cortex, thus producing excessive motor output, particularly during movement.[11] Ridding et al.[139] have reported that ipsilateral corticocortical inhibition is abnormal in patients with WC, which could represent a disturbance in the excitability of local intracortical inhibitory interneurons. In a patient with unilateral focal dystonia resulting from a lesion of the contralateral putamen, Hanjima et al.[140] detected, using double cortical stimulation techniques, hyperexcitability of the motor cortex ipsilateral to the putaminal lesion, with normal excitability of the sensory cortex. In a study investigating cortical excitability using high-intensity transcortical magnetic stimulation, Curra et al.[141] elicited an abnormally short cortical silent period in facial muscles in patients with cranial dystonia, suggesting a reduced excitability of cortical inhibitory interneurons in the motor cortex.

In addition to these alterations in the cortex, many reflex abnormalities have been described in dystonic patients, and these are greatest in muscles affected by dystonia. In cranial, laryngeal, and cervical dystonia, blink reflex and masseter inhibitory reflex abnormalities have been clearly documented (Fig. 31-2), suggesting that both excitatory and inhibitory interneuronal pathways in the brainstem are perturbed.[142–144] In many of the focal dystonias, such as ST or spasmodic dysphonia, subclinical abnormalities of the blink reflexes generally occur, suggesting that the clinical abnormalities are not a consequence of the abnormalities observed in these tests. Also, treatment with botulinum toxin markedly improves BSP and ST, but clinical improvement is not accompanied by a concomitant normalization of the blink reflex excitability curve in these patients.[145,146]

Another example of abnormal brain stem interneuronal excitability is the finding of reduced exteroceptive inhibition of the sternocleidomastoid muscle after a supra- or infraorbital nerve stimulus.[147,148] Vestibular abnormalities have also been reported in ST, but they could be secondary to the abnormal head position.[149,150] Reciprocal inhibition has been extensively studied in dystonia. It refers to the active inhibition of activity in antagonist muscles during voluntary contraction of the agonist. In limb dystonia, reciprocal inhibition studied in the flexor and extensor muscles of the forearm is reduced.[151,152] A similar abnormality has been detected in patients with ST and with BSP, even though there was no clinical involvement of forearm muscles.

Although there is no deficit of sensation in dystonia, there are some phenomena relating to the sensory system, such as overuse or trauma preceding dystonia, which could indicate that there are sensory disturbances in dystonia that can contribute to generate, maintain or suppress the dystonic movements. In a study investigating how sensory tricks diminish the dystonic symptoms, we examined the effects on blink reflex and its recovery curve by touching the face with the finger in 8 patients with BSP.[153] This maneuver increased the amplitude of R_1 and reduced the area of R_2. This reduction of R_2 could be caused by sensory gating of trigeminal afferents, thereby lowering the gain of trigeminofacial reflexes and contributing to transit benefit induced by sensory tricks. Stimulation of spindle afferents obtained by tonic vibration of the tendon or the belly muscle can induce dystonia in patients with WC, which can be improved with partial lidocaine block of the muscle.[154]

The picture that emerges from all of these physiological studies is that the brainstem and spinal interneuron circuitry are functioning abnormally in patients with focal dystonias, resulting in a change in the tonic control of reflex excitability. An abnormal input from the basal ganglia via cortical or subcortical connections on brainstem and spinal interneurons could result in these static abnormalities. Such changes might produce particular problems during movement, when activity in specific reflex pathways is normally well regulated according to the task being performed.[72]

Differential Diagnosis and Investigations in Patients with Focal Dystonias

The focal dystonias are usually idiopathic, regardless of the location. Occasionally, they have a known cause. Although the list of such secondary or symptomatic dystonias is quite extensive,[58,155] symptomatic focal dystonias clinically similar to idiopathic ones are not common. Nevertheless, the distinction between idiopathic and symptomatic forms is important to give patients an appropriate prognosis and genetic counseling. Most importantly, adequate treatment of some of the symptomatic dystonias, when appropriately diagnosed, can result in a cure or avoid progression to a more generalized disorder, as could be the case in dystonia associated with Wilson's disease.

The most common cause of symptomatic AOFD is tardive dystonia induced by chronic neuroleptic administration.[156,157] Cases of tardive dystonia can be identical to those of BSP, OMD, cervical dystonia, spasmodic dysphonia, or idiopathic truncal dystonia, and can sometimes only be differentiated from the idiopathic dystonias by the history of neuroleptic use.[28] Tardive dystonia does not usually lead to WC.

Also relatively common in movement disorder clinics are focal dystonias induced by L-dopa in Parkinson's disease,[158] and those occurring in the setting of the various degenerative parkinsonian syndromes. Kinesigenic foot dystonia can be the presenting manifestation of untreated young-onset Parkinson's disease,[159,160] and WC, torticollis, OMD, and BSP have been described as preceding the onset of otherwise typical Parkinson's disease by variable periods of time, from months up to several years (see Ref. 105 for review). LD and BSP can also be the presenting manifestations of progressive supranuclear palsy,[161] and focal dystonia was described as a prominent presenting feature in a group of patients with hereditary or sporadic cerebellar ataxia.[162] When a focal dystonia is the presenting feature of one of these syndromes, when other neurological findings are not yet present, it is usually impossible to differentiate it from one of the "idiopathic" dystonias on clinical grounds.

Focal dystonic spasms similar to the primary ones have been described secondary to focal hemispheric brain pathology and to brainstem/diencephalic lesions in patients with stroke, multiple sclerosis, or hydrocephalus. We have also seen prominent focal dystonia, either as the initial manifestation or during the course of disorders such as head trauma, kernicterus, delayed-onset dystonia, Hallervorden-Spatz disease, Tourette's syndrome, Huntington's disease, Wilson's disease and acquired nonwilsonian hepatocerebral degeneration and the degenerative cerebellar ataxias.[105,163] Focal limb dystonia has also been encountered in patients with cerebellar lesions.[164,165]

A large part of the clinical investigations in a patient with AOFD is directed to uncover a possible cause for the disorder. Historical features can be quite useful in ruling out certain etiological factors. A history of exposure to drugs or toxins must be sought diligently. Antidopaminergic drugs, such as the neuroleptics, antiemetics, or some antivertiginous agents, can cause tardive focal dystonias that can be otherwise indistinguishable from idiopathic ones. Toxins such as manganese and methanol can cause similar symptoms, usually after an initial neurological insult. In a number of instances, symptomatic dystonia appears months to years after the initial cerebral insult.[166,167] Delayed-onset dystonias can occur in adolescence that are related to birth asphyxia,[168] but this phenomenon can be observed also with central pontine myelinolysis[169] and cyanide intoxication.[170] A history of recent trauma, in the same body region as the focal dystonia, or head trauma, suggests a posttraumatic dystonia.[108,118] Details of the onset, distribution, and clinical characteristics of the dystonic spasms is sometimes helpful in diagnosing a symptomatic dystonia. A focal dystonia of abrupt onset suggests a structural nervous system lesion or a psychogenic etiology. Idiopathic dystonias are typically action-induced at onset, followed by overflow dystonia and, eventually, are present at rest. Dystonia at rest, even from the beginning, strongly suggests a secondary dystonia.

In idiopathic dystonia, the only neurological abnormality is the presence of dystonic postures and movements.

Such movements are tremoric at times and exceptionally myoclonic. There is no associated oculomotor abnormality, ataxia, dementia, seizures, weakness, atrophy, or spasticity. However, many of the symptomatic dystonias are associated with some of these neurological findings and, therefore, their presence strongly suggests that one is dealing with such a case. The presence of stereotypes—repetitive, patterned, seemingly purposeful but purposeless movements, such as repetitive tongue protrusion ("fly-catching" tongue movements) or the "bon-bon" sign (roving movements of the tongue inside the mouth)—in patients with otherwise typical BSP, for example, strongly suggests the diagnosis of tardive dystonia. The absence of such neurological abnormalities, however, does not exclude the possibility of symptomatic dystonia, which may present as pure dystonia. Equally important in the evaluation of a patient with focal dystonia are the findings on general physical examination, which can even be diagnostic of a specific disorder; for example, the presence of a Kayser-Fleischer ring indicates Wilson's disease.

Careful clinical evaluation of the dystonic spasm is always necessary, particularly if the patient is a candidate for botulinum toxin treatment. In some patients, diagnosis may not be possible on simple inspection, because dystonia may not be present at all times. In these cases, certain clinical maneuvers may bring out the dystonic spasms and allow for a precise diagnosis. Shining a bright light in front of the patient's eyes or asking the patient to open and close the eyes repeatedly[27] may, for example, trigger BSP. Dystonic tremor, which may be treated successfully with botulinum toxin, may have to be brought out by asking the patient to adopt a certain position (e.g., trying to oppose the dystonic spasms). In general, an attempt has to be made to find the position with the most severe dystonia, instructing the patient to position the affected body region so as to show maximal abnormality. The patient should always be examined while standing, walking, sitting, and lying down. In patients with LD or cervical dystonia, passive movements of the affected region may help in localizing the contracting muscles and in determining the full range of motion or the presence of contractures.

Palpation of the contracting muscles is also useful in localizing involved muscles and in estimating muscle mass, and it helps in detecting points of tenderness.

Nonorganic psychogenic dystonia can be most difficult to diagnose in an adult, but it can occur, particularly in certain subsets of dystonia, such as adult-onset lower LD, paroxysmal dystonia, and adductor laryngeal dystonia. Certain historical or examination features, such as a large number of somatic complaints, abrupt onset, presence of false weakness, or incongruous movements not fitting with typical organic dystonia, provide clues that suggest a psychogenic etiology[171] (see Chap. 56).

In addition to psychogenic causes, a number of other disorders in which abnormal postures occur but are not associated with underlying inappropriate muscle contraction should be differentiated from dystonia. Conditions simulating focal dystonia[55] can be orthopedic (an atlantoaxial subluxation, for example, can lead to an abnormal head posture that mimics torticollis), or neurological (such as posterior fossa tumors, syringomyelia, or extraocular muscle palsies), producing abnormal head or spine postures. Muscle contractures occurring in neurological patients or after orthopedic injuries may also pose difficult diagnostic problems, and infectious, inflammatory, and neoplastic involvement of the soft-tissue structures of the head and neck may simulate cervical dystonia.[172]

In the investigation of patients with AOFD presumed to be idiopathic, there is little need for laboratory or neuroimaging tests, because a symptomatic cause is almost never found. When the patient is under 40 years of age, investigations for Wilson's disease should be conducted (see Chap. 49), but older patients with typical focal dystonias require no further workup unless new or atypical features appear on follow-up, particularly when the disorder has been present for several months or longer.

References

1. Kramer PL, DeLeon D, Ozelius L, et al: Dystonia gene in Ashkenazi Jewish population is located on chromosome 9q32-34. *Ann Neurol* 27:114–120, 1990.
2. Opal P, Tintner R, Jankovic J et al: Intrafamilial phenotypic variability of the DYT1 dystonia: From asymptomatic TORIA gene carrier status to dystonic storm. *Mov Disord* 17:339–345, 2002.
3. Chinnery PF, Reading PJ, McCarthy EL, et al: Late-onset axial jerky dystonia due to DYT1 deletion. *Mov Disord* 17:196–198, 2002.
4. Holmgren G, Ozelius L, Forsgren L, et al: Adult onset idiopathic torsion dystonia is excluded from the DYT1 region (9q34) in a Swedish family. *J Neurol Neurosurg Psychiatry* 59:178–181, 1995.
5. Lee LV, Kupke KG, Caballar-Gonzaga F, et al: The phenotype of the X-linked dystonia-parkinsonism syndrome: An assessment of 42 cases in the Philippines. *Medicine (Baltimore)* 70:179–187, 1991.
6. Lew MF, Shindo M, Moskowitz CB, et al: Adductor laryngeal breathing dystonia in a patient with Lubag (X-linked dystonia-parkinsonism syndrome). *Mov Disord* 9:318–320, 1994.
7. Kramer PL, Mineta M, Klein C, et al: Rapid-onset dystonia-parkinsonism: Linkage to chromosome 19q13. *Ann Neurol* 46:176–182, 1999.
8. Nutt JG, Muenter MD, Aronson A, et al: Epidemiology of focal and generalized dystonia in Rochester, Minnesota. *Mov Disord* 3:188–194, 1988.
9. Nakashima K, Kusumi M, Inoue Y, Takahashi K: Prevalence of focal dystonias in the Western area of Tottori prefecture in Japan. *Mov Disord* 10:440–443, 1995.
10. The Epidemiological Study of Dystonia in Europe (ESDE) Collaborative Group: A prevalence study of primary dystonia in eight European countries. *J Neurol* 247:787–792, 2000.
11. Fahn S: Generalized dystonia, in Tsui JK, Calne DB (eds): *Handbook of Dystonia*. New York: Marcel Dekker, 1995, pp 193–211.
12. Jankovic J, Fahn S: Dystonic disorders, in Jankovic J, Tolosa E (eds): *Parkinson's Disease and Movement Disorders*, 2d ed. Baltimore: Williams & Wilkins, 1993, pp 337–374.

13. Fahn S: Dystonia, in Jankovic J, Hallett M (eds): *Therapy with Botulinum Toxin*. New York: Marcel Dekker, 1994, pp 173–189.

14. Marsden CD: The focal dystonias. *Clin Neuropharmacol* 9(suppl 2): 49–60, 1986.

15. Friedman A, Fahn S: Spontaneous remissions in spasmodic torticollis. *Neurology* 36:398–400, 1986.

16. Rothwell JC, Obeso JA, Day BL, Marsden CD: Pathophysiology of dystonias, in Desmedt JE (ed): *Motor Control Mechanisms in Health and Disease*. New York: Raven Press, 1983, pp 851–863.

17. Obeso JA, Rothwell JC, Lang AE, Marsden CD: Myoclonic dystonia. *Neurology* 33:825–830, 1983.

18. Cleeves L, Findley J, Marsden D: Odd tremors, in Marsden D, Fahn S (eds): *Movement Disorders 3*. Oxford: Butterworth-Heinemann, 1994, pp 434–453.

19. Rivest J, Marsden D: Trunk and head tremor as isolated manifestation of dystonia. *Mov Disord* 5:60–65, 1990.

20. Patterson RM, Little SC: Spasmodic torticollis. *J Nerv Ment Dis* 98:571–599, 1943.

21. Sheehy MP, Marsden CD: Writer's cramp: A focal dystonia. *Brain* 105:461–480, 1982.

22. Conway D, Bain PG, Warner TT, et al: Linkage analysis with chromosome-9 markers in hereditary essential tremor. *Mov Disord* 8:374–376, 1993.

23. Tolosa ES: Clinical features of Meige's disease (idiopathic orofacial dystonia): A report of 17 cases: *Arch Neurol* 38:147–151, 1981.

24. Tolosa ES, Klawans HL: Meige's disease: A clinical form of facial convulsion bilateral and medial. *Arch Neurol* 36:635–637, 1979.

25. Grandas F, Elston JS, Quinn N, Marsden CD: Blepharospasm: A review of 264 patients. *J Neurol Neurosurg Psychiatry* 51:767–772, 1988.

26. Marsden CD: The problem of adult-onset idiopathic torsion dystonia and other isolated dyskinesias in adult life (including blepharospasm, oromandibular dystonia, dystonic writer's cramp and torticollis, or axial dystonia). *Adv Neurol* 14:259–276, 1976.

27. Jankovic J, Ford J: Blepharospasm and orofacial-cervical dystonia: Clinical and pharmacological findings in 100 patients. *Ann Neurol* 13:402–411, 1983.

28. Tolosa E, Martí MJ: Blepharospasm-oromandibular dystonia syndrome (Meige's syndrome): Clinical aspects. *Adv Neurol* 49:73–84, 1988.

29. Tolosa E, Kulisevsky J, Martí MJ: Apraxia of lid opening in dystonic blepharospasm. IV International Meeting of the Benign Essential Blepharospasm Research Foundation, Barcelona, Spain, 1986.

30. Tolosa E, Kulisevsky J, Martí MJ: "Apraxia" of lid opening in essential blepharospasm. XXXVIIII Reunión de la American Academy of Neurology, New York, 1987.

31. Elston JS: A new variant of blepharospasm. *J Neurol Neurosurg Psychiatry* 55:369–371, 1992.

32. Obeso JA, Artieda J, Marsden CD: Stretch reflex blepharospasm. *Neurology* 35:1378–1380, 1985.

33. Defazio G, Berardelli A, Abbruzzese G, et al: Risk factors for spread of primary adult onset blepharospasm: A multicentre investigation of the Italian movement disorders study group. *J Neurol Neurosurg Psychiatry* 67:613–619, 1999.

34. Marsden CD: Blepharospasm-oromandibular dystonia syndrome (Breughel's syndrome): A variant of adult-onset torsion dystonia? *J Neurol Neurosurg Psychiatry* 39:1204–1209, 1976.

35. Cardoso F, Jankovic J: Oromandibular dystonia, in Ching Tsiu JK, Calne DB (eds): *Handbook of Dystonia*. New York: Marcel Dekker, 1995, pp 181–192.

36. Brin MF, Blitzer A, Herman S, Stewart C: Oromandibular dystonia: Treatment of 96 patients with botulinum toxin type A, in Jankovic J, Hallett M (eds): *Therapy with Botulinum Toxin*. New York: Marcel Dekker, 1994, pp 429–436.

37. Traube L: *Zur Lehre von den Larynxaffectionen beim Ileotyphus*. Berlin: Verlag Von August Hirschwald, 1871.

38. Ludlow CL: The spasmodic dysphonias: Speech, movement, and physiological characteristics, in Ching Tsui JK, Calne DB (eds): *Handbook of Dystonia*. New York: Marcel Dekker, 1995, pp 159–180.

39. Aronson AE: *Clinical Voice Disorders*. New York: Thieme, 1985.

40. Blitzer A, Brin MF, Fahn S, Lovelace RE: Clinical and laboratory characteristics of focal laryngeal dystonia: Study of 110 cases. *Laryngoscope* 98:636–640, 1988.

41. Rosenfield DB: Spasmodic dysphonia. *Adv Neurol* 49:317–328, 1988.

42. Ludlow CL, Naunton RF, Terada S, Anderson BJ: Successful treatment of selected cases of abductor spasmodic dysphonia using botulinum toxin injection. *Otolaryngol Head Neck Surg* 104:849–855, 1991.

43. Hartman DE, Aronson AE: Clinical investigations of intermittent breathy dysphonia. *J Speech Hear Disord* 46:428–432, 1991.

44. Izdebski K, Dedo HH, Boles L: Spastic dysphonia: A patient profile of 200 cases. *Am J Otolaryngol* 5:7–14, 1984.

45. Aronson AB, Petersen HW, Litin EM: Voice symptomatology in functional dysphonia and aphonia. *J Speech Hear Disord* 29:367–380, 1964.

46. Tsui JKC: Cervical dystonia, in Tsui JKC, Calne DB (eds): *Handbook of Dystonia*. New York: Marcel Dekker, 1995, pp 115–127.

47. Jankovic J, Leder S, Warner D, Schwartz K: Cervical dystonia: Clinical findings and associated movement disorders. *Neurology* 41:1088–1091, 1991.

48. Chan J, Brin MF, Fahn S: Idiopathic cervical dystonia: Clinical characteristics. *Mov Disord* 6:119–126, 1991.

49. Couch JR: Dystonia and tremor in spasmodic torticollis. *Adv Neurol* 14:245–258, 1976.

50. Duane DD: Spasmodic torticollis: Clinical and biologic features and their implications for focal dystonia. *Adv Neurol* 50:473–492, 1988.

51. Duane DD: Spasmodic torticollis. *Adv Neurol* 49:135–150, 1988.

52. Truong DD, Dubinsky R, Hermanowicz N, et al: Posttraumatic torticollis. *Arch Neurol* 48:221–223, 1991.

53. Schott GD: The relationship of peripheral trauma and pain to dystonia. *J Neurol Neurosurg Psychiatry* 48:698–701, 1985.

54. Lowenstein DH, Aminoff MJ: The clinical course of spasmodic torticollis. *Neurology* 38:530–532, 1988.

55. Jahanshahi M, Marion MH, Marsden CD: Natural history of adult-onset idiopathic torticollis. *Arch Neurol* 47:548, 1990.

56. Friedman A, Fahn S: Spontaneous remission in spasmodic torticollis. *Neurology* 36:398–400, 1986.

57. Uitti RJ, Vingerhoets FJG, Tsui JKC: Limb dystonia, in Tsui JKC, Calne DB (eds): *Handbook of Dystonia*. New York: Marcel Dekker, 1995, p 143–158.

58. Fahn S, Marsden CD, Calne DB: Classification and investigation of dystonia, in Marsden CD, Fahn S (eds): *Movement Disorders 2*. London: Butterworth, 1987, pp 332–358.

59. Lockwood AH: Medical problems in musicians. *N Engl J Med* 320:221–227, 1989.
60. Newmark J, Hochberg FH: Isolated painless manual incoordination in 57 musicians. *J Neurol Neurosurg Psychiatry* 50:291–295, 1987.
61. McDaniel KD, Cummings JL, Shain S: The "yips": A focal dystonia in golfers. *Neurology* 39:192–195, 1989.
62. Sheehy MP, Marden CD: Writer's cramp: A focal dystonia. *Brain* 105:462–480, 1982.
63. Marsden CD, Sheehy MP: Writer's cramp. *Trends Neurosci* 13:148–153, 1990.
64. Sheehy MP, Rothwell JC, Marsden CD: Writer's cramp. *Adv Neurol* 50:457–472, 1988.
65. Ludolph AC, Windgassen K: Klinische Untersuchungen zum Schreibkrampf bei 30 Patienten. *Nervenarzt* 8:462–466, 1992.
66. Rothwell JC, Traub MM, Marsden CD: Primary writing tremor. *J Neurol Neurosurg Psychiatry* 42:1106–1114, 1979.
67. Rosenbaum F, Jankovic J: Focal task-specific tremor and dystonia: Categorization of occupational movement disorders. *Neurology* 38:522–527, 1988.
68. Quinn N, Critchley P, Marsden CD: Young onset Parkinson's disease. *Mov Disord* 2:73–91, 1987.
69. Poewe WH, Lees AJ, Stern GM: Dystonia in Parkinson's disease: Clinical and pharmacological features. *Ann Neurol* 23:73–78, 1988.
70. Rivest J, Quinn N, Marsden CD: Dystonia in Parkinson's disease, multiple system atrophy, and progressive supranuclear palsy. *Neurology* 40:1571–1578, 1990.
71. Rafal RD, Friedman JH: Limb dystonia in progressive supranuclear palsy. *Neurology* 37:1546–1549, 1987.
72. Rothwell JC: The physiology of dystonia, in Tsui JKC, Calne DB (eds): *Handbook of Dystonia*. New York: Marcel Dekker, 1995, pp 59–76.
73. Marsden CD, Harrison MJG, Bundey S: Natural history of idiopathic torsion dystonia, in Eldridge R, Fahn S (eds): *Dystonia*. New York: Raven Press, 1976, pp 177–187.
74. Gowers WR: *A Manual of Diseases of the Nervous System*. London: Churchill, 1888, p 656.
75. Ferguson D: An Australian study of telegraphist's cramp. *Br J Int Med* 28:280–285, 1971.
76. Frucht SJ, Fahn S, Greene PE, et al: The natural history of embouchure dystonia. *Mov Disord* 16:899–906, 2001.
77. Cohen A: Putting on the agony. *Nurs Mirror Midwives J* 143:72, 1976.
78. Marsden CD: The focal dystonias. *Clin Neuropharmacol* 9(suppl 2):S49–S60, 1986.
79. Marsden CD: Dystonia: The spectrum of the disease, in Yahr M (ed): *The Basal Ganglia*. New York: Raven Press, 1976, pp 351–367.
80. Marsden CD: Blepharospasm-oromandibular dystonia syndrome (Breughel's syndrome). *J Neurol Neurosurg Psychiatry* 39:1204–1209, 1976.
81. Robertson-Hoffman DE, Mark MH, Sage JL: Isolated lingual-palatal dystonia. *Mov Disord* 6:177–179, 1991.
82. Iliceto G, Thompson PD, Day BL, et al: Diaphragmatic flutter, the moving umbilicus syndrome, and "belly dancer's" dyskinesia. *Mov Disord* 5:1522, 1990.
83. Caviness JN, Gabellini A, Kneebone CS, et al: Unusual focal dyskinesias: The ears, the shoulders, the back, and the abdomen. *Mov Disord* 9:531–538, 1994.
84. Ozelius L, Kramer PL, Moskowitz CB, et al: Human gene for torsion dystonia on chromosome 9q32-34. *Neuron* 2:1427–1434, 1989.
85. Fletcher NA, Harding AE, Marsden CD: A genetic study of idiopathic torsion dystonia in the UK. *Brain* 113:379–395, 1990.
86. Bressman SB, De Leon D, Brin MF, et al: Idiopathic torsion dystonia among Ashkenazi Jews: Evidence for autosomal dominant inheritance. *Ann Neurol* 26:612–620, 1989.
87. Risch NJ, Bressman SB, De Leon D, et al: Segregation analysis of idiopathic torsion dystonia in Ashkenazi Jews suggests autosomal dominant inheritance. *Am J Hum Genet* 46:533–538, 1990.
88. Gasser T, Windgassen K, Bereznai B, et al: Phenotypic expression of the DYT1 mutation: A family with writer's cramp of juvenile onset. *Ann Neurol* 44:126–128, 1998.
89. Chan J, Brin MF, Fahn S: Idiopathic cervical dystonia: Clinical characteristics. *Mov Disord* 6:119–126, 1991.
90. De Leon D, Heiman G, Brin MF, et al: Genetic factors in spastic dysphonia. *Neurology* 40(suppl 1):142, 1990.
91. Comella CL, Klawans HL: Meige's syndrome in twins. *Neurology* 38(suppl 1):315, 1988.
92. Kramer PL, Bressman SB, Fahn S, et al: The genetics of dystonia, in Tsui JKC, Calne DB (eds): *Handbook of Dystonia*. New York: Marcel Dekker, 1995, pp 43–58.
93. Waddy HM, Fletcher NA, Harding AE, Marsden CD: A genetic study of idiopathic focal dystonias. *Ann Neurol* 29:320–324, 1991.
94. Defazio G, Livrea P, Leon A, Dal Toso R: Antineuronal antibodies in cranial dystonia. *Mov Disord* 6:183–184, 1991.
95. Leube B, Rudnicki D, Ratzlaff T, et al: Idiopathic torsion dystonia: Assignment of a gene to chromosome 18p in a German family with adult onset, autosomal dominant inheritance and purely focal distribution. *Hum Mol Genet* 5:1673–1677, 1996.
96. Almasy L, Bressman SB, Raymond D, et al: Idiopathic torsion dystonia linked to chromosome 8 in two mennonite families. *Ann Neurol* 42:670–673, 1997.
97. Bentivoglio AR, Del Grosso N, Valente EM: Non DTY1 dystonia in a large Italian family. *J Neurol Neurosurg Psychiatry* 62:357–360, 1997.
98. Valente EM, Bentivoglio AR, Cassetta E, et al: Identification of a novel primary torsion dystonia locus (DYT13) on chromosome 1p36 in an Italian family with cranial-cervical or upper limb onset. *Neurol Sci* 22:95–96, 2001.
99. Steinberger D, Topka H, Fisher D, Muller U: CGH1 mutation in a patient with adult-onset oromandibular dystonia. *Neurology* 52:877–879, 1999.
100. Plazcek MR, Misbauddin A, Chaudhuri KR, et al: Cervical dystonia is associated with a polymorphism in the dopamine (D5) receptor gene. *J Neurol Neurosurg Psychiatry* 71:262–264, 2001.
101. Bathia KP, Warner TT: A polymorphism in the dopamine receptor DRD5 is associated with blepharospasm. *Neurology* 58:124–126, 2002.
102. Jankovic J, Patten BM: Blepharospasm and autoimmune diseases. *Mov Disord* 2:159–163, 1987.
103. Nilaver G, Whitling S, Nutt JG: Autoimmune etiology for cranial dystonia. *Mov Disord* 5:179–180, 1990.
104. Ramachandran V, Church A, Giovannoni G, Bhatia KP: Antibasal ganglia antibodies are absent in patients with primary blepharospasm. *Neurology* 58:150, 2002.
105. Tolosa E, Kulisevski J: The pathophysiology of dystonia, in Quinn NP, Jenner PG (eds): *Disorders of Movement. Clinical, Pharmacological and Physiological Aspects*. London: Academic Press, 1989, pp 251–262.

106. Fletcher NA, Harding AE, Marsden CD: The relationship between trauma and idiopathic torsion dystonia. *J Neurol Neurosurg Psychiatry* 54:713–717, 1991.

107. Grandas F, Elston J, Quinn N, Marsden CD: Blepharospasm: A review of 264 patients. *J Neurol Neurosurg Psychiatry* 51:767–772, 1988.

108. Jankovic J, Van Der Linden C: Dystonia and tremor induced by peripheral trauma: Predisposing factors. *J Neurol Neurosurg Psychiatry* 51:1512–1519, 1988.

109. Truong DD, Dubinsky R, Hermanowicz N, et al: Posttraumatic torticollis. *Arch Neurol* 48:221–223, 1991.

110. Brin MF, Fahn S, Bressman SB, Burke RE: Dystonia precipitated by peripheral trauma. *Neurology* 36(suppl 1):119, 1986.

111. Ludlow CL: The spasmodic dysphonias: Speech, movement, and physiological characteristics, in Tsui JKC, Calne DB (eds): *Handbook of Dystonia.* New York: Marcel Dekker, 1995, pp 159–180.

112. Tarsy D, Sudarsky L, Charness ME: Limb dystonia following electrical injury. *Mov Disord* 9:230–232, 1994.

113. Schott GD: Induction of involuntary movements by peripheral trauma: An analogy with causalgia. *Lancet* ii:712–715, 1986.

114. Bhatia KP, Bhatt MH, Marsden CD: The causalgia-dystonia syndrome. *Brain* 116:834–851, 1993.

115. Scolding NJ, Smith SM, Sturman S, et al: Auctioneer's jaw: A case of occupational oromandibular dystonia. *Mov Disord* 10:508–509, 1995.

116. Inzelberg R, Zilber N, Kahana E, Korczyn AD: Laterality of onset in idiopathic torsion dystonia. *Mov Disord* 8:327–330, 1993.

117. Fletcher NA, Harding AE, Marsden CD: A case-control study of idiopathic torsion dystonia. *Mov Disord* 6:304–309, 1992.

118. Marsden CD: Peripheral movement disorders, in Marsden CD, Fahn S (eds): *Movement Disorders 3.* Oxford: Butterworth-Heinemann, 1994, pp 406–417.

119. Schicatano EJ, Basso MA, Evinger C: Animal model explains the origins of the cranial dystonia benign essential blepharospasm. *J Neurophysiol* 77:2842–2846, 1997.

120. Lang AE, Fahn S: Movement disorders of RSD. *Neurology* 40:1476–1477, 1990.

121. Garcia-Albea E, Franch O, Muñoz D: Breughel's syndrome: Report of a case with postmortem studies. *J Neurol Neurosurg Psychiatry* 44:437–440, 1981.

122. Jankovic J: Pharmacologic approach to blepharospasm and cranial-cervical dystonia. *Adv Ophthalmol Plast Reconstr Surg* 4:211–217, 1985.

123. Altrocchi PH, Forno LS: Spontaneous oral-facial dyskinesia: Neuropathology of a case. *Neurology* 33:802–805, 1983.

124. Kulisevsky J, Marti MJ, Ferrer I, Tolosa E: Meige syndrome: Neuropathology of a case. *Mov Disord* 3:170–175, 1988.

125. Zweig RM, Hedreen JC, Jankel WR: Pathology in brainstem regions of individuals with primary dystonia. *Neurology* 38:702–706, 1988.

126. Rothwell JC, Obeso JA: The anatomical and physiological basis of torsion dystonia, in Marsden CD, Fahn S (eds): *Movement Disorders 2.* London: Butterworths, 1987, pp 313–331.

127. Jankovic J: Blepharospasm with basal ganglia lesions. *Arch Neurol* 43:866–868, 1986.

128. Karbe H, Holthoff VA, Rudolf J: Positron emission tomography demonstrates frontal cortex and basal ganglia hypometabolism in dystonia. *Neurology* 42:1540–1544, 1992.

129. Fife TD, Hutchinson M, Woods RP, et al: Motor system hypermetabolism in Meige's syndrome. *Neurology* 43(suppl 4):A409–410, 1993.

130. Hutchinson M, Fife TD, Woods RP, et al: Glucose metabolism in Meige's syndrome in wakefulness and sleep. *J Cereb Blood Flow Metab* 13(suppl 1):S370, 1993.

131. Ceballos-Baumann O, Passingham RE, Warner T, et al: Overactive prefrontal and underactive motor cortical areas in idiopathic dystonia. *Ann Neurol* 37:363–372, 1995.

132. Ibañez V, Sadato N, Karp B, et al: Deficient activation of the motor cortical network in patients with writer's cramp. *Neurology* 53:96–105, 1999.

133. Feiwell RJ, Black KJ, McGee-Minnich LA, et al: Diminished regional cerebral blood flow response to vibration in patients with blepharospasm. *Neurology* 52:291–297, 1999.

134. Hutchinson M, Nakamura T, Moeller JR, et al: The metabolic topography of essential blepharospasm. A focal dystonia with general implications. *Neurology* 55:673–677, 2000.

135. Perlmutter JS, Stambuk MK, Markham J, et al: Decreased [18F] spiperone binding in putamen in idiopathic focal dystonia. *J Neurosci* 17:843–850, 1997.

136. Federico F, Simone IL, Lucivero V, et al: Proton magnetic resonance spectroscopy in primary blepharospasm. *Neurology* 51:892–895, 1998.

137. Federico F, Lucivero V, Simone IL, et al: Proton MR spectroscopy in idiophatic spasmodic torticollis. *Neuroradiology* 43:532–536, 2001.

138. Naumann M, Warmuth-Metz M, Hillerer C, et al: Magnetic resonance spectroscopy of lentiform nucleus in the primary focal hand dystonia. *Mov Disord* 13:929–933, 1998.

139. Ridding MC, Sheean G, Rothwell JC, et al: Changes in the balance between motor cortical excitation and inhibition in focal, task specific dystonia. *J Neurol Neurosurg Psychiatry* 59:493–498, 1995.

140. Hanajima R, Ugawa Y, Masuda N, Kanazawa I: Changes of motor cortical excitability in a patient with unilateral focal dystonia due to a lesion of the contralateral putamen. *Mov Disord* 9(suppl 1):43, 1994.

141. Curra A, Romaniello A, Berardelli A, et al: Shortened cortical silent period in facial muscles of patients with cranial dystonia. *Neurology* 54:130–135, 2000.

142. Tolosa ES, Montserrat L: Depressed blink reflex habituation in dystonia blepharospasm. *Neurology* 35:271, 1985.

143. Berardelli A, Rothwell JC, Day BL, Marsden CD: Pathophysiology of blepharospasm and oromandibular dystonia. *Brain* 108:593–608, 1985.

144. Tolosa E, Montserrat L, Bayes A: Blink reflex studies in focal dystonias: Enhanced excitability of brainstem interneurones in cranial dystonia and spasmodic torticollis. *Mov Disord* 3:61–69, 1988.

145. Valls J, Tolosa E, Ribera G: Neurophysiological observation on the effects of botulinum toxin treatment in patients with dystonic blepharospasm. *J Neurol Neurosurg Psychiatry* 54:310–313, 1991.

146. Valls J, Tolosa E, Martí MJ, Allam N: Treatment with botulinum toxin injection does not change brainstem interneuronal excitability in patients with cervical dystonia. *Clin Neuropharmacol* 17:229–235, 1994.

147. Carella F, Ciano C, Musicco M, Scaioli V: Exteroceptive reflexes in dystonia: A study of the recovery cycle of the R2 component of the blink reflex and of the exteroceptive suppression of the

contracting sternocleidomastoid muscle in blepharospasm and torticollis. *Mov Disord* 9:183–187, 1994.

148. Quartarone A, Girlanda P, Di Lazzaro V, et al: Short latency trigemino-sternocleidomastoid response in muscles in patients with spasmodic torticollis and blepharospasm. *Clin Neurophysiol* 111:1672–1677, 2000.

149. Münchau A, Bronstein AM: Role of the vestibular system in the pathophysiology of spasmodic torticollis. *J Neurol Neurosurg Psychiatry* 71:285–288, 2001.

150. Colebatch JG, Di Lazzaro V, Quartarone A, et al: Click-evoked vestibulocollic reflexes in torticollis. *Mov Disord* 10:455–459, 1995.

151. Nakashima K, Rothwell JC, Day BL, et al: Reciprocal inhibition in writer's and other occupational cramps and hemiparesis due to stroke. *Brain* 112:681–697, 1989.

152. Panizza ME, Hallett M, Nilson J: Reciprocal inhibition in patients with hand cramps. *Neurology* 41:553–556, 1991.

153. Gomez-Wong E, Marti MJ, Cossu G, et al: The "geste antagonistique" induces transient modulation of the blink reflex in human patients with blepharospasm. *Neurosci Lett* 252:125–128, 1998.

154. Kaji R, Rothwell JC, Katayama M, et al: Tonic vibration reflex and muscle afferent block in writer's cramp. *Ann Neurol* 38:155–162, 1995.

155. Calne DB, Lang AE: Secondary dystonia. *Adv Neurol* 50:9–34, 1988.

156. Weiner WJ, Nausieda PA, Glanz RH: Meige syndrome (blepharospasm-oromandibular dystonia) after long term neuroleptic therapy. *Neurology* 31:1555–1556, 1981.

157. Burke RE, Fahn S, Jankovic J, et al: Tardive dystonia: Late onset and persistent dystonia caused by antipsychotic drugs. *Neurology* 32:1335–1346, 1982.

158. Weiner W, Nausieda P: Meige's syndrome during long-term dopaminergic therapy in Parkinson's disease. *Arch Neurol* 39:451–452, 1982.

159. Gershanik OS, Leist A: Juvenile onset Parkinson's disease. *Adv Neurol* 45:213–216, 1986.

160. Poewe WH, Lees AJ, Stern GM: Dystonia in Parkinson's disease: Clinical and pharmacological features. *Ann Neurol* 23:73–79, 1988.

161. Leger JM, Girault JA, Bolgert F: Deux cas de dystonie isolee d'un membre superieur inagurant une maladie de Steele-Richardson-Olszweski. *Rev Neurol (Paris)* 143:140–142, 1987.

162. Fletcher NA, Stell R, Harding A, Marsden CD: Degenerative cerebellar ataxia and focal dystonia. *Mov Disord* 3:336–342, 1988.

163. Tolosa E, Kulisevsky J, Fahn S: Meige syndrome: Primary and secondary forms. *Adv Neurol* 50:509–516, 1988.

164. Muñoz E, Tolosa E: Upper-limb dystonia secondary to a midbrain hemorrhage. *Mov Disord* 11:96–99, 1996.

165. Alarcon F, Muñoz E, Tolosa E: Focal limb dystonia in a patient with a cerebellar mass. *Arch Neurol* 58:1125–1227, 2001.

166. Chu Nai-Shin, Huang Chin-Chang, Lu Chin-Song, Calne DB: Dystonia caused by toxins, in Ching Tsui JK, Calne BC (eds): *Handbook of Dystonia*. New York: Marcel Dekker, 1995, pp 241–265.

167. LeWitt PA, Martin SD: Dystonia and hypokinesia with putaminal necrosis after methanol intoxication. *Clin Neuropharmacol* 11:61, 1988.

168. Burke RE, Fahn S, Gold AP: Delayed-onset dystonia in patients with "static" encephalopathy. *J Neurol Neurosurg Psychiatry* 43:789, 1980.

169. Maraganore DM, Folger WN, Swanson JW, Ahlskog JE: Movement disorders as sequelae of central pontine myelinolysis: Report of three cases. *Mov Disord* 7:142–148, 1992.

170. Grandas F, Artieda J, Obeso JA: Clinical and CT scan findings in a case of cyanide intoxication. *Mov Disord* 4:188, 1989.

171. Fahn S, Williams DT: Psychogenic dystonia. *Adv Neurol* 50:431–455, 1988.

172. Lang AE, Weiner WJ: Symptomatic dystonia, in Lang E, Weiner WJ (eds): *Movement Disorders: A Comprehensive Survey*. Mount Kisko, NY: Futura, 1989.

TREATMENT OF DYSTONIA

JOSEPH JANKOVIC

PHYSICAL AND SUPPORTIVE THERAPY 527
PHARMACOLOGIC THERAPY 528
    Dopaminergic Therapy 528
    Antidopaminergic Therapy 529
    Anticholinergic Therapy 529
    Other Pharmacologic Therapies 530
    Botulinum Toxin (BTX) 531
SURGICAL TREATMENT OF DYSTONIA 534
    Central Ablative Procedures and High-Frequency
        Stimulation 534
    Peripheral Surgery 535
SUMMARY: THERAPEUTIC GUIDELINES 535

The symptomatic treatment of dystonia has markedly improved, particularly since the introduction of botulinum toxin (BTX) and as a result of improved surgical treatments, including deep brain stimulation (DBS). In most cases, the treatment is merely symptomatic, designed to improve posture and function and to relieve associated pain. In rare patients, however, dystonia may be so severe that it can compromise respiration and lead to a muscle breakdown, rhabdomyolysis, and myoglobinuria.[1]

The assessment of various therapeutic interventions in dystonia is problematic for the following reasons: (1) dystonia and its effects on function are difficult to quantitate and, therefore, most trials utilize crude clinical rating scales many of which have not been properly evaluated or validated; (2) dystonia is a syndrome with different etiologies, anatomic distributions, and heterogeneous clinical manifestations producing variable disability; (3) some patients, perhaps up to 15 percent, may have spontaneous, albeit transient, remissions; (4) the vast majority of therapeutic trials in dystonia are not double-blind, placebo-controlled; and (5) most studies, even those that have been otherwise well designed and controlled, have utilized small sample sizes, which makes the results difficult to interpret, particularly in view of a large placebo effect demonstrated in dystonia. For these and other reasons, the selection of a particular choice of therapy is largely guided by personal clinical experience and by empirical trials.[2,3] The age of the patient, the anatomic distribution of dystonia and the potential risk of adverse effects are also important determinants of choice of therapy (Table 32-1). The identification of a specific cause of dystonia, such as drug-induced dystonias or Wilson's disease, may lead to a treatment that is targeted to the particular etiology. It is, therefore, prudent to search for identifiable causes of dystonia, particularly when some atypical features are present. It is beyond the scope of this chapter to discuss the diagnostic approaches to patients with dystonia; this topic is covered elsewhere in this volume and in other reviews.[2]

Physical and Supportive Therapy

Before reviewing pharmacologic and surgical therapy of dystonia, it is important to emphasize the role of patient education and supportive care as these are integral components of a comprehensive approach to patients with dystonia. Physical therapy and well-fitted braces are designed primarily to improve posture and to prevent contractures. Although braces are often poorly tolerated, particularly by children, in some cases they may be used as a substitute for a "sensory trick." For example, in some of our patients with cervical dystonia we were able to construct neck-head braces that seem to provide sensory input by touching certain portions of the neck or head in a fashion similar to the patient's own sensory trick, thus enabling the patient to maintain a desirable head position. Various hand devices have been developed in an attempt to help patients with writer's cramp to use their hands more effectively and comfortably.[4] In one small study of 5 professional musicians with focal dystonia, Candia et al.[5] reported success with immobilization by splints of one or more of the digits other than the dystonic finger, followed by intensive repetitive exercises of the dystonia finger. It is not clear, however, whether this therapy provides lasting benefits. In another study involving 8 patients with idiopathic occupational focal dystonia of the upper limb, immobilization with a splint for 4–5 weeks resulted in a significant improvement at a 24-week follow-up visit, based on Arm Dystonia Disability Scale (0 = normal, 3 = marked difficulty in playing) and the Tubiana and Champagne Score (0 = unable to play, 5 = returns to concert performances), and was considered marked in 4, moderate in 3 and the initial improvement disappeared in 1.[6] The splint was applied for 24 hours every day, except for 10 minutes once a week when it was removed for brief local hygiene. Immediately upon removal of the splint, all patients reported marked clumsiness and weakness, which resolved in 4 weeks. There was also some local subcutaneous and joint edema and pain in the immobilized joint, and nail growth stopped; no patient developed contractures. While the mechanisms of action of immobilization are unknown, the authors have postulated that removing all motor and sensory input to a limb may allow the cortical map to "reset" to the previous normal topography. One major concern about immobilization of a limb, particularly dystonic limb, is that such immobilization can actually increase the risk of exacerbating or even precipitating dystonia, as has been well demonstrated in dystonia following casting or other peripheral causes of dystonia.[7] A variation of the immobilization therapy, "constraint-induced movement therapy," has been used

TABLE 32-1 Treatment of Dystonia

Focal Dystonias

Blepharospasm
1. Clonazepam, lorazepam
2. Botulinum toxin injections
3. Trihexyphenidyl
4. Orbicularis oculi myectomy

Oromandibular dystonia
1. Baclofen
2. Trihexyphenidyl
3. Botulinum toxin injections

Spasmodic dysphonia
1. Botulinum toxin injections
2. Voice and supportive therapy

Cervical
1. Trihexyphenidyl
2. Diazepam, lorazepam, clonazepam
3. Botulinum toxin injections
4. Tetrabenazine
5. Cyclobenzaprine
6. Carbamazepine
7. Baclofen (oral)
8. Peripheral surgical denervation

Task-specific dystonias (e.g., writer's cramp)
1. Benztropine, trihexyphenidyl
2. Botulinum toxin injections
3. Occupational therapy

Segmental and Generalized Dystonias
1. L-Dopa (in children and young adults)
2. Trihexyphenidyl, benztropine
3. Diazepam, lorazepam, clonazepam
4. Baclofen (oral, intrathecal)
5. Carbamazepine
6. Tetrabenazine (with lithium)
7. Triple therapy: tetrabenazine, fluphenazine, trihexyphenidyl
8. Intrathecal baclofen infusion (axial dystonia)
9. Thalamotomy (in distal dystonia or hemidystonia)

successfully in rehabilitation of patients after stroke and other brain insults, and the observed benefit has been attributed to cortical reorganization. Some patients find various muscle relaxation techniques and sensory feedback therapy useful adjuncts to medical or surgical treatments. Since some patients with dystonia have impaired sensory perception, it has been postulated that sensory training may relieve dystonia. In a study of 10 patients with focal hand dystonia, Zeuner et al.[8] showed that reading braille for 30–60 minutes daily for 8 weeks improved spatial acuity and dystonia. Sensory training to restore sensory representation of the hand, along with mirror imagery and mental practice techniques, has also been reported to be useful in the treatment of focal hand dystonia.[9]

Using repetitive transcranial magnetic stimulation delivered at low frequencies ($\leq$1 Hz) for 20 minutes, Siebner et al.[10] showed that this technique may temporarily (8 of 16 patients reported improvement that lasted longer than 3 hours) improve handwriting impaired by dystonic writer's cramp, presumably by increasing inhibition (and thus reducing excitability) of the underlying cortex. Finally, long-term neck muscle vibration of the contracting muscle may have a therapeutic value in patients with cervical dystonia. This is suggested by transient (minutes) improvement in head position in 1 patient treated for 15 minutes with muscle vibration.[11] Such observation is consistent with the notion that proprioceptive sensory input affects cervical dystonia.

Pharmacologic Therapy

DOPAMINERGIC THERAPY

Pharmacologic treatment of dystonia is largely based on empirical, rather than scientific, rationale (Table 32-2). Unlike Parkinson's disease, in which therapy with L-dopa replacement is based on the finding of depletion of dopamine in the brains of parkinsonian animals and humans, our knowledge of biochemical alterations in idiopathic dystonia is very limited. One exception is dopa-responsive dystonia (DRD), in which the biochemical and genetic mechanisms have been elucidated by studies of postmortem brains and by molecular DNA and biochemical studies. Decreased neuromelanin in the substantia nigra with otherwise normal nigral cell count and morphology and normal tyrosine hydroxylase immunoreactivity were found in the brain of one patient with classic DRD.[12] There was a marked reduction in dopamine in the substantia nigra and striatum. These findings suggested that, in DRD, the primary abnormality is a defect in dopamine synthesis. This proposal is supported by the finding of a mutation in the GTP cyclohydrolase I gene on chromosome 14q which indirectly regulates the production of tetrahydrobiopterin, a cofactor for tyrosine hydroxylase, the rate-limiting enzyme in the synthesis of dopamine.[13,14]

Most patients with DRD improve dramatically, even with small doses of L-dopa (100 mg of L-dopa with 25 mg of decarboxylase inhibitor), but some may require doses of L-dopa as high as 1000 mg/day. In contrast to patients with juvenile Parkinson's disease,[15] DRD patients usually do not develop L-dopa-induced fluctuations or dyskinesias. If no clinically evident improvement is noted after 3 months of therapy, the diagnosis of DRD is probably in error and L-dopa can be discontinued. In addition to L-dopa, patients with DRD also improve with dopamine agonists, with anticholinergic drugs, and with carbamazepine. In contrast to patients with DRD, patients with idiopathic or other types of dystonia rarely improve with dopaminergic therapy. While dopaminergic therapy is remarkably effective in DRD, this strategy is not useful in the treatment of idiopathic dystonia. Apomorphine, however, perhaps by decreasing dopamine as well as serotonin release, may ameliorate dystonia.[16]

TABLE 32-2 Therapeutic Options for Patients with Dystonia

Generic Name	Trade Name	Daily Dosage*	Mechanism of Action
Trihexyphenidyl	Artane	6–100	Anticholinergic
Benztropine	Cogentin	4–15	Anticholinergic
Orphenadrine	Norflex	200–800	Anticholinergic
Clonazepam	Klonopin	1–12	Serotonergic, relaxant
Lorazepam	Ativan	1–16	Relaxant
Diazepam	Valium	10–100	Relaxant
Cyclobenzaprine	Flexeril	20–60	Relaxant
Chlordiazepoxide	Librium	10–100	Relaxant
Baclofen	Lioresal	40–120	Antispastic, GABA agonist, substance P antagonist
Baclofen intrathecal infusion	Lioresal	200–1500 µg/day	
Primidone	Mysoline	50–800	Antiepileptic, antitremor
Valproate	Depakote	500–1500	Antiepileptic, GABA-T inhibitor
Carbamazepine	Tegretol	1600–1600	Antiepileptic
L-Dopa/carbidopa	Sinemet (CR)	75/300–200/2000	Dopamine precursor
Lithium	Lithobid	600–1800	Antidopaminergic
Tetrabenazine	Xenazine 25	50–300	Monoamine depleter and blocker
Botulinum toxin A	BOTOX	5–400 mouse units	Blocks acetylcholine release at the neuromuscular junction by cleaving SNAP-25
Botulinum toxin B	MYOBLOC	100–15,000 mouse units	Blocks acetylcholine release at the neuromuscular junction by cleaving synaptobrevin (VAMP)

Surgery: Peripheral denervation, myectomy, thalamotomy, pallidotomy, pallidal deep brain stimulation

*Dose in mg unless otherwise specified.

ANTIDOPAMINERGIC THERAPY

Although used extensively in the past, most clinical trials have produced mixed results with dopamine receptor blocking drugs. Because of the poor response and the possibility of undesirable side-effects, particularly sedation, parkinsonism and tardive dyskinesia, the use of these drugs in the treatment of dystonia should be discouraged.[17] Clozapine, an atypical neuroleptic, has been reported in a small, open trial to be moderately effective in the treatment of segmental and generalized dystonia, but its usefulness was limited by potential side-effects.[18] Although antidopaminergic drugs have been reported to be beneficial in the treatment of dystonia, the potential clinical benefit is usually limited by the development of side-effects. Dopamine-depleting drugs, however, such as tetrabenazine, have been found useful in some patients with dystonia, particularly in those with tardive dystonia.[19] Tetrabenazine has the advantage over other antidopaminergic drugs in that it does not cause tardive dyskinesia, although it may cause transient acute dystonic reaction. The drug is not readily available in the US, but it is dispensed by prescription under the trade name Nitoman in other countries. It is possible that some of the new atypical neuroleptic drugs will be useful not only as antipsychotics, but also in the treatment of hyperkinetic movement disorders. Risperidone, a D2 dopamine receptor blocking drug with a high affinity for $5HT_2$ receptors, has been reported to be useful in a 4-week trial of 5 patients with various forms of dystonia.[16] Clozapine, a D4 dopamine receptor blocker with relatively low affinity for the D2 receptors and high affinity for the $5\text{-}HT_{2A}$ receptors, has been reported to ameliorate the symptoms of tardive dystonia.[20] The treatment of tardive dystonia and other tardive syndromes is discussed elsewhere in this volume and in other reviews.[17]

ANTICHOLINERGIC THERAPY

Anticholinergic medications such as trihexyphenidyl have been found to be most useful in the treatment of generalized and segmental dystonia.[21] In the experience of Greene et al.,[22] patients with blepharospasm, generalized dystonia, tonic (in contrast to clonic) dystonia, and with onset of dystonia at age younger than 19 years seemed to respond better to anticholinergic drugs than other subgroups, but this difference did not reach statistical significance. Except for short duration of symptoms before onset of therapy, there was no other variable, such as gender or severity, that reliably predicted a favorable response. This therapy is generally well tolerated when the dose is increased slowly. We recommend starting with a 2-mg preparation, half a tablet at bedtime and advancing up to 12 mg/day over the next 4 weeks, eventually switching to sustained-release preparations such as Artane Sequels (5 mg). Some patients require up to 60–100 mg/day, but may experience dose-related drowsiness, confusion, memory difficulty, and hallucinations. In one study of 20 cognitively intact patients with dystonia, only 12 of whom could tolerate 15–74 mg of daily trihexyphenidyl, drug-induced impairments of recall and slowing of mentation was noted, particularly in the older patients.[23] Diphenhydramine, an anticholinergic with H_1 antagonist properties, was reported to have an antidystonic effect in 3 of 5 patients.[24] The drug, however, was not effective in 10 other patients with cervical dystonia, and it was associated with sedation and other anticholinergic side-effects in most patients. Pyridostigmine, peripherally acting anticholinesterase, and eye drops of pilocarpine (a muscarinic agonist) often ameliorate at least some of the peripheral side-effects, such as urinary retention and blurred vision. Pilocarpine (Salagen) 5 mg 4 times per day, cevimeline (Evoxac) 30 mg 3 times per day, and synthetic saliva (Salivart, Salix) have been found effective in the treatment of dry mouth.

OTHER PHARMACOLOGIC THERAPIES

Many patients with dystonia require a combination of several medications and treatments[25] (Table 32-2). Benzodiazepines (diazepam, lorazepam, clonazepam) may provide additional benefit for patients whose response to anticholinergic drugs is unsatisfactory. Clonazepam may be particularly useful in patients with blepharospasm and with myoclonic dystonia.

TABLE 32-3 Clinical Applications of Botulinum Toxin

Focal dystonia
  Blepharospasm
  Lid "apraxia"
  Oromandibular-facial-lingual dystonia
  Cervical dystonia (torticollis)
  Laryngeal dystonia (spasmodic dysphonia)
  Task-specific dystonia (occupational cramps)
  Other focal dystonias (idiopathic, secondary)

Other involuntary movements
  Voice, head, and limb tremor
  Palatal myoclonus
  Hemifacial spasm
  Tics

Inappropriate contractions
  Strabismus
  Nystagmus
  Myokymia
  Bruxism (temporomandibular joint)
  Stuttering
  Painful rigidity
  Muscle contraction headaches
  Lumbosacral strain and back spasms
  Radiculopathy with secondary muscle spasm
  Spasticity
  Spastic bladder
  Achalasia (esophageal, pelvirectal)
  Other spasmic disorders

Other potential applications
  Protective ptosis
  Cosmetic (wrinkles, facial asymmetry)
  Debarking dogs
  Other

Tizanidine hydrochloride (Zanaflex) has been approved for the treatment of spasticity, but it is not yet known whether the drug will be also useful in the treatment of dystonia.[26] A centrally acting alpha 2-adrenergic agonist, its postulated mechanism of action involves increased presynaptic inhibition of motor neurons. Other muscle relaxants useful in the treatment of dystonia include cyclobenzaprine (Flexeril, 30–40 mg/day), metaxalone (Skelaxin, 800 mg 2–3 times/day), carisoprodol (Soma), orphenadrine (Norflex), and chlorzoxazone (Parafonforte). Structurally and pharmacologically similar to amitriptyline, cyclobenzaprine has been found at doses of 30–40 mg/day to be superior to placebo but equal to diazepam.

Oral baclofen may be occasionally helpful, particularly in the treatment of oromandibular dystonia. This $GABA_B$ autoreceptor agonist has been found to produce substantial and sustained improvement in 29 percent of children at a mean dose of 92 mg/day (range 40–180).[27] Although initially effective in 28 of 60 (47 percent) adults with cranial dystonia, only 18 percent continued baclofen at a mean dose of 105 mg/day after a mean of 30.6 months.[28] Narayan et al.[29] first suggested that intrathecal baclofen (ITB) may be effective in the treatment of dystonia in 1991 in a report of an 18-year-old man with severe cervical and truncal dystonic spasms who was refractory to all forms of oral therapy and to large doses of paraspinal BTX injections. Muscle-paralyzing agents were necessary to relieve these spasms, which compromised his respiration. Within a few hours after the institution of ITB infusion, the patient's dystonia markedly improved and he was able to be discharged from the ICU within 1–2 days. The subsequent experience with intrathecal infusions has been quite encouraging, and studies are currently in progress to further evaluate this form of therapy in patients with dystonia and other motor disorders.[30] In some patients treated with ITB for spasticity, the benefits persisted even after the infusion was stopped.[31] Ford et al.[32] reviewed the experience with ITB in 25 patients and concluded that this form of therapy may be "more effective when dystonia is associated with spasticity or pain." ITB may have a role in selected patients with dystonic storm and in secondary dystonias associated with pain and spasticity.[33] For example, Albright et al.[34] found improvement in dystonia scores in 10 of 12 patients with cerebral palsy using an average daily dose of ITB of 575 µg; the improvement was sustained in 6 patients. In a subsequent study involving 86 patients ages 3–42 (mean 13) years with generalized dystonia (secondary to cerebral palsy in 71 percent of patients), external infusion or bolus-dose screening was positive in approximately 90 percent of patients.[35] Programmable pumps were implanted in 77 patients. Infusion began at 200 µg/day, and increased by 10–20 percent/day until the best dose was achieved. Median duration of ITB therapy was 26 months. Mean dose increased over time, from 395 µg at 3 months, to 610 at 24 months, to 960 at 36 months. Quality of life and ease of care rated by patients and caregiver were improved in approximately 85 percent of patients. Seven patients, including 4 with cerebral palsy, lost their response to ITB during the study, usually during the first year. The most common side-effects were increased constipation (19 percent), decreased neck/trunk control, and drowsiness. Surgical and device complications occurred in 38 percent of patients, including infections, and catheter breakage and disconnection. Complication rates decreased over time. The authors conclude: "In our opinion, ITB is the treatment of choice for severe, generalized secondary dystonia after oral medications have been shown to be ineffective." In a long-term (6 years) follow-up of 14 patients, 5 were found to have improvement in their rating scale scores, although only 2 had sustained "clear clinical benefit."[36] Continuous ITB has been found to be safe and effective in some patients with reflex sympathetic dystrophy and dystonia.[37] It is not yet clear whether ITB can induce lasting remissions in patients with dystonia. The American Academy for Cerebral Palsy and Developmental Medicine has published a systematic review of the use of ITB for spastic and dystonic cerebral palsy.[38] The limited published data show that ITB reduced spasticity and dystonia, particularly in the lower extremities.

There are other medications used in the treatment of dystonia. For example, slow-release morphine sulfate has been shown to improve not only pain but also dystonic movement in some patients with primary and tardive dystonia.[39] Besides clonazepam, gamma-hydroxybutyrate, used in the treatment of alcohol abuse, has been found beneficial in the treatment of myoclonus-dystonia syndrome.[40] It is not known whether acamprosate, another drug used in the treatment of alcohol abuse, is useful in the treatment of myoclonus-dystonia.

Anticonvulsants such as levetiracetam (Keppra) and zonisamide (Zonegran) have been reported to be effective in the treatment of cortical myoclonus, but it is not clear whether these drugs play a role in the treatment of dystonia.

Peripheral deafferentation with anesthetic was previously reported to improve tremor, but this approach may also be useful in the treatment of focal dystonia such as writer's cramp,[41] or oromandibular dystonia[42] unresponsive to other pharmacologic therapy. An injection of 5–10 mL of 0.5 percent lidocaine into the target muscle improved focal dystonia for up to 24 hours. This short effect can be extended for up to several weeks if ethanol is simultaneously injected. Mexiletine, an oral derivative of lidocaine, has been found effective in the treatment of cervical dystonia at doses ranging from 450 to 1200 mg/day.[43] Two-thirds of the patients, however, experienced adverse effects, such as heartburn, drowsiness, ataxia, tremor, and other side-effects. Based on a review and a rating of videotapes by a "blind" rater, Lucetti et al.[44] reported a significant improvement in 6 patients with cervical dystonia treated with mexiletine.

Local EMG-guided injections of phenol is currently being investigated as a potential treatment of cervical dystonia, but the results have not been very encouraging because of pain associated with the procedure and unpredictable response.[45,46] Chemomyectomy with muscle-necrotizing drugs, such as doxorubicin, has been tried in some patients

with blepharospasm and hemifacial spasm,[47] but, because of severe local irritation, it is doubtful that this approach will be adopted in clinical practice.

Attacks of kinesigenic paroxysmal dystonia may be controlled with anticonvulsants (e.g., carbamazepine, phenytoin). The nonkinesigenic forms of paroxysmal dystonia are less responsive to pharmacologic therapy, although clonazepam and acetazolamide may be beneficial. Treatment of paroxysmal dyskinesias is covered in other chapters in this book and in other reviews.[48]

BOTULINUM TOXIN (BTX)

The introduction of BTX into clinical practice in the late 1980s revolutionized treatment of dystonia. The most potent biologic toxin, BTX has become a powerful therapeutic tool in the treatment of a variety of neurologic, ophthalmic, and other disorders manifested by abnormal, excessive, or inappropriate muscle contractions.[49,50] In December 1989, after extensive laboratory and clinical testing, the Food and Drug Administration (FDA) approved BTX-A (or BOTOX) as a therapeutic agent in patients with strabismus, blepharospasm, and other facial nerve disorders, including hemifacial spasm. In December 2000, the FDA approved BOTOX and BTX-B (MYOBLOC) as treatments for cervical dystonia. Although its widest application is still in the treatment of disorders manifested by abnormal, excessive, or inappropriate muscle contractions, the use of BTX is rapidly expanding to include treatment of a variety of ophthalmologic, gastrointestinal, urologic, orthopedic, dermatologic, secretory, painful, and cosmetic disorders[51,52] (Table 32-3).

Few therapeutic agents have been better understood in terms of their mechanism of action before their clinical application or have had greater impact on patients' functioning than BTX (Table 32-4). The therapeutic value of BTX is due to its ability to cause chemodenervation and to produce local paralysis when injected into a muscle. There are 7 immunologically distinct toxins that share structurally homologous subunits. Synthesized as single-chain polypeptides (molecular weight 150 kDa), these toxin molecules have relatively little potency until they are cleaved by trypsin or bacterial enzymes into a heavy chain (100 kDa) and a light chain (50 kDa). The 150-kDa protein, the active portion of the molecule, complexes with one or more nontoxin proteins that support its structure and protect it from degradation. BTX-A has been studied the most intensively and most widely used,

TABLE 32-4 Botulinum Neurotoxins

BTX type	Substrate	Localization
A, E	SNAP-25	Presynaptic plasma membrane
B, D, F	VAMP/synaptobrevin	Synaptic vesicle membrane
C	Syntaxin	Presynaptic plasma membrane

but the clinical applications of other types of toxins, including B and F, are also expanding.[53]

A small percentage of patients receiving repeated injections develop antibodies against BTX, causing them to be completely resistant to the effects of subsequent BTX injections.[54] In addition to high and frequent dosages, young age may also be a potential risk factor for the development of immunoresistance to BTX-A.[55–57] Some of the patients who have developed BTX-A antibodies have benefited from injections by immunologically distinct preparations, such as BTX-F and BTX-B.[58] After 1–3 years, some patients become antibody-negative and when re-injected with the same type of toxin they may again experience transient benefit.[59] The original preparation of BOTOX contained 25 ng of neurotoxin complex protein per 100 units, but in 1997 the FDA approved a new preparation containing only 5 ng per 100 units, which presumably should have lower antigenicity.[60] In fact, in a 3-year follow-up of patients treated with the current BOTOX, we have found no evidence of blocking antibodies as compared with 9.4 percent frequency of blocking antibodies in patients treated with the original BOTOX for the same period of time.[61] The preliminary data suggest that BTX-B provides clinical effects similar to BTX-A, but the benefits of BTX-F seem to last only 1 month.

BLEPHAROSPASM

The effectiveness of BTX in blepharospasm was first demonstrated in a double-blind, placebo-controlled trial in 1987.[62] In a subsequent report of our experience with BTX in 477 patients with various dystonias and hemifacial spasm, Jankovic et al.[63] reviewed the results in 90 patients injected with BTX for blepharospasm. Moderate or marked improvement was noted in 94 percent of the blepharospasm patients. The average latency from the time of the injection to the onset of improvement was 4.2 days; the average duration of maximum benefit was 12.4 weeks, but the total benefit lasted considerably longer (average 15.7 weeks). While 41 percent of all treatment sessions were followed by some side-effects (ptosis, blurring of vision or diplopia, tearing, and local hematoma), only 2 percent affected patients' functioning. One controlled study showed that an injection into the pretarsal rather than the preseptal portion of the orbicularis oculi is associated with a significantly lower frequency of ptosis.[64] Ptosis can be prevented also by injecting initially only the lateral and medial portion of the upper lid, thus avoiding the midline levator muscle. This finding has been confirmed by others.[2,65]

BTX injections are now considered by many as the treatment of choice for blepharospasm. In addition to idiopathic blepharospasm, BTX injections have been used effectively in the treatment of blepharospasm induced by drugs (e.g., L-dopa in parkinsonian patients, or neuroleptics in patients with tardive dystonia), dystonic eyelid and facial tics in patients with Tourette's syndrome, and in patients in whom blepharospasm was associated with "apraxia of eyelid opening."[66,67]

OROMANDIBULAR DYSTONIA

Oromandibular dystonia is among the most challenging forms of focal dystonia to treat with BTX; it rarely improves with medications, there are no surgical treatments, and BTX therapy can be complicated by swallowing problems. The masseter muscles are usually injected in patients with jaw-closure dystonia; in patients with jaw-opening dystonia, either the submental muscle complex or the lateral pterygoid muscles are injected. Of a total of 91 patients treated in 271 visits, the overall improvement was rated as 2.6 (0 = no response, 4 = marked improvement in spasms and function).[68] A meaningful reduction in the oromandibular-lingual spasms and an improvement in chewing and speech was achieved in more than 70 percent of all patients. BTX can provide lasting improvement not only in patients with primary (idiopathic) dystonia but also in oromandibular-lingual tardive dystonia. Clenching and bruxism are frequent manifestations of oromandibular dystonia, although nocturnal and diurnal bruxism can occur even without evident dystonia.[69,70] Oromandibular involuntary movements caused by hemimasticatory spasms and other disorders such as Satoyoshi syndrome have been also successfully treated with BTX.[71]

LARYNGEAL DYSTONIA (SPASMODIC DYSPHONIA)

Until the introduction of BTX, the therapy for spasmodic dysphonia was disappointing. Unilateral transection of the recurrent laryngeal nerve, although effective in most patients, frequently causes unacceptable complications and the voice symptoms often recur. A more recent procedure, which involves denervation of the adductor branch of the recurrent laryngeal nerve with reinnervation of the distal sumps with branches of the ansa cervicalis nerve, was reported to produce marked improvement in patients with adductor spasmodic dysphonia.[72] Several studies have established the efficacy and safety of BTX in the treatment of laryngeal dystonia, and this approach is considered by most to be the treatment of choice for spasmodic dysphonia.[73] Before a patient can be considered a potential candidate for BTX injections, the diagnosis of spasmodic dysphonia must be confirmed by detailed neurologic, otolaryngologic, and voice assessment, and documented by video and voice recordings. There are three approaches currently used in the BTX treatment of spasmodic dysphonia: (1) unilateral EMG-guided injection of 5–30 units;[63] (2) bilateral approach, injecting, with EMG-guidance, 1.25–4 units in each vocal fold;[74] and (3) an injection via indirect laryngoscopy without EMG.[75] Irrespective of the technique, most investigators report about 75–95 percent improvement in voice symptoms. One controlled study, however, concluded that unilateral injections "may provide both superior and longer lasting benefits" than bilateral injections.[76] The dosage can be adjusted depending on the severity of glottal spasms and the response to previous injections. Adverse experiences include transient breathy hypophonia, hoarseness and rare dysphagia with aspiration.

Although more complicated and less effective, BTX injections into the posterior cricoarytenoid muscle, with the EMG needle placed posterior to the thyroid lamina, may be used in the treatment of the abductor form of spasmodic dysphonia.[74] Using a multidisciplinary team approach, consisting of an otolaryngologist experienced in laryngeal injections and a neurologist knowledgeable about motor disorders of speech and voice, BTX injections can provide effective relief for most patients with spasmodic dysphonia. Outcome assessments clearly show that BTX injections for spasmodic dysphonia produce measurable improvements in the quality of life of patients with this disorder.[77] BTX may be useful in the treatment of voice tremor and stuttering, but the results are less predictable.[78]

CERVICAL DYSTONIA

The goal of therapy of cervical dystonia is not only to improve abnormal posture of the head and associated neck pain, but also to prevent the development of secondary complications, such as contractures, cervical radiculopathy, and cervical myelopathy. A variety of instruments have been used to assess the response in patients with cervical dystonia, but the Toronto Western Spasmodic Torticollis Rating Scale (TWSTRS)[79,80] is being used most frequently. The TWSTRS (range 0–87) consists of three subscales: severity (range 0–35), disability (0–23), and pain (0–20). In addition, visual analog scale, global assessment of change, and pain analog assessments have been used in various clinical trials. The most important determinants of a favorable response to BTX treatments are a proper selection of the involved muscles and an appropriate dosage (Table 32-5). EMG may be helpful in some patients with obese necks or in whom the involved muscles are difficult to identify by palpation.[81]

TABLE 32-5 Examination of Patients with Cervical Dystonia

1. Find the most uncompensated position
   —the patient is instructed to allow the head to "draw" into the maximal abnormal posture without resisting the dystonic "pulling" (with eyes open and closed)
   —examine while standing, walking, sitting, and writing

2. Passively move the head
   —to define the dystonic posture
   —to localize the contracting muscles
   —to determine the full range of motion
   —to determine if there are contractures

3. Palpate contracting muscles
   —to localize the involved muscles
   —to estimate the muscle mass
   —to find points of tenderness

4. EMG (needed rarely)
   —to localize involved muscles that cannot be palpated
   —to guide the injection into the muscles that are difficult to access

Using these and other scales, the efficacy and safety of BTX in the treatment of cervical dystonia has been demonstrated in several controlled and open trials.[3,82] Open-label studies generally report a more dramatic improvement, partly because of a "placebo effect" and, more importantly, because of greater flexibility in selecting the proper dosage and site of injection. Most trials report that about 90 percent of patients experience improvement in both function and control of head-neck, and pain. The average latency between injection and onset of improvement (and muscle atrophy) is 1 week; the average duration of maximum improvement is 3–4 months. On average, injections are repeated every 4–6 months. Complications are usually related to local spread, leading to transient dysphagia and neck weakness, although distant and systemic subclinical and clinical effects, such as generalized weakness and malaise, rarely occur, possibly as a result of blood distribution or retrograde axonal transport to the spinal motor neurons. Most complications resolve spontaneously, usually within 2 weeks. There have been only a few long-term studies of BTX treatment in cervical dystonia.[83,84] Brashear et al.[84] showed that two-thirds of patients receiving BTX reported that the injections always helped.

Results similar to those obtained with BTX-A have been obtained in patients treated for cervical dystonia with BTX-B.[53] In a double-blind, controlled trial of 122 patients with cervical dystonia treated with BTX-B, we observed a dose-response effect, particularly at doses of 10,000 units.[85] Using the TWSTRS, 77 percent of patients were found to respond at week 4. Other studies have subsequently confirmed the efficacy of BTX-B,[86] even in patients who are resistant to BTX-A.[58] In a 16-week, randomized, multicenter, double-blind, placebo-controlled trial of BTX-B, 109 patients, who previously responded well to BTX-A, were randomized into one of the treatment groups: placebo, 5000 U and 10,000 U administered into 2–4 cervical muscles.[86] At week 4, the total TWSTRS score improved by 4.3, 9.3 ($P = 0.01$), and 11.7 ($P = 0.0004$), respectively, when compared to baseline, and this was accompanied by significant improvements in pain, disability, and severity. The estimated median time until the total TWSTRS score returned to baseline was 63, 114, and 111 days, respectively. The most frequent side-effects associated with BTX-B included dysphagia and dry mouth.

WRITER'S CRAMP AND OTHER LIMB DYSTONIAS

Treatments of writer's cramp with muscle relaxation techniques, physical and occupational therapy, and medical and surgical therapies, have been disappointing. Several open and double-blind controlled trials have concluded that BTX injections into selected hand and forearm muscles probably provide the most effective relief in patients with these task-specific occupational dystonias. In some studies, fine wire electrodes were used to localize bursts of muscle activation during the task, and the toxin was injected through a hollow EMG needle into the belly of the most active muscle.[87] Similar beneficial results, however, were obtained in other studies without complex EMG studies.[88] Several lines of evidence support the notion that an intramuscular injection of BTX into the forearm muscles corrects the abnormal reciprocal inhibition.[89] Although one study showed that only 14 of 38 (37 percent) of needle placement attempts reached the proper hand muscles in the absence of EMG guidance, this does not mean that placement with EMG guidance correlates with better results, since the selection of the muscle involved in the hand dystonia is based on clinical examination and not on EMG.[90] Voluntary activity of the hand immediately after treatment for 30 minutes may enhance the weakness produced by the injection.[91]

In addition to improving writer's cramp, BTX may provide relief in other task-specific disorders affecting typists, draftsmen, musicians, sportsmen, and other people who depend on skilled movements of their hands. Other focal distal dystonias, besides those involving the hands, may be amenable to treatment with BTX. Patients with Parkinson's disease, progressive supranuclear palsy, corticobasal degeneration and other forms of parkinsonism or stroke-related hemiplegia occasionally develop secondary fixed dystonia of the hand ("dystonic clenched fist") which may benefit in terms of pain and hygiene from local BTX injections.[92] Patients with foot dystonia as a manifestation of primary (idiopathic) dystonia and patients with parkinsonism who may experience foot dystonia as an early symptom of their disease, or, more commonly, as a complication of L-dopa therapy, may benefit from local BTX infections.[93] BTX injections into the foot-toe flexors or extensors may not only alleviate the disability, pain, and discomfort often associated with such dystonia, but may also improve gait. Whether BTX injections will play an important role in the treatment of recurrent painful physiologic foot and calf cramps is yet to be determined.

OTHER INDICATIONS FOR BTX

It is beyond the scope of this chapter to review the rapidly broadening indications for BTX therapy (Table 32-3). The reader is referred to some recent reviews on this topic.[50,52]

Surgical Treatment of Dystonia

Although surgery has been used in the treatment of dystonia for a long time, there has been a recent resurgence in this approach, largely because of improved surgical and imaging techniques and as a result of surgical benefits observed in patients with tremor and Parkinson's disease.[94−96]

CENTRAL ABLATIVE PROCEDURES AND HIGH-FREQUENCY STIMULATION

Improved understanding of the functional anatomy of the basal ganglia and physiologic mechanisms underlying movement disorders, coupled with refinements in imaging and

surgical techniques, has led to a resurgence of interest in thalamotomy in patients with disabling tremors, dystonia, and other hyperkinetic movement disorders.[96] The observation, supported by both physiologic and positron emission tomographic (PET) studies, that in dystonia there is a disruption of pallidothalamocortical projections provides some rationale for treating dystonia by interrupting the abnormal outflow from the thalamus to the overactive prefrontal motor cortex.[97] In a longitudinal study of 17 patients with severe dystonia, 8 (47 percent) had a moderate to marked improvement in their abnormal postures and functional disability.[98] Patients with primary and secondary dystonia had similar response, but 43 percent of the patients with primary dystonia deteriorated during a mean follow-up of 32.9 months, whereas only 30 percent of patients with secondary dystonia deteriorated during a mean follow-up of 41.0 months. Neurological complications were observed in 6 of 17 patients (35 percent) immediately after surgery, but deficits (contralateral weakness, dysarthria, pseudobulbar palsy) persisted in only 1 subject. Mild weakness contralateral to the surgery was the most common complication, noted in 3 patients immediately following the procedure. One patient who underwent bilateral procedures had no detectable dysarthria. These results are consistent with other studies that have reported improvement in 34–70 percent of patients with dystonia following thalamotomy.[99]

The role of pallidotomy in the treatment of dystonia is currently being re-evaluated in view of emerging use of deep brain stimulation (DBS).[100] In one study of 8 patients with severe generalized dystonia, we showed 59 percent and 62.5 percent improvement in the Burke-Marsden-Fahn Dystonia Scale (BMFDS) and in the Unified Dystonia Rating Scale (UDRS), respectively, following pallidotomy.[101] Our experience with pallidotomy continues to show favorable long-term effects, particularly in patients with primary dystonia.[96,102] Although the surgery does not slow or halt the progression of the underlying disease, most patients continue to benefit. The procedure was well tolerated and the benefits have persisted during more than 10 years in most patients with primary dystonia. Pallidotomy has been also reported to be effective in a 47-year-old-woman with paroxysmal dystonia induced by exercise.[103]

Although there are no data from normal humans, microelectrode recordings from patients with generalized dystonia indicate that the mean discharge rates (about 50 Hz) in the globus pallidus internum (GPi) are lower than those in patients with Parkinson's disease (80–85 Hz)[104] or parkinsonian primates (70–75 Hz), but higher than in hemiballism,[105] and that the proportion of GPi cells that respond to stimulation is higher in patients with dystonia than in those with hemiballism.[106] In comparison to normal or parkinsonian primates, the GPi discharges in patients with dystonia seem to be more irregular with more bursting and pauses, and the receptive fields to passive and active movements seem to be widened.[107] We compared intraoperative neurophysiologic recordings in 15 patients with dystonia and 78 patients with

Parkinson's disease undergoing pallidotomy and found that the discharge rates were lower in frequency and more irregular in GPi and GPe of patients with dystonia.[108] Although the physiological studies, based on lower mean discharge rates in GPe and Gpi,[105,109] suggest an overactivity of both direct (striatum-GPi) and indirect (striatum-GPe-GPi) pathways, the dopamine receptor ligand studies[110] suggest increased activity in the direct pathway and decreased activity in the indirect pathway. In either case, pallidotomy[101,104,105] and GPi DBS[107,111–116] appear to be an effective procedure for patients with dystonia, perhaps because they disrupt the abnormal GPi pattern and thus reduce cortical overactivation, characteristic of dystonia. The procedure has been reported also to be effective in patients with tardive dystonia.[117] Vercueil et al.[115] described 10 patients with bilateral GPi DBS, 5 of whom had a major improvement, 2 had a moderate improvement, and 1 had a minor improvement after 14 months. They concluded that GPi DBS is much more effective than thalamic DBS for the treatment of dystonia. Since an ablative lesion or high-frequency stimulation of the GPi can both produce as well as improve dystonia, this suggests that it is the pattern of discharge in the basal ganglia rather than the actual location or frequency of discharge that is pathophysiologically relevant to dystonia.[118]

PERIPHERAL SURGERY

Peripheral denervation procedures have been used extensively prior to the advent of BTX therapy. In our series of patients with cervical dystonia seen before 1990, 40 of 300 (13 percent) elected to have surgery.[119] While 10 percent of the patients noted worsening after the surgery, 38 percent experienced a noticeable improvement in the ability to control their head position or in reduction of the neck pain. Three procedures have been used in the treatment of cervical dystonia: (1) extradural selective sectioning of posterior (dorsal) rami (posterior ramisectomy) with or without myotomy, (2) intradural sectioning of anterior cervical roots (anterior cervical rhizotomy), and (3) microvascular decompression of the spinal accessory nerve. Although the first procedure, championed by Bertrand,[120] is considered by many clinicians to be the procedure of choice, no study has compared the different surgical approaches. Bertrand and Molina-Negro[120] reported that 97 of 111 (87 percent) patients had "excellent" or "very good" results. In a smaller series, 5 of 9 (56 percent) patients had moderate benefit, which was sustained during up to 21 months of follow-up.[121] The procedure is performed under general anesthesia without a paralyzing agent so that intraoperative nerve root stimulation can be used to identify the innervation to the dystonic muscles. This information, coupled with preoperative EMG, is used to avulse selected nerve roots, usually the branches of the spinal accessory nerve and the posterior rami of C1-C6. Thorough avulsion of the peripheral branches is felt to be essential in preventing recurrences. Pain seems to improve more than the abnormal posture following the cervical muscle denervation, although

some patients complain of "stiff neck," sometimes lasting several months after the surgery. Other complications may include local numbness, neck weakness, and, rarely, dysphagia. The chief disadvantage of anterior rhizotomy compared to posterior primary ramisectomy is that the former procedure causes denervation of both involved and uninvolved muscles and it cannot be carried out at or below C4 level because of the potential for involvement of the roots to the phrenic nerve leading to paralysis of the diaphragm. The posterior ramisectomy (C2-C6) allows more selective denervation of the involved muscles. We reported the effects of 70 intradural or extradural approaches in 46 patients with severe cervical dystonia.[122] During a mean duration of follow-up of 6.5 years, 21 (46 percent) of the patients reported excellent or marked improvement on a global outcome scale. There was no difference in the distribution of outcome when patients who still responded to BTX were compared with the BTX nonresponders. Using modified TWSTRS scale, we found statistically significant improvements, not only in the severity of dystonia, but also in occupational and domestic work, as well as in various activities of daily living. The results of this study are comparable with those of Ford et al.,[123] who reported an open-label, retrospective study of a selective denervation for severe cervical dystonia (torticollis) in 16 patients refractory to injections with BTX- A. Using functional capacity scales, they concluded that 6 (37.5 percent) patients had "a moderate or complete return of normal neck function." Despite some improvement in 12 of 14 (85.7 percent) patients on the TWSTRS dystonia rating scale applied to "blinded" ratings of videotaped examinations, the surgery failed to return patients to their occupations. Based on the reported experience, we conclude that surgical treatment tailored to the specific pattern of dystonic activity in the individual patient is a valuable alternative in the long-term management of cervical dystonia.

Surgical treatments, such as facial nerve lysis and orbicularis oculi myectomy, once used extensively in the treatment of blepharospasm, have been essentially abolished because BTX treatment is usually very effective, and postoperative complications, such as ectropion, exposure keratitis, facial droop, and postoperative swelling and scarring are common.[124] Likewise, recurrent laryngeal nerve section, once used in the treatment of spasmodic dysphonia,[125] is used rarely and only when BTX fails to provide a satisfactory relief. Another once popular procedure, spinal cord stimulation for cervical dystonia, has been shown to be ineffective by a controlled trial.[126]

Summary: Therapeutic Guidelines

In summary, patients with segmental or generalized dystonia beginning in childhood or adolescence should be initially tried on L-dopa/carbidopa up to 1000 mg of L-dopa/day. If this therapy is successful, it should be maintained at a lowest possible dose. If ineffective after 3 months, then high-dose anticholinergic (e.g., trihexyphenidyl, diphenhydramine) therapy should be instituted and the dosage increased to highest tolerated level. If the results are poor, then baclofen, benzodiazepines, carbamazepine, and tetrabenazine should be tried. Some patients may require "triple therapy" consisting of an anticholinergic agent (e.g., trihexyphenidyl), monoamine depleting drug (e.g., tetrabenazine), and a dopamine receptor blocking drug (e.g., fluphenazine, pimozide, risperidol, or clozapine). Tetrabenazine alone or with anticholinergic drugs is particularly useful in the treatment of tardive dystonia. In some patients, BTX injections may be helpful to control the most disabling symptom of the segmental or generalized dystonia. In most patients with adult-onset dystonia, the distribution is usually focal and, therefore, BTX injections are usually considered the treatment of choice. Besides the abnormal movement, posture, and pain, associated depression, anxiety and other psychological comorbidities may have an important impact on the quality of life of patients with cervical dystonia and must be appropriately treated.[127] In some patients, this treatment may need to be supplemented by other drugs noted above or by surgical peripheral denervation. Thalamotomy should be reserved only for patients whose symptoms continue to be disabling despite optimal medical therapy. Any form of therapy should, of course, be preceded by a thorough evaluation designed to rule out secondary causes of dystonia. Finally, it is important to emphasize that patient education and counseling are essential components of a comprehensive therapeutic approach to all patients with dystonia (Table 32-6).

TABLE 32-6 Patient Organizations

There are several organizations, some listed below, that are dedicated to the education of patients and their families about dystonia. They provide guidance to local support groups and they are instrumental in increasing public awareness about dystonia. Another major aim is to raise funds to support research dedicated to finding the cause, cure and new symptomatic treatments for this disorder.

Dystonia Medical Research Foundation
One East Wacker Drive, Suite 2430
Chicago, IL 60601-1905
USA
Tel: (312) 755-0198 in Canada (800) 361-8061
Fax: (312) 803-0138
Email: dystonia@dystonia-foundation.org
Web site: http://www.dystonia-foundation.org/

National Spasmodic Torticollis Association
9920 Talbert Avenue #233
Fountain Valley, CA 92708TEL: 800-HURTFUL
Email: nstamail@aol.com
Web site: http://www.torticollis.org

The Bachmann-Strauss Dystonia & Parkinson Foundation, Inc.
One Gustave L. Levy Place, Box 1490

TABLE 32-6—(continued)

New York, NY 10029
USA
Tel: (212) 241-5614
Fax: (212) 987-0662
Email: Bachmann.Strauss@mssm.edu
Web site: http://www.dystonia-parkinsons.org

Spasmodic Torticollis/Dystonia, Inc.
P.O. Box 28
Mukwonago, WI 53149
USA
Tel: 1-888-445-4598
Email: info@spasmodictorticollis.org
Web site: http://www.spasmodictorticollis.org

Care4Dystonia, Inc
440 East 78th Street
New York, NY 10021
USA
Tel: 212-249-2808
Email: bekadys@aol.com
Web site: http://www.care4dystonia.org/

Benign Essential Blepharospasm
Research Foundation, Inc.
P.O. Box 12468
Beaumont, TX 77726-2468
Tel: 409-832-0788
Fax: 409-832-0890
Email: bebrf@ih2000.net

For further information about movement disorders contact:
WE MOVE—A Worldwide Education and Awareness for
    Movement Disorders
204 West 84th Street
New York, NY 10024
Tel: 800-437-6682 (MOV2)
Fax: 212-875-8389
Email: jblazer@wemove.org
Web site: www.wemove.org

References

1. Opal P, Tintner R, Jankovic J, et al: Intrafamilial phenotypic variability of the DYT1 dystonia: From asymptomatic TOR1A gene carrier status to dystonic storm. *Mov Disord* 17:339–345, 2002.
2. Jankovic J, Fahn S: Dystonic disorders, in Jankovic J, Tolosa E (eds): *Parkinson's Disease and Movement Disorders*, 4th ed. Philadelphia: Lippincott Williams & Wilkins, 2002:331–357.
3. Jankovic J: Treatment of cervical dystonia with botulinum toxin. *Mov Disord* 19 (suppl 1), 2004 (in press).
4. Tas N, Karatas K, Sepici V: Hand orthosis as a writing aid in writer's cramp. *Mov Disord* 16:1185–1189, 2001.
5. Candia V, Elbert T, Altenmüller E, et al: Constraint-induced movement therapy for focal hand dystonia in musicians. *Lancet* 53:42, 1999.
6. Priori A, Pesenti A, Cappellari A, et al: Limb immobilization for the treatment of focal occupational dystonia. *Neurology* 57:405–409, 2001.

7. Jankovic J: Can peripheral trauma induce dystonia and other movement disorders? Yes! *Mov Disord* 16:7–12, 2001.

8. Zeuner KE, Bara-Jimenez W, Noguchi PS, et al: Sensory training for patients with focal hand dystonia. *Ann Neurol* 51:593–598, 2002.

9. Byl NN, McKenzie A: Treatment effectiveness for patients with a history of repetitive hand use and focal hand dystonia: A planned, prospective follow-up study. *J Hand Ther* 13:289–301, 2000.

10. Siebner HR, Tormos JM, Ceballos-Baumann AO, et al: Low-frequency repetitive transcranial magnetic stimulation of the motor cortex in writer's cramp. *Neurology* 52:529–537, 1999.

11. Karnath H-O, Konczak J, Dichgans J: Effect of prolonged neck muscle vibration on lateral head tilt in severe spasmodic torticollis. *J Neurol Neurosurg Psychiatry* 69:658-660, 2000.

12. Rajput AH, Gibb WRG, Zhong XH, et al: DOPA-responsive dystonia: Pathological and biochemical observations in a case. *Ann Neurol* 35:396–402, 1994.

13. Ichinose H, Ohye T, Takahi E, et al: Hereditary progressive dystonia with marked diurnal fluctuation caused by mutations in the GTP cyclohydrolase I gene. *Nat Gen* 8:236–242, 1994.

14. Segawa M: Hereditary progressive dystonia with marked diurnal fluctuation. *Brain Dev* 22 (suppl):S65–S80, 2000.

15. Ishikawa A, Miyatake T: A family with hereditary juvenile dystonia-parkinsonism. *Mov Disord* 10:482–488, 1995.

16. Zudas A, Cianchetti C: Efficacy of risperidone in idiopathic segmental dystonia. *Lancet* 347:127–128, 1996.

17. Jankovic J: Tardive syndromes and other drug-induced movement disorders. *Clin Neuropharmacol* 18:197–214, 1995.

18. Karp BI, Goldstein SR, Chen R, et al: An open trial of clozapine for dystonia. *Mov Disord* 14:652–657, 1999.

19. Jankovic J, Beach J: Long-term effects of tetrabenazine in hyperkinetic movement disorders. *Neurology* 48:358–362, 1997.

20. Trugman JM, Leadbetter R, Zalis M, et al: Treatment of severe axial tardive dystonia with clozapine: Case report and hypothesis. *Mov Disord* 9:441–446, 1994.

21. Hoon AH Jr, Freese PO, Reinhardt EM, et al: Age-dependent effects of trihexyphenidyl in extrapyramidal cerebral palsy. *Pediatr Neurol* 25:55–58, 2001.

22. Greene P, Shale H, Fahn S: Analysis of open-label trials in torsion dystonia using high dosage of anticholinergics and other drugs. *Mov Disord* 3:46–60, 1988.

23. Taylor AE, Lang AE, Saint-Cyr JA, et al: Cognitive processes in idiopathic dystonia treated with high-dose anticholinergic therapy: Implications for treatment strategies. *Clin Neuropharmacol* 14:62–77, 1991.

24. Truong DD, Sandromi P, van der Noort S, Matsumoto RR: Diphenhydramine is effective in the treatment of idiopathic dystonia. *Arch Neurol* 52:405–407, 1995.

25. Jankovic J: Dystonia: Medical therapy and botulinum toxin in dystonia. *Adv Neurol* 78:169–184, 1998.

26. Nance PW, Bugaresti J, Shellenberger K, et al: Efficacy and safety of tizanidine in the treatment of spasticity in patients with spinal cord injury. *Neurology* 44(suppl 9):S44–S52, 1994.

27. Greene P: Baclofen in the treatment of dystonia. *Clin Neuropharmacol* 15:276–288, 1992.

28. Fahn S, Henning WA, Bressman S, et al: Long-term usefulness of baclofen in the treatment of essential blepharospasm. *Adv Ophthalmol Plast Reconstr Surg* 4:219–226, 1985.

29. Narayan RK, Loubser PG, Jankovic J, et al. Intrathecal baclofen for intractable axial dystonia. *Neurology* 41:1141–1142, 1991.

30. van Hilten JJ, Hoff JI, Thang MC, et al: Clinimetric issues of screening for responsiveness to intrathecal baclofen in dystonia. *J Neural Transm* 106:931–941, 1999.

31. Dressnandt J, Conrad B: Lasting reduction of severe spasticity after ending chronic treatment with intrathecal baclofen. *J Neurol Neurosurg Psychiatry* 60:168–173, 1996.

32. Ford B, Greene P, Louis ED, et al: Use of intrathecal balcofen in the treatment of patients with dystonia. *Arch Neurol* 53:1241–1246, 1996.

33. Ford B, Greene PE, Louis ED, et al: Intrathecal baclofen in the treatment of dystonia. *Adv Neurol* 78:199–210, 1998.

34. Albright AL, Barry MJ, Painter MJ, Shultz B: Infusion of intrathecal baclofen for generalized dystonia in cerebral palsy. *J Neurosurg* 88:73–76, 1998.

35. Albright AL, Barry MJ, Shafron DH, Ferson SF: Intrathecal baclofen for generalized dystonia. *Dev Med Child Neurol* 43:652–657, 2001.

36. Walker RH, Danisi FO, Swope DM, et al: Intrathecal baclofen for dystonia: Benefits and complications during six years of experience. *Mov Disord* 15:1242–1247, 2000.

37. van Hilten BJ, Willem-Johan T, van de Beek, et al: Intrathecal baclofen for the treatment of dystonia in patients with reflex sympathetic dystrophy. *N Engl J Med* 343:625–630, 2000.

38. Butler C, Campbell S, AACPDM Treatment Outcomes Committee Review Panel. Evidence of the effects of intrathecal baclofen for spastic and dystonic cerebral palsy. *Dev Med Child Neurol* 42:634–645, 2000.

39. Berg D, Becker G, Naumann M, Reiners K: Morphine in tardive and idiopathic dystonia. *J Neural Transm* 108:1035–1041, 2001.

40. Priori A, Bertolasi L, Pesenti A, et al: Gamma-hydroxybutyric acid for alcohol-sensitive myoclonus in dystonia. *Neurology* 54:1706, 2000.

41. Kaji R, Kohara N, Katayama M, et al: Muscle afferent block by intramuscular injection of lidocaine for the treatment of writer's cramp. *Muscle Nerve* 18:234–235, 1995.

42. Yoshida K, Kaji R, Kubori T, et al: Muscle afferent block for the treatment of oromandibular dystonia. *Mov Disord* 13:699–705, 1998.

43. Ohara S, Hayashi R, Momoi H, et al: Mexiletine in the treatment of spasmodic torticollis. *Mov Disord* 13:934–940, 1998.

44. Lucetti C, Nuti A, Gambaccini G, et al: Mexiletine in the treatment of torticollis and generalized dystonia. *Clin Neuropharmacol* 23:186–189, 2000.

45. Ruiz PJG, Bernardos VS: Intramuscular phenol injection for severe cervical dystonia. *J Neurol* 247:146–147, 2000.

46. Massey JM: Electromyography-guided chemodenervation with phenol in cervical dystonia (Spasmodic Torticollis), in Brin MF, Hallett M, Jankovic J (eds): *Scientific and Therapeutic Aspects of Botulinum Toxin.* Philadelphia: Lippincott Williams & Wilkins, 2002:459–462.

47. Wirtschafeter JD: Clinical doxorubicin chemomyectomy. An experimental treatment for benign essential blepharospasm and hemifacial spasm. *Ophthalmology* 98:357–366, 1991.

48. Jankovic J, Demirkiran M: Classification of paroxysmal dyskinesias and ataxias. In: Frucht S, Fahn S(eds.): Myoclonus and Paroxysmal Dyskinesias. *Adv Neurol* 89:387–400, 2002.

49. Jankovic J, Hallett M (eds): *Therapy with Botulinum Toxin.* New York: Marcel Dekker, 1994.

50. Brin MF, Hallett M, Jankovic J (eds): *Scientific and Therapeutic Aspects of Botulinum Toxin.* Philadelphia: Lippincott Williams & Wilkins, 2002.

51. Tintner R, Jankovic J: Focal dystonia: The role of botulinum toxin. *Curr Neurol Neurosci Rep* 1:337–345, 2001.

52. Jankovic J, Brin M: Botulinum toxin: Historical perspective and potential new indications, in Simpson DM, Mayer NH (eds): WE MOVE, 2002, pp 100–109.

53. Figgitt DP, Noble S: Botulinum toxin B. A review of its therapeutic potential in the management of cervical dystonia. *Drugs* 62:705–755, 2002.

54. Jankovic J: Botulinum toxin: Clinical implications of antigenicity and immunoresistance, in Brin MF, Hallett M, Jankovic J (eds): *Scientific and Therapeutic Aspects of Botulinum Toxin*. Philadelphia: Lippincott Williams & Wilkins, 2002, pp 409–416.

55. Jankovic J, Schwartz K: Response and immunoresistance to botulinum toxin injections. *Neurology* 45:1743–1746, 1995.

56. Hanna PA, Jankovic J: Mouse bioassay versus Western blot assay for botulinum toxin antibodies: Correlation with clinical response. *Neurology* 50:1624–1629, 1998.

57. Hanna PA, Jankovic J, Vincent A: Comparison of mouse bioassay and immunoprecipitation assay for botulinum toxin antibodies. *J Neurol Neurosurg Psychiatry* 66:612–616, 1999.

58. Brin MF, Lew MF, Adler CH, et al: Safety and efficacy of NeuroBloc (botulinum toxin type B) in type A-resistant cervical dystonia. *Neurology* 53:1431–1438, 1999.

59. Sankhla C, Jankovic J, Duane D: Variability of the immunologic and clinical response in dystonic patients immunoresistant to botulinum toxin injections. *Mov Disord* 13:150–154, 1998.

60. Aoki KR, Guyer B: Botulinum toxin type A and other botulinum toxin serotypes: A comparative review of biochemical and pharmacological actions. *Eur J Neurol* 8(suppl 5):21–29, 2001.

61. Jankovic J: Dystonia: Medical therapy and botulinum toxin. In Fahn S, Hallett M, DeLong DR (eds): Dystonia 4. *Adv Neurol* 94:275–863, 2004.

62. Jankovic J, Orman J: Botulinum A toxin for cranial-cervical dystonia: A double-blind, placebo-controlled study. *Neurology* 37:616–623, 1987.

63. Jankovic J, Schwartz K, Donovan DT: Botulinum toxin treatment of cranial-cervical dystonia, spasmodic dysphonia, other focal dystonias and hemifacial spasm. *J Neurol Neurosurg Psychiatry* 53:633–639, 1990.

64. Jankovic J: Apraxia of eyelid opening [letter]. *Mov Disord* 10:686–687, 1995.

65. Cakmur R, Ozturk V, Uzunel F, et al: Comparison or preseptal and pretarsal injections of botulinum toxin in the treatment of blepharospasm and hemifacial spasm. *J Neurol* 249:64–68, 2002.

66. Jankovic J: Pretarsal injection of botulinum toxin for blepharospasm and apraxia of eyelid opening. *J Neurol Neurosurg Psychiatry* 60:704, 1996.

67. Forget R, Tozlovanu V, Iancu A, Boghen D: Botulinum toxin improves lid opening in blepharospasm-associated apraxia of lid opening. *Neurology* 58:1843–1846, 2002.

68. Jankovic J, Schwartz KS: Clinical correlates of response to botulinum toxin injections. *Arch Neurol* 48:1253–1256, 1991.

69. Tan E-K, Jankovic J: Botulinum toxin A in patients with oromandibular dystonia: Long-term follow-up. *Neurology* 53:2102–2105, 1999.

70. Tan E-K, Jankovic J: Treating severe bruxism with botulinum toxin. *Journal of American Dental Association* 131:211–216, 2000.

71. Merello M, Garcia H, Nogues M, Leiguarda R: Masticatory muscle spasm in non-Japanese patient with Satoyoshi syndrome successfully treated with botulinum toxin. *Mov Disord* 9:104–105, 1994.

72. Berke GS, Blackwell KE, Gerratt BR, et al: Selective laryngeal adductor denervation-reinnervation: A new surgical treatment for adductor spasmodic dysphonia. *Ann Otol Rhinol Laryngol* 108:227–237, 1999.

73. Blitzer A, Zalvan C, Gonzalez-Yanez O, Brin MF: Botulinum toxin type A injections for the management of the hyperfunctional larynx, in Brin MF, Hallett M, Jankovic J (eds): *Scientific and Therapeutic Aspects of Botulinum Toxin*. Philadelphia: Lippincott Williams & Wilkins, 2002, pp 207–216.

74. Brin MF, Blitzer A, Stewart C, Fahn S: Treatment of spasmodic dysphonia (laryngeal dystonia) with local injections of botulinum toxin: Review and technical aspects, in Blitzer A, Brin MF, Sasaki CT, et al (eds): *Neurologic Disorders of the Larynx*. New York: Thieme, 1992, pp 214–228.

75. Ford CN, Bless DM, Lowery JD: Indirect laryngoscopic approach for injection of botulinum toxin in spasmodic dysphonia. *Otolaryngol Head Neck Surg* 103:752–758, 1990.

76. Adams SG, Hunt EJ, Charles DA, Lang AE: Unilateral versus bilateral botulinum toxin injections in spasmodic dysphonia: Acoustic and perceptual results. *J Otolaryngol* 22:171–175, 1993.

77. Courey MS, Garrett CG, Billante CR, et al: Outcomes assessment following treatment of spasmodic dysphonia with botulinum toxin. *Ann Otol Rhinol Laryngol* 109:819–822, 2000.

78. Warrick P, Dromey C, Irish JC, et al: Botulinum toxin for essential tremor of the voice with multiple anatomical sites of tremor: A crossover design study of unilateral versus bilateral injection. *Laryngoscope* 110:1366–1374, 2000.

79. Consky ES, Lang AE: Clinical assessments of patients with cervical dystonia, in Jankovic J, Hallett M (eds): *Therapy with Botulinum Toxin*. New York: Marcel Dekker, 1994, pp 211–237.

80. Comella CL, Stebbins GT, Goetz CG, et al: Teaching tape for the motor section of the Toronto Western Spasmodic Torticollis Scale. *Mov Disord* 12:570–575, 1997.

81. Jankovic J: Needle EMG guidance is rarely required. *Muscle Nerve* 24:1568–1570, 2001.

82. Tintner R, Jankovic J: Botulinum toxin for the treatment of cervical dystonia. *Expert Opin Pharmacother* 2:1985–1994, 2001.

83. Jankovic J, Schwartz K: Longitudinal experience with botulinum toxin injections for treatment of blepharospasm and cervical dystonia. *Neurology* 43:834–836, 1993.

84. Brashear A, Bergan K, Wojcieszek J, et al: Patients' perception of stopping or continuing treatment of cervical dystonia with botulinum toxin type A. *Mov Disord* 15:150–153, 2000.

85. Lew MF, Adomato BT, Duane DD, et al: Botulinum toxin type B: A double-blind, placebo-controlled, safety and efficacy study in cervical dystonia. *Neurology* 49:701–707, 1997.

86. Brashear A, Lew MF, Dykstra DD, et al: Safety and efficacy of Neurobloc (botulinum toxin type B) in type A-responsive cervical dystonia. *Neurology* 53:1439–1446, 1999.

87. Cole R, Hallett M, Cohen LG: Double-blind trial of botulinum toxin for treatment of focal hand dystonia. *Mov Disord* 10:466–471, 1995.

88. Rivest J, Lees AJ, Marsden CD: Writer's cramp: Treatment with botulinum toxin injections. *Mov Disord* 6:55–59, 1990.

89. Priori A, Berardelli A, Mercuri B, Mafredi M: Physiological effects produced by botulinum toxin treatment of upper limb dystonia. Changes in reciprocal inhibition between forearm muscles. *Brain* 118:801–807, 1995.

90. Molloy FM, Shill HA, Kaelin-Lang A, Karp BI: Accuracy of muscle localization without EMG: Implications of limb dystonia. *Neurology* 58:805–807, 2002.

91. Chen R, Karp BI, Goldstein SR, et al: Effect of muscle activity immediately after botulinum toxin injection for writer's cramp. *Mov Disord* 14:307–312, 1999.

92. Cordivari C, Misra P, Catania S, Lees AJ: Treatment of dystonic clenched fist with botulinum toxin. *Mov Disord* 16:907–913, 2001.

93. Pacchetti C, Albani G, Martignoni E, et al: "Off'' painful dystonia in Parkinson's disease treated with botulinum toxin. *Mov Disord* 10:333–336, 1995.

94. Lang AE: Surgical treatment of dystonia. *Adv Neurol* 78:185–198, 1998.

95. Jankovic J: Re-emergence of surgery for dystonia. *J Neurol Neurosurg Psychiatry* 65:434, 1998.

96. Ondo WG, Desalom JM, Jankovic J, Grossman RG: Pallidotomy and thalamotomy for dystonia, in Krauss JK, Jankovic J, Grossman RG (eds): *Surgery for Parkinson's Disease and Movement Disorders*. Philadelphia: Lippincott Williams & Wilkins, 2001, pp 299–306.

97. Ceballos-Baumann AO, Passingham RE, Warner T, et al: Overactive prefrontal and underactive motor cortical areas in idiopathic dystonia. *Ann Neurol* 37:363–372, 1995.

98. Cardoso F, Jankovic J, Grossman R, Hamilton W: Outcome after stereotactic thalamotomy for dystonia and hemiballismus. *Neurosurgery* 36:501–508, 1995.

99. Tasker RR, Doorly T, Yamashiro K: Thalamotomy in generalized dystonia. *Adv Neurol* 50:615–631, 1988.

100. Jankovic J, Hamilton W, Grossman RG: Thalamic surgery for movement disorders. *Adv Neurol* 74:221–233, 1997.

101. Ondo WG, Desaloms M, Jankovic J, Grossman R: Surgical pallidotomy for the treatment of generalized dystonia. *Mov Disord* 13:693–698, 1998.

102. Yoshor D, Hamilton WJ, Ondo W, et al: Comparison of thalamotomy and pallidotomy for the treatment of dystonia. *Neurosurgery* 48:818–824, 2001.

103. Bhatia KP, Marsden CD, Thomas DGT: Posteroventral pallidotomy can ameliorate attacks of paroxysmal dystonia induced by exercise. *J Neurol Neurosurg Psychiatry* 65:604–615, 1998.

104. Lozano AM, Kumar R, Gross RE, et al: Globus pallidus internus pallidotomy for generalized dystonia. *Mov Disord* 12:865–870, 1997.

105. Vitek JL, Chockkan V, Zhang J-Y, et al: Neuronal activity in the basal ganglia in patients with generalized dystonia and hemiballism. *Ann Neurol* 46:22–35, 1999.

106. Lenz FA, Suarez JI, Verhagen Metman L, et al: Pallidal activity during dystonia: Somatosensory reorganization and changes with severity. *J Neurol Neurosurg Psychiatry* 65:767–770, 1998.

107. Kumar R, Dagher A, Hutchison WD, et al: Globus pallidus deep brain stimulation (DBS) for generalized dystonia: Clinical efficacy and reversal of the abnormal PET activation pattern. *Neurology* 53:871–874, 1999.

108. Sanghera M, Grossman RG, Kalhorn CG, et al: Basal ganglia neuronal discharge in primary and secondary dystonia in patients undergoing pallidotomy. *Neurosurgery* 52:1358–1373, 2003.

109. Vitek JL, Zhang J, Evatt M, et al: GPi pallidotomy for dystonia: Clinical outcome and neuronal activity. *Adv Neurol* 78:211–219, 1998.

110. Perlmutter JS, Stambuk MK, Markham J, et al: Decreased [^{18}F]spiperone binding in putamen in idiopathic focal dystonia. *J Neurosci* 17:843–850, 1997.

111. Krauss JK, Pohle T, Weber S, et al: Bilateral stimulation of globus pallidus internus for treatment of cervical dystonia. *Lancet* 354:837–838, 1999.

112. Krauss JK, Loher TJ, Pohle T, et al: Pallidal deep brain stimulation in patients with cervical dystonia and severe cervical dyskinesias with cervical myelopathy. *J Neurol Neurosurg Psychiatry* 72:249–256, 2002.

113. Tronnier VM, Fogel W: Pallidal stimulation for generalized dystonia. Report of three cases. *J Neurosurg* 92:453–456, 2000.

114. Coubes P, Roubertie A, Vayssiere N, et al: Treatment of DYT1-generalised dystonia by stimulation of the internal globus pallidus. *Lancet* 355:2220–2221, 2000.

115. Vercueil L, Pollak P, Fraix V, et al: Deep brain stimulation in the treatment of severe dystonia. *J Neurol* 248:695–700, 2001.

116. Bereznai B, Steude U, Seelos K, Botzel K: Chronic high-frequency globus pallidus internus stimulation in different types of dystonia: A clinical, video, and MRI report of six patients presenting with segmental, cervical, and generalized dystonia. *Mov Disord* 17:138–144, 2002.

117. Trottenberg T, Paul G, Meissner W, et al: Pallidal and thalamic neurostimulation in severe tardive dystonia. *J Neurol Neurosurg Psychiatry* 70:557–559, 2001.

118. Münchau A, Mathen D, Cox T, et al: Unilateral lesions of the globus pallidus: report of four patients presenting with focal or segmental dystonia. *J Neurol Neurosurg Psychiatry* 69:494–498, 2000.

119. Jankovic J, Leder S, Warner D, Schwartz K: Cervical dystonia: Clinical findings and associated movement disorders. *Neurology* 41:1088–1091, 1991.

120. Bertrand CM, Molina-Negro P: Selective peripheral denervation in 111 cases of spasmodic torticollis: Rationale and results. *Adv Neurol* 50:637–643, 1988.

121. Davis DH, Ahlskog JE, Litchy WJ, Root LM: Selective peripheral denervation for torticollis: Preliminary results. *Mayo Clin Proc* 66:365–371, 1991.

122. Krauss JK, Toops EG, Jankovic J, Grossman RG: Symptomatic and functional outcome of surgical treatment of cervical dystonia. *J Neurol Neurosurg Psychiatry* 63:642–648, 1997.

123. Ford B, Louis ED, Greene P, Fahn S: Outcome of selective ramisectomy for botulinum toxin resistant torticollis. *J Neurol Neurosurg Psychiatry* 65:472–478, 1998.

124. Chapman KL, Bartley GB, Waller RR, Hodge DO: Follow-up of patients with essential blepharospasm who underwent eyelid protractor myectomy at the Mayo Clinic from 1980 through 1995. *Ophthalmol Plast Reconstr Surg* 15:106–110, 1999.

125. Dedo HH, Izdebski K: Intermediate results of 306 recurrent laryngeal nerve sections for spastic dysphonia. *Laryngoscope* 93:9–15, 1983.

126. Goetz CG, Penn RD, Tanner CM: Efficacy of cervical cord stimulation in dystonia. *Adv Neurol* 50:645–649, 1988.

127. Ben-Shlomo Y, Camfield L, Warner T: What are the determinants of quality of life in people with cervical dystonia? *J Neurol Neurosurg Psychiatry* 72:608–614, 2002.

Chapter 33

SYMPTOMATIC DYSTONIAS

J.G. DE YÉBENES, S. CANTARERO, C. TABERNERO and A.V. VÁZQUEZ

DEFINITION OF SECONDARY OR SYMPTOMATIC
   DYSTONIA   541
SYMPTOMATIC DYSTONIA RELATED TO FOCAL
   BRAIN LESIONS   541
   Relevant Brain Structures Involved in Dystonia   544
   Type of Brain Lesion   545
   Anatomicoclinical Correlation   546
   Delayed Onset and Independent Progression   546
DYSTONIA RELATED TO PERIPHERAL INJURY   546
DYSTONIA IN NEURODEGENERATIVE
   DISORDERS   547
   Dystonia in Akinetic-Rigid Syndromes   547
   Dystonia in Choreic Syndromes   548
   Dystonia in Basal Ganglia Disorders   549
   Dystonia in Hereditary Ataxias   551
   Dystonia in other Neurodegenerations   551
DYSTONIA IN METABOLIC DISORDERS   552
   Disorders of Lipid Metabolism   552
   Disorders of Energy Production   554
   Disorders of Organic and Amino Acid
     Metabolism   554
   Abnormalities of Purine Metabolism   555
DYSTONIA DUE TO PHYSICAL AND CHEMICAL
   AGENTS   556
PSYCHOGENIC DYSTONIAS   557
PSEUDODYSTONIAS OF ORGANIC ORIGIN   558

Definition of Secondary or Symptomatic Dystonia

The concept of symptomatic or secondary dystonia, as opposed to primary or idiopathic dystonia, emerged in the medical literature as a class of dystonias of known etiology. Perinatal brain injury was the most representative cause of symptomatic dystonia. More recently, different focal brain lesions, neurodegenerations, metabolic disorders of the nervous system, and drugs and chemicals have been recognized as causes of dystonia. In addition, several genes or gene markers of the formerly considered primary or idiopathic dystonias have been discovered and, in some cases, the mechanism of production is better known for the idiopathic dystonias than for the symptomatic dystonias. Thus, although it is a time- honored tradition, the distinction between primary and secondary dystonias caused by different gene defects has lost some of its conceptual background. However, it is rather useful for the purpose of differential diagnosis to maintain the separation between primary and secondary dystonias. We will include in the group of primary dystonias, and therefore exclude from our discussion, the sporadic cases of unknown origin and the familial cases of autosomal-dominant idiopathic torsion dystonia linked to chromosome 9 (mutations of the torsin gene), and other loci of unknown genes at chromosomes 18 and 19, as well as myoclonic dystonia of unknown genetic origin, L-dopa-responsive dystonias, parkinsonism related to mutations of the GTP hydrolase and tyrosine hydroxylase genes, and X-linked dystonia and parkinsonism (Table 33-1).

As opposed to primary dystonia, secondary dystonia is considered to be "often accompanied by other neurological deficits,"[1,2] to "begin suddenly at rest and occur at rest from the onset,"[3] and to be associated with different known hereditary and environmental causes.[4] These differential criteria are relative since there is a great clinical diversity of secondary dystonias; in addition, primary dystonias are subdivided into different clinical syndromes. In this chapter we discuss the dystonic syndromes secondary to focal, degenerative, metabolic, or chemical insult to the nervous system as well as the pseudodystonias of organic and psychogenic origin. The main clinical characteristics of secondary dystonia, as well as clues for the differential diagnosis, are summarized in Tables 33- 2 and 33-3.

Symptomatic Dystonia Related to Focal Brain Lesions

In spite of recent improvements in prenatal care and delivery throughout the world, the most frequent cause of dystonia secondary to focal brain lesions is cerebral palsy (Fig. 33-1).[5,6] With modern neuroimaging techniques it is not uncommon to find focal brain lesions, frequently perinatal vascular injury, in patients with dystonia, occasionally unaware of perinatal brain damage. Focal brain lesions are responsible for the great majority of cases of hemidystonia.[7–16]

TABLE 33-1 Etiologic Classification of Dystonia

I. Primary Dystonias
   A. Hereditary
      1. Autosomal-dominant idiopathic torsion dystonia linked to chromosome 9
      2. Autosomal-dominant, L-dopa-responsive dystonia related to GTP hydrolase deficiency
      3. Autosomal-dominant myoclonic dystonia
      4. X-linked dystonia-parkinsonism
   B. Sporadic idiopathic dystonias
II. Secondary Dystonias
   A. Caused by focal brain lesions
   B. Associated with degeneration of the central nervous system
   C. Resulting from metabolic disorders of the central nervous system
   D. Produced by drugs and chemicals

TABLE 33-2 Differential Diagnosis of Symptomatic Dystonias

Disease	Inheritance	Type of Dystonia	Age at Onset	Clinical Findings	Neuroimaging	Diagnosis
Focal brain lesions	Sporadic	Hemidystonia, focal	Children, young adults	Corticospinal and brainstem signs	Focal lesion	Clinical/MRI
PD	Mostly sporadic	Focal	Adults	Tremor, ARS	Normal (nigral T_2 shortening)	Clinical
PSP	Mostly sporadic	Axial	Mature senile	Gaze palsy, ARS	Midbrain tectal atrophy	Clinicopathological
CBD	Sporadic	Limb	Mature senile	Apraxia, myoclonus, alien limb	Asymmetric cerebral atrophy	Clinicopathological
MSA	Sporadic	Axial	Mature senile	ARS, autonomic, cerebellar	OPCA, T_2 putaminal hypointensity in SDS and SND	Pathology
Huntington's disease	AD	Generalized	Young adults	Chorea, dementia	Candate and cortical atrophy	Genetic, IT_{15} CAG expansion
Neuroacanthocytosis	AR sporadic	Orolingual, generalized	Young adults	Chorea, amyotrophy, epilepsy	Caudate atrophy	Acanthocytes
Wilson's disease	AR	Generalized	Children, young adults	Tremor, psychiatric, dysarthria	Putaminal, thalamic, dentate, brainstem, T_2 high signal	K-F rings, Cu^{2+} levels, ceruloplasmin gene defects of chromosome 13
Hallervorden–Spatz	AR	Multifocal, generalized	Children, young adults	Corticospinal, dementia	Pallidal T_2 hypointensity ("eye of the tiger" sign)	Pathology
Fahr's syndrome	AD/AR/sporadic	Generalized hemidystonia	Adults	ARS, corticospinal, ataxia, dementia	Basal ganglia striking calcifications	Imaging (exclusion diagnosis)
Ataxia telangiectasia	AR	Generalized	Children	Ataxia, neuropathy	Cerebellar atrophy	Clinical, low levels IgA
Machado-Joseph	AD	Multifocal, generalized	Children, young adults	Ataxia, ophthalmoplegia, amyotrophy	Cerebellar atrophy	Genetic, CAG expansion 14q
Dentatorubro-pallidoluysian atrophy	AD	Generalized	Adults	Ataxia, dementia, myoclonus	Brainstem, cerebellum Alt signal	Genetic, CAG expansion 21p
Intraneuronal inclusion	Sporadic	Focal, generalized	Children, young adults	Corticospinal, ataxia, dementia		Pathology (rectal biopsy)
Rett syndrome	Sporadic (females)	Focal	Children	Autism, stereotypy, epilepsy	Brain atrophy	Clinical
GM1 gangliosidosis, type 3	AR	Generalized	Children, young adults	Ataxia, corticospinal (no dementing)	Basal ganglia lesions	Beta-D-galactosidase
GM2 gangliosidosis	AR	Generalized	Children, young adults	Corticospinal, epilepsy, blindness	T_2 high signal in the basal ganglia, severe atrophy	Hexosaminidase

Disease	Inheritance	Distribution	Onset	Clinical features	Neuroimaging	Diagnostic test
Niemann-Pick type C	AR	Generalized	Children	Dementia, gaze palsy, epilepsy		Defective cholesterol esterification/sphingomyelinase
Metachromatic leukodystrophy	AR	Generalized	Children	Dementia, psychiatric symptoms	White matter, diffuse confluent T_2 high signal	Aryl sulfatase A
Ceroid lipofuscinosis/Kufs disease	AR	Focal (cranial) hemidystonia	Children, young adults	Dementia, ataxia, epilepsy	T_2 low signal in thalami and striata	Pathology (rectal biopsy)
Leigh's syndrome	AR	Generalized	Children	Hypotonia, ataxia, optic atrophy	Striatal lucencies (T_2 basal ganglia hyperintensities)	Pyruvic acid and alanine levels, mtDNA mutations, cytochrome *c* oxidase activity
Glutaric aciduria I	AR	Generalized	Children	Encephalopathic crisis, mental retardation	Frontotemporal atrophy, enlarged Sylvian fissures	Glutaric acid in urine, glutaryl-CoA dehydrogenase
Methylmalonic aciduria	AR	Generalized	Children	Acute encephalopathy	Pallidal T_2 hyperintensity	Chromatography of organic acids, methylmalonyl-CoA mutase
Homocystinuria	AR	Generalized	Children	Focal deficits, mental retardation	Focal ischemic lesions, sinus thrombosis	AA chromatography
Hartnup disease	AR	Generalized, paroxysmal	Children	Mental retardation, recurrent ataxia, and behavioral alterations	White matter T_2 hyperintensity	AA chromatography
Lesch-Nyhan syndrome	X-linked	Generalized	Children	Mental retardation, self-mutilation		Hypoxanthine-guanine phosphoribosyl transferase

ARS, akinetic-rigid syndrome; OPCA, olivopontocerebellar atrophy; SDS, Shy-Drager syndrome; SND, Striatonigral degeneration; CBD, corticobasal degeneration; AR, autosomal-recessive inheritance; AD, autosomal-dominant inheritance; AA, amino acid; K-F rings, Kayser-Fleisher rings; MRI, magnetic resonance imaging; mtDNA, mitochondrial DNA.

TABLE 33-3 Dignostic Clues to Secondary Dystonia

Clinical Clues in the Most Common Symptomatic Dystonias	Most Likely Clinical Diagnosis
I. Dystonia in Children	
A. Dystonia associated with focal neurological signs and perinatal brain injury, ectopia lentis, skeletal deformities, mental retardation	Dystonic cerebral palsy, homocystinuria
B. Dystonia after acute encephalopathy associated with macrocephaly, tetraparesis, dysphagia, dysarthria, optic atrophy, hypotonia, tetraparesis, ataxia, dysphagia, dysarthria	Glutaric aciduria, methylmalonic aciduria, Leigh's syndrome
C. Acute dystonia, without any other neurological symptoms	Intake of neuroleptics, antiemetics, catecholamine releasers, antiepileptics, and other drugs and chemicals
D. Fixed congenital focal dystonia	Musculoskeletal deformities
E. Dystonia associated with other neurological deficits, spinocerebellar deficits, tetraparesis, blindness, and seizures	GM1 gangliosidosis
F. Dystonia associated with spasticity, exaggerated startle reaction and seizures, skeletal deformities, mental retardation associated with automutilation, urinary stones, and hyperuricemia	GM2 gangliosidosis, Niemann-Pick disease, Lesch-Nyhan syndrome
II. Dystonia in Youngsters and Adults	
A. Dystonia associated with akinetic-rigid syndromes, foot dystonia, axial dystonia mostly in extension, gaze palsy, dysphagia, dysarthria, gait disturbance, anterocollis, poor response to L-dopa, autonomic disturbances, asymmetric hand dystonia with myoclonus, generalized dystonia with akinetic-rigid syndrome in children and young adults	PD, PSP MSA, CBD, mitochondrial, encephalopathy
B. Dystonia associated with chorea and oromandibular dystonia	Neuroacanthocytosis
C. Dystonia associated with ataxia, Autosomal-dominant disease with ataxia, dementia, dysarthria, ophthalmoplegia, dystonia and akinetic-rigid syndromes, rhythmic dystonia, and hemidystonia	Machado-Joseph disease, OPCA, drug-induced, focal putaminal lesions

III. MRI Findings	Most likely Clinical Diagnosis
A. Pattern of atrophy	
Frontotemporal atrophy with Sylvian enlargement, cerebellar atrophy, caudate atrophy, midbrain atrophy, asymmetric frontoparietal atrophy	Glutaric aciduria, OPCA, Machado-Joseph, ataxia telangiectasia, HD, neuroacanthocytosis, PSP, CBD
B. T_2 high-intensity signal	
1. Putaminal	Focal vascular lesion, WD, Leigh's disease, GM2 gangliosidosis, cyanide
2. Pallidal	Methylmalonic aciduria, carbon monoxide, methyl alcohol
3. White matter	Metachromatic leukodystrophy, homocystinuria, Hartnup disease
C. Low-intensity signal	
1. Putaminal	MSA, Kufs' disease, calcification of the basal ganglia
2. Pallidal	Hallervorden-Spatz disease

RELEVANT BRAIN STRUCTURES INVOLVED IN DYSTONIA

Identification of the brain structures involved in dystonia is based on neuroimaging and pathology.[7,9,10,13,15] Magnetic resonance imaging (MRI) and positron emission tomography (PET) are more sensitive than computed tomography (CT).[12–15] Three regions are most often involved: the basal ganglia, thalamus, and brainstem.[7–9] Focal dystonia has been also rarely described in patients with lesions of the parietal cortex,[17,18] and the cerebellum.[19]

The role of basal ganglia damage in dystonia is firmly established. Putaminal lesions are the most frequent cause of hemidystonia (Fig. 33-2).[7–9,12,20–22] Even some patients with idiopathic dystonia have a T_2 signal alteration in the putamen in high-field MRI.[23] The caudate nucleus is occasionally involved in limb dystonia. Pallidal lesions with gliosis due to kernicterus cause symptomatic dystonia in childhood.[12]

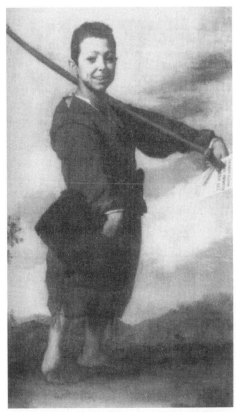

FIGURE 33-1 The limp child. Hemidystonia in cerebral palsy, documented by J. Ribera (1591–1652) in 1642. (*The Louvre, Paris, resonance.*)

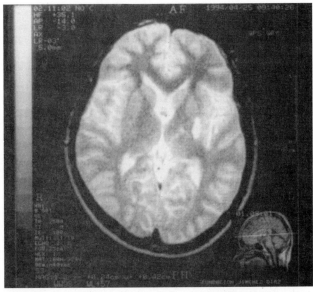

FIGURE 33-2 MRI scan showing left perinatal putaminal hemorrhage in a patient with right hemiparesis and right hemidystonia.

Thalamic lesions are also a cause of secondary dystonia. Limb dystonia may appear after stereotaxic thalamotomy for the treatment of tremor,[24] and dystonia.[25] In summary, symptomatic dystonia due to focal brain lesions suggests that the structural basis of dystonia lies in the basal ganglia-thalamocortical motor circuit; this has led to the current concept of dystonia as a dysfunction of this loop.

Evidence of brainstem lesions inducing dystonia (i.e., cranial dystonia) is supported by neuroimaging, neurophysiological studies, and clinical physiopathological associations.[26–33] Neuropathological results are not consistent.[34–40] Although it has not yet been possible to localize accurately a responsible nucleus or neuronal circuit, brainstem projections to and from the basal ganglia are most probably involved.

TYPE OF BRAIN LESION

Dystonia may appear after almost any properly placed focal lesion (i.e., in the basal ganglia, thalamus, or brainstem) (Table 33-4), although the most common cause of dystonia of focal origin is vascular injury. Diffuse brain injuries (anoxia, kernicterus, hydrocephalus, etc.) may produce a selective involvement of the structures mentioned above (Fig. 33-3).

TABLE 33-4 Symptomatic Dystonia Resulting from Focal Lesions of the Nervous System

A. Focal lesion of the basal ganglia, thalamus, and brainstem
  1. Vascular
    a. Infarction
    b. Hemorrhage
    c. Vascular malformation
    d. Vasculitis (systemic lupus erythematosus, primary antiphospholipid syndrome, Behçet's syndrome, Sjögren syndrome, isolated angiitis of the central nervous system)
    e. Migraine
  2. Head trauma
  3. Tumor and cysts: astrocytoma, lymphoma, glioma, porencephalic cyst, subarachnoid cyst, metastasis
  4. Infection: HIV and related infections, tuberculosis, viral
  5. Multiple sclerosis
  6. Syringomyelia, cerebellar ectopia
B. Diffuse lesions with prominent damage of the basal ganglia, thalamus, or brainstem
  1. Anoxia and energy failure: perinatal asphyxia, cardiac arrest, toxins
  2. Kernicterus
  3. Hydrocephalus
  4. Metabolic disorders: hyponatremia, hypernatremia, dehydration, hypoparathyroidism, hypoglycemia
  5. Hepatocerebral degeneration
  6. Paraneoplastic syndrome
  7. Hemiparkinsonism-hemiatrophy syndrome
C. Superficial lesions, with unclear effects on the basal ganglia, thalamus or brainstem
  1. Subdural hematoma
  2. Pachygyria

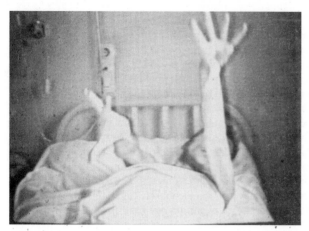

FIGURE 33-3 Generalized dystonia in a patient with AIDS and cerebral toxoplasmosis.

Focal lesions (vascular malformation, tumor) located away from these regions (basal ganglia, thalami, brainstem) may produce dystonia by indirect mechanisms, most probably related to compression or steal phenomena.[12–18] Demyelinating lesions inducing dystonia are most often located at the brainstem level.

Individual features, including age and genetic susceptibility, are distinctly relevant for the different phenotypic expression of similar lesions.[8,12]

Secondary dystonia due to basal ganglia and thalamic injuries is much more frequent when the insult takes place in the perinatal period and earlier years of life than in adulthood (Fig. 33-4).[2,41–45] Brain injury in young children is associated with longer latency to onset of subsequent movement disorder, a greater tendency to development of generalized dystonia, and a greater probability of altered handedness.[46]

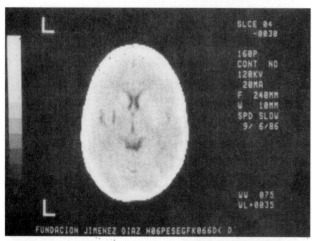

FIGURE 33-4 CT scan showing right putaminal infarction in an 8-year-old girl with acute lymphocytic leukemia and left hemidystonia.

An increased vulnerability of the striatum during development, related to different arrangement of matrix/striosomes or to a high level of excitatory neurotransmission at this stage, could be a possible explanation. Age-related differences reflect different grades of neuronal plasticity and different compensatory potential of particular neuronal circuits. The role of genetic susceptibility is well documented in drug-induced dystonia, but unknown in dystonia induced by focal lesions.

ANATOMICOCLINICAL CORRELATION

There is a certain correlation between the topographic localization of the lesion and the pattern of dystonia:

- Putaminal lesion: hemidystonia or limb dystonia
- Thalamic lesion: hand dystonia
- Brainstem lesion: blepharospasm, Meige's syndrome

However, in some cases, it is difficult to establish which is the most relevant lesion.[47] Cranial dystonia with putaminal lesions,[37,43,48] cranial dystonia and hemidystonia with thalamic lesions,[30,49] and oromandibular dystonia with lesion in head of caudate nucleus[10] are some of the exceptions to this oversimplified scheme. Unilateral diencephalic or brainstem lesions produce bilateral symmetric blepharospasm,[30] although a case of a left rostral diencephalic-brainstem lesion with ipsilateral blepharospasm and contralateral hemidystonia has been reported.[33]

DELAYED ONSET AND INDEPENDENT PROGRESSION

Some of the most characteristic and intriguing features of dystonia secondary to focal brain lesions are the time delay from injury to the appearance of the movement disorder and its posterior independent progression.

It is unlikely that delayed onset is related to the recovery of an associated corticospinal tract lesion[12,50] since in many cases dystonia appears without previous hemiparesis. Three alternative physiopathological mechanisms—denervation hypersensitivity,[26] aberrant sprouting of the damaged neurons,[51,52] and secondary retrograde degeneration[53]—have been proposed.

Dystonia Related to Peripheral Injury

The relationship between peripheral trauma and dystonia is quite controversial.[54,55] In genetically predisposed individuals (i.e., asymptomatic carriers of the gene for idiopathic torsion dystonia), peripheral trauma may trigger the onset of the dystonia.[56–58] However, it is not proved that peripheral injury induces dystonia through alteration of the sensory input to the central nervous system (CNS) or changes of the central processing. Some peculiarities of peripherally induced dystonia[59-64] set it apart from other symptomatic dystonias:

- Short latency of onset (days)
- Present at rest from the start and persists during sleep
- No "geste antagonistique"
- No overflow
- Fixed postures with limitation of range of motion
- Little response to anticholinergics or botulinum toxin
- Associated causalgia and reflex sympathetic dystrophy
- Associated hypertrophy of individual muscles[55]

Direct nerve injury or surgery, entrapment neuropathies, and electrical injury have been related to the onset of dystonia. Usually, the same region that receives the injury develops the dystonia;[64] hence, local ocular disease is associated to blepharospasm, dental procedures to oromandibular dystonia,[57] whiplash and other neck injuries to cervical dystonia, limb injury to limb dystonia, and posttraumatic abnormal postures and muscle hypertrophy in shoulder after local minor injury.[65] In some cases, occupational cramps may be related to repetitive microtraumatisms; hence, they could be considered as a kind of peripherally induced dystonia. The role of peripheral trauma in dystonia may be underlined by the frequency of occupational dystonia in certain professionals (laryngeal dystonia in teachers, hand dystonia in string or piano players, oromandibular dystonia in wind players). In most cases, these professionals do not record important trauma but only excessive use of the muscles involved in the dystonic phenomenon. It has been recently reported that in some cases of occupational dystonia there is an abnormal lack of physiological inhibition of somatosensory evoked potentials in the parietal cortex.[66] It has also been shown that prolonged immobilization of the dystonic extremity produces persistent improvement in occupational dystonia.[67] These data may support the hypothesis of excessive facilitation of muscle contraction in dystonia triggered by lack of inhibition or plasticity of neuronal circuits in response to trauma or overuse of certain muscles.

Dystonia in Neurodegenerative Disorders

Dystonia is a common symptom of neurodegenerative disorders, especially those involving the basal ganglia. In most of these diseases, dystonia is associated with other manifestations of the clinical picture. However, in some instances, dystonia may be the unique, most relevant, or first clinical symptom of the neurodegenerative disorder and, therefore, it may be misdiagnosed as idiopathic torsion dystonia.

DYSTONIA IN AKINETIC-RIGID SYNDROMES

PARKINSON'S DISEASE (PD)
Three points deserve discussion regarding dystonia and PD: (1) the presence of dystonia in untreated PD, (2) the evidence

of dystonia and parkinsonism as different phenotypic expressions of the same disorders, and (3) the appearance of dystonia as a complication of therapy in PD.

Dystonia is not uncommon in untreated PD, especially in patients with early onset of clinical symptoms. Adult-onset foot dystonia should raise the possibility of PD.[68,69] The foot is often deviated in equinovarus, with 2nd to 5th toes flexed and the great toe dorsiflexed (the so-called striatal toe); this is a typical action dystonia or kinesogenic dystonia, and the deviation worsens with walking (see Chap. 14). Less frequently, dystonia occurs in the upper extremity in untreated patients with PD, and it is most frequently characterized by cubital deviation, metacarpophalangeal flexion, proximal interphalangeal extension, and distal interphalangeal extension. There are some isolated clinical reports of untreated patients suffering blepharospasm, oromandibular dystonia, hemidystonia, writer's cramp, and cervical dystonia,[70,71] and there is a neuropathologically confirmed case of PD with Meige's syndrome.[72] If we consider isolated scoliosis as a symptom of dystonia, then this disorder would be even more frequent in patients with PD.[73] Some authors consider anismus, which is a result of abnormal puborectalis muscle contraction, as a form of dystonia[74] common in PD.

Dystonia and parkinsonism coexist as different clinical manifestations of the same disease in a number of hereditary conditions, including autosomal-dominant familial parkinsonism related to synuclein mutations,[75] L-dopa-responsive dystonia,[76,77] juvenile parkinsonism,[78,79] early-onset parkinsonism with gliosis of the substantia nigra,[80] and other conditions. Recently a patient was identified with typical L-dopa-responsive dystonia due to a hemizygous mutation of the gene Park 2 (Vidal et al., unpublished).

In addition, dystonia occurs in patients under treatment for PD as a complication of the treatment. Off-period dystonia occurs more frequently in the morning (early-morning dystonia), after the nocturnal period of L-dopa deprivation, or at moments when the patient is akinetic in the interval between two doses of medication (off-period dystonia). Dystonia also occurs as a side-effect of L-dopa treatment at times when the antiparkinsonian effect is present. Peak-effect dyskinesia and, more frequently, biphasic dyskinesia are occasionally characterized by repetitive dystonia of the extremities (see Chap. 15).

PROGRESSIVE SUPRANUCLEAR PALSY (PSP)
Oculofaciocervical dystonia[81] is frequent in PSP, which is characterized by akinetic-rigid syndrome, supranuclear gaze palsy, early gait problems, dysphagia, dysarthria, and a variable disturbance of cognitive function, most frequently consistent with apathy and frontal lobe dysfunction. Familial PSP has been described,[82,83] but the gene that causes it is unknown since the PSP-like families already described and related to mutations of tau gene in chromosome 17[84] are better classified as familial frontotemporal dementia with parkinsonism. Axial dystonia is characterized by hyperextended

neck and trunk. Facial expression[85] is related to tonic-dystonic contraction of frontal and oromandibular muscles which, together with the fixed eyes, make the patients exhibit "stare gaze." Facial dystonia is often induced by speech. Blepharospasm, often associated with eyelid apraxia, has been described in PSP.[86] Upper limb dystonia, although less typical in PSP, was present in some autopsy-proven cases,[81,84,87–91] as well as in another pathologically confirmed patient from our group[82] (see Chap. 20).

CORTICOBASAL DEGENERATION (CBD)

Since the original report by Rebeiz et al.,[92] increasing numbers of patients are being described. The disorder characteristically combines an asymmetric akinetic-rigid syndrome, dystonia, and myoclonus with focal cortical dysfunction. The pathological examination discloses frontoparietal and basal ganglia asymmetrical atrophy, and swollen achromatic neurons (see Chap. 46).

Dystonia was present in 83 percent of 36 patients suspected of having CBD, after a mean evolution of 5.2 years.[93] In CBD, contrary to PSP, dystonia is fairly asymmetric and involves mainly the most affected arm, leading to an adducted and flexed posture with clawed fingers.

MULTIPLE-SYSTEM ATROPHY (MSA)

MSA is characterized by a varied combination of clinical symptoms related to the degeneration of several neuronal systems, including the nigrostriatal pathway, striatum, cerebellum, autonomic nervous system. Three subtypes of MSA are currently recognized: striatonigral degeneration, characterized by akinetic-rigid syndrome with poor or short-lasting response to dopaminomimetic agents; Shy-Drager syndrome, characterized by akinetic-rigid syndrome and autonomic failure; and olivopontocerebellar atrophy (OPCA), characterized by ataxia, akinetic-rigid syndrome, different movement disorders, dementia, corticospinal tract signs, and ophthalmoplegia (see Chap. 21).

The frequency of dystonia in MSA is variable. Quinn suggests that around 50 percent of his patients with MSA, as confirmed by pathology, had anterocollis.[74] Berciano[94] reported the presence of "involuntary movements" in 40 percent of patients with familial OPCA and 18 percent with sporadic OPCA. Description of these involuntary movements lacks precise details for most of these patients. Some of them had chorea, probably related to lesions of the subthalamic nucleus; others, including the initial patient described by Menzel,[95] had torticollis. In 1 case, this torticollis was attributed to atrophy of the vestibuloreticular system.[96]

DYSTONIA IN CHOREIC SYNDROMES

HUNTINGTON'S DISEASE (HD)

Dystonia is a frequent clinical symptom in (HD). In patients with late-onset and rapid chorea, dystonia occurs most often as a complication of treatment with neuroleptics.

In juvenile patients, hypokinesia, rigidity, hypomimia, bradykinesia, and dystonia are the motor signs.[97] In many patients with classical forms, initial rapid chorea disappears with the progression of the illness and is substituted for or accompanied by dystonia. In an epidemiological study, dystonia occurred in 95 percent of patients and was directly related to the disease progression and antidopaminergic drugs. In 12 percent of 127 adult-onset HD patients, dystonia was the main finding, and it appeared mainly in those with younger age of onset (see Chap. 35).

OTHER HUNTINGTON-LIKE DISORDERS

Several diseases resemble HD but have no alteration in gene IT15. A dominantly inherited disease due to mutations of the gene encoding the ferritin light polypeptide produces choreoathetosis, dystonia, spasticity, and rigidity, with onset between ages of 40 and 55. Cavitation of basal ganglia is found on MRI.[98]

In so-called Huntington disease-like 3 (HDL-3), an autosomal-recessive early-onset disease develops in the first decade, with dystonia as a feature.[99,100]

Benign hereditary chorea is an autosomal-dominant disorder with chorea and dystonia in some cases not associated with intellectual deterioration.[101] It has been mapped to chromosome 14q.[102]

NEUROACANTHOCYTOSIS

Three neurological disorders associate with acanthocytosis: hypobetalipoproteinemia or Basen-Kornzweig disease, McLeod syndrome, and choreoacanthocytosis.

Hypobetalipoproteinemia is mainly a spinocerebellar syndrome associated with peripheral neuropathy and retinitis pigmentosa.

McLeod syndrome is usually considered a red blood cell disorder in which X chromosome mutations cause a dysfunction of an erythrocyte membrane protein Kx. It associates to a benign myopathy. However, the phenotype can be similar to choreoacanthocytosis, including dystonia. Caudate atrophy can be found in late disease, but early presymptomatic hypometabolism in caudate nucleus has been found.[103] The clinical manifestations of neuroacanthocytosis usually start in the 3rd decade as orobuccolinguofacial hyperkinesia, lip smacking, vocalizations, and even orolingual action dystonia, leading to lip and tongue automutilation. Thereafter, a generalized chorea develops, often a mixture of chorea and dystonia. In 30 percent of patients, there is no cognitive deterioration. About one-half of patients suffer epileptic seizures. Most of them present a motor polyneuropathy with distal amyotrophy and pes cavus. The clinical diagnosis is confirmed by the finding of acanthocytes, usually more than 20 percent of red blood cells, in fresh or saline-incubated blood smears. The neuropathology shows atrophy of the basal ganglia, maximal in caudate nucleus and preferentially affecting small neurons.[104] Neuronal loss also involves the anterior horn of the spinal cord in some cases. The muscle shows denervation, and peripheral nerve shows axonal degeneration with demyelination.

Kito et al.[105] described increased norepinephrine in the cerebrospinal fluid and low urinary excretion of dihydroxyphenylacetic acid. De Yebenes et al.[106,107] found moderately decreased striatal levels of dopamine, as well as a great elevation of norepinephrine levels, suggesting that dystonia may be related to disequilibrium of dopamine/norepinephrine neurotransmission in the basal ganglia. Choreoacanthocytosis is inherited in most cases as an autosomal-recessive complex movement disorder. Linkage has been found to chromosome 9q21.[108] The gene responsible for this disease has been recently identified, independently, by two groups;[109,110] the protein, called chorein, is considered to play a key role in protein sorting.

DENTATORUBROPALLIDOLUYSIAN ATROPHY

In this disease, there is degeneration of cerebellar efferent (dentatorubral) and pallidoluysian systems. It is an unusual disease, initially described in Europe by Titica and Van Bogaert in 1946,[111] but most of the actual cases are from Japan. The genetic defect has been located on chromosome 12p as an expansion of the trinucleotide CAG.[112] Iizuka[113] described three clinical types: an ataxochoreoathetoid, a pseudo-Huntington, and a third type combining myoclonic epilepsy with ataxia. Now that genetic diagnosis is possible, two main clinical groups have been described: adult-onset (at 20 years or older) with ataxia, choreoathetosis, and dementia; and juvenile-onset (before 20 years), with a progressive myoclonic epilepsy added to the previous symptoms.[114] As in HD, paternal transmission correlates with larger expansions of the repeat and earlier presentation.[115] Dystonia has been described, but not as an isolated or prominent manifestation.

DYSTONIA IN BASAL GANGLIA DISORDERS

WILSON'S DISEASE (WD)

This is an autosomal-recessive systemic disease related to abnormal metabolism of copper with mutations of an ATPase, located on chromosome 13q; ATPase plays a very important role in the metabolism of copper, transferring copper ions from apoceruloplasmin to ceruloplasmin. Tissue damage is a result of copper accumulation. In 217 patients reviewed by Walshe,[116] 43 percent started with hepatic disease and 42 percent with CNS involvement, including 2 patients with initial psychiatric symptoms. In the patients with neurological onset, tremor in the upper extremities, dysarthria, dystonia, and athetosis were, in that order, the most frequent presenting manifestations. Dystonia also appears during the evolution of the disease, producing bizarre posturing that may affect the four limbs and the trunk (Fig. 33-5). In a clinicoradiological correlation study of 16 symptomatic patients with WD, 11 of them, presenting with dystonia, had putaminal lesions in MRI.[117] When considering the differential diagnosis of a patient with dystonia, it is of prime importance

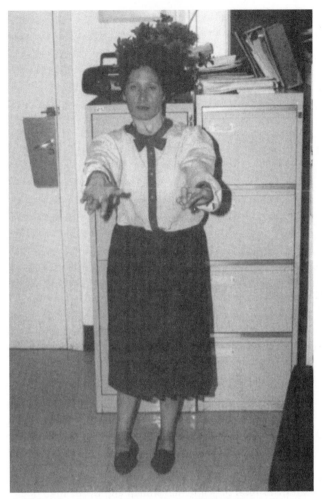

FIGURE 33-5 Generalized dystonia in Wilson's disease.

to consider and screen for WD, because it is a treatable condition in which the reversibility of the clinical symptoms may depend on when definitive therapy is initiated (see also Chap. 47).

HALLERVORDEN-SPATZ DISEASE (HSD)

Seitelberger classified the primary neuroaxonal dystrophies, including HSD, infantile neuroaxonal dystrophy (INAD), late infantile and juvenile neuroaxonal dystrophy, and neuroaxonal leukodystrophy. The pathological marker in this group of related disorders is neuroaxonal dystrophy or axonal spheroid.

In INAD, the clinical symptoms develop at the end of the first year or during the second year of life, and are characterized by psychomotor retardation, spasticity and rigidity, loss of vision and hearing, autonomic signs, and death between 3 and 6 years of age. Dystonia may occur with the progression of the disease, especially in cases with long evolution.[118] Pathological involvement is widespread but is most prominent in the posterior spinal horns and the dorsal

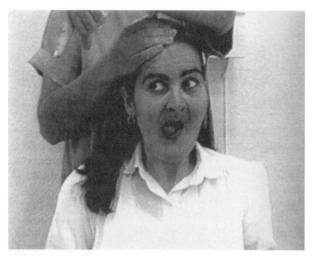

FIGURE 33-6 Orolinguomandibular dystonia in a patient with Hallervorden-Spatz disease and generalized dystonia.

bulbomedullary nuclei, the pallidum, substantia nigra and other brainstem nuclei, and cerebellar cortex. There is an excess of ferric pigment. Gliosis and long tract degeneration take place.

HSD is an autosomal-recessive disorder related to a mutation in the pantothenate kinase gene.[119] Neuropathology is characterized by iron deposition in the pallidum and substantia nigra, pars reticularis, and widespread axonal spheroid formation neuroaxonal dystrophy. Of 64 pathologically confirmed cases, 8 presented with dystonia, and 41 more suffered dystonia during evolution of the disease.[120] Generalized dystonia was the most frequent presentation, but it could appear as focal or segmental cranial and upper limb dystonia (Fig. 33-6). Dystonia may be associated with tics and other movement disorders in HSD.[121] An isolated case of treatment of dystonia in HSD with stereotactic pallidotomy has been described.[122]

CALCIFICATION OF THE BASAL GANGLIA (CBG)

CBG occurs in up to 30 sporadic and hereditary diseases, and is often associated with different movement disorders, including parkinsonism, chorea, and dystonia. Abnormal parathyroid function is frequently associated with CBG, but there are cases without any evidence of biochemical or humoral abnormalities of calcium and phosphorus metbolism. These idiopathic cases are often called Fahr's disease; this can be hereditary or sporadic and diagnosis is by exclusion. A long series of familial and sporadic cases found movement disorders the most frequent neurological manifestation of CBG: parkinsonism accounted for 57 percent, chorea 19 percent, tremor 8 percent, dystonia 8 percent, athetosis 5 percent, and orofacial dyskinesia 3 percent. This study found a relationship between volume of calcification and clinical status.[123] There are reports of familial dystonia as the main manifestation of this disease. The patients reported by

Caraceni et al.[124] were two brothers with cranial dystonia or limb dystonia. Larsen et al.[125] reported a family with idiopathic CBG and autosomal-dominant segmental dystonia.

Two sporadic cases with isolated calcification of the globus pallidus have been described.[126] Both patients had cognitive dysfunction, amnesia state, perceptual distortions, complex visual hallucinations, and myoclonus. Patient 1 manifested depression, auditory hallucinations, anxiety, paranoia, and postural tremor; patient 2 manifested multifocal dystonia with dystonic tremor. These cases suggest specific involvement of the pallidal pathways in hallucinations, myoclonus, and dystonia.

In a family with CBG, a linkage to chromosome 14q and genetic anticipation have beeen found. Interestingly the proband started with writing tremor and hand dystonia.[127]

No specific therapy (aside from symptomatic) exists for Fahr's disease, but there is an incidental case that benefited from etidronate.[128]

PROGRESSIVE PALLIDAL DEGENERATIONS

These rare diseases have been subdivided into four groups according to the pathological findings:[129] (1) "pure" pallidal atrophy, (2) "pure" pallidoluysian atrophy, (3) "extended" forms with nigral, striatal, or dentate nucleus involvement, including pallidoluysionigral atrophy, (4) combinations of (1) and (2), with thalamic, pyramidal, or spinal motor lesion.

Given the small number of cases, precise clinicopathological correlation has not been possible, but prominent generalized or focal dystonia, together with akinetic-rigid syndromes, is the most common clinical manifestation. Dystonia was described in patients with pure pallidal and pallidoluysian atrophies by Van Bogaert.[130] A patient reported by Wooten et al.[131] had progressive generalized dystonia, dysarthria, and supranuclear gaze palsy. Pathological examination disclosed a pure pallidoluysian atrophy; hence, the authors attributed the symptoms to damage of the indirect pathway and increased inhibition of internal pallidum.

INTRANUCLEAR NEURONAL INCLUSION DISEASE

This is a rare disorder characterized by developmental delay and movement disorders, including dystonia and parkinsonism, with onset from 3 to 30 years of age, most frequently in childhood,[132] but also in adults.[133] The pathological marker is a round autofluorescent eosinophilic inclusion body found in neurons of different regions, more abundant in the basal ganglia but also involving other structures such as the motor neurons, autonomic system, and myenteric plexus. Antemortem diagnosis is possible by means of rectal biopsy.[134]

RETT SYNDROME

This disease characteristically combines psychomotor regression, loss of purposeful use of the hands and stereotypia, ataxia and apraxia of gait, and acquired microcephaly. Mutations in the X chromosome gene encoding methyl-CpG-binding protein 2 are the cause of Rett syndrome.[135]

Phenotypical variability in females is explained by skewed X chromosome inactivation and by the type of mutations. It was previously considered that only females were affected, but there are a few affected males whose phenotype is more severe as in neonatal encephalopathy.[136]

Abnormal levels of 5-hydroxyindoleacetic acid and catecholamine metabolites are found in the cerebrospinal fluid. Dystonia is included among the diagnostic criteria.[137] Fitzgerald et al.[138] found that the presence of movement disorders in 32 patients with Rett syndrome was common, and increased with age. The disease usually evolves with age from hyperkinetic to hypokinetic patterns. Dystonia, most frequently crural, was present in 59 percent of patients. Bruxism was the most common movement disorder after gait abnormality and stereotyped movements of the hands. Oculogyric crises occurred in 63 percent of cases (see Chap. 26).

DYSTONIA IN HEREDITARY ATAXIAS

Dystonia can be found in some hereditary ataxias and can aid specific diagnosis.[139] In autosomal-dominant ataxias, dystonia is very suggestive of spinocerebellar atrophy type 3 (SCA-3) and DRPLA, but it could occur in other SCA subtypes. Two young patients of the only SCA-12 family reported suffered lower extremity dystonia.[140] In recessive ataxia, dystonia is common in ataxia telangiectasia but not found in the more frequent Friedreich ataxia, although there is some report of head dystonic tremor.[141] Dystonia is also common in non-Friedreich recessive ataxia with ocular apraxia.[142]

MACHADO-JOSEPH DISEASE

This is an autosomal-dominant spinocerebellar degeneration, mainly affecting families descending from ancestors in the Portuguese islands of the Azores. The clinical manifestations have been classified into different phenotypes. Coutinho and Andrade[143] suggested three clinical subtypes according to the clinical symptoms present, in addition to a common ataxic disorder: type I with earliest onset and predominant pyramidal-extrapyramidal signs; type II, the most common, with middle-aged onset and cerebellar plus pyramidal manifestations; and type III of later onset, with cerebellar features and distal amyotrophy. Barbeau et al.[144] reviewed 138 patients with this disease and concluded, based on the continuity of the clinical symptoms in the three subtypes, that this disease was a single clinical entity. The pathological examination usually discloses spinal degeneration affecting anterior horn cells and Clarke's column, and neuronal loss in the dentate nucleus and substantia nigra pars compacta (hence, the name nigrospinodentatal degeneration).[145] A GAG expansion has been found on chromosome 14q in Japanese cases.[146,147] Dystonia was present in 20 percent of the 82 patients reported by Freire Gonzalves et al.,[148] and involved the hands, feet, face, or neck most commonly, but it was rarely generalized and severe. Dystonia appeared mostly in the younger group. The patient of Lang et al.[149] with a double genetic load, also had an early onset with generalized dystonia.

The presence of dystonia in Machado-Joseph disease is much more common than in other familial spinocerebellar degenerations.[150] This is attributed to the much more frequent involvement of subthalamopallidal pathways in Machado-Joseph disease, in comparison to other degenerative ataxias.

ATAXIA TELANGIECTASIA

This is an autosomal-recessive hereditary disorder associated with abnormalities of DNA repair. It is clinically characterized by progressive ataxia in childhood, ocular and auricular telangiectasia, increased frequency of respiratory infections resulting from absent or low IgA levels, and increased frequency of malignancies. In most of these patients, dystonia is severe, although often not recognized because of the severity of the cerebellar symptoms.[151] After a few years of normal development, affected children develop progressive ataxia of gait, which progressively involves the trunk and upper extremities. Independent gait is progressively more difficult and requires special walkers. Dystonia appears early in the course of the disease,[152–155] but usually after the ataxia; most frequently, it is generalized and further disturbs ambulation (Fig. 33-7). Ocular apraxia, slow saccades, and polyneuropathy may complicate the clinical picture. Severe intellectual deterioration is not typical of this disorder. Telangiectatic lesions appear at about 3–5 years of age, and may disappear after several years of progression of the disease. Therefore, there may be patients with ataxia telangiectasia with severe dystonia and no prominent telangiectasia in late stages of the disease. Death occurs as a complication of bronchopulmonary infection or neoplasm, usually a lymphoma.

The pathology of ataxia telangiectasia involves mainly the cerebellar cortex, in which there is a loss of neurons, and the pigmented brainstem nuclei, including the substantia nigra and locus ceruleus, which occasionally show Lewy bodies.[156] There is demyelinating neuropathy and loss of fibers in the posterior columns and spinocerebellar tracts.

DYSTONIA IN OTHER NEURODEGENERATIONS

XERODERMA PIGMENTOSUM

The main manifestations of this entity are dermatological, with photosensitivity and skin malignancies, but in some patients neurological manifestations appear with combinations of mental retardation, seizures, spasticity, deafness, ataxia, chorea, dystonia, and axonal sensory neuropathy.[157] There is a defect in DNA repair, as in ataxia telangiectasia. The inheritance is autosomal-recessive. The gene locus has been mapped to 9q in the xeroderma pigmentosum gene.

WOLFRAM'S SYNDROME

Although mainly described as an association of diabetes mellitus, diabetes insipidus, optic atrophy, and deafness, with

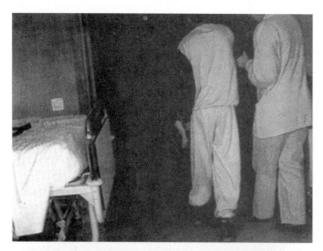

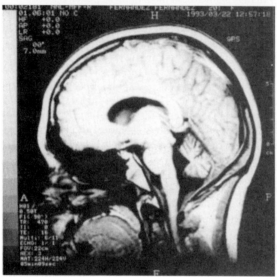

FIGURE 33-7 *Top:* **Generalized dystonia in ataxia telangiectasia.** *Bottom:* **MRI scan showing cerebellar atrophy in ataxia telangiectasia.**

autosomal-recessive transmission, Wolfram's sydrome can also be associated with several neurological manifestations. These occur usually late in the course, and consist of ataxia, dizziness, mental and conduct alterations, seizures, tremor and dystonia, areflexia, tonic pupils, and neurogenic bladder.[158] A specific gene in chromosome 4p16.1 has been found with different mutations.[159]

Dystonia in Metabolic Disorders

DISORDERS OF LIPID METABOLISM

GM1 GANGLIOSIDOSIS

Dystonia can appear in disorders of lipid metabolism in children and adults. GM1 gangliosidosis is an autosomal-recessive disorder related to a deficiency in beta-galactosidase, leading

to intraneuronal storage of GM1 and visceral deposit of compounds with a beta-galactose terminal. GM1 gangliosidosis is clinically characterized by visceromegaly, intellectual impairment, dysmorphism, and a cherry-red spot in the macular region in children. The infantile form, or GM1 type 1, begins at birth or in the first months of life. Affected infants display coarse facial features, and skeletal deformities similar to those seen in Hurler's disease. They develop blindness, quadriplegia, and seizures, and they usually die before 2 years of age. Type 2 GM1 begins between 6 and 18 months of age. The course is slower, with gait disturbance, mental deterioration, seizures, optic atrophy with a macular cherry-red spot, and late acoustic startle. No marked skeletal deformities are present. Type 3 GM1 gangliosidosis presents between 2 and 27 years of age, with variable manifestations, including a spinocerebellar deficit, dystonia, and myopathy.[160–162]

In adults, GM1 gangliosidosis is characterized by dystonia and early-onset parkinsonism, lack of mental deterioration, and prolonged survival.[163] Atrophy of the head of the caudate nucleus was found in CT scans of two patients,[161,162] and bilateral putaminal lesions on MRI were seen in other patients.[162] Pathological examination of 1 patient revealed depletion of neurons and intracytoplasmic accumulation of storage material in the basal ganglia, amygdala, and cerebellum.[161] Adult GM1 gangliosidosis occurs with partial deficiencies of beta-galactosidase activity (total lack of activity is associated with the infantile phenotype; partial, 5–15 percent, enzyme activity is associated with adult forms; activity above 15 percent does not produce neurological symptoms).

GM2 GANGLIOSIDOSIS

This disease is due to intraneuronal accumulation of GM2 to 100–300 times the normal levels. The cause of the disease is a deficiency in lysosomal hexosaminidase inherited as an autosomal-recessive trait. It is more frequent among Ashkenazis from East Europe.

The symptoms start in infancy. The first symptoms are jerks in response to loud and sudden noises. Quick deterioration of developmental acquisitions takes place and few infants reach sitting position. Blindness, spasticity, and convulsions appear, and about 90 percent of these children have a cherry-red spot uni- or bilaterally. Some children develop macrocephaly related to neuronal storage. Survival after the second year of life is rare.

Diagnosis is made by measuring blood and leukocyte hexosaminidase activity. This test shows the heterogeneity of the disease. There are three isoenzymes (A, B, and S), differing in their quaternary structure: hexosaminidiase A is a trimer (a1 b2), hexosaminidase B a tetramer (b2 b2), and hexosaminidase S a dimer (a2). There are different mutations of the locus. In classic Tay-Sachs, or B variant, A and S isoenzymes are not functional, and normal hexosaminidase B is unable to hydrolyze gangliosides. In Sandhoff's disease (O variant), a mutation of the gene coding for B chain on chromosome 5 (5q13) reduces both A and B isoenzymes. In the AB variant, hexosaminidase A and B levels are normal but the disease is related to a deficit in an activator protein. Individuals with the same enzymatic variants present with similar phenotypes.[163] The parents are heterozygous and it is possible to do a prenatal diagnosis through chorionic biopsy. There is another variant, B1, which is a rare form characterized by the presence of a mutation in the hexosaminidase A gene, leading to a defect in the catalytic region of the alpha-subunit of hexosaminidase A (heterodimer). The mutated hexosaminidase A has almost normal activity against the natural synthetic substrates but is unable to hydrolyse GM2 ganglioside and sulfated synthetic substrates. There is a report that describes two cases of this variant; both cases presented regression of mental skills, leading to dementia, epilepsy, quadriplegia, and dystonic involuntary movements.[164] There is no effective treatment available, although transplantation of bone marrow and genetic engineering have been attempted.

Most children with classic infantile GM2 gangliosidosis develop an aggressive disease, with spastic tetraparesis, seizures and, blindness. Dystonia may appear late in the course of the disease. In juvenile GM2 and in chronic GM2, or adult form, dystonia may appear as the presenting clinical feature,[165–168] and, if so, dystonia involves primary the legs (Fig. 33-8). Some of the juvenile and chronic forms present clinical pictures resembling spinocerebellar degeneration and motor neuron disease.[169]

NIEMANN-PICK DISEASE AND RELATED DISORDERS
This is a heterogeneous group of conditions linked by an accumulation of sphingomyelin in the reticuloendothelial system. Spence and Callahan[170] divided it into group I, including former types A and B, with sphingomyelinase deficiency, and group II, including types C, D and E without precise enzymatic deficit.

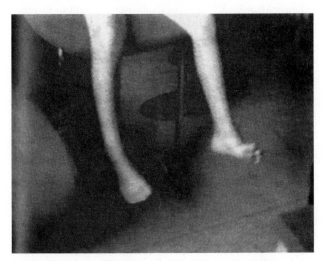

FIGURE 33-8 Foot dystonia in an 8-year-old patient with generalized dystonia resulting from GM2 gangliosidosis.

The main neurological manifestations in Niemann-Pick type A are myoclonic seizures, spasticity, and blindness. Type B disease is also termed visceral or not neuronopathic because only occasionally do neurological signs develop. No primary metabolic defect has been identified for types C and D. Sphingomyelinase activity is normal in most tissues and only in three-quarters of patients is it decreased in cultured fibroblasts. However, there is a constant defective cholesterol esterification[171] and excessive lysosomal filipin staining in cultured skin fibroblasts.[172,173] The initial manifestation is transient neonatal cholestatic icterus which relapses in 20 percent of patients, returns in the first months of life, and leads to death. Surviving patients develop neurological symptoms. Severe cases with onset before 3 years suffer a devastating neurological deterioration and may not develop ophthalmoplegia. Patients with later onset present with a very characteristic supranuclear or vertical gaze palsy, mental deterioration, gait disorder, cerebellar ataxia, and dystonia. So-called juvenile dystonic lipidosis may be included in type C Niemann-Pick.[174]

METACHROMATIC LEUKODYSTROPHY
Deficiency of cerebroside sulfatase leads to sulfatide accumulation. Different mutations underlie the late infantile and adult forms; the juvenile form seems to be related to compound heterozygosity.[175] Rare cases due to mutation in an activator protein[176] have also been reported. Juvenile forms present between 4 and 10 years of age, with schizophrenia-like psychosis, deterioration of the cognitive functions, personality changes, depression, and dementia.[177] Nerve conduction velocity may be normal and a dystonic phenotype has been described.[178]

CEROID LIPOFUSCINOSIS
This group of diseases is marked by the storage of lipopigments in nervous and other tissues.[178] So far, eight subtypes have been described with different clinical features, age at onset, and gene defects, identified so far in five of these subtypes. Accumulation takes place in lysosomal-like structures, and the finding of a high concentration of dolichols is supportive of the lysosomal nature of these cytosomes. The infantile form (Santavuori-Haltia disease), rare outside Finland, has been mapped to chromosome 1p32, and the gene defect is related to palmitoyl thiol esterase. Other clinical forms include a late infantile form, a juvenile form (Vogt-Spielmeyer or Batten disease), and an adult form (Kufs' disease), without visual failure and presenting with myoclonic epilepsy, dementia and behavioral disturbances, and extrapyramidal signs, mainly facial dyskinesias.[179]

PELIZAEUS-MERZBACHER DISEASE
This disorder has been related to a severe deficiency in myelin-specific lipids caused by a lack of two types of lipoproteins: proteolipid protein, and DM20 transcripts from the

proteolipid protein gene. The mutations of these genes are very varied: deletions, loss of function, and missense mutations to additional copies of the gene.[180] Two clinical forms of the disorder have been described: type I is X-linked and starts in infancy; type II is X-linked or autosomal-recessive. The pathology shows a partial to total absence of myelination. In type I, myelin is preserved in internal capsule and subcortical U fibers. Clinical manifestations include ataxia, nystagmus and hypotonia, and later dystonia progressing slowly. In type II, there is a severe psychomotor retardation.[181]

DISORDERS OF ENERGY PRODUCTION

MITOCHONDRIAL ENCEPHALOMYOPATHIES

Movement disorders, including dystonia, are present in patients with mitochondrial encephalopathies.[182,183] Truong et al.[184] reviewed 85 patients with mitochondrial myopathies and found that 9 had movement disorders, most frequently myoclonus,[183] but there was generalized dystonia preceded by mild parkinsonism in 1 case, and associated with strokes in another patient.

Generalized dystonia was reported in a patient with suspected mitochondrial myopathy and putaminal hypodensities,[185] in some individuals of a family with patients affected by Leber's hereditary optic neuropathy, and others with childhood-onset dystonia.[186] There is a report of 1 patient with writer's cramp who progressed over 5 years to dystonia in facial muscles and lower limbs with a 3243 mitochondrial DNA mutation.[187]

SUBACUTE NECROTIZING ENCEPHALOMYELOPATHY, OR LEIGH'S SYNDROME

Leigh's disease is characterized by intermittent or progressive neurological deterioration after normal development during the first year of life. Children lose their motor acquisitions and develop hypotonia, ataxia, corticospinal tract signs, optic atrophy, dystonia, dysphagia, and dysarthria with relative intellectual preservation. Dystonia is the most common movement disorder in Leigh's disease.[188,189] It may be the principal clinical manifestation in infants,[190] and it is occasionally associated with other movement disorders, including rigidity, tremor, chorea, hypokinesia, myoclonus, and tics. Some patients resemble the primary torsion dystonia phenotype. Neuroradiologic studies show basal ganglia lesions[189] in putamen, caudate, substantia nigra, and globus pallidus, in the majority of the patients. MRI is very helpful since it shows in nearly all cases the symmetric lesions of basal ganglia and brainstem. This pattern of striatal lucencies is consistent with the pathologic findings. The pathology of Leigh's disease is characterized by extensive damage of the brainstem and basal ganglia. There is spongiosis of the neuropil and capillary proliferation, but extensive leukoencephalopathy or gray cortical damage are uncommon. Leigh's disease is an autosomal-recessive disorder related to abnormalities of the pyruvate kinase complex. The activity of this enzyme in fibroblasts is low, and the blood levels of pyruvate and alanine are usually high. The most common enzymatic defect found in these patients is a reduction of the activity of cytochrome *c* oxidase. The juvenile forms present dystonia and movement disorders as protagonistic clinical elements.[191]

Two other disorders related to energy production, Leber's disease and bilateral striatal necrosis, occasionally overlap with Leigh's disease. Therefore it has been suggested that a variety of energy production disorders, including subacute necrotizing encephalomyelopathy, bilateral striatal necrosis, and Leber's disease, may be grouped under the title of Leigh's syndrome.[192,193] Leber's hereditary optic neuropathy is an X-linked inherited disorder related to different mutations of the mitochondrial genome. Striatal lucencies are present in dystonic patients with Leigh's disease, Leber's hereditary optic neuropathy, and other conditions. In some cases, no biochemical abnormality is found, although some of these may be variants of Leigh's disease. Mutations at point 14459 of the NADH dehydrogenase subunit 6 gene are associated with maternally inherited Leber's hereditary optic neuropathy and dystonia,[194] but there is a report that describes 3 complex I-deficient patients from two separate pedigrees who presented with Leigh's disease, with no evidence of family history of Leber's hereditary optic neuropathy or dystonia.[195]

There is a wide variety of clinical presentations, ranging from adult-onset blindness to pediatric dystonia and basal ganglial degeneration in patients with this mutation. Severe nucleotide substitutions are generally new mutations that cause pediatric diseases such as Leigh's syndrome and dystonia. Mitochondrial DNA rearrangements also cause a variety of phenotypes.[196,197]

MOHR-TRANEBJAERG SYNDROME

This is an X-linked recessive disorder with childhood-onset deafness and adult-onset progressive dystonia, spasticity, and optic atrophy.[198] It has been related to mutations in a protein (DDP) related to protein import to mitochondria.[199,200]

DISORDERS OF ORGANIC AND AMINO ACID METABOLISM

GLUTARIC ACIDURIA TYPE I

Glutaric aciduria type I is a rare autosomal-recessive disease due to a deficiency in glutaryl-CoA dehydrogenase. Homozygous patients have an abnormal degradation of tryptophan, lysine, and hydroxylysine; some of these homozygotes may be clinically asymptomatic. Patients develop their symptoms in infancy. Many of these individuals present generalized dystonia, which occasionally may appear after recovery from an acute episode of diffuse encephalopathy. Other patients follow a progressive course leading to similar manifestations. Generalized dystonia is the main manifestation, being present in 77 percent of 57 cases.[201] Imaging studies show a characteristic frontotemporal atrophy with enlargement of the Sylvian fissures.[202] MRI shows involvement of the putamina. PET shows lesions in the head of the caudate nuclei and decreased uptake in the cerebral cortex and thalamus.[203] The pathology reveals a severe loss of cells in the basal ganglia, especially in the putamen.[204] Diagnosis is made by measurement of glutaric acid in urine or cerebrospinal fluid. Dietetic treatment with restriction of tryptophan and lysine reduces the levels of glutaric acid; if recognized in the presymptomatic stage, early institution of treatment may prevent the onset of neurological symptoms.[205,206]

METHYLMALONIC ACIDURIA

This is an autosomal-recessive aciduria due to abnormal catabolism of methylmalonic acid. Acute neurological symptoms develop during the first years of life, including generalized dystonia, dysphagia, dysarthria, and different degrees of tetraparesis. These symptoms are considered to be a metabolic stroke involving the globus pallidus and the internal capsule.[207–211] Recent reports on the neurological deficits present in children with different mutations of the enzyme methylmalonyl-CoA mutase suggest that there is a phenotypic pleomorphism without a consistent pattern of neurological injury, and that acidosis and metabolic imbalance are not necessary preconditions for significant neurological morbidity in methylmalonic aciduria. Analysis of urinary organic acids reveals a massive amount of methylmalonic acid. Some patients obtain relief from dystonic symptoms with L-dopa.[210]

FUMARASE DEFICIENCY

This is an inborn error of the tricarboxylic acid cycle characterized by progressive encephalopathy, dysmorphic facial features,[212] dystonia, leukopenia, and neutropenia. MRI shows multiple abnormalities, including diffuse polymicrogyria, decreased cerebral white matter, large ventricles, and open opercula. Elevation of lactate in the cerebrospinal fluid and high fumarate excretion in the urine provide clues for the investigation of the cytosolic and mitochondrial fumarase isoenzymes. In 2 recently reported cases,[213] the analysis of fumarase cDNA demonstrated that both patients were homozygous for a missense mutation, a G955-C transversion, predicting a Glu319-Gln substitution. This substitution occurred in a highly conserved region of the fumarase cDNA. Both parents exhibited half the expected fumarase activity in their lymphocytes and were found to be heterozygous for this substitution.

HOMOCYSTINURIA

Homozygous patients for cystathionine beta-synthase deficiency present ectopia lentis, ocular and skeletal deformities, mental retardation, and vascular occlusions sometimes affecting the brain vessels. Occasionally dystonia has been described in homocystinuria,[214–218] sometimes in adulthood,[219]

and could be due to vascular damage to the basal ganglia. It is also possible that dystonia develops as a metabolic complication[216] through enhanced excitotoxic neurotransmission via stimulation of the glutamate receptors by homocysteinic acid or by alteration of the levels of taurine in the basal ganglia.

HARTNUP DISEASE

This disease is characterized by a recurrent personality disorder and cerebellar ataxia, together with a failure to thrive and an intermittent cutaneous rash resembling pellagra. Onset occurs in late infancy and early childhood. Darras et al.[220] described a patient with intermittent focal dystonia. Tamoush et al. reported 2 patients with dystonic features.[221] The biochemical deficit is characterized by a defect in the transport of large neutral amino acids.

ABNORMALITIES OF PURINE METABOLISM

LESCH-NYHAN SYNDROME

This is an X-linked disorder of purine metabolism related to reduced activity of the enzyme hypoxanthine-guanine phosphoribosyl transferase (HGPRT). The clinical features are characterized by normal development up to the age of 6–12 months, followed by developmental delay, mental retardation, spasticity, a variety of movement disorders, most prominently dystonia, and automutilation. The patients have high blood levels of uric acid and enhanced urinary elimination of uric acid, which often produces "sandy urine" and urinary stones. Frequent complications of hyperuricemia include gout and tophus. The diagnosis is performed by measurement of HGPRT activity in fibroblasts or red blood cells.

HGPRT deficiency may be complete (Lesch-Nyhan syndrome) or partial (Kelley-Seegmiller syndrome). In a recent series[222] of 8 patients with complete HGPRT deficiency and 4 with incomplete enzymatic defect, it was found that the 8 patients with Lesch-Nyhan syndrome presented choreoathetosis, corticospinal motor system dysfunction, mental retardation, and signs of self-mutilation. The patients with Kelley-Seegmiller syndrome were heterogeneous: 2 patients had psychomotor retardation with spasticity, 1 was mentally retarded with generalized dystonia, and 1 patient had only gout with no neurologic manifestations. There is a report that describes a Lesch-Nyhan variant that presented with dystonia, ataxia, near-normal intelligence, and no self-mutilation.[223] A mutation was identified in exon 3 of the gene coding for HGPRT (substitution of guanine with thymine), conditioning the substitution of the normal glycine by valine (HGPRT Madrid).[224] Affected patients have abnormally few dopaminergic nerve terminals and cell bodies; this includes all dopaminergic pathways and is not restricted to the basal ganglia. These dopaminergic deficits contribute to the characteristic neuropsychiatric manifestations of the disease.[225]

Dystonia Due to Physical and Chemical Agents

Head trauma, which can produce dystonia secondary to focal lesions of the nervous system, and peripheral trauma, which can trigger the development of focal dystonias in individuals at risk, are physical injuries that can produce dystonia. In addition, other physical agents have been reported to induce dystonia. Electrical injuries may produce dystonia, often located in limbs but also in other locations.[226–229] Dystonia induced by physical agents has also been described as an occupational disease in users of lasers and in survivors of the Chernobyl radiation leakage.[230,231] The pathogenesis of dystonia in these cases has been attributed to radiation-induced lesions of small blood vessels in the brain; the clinical description of these cases is far from clear. Most of these reports are in the Russian literature and the word "dystonia" is used with different meanings, including disturbances compatible with dystonia, others with autonomic symptoms, as well as psychogenic disorders.

Dystonia induced by chemicals is common.[232–235] Therapeutic agents, with a variety of pharmacological actions, produce dystonia as an acute side-effect of the pharmacological treatment, or as a persistent, and often permanent, complication. Many of these compounds modify the metabolism of the brain monoamines dopamine, norepinephrine, serotonin, and acetylcholine. Most frequently, dopamine-stimulating agents, such as L-dopa and dopamine agonists, induce acute dystonia, particularly in patients with akinetic-rigid syndromes, but there are reports of persistent, and occasionally paroxysmal, dystonia after intake of cocaine, amphetamine, and related compounds.[236,237] Dopamine receptor blockers produce acute and persistent dystonia. Acute dystonic reactions occur frequently with typical neuroleptics, less frequently with atypical neuroleptics, and with frequently used benzamide derivatives, and antihistaminics. These acute dystonic reactions, which are occasionally life-threatening and always alarming, respond very well to treatment with anticholinergics, which sometimes should be administered intravenously. Persistent dystonia was described in the French literature of the 1950s as a late (hence the name "tardive") complication of the treatment of schizophrenic patients with chlorpromazine, and is a frequent complication of long-term neuroleptic treatment (Fig. 33-9). However, the adjective "tardive" meaning "late" is misleading since the condition occasionally occurs very early. The mechanism usually proposed is dopamine receptor blockage, especially D2 receptors, but other neurotransmitters and neuropeptides have also been implicated.[235,238–240] Persistent dystonia is very difficult to treat.[241–245] Not infrequently, it is produced by drugs of doubtful indication. Therefore, prevention, early recognition of symptoms, and discontinuation of the offending medication, whenever possible, are the first steps in the treatment of drug-induced dystonia. Other drugs implicated in producing dystonia are some

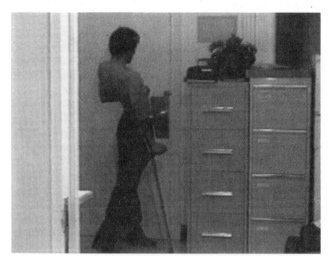

FIGURE 33-9 Generalized persistent dystonia induced by neuroleptics.

antiepileptic drugs, anxiolytics, and others (usually sporadic or isolated reports). A list of drugs that produce dystonia is given in Table 33-5.

Dystonia is produced by toxic environmental agents. Manganese produces dystonia and parkinsonism, related to degeneration of the striatum and pallidum, in miners as well as in patients with chronic liver disease.[246,247] Dystonia has also been attributed to high copper levels in 1 patient with cholestatic liver disease.[248] Organic mercury poisoning produces choreoathetosis, parkinsonism, and occasionally dystonic reactions.[249] Organic compounds, including methanol,[250] cyanide,[251–253] and carbon monoxide,[254,255] also produce dystonia. The mechanism usually implicated is cellular hypoxia from mitochondrial damage, or generation of free radicals.

Dystonia may be caused by plant derivatives. The best known of these diseases is epidemic ergotism, which associates to focal and generalized dystonia, epilepsy, stroke, and peripheral ischemia of the limbs (Fig. 33-10).[256,257] Mycotoxin poisoning (3-nitropropionic acid) from mildew-infected sugar cane produces encephalopathy and dystonia[258,259] in the developing world.

Psychogenic Dystonias

Although about 40 percent of patients with dystonia are misdiagnosed with psychogenic disorders at a certain stage, less than 3 percent of our patients have dystonia of psychogenic etiology. This distinction is especially difficult in psychotic patients.[260] These patients do not belong to a single group, but can be subdivided into different subtypes which occasionally overlap.

Munchausen's syndrome simulating dystonia[261] is characterized by a chronic factitious disorder consistent with clinical symptoms that are under the patient's voluntary control and depend on the medical knowledge of the subject.

TABLE 33-5 Drugs and Chemicals Implicated in Drug-Induced Dystonia

	Acute Dystonia	Persistent Dystonia
I. THERAPEUTIC AGENTS		
A. Dopamine receptor blockers		
Classic neuroleptics[235,238–240]	•••	••
Atypical neuroleptics[265–290]	•	•
Substituted benzamides[291–303]	•••	•
Catecholamine depletors[304,305]	•	
B. Antihistaminics (with dopamine receptor blocking properties)		
Thiethylperazine[306]	•	
Prochlorperazine[307]	•	
Diphenhydramine[303–309]	•	
C. Catecholamine stimulating agents		
L-Dopa[310–316]	•	•
Dopamine agonists[317–319]	•	
Cocaine[320–323]	•	
Catecholamine releasers[324–327]	•	•
Tricyclic antidepressants[328–330]	•	•
Monoamine oxidase inhibitors[331]	•	
Ergotamine[332,333]	•	•
D. 5-HT stimulating agents		
Selective serotonin reuptake inhibitors[334–344]	•	•
m-chlorophenyl-piperazine[345]	•	
E. Acetylcholine stimulators		
Acetylcholinesterase inhibitors[346,347]	•	
F. Anxiolytics		
Buspirone[348,349]	•	
Fluspirene[350,353]	•	
Bromazepam[354]	•	
Midazolam[355]	•	
Diazepam[356]	•	
G. Antiepileptic drugs		
Carbamazepine[357,358]	•	•
Phenytoin[359,360]	•	•
Phenobarbital[361]	•	
Gabapentine[362,363]	•	
Tiagabine[364]	•	
H. Other		
Anesthetics[365–368]	•	
Disulfiram[369–371]	•	•
Erythromycin[372]	•	
Chloroquine[373]	•	
Flecainide[374]	•	•
Ranitidine[375–376]	•	
Cimetidine[377]	•	
Sumatriptan[378,379]	•	
Meperidine[380]	•	
Flunarizine and cinnarizine[381]		•
Bromvalerylurea[382]		•
5-Fluorouracil and doxorubicin[383]		•
Lithium[384]		•
Betahistine[385]	•	

TABLE 33-5—*(continued)*

	Acute Dystonia	Persistent Dystonia
II. NEUROTOXIC CHEMICALS		
A. Minerals		
Manganese[246,247]	•	
Copper[248]	•	
Mercury[249]	•	
B. Organic compounds		
Methyl alcohol[250]	•	
Cyanide[251,253]	•	
Carbon monoxide[254,255]	•	
Carbon disulfide[386]	•	
C. Plant derivatives and pesticides		
Ergotmycotoxin[256,257]	•	
Poisoning from mildew-infected sugar cane[258,259]	•	
Fenthion	•	

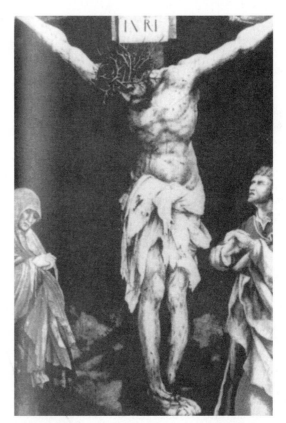

FIGURE 33-10 Foot dystonia in a patient with epidemic ergotism. The painting was done by M. Grunewald (c 1455–1528), about 1523. The model was probably a patient with epidemic ergotism contacted by Grunewald during his work for the Antonin friars at the Monastery of Issenheim. *(Tauberbischofstein Museum, Karlsruhe, Germany.)*

TABLE 33-6 Clinical Characteristics of Genuine Dystonia, Psychogenic Dystonia, and Pseudodystonia

	Dystonia	Psychogenic Dystonia	Pseudodystonia
Socioeconomic benefit	+/−	+++	+/−
Atypical symptoms (weakness, sensory complaints)	+/−	+++	+/−
Triggered/worsened by action	+++	−	−
Triggered/worsened by stress	++	+++	+/−
Fixed dystonia	+	+++	+++
Improved by sensory tricks or geste antagonistic	+++	−	−
Improved by relaxation	++	+++	−
Abnormal imaging findings	+/−	−	++

−, negative; +/−, questionable; +, positive; ++, very positive; +++, very characteristic.

This behavior is intended to ensure that the affected individual is permanently dependent on medical care, and may cause unjustified, aggressive, and occasionally risky, medical treatments. Malingering is characterized by consciously simulated illness in order to obtain social or economic compensation. Hysteria or conversion disorders are characterized by no conscious production of symptoms.

In general, psychogenic dystonia can be differentiated from genuine dystonia by several clinical characteristics, including the presence of associated atypical weakness or sensory complaints, fixed postures, and lack of modification of the movement disorder by action or sensory tricks. The pattern of movement changes inconsistently in different situations and in the presence or absence of medical and nursing staff or, at times, when the patient believes they are not being observed. There is worsening by stress, improvement by relaxation and psychotherapy, and disappearance by revelation of the nature of the disorder.[262–264] Such disorders can persist for a long time (Table 33-6).

Pseudodystonias of Organic Origin

These disorders are characterized by abnormal postures or movements related to musculoskeletal deformities, or are performed to compensate for pain or abnormal function of different elements of the central or peripheral nervous system. These disorders may be confounded with focal or segmental dystonias since they are restricted to a part of the body. The correct diagnosis can be made by taking into consideration the fixed nature of the abnormality, the lack of improvement with sensory tricks, and the absence of aggravation by action. A list of organic disorders simulating dystonias is given in Table 33-7.

TABLE 33-7 Pseudodystonia of Organic Origin

A. Disorders simulating blepharospasm
    Eyelid apraxia
    Palpebral ptosis
B. Disorders simulating oromandibular dystonia
    Trismus
C. Disorders simulating cervical dystonia
    1. Osteoarticular
        Subluxation of the atlantoaxial articulation
        Klippel-Feil abnormality
        Platybasia and basilar imprecision
        Cervical hemivertebra
        Damage, absence or laxity of the cervical ligaments
    2. Muscular
        Congenital or acquired muscle weakness
        Muscle fibrosis following local radiation therapy
    3. Soft tissue
        Neck mass
    4. Neurological
        Posterior fossa tumor or cyst
        Diplopia, mainly cranial nerve IV palsy
        Vestibular lesions
        Syringomyelia, syringobulbia
        Tonsillar herniation of any cause, including
          Arnold-Chiari syndrome
D. Disorders simulating brachial dystonia
    Carpal tunnel syndrome and other painful neuropathies
    Hyperventilation
E. Disorders simulating trunk dystonia
    1. Osteoarticular
        Bony abnormalities causing kyphosis, lordosis or scoliosis
    2. Neuromuscular
        Myopathies or neuropathies
        Opisthotonos
        Muscle cramps
        Stiff-person syndrome
        Isaac's syndrome
        Compensatory postures due to visceral or anorectal pain
F. Disorders simulating leg dystonia
    1. Osteoarticular
        Asymmetry, bony abnormalities
    2. Neuromuscular
        Spasticity, muscle cramps
        Restless legs
        Focal tetanus

References

1. Calne DB, Lang AE: Secondary dystonia. *Adv Neurol* 50:9–33, 1988.
2. Hartmann A, Pogarell O, Oertel WH: Secondary dystonias. *J Neurol* 245:511-518, 1998.
3. Jankovic J, Fahn S: Dystonic disorders, in Jankovic J, Tolosa E (eds): *Parkinson's Disease and Movement Disorders*. Baltimore: Williams & Wilkins, 1993, pp 337–374.
4. Fahn S: Dystonia: Where next? in Quinn NP, Jenner PG (eds): *Disorders of Movement*. New York: Academic Press, 1989, pp 349–357.

5. Dooling EC, Adams RD: The pathologic anatomy of posthemiplegic athetosis. *Brain* 98:29–48, 1975.

6. Gracia Cruz A, Ortega Perez M, Hernandez Lara J: Cerebral palsy with dystonic components. A presentation of nine cases. *Rev Neurol* 29:591, 1999.

7. Marsden CD, Obeso JA, Zarranz JJ: The anatomical basis of symptomatic dystonia. *Brain* 108:463–483, 1985.

8. Pettigrew LC, Jankovic J: Hemidystonia: A report of 22 cases and a review of the literature. *J Neurol Neurosurg Psychiatry* 48:650–657, 1985.

9. Obeso JA, Giménez-Roldán S: Clinicopathological correlation in symptomatic dystonia. *Adv Neurol* 50:113–122, 1988.

10. Kostiæ VS, Stpkampvoc-Svetel M, Kacar A: Symptomatic dystonias associated with structural brain lesions: Report of 16 cases. *Can J Neurol Sci* 23:53–56, 1996.

11. Demierre B, Rondot P: Dystonia caused by putamino-capsulo-caudate vascular lesions. *J Neurol Neurosurg Psychiatry* 46:404–409, 1983.

12. Burton K, Farrel K, Li D, Calne DB: Lesions of the putamen and dystonia: Computed tomography and magnetic resonance imaging. *Neurology* 34:962–965, 1984.

13. Perlmutter JS, Raichle ME: Pure hemidystonia with basal ganglion abnormalities on positron emission tomography. *Ann Neurol* 15:228–233, 1984.

14. Quinn N, Bydder G, Leenders N, Marsden CD: Magnetic resonance imaging to detect deep basal ganglia lesions in hemidystonia that are missed by computerized tomography [letter]. *Lancet* 2:1007–1008, 1985.

15. Cho C, Samkoff LM: A lesion of the anterior thalamus producing dystonic tremor of the hand. *Arch Neurol* 57:1353–1355, 2000.

16. Fross RD, Martin WRW, Li D, et al. Lesions of the putamen: their relevance to dystonia. *Neurology* 37:1125–1129, 1987.

17. Krauss JK, Mohakjer M, Nobbe F, Scheremet R: Hemidystonia due to a contralateral parietooccipital metastasis: Disappearance after removal of the mass lesion. *Neurology* 41:1519–1520, 1991.

18. Coria F, Blanco Martin AI, Rivas Vilas MD: Pseudodystonic hand posturing contralateral to a metastasis of the parietal association cortex. *Neurologia* 15:362–365, 2000.

19. Alarcon F, Tolosa E, Muñoz E: Focal limb dystonia in a patient with a cerebellar mass. *Arch Neurol* 58:1125–1127, 2001.

20. Menkes JH, Curren J: Clinical and MR correlates in children with extrapyramidal cerebral palsy. *Am J Neuroradiol* 15:451–457, 1994.

21. Krystkowiak P, Martinat P, Defebvre L, et al: Dystonia after striatopallidal and thalamic stroke: Clinicoradiological correlations and pathophysiological mechanisms. *J Neurol Neurosurg Psychiatry* 65:703–708, 1998.

22. Kelley RE, Jain PK: Hyperkinetic movement disorders caused by corpus striatum infarcts: brain MRI/CT findings in three cases. *J Neuroimaging* 10:22–26, 2000.

23. Schneider S, Feifel E, Ott D, et al: Prolonged MRI T2 times of the lentiform nucleus in idiopathic spasmodic torticollis. *Neurology* 44:846–850, 1994.

24. Krauss JK, Mohadjer M, Nobbe F, Mundinger F: The treatment of post traumatic tremor by stereotactic surgery. Symptomatic and functional outcome in a series of 35 patients. *J Neurosurg* 80:810–819, 1994.

25. Yamashiro K, Tasker RR: Stereotactic thalamotomy for dystonic patients. *Stereotact Funct Neurosurg* 60:81–85, 1993.

26. Jankovic J, Patel SC: Blepharospasm associated with brainstem lesions. *Neurology* 33:1237–1240, 1983.

27. Lang AE, Sharpe JA: Blepharospasm associated with palatal myoclonus [letter]. *Neurology* 34:1522, 1984.

28. Sandyk R, Gillman MA: Blepharospasm associated with communicating hydrocephalus [letter]. *Neurology* 34:1522–1523, 1984.

29. Jankovic J: Blepharospasm associated with palatal myoclonus and communicating hydrocephalus [letter]. *Neurology* 34:1523–1525, 1984.

30. Powers JM: Blepharospasm due to unilateral diencephalon infarction. *Neurology* 35:283–284, 1985.

31. Jankovic J: Blepharospasm with basal ganglia lesions [letter]. *Arch Neurol* 43:866–868, 1986.

32. Day TJ, Lefroy RB, Mastaglia FL: Meige's syndrome and palatal myoclonus associated to brainstem stroke. A common mechanism? *J Neurol Neurosurg Psychiatry* 48:1324–1325, 1986.

33. Leenders KL, Frackowiack RSJ, Quinn N, et al: Ipsilateral blepharospasm and contralateral hemidystonia and parkinsonism in a patient with a unilateral rostral brainstem-thalamic lesion: Structural and functional abnormalities studied with CT, MRI and PET scanning. *Mov Disord* 1:151–158, 1986.

34. Salerno SM, Kurlan R, Joy SE, Shoulson I: Dystonia in central pontine myelinolysis without evidence of extrapontine myelinolysis. *J Neurol Neurosurg Psychiatry* 56:1221–1223, 1993.

35. García-Albea E, Franch O, Muñoz D, Ricoy JR: Brueghel's syndrome, report of a case with post-mortem study. *J Neurol Neurosurg Psychiatry* 44:437–440, 1981.

36. Gibb WRG, Lees AJ, Marsden CD: Pathological report of four patients presenting with cranial dystonias. *Mov Disord* 3:211–221, 1988.

37. Altrocchi PH, Forno LS: Spontaneous oral-facial dyskinesia: Neuropathology of a case. *Neurology* 33:802–805, 1983.

38. Zweigg RM, Jankel WR, Whitehouse MF, et al: Brainstem pathology in dystonia. *Neurology* 36(suppl 1):74–75, 1986.

39. Kulisevsky J, Marti MJ, Ferrer I, Tolosa E: Meige syndrome: Neuropathology of a case. *Mov Disord* 3:170–175, 1988.

40. Mark MH, Sage JI, Dickson DW, et al: Meige syndrome in the spectrum of Lewy body disease. *Neurology* 44:1432–1436, 1994.

41. Grimes JD, Hassan MN, Quarrington AM, D'Alton J: Delayed-onset post-hemiplegic dystonia: CT demonstration of basal ganglia pathology. *Neurology* 32:1033–1035, 1982.

42. Russo LS: Focal dystonia and lacunar infarction of the basal ganglia. *Arch Neurol* 40:61–62, 1983.

43. Keane JR, Young JA: Blepharospasm with bilateral basal ganglia infarction. *Arch Neurol* 42:1206–1208, 1985.

44. Giroud M, Dumas R: Dystonie secondaire, un infarctus putamino-capsulo-caud chez l'enfant. *Rev Neurol (Paris)* 144:375–377, 1988.

45. Picard A, Elghozi D, Schuman-Clacy E, Lacert P: Troubles du langage de type sous-cortical et hemidystonie sequelles d'un infarctus putamino-caude datant de la premiere enfance. *Rev Neurol (Paris)* 145:73–75, 1989.

46. Burton L, Scott PhD, Jankovic J: Delayed-onset progressive movement disorders after static brain lesions. *Neurology* 46:68–74, 1996.

47. Bhatt MH, Obeso JA, Marsden CD: Time course of post anoxic dystonic syndromes. *Neurology* 43:314–317, 1993.

48. Larumbe R, Vaamonde J, Artieda J, et al: Blepharospasm associated with anoxic damage of the basal ganglia during cardiac surgery. *Mov Disord* 8:198–200, 1993.

49. Chiang CY, Lu CS: Delayed-onset posthemiplegic dystonia and imitation synkinesia [letter]. *J Neurol Neurosurg Psychiatry* 53:623, 1990.

50. Factor SA, Sanchez-Ramos J, Weiner WJ: Delayed-onset dystonia associated with corticospinal tract dysfunction. *Mov Disord* 3:201–210, 1988.

51. Burke RE, Fahn S, Gold AP: Delayed-onset dystonia in patients with "static" encephalopathy. *J Neurol Neurosurg Psychiatry* 43:789–797, 1982.

52. Saint Hilaire MH, Burke RE, Bressman SB, et al: Delayed-onset dystonia due to perinatal or early chilhood asphyxia. *Neurology* 41:216–222, 1991.

53. Münchau A, Mathen D, Cox T, et al: Unilateral lesions of the globus pallidus: Report of four patients presenting with focal or segmental dystonia. *J Neurol Neurosurg Psychiatry* 69:494–498, 2000.

54. Jankovic J: Can peripheral trauma induce dystonia and other movement disorders? Yes! *Mov Disord* 16:7–12, 2001.

55. Weiner WJ: Can peripheral trauma induce dystonia? No! *Mov Disord* 16:13–22, 2001.

56. Fletcher NA, Harding AE, Marsden CD: The relationship between trauma and idiopathic torsion dystonia. *J Neurol Neurosurg Psychiatry* 54:713–717, 1991.

57. Sankhla C, Lai EC, Jankovic J: Peripherally induced oromandibular dystonia. *J Neurol Neurosurg Psychiatry* 65:722–728, 1998.

58. Frucht S, Fahn S, Ford B: Focal task-specific dystonia induced by peripheral trauma. *Mov Disord* 15:348–350, 2000.

59. Schott GD: The relationship of peripheral trauma and pain to dystonia. *J Neurol Neurosurg Psychiatry* 48:698–701, 1985.

60. Jankovic J, Van der Linden C: Dystonia and tremor induced by peripheral trauma: predisposing factors. *J Neurol Neurosurg Psychiatry* 51:1512–1519, 1988.

61. Truong DD, Dubinsky R, Hermanowicz N, et al: Posttraumatic torticollis. *Arch Neurol* 48:221–223, 1991.

62. Goldman S, Ahlskog JE: Posttraumatic cervical dystonia. *Mayo Clin Proc* 68:443–448, 1993.

63. Foley-Nolan D, Kinirons M, Coughlan RJ, O'Connor P: Post-whiplash dystonia well controlled by transcutaneous electrical nervous stimulation (TENS): Case report. *J Trauma* 30: 909–910, 1990.

64. Jankovic J: Post-traumatic movement disorders: Central and peripheral mechanisms. *Neurology* 44:2006–2014, 1994.

65. Thyagarajan D, Kompoliti K, Ford B: Post-traumatic shoulder dystonia: persistent abnormal postures of the shoulder after minor trauma. *Neurology* 51:1205–1207, 1998.

66. Murase N, Kaji R, Shimazu H, et al: Abnormal premovement gating of somatosensory input in writer's cramp. *Brain* 123:1813–1829, 2000.

67. Priori A, Pescuti A, Cappelari A, et al: Limb immobilization for the treatment of focal occuptional dystonia. *Neurology* 57:405–409, 2001.

68. Lees AJ, Hardie RJ, Stern GM: Kinesigenic foot dystonia as a presenting feature of Parkinson's disease. *J Neurol Neurosurg Psychiatry* 47:885, 1984.

69. Poewe W, Lees AJ, Steiger D, Stern GM: Foot dystonia in Parkinson's disease: Clinical phenomenology and neuropharmacology. *Adv Neurol* 45:357–360, 1986.

70. LeWitt PA, Burns RS, Newman RP: Dystonia in untreated Parkinsonism. *Clin Neuropharmacol* 9:293–297, 1986.

71. Katchen M, Duvoisin RC: Parkinsonism following dystonia in three patients. *Mov Disord* 1:151–157, 1986.

72. Grimes JD, Hassan MN, Halle D, Armstrong GWD: Clinical and radiographic features of scoliosis in Parkinson's disease. *Adv Neurol* 45:353–355, 1986.

73. Mathers SE, Kempster PA, Swash M, Lees AJ: Constipation and paradoxical puborectalis contraction in anismus and Parkinson's disease: A dystonic phenomenon? *J Neurol Neurosurg Psychiatry* 51:1503–1507, 1988.

74. Quinn NP: Parkinsonism and dystonia, pseudo-parkinsonism and pseudodystonia. *Adv Neurol* 60:540–543, 1993.

75. Golbe LI, Di Iorio G, Bonavita V, et al: A large kindred with autosomal dominant Parkinson's disease. *Ann Neurol* 27:276–282, 1990.

76. De Yebenes JG, Moskowitz C, Fahn S, Saint-Hilare MH: Long-term treatment with levodopa in a family with autosomal dominant torsion dystonia. *Adv Neurol* 50:101–111, 1988.

77. Nygaard TG, Trugman JM, de Yebenes JG, Fahn S: DOPA responsive dystonia: The spectrum of clinical manifestations in a large North American family. *Neurology* 40:253–257, 1990.

78. Yokochi M: Nosological concept of juvenile parkinsonism with reference to the DOPA-responsive syndrome. *Adv Neurol* 60:548–552, 1993.

79. Bastos Lima A, Levy A, Castro Galdas A, et al: Parkinson's disease before age 30. *Adv Neurol* 60:553–561, 1993.

80. Dwork AJ, Balmaceda C, Fazzini EA, et al: Dominantly inherited, early-onset parkinsonism: Neuropathology of a new form. *Neurology* 43:69–74, 1993.

81. Probst A, Dufresne JJ: Paralysie supranuclaire progressive ou dystonie oculo facio cervicale. *Schweiz Arch Neurol Neurochir Psychiatr* 116:107–134, 1975.

82. Constantino A, Bolton CF: The face in progressive supranuclear palsy. *Neurology* 35(suppl 1):161, 1985.

83. Jackson JA, Jankovic J, Ford J: Progressive supranuclear palsy: Clinical features and response to treatment in 16 patients. *Ann Neurol* 13:237–278, 1983.

84. Steele JC, Richardson JC, Olszewsky J: Progressive supranuclear palsy. *Arch Neurol* 10:333–359, 1964.

85. Weimann RL: Heterogeneous degeneration of the central nervous system associated with peripheral neuropathy. *Neurology* 17:507–603, 1967.

86. Steele JC: Progressive supranuclear palsy. *Brain* 95:693–704, 1972.

87. Ratal RD, Fredman JH: Limb dystonia in progressive supranuclear palsy. *Neurology* 37:1546–1548, 1987.

88. Kurihara T, Landau WM, Torack RM: Progressive supranuclear palsy with action myoclonus, seizures. *Neurology* 24:219–223, 1974.

89. Leger JM, Girault JA, Bolgert F: Deux cas de dystonie isole d'un membre superieur inagurant una maladie de Steele Richardson Olszewsky. *Rev Neurol (Paris)* 143:140–142, 1987.

90. Fenelon G, Guillard A, Romanet S, et al: Les signes parkinsoniens du syndrome de Steele-Richardson-Olszewsky. *Rev Neurol (Paris)* 149:69–64, 1993.

91. De Yebenes JG, Sarasa JL, Daniel SE, Lees AJ: Familial progressive supranuclear palsy. *Brain* 118:1095–1103, 1995.

92. Rebeiz JJ, Kolondy EH, Richardson EP: Corticodentatonigral degeneration with neuronal achromasia. *Arch Neurol* 18:20–33, 1968.

93. Lee MS, Thompson PD, Marsden CD: Corticobasal degeneration: a clinical study of 36 cases. *Brain* 117:1183–1196, 1994.

94. Berciano J: Olivopontocerebellar atrophy. In Jancovic J, Tolosa E (eds): *Parkinson's Disease and Movement Disorders*. Baltimore: Williams & Wilkins, 1993, pp 163–189.

95. Menzel P: Beitrage zur Kenntnigs der hereditarien Ataxie und Kleinhinrnatrophie. *Arch Psychiatr Nervenkr* 22:160–190, 1891.

96. Neumann MA: Pontocerebellar atrophy combined with vestibular reticular degeneration. *J Neuropathol Exp Neurol* 36:321–337, 1977.

97. Bruyn GW, Went LN: Huntington's chorea, in Vinken PJ, Bruyn GW, Klawans HL (eds): *Handbook of Clinical Neurology: Extrapyramidal Disorders*. Amsterdam: Elsevier, 1986, vol 5, pp 255–266.

98. Curtis ARJ, Fey C, Morris C, et al: Mutation in the gene encoding ferritin light polypeptide causes dominant adult-onset basal ganglia disease. *Nat Genet* 28:350–354, 2001.

99. Al-Tahan AY, Divarkaran MP, Kambouris M, et al: A novel autosomal recessive "Huntington's disease-like" neurodegenerative disorder in a Saudi family. *Saudi Med J* 20:85–89, 1999.

100. Kambouris M, Bohlega S, Al T, Meyer BF: Localization of the gene for a novel autosomal recessive neurodegenerative Huntington-like disorder to 4p15.3. *Am J Hum Genet* 66:445–452, 2000.

101. Schady W, Meara RJ: Hereditary progressive chorea without dementia. *J Neurol Neurosurg Psychiatry* 51:295–297, 1988.

102. de Vries BBA, Arts WFM, Breedveld G, et al: Benign hereditary chorea of early onset maps to chromosome 14q. *Am J Hum Genet* 66:136–142, 2000.

103. Oechsner M, Buchert R, Beyer W, Danek A: Reduction of striatal glucose metabolism in McLeod choreoacanthocytosis. *J Neurol Neurosurg Psychiatry* 70:517–520, 2001.

104. Rinne JO, Daniels E, Scaravilli F, et al: Neuropathological features of neuroacanthocytosis. *Mov Disord* 9:297–304, 1994.

105. Kito S, Itoga E, Hiroshige Y, Matsumoto N: A pedigree of amyotrophic chorea with acanthocytosis. *Arch Neurol* 37:514–517, 1980.

106. De Yebenes JG, Vazquez A, Martinez A, et al: Biochemical findings in symptomatic dystonias. *Adv Neurol* 50:167–175, 1988.

107. de Yebenes JG, Brin MF, Mena MA, et al: Neurochemical findings in neuroacanthocytosis. *Mov Disord* 3:300–312, 1988.

108. Rubio JP, Danek A, Stone C, et al: Chorea-acanthocytosis: Genetic linkage to chromosome 9q21. *Am J Hum Genet* 61:899–908, 1997.

109. Rampoldi L, Dobson-Stone C, Rubio JP, et al: A conserved sorting-associated protein is mutant in chorea-acanthocytosis. *Nat Genet* 28:119–120, 2001.

110. Ueno S, Maruki Y, Nakamura M, et al: The gene encoding a newly discovered protein, chorein, is mutated in chorea-acanthocytosis. *Nat Genet* 28:121–122, 2001.

111. Titica J, Van Bogaert L: Heredodegenerative hemiballismus: A contribution to the question of primary atrophy of the corpus Luysii. *Brain* 69:251–263, 1946.

112. Nagafuchi S, Yanagisawa H, Sato K: Dentatorubral and pallidoluysian atrophy expansion of an unstable CAG trinucleotide on chromosome 12p. *Nat Genet* 6:14–18, 1994.

113. Iizuka R, Hirayama K, Maehara K: Dentato-rubro-pallidoluysian atrophy: A clinico-pathological study. *J Neurol Neurosurg Psychiatry* 47:1288–1298, 1984.

114. Komure O, Sano A, Nishino N: DNA analysis in hereditary dentatorubral-pallidoluysian atrophy: Correlation between CAG repeat length and phenotypic variation and the molecular basis of anticipation. *Neurology* 45:143–149, 1995.

115. Sano A, Yamamuchi N, Kakimoto Y: Anticipation in hereditary dentatorubral-pallidoluysian atrophy. *Hum Genet* 93:699–702, 1994.

116. Walshe JM: Wilson's disease, in Vinken PJ, et al (eds): *Handbook of Clinical Neurology*. Amsterdam: Elsevier, 1986, pp 223–238.

117. Magalhaes AC, Caramelli P, Menezes JR, et al. Wilson's disease: MRI with clinical correlation. *Neuroradiology* 36:97–100, 1994.

118. Simonati A, Trevisan C, Salviati A, Rizzuto N: Neuroaxonal dystrophy with dystonia and pallidal involvement. *Neuropediatrics* 30:151–154, 1999.

119. Zhou B, Westaway SK, Levinson B, et al: A novel pantothenate kinase gene (PANK2) is defective in Hallervorden-Spatz syndrome. *Nat Genet* 28:345–349, 2001.

120. Dooling EC, Schoene WC, Richardson EP: Hallervorden-Spatz syndrome. *Arch Neurol* 30:70–83, 1974.

121. Nardocci N, Rumi V, Combi ML, et al: Complex tics, stereotypies, and compulsive behavior as clinical presentation of a juvenile progressive dystonia suggestive of Hallervorden-Spatz disease. *Mov Disord* 9:369–371, 1994.

122. Justesen CR, Penn RD, Kroin JS, Egel RT: Stereotactic pallidotomy in a child with Hallervorden-Spatz disease. Case report. *J Neurosurg* 90:551–554, 1999.

123. Manyam BV, Walters AS, Narla KR: Bilateral striopallidodentate calcinosis: Clinical characteristics of patients seen in a registry. *Mov Disord* 16:258–264, 2001.

124. Caraceni T, Broggi G, Avanzini G: Familial idiopathic basal ganglia calcifications exhibiting "dystonia musculorum deformans". *Eur Neurol* 12:351–359, 1974.

125. Larsen TA, Dunn HG, Jan JE, Calne DA: Dystonia and calcification of the basal ganglia. *Neurology* 35:533–537, 1985.

126. Lauterbach EC, Spears TE, Prewett MJ, et al: Neuropsychiatric disorders, myoclonus, and dystonia in calcification of basal ganglia pathways. *Biol Psychiatry* 35:345–351, 1994.

127. Geschwind DH, Loginov M, Stern JM: Identification of a locus on chromosome 14q for idiopathic basal ganglia calcification (Fahr disease). *Am J Hum Genet* 65:764–772, 1999.

128. Loeb JA: Functional improvement in a patient with cerebral calcinosis using a bisphosphonate. *Mov Disord* 13:345–349, 1998.

129. Jellinger K: Pallidal, pallidonigral and pallidoluysonigral degeneration including association with thalamic and dentate degeneration, in Vinken PJ, Bruyn GW, Klawans HL (eds): *Handbook of Clinical Neurology: Extrapyramidal Disorders*. Amsterdam: Elsevier, 1986, vol 5, pp 445–464.

130. Van Bogaert L: Aspects cliniques et pathologiques des atrophies pallidales et pallido-luysiennes progressives. *J Neurol Neurosurg Psychiatry* 9:125–157, 1946.

131. Wooten GF, Lopes MB, Harris WO, et al: Pallidoluysian atrophy: Dystonia and basal ganglia functional anatomy. *Neurology* 43:1764–1768, 1993.

132. Haltia M, Somer H, Palo J: Neuronal intranuclear inclusion disease in identical twins. *Ann Neurol* 15:316–321, 1984.

133. Muñoz-García D, Ludwin SK: Adult onset neuronal intranuclear hyaline inclusion disease. *Neurology* 36:785–790, 1986.

134. Goutieres F, Mikol F, Aicardi J: Neuronal intranuclear inclusion disease in a child: Diagnoses by rectal biopsy. *Ann Neurol* 27:103–106, 1990.

135. Amir RE, Wan M, van den Veyver IB, et al: Rett syndrome is caused by mutations in X-linked MECP2, encoding methyl-CpG-binding protein 2. *Nat Genet* 23:185–188, 1999.

136. Shahbazian MD, Zoghbi HY: Molecular genetics of Rett syndrome and clinical spectrum of MECP2 mutations. *Curr Opin Neurol* 14:171–176, 2001.

137. The Rett syndrome Diagnostic Criteria Study Group: Diagnostic criteria for Rett syndrome. *Ann Neurol* 23:425–428, 1988.

138. Fitzgerald PM, Jankovic J, Percy AK: Rett syndrome and associated movement disorders. *Mov Disord* 5:195–202, 1990.

139. Subramony SH, Filla A: Autosomal dominant spinocerebellar ataxias ad infinitum? *Neurology* 56:287–289, 2001.

140. Hearn E, Holmes SE, Calvert PC, et al: SCA-12: Tremor with cerebellar and cortical atrophy is associated with a CAG repeat expansion. *Neurology* 56:299–303, 2001.

141. Wali GM: Friedreich ataxia associated with dystonic head tremor provoked by prolonged exercise. *Mov Disord* 15:1298–1299, 2000.

142. Barbot C, Coutinho P, Chorao R, et al. Recessive ataxia with ocular apraxia: review of 22 Portuguese patients. *Arch Neurol* 58:201–205, 2001.

143. Coutinho P, Andrade C: Autosomal dominant system degeneration in Portuguese families of the Azores islands. *Neurology* 28:703–709, 1978.

144. Barbeau A, Roy M, Cunha L: The natural history of Machado-Joseph disease. *Can J Neurol Sci* 11:510–525, 1984.

145. Woods B, Schaumburg H: Nigro-spino-dentatal degeneration with nuclear ophthalmoplegia: A unique and partially treatable clinicopathological entity. *J Neurol Sci* 17:149–166, 1972.

146. Takiyama Y, Oyanagi S, Kawashima S, et al: A clinical and pathologic study of a large Japanese family with Machado-Joseph disease tightly linked to the DNA markers on chromosome 14q. *Neurology* 44:1302–1308, 1994.

147. Kawaguchi Y, Okamoto T, Taniwaki M: CAG expansions in a novel gene for Machado-Joseph disease at chromosome 14q32.1. *Nat Genet* 8:221–227, 1994.

148. Freire Gonzalves A, Dinis M, Ferro MA: Machado-Joseph disease, in Berciano J (ed): *Ataxias y Paraplegias Hereditarias: Aspectos Clínicos y Genéticos*. Madrid: Ergon, 1993, pp 189–202.

149. Lang AE, Rogaeva EA, Tsuda T, et al: Homozygous inheritance of the Machado-Joseph disease gene. *Ann Neurol* 36:443–447, 1994.

150. Schols L, Peters S, Szymanski S, et al: Extrapyramidal motor signs in degenerative ataxias. *Arch Neurol* 57:1495–1500, 2000.

151. Bodesteiner JB, Goldblum RM, Goldman AS: Progressive dystonia masking ataxia telangiectasia. *Arch Neurol* 37:464–465, 1980.

152. Aguilera T, Negrete O: Un caso de ataxia telangiectasia. *Rev Clin Esp* 107:51–54, 1967.

153. Castroviejo P, Rodriguez-Costa T, Ojeda Casas A: Ataxia telangiectasia, presentacion de dos casos con agammaglobulinemia. *Rev Clin Esp* 109:439–444, 1968.

154. Garcia-Urra D, Campos J, Varela de Seijas E, de Yebenes JG: Movement disorders in ataxia telangiectasia. *Neurology* 39:321, 1989.

155. Garcia-Ruiz P, Garcia-Urra D, Jimenez-Jimenez FJ: Movimientos anormales en ataxia telangiectasia. *Arch Neurobiol* 56:30–33, 1993.

156. Agamanolis DP, Greenstein JI: Ataxia telangiectasia. *J Neuropathol Exp Neurol* 38:475, 1979.

157. Robbins JH, Kraemer KH, Lutzer MA: Xeroderma pigmentosum: An inherited disease with sun sensitivity, multiple cutaneous neoplasm and abnormal DNA repair. *Ann Intern Med* 80:221–248, 1974.

158. Rando TA, Horton JL, Layder BB: Wolfram syndrome: Evidence of a neurodegenerative disease by magnetic resonance imaging. *Neurology* 36:438–440, 1986.

159. Hardy EL, Khanim F, Torres R, et al: Clinical and molecular genetic analysis of 19 Wolfram syndrome kindreds demonstrating a wide spectrum of mutations in WFS1. *Am J Hum Genet* 65:1279–1290, 1999.

160. Goldman JE, Katz D, Rapin I: Chronic GM1 gangliosidosis presenting as dystonia: I. Clinical and pathological features. *Ann Neurol* 9:465–475, 1981.

161. Guazzi GC, D'Amore I, Van Hoff F, Fruschelli C: Type 3 (chronic) GM1 gangliosidosis presenting as infanto choreo athetotic dementia, without epilepsy in three sisters. *Neurology* 38:1124–1127, 1988.

162. Uyama E, Terasaki T, Watanabe S, et al: Type 3 GM1 gangliosidosis: Characteristic MRI findings correlated with dystonia. *Acta Neurol Scand* 86:609–615, 1992.

163. Federico A, Palmeri S, Malandrini A, et al: The clinical aspects of adult hexosaminidase deficiencies. *Dev Neurosci* 13:280–287, 1991.

164. Eirís J, Chabás A, Coll MJ, Castro-Gago: Fenotipo infantil tardío y juvenil de la variante B1 de gangliosidosis GM2. *Rev Neurol* 29:435–438, 1999.

165. Meek D, Wolfe LS, Andermann E, Andermann F: Juvenile progressive dystonia: A new phenotype of GM2 gangliosidosis. *Ann Neurol* 15:348–352, 1984.

166. Hardie RJ, Young EP, Morgan-Hughes JA: Hexosaminidase A deficiency presenting as juvenile progressive dystonia. *J Neurol Neurosurg Psychiatry* 51:446–447, 1988.

167. Hardie RJ, Morgan-Hughes JA: Dystonia in GM2 gangliosidosis. *Mov Disord* 7:390–391, 1992.

168. Nardocci N, Bertagnolio B, Rumi V, Angelini L: Progressive dystonia symptomatic of juvenile GM2 gangliosidosis. *Mov Disord* 7:64–67, 1992.

169. Johnson WG: The clinical spectrum of hexosaminidase deficiency diseases. *Neurology* 31:1453–1456, 1981.

170. Spence MW, Callahan JW: Sphingomyelin cholesterol lipidoses: The Niemann Pick group of diseases, in Scriver CR, Beaudet Al, Sly WS, Valle D (eds): *The Metabolic Basis of Inherited Disease*, 6th ed. New York: McGraw-Hill, 1989, pp 1655–1676.

171. Varier MT, Wenger DA, Comly ME, et al: Niemann Pick disease group C: Clinical variability and diagnosis based on defective cholesterol sterification: A collaborative study of 70 patients. *Clin Genet* 33:311–348, 1988.

172. Uc EY, Wenger DA, Jankovic J: Niemann-Pick disease type C: Two cases and an update. *Mov Disord* 15:1199–1203, 2000.

173. Watanabe Y, Akoboshi S, Ishida G, et al: Increased levels of GM2 ganglioside in fibroblasts from a patient with juvenile Niemann-Pick disease type C. *Brain Dev* 20:95–97, 1998.

174. Martin JJ, Loventhal A, Luteric C, Varier MT: Juvenile dystonic lipidosis (variant of Niemann Pick disease type C). *J Neurol Sci* 66:33–45, 1984.

175. Pollen A, Fluharty AL, Fluharty EB, et al: Molecular basis of different forms of metachromatic leucodystrophy. *N Engl J Med* 324:18–22, 1991.

176. Inui K, Emmett M, Wenger DA: Immunological evidence for deficiency in an activator protein for sulfatide sulfatase in a variant form of metachromatic leukodystrophy. *Proc Natl Acad Sci U S A* 80:3074–3076, 1983.

177. Mihaljevic-Peles A, Jakkovljevis M, Milicevic Z, Kracun I: Low arylsulphatase A activity in the development of psychiatric disorders. *Neuropsychobiology* 43:75–78, 2001.

178. Berkovic SF, Carpenter S, Andermann F, et al: "Kufs" disease: A critical reappraisal. *Brain* 111:27–62, 1988.

179. Simonati A, Santorum E, Tessa A, et al: A CLN2 gene nonsense mutation is associated with severe caudade atrophy and dystonia in LINCL. *Neuropediatrics* 31:199–201, 2000.

180. Yool DA, Edgar JM, Montague P, Malcolm S: The proteolipid protein gene and myelin disorders in man and animal models. *Hum Mol Genet* 9:987–992, 2000.

181. Boulloche J, Aicardi A: Pelizaeus-Merzbacher disease: Clinical and nosological study. *J Child Neurol* 1:233–239, 1986.

182. Harding AE, Shapira A: Mitochondrial disease and movement disorders, in Jankovic J, Tolosa E (eds): *Parkinson's Disease and Movement Disorders*. Baltimore: Williams & Wilkins, 1993, pp 569–583.

183. Hanna MG, Bhatia KP: Movement disorders and mitochondrial dysfunction. *Curr Opin Neurol* 10:351–356, 1997.

184. Truong DD, Harding AE, Scaravilli F: Movement disorders in mitochondrial myopathies: A report of nine cases with two autopsy studies. *Mov Disord* 5:109–117, 1990.

185. Bercovic SF, Karpati G, Carpenter S, Lang AE: Progressive dystonia with bilateral putaminal hypodensities. *Arch Neurol* 44:1184–1187, 1987.

186. Novotny EJ, Singh G, Wallace DC, et al: Leber's disease and dystonia: A mitochondrial disease. *Neurology* 36:1053–1060, 1986.

187. Sudarski L, Plotkin GM, Logigian EL, Johns DR: Dystonia as a presenting feature of the 3243 mitochondrial DNA mutation. *Mov Disord* 14:488–491, 1999.

188. Macaya A, Munell F, Burke RE, De Vivo DC: Disorders of movement in Leigh syndrome. *Neuropediatrics* 24:60–67, 1993.

189. Lera G, Bhatia K, Marsden CD: Dystonia as the major manifestation of Leigh's syndrome. *Mov Disord* 9:642–649, 1994.

190. Munoz-Hiraldo ME, Martinez-Bermejo A, Gutierrez-Molina M, et al: Distonia como manifestacion principal en el sindrome de Leigh del lactante. *An Esp Pediatr* 38:348–350, 1993.

191. Whetsell WO, Plaitakis A: Leigh's disease in an adult: Evidence of an "inhibitory factor" in family members. *Ann Neurol* 3:529–534, 1978.

192. Leuzzi V, Bertini E, De Negri AM, et al: Bilateral striatal necrosis, dystonia and optic atrophy in two siblings. *J Neurol Neurosurg Psychiatry* 55:16–19, 1992.

193. Bruyn GW, Bots GTAM, Went LN, Klinkhamer PJJM: Hereditary optic neuropathy: Neuropathological findings. *J Neurol Sci* 113:55–61, 1992.

194. Jun AS, Brown MD, Walance DC: A mitochondrial DNA mutation at nucleotide pair 14459 of the NADH dehydrogenase subunit 6 gene associated with maternally inherited Leber hereditary optic neuropathy and dystonia. *Proc Natl Acad Sci U S A* 91:6206–6210, 1994.

195. Kirby DM, Hons BS, Kahler SG, et al: Leigh disease caused by the mitochondrial DNA G14459A mutation in unrelated families. *Ann Neurol* 48:102–104, 2000.

196. Walance DC: Mitochondrial DNA mutations in diseases of energy metabolism. *J Bioeneg Biomembr* 26:241–250, 1994.

197. Walance DC: Mitochondrial DNA sequence variation in human evolution and disease. *Proc Natl Acad Sci U S A* 91:8739–8746, 1994.

198. Tranebjaerg L, Schwartz C, Eriksen H, et al: A new X linked recessive deafness syndrome with blindness, dystonia, fractures, and mental deficiency is linked to Xq22. *J Med Genet* 32: 257–263, 1995.

199. Jin H, Kendall E, Freeman TC, et al: The human family of deafness dystonia peptide (DDP) related mitochondrial import proteins. *Genomics* 61:259–267, 1999.

200. Koehler CM, Leuenberger D, Merchant S, et al: Human deafness dystonia syndrome is a mitochondrial disease. *Proc Natl Acad Sci U S A* 96:2141–2146, 1999.

201. Kyllerman M, Skjeldal OH, Lundberg M, et al: Dystonia and dyskinesia in glutaric aciduria type I: Clinical heterogeneity and therapeutic considerations. *Mov Disord* 9:22–30, 1994.

202. Voll R, Hoffmann GF, Lipinski CG, et al: Die Glutarazidamie/Glutaraziurie I as differential Diagnose der Chorea Minor. *Klin Peadiatr* 205:124–126, 1993.

203. Al-Essa M, Bakheet S, Patay Z, et al: Fluoro-2-deoxyglucose (18FDG) PET scan of the brain in glutaric aciduria type 1: Clinical and MRI correlations. *Brain Dev* 20:295–301, 1998.

204. Chow CW, Haan EA, Goodman SI, et al: Neuropathology of glutaric acidemia type I. *Acta Neuropathol (Berl)* 75:590–594, 1988.

205. Lawrence Wolf B, Herberg KP, Hoffmann GF, et al: Entwicklung der Hirnatrophie. Therapie und Therapieuberwachung bei Glutarazidurie Typ 1 (Glutaryl-CoA Dehydrogenase-Mangel). *Klin Paediatr* 205:23–29, 1993.

206. Hauser SE, Peters H: Glutaric aciduria type I: An underdiagnosed cause of encephalopathy and dystonia-dyskinesia syndrome in children. *J Paediatr Child Health* 34:302–304, 1998.

207. Heindenreich R, Natowicz M, Hainline BE, et al: Acute extrapyramidal syndrome in methylmalonic acidemia: "Metabolic stroke" involving the globus pallidus. *J Pediatr* 113: 1022–1027, 1988.

208. Roodhooft AM, Baumgartner ER, Martin JJ, et al: Symmetrical necrosis of the basal ganglia in methylmalonic acidemia. *Eur J Pediatr* 149:582–584, 1990.

209. de Sousa C, Piesowicz AT, Brett EM, Leonard JV: Focal changes in the globi pallidi associated with neurological dysfunction in methylmalonic acidemia. *Neuropediatrics* 20:119–201, 1989.

210. Shimoizumi H, Okabe I, Kodama H, Yanagisawa M. [Methylmalonic acidemia with bilateral MRI high intensities of the globus pallidus]. *No To Hattatsu* 25:554–557, 1993.

211. Andreula CF, Blasi RD, Carella A: CT and MR studies of methylmalonic acidemia. *Am J Neuroradiol* 12:410–412, 1991.

212. Kerrigan JF, Aleck KA, Tarby TJ, et al: Fumaric aciduria: Clinical and imaging features. *Ann Neurol* 47:583–588, 200

213. Bourgeron T, Chretien D, Poggi Bach J, et al: Mutation of the fumarase gene in two siblings with progressive encephalopathy and fumarase deficiency. *J Clin Invest* 93:2514–2518, 1994.

214. Hagberg B, Hambraeus L, Bensch K: A case of homocystinuria with a dystonia neurological syndrome. *Neuropadiatrie* 1:337–343, 1970.

215. Davous P, Rondot P: Homocystinuria and dystonia. *J Neurol Neurosurg Psychiatry* 46:283–286, 1983.

216. Arbour L, Rosenblatt B, Clow C, Wilson GN: Postoperative dystonia in a female patient with homocystinuria. *J Pediatr* 113:863–864, 1988.

217. Kempster PA, Brenton DP, Gale AN, Stern GM: Dystonia in homocystinuria. *J Neurol Neurosurg Psychiatry* 51:859–862, 1988.

218. Bernardelli A, Thompson PD, Zacagnini M, et al: Two sisters with generalized dystonia associated with homocystinuria. *Mov Disord* 6:163–165, 1991.

219. Wada Y, Kita Y, Yamamoto T, et al: Homocystinuria with generalized chorea and other movement disorders: A case report. *No To Shinkei* 52:629–631, 2000.

220. Darras BT, Ampola MG, Dietz WH, Gilmore HE: Intermittent dystonia in Hartnup disease. *Pediatr Neurol* 5:118–120, 1989.

221. Tamoush A, Alpers PH, Feigin RD, et al: Hartnup disease: Clinical, pathological and biochemical observations. *Arch Neurol* 33:797–807, 1976.

222. Jankovic J, Caskey TC, Stout JT, Butler T: Lesch Nyhan syndrome: A study of motor behavior and CSF monoamine turnover. *Ann Neurol* 23:466–469, 1988.

223. Adler CH, Wrabetz L: Lesch-Nyhan variant: Dystonia, ataxia, near-normal intelligence, and no self mutilation. *Mov Disord* 11:583–584, 1996.

224. Garcia Puig J, Mateos FA, Jimenez ML, et al: Espectro clinico de la deficiencia de hipoxantina-guanina fosforribosiltransferasa: Estudio de 12 pacientes. *Med Clin (Barc)* 14; 102:681–687, 1994.

225. Ernst M, Zametkin AJ, Matochik JA, et al: Presynaptic dopaminergic deficits in Lesch-Nyhan disease. *N Engl J Med* 334:1568–1572, 1996.

226. Adler CH, Caviness JN: Dystonia secondary to electrical injury: Surface electromyographic evaluation and implications for the organicity of the condition. *J Neurol Sci* 148:187–192, 1997.

227. Ondo W: Lingual dystonia following electrical injury. *Mov Disord* 12:253, 1997.

228. Boonkongchuen P, Lees A: Case of torticollis following electrical injury. *Mov Disord* 11:109, 1996.

229. Tarsy D, Sudarsky L, Charness ME: Limb dystonia following electric injury. *Mov Disord* 9:230–232, 1994.

230. Panchenko EN, Kazakova SE, Safonova EF: Nervnye narusheniia u likvidatorov avarii na Chernobyl'skoi AES, podvergavshikhsia vozdeistviiu ioniziruiushchego izlucheniia v malykh dozakh. *Vrach Delo* 8:13–16, 1993.

231. Ushkova IN, Koshelev NF: Kliniko-gigienicheskie i eksperimental'nye obosnovaniia nozologii lazernoi bolezni. *Vrach Delo* 2:63–68, 1994.

232. Friedman J, Standaert DG: Dystonia and its disorders. *Neurol Clin* 19:681–705, 2001.

233. Van Harten P, Hoek HW, Kahn RS: Acute dystonia induced by drug treatment. *BMJ* 319:623–626, 1999.

234. Llau ME, Senard JM, Rascol O, Montasstruc JL: *Therapie* 50:425–427, 1995.

235. Jankovic J: Tardive syndromes and other drug-induced movement disorders. *Clin Neuropharmacol* 18:197–214, 1995.

236. Gay CT, Ryan SG: Paroxysmal kinesigenic dystonia after methylphenidate administration. *J Child Neurol* 9:45–46, 1994.

237. Humphreys A, Tanner AR: Acute dystonic drug reaction or tetanus? An unusual consequence of a 'Whizz' overdose. *Hum Exp Toxicol* 13:311–312, 1994.

238. Saltz B, Woerner MG, Robinson DG, Kane JM: Side effects of antipsychotic drugs. *Postgrad Med* 107:169–178, 2000.

239. Kiriakakis V, Bhatia KP, Quinn NP, Marsden D: The natural history of tardive dystonia. A long -term follow up study of 107 cases. *Brain* 121:2053–2066, 1998.

240. Van Harten PN, Hoek HW, Matroos GE, et al: Intermittent neuroleptic treatment and risk for tardive dyskinesia: Curaçao Extrapyramidal Syndromes Study III. *Am J Psychiatry* 155:565–567, 1998.

241. Soares KVS, McGrath JJ: Anticholinergic medication for neuroleptic-induced tardive dyskinesia. *Cochrane Library,* Issue 1, 2001.

242. Caligiuri MR, Jeste DV, Lacro JP: Antipsychotic-induced movement disorders in the elderly: epidemiology and treatment recommendations. *Drugs Aging* 17:363–384, 2000.

243. Simpson GM: The treatment of tardive dyskinesia and tardive dystonia. *J Clin Psychiatry* 61(suppl 4):39–44, 2000.

244. Burke RE, Fahn S, Jankovic J, et al: Tardive dystonia: Late onset and persistent dystonia caused by antipsychotic drugs. *Neurology* 32:1335–1346, 1982.

245. Giménez Roldán S, Mateo D, Bartolome P: Tardive dystonia and severe tardive dyskinesia. *Acta Psychiat Scand* 71:488–494, 1985.

246. Barbeau A, Inoue N, Cloutier T: Role of manganese in dystonia. *Adv Neurol* 14:339–352, 1976.

247. Pal PK, Samii A, Calne DB: Manganese neurotoxicity: A review of clinical features, imaging and pathology. *Neurotoxicology* 20:227–238, 1999.

248. Danks DM: Copper-induced dystonia secondary to cholestatic liver disease. *Lancet* 335:410, 1990.

249. Janavs JL, Aminoff MJ: Dystonia and chorea in acquired systemic disorders. *J Neurol Neurosurg Psychiatry* 65:436–444, 1998.

250. Ross. Methanol induced dystonia. *Can J Neurol Sci* 97:155–162, 1990.

251. Borgohain R, Singh AK, Radhakrishna H, et al: Delayed onset generalised dystonia after cyanide poisoning. *Clin Neurol Neurosurg* 97:213–215, 1995.

252. Valenzuela R, Court J, Godoy J: Delayed cyanide induced dystonia. *J Neurol Neurosurg Psychiatry* 55:198–199, 1992.

253. Carella F, Grassi MP, Savoiardo M, et al: Dystonic-parkinsonian syndrome after cyanide poisoning: Clinical and MRI findings. *J Neurol Neurosurg Psychiatry* 51:1345–1348, 1988.

254. Choi IS, Cheon HY: Delayed movement disorders after carbon monoxide poisoning. *Eur Neurol* 42:141–144, 1999.

255. Choi IS: Delayed neurologic sequelae in carbon monoxide intoxication. *Arch Neurol* 40:433–435, 1983.

256. De Yebenes JG, de Yebenes PG: La distonia en la pintura de Matias Grunewald. El ergotismo epidemico en la baja Edad Media. *Arch Neurobiol* 54:37–40,1991.

257. Quinn NP: Dystonia in epidemic ergotism. *Neurology* 33:1267, 1983.

258. He F, Zhang S, Quian F, Zhang C: Delayed dystonia with striatal CT lucencies induced by a mycotoxin (3-nitropropionic acid). *Neurology* 45:2178–2183, 1995.

259. Spencer PS, Ludolph AC, Kisby GE: Neurologic diseases associated with use of plant components with toxic potential. *Environ Res* 62:106–113, 1993.

260. Thornton A, McKenna PJ: Acute dystonic reaction complicated by psychotic phenomena. *Br J Psychiatry* 164:115–118, 1994.

261. Batshaw ML, Wachtel RC, Deckel AW, et al: Munchausen's syndrome simulating torsion dystonia. *N Engl J Med* 312:1437–1439, 1985.

262. Marsden D: Psychogenic problems associated with dystonia. *Adv Neurol* 65:319–326, 1995.

263. Factor SA, Podskalny GD, Molho ES: Psychogenic movement disorders: Frequency, clinical profile, and characteristics. *J Neurol Neurosurg Psychiatry* 59:406–412, 1995.

264. Feinstein A, Stergiopoulos V, Fine J, Lang AE: Psychiatric outcome in patients with a psychogenic movement disorder: A prospective study. *Neuropsychiatry Neuropsychol Behav Neurol* 14:169–176, 2001.

265. Owens DG: Extrapyramidal side effects and tolerability of risperidone: A review. *J Clin Psychiatry* 55(suppl):29–35, 1994.

266. Casey DE: Motor and mental aspects of acute extrapyramidal syndromes. *Acta Psychiatr Scand Suppl* 380:14–20, 1994.

267. Khanna R, Damodaran SS, Chakraborty SP: Overflow movements may predict neuroleptic-induced dystonia. *Biol Psychiatry* 35:491–492, 1994.

268. Malhotra AK, Litman RE, Pickar D: Adverse effects of antipsychotic drugs. *Drug Saf* 9:429–436, 1993.

269. Sachdev P: Risk factors for tardive dystonia: A case control comparison with tardive dyskinesia. *Acta Psychiatr Scand* 88:98–103, 1993.

270. Sachdev P: Clinical characteristics of 15 patients with tardive dystonia. *Am J Psychiatry* 150:498–500, 1993.

271. Meltzer LT, Christoffersen CL, Serpa KA, et al: Lack of involvement of haloperidol-sensitive sigma binding sites in modulation of dopamine neuronal activity and induction of dystonias by antipsychotic drugs. *Neuropharmacology* 31:961–967, 1992.

272. Yassa R, Nastase C, Dupont D, Thibeau M: Tardive dyskinesia in elderly psychiatric patients: A 5-year study. *Am J Psychiatry* 149:1206–1211, 1992.

273. Chiu H, Shum P, Lau J, et al: Prevalence of tardive dyskinesia, tardive dystonia, and respiratory dyskinesia among Chinese psychiatric patients in Hong Kong. *Am J Psychiatry* 149:1081–1085, 1992.

274. Khanna R, Das A, Damodaran SS: Prospective study of neuroleptic-induced dystonia in mania and schizophrenia. *Am J Psychiatry* 149:511–513, 1992.

275. Wojcik JD, Falk WE, Fink JS, et al: A review of 32 cases of tardive dystonia. *Am J Psychiatry* 148:1055–1059, 1991.

276. Matsumoto RR, Hemstreet MK, Lai NL: Drug specificity of pharmacological dystonia. *Pharmacol Biochem Behav* 36:151–155, 1990.

277. Shorten GD, Srithran S, Hendron M: Pseudo-tetanus following trifluoperazine. *Ulster Med J* 59:221–222, 1990.

278. Ernst M, Gonzalez NM, Campbell M: Acute dystonic reaction with low-dose pimozide. *J Am Acad Child Adolesc Psychiatry* 32:640–642, 1993.

279. Vaamonde J, González JM, Hernández A, et al: Writer's cramp induced by olanzapine. *J Neurol* 248:422, 2001.

280. Jonnalagada JR, Norton JW: Acute dystonia with quetiapine. *Clin Neuropharmacol* 23:229–230, 2000.

281. Dunayevich E, Strakowski S: Olanzapine-induced tardive dystonia. *Am J Psychiatry* 156:1662, 1999.

282. Vercueil L, Foucher J: Risperidone-induced tardive dystonia and psychosis. *Lancet* 353:981, 1999.

283. Krebs MO, Olie JP: Tardive dystonia induced by risperidone. *Can J Psychiatry* 44:507–508, 1999.

284. Simpson GM, Lindemayer JP: Extrapyramidal symptoms in patients treated with risperidone. *J Clin Psychopharmacol* 17:194–201, 1997.

285. Tollefson GD, Beasley CM, Tamura RN, et al: Blind, controlled, long-term study of the comparative incidence of treatment-emergent tardive dyskinesia with olanzapine or haloperidol. *Am J Psychiatry* 154:1248–1253, 1997.

286. Faulk R, Gilmore JH, Jensen EW, Perkins DO: Risperidone-induced dystonic reaction. *Am J Psychiatry* 153:577, 1996.

287. Miller LG, Jankovic J: Neurologic approach to drug-induced movement disorders: A study of 125 patients. *South Med J* 83:525–532, 1990.

288. Dickson R, Williams R, Dalby JT: Dystonic reaction and relapse with clozapine discontinuation and risperidone intitiation. *Can J Psychiatry* 39:184, 1994.

289. Thomas P, Lalaux N, Vaiva G, Goudemand M: Dose-dependent stuttering and dystonia in a patient taking clozapine. *Am J Psychiatry* 151:1096, 1994.

290. Kastrup O, Gastpar M, Schwarz M: Acute dystonia due to clozapine. *J Neurol Neurosurg Psychiatry* 57:119, 1994.

291. Ganzini L, Casey DE, Hoffman F, et al: The prevalence of metoclopramide-induced tardive dyskinesia and acute extrapyramidal movement disorders. *Arch Intern Med* 153:1469–1475, 1993.

292. Sempere AP, Mola S, Flores J: Distonia tardia tras la administración de cleboprida. *Rev Neurol* 25:2060, 1997.

293. Angelini L, Zorzi G, Rumi V, et al: Transient paroxysmal dystonia in an infant possibly induced by cisapride. *Ital J Neurol Sci* 17:157–159, 1996.

294. Cory DA: Adverse reaction to metoclopramide during enteroclysis. *AJR Am J Roentgenol* 163:480, 1994.

295. Guala A, Mittino D, Ghini T, Quazza G: Le distonie da metoclopramide sono familiari? *Pediatr Med Chir* 14:617–618, 1992.

296. Guala A, Mittino D, Fabbrocini P, Ghini T: Familial metoclopramide-induced dystonic reactions. *Mov Disord* 7:385–386, 1992.

297. Lauterbach EC: Haloperidol-induced dystonia and parkinsonism on discontinuing metoclopramide: Implications for differential thalamocortical activity. *J Clin Psychopharmacol* 12:442–443, 1992.

298. Gabellini AS, Pezzoli A, De Massis P, Sacquegna T: Veralipride-induced tardive dystonia in a patient with bipolar psychosis. *Ital J Neurol Sci* 13:621–623, 1992.

299. Linazasoro G, Marti Masso JF, Olasagasti B: Acute dystonia induced by sulpiride. *Clin Neuropharmacol* 14:463–464, 1991.

300. Factor SA, Matthews MK: Persistent extrapyramidal syndrome with dystonia and rigidity caused by combined metoclopramide and prochlorperazine therapy. *South Med J* 84:626–628, 1991.

301. Bonuccelli U, Nocchiero A, Napolitano A, et al: Domperidone-induced acute dystonia and polycystic ovary syndrome. *Mov Disord* 6:79–81, 1991.

302. Miller LG, Jankovic J: Sulpiride-induced tardive dystonia. *Mov Disord* 5:83–84, 1990.

303. Tait P, Balzer R, Buchanan N: Metoclopramide side effects in children. *Med J Aust* 152:387, 1990.

304. McCann UD, Penetar DM, Belenky G: Acute dystonic reaction in normal humans caused by catecholamine depletion. *Clin Neuropharmacol* 13:565–568, 1990.

305. Burke RE, Reches A, Traub MM, et al: Tetrabenazine induces acute dystonic reactions. *Ann Neurol* 17:200–202, 1985.

306. Jimenez Jimenez FJ, Vazquez A, Garcia Ruiz P, et al: Chronic hemidystonia following acute dystonic reaction to thiethylperazine. *J Neurol Neurosurg Psychiatry* 54:562, 1991.

307. Olsen JC, Keng JA, Clark JA: Frequency of adverse reactions to prochlorperazine in the ED. *Am J Emerg Med S* 18:609–611, 2000.

308. Joseph MM, King WD: Dystonic reaction following recommended use of cold syrup. *Ann Emerg Med* 26:749–751, 1995.

309. Etzel JV: Diphenhydramine-induced acute dystonia. *Pharmacotherapy* 14:492–496, 1994.

310. Fahn S: The spectrum of levodopa-induced dyskinesias. *Ann Neurol* 47(suppl 1):S1–S11, 2000.

311. Bejjani BB, Arnulf I, Damier P, et al: Levodopa-induced dyskinesias in Parkinson's disease: Is sensitization reversible? *Ann Neurol* 47:655–658, 2000.

312. Zimmerman TR Jr, Sage JI, Lang AE, Mark MH: Severe evening dyskinesias in advanced Parkinson's disease: Clinical description, relation to plasma levodopa, and treatment. *Mov Disord* 9:173–177, 1994.

313. Marconi R, Lefebvre Caparros D, Bonnet AM, et al: Levodopa-induced dyskinesias in Parkinson's disease: Phenomenology and pathophysiology. *Mov Disord* 9:2–12, 1994.

314. Bravi D, Mouradian MM, Roberts JW, et al: End-of-dose dystonia in Parkinson's disease. *Neurology* 43:2130–2131, 1993.

315. Rupniak NM, Boyce S, Steventon MJ, et al: Dystonia induced by combined treatment with L-DOPA and MK-801 in parkinsonian monkeys. *Ann Neurol* 32:103–105, 1992.

316. Mark MH, Sage JI: Levodopa-associated hemifacial dystonia. *Mov Disord* 6:383, 1991.

317. Leiguarda R, Merello M, Sabe L, Starkstein S: Bromocriptine-induced dystonia in patients with aphasia and hemiparesis. *Neurology* 43:2319–2322, 1993.

318. Peacock L, Lublin H, Gerlach J: The effects of dopamine D1 and D2 receptor agonists and antagonists in monkeys withdrawn from long-term neuroleptic treatment. *Eur J Pharmacol* 186:49–59, 1990.

319. Mitchell IJ, Luquin R, Boyce S, et al: Neural mechanisms of dystonia: Evidence from a 2-deoxyglucose uptake study in a primate model of dopamine agonist-induced dystonia. *Mov Disord* 5:49–54, 1990.

320. Van Harten N, Van Trier J, Horwitz EH, et al: Cocaine as a risk factor of neuroleptic-induced acute dystonia. *J Clin Psychiatry* 59:128–130, 1998.

321. Cardoso FE, Jankovic J: Cocaine-related movement disorders. *Mov Disord* 8:175–178, 1993.

322. Hegarty AM, Lipton RB, Merriam AE, Freeman K: Cocaine as a risk factor for acute dystonic reactions. *Neurology* 41:1670–1672, 1991.

323. Farrell PE, Diehl AK: Acute dystonic reaction to crack cocaine. *Ann Emerg Med* 20:322, 1991.

324. Heath HW, Allen JK: Acute dystonia following standard doses of cold medicine containing phenylpropanolamine. *Clin Pediatr* 36:57–58, 1997.

325. Prior A, Bertolasi L, Berardelli A, Manfredi M: Acute dystonic reactions to ecstasy. *Mov Disord* 10:353, 1995.

326. Thiel A, Dressler D: Dyskinesias possibly induced by norpseudoephedrine. *J Neurol* 241:167–169, 1994.

327. Capstick C, Checkley S, Gray J, Dawe S: Dystonia induced by amphetamine and haloperidol. *Br J Psychiatry* 165:276, 1994.

328. Vandel P, Bonin B, Leveque E, et al: Tricyclic antidepressant-induced extrapyramidal side effects. *Eur Neuropsychopharmacol* 7:207–212, 1997.

329. Ornadel D, Barnes EA, Dick DJ: Acute dystonia due to amitryptiline. *J Neurol Neurosurg Psychiatry* 55:414, 1992.

330. Matot JP, Ziegler M, Olie JP, Rondot P: Amoxapine. An antidepressant responsible for extrapyramidal side effects? *Therapie* 40:187–190, 1985.

331. Jarecke CR, Reid PJ: Acute dystonic reaction induced by a monoamine oxidase inhibitor. *J Clin Psychopharmacol* 10:144–145, 1990.

332. Olson WL: Dystonia and reflex sympathetic dystrophy induced by ergotamine. *Mov Disord* 7:188–189, 1992.

333. Merello MJ, Nogues MA, Leiguarda RC, Lopez Saubidet C: Dystonia and reflex sympathetic dystrophy induced by ergotamine. *Mov Disord* 7:188–189, 1992.

334. Gerber PE, Lynd LD: Selective serotonin-reuptake inhibitor-induced movement disorders. *Ann Pharmacother* 32:692–698, 1998.

335. Lauterbach EC, Meyer JM, Simpson GM: Clinical manifestations of dystonia and dyskinesia after SSRI administration. *J Clin Psychiatry* 58:403–404, 1997.

336. Poyurovsky M, Schneidman M, Weizman A: Successful treatment of fluoxetin-induced dystonia with low dose mianserin. *Mov Disord* 12:1102–1104, 1997.

337. Pies RW: Must we now consider SRIs as neuroleptics? *J Clin Psychopharmacol* 17:443–445, 1997.

338. Leo RJ: Movement disorders associated with the serotonin selective reuptake inhibitors. *J Clin Psychiatry* 57:449–454, 1996.

339. Shihabuddin L, Rapport D: Sertraline and extrapyramidal side effects. *Am J Psychiatry* 151:288, 1994.

340. Dave M: Fluoxetine-associated dystonia. *Am J Psychiatry* 151:149, 1994.

341. George MS, Trimble MR: Dystonic reaction associated with fluvoxamine. *J Clin Psychopharmacol* 13:220–221, 1993.

342. Rio J, Molins A, Viguera ML, Codina A: Distonia aguda por fluoxetina. *Med Clin (Barc)* 99:436–437, 1992.

343. Lock JD, Gwirtsman HE, Targ EF: Possible adverse drug interactions between fluoxetine and other psychotropics. *J Clin Psychopharmacol* 10:383–384, 1990.

344. Reccoppa L, Welch WA, Ware MR: Acute dystonia and fluoxetine. *J Clin Psychiatry* 51:487, 1990.

345. Adityanjee, Lindenmeyer JP: Precipitation of dystonia by m-CPP in a schizophrenic patient treated with haloperidol. *Am J Psychiatry* 150:837–838, 1993.

346. Miyaoka T, Seno H, Yamamori C, et al: Pisa syndrome due to a cholinesterase inhibitor (donepezil): A case report. *J Clin Psychiatry* 62:573–574, 2001.

347. Kwak YT, Han IW, Baik J: Relation between cholinesterase inhibitor and Pisa syndrome. *Lancet* 355:2222, 2000.

348. LeWitt PA, Walters A, Hening W, McHale D: Persistent movement disorders induced by buspirone. *Mov Disord* 8:331–334, 1993.

349. Boylan K: Persistent dystonia associated with buspirone. *Neurology* 40:1904, 1990.

350. Kappler J, Menges C, Ferbert A, Ebel H: Schwere "Spat" Dystonie nach "Neuroleptanxiolyse" mit Fluspirilen. *Nervenarzt* 65:668, 1994.

351. Stones M, Kennie DC, Fulton JD: Dystonic dysphagia associated with fluspirilene. *BMJ* 301:668–669, 1990.

352. Rittmann M, Steegmanns Schwarz I: Schwere Spatdystonie unter Fluspirilen. *Dtsch Med Wochenschr* 116:1613, 1991.

353. Laux G, Gunreben G: Schwere Spatdystonie unter Fluspirilen. *Dtsch Med Wochenschr* 116:977–980, 1991.

354. Perez Trullen JM, Modrego Pardo PJ, Vazquez Andre M, Lopez Lozano JJ: Bromazepam-induced dystonia. *Biomed Pharmacother* 46:375–376, 1992.

355. Tolarek IH, Ford MJ: Acute dystonia induced by midazolam and abolished by flumazenil. *BMJ* 300:614, 1990.

356. Hooker EA, Danzl DF: Acute dystonic reaction due to diazepam. *J Emerg Med* 6:491–493, 1988.

357. Lee JW: Persistent dystonia associated with carbamazepine therapy: A case report. *N Z Med J* 107:360–361, 1994.

358. Soman P, Jain S, Rajsekhar V, et al: Dystonia: A rare manifestation of carbamazepine toxicity. *Postgrad Med J* 70:54–55, 1994.

359. Reynolds EH, Trimble MR: Adverse neuropsychiatric effects of anticonvulsant drugs. *Drugs* 29:570–581, 1985.

360. Moss W, Ojukwu C, Chiriboga CA: Phenytoin-induced movement disorder. Unilateral presentation in a child and response to diphenhydramine. *Clin Pediatr (Phila)* 33:634–638, 1994.

361. Lacayo A, Mitra N: Report of a case of phenobarbital-induced dystonia. *Clin Pediatr (Phila)* 31:252, 1992.

362. Palomeras E, Sanz P, Cano A, Fossas P: Dystonia in a patient treated with propranolol and gabapentin. *Arch Neurol* 57:570–571, 2000.

363. Reeves AL, So EL, Sharbrough FW, Krahn LE: Movement disorder associated with the use of gabapentin. *Epilepsia* 37:988–990, 1996.

364. Wolanczyk T, Grabowska A: Transient dystonia in three patients treated with tiagabine. *Epilepsia* 42:944–946, 2001.

365. Bernard JM, Le Roux D, Pereon Y: Acute dystonia during sevofluorane induction. *Anesthesiology* 90:1215–1216, 1999.

366. Hussein G, Olejniczak P, Carey M, et al: Propofol-induced dystonia: A case report and a review of the literature. *Clin Res Regul Affairs* 16:175–181, 1999.

367. Reddy RV, Moorthy SS, Dierdorf SF, et al: Excitatory effects and electroencephalographic correlation of etomidate, thiopental, methohexital, and propofol. *Anesth Analg* 77:1008–1011, 1993.

368. Mets B: Acute dystonia after alfentanil in untreated Parkinson's disease. *Anesth Analg* 72:557–558, 1991.

369. Riley D: Disulfiram induced dystonia. *Mov Disord* 7:188–192, 1992.

370. Riley D: Pallidal and putaminal lesions resulting from disulfiram intoxication. *Mov Disord* 6:166–170, 1991.

371. Krauss JK, Mohadjer M, Wakhlo AK, et al: Dystonia and akinesia due to pallidoputaminal lesions after disulfiram intoxication. *Mov Disord* 6:166–170, 1991.

372. Brady W, Hall K: Erythromycin-related dystonic reaction. *Am J Emerg Med* 10:616, 1992.

373. Achumba JI, Ette E, Thomas WO, Essien EE: Chloroquine-induced acute dystonic reactions in the presence of metronidazole. *Drug Intell Clin Pharm* 22:308–310, 1988.

374. Miller LG, Jankovic J: Persistent dystonia possibly induced by flecainide. *Mov Disord* 7:62–63, 1992.

375. Kapur V, Barber KR, Peddireddy R: Ranitidine-induced acute dystonia. *Am J Emerg Med* 17:258–260, 1999.

376. Davis BJ, Aull EA, Granner MA, Rodnitzky RL: Ranitidine-induced cranial dystonia. *Clin Neuropharmacol* 17:489–491, 1994.

377. Peiris RS, Peckler BF: Cimetidine-induced dystonic reaction. *J Emerg Med* 21:27–29, 2001.

378. Oterino A, Pascual J: Sumatriptan-induced axial dystonia in a patient with cluster headache. *Cephalalgia* 18:360–361, 1998.

379. Lopez M, Ferrer C, Bernacer B: Akathisia and acute dystonia induced by sumatriptan. *J Neurol* 244:131–133, 1997.

380. Saneto RP, Fitch JA, Cohen BH: Acute neurotoxicity of meperidine in an infant. *Pediatr Neurol* 14:339–341, 1996.

381. Micheli FE, Fernandez MM, Giannaula R: Movement disorders and depression due to flunarizine and cinnarizine. *Mov Disord* 4:139–146, 1989.

382. Kawakami T, Takiyama Y, Yanaka I, et al: Chronic bromvalerylurea intoxication: Dystonic posture and cerebellar ataxia due to nonsteroidal anti-inflammatory drug abuse. *Intern Med* 37:788–791, 1998.

383. Brashear A, Siemers E: Focal dystonia after chemotherapy: A case series. *J Neurooncol* 34:163–167, 1997.

384. Ghadirian A, Annable L, Belanger MC, Chouinard G: A cross-sectional study of parkinsonism and tardive dyskinesia in lithium-treated affective disordered patients. *J Clin Psychiatry* 57:22–28, 1996.

385. Mascias J, Perez OS, Chaverri D, Mora JS: Distonia aguda secundaria a tratamiento ccon betahistina. *Neurologia* 15:417, 2000.

386. Frumkin H: Multiple system atrophy following chronic carbon disulfide exposure. *Environ Health Perspect* 106:611–613, 1998.

IV. CHOREATIC DISORDERS

HUNTINGTON'S DISEASE

Chapter 34

GENETICS AND MOLECULAR BIOLOGY OF HUNTINGTON'S DISEASE

JAMES F. GUSELLA and MARCY E. MACDONALD

HISTORY AND EPIDEMIOLOGY   571
GENETIC LINKAGE APPROACH   571
GENETIC AND PHYSICAL MAPPING OF THE
   HD REGION   572
MINIMIZING THE CANDIDATE REGION
   WITH HISTORICAL RECOMBINATIONS   574
IDENTIFICATION OF THE HD DEFECT   575
CHARACTERISTICS OF THE CAG REPEAT   575
CLINICAL CORRELATES OF CAG REPEAT
   LENGTH   576
STRUCTURE AND EXPRESSION OF THE
   HD GENE   578
OTHER POLYGLUTAMINE
   NEURODEGENERATIVE DISORDERS   579
MECHANISM OF ACTION OF THE HD
   DEFECT   580
HD AS A CONFORMATIONAL DISORDER   580
MODELING THE GENETICS OF HD IN THE
   MOUSE   581
CLINICAL CONSEQUENCES: DIAGNOSIS   581
CLINICAL CONSEQUENCES: PROSPECTS
   FOR THERAPY   583

History and Epidemiology

In 1872, George Huntington described a unique ailment involving characteristic involuntary movements that begin insidiously, usually in middle age, and progress gradually until the victim is consumed by full-blown chorea.[1] His description was based on his observations of families with the disorder in his clinical practice as a family physician in East Hampton, on Long Island, New York. As members of the same families had been cared for by his father and grandfather, who were also physicians, Huntington was attuned to the inherited nature of the peculiar disorder. He described frequent transmission of the defect from either an affected mother or an affected father to offspring, with no skipping of generations. Huntington also noted that "if by any chance these children go through life without it, the thread is broken and the children and great grandchildren of the original shakers may rest assured that they are free from the disease." This pattern of transmission was recognized as the result of

a Mendelian autosomal-dominant defect by Osler in 1908.[2] Indeed, Vessie[3] later traced many of the Long Island families to immigrants from Bures, England, who landed in New England in 1649, confirming Huntington's description of this hereditary chorea as "an heirloom from generations away back in the dim past." George Huntington's accurate, lucid, and succinct description of this nightmarish affliction led to its appellation of Huntington's chorea, subsequently changed to Huntington's disease (HD), as its manifestations are not limited to loss of motor control.

Although Huntington believed that the disorder existed only in eastern Long Island, it is now known to be widespread throughout the world. The prevalence is highest in populations of western European ancestry, in which 4–7 persons/100,000 are affected.[4] However, the actual disease gene frequency is 2.5–3 times higher, as HD typically has its onset only in midlife, and, at any given time, two-thirds of gene carriers have yet to become symptomatic. The prevalence is relatively consistent across Europe and in other regions of the world that have populations of western European descent, with the exception of Finland, where a significantly lower rate reflects this population's restricted genetic origin. HD is also seen in Africans and Asians, although with a much lower prevalence.

Many of the early studies of HD concentrated on its familial nature, documenting large kindreds in which the defect was passed from generation to generation. HD, as an autosomal-dominant disorder, is transmitted equally from males and females, and both sexes have a 50:50 chance of inheriting the defect. The disease gene is highly penetrant, but onset is variable, ranging from early childhood to late in life. As most cases manifest in middle age, the HD gene is often passed on to children before the parent is aware of the disorder. The rare cases of juvenile onset (<15 years of age) are usually inherited from an affected father.[5,6]

HD is untreatable, and its victims are condemned to slow, inexorable progression of their disease that ends in death 10–20 years after onset. The progression of the motor symptoms of HD is accompanied by intellectual decline and psychiatric alterations, all of which are ultimately due to a selective loss of neurons in the brain. The most prominent region affected is the striatum, where medium-sized spiny neurons are lost along the posteroanterior, dorsoventral, and mediolateral axes, leading to destruction of the archictecture of the caudate nucleus.[7]

Genetic Linkage Approach

The high penetrance, late onset, and characteristic clinical manifestations, which combine to produce large identifiable disease families (Fig. 34-1), made this disorder the ideal candidate for pioneering a novel strategy that emerged in the early 1980s for establishing the chromosomal location of a genetic defect.[8] This approach relied on merging the tenets of Mendelian inheritance with the power of recombinant DNA technology, using naturally occurring variations in

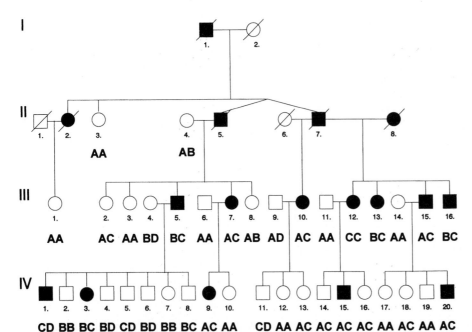

FIGURE 34-1 An idealized HD pedigree showing cosegregation of *D4S10* with the disorder. An imaginary four generation (I-IV) HD pedigree is shown with genotypes for the *D4S10* marker (4 alleles: A, B, C, D) shown under the symbol for each living family member. In each generation, the family members are numbered sequentially. Circles and squares denote females and males, respectively. Slashed symbols indicate deceased individuals. Filled symbols represent those individuals clinically diagnosed with HD. Individuals II-5 and II-7 are monozygotic twins. The disorder is segregating in this pedigree with the C allele of *D4S10*. As this marker displays 4 percent recombination with HD, all individuals who inherit the C allele from their affected parent have a 96 percent chance of also having inherited the HD defect. Individual II-8 is an HD-affected individual who married into the pedigree and, with II-7, produced progeny at risk of having two copies of the HD defect.

DNA sequence as highly informative genetic markers to search for genetic linkage with the disease gene. The goal was to discover a polymorphic DNA marker that co-segregates with the disorder in families and thereby infers the presence of the disease gene in the same chromosomal vicinity. It would then be possible to identify the genetic defect on the basis of its chromosomal location, without any additional knowledge of its biochemical nature.

Previous genetic linkage studies of HD had used a limited panel of expressed polymorphic systems, blood group antigens, and serum enzymes that permitted only 15 percent of the autosomal genome to be searched.[9] The concept of DNA markers offered a potential route to making the remaining 85 percent of the genome accessible to examination, but only a handful of DNA markers had been described. These were restriction fragment-length polymorphisms (RFLP), detected by using single-copy human DNA clones to probe genomic DNA blots for variations in restriction fragment size that reflected differences in the primary DNA sequence. As RFLP markers were generated, they were tested for genetic linkage to HD in two large pedigrees, one of American and one of Venezuelan origin. In 1983, success came quickly, as one of the initial 13 RFLP markers tested revealed strong genetic linkage to the disorder[10] (see Fig. 34-1). This marker, *D4S10*, consisting of two *Hind*III polymorphisms detected by an

anonymous DNA probe (G8), placed *HD* (the Huntington's disease gene) on the short arm of chromosome 4 (Fig. 34-2). There were no crossovers between the marker and *HD*, either in a large section of the Venezuela pedigree or in the independent American HD family with 14 affected members, producing odds of greater than 100 million to 1 in favor of genetic linkage. This was the first example of mapping a genetic defect to a human chromosome using only genetic linkage to a DNA polymorphism, without any prior clue to the disease gene's location. This approach has been replicated subsequently in a host of different disorders and has become increasingly sophisticated as newer and more informative markers have been elaborated, and the human genetic map has become increasingly detailed. The success of the linkage strategy, and the opportunities that it created for isolating disease genes via their chromosomal location, provided a major impetus for undertaking the Human Genome Initiative to map and sequence the human genome.

Genetic and Physical Mapping of the HD Region

The anonymous DNA marker, *D4S10*, genetically linked to *HD*, was initially assigned to chromosome 4 by hybridization

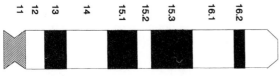

Chromosome 4 Short Arm

D4S10 linkage	1983
D4S10 mapping	1985
Linkage with 4p16.1 markers	1987
Contradictory recombinants	1989
Linkage disequilibrium	1991
Haplotype analysis	1992
HD gene identification	*HD* 1993

FIGURE 34-2 Progressive narrowing of the HD gene search. In 1983, genetic linkage with *D4S10* assigned the HD gene to chromosome 4. The horizontal lines below the schematic diagram of the chromosome 4 short arm depict the chronology of the HD search (1983–1993), as the candidate region was progressively narrowed using the techniques listed and described in the text.

of the G8 probe to a panel of human × mouse somatic cell hybrid lines that had segregated various human chromosomes.[10] The marker was then regionally assigned to the terminal cytogenetic band of the chromosome 4 short arm, because it was hemizygous (present in a single copy) in patients with Wolf-Hirschhorn syndrome, a congenital anomaly caused by heterozygous deletion on 4p.[11] Several groups later confirmed this assignment by in situ hybridization to metaphase chromosomes.[12–14] Genotyping of HD families revealed that the HD gene is located on chromosome 4 in all of the families tested, yielding no evidence of other genes that can cause both the clinical symptoms and neuropathological correlates of HD (nonallelic heterogeneity).[15] These same investigations made HD the first genetic disorder in man established to be completely dominant. Several individuals who were homozygous for the HD defect, having inherited a disease allele from both parents, were found to be clinically indistinguishable from typical heterozygous HD gene carriers.[16,17] This surprising result indicated that, in HD heterozygotes, the remaining normal allele does not act to delay the disease process or to alter its manifestation, and two doses of the defective gene are not significantly more damaging than a single dose.

The position of the HD defect relative to the cytogenetic map could be determined only indirectly, by linkage analysis with *D4S10* and other surrounding DNA markers. *HD* and *D4S10* displayed 4 percent recombination, placing the disease gene within about 4×10^6 base pairs (bp) of DNA either centromeric or telomeric to the DNA marker (Fig. 34-2). DNA markers were identified centromeric to *D4S10* in 4p16, using Wolf-Hirschhorn patients with different extents of 4p16 deletion. When the highly polymorphic 4p16.1 marker

RAF1P1 (then known as *RAF2*) was typed in the same HD kindreds as *D4S10*, it revealed additional crossovers, indicating that the disease gene must be located telomeric to both DNA markers.[18] This assigned the HD gene to the 4p16.3 subband, between *D4S10* and the short-arm telomere, a segment corresponding to about 0.2 percent of the genome, or 6 million bp of DNA (Fig. 34-2).

The chromosomal localization of the HD gene, and, subsequently, many other genetic defects, created the need to improve standard mapping methods and to develop new techniques to clone genes based on their map location, without a knowledge of the protein defect involved. As with the DNA marker linkage approach, the search for the HD gene also acted as the proving ground for several of these technologies. The initial stages of more detailed mapping in 4p16.3 were aided by the construction of regional somatic cell hybrid panels that permitted rapid assignment and ordering of new DNA probes to several regions of 4p16.[19,20] These hybrid panels acted as a backbone on which more sophisticated approaches, such as radiation hybrid mapping[21,22] and pulsed-field gel electrophoresis,[23] could be appended. Numerous novel sources of DNA probes, including phage libraries of flow-sorted chromosome 4 DNA, chromosome 4-enriched somatic cell hybrid genomic libraries, chromosome "jumping" libraries, *Not*I "linking" clones, P1 clones, yeast artificial chromosome clones, combined with pulsed-field gel electrophoresis, and somatic cell hybrid mapping eventually produced a physical map that spanned 5×10^6 bp in 4p16.3 (Fig. 34-2).[24–26]

Because the HD gene had been assigned to 4p16.3, using only genetic linkage techniques, and because there was no physical rearrangement of the region associated with the disorder, the only means of locating the defect on the physical map was to construct a parallel genetic map by tracking the inheritance of informative DNA markers through normal and HD pedigrees. Although RFLP markers, like *D4S10*, were used initially, successive generations of newer, more informative markers were added to the map as they emerged. First, variable numbers of tandem repeat (VNTR) markers, detected like RFLPs by DNA blotting but displaying many different potential restriction fragment sizes as a result of variation in the copy number and, therefore, length, of a repeated DNA motif located between two restriction sites, were found to be particularly frequent in telomeric regions like 4p16.[27,28] Later, the advent of the polymerase chain reaction permitted the easy use of simple-sequence repeats (SSR), di-, tri-, and tetranucleotide repeat, varying in repeat unit number, as highly informative multi-allele polymorphisms.[29,30] The genetic map of 4p16.3 was anchored to the physical map by DNA sites common to both, revealing that the 5×10^6 bp of DNA between *D4S10* and *D4S90* in 4p16.3 spanned 6 percent recombination.[31–33] However, there was a striking difference between the apparent distance between markers suggested by the genetic map and their actual separation on the physical map. Markers located within a 300–400-kb genetic "hot spot" immediately telomeric to *D4S10* revealed far more recombination than expected, such that this small physical interval accounted for more than one-half of the genetic distance of the entire 4p16.3 genetic map.[32] The remaining segment between *D4S125* and the telomere spans at least 4 Mb of physical distance but shows only 2.6 percent recombination.

In the absence of a physical benchmark, such as a deletion or translocation, to precisely position the disease gene within the linked segment, genetic crossovers between 4p16.3 DNA markers and the disease gene in HD families remained the only potential route to defining the DNA segment containing the defect. The success of this strategy depends on unequivocal diagnosis of the disorder in affected individuals, on accurate DNA typing, and on the frequency of double, as opposed to single, crossovers on HD chromosomes. *HD* was readily mapped beyond the "hot spot" of increased recombination telomeric to *D4S10*, as most crossovers with the defect occurred within this interval. However, the position of the disease gene in the remaining 3.5×10^6 of the physical map was not so easily discerned, as several genetic events in well-defined HD pedigrees yielded contradictory implications concerning its location.[31,34] Initially, a few diagnosed individuals in well-defined HD pedigrees were found to possess only marker alleles characteristic of the affected parent's normal chromosome. These events, in which no evidence of marker-marker crossover was seen, suggested that *HD* must be located in the telomeric 100-kb segment of the chromosome, beyond all informative DNA markers then available. However, several other HD cases were subsequently discovered that predicted a location closer to *D4S10*, as markers in the terminal 1.5×10^6 bp of the chromosome showed crossover with *HD*, whereas markers in the 2.5×10^6 bp telomeric to *D4S10* did not. Thus, the two classes of apparent recombination events implied mutually exclusive locations for the defect (Fig. 34-2).

One explanation for this genetic conundrum was the possibility of double recombination in the latter cases, with the chromosome switching back to the HD version telomeric to the final marker (*D4S142*) in the terminal 100 kb predicted by former events. This scenario led to the isolation of the entire segment between *D4S142* and the telomere of an HD chromosome as a yeast artificial chromosome (YAC).[35] Analysis of this DNA was complicated by the presence of subtelomeric repeat sequences and by sequence similarities to acrocentric chromosomes.[36] No evidence was found for a double crossover or for the presence of genes that could cause HD. Mounting evidence (see below) gradually favored the internal region of 4p16.3 as the site of the HD gene, but an explanation for the apparent crossovers that predicted this telomeric location had to await the identification of the genetic defect. Pulsed-field gel mapping initially produced a long-range physical map spanning the 2.5×10^6 bp of this internal region, which was subsequently isolated as overlapping clone sets, first of YACs and later of cosmids.[23–26]

Minimizing the Candidate Region with Historical Recombinations

With genetic recombination having failed to provide a single, unequivocal site for the HD gene, innovative genetic strategies were required to progress with the search. The observation that some markers in the internal 4p16.3 segment displayed allele association with HD implicated this region as the site of the defect and provided the opportunity for a more powerful approach to localizing it.[37,38] Certain alleles for *D4S95* and *D4S98* RFLPs were frequently represented on HD chromosomes than expected from their frequency on normal chromosomes. This was presumed to be a result of the presence of these alleles on the original chromosome 4 that underwent an HD mutation, with an insufficient number of subsequent generations to return the markers to their equilibrium frequencies. A comprehensive analysis of 4p16.3 DNA markers revealed the patterns of allele association to be quite complex.[39] Markers with evident allele association were interspersed on the physical map with sites that showed no association with HD. This supported the view that the current pool of HD chromosomes reflects more than one independent HD mutation or primordial chromosome. It also suggested that if HD chromosomes could be grouped based on their mutational ancestry, the identification of a minimum cluster of shared marker alleles of 4p16.3 might pinpoint the location of the genetic defect.

The implementation of this novel approach was feasible because of the emergence of VNTR and SSR markers with a sufficiently large array of alleles to discriminate many potential primordial haplotypes.[40] Haplotype analysis unearthed evidence for a multitude of independent HD

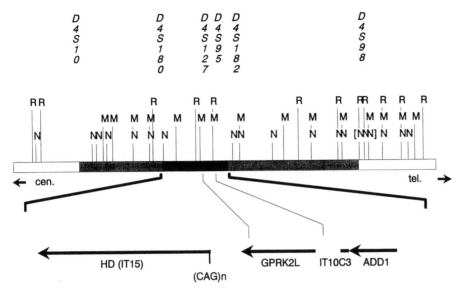

FIGURE 34-3 Isolation of HD candidate gene from the region of haplotype sharing. The long-range restriction enzyme map of $\sim 3 \times 10^6$ bp of the central portion of 4p16.3 is shown, with the progressively narrowing candidate region denoted by increasing intensity of shading. The unshaded region was eliminated by recombination events in HD families, placing the defect within the region between the DNA markers *D4S10* and *D4S98*. Initial haplotype analysis placed the defect in the 500-kb segment between DNA markers *D4S180* and *D4S182*. Candidate genes from this region are depicted below the map. Detailed haplotype analysis eventually narrowed the search to the interval of darkest shading, targeting the search to the 5' end of the IT15 gene. This proved to contain the HD defect as an unstable, expanded CAG trinucleotide repeat (CAG)n. R, *Nru*I site; M, *Mlu*I site; N, *Not*I site; cen., centromeric direction; tel., telomeric direction.

mutations, with 78 HD chromosomes exhibiting 26 different haplotypes within the region of maximal linkage disequilibrium, around *D4S127* and *D4S95*. The most frequent HD haplotype accounted for about one-third of HD chromosomes, and the initial assessment of decay in strength of linkage disequilibrium within this class of chromosomes predicted a most likely location for *HD* in the 500-kb region between *D4S180* and *D4S182* (Figs. 34-2 and 34-3).

Identification of the HD Defect

A set of overlapping cosmid clones between *D4S180* and *D4S182* acted as the source of genomic DNA for exon amplification, a novel approach for identifying candidate genes that takes advantage of the splicing signals bordering exons to permit rapid and efficient isolation of the small proportion of genomic DNA that codes for proteins. This strategy identified a number of candidate genes:[41–43] *ADD1*, encoding alpha-adducin, a protein that participates in organizing the actin-spectrin cytoskeletal lattice; *IT10C3*, a probable small-molecule transporter with similarity to the tetracycline efflux proteins of *Escherichia coli*; *GPRK2L*, a G protein-coupled receptor kinase; and several anonymous genes with no similarity to previously described sequences (Fig. 34-3). Scanning of the full coding sequence of the first three candidates revealed no evidence of abnormalities or sequence differences specific to HD. Similarly, examination of the genomic

segment spanned by each of these genes failed to disclose any alteration on disease chromosomes, with the exception of one report that mistakenly interpreted a rare Alu repeat sequence insertion within an intron of *ADD1* in two individuals as causative of HD.[44] This change was relegated to the status of a rare polymorphism by the discovery of the actual HD defect that had emerged from investigation of IT15, one of the anonymous candidate genes.[45]

Continued haplotype analysis with markers in the *D4S180*-*D4S182* interval, particularly a codon deletion polymorphism in the very long IT15 transcript, refined the size of the candidate region as additional HD chromosomes, previously thought to be unrelated, were exposed to belong to the most common haplotype class, based on sharing of a small segment of 150 kb immediately centromeric to *D4S95* (Fig. 34-3). This finding, which represented the ultimate distillation of the genetic approach, targeted the search for the defect to the extreme 5' end of IT15. The culmination of the location cloning strategy came in 1993 with the discovery of an expanded, unstable trinucleotide repeat with the sequence CAG as the cause of HD (Fig. 34-4).[46]

Characteristics of the CAG Repeat

The IT15 CAG repeat on normal chromosomes is polymorphic, ranging from 6 to 34 units (Fig. 34-5), and is inherited in a Mendelian fashion.[47,48] Adjacent to the CAG trinucleotide

```
Normal HD cDNA sequence          ATGGCGACCCTGGAAAAGCTGATGAAGGCCTTCGAGTCCCTCAAGTCCTTCCAGCAGCAGCAG
Normal huntingtin sequence    1  MetAlaThrLeuGluLysLeuMetLysAlaPheGluSerLeuLysSerPheGlnGlnGlnGln


Expanded disease CAG segment     CAGCAGCAGCAGCAGCAGCAGCAGCAGCAGCAGCAGCAGCAGCAGCAGCAGCAGCAGCAGCAG
Insert in disease huntingtin     GlnGlnGlnGlnGlnGlnGlnGlnGlnGlnGlnGlnGlnGlnGlnGlnGlnGlnGlnGlnGln


Normal HD cDNA sequence          CAGCAGCAGCAGCAGCAGCAGCAGCAGCAGCAGCAGCAGCAGCAGCAACAGCCGCCACCG
Normal huntingtin sequence   22  GlnGlnGlnGlnGlnGlnGlnGlnGlnGlnGlnGlnGlnGlnGlnGlnGlnGlnProProPro


Normal HD cDNA sequence          CCGCCGCCGCCGCCGCCGCCTCCTCAGCTTCCTCAGCCGCCGCCGCAGGCACAGCCGCTGCTG
Normal huntingtin sequence   43  ProProProProProProProProGlnLeuProGlnProProProGlnAlaGlnProLeuLeu


Normal HD cDNA sequence          CCTCAGCCGCAGCCGCCCCCGCCGCCGCCCCCGCCGCCACCCGGCCCGGCTGTGGCTGAGGAG
Normal huntingtin sequence   64  ProGlnProGlnProProProProProProProProProGlyProAlaValAlaGluGlu


Normal HD cDNA sequence          CCGCTGCACCGACCAAAGAAAGAACTTTCAGCTACC-->+ 9,141 bases
Normal huntingtin sequence   85  ProLeuHisArgProLysLysGluLeuSerAlaThr-->+ 3,047 amino acids
```

FIGURE 34-4 The N-terminal sequence of huntingtin encoded by the 5′ end of the HD gene. The huntingtin cDNA 5′ coding sequence for a normal allele is shown above the amino acids (1–96) specified by each codon. This normal allele produces a huntingtin protein with 22 consecutive glutamine (Gln) residues. The effect of the HD mutation is shown as an inserted sequence of an additional 21 CAG repeats, encoding 21 Gln residues.

stretch is a segment of consecutive CCG codons that is also polymorphic, varying from 6 to 12 repeat units.[49] The CCG alleles are also inherited in a Mendelian fashion but show strong linkage disequilibrium in HD, as more than 90 percent of disease chromosomes have 7 CCG units.[50] The CAG repeat of disease chromosomes is expanded, ranging from 37 to more than 100 units (Fig. 34-5). By contrast with the normal CAG alleles and with the CCG repeat, the HD CAG alleles do not show Mendelian inheritance. Rather, they change in length, becoming either shorter or longer, when passed to progeny from either a male or a female parent (Fig. 34-6). In most cases,

the magnitude of the changes is small (<6 repeat units), with a bias toward repeat length increases, but fathers sometimes transmit alleles with larger expansions, up to a doubling or more in the number of CAG units.[47] The different allele sizes among progeny of an HD gene carrier are reflected in similar variation in DNA prepared from sperm, although the normal alleles in these individuals remain identical in somatic and sperm DNA.[51] It has not yet been established at what stage in spermatogenesis this HD-specific variation occurs, what biological parameters (e.g., parental age, disease status, etc.) may affect it, whether all HD alleles of a given CAG length are equally unstable, and whether the degree of instability can be altered by the surrounding haplotype. Similar CAG repeat variation, albeit of reduced magnitude, is expected to occur in HD oogenesis but has not yet been demonstrated directly.

By contrast with gametic variation, the expanded HD CAG repeat exhibits very limited somatic alteration for most repeat lengths.[51–54] For example, several pairs of identical twins have been shown to possess repeats of identical length. For the very longest HD alleles (>60 CAG units), somatic changes may be more frequent, but these do not correlate with neuropathology. Surprisingly, decreases in the number of CAG units in these cases may be most pronounced in the cerebellum, although this region is relatively insensitive to the pathological effects of the mutation.

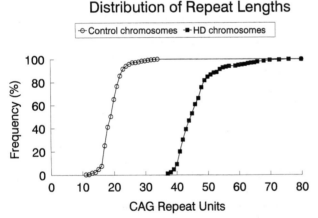

FIGURE 34-5 The cumulative distribution of CAG repeat lengths on HD and normal chromosomes. The frequency of CAG allele sizes on normal (circles) and disease (squares) chromosomes determined in Ref. 154 is depicted as a cumulative distribution for each.

Clinical Correlates of CAG Repeat Length

After the cloning of the HD gene, a plethora of reports analyzed the CAG repeat in cohorts of individuals with a clinical

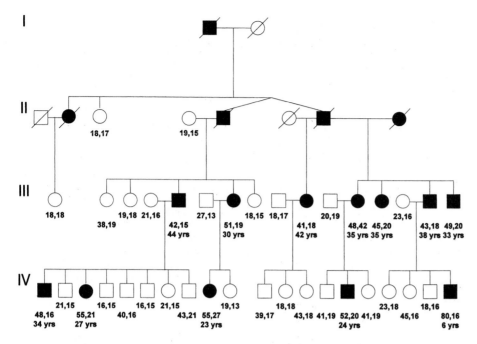

FIGURE 34-6 CAG repeat lengths and age of onset in the idealized HD pedigree. The same pedigree shown in Fig. 34-1 is displayed with CAG repeat length for both alleles (larger allele shown first by convention) under each symbol. For those individuals who are symptomatic, age of onset (in years) is also shown. Of the 4 progeny who were potential HD homozygotes, only the eldest possesses two HD alleles with CAG repeat lengths of 48 and 42, respectively. Juvenile onset has occurred in the youngest member of the pedigree in generation IV, because of an HD allele with 80 CAG units, whereas the eldest member of generation III remains asymptomatic with an HD allele of 38 CAG repeats.

diagnosis of HD.[48] In all studies, the vast majority of patients possessed a CAG repeat in the expanded size range, attesting to the universality of this mutational mechanism of HD in many races, nationalities, and ethnic groups. In some studies, a number of HD-diagnosed individuals did not possess an expanded CAG allele, but careful analysis of one such data set showed that the majority of these can be explained as sample mix-ups, laboratory errors, or erroneous diagnoses based on atypical features.[55] The latter category is well-established to exist, based on the absence of HD-like neuropathology in a small percentage of postmortem brains from individuals with a clinical diagnosis of HD.

As almost all cases of HD are familial, the disorder has traditionally been viewed as having a very low rate of new mutation. Support for this notion came in the failure of the few sporadic cases to meet stringent criteria for new mutation status, including absence of disease in elderly parents, proof of paternity, and disease transmission. The linkage disequilibrium approach used in the search for the HD gene provided the first evidence that new mutations to HD do occur, as the many different 4p16.3 haplotypes on HD chromosomes indicated independent origins for some chromosomes.[40] Identification of the HD CAG repeat has provided a direct genetic test of whether sporadic cases of HD-like symptoms are a result of new mutations. Indeed, sporadic cases with classic HD symptoms display an expanded CAG repeat in the HD size range.[46,56,57] Interestingly, their unaffected relatives who have the same chromosome possess a CAG repeat that is intermediate between the size ranges associated with normal and HD chromosomes. Several cases of HD new mutation have occurred on a chromosome bearing the major HD haplotype, that shared by one-third of HD

chromosomes. This indicates that many of the HD families with this major haplotype may share a common ancestor who was not in fact affected with the disorder. Chromosomes with intermediate alleles on this and other haplotype backgrounds thus represent a reservoir from which new sporadic HD cases may arise.

The complement of the clinical HD studies is the analysis of postmortem brain tissue, in which HD neuropathology has been documented. In a study of 310 brains assessed for HD neuropathology, using the grading system of Vonsattel et al.,[7] only 3 were found not to have an expanded CAG repeat.[58] Examination of the clinical records in these 3 cases revealed numerous features atypical of HD, suggesting a distinct disorder. Consequently, use of a combination of clinical and neuropathological criteria to assign a diagnosis of HD yields a collection of cases that all display an expanded CAG allele. If another type of mutation, either at the *HD* locus or elsewhere in the genome, can cause the same constellation of clinical and neuropathological features typically associated with HD, then it is quite rare.

Before the identification of the HD defect, family studies had established that inheritance of the HD defect invariably produced the disorder but with significant variation in clinical presentation. The most dramatic example is the manifestation of HD in juveniles in some cases of paternal transmission of the defect. The nature of the HD mutation has explained much of this variation, including the effect of paternal inheritance, as there is a strong inverse correlation between CAG repeat length and age at onset of neurological symptoms (Fig. 34-7) in all populations examined.[48] The increased magnitude of size changes in spermatogenesis dictates that paternal transmissions are the

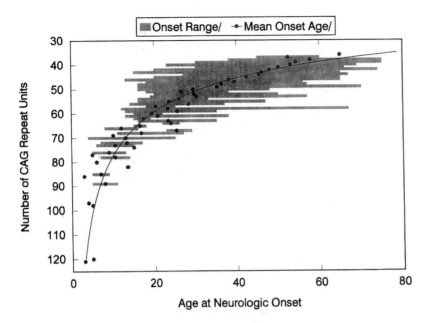

FIGURE 34-7 Inverse correlation between onset age and CAG repeat length. Published age at onset data for 1070 HD patients were used to calculate the average age at onset associated with any given repeat length. This mean age at onset (filled circles) and the associated range of onset ages (shaded bars) are plotted against CAG repeat length with curve fitting by power regression. A highly significant inverse correlation ($r = -0.87$, $P < 0.00001$) between age at onset of neurological symptoms and CAG repeat length occurs across all HD alleles. However, in the adult-onset age group, there is a very wide range of possible ages of onset associated with any given repeat length, precluding its use in predicting the timing of the disorder in individual cases.

major source of the long CAG repeats that underlie juvenile onset.

The assessment of neurological onset and, to an even greater degree, psychiatric onset, has been viewed as prone to considerable subjective error. However, inverse correlations of CAG repeat length with age at onset of both neurological and psychiatric symptoms and with the objective parameter, age at death, are evident even when clinical data are contributed by many independent reporting physicians from different areas.[58] About one-half of the variation in age at onset and death is explained by CAG repeat length, as there can be significant differences between individual patients with identical HD alleles, presumably because of modifying factors, such as interacting genes, environmental influences, or stochastic events. Indeed, normal genetic variation at the GRIK2 locus, encoding a glutamate receptor subunit, has been reported in three independent studies to explain a small amount of the variance in HD age at onset.[59–61] The question as to whether rate of progression also varies with repeat length is more complicated, as studies comparing CAG repeat with functional decline have been in conflict.[62–66] The result may depend on the particular measures of progression that are used as neuropathological severity clearly increases with CAG repeat length.[67,68] However, if duration from onset of motor symptoms to patient death is used as a measure, CAG length has little or no effect.[69]

Structure and Expression of the HD Gene

The HD CAG repeat is located in exon 1 of a 67-exon gene, 17 codons downstream from the initiator ATG.[45] The gene is transcribed in a telomere-to-centromere orientation and encodes a protein of more than 3140 amino acids named huntingtin.[46] The CAG repeat produces a polymorphic segment of consecutive glutamine residues, adjacent to a set of proline residues encoded by the CCG repeat. Huntingtin's function is not known. Its sequence is not closely related to other proteins but shows a high degree of evolutionary conservation relative to mouse, rat, pig, zebrafish, and pufferfish homologs[70–75] and a much lower similarity to the homolog in the fruitfly.[76,77] No huntingtin homologs have been discovered in yeast or nematodes. Pufferfish huntingtin, for example, is 73 percent identical to human huntingtin, with the homology segregated into numerous patches likely to represent regions most critical for function. Interestingly, the most evolutionarily divergent segment is the polyglutamine-polyproline stretch, encoded by the adjacent CAG and CCG repeats. The normal human gene encodes 12–36 glutamines, whereas the pig, rat, mouse, zebrafish, and pufferfish genes, respectively, encode 18, 8, 7, 4, and 4 glutamines at the equivalent location in the protein. The human glutamine segment is followed by a region of 42 amino acids that includes 29 prolines. The corresponding regions of pig, rat, and mouse huntingtins have 27, 28, and 27 prolines of 35, 36, and 35 residues, respectively, while zebrafish and pufferfish huntingtins have only 1 or 2 prolines, respectively, out of 4 residues. The Drosophila huntingtin has no glutamine or proline repeats in the region. These comparisons suggest that the long polyglutamine and polyproline segments are not essential for huntingtin's most fundamental normal functions.

The sequence of huntingtin protein contributed to the definition of a new protein domain, termed HEAT for its presence in huntingtin, elongation factor 3, protein phosphatase 2A, and yeast TOR1.[78] HEAT motifs do not show strong sequence conservation, but appear structurally to represent two alpha-helices separated by a nonhelical linker. They are typically found in tandem arrays, such as in the PP2A PR65/A subunit and β-importin, which are entirely composed of 15 and 19 HEAT repeats, respectively. The crystal structures of these proteins reveal that tandem HEATs can form a flexible solenoid structure that provides a binding surface to act as a scaffold in bringing together interacting proteins.[79–84] Huntingtin was originally reported to have 10 HEAT repeats in three different locations in the protein, with the three near its N-terminus being the most evolutionarily conserved.[78] However, recent analysis has revealed that all huntingtins are largely made up of HEAT-like sequences, perhaps explaining the absence of other notable functional domains, and suggesting that huntingtin's normal function is as a scaffold or carrier of multiple protein partners.[77] Indeed, molecular biological and biochemical analyses have indicated that huntingtin, especially at its N-terminus, can interact with more than three dozen different proteins, including transcription factors, cytoskeletal components, and a variety of proteins involved in intracellular trafficking.[85–99] However, huntingtin's precise normal functions remain uncertain.

Huntingtin is expressed widely in both neural and nonneural (e.g., kidney, liver, lymphoblast, lung, heart, etc.) tissues based on studies of both mRNA and protein, suggesting that its normal function is not confined to cells in the areas of HD neuropathology.[100–108] Antisera against the N-terminal peptide encoded 5′ to the CAG stretch have provided direct evidence that the CAG repeat is translated, as they react with the same large ~350-kDa Western blot band detected by antisera raised against C-terminal regions.[104,106–108] The size change caused by the expanded CAG of the disease allele permits normal and HD isoforms of huntingtin to be distinguished by sodium dodecyl sulfate (SDS)-polyacrylamide gel electrophoresis. Cell fractionation experiments have indicated that huntingtin is a protein principally found in the cytoplasm, although it is capable of shuttling to and from the nucleus.[107,109]

Different antihuntingtin antibodies reveal different patterns of localization, suggesting that either the corresponding epitopes may be accessible or hidden, depending on the protein complex containing huntingtin, or that the protein can undergo conformational changes, consistent with a flexible solenoid structure, depending on its modifications or binding partners.[109,110] Immunocytochemical localization of huntingtin in rat, monkey, and human brain tissues, has shown that the pattern of huntingtin expression does not parallel the regions of HD neuropathology.[104,105,108] Thus, the neuronal target cells that succumb to the effects of the HD defect represent only a small subset of the neural and nonneural cell populations that actually express the mutant protein.

Other Polyglutamine Neurodegenerative Disorders

Several other neurodegenerative disorders (Fig. 34-8) are also caused by expanded trinucleotide repeats and show striking

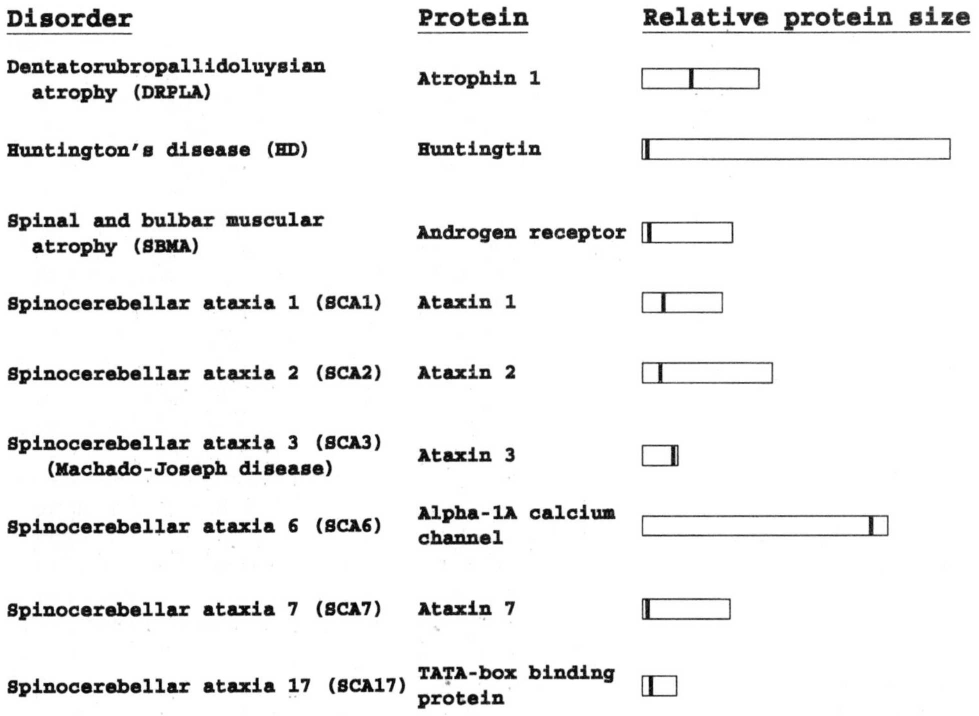

Disorder	Protein	Relative protein size
Dentatorubropallidoluysian atrophy (DRPLA)	Atrophin 1	
Huntington's disease (HD)	Huntingtin	
Spinal and bulbar muscular atrophy (SBMA)	Androgen receptor	
Spinocerebellar ataxia 1 (SCA1)	Ataxin 1	
Spinocerebellar ataxia 2 (SCA2)	Ataxin 2	
Spinocerebellar ataxia 3 (SCA3) (Machado-Joseph disease)	Ataxin 3	
Spinocerebellar ataxia 6 (SCA6)	Alpha-1A calcium channel	
Spinocerebellar ataxia 7 (SCA7)	Ataxin 7	
Spinocerebellar ataxia 17 (SCA17)	TATA-box binding protein	

FIGURE 34-8
Neurodegenerative disorders caused by translated expanded CAG trinucleotide repeats. Nine polyglutamine neurodegenerative disorders are listed with the name of the corresponding protein. The relative size of each protein is shown as a box to the right, with the location of the polyglutamine tract denoted by a vertical black line.

genetic similarities with HD.[111] In each case, a normally poly-morphic CAG repeat is expanded and unstable on disease chromosomes, with the onset of the neurological symptoms beginning only above a threshold CAG repeat length, which can be lower or higher than the ~35 CAGs required in HD. The CAG repeat is located within the coding sequence of the respective gene, predicting an altered protein with an extended stretch of consecutive glutamine residues. Hence, these disorders have been grouped with HD under the term "polyglutamine neurodegenerative disorders." In each, a different pattern of neuronal cell loss results from the CAG expansion mutation. Most strikingly, in every disorder there is a strong negative correlation between CAG repeat length and age at onset of neurological symptoms, supporting a common fundamental mechanism.

Mechanism of Action of the HD Defect

While the precise mechanism of action of the HD defect is not certain, much has been learned since the cloning of the disease gene and some significant possibilities have been ruled out. The expanded CAG repeat does not drastically alter tran-scription of the HD gene, as huntingtin mRNA is expressed at comparable levels from the disease and normal alleles.[45,112] Similarly, the ability to distinguish HD and normal huntingtin based on electrophoretic mobility has revealed that the defect does not prevent translation of the mRNA. Thus, the lack of transcriptional and translational effects suggests that the HD defect acts through the altered structure of huntingtin and its extended polyglutamine segment.

The lengthened polyglutamine stretch does not cause HD by simply eliminating huntingtin's activity, as there is direct genetic evidence in both man and mouse that disruption of this gene does not produce disease symptoms. In humans, individuals with an HD gene translocation that eliminates 50 percent of huntingtin production do not develop HD.[45] Similarly, mice with one copy of the HD gene homolog (Hdh) inactivated by targeted mutagenesis show no abnormality.[113,114] Interestingly, transgenic mice expressing a novel truncated version of murine huntingtin's N-terminus display pathology in the subthalamic nucleus and develop behavioral anxieties, suggesting that truncated versions of normal huntingtin may have neuronal consequences.[115] However, homozygosity for complete inactivation of the mouse gene results in early embryonic death, before develop-ment of the nervous system, which is in sharp contrast with the adult-onset neuropathology in humans.[113,114] The mouse experiments establish that huntingtin activity is essential for normal development. Thus, the existence of adult individuals homozygous for an expanded CAG allele indicates that the HD mutation does not simply remove huntingtin's normal activity.

The most probable mechanism of HD pathogene-sis is a "gain of function," in which the lengthened polyglutamine segment confers a new property on the protein. Genotype-phenotype studies relating CAG repeat length with age at neurological onset in HD patients dic-tate a number of criteria for this "gain of function" and the fundamental mechanism that triggers the disorder.[111] Investigations of heterozygous HD patients indicate that the disease-initiating mechanism requires a threshold glutamine tract length, is progressively more severe above that length, and is dominant over normal huntingtin. As individuals who possess two mutant HD alleles (HD homozygotes), and conse-quently no normal HD allele, do not show earlier onset than equivalent HD heterozygotes, the "gain of function" mech-anism is insensitive to the presence or absence of normal huntingtin and is much more sensitive to increasing poly-glutamine length than huntingtin concentration. Finally, the comparison of HD with the other polyglutamine neurode-generative disorders indicates that the deleterious effect of the polyglutamine tract achieves its neuronal specificity due to its being presented in the context of the huntingtin protein, either because of the protein's structure, localization/interactions or inherent activity.

HD as a Conformational Disorder

Evidence has accumulated that the "gain of function" in HD is a novel conformational property of the huntingtin protein that matches the genetic criteria described above. This con-formational property has been most extensively studied in model systems in the context of a small N-terminal fragment of huntingtin, but it probably acts in the human patient at the level of the full-length mutant huntingtin protein.[111,116]

That polyglutamine tracts are predisposed to form beta-sheet structures was first proposed on theoretical grounds by Perutz et al.[117] It was later demonstrated experimentally that an N-terminal fragment of mutant huntingtin corresponding to exon 1 of the HD gene had the capacity to form insoluble aggregates with the characteristics of amyloid.[118,119] A sim-ilar fragment, when expressed in transgenic mice, produced large intranuclear inclusions in neurons throughout the brain and in cells in the periphery and resulted in premature death of the animal.[120,121] These observations have led to a massive literature exploring the effects of forced expression of poly-glutamine and various polyglutamine-containing fragments on a variety of cultured cells, yeast, worms, flies, and mice.[122] Polyglutamine itself has typically been directly toxic, whereas its inclusion in a short huntingtin fragment has led to intracel-lular aggregates, either in the cytoplasm or in the nucleus, but not always to outright toxicity. In the heavily studied R6/2 line of transgenic mice, which express an HD exon 1 fragment encoding more than 125 glutamines, neuronal loss compa-rable to HD does not occur, although various measures of neuronal dysfunction and the early death of the mouse signify a significant toxic effect of the transgene. The demonstration that cultured cells expressing similar fragments can con-tain visible inclusions that are not always SDS-insoluble and may have different staining characteristics using huntingtin antibodies indicates that there are different routes by which the polyglutamine can lead to inclusion formation.[111]

Interestingly, in vitro, the conversion from soluble to insoluble fragment involves a conformational change in the fragment that is dependent on having a polyglutamine tract length greater than the threshold characteristic of HD disease alleles.[119] The rate and extent of aggregate formation also increases with polyglutamine length, is relatively more responsive to increased glutamine length than to fragment concentration, and is dominant over fragment with normal CAG tract lengths, incorporating some of the normal fragment into mutant-initiated aggregates. The fulfillment of the genetic criteria suggests that the conformational property of polyglutamine that promotes aggregation in the context of a small fragment is the same property that causes the disease. In at least one cell system, the criteria are also met for inclusion formation by overexpressed N-terminal fragment.[123] These observations suggest that the conformational property participates in the triggering of pathogenesis in HD patients. However, in vivo, the property probably first acts when the polyglutamine tract is still contained within the full-length huntingtin protein where it is restricted from producing aggregates but may alter protein-protein interactions that lead to the specific vulnerability of striatal neurons.[111,116,124]

Modeling the Genetics of HD in the Mouse

The well-defined genetic lesion in HD has permitted the construction by a number of laboratories of precise genetic models of HD, in which the expanded CAG tract has been inserted by "knock-in" technology into the homologous mouse gene (*Hdh*).[125–129] Longer CAG alleles in the endogenous mouse gene display gametic instability, although the distribution of size changes is somewhat different from that seen in human gametogenesis.[126,129,130] The precise genetic models express full-length mutant huntingtin at normal physiological levels in a tissue pattern comparable to wild-type huntingtin. The mutant huntingtin is functional in development, as it fully rescues the embryonic lethality of *Hdh* null "knock-out" alleles.[125] Moreover, other engineered mice displaying either globally reduced huntingtin expression or elimination of huntingtin expression in selected populations of adult neurons have revealed a postembryonic role for huntingtin in neurogenesis,[125,131] and in the maintenance of adult neurons.[132] Defects in neither of these are seen in mice either heterozygous or homozygous for mutant *Hdh* alleles expressing full-length mutant huntingtin with glutamine tract lengths that are associated with adult onset or juvenile onset in man.

While the mutant huntingtin in these mice effectively replaces the function of wild-type huntingtin, it also appears to possess a "gain of function" property that fulfills all of the genetic criteria for participation in the initiation of HD pathogenesis, including striatal specificity.[116,133–135] The knock-in

mice display a series of subtle, progressive phenotypes staged across the entire lifespan. At a few weeks of life, a subset of the huntingtin protein in striatal neurons becomes more apparent in the nucleus and begins to disappear from the cytoplasm. This redistribution of huntingtin staining progresses, with apparent accumulation of full-length huntingtin in the nucleus and is followed over the ensuing 2 years by a series of histological and biochemical changes that include alterations in gene expression, energy metabolism, cellular signaling, eventual appearance of N-terminal huntingtin fragment and nuclear inclusions, and, late in life, evidence for dysfunctional degenerating neurons. Similar findings have been derived with transgenic mice expressing full-length human mutant huntingtin from a modified YAC clone.[136,137]

These precise genetic knock-in models of HD argue that the process of pathogenesis is a long one that is time-dependent, rather than developmental-stage dependent, and that the lifespan of the mouse is insufficient to reproduce the full 1–2 decade course of the disorder in humans. Rather, these mice appear to model presymptomatic HD, with deleterious consequences first resulting from expression of full-length mutant huntingtin. Interestingly, the progressive phenotypes that the mice display raise the likelihood that other features of huntingtin may participate downstream in the pathogenic pathway to accelerate the demise of the vulnerable neuronal cells. For example, in vulnerable neurons CAG repeat instability is eventually detected that would be expected to produce mutant huntingtin with even longer polyglutamine tracts than those in the inherited allele.[133,138] This potential for increasing the severity of the triggering mechanism has received some support from CAG instability measured in post-mortem HD brain,[139] and from the demonstration that, in the mice, the DNA repair enzyme MSH2 is a genetic modifier of the progressive phenotypes.[140] Similarly, the eventual appearance of nuclear inclusions suggests that cleavage of huntingtin later in the disease process may reduce the beneficial effects of its normal activities,[141–144] which have been suggested to be antiapoptotic, and introduce the deleterious effects of N-terminal mutant fragment. The former is consistent with the suggestion that symptomatic progression may be accelerated in HD homozygotes.[145] Evidence supporting the latter comes from the accelerated appearance of phenotypes in mice with both a knock-in *Hdh* mutant allele and an N-terminal mutant transgene,[133] from the implication of a ubiquitin hydrolase gene as a genetic modifier of onset age in man,[61] and from the detection of inclusions and insoluble aggregate in HD brain.[146]

Clinical Consequences: Diagnosis

The major impact of molecular biology on clinical care of HD has so far been the capacity to perform predictive testing, determining whether asymptomatic individuals born "at risk" because of a parent with HD have, in fact, inherited the defect. The discovery of DNA markers for HD in 1983

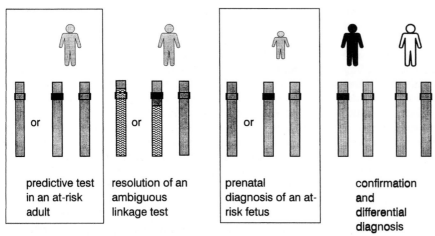

predictive test
in an at-risk
adult

resolution of an
ambiguous
linkage test

prenatal
diagnosis of an at-
risk fetus

confirmation
and
differential
diagnosis

FIGURE 34-9 Applications of molecular diagnosis. A schematic diagram is shown to illustrate the clinical uses of direct measurement of CAG repeats. An expanded CAG repeat is depicted by a black box on one chromosome. The normal allele is denoted by an unfilled box. CAG repeat measurement distinguishes between normal and HD chromosomes in predictive testing of "at-risk" individuals, including those who have received an ambiguous result from the HD linkage test because of recombination between the markers and the disease gene. CAG repeat length can also provide prenatal diagnosis in at-risk pregnancies and is of value in confirming or refuting the clinical diagnosis of HD in atypical or difficult cases.

made it possible to perform presymptomatic or prenatal diagnostic testing for some interested individuals. However, the test was cumbersome and prone to various forms of inaccuracy, as it required tracing genetically linked markers through several related family members, at least one of whom was clinically affected. Thus, it was only applicable to at-risk individuals for whom several family members were able and willing to donate their DNA. This newfound ability to predict the future presence of a devastating, untreatable neurological disorder in a currently unaffected individual raised numerous ethical dilemmas that were debated at length. Pilot testing programs began cautiously, with a heavy emphasis on counseling both before and after delivery of the test result.[147–149] A high level of psychological and emotional support was built in because of the potentially calamitous consequences of a positive test result in a disorder with psychiatric disturbances and the lack of a precedent for determining ability to cope with such information. This experience led to the establishment of formal guidelines sanctioned by the International Huntington Association (IHA) and by the World Federation of Neurology (WFN) to ensure ethical administration of predictive testing.[150] This precedent has become an increasingly important guide, as genetic defects have been found in numerous other late-onset human disorders, including the other CAG repeat diseases referred to above.

The discovery of the nature of the genetic defect in HD has revolutionized the technical aspects of predictive testing, providing an inexpensive method that can be applied to any at-risk individual, without the critical need for DNA from relatives. CAG repeat measurement can also be applied to prenatal testing for confirmation of a clinical diagnosis of HD and for differential diagnosis in difficult cases (Fig. 34-9).

Although direct assay of CAG length is more accurate and more widely applicable than the former linkage test, the essential nature of the information being obtained remains the same. Thus, the IHA-WFN guidelines remain in force, revised to take into account the nature of direct testing.[151]

Despite the improvement in the testing procedure, there remain complicating factors that must be considered in applying CAG repeat measurement to disease prediction. Alleles low in the HD range are sometimes nonpenetrant within a typical lifespan.[152] Moreover, chromosomes from unaffected members of the rare "new mutation" families can possess high "normal" alleles whose potential for causing HD symptoms if these individuals have a sufficiently long life.[46,55,56] Indeed, there may be no precise border between chromosomes that cause HD and those that do not, as modifying factors become paramount in determining onset for alleles low in the HD range. Moreover, potential gametic instability of alleles high in the "normal" range must be taken into account in counseling potential parents with such alleles. Thus, alleles in the high "normal" and low HD ranges represent dilemmas for predictive testing of at-risk individuals and for assessing the potential risk of transmitting HD.[153]

A second consideration in using the CAG assay for predictive testing derives from the linkage studies aimed at delineating the HD candidate region. As noted above, several clinically diagnosed individuals in different HD pedigrees yielded marker genotypes characteristic of the normal chromosome from the corresponding affected parent, confusing the localization of the defect by predicting a second candidate region.[31,34] Discovery of the HD CAG mutation permitted resolution of this genetic conundrum. Despite the presence of expanded trinucleotide repeats in all other affected members of these HD families, the exceptional individuals had only normal alleles. Thus, these individuals appear to have another movement disorder mistakenly diagnosed as HD because of an extensive family history. Such cases can be expected to occur at a low frequency in families undergoing presymptomatic testing. The fact that a negative HD test does not exclude the future occurrence of another movement disorder should be conveyed to at-risk individuals.

Finally, the strong inverse correlation between age at onset and CAG repeat length raises special problems in delivering the results of the HD CAG test.[154] Every HD test that yields an allele in the established disease range can be considered diagnostic of the future onset of the disorder. However, despite the precision with which the number of CAG units can be measured, the CAG length cannot be considered an accurate predictor of age at onset in any individual case, because the range of ages at onset observed for any particular repeat length is far too extensive to make such predictions meaningful. Effective communication of the dubious prognostic value of CAG length for each at-risk individual represents another significant challenge for genetic counselors dealing with this disorder.

Although delivery of the HD predictive test has become more practical and experience with its associated genetic counseling has grown, many at-risk individuals choose not to undergo testing. Despite its reduced cost, increased accuracy, and wider applicability, the CAG repeat test shares the major drawback of the linkage test: nothing can yet be done to prevent the disease in those found to carry the defective gene. Without an effective treatment, the predictive test is a mixed blessing.

Clinical Consequences: Prospects for Therapy

Over the past 20 years, molecular biology has brought us to identification of HD's primary defect, and, while it has yet to define precisely its biochemical mechanism, it has revealed numerous targets for development of potential therapies. Overall, the findings are consistent with a disease course in which the first abnormality, which remains to be identified, is triggered by expression of full-length mutant protein and leads over a long period of time to progressive debilitation of individual neurons which eventually begin to cleave retained nuclear huntingtin and accumulate nuclear inclusions prior to neuronal death.[111,116,124,133–135] Consequently, potential rational treatments can be considered at various levels. If possible, eliminating the expression of mutant huntingtin would clearly be effective, but would require continued expression of wild-type huntingtin for neuronal maintenance. Interfering directly with the conformational property conferred by the expanded polyglutamine might also prevent triggering of the pathogenic pathway. Once triggered, treatments aimed at correcting the biochemical alterations that

occur require precisely defining these targets, but might include boosting mitochondrial energy metabolism, providing general neuroprotectants, modulating proteosome-mediated protein degradation, and inhibiting the enzymes that lead to huntingtin cleavage and apoptosis. Once neuronal cells have been lost, treatment options would appear to be limited to preventing further damage and possibly replacing function via neuronal implants.

Recently, there has been an increasing recognition that screening for small molecules as potential therapeutics, formerly the province mainly of industry, must also occur in academia, particularly for rare disorders.[155,156] The use of screening assays based on targets emerging from HD research to identify small molecules for testing in preclinical models and eventually in HD gene carriers is the best hope for translating the advances in our understanding of the disorder into effective treatments. The recognition that the conformational property of expanded polyglutamine tracts can be measured by its capacity to promote aggregation of small fragments[118,119] has led to assays to identify drugs that block the fundamental "gain of function" in HD.[157,158] Although none of these has yet reached clinical testing, they represent a major hope for delaying or preventing the neuronal loss in this devastating disorder and in the other polyglutamine disorders that are triggered by the same conformational property.

References

1. Huntington G: On chorea. *Med Surg Rep* 26:317, 1872.
2. Osler W: Historical note on hereditary chorea, in Browning W (ed): *Neurographs*. Brooklyn, NY: Albert C Huntington Publishing, 1908, vol 1, pp 113–116.
3. Vessie PR: On the transmission of Huntington's chorea for 300 years: The Bures family group. *J Nerv Ment Dis* 76:553, 1932.
4. Harper PS: The epidemiology of Huntington's disease. *Hum Genet* 89:365, 1992.
5. Merritt AD, Conneally PM, Rahman NF, Drew AL: Juvenile Huntington's chorea, in Barbeau A, Brunette TR (eds): *Progress in Neurogenetics*. Amsterdam: Excerpta Medica Foundation, 1969, pp 645–650.
6. Bird ED, Caro AJ, Pilling JB: A sex related factor in the inheritance of Huntington's chorea. *Ann Hum Genet* 37:255, 1974.
7. Vonsattel JP, Myers RH, Stevens TJ, et al: Neuropathologic classification of Huntington's disease. *J Neuropathol Exp Neurol* 44:559, 1985.
8. Gusella JF: DNA polymorphism and human disease. *Annu Rev Biochem* 55:831, 1986.
9. Pericak-Vance MA, Conneally PM, Merritt AD, et al: Genetic linkage studies in Huntington disease. *Cytogenet Cell Genet* 22:640, 1978.
10. Gusella JF, Wexler NS, Conneally PM, et al: A polymorphic DNA marker genetically linked to Huntington's disease. *Nature* 306:234, 1983.
11. Gusella JF, Tanzi RE, Bader PI, et al: Deletion of Huntington's disease-linked G8 (*D4S10*) locus in Wolf-Hirschhorn syndrome. *Nature* 318:75, 1985.

12. Zabel BU, Naylor SL, Sakaguchi AY, Gusella JF: Mapping of the DNA locus *D4S10* and the linked Huntington's disease gene to 4p16-p15. *Cytogenet Cell Genet* 42:187, 1986.

13. Wang HS, Greenberg CR, Hewitt J, et al: Subregional assignment of the linked marker G8 (*D4S10*) for Huntington's disease to chromosome 4p16.1-16.3. *Am J Hum Genet* 39:392, 1986.

14. Landegent JE, Jansen IN, De Wal N, et al: Fine mapping of the Huntington disease linked D4S20 locus by non-radioactive in situ hybridization. *Hum Genet* 73:354, 1986.

15. Conneally PM, Haines JL, Tanzi RE, et al: Huntington disease: No evidence for locus heterogeneity. *Genomics* 5:304, 1989.

16. Wexler NS, Young AB, Tanzi RE, et al: Homozygotes for Huntington's disease. *Nature* 326:194, 1987.

17. Myers RH, Leavitt J, Farrer LA, et al: Homozygote for Huntington's disease. *Am J Hum Genet* 45:615, 1989.

18. Gilliam TC, Tanzi RE, Haines JL, et al: Localization of the Huntington's disease gene to a small segment of chromosome 4 flanked by D4S10 and the telomere. *Cell* 50:565, 1987.

19. Smith B, Skarecky D, Bengtsson U, et al: Isolation of DNA markers in the direction of the Huntington disease gene from the G8 locus. *Am J Hum Genet* 42:335, 1988.

20. MacDonald ME, Anderson MA, Gilliam TC, et al: A somatic cell hybrid panel for localizing DNA segments near the Huntington's disease gene. *Genomics* 1:29, 1987.

21. Doucette-Stamm LA, Riba L, Handelin B, et al: Generation and characterization of irradiation hybrids of human chromosome 4. *Somat Cell Mol Genet* 17:471, 1991.

22. Altherr MR, Plummer S, Bates GP, et al: Radiation hybrid map spanning the Huntington disease gene region of chromosome 4. *Genomics* 13:1040, 1992.

23. Bucan M, Zimmer M, Whaley WL, et al: Physical maps of 4p16.3, the area expected to contain the Huntington's disease mutation. *Genomics* 6:1, 1990.

24. Bates GP, MacDonald ME, Baxendale S, et al: Defined physical limits of the Huntington disease gene candidate region. *Am J Hum Genet* 49:7, 1991.

25. Bates GP, Valdes J, Hummerich H, et al: Characterisation of a YAC contig spanning the Huntington's disease gene candidate region. *Nat Genet* 1:180, 1992.

26. Baxendale S, MacDonald ME, Mott R, et al: Construction of cosmid contigs and high resolution restriction maps of a 2 megabase region containing the Huntington's disease gene. *Nat Genet* 4:181, 1993.

27. Wasmuth JJ, Hewitt J, Smith B, et al: A highly polymorphic locus very tightly linked to the Huntington's disease. *Nature* 332:73, 1988.

28. MacDonald ME, Cheng SV, Zimmer M, et al: Clustering of multi-allele DNA markers near the Huntington's disease gene. *J Clin Invest* 84:1013, 1989.

29. Taylor SAM, Barnes GT, MacDonald ME, Gusella JF: A dinucleotide repeat polymorphism at the D4S127 locus. *Hum Mol Genet* 1:147, 1992.

30. Tagle DA, Blanchard-McQuate L, Valdes J, et al: Dinucleotide repeat polymorphism in the Huntington's disease region at the D4S182 locus. *Hum Mol Genet* 2:489, 1993.

31. MacDonald ME, Haines JL, Zimmer M, et al: Recombination events suggest possible locations for the Huntington's disease gene. *Neuron* 3:183, 1989.

32. Allitto BA, MacDonald ME, Bucan M, et al: Increased recombination adjacent to the Huntington's disease-linked *D4S10* marker. *Genomics* 9:104, 1991.

33. Youngman S, Sarafarazi M, Bucan M, et al: A new DNA marker (*D4S90*) is terminally located on the short arm of chromosome 4 close to the Huntington's disease gene. *Genomics* 5:802, 1989.

34. Robbins C, Theilmann J, Youngman S, et al: Evidence from family studies that the gene causing Huntington disease is telomeric to *D4S95* and *D4S90*. *Am J Hum Genet* 44:422, 1989.

35. Bates GP, MacDonald ME, Baxendale S, et al: A YAC telomere clone spanning a possible location of the Huntington's disease gene. *Am J Hum Genet* 46:762, 1990.

36. Youngman S, Bates GP, Williams S, et al: The telomeric 60 kb of chromosome arm 4p is homologous to telomeric regions on 13p, 15p, 21p and 22p. *Genomics* 14:350, 1992.

37. Snell RG, Lazarou L, Youngman S, et al: Linkage disequilibrium in Huntington's disease: An improved localization for the gene. *J Med Genet* 26:673, 1989.

38. Theilmann J, Kanani S, Shiang R, et al: Non-random association between alleles detected at *D4S95* and *D4S98* and the Huntington's disease gene. *J Med Genet* 26:676, 1989.

39. MacDonald ME, Lin C, Srinidhi L, et al: Complex patterns of linkage disequilibrium in the Huntington disease region. *Am J Hum Genet* 49:723, 1991.

40. MacDonald ME, Novelletto A, Lin C, et al: The Huntington's disease candidate region exhibits many different haplotypes. *Nat Genet* 1:99, 1992.

41. Taylor SAM, Snell RG, Buckler A, et al: Cloning of the alpha-adducin gene from the Huntington's disease candidate region of chromosome 4 by exon amplification. *Nat Genet* 2:223, 1992.

42. Duyao MP, Taylor SAM, Buckler AJ, et al: A gene from the Huntington's disease candidate region with similarity to a superfamily of transporter proteins. *Hum Mol Genet* 2:673, 1993.

43. Ambrose C, James M, Barnes G, et al: A novel G protein-coupled receptor kinase cloned from 4p16.3. *Hum Mol Genet* 1:697, 1992.

44. Goldberg PY, Rommens JM, Andrew SE, et al: Identification of an Alu retrotransposition event in close proximity to a strong candidate gene for Huntington's disease. *Nature* 362:370, 1993.

45. Ambrose CM, Duyao MP, Barnes G, et al: Structure and expression of the Huntington's disease gene: Evidence against simple inactivation due to an expanded CAG repeat. *Somat Cell Mol Genet* 20:27, 1994.

46. Huntington's Disease Collaborative Research Group: A novel gene containing a trinucleotide repeat that is expanded and unstable on Huntington's disease chromosomes. *Cell* 72:971, 1993.

47. Gusella JF, MacDonald ME: Huntington's disease. *Semin Cell Biol* 6:21, 1995.

48. Gusella JF, MacDonald ME: Huntington's disease: CAG genetics expands neurobiology. *Curr Opin Neurobiol* 5:656, 1995.

49. Rubinsztein DC, Barton DE, Davison BCC, Ferguson-Smith MA: Analysis of the Huntington gene reveals a trinucleotide-length polymorphism in the region of the gene that contains two CCG-rich stretches and a correlation between decreased age of onset of Huntington's disease and CAG repeat number. *Hum Mol Genet* 2:1713, 1993.

50. Andrew SE, Goldberg YP, Theilmann J, et al: A CCG repeat polymorphism adjacent to the CAG repeat in the Huntington disease gene: Implications for diagnostic accuracy and predictive testing. *Hum Mol Genet* 3:65, 1994.

51. MacDonald ME, Barnes G, Srinidhi J, et al: Gametic but not somatic instability of CAG repeat length in Huntington's disease. *J Med Genet* 30:982, 1993.

52. De Rooij KE, De Konig Gans PA, et al: Somatic expansion of the (CAG)*n* repeat in Huntington disease brains. *Hum Genet* 95:270, 1995.

53. Zuhlke C, Riess O, Bockel B, et al: Mitotic stability and meiotic variability of the (CAG)*n* repeat in the Huntington disease gene. *Hum Mol Genet* 2:2063, 1993.

54. Telenius H, Kremer B, Goldberg YP, et al: Somatic and gonadal mosaicism of the Huntington disease gene CAG repeat in brain and sperm. *Nat Genet* 6:409, 1994; published erratum appears in *Nat Genet* 7:113, 1994.

55. Andrew SE, Goldberg YP, Kremer B, et al: Huntington disease without CAG expansion: Phenocopies or errors in assignment? *Am J Hum Genet* 54:852, 1994.

56. Myers RH, MacDonald ME, Koroshetz WJ, et al: De novo expansion of a (CAG)*n* repeat in sporadic Huntington's disease. *Nat Genet* 5:168, 1993.

57. Goldberg YP, Kremer B, Andrew SE, et al: Molecular analysis of new mutations for Huntington's disease: Intermediate alleles and sex of origin effects. *Nat Genet* 5:174, 1993.

58. Persichetti F, Srinidhi J, Kanaley L, et al: Huntington's disease CAG trinucleotide repeats in pathologically confirmed post-mortem brains. *Neurobiol Dis* 1:159, 1994.

59. Rubinsztein DC, Leggo J, Chiano M, et al: Genotypes at the GluR6 kainate receptor locus are associated with variation in the age of onset of Huntington disease. *Proc Natl Acad Sci U S A* 94:3872, 1997.

60. MacDonald ME, Vonsattel JP, Shrinidhi J, et al: Evidence for the GluR6 gene associated with younger onset age of Huntington's disease. *Neurology* 53:1330, 1999.

61. Wintermeyer P, Kruger R, Kuhn W, et al: Mutation analysis and association studies of the UCHL1 gene in German Parkinson's disease patients. *Neuroreport* 11:2079, 2000.

62. Kieburtz K, MacDonald M, Shih C, et al: Trinucleotide repeat length and progression of illness in Huntington's disease. *J Med Genet* 31:872, 1994.

63. Illarioshkin SN, Igarashi S, Onodera O, et al: Trinucleotide repeat length and rate of progression of Huntington's disease. *Ann Neurol* 36:630, 1994.

64. Squitieri F, Cannella M, Simonelli M: CAG mutation effect on rate of progression in Huntington's disease. *Neurol Sci* 23(suppl 2):S107, 2002.

65. Brandt J, Bylsma FW, Gross R, et al: Trinucleotide repeat length and clinical progression in Huntington's disease. *Neurology* 46:527, 1996.

66. Marder K, Sandler S, Lechich A, et al: Relationship between CAG repeat length and late-stage outcomes in Huntington's disease. *Neurology* 59:1622, 2002.

67. Penney JB Jr, Vonsattel JP, MacDonald ME, et al: CAG repeat number governs the development rate of pathology in Huntington's disease. *Ann Neurol* 41:689, 1997.

68. Furtado S, Suchowersky O, Rewcastle B, et al: Relationship between trinucleotide repeats and neuropathological changes in Huntington's disease. *Ann Neurol* 39:132, 1996.

69. Gusella JF, McNeil S, Persichetti F, et al: Huntington's disease. *Cold Spring Harb Symp Quant Biol* 61:615, 1996.

70. Barnes GT, Duyao MP, Ambrose CM, et al: Mouse Huntington's disease gene homolog (*Hdh*). *Somat Cell Mol Genet* 20:87, 1994.

71. Lin B, Nasir J, MacDonald H, et al: Sequence of the murine Huntington disease gene: Evidence for conservation, alternate splicing and polymorphism in a triplet (CCG) repeat. *Hum Mol Genet* 3:85, 1994; published erratum appears in *Hum Mol Genet* 3:530, 1994.

72. Schmitt I, Baechner D, Megow D, et al: Expression of the Huntington disease gene in rodents: Cloning the rat homologue and evidence for down regulation in non-neuronal tissues during development. *Hum Mol Genet* 4:1173, 1995.

73. Matsuyama N, Hadano S, Onoe K, et al: Identification and characterization of the miniature pig Huntington's disease gene homolog: Evidence for conservation and polymorphism in the CAG triplet repeat. *Genomics* 69:72, 2000.

74. Karlovich CA, John RM, Ramirez L, et al: Characterization of the Huntington's disease (HD) gene homologue in the zebrafish *Danio rerio. Gene* 217:117, 1998.

75. Baxendale S, Abdulla S, Elgar G, et al: Comparative sequence analysis of the human and pufferfish Huntington's disease genes. *Nat Genet* 10:67, 1995.

76. Li Z, Karlovich CA, Fish MP, et al: A putative *Drosophila* homolog of the Huntington's disease gene. *Hum Mol Genet* 8:1807, 1999.

77. Takano H, Gusella JF: The predominantly HEAT-like motif structure of huntingtin and its association and coincident nuclear entry with dorsal, an NF-κB/Rel/dorsal family transcription factor. *BMC Neurosci* 3:15, 2002.

78. Andrade MA, Bork P: HEAT repeats in the Huntington's disease protein. *Nat Genet* 11:115, 1995.

79. Vetter IR, Arndt A, Kutay U, et al: Structural view of the Ran-Importin beta interaction at 2.3 Å resolution. *Cell* 97:635, 1999.

80. Cingolani G, Lashuel HA, Gerace L, Muller CW: Nuclear import factors importin alpha and importin beta undergo mutually induced conformational changes upon association. *FEBS Lett* 484:291, 2000.

81. Cingolani G, Petosa C, Weis K, Muller CW: Structure of importin-beta bound to the IBB domain of importin-alpha. *Nature* 399:221, 1999.

82. Groves MR, Hanlon N, Turowski P, et al: The structure of the protein phosphatase 2A PR65/A subunit reveals the conformation of its 15 tandemly repeated HEAT motifs. *Cell* 96:99, 1999.

83. Groves MR, Barford D: Topological characteristics of helical repeat proteins. *Curr Opin Struct Biol* 9:383, 1999.

84. Chook YM, Blobel G: Structure of the nuclear transport complex karyopherin-beta2-Ran × GppNHp. *Nature* 399:230, 1999.

85. Gusella JF, MacDonald ME: Huntingtin: A single bait hooks many species. *Curr Opin Neurobiol* 8:425, 1998.

86. Faber PW, Barnes GT, Srinidhi J, et al: Huntingtin interacts with a family of WW domain proteins. *Hum Mol Genet* 7:1463, 1998.

87. Passani LA, Bedford MT, Faber PW, et al: Huntingtin's WW domain partners in Huntington's disease post-mortem brain fulfill genetic criteria for direct involvement in Huntington's disease pathogenesis. *Hum Mol Genet* 9:2175, 2000.

88. Modregger J, DiProspero NA, Charles V, et al: PACSIN 1 interacts with huntingtin and is absent from synaptic varicosities in presymptomatic Huntington's disease brains. *Hum Mol Genet* 11:2547, 2002.

89. Holbert S, Dedeoglu A, Humbert S, et al: Cdc42-interacting protein 4 binds to huntingtin: Neuropathologic and biological evidence for a role in Huntington's disease. *Proc Natl Acad Sci U S A* 100:2712, 2003.

90. Holbert S, Denghien I, Kiechle T, et al: The Gln-Ala repeat transcriptional activator CA150 interacts with huntingtin: Neuropathologic and genetic evidence for a role in Huntington's

disease pathogenesis. *Proc Natl Acad Sci U S A* 98:1811, 2001.

91. Kegel KB, Meloni AR, Yi Y, et al: Huntingtin is present in the nucleus, interacts with the transcriptional corepressor C-terminal binding protein, and represses transcription. *J Biol Chem* 277:7466, 2002.

92. Wanker EE, Rovira C, Scherzinger E, et al: HIP-I: A huntingtin interacting protein isolated by the yeast two-hybrid system. *Hum Mol Genet* 6:487, 1997.

93. Hattula K, Peranen J: FIP-2, a coiled-coil protein, links Huntingtin to Rab8 and modulates cellular morphogenesis. *Curr Biol* 10:1603, 2000.

94. Li SH, Cheng AL, Zhou H, et al: Interaction of Huntington disease protein with transcriptional activator Sp1. *Mol Cell Biol* 22:1277, 2002.

95. Sittler A, Walter S, Wedemeyer N, et al: SH3GL3 associates with the Huntingtin exon 1 protein and promotes the formation of polygln-containing protein aggregates. *Mol Cell* 2:427, 1998.

96. Li XJ, Li SH, Sharp AH, et al: A huntingtin-associated protein enriched in brain with implications for pathology. *Nature* 378:398, 1995.

97. Bao J, Sharp AH, Wagster MV, et al: Expansion of polyglutamine repeat in huntingtin leads to abnormal protein interactions involving calmodulin. *Proc Natl Acad Sci U S A* 93:5037, 1996.

98. Boutell JM, Wood JD, Harper PS, Jones AL: Huntingtin interacts with cystathionine beta-synthase. *Hum Mol Genet* 7:371, 1998.

99. Peters MF, Ross CA: Isolation of a 40-kDa Huntingtin-associated protein. *J Biol Chem* 276:3188, 2001.

100. Li SH, Schilling G, Young WS III, et al: Huntington's disease gene (IT15) is widely expressed in human and rat tissues. *Neuron* 11:985, 1993.

101. Strong TV, Tagle DA, Valdes JM, et al: Widespread expression of the human and rat Huntington's disease gene in brain and nonneural tissues. *Nat Genet* 5:259, 1993.

102. Landwehrmeyer GB, McNeil SM, Dure LS IV, et al: Huntington's disease gene: Regional and cellular expression in brain of normal and affected individuals. *Ann Neurol* 37:218, 1995.

103. Hoogeveen AT, Willemsen R, Meyer N, et al: Characterization and localization of the Huntington disease gene product. *Hum Mol Genet* 2:2069, 1993.

104. Sharp AH, Loev SJ, Schilling G, et al: Widespread expression of Huntington's disease gene (IT15) protein product. *Neuron* 14:1065, 1995.

105. DiFiglia M, Sapp E, Chase K, et al: Huntingtin is a cytoplasmic protein associated with vesicles in human and rat brain neurons. *Neuron* 14:1075, 1995.

106. Jou YS, Myers RM: Evidence from antibody studies that the CAG repeat in the Huntington disease gene is expressed in the protein. *Hum Mol Genet* 4:465, 1995.

107. Persichetti F, Ambrose CM, Ge P, et al: Normal and expanded Huntington's disease alleles produce distinguishable proteins due to translation across the CAG repeat. *Mol Med* 1:374, 1995.

108. Trottier Y, Devys D, Imbert G, et al: Cellular localization of the Huntington's disease protein and discrimination of the normal and mutated form. *Nat Genet* 10:104, 1995.

109. Trettel F, Rigamonti D, Hilditch-Maguire P, et al: Dominant phenotypes produced by the HD mutation in STHdh(Q111) striatal cells. *Hum Mol Genet* 9:2799, 2000.

110. Persichetti F, Trettel F, Huang CC, et al: Mutant huntingtin forms in vivo complexes with distinct context-dependent conformations of the polyglutamine segment. *Neurobiol Dis* 6:364, 1999.

111. Gusella JF, MacDonald ME: Molecular genetics: Unmasking polyglutamine triggers in neurodegenerative disease. *Nat Rev Neurosci* 1:109, 2000.

112. Stine OC, Li SH, Pleasant N, et al: Expression of the mutant allele of *IT-15* (the HD gene) in striatum and cortex of Huntington's disease patients. *Hum Mol Genet* 4:15, 1995.

113. Duyao MP, Auerbach AB, Ryan A, et al: Homozygous inactivation of the mouse Hdh gene does not produce a Huntington's disease-like phenotype. *Science* 269:407, 1995.

114. Zeitlin S, Liu JP, Chapman DL, et al: Increased apoptosis and early embryonic lethality in mice nullizygous for the Huntington's disease gene homologue. *Nat Genet* 11:155, 1995.

115. Nasir J, Floresco JB, O'Kusky JR, et al: Targeted disruption of the Huntington's disease gene results in embryonic lethality and behavioral and morphological changes in heterozygotes. *Cell* 81:811, 1995.

116. Wheeler VC, White JK, Gutekunst CA, et al: Long glutamine tracts cause nuclear localization of a novel form of huntingtin in medium spiny striatal neurons in HdhQ92 and HdhQ111 knock-in mice. *Hum Mol Genet* 9:503, 2000.

117. Perutz MF, Johnson T, Suzuki M, Finch JT: Glutamine repeats as polar zippers: Their possible role in inherited neurodegenerative diseases. *Proc Natl Acad Sci U S A* 91:5355, 1994.

118. Scherzinger E, Lurz R, Turmaine M, et al: Huntingtin-encoded polyglutamine expansions form amyloid-like protein aggregates in vitro and in vivo. *Cell* 90:549, 1997.

119. Huang CC, Faber PW, Persichetti F, et al: Amyloid formation by mutant huntingtin: Threshold, progressivity and recruitment of normal polyglutamine proteins. *Somat Cell Mol Genet* 24:217, 1998.

120. Mangiarini L, Sathasivam K, Seller M, et al: Exon 1 of the HD gene with an expanded CAG repeat is sufficient to cause a progressive neurological phenotype in transgenic mice. *Cell* 87:493, 1996.

121. Davies SW, Turmaine M, Cozens BA, et al: Formation of neuronal intranuclear inclusions underlies the neurological dysfunction in mice transgenic for the HD mutation. *Cell* 90:537, 1997.

122. Sipione S, Cattaneo E: Modeling Huntington's disease in cells, flies, and mice. *Mol Neurobiol* 23:21, 2001.

123. Narain Y, Wyttenbach A, Rankin J, et al: A molecular investigation of true dominance in Huntington's disease. *J Med Genet* 36:739, 1999.

124. Gusella J, MacDonald M: No post-genetics era in human disease research. *Nat Rev Genet* 3:72, 2002.

125. White JK, Auerbach W, Duyao MP, et al: Huntingtin is required for neurogenesis and is not impaired by the Huntington's disease CAG expansion. *Nat Genet* 17:404, 1997.

126. Ishiguro H, Yamada K, Sawada H, et al: Age-dependent and tissue-specific CAG repeat instability occurs in mouse knock-in for a mutant Huntington's disease gene. *J Neurosci Res* 65:289, 2001.

127. Lin CH, Tallaksen-Greene S, Chien WM, et al: Neurological abnormalities in a knock-in mouse model of Huntington's disease. *Hum Mol Genet* 10:137, 2001.

128. Menalled LB, Sison JD, Wu Y, et al: Early motor dysfunction and striosomal distribution of huntingtin microaggregates in Huntington's disease knock-in mice. *J Neurosci* 22:8266, 2002.

129. Shelbourne PF, Killeen N, Hevner RF, et al: A Huntington's disease CAG expansion at the murine Hdh locus is unstable and associated with behavioural abnormalities in mice. *Hum Mol Genet* 8:763, 1999.

130. Wheeler VC, Auerbach W, White JK, et al: Length-dependent gametic CAG repeat instability in the Huntington's disease knock-in mouse. *Hum Mol Genet* 8:115, 1999.

131. Auerbach W, Hurlbert MS, Hilditch-Maguire P, et al: The HD mutation causes progressive lethal neurological disease in mice expressing reduced levels of huntingtin. *Hum Mol Genet* 10:2515, 2001.

132. Dragatsis I, Levine MS, Zeitlin S: Inactivation of Hdh in the brain and testis results in progressive neurodegeneration and sterility in mice. *Nat Genet* 26:300, 2000.

133. Wheeler VC, Gutekunst CA, Vrbanac V, et al: Early phenotypes that presage late-onset neurodegenerative disease allow testing of modifiers in Hdh CAG knock-in mice. *Hum Mol Genet* 11:633, 2002.

134. Fossale E, Wheeler VC, Vrbanac V, et al: Identification of a presymptomatic molecular phenotype in Hdh CAG knock-in mice. *Hum Mol Genet* 11:2233, 2002.

135. Gines S, Seong IS, Fossale E, et al: Specific progressive cAMP reduction implicates energy deficit in presymptomatic Huntington's disease knock-in mice. *Hum Mol Genet* 12:497, 2003.

136. Hodgson JG, Agopyan N, Gutekunst CA, et al: A YAC mouse model for Huntington's disease with full-length mutant huntingtin, cytoplasmic toxicity, and selective striatal neurodegeneration. *Neuron* 23:181, 1999.

137. Hodgson JG, Smith DJ, McCutcheon K, et al: Human huntingtin derived from YAC transgenes compensates for loss of murine huntingtin by rescue of the embryonic lethal phenotype. *Hum Mol Genet* 5:1875, 1996.

138. Kennedy L, Shelbourne PF: Dramatic mutation instability in HD mouse striatum: Does polyglutamine load contribute to cell-specific vulnerability in Huntington's disease? *Hum Mol Genet* 9:2539, 2000.

139. Kono Y, Agawa Y, Watanabe Y, et al: Analysis of the CAG repeat number in a patient with Huntington's disease. *Intern Med* 38:407, 1999.

140. Wheeler VC, Lebel LA, Vrbanac V, et al: Mismatch repair gene Msh2 modifies the timing of early disease in Hdh (Q111) striatum. *Hum Mol Genet* 12:273, 2003.

141. Rigamonti D, Bauer JH, De-Fraja C, et al: Wild-type huntingtin protects from apoptosis upstream of caspase-3. *J Neurosci* 20:3705, 2000.

142. Rigamonti D, Sipione S, Goffredo D, et al: Huntingtin's neuroprotective activity occurs via inhibition of procaspase-9 processing. *J Biol Chem* 276:14545, 2001.

143. Zuccato C, Ciammola A, Rigamonti D, et al: Loss of huntingtin-mediated BDNF gene transcription in Huntington's disease. *Science* 293:493, 2001.

144. Hilditch-Maguire P, Trettel F, Passani LA, et al: Huntingtin: An iron-regulated protein essential for normal nuclear and perinuclear organelles. *Hum Mol Genet* 9:2789, 2000.

145. Squitieri F, Gellera C, Cannella M, et al: Homozygosity for CAG mutation in Huntington disease is associated with a more severe clinical course. *Brain* 126:946, 2003.

146. DiFiglia M, Sapp E, Chase KO, et al: Aggregation of huntingtin in neuronal intranuclear inclusions and dystrophic neurites in brain. *Science* 277:1990, 1997.

147. Meissen GJ, Myers RH, Mastromauro CA, et al: Predictive testing for Huntington's disease with use of a linked DNA marker. *N Engl J Med* 318:535, 1988.

148. Brandt J, Quaid KA, Folstein SE, et al: Presymptomatic diagnosis of delayed-onset disease with linked DNA markers: The experience in Huntington's disease. *JAMA* 261:3108, 1989.

149. Wiggins S, Whyte P, Huggins M, et al: The psychological consequences of predictive testing for Huntington's disease. *N Engl J Med* 327:1401, 1992.

150. World Federation of Neurology Research Group on Huntington's Disease: Ethical issues policy statement on Huntington's disease molecular genetics predictive test. *J Med Genet* 27:34, 1990.

151. International Huntington Association and World Federation of Neurology Research Group on Huntington's Chorea: Guidelines for the molecular genetics predictive test in Huntington's disease. *Neurology* 44:1533, 1994.

152. McNeil SM, Novelletto A, Srinidhi J, et al: Reduced penetrance of the Huntington's disease mutation. *Hum Mol Genet* 6:775, 1997.

153. Gasser T, Bressman S, Durr A, et al: State of the art review: Molecular diagnosis of inherited movement disorders. Movement Disorders Society task force on molecular diagnosis. *Mov Disord* 18:3, 2003.

154. Duyao M, Ambrose C, Myers R, et al: Trinucleotide repeat length instability and age of onset in Huntington's disease. *Nat Genet* 4:387, 1993.

155. Heemskerk J, Tobin AJ, Bain LJ: Teaching old drugs new tricks. Meeting of the Neurodegeneration Drug Screening Consortium, 7–8 April 2002, Washington, DC, USA. *Trends Neurosci* 25:494, 2002.

156. Heemskerk J, Tobin AJ, Ravina B: From chemical to drug: Neurodegeneration drug screening and the ethics of clinical trials. *Nat Neurosci* 5(suppl):1027, 2002.

157. Heiser V, Engemann S, Brocker W, et al: Identification of benzothiazoles as potential polyglutamine aggregation inhibitors of Huntington's disease by using an automated filter retardation assay. *Proc Natl Acad Sci U S A* 99(suppl 4):16400, 2002.

158. Heiser V, Scherzinger E, Boeddrich A, et al: Inhibition of huntingtin fibrillogenesis by specific antibodies and small molecules: Implications for Huntington's disease therapy. *Proc Natl Acad Sci U S A* 97:6739, 2000.

Chapter 35

CLINICAL FEATURES AND TREATMENT OF HUNTINGTON'S DISEASE

FREDERICK J. MARSHALL

EPIDEMIOLOGY   589
NATURAL HISTORY   589
CLINICAL FEATURES   590
    Movement Disorder   590
    Cognitive Disorder   591
    Behavioral Disorder   592
    Progressive Functional Decline   592
DIAGNOSIS   593
    Positive Family History 593
    Negative or Absent Family History   594
    Technological Approaches 594
    Genetic Testing   594
TREATMENT   594
    Symptomatic Intervention 594
    Experimental Therapeutics 596

George Huntington first described the cardinal features of "hereditary chorea" in 1872, culling from his own clinical experience and that of his father and grandfather, who preceded him in the rural practice of medicine on Long Island.[1] Huntington's disease (HD) is an autosomal-dominant neurodegenerative disorder characterized clinically by abnormal movements, cognitive decline, behavioral disturbances, and progressive functional deterioration. Gene carriers typically manifest illness in adulthood after normal birth and development.

A cooperative investigative effort beginning in the early 1980s culminated in the characterization of the HD gene (IT15), located near the telomere of the short arm of chromosome 4.[2] The mutant gene contains an excessive number of trinucleotide CAG repeats that code for a polyglutamine stretch in the 348-kDa protein product, referred to as huntingtin. The protein product is widely expressed in both neuronal and nonneuronal tissues.[3–5] Deletions within the region of chromosome 4 encompassing IT15, such as occur in Wolf-Hirschhorn syndrome, do not give rise to the HD phenotype, suggesting that the expanded gene codes for a protein resulting in an abnormal gain of function.[6] A number of transgenic animal models of HD have now been developed,[7–9] and current research on the genetics and pathophysiology of HD is reviewed in detail elsewhere in this volume (Chaps. 34 and 36). This chapter focuses on the clinical features and treatment of HD.

Epidemiology

HD occurs with a worldwide prevalence of approximately 5–10 per 100,000 population.[10] Northern and Southern European, as well as Indian and Central Asian populations, are similarly affected.[11] Some areas have a low frequency of HD, notably Japan (0.1 per 100,000),[12] and Finland (0.5 per 100,00).[13] The highest known concentration of HD is in the state of Zulia, in Venezuela, where a single large family, now numbering more than 10,000 individuals, is thought to be descended from a progenitor who lived on the shores of Lake Maracaibo approximately 200 years ago.[14]

In the US, approximately 25,000 individuals have clinical features of HD, with an additional 125,000 people at risk of developing HD.[10,15] Although analysis of restriction fragment length polymorphisms (RFLP) to determine carrier status became available by the mid-1980s,[16] and direct testing for CAG repeat length has been conducted since 1993,[2] the vast majority of asymptomatic at-risk individuals have not been tested.[17] In the past two decades, nondirective and supportive genetic counseling appears to have lowered the frequency of the HD gene.[18,19]

Natural History

The age at onset of symptoms and the initial clinical manifestations of illness vary widely. The majority of patients have onset of symptoms normally distributed around a mean age of 39 years.[20] Juvenile HD, as defined by onset of illness before age 20 years, accounts for about 5–10 percent of all affected patients.[21,22] Rigidity, dystonia, and bradykinesia are the predominant motor features in juvenile-onset patients, in whom paternal inheritance of the HD gene is more common than in the more typical adult-onset form.[20,23–25]

It is difficult to date the onset of illness precisely, and there is typically a delay of months to years between symptom onset and diagnosis. Patients from the Venezuelan family who were examined annually often showed subtle "soft" neurological signs as much as 5 years or more before manifest illness could be diagnosed.[14,26] Even at an early stage of the disease, subjects with HD have a lower body mass index than matched controls.[27] Subtle psychological and motor deficits and personality changes have been described in "presymptomatic" individuals,[28–31] and there is now evidence for progressive caudate atrophy prior to symptom onset.[32]

Duration of illness also varies considerably around a mean of about 19 years. Most patients survive for 10–25 years after onset of illness.[22] Although juvenile-onset HD may be a risk factor for rapid progression,[33] Roos et al. found no relationship between duration of illness and age at onset in

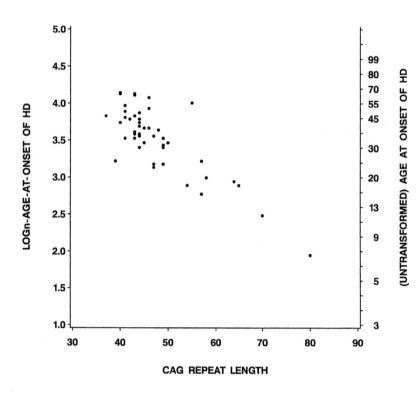

FIGURE 35-1 Relationship between $\log_n$ age-at-onset or untransformed age-at-onset and CAG repeat length in 50 patients with HD. For $\log_n$ age-at-onset versus CAG repeat length, $r = -0.82$, $P < 0.0001$. For untransformed age-at-onset versus-CAG repeat length, $r = -0.69$, $P < 0.001$. *Adapted from Kieburtz et al.*[40]

a retrospective study of 1106 patients.[34] Male patients with affected fathers progressed the fastest in this large study population.

An inverse relationship between CAG repeat length and age at onset of HD has been reported and confirmed.[35-39] This relationship accounts for about 50 percent of the variance in age at onset. A strong correlation persists between very high CAG repeat lengths and juvenile presentation. However, for the majority of gene carriers with CAG repeat lengths ranging from 37 to 52, age at onset varies considerably from 15 to 75 years of age. Therefore, CAG repeat length by itself is not an accurate or sufficient predictor of HD onset.[35] Interestingly, the correlation between the degree of CAG expansion and $\log_n$ age-at-onset appears stronger, suggesting a higher-order relationship between symptom onset and CAG length[40] (Fig. 35-1). There is a clear familial influence on age of onset which is independent from the effect of CAG repeat length.[41]

The relationship between CAG repeat length and clinical progression of illness remains unsettled. Several studies have failed to show a link between CAG repeat length and the mode of presentation or pace of deterioration in HD.[42-44] Others have reported a strong relationship between CAG repeat length and selected clinical outcomes.[45] CAG repeat length was inversely correlated with time to nursing home placement and age at percutaneous endoscopic gastrostomy, independent of age at onset.[46]

As HD advances, patients experience progressive debility and weight loss. Heightened immobility and dysphagia often lead to aspiration pneumonia, a common cause of death. Palliative care plays an important role for people in the late stages of illness.[47] Among 395 affected patients in a Danish study, pneumonia and cardiovascular disease were the most common primary causes of death.[48]

Clinical Features

MOVEMENT DISORDER

CHOREA

The term "chorea" derives from the Greek verb meaning "to dance." Chorea is reminiscent of the continuous, irregular, and fleeting movements of a marionette. In less dramatic forms, chorea may pass for fidgetiness. These movements eventually occur throughout the body, including respiratory, pharyngeal, and laryngeal musculature. Patients may incorporate involuntary choreiform movements into apparently purposeful gestures, a phenomenon referred to as parakinesia. In some patients, chorea may appear as severe uncontrollable flailing of the extremities, or ballism, interfering with the patient's ability to feed, sit in a chair, or sleep in a bed.

Although conspicuous and of cosmetic concern, chorea is not usually disabling. Individuals with relatively severe chorea may be able to function, ambulate, and care for themselves surprisingly well. Bradykinesia, rigidity, dystonia, and postural instability more commonly impair function.

DYSTONIA AND PARKINSONISM

As HD progresses, chorea often gives way to axial posturing (dystonia) and parkinsonian features of bradykinesia, rigidity, and postural instability.[14,49,50] Mild dystonia in combination with chorea gives the writhing appearance of choreoathetosis. Sustained dystonic posturing affecting the neck, trunk, or limbs may result in contractures, immobility, and skin breakdown. Bradykinesia and dystonia, with or without significant rigidity, are often heralding features of juvenile- onset HD.[50]

Progressive postural instability occurs in both juvenile-onset and advanced adult-onset HD. Severe chorea, dystonia, rigidity, postural sway, and disruption of central vestibular reflexes contribute to the progressive balance problems attending HD.[51]

In the terminal stages of illness, patients may become akinetic and rigid, with little or no evidence of chorea. Pyramidal tract signs, such as spasticity, clonus, and extensor plantar responses, may appear.

DYSARTHRIA AND DYSPHAGIA

Deterioration in communication abilities and swallowing also characterizes the advanced stages of illness. Initially, speech may be hypophonic, with irregular rate, rhythm, and pitch in the setting of impaired respiratory coordination. HD patients show variability of utterance duration and/or voice-onset time in tests of acoustic speech signals.[52] As articulation disturbances progress from understandable to unintelligible, the ability to sustain voluntary tongue protrusion is lost.

EYE MOVEMENT ABNORMALITIES

Disordered ocular motility is one of the earliest motor signs of HD.[53,54] Voluntary initiation of ocular saccades becomes slowed and uncoordinated. Patients find it more difficult to suppress head movements, and often blink in order to break fixation and generate a saccadic burst.[55] Smooth pursuit movements are frequently disrupted by saccadic intrusions and impersistence. Initiation of internally generated saccades is more difficult than initiation of externally triggered ones, suggesting a relative sparing of parietosuperior collicular pathways in the setting of extensive damage to frontostriatal circuits.[56] Opticokinetic nystagmus is impaired both vertically and horizontally, although vertical movements are generally affected earlier.[57] Presymptomatic gene carriers exhibit significantly more abnormalities than nongene carriers in overall oculomotor function, saccade velocity and opticokinetic nystagmus,[30] but quantitative oculomotor assessment does not appear to be sufficiently sensitive or specific to distinguish accurately between asymptomatic gene carriers and nongene carriers at risk for HD.[58]

OTHER HYPERKINESIAS

Patients with HD may manifest other movement disorders, such as tics and involuntary vocalizations resembling Tourette's syndrome.[59,60] Some individuals may exhibit myoclonus as a dominant feature of their movement disorder.[61–63] Increasing variability in grip strength has been identified as a marker of disease progression.[64]

COGNITIVE DISORDER

The cognitive and psychiatric features of HD are perhaps the earliest and most important indicators of functional decline.[28,29,65,66] The dementia of HD has been characterized as "subcortical" because of the prominence of bradyphrenia (slowed thinking), and because of attentional and sequencing impairments in the absence of cortical deficits such as aphasia, agnosia, and apraxia.[67,68] Executive function (the ability to plan, sequence, and carry out complex tasks) is thought to be selectively lost, perhaps related to damage to frontostriatal circuits.[69,70]

Paulsen et al. have emphasized that the memory impairment in cortical dementias typically involves deficits of both recognition and recall, whereas recognition is generally spared in patients with subcortical dementia. They found that Alzheimer patients performed poorly on tests of memory function, regardless of the severity of dementia, whereas HD patients performed poorly on tests of initiation (e.g., the double alternating movement task of the Mattis Dementia Rating Scale).[71] These observations are consistent with the findings of other investigators.[72–75] Registration and immediate memory recall are relatively spared in HD patients, whereas retrieval of recent and remote memories is impaired.[76–78] Semantic memory is differentially impacted in Alzheimer's disease and HD.[79]

Neuropsychological tests that appear to be sensitive indicators of disease progression include the Symbol Digit Modalities Test,[80] the Verbal Fluency Subtest of the Multilingual Aphasia Examination,[81] and the Stroop Interference Test.[82] These tests are part of the Unified Huntington's Disease Rating Scale (UHDRS), a battery of motor, cognitive, behavioral, and functional assessments used primarily as a clinical research tool.[83] The Trail Making Test Part B, designed to assess executive functions, may also be useful in characterizing the progressive dementia of HD.[84]

Several investigators have examined the cognitive profile of asymptomatic persons at risk for HD.[31,85,86] Foroud and coworkers administered the Wechsler Adult Intelligence Scale–Revised (WAIS-R) to 394 at-risk individuals who denied symptoms referable to HD. After cognitive testing was complete, CAG repeat length measures revealed that gene carriers generally scored lower on all portions of the WAIS-R than noncarriers. There was an inverse correlation between CAG repeat length in gene carriers and scores on the WAIS-R.[85] These findings suggest that subtle intellectual impairment may antedate overt signs or symptoms of illness.

Cognitive decline is characteristic of HD, but the pace of progression among patients varies considerably.[87,88] Some individuals may remain cognitively intact despite many years of motor impairment. Insight and central language function generally remain preserved, even in the advanced stages of illness.[68,89]

BEHAVIORAL DISORDER

AFFECTIVE ILLNESS

Affective illness is a common presentation for HD,[90] and occurs in as many as 30–50 percent of patients during the course of the illness.[90–93] Individuals at risk for HD are vulnerable to depression, and presymptomatic gene carriers may have subtle impairments of working memory in the context of depression.[94] Depressed patients experience enduring feelings of sadness, worthlessness, or guilt. Anhedonia (the loss of pleasure in activities) is commonly associated with poor concentration, decreased libido, hypersomnia, and psychomotor retardation. Affective disorder may be more prevalent in some families, particularly in those with a relatively late age at onset.[95] Only 10 percent of depressed HD patients experience episodic bouts of mania and agitation characteristic of bipolar disorder.[96]

SUICIDE

George Huntington was aware of the risk of suicide in HD. He noted that "the tendency to insanity, and sometimes that form of insanity which leads to suicide, is marked. I know of several instances of suicide of people suffering from this form of chorea, or who belonged to families in which the disease existed."[1] Suicide is influenced not only by the severity of the affective disorder but also by the degree of functional capacity retained, the level of insight remaining, and the extent of social supports available. Identified risk factors (many of which are interrelated) include childlessness, depression, single marital status, living alone, and other suicides in the family.[97] An increased rate of suicide has also been reported in those at risk for HD.[98–100] In a retrospective study, suicide was nearly as common in 282 asymptomatic siblings (5.3 percent) as it was in 395 HD patients (5.6 percent).[48] Individuals undergoing presymptomatic genetic testing may be at an increased risk of suicide.[101]

PSYCHOSIS

The lifetime prevalence of psychosis in HD has been estimated at about 10 percent.[102] Impaired reality testing may occur at any time in the course of the illness, and patients may display psychotic features long before they manifest motor signs. When HD presents as an isolated thought disorder in a young person, it may be misdiagnosed as schizophrenia.[102] There appears to be a familial influence on incidence of psychosis in HD.[103]

Apathy is a common manifestation of affective illness in HD. Extreme social withdrawal may also represent an underlying thought disorder. Other psychotic features include paranoid delusions (typically, of spousal infidelity), thought broadcasting (the feeling that one's thoughts are immediately accessible to others), thought insertion (the feeling that others' thoughts are forcing their way into one's mind), and hallucinations, most commonly auditory or visual.[102]

OBSESSIVE-COMPULSIVE SYMPTOMS

Current theories implicate the basal ganglia and frontal lobes in obsessive-compulsive disorders, and compulsive handwashing and other ritualistic behaviors may occur in HD patients who have no other affective illness.[104]

PERSONALITY AND BEHAVIOR CHANGES

Personality changes occur commonly in HD patients, often beginning years before the onset of cognitive or motor manifestations.[28,29,93] Irritability, apathy, or anxiety may be the first signs of personality change.[105] Conduct disorder and antisocial personality disorder occur in about 5 percent of patients with HD, but their presence in at-risk teens does not accurately predict gene carrier status.[95,102] Although the prevalence of alcohol abuse in HD is similar to that in the population at large, alcohol and other substance abuse no doubt contributes to the social disruption and turmoil in many HD families.[106]

In general, psychiatric illness among individuals at risk for HD does not predict gene carrier status. The risk of developing major depressive disorder increases when HD patients begin to show motor manifestations of the illness.[107] However, no differences in the incidence of depression, psychosis, or behavioral disorders reliably distinguish between asymptomatic gene-positive and gene-negative individuals. Major psychiatric illness is common in at-risk individuals, regardless of gene carrier status, suggesting that childhood and adolescent environments, as well as the HD gene, predispose a patient to behavioral disturbances.[103,108]

SLEEP DISORDERS

HD patients frequently experience daytime hypersomnolence and nocturnal insomnia. Increased latency to nocturnal sleep onset, frequent awakenings, and decreased slow-wave sleep on polysomnography have been correlated with severity of motor impairment, duration of illness, and extent of caudate atrophy as shown by computed tomography (CT).[109] Underlying affective illness remains a major and remediable cause of sleep disruption in HD.

PROGRESSIVE FUNCTIONAL DECLINE

As motor, cognitive, and behavioral problems come to the surface, accustomed functions become compromised.[110] A number of rating scales provide quantitative assessments of the functional impact of HD.[33,111,112] The total functional capacity (TFC) score derived from the HD Functional Capacity Scale[111] (Tables 35-1 and 35-2) has been validated against radiographic measures of disease progression, including CT and magnetic resonance imaging (MRI) measures of striatal volume, as well as fluorodeoxyglucose

TABLE 35-1 Criteria for Quantified Staging of Functional Activities in HD

A. Engagement in occupation
    3 = *Usual level*—Full-time salaried employment, actual or potential (e.g., job offer or qualified), with normal work expectations and satisfactory performance.
    2 = *Lower level*—Full- or part-time salaried employment, actual or potential, with a lower-than-usual work expectation (relative to patient's training and education) but with satisfactory performance.
    1 = *Marginal level*—Part-time voluntary or salaried employment, actual or potential, with lower expectation and less-than-satisfactory work performance.
    0 = *Unable*—Totally unable to engage in voluntary or salaried employment.
B. Capacity to handle financial affairs
    3 = *Full*—Normal capacity to handle personal and family finances (income tax, balancing checkbook, paying bills, budgeting, shopping).
    2 = *Requires slight assistance*—Mildly impaired ability to handle financial affairs, such that accustomed routine responsibilities require some organization and assistance from family member or financial advisor.
    1 = *Requires major assistance*—Moderately impaired ability to handle financial affairs, such that patient comprehends the nature and purpose of routine financial procedures and is competent to handle funds but requires major assistance in the performance of these tasks.
    0 = *Unable*—Patient is unable to comprehend the financial process and is totally unable to perform task-related routine financial procedures.
C. Capacity to manage domestic responsibilities
    2 = *Full*—No impairment in performance of routine domestic tasks (cleaning, laundering, dishwashing, table setting, recipes, lawn care, answering mail, civic responsibilities).
    1 = *Impaired*—Moderate impairment in performance of routine domestic tasks, such that patient requires some assistance in carrying out these tasks.
    0 = *Unable*—Marked impairment in function and marginal performance; requires major assistance.
D. Capacity to perform activities of daily living
    3 = *Full*—Complete independence in eating, dressing, and bathing.
    2 = *Mildly impaired*—Somewhat labored performance in eating (avoids certain foods that cause chewing and swallowing problems), in dressing (difficulty in fine tasks only, e.g., buttoning or tying shoes), in bathing (difficulty in fine performance only, e.g., brushing teeth); requires only slight assistance.
    1 = *Moderately impaired*—Substantial difficulty in eating (swallows only liquid or soft foods and requires considerable assistance), in dressing (performs only gross dressing activities and requires assistance with everything else), in bathing (performs only gross bathing tasks; otherwise, requires assistance).
    0 = *Severely impaired*—Requires total care in activities of daily living.
E. Care can be provided at:
    2 = *Home*—Patient living at home and family readily able to meet care needs.
    1 = *Home or extended care facility*—Patient may be living at home, but care needs would be better provided at an extended care facility.
    0 = *Total care facility only*—Patient requires full-time, skilled nursing care.

SOURCE: *From Shoulson et al.[115] Used with permission.*

positron emission tomography (PET) measures of striatal metabolism.[69,70,113,114] Reliability has been demonstrated among a variety of health professionals.[115] A prospective evaluation of 129 HD patients by a single examiner demonstrated an overall TFC decline of 0.63 ± 0.75 (mean ± SD) units per year.[116] The pace of functional decline was not reliably predicted by age at onset, body weight, gender of affected parent, or neuroleptic use.[116] No association between

CAG repeat length and the rate of functional deterioration was found among patients followed prospectively by a single examiner who was kept unaware of CAG repeat length.[40]

The UHDRS includes standardized assessments of motor, cognitive, and behavioral performance, as well as the TFC and other functional measures of illness.[83] The UHDRS appears to be a reliable and internally consistent tool in assessing the progression of illness and the impact of therapeutic interventions.[83,117–121] The UHDRS has been incorporated into the Core Assessment Program for Intercerebral Transplantation in HD (CAPIT-HD).[122]

TABLE 35-2 Relationships of Stage of Illness to TFC Scores in HD

Stage	Corresponding TFC Score
I	11–13
II	7–11
III	3–6
IV	1–2
V	0

SOURCE: *Adapted from Shoulson et al.[115]*

Diagnosis

POSITIVE FAMILY HISTORY

Diagnosis is relatively straightforward when a characteristic movement disorder occurs in the setting of a clear-cut family history of HD. The failure to obtain a complete and accurate family history is the most common cause of misdiagnosis in patients who present primarily with psychiatric features.[105]

There are other heritable neurological disorders that may present with chorea, progress inexorably, and involve cognitive and behavioral changes.[123] Dentatorubropallidoluysian atrophy (DRPLA) is an autosomal-dominant disorder, phenotypically similar to HD, which results from CAG repeat expansion in a gene located on chromosome 12.[124] Ataxia is a prominent presenting feature of DRPLA, with oculomotor abnormalities, chorea, and dementia developing as the disease progresses.[125,126] Genetic testing is available for both HD and DRPLA and may be helpful when clinical features alone are insufficient to establish the diagnosis.

Neuroacanthocytosis may present in adulthood with progressive dementia and chorea accompanied by seizures, orolingual dystonia with self-mutilation, progressive muscle wasting, elevated creatine kinase, and peripheral neuropathy. Neuroacanthocytosis can occur in dominant, recessive, or sporadic patterns. The diagnosis may be confirmed by the presence of acanthocytes on peripheral blood smear.[127,128]

Rarely, patients may have the clinical phenotype of HD and a positive family history, but fail to show CAG repeat expansion.[129,130]

NEGATIVE OR ABSENT FAMILY HISTORY

When characteristic abnormalities of movement, cognition, and behavior occur in the absence of a family history of progressive neurodegenerative disease, a broader differential diagnosis should be considered (see Chap. 38). Identification of the mutation causing HD has made definitive diagnosis possible in the absence of a family history. In a study of apparently sporadic cases, 25 of 28 patients with signs and symptoms typical of HD showed expanded CAG repeats on chromosome 4, whereas only 5 of 16 patients with atypical clinical features (e.g., static illness, history of cerebrovascular disease, or Sydenham's chorea) tested positive for the expansion.[131,132]

There are several reasons why a patient with confirmed HD might not have a positive family history of this highly penetrant disease. Nonpaternity or ancestral death before manifestation of the disease may obscure the history. Alternatively, expansion of an unstable intermediate CAG length paternal allele into the HD range (>36 CAG repeats) may occur during spermatogenesis, giving rise to an affected individual whose father was unaffected.[133] Goldberg et al. have explored the genetic risk to siblings of sporadic cases, identifying a family with "pseudorecessive" HD on the basis of this type of expansion.[134] While the frequency of de novo HD mutations has traditionally been considered quite low,[135] more recent evidence suggests that the underlying rate is higher than previously suspected.[136] Almqvist et al. have reported absent family histories in up to one-quarter of newly diagnosed HD patients in British Columbia.[137]

TECHNOLOGICAL APPROACHES

A number of imaging methods have been used in the investigation of patients with HD. Advances in neuroimaging techniques in HD using volumetric MRI, PET, and MR spectroscopy are reviewed extensively in Chap. 3.

Several investigators have reported the variable loss of frontal somatosensory evoked potentials (SEPs) in HD, but these findings are nonspecific and are frequently encountered in other disorders of the basal ganglia.[138–140] More recently, Lefaucheur et al. reported that alterations of electrophysiological results, including SEPs, palmar sympathetic skin responses, and blink reflexes (but not thenar long-latency responses), increased in parallel to the evolution of the disease.[141]

GENETIC TESTING

An international study has evaluated the sensitivity and specificity of CAG repeat analysis in patients who were diagnosed with HD on the basis of characteristic clinical features. Of the 1007 clinically diagnosed patients, 995 had expanded CAG repeats (sensitivity 98.8 percent). None of the 113 patients with other neuropsychiatric illnesses showed repeat expansion (specificity 100 percent).[142] Therefore, clinical assessment of symptomatic individuals remains a very accurate means of diagnosis.

The ethical, psychological, and social implications of presymptomatic testing for HD have received wide attention.[143–145] There were no differences with regard to gender, average age, stability of relationship, or level of education between nonparticipants and participants in a predictive testing program.[146] Nonparticipants tended to have learned of their at-risk status during adolescence, whereas participants had done so in adulthood. The World Federation of Neurology–International Huntington Association Research Group on Huntington's Chorea has published guidelines for predictive testing that emphasize the importance of confidentiality, informed consent, and multidisciplinary supportive counseling both before and after reporting of test results. The guidelines stress that predictive testing should not be performed on minors.[147] While it was widely assumed that the discovery of the gene for HD would lead to widespread predictive testing, only 3 percent of at-risk individuals have chosen to be tested, and only 500 or so predictive DNA tests are performed annually in the US.[148]

Treatment

SYMPTOMATIC INTERVENTION

George Huntington said of HD in 1872:

> I have never known a recovery or even an amelioration of symptoms in this form of chorea; when once it begins it clings

TABLE 35-3 Huntington's Disease Organizations

HUNTINGTON'S DISEASE SOCIETY OF AMERICA
140 West 22nd St., 6th Floor
New York, NY 10011-2420
Phone: (212) 242-1968; (800) 345-HDSA
Fax: (212) 243-2443

FOUNDATION FOR THE CARE AND CURE OF
  HUNTINGTON'S DISEASE, INC.
PO Box 1084
32681 Overseas Highway
Islamorada, FL 33036
Phone: (305) 664-5044
Fax: (305) 664-8524

INTERNATIONAL HUNTINGTON ASSOCIATION
c/o Gerritt Dommerholt
Callunahof 8
7217 ST
Harfsen
NETHERLANDS
Phone: 31-573-43-1595

HUNTINGTON SOCIETY OF CANADA
13 Water Street North, Suite 3
PO Box 1269
Cambridge, Ontario N1R 7G6
CANADA
Phone: (519) 622-1002
Fax: (519) 622-7370

HEREDITARY DISEASE FOUNDATION
1427 7th St., Suite 2
Santa Monica, CA 90401
Phone: (310) 458-4183
Fax: (310) 458-3937

to the bitter end. No treatment seems to be of any avail, and indeed nowadays its end is so well known to the sufferer and his friends, that medical advice is seldom sought. It seems at least to be one of the incurables.

Despite the therapeutic nihilism so prevalent since HD was first described, several interventions may appreciably improve the quality of life for patients and their families. Although pharmacotherapies are available for the amelioration of some of the motor and psychiatric manifestations of HD, the provision of clear and accurate information and psychosocial support measures remains central to the care of HD patients and families.

Psychosocial support aimed at the family and the patient should ensure the availability of compassionate care providers, psychological and genetic counseling and referral, and access to social and legal services, including concrete assistance with long-term planning, facilitation of disability reviews, and support groups. Several clinical support and research organizations may be of help to the patient, family, and clinicians in their efforts to ease the burden of illness (see Table 35-3 and Appendix). Awareness of active research into the cause and treatment of HD is an important component of comprehensive care.

TREATING THE MOVEMENT DISORDER

There is little evidence that treatment of chorea or other hyperkinetic manifestations of HD results in functional improvement. Occasionally, patients with disabling chorea may benefit temporarily from antichoreic pharmacotherapy to facilitate self-care. Reduction of heightened dopaminergic activity by use of dopamine receptor antagonists

(e.g., phenothiazines, butyrophenones, thioxanthines)[149–151] or dopamine-depleting agents (e.g., reserpine, tetrabenazine)[152–155] may suppress chorea in the short term. Use of these neuroleptic agents may exacerbate bradykinesia and rigidity and may also lead to further functional decline from drug-induced sedation, apathy, akathisia, depression, dysarthria, or dysphagia. When chorea is sufficiently disabling, neuroleptic agents should be initiated, using the smallest effective dosage. Because the severity of chorea tends to diminish over time as HD progresses, continued use of dopamine antagonists or dopamine depletors requires frequent reassessment. The routine use of neuroleptics in juvenile-onset illness or in patients with advanced illness should be avoided.

The antichoreic effect of neuroleptics is thought to be mediated primarily by their blockade of D2 receptors on neurons projecting to the lateral globus pallidus via the indirect pathway of basal ganglia transmission (see Chap. 36). The selective D4 receptor antagonist, clozapine, has been found to exert antichoreic effects in a small open-label study,[156] but controlled trials have not been done.

Antiglutamatergic agents, including riluzole,[157–159] amantadine,[160] remacemide[161] and lamotrigine,[162] have all demonstrated antichoreic effects, but the cost-benefit of these approaches is not established.

HD patients with predominant features of bradykinesia and rigidity may benefit from treatment with L-dopa or direct-acting dopamine agonists,[163] but caution should be used with such agents because they can exacerbate chorea and dystonia and provoke hallucinations and psychosis. There are no effective pharmacotherapies for treating the disabling dystonic features of HD.

TREATMENT OF THE PSYCHIATRIC AND BEHAVIORAL DISORDER

Depression represents the single most remediable feature of HD.[91,102] The relative efficacies of various tricyclic compounds, monoamine oxidase inhibitors, and selective serotonin reuptake inhibitors have not been established. In patients for whom sedation is a concern, antidepressants with minimal anticholinergic effects (e.g., nortriptyline, desipramine) may be useful. Alternatively, if agitation and irritability predominate, using agents with more anticholinergic effects (e.g., amitriptyline, imipramine) may be appropriate. Fluoxetine may be beneficial as a first-line therapy for depression or as an alternative if tricyclics have failed. A controlled trial of fluoxetine in nondepressed HD patients did not show functional benefits.[164] Other serotonin reuptake inhibitors have not been examined systematically in HD. Electroconvulsive therapy may be effective in treating selected patients with HD who suffer from depression that is otherwise unresponsive to pharmacotherapeutic interventions.[165]

HD patients with bipolar affective illness may benefit from supervised trials of carbamazepine, valproate, or lithium, but there are no studies that have examined this problem systematically.

Frank psychosis with agitation and behavioral aggression usually requires antipsychotic neuroleptic medications for short-term and often long-term treatment. When required, atypical neuroleptics should be used in the lowest possible dosage, with attention to the risks of a patient developing extrapyramidal side-effects. The possible use of clozapine for treatment of psychosis in HD has been advocated,[166] but no controlled studies have been reported.

The novel tricyclic compound, clomipramine, as well as other serotonin reuptake inhibitors, may be useful in treating patients with compulsive behaviors or obsessive preoccupations.

EXPERIMENTAL THERAPEUTICS

REPLACEMENT STRATEGIES

Given the complexity of neurochemical changes in HD (see Chap. 36), it appears extremely unlikely that replacing neurotransmitter loss (as L-dopa restores dopamine for Parkinson's disease) will be a successful treatment strategy for HD. The loss of gamma-aminobutyric acid (GABA)-ergic neurons in the striatum has prompted several unsuccessful pharmacological efforts to increase GABA activity.[167,168] Increasing cholinergic activity has also proved to be of little benefit.[169] Attempts to reduce the increased concentration of somatostatin in the HD basal ganglia using cysteamine have not produced clinical benefits.[170] Although there is a decrease in the number of cannabinoid receptors in HD,[171] there was no difference between placebo and cannabidiol (a nonpsychotropic constituent of cannabis that stimulates cannabinoid receptors) in a 6-week, double-blind, crossover trial of efficacy and safety for the treatment of chorea.[172]

NEUROPROTECTIVE STRATEGIES

A number of strategies are being aimed at slowing the progression of HD based on the emerging knowledge of pathogenesis (see Chap. 36). While antiglutamatergic agents have shown promise in excitotoxic and transgenic animal models,[173,174] they have not slowed functional decline in human clinical trials.[161,162,175,176] Riluzole is currently undergoing Phase III assessment for HD in Europe.

Cellular energy-enhancing agents such as creatine,[177,178] and coenzyme Q10,[179,180] have shown promise in animal models and are being studied in humans. A large scale trial of coenzyme Q10 at 600 mg/day failed to demonstrate a definitive neuroprotective effect, although there was a trend towards slowing of functional decline.[161] Minocycline inhibits caspase-1 and caspase-3, and prolongs survival in a transgenic mouse model of HD.[181] A Phase II trial of minocycline in 63 patients with HD followed for 8 weeks is currently being analyzed.

A number of other compounds show efficacy in animal models, including interleukin 6,[182] lipoic acid,[183] dichloroacetate,[184] and lithium.[185] Environmental enrichment has also been reported to slow disease progression in a transgenic mouse model.[186]

A 12-month, double-blinded, placebo-controlled trial of alpha-trocopherol in 73 HD patients failed to show consistent benefit, although patients in the earlier stages of illness responded more favorably.[187]

Based on the contention that the primary degenerative process in HD is linked to intrinsic striatal vulnerabilities, implantation of normal fetal striatal tissue is under investigation as a possible method of intervention for HD.[188,189] Another promising strategy involves the provision of neurotrophic factors directly to the striatum via genetically modified polymer-encapsulated cell lines.[190]

To date, the early experimental therapeutics of HD has little to show in tangible terms. Rapidly increasing knowledge of etiology and pathogenesis, however, has expanded the options for rational therapeutic interventions and the prospects for substantive benefits for persons affected by, and at risk for, HD.

References

1. Huntington G: On chorea. *Med Surg Rep* 26:320, 1872.
2. The Huntington's Disease Collaborative Research Group: A novel gene containing a trinucleotide repeat that is expanded and unstable on Huntington's disease chromosomes. *Cell* 72:971–983, 1993.
3. Sharp AH, Loev SJ, Schilling G, et al: Widespread expression of Huntington's disease gene (*IT15*) protein product. *Neuron* 4:1065–1074, 1995.
4. Strong TV, Tagle DA, Valdes JM, et al: Widespread expression of the human and rat Huntington's disease gene in brain and nonneural tissues. *Nat Genet* 5:259–265, 1993.
5. Li SH, Schilling G, Young WS, et al: Huntington's disease gene (*IT15*) is widely expressed in human and rat tissues. *Neuron* 1:985–993, 1993.

6. Albin RL, Tagle DA: Genetics and molecular biology of Huntington's disease. *Trends Neurosci* 8:11–14, 1995.

7. Mangiarini L, Sathasivam K, Seller M, et al: Exon 1 of the HD gene with an expanded CAG repeat is sufficient to cause a progressive neurological phenotype in transgenic mice. *Cell* 87:493–506, 1996.

8. Jackson GR, Salecker I, Dong X, et al: Polyglutamine-expanded human huntingtin transgenes induce degeneration of *Drosophila* photoreceptor neurons. *Neuron* 21:633–642, 1998.

9. Faber PW, Alter JR, MacDonald ME, Hart AC: Polyglutamine-medicated dysfunction and apoptotic death of a *Caenorhabditis elegans* sensory neuron. *Proc Natl Acad Sci U S A* 96:179–184, 1999.

10. Conneally PM: Huntington's disease: Genetics and epidemiology. *Am J Hum Genet* 36:506–526, 1984.

11. Harper PS: The epidemiology of Huntington's disease. *Hum Genet* 89:365–376, 1992.

12. Narabayashi H: Huntington's chorea in Japan: Review of the literature. *Adv Neurol* 1:253–259, 1973.

13. Palo J, Somer H, Ikonen EM: Low prevalence of Huntington's disease in Finland. *Lancet* ii:805–806, 1987.

14. Penney JB, Young AB, Shoulson I, et al: Huntington's disease in Venezuela: 7-year follow-up on symptomatic and asymptomatic individuals. *Mov Disord* 5:93–99, 1990.

15. Tanner CM, Goldman SM: Epidemiology of movement disorders. *Curr Opin Neurol* 7:325–332, 1994.

16. Gusella JF, Wexler NS, Conneally PM, et al: A polymorphic DNA marker linked to Huntington's disease. *Nature* 306:234–238, 1983.

17. Quaid KA, Morris M: Reluctance to undergo predictive testing: The case of Huntington's disease. *Am J Med Genet* 45:41–45, 1993.

18. Harper PS, Tyler A, Smith S, et al: Decline in the predicted incidence of Huntington's chorea associated with systematic genetic counseling and family support. *Lancet* ii:411–413, 1981.

19. Carter CO, Evans KA, Baraitser M: Effect of genetic counseling on the prevalence of Huntington's chorea. *Br Med J* 286:281–283, 1983.

20. Riley DE, Lang A: Movement disorders, in Bradley WG, Daroff RB, Fenichel GM, Marsden CD (eds): *Neurology in Clinical Practice: The Neurological Disorders.* Boston: Butterworth-Heinemann, 1991, vol 2, pp 1563–1601.

21. Adams P, Falek A, Arnold J: Huntington's disease in Georgia: Age at onset. *Am J Hum Genet* 43:695–704, 1988.

22. Oliver JE: Huntington's chorea in Northamptonshire. *Br J Psychiatry* 116:241–253, 1970.

23. Bruyn GW: Huntington's chorea: Historical clinical and laboratory synopsis, in Vinken PJ, Bruyn GW (eds): *Handbook of Clinical Neurology.* Amsterdam: North-Holland, 1968, vol 16, pp 298–378.

24. Merrit AD, Conneally PM, Rahman NF, Drew AL: Juvenile Huntington's chorea, in Barbeau A, Brunette JR (eds): *Progress in Neurogenetics 1.* Amsterdam: Excerpta Medica, 1969, pp 645–650.

25. Louis ED, Anderson KE, Moskowitz C, et al: Dystonia-predominant adult-onset Huntington disease: Association between motor phenotype and age of onset in adults. *Arch Neurol* 57:1326–1330, 2000.

26. Young AB, Shoulson I, Penney JB, et al: Huntington's disease in Venezuela: Neurologic features and functional decline. *Neurology* 36:244–249, 1986.

27. Djousse L, Knowlton B, Cupples LA, et al: Weight loss in early stage of Huntington's disease. *Neurology* 59:1325–1330, 2002.

28. Kirkwood SC, Siemers E, Viken RJ, et al: Evaluation of psychological symptoms among presymptomatic HD gene carriers as measured by selected MMPI scales. *J Psychiatri Res* 36:377–382, 2002.

29. Kirkwood SC, Siemers E, Viken R, et al: Longitudinal personality changes among presymptomatic Huntington disease gene carriers. *Neuropsychiatry Neuropsychol Behav Neurol* 15:192–197, 2002.

30. Kirkwood SC, Siemers E, Bond C, et al: Confirmation of subtle motor changes among presymptomatic carriers of the Huntington disease gene. *Arch Neurol* 57:1040–1044, 2000.

31. Kirkwood SC, Siemers E, Stout JC, et al: Longitudinal cognitive and motor changes among presymptomatic Huntington disease gene carriers. *Arch Neurol* 56:563–568, 1999.

32. Aylward EH, Codori AM, Rosenblatt A, et al: Rate of caudate atrophy in presymptomatic and symptomatic stages of Huntington's disease. *Mov Disord* 15:552–560, 2000.

33. Myers RH, Sax DS, Koroshetz WJ, et al: Factors associated with slow progression in Huntington's disease. *Arch Neurol* 48:800–804, 1991.

34. Roos RA, Hermans J, Vegter-van der Vlis M, et al: Duration of illness in Huntington's disease is not related to age at onset. *J Neurol Neurosurg Psychiatry* 56:98–100, 1993.

35. Duyao M, Ambrose C, Myers R, et al: Trinucleotide repeat length instability and age of onset in Huntington's disease. *Nat Genet* 4:387–392, 1993.

36. Stine OC, Pleasant N, Franz ML, et al: Correlation between the onset age of Huntington's disease and length of the trinucleotide repeat in IT-15. *Hum Mol Genet* 2:1547–1549, 1993.

37. Craufurd D, Dodge A: Mutation size and age at onset in Huntington's disease. *J Med Genet* 30:1008–1011, 1993.

38. Simpson SA, Davidson MJ, Barron LH: Huntington's disease in Grampian region: Correlation of the CAG repeat number and the age of onset of the disease. *J Med Genet* 30:1014–1017, 1993.

39. Andrew SE, Goldberg YP, Kremer B, et al: The relationship between trinucleotide (CAG) repeat length and clinical features of Huntington's disease. *Nat Genet* 4:398–403, 1993.

40. Kieburtz K, MacDonald M, Shih C, et al: Trinucleotide repeat length and progression of illness in Huntington's disease. *J Med Genet* 31:872–874, 1994.

41. Rosenblatt A, Brinkman RR, Liang KY, et al: Familial influence on age of onset among siblings with Huntington disease. *Am J Med Genet* 105:399–403, 2001.

42. Ashizawa T, Wong LJ, Richards CS, et al: CAG repeat size and clinical presentation in Huntington's disease. *Neurology* 44:1137–1143, 1994.

43. Claes S, Van Zand K, Legius E, et al: Correlations between triplet repeat expansion and clinical features in Huntington's disease. *Arch Neurol* 52:749–753, 1995.

44. Marshall FJ, Kieburtz K, MacDonald M, et al: Lack of correlation between CAG-repeat length and rate of motor decline in Huntington disease, in Cassiman JJ (ed): Proceedings of the 16th International Meeting of the World Federation of Neurology Research Group on Huntington's Disease, July 15–18, 1995. University of Leuven, Belgium, 1995, p 19.

45. Illarioshkin SN, Igarashi S, Onodera O, et al: Trinucleotide repeat length and rate of progression of Huntington's disease. *Ann Neurol* 36:360–365, 1994.

46. Marder K, Sandler S, Lechich A, et al: Relationship between CAG repeat length and late-stage outcomes in Huntington's disease. *Neurology* 59:1622–1624, 2002.

47. Moskowitz CB, Marder K: Palliative care for people with late-stage Huntington's disease. *Neurol Clin* 19:849–865, 2001.

48. Sorensen SA, Fenger K: Causes of death in patients with Huntington's disease and in unaffected first degree relatives. *J Med Genet* 29:911–914, 1992.

49. Kremer B, Weber B, Hayden MR: New insights into the clinical features, pathogenesis and molecular genetics of Huntington's disease. *Brain Pathol* 2:321–335, 1992.

50. Shoulson I: Care of patients and families with Huntington's disease, in Marsden CD, Fahn S (eds): *Movement Disorders*. London: Butterworth, 1982, pp 277–290.

51. Tian JR, Herman SJ, Zee DS, Folstein SE: Postural control in Huntington's disease (HD). *Acta Otolaryngol Suppl (Stockh)* 481:333–336, 1991.

52. Hertrich I, Ackermann H: Acoustic analysis of speech timing in Huntington's disease. *Brain Lang* 47:182–196, 1994.

53. Leigh RJ, Newman SA, Folstein SE, Lasker AG: Abnormal ocular motor control in Huntington's disease. *Neurology* 33:1268–1275, 1983.

54. Collewijn H, Went LN, Tomminga EP, Vegter-van de Vlis M: Oculomotor defects in patients with Huntington's disease and their offspring. *J Neurol Sci* 86:307–320, 1988.

55. Lasker AG, Zee DA, Hain TC, et al: Saccades in Huntington's disease: Initiation defects and distractability. *Neurology* 37:364–370, 1987.

56. Tian JR, Zee DS, Lasker AG, Folstein SE: Saccades in Huntington's disease: Predictive tracking and interaction between release of fixation and initiation of saccades. *Neurology* 41:875–881, 1991.

57. Rubin AJ, King WM, Reinbold KA, Shoulson I: Quantitative longitudinal assessment of saccades in Huntington's disease. *J Clin Neuroophthalmol* 13:59–66, 1993.

58. Rothlind JC, Brandt J, Zee D, et al: Unimpaired verbal memory and oculomotor control in asymptomatic adults with the genetic marker for Huntington's disease. *Arch Neurol* 50:799–802, 1993.

59. Jankovic J, Ashizawa T: Tourettism associated with Huntington's disease. *Mov Disord* 10:103–105, 1995.

60. Kerbeshian J, Burd L, Leech C, Rorabaugh A: Huntington disease and childhood onset Tourette syndrome. *Am J Med Genet* 39:1–3, 1991.

61. Thompson PD, Bhatia KP, Brown P, et al: Cortical myoclonus in Huntington's disease. *Mov Disord* 9:633–641, 1994.

62. Carella F, Scaioli V, Ciano C, et al: Adult onset myoclonic Huntington's disease. *Mov Disord* 8:201–205, 1993.

63. Vogul CM, Drury I, Terry LC, Young AB: Myoclonus in adult Huntington's disease. *Ann Neurol* 29:213–215, 1991.

64. Reilmann R, Kirsten F, Quinn L, et al: Objective assessment of progression in Huntington's disease: A 3-year follow-up study. *Neurology* 57:920–924, 2001.

65. Feigin A, Kieburtz K, Shoulson I: Treatment of Huntington's disease and other choreic disorders, in Kurlan R (ed): *Treatment of Movement Disorders*. Philadelphia: Lippincott, 1995, pp 337–364.

66. Paulsen JS, Ready RE, Hamilton JM, et al: Neuropsychiatric aspects of Huntington's disease. *J Neurol Neurosurg Psychiatry* 71:310–314, 2001.

67. Kennedy JS, Kenny JT: Cognitive disorders associated with psychiatric illnesses, in Thal LJ, Moos WJ, Gamzu ER (eds): *Cognitive Disorders*. New York: Marcel Dekker, 1992, p 138.

68. Shoulson I: Huntington's disease: Cognitive and psychiatric features. *Neuropsychiatry Neuropsychol Behav Neurol* 3:15–22, 1990.

69. Bamford KA, Caine ED, Kido DK, et al: Clinical-pathological correlation in Huntington's disease: A neuropsychological and computed tomography study. *Neurology* 39:796–801, 1989.

70. Bamford KA, Caine ED, Kido DK, et al: A prospective evaluation of cognitive decline in early Huntington's disease: Functional and radiographic correlates. *Neurology* 45:1867–1873, 1995.

71. Paulsen JS, Butters N, Sadek JR, et al: Distinct cognitive profiles of cortical and subcortical dementia in advanced illness. *Neurology* 45:951–956, 1995.

72. Lange KW, Sahakian BJ, Quinn NP, et al: Comparison of executive and visuospatial memory function in Huntington's disease and dementia of Alzheimer type matched for degree of dementia. *J Neurol Neurosurg Psychiatry* 58:598–606, 1995.

73. Rosser AE, Hodges JR: The dementia rating scale in Alzheimer's disease, Huntington's disease and progressive supranuclear palsy. *J Neurol* 241:531–536, 1994.

74. Mohr E, Brouwers P, Claus JJ, et al: Visuospatial cognition in Huntington's disease. *Mov Disord* 6:127–132, 1991.

75. Brandt J, Folstein SE, Folstein MF: Differential cognitive impairment in Alzheimer's and Huntington's disease. *Ann Neurol* 23:555–561, 1988.

76. Aminoff MJ, Marshall J, Smith EM, Wyke MA: Pattern of intellectual impairment in Huntington's chorea. *Psychol Med* 5:169–172, 1975.

77. Caine ED, Ebert MH, Weingartner H: An outline for the analysis of dementia: The memory disorder of Huntington's disease. *Neurology* 27:1087–1092, 1977.

78. Brandt J: Access to knowledge in dementia of Huntington's disease. *Dev Neuropsychol* 1:335–348, 1985.

79. Rohrer D, Salmon DP, Wixted JT, Paulsen JS: The disparate effects of Alzheimer's disease and Huntington's disease on semantic memory. *Neuropsychology* 13:381–388, 1999.

80. Smith A: *Symbol Digit Modalities Test Manual*. Los Angeles: Western Psychological Services, 1973.

81. Benton AL, Hamsher K: *Multilingual Aphasia Examination Manual*. Iowa City: University of Iowa, 1978.

82. Stroop JR: Studies of interference in serial verbal reactions. *J Exp Psychol* 18:643–662, 1935.

83. Huntington Study Group: Unified Huntington's Disease Rating Scale: Reliability and consistency. *Mov Disord* 11:136–142, 1996.

84. Lezak MD: *Neuropsychological Assessment*. New York: Oxford University Press, 1983.

85. Foroud T, Siemers E, Kleindorfer D, et al: Cognitive scores in carriers of Huntington's disease gene compared to noncarriers. *Ann Neurol* 37:657–664, 1995.

86. Diamond R, White RF, Myers RH, et al: Evidence of presymptomatic cognitive decline in Huntington's disease. *J Clin Exp Neuropsychol* 14:961–975, 1992.

87. MacMillan JC, Morrison PJ, Nevin NC, et al: Identification of an expanded CAG repeat in the Huntington's disease gene (*IT15*) in a family reported to have benign hereditary chorea. *J Med Genet* 30:1012–1013, 1993.

88. Britton JW, Uitti RJ, Ahlskog JE, et al: Hereditary late-onset chorea without dementia: Genetic evidence for substantial phenotypic variation in Huntington's disease. *Neurology* 45:443–447, 1995.

89. Caine ED, Hunt RD, Weingartner H, Ebert MH: Huntington's dementia: Clinical and neuropsychological features. *Arch Gen Psychiatry* 35:377–384, 1978.

90. Di Maio L, Squitieri F, Napolitano G, et al: Onset symptoms in 510 patients with Huntington's disease. *J Med Genet* 30:289–292, 1993.

91. Caine ED, Shoulson I: Psychiatric syndromes in Huntington's disease. *Am J Psychiatry* 140:728–733, 1983.

92. Folstein SE, Folstein MF: Psychiatric features of Huntington's disease: Recent approaches and findings. *Psychiatr Dev* 2:193–205, 1983.

93. Shiwach R: Psychopathology in Huntington's disease patients. *Acta Psychiatr Scand* 90:241–246, 1994.

94. Nehl C, Ready RE, Hamilton J, Paulsen JS: Effects of depression on working memory in presymptomatic Huntington's disease. *J Neuropsychiatry Clin Neurosci* 13:342–346, 2001.

95. Folstein SE: The psychopathology of Huntington's disease, in McHugh RR, McKurick VA (eds): *Genes, Brain and Behavior.* New York: Raven Press, 1991.

96. Folstein SE, Chase GA, Wahl WE, et al: Huntington's disease in Maryland: Clinical aspects of racial variation. *Am J Hum Genet* 41:168–171, 1987.

97. Lipe H, Schultz A, Bird TD: Risk factors for suicide in Huntington's disease: A retrospective case controlled study. *Am J Med Genet* 48:231–233, 1993.

98. Schoenfeld M, Myers RH, Cupples LA, et al: Increased rate of suicide among patients with Huntington's disease. *J Neurol Neurosurg Psychiatry* 47:1283–1287, 1984.

99. Farrer LA: Suicide and attempted suicide in Huntington's disease: Implications for preclinical tests of persons at risk. *Am J Med Genet* 24:305–311, 1986.

100. Wong MT, Chang PC, Yu YL, et al: Psychosocial impact of Huntington's disease on Hong Kong Chinese families. *Acta Psychiatr Scand* 90:16–18, 1994.

101. Almqvist EW, Bloch M, Brinkman R, et al: A worldwide assessment of the frequency of suicide, suicide attempts, or psychiatric hospitalization after predictive testing for Huntington disease. *Am J Hum Genet* 64:1293–1304, 1999.

102. Folstein SE: *Huntington's Disease: A Disorder of Families.* Baltimore: Johns Hopkins University Press, 1989.

103. Tsuang D, Almqvist EW, Lipe H, et al: Familial aggregation of psychotic symptoms in Huntington's disease. *Am J Psychiatry* 157:1955–1959, 2000.

104. Cummings JL, Cunningham K: Obsessive-compulsive disorder in Huntington's disease. *Biol Psychiatry* 31:263–270, 1992.

105. Pflanz S, Besson JA, Ebmeier KP, Simpson S: The clinical manifestation of mental disorder in Huntington's disease: A retrospective case record study of disease progression. *Acta Psychiatr Scand* 83:53–60, 1991.

106. King M: Alcohol abuse and Huntington's disease. *Psychol Med* 15:815–819, 1985.

107. Watt DC, Seller A: A clinico-genetic study of psychiatric disorder in Huntington's chorea. *Psychol Med* 23(suppl 1):1–46, 1993.

108. Shiwach RS, Norbury CG: A controlled psychiatric study of individuals at risk for Huntington's disease. *Br J Psychiatry* 165:500–505, 1994.

109. Wiegand M, Moller AA, Lauer CJ, et al: Nocturnal sleep in Huntington's disease. *J Neurol* 238:203–208, 1991.

110. Biglan KM, Shoulson I: Huntington's disease, in Jankovic JJ, Tolosa E (eds.): *Parkinson's Disease and Movement Disorders*, 4th ed. Philadelphia: Lippincott Williams & Wilkins, 2002.

111. Shoulson I, Fahn S: Huntington's disease: Clinical care and evaluation. *Neurology* 29:1–3, 1979.

112. Blysma FW, Rothlind J, Hall MR, et al: Assessment of adaptive functioning in Huntington's disease. *Mov Disord* 8:183–190, 1993.

113. Kido DK, Shoulson I, Manzione JV, Harnish PP: Measurements of caudate and putamen atrophy in patients with Huntington's disease. *Neuroradiology* 33(suppl 1):604–606, 1991.

114. Young AB, Penney JB, Starosta-Rubenstein S, et al: PET scan investigations of Huntington's disease: Cerebral metabolic correlates of neurological features and functional decline. *Ann Neurol* 20:296–303, 1986.

115. Shoulson I, Kurlan R, Rubin AJ, et al: Assessment of functional capacity in neurodegenerative movement disorders: Huntington's disease as a prototype, in Munsat TL (ed): *Quantification of Neurological Deficit*. Boston: Butterworth, 1989, pp 271–283.

116. Feigin A, Kieburtz K, Bordwell K, et al: Functional decline in Huntington's disease. *Mov Disord* 10(suppl 2):211–214, 1995.

117. Kieburtz K, Feigin A, Como P, et al: A controlled trial of the glutamate antagonist remacemide hydrochloride in Huntington's disease. *Soc Neurosci Abstr* 20:1256, 1994.

118. Feigin A, Kieburtz K, Como P, et al: An open-label trial of coenzyme Q10 (CoQ) in Huntington's disease (HD). *Neurology* 44(suppl 2):A398–A399, 1994.

119. Marder K, Zhao H, Myers RH, et al: Rate of functional decline in Huntington's disease. Huntington Study Group. *Neurology* 54:452–458, 2000.

120. Siesling S, Zwinderman AH, van Vugt JP, et al: A shortened version of the motor section of the Unified Huntington's Disease Rating Scale. *Mov Disord* 12:229–234, 1997.

121. Siesling S, van Vugt JP, Zwinderman KA, et al: Unified Huntington's disease rating scale: A follow up. *Mov Disord* 13:915–919, 1998.

122. Quinn N, Brown R, Craufurd D, et al: Core Assessment Program for Intracerebral Transplantation in Huntington's Disease (CAPIT-HD). *Mov Disord* 11:143–150, 1996.

123. Greenamyre JT, Shoulson I: Huntington's disease, in Calne D (ed): *Neurodegenerative Diseases*. Philadelphia: WB Saunders, 1994, pp 684–704.

124. Koide R, Ikeuchi T, Onodera O, et al: Unstable expansion of CAG repeat in hereditary dentatorubral-pallidoluysian atrophy (DRPLA). *Nat Genet* 6:9–13, 1994.

125. Warner TT, Lennox GG, Janota I, Harding AE: Autosomal-dominant dentatorubropallidoluysian atrophy in the United Kingdom. *Mov Disord* 9:289–296, 1994.

126. Iazuka R, Hirayama K, Machara K: Denatato-rubro-pallidoluysian atrophy: A clinico-pathological study. *J Neurol Neurosurg Psychiatry* 47:1288–1298, 1984.

127. Hardie RJ, Pullon HWH, Harding AE, et al: Neuroacanthocytosis: A clinical haematological and pathological study of 19 cases. *Brain* 114:13–49, 1991.

128. Rinne JO, Daniel SE, Scaravilli F, et al: The neuropathological features of neuroacanthyocytosis. *Mov Disord* 9:297–304, 1994.

129. Rosenblatt A, Ranen N, Rubinsztein DC, et al: Patients with features similar to Huntington's disease, without CAG expansion in huntingtin. *Neurology* 51:215–220, 1998.

130. Fernandez M, Raskind W, Matsushita M, et al: Hereditary benign chorea: Clinical and genetic features of a distinct disease. *Neurology* 57:106–110, 2001.

131. Bateman D, Boughey AM, Scaravilli F, et al: A follow-up study of isolated cases of suspected Huntington's disease. *Ann Neurol* 31:2983–2987, 1992.

132. David MB, Bateman D, Quinn NP, et al: Mutation analysis in patients with possible but apparently sporadic Huntington's disease. *Lancet* 344:714–717, 1994.

133. MacDonald ME, Barnes G, Srinidhi J, et al: Gametic but not somatic instability of CAG repeat length in Huntington's disease. *J Med Genet* 30:982–986, 1993.

134. Goldberg YP, Andrew SE, Theilmann J, et al: Familial predisposition to recurrent mutations causing Huntington's disease: Genetic risk to sibs of sporadic cases. *J Med Genet* 30:987–990, 1993.

135. Vogel F, Motulsky AG: *Human Genetics: Problems and Approaches.* Berlin, Springer-Verlag, 1986, p 419.

136. Falush D, Almqvist EW, Brinkmann RR, et al: Measurement of mutational flow implies both a high new-mutation rate for Huntington disease and substantial under ascertainment of late-onset cases. *Am J Hum Genet* 68:373–385, 2001.

137. Almqvist EW, Elterman DS, MacLeod PM, Hayden MR: High incidence rate and absent family histories in one quarter of patients newly diagnosed with Huntington disease in British Columbia. *Clin Genet* 60:198–205, 2001.

138. Topper R, Schwarz M, Podoll K, et al: Absence of frontal somatosensory evoked potentials in Huntington's disease. *Brain* 116:87–101, 1993.

139. Yamada T, Rodnitzky RL, Kameyama S, et al: Alternation of SEP topography in Huntington's patients and their relatives at risk. *Electroencephalogr Clin Neurophysiol* 80:251–261, 1991.

140. Kuwert T, Noth J, Scholz D, et al: Comparison of somatosensory evoked potentials with striatal glucose consumption measured by positron emission tomography in the early diagnosis of Huntington's disease. *Mov Disord* 8:98–106, 1993.

141. Lefaucheur JP, Bachoud-Levi AC, Bourdet C, et al: Clinical relevance of electrophysiological tests in the assessment of patients with Huntington's disease. *Mov Disord* 17:1294–1301, 2002.

142. Kremer B, Goldberg P, Andrew SE, et al: A worldwide study of the Huntington's disease mutation: The sensitivity and specificity of measuring CAG repeats. *N Engl J Med* 330:1401–1406, 1994.

143. Terrenoire G: Huntington's disease and the ethics of genetic prediction. *J Med Ethics* 18:79–95, 1992.

144. Hayden MR, Bloch M, Wiggens S: Psychological effects of predictive testing for Huntington's disease. *Adv Neurol* 65:201–210, 1995.

145. Tibben A, Duivenvoorden HJ, Niermeijer MF, et al: Psychological effects of presymptomatic DNA testing for Huntington's disease in the Dutch program. *Psychosom Med* 56:526–532, 1994.

146. van der Steenstraten IM, Tibben A, Roos RA, et al: Predictive testing for Huntington's disease: Nonparticipants compared with participants in the Dutch program. *Am J Med Genet* 55:618–625, 1994.

147. World Federation of Neurology and International Huntington Association Research Group on Huntington's Chorea: Guidelines for the molecular genetics predictive test in Huntington's disease. *Neurology* 44:1533–1536, 1994.

148. Nance MA, Myers RH, the US Huntington Disease Genetic Testing Group: Trends in predictive and prenatal testing for Huntington's disease 1993–1999. *Am J Hum Genet* 65:A406, 1999.

149. Shoulson I: Huntington's disease: Functional capacities in patients treated with neuroleptic and antidepressant drugs. *Neurology* 31:1333–1335, 1981.

150. Girotti F, Carella F, Scigliano G, et al: Effect of neuroleptic treatment of involuntary movements and motor performances in Huntington's disease. *J Neurol Neurosurg Psychiatry* 47:848–852, 1984.

151. Barr AN, Fischer JH, Koller WC, et al: Serum haloperidol concentration and choreiform movements in Huntington's disease. *Neurology* 38:84–88, 1988.

152. Kempinski WH, Boniface WR, Morgan PP, et al: Reserpine in Huntington's chorea. *Neurology* 10:38–42, 1960.

153. Friedman JH: A case of progressive hemichorea responsive to high-dose reserpine. *J Clin Psychiatry* 47:149–150, 1986.

154. Jankovic J, Orman J: Tetrabenazine therapy of dystonia, chorea, tics and other dyskinesias. *Neurology* 38:391–394, 1988.

155. Jankovic J, Beach J: Long-term effects of tetrabenazine in hyperkinetic movement disorders. *Neurology* 48:358–362, 1997.

156. Bonuccelli U, Ceravolo R, Maremmani C, et al: Clozapine in Huntington's chorea. *Neurology* 44:821–823, 1994.

157. Rosas HD, Koroshetz W, Jenkins BG, et al: Riluzole therapy in Huntington's disease (HD). *Mov Disord* 14:326–330, 1999.

158. Marshall FJ: Riluzole dosing in Huntington's disease (RID-HD): Results of an 8-week double-blind, placebo-controlled, multi-center study by the Huntington Study Group. Proceedings of the 19th International Meeting of the World Federation of Neurology Research Group on Huntington's Disease, 2001, pp 29–30.

159. Seppi K, Mueller J, Bodner T, et al: Riluzole in Huntington's disease (HD): An open label study with one year follow up. *J Neurol* 248:866–869, 2001.

160. Verhagen L, Morris M, Farmer C, et al: A double-blind placebo-controlled crossover study of the effect of amantadine on chorea in Huntington's disease. *Neurology* 56:A386, 2001.

161. Huntington Study Group: A randomized, placebo-controlled trial of coenzyme Q10 and remacemide in Huntington's disease. *Neurology* 57:397–404, 2001.

162. Kremer B, Clark CM, Almqvist EW, et al: Influence of lamotrigine on progression of early Huntington disease: A randomized clinical trial. *Neurology* 53:1000–1011, 1999.

163. Jongen PJ, Renier WO, Gabreels FJ: Seven cases of Huntington's disease in childhood and L-dopa-induced improvement in the hypokinetic-rigid form. *Clin Neurol Neurosurg* 82:251–261, 1980.

164. Como PG, Rubin AJ, O'Brien CF, et al: A controlled trial of fluoxetine in nondepressed patients with Huntington's disease. *Mov Disord* 12:397–401, 1997.

165. Ranen NG, Peyser CE, Folstein SE: ECT as a treatment for depression in Huntington's disease. *J Neuropsychiatry Clin Neurosci* 6:154–159, 1994.

166. Sajotovic M, Verbanac P, Ramirez LF, Meltzer HY: Clozapine treatment of psychiatric symptoms resistant to neuroleptic treatment in patients with Huntington's chorea. *Neurology* 41:156, 1991.

167. Shoulson I, Goldblatt D, Charlton M, Joynt RJ: Huntington's disease: Treatment with muscimol, a GABA-mimetic drug. *Ann Neurol* 4:279–284, 1978.

168. Manyam N, Hare T, Katz L: Effect of isoniazid on CSF and plasma GABA levels in Huntington's disease. *Life Sci* 26:1303–1308, 1980.

169. Nutt JG, Rosin A, Chase TN: Treatment of Huntington's disease with a cholinergic agonist. *Neurology* 28:1061–1064, 1978.

170. Schults C, Steardo L, Barone P, et al: Huntington's disease: Effect of cysteamine, a somatostatin-depleting agent. *Neurology* 36:1099–1102, 1986.

171. Glass M, Faull RL, Dragunow M: Loss of cannabinoid receptors in the substantia nigra in Huntington's disease. *Neuroscience* 56:523–527, 1993.

172. Consroe P, Laguna J, Allender J, et al: Controlled clinical trial of cannabidiol in Huntington's disease. *Pharmacol Biochem Behav* 40:701–708, 1991.

173. Greenamyre JT: The role of glutamate in neurotransmission and neurologic disease. *Arch Neurol* 43:1058–1063, 1986.

174. Feigin A, Zgaljardic D: Recent advances in Huntington's disease: Implications for experimental therapeutics. *Curr Opin Neurol* 15:483–489, 2002.

175. Shoulson I, Odoroff C, Oakes D, et al: A controlled clinical trial of baclofen in Huntington's disease. *Ann Neurol* 25:252–259, 1989.

176. Walker FO, Hunt VP: An open label trial of dextromethorphan in Huntington's disease. *Clin Neuropharmacol* 12:322–330, 1989.

177. Andreassen OA, Dedeoglu A, Ferrante RJ, et al: Creatine increase survival and delays motor symptoms in a transgenic animal model of Huntington's disease. *Neurobiol Dis* 8:479–491, 2001.

178. Ferrante RJ, Andreassen OA, Jenkins BG, et al: Neuroprotective effects of creatine in a transgenic mouse model of Huntington's disease. *J Neurosci* 20:4389–4397, 2000.

179. Schilling G, Coonfield ML, Ross CA, Borchelt DR: Coenzyme Q10 and remacemide hydrochloride ameliorate motor deficits in a Huntington's disease transgenic mouse model. *Neurosci Lett* 315:149–153, 2001.

180. Ferrante RJ, Andreassen OA, Dedeoglu A, et al: Therapeutic effects of coenzyme Q10 and remacemide in transgenic mouse models of Huntington's disease. *J Neurosci* 22:1592–1599, 2002.

181. Chen M, Ona VO, Li M, et al: Minocycline inhibits caspase-1 and caspase-3 expression and delays mortality in a transgenic mouse model of Huntington disease. *Nat Med* 6:797–801, 2000.

182. Bensadoun JC, De Almeida LP, Dreano M, et al: Neuroprotective effect of interleukin-6 and IL6/IL6R chimera in the quinolinic acid rat model of Huntington's syndrome. *Eur J Neurosci* 14:1753–1761, 2001.

183. Andreassen OA, Ferrante RJ, Dedeoglu A, Beal MF: Lipoic acid improves survival in transgenic mouse models of Huntington's disease. *Neuroreport* 12:3371–3373, 2001.

184. Andreassen OA, Ferrante RJ, Huang HM, et al: Dichloroacetate exerts therapeutic effects in transgenic mouse models of Huntington's disease. *Ann Neurol* 50:112–117, 2001.

185. Wei H, Qin ZH, Senatorov VV, et al: Lithium suppresses excitotoxicity-induced striatal lesions in a rat model of Huntington's disease. *Neuroscience* 106:603–612, 2001.

186. Hockly E, Cordery PM, Woodman B, et al: Environmental enrichment slows disease progression in R6/2 Huntington's disease mice. *Ann Neurol* 51:235–242, 2002.

187. Peyser CE, Folstein M, Chase GA, et al: Trial of d-alpha tocopherol in Huntington's disease. *Am J Psychiatry* 152:1771–1775, 1995.

188. Schumacher JM, Hantraye P, Brownell AL, et al: A primate model of Huntington's disease: Functional neural transplantation and CT-guided stereotactic procedures. *Cell Transplant* 1:313–322, 1992.

189. Bachoud-Levi AC, Remy P, Nguyen JP, et al: Motor and cognitive improvements in patients with Huntington's disease after neural transplantation. *Lancet* 356:1975–1979, 2000.

190. Bachoud-Levi AC, Deglon N, Nguyen JP, et al: Neuroprotective gene therapy for Huntington's disease using a polymer encapsulated BHK cell line engineered to secrete human CNTF. *Hum Gene Ther* 11:1723–1729, 2000.

Chapter 36

NEUROPATHOLOGY AND PATHOPHYSIOLOGY OF HUNTINGTON'S DISEASE

STEVEN M. HERSCH, H. DIANA ROSAS,
and ROBERT J. FERRANTE

NEUROPATHOLOGY   603
    Striatum   603
    Globus Pallidus   608
    Substantia Nigra   608
    Thalamus   609
    Subthalamus   610
    Hypothalamus   610
    Cerebral Cortex   610
    Cerebellum and Brainstem   612
    In Vivo Imaging of Neuropathology   613
MOLECULAR PATHOLOGY
  AND PATHOPHYSIOLOGY   615
    Excitotoxic Stress   615
    Energy Depletion and Oxidative Stress   615
    Role of Normal and Mutant Huntingtin
        Proteins in Pathogenesis   616

Huntington's disease (HD) is a neurodegenerative disorder related to a mutation occurring in the coding region of the IT15 gene on chromosome 4. The average age of onset is about 40 years of age; however, the range is extremely broad, with pediatric and late-life onsets not infrequent. The genetic mutation consists of expansion of a polymorphic trinucleotide (CAG) repeat, near the 5' end of the gene, that normally ranges from about 17 to 30 copies. Individuals with more than 37 repeats develop HD, with the largest numbers (greater than 60) correlating with juvenile onset of HD. Genetic anticipation occurs such that the affected offspring of males have an increased probability of developing the disease at an earlier age than their fathers. The IT15 gene codes for a normal protein, named huntingtin, which is of unknown function. In individuals heterozygous for HD, both normal huntingtin and huntingtin containing an expanded polyglutamine tract, transcribed by the CAG expansion, are expressed. The relationship between this abnormal protein and neuropathology has been studied extensively since the gene was discovered and it seems likely that its aberrant protein-protein interactions lead to neuronal degeneration and death. A hallmark of HD is the presence of insoluble aggregates of huntingtin[1] which can occur in neuronal nuclei, cytoplasm, and processes[2] and which consists of heterogeneous mixtures of mutant and normal huntingtin and a variety of other proteins. While much has been learned, many questions remain, particularly which interactions of mutant huntingtin are most important for pathogenesis. The clinical expression of HD is characteristic and consists of progressively disordered movement, behavior, and cognition. The specific symptoms and progression of HD can be related to its neuropathology, which is characterized by relatively selective loss of specific neuronal populations in a variety of brain regions. Basal ganglia pathology has been the most thoroughly characterized and has been central to the development of animal models and hypotheses about the circuitry involved in chorea and about potential mechanisms of neuronal death in HD. Pathology in other brain regions has not been studied as extensively but is more widespread than the customary focus on basal ganglia might suggest and undoubtedly contributes to disease phenotype. Pathology outside the brain has neither been positively identified nor excluded. This review focuses on research occurring in the last 25 years, during which the identification of the causative genetic mutation and new methods in quantitative anatomy, neuroimaging, immunocytochemistry, biochemistry, and molecular biology have converged to produce an explosion of new knowledge and ideas about HD.

Neuropathology

STRIATUM

GROSS AND HISTOLOGIC PATHOLOGY

The most striking neuropathology in HD occurs within the neostriatum, in which there is gross atrophy of the caudate nucleus and putamen, accompanied by marked neuronal loss, astrogliosis (Fig. 36-1), and reactive microgliosis.[3–6] The striatal astrogliosis appears to reflect relative astrocyte survival in a shrinking striatum,[7] rather than a primary or reactive astrocytosis. Oligodendrogliosis also accompanies neuronal loss,[8] most likely an artifact of their relative preservation. The extent of gross striatal pathology, neuronal loss, and gliosis provides a basis for grading the severity of HD pathology (grades 0–4),[9] which also correlates to the extent of clinical disability (Fig. 36-2). Grade 0 cases have a strong clinical and familial history suggesting HD but no detectable histological neuropathology at autopsy. In grade 1 cases, neuropathological changes can be detected microscopically with as much as 50 percent depletion of striatal neurons but without gross atrophy. In more severe grades (2–4), gross atrophy, neuronal depletion, and gliosis are progressively more pronounced, and pallidal pathology becomes evident. In the most severe grade (4), more than 90 percent of striatal neurons are lost, and microscopy predominantly reveals astrocytes. There is a dorsal-to-ventral, anterior-to-posterior, and medial-to-lateral progression of neuronal death, with the dorsomedial striatum affected earliest and relative sparing of the ventral striatum and nucleus accumbens.[9,10] Increasing data suggest

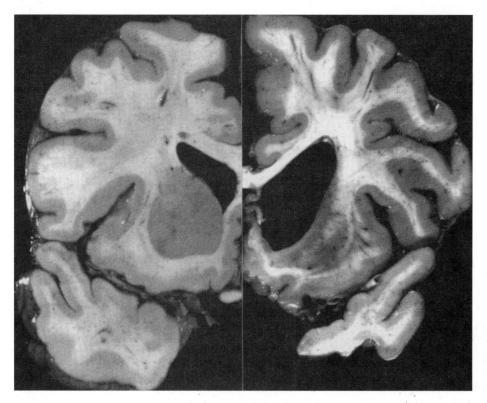

FIGURE 36-1 Photomicrographs of fixed cerebral hemispheres from a 58-year-old female with HD (*right*) and an age-matched normal specimen (*left*) at a coronal level through the rostral striatum. Note the marked atrophy of the caudate nucleus and putamen, along with cortical atrophy and white matter loss in HD.

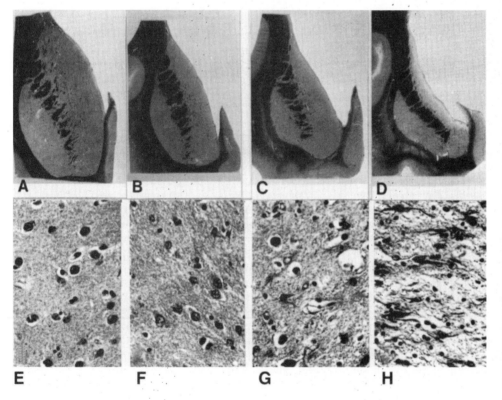

FIGURE 36-2 Coronal sections through the level of the caudate nucleus and putamen, demonstrating the grades of severity of striatal involvement. A normal specimen is represented in *A*. No gross striatal atrophy is observed in grades 0 and 1. In grade 2 (*B*), there is striatal atrophy, but the caudate nucleus remains convex. In grade 3 (*C*), striatal atrophy is more severe, with the caudate nucleus flat. In grade 4 (*D*), striatal atrophy is most severe, with the medial surface concave. Concomitant with the severity of gross atrophy observed in grades 2, 3, and 4, progressive neuronal loss and astrogliosis occur within the caudate nucleus and putamen in *F*, *G*, and *H*, respectively. There is a dorsoventral gradient of cell death, with the dorsal striatum most severely involved.

that neuropathology can predate symptoms by many years. Postmortem evaluations of individuals at risk for HD who died prior to the onset of symptoms has revealed striatal atrophy, widespread huntingtin aggregation, and oligodendrogliosis in the presence of neuronal loss.[2,11] Similarly, quantitative magnetic resonance imaging (MRI) analysis has indicated striatal volume atrophy in presymptomatic individuals at known genetic risk for developing HD.[12–14] The magnitude of the CAG repeat expansion correlates with the magnitude of striatal volume loss, suggesting that the rate of progression of striatal pathology is faster in individuals with higher numbers of repeats.[15–17]

SELECTIVE NEURONAL LOSS AND PRESERVATION

Quantitative microscopic studies demonstrating relative preservation of large striatal neurons and severe loss of medium-sized striatal neurons provided early evidence for selective neuronal degeneration in the neostriatum.[7,18] Since then, extensive biochemical, tissue-binding, and immunocytochemical studies of HD brain tissue have demonstrated marked disparities, with loss versus preservation of a variety of neurochemical substances within the basal ganglia, suggesting that the destructive process is not equally expressed in all striatal neurons and that there is a selective pattern of neuronal vulnerability.

Medium spiny neurons are inhibitory projection neurons that use gamma-aminobutyric acid (GABA) as their primary neurotransmitter, and they comprise more than 80 percent of all striatal neurons. Reductions in GABA, its synthetic enzyme glutamic acid decarboxylase, and its degradative enzyme GABA transaminase in the neostriatum were among the earliest neurochemical changes detected in HD and could be correlated with loss of medium spiny neurons.[19–23] Medium spiny neurons have further been shown to be depleted in HD based on the loss of substance P,[24] enkephalin,[24] calcineurin,[25] calbindin,[26–28] histamine H_2 receptors,[30] dopamine receptors,[31,32] cannabinoid receptors,[33] and adenosine A_{2A} receptors[29] (Fig. 36-3). Medium spiny neurons can be divided into two populations based upon both connectional and neurochemical differences. One subpopulation expresses D1 dopamine receptors and the cotransmitter substance P, and projects primarily to the internal segment of the globus pallidus (GPi) and the substantia nigra pars reticulata (SNr). The other population expresses the D2 dopamine receptor and enkephalin and projects primarily to the external segment of the globus pallidus (GPe).[34] All of these markers of striatal projection neurons and their axonal projections are progressively lost in HD, correlating with the degeneration and loss of medium spiny neurons.[24,25,31,35–40] The earliest changes seem to be losses in cannabinoid CB1, D2 and adenosine A_{2A} receptors

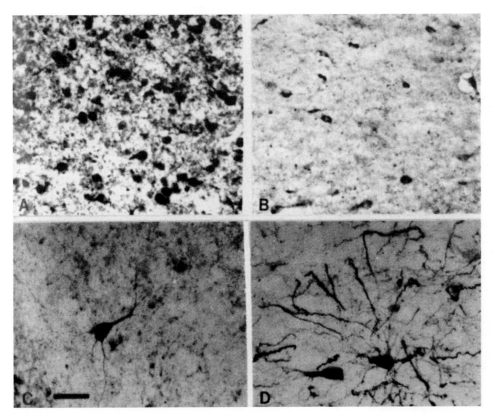

FIGURE 36-3 Calbindin-positive spiny striatal neurons in normal (*A* and *C*) and HD (*B* and *D*) caudate nucleus. The number of immunoreactive neurons is significantly reduced in HD. Degenerative alterations of this neuronal population, as demonstrated in Golgi preparations (see Fig. 36-5), are observed in *D*. There is a distal shift in dendritic staining in HD.

in the striatum and GPe, followed later by a loss of D1, with all of these receptors being profoundly lost as HD progresses.[41] Recent evidence, especially in transgenic mouse models of HD, suggests that there are many selective neurochemical alterations due to transcriptional dysfunction that predates neuronal loss and provides neurochemical bases for neuronal dysfunction prior to neuronal loss.[42]

Although both populations of medium spiny neurons are lost, there is evidence that, particularly in the early stages of HD, striatal neurons projecting to the GPe are preferentially lost in comparison to striatal neurons projecting to the GPi.[43–45] It has been suggested that this differential loss of striatal projections leads to imbalanced activity in the so-called direct and indirect pathways, causing chorea.[46–48] More specifically, the release of the GPe from inhibitory striatal input is hypothesized to result in excessive inhibition of the subthalamic nucleus which, in turn, causes decreased activation of the GPi and reduced inhibition of the thalamus, leading to increased cortical excitation and chorea. Consistent with this hypothesis, bicuculline blockade of the GABAergic input to the GPe causes chorea in primates.[49]

Furthermore, more equal loss of neurons projecting to both GPi and GPe may be associated with the occurrence of the rigid-akinetic variant of HD,[44] which usually occurs in juveniles. This model has been very useful but is probably oversimplified, because it does not account for such findings as increased thalamic levels of GABA,[45] for simultaneous pathology in other parts of the circuit, or for the finding that the D1 dopamine receptor is reduced more than D2 in the striatum and in the termination zones of striatal afferents.[31,32] This latter finding is contrary to what would be predicted, based on the changes in substance P and enkephalin.

In addition to medium spiny neurons, there are a variety of interneurons in the striatum, expressing other neuroactive substances. Those interneurons that have been studied appear resistant to the neurodegeneration that occurs in HD (Fig. 36-4). These include several types of large- and medium-sized aspiny or sparsely spiny neurons, including one type that expresses somatostatin and neuropeptide Y and can be visualized by NADPH-diaphorase histochemistry,[50] a type of substance P-expressing neuron,[51] large cholinergic interneurons,[52] and calretinin-expressing interneurons.[53]

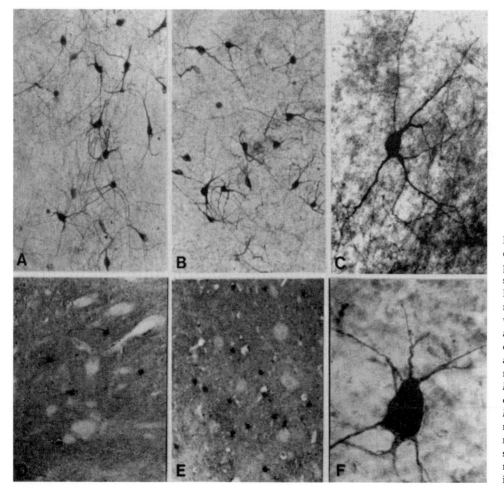

FIGURE 36-4 Photomicrographs of aspiny striatal neuron populations, which are relatively spared in HD. Medium-sized NADPH-diaphorase striatal neurons are represented in *A–C*, with normal staining found in *A* and preservation in an HD case demonstrated in *B*. Large acetylcholinesterase striatal neurons are demonstrated in *D–F*. *D* demonstrates the normal density of these neurons, while *E* demonstrates that their numbers increase in HD as a result of survival in a shrinking striatum. The density of both neuronal types is significantly increased in HD.

There is a striking persistence of somatostatin and neuro-peptide Y,[54,55] and of the somatostatin/neuropeptide Y/NADPH-diaphorase neurons that express them in both caudate nucleus and putamen in HD.[56−59] The density of these neurons is actually increased 4–5-fold, reflecting the combined effects of both neuronal sparing and tissue shrinkage. The preservation of large cholinergic interneurons likely accounts for the increased ratio of large to small neurons seen in morphometric studies[7,18] of the striatum in HD and also for the preservation of acetylcholinesterase activity.[60] Levels of choline acetyltransferase, the synthetic enzyme for acetylcholine, by contrast, are progressively reduced.[21,52] This may be a result of loss of local postsynaptic targets for cholinergic neurons, most of which are spiny dendrites,[61] and of subsequent reduction in their axons and in acetylcholine synthesis. The preservation of classes of neurons has been invaluable experimentally, providing a means for determining whether animal models of HD reproduce the selective vulnerability that occurs in human HD.

NEURONAL REMODELING AND DEGENERATION

Alterations in the dendritic structure of several types of neurons vulnerable in HD have suggested that both proliferative and degenerative alterations occur in a prolonged process before cell death finally ensues. Whether these alterations reflect a primary abnormality in the regulation of dendritic architecture or a secondary compensation and decompensation for altered striatal circuitry is unknown; however, they likely represent significant functional changes in the neurophysiology of striatal neurons. Early morphological alterations of spiny striatal neurons have been described using Golgi and calbindin immunocytochemical methods (Fig. 36-5).[62,63] Proliferative changes, found primarily in moderate grades of HD, include prominent recurving of distal dendritic segments, short-segment branching along the length of dendrites, and increased numbers and size of dendritic spines. Degenerative alterations, found primarily in more severe cases, consist of truncated dendritic arbors, focal dendritic swelling, and marked spine loss. The relative extent to which enkephalin and substance P subsets develop proliferative changes is not known. It is also not known whether such alterations also occur in striatal interneurons that are spared in HD. These newly formed dendritic arbors and increased numbers of dendritic spines may form functional connections and represent a plastic increase in postsynaptic surfaces in compensation for lost neurons. It has been suggested that the resulting increase in synapses could facilitate neuronal excitability and exacerbate excitotoxic cell death. [63] Plastic degenerative alterations in dendritic structure have also been reported in transgenic mouse models of HD.[64−66] Once neurons become unable to compensate for the stresses they undergo, they degenerate in a process with some similarities to apoptosis.[67−69] The morphology of the cell death, which has been best examined in HD transgenic mouse models (Fig. 36-6), includes shrinkage, irregular cell and nuclear envelopes, chromatin clumping, mild endoplasmic reticulum swelling, and mitochondrial degeneration. Unlike neuronal apoptosis or excitotoxic cell death, the nuclear membrane does not break down until very late, smooth

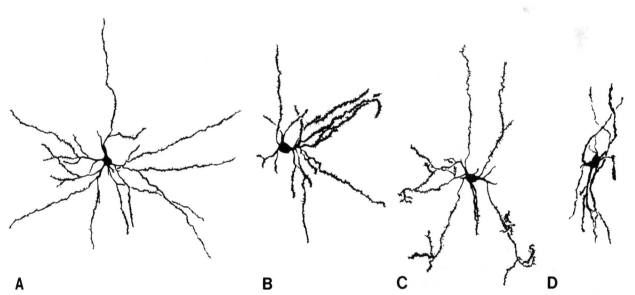

A **B** **C** **D**

FIGURE 36-5 Camera lucida drawings of representative spiny striatal neurons in normal (*A*), moderate grades of HD (*B* and *C*), and severe grades of HD (*D*). Normal spiny neurons have 3–7 primary dendrites, which centrifugally radiate from the soma. In moderate grades of HD, the dysmorphic alterations are proliferative. There is an increase in spine density with short-segment branching and terminal dendritic curving. In severe grades of HD, the changes are degenerative, consisting of truncated dendritic arbors, focal swellings, and marked spine loss.

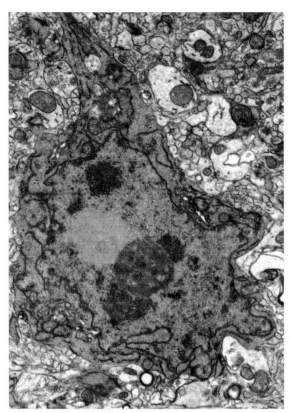

FIGURE 36-6 Electron micrograph of a degenerating striatal neuron from the R6/2 transgenic mouse, demonstrating typical features of cell death in HD models with shrinkage, loss of round cellular and nuclear contours, nuclear invaginations, chromatin clumping, and mild swelling of organelles. The pale nuclear mass is a nuclear aggregate.

dense spherical chromatin balls are not formed, and apoptotic bodies are not seen.[70] Perhaps transcriptional dysfunction (see below) prevents the complete expression of genetic cell death programs.

STRIOSOME AND MATRIX PATHOLOGY

The striatum is also composed of chemically and connectionally heterogeneous compartments termed patches or striosomes and matrix.[34,71] Striosomes consist of discrete areas distributed throughout the striatum in which opiate receptors, substance P, met-enkephalin, and cholecystokinin are concentrated. The intervening matrix is enriched in somatostatin, neuropeptide Y, NADPH-diaphorase, calbindin, choline acetyltransferase, acetylcholinesterase, and cytochrome oxidase. Although the striosome-matrix compartments, as determined by acetylcholinesterase[72,73] or by calbindin immunocytochemistry,[27,74] persist in the striatum in HD, the total area of the matrix is reduced, whereas the total area of striosomes is unchanged (Fig. 36-7). These findings are consistent with the preferential loss of striatal D1

receptors[31,32] but would be unexpected when striatal neurons projecting to the GPe are preferentially lost. Because both types of projection neurons are actually admixed in the striatum,[75] patterns of connectivity may not relate quite exactly to striosome/matrix organization.

GLOBUS PALLIDUS

Pallidal atrophy and gliosis have long been recognized to occur in HD;[9,76] however, its extent is probably underappreciated. In a standard-setting quantitative study,[7] Lange et al. determined that both the GPe and GPi can lose more than 50 percent of volume and more than 40 percent of neurons, while glia increase both in concentration and in absolute number (Fig. 36-8). These authors felt that pallidal degeneration is more likely a result of primary degeneration of pallidal neurons than of a transneuronal consequence of striatal atrophy. As they also pointed out, pallidal degeneration and loss of pallidal projections has not been sufficiently considered in models attempting to explain chorea. Most recent studies concerned with pallidal pathology in HD have focused more on striatopallidal afferents than on pallidal neurons or their projections. Inhibitory striatal afferents project differentially to the GPi and GPe and coat pallidal dendrites with terminals. Striatopallidal neurons expressing substance P project primarily to the GPi, whereas those expressing enkephalin project primarily to the GPe.[34] As discussed above, there has been some evidence of preferential loss of GPe afferents in choreatic HD, based primarily on the differential loss of substance P and enkephalin immunoreactivity.[43–45,77] Whether these results were in any way affected by pallidal neuron loss is unknown.

SUBSTANTIA NIGRA

Loss of striatonigral fibers, as well as nigral neurons, has previously been reported to occur in HD.[6,78,79] There have been two recent quantitative studies of nigral pathology in HD, using distinct methods that may explain the differences in their results.[80,81] Both studies found substantial atrophy and gliosis of both the pars compacta (SNc) and pars reticulata (SNr), with a loss in cross-sectional area of as much as 40 percent (Fig. 36-9). Ferrante et al. observed that the SNr, however, had a greater area loss than the SNc.[81] Both studies also reported that nonpigmented neurons were reduced in both nigral zones and by as much as 45 percent. Oyanagi et al. found that pigmented neurons were reduced by about 50 percent medially and laterally but were preserved centrally,[80] whereas Ferrante et al. found pigmented neurons to be relatively spared with an increase in number resulting from their preservation in a shrinking SNc.[81] The loss of nonpigmented cells may be quite relevant to the development of motor symptoms, because these neurons are the source of nigral afferents to the thalamus, superior colliculus, and brainstem. The relative preservation of pigmented neurons is consistent with some preservation of dopaminergic

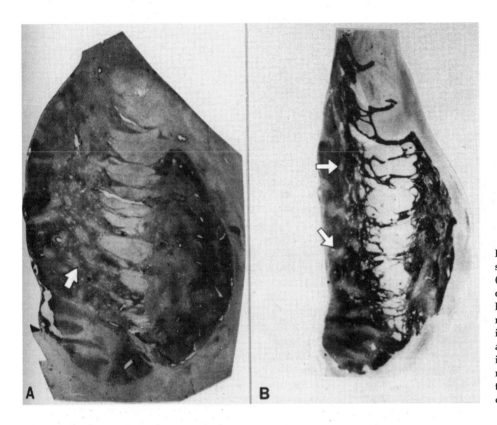

FIGURE 36-7 Acetylcholinesterase staining in the striatum in normal (*A*) and severe (*B*) HD. The intensity of staining is heterogeneous, with lighter-stained areas (arrows) referred to as patches, and the intervening more intensely stained area referred to as the matrix. There is a significant reduction in the matrix compartment, in comparison to that of the total area of patch compartments in HD.

nigrostriatal projections,[54] although there is evidence of significant loss of nigrostriatal terminals, especially in HD patients with a rigid-akinetic syndrome.[82] The topography of nigral atrophy did not correlate with the dorsomedial-to-ventrolateral pattern of striatal atrophy,[80] suggesting that nigral cell loss cannot be fully explained by loss of striatonigral afferents. However, the possibility of

transneuronal degeneration remains, because striatal excitotoxic lesions in rodents can cause subsequent neuronal degeneration in the SNr.[83] Interestingly, because the neuronal loss can be prevented by administration of a specific GABA agonist, neuronal death may be related to the loss of inhibitory GABAergic input with subsequent excessive excitation of SNr neurons.

THALAMUS

Until recently, there has been limited study of thalamic pathology in HD, although its presence has been acknowledged. Dom et al.,[84] who examined the ventrolateral thalamus in 7 cases of HD, performed the first specific study. Because the basal ganglia outflow directed to the frontal cortex is relayed by the ventrolateral thalamus, pathology in this nucleus may be quite relevant to the movement disorders occurring in HD. These investigators found that 50 percent of small neurons disappeared, whereas large neurons were not altered. If these small thalamic neurons are inhibitory interneurons, their loss could be related to thalamic disinhibition. Increased levels of thalamic GABA in HD,[45] however, are not consistent with this hypothesis, unless it can somehow be viewed as a compensatory upregulation of GABA. The centromedian-parafascicular complex, which is the major source of thalamostriatal afferents, was found to undergo a loss of 55 percent of neurons along with marked astrogliosis.[85]

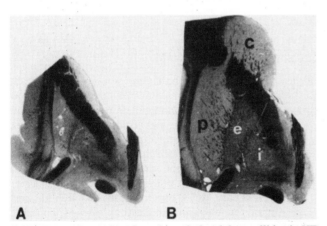

FIGURE 36-8 Coronal sections through the globus pallidus in HD (*A*) and a normal age-matched specimen (*B*) stained for myelin. The caudate nucleus (c) is reduced to a thin ribbon, whereas the putamen (p), GPi (i) and GPe (e) are severely atrophic in HD.

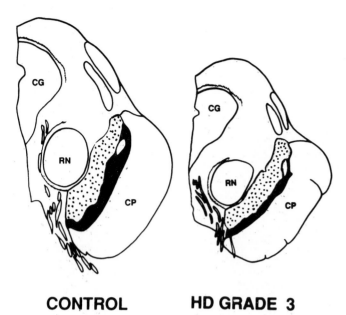

CONTROL   **HD GRADE 3**   **HD GRADE 4**

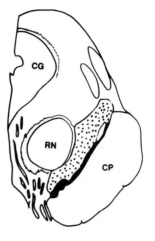

FIGURE 36-9 Sections through the substantia nigra at the level of the red nucleus (RN) and third nerve in normal control and grades 3 and 4 HD. The total area of the SNc (stippled area) and SNr (solid black area) is significantly reduced in HD, with the SNr most severely involved and the SNc relatively spared.

In contrast, the mediodorsal nucleus, which is not directly connected to the striatum but projects to the frontal cortex, was found to undergo a loss of 23.8 percent of neurons and a modest gliosis.[86] Perhaps these differences reflect the relative severity of neuropathology affecting striatal and frontal cortex circuitry. Clearly, further study of thalamic neuropathology is needed to clarify its contribution to HD symptoms.

SUBTHALAMUS

The subthalamus is an extremely interesting nucleus in regard to HD. Subthalamic strokes have long been known to cause ballistic involuntary movements that are very similar to those of chorea. The subthalamus is also postulated to be excessively inhibited in HD, leading to alterations in pallidothalamic excitation, as previously outlined, which may be the basis for chorea. Furthermore, the subthalamus gives rise to one of the few excitatory pathways in the basal ganglia and thus may be relevant in excitotoxic cell death (see section on pathophysiology). Nevertheless, little has been added to knowledge of subthalamic pathology in HD since the morphometric study by Lange et al., who found that subthalamic volume and neuron number are reduced by about 25 percent.[7] Studies examining how neurotransmitters and receptors are altered in the subthalamus have not been performed, but may help elucidate its role in the pathogenesis of chorea.

HYPOTHALAMUS

Hypothalamic pathology has been postulated to be related to the cachexia and autonomic disturbance that occurs in HD patients. Bruyn noted significant neuronal loss and gliosis in the supraoptic nucleus and lateral hypothalamic nucleus.[76]

In the only quantitative studies of hypothalamic pathology, Kremer et al.[87,88] found up to 90 percent neuronal loss in the lateral tuberal nucleus, which was worse in patients developing motor symptoms at an early age. The percentage of astrocytes did not change, whereas oligodendrocytes were reduced by 40 percent. It was further postulated that the high levels of glutamate receptors normally present in the lateral tuberal nucleus render these neurons selectively susceptible to excitotoxic cell death.[87] Although little is known about the normal function of the lateral tuberal nucleus, the possibility that its degeneration underlies the catabolic state that frequently occurs in HD patients is intriguing. Furthermore, because cell loss is so severe, this nucleus may have value in experimental investigations of cell death and neuroprotection in HD.

CEREBRAL CORTEX

Cortical atrophy has long been recognized as occurring in HD.[89,90] Its extent, clinical significance, and relationship to striatal degeneration have emerged as important issues in understanding and treating HD. For example, the cortex is the most important source of glutamatergic projections to the striatum, which have been implicated in excitotoxic contributions to degeneration, and it is also the source of trophic factors, particularly brain-derived neurotrophic factor (BDNF), critical for maintaining striatal neurons and which huntingtin may play a direct role in regulating.[91] Although the relative roles of the cerebral cortex and basal ganglia in psychiatric, behavioral, and cognitive symptoms of HD are difficult to separate, there should be little doubt that cortical degeneration is at least involved in personality change, dementia, and spasticity. If cortical atrophy contributes significantly to these symptoms, as seems likely from its extent, this may be a crucial area for further research. Because the entire cerebral cortex projects to the striatum and much of the frontal lobe receives the outflow of striatopallidothalamocortical circuits,[92,93] cortical and basal ganglia pathology may not be very separable clinically. Most studies related to potential medical and surgical therapies have focused on the striatum; however, when treatments preserve the striatum but not the cortex, many of the worst symptoms of the disease might still occur. Thus, understanding whether cortical degeneration is a primary process or a secondary retrograde phenomenon related to loss of a major cortical afferent target, the neostriatum, and whether cortical and striatal cell death occur by similar cellular mechanisms, may be of great importance.

GROSS AND REGIONAL NEUROPATHOLOGY

Generalized cortical atrophy is frequently apparent at autopsy (Fig. 36-1) and accounts for the majority of the 15–30 percent loss in brain weight that occurs in HD.[94,95] Gross and regional cortical atrophy has been studied planimetrically by several investigators. Lange[94] reported an overall cortical shrinkage of 15 percent in 5 cases of HD, and noted that atrophy occurred the least in frontal regions and the most in occipital association areas (30 percent). De la Monte et al.[95] studied 30 HD brains and demonstrated a 20–30 percent overall reduction in the cross-sectional area of cerebral cortex, accompanied by a 29–34 percent reduction in subcortical white matter. Thinning of the cortical gray matter ranged from 9 percent to 16 percent, perhaps explaining why obvious cortical pathology is easily missed when one is examining individual sections. The severity of atrophy occurring in the cortex, as well as in the striatum and thalamus, correlated with the clinical progression of the disease.[9,95] With increasing pathological grades of HD, brain weight declined, ventricular volume increased, cerebral atrophy increased, and the cortical ribbon thinned. Depression and dementia corresponded to the extent of both cortical and basal ganglia atrophy. It is not clear to what extent any cortical areas undergo more atrophy than others, and new MRI technology capable of detecting cortical thinning suggests a mixture of areas predictably affected and areas more variably affected.[96] However, pronounced degenerative changes occur in medial postcentral cortex, occipital isocortex (areas 18 and 19), prepyriform cortex, cingulate cortex,[94] primary motor cortex,[97] dorsolateral prefrontal cortex (areas 8, 9, 10, and 46),[98–100] and perihippocampal cortex, including entorhinal and transentorhinal regions.[101,102] A more recent volumetric study of 7 late-stage cases found shrinkage of all cortical lobes, averaging 19 percent, with sparing of the medial temporal lobe.[103] Gray matter volume loss averaged 23 percent and white matter 13 percent. In contrast to a previous study,[104] the CAG repeat number in these cases correlated with cortical atrophy divided by age of death but not with striatal

atrophy, suggesting that cortical atrophy may be a better marker for disease progression than striatal atrophy, which likely loses linearity because it is so severe early in the disease.

LAMINAR AND CELLULAR NEUROPATHOLOGY

The laminar pattern of cerebral cortical degeneration in HD has been studied qualitatively, with varying results. McCaughey[105] described diffuse degeneration through layers III, V, and VI, with some patchy involvement of IV. In 4 pediatric cases,[106] cortical degeneration appeared panlaminar. Forno and Jose[78] observed layer III to be the most severely affected in a series of adults. Roizin et al.[107] found that the middle layers of cortex were most affected in some cases, whereas the deeper layers were most affected in others. Bruyn et al.[6] later reported that layers III and V, and sometimes IV, had the most neuronal loss.

Quantitative studies have been performed more recently in a variety of brain regions, mostly in the frontal lobes.[97–100,108,109] The most consistent findings have been loss of volume and neurons in layers III, V, and VI. The concentration of neurons in these layers may not change,[98–100] however, indicating that cortical neuronal loss is proportional to cortical volume loss. Only one study has used unbiased counting methods, which permit estimating total numbers of neurons and glia.[108] The mean neuronal loss in the entire left cortical hemisphere was 33 percent, and was most pronounced in the supragranular layers. Interestingly, regional atrophy varied, with the primary sensory areas seemingly most affected, followed by prefrontal and premotor areas, while temporal association areas were only subtly affected. Astrocyte and oligodendrocyte concentrations, though not necessarily absolute numbers,[108] increase dramatically, especially in layers III–VI (Fig. 36-10). These increases likely indicate glial survival in a shrinking cortex and not reactive gliosis, because cortical glial fibrillary acidic protein staining does not increase.[110] The size of cortical neurons also declines in HD, suggesting selective loss or shrinkage of larger pyramidal cells (Fig. 36-10). Although there have been differing interpretations of these data, cortical cell loss is clearly not confined to neurons projecting to the striatum, which consist of a limited population of medium-sized pyramidal cells located deep in layer III and superficially in layer V. Thus, retrograde degeneration of corticostriatal neurons cannot readily account for cortical atrophy. These studies also suggest that there is relative sparing of cortical interneurons, which typically are small neurons. Further evidence for this includes data indicating that substance P-expressing interneurons are spared,[111] and that cortical concentrations of GABA, somatostatin, neuropeptide Y, cholecystokinin, and vasoactive intestinal polypeptide, which are expressed by interneurons, are all elevated in HD.[112–114] Cerebral cortical pyramidal cells have also been shown, by means of Golgi staining, to develop increased numbers of dendrites and dendritic spines whereas others appear to have degenerative

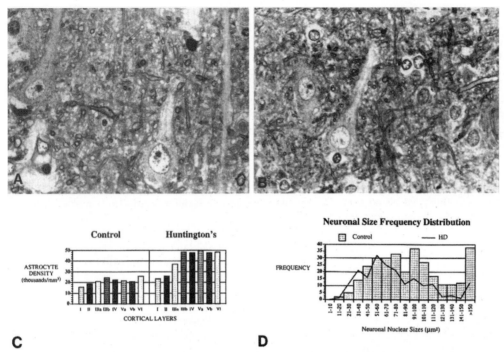

FIGURE 36-10 Toluidine blue-stained 2-μm sections from control (*A*) and HD (*B*) primary motor cortex. Normal-appearing pyramidal cells are visible in each. The HD case, however, contains many more astrocytes, as well as nuclear ghosts from degenerated neurons. Quantitative data (*C*) demonstrate that the density of astrocytes is more than doubled in layers III–VI. Measurement of nuclear diameters demonstrates that surviving neurons are smaller than control neurons and that the largest neurons seem to have disappeared.

changes,[115] suggesting that proliferative and degenerative changes occur in these neurons before cell death.

NEUROCHEMISTRY

Neurochemical alterations in the cerebral cortex in HD have been identified, although findings have been inconsistent. Two laboratories[23,116] have found that glutamate, the putative neurotransmitter of pyramidal cells, and GABA, a marker for inhibitory cortical interneurons, are reduced in the cerebral cortex. In contrast, Storey et al. showed glutamate and aspartate to increase in most areas of cortex that they examined.[114] Unlike the striatum, *N*-methyl-D-aspartate (NMDA) receptor binding is unchanged in cortex, whereas oc-amino-3-hydroxy-5-methyl-4-isoxazole propionic acid (AMPA) and kainate receptor binding is reduced in layer VI.[117] Such studies may offer evidence of selective vulnerability of distinct neuronal types; however, biochemical changes can be difficult to interpret without a detailed understanding of the underlying anatomic changes. For example, glutamate could be reduced from loss of neurons, loss of glutamatergic afferents, or alteration of glutamate transport, or metabolism in the absence of degenerative change. Understanding how the expression of glutamate receptors is altered in the cortex in HD may help explain altered cortical levels of glutamate. Whether cortical alterations in glutamate levels or glutamate

receptors play a role in excitotoxic cell death in the cerebral cortex or in the striatum, via corticostriatal projections, is an interesting question, about which there has been recent speculation fueled by the much greater concentration of huntingtin aggregates occurring in cortex than in striatum. Neurochemical markers of cortical interneurons have also been studied, including cholecystokinin, vasoactive intestinal peptide, neuropeptide Y, and somatostatin, which remain stable or increase, suggesting relative preservation of the interneurons expressing them.[118]

CEREBELLUM AND BRAINSTEM

Reports of cerebellar involvement in HD have been variable, with cerebellar atrophy being reported in some pediatric and adult cases.[106,119–121] At a cellular level, Purkinje cell loss has been the primary consistent finding;[6] however, thinning of the granule cell layer has also been observed and has been taken to indicate loss of this cell type as well.[121] One quantitative study[122] examined Purkinje cell loss in 17 HD cases of unknown grade. More than one-half had a reduction in Purkinje cell density greater than 50 percent. With huntingtin immunocytochemistry, we have also noted severe loss of Purkinje cells in advanced grades of HD (Fig. 36-11). In addition, proliferative and degenerative changes are visible

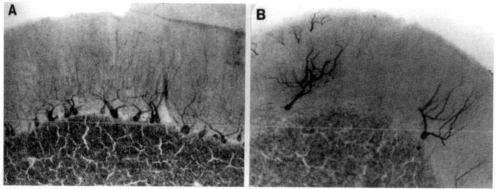

FIGURE 36-11 Immunocytochemistry in control (*A*) and HD cerebellum (*B*), using antihuntingtin antibodies. Purkinje cell drop-out is evident in the HD case (*B*), as is remodeling of the dendritic trees of those that survive.

in Purkinje cells. Dentate cell loss and gliosis and involvement of cerebellar efferent and afferent pathways have also been noted.[6,121] The clinical significance of cerebellar atrophy is difficult to gauge, as involuntary movements and dystonia may obscure the cardinal signs of cerebellar dysfunction. Nevertheless, contributions to gait ataxia, postural instability, dysrhythmic voluntary movements, altered speech cadence, and disordered eye movements are all possible.

Brainstem alterations in HD have received almost no attention in the last two decades, so there is little to add to the review of Bruyn et al.[6] from 1979, in which severe degeneration of the superior and inferior olivary, lateral vestibular, dorsal vagal, and hypoglossal nuclei was noted. Additional significant regions of neuropathology from the earlier literature include the red nucleus, the basis pontis, and the spinal cord.[5,6,78,120,123]

IN VIVO IMAGING OF NEUROPATHOLOGY

Novel neuroimaging methodologies are providing new opportunities to study brain changes in vivo, and to understand the progressive changes that occur during the course of disease. Several methods have thus far been applied in HD, including MRI, magnetic resonance spectroscopy (MRS), single-photon emission computed tomography, and positron emission tomography (PET). Each methodology provides unique information which, in concert, may provide insights into pathophysiological mechanisms.

High-resolution MRI has been used to obtain accurate measurements of brain atrophy. Although a significant body of research has focused on the striatum,[17,124,125] the brain region most severely affected in HD, more recent work using newly available techniques has demonstrated that measurable changes are present more globally in the brain even in early stages of disease, and that these changes may be present presymptomatically. Regional cortical thinning has been demonstrated in frontal, parietal, posterior temporal, parahippocampal, and occipital regions; some of

these changes have been found even presymptomatically.[14,96] As demonstrated in Fig. 36-12, cortical thinning appears to be both regionally and individually variable, suggesting that, not only is the cortex involved early in the disease, but that it may explain some of the variability in the clinical symptoms that occur in HD. Using semiautomated morphometric tools, more extensive loss of volumes of other brain structures, including the hippocampus, amygdala, hypothalamus, globus pallidus, and brainstem, in addition to the striatum, has recently been demonstrated in individuals in stages I and II of disease (Fig. 36-13). Selective structural volume loss was also shown to correlate with total functional capacity and duration of symptoms.[126] In summary, these studies

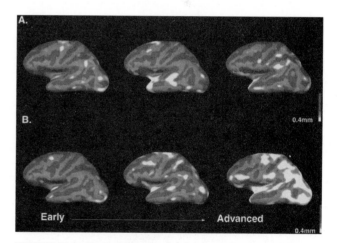

FIGURE 36-12 Cortical thinning in vivo in patients with HD determined in the left hemisphere by MRI. *A* demonstrates heterogeneity of regional involvement. All three individual subjects were in similar stages of disease. The left and middle mean thickness maps are from a set of twins. *B* demonstrates the progression of cortical thinning with advancing disease. Full yellow corresponds to >0.4 mm of cortical thinning. The mean thickness of the cortex normally varies from 2.5 to 4 mm. See Color Plate Section.

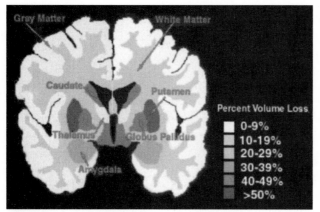

FIGURE 36-13 MRI brain segmentation. Composite representation of volume loss occurring in the brains of 18 individuals in the early stages of HD. In addition to the expected marked atrophy of the striatum, significant volume loss is also evident in the globus pallidus, amygdala, hypothalamus, and cortical white and gray matters. See Color Plate Section.

suggest that (1) more global, measurable atrophy is present in even early stages of disease, and (2) at least some of the phenotypic heterogeneity (i.e., some individuals have more prominent early cognitive or early psychiatric symptoms, rather than motor symptoms) may be explained by extrastriatal degeneration. As these types of analyses are extended to the determination of longitudinal changes that occur in the same subject, there is great potential to learn more about the precise nature of the altered structure-function relationships that occur throughout the course of disease in HD.

^{1}H-MRS has emerged as a tool for the measurement of brain metabolites and has been particularly useful in the determination of key substrates in oxidative and intermediary metabolism. Increased concentrations of lactate (Fig. 36-14), a marker of energetic defects, and choline, a glial marker, which may represent neuronal membrane breakdown and liberation of glycerylphosphocholine, have been reported in the striatum, occipital and frontal regions.[127] Decreased levels of *N*-acetyl-aspartate (NAA, a neuronal marker) have been reported in the striatum, most likely reflecting neuronal loss, or which may reflect impaired mitochondrial energy production as inhibitors of the mitochondrial respiratory chain have been shown to result in lower NAA concentrations. Increases in glutamine have been postulated in humans and reported in transgenic mouse models of HD; however, it is impossible to separate glutamate from glutamine using 1.5-T field strengths, but this could likely be done using higher field strengths. [31]P studies of skeletal muscle have shown reduced phosphocreatine/inorganic phosphate ratios in symptomatic HD, supporting a role for a more global mitochondrial dysfunction in HD.[128] [13]C studies have been performed in transgenic mouse models, with potential to provide important information on the specific nature of the metabolic defect in humans with HD.

In PET, radioactive tracers are used to measure glucose metabolism or receptor density. Reductions of ^{18}F-fluorodeoxyglucose and in postsynaptic D1 and D2 receptor densities, as measured by radiolabeled ^{11}C-raclopride or ^{11}C-beta-CIT, respectively, have been reported in the striatum and in areas of cortex, and were found to correlate with duration of symptoms or with cognitive performance.[129]

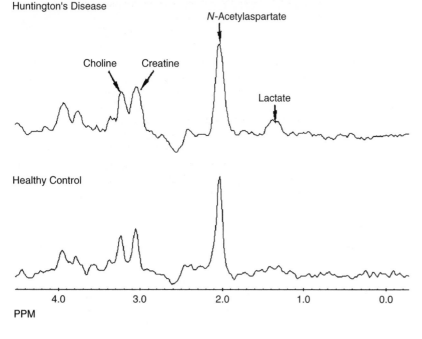

FIGURE 36-14 ^{1}H-MRS spectra of supplementary motor cortex, comparing an individual with HD (*top*) and a control subject (*bottom*). Lactate is elevated in the HD subject compared to the healthy control, suggesting an energetic defect.

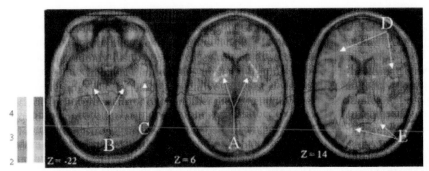

FIGURE 36-15 Voxel-based network analysis utilizing a principal component analysis applied to flourodeoxyglucose/PET scans from a group of 12 presymptomatic HD gene carriers and 11 age-matched controls. The first principal component discriminated the HD gene carriers from controls (*P* < 0.005), and was characterized by hypometabolism in bilateral striatum (A), covarying with hypermetabolism in bilateral hippocampi (B), right superior temporal gyrus (C), bilateral insula (D), and cuneus (E). *Courtesy of Andy Feigin.* **See Color Plate Section.**

Similar alterations have been reported in individuals who were known genetic carriers but who did not have motor symptoms and in whom there was no measurable change in striatal volumes,[130–132] suggesting that neuronal dysfunction occurs prior to measurable morphometric changes and may be used to identify transition to clinical symptoms. This is illustrated in Fig. 36-15, which utilizes a statistical modeling approach, the scaled subprofile model, and principal components analysis, to identify significant patterns of regional metabolic covariation in regional cerebral metabolic rates for glucose in presymptomatic as compared to healthy control groups.

Functional MRI also holds promise to provide important information on the nature of the structure-function alterations, especially in the earliest stages of disease, when neurons are at risk and dysfunctional, but where there is no measurable atrophy. Altered patterns of activation have been reported in the few studies published to date,[133,134] and may provide additional information about the neural processes in HD.

In summary, novel imaging tools are providing important insights into basic disease mechanisms, in vivo, in a noninvasive and reproducible fashion. Much work remains to be done. Nevertheless, they may provide reliable and sensitive biomarkers for use in future neuroprotective interventions in both individuals at risk for developing disease and for those already symptomatic, and may enable us to disentangle the altered structure-function relationships that develop in HD.

Molecular Pathology and Pathophysiology

EXCITOTOXIC STRESS

The initial observations suggesting that excitotoxicity may play a role in HD was made by the McGeers[60] and Coyle and Schwarcz.[135] Both sets of investigators showed that injections of the glutamate agonist kainic acid produced axon-sparing lesions of the striatum resembling HD. This model was refined by the use of selective NMDA agonists, such as quinolinic acid,[54,136,137] which cause medium spiny neurons to degenerate (astrogliosis) but are sparing of NADPH-diaphorase and cholinergic interneurons. Chronic lesions result in significantly increased striatal atrophy, more closely replicating the neuropathology of HD.[138,139] Furthermore, in the monkey, quinolinic acid excitotoxic lesions lead to hyperkinesis and dopamine agonist-induced chorea.[114] The close match of these models with HD neuropathology strongly suggests an excitotoxic mechanism of cell death. Selective depletion of NMDA receptors in the putamen in HD suggested that neurons expressing this glutamate receptor are selectively vulnerable.[140] However, alterations in other types of glutamate receptors also occur.[141,142] Because increased glutamate levels, abnormal functioning of glutamate receptors, or the significant presence of endogenous excitotoxins have not been demonstrated in the striatum in HD, a basis for why excitotoxicity should occur has been elusive. Recent studies using transgenic mouse models of HD have identified increased NMDA receptor sensitivity,[143,144] possible alterations in glutamate transporter function,[145] and altered corticostriatal physiology as possible mechanisms.[146] Neurons weakened by the toxic effects of mutant huntingtin may simply be unable to tolerate the stress of normal synaptic activity. Importantly, glutamate antagonists had been neuroprotective in transgenic mouse models of HD.[147–149] The evidence for excitotoxicity contributing to the pathogenesis of HD remains compelling enough to justify medication trials with glutamate antagonists,[150] despite the recent failure of remacemide to be neuroprotective in one such trial.[151]

ENERGY DEPLETION AND OXIDATIVE STRESS

An hypothesis explaining the pattern of degeneration in HD has evolved that suggests that impaired energy metabolism may be involved in the degenerative process.[152–155] Several studies have suggested that altered energy metabolism occurs in HD. Cytochrome oxidase (complex IV) activity is reduced in striatum;[156] complex I activity is reduced in platelets[157] and muscle;[158] complex II/III activity is reduced in the caudate nucleus and putamen.[156,159] Levels of oxidative damage to DNA, proteins, and lipids are also increased in the HD striatum.[156,160] Increased lactate, a marker for metabolic stress, has been demonstrated in HD cortex and striatum in vivo by means of MRS.[161] These studies in HD suggest that metabolic dysfunction does occur, but it has been difficult to discern whether it is a secondary marker of degeneration or related to the pathophysiology of neuronal death. New studies in lymphoblasts from HD patients are suggesting that early mitochondrial dysfunction due to the presence of mutant huntingtin precedes degeneration.[162,163] Experimentally, energy (adenosine triphosphatase) depletion, which has recently been demonstrated to occur in a presymptomatic knock-in mouse model of HD,[164] can produce partial membrane depolarization and removal of the voltage-dependent magnesium block of the NMDA-linked calcium channel.[165] The open calcium channel could then permit normal amounts of glutamate to produce a heightened NMDA receptor response, which, in turn, could cause excitotoxic cell death. Animal studies show that striatal injection of mitochondrial toxins, such as the succinic dehydrogenase inhibitors 3-nitropropionic acid (3-NP) and malonic acid, produces selective neuronal loss identical to that produced by NMDA agonists and identical to the neuropathological pattern in HD, as well as analogous motor symptoms (Fig. 36-16 and Table 36-1).[166–168] Importantly, mitochondrial toxin-induced striatal pathology is dramatically reduced by NMDA receptor blockade, as well as by antioxidants and free radical scavengers.[169,170] This further strengthens the hypothesis of a metabolic defect underlying selective excitotoxicity,[165,171] and provides a rationale for treating HD with protectants against oxygen free-radical activity, such as OPC-14117 and coenzyme Q_{10},[151,172] as well as energy buffers such as creatine.[173]

ROLE OF NORMAL AND MUTANT HUNTINGTIN PROTEINS IN PATHOGENESIS

HUNTINGTIN mRNA

Huntingtin mRNA is normally distributed in diverse tissues in humans and rats and is expressed predominantly in neurons within the brain.[174–176] All neurons appear to express huntingtin mRNA, and there is no apparent correlation within particular types of neurons between levels of mRNA and their vulnerability to cell death. Because mRNA for both the normal and mutant alleles is produced by individuals with HD, and because known "knockout" mutations affecting one HD allele do not cause the HD phenotype,[177–179] simple gene inactivation is unlikely to underlie disease pathogenesis. Because mRNA for the mutant allele is expressed in HD brain in amounts similar to that of the normal allele,[175,180] an alteration in transcription is also unlikely to be pathogenic. The remaining possibilities are that the genetic mutation

affects ribosomal translation, or that it acts at the protein level to alter the normal function of huntingtin. RNA-binding proteins, which are tissue-specific and have been demonstrated to interact with the huntingtin CAG repeat,[181] could affect translation and also the intracellular localization of huntingtin mRNA. Nevertheless, inactivation of one allele does not cause HD, and so it would be difficult for a translational block to account for disease pathogenesis.

HUNTINGTIN PROTEIN

The normal functions of huntingtin remain uncertain. Current hypotheses have been based on its subcellular localization and on its interactions with a variety of known proteins. Subcellular fractionation reveals that huntingtin is found primarily in soluble fractions, and its relative levels in various tissues and brain areas correspond to the levels of its mRNA.[182] Both normal and mutant proteins are expressed in cell lines and tissues from HD patients (Fig. 36-17). Immunocytochemistry[182–186] (Fig. 36-18) indicates that huntingtin is located in neurons throughout the brain, with high levels evident in cortical pyramidal cells, cerebellar Purkinje cells, and large striatal interneurons, among others. Striatal medium spiny neurons are also well labeled, whereas medium-sized neurons in other brain regions may be quite variable. There are significant levels of huntingtin in the striatum, with heterogeneous expression evident both in medium spiny neurons and in interneurons such that more vulnerable neuronal populations appear to have relatively higher levels of huntingtin protein.[187] Subcellular localization of huntingtin is consistent with a primarily cytosolic protein found most abundantly in somatodendritic regions, but with some presence in axons as well as in the nucleus (Fig. 36-19). Huntingtin appears to associate particularly with dendritic microtubules and membrane-bound organelles, including mitochondria, transport vesicles, synaptic vesicles, and components of the endocytic system.[182,184,188,189] These localization studies suggested a possible role for huntingtin in the transport or function of these organelles, with mitochondrial, synaptic, and endosomal-lysosomal systems all being of potential interest. Dysfunction in these pathways could conceivably impair their cytoskeletal anchoring, transport, function, or degradation. The availability of mutant huntingtin at these functional sites, however, is not well understood and it is possible that mutant huntingtin is largely redistributed.

MUTANT HUNTINGTIN AGGREGATION AND HD PATHOGENESIS

The polyglutamine expansion causes a conformational change in huntingtin, as shown by the ability of antibodies to completely discriminate the normal and mutated forms.[190,191] It had been hypothesized that long polyglutamine stretches self-associate, either internally by forming hairpin loops or with other polyglutamine-containing

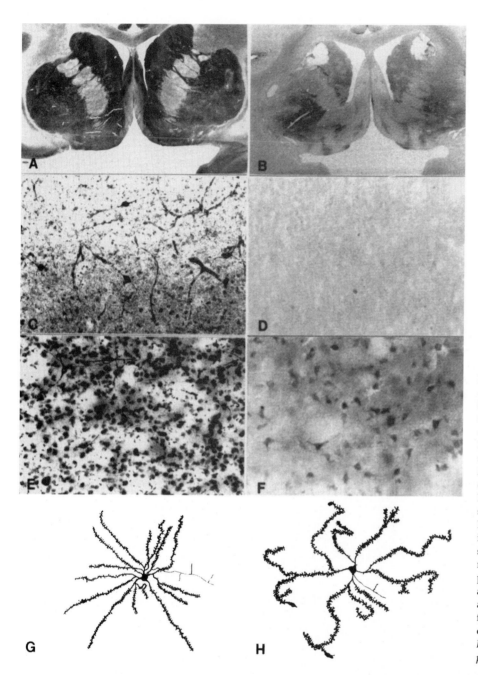

FIGURE 36-16 Histopathological alterations observed in a 3-NP-treated primate. Gross lesions are found in the dorsal aspect of the caudate nucleus and putamen in Nissl- and calbindin-stained sections through the striatum (*A* and *B*, respectively). There is a dorsoventral gradient of neuronal loss, with the dorsal striatum more severely involved. Only aspiny NADPH-diaphorase neurons persist in the dorsal striatum (*C*), with few spiny calbindin neurons (*D*). All neuronal populations are better preserved in the ventral striatum (*E* and *F*). Similar dysmorphic alterations, as observed in HD, are found in treated animals (*H*) in comparison to controls (*G*). (*From Brouillet et al.* [168] *Used with permission.*)

molecules,[192] and thereby engage in aberrant molecular interactions. Mutant huntingtin also undergoes proteolytic processing, releasing persistent N-terminal fragments containing the polyglutamine tract, which may be more toxic than the holoprotein. These fragments form macromolecular aggregates with themselves and with other proteins, which become ubiquitinated (targeting them for proteasomal degradation), insoluble, and large enough to be visible in the processes, cytoplasm, and nuclei of neurons.[1] Huntingtin aggregates are readily detected in histologic sections by antibodies against polyglutamines, N-terminal huntingtin epitopes, or ubiquitin. They have not been observed to persist in the extracellular space after the degeneration of the neurons containing them. They can be found all over the brain and are especially frequent in cortical regions and relatively infrequent in the striatum (Fig. 36-20).[188,193] The great majority of huntingtin aggregates are in dendrites, dendritic spines, and axons with a small proportion in neuronal somata and nuclei (Fig. 36-21).[188] Few are identifiable in glia. Many of the proteins that interact with huntingtin can also be

TABLE 36-1 Comparison of HD and 3-NP Striatal Lesions

Huntington's Disease	3-NP Striatal Lesion
Young-adult onset	Vulnerability in young adult animals
Striatal vulnerability	Striatal vulnerability
Dorsal-ventral gradient	Dorsal-ventral gradient
Movement disorder	Movement disorder
Chorea	Dystonia in rats, chorea in primates
Loss of medium spiny projection neurons	Loss of medium spiny projection neurons
Sparing of NADPH-diaphorase neurons	Sparing of NADPH-diaphorase neurons
Dendritic remodeling in spiny neurons	Dendritic remodeling in spiny neurons
Sparing of striatal afferents	Sparing of striatal afferents

found sequestered in the aggregates, and this sequestration is a potential means of lowering functional levels of needed proteins.

Aggregation of the N-terminus fragments of huntingtin is CAG length-dependent, occurring once the polyglutamine tract is about 39 amino acids long and increasing with greater lengths.[190,194,195] Thus it has been hypothesized that

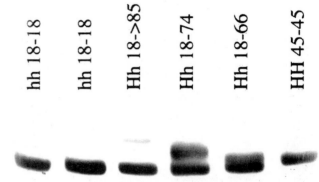

FIGURE 36-17 Western blot, using monoclonal antihuntingtin antibodies of lymphoblast lysates from control (hh) patients, heterozygote HD patients (Hh), and a homozygote HD patient (HH). The numbers correspond to the number of CAG repeats contained in each huntingtin allele. A single band is detected in control and homozygote cases, because the alleles have identical numbers of repeats; however, the homozygote is at a higher molecular weight. Two bands are visible in each of the heterozygote cases, corresponding to the differing molecular weights of normal and mutant huntingtin. This immunoblot demonstrates that both normal and mutant forms of huntingtin are expressed in tissue from HD patients. (*From Gutekunst et al.[184] Used with permission.*)

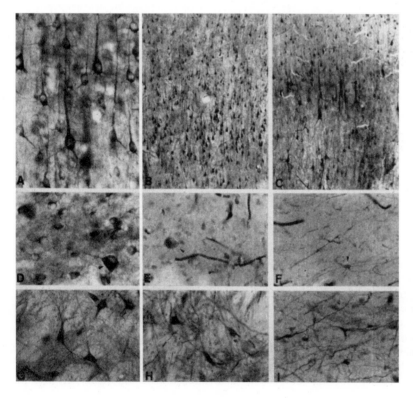

FIGURE 36-18 Immunocytochemistry using monoclonal antihuntingtin antibodies in sections from monkey (first column), from human controls (middle column), and from human HD cases (last column). The first row is from frontal cortex (*A–C*), the second row is from caudate nucleus (*D–F*), and the third row is from globus pallidus (*G–I*). As a result of optimal fixation, the monkey tissue is better stained and permits better resolution of cellular detail. In each region, neurons are well-stained, glia are unstained, nuclei are not labeled, and most label is somatodendritic, with some additional staining of axons and more diffuse staining of the neuropil. In cerebral cortex (*A–C*), pyramidal cells are most prominently stained. In normal monkey (*D*) and human (*E*) caudate nucleus, medium-sized neurons and large interneurons (arrows) are visible. In HD (*F*), only one neuron (arrow) is visible, which appears to be an aspiny interneuron. GPe and GPi neurons are also well-stained in monkey (*G*) and human (*H*), although they appear shrunken in HD (*I*). (Several of these micrographs were from *Gutekunst et al.[184] Used with permission.*)

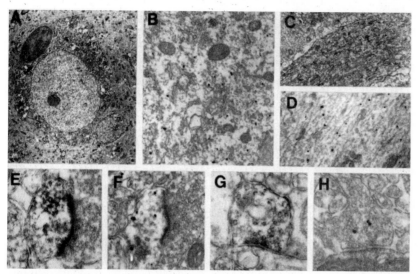

FIGURE 36-19 Electron-microscopic immunocytochemistry of huntingtin in monkey, using the diffusible reaction product, diaminobenzidine (DAB) (*A, C, E, G*) and immunogold (*B, D, F, H*), which permits much higher spatial resolution. DAB reaction product is visible in the perikaryon of a cortical pyramidal cell (center), but not in an adjacent astrocyte (bottom right) or oligodendrocyte (top left). All nuclei are unlabeled. At a higher magnification, immunogold particles are primarily free in the cytoplasm and are not associated with endoplasmic reticulum or Golgi apparatus, suggesting that the protein is synthesized by free ribosomes. A Purkinje cell dendrite (*C*), in longitudinal section, is filled with reaction product, which coats all its organelles but appears to associate particularly with its microtubules. Immunogold labeling of another Purkinje cell dendrite (*D*) shows many immunogold particles contacting microtubules. A DAB-labeled dendritic spine (*E*) from the putamen is diffusely filled with reaction product, which also appears to label the postsynaptic density; however, with immunogold labeling (*F*), neither plasma membrane nor postsynaptic density labeling is seen. Axon terminals from the cerebellum (*G*) and cerebral cortex (*H*) are also shown. DAB coats the membrane, synaptic vesicles, and presynaptic density. In contrast, immunogold particles appear to associate primarily with synaptic vesicles but not with the presynaptic density or membrane. (Several of these micrographs were reproduced from *Gutekunst et al.*[184] and were *used with permission*.)

aggregation may be the trigger for a toxic gain of function leading to neurodegeneration. Since similar inclusions have been seen in other triple repeat disorders, including dentatorubropallidoluysian atrophy,[196] spinocerebellar ataxia (SCA) types SCA1,[197] SCA3,[198] and SCA7,[199] and spinal and bulbar muscular atrophy,[200] protein aggregates have been proposed to be the common cause of neurodegeneration.[201,202] Many studies, however, have cast doubt on whether insoluble aggregates directly cause neurodegeneration. Huntingtin aggregates are relatively infrequent in the striatum in cases of HD compared to other brain regions.[2] Striatal interneurons resistant to neurodegeneration are far more likely to have huntingtin aggregates than

the vulnerable medium spiny neurons.[203] It has been relatively difficult to show neuronal death in the R6/2 transgenic mouse model of HD in which huntingtin aggregates appear early and are extraordinarily large and frequent.[204] In a transgenic model utilizing a polyglutamine expansion to cause an unrelated cytoplasmic protein to translocate to the nucleus and aggregate, there was no evidence for neuronal death.[205] A variety of in vitro studies have dissociated the presence of huntingtin aggregates from cell death.[206–208] In transgenic models of SCA1, nuclear but not aggregated ataxin-1 is responsible for the neurodegenerative phenotype.[209] Thus, it is possible that macroscopic huntingtin aggregates represent a relatively benign cellular sequestration of a protein

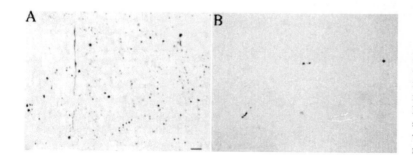

FIGURE 36-20 Huntingtin immunocytochemistry in the cerebral cortex and striatum of a presymptomatic individual using an antibody selective for aggregated mutant protein (EM48). There are many more huntingtin aggregates in the cortex (*A*) than in the striatum (*B*). Most aggregates are in neuronal processes, which they appear to loosely fill before condensing into more punctate forms.

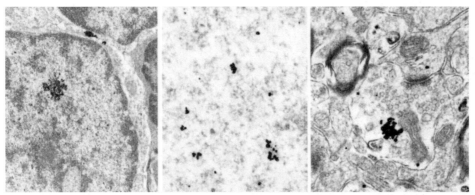

FIGURE 36-21 Electron micrographs of huntingtin aggregates in HD transgenic mice labeled with EM48 immunogold. *Left*: nuclear and cytoplasmic aggregates in a cerebellar granule cell. *Center*: microaggregates in the nucleus of striatal neuron that might still represent soluble intermediates. *Right*: a neuropil aggregate in an axon terminal.

fragment that cannot be readily broken down and might even be protective.[188,205] Aggregation of huntingtin N-terminal fragments, however, has not yet been ruled out as a cause of cell death, particularly since both the human disease and aggregation occur when the CAG length reaches about 38.[210] One possibility is that there are soluble aggregated intermediates (microaggregates) (Fig. 36-22) that are toxic but which do not correlate with the presence of macroscopic insoluble aggregates.[211,212] Moreover, aggregation may not be the only new property of huntingtin triggered at the 38 CAG transition.

PROTEIN-PROTEIN INTERACTIONS OF MUTANT HUNTINGTIN AND PATHOGENESIS

It is widely assumed that the toxic effects of mutant huntingtin are exerted through abnormal interactions that it has with proteins that it normally relates to or with proteins that unexpectedly relate to it as a result of its altered conformation. A variety of proteins that huntingtin normally interacts with have been identified. A number of these can be related to intracellular transport of organelles, including huntingtin-associated protein 1,[188,213–216] a protein analogous to the yeast cytoskeleton-associated protein Sla2p (huntingtin-interacting protein 1, or HIP1),[217–219] and HIP14, a protein related to endocytosis and endosome transport.[220] Other interacting proteins, such as glyceraldehyde phosphate dehydrogenase,[221] an unidentified calmodulin-associated protein,[222] and CIP4,[223] play roles in signal transduction and metabolism.

An emerging and important group of huntingtin interactions are with proteins related to gene transcription.[224–230] Some of these interactions may primarily be with insoluble aggregated huntingtin, while others are with

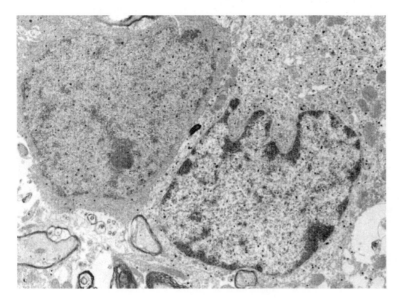

FIGURE 36-22 Electron micrograph of degenerating striatal neurons from a transgenic mouse model of HD containing nuclear and cytoplasmic microaggregates labeled by EM48 immunogold.

soluble huntingtin. There is growing evidence of early transcriptional dysfunction in cellular and animal models of HD,[231] and reversing this has become a major therapeutic focus. Additional interactions are with processive or proteolytic enzymes, such as a ubiquitin-conjugating enzyme,[232] transglutaminases which can crosslink glutamine residues,[233] and caspases[234–236] and calpains,[237,238] which have been implicated in the production of toxic fragments of mutant huntingtin,[239] all of which are also being considered as therapeutic targets. Additionally, polyglutamines may impair proteasome function and their own proteolysis,[240,241] further perturbing cellular homeostasis. Some of the huntingtin protein-protein interactions vary with the length of the huntingtin polyglutamine tract and are thus stronger candidates for being affected by the HD genetic mutation. Huntingtin therefore has a number of possible molecular interactions, the disruption of which might be relevant to neurodegeneration. While a toxic gain of function due to mutant huntingtin has been considered to be a means through which the HD genetic mutation causes neurotoxicity, there is also increasing evidence that a loss of the normal functions of huntingtin may also play roles in the pathogenesis of HD. Wild-type huntingtin is itself protective,[242–244] and its reduction might reduce levels of needed neurotrophic factors, such as BDNF,[91] or compromise some of its normal functions.

References

1. DiFiglia M, Sapp E, Chase KO, et al: Aggregation of huntingtin in neuronal intranuclear inclusions and dystrophic neurites in brain. *Science* 277:1990–1993, 1997.
2. Gutekunst CA, Li SH, Yi H, et al: Nuclear and neuropil aggregates in Huntington's disease: Relationship to neuropathology. *J Neurosci* 19:2522–2534, 1999.
3. Sapp E, Kegel KB, Aronin N, et al: Early and progressive accumulation of reactive microglia in the Huntington disease brain. *J Neuropathol Exp Neurol* 60:161–172, 2001.
4. Singhrao SK, Neal JW, Morgan BP, et al: Increased complement biosynthesis by microglia and complement activation on neurons in Huntington's disease. *Exp Neurol* 159:362–376, 1999.
5. Bruyn GW: Huntington's chorea. Historical, clinical and laboratory synopsis, in Vinken PJ, Bruyn GW (eds): *Handbook of Clinical Neurology*, Vol. 6. Amsterdam: Elsevier, 1968, pp 298–378.
6. Bruyn G, Bots G, Dom R: Huntington's chorea: current neuropathological status. *Adv Neurol* 23:83–93, 1979.
7. Lange H, Thorner G, Hopf A, et al: Morphometric studies of the neuropathological changes in choreatic diseases. *J Neurol Sci* 28:401–425, 1976.
8. Myers RH, Vonsattel JP, Paskevich PA, et al: Decreased neuronal and increased oligodendroglial densities in Huntington's disease caudate nucleus. *J Neuropathol Exp Neurol* 50:729–742, 1991.
9. Vonsattel JP, Myers RH, Stevens TJ, et al: Neuropathological classification of Huntington's disease. *J Neuropathol Exp Neurol* 44:559–577, 1985.
10. Roos RA, Pruyt JF, de Vries J, et al: Neuronal distribution in the putamen in Huntington's disease. *J Neurol Neurosurg Psychiatry* 48:422–425, 1985.
11. Gomez-Tortosa E, MacDonald ME, Friend JC, et al: Quantitative neuropathological changes in presymptomatic Huntington's disease. *Ann Neurol* 49:29–34, 2001.
12. Aylward EH, Codori AM, Rosenblatt A, et al: Rate of caudate atrophy in presymptomatic and symptomatic stages of Huntington's disease. *Mov Disord* 15:552–560 2000.
13. Aylward EH, Codori AM, Barta PE, et al: Basal ganglia volume and proximity to onset in presymptomatic Huntington disease. *Arch Neurol* 53:1293–1296, 1996.
14. Thieben MJ, Duggins AJ, Good CD, et al: The distribution of structural neuropathology in pre-clinical Huntington's disease. *Brain* 125(Pt 8):1815–1828, 2002.
15. Furtado S, Suchowersky O, Rewcastle B, et al: Relationship between trinucleotide repeats and neuropathological changes in Huntington's disease. *Ann Neurol* 39:132–136, 1996.
16. Penney JB Jr, Vonsattel JP, MacDonald ME, et al: CAG repeat number governs the development rate of pathology in Huntington's disease. *Ann Neurol* 41:689–692, 1997.
17. Rosas HD, Goodman J, Chen YI, et al: Striatal volume loss in HD as measured by MRI and the influence of CAG repeat. *Neurology* 57:1025–1028, 2001.
18. Dom R, Baro F, Brucher JM: A cytometric study of the putamen in different types of Huntington's chorea. *Adv Neurol* 1:369–385, 1973.
19. Perry TL, Hansen S, Kloster M: Huntington's chorea. Deficiency of gamma-aminobutyric acid in brain. *N Engl J Med* 288:337–342, 1973.
20. Bird ED, Iversen LL: Huntington's chorea. Post-mortem measurement of glutamic acid decarboxylase, choline acetyltransferase and dopamine in basal ganglia. *Brain* 97:457–472, 1974.
21. Spokes EGS: Neurochemical alterations in Huntington's chorea. A study of post-mortem brain tissue. *Brain* 103:179–210, 1980.
22. Carter CJ: Reduced GABA transaminase activity in the Huntington's disease putamen. *Neurosci Lett* 48:339–342, 1984.
23. Reynolds GP, Pearson SJ: Decreased glutamic acid and increased 5-hydroxytryptamine in Huntington's disease brain. *Neurosci Lett* 78:233–238, 1987.
24. Marshall P, Landis D, Zalneraitis E: Immunocytochemical studies of substance P and leucine-enkephalin in Huntington's disease. *Brain Res* 289:11–26, 1983.
25. Goto S, Hirano A, Rojas-Corona RR: An immunohistochemical investigation of the human neostriatum in Huntington's disease. *Ann Neurol* 25:298–304, 1989.
26. Ferrante R, Kowall N, Richardson E Jr: Immunocytochemical localization of calcium binding protein in normal and Huntington's disease striatum. *J Neuropathol Exp Neurol* 47:352, 1988.
27. Seto-Ohshima A, Emson PC, Lawson E, et al: Loss of matrix calcium-binding protein-containing neurons in Huntington's disease. *Lancet* i:1252–1255, 1988.
28. Augood SJ, Faull RL, Emson PC: Dopamine D1 and D2 receptor gene expression in the striatum in Huntington's disease. *Ann Neurol* 42:215–221, 1997.
29. Martinez-Mir MI, Probst A, Palacios JM: Adenosine A2 receptors: Selective localization in the human basal ganglia and alterations with disease. *Neuroscience* 42:697–706, 1991.
30. Martinez-Mir MI, Pollard H, Moreau J, et al: Loss of striatal histamine H2 receptors in Huntington's chorea but not in

Parkinson's disease: comparison with animal models. *Synapse* 15:209–220, 1993.

31. Joyce JN, Lexow N, Bird E, et al: Organization of dopamine D1 and D2 receptors in human striatum: Receptor autoradiographic studies in Huntington's disease and schizophrenia. *Synapse* 2:546–557, 1988.

32. Richfield EK, O'Brien CF, Eskin T, et al: Heterogeneous dopamine receptor changes in early and late Huntington's disease. *Neurosci Lett* 132:121–126, 1991.

33. Richfield EK, Herkenham M: Selective vulnerability in Huntington's disease: Preferential loss of cannabinoid receptors in lateral globus pallidus. *Ann Neurol* 36:577–584, 1994.

34. Gerfen C: The neostriatal mosaic: multiple levels of compartmental organization in the basal ganglia. *Annu Rev Neurosci* 15:285–320, 1992.

35. Kanazawa I, Bird E, O'Connell R, et al: Evidence for the decrease in substance P content of substantia nigra in Huntington's chorea. *Brain Res* 120:387–392, 1977.

36. Gale J, Bird E, Spokes E, et al: Human brain substance P: Distribution in controls and Huntington's chorea. *J Neurochem* 30:633–634, 1978.

37. Emson P, Arregui A, Clement-Jones V, et al: Regional distribution of met-enkephalin and substance P immunoreactivity in normal human brain and in Huntington's disease. *Brain Res*, 199:147–160, 1980.

38. Grafe MR, Forno LS, Eng LF: Immunocytochemical studies of substance P and Met-enkephalin in the basal ganglia and substantia nigra in Huntington's, Parkinson's and Alzheimer's diseases. *J Neuropathol Exp Neurol* 44:47–59, 1985.

39. Waters CM, Peck R, Rossor M, et al: Immunocytochemical studies on the basal ganglia and substantia nigra in Parkinson's disease and Huntington's chorea. *Neuroscience* 25:419–438 1988.

40. Beal MF, Ellison DW, Mazurek MF, et al: A detailed examination of substance P in pathologically graded cases of Huntington's disease. *J Neurol Sci* 84:51–61, 1988.

41. Glass M, Dragunow M, Faull RL: The pattern of neurodegeneration in Huntington's disease: A comparative study of cannabinoid, dopamine, adenosine and GABA(A) receptor alterations in the human basal ganglia in Huntington's disease. *Neuroscience* 97:505–519, 2000.

42. Cha JH, Frey AS, Alsdorf SA, et al: Altered neurotransmitter receptor expression in transgenic mouse models of Huntington's disease. *Philos Trans R Soc Lond B Biol Sci* 354: 981–989, 1999.

43. Reiner A, Albin RL, Anderson KD, et al: Differential loss of striatal projection neurons in Huntington disease. *Proc Natl Acad Sci U S A* 85:5733–5737, 1988.

44. Albin RL, Young AB, Penney JB, et al: Abnormalities of striatal projection neurons and N-methyl-D-aspartate receptors in presymptomatic Huntington's disease. *N Engl J Med* 322: 1293–1298, 1990.

45. Storey E, Beal MF: Neurochemical substrates of rigidity and chorea in Huntington's disease. *Brain* 116(Pt 5):1201–1222, 1993.

46. Crossman AR: Primate models of dyskinesia: The experimental approach to the study of basal ganglia-related involuntary movement disorders. *Neuroscience* 21:1–40, 1987.

47. Albin R, Young A, Penney J: The functional anatomy of basal ganglia disorders. *Trends Neurosci* 12:366–375, 1989.

48. DeLong M: Primate models of movement disorders of basal ganglia origin. *Trends Neurosci* 13:281–285, 1990.

49. Crossman A, Mitchell I, Sambrook M, et al: Chorea and myoclonus in the monkey induced by gamma-aminobutyric acid antagonism in the lentiform complex. *Brain* 111:1211–1233, 1988.

50. Kowall N, Ferrante R, Martin J: Patterns of cell loss in Huntington's disease. *Trends Neurosci* 10:24–29, 1987.

51. Ferrante R, Kowall N, Martin J, et al: Substance P-containing striatal neurons in Huntington's disease. *Exp Neurol* 46:375, 1987.

52. Ferrante RJ, Beal MF, Kowall NW, et al: Sparing of acetylcholinesterase-containing striatal neurons in Huntington's disease. *Brain Res* 411:162–166, 1987.

53. Cicchetti F, Gould PV, Parent A: Sparing of striatal neurons coexpressing calretinin and substance P (NK1) receptor in Huntington's disease. *Brain Res* 730:232–237, 1996.

54. Beal M, Kowall N, Ellison D, et al: Replication of the neurochemical characteristics of Huntington's disease by quinolinic acid. *Nature* 321:168–171, 1986.

55. Aronin N, Cooper PE, Lorenz LJ, et al: Somatostatin is increased in the basal ganglia in Huntington's disease. *Ann of Neurol* 13:519–526, 1983.

56. Albin RL, Reiner A, Anderson KD, et al: Striatal and nigral neuron subpopulations in rigid Huntington's disease: Implications for the functional anatomy of chorea and rigidity akinesia. *Ann Neurol* 27:357–365, 1990.

57. Ferrante RJ, Kowall NW, Beal MF, et al: Morphologic and histochemical characteristics of a spared subset of striatal neurons in Huntington's disease. *J Neuropathol Exp Neurol* 46:12–27, 1987.

58. Ferrante RJ, Kowall NW, Beal MF, et al: Selective sparing of a class of striatal neurons in Huntington's disease. *Science* 230:561–563, 1985.

59. Dawbarn D, De Quidt ME, Emson PC: Survival of basal ganglia neuropeptide Y-somatostatin neurones in Huntington's disease. *Brain Res* 340:251–260, 1985.

60. McGeer E, McGeer P: Duplication of biochemical changes of Huntington's chorea by intrastriatal injections of glutamic and kainic acids. *Nature* 263:517–519, 1976.

61. Hersch S, Gutekunst C-A, Rees H, et al: Distribution of m1–4 muscarinic receptor proteins in the rat striatum: Light and electron microscopic immunocytochemistry using subtype specific antibodies. *J Neurosci* 14:3351–3363, 1994.

62. Graveland GA, Williams RS, DiFiglia M: Evidence for degenerative and regenerative changes in neostriatal spiny neurons in Huntington's disease. *Science* 227:770–773, 1985.

63. Ferrante RJ, Kowall NW, Richardson EP Jr: Proliferative and degenerative changes in striatal spiny neurons in Huntington's disease: A combined study using the section-Golgi method and calbindin D28k immunocytochemistry. *J Neurosci* 11:3877–3887, 1991.

64. Guidetti P, Charles V, Chen EY, et al: Early degenerative changes in transgenic mice expressing mutant huntingtin involve dendritic abnormalities but no impairment of mitochondrial energy production. *Exp Neurol* 169:340–350, 2001.

65. Laforet GA, Sapp E, Chase K, et al: Changes in cortical and striatal neurons predict behavioral and electrophysiological abnormalities in a transgenic murine model of Huntington's disease. *J Neurosci* 21:9112–9123, 2001.

66. Klapstein GJ, Fisher RS, Zanjani H, et al: Electrophysiological and morphological changes in striatal spiny neurons in R6/2 Huntington's disease transgenic mice. *J Neurophysiol* 86:2667–2677, 2001.

67. Portera-Cailliau C, Hedreen JC, Price DL, et al: Evidence for apoptotic cell death in Huntington disease and excitotoxic animal models. *J Neurosci* 15(5 Pt 2):3775–3787, 1995.

68. Butterworth NJ, Williams L, Bullock JY, et al: Trinucleotide (CAG) repeat length is positively correlated with the degree of DNA fragmentation in Huntington's disease striatum. *Neuroscience* 87:49–53, 1998.

69. Kiechle T, Dedeoglu A, Kubilus J, et al: Cytochrome C and caspase-9 expression in Huntington's disease. *Neuromol Med* 1:183–195, 2002.

70. Dikranian K, Ishimaru MJ, Tenkova T, et al: Apoptosis in the in vivo mammalian forebrain. *Neurobiol Dis* 8:359–379, 2001.

71. Graybiel A: Neurotransmitters and neuromodulators in the basal ganglia. *Trends Neurosci* 13:244–254, 1990.

72. Ferrante RJ, Kowall NW, Richardson EP Jr, et al: Topography of enkephalin, substance P and acetylcholinesterase staining in Huntington's disease striatum. *Neurosci Lett* 71:283–288, 1986.

73. Ferrante RJ, Kowall NW: Tyrosine hydroxylase-like immunoreactivity is distributed in the matrix compartment of normal human and Huntington's disease striatum. *Brain Res* 416:141–146, 1987.

74. Kiyama H, Seto-Ohshima A, Emson PC: Calbindin D28K as a marker for the degeneration of the striatonigral pathway in Huntington's disease. *Brain Res* 525:209–214, 1990.

75. Hersch S, Ciliax B, Gutekunst C-A, et al: Electron microscopic analysis of D1 and D2 dopamine receptor proteins in the dorsal striatum and their synaptic relationships with motor corticostriatal afferents. *J Neurosci* 15:5222–5237, 1995.

76. Bruyn G: Neuropathological changes in Huntington's chorea. *Adv Neurol* 1:399–403, 1973.

77. Sapp E, Ge P, Aizawa H, et al: Evidence for a preferential loss of enkephalin immunoreactivity in the external globus pallidus in low grade Huntington's disease using high resolution image analysis. *Neurosci* 64:397–404, 1995.

78. Forno LS, Jose C: Huntington's chorea: A pathological study. *Adv Neurol* 1:453–470, 1973.

79. Bugiani O, Tabaton M, Cammarata S: Huntington's disease: Survival of large striatal neurons in the rigid variant. *Ann Neurol* 15:154–156, 1984.

80. Oyanagi K, Takeda S, Takahashi H, et al: A quantitative investigation of the substantia nigra in Huntington's disease. *Ann Neurol* 26:13–19, 1989.

81. Ferrante R, Kowall N, Richardson EJ: Neuronal and neuropil loss in the substantia nigra in Huntington's disease. *J Neuropathol Exp Neurol* 48:380, 1989.

82. Bohnen NI, Koeppe RA, Meyer P, et al: Decreased striatal monoaminergic terminals in Huntington disease. *Neurology* 54:1753–1759, 2000.

83. Saji M, Reis D: Delayed transneuronal death of substantia nigra neurons prevented by gamma-aminobutyric acid. *Science* 235:66–67, 1987.

84. Dom R, Malfroid M, Baro F: Neuropathology of Huntington's chorea. Studies of the ventrobasal complex of the thalamus. *Neurology* 26:64–68, 1976.

85. Heinsen H, Rub U, Gangnus D, et al: Nerve cell loss in the thalamic centromedian-parafascicular complex in patients with Huntington's disease. *Acta Neuropathol (Berl)* 91:161–168, 1996.

86. Heinsen H, Rub U, Bauer M, et al: Nerve cell loss in the thalamic mediodorsal nucleus in Huntington's disease. *Acta Neuropathol (Berl)* 97:613–622, 1999.

87. Kremer HP, Roos RA, Dingjan GM, et al: The hypothalamic lateral tuberal nucleus and the characteristics of neuronal loss in Huntington's disease. *Neurosci Lett* 132:101–104, 1991.

88. Kremer HP, Roos RA, Dingjan G, et al: Atrophy of the hypothalamic lateral tuberal nucleus in Huntington's disease. *J Neuropathol Exp Neurol* 49:371–382, 1990.

89. Alzheimer A: Über die anatomische Grunglage der Huntingtonschen Chorea und der choreatischen bewegungen Überhaupt. *Neurol Zentral* 30:891–892, 1911.

90. Hallervorden J: Huntingtonsche chorea (chorea chronica progressiva herditaria), in Lubarsch O, et al (eds): *Handbuch der speziellen pathologischen Anatomie und Histologie.* Springer: Berlin, 1957, pp 793–822.

91. Zuccato C, Ciammola A, Rigamonti D, et al: Loss of huntingtin-mediated BDNF gene transcription in Huntington's disease. *Science* 293: 493–498, 2001.

92. Alexander GE, Delong MR, Strick PL: Parallel organization of functionally segregated circuits linking basal ganglia and cortex. *Annu Rev Neurosci* 9:357–381, 1986.

93. Alexander GE, Crutcher MD, DeLong MR: Basal ganglia-thalamocortical circuits: Parallel substrates for motor, oculomotor, "prefrontal" and "limbic" functions. *Prog Brain Res* 85:119–146, 1990.

94. Lange HW: Quantitative changes of telencephalon, diencephalon, and mesencephalon in Huntington's chorea, postencephalic, and idiopathic Parkinson's disease. *Verh Anat Ges* 75:923–925, 1981.

95. De la Monte SM, Vonsattel JP, Richardson EP Jr: Morphometric demonstration of atrophic changes in the cerebral cortex, white matter, and neostriatum in Huntington's disease. *J Neuropathol Exp Neurol* 47:516–525, 1988.

96. Rosas HD, Liu AK, Hersch S, et al: Regional and progressive thinning of the cortical ribbon in Huntington's disease. *Neurology* 58:695–701, 2002.

97. Hersch S, Gutekunst C-A, Rosenfeld V, et al: *A Quantitative Morphometric Study of the Cerebral Cortex in Huntington's Disease.* World Fed Neurol (Abs), 1991.

98. Sotrel A, Paskevich PA, Kiely DK, et al: Morphometric analysis of the prefrontal cortex in Huntington's disease. *Neurology* 41:1117–1123, 1991.

99. Hedreen JC, Peyser CE, Folstein SE, et al: Neuronal loss in layers V and VI of cerebral cortex in Huntington's disease. *Neurosci Lett* 133:257–261, 1991.

100. Rajkowska G, Selemon L, Goldman-Rakic P: Morphometric evidence for prefrontal cellular atrophy in advanced Huntington's disease. *Soc Neurosci Abstr* 19:838, 1993.

101. Braak H, Braak E: Allocortical involvement in Huntington's disease. *Neuropathol Appl Neurobiol* 18:539–547, 1992.

102. Braak H, Del Tredici K, Bohl J, et al: Pathological changes in the parahippocampal region in select non-Alzheimer's dementias. *Ann N Y Acad Sci* 911:221–239, 2000.

103. Halliday GM, McRitchie DA, Macdonald V, et al: Regional specificity of brain atrophy in Huntington's disease. *Exp Neurol* 154:663–672, 1998.

104. Sieradzan K, Mann DM, Dodge A: Clinical presentation and patterns of regional cerebral atrophy related to the length of trinucleotide repeat expansion in patients with adult onset Huntington's disease. *Neurosci Lett* 225:45–48, 1997.

105. McCaughey W: The pathologic spectrum of Huntington's chorea. *J Nerv Ment Dis* 133:91–103, 1961.

106. Byers RK, Gilles FH, Fung C: Huntington's disease in children. Neuropathologic study of four cases. *Neurology* 23:561–569, 1973.

107. Roizin L, Kaufman M, Wilson N, et al: Neuropathologic observations in Huntington's chorea, in Zimmerman H (ed): *Progress in Neuropathology*. New York: Grune & Stratton, 1976, pp 447–488.

108. Heinsen H, Strik M, Bauer M, et al: Cortical and striatal neurone number in Huntington's disease. *Acta Neuropathol* 88:320–333, 1994.

109. Selemon LD, Rajkowska G, Goldman-Rakic PS: Elevated neuronal density in prefrontal area 46 in brains from schizophrenic patients: Application of a three-dimensional, stereologic counting method. *J Comp Neurol* 392:402–412, 1998.

110. Zalneraitis EL, Landis DMA, Richardson EPJ, et al: A comparison of astrocytic structure in cerebral cortex and striatum in Huntington's disease. *Neurology* 31:151, 1981 (abstract).

111. Cudkowicz M, Kowall NW: Degeneration of pyramidal projection neurons in Huntington's disease cortex. *Ann Neurol* 27:200–204, 1990.

112. Beal MF, Swartz KJ, Finn SF, et al: Amino acid and neuropeptide neurotransmitters in Huntington's disease cerebellum. *Brain Res* 454: 393–396, 1988.

113. Mazurek MF, Beal MF, Knowlton SF, et al: Elevated concentrations of cholecystokinin and vasoactive intestinal peptide in Huntington's disease postmortem cerebral cortex. *Neurology* 39(Suppl 1):203, 1989.

114. Storey E, Kowall NW, Finn SF, et al: The cortical lesion of Huntington's disease: Further neurochemical characterization, and reproduction of some of the histological and neurochemical features by *N*-methyl-D-aspartate lesions of rat cortex. *Ann Neurol* 32:526–534, 1992.

115. Sotrel A, Paskevich P, Kiely D, et al: Morphometric analysis of the prefrontal cortex in Huntington's disease. *Neurology* 41:1117–1123, 1991.

116. Ellison DW, Beal MF, Mazurek MF, et al: Amino acid neurotransmitter abnormalities in Huntington's disease and in the quinolinic acid animal model of Huntington's disease. *Brain* 110:1657–1673, 1987.

117. Wagster MV, Hedreen JC, Peyser CE, et al: Selective loss of [3H]kainic acid and [3H]AMPA binding in layer VI of frontal cortex in Huntington's disease. *Exp Neurol* 127:70–75, 1994.

118. Mazurek MF, Garside S, Beal MF: Cortical peptide changes in Huntington's disease may be independent of striatal degeneration. *Ann Neurol* 41:540–547, 1997.

119. Markham C, Knox J: Observations on Huntington's chorea in childhood. *J Pediatr* 67:46–57, 1965.

120. Jervis G: Huntington's chorea in childhood. *Arch Neurol* 9:50–63, 1963.

121. Rodda R: Cerebellar atrophy in Huntington's disease. *J Neurol Sci* 50:147–157, 1981.

122. Jeste DV, Barban L, Parisi J: Reduced Purkinje cell density in Huntington's disease. *Exp Neurol* 85:78–86, 1984.

123. McCaughey WTE: The pathologic spectrum of Huntington's chorea. *J Nerv Ment Dis* 133:91–103, 1961.

124. Aylward EH, Brandt J, Codori AM, et al: Reduced basal ganglia volume associated with the gene for Huntington's disease in asymptomatic at-risk persons. *Neurology* 44:823–828, 1994.

125. Aylward EH, Li Q, Stine OC, et al: Longitudinal change in basal ganglia volume in patients with Huntington's disease. *Neurology* 48:394–399, 1997.

126. Rosas H, Koroshetz W, Chen Y, et al: Evidence for more widespread cerebral pathology in early HD: an MRI-based morphometric analysis. *Neurology* 60:1615–1619, 2003.

127. Jenkins BG, Koroshetz WJ, Beal MF, et al: Evidence for impairment of energy metabolism in vivo in Huntington's disease using localized 1H NMR spectroscopy. *Neurology* 43: 2689–2695, 1993.

128. Lodi R, Schapira AH, Manners D, et al: Abnormal in vivo skeletal muscle energy metabolism in Huntington's disease and dentatorubropallidoluysian atrophy. *Ann Neurol* 48:72–76, 2000.

129. Backman L, Robins-Wahlin TB, Lundin A, et al: Cognitive deficits in Huntington's disease are predicted by dopaminergic PET markers and brain volumes. *Brain* 120(Pt 12):2207–2217, 1997.

130. Feigin A, Leenders KL, Moeller JR, et al: Metabolic network abnormalities in early Huntington's disease: an [(18)F]FDG PET study. *J Nucl Med* 42: 1591–1595, 2001.

131. Antonini A, Leenders KL, Spiegel R, et al: Striatal glucose metabolism and dopamine D2 receptor binding in asymptomatic gene carriers and patients with Huntington's disease. *Brain* 119(Pt 6): 2085–2095, 1996.

132. Ginovart N, Lundin A, Farde L, et al: PET study of the pre- and post-synaptic dopaminergic markers for the neurodegenerative process in Huntington's disease. *Brain* 120(Pt 3):503–514, 1997.

133. Clark VP, Lai S, Deckel AW: Altered functional MRI responses in Huntington's disease. *Neuroreport* 13:703–706, 2002.

134. Aron AR, Schlaghecken F, Fletcher PC, et al: Inhibition of subliminally primed responses is mediated by the caudate and thalamus: Evidence from functional MRI and Huntington's disease. *Brain* 126(Pt 3):713–723, 2003.

135. Coyle J, Schwarcz R: Lesions of striatal neurons with kainic acid provides a model for Huntington's chorea. *Nature* 263:244–246, 1976.

136. Ferrante RJ, Kowall NW, Cipolloni PB, et al: Excitotoxin lesions in primates as a model for Huntington's disease: Histopathologic and neurochemical characterization. *Exp Neurol* 119:46–71, 1993.

137. Beal MF, Kowall NW, Ferrante RJ, et al: Quinolinic acid striatal lesions in primates as a model of Huntington's disease. *Ann Neurol* 26:137, 1989.

138. Beal MF, Ferrante RJ, Swartz KJ, et al: Chronic quinolinic acid lesions in rats closely resemble Huntington's disease. *J Neurosci* 11:1649–1659, 1991.

139. Bazzett TJ, Becker JB, Kaatz KW, et al: Chronic intrastriatal dialytic administration of quinolinic acid produces selective neural degeneration. *Exp Neurol* 120:177–185, 1993.

140. Young AB, Greenamyre JT, Hollingsworth Z, et al: NMDA receptor losses in putamen from patients with Huntington's disease. *Science* 241: 981–983, 1988.

141. Dure LS, Young AB, Penney JB: Excitatory amino acid binding sites in the caudate nucleus and frontal cortex of Huntington's disease. *Ann Neurol* 30:785–793, 1991.

142. Gutekunst C-A, Hersch S, Wimpey T, et al: *Western Blot Analysis of Glutamate Receptor Subunits in Huntington's Disease*. Society for Neuroscience, 1993.

143. Levine MS, Klapstein GJ, Koppel A, et al: Enhanced sensitivity to *N*-methyl-D-aspartate receptor activation in transgenic and knockin mouse models of Huntington's disease. *J Neurosci Res* 58:515–532, 1999.

144. Zeron MM, Hansson O, Chen N, et al: Increased sensitivity to N-methyl-D-aspartate receptor-mediated excitotoxicity in a mouse model of Huntington's disease. *Neuron* 33:849–860, 2002.

145. Behrens PF, Franz P, Woodman B, et al: Impaired glutamate transport and glutamate-glutamine cycling: Downstream effects of the Huntington mutation. *Brain* 125(Pt 8):1908–1922, 2002.

146. Cepeda C, Hurst RS, Calvert CR, et al: Transient and progressive electrophysiological alterations in the corticostriatal pathway in a mouse model of Huntington's disease. *J Neurosci* 23:961–969, 2003.

147. Ferrante RJ, Andreassen OA, Dedeoglu A, et al: Therapeutic effects of coenzyme Q10 and remacemide in transgenic mouse models of Huntington's disease. *J Neurosci* 22:1592–1599, 2002.

148. Schiefer J, Landwehrmeyer GB, Luesse HG, et al: Riluzole prolongs survival time and alters nuclear inclusion formation in a transgenic mouse model of Huntington's disease. *Mov Disord* 17:748–757, 2002.

149. Schilling G, Coonfield ML, Ross CA, et al: Coenzyme Q10 and remacemide hydrochloride ameliorate motor deficits in a Huntington's disease transgenic mouse model. *Neurosci Lett* 315:149–153, 2001.

150. Kieburtz K: Antiglutamate therapies in Huntington's disease. *J Neural Transm Suppl* 55:97–102, 1999.

151. Group HS: A randomized, placebo-controlled trial of coenzyme Q10 and remacemide in Huntington's disease. *Neurology* 57:397–404, 2001.

152. Beal M: Does impairment of energy metabolism result in excitotoxic neuronal death in neurodegenerative illnesses? *Ann Neurol* 31:119–130, 1992.

153. Beal MF, Hyman BT, Koroshetz W: Do defects in mitochondrial energy metabolism underlie the pathology of neurodegenerative diseases? *Trends Neurosci* 16:125–131, 1993.

154. Albin R, Greenamyre J: Alternative excitotoxic hypotheses. *Neurology* 42:733–738, 1992.

155. Beal MF: Aging, energy, and oxidative stress in neurodegenerative diseases. *Ann Neurol* 38:357–366, 1995.

156. Browne SE, Bowling AC, MacGarvey U, et al: Oxidative damage and metabolic dysfunction in Huntington's disease: Selective vulnerability of the basal ganglia. *Ann Neurol* 41:646–653, 1997.

157. Parker WJ, Boyson SJ, Luder AS, et al: Evidence for a defect in NADH: Ubiquinone oxidoreductase (complex I) in Huntington's disease. *Neurology* 40:1231–1234, 1990.

158. Arenas J, Campos Y, Ribacoba R, et al: Complex I defect in muscle from patients with Huntington's disease. *Ann Neurol* 43:397–400, 1998.

159. Brennan WA Jr, Bird ED, Aprille JR: Regional mitochondrial respiratory activity in Huntington's disease brain. *J Neurochem* 44:1948–1950, 1985.

160. Browne SE, Ferrante RJ, Beal MF: Oxidative stress in Huntington's disease. *Brain Pathol* 9:147–163, 1999.

161. Jenkins B, Koroshetz W, Beal M, et al: Localized proton-NMR spectroscopy in patients with Huntington's disease (HD) demonstrates abnormal lactate levels in occipital cortex: Evidence for compromised metabolism in HD. *Neurology* 42:223–229, 1992.

162. Panov AV, Burke JR, Strittmatter WJ, et al: In vitro effects of polyglutamine tracts on Ca2+-dependent depolarization of rat and human mitochondria: Relevance to Huntington's disease. *Arch Biochem Biophys* 410:1–6, 2003.

163. Panov AV, Gutekunst CA, Leavitt BR, et al: Early mitochondrial calcium defects in Huntington's disease are a direct effect of polyglutamines. *Nat Neurosci* 5:731–736, 2002.

164. Gines S, Seong IS, Fossale E, et al: Specific progressive cAMP reduction implicates energy deficit in presymptomatic Huntington's disease knock-in mice. *Hum Mol Genet* 12:497–508, 2003.

165. Novelli A, Reilly J, Lysko P, et al: Glutamate becomes neurotoxic via the N-methyl-D-aspartate receptor when intracellular energy levels are reduced. *Brain Res* 451:205–212, 1988.

166. Greene J, Porter R, Eller R, et al: Inhibition of succinate dehydrogenase by malonic acid produces an "excitotoxic" lesion in rat striatum. *J Neurochem* 61:1151–1154, 1993.

167. Beal MF, Brouillet E, Jenkins B, et al: Neurochemical and histologic characterization of striatal excitotoxic lesions produced by the mitochondrial toxin 3-nitropropionic acid. *J Neurosci* 13:4181–4192, 1993.

168. Brouillet E, Hantraye P, Ferrante RJ, et al: Chronic mitochondrial energy impairment produces selective striatal degeneration and abnormal choreiform movements in primates. *Proc Natl Acad Sci U S A* 92:7105–7109, 1995.

169. Greene J, Greenamyre J: Characterization of the excitotoxic potential of the reversible succinate dehydrogenase inhibitor malonate. *J Neurochem* 64:430–436, 1995.

170. Beal M, Henshaw D, Jenkins B, et al: Coenzyme Q10 and nicotinamide block striatal lesions produced by the mitochondrial toxin malonate. *Ann Neurol* 36:882–888.

171. Henshaw R, Jenkins B, Schulz J, et al: Malonate produces striatal lesions by indirect NMDA receptor activation. *Brain Res* 647:161–166, 1994.

172. Huntington Study Group: Safety and tolerability of the free-radical scavenger OPC-14117 in Huntington's disease. *Neurology* 50:1366–1373, 1998.

173. Ferrante RJ, Andreassen OA, Jenkins BG, et al: Neuroprotective effects of creatine in a transgenic mouse model of Huntington's disease. *J Neurosci* 20: 4389–4397, 2000.

174. Huntington's Disease Collaborative Research Group: A novel gene containing a trinucleotide repeat that is expanded and unstable on Huntington's disease chromosomes. *Cell* 72:971–983, 1993.

175. Li SH, Schilling G, Young WS, et al: Huntington's disease gene (IT15) is widely expressed in human and rat tissues. *Neuron* 11:985–993, 1993.

176. Strong TV, Tagle DA, Valdes JM, et al: Widespread expression of the human and rat Huntington's disease gene in brain and nonneural tissues. *Nat Genet* 5:259–265, 1993.

177. Ambrose CM, Duyao MP, Barnes G, et al: Structure and expression of the Huntington's disease gene: Evidence against simple inactivation due to an expanded CAG repeat. *Somat Cell Mol Genet* 20:27–38, 1994.

178. Duyao MP, Auerbach AB, Ryan A, et al: Inactivation of the mouse Huntington's disease gene homolog Hdh. *Science* 269:407–410, 1995.

179. Nasir J, Floresco SB, O'Kusky JR, et al: Targeted disruption of the Huntington's disease gene results in embryonic lethality and behavioral and morphological changes in heterozygotes. *Cell* 81:811–823, 1995.

180. Landwehrmeyer GB, McNeil SM, Dure LS, et al: Huntington's disease gene: Regional and cellular expression in brain of normal and affected individuals. *Ann Neurol* 37:218–230, 1995.

181. Eberwine J, McLaughlin B: Striatal RNA-binding proteins interact with huntingtin mRNA, in Ariano M, Surmeier D

(eds): *Molecular and Cellular Mechanisms of Neostriatal Function.* Austin: RG Landes, 1995, pp 143–149.

182. DiFiglia M, Sapp E, Chase K, et al: Huntingtin is a cytoplasmic protein associated with vesicles in human and rat brain neurons. *Neuron* 14:1075–1081, 1995.

183. Hoogeveen AT, Willemsen R, Meyer N, et al: Characterization and localization of the Huntington disease gene product. *Hum Mol Genet* 2: 2069–2073, 1993.

184. Gutekunst CA, Levey AI, Heilman CJ, et al: Identification and localization of huntingtin in brain and human lymphoblastoid cell lines with anti-fusion protein antibodies. *Proc Natl Acad Sci U S A* 92:8710–8714, 1995.

185. Sharp AH, Loev SJ, Schilling G, et al: Widespread expression of Huntington's disease gene (*IT15*) protein product. *Neuron* 14:1065–1074, 1995.

186. Trottier Y, Devys D, Imbert G, et al: Cellular localization of the Huntington's disease protein and discrimination of the normal and mutated form. *Nat Genet* 10:104–110, 1995.

187. Ferrante R, Gutekunst C-A, Persichetti F, et al: Heterogeneous topographic and cellular distribution of huntingtin expression in the normal human neostriatum. *J Neurosci* 17:3052–3063, 1997.

188. Gutekunst CA, Li SH, Yi H, et al: The cellular and subcellular localization of huntingtin-associated protein 1 (HAP1): Comparison with huntingtin in rat and human. *J Neurosci* 18: 7674–7686, 1998.

189. Kegel KB, Kim M, Sapp E, et al: Huntingtin expression stimulates endosomal-lysosomal activity, endosome tubulation, and autophagy. *J Neurosci* 20: 7268–7278, 2000.

190. Li SH, Li XJ: Aggregation of N-terminal huntingtin is dependent on the length of its glutamine repeats. *Hum Mol Genet* 7:777–782, 1998.

191. Trottier Y, Lutz Y, Stevanin G, et al: Polyglutamine expansion as a pathological epitope in Huntington's disease and four dominant cerebellar ataxias. *Nature* 378:403–406, 1995.

192. Perutz MF, Johnson T, Suzuki M, et al: Glutamine repeats as polar zippers: Their possible role in inherited neurodegenerative diseases. *Proc Natl Acad Sci U S A* 91:5355–5358, 1994.

193. Maat-Schieman ML, Dorsman JC, Smoor MA, et al: Distribution of inclusions in neuronal nuclei and dystrophic neurites in Huntington disease brain. *J Neuropathol Exp Neurol*, 58:129–137, 1999.

194. Scherzinger E, Lurz R, Turmaine M, et al: Huntingtin-encoded polyglutamine expansions form amyloid-like protein aggregates in vitro and in vivo. *Cell* 90:549–558, 1997.

195. Martindale D, Hackam A, Wieczorek A, et al: Length of huntingtin and its polyglutamine tract influences localization and frequency of intracellular aggregates. *Nat Genet* 18:150–154, 1998.

196. Becher MW, Kotzuk JA, Sharp AH, et al: Intranuclear neuronal inclusions in Huntington's disease and dentatorubral and pallidoluysian atrophy: Correlation between the density of inclusions and IT15 CAG triplet repeat length. *Neurobiol Dis* 4:387–397, 1998.

197. Skinner P, Koshy B, Cummings C, et al: Ataxin-1 with an expanded glutamine tract alters nuclear matrix-associated structures. *Nature* 389:971–974, 1997.

198. Paulson H, Perez M, Trottier Y, et al: Intranuclear inclusions of expanded polyglutamine protein in spinocerebellar ataxia type 3. *Neuron* 19:333–344, 1997.

199. Holmberg M, Duyckaerts C, Durr A, et al: Spinocerebellar ataxia type 7 (SCA7): A neurodegenerative disorder with neuronal intranuclear inclusions. *Hum Mol Genet* 7:913–918, 1998.

200. Li M, Miwa S, Kobayashi Y, et al: Nuclear inclusions of the androgen receptor protein in spinal and bulbar muscular atrophy. *Ann Neurol* 44:249–254, 1998.

201. Ross CA: Intranuclear neuronal inclusions: A common pathogenic mechanism for glutamine-repeat neurodegenerative diseases? *Neuron* 19:1147–1150, 1997.

202. Davies SW, Beardsall, K, Turmaine M, et al: Are neuronal intranuclear inclusions the common neuropathology of triplet-repeat disorders with polyglutamine-repeat expansions? *Lancet* 351:131–133, 1998.

203. Kuemmerle S, Gutekunst CA, Klein AM, et al: Huntington aggregates may not predict neuronal death in Huntington's disease. *Ann Neurol* 46:842–849, 1999.

204. Davies SW, Turmaine M, Cozens BA, et al: Formation of neuronal intranuclear inclusions underlies the neurological dysfunction in mice transgenic for the HD mutation. *Cell* 90: 537–548, 1997.

205. Ordway J, Tallaksen-Greene S, Gutekunst C-A, et al: Ectopically expressed CAG repeats cause intranuclear inclusions and a progressive late onset neurological phenotype in the mouse. *Cell* 91:753–763, 1997.

206. Saudou F, Finkbeiner S, Devys D, et al: Huntingtin acts in the nucleus to induce apoptosis but death does not correlate with the formation of intranuclear inclusions. *Cell* 95:55–66, 1998.

207. Chun W, Lesort M, Lee M, et al: Mutant huntingtin aggregates do not sensitize cells to apoptotic stressors. *FEBS Lett* 515:61–65, 2002.

208. Kim M, Lee HS, LaForet G, et al: Mutant huntingtin expression in clonal striatal cells: Dissociation of inclusion formation and neuronal survival by caspase inhibition. *J Neurosci* 19:964–973, 1999.

209. Klement I, Skinner P, Kaytor M, et al: Ataxin-1 nuclear localization and aggregation: Role in polyglutamine-induced disease in SCA1 transgenic mice. *Cell* 95:41–53, 1998.

210. Chen S, Berthelier V, Yang W, et al: Polyglutamine aggregation behavior in vitro supports a recruitment mechanism of cytotoxicity. *J Mol Biol* 311:173–182, 2001.

211. Poirier MA, Li H, Macosko J, et al: Huntingtin spheroids and protofibrils as precursors in polyglutamine fibrilization. *J Biol Chem* 277:41032–41037, 2002.

212. Hodgson J, Agopyan N, Gutekunst C-A, et al: A YAC mouse model for Huntington's disease with full-length mutant huntingtin, cytoplasmic toxicity, and selective striatal neurodegeneration. *Neuron* 23:181–192, 1999.

213. Li XJ, Li SH, Sharp AH, et al: A huntingtin-associated protein enriched in brain with implications for pathology. *Nature* 378:398–402, 1995.

214. Li Y, Chin LS, Levey AI, et al: Huntingtin-associated protein 1 interacts with hepatocyte growth factor-regulated tyrosine kinase substrate and functions in endosomal trafficking. *J Biol Chem* 277:28212–28221, 2002.

215. Li SH, Gutekunst CA, Hersch SM, et al: Interaction of huntingtin-associated protein with dynactin P150Glued. *J Neurosci* 18:1261–1269, 1998.

216. Sittler A, Walter S, Wedemeyer N, et al: SH3GL3 associates with the Huntingtin exon 1 protein and promotes the formation of polygln-containing protein aggregates. *Mol Cell* 2:427–436, 1998.

217. Kalchman M, Koide H, McCutcheon K, et al: HIP1, a human homolog of S. *cerevisiae* Sla2p, interacts with membrane associated huntingtin in the brain. *Nat Genet* 16:44–53, 1997.
218. Wanker EE, Rovira C, Scherzinger E, et al: HIP-I: A huntingtin interacting protein isolated by the yeast two-hybrid system. *Hum Mol Genet* 6:487–495, 1997.
219. Metzler M, Legendre-Guillemin V, Gan L, et al: HIP1 functions in clathrin-mediated endocytosis through binding to clathrin and adaptor protein 2. *J Biol Chem* 276:39271–39276, 2001.
220. Singaraja RR, Hadano S, Metzler M, et al: HIP14, a novel ankyrin domain-containing protein, links huntingtin to intracellular trafficking and endocytosis. *Hum Mol Genet* 11:2815–2828, 2002.
221. Burke, JR, Enghild JJ, Martin ME, et al: Huntingtin and DRPLA proteins selectively interact with the enzyme GAPDH. *Nat Med* 2:347–350, 1996.
222. Bao J, Sharp AH, Wagster MV, et al: Expansion of polyglutamine repeat in huntingtin leads to abnormal protein interactions involving calmodulin. *Proc Natl Acad Sci U S A* 93:5037–5042, 1996.
223. Holbert S, Dedeoglu A, Humbert S, et al: Cdc42-interacting protein 4 binds to huntingtin: Neuropathologic and biological evidence for a role in Huntington's disease. *Proc Natl Acad Sci U S A* 100:2712–2717, 2003.
224. Gerber H-P, Seipel K, Georgiev O, et al: Transcriptional activation modulated by homopolymeric glutamine and proline stretches. *Science* 263:808–811, 1994.
225. Passani LA, Bedford MT, Faber PW, et al: Huntingtin's WW domain partners in Huntington's disease post-mortem brain fulfill genetic criteria for direct involvement in Huntington's disease pathogenesis. *Hum Mol Genet* 9:2175–2182, 2000.
226. Boutell JM, Thomas P, Neal JW, et al: Aberrant interactions of transcriptional repressor proteins with the Huntington's disease gene product, huntingtin. *Hum Mol Genet* 8:1647–1655, 1999.
227. Steffan JS, Kazantsev A, Spasic-Boskovic O, et al: The Huntington's disease protein interacts with p53 and CREB-binding protein and represses transcription. *Proc Natl Acad Sci U S A* 97:6763–6768, 2000.
228. Li SH, Cheng AL, Zhou H, et al: Interaction of Huntington disease protein with transcriptional activator Sp1. *Mol Cell Biol* 22:1277–1287, 2002.
229. Holbert S, Denghien I, Kiechle T, et al: The Gln-Ala repeat transcriptional activator CA150 interacts with huntingtin: Neuropathologic and genetic evidence for a role in Huntington's disease pathogenesis. *Proc Natl Acad Sci U S A* 98:1811–1816, 2001.
230. Dunah AW, Jeong H, Griffin A, et al: Sp1 and TAFII130 transcriptional activity disrupted in early Huntington's disease. *Science* 296:2238–2243, 2002.
231. Cha JH: Transcriptional dysregulation in Huntington's disease. *Trends Neurosci* 23:387–392, 2000.
232. Kalchman MA, Graham RK, Xia G, et al: Huntingtin is ubiquitinated and interacts with a specific ubiquitin-conjugating enzyme. *J Biol Chem* 271:19385–19394, 1996.
233. Cooper AJ, Jeitner TM, Gentile V, et al: Cross linking of polyglutamine domains catalyzed by tissue transglutaminase is greatly favored with pathological-length repeats: Does transglutaminase activity play a role in (CAG)(n)/Q(n)-expansion diseases? *Neurochem Int* 40:53–67, 2002.
234. Goldberg YP, Nicholson DW, Rasper DM, et al: Cleavage of huntingtin by apopain, a proapoptotic cysteine protease, is modulated by the polyglutamine tract. *Nat Genet* 13:442–449, 1996.
235. Wellington CL, Singaraja R, Ellerby L, et al: Inhibiting caspase cleavage of huntingtin reduces toxicity and aggregate formation in neuronal and nonneuronal cells. *J Biol Chem* 275:19831–19838, 2000.
236. Wellington CL, Ellerby LM, Gutekunst CA, et al: Caspase cleavage of mutant huntingtin precedes neurodegeneration in Huntington's disease. *J Neurosci* 22:7862–7872, 2002.
237. Kim YJ, Yi Y, Sapp E, et al: Caspase 3-cleaved N-terminal fragments of wild-type and mutant huntingtin are present in normal and Huntington's disease brains, associate with membranes, and undergo calpain-dependent proteolysis. *Proc Natl Acad Sci U S A* 98:12784–12789, 2001.
238. Gafni J and Ellerby LM: Calpain activation in Huntington's disease. *J Neurosci* 22:4842–4849, 2002.
239. Lunkes A, Lindenberg KS, Ben-Haiem L, et al: Proteases acting on mutant huntingtin generate cleaved products that differentially build up cytoplasmic and nuclear inclusions. *Mol Cell* 10:259–269, 2002.
240. Jana NR, Zemskov EA, Wang G, et al: Altered proteasomal function due to the expression of polyglutamine-expanded truncated N-terminal huntingtin induces apoptosis by caspase activation through mitochondrial cytochrome c release. *Hum Mol Genet* 10:1049–1059, 2001.
241. Waelter S, Boeddrich A, Lurz R, et al: Accumulation of mutant huntingtin fragments in aggresome-like inclusion bodies as a result of insufficient protein degradation. *Mol Biol Cell* 12:1393–1407, 2001.
242. Rigamonti D, Bauer JH, De-Fraja C, et al: Wild-type huntingtin protects from apoptosis upstream of caspase-3. *J Neurosci* 20:3705–3713, 2000.
243. Leavitt BR, Guttman JA, Hodgson JG, et al: Wild-type huntingtin reduces the cellular toxicity of mutant huntingtin in vivo. *Am J Hum Genet* 68:313–324, 2001.
244. Ho LW, Brown R, Maxwell M, et al: Wild type huntingtin reduces the cellular toxicity of mutant huntingtin in mammalian cell models of Huntington's disease. *J Med Genet* 38:450–452, 2001.

Chapter 37 _____

TARDIVE DYSKINESIA

CHRISTOPHER G. GOETZ and STACY HORN

PHENOMENOLOGY 629
EPIDEMIOLOGY AND NATURAL HISTORY 630
PATHOPHYSIOLOGY 630
NEUROIMAGING AND NEUROPATHOLOGY 631
PREVENTION AND TREATMENT:
    GENERAL CONSIDERATIONS 631
      Conservative Use of Neuroleptics 631
      Choice of Neuroleptics 632
      Treatment with Other Drugs 632
TREATMENT OF SPECIFIC FORMS OF TARDIVE
    DYSKINESIA 632
      Choreic-Stereotypic Movements 633
      Dystonic Movements 634
      Tardive Akathisia 635
FUTURE PERSPECTIVES 635

The term "tardive dyskinesia" (TD) applies only to abnormal involuntary movements resulting from chronic treatment with agents that block central dopamine receptors. In most instances, these drugs are antipsychotic neuroleptic agents. Nonetheless, other dopaminergic receptor blockers such as metoclopramide are associated with the same disorder.[1] Schoenecker associated oral-facial dyskinesia with chlorpromazine treatment in 1957, yet three decades later a cause-and-effect relationship between neuroleptic therapy and involuntary movements was still questioned.[2,3] The controversy persisted in part because neuroleptics are most commonly used to treat psychosis and agitated senile depression; mannerisms resembling the movements of TD can occur spontaneously in some persons with psychosis and in normal elderly patients.[4]

Nonetheless, the unequivocal occurrence of involuntary movements after chronic neuroleptic therapy in nonpsychotic young adults without other cause for movement disorders[5] leaves no doubt that TD does occur. The 1980 American Psychiatric Association Task Force provided a useful definition of TD as "an abnormal involuntary movement, not including tremor, resulting from treatment with a neuroleptic drug for 3 months in persons with no other identifiable cause for movement disorder."[6] New descriptions add the possibility that tremor might need to be included as a form of TD. This discussion focuses on four topics: phenomenology, epidemiology and natural history, pathophysiology, and treatment of TD.

Phenomenology

A variety of movements occur in TD. Most common are rapid unsustained movements variously described as choreic or stereotypic.[7,8] The former term refers to movements that are unpredictable and flow from one body region to another, whereas stereotypic movements are reproducible and regular, remaining generally restricted in their anatomic distribution. Controversy exists currently as to which term is best for most rapid TD movements and the authors have personally seen instances of both, sometimes in the same patient. Any body area may be affected, but the mouth is commonly involved, producing lip-smacking, tongue protrusion, or grimacing. In addition to facial movements, rapid movements of the fingers, hands or more proximal arm, nodding or head-bobbing, pelvic rocking motions, fine movements of the toes, or a nonrhythmic motion of both legs may develop. TD may involve the trunk and diaphragm, sometimes leading to speech disorders[9,10] or even respiratory distress,[11,12] which may rarely be life-threatening.[13,14]

Dystonic movements also occur in TD, either alone or in combination with choreic or stereotypic movements. Dystonic movements are sustained abnormal postures of a body part or parts, induced or increased with use of the affected part, often with superimposed spasm. Although axial dystonia was first reported as a sequel of chronic neuroleptic treatment in 1962,[15] the term "tardive dystonia" was only recently applied to a series of neuroleptic-treated patients,[16] most suffering primarily from axial dystonias.

"Tardive akathisia" is an unpleasant sensation of internal restlessness that is partially relieved by volitional movements occurring in a patient who has received chronic neuroleptics. These movements typically involve the lower extremities.[17] Tardive akathisia is phenomenologically indistinguishable from acute or subacute akathisia, but these latter entities occur when a patient's normal dose is increased, and akathisia occurs within days or weeks. Tardive akathisia occurs after chronic exposure to neuroleptics and a steady or decreasing drug dosage.

Tics and myoclonic movements are also within the potential repertoire of TD, as well as "tardive tremor."[8,18,19] This latter movement disorder is a parkinsonian tremor that develops in the context of a constant or decreasing dose of neuroleptic. Importantly, it does not refer to parkinsonism or mouth tremor (rabbit syndrome) seen with starting neuroleptic medication or with a recent increase in neuroleptic dose. As a group, tardive movements often represent combinations of various movement disorders, so that dystonia and chorea, myoclonus and stereotypy, or dystonia and myoclonus occur together, rather than as isolated phenomena. When a physician encounters a patient with such mixed disorders, drug-induced, and specifically TD, should be carefully considered.

Epidemiology and Natural History

Despite methodological differences, recent reviews have shown a striking consistency in prevalence estimates of TD.[20] Jeste and Wyatt[21] reviewed 37 studies and, using a weighted mean methodology, found a prevalence of 17.6 percent. Kane and Smith[22] reviewed 56 studies and found a prevalence of 20 percent. Although more recent estimates (1981–1986) have been higher, with an average prevalence of 30 percent, overall, the average prevalence of TD is 15–20 percent.[23]

Another condition termed spontaneous dyskinesia resembles TD, but occurs independently of neuroleptic treatment. To estimate the true prevalence of TD, the frequency of this movement disorder should be subtracted from those for TD. The prevalence of spontaneous dyskinesia ranges from 0 percent to 53 percent.[24] Based on a series of 18 studies carried out between 1966 and 1983, Casey and Gerlach[25] calculated the prevalence rate of TD to be 19.8 percent and spontaneous dyskinesia as 5.9 percent. The net difference of 13.9 may, therefore, be a better estimate of the prevalence of TD. A small prospective study of schizophrenic patients attempted to answer the question of prevalence of spontaneous dyskinesia. In this small sample, 27 neuroleptic-naïve patients were compared to 36 age-matched controls with neuroleptic exposure. Using the Abnormal Involuntary Movements Scale (AIMS), these investigators found an incidence of spontaneous dyskinesia in 4–11 percent of patients depending upon the stringency of diagnostic criteria.[26]

Gardos and Cole estimate that the risk for a schizophrenic inpatient developing TD during 1 year of continuous neuroleptic exposure is 4–5 percent.[27] Cumulative incidence of TD is approximately 10 percent after 2 years, 15 percent after 3 years, and 19 percent after 4 years. This linear increase over the first years of neuroleptic exposure argues against the idea of a period of maximal risk. Incidence estimates in other prospective studies range from 3 percent to 7 percent, with an average of approximately 5 percent.[28]

The above figures do not take into account several putative risk factors related to either the patient or the neuroleptic treatment. The most consistently observed risk factors are age and gender. Several studies have shown that the prevalence of TD is higher in women,[29,30] particularly when they are elderly.[31] Patients with affective disorders appear to be more susceptible to TD than patients with schizophrenia.[32,33] Crane first suggested that TD was more likely to develop in patients with neuroleptic-induced parkinsonism,[34] but this issue has been debated. Likewise, early studies suggested an association between TD and prior brain injury, electroconvulsive therapy (ECT), and lobotomy, but more recent studies have been less certain.[35]

Treatment-related variables such as type of neuroleptic, dose, duration of treatment, and concurrent drug treatment have additionally been studied as putative risk factors for TD. Early reports suggested that piperazine phenothiazines were most likely to result in TD,[36] but subsequent studies[37] have not confirmed this observation. Several studies[38] found that depot fluphenazine increased the prevalence of TD. Dose and duration of neuroleptic exposure have not been established as definite risk factors, but recent studies suggest that high dose[39] and high cumulative dose[40] are risk factors for eventual TD. Other drug exposure, including antiparkinson agents such as anticholinergics, have not been consistently related to an increased risk of TD.[20]

Whereas most of the risk factors appear to relate to TD regardless of phenomenologic form, for tardive dystonia, special risk factor analyses have been performed with case-control methodology. In one study, tardive dystonia was more likely in patients with a prior history of acute neuroleptic-induced dystonia.[41]

If neuroleptics can be discontinued, the signs of TD resolve spontaneously in some patients,[6] transiently worsen in others, and persist in some. Predicting which symptomatic patients have "reversible" rather than "persistent" dyskinesias is at present impossible.[7] Approximately one-third of patients with TD on neuroleptics remit within 3 months of discontinuation.[42] Resolution of movements can occur as long as 5 years after neuroleptic withdrawal.[29,43] Some studies suggested that discontinuation shortly after the onset of dyskinesias makes remission more likely, and that remissions are less likely in persons over the age of 60.[44]

In patients who remain on neuroleptics, there is little difference in overall prevalence over a 10-year period. In 63 patients examined at baseline, 5 and 10 years, most TD patients continued to have involuntary movements at all time points. Some patients (15 percent), however, remitted completely in spite of continued therapy.[45]

Pathophysiology

The pathophysiology of TD remains unknown, but interaction between dopamine, acetylcholine, gamma-aminobutyric acid (GABA) and glutamate systems may be important. In 1973, Klawans[46] proposed that the hyperkinetic movements of TD reflected a relative overactivity of striatal dopaminergic systems and that a reciprocal antagonism existed between striatal cholinergic and dopaminergic systems. He suggested that TD related to denervation hypersensitivity of striatal dopamine receptors, resulting from the "chemical denervation" by the neuroleptic. This behavior was suggested to lead to increased numbers and affinity of D2 receptors.

In spite of its usefulness, this hypothesis met several problems. For example, in laboratory studies, neuroleptic-induced receptor changes occur within days,[47] while movements in TD typically develop after months or years. Second, only about 15–20 percent of neuroleptic-exposed individuals develop TD,[20] while the neuroleptic-related increases in receptor density and sensitivity observed in animals was essentially a universal phenomenon.[48] In animals, neuroleptic-induced changes in motor behavior rarely persisted after drug withdrawal.[48] Finally, attempts to identify receptor changes specifically associated with TD in humans were uniformly inconclusive.

Gunne and Haggstrom[49] proposed that an abnormality of GABA-related striatal neurons caused TD. They observed changes in the GABA-synthesizing enzyme glutamic acid decarboxylase in animals treated with neuroleptics and noted similar changes in humans with TD.[50,51] Although they suggested that neuroleptics specifically injured GABAergic neurons, others have not replicated these findings.[52] Even if GABA changes occur, these changes could reflect increased dopaminergic activity, and thereby be only secondary phenomena.

New interest focuses on the glutamate system and theories of excitotoxins. Basal ganglia function is mediated in part by cortical glutaminergic afferents, which innervate two putaminal GABAergic neuronal populations.[53] Anatomic, physiologic, and pharmacologic studies suggest that these neuronal populations form specific, parallel efferent pathways that function with peptide cotransmitters.[54] These peptide-specific pathways have been termed "direct" and "indirect" by DeLong, and the "indirect" system[55] has been shown to be dysfunctional in some hyperkinetic disorders. In the "indirect" basal ganglia-thalamocortical circuit, somatotopically organized input from specific cortical areas facilitates striatal GABA/enkephalin (and possibly neurotensin) neurons. These putaminal neurons contain D2 receptors and are inhibited by nigral dopamine input. They inhibit a second population of GABAergic neurons in the external portion of the globus pallidus. The pallidal GABAergic neurons in turn inhibit excitatory glutaminergic outflow from the subthalamic nucleus to GABA/substance P (and possibly dynorphin) neurons in the internal portion of the globus pallidus. These GABA/substance P/dynorphin cells inhibit thalamic outflow. A parallel "direct" system involves putaminal GABA/substance P neurons and does not include subthalamic nucleus. Studies using 2-deoxyglucose autoradiography in primates suggest that chronic neuroleptics lead to underactivity of the pathway from the subthalamic nucleus to the medial pallidal segment and substantia nigra (pars reticulata), leading ultimately to facilitation of thalamic outflow.[56]

Dysfunction of "indirect" striatal outflow may be consistent with the dopaminergic hypothesis of TD and other forms of chorea.[57] A drug-induced overactivity of dopaminergic function, perhaps via neuroleptic-induced changes in D2 receptors, could cause excessive inhibition of subthalamic nucleus neurons and functional disinhibition of pallidothalamic outflow. Indirectly, blockade of dopamine receptors and resultant striatal changes could thereby alter expression of peptide cotransmitters. Haloperidol is known to cause alterations of concentrations of several peptide neurotransmitters, including enkephalins and neurotensin, although the clinical sign of such changes is unknown. The unusual temporal course of TD, becoming evident after prolonged exposure and persisting long after drug withdrawal, could in part reflect alterations of these peptide systems. A neurotransmitter system under greater current scrutiny is the cholinergic interneuron pathway in the striatum. Miller and Chouinard[58] reviewed clinical and laboratory evidence to suggest that primary attention to this cell population should not be overshadowed by studies of the dopaminergic system.

Neuroimaging and Neuropathology

Magnetic resonance (MR) studies have not revealed differences in size or configuration of basal ganglia or other structures in TD subjects.[59] In one study of 8 patients with TD using positron emission tomography (PET), D2 receptor density was not greater than that in age-matched controls.[60] Nine subjects with chronically treated schizophrenia were compared with 9 age-matched never-treated controls with schizophrenia for a PET study. The neuroleptic-treated patients were given a 2-week washout period. Each group underwent PET imaging to examine D2 receptor binding potentials. This small study found a difference in the binding potential in that patients treated with neuroleptic medications had higher D2 binding.[61] Whereas most subjects receiving neuroleptic medications have significant psychiatric illness and those not requiring neuroleptic medications are either less severely impaired or have shorter disease duration, additional control groups are needed for full interpretation of these findings. A nonpsychotic group, for instance patients with TD due to other dopamine-blocking agents such as metoclopromide or prochlorperazine used for gastrointestinal illness, may serve as a useful comparison group. TD is not associated with a characteristic pathologic finding. In some reports, the brains are normal,[61] whereas other reports show inferior olive damage, substantia nigra or nigrostriatal degeneration, or swelling of large neurons of the caudate.[62] In two studies comparing the brains of TD patients to those of controls with similar psychiatric and treatment histories, nonspecific abnormalities were more common in TD.[63,64] Postmortem neurochemical studies found alterations in dopamine concentrations and receptor binding in the brains of persons with schizophrenia, but no specific change correlated with TD.[64]

Prevention and Treatment: General Considerations

CONSERVATIVE USE OF NEUROLEPTICS

TD has no universally effective therapy, and therefore prevention of its development must be the cornerstone of therapy. The first tenet of prevention is to use neuroleptics only when necessary (see Table 37-1). The American Psychiatric Association[6] has published useful guidelines. Indications for the short-term use of neuroleptics (6 months or less) included the management of acute psychosis, preoperative medication, control of nausea, and treatment

TABLE 37-1 Treatment of TD Regardless of Phenomenology

Use neuroleptics only when needed
Withdraw neuroleptics as soon as medically possible
Use lowest possible doses

TABLE 37-2 Drugs Associated with TD

Antipsychotic agents (e.g., neuroleptic drugs)
Antidepressants with dopamine-receptor blockade (e.g., amoxapine)
Antinausea medications with dopamine receptor blockade (e.g., metoclopramide)

of primary neurologic disorders such as Huntington's disease and Tourette's syndrome. Treatment for longer than 6 months was recommended for psychotic patients with objective evidence of continuing psychosis, recurrent psychosis with neuroleptic withdrawal, disabling neurologic illnesses requiring chronic treatment, and demonstrated responsiveness to therapy. The continued need for chronic neuroleptic treatment should be regularly reassessed. Neuroleptics should be discontinued when their efficacy is uncertain, and should not be used if other agents can be substituted.

Although never evaluated in a clinical trial, simple precautions, such as using the lowest effective neuroleptic dose and regularly re-evaluating the need for treatment, make intuitive sense.

CHOICE OF NEUROLEPTICS

For decades pharmacologists have searched for a specific antipsychotic drug that acts only at receptors mediating psychosis, without any dopamine-blocking effects elsewhere. This goal has not been achieved, but several "atypical" neuroleptics, most notably, clozapine, have relatively greater effects on limbic than striatal dopamine neurons, and appear to be less associated with TD.[65] Sokoloff et al.,[66] using molecular genetic techniques, proposed that a third dopamine receptor (D3) distributed primarily in anterior, limbic, striatal regions may be important. "Typical" neuroleptics have much stronger affinities for D2 than for D3 receptors, while "atypical" neuroleptics have only a slightly greater preference for D2 than for D3 receptors.[67] If D3 receptors primarily mediate behavior, rather than motoric function, specific D3 antagonists should have minimal motoric adverse effects. Although a specific D3 antagonist is not yet available, use of agents with high D3 affinity, such as clozapine, sulpiride, thioridazine, olanzepine, and quitiapine may lower the relative risk of TD compared to other neuroleptics. With clozapine, frequent blood counts are necessary to monitor for the possibility of aplastic anemia. It is important to recognize that atypical neuroleptics too can cause TD, and that no neuroleptic is entirely safe.

If a patient is on a neuroleptic and develops early signs of TD, ideally the drug should be stopped immediately. Unfortunately, withdrawal of neuroleptic agents is impossible in the case of many psychotic patients or in disorders like severe Tourette syndrome where neuroleptics play a specific therapeutic role. In these cases, the behavioral benefit of continuing neuroleptics must be weighed against the relative neurologic risk of TD. Specific data on this question

are unclear. In many patients, the movement disorder may not progressively worsen, despite continued therapy.[6] It is well established that TD symptoms will diminish if the neuroleptic dose is increased, since higher medication doses increase blockade of striatal dopamine receptors. The use of the pathogenetic agent, however, for the treatment of TD is advised only in life-threatening situations in which all other treatments have failed.

TREATMENT WITH OTHER DRUGS

Since many patients do not have spontaneous remissions of TD, and severe psychosis precludes neuroleptic discontinuation in others, a variety of therapeutic agents have been studied in TD (Table 37-2). Evaluations of all therapeutic regimens are confounded by the inability to distinguish spontaneous remission from treatment-related resolution, the wide variation in age, sex, duration and severity of movements, the lack of universal diagnostic techniques, and the absence of a single standardized rating scale. Also, some studies have treated only patients receiving concurrent neuroleptics, others have treated those no longer taking neuroleptics, and others have mixed the two groups.

Treatment of Specific Forms of Tardive Dyskinesia

The movements of TD are generally choreic-stereotypic or dystonic, and drug treatment protocols have primarily focused attention on one or the other (see Table 37-3). Since many TD patients have a combination of movement types, the treating physician may need to weigh the relative impact of medications on each component of the movement disorder in a patient. Some treatments ameliorate one type of movement disorder while aggravating another.

TABLE 37-3 Treatment of TD Based on Phenomenology

Stereotypies, chorea, tics: reserpine, tetrabenazine, baclofen, benzodiazepines
Dystonia: reserpine, tetrabenazine, anticholinergics, botulinum toxin
Akathisia: reserpine, tetrabenazine, propranolol, opioids

CHOREIC-STEREOTYPIC MOVEMENTS

TREATMENTS INVOLVING THE DOPAMINE SYSTEM

The dopamine-depleting agents, reserpine and tetrabenazine, are the treatment of choice for the choreic or stereotypic movements of typical TD.[68] Reserpine depletes presynaptic stores of biogenic amines and is not believed to cause TD. Tetrabenazine, an experimental agent in the US, also depletes presynaptic stores of biogenic amines but in addition blocks postsynaptic dopamine receptors. Because of this latter action, it could theoretically cause TD. A recent study attempted to answer the question of the efficacy and tolerability of tetrabenazine in the treatment of patients with refractory TD. Twenty patients were studied in this protocol. Each patient was videotaped before and after treatment with tetrabenazine. One patient could not tolerate tetrabenazine due to sedation and was withdrawn from the study. The remaining patients were treated for a mean of 20.3 weeks. The videotapes were then randomized and studied by a blinded rater using AIMS. Videotapes performed after treatment had a significant improvement over pretreatment videotapes. The mean dosage used in this study was 57.9 mg/day. All patients elected to continue treatment with tetrabenazine at the conclusion of the study.[69] Reserpine and tetrabenazine control the movements of TD in the majority of patients and, in some cases, treatment is followed by complete remission of TD.[70] The major side-effects of these agents are orthostatic hypotension, depression, and drug-induced parkinsonism. Orthostatic hypotension occurs most commonly in older patients and may be avoided or minimized through the gradual introduction of the drug. Reserpine can be instituted at 0.125–0.25 mg daily and increased by 0.124–0.25 mg weekly, while tetrabenazine can be instituted at 25 mg daily and increased by 25 mg weekly or biweekly while monitoring blood pressure. Depression occurs commonly after prolonged (months to years) continuous therapy and generally requires drug discontinuation. Concurrent or latent depression can be severely exacerbated by reserpine and tetrabenazine. The full therapeutic response to a given dose of these agents is not apparent for several weeks and doses as high as 6 mg/day of reserpine may be necessary. Sometimes a neuroleptic will be needed for short-term control of TD during the few weeks when reserpine is being introduced.[71]

Low doses of dopamine agonists designed to activate presynaptic autoreceptors and thereby decrease dopamine release have not been consistently successful.[72] "Desensitizing" dopamine receptors by using increasing doses of L-dopa has not proved regularly beneficial.[73] The monoamine oxidase B inhibitor, selegiline, with putative antioxidant properties along with its dopaminergic facilitation, was tried in a placebo-controlled sample of TD patients, but drug-treated patients fared worse than those receiving placebo.[74] Calcium channel-blocking agents, usually used in cardiac patients, have been suggested to have dopamine-blocking properties, but, in one placebo-controlled study, diltiazem had no efficacy in treated TD.[75] Other studies have suggested that nifedipine and verapamil may be more effective,[76] but better placebo-controlled, and blinded protocols are needed to evaluate this drug class.

In severely disabled patients, particularly those with respiratory or oropharyngeal dyskinesias, withdrawal of the neuroleptic agent may be potentially life-threatening. In such severe cases, a return to neuroleptic medication may be the only feasible therapy. On the other hand, reserpine may be added to a stable dose of the neuroleptic and increased until the movements abate. When movements decrease, the neuroleptic may be slowly withdrawn in order to keep the dose of the causative agent at its very lowest level. Novel or atypical neuroleptics like clozapine have been tried at high doses in treating TD, but side-effects in the elderly (primarily sedation) preclude its general use.[77] In low doses (50–250 mg/day), clozapine has no significant effect on TD.

TREATMENTS INVOLVING THE GABA SYSTEM

Based on observations that prograbide co-administration with chronic haloperidol can reduce vacuous chewing movements in experimental animals, agents with effects on the GABA system have been tried in TD. The magnitude of benefit achieved with agents that are designed to augment GABA function is generally less than with drugs affecting dopamine systems. However, the therapeutic index is generally greater, so that a short trial with a GABAergic agent is often indicated in mild or moderate TD, before attempting treatment with dopamine-depleting agents. Respiratory depression may accompany overdose with this class of drugs, and the respiratory depressant effect may be additive with other central nervous system depressants, including ethanol. The physician must carefully consider suicide risk and concurrent medications when prescribing these agents.

Small studies have suggested that baclofen,[78] sodium valproate,[79] and gamma-vinyl-GABA[80] produce mild improvement in TD, but the effects were inconsistent, short-lasting, or limited by side-effects. Of these, baclofen, starting at 5 or 10 mg daily and increasing in 5–10 mg/day increments up to a maximum daily dose of 60–80 mg/day in three or four doses is most likely to be beneficial. In patients receiving concurrent neuroleptics, baclofen may aggravate drug-induced parkinsonism. Sedation is a common adverse effect, and ataxia, confusion, and auditory or visual hallucinations may rarely occur. Abrupt discontinuation should be avoided, since anxiety or hallucinations may occur. Coma, respiratory depression, and seizures may follow severe overdosage.

Benzodiazepines may potentiate central GABA transmission, and are mildly beneficial in TD, especially clonazepam, and diazepam.[81] Sedation, a common dose-limiting side-effect of clonazepam, can be minimized by gradual drug introduction, beginning with 0.5 mg daily and increasing in 0.5–1 mg/week increments. Tolerance for the antidyskinetic effect is common after months of therapy, but Thaker et al.[81] found gradual withdrawal followed by a 2-week drug-free period to be associated with renewed efficacy when the drug was reintroduced.

ANTIOXIDANT AND OTHER PHARMACOLOGIC STRATEGIES

A recent focus for studying the pathophysiology of several movement disorders is membrane damage due to free radical formation.[82,83] The antioxidant vitamin, tocopherol, a free radical scavenger, was found to be useful in several short trials of TD,[84,85] but not in all.[86] Since the doses used (400–1200 IU/day) are not associated with adverse effects, tocopherol could become an important therapeutic agent if further trials replicate these results. A recent study of 20 patients looked at higher dosages of tocopherol over a 7-month period. In this protocol, 9 patients were treated with tocopherol and 11 patients served as controls using improvement of AIMS scoring as an endpoint. The treatment group was started at 600 mg/day of tocopherol and increased to 1600 mg/day over 7 months. No significant difference in AIMS scores were found until treated patients reached 1600 mg/day.[87] High doses of tocopherol can be associated with coagulation alterations and careful consideration of patient compliance must be balanced with anticipated clinical benefit in prescribing a high dose of tocopherol. At present, a 2- or 3-week trial of tocopherol in mildly to moderately affected patients could be attempted before other therapeutic regimens, since no risk of treatment-related adverse effects is associated. Higher doses have also been studied with positive effects, but coagulation status and cholesterol levels need to be monitored.[87,88] The effect is not due to changes in neuroleptic drug levels.[88] Whereas most studies are short term, one has shown maintained improvement for as long as 36 weeks.[89]

Another vitamin therapy under study in tardive dyskinesia is pyridoxine (B_6). Five patients with TD underwent a 4-week open-label trial of pyridoxine at 100 mg/day. Severity of movements was rated using AIMS, Barnes Akathisia Rating Scale (BARS), and the Simpson-Angus Scale (SAS). Four patients had clinically significant improvement using the AIMS scale. No patients had significant side-effects from the pyridoxine.[90] A second study was performed testing the efficacy of vitamin B_6 for the treatment of tardive dyskinesia. Fifteen patients with schizophrenia and TD were randomly assigned to treatment or placebo groups and treated for 4 weeks with either placebo or vitamin B_6 in escalating dosages to 400 mg/day. A washout period of 1 week was then instituted with a crossover to treatment or placebo. Patients were evaluated by a blinded rater using the Extrapyramidal Symptom Rating Scale (ESRS). The treatment group had significant improvement in dyskinesia scores with vitamin B_6 at dosages of 300–400 mg/day.[91] A large double-blind placebo-controlled trial will be needed to determine if pyridoxine is effective therapy for TD.

In uncontrolled studies of small numbers of patients, several other agents have been reported to have minimal benefit in TD, including propranolol,[92] clonidine,[93] tryptophan,[94] cyproheptadine,[95] opiates,[96] manganese and niacin,[97]

gabapentin,[98] and GM1 ganglioside.[99] Lithium was beneficial in some studies,[94] but not in others.[100] Agents affecting the cholinergic system have not had consistent benefit.[7] Buspirone has been used in an open-label trial with statistically significant improvement.[101] With the new interest in neuropeptides, ceruletide has been examined with clinical improvement. The putative advantage to such therapy is its once-weekly administration.[102]

Finally, ECT was reported to both ameliorate TD and increase its occurrence.[103] Since others have noted mood fluctuations to alter the expression of TD,[103,104] these observations may relate to ECT effects on mood more than movement disorders.

DYSTONIC MOVEMENTS

Some drugs are useful for dystonic, as well as choreic-stereotypic TD.[16] Like patients with unusual TD, those with tardive dystonia are helped by dopamine-depleting agents such as reserpine and tetrabenazine.[105] Clonazepam,[81] and ECT[104] have been reported to be beneficial in a few patients.

In contrast, however, centrally active anticholinergic drugs (muscarinic receptor blockers) are a major therapeutic tool in tardive dystonia,[16] whereas in typical choreic-stereotypic TD, movements worsen when an anticholinergic is given.[46] In patients with both dystonia and typical TD, use of anticholinergics may improve dystonia but worsen other signs. In such cases, the physician should analyze which movements are causing the most pronounced disability. In most instances, other than cosmetic, dystonic movements are more disabling than choreic-stereotypic.

A treatment primarily designed for idiopathic dystonia, but recently applied to other dystonic syndromes, is botulinum toxin (BTX) injection. This biologic toxin, when injected directly into overactive muscles, weakens them by decreasing acetylcholine release at the neuromuscular junction. For patients whose tardive dystonia affects primarily one body region, this treatment could be considered.[106] Two serotypes of BTX are currently available for widespread use: BTX-A, and BTX-B. BTX-A has been available since the late 1980s and the majority of our clinical experience is with this agent. BTX-B has only been approved since 2000, so our clinical experience with this agent is limited. In patients with combined tardive dystonia and choreic TD movements, BTX can abate the dystonia, while other medications focus on the dyskinesias.[107]

In setting an order for medication trials in tardive dystonia, clonazepam or baclofen may be selected first if the dystonia is painful. A trial of anticholinergic agents may be useful in those without prominent choreic or stereotypic movements. Dopamine-depleting agents may be tried as more aggressive treatment in patients without depression. In persons with extreme disability, as is often the case in those with predominantly axial dystonias, neuroleptic agents may be necessary. In this case, careful explanation of the potential for the treatment to aggravate the tardive disorder is recommended.

BTX is usually an adjunct medication, supplementing other drugs, and used to focus specific attention to one or two prominently involved body areas.

TARDIVE AKATHISIA

Tardive akathisia is phenomenologically indistinguishable from subacute akathisia accompanying neuroleptic treatment; hence, in patients requiring continued use of neuroleptic agents, a distinction between the two is particularly problematic. Dopamine-depleting agents are useful in tardive akathisia, in doses similar to those used in typical TD.[17] In a few persons, agents useful in treating subacute akathisia may be helpful, such as propranolol (60 mg daily)[108] and opiates (propoxyphene up to 100 mg daily or codeine up to 60 mg daily).[109] In contrast to subacute akathisia, anticholinergic agents are not helpful in tardive akathisia.

Future Perspectives

The development of functional MR scanning and PET technology may provide clearer evidence of the pathophysiologic changes that occur with the introduction of neuroleptic drugs in humans and the progressive, long-term consequences of their use. The appreciation of receptor subtypes for the dopaminergic system provides solid evidence that TD occurs when striatal dopaminergic receptors are blocked, and such studies support the concept that TD may be avoided by selective antagonists that avoid striatal dopaminergic receptor antagonism. More complete understanding of neurotransmitter systems other than the dopaminergic promises direct clinical impact for treatment and prevention, especially related to the GABAergic pathways. Finally, new discoveries on oxidative metabolism in the central nervous system and the role of such chemical reactions in neurodegenerative and neurotoxic syndromes may lead to significant treatment breakthrough that does not necessarily relate to specific neurotransmitters systems, but rather to general chemical reactions affecting neuronal and glial function.

References

1. Sewell DD, Jeste DV: Metoclopramide-associated tardive dyskinesia: An analysis of 67 cases. *Arch Fam Med* 1:271–278, 1992.
2. Schoenecker VM: Ein eigentümliches Syndrom in oralen Bereich bei megphen Application. *Nervenarzt* 28:35–43, 1957.
3. Waddington JL: Tardive dyskinesia: A critical re-evaluation of the causal role of neuroleptics and of the dopamine receptor supersensitivity hypothesis, in Callaghan N, Galvin R (eds): *Recent Researches in Neurology*. London: Pitman, 1984, pp 34–48.
4. Marsden CD, Tarsy D, Baldessarini RJ: Spontaneous and drug-induced movement disorders in psychotic patients, in Benson DF, Blumer D (eds): *Psychiatric Aspects of Neurologic Disease*. New York: Grune & Stratton, 1975, pp 219–265.
5. Klawans HL, Bergen D, Bruyn GW, Paulson GW: Neuroleptic-induced tardive dyskinesia in nonpsychotic patients. *Arch Neurol* 30:338–339, 1974.
6. Baldessarini RJ, Cole JO, Davis JM, et al: Tardive dyskinesia: Summary of a Task Force Report of the American Psychiatric Association. *Am J Psychiatry* 137:1163–1172, 1980.
7. Tanner CM: Drug-induced movement disorders (tardive dyskinesia and dopa-induced dyskinesia), in Vinken PJ, Bruyn GW, Klawans HL (eds): *Handbook of Clinical Neurology*. Amsterdam: Elsevier, 1986, pp 185–212.
8. Stacy M, Jankovic J: Tardive dyskinesia. *Curr Opin Neurol Neurosurg* 4:343–349, 1991.
9. Feve A, Angelard B, Benelon G, et al: Postneuroleptic laryngeal dyskinesias: A cause of upper airway obstructive syndrome improved by local injections of botulinum toxin. *Mov Disord* 7:217–219, 1993.
10. Gerratt BR, Goetz CG, Fisher HB. Speech abnormalities in tardive dyskinesia. *Arch Neurol* 41:273–276, 1984.
11. Weiner WJ, Goetz CG, Nausieda PA, Klawans HL: Respiratory dyskinesias: Extrapyramidal dysfunction and dyspnea. *Am J Intern Med* 88:327–331, 1978.
12. Wilcos PG, Bassett A, Jones B, Fleetham JA: Respiratory arrhythmias in patients with tardive dyskinesia. *Chest* 105:203–207, 1994.
13. Casey DE, Rabins P: Tardive dyskinesias as a life-threatening illness. *Am J Psychiatry* 135:486–488, 1978.
14. Feve A, Angelard B, Fenelon G, et al: Postneuroleptic laryngeal dyskinesias: A cause of upper airway obstructive syndrome improved by local injections of botulinum toxin. *Mov Disord* 8:217–219, 1993.
15. Druckman R, Seelinger D, Thulin B: Chronic involuntary movements induced by phenothiazines. *J Nerv Ment Dis* 135:69–76, 1962.
16. Burke RE, Fahn S, Jankovic J, et al: Tardive dystonia: Late-onset and persistent dystonia caused by anti-psychotic drugs. *Neurology* 32:1335–1346, 1982.
17. Christiansen E, Moller JE, Faurbye A: Neurological investigation of 28 brains from patients with dyskinesia. *Acta Psychiatr Scand* 46:14–23, 1970.
18. Stacy M, Jankovic J: Tardive tremor. *Mov Disord* 7:75–77, 1992.
19. Adler LA, Peselow E, Duncan E, et al: Vitamin E in tardive dyskinesia: Time course of effect after placebo substitution. *Psychopharmacol Bull* 39:371–374, 1993.
20. Khot V, Egan MF, Hyde TM, Wyatt J: Neuroleptics and classic tardive dyskinesia, in Lang AE, Weiner WJ (eds): *Drug-Induced Movement Disorders*. Kisco: Futura, 1982, pp 121–166.
21. Jeste DV, Wyatt RJ: *Understanding and Treating Tardive Dyskinesia*. New York: Guilford Press, 1982.
22. Kane JM, Smith JM: Tardive dyskinesia. *Arch Gen Psychiatry* 39:473–481, 1982.
23. Baldessarini RJ, Cole JO, Davis JM, et al: *Tardive Dyskinesia: A Task Force Report*. Washington, DC: American Psychiatric Association, 1980.
24. Casey DE, Hansen TE: Spontaneous dyskinesia, in Jeste DV, Wyatt RJ (eds): *Neuropsychiatric Movement Disorders*. Washington, DC: American Psychiatric Press, 1984, pp 68–95.
25. Casey DE, Gerlach J: Tardive dyskinesia. *Acta Psychiatr Scand* 77:369–378, 1988.
26. Puri BK, Barnes TR, Chapman JM, et al: Spontaneous dyskinesia in first episode schizophrenia. *J Neurol Neurosurg Psychiatry* 66:76–78, 1999.

27. Gardos G, Cole JO: Overview: Public health issues in tardive dyskinesia. *Am J Psychiatry* 137:776–781, 1980.

28. Chouinard G, Annable L, Ross-Chouinard A, Mercier P: A 5-year prospective longitudinal study of tardive dyskinesia: Factors predicting appearance of new cases. *J Clin Psychopharmacol* 8(suppl):21–26, 1988.

29. Jeste DV, Wyatt RJ: *Understanding and Treating Tardive Dyskinesia.* New York: Guilford Press, 1982.

30. Byne W, White L, Parella. Tardive dyskinesias in a chronically instutionalized population of elderly schizophrenic patients. *Int J Geriatr Psychiat* 13:473–479, 1998.

31. Smith JM, Oswald WT, Kucharski LT, Waterman LJ: Tardive dyskinesia: Age and sex differences in hospitalized schizophrenics. *Psychopharmacology* 58:207–211, 1978.

32. Gardos G, Casey D (eds): *Tardive Dyskinesia and Affective Disorders.* Washington, DC: American Psychiatric Press, 1983.

33. Yassa R, Nastase C, Dupont D, Thibeau M: Tardive dyskinesia in elderly psychiatric patients: A 5-year study. *Am J Psychiatry* 149:1206–1211, 1992.

34. Crane GE: Persistent dyskinesia. *Br J Psychiatry* 122:395–405, 1973.

35. Gupta S, Egan MF, Hyde TM: An unusual presentation of tardive dyskinesia with prominent involvement of the pectoral musculature. *Biol Psychiatry* 33:291–292, 1993.

36. Gershanik OS: Drug-induced movement disorders. *Curr Opin Neurol Neurosurg* 6:369–376, 1993.

37. Klawans HL, Goetz CG, Perlik S: Tardive dyskinesia: Review and update. *Am J Psychiatry* 137:900–908, 1980.

38. Gardos G, Cole JO, LaBrie RA: Drug variables in the etiology of tardive dyskinesia: Application of discriminant function analysis, in Fahn WE, Smith RC, Davis JM, Domino EF (eds): *Tardive Dyskinesia: Research and Treatment.* New York: SP Medical and Scientific Books, 1980, pp 291–296.

39. Morgernstern H, Glazer WM: Identify risk factors for tardive dyskinesia among long-term outpatients maintained with neuroleptic medications. Results of the Yale Tardive Dyskinesia Study. *Arch Gen Psychiatry* 50:723–733, 1993.

40. Cavallaro R, Regazzetti MG, Mundo E, et al: Tardive dyskinesia outcomes: Clinical and pharmacologic correlates of remission and persistence. *Neuropsychopharmacology* 8:233–239, 1993.

41. Sachdev P: Risk factors for tardive dystonia: A case-control comparison with tardive dyskinesia. *Acta Psychiatr Scand* 88:98–103, 1993.

42. Jeste DV, Jeste SD, Wyatt RJ: Reversible tardive dyskinesia: Implications for therapeutic strategy and prevention of tardive dyskinesia. *Mod Probl Pharmacopsychiatry* 21:34–48, 1983.

43. Klawans HL, Tanner CM: The reversibility of permanent tardive dyskinesia. *Neurology* 33(suppl 2):163, 1983.

44. Quitkin F, Rifkin A, Gochfeld L, Klein DF: Tardive dyskinesia: Are first signs reversible? *Am J Psychiatry* 134:84–87, 1977.

45. Gardos G, Casey DE, Cole HO, et al: Ten-year outcome of tardive dyskinesia. *Am J Psychiatry* 151:836–841, 1994.

46. Klawans HL: *The Pharmacology of Extrapyramidal Movement Disorders.* Basel: Karger, 1973.

47. Klawans HL, Rubovits R: The effect of cholinergic and anticholinergic agents on tardive dyskinesias. *J Neurol Neurosurg Psychiatry* 37:941–947, 1974.

48. Goetz CG, Klawans HL: Controversies in animal models of tardive dyskinesia, in Marsden CD, Fahn S (eds): *Movement Disorders.* Boston: Butterworth, 1982, pp 263–276.

49. Gunne LM, Haggstrom JE: Pathophysiology of tardive dyskinesia. *Psychopharmacol* (suppl 2):191–193, 1985.

50. Gunne LM, Haggstrom JE, Sjoquist B: Association with persistent neuroleptic-induced dyskinesia of regional changes in brain: GABA synthesis. *Nature* 309:347–349, 1984.

51. Andersson U, Haggstrom JE, Levin ED, et al: Reduced glutamate decarboxylase activity in the subthalamic nucleus in patients with tardive dyskinesia. *Mov Disord* 4:37–46, 1989.

52. Mithani S, Atmada S, Baimbridge KG, Fubuger HC: Neuroleptic-induced oral dyskinesias: Effects of progabide and lack of correlation with regional changes in glutamic acid decarboxylase and choline acetyl transferase activities. *Psychopharmacology* 93:94–100, 1987.

53. Alexander GE, Crutcher MD: Functional architecture of basal ganglia circuits: Neural substrates of parallel processing. *Trends Neurosci* 13:266–271, 1990.

54. Graybiel AM: Neurotransmitters and neuromodulators in the basal ganglia. *Trends Neurosci* 13:244–254, 1990.

55. DeLong MR: Primate model of movement disorders of basal ganglia origin. *Trends Neurosci* 13:281–285, 1990.

56. Feve A, Angelard B, Fenelon G, et al: Neuroleptic-induced tardive dyskinesia in the Cebus monkey. *Mov Disord* 7:32–37, 1992.

57. Reiner A, Albin RL, Anderson KD, et al: Differential loss of striatal projection neurons in Huntington disease. *Proc Natl Acad Sci U S A* 85:5733–5737, 1988.

58. Miller R, Chouinard G: Loss of striatal cholinergic neurons as a basis for tardive and L-dopa-induced dyskinesias, neuroleptic-induced supersensitivity psychosis and refractory schizophrenia. *Biol Psychiatry* 34:713–738, 1993.

59. Buckley P, O'Callaghan E, Mulvany E: Basal Ganglia T2 relaxation times in schizophrenia: a quantitative magnetic resonance imaging study in relation to tardive dyskinesia. *Psychiatry Res* 61:95–102, 1995.

60. Blin J, Baron JC, Cambon H, et al: Dyskinesia: PET study. *J Neurol Neurosurg Psychiatry* 52:1248–1252, 1989.

61. Hunter R, Blackwood W, Smith MC: Neuropathological findings in three cases of persistent dyskinesias following phenothiazines. *J Neurol Sci* 7:263–273, 1968.

62. Silverstri S, Seeman MV, Negrete JC, et al: Increased dopamine D2 receptor binding after long-term treatment with antipsychotics in humans: A clinical PET study. *Psychopharmacology* 152:174–180, 2000.

63. Christiansen E, Moller JE, Faurbye A: Neurological investigation of 28 brains from patients with dyskinesia. *Acta Psychiatr Scand* 46:14–23, 1970.

64. Jellinger K: Neuropathologic findings after neuroleptic long-term therapy, in Roizin L, Shiraki H, Grecevic N (eds): *Neurotoxicology.* New York: Raven Press, 1977, pp 25–42.

65. Lieberman J, Johns C, Cooper T, et al: Clozapine pharmacology and tardive dyskinesia. *Psychopharmacology* 99:S54–S59, 1989.

66. Sokoloff P, Giros B, Mrtres MP, et al: Molecular cloning and characterization of a novel dopamine receptor (D3) as a target for neuroleptics. *Nature* 347:146–151, 1990.

67. Strange PG: Interesting times for dopamine receptors. *Trends Neurosci* 14:43–45, 1991.

68. Jankovic J, Orman J: Tetrabenazine therapy of dystonia, chorea, tics and other dyskinesias. *Neurology* 38:391–394, 1988.

69. Ondo WG, Hanna PA, Jankovic J: Tetrabenazine treatment for tardive dyskinesia: Assessment by randomized videotape protocol. *Am J Psychiatry* 156: 1279–1281, 1999

70. Lang AE, Marsden CD: Alphamethylparatyrosine and tetrabenazine in movement disorders. *Clin Neuropharmacol* 5:375–387, 1982.

71. Stacy M, Francisco C, Jankovic J: Tardive stereotypy and other movement disorders in tardive dyskinesia. *Neurology* 43:937–941, 1993.

72. Tamminga CA, Chase TN: Bromocriptine and CF 25–396 in the treatment of tardive dyskinesia. *Arch Neurol* 37:204–205, 1980.

73. Alpert M, Friedhoff A: Clinical application of receptor modification treatment, in Fann WE, Smith RC, Davis JM, Domino EF (eds): *Tardive Dyskinesia: Research and Treatment*. New York: Spectrum, 1980, pp 471–474.

74. Goff DC, Renshaw PF, Sarid-Segal O, et al: A placebo-controlled trial of selegiline (L-deprenyl) in the treatment of tardive dyskinesia. *Biol Psychiatry* 33:700–706, 1993.

75. Loonen AJ, Verwey HA, Roels PR, et al: Is diltiazem effective in treating the symptoms of (tardive) dyskinesia in chronic psychiatric inpatients? A negative, double-blind, placebo-controlled trial. *J Clin Psychopharmacology* 12:39–42, 1992.

76. Cates M, Lusk K, Wells BG: Are calcium-channel blockers effective in the treatment of tardive dyskinesia? *Ann Pharmacother* 27:191–196, 1993.

77. Simpson CM, Lee JH, Shrivastava RK: Clozapine and tardive dyskinesia. *Psychopharmacologia* 56:75–80, 1978.

78. Stewart RM, Rollins J, Beckham B, Roffman M: Baclofen in tardive dyskinesia patients maintained on neuroleptics. *Clin Neuropharmacol* 5:365–373, 1982.

79. Nair NPV, Lal S, Schwartz G, Tharundayil JX: Effects of sodium valproate and baclofen in tardive dyskinesia: Clinical and neuroendocrine studies. *Adv Biochem Psychopharmacol* 24:437–441, 1980.

80. Tell GP, Schecter PJ, Koch-Weser J, et al: Effects of gamma vinyl GABA [letter]. *N Engl J Med* 305:581–582, 1981.

81. Thaker GK, Nguyen JA, Strauss ME, et al: Clonazepam treatment of tardive dyskinesia: A practical GABA mimetic strategy. *Am J Psychiatry* 147:445–451, 1990.

82. Lohr JB, Kuczenski R, Bracha HS, et al: Increased indices of free radical activity in the cerebrospinal fluid of patients with tardive dyskinesia. *Biol Psychiatry* 28:535–539, 1990.

83. Cadet JL: Movement disorders: Therapeutic role of vitamin E. *Toxicol Ind Health* 9:337–347, 1993.

84. Elkashef AM, Ruskin PE, Bacher N, Barrett D: Vitamin E and the treatment of tardive dyskinesia. *Am J Psychiatry* 147:505–506, 1990.

85. Dabiri LM, Pasta D, Darby JK, Mosbacher D: Effectiveness of vitamin E for treatment of long-term tardive dyskinesia. *Am J Psychiatry* 151:925–926, 1994.

86. Shriqui CL, Bradwejn J, Annable L, Jones BD: Vitamin E in the treatment of tardive dyskinesia: A double-blind placebo-controlled study. *Am J Psychiatry* 149:391–393, 1992.

87. Adler LA, Peselow E, Rotrosen J, et al: Vitamin E treatment of tardive dyskinesia. *Am J Psychiatry* 150:1405–1407, 1993.

88. Egan MF, Hyde TM, Albers GW, et al: Treatment of tardive dyskinesia with vitamin E. *Am J Psychiatry* 149:773–777, 1992.

89. Sajjad SH: Vitamin E in the treatment of tardive dyskinesia: A preliminary study over 7 months at different doses. *International Clinical Psychopharmacology* 13(4):147–155, 1998.

90. Lerner V, Kaptsan A, Miodownik, et al: Vitamin B_6 in treatment of tardive dyskinesia: A preliminary case series study. *Clin Neuropharmacol* 22:241–243, 1999.

91. Lerner V, Miodownik C, Kaptsan A, et al: Vitamin B_6 in the treatment of tardive dyskinesia: A double-blind, placebo-controlled, crossover study. *Am J Psychiatry* 159:1511–1514, 2001.

92. Bacher NM, Lewis HA: Low dose propranolol in tardive dyskinesia. *Am J Psychiatry* 137:495–497, 1980.

93. Freedman R, Bell J, Kirch D: Clonidine therapy for coexisting psychosis and tardive dyskinesia. *Am J Psychiatry* 137:629–630, 1980.

94. Prange AJ Jr, Wilson IC, Morris CE: Preliminary experience with tryptophan and lithium in the treatment of tardive dyskinesia. *Psychopharmacol Bull* 9:36–37, 1973.

95. Gardos G, Cole JO: Pilot study of cyproheptadine (Periactin) in tardive dyskinesia. *Psychopharmacol Bull* 14:18–20, 1978.

96. Stoessl AJ, Polanski E, Frydryszak H: The opiate antagonist naloxone suppresses a rodent model of tardive dyskinesia. *Mov Disord* 8:445–452, 1993.

97. Kunin RA: Manganese and niacin in the treatment of drug-induced dyskinesia. *J Orthomol Psychiatry* 5:4–27, 1976.

98. Hardoy MC, Hardoy MJ, Carta MG, et al: Gabapentin as a promising treatment for antipsychotic-induced movement disorders in schizoaffective and bipolar patients. *J Affect Dis* 54:315–317, 1999.

99. Peselow ED, Irons S, Rotrosen J, et al: GM1 ganglioside as a potential treatment in tardive dyskinesia. *Psychopharmacology* 25:277–280, 1989.

100. Reda FA, Scanlan JM, Escobar JI, et al: Lithium Carbonate in the treatment of tardive dyskinesia, *Am J Psychiatry* 132:560–562, 1975.

101. Simpson GM, Branchez MH, Lee HJ: Lithium in tardive dyskinesia. *Pharmakopsychiatr Neuropsychopharmakol* 9:76–80, 1976.

102. Moss LE, Neppe VM, Drevets WC: Buspiron in the treatment of tardive dyskinesia. *J Clin Psychopharmacol* 13:204–209, 1993.

103. Kojima T, Yamauchi T, Miyasaka M, et al: Treatment of tardive dyskinesia with ceruletide: A double-blind, controlled study. *Psychiatry Res* 43:129–136, 1992.

104. Price TRP, Levin R: Effects of electroconvulsive therapy on tardive dyskinesia. *Am J Psychiatry* 135:991–993, 1978.

105. Unrbrand L, Faurbye A: Reversible and irreversible dyskinesia after treatment with perphenazine, chlorpromazine, reserpine and ECT therapy. *Psychopharmacologia* 1:408–418, 1960.

106. Kang JU, Burke RE, Fahn S: Natural history and treatment of tardive dystonia. *Mov Disord* 1:193–208, 1986.

107. Jankovic J, Brin MF: Therapeutic uses of botulinum toxin. *N Engl J Med* 324:1186–1194, 1991.

108. Stip E, Faughnan M, Desjardin I, Labrecque R: Botulinum toxin in a case of severe tardive dyskinesia mixed with dystonia. *Br J Psychiatry* 161:867–868, 1992.

Chapter 38

OTHER CHOREATIC DISORDERS

MARGERY H. MARK

CHOREA   639
THE IMMUNE SYSTEM, HORMONES, AND
    CHOREA   639
    Sydenham's Chorea (SC)   639
    Chorea Gravidarum   640
    Systemic Lupus Erythematosus (SLE), and the
       Primary Antiphospholipid Antibody
       Syndrome (PAPS)   640
    Pathophysiology: Immune-Mediated Mechanism?   641
HEREDITARY CHOREAS   641
    Neuroacanthocytoses: Choreoacanthocytosis (CA)
       and McLeod Syndrome   641
    Benign Hereditary Chorea (BHC)   642
    Dentatorubropallidoluysian Atrophy (DRPLA)   642
SENILE CHOREA   643
VASCULAR CHOREA, HEMICHOREA, AND
    HEMIBALLISMUS   643
OTHER NEUROLOGIC AND SYSTEMIC DISEASES   644
    Hyperthyroidism   644
    Polycythemia Vera   644
    Metabolic Disorders   644
    Multiple Sclerosis   644
    Postpump Chorea   644
OTHER CAUSES   645
    Drugs, Toxins, Infections, Neoplasms,
       Degenerative Disorders   645
PAROXYSMAL DYSKINESIAS   645
PAINFUL LEGS AND MOVING TOES   647
CONCLUSIONS   648

Chorea

Chorea (Greek for "dance") consists of irregular, unpredictable, brief movements that flow from one body part to another in a nonstereotyped fashion. They may be incorporated, especially in milder cases, into more purposeful movements. They may consist of small twitches or larger jerks of any body part. Choreiform movements rarely occur in isolation; rather, they may often be seen in a spectrum with slower, distal, writhing, sinuous movements called athetosis, and described as choreoathetosis. In many disorders in which chorea is a feature, it is not uncommon to see other movement disorders as well, particularly dystonia. The converse of speed and amplitude from athetoid movements are ballistic movements, which are usually seen unilaterally as

hemiballism, although bilateral movements (paraballism or biballism) may be encountered. Ballistic movements, the most extreme type of movement disorder, are large-amplitude, usually proximal, flinging of a limb or body part. Although some investigators separate these disorders, others (including the present author) consider ballism to be a severe form of chorea, and in fact many cases of resolving ballistic movements taper down to chorea.[1]

The prototypic choreic disorder is Huntington's disease (HD), discussed in detail in the preceding chapters. The phenomenology of chorea in other disorders, both primary and secondary, is essentially the same as in HD. Likewise, theories of the pathophysiology of the choreas, for the most part, are very similar. Similarly, Wilson's disease (Chap. 49), tardive dyskinesia (Chap. 39), and treated Parkinson's disease (Chap. 15) may also demonstrate chorea; the reader is referred to those chapters for more details. In this chapter, we focus on several clinical entities in which chorea plays a significant role. Other related movement disorders will also be discussed.

The Immune System, Hormones, and Chorea

It has long been recognized that several seemingly unrelated conditions have been uncommonly associated with chorea: rheumatic fever, systemic lupus erythematosus (SLE), and pregnancy (and its flip side, use of oral contraceptives). The pathophysiology of chorea in these conditions may be similar, and will be explored below.

SYDENHAM'S CHOREA (SC)

In 1686, Thomas Sydenham described the clinical syndrome that now bears his name.[2] Originally called St Vitus dance, as well as chorea minor, acute chorea, and rheumatic chorea, Sydenham's chorea (SC) not uncommonly follows rheumatic fever in children and adolescents. Antecedent infection with group A streptococcus is usual, although many patients do not give a history of streptococcal infection; also, as the chorea may occur 6 months or more after infection, antistreptolysin and antistreptococcal antibodies may not be elevated. Adequate antibiotic therapy in the US has dramatically reduced the occurrence of rheumatic fever, and thus of SC,[3] although it may still be found. It may be seen more often in children from developing countries who lack routine antibiotic care. In fact, a recent series from Turkey showed that acute rheumatic fever is not only still very prevalent in that country, but remains a significant cause of morbidity, and revealed that 20 percent of patients (45/228) admitted to hospital with rheumatic fever had chorea.[4] Another series of admissions to one hospital in Chile during 1976–1989 demonstrated that 16 percent of attacks of acute rheumatic fever (70/438 in 402 patients) presented with SC.[5]

The clinical syndrome of SC, in addition to the chorea, is characterized by a semi-acute illness involving muscular weakness, hypotonia, dysarthria, and behavioral abnormalities. The most common behavioral problem is obsessive-compulsive symptomatology, with 82 percent of individuals affected in one series; nearly half of these children met criteria for frank obsessive-compulsive disorder.[6,7] They also demonstrate increased emotional lability, motoric hyperactivity, irritability, distractibility, and age-regressed behavior. Behavioral symptoms may begin several days to weeks prior to onset of chorea, and wax and wane with motor signs.[6] The chorea is usually bilateral, but may be unilateral in about 20 percent of patients. It may begin either abruptly or insidiously, worsen over 2–4 weeks, and usually resolves spontaneously in 3–6 months, although some patients may have residual chorea. Recurrences may occur in about 20 percent of patients, usually within about 2 years.[3,8] The vast majority of patients are between 5 and 15 years of age at first occurrence; girls are affected about twice as frequently as boys, especially in the peripubescent ages, suggesting a role for sex hormones in this disorder.[9]

The EEG is often abnormal, with slowing, particularly irregular occipital slowing.[10,11] Neuroimaging studies may shed some light on the pathophysiology (discussed below). Magnetic resonance imaging (MRI) in two cases revealed increased signal on T_2-weighted images in the striatum and globus pallidus, with resolution of signal intensity upon clinical improvement,[12,13] whereas another showed permanent basal ganglia injury.[14] Yet another case demonstrated multiple areas of abnormal signal on MRI, with resultant angiography revealing vasculitis attributed directly to her SC.[15] One analysis of MRI of 24 subjects with SC demonstrated increased size of caudate, putamen, and globus pallidus,[16] suggesting an inflammatory process. Functional neuroimaging, evaluating regional cerebral glucose metabolism using fluorodeoxyglucose positron emission tomography (FDG-PET), in SC differs from HD and other hereditary choreas. In HD, there is striatal hypometabolism;[17] in SC, increased glucose metabolism has been demonstrated in bilateral striatum in two girls with SC, and contralaterally in an elderly woman with hemichorea as a residual to adolescent-onset SC.[18,19] The abnormality on PET was reversible in the girls following clinical improvement. A recent report of single photon emission computed tomographic (SPECT) scanning in 10 patients with SC demonstrated basal ganglia hyperperfusion in the 6 most acute cases; the rest were normal.[20]

The chorea in SC responds to dopaminergic blockers (pimozide may be less sedating than haloperidol)[21] or depleters,[22] but, as it tends to be self-limited, should be restricted to those in whom the chorea is so severe as to interfere with function. More recent studies showed more efficacy obtained from valproate and carbamazepine than with halperidol.[23,24] Corticosteroids, intravenous immunoglobulin, and plasmapheresis may also have a role in the treatment of SC.[11] Antibiotic therapy with penicillin to prevent cardiac dysfunction may be indicated as well.

CHOREA GRAVIDARUM

Pregnancy is another nonneurologic condition that may rarely present with chorea as chorea gravidarum (CG). It is more frequently seen in women with a prior history of SC, or the chorea may be secondary to other conditions (e.g., SLE[25]). It is far less common than when first reviewed in 1932,[26] and morbidity and maternal and fetal mortality have continued to drop with each subsequent decade.[27,28] In the original reports, approximately 60 percent of women with CG had an antecedent episode of chorea in childhood, almost certainly SC. CG may also herald HD[29] or SLE.[30] It usually resolves without sequelae following delivery. In a single report of a fatal case,[31] neuronal loss and astrocytosis in the striatum, especially the caudate, was found. Although this pathology was nonspecific for CG, it suggests that the chorea has a structural basis in some cases.

Similarly, chorea may occur with the use of estrogens. Chorea following oral contraceptive use has been reported.[32–35] An interesting report[36] describes recurrent chorea in a 61-year-old woman following the use of a topical vaginal cream that contained conjugated estrogen. She had CG when she was younger. As estrogen may affect dopamine receptor sensitivity by upregulating receptors in experimental animals, these reports suggest a role for hormone-induced chorea, especially in the setting of previously damaged basal ganglia.[9,32,37] As with CG, chorea with oral contraceptive use may be the presenting symptom of SLE.[38]

SYSTEMIC LUPUS ERYTHEMATOSUS (SLE), AND THE PRIMARY ANTIPHOSPHOLIPID ANTIBODY SYNDROME (PAPS)

Of the other systemic disorders that cause chorea, SLE is the most common, although only about 2 percent of SLE patients have chorea.[39] As with SLE in general, it tends to occur primarily in girls and women, and it occurs more commonly in those with younger onset of their SLE. Chorea may be the sole neurologic manifestation, preceding the diagnosis of SLE in nearly one-quarter of those afflicted.[40] The chorea may last from days to years; it may be episodic and recurrent. It is often unilateral, although it may be generalized. Other neurologic manifestations of SLE include stroke, transient ischemic attacks, seizures, migraine, psychosis, and dementia. Diagnosis of SLE is important because of treatment aimed at the more serious and life-threatening complications of this disease. Treatment of the chorea, as in other disorders, may occasionally require antidopaminergics. Steroids and antithrombotic agents such as aspirin and warfarin have also been found to be effective.[41]

A related disorder, primary antiphospholipid antibody syndrome (PAPS), has also been associated with chorea.[42]

These patients do not fit criteria for SLE. Clinically, PAPS is also associated with, among other things, stroke, transient cerebral ischemia, migraines, recurrent spontaneous abortions, venous thrombosis, cardiac valvular dysfunction, and thrombocytopenia.[43–47] The hallmark is the presence of antiphospholipid antibodies (aPL), consisting of false-positive VDRL, anticardiolipin antibody, and lupus anticoagulant, all of which are also associated with (and were first described in) SLE. These antibodies, both IgG and IgM, inhibit coagulation by interfering with phospholipid-dependent coagulation tests and prolong activated partial thromboplastin time in vitro, but are paradoxically associated with thrombosis rather than with bleeding.[48] As with SLE, chorea is more frequently associated with younger age of onset (under 15 in a pan-European cohort of 1000 patients), and female gender.[47]

PATHOPHYSIOLOGY: IMMUNE-MEDIATED MECHANISM?

Most interesting is the occurrence of chorea in SC, CG, SLE, PAPS, or without such associations in the presence of aPL.[49] Although thrombotic vascular occlusion is implicated in some cases,[50–52] the current theory of the pathophysiology of chorea in all these disorders is immunological; this is further supported by an MRI study of 8 patients with SLE 7 of whom had scans that were negative for lesions in the basal ganglia in the presence of chorea.[53] Many cases of chorea have now been reported with the presence of aPL in SLE,[51,54] and PAPS.[55] Interestingly, there are now also cases of SC (or rheumatic fever)[56] and CG and/or oral contraceptive use[57,58] with evidence of aPL, and others with isolated aPL[59,60] who do not meet criteria for either SLE or PAPS. There are further cases with combination of SC, SLE, and aPL with chorea.[61]

As with SC, increased striatal/cortical FDG metabolism measured with PET was found in SLE patients,[62] and, in a woman with alternating hemichorea with PAPS, evidence was found on PET for contralateral striatal hypermetabolism.[63] These findings, along with similar results in SC,[18,19] suggest that hypermetabolism in these disorders reflects an autoimmune process, with antibodies directly affecting basal ganglia neurons.[49,63] This hypothesis was first supported by the work of Husby et al.,[64] who showed that antibodies from both serum and spinal fluid from SC patients crossreacted with antigens in the cytoplasm of caudate and subthalamic nucleus neurons, and most recently confirmed by Church et al.,[65] who demonstrated the presence of antibasal ganglia antibodies in acute and persistent SC using Western immunoblotting and immunofluorescence techniques. Streptococcal antigens have also been shown to crossreact to neuronal epitopes[66,67] as well as to cardiolipin,[66] further supporting the hypothesis of crossreactive antibody-mediated inflammation or hypermetabolic dysfunction in these conditions.

Hereditary Choreas

NEUROACANTHOCYTOSES: CHOREA-ACANTHOCYTOSIS (CA) AND MCLEOD SYNDROME

Chorea-acanthocytosis (CA) is an uncommon autosomal-recessive disorder recognized since the mid-1960s; it has also been called familial amyotrophic chorea, amyotrophic chorea with acanthocytes, and Levine-Critchley syndrome.[68–74] The more general nomenclature, neuroacanthocytosis (NA), was employed as well, given the wide variety of neurological abnormalities involved, but now should be used more as an umbrella term encompassing CA and the related McLeod syndrome.[75] CA is characterized by acanthocytosis, normal beta-lipoproteins, and multiple movement disorders. Chorea is the most prominent finding, but dystonia (especially lingual action dystonia), motor and vocal tics, and parkinsonism all occur, and may occur in the same individual. Linguolabial dyskinesias may be so severe as to cause self-mutilation. An axonal sensorimotor polyneuropathy, mostly affecting the distal portion of nerves,[76] is common, along with attendant amyotrophy and, consequently, elevated creatine phosphokinase. Autonomic nervous system involvement, both sympathetic and parasympathetic, has been reported.[77] Decreased or absent reflexes, dysarthria, and dysphagia also occur. Generalized seizures occur in more than half the cases. Cognitive impairment, on the other hand, has been less commonly reported, but mild frontal lobe dysfunction probably exists in at least half of affected individuals.[78–80] Onset is usually in the twenties to thirties, and death occurs, on average, in about 9 years.[79] Some authors propose that NA is, in fact, a heterogeneous group of neurodegenerative disorders, as unusual families have been described, including an autosomal-dominant family with cortical intranuclear inclusions.[81] Further, association of some cases with the McLeod phenotype (a weak expression of Kell blood group antigens), which is X-linked, raised the issue of whether some patients with apparent CA and McLeod syndrome had the same disease.[82–84] Phenotypically, in McLeod syndrome, chorea generally occurs in the 5th decade. Facial grimacing and involuntary vocalizations may be present, but lip-biting and facial tics are uncommon, as opposed to CA. Dysphagia is notably absent.[85] Psychiatric signs and symptoms may occur.[86]

As with other disorders, recent elucidation of genetics has clarified the diagnostic dilemma. Linkage to chromosome 9q21[87] was found in CA, followed by discovery of autosomal-recessive mutations of the gene coding for a new protein, chorein.[88] McLeod syndrome, long known to be X-linked, has more recently been characterized as a disorder in which there is absence of the Kell-binding erythrocyte membrane protein Kx. Kx is encoded by the XK gene; several mutations are responsible for the phenotype.[85,86] Molecular genetic analysis, finally, now allows the two syndromes to be distinguished despite phenotypic heterogeneity.[75]

Treatment is symptomatic; the chorea may respond to reduction of dopaminergic transmission (although concomitant parkinsonism may worsen), and seizures should be treated with appropriate anticonvulsants. More recently, some patients with CA have responded successfully to treatment with deep brain stimulation (DBS) of the thalamus.[89]

Pathologically, the findings in the central nervous system are principally confined to the basal ganglia. The caudate and putamen are primarily affected, with neuronal loss and gliosis. The globus pallidus is almost as severely involved. Cortex, subthalamic nucleus, cerebellum, pons, and medulla are generally spared.[79] In cases with prominent parkinsonism, reduced neuronal density in the substantia nigra, primarily the ventrolateral region, has been reported.[90] The pathology of the peripheral nerves reveals a distal axonal neuropathy.[76,91] In a study of the neurochemical findings in the brains of patients with NA, the main abnormality was depletion of dopamine and its metabolites, particularly in the striatum; there were also increases in norepinephrine in putamen and globus pallidus, and marked reduction in substance P in striatum and substantia nigra.[92]

Functional neuroimaging with PET in patients with CA[93,94] and McLeod syndrome[86,95] has demonstrated striatal hypometabolism with FDG, similar to findings in HD.[17] Brooks et al. evaluated the presynaptic and postsynaptic dopaminergic system in CA.[96] They found ^{18}F-fluorodopa uptake to be normal in caudate and anterior putamen but significantly reduced (in the range of patients with Parkinson's disease) in the posterior putamen. Using ^{11}C-raclopride to evaluate the integrity of striatal D2 receptors, they found reduction in both caudate and putamen/cerebellum uptake ratios, reflecting a 65 percent (caudate) and 53 percent (putamen) loss of D2 receptor binding sites. Their findings indicate a loss of nigrostriatal dopaminergic projections and of D2 receptor neurons, and are consistent with a clinical picture of both chorea and parkinsonism in CA.

The erythrocyte abnormalities in CA have been a subject of scrutiny, and some feel that the red cell membrane dysfunction may hold the key to understanding the pathophysiology of this disorder. Although acanthocytes define the disorder (as well as McLeod syndrome), they are variably seen in CA, and they may be absent in an occasional patient.[91] They are also frequently seen, or can be induced, in obligate heterozygotes.[97] The red blood cells of patients with CA can be induced to form spiny or rounded projections by dilution in normal saline, in vitro aging, or contact with glass.[98] Interestingly, echinocytic transformation is completely reversible by incubation with chlorpromazine. CA erythrocytes also have abnormal membrane-bound fatty acid structures, with increases in palmitic (C16:0) and docosahexaenoic (C22:6) acids and reduction in stearic acid (C18:0).[99] Bosman et al.[100,101] have demonstrated abnormal erythrocyte band 3 structure and sulfate flux measurements, indicating anion transport activity is reduced in the erythrocytes of patients with definite CA and with likely CA but without acanthocytes. Their plasma also showed distinct antibrain immunoreactivity. Moreover, band 3 serves as a membrane substrate for tissue transglutaminase, products of which are increased in erythrocytes and muscle in CA patients.[102]

BENIGN HEREDITARY CHOREA (BHC)

Benign hereditary chorea (BHC), also called hereditary nonprogressive chorea, is another rare disorder. It is primarily symmetric and distal, with onset in childhood and little if any progression beyond adolescence, which may help differentiate it from HD.[103,104] Few other neurologic abnormalities are present, with the occasional exception of ataxia, dysarthria, pyramidal tract signs, and postural-action tremor.[105] Although cognitive processes are generally normal, intellectual impairment has been reported in one family.[106] Occasionally, the chorea has been found to be progressive.[107,108] In another sibship in which the basic disorder was compatible with a diagnosis of BHC, monocular horizontal nystagmus (beginning in infancy and remitting in childhood, along with the chorea) and peripheral cataracts were also found. It is questioned whether this is a form of BHC or another familial illness.[109] Functional neuroimaging has not been helpful in differentiating this form of chorea from others. Striatal FDG metabolism was found to be decreased in one study[110] and normal in another.[111]

The very existence of BHC as a distinct entity has been questioned even through the new millennium.[112] It is very likely that some families may, in fact, have HD, as in some of the cases with progressive chorea. One family was reported to have the expanded CAG repeat in the HD gene, suggesting that some families with so-called "benign" chorea may in fact be a phenotypic variant of HD.[113] But the finding in 2000 by de Vries et al. of linkage to chromosome 14q,[114] along with subsequent confirmation of the locus in several more autosomal-dominant families both in the US[115] and Europe,[116] has put most doubts to rest. Further analysis revealed a mutation in the TITF-1 gene, a homeodomain-containing transcription factor essential for the organogenesis of the lung, thyroid, and basal ganglia.[117]

DENTATORUBROPALLIDOLUYSIAN ATROPHY (DRPLA)

An extremely rare autosomal-dominant disorder, dentatorubropallidoluysian atrophy (DRPLA), is characterized by its distinctive pathology with extensive cell loss and gliosis in (as its name implies) the dentate nucleus, the red nucleus, the external globus pallidus, and the subthalamic nucleus.[118] DRPLA has a variable phenotypic picture, including chorea, myoclonus, epilepsy, cerebellar ataxia, and dementia, and comprising both juvenile and adult onset. Three clinical subtypes have been proposed: type I, ataxochoreoathetoid type; type II, the pseudo-Huntington type; type III, the myoclonic-epileptic type.[119] Warner et al.,[118] however, suggest that, as phenotypic variation is the rule rather than the exception in autosomal-dominantly inherited diseases (as in the hereditary ataxias and the probably mislabeled olivo-pontocerebellar atrophies[120]), the clinical subclassification is inappropriate and misleading.

The molecular genetic defect of DPRLA is, like HD, a trinucleotide repeat of CAG, with a locus on chromosome 12p, encoding the gene CTG-B37, and producing mutations in the protein named atrophin-1.[121–125] Anticipation is a feature of this disorder, as it is in HD, and accounts for the differences in juvenile and adult onsets.[121] The molecular genetics of this disorder become key information in defining syndromes, as in the case of a kindred with the so-called Haw River syndrome,[126] which underwent molecular re-evaluation; expanded DRPLA alleles were discovered in this family.[127] Since then, while initial reports of families were not uncommon in Japan, multiple North American and European families have been confirmed by genetic testing.[128–130] Molecular genetic studies suggest that cleavage of atrophin-1 into a toxic fragment,[131] possibly by caspases (as has been implicated in HD),[132] may be responsible for the pathogenesis of DPRLA.

Senile Chorea

Senile chorea is an insidiously developing generalized choreic disorder, primarily involving the limbs, occurring in individuals over 60 with normal mentation, no family history, and no other apparent etiology. It is another unusual and controversial entity, with opinion divided over whether it is a single disorder or a syndrome with multiple etiologies.[133] Few pathologic reports exist. A very early study by Alcock[134] described atrophy and cell loss in both the caudate and putamen to a lesser degree than that seen in HD, whereas a more recent case examined by Friedman and Ambler demonstrated primarily putaminal cell loss and gliosis, but with caudate sparing.[133]

Some authors have considered senile chorea to be a variant of late-onset HD, while others argue that senile chorea is a separate and distinct nosologic entity. One study by Shinotoh et al.,[135] in which they measured CAG trinucleotide repeat expansion in the HD gene in 4 patients with senile chorea, demonstrated normal repeat lengths, supporting the latter theory. On the other hand, in a prospective study by Warren et al.,[136] of 12 patients followed over a 3-year period, half were ultimately confirmed to have HD, 2 were found to have PAPS, and 1 each with hypocalcemia, tardive dyskinesia, and basal ganglia calcification. Only 1 patient remained undiagnosed after extensive evaluation, leading these authors to conclude that HD remains the most likely cause of senile chorea, even in the absence of a family history.

Vascular Chorea, Hemichorea, and Hemiballismus

Both generalized chorea and, more commonly, hemichorea and hemiballismus may occur as a result of vascular disease.

Classically, hemiballismus was described as a result of a lesion of the subthalamic nucleus.[137–139] It is now known that a variety of lesions in the basal ganglia (and in corticostriatal pathways as well) that interrupt both afferent and efferent subthalamopallidal pathways, detected both at autopsy and with modern neuroimaging, may cause persistent or paroxysmal choreic or ballistic movements, and vascular insults in many areas, including caudate, putamen, thalamus, and corona radiata, have been reported.[50,140–154] Vascular etiologies include ischemia, infarction, hemorrhage, and vascular malformations (arteriovenous malformations,[155,156] venous angiomas,[157] and cavernous angiomas[158,159]). Both hyperglycemia and hypoglycemia may produce hemichorea-hemiballism, generalized chorea, and paroxysmal chorea, presumably also on a vascular basis.[160–169] We will consider the generation of all these types of movements interchangeable. In fact, early authors, including Martin and Alcock,[138] argued that hemiballism was really just an intense, more violent, form of hemichorea, and that the ballistic movements generally were more proximal than the choreiform movements. More recent evidence shows that experimental chorea and ballism from different lesions may result in the same reduction in subthalamopallidal activity,[170,171] and may also be produced by the same lesion as well,[172,173] further supporting the notion that they result from a common neural mechanism.

Clinically, in the majority of patients with chorea or ballism of vascular etiology, the onset is abrupt. The face is usually spared. Most patients recover spontaneously within 2–4 weeks, although some do continue to have choreic movements of long duration. In the interim, if the movements interfere with function, they may respond very well to neuroleptics (low-dose haloperidol) or dopamine depleters in the short term. Nevertheless, as many of these patients may be elderly, they may be more susceptible to side-effects of these drugs such as parkinsonism and tardive dyskinesia. A safer (from the perspective of extrapyramidal adverse effects) and possibly equally effective therapeutic choice is clozapine,[174] or other newer atypical antipsychotics such as quetiapine, olanzapine,[175] and risperidone.[176] Similarly, ondansetron has also been reported to provide favorable results.[177] Unlike SC, the response to valproate in vascular hemichorea-hemiballism is variable.[178–180] In children with chorea from vascular lesions, thalamic DBS has been successful in reducing movements and improving upper extremity function.[181]

As mentioned above, neuroimaging (computed tomography [CT], and especially MRI) is particularly helpful in localizing an anatomic lesion. PET, however, has not shown specific abnormalities. In one study of hemichorea, the contralateral striatum had decreased glucose metabolism and striatal ^{18}F-fluorodopa uptake was normal.[182] Similarly, a SPECT study of 1 patient with hemichorea-hemiballism in nonketotic hyperglycemia revealed decreased perfusion.[183]

Other Neurologic and Systemic Diseases

HYPERTHYROIDISM

Chorea secondary to hyperthyroidism, an eminently treatable disorder, is rare but may affect about 2 percent of individuals with hyperthyroidism,[184] although this may be an overestimation. It may be clinically indistinguishable from the chorea of other etiologies, and may be bilateral or unilateral, persistent,[185–191] or paroxysmal.[192,193] It is generally reversible with normalization of thyroid hormone levels, but may also respond (while still in the hyperthyroid state) to dopaminergic blocking agents.[194] The pathophysiology of hyperthyroid chorea is not understood, but theories include altered function rather than altered structure of the striatum.[1] In view of the seriousness of the disease and the ease of evaluation and treatment, a thyroid screen should be checked in adults who develop chorea, including paroxysmal choreic movements, of otherwise undetermined cause.

POLYCYTHEMIA VERA

Polycythemia vera, a hematologic disorder which is more prevalent in men, can rarely be the cause of chorea; interestingly, when it occurs (in less than 1 percent of cases), it is more common in women (again, invoking a hormonal influence?) and may be the presenting sign of polycythemia in about two-thirds of patients.[195] Patients may also demonstrate facial erythrosis or splenomegaly.[196] Onset is usually after age 50 years, and the chorea is generally bilateral and symmetric. It responds to treatment with both reduction of hyperviscosity and antidopaminergics.[197–199] Pathophysiologically, the hyperviscosity may lead to reduced cerebral blood flow with resultant localized ischemia, and the results may be similar to other vascular choreas. As with hyperthyroidism, presentation of chorea in later adulthood should trigger a hematologic work-up.

METABOLIC DISORDERS

Other metabolic causes of chorea, besides hyperglycemia,[160–164,167–169] hypoglycemia,[165–167] and hyperthyroidism,[183–193] include hyponatremia,[200] hypernatremia,[201] hypocalcemia,[202] hypomagnesemia,[203] hypoparathyroidism,[204–207] hyperparathyroidism,[208] and hepatic encephalopathy (acquired hepatocerebral degeneration).[209–213] Rapid correction of hyponatremia with resultant central pontine myelinolysis has also been reported to be associated with chorea.[214,215]

MULTIPLE SCLEROSIS

Although it too is rare, movement disorders have been reported as a complication of multiple sclerosis. Paroxysmal dyskinesias may be the most common presentation, and may include choreic movements.[216] Persistent chorea (bilateral or hemichorea) and hemiballism have also been noted to be infrequent accompaniments to multiple sclerosis.[217–221] Demyelinating plaques in the basal ganglia have occasionally been seen.[217,221]

POSTPUMP CHOREA

A little-known entity outside of pediatric cardiovascular services, postpump chorea is a not infrequent accompaniment to cardiopulmonary bypass surgery with deep hypothermia for congenital heart disease in children. It was first recognized in 1960,[222] and described fully the following year by Bergouignan et al.[223] There have been a number of other reports since, with the incidence of chorea within 2 weeks of surgery varying from 1.2 percent to 18 percent, depending on the center.[224–232] Children are from a few months to 3 years old at the time of surgery. They undergo deep hypothermia and there is an association with circulatory arrest. The chorea may resolve within a few months,[227,230] or may persist (the longest follow-up of a child with irreversible chorea is >10 years).[230] Most patients with postpump chorea syndrome develop other neurological abnormalities, including seizures (postoperative, occasionally persistent), and developmental delay and cognitive deficits.[226,228,230] The persistent chorea does not respond well to most treatment modalities.[230] Most reports of CT and MRI scans have been normal or show diffuse cerebral atrophy, but a single study with FDG-PET demonstrated hypometabolism in the left frontal lobe.[230] Interestingly, a SPECT evaluation of another child showed nonspecific hypoperfusion of frontal lobe and cerebellum; this child had an unremarkable CT and MRI as well.[231] One long-term follow-up study (from 1986 to 1995)[233] demonstrated a sudden, transient increase in postoperative chorea that disappeared as treatment strategies in perioperative care were modified. Fifteen patients were followed up and were found to have pervasive deficits in memory, attention, and language; 7 of the 15 had persistent chorea.

The pathophysiology of this intriguing disorder is, not surprisingly, unknown. Hypoxic-ischemic damage and thromboembolic infarction in the basal ganglia circuitry has been proposed, especially as this is not uncommon in the setting of cardiac bypass surgery.[230] Medlock et al. concluded that the absence of structural lesions in the basal ganglia following prolonged chorea suggested a biochemical or microembolic etiology.[230] Another study by Curless et al.[232] of 3 children with postpump chorea, found that none had significant intraoperative hypoxemia or hypotension, but all 3 had hypocapnia and respiratory alkalosis during the rewarming period; they hypothesize that hypocapnia-induced cerebral vasoconstriction may contribute to ischemic damage in critical focal brain areas. In a recent neuropathologic examination of 2 patients, Kupsky et al.[234] demonstrated selective neuronal loss and gliosis of the external globus pallidus; areas of the brain usually susceptible to hypoxic-ischemic necrosis were spared. This finding correlates with the older evidence that the globus pallidus bears the brunt of the damage in children who die after cardiac surgery.[222] One other theory proposed for the mechanism of injury here is autoimmune;[230] as with the situation in rheumatic disease,[64] could there be antibodies directed against the basal ganglia in these children? In a slightly different but related story,[235] a child with congenital heart disease received a heart transplant, with deep hypothermia and circulatory arrest, at age 12. Four weeks later, she developed generalized chorea which responded dramatically to corticosteroids, which makes an autoimmune mechanism a reasonable hypothesis. It is unclear if there is a connection between this case of cardiac transplantation and the chorea developing following bypass surgery. There are no reports of specific aPL being evaluated in any of these cases, which may shed more light on the situation.

Other Causes

DRUGS, TOXINS, INFECTIONS, NEOPLASMS, DEGENERATIVE DISORDERS

A plethora of case reports exist describing the association of chorea with drugs, degenerative disorders, medical conditions, infections, and a variety of other situations. In some instances, there is only a single report to document the connection. Previous authors have compiled extensive lists.[1,236,237] Here, Table 38-1 serves to amend and to expand those before it with more recent references (those previously mentioned in text, and Refs. 238–312). (Accordingly, only those new references will be noted; all others are to be understood as referred to in the lists of Weiner and Lang,[1] Duvoisin,[236] and Shoulson.[237]) As with other conditions, treatment of the underlying disease process should be the primary goal in correcting the cause of the chorea.

Paroxysmal Dyskinesias

Paroxysmal dyskinesias are movement disorders occurring as "attacks" without loss of consciousness, with recovery between attacks. Many of the etiologic factors already discussed as the causes of choreic and/or ballistic movements can result in paroxysmal chorea as well as persistent movements. Nonepileptic causes of symptomatic paroxysmal chorea include vascular causes,[187,189] hypoglycemia,[199] hyperglycemia,[202] hyperthyroidism,[225,226] hypoparathyroidism,[238,239] multiple sclerosis,[255] direct infection with human immunodeficiency virus type 1 (HIV),[288] as well as other infections, central and peripheral trauma, kernicterus, and migraine.[282]

The original nomenclature of the two major primary forms of paroxysmal dyskinesias, paroxysmal kinesigenic choreoathetosis and paroxysmal dystonic choreoathetosis, have given way to the newer, preferred terms of paroxysmal kinesigenic dyskinesia (PKD) and paroxysmal nonkinesigenic

TABLE 38-1 Conditions Associated with Chorea and Ballism

Drugs
- Neuroleptics, dopamine receptor blockers
  - Phenothiazines (e.g., chlorpromazine)
  - Butyrophenones (e.g., haloperidol)
  - Thioxanthines (e.g., thiothixene)
  - Benzamides (e.g., metoclopramide)
- Antiparkinson agents
  - L-Dopa
  - Dopamine agonists (bromocriptine, pergolide)
  - Amantadine
  - Anticholinergics (including atropine)[238,239]
- Anticonvulsants
  - Phenytoin[240]
  - Carbamazepine
  - Phenobarbital
  - Ethosuximide
  - Valproate[241]
  - Lamotrigine[242]
  - Gabapentin[243]
- Stimulants
  - Methamphetamine,[244] other amphetamines[245]
  - Methylphenidate
  - Cocaine, crack cocaine ("crack dancing")[246]
  - Caffeine
  - Pemoline
  - Aminophylline
  - Theophylline[247]
- Steroids
  - Anabolic steroids
  - Conjugated topical estrogens[36]
  - Oral contraceptives
- Opiates
  - Methadone[248]
- Calcium-channel blockers
  - Cinnarizine
  - Flunarizine
  - Verapamil[249]
- Serotonin reuptake inhibitors
  - Fluoxetine[250]
  - Paroxetine[251]
- Other drugs
  - Alcohol (intoxication and withdrawal)
  - Amoxapine
  - Baclofen[252]
  - Cyclizine
  - Cyclosporine[253]
  - Cyproheptadine,[254] other antihistamines
  - Diazepam-pentobarbital withdrawal[255]
  - Diazoxide
  - Digoxin[256]
  - Interferon-alpha[257]
  - Isoniazid
  - Lithium[249,258,259]
  - Methyldopa
  - Pentamidine[260]
  - Ranitidine, cimetidine[261]
  - Reserpine

Continued

TABLE 38-1—*(continued)*

Triazolam
Tricyclic antidepressants[262]

Hereditary/Degenerative Disorders
Alzheimer's disease[263]
Amino acid disorders (glutaric acidemia/aciduria type I,[264] propionic acidemia,[265] cystinuria, homocystinuria, phenylketonuria, Hartnup disease, argininosuccinic aciduria, ornithine carbamoyltransferase deficiency[266])
Ataxia telangiectasia[267]
Benign hereditary chorea[104,108,111]
Carbohydrate metabolism (galactosemia, mucopolysacchari-doses, mucolipidoses, pyruvate dehydrogenase deficiency)
Dentatorubropallidoluysian atrophy[118,121–130]
Familial striatal necrosis
Friedreich's ataxia[268,269]
Gilles de la Tourette syndrome
Hallervorden-Spatz
Hereditary spinocerebellar ataxias (SCA), including Machado-Joseph disease and SCA type 1[270])
Huntington's disease
Idiopathic basal ganglia calcinosis (Fahr's disease)[271]
Leigh's disease
Lesch-Nyhan syndrome
Lipidoses (GM1 and GM2 gangliosidosis, sphingolipidosis, Gaucher's disease, globoid cell leukodystrophy, metachromatic leukodystrophy, ceroid lipofuscinosis)
Mitochondrial encephalomyopathy[272,273]
Multiple system atrophy[274]
Myoclonus epilepsy
Neuroacanthocytoses (chorea-acanthocytosis, McLeod syndrome)[80–102]
Paroxysmal dyskinesias (PKO,PNKO)
Pelizaeus-Merzbacher disease
Pick's disease
Progressive supranuclear palsy[275]
Progressive systemic sclerosis[276]
Sea-blue histiocytosis
Sturge-Weber syndrome
Sulfite oxidase deficiency
Tuberous sclerosis[277]
Wilson's disease
Xeroderma pigmentosum

Autoimmune/Collagen Vascular
Systemic lupus erythematosus[43,62]
Primary antiphospholipid syndrome[43–47,63]
Rheumatoid arthritis
Behçet's disease[278]
Henoch-Schonlein syndrome
Periarteritis nodosa
Churg-Straus syndrome[279]
Hashimoto's thyroiditis[280]

Autoimmune Parainfectious
Sydenham's chorea (post-streptococcal)[6,7,11–16,18–24]
Other infections (pertussis, varicella, diphtheria)
Serum sickness reaction to tetanus toxoid

Infectious Disease, including Prion-Related
Scarlet fever (streptococcal)
Bacterial endocarditis
Typhoid fever
Legionnaire's disease
Lyme disease
Neurosyphilis,[281] meningovascular syphilis[282]
Mycoplasma pneumoniae encephalitis[283]
Encephalitis lethargica (Von Economo's encephalitis)
Viral meningoencephalitis[284] (mumps, measles, varicella, influenza)
Postvaccinial
Infectious mononucleosis
Herpes simplex encephalitis relapse[285,286]
Creutzfeld-Jakob disease[262]
Subacute sclerosing panencephalitis
Cysticercosis[287]

Human immunodeficiency virus (HIV)-related
HIV-1[288–290]
Cryptococcal granuloma[291]
Toxoplasmosis[289,292–294]
Cytomegalovirus encephalitis[282]
Progressive multifocal leukoencephalopathy[289]

Other Systemic
Acute intemittent porphyria
Polycythemia vera[197–199]
Sarcoidosis
Sickle cell anemia
Transitional myeloproliferative disease

Metabolic
Hypoglycemia,[165,167] and hyperglycemia[161–164,167–169]
Hyponatremia, and hypernatremia (and central pontine myelinolysis[214,215])
Hypocalcemia
Hypomagnesemia
Hepatic failure, acquired hepatocerebral degeneration[213]
Renal failure

Endocrine
Hyperthyroidism[187–191,193]
Hypoparathyroidism,[206] pseudohypoparathyroidism, and hyperparathyroidism
Chorea gravidarum
Addison's disease

Nutritional
Beriberi (thiamine deficiency)
Wernicke's encephalopathy[295]
Pellagra (niacin deficiency)
B_{12} deficiency[296]

Toxins
Carbon monoxide[297]
Manganese[298]
Mercury
Organophosphate poisoning[299]
Thallium
Toluene (glue-sniffing)

Continued

TABLE 38-1—*(continued)*

Neoplastic
  Primary brain tumor
  Metastatic brain tumor
  Primary CNS lymphoma[300,301]
  Acute lymphoblastic leukemia (with lupus anticoagulant)[302]
  Paraneoplastic[303,304]

Cerebrovascular
  Basal ganglia, subcortical infarcts[147–149,152,164]
  Basal ganglia, subcortical ischemia[151] (including secondary to hypotension[305])
  Basal ganglia, thalamic hemorrhage[146,150]
  Epidural hematoma
  Subdural hematoma
  Moyamoya disease[306–308]
  Vascular malformations (arteriovenous malformations,[155,156] venous angioma,[157] cavernous angioma[158,159])

Other Neurologic and Miscellaneous Disorders
  Head trauma
  Peripheral trauma[282]
  Cervical disc prolapse/spinal cord compression[309]
  Migraine[281]
  Multiple sclerosis[216,221,310]
  Orobuccolingual dyskinesias of aging
  Post-status epilepticus[311]
  Senile chorea[133,135,136]
  Cerebral palsy
  Infantile chorea in bronchopulmonary dysplasia[312]
  Kernicterus[282]
  Physiological chorea of infancy
  Postpump chorea[225–235]

New additions or updated references only are noted. More than one category may apply to a single condition (e.g., Autoimmune and Endocrine for chorea gravidarum, Autoimmune and Neoplastic for acute lymphoblastic leukemia with antiphospholipid antibodies), and some are just difficult to classify (e.g., postpump chorea), but each item will only be listed once.
SOURCE: *Adapted from Weiner and Lang,[1] Duvoisin,[202] and Shoulson.[203]*

dyskinesia (PNKD),[313] as the movements may not necessarily be choreoathetotic; in fact, they may be primarily dystonic syndromes, but will be described briefly here nonetheless. Other types of paroxysmal dyskinesias include an intermediate form between PKD and PNKD,[1] the rare paroxysmal exercise-induced dyskinesia (PED), and paroxysmal nocturnal dyskinesia (PND).

PKD is precipitated by sudden movements, particularly after coming from a rest position, and by focal movements, stress, excitement, or hyperventilation. Abnormal involuntary movements may span the spectrum of dystonic to choreic to ballistic, but dystonic movements probably predominate; they may be bilateral or unilateral. They usually begin in youth and diminish with age. Attacks may be frequent (100/day) or rare (2/year). Consciousness is spared. The attacks usually do not last longer than 2 minutes, and never more than 5 minutes. There is often a prodromal sensation of tightness or tingling, and may warn the individual to allow avoidance of the attacks. Although the EEG is normal, patients respond well to low doses of carbamazepine or other anticonvulsants.[1,314,315]

PNKD has similarities to PKD, but differs in that onset is younger (infancy), and duration of the attacks is longer (up to hours). The movements are mostly dystonic, but may be choreic as well. They also differ in precipitating events: in PNKD, it is alcohol and caffeine, as well as sometimes fatigue, stress, or excitement. Frequency is also less than in PKD. Treatment also differs. Anticonvulsants do not usually help, but there is one report of a child improving with gabapentin.[316] In PNKD, benzodiazepines are the treatment of choice. Also reportedly effective are acetazolamide and low-dose haloperidol,[1] as well as anticholinergics for more dystonic features of PNKD.

Most recently, genetic linkage has been found for both PKD and PNKD. PKD is associated in some families with benign familial infantile convulsions (BFIC) in a syndrome termed ICCA, and linkage has been found on the centromeric region of chromosome 16 (16p12-q12).[317,318] This locus is also responsible for the occurrence of familial PKD without BFIC.[319] PNKD has been linked in several families to 2q31-36.[320] The pathophysiology of these disorders has been identified as channelopathies, with linkage in the region of ion channel genes for both PKD and PNKD.[314] A mouse model for paroxysmal dyskinesias has recently been described.[321] The lethargic mouse mutant, which carries a mutation in the CCHB4 gene, encoding the beta4-subunit of voltage-regulated calcium channels, has been shown to have transient attacks of severe dyskinetic behavior, often triggered by environmental or chemical influences. This model provides further evidence for channelopathies producing paroxysmal dyskinesias.[321]

PED is characterized as episodes of dystonia, particularly of the feet, induced by continuous exercise (e.g., walking or running). The pathophysiology of PED is unknown and antiepileptic drugs are generally unhelpful.[314] PND is now considered a form of frontal lobe epilepsy and is linked to mutations of the neuronal nicotinic acetylcholine receptor genes on chromosomes 20 and 15.[314]

Painful Legs and Moving Toes

Although not a true choreic disorder, we will include the uncommon entity painful legs and moving toes in this chapter. First described in 1971,[322] this condition appears to be a peripherally-derived movement disorder. The syndrome consists of pain in the affected limb associated with spontaneous, involuntary, wriggling movements of the toes. The movements may be bilateral or unilateral, continuous or intermittent, occasionally stopping completely for minutes.[322–327] Rarely, the upper limbs may be involved instead of the legs and toes (painful arms and moving fingers),[328,329] or even in addition to the lower limbs.[330] The disability here is largely from the pain, and rarely from the digit movements. Unfortunately, all treatment modalities, both for hyperkinetic movements and for pain, have been fruitless, with the occasional exception of sympathetic block. There have been occasional recent reports of success in treating both the pain and the movements with lumbar epidural block with mepivacaine[331] and epidural spinal cord stimulation.[332]

Painful legs and moving toes frequently occurs in individuals with a history of lumbosacral disease, including spinal nerve root injury, peripheral trauma, or peripheral neuropathy (including HIV-related axonal neuropathy[333,334]), suggesting a peripheral origin for the disorder, but with postulated central nervous system alterations in segmental motor pathways.[335] The severe and unrelenting pain makes the diagnosis clear, despite the disorder's rarity. There also exists a variant, painless legs and moving toes, in which the characteristics of the movements are the same, but pain is absent.[335,336] In these patients, the digit movements may be bothersome, and partial relief may be had with injection of botulinum toxin into the toe extensor and flexor muscles (author's personal observations).

Conclusions

Chorea is a rare manifestation of some very common diseases (vascular disease, hyperthyroidism) as well as a common finding in very rare disorders (chorea-acanthocytosis, DRPLA, benign hereditary chorea). Choreiform movements should alert the physician that any one of a legion of conditions may be responsible, and a thorough physical examination with appropriate laboratory tests are in order. The pathophysiology of chorea is still not understood, but both animal studies and careful observation of clinical phenomena are bringing us closer to elucidating the elusive puzzle of the choreas.

References

1. Weiner WJ, Lang AE: *Movement disorders: A Comprehensive Survey.* Mount Kisco, NY: Futura, 1989.
2. Sydenham T: *The Entire Works of Thomas Sydenham.* London: Sydenham Society, 1848–1850.
3. Nausieda PA, Grossman BJ, Koller WC, et al: Sydenham's chorea: An update. *Neurology* 30:331–334, 1980.
4. Karademir S, Demirceken F, Atalay S, et al: Acute rheumatic fever in children in the Ankara area in 1990–1992 and comparison with a previous study in 1980–1989. *Acta Paediatr* 83:862–865, 1994.
5. Figueroa F, Berríos X, Gutiérrez M, et al: Anticardiolipin antibodies in acute rheumatic fever. *J Rheumatol* 19:1175–1180, 1992.
6. Swedo SE, Leonard HL, Schapiro MB, et al: Sydenham's chorea: Physical and psychological symptoms of St Vitus dance. *Pediatrics* 91:706–713, 1993.
7. Swedo SE, Leonard HL: Childhood movement disorders and obsessive compulsive disorder. *J Clin Psychiatry* 55(suppl): 32–37, 1994.
8. Bird MT, Palkes H, Prensky AL: A follow up study of Sydenham's chorea. *Neurology* 26:601–606, 1976.
9. Schipper HM: Sex hormones in stroke, chorea, and anticonvulsant therapy. *Sem Neurol* 8:181–186, 1988.
10. Ch'ien LT, Economides AN, Lemmi H: Sydenham's chorea and seizures: Clinical and electroencephalographic studies. *Arch Neurol* 35:382–385, 1978.
11. Swedo SE: Sydenham's chorea: A model for childhood autoimmune neuropsychiatric disorders. *JAMA* 272:1788–1791, 1994.
12. Kienzle GD, Breger RK, Chun RW, et al: Sydenham chorea: MR manifestations in two cases. *Am J Neuroradiol* 12:73–76, 1991.
13. Traill Z, Pike M, Byrne J: Sydenham's chorea: A case showing reversible striatal abnormalities on CT and MRI. *Dev Med Child Neurol* 37:270–273, 1995.
14. Emery ES, Vieco PT: Sydenham chorea: Magnetic resonance imaging reveals permanent basal ganglia injury. *Neurology* 48:531–533, 1997.
15. Ryan MM, Antony JH: Cerebral vasculitis in a case of Sydenham's chorea. *J Child Neurol* 14:815–818, 1999.
16. Giedd JN, Rapoport JL, Kruesi MJP, et al: Sydenham's chorea: Magnetic resonance imaging of the basal ganglia. *Neurology* 45:2199–2202, 1995.
17. Grafton ST, Mazziotta JC, Pahl JJ, et al: Serial changes of cerebral glucose metabolism and caudate size in persons at risk for Huntington's disease. *Arch Neurol* 49:1161–1167, 1992.
18. Goldman S, Amrom D, Szliwowski HB, et al: Reversible striatal hypermetabolism in a case of Sydenham's chorea. *Mov Disord* 8:355–358, 1993.
19. Weindl A, Kuwert T, Leenders KL, et al: Increased striatal glucose consumption in Sydenham's chorea. *Mov Disord* 8:437–444, 1993.
20. Barsottini OG, Ferraz HB, Seviliano MM, Barbieri A: Brain SPECT imaging in Sydenham's chorea. *Braz J Med Biol Res* 35: 431–436, 2002.
21. Shannon KM, Fenichel GM: Pimozide treatment of Sydenham's chorea. *Neurology* 40:186, 1990.
22. Jankovic J, Orman J: Tetrabenazine therapy of dystonia, chorea, tics, and other dyskinesias. *Neurology* 38:391–394, 1988.
23. Pena J, Mora E, Cardozo J, et al: Comparison of the efficacy of carbamazepine, haloperidol and valproic acid in the treatment of children with Sydenham's chorea: Clinical follow-up of 18 patients. *Arq Neuropsiquiatr* 60:374–377, 2002.
24. Genel F, Arslanoglu S, Uran N, Saylan B: Sydenham's chorea: Clinical findings and comparison of the efficacies of sodium valproate and carbamazepine regimens. *Brain Dev* 24:73–76, 2002.
25. Wolf RE, McBeath JG: Chorea gravidarum in systemic lupus erythematosus. *J Rheumatol* 12:992–993, 1985.
26. Willson P, Preece AA: Chorea gravidarum: A statistical study of 951 collected cases, 846 from the literature and 105 previously unreported. *Arch Intern Med* 49:471–533, 1932.
27. Beresford OD, Graham AM: Chorea gravidarum. *J Obstet Gynaecol Br Emp* 57:616–625, 1950.
28. Lewis BV, Parsons M: Chorea gravidarum. *Lancet* i:284–288, 1966.
29. Bolt JM: Abortion and Huntington's chorea. *Br Med J* 1:840, 1968.
30. Donaldson IM, Espiner EA: Disseminated lupus erythematosus presenting as chorea gravidarum. *Arch Neurol* 25:240–244, 1971.

31. Ishikawa K, Kim RC, Givelber H, Collins GH: Chorea gravidarum. Report of a fatal case with neuropathological observations. *Arch Neurol* 37:429–432, 1980.

32. Nausieda PA, Koller WC, Weiner WJ, Klawans HL: Chorea induced by oral contraceptives. *Neurology* 29:1605–1609, 1979.

33. Galimberti D: Chorea induced by the use of oral contraceptives. Report of a case and review of the literature. *Ital J Neurol Sci* 8:383–386, 1987.

34. Leys D, Destee A, Petit H, Warot P: Chorea associated with oral contraception. *J Neurol* 235:46–48, 1987.

35. Driesen JJ, Wolters EC: Oral contraceptive induced paraballism. *Clin Neurol Neurosurg* 89:49–51, 1987.

36. Caviness JN, Muenter MD: An unusual cause of recurrent chorea. *Mov Disord* 6:355–357, 1991.

37. Hruska RE, Silbergeld EK: Increased dopamine receptor sensitivity after estrogen treatment using the rat rotation model. *Science* 208:1466–1468, 1980.

38. Iskander MK, Khan M: Chorea as the initial presentation of oral contraceptive related systemic lupus erythematosus. *J Rheumatol* 16:850–851, 1989.

39. Gibson T, Myers AR: Nervous system involvement in systemic lupus erythematosus. *Ann Rheum Dis* 35:398–406, 1976.

40. Bruyn GW, Padberg G: Chorea and systemic lupus erythematosus. *Eur Neurol* 23:278–290, 1984.

41. Feigin A, Kieburtz K, Shoulson I: Treatment of Huntington's disease and other choreic disorders, in Kurlan R (ed): *Treatment of Movement Disorders*. Philadelphia: Lippincott, 1995, pp 337–364.

42. Hughes GRV: Thrombosis, abortion, cerebral disease and the lupus anticoagulant. *Br Med J* 287:1088–1089, 1983.

43. Asherson RA, Khamashta MA, Gil A, et al: Cerebrovascular disease and antiphospholipid antibodies in systemic lupus erythematosus, lupus-like disease, and the primary antiphospholipid syndrome. *Am J Med* 86:391–399, 1989.

44. Asherson RA, Khamashta MA, Ordi-Ros J, et al: The "primary" antiphospholipid syndrome: Major clinical and serological features. *Medicine* 68:366–374, 1989.

45. Levine SR, Welch KM: The spectrum of neurologic disease associated with antiphospholipid antibodies. Lupus anticoagulants and anticardiolipin antibodies. *Arch Neurol* 44:876–883, 1987.

46. Levine SR, Deegan MJ, Futrell N, Welch KMA: Cerebrovascular and neurologic disease associated with antiphospholipid antibodies: 48 cases. *Neurology* 40:1181–1189, 1990.

47. Cervera R, Piette JC, Font J, et al: Antiphospholipid syndrome: Clinical and immunologic manifestations and patterns of disease expression in a cohort of 1,000 patients. *Arthritis Rheum* 46:1019–1027, 2002.

48. Boey ML, Colaco CB, Gharavi AE, et al: Thrombosis in SLE: Striking association with the presence of circulating "lupus" anticoagulant. *Br Med J* 287:1021–1023, 1983.

49. Bouchez B, Arnott G, Hatron PY, et al: Chorée et lupus erythemateux disséminé avec anticoagulant circulant. Trois cas. *Rev Neurol* 141:571–577, 1985.

50. Kirk A, Harding SR: Cardioembolic caudate infarction as a cause of hemichorea in lupus anticoagulant syndrome. *Can J Neurol Sci* 20:162–164, 1993.

51. Asherson RA, Derksen RH, Harris EN, et al: Chorea in systemic lupus erythematosus and "lupus-like" disease: Association with antiphospholipid antibodies. *Semin Arthritis Rheum* 16:253–259, 1987.

52. Kashihara K, Nakashima S, Kohira I, et al: Hyperintense basal ganglia on T1-weighted MR images in a patient with central nervous system lupus and chorea. *Am J Neuroradiol* 19:284–286, 1998.

53. Galanaud D, Dormont D, Marsault C, et al: Brain MRI in patients with past lupus-associated chorea. *Stroke* 31:3080–3081, 2000.

54. Khamashta MA, Gil A, Anciones B, et al: Chorea in systemic lupus erythematosus: Association with antiphospholipid antibodies. *Ann Rheum Dis* 47:681–683, 1988.

55. Vlachoyiannopoulos PG, Dimou G, Siamopoulou-Mavridou A: Chorea as a manifestation of the antiphospholipid syndrome in childhood. *Clin Exp Rheumatol* 9:303–305, 1991.

56. de la Fuente Fernandez R: Rheumatic chorea and lupus anticoagulant. *J Neurol Neurosurg Psychiatry* 57:1545, 1994.

57. Lubbe WF, Walker EB: Chorea gravidarum associated with circulating lupus anticoagulant: Successful outcome of pregnancy with prednisone and aspirin therapy. Case report. *Br J Obstet Gynaecol* 90:487–490, 1983.

58. Omdal R, Roalso S: Chorea gravidarum and chorea associated with oral contraceptives: Diseases due to antiphospholipid antibodies? *Acta Neurol Scand* 86:219–220, 1992.

59. Okseter K, Sirnes K: Chorea and lupus anticoagulant: A case report. *Acta Neurol Scand* 78:206–209, 1988.

60. Shimomura T, Takahashi S, Takahashi S: Chorea associated with antiphospholipid antibodies. *Clin Neurol* 32:989–993, 1992.

61. Besbas N, Damarguc I, Ozen S, et al: Association of antiphospholipid antibodies with systemic lupus erythematosus in a child presenting with chorea: A case report. *Eur J Pediatr* 153:891–893, 1994.

62. Guttman M, Lang AE, Garnett ES, et al: Regional cerebral glucose metabolism in SLE chorea: Further evidence that striatal hypometabolism is not a correlate of chorea. *Mov Disord* 2:201–210, 1987.

63. Furie R, Ishikawa T, Dhawan V, Eidelberg D: Alternating hemichorea in primary antiphospholipid syndrome: Evidence for contralateral striatal hypermetabolism. *Neurology* 44:2197–2199, 1994.

64. Husby G, van de Rijn I, Zabriskie JB, et al: Antibodies reacting with cytoplasm of subthalamic and caudate nuclei neurons in chorea and acute rheumatic fever. *J Exp Med* 144:1094–1110, 1976.

65. Church AJ, Cardoso F, Dale RC, et al: Anti-basal ganglia antibodies in acute and persistent Sydenham's chorea. *Neurology* 59:227–231, 2002.

66. Cunningham MW, Swerlick RA: Polyspecificity of antistreptococcal murine monoclonal antibodies and their implications in autoimmunity. *J Exp Med* 164:998–1012, 1986.

67. Bronze MS, Dale JB: Epitopes of streptococcal M proteins that evoke antibodies that cross-react with human brain. *J Immunol* 151:2820–2828, 1993.

68. Levine IM, Estes JW, Looney JM: Hereditary neurological disease with acanthocytosis. *Arch Neurol* 19:403–409, 1968.

69. Critchley EMR, Clark DB, Wikler A: Acanthocytosis and neurological disorder without abetalipoproteinemia. *Arch Neurol* 18:134–140, 1968.

70. Kito S, Itoga E, Hiroshige Y, et al: A pedigree of amyotrophic chorea with acanthocytosis. *Arch Neurol* 37:514–517, 1980.

71. Sakai T, Mawatari S, Iwashita H, et al: Choreoacanthocytosis. Clues to clinical diagnosis. *Arch Neurol* 38:335–338, 1981.

72. Sotaniemi KA: Chorea-acanthocytosis. Neurological disease with acanthocytosis. *Acta Neurol Scand* 68:53–56, 1983.

73. Sakai T, Iwashita H, Goto I, Kakugawa M: Neuroacanthocytosis syndrome and choreoacanthocytosis (Levine-Critchley syndrome). *Neurology* 35:1679, 1985.

74. Hardie RJ: Acanthocytosis and neurological impairment: A review. *Q J Med* 71:291–306, 1989.

75. Danek A: Progress in molecular chorea diagnosis. McLeod syndrome and chorea acanthocytosis. *Nervenarzt* 73:564–569, 2002.

76. Vita G, Serra S, Dattola R, et al: Peripheral neuropathy in amyotrophic chorea-acanthocytosis. *Ann Neurol* 26:583–587, 1989.

77. Kihara M, Nakashima H, Taki M, et al: A case of chorea-acanthocytosis with dysautonomia: Quantitative autonomic deficits using CASS. *Autonom Neurosci Basic Clin* 97:42–44, 2002.

78. Delecluse F, Deleval J, Gérard J-M, et al: Frontal impairment and hypoperfusion in neuroacanthocytosis. *Arch Neurol* 48:232–234, 1991.

79. Rinne JO, Daniel SE, Scaravilli F, et al: The neuropathological features of neuroacanthocytosis. *Mov Disord* 9:297–304, 1994.

80. Hardie RJ, Pullon HWH, Harding AE, et al: Neuroacanthocytosis: A clinical, haematological and pathological study of 19 cases. *Brain* 114:13–49, 1991.

81. Walker RH, Morgello S, Davidoff-Feldman B, et al: Autosomal dominant chorea-acanthocytosis with polyglutamine-containing neuronal inclusions. *Neurology* 58:1031–1037, 2002.

82. Witt TN, Danek A, Reiter M, et al: McLeod syndrome: A distinct form of neuroacanthocytosis. Report of 2 cases and literature review with emphasis on neuromuscular manifestations. *J Neurol* 239:302–306, 1992.

83. Takashima H, Sakai T, Iwashita H, et al: A family of McLeod syndrome, masquerading as chorea-acanthocytosis. *J Neurol Sci* 124:56–60, 1994.

84. Malandrini A, Fabrizi GM, Truschi F, et al: Atypical McLeod syndrome manifested as X-linked chorea-acanthocytosis, neuromyopathy and dilated cardiomyopathy: Report of a family. *J Neurol Sci* 124:89–94, 1994.

85. Danek A, Tison F, Rubio J, et al: The chorea of McLeod syndrome. *Mov Disord* 16:882–889, 2001.

86. Jung HH, Hergersberg M, Kneifel S, et al: McLeod syndrome: A novel mutation, predominant psychiatric manifestations, and distinct striatal imaging findings. *Ann Neurol* 49:384–392, 2001.

87. Rubio JP, Danek A, Stone C, et al: Chorea-acanthocytosis: Genetic linkage to chromosome 9q21. *Am J Hum Genet* 61:899–908, 1997.

88. Ueno S, Maruki Y, Nakamura M, et al: The gene encoding a newly discovered protein, chorein, is mutated in chorea-acanthocytosis. *Nat Genet* 28:121–122, 2001.

89. Burbaud P, Vital A, Rougier A, et al: Minimal tissue damage after stimulation of the motor thalamus in a case of chorea-acanthocytosis. *Neurology* 59:1982–1984, 2002.

90. Rinne JO, Daniel SE, Scaravilli F et al: Nigral degeneration in neuroacanthocytosis. *Neurology* 44:1629–1632, 1994.

91. Malandrini A, Fabrizi GM, Palmeri S, et al: Choreo-acanthocytosis-like phenotype without acanthocytes: Clinicopathological case report. A contribution to the knowledge of the functional pathology of the caudate nucleus. *Acta Neuropathol* 86:651–658, 1993.

92. de Yebenes JG, Brin MF, Mena MA, et al: Neurochemical findings in neuroacanthocytosis. *Mov Disord* 3:300–312, 1988.

93. Dubinsky RM, Hallett M, Levey R, Di Chiro G: Regional brain glucose metabolism in neuroacanthocytosis. *Neurology* 39:1253–1255, 1989.

94. Hosokawa S, Ichiya Y, Kuwabara Y, et al: Positron emission tomography in cases of chorea with different underlying diseases. *J Neurol Neurosurg Psychiatry* 50:1284–1287, 1987.

95. Oechsner M, Buchert R, Beyer W, Danek A: Reduction of striatal glucose metabolism in McLeod choreoacanthocytosis. *J Neurol Neurosurg Psychiatry* 70:517–520, 2001.

96. Brooks DJ, Ibanez V, Playford ED, et al: Presynaptic and postsynaptic striatal dopaminergic function in neuroacanthocytosis: A positron emission tomographic study. *Ann Neurol* 30:166–171, 1991.

97. Brin MF, Bressman SB, Fahn S, et al: Chorea-acanthocytosis: Clinical and laboratory features in five cases (abstract). *Neurology* 35(suppl 1):110, 1985.

98. Feinberg TE, Cianci CD, Morrow JS, et al: Diagnostic tests for choreoacanthocytosis. *Neurology* 41:1000–1006, 1991.

99. Sakai T, Antoku Y, Iwashita H, et al: Chorea-acanthocytosis: Abnormal composition of covalently bound fatty acids of erythrocyte membrane proteins. *Ann Neurol* 29:664–669, 1991.

100. Kay MM, Goodman J, Lawrence C, Bosman G: Membrane channel protein abnormalities and autoantibodies in neurological disease. *Brain Res Bull* 24:105–111, 1990.

101. Bosman GJ, Bartholmeus IG, De Grip WJ, Horstink MW: Erythrocyte anion transporter and antibrain immunoreactivity in chorea-acanthocytosis. A contribution to etiology, genetics, and diagnosis. *Brain Res Bull* 33:523–528, 1994.

102. Melone MA, Di Fede G, Peluso G, et al: Abnormal accumulation of tTGase products in muscle and erythrocytes of chorea-acanthocytosis patients. *J Neuropathol Exp Neurol* 61:841–848, 2002.

103. Haerer AF, Currier RD, Jackson JF: Hereditary nonprogressive chorea of early onset. *N Engl J Med* 276:1220–1224, 1967.

104. Wheeler PG, Weaver DD, Dobyns WB: Benign hereditary chorea. *Pediatr Neurol* 9:337–340, 1993.

105. Pincus JH, Chutorian A: Familial benign chorea with intention tremor: A clinical entity. *J Pediatr* 70:724–729, 1967.

106. Leli DA, Furlow TW, Falgout JC: Benign familial chorea: An association with intellectual impairment. *J Neurol Neurosurg Psychiatry* 47:471–474, 1984.

107. Behan PO, Bone I: Hereditary chorea without dementia. *J Neurol Neurosurg Psychiatry* 40:687–691, 1977.

108. Schady W, Meara RJ: Hereditary progressive chorea without dementia. *J Neurol Neurosurg Psychiatry* 51:295–297, 1988.

109. Wheeler PG, Dobyns WB, Plager DA, Ellis FD: Familial remitting chorea, nystagmus, cataracts. *Am J Med Genetics* 47:1215–1217, 1993.

110. Suchowersky O, Hayden MR, Martin WRW, et al: Cerebral metabolism of glucose in benign hereditary chorea. *Mov Disord* 1:33–45, 1986.

111. Kuwert T, Lange HW, Langen KJ, et al: Normal striatal glucose consumption in two patients with benign hereditary chorea as measured by positron emission tomography. *J Neurol* 237:80–84, 1990.

112. Schrag A, Quinn NP, Bhatia KP, Marsden CD: Benign hereditary chorea: Entity or syndrome? *Mov Disord* 15:280–288, 2000.

113. MacMillan JC, Morrison PJ, Nevin NC, et al: Identification of an expanded CAG repeat in the Huntington's disease gene (*IT15*) in a family reported to have benign hereditary chorea. *J Med Genet* 30:1012–1013, 1993.

114. de Vries BB, Arts WF, Breedveld GJ, et al: Benign hereditary chorea of early onset maps to chromosome 14q. *Am J Hum Genet* 66:136–142, 2000.

115. Fernandez M, Raskind W, Matsushita M, et al: Hereditary benign chorea: Clinical and genetic features of a distinct disease. *Neurology* 57:106–110, 2002.

116. Breedveld GJ, Percy AK, MacDonald ME, et al: Clinical and genetic heterogeneity in benign hereditary chorea. *Neurology* 59:579–584, 2002.

117. Breedveld GJ, van Dongen JW, Danesino C, et al: Mutations in TITF-1 are associated with benign hereditary chorea. *Hum Mol Genet* 11:971–979, 2002.

118. Warner TT, Lennox GG, Janota I, Harding AE: Autosomal-dominant dentatorubropallidoluysian atrophy in the United Kingdom. *Mov Disord* 9:289–296, 1994.

119. Iizuka R, Hirayama K, Machara K: Dentato-rubro-pallido-luysian atrophy. A clinico-pathological study. *J Neurol Neurosurg Psychiatry* 47:1288–1298, 1984.

120. Mark MH, Sage JI: Olivopontocerebellar atrophy, in Stern MB, Koller WC (eds): *Parkinsonian Syndromes*. New York: Marcel Dekker, 1993, pp 43–67.

121. Potter NT, Meyer MA, Zimmerman AW, et al: Molecular and clinical findings in a family with dentatorubral-pallidoluysian atrophy. *Ann Neurol* 37:273–277, 1995.

122. Koide R, Ikeuchi T, Onodera O, et al: Unstable expansion of CAG repeat in hereditary dentatorubral-pallidoluysian atrophy (DRPLA). *Nat Genet* 6:9–13, 1994.

123. Nagafuchi S, Yanagisawa H, Sato K, et al: Dentatorubral and pallidoluysian atrophy expansion of an unstable CAG trinucleotide on chromosome 12p. *Nat Genet* 6:14–18, 1994.

124. Nagafuchi S, Yanagisawa H, Ohsaki E, et al: Structure and expression of the gene responsible for the triplet repeat disorder, dentatorubral and pallidoluysian atrophy (DRPLA). *Nat Genet* 8:177–182, 1994.

125. Margolis RL, Li SH, Young WS, et al: DRPLA gene (atrophin-1) sequence and mRNA expression in human brain. *Mol Brain Res* 36:219–226, 1996.

126. Farmer TW, Wingfield MS, Lynch SA, et al: Ataxia, chorea, seizures, and dementia. Pathologic features of a newly defined familial disorder. *Arch Neurol* 46:774–779, 1989.

127. Burke JR, Wingfield MS, Lewis KE, et al: The Haw River syndrome: Dentatorubropallidoluysian atrophy (DRPLA) in an African-American family. *Nat Genet* 7:521–524, 1994.

128. Munoz E, Mila M, Sanchez A, et al: Dentatorubropallidoluysian atrophy in a Spanish family: A clinical, radiological, pathological, and genetic study. *J Neurol Neurosurg Psychiatry* 67:811–814, 1999.

129. Becher MW, Rubinsztein DC, Leggo J, et al: Dentatorubral and pallidoluysian atrophy (DRPLA). Clinical and neuropathological findings in genetically confirmed North American and European pedigrees. *Mov Disord* 12:519–530, 1997.

130. Nielesen JE, Sorensen SA, Hasholt L, Norremolle A: Dentatorubral-pallidoluysian atrophy. Clinical features of a five-generation Danish family. *Mov Disord* 11:533–541, 1996.

131. Schilling G, Wood JD, Duan K, et al: Nuclear accumulation of truncated atrophin-1 fragments in a transgenic mouse model of DRPLA. *Neuron* 24:275–286, 1999.

132. Ellerby LM, Andrusiak RL, Wellington CI, et al: Cleavage of atrophin-1 at caspase site aspartic acid 109 modulates cytotoxicity. *J Biol Chem* 274:8730–8736, 1999.

133. Friedman JH, Ambler M: A case of senile chorea. *Mov Disord* 5:251–253, 1990.

134. Alcock NS: A note on the pathology of senile chorea (nonhereditary). *Brain* 59:376–387, 1936.

135. Shinotoh H, Calne DB, Snow B, et al: Normal CAG repeat length in the Huntington's disease gene in senile chorea. *Neurology* 44:2183–2184, 1994.

136. Warren JD, Firgaira F, Thompson EM, et al: The causes of sporadic and 'senile' chorea. *Aust N Z J Med* 28:429–431, 1998.

137. Jakob A: *Die extrapyramidalen Enkrankungen*. Berlin: Springer, 1923.

138. Martin JP, Alcock NS: Hemichorea associated with a lesion of the corpus luysii. *Brain* 504–516, 1934.

139. Melamed E, Korn-Lubetzki I, Reches A, Siew F: Hemiballismus: Detection of focal hemorrhage in subthalamic nucleus by CT scan. *Ann Neurol* 4:582, 1978.

140. Martin JP: Hemichorea (hemiballismus) without lesions in the corpus luysii. *Brain* 80:1–10, 1957.

141. Kase CS, Maulsby GO, deJuan E, Mohr JP: Hemichorea-hemiballism and lacunar infarction of the basal ganglia. *Neurology* 31:452–455, 1981.

142. Folstein S, Abbott M, Moses R, et al: A phenocopy of Huntington's disease: Lacunar infarcts of the corpus striatum. *Johns Hopkins Med J* 148:104–113, 1981.

143. Saris S: Chorea caused by caudate infarction. *Arch Neurol* 40:590–591, 1983.

144. Tabaton M, Mancardi G, Loeb C: Generalized chorea due to bilateral small, deep cerebral infarcts. *Neurology* 35:588–589, 1985.

145. Sethi KD, Nichols FT, Yaghmai F: Generalized chorea due to basal ganglia lacunar infarcts. *Mov Disord* 2:61–66, 1987.

146. Altafullah I, Pascual-Leone A, Duvall K, et al: Putaminal hemorrhage accompanied by hemichorea-hemiballism. *Stroke* 21:1093–1094, 1990.

147. Defebvre L, Destee A, Cassim F, et al: Transient hemiballism and striatal infarction. *Stroke* 21:967–968, 1990.

148. Destee A, Muller JP, Vermersch P, et al: Hemiballismus, hemichorea, striatal infarction. *Rev Neurol* 146:150–152, 1990.

149. Bhatia KP, Lera G, Luthert PJ, Marsden CD: Vascular chorea: Case report with pathology. *Mov Disord* 9:447–450, 1994.

150. Freilich RJ, Chambers BR: Choreoathetosis and thalamic haemorrhage. *Clin Exp Neurol* 25:115–120, 1988.

151. Fukui T, Hasegawa Y, Seriyama S, et al: Hemiballism-hemichorea induced by subcortical ischemia. *Can J Neurol Sci* 20:324–328, 1993.

152. Barinagarrementeria F, Vega F, DelBrutto OH: Acute hemichorea due to infarction in the corona radiata. *J Neurol* 236:371–372, 1989.

153. Vidakovic A, Dragasevic N, Kostic VS: Hemiballism: Report of 25 cases. *J Neurol Neurosurg Psychiatry* 57:945–949, 1994.

154. Calzetti S, Moretti G, Gemignani F, et al: Transient hemiballismus and subclavian steal syndrome. *Acta Neurol Belg* 80:329–335, 1980.

155. Tamaoka A, Sakuta M, Yamada H: Hemichorea-hemiballism caused by arteriovenous malformations in the putamen. *J Neurol* 234:124–125, 1987.

156. Shintani S, Shiozawa Z, Tsunoda S, Shiigai T: Paroxysmal choreoathetosis precipitated by movement, sound and photic stimulation in a case of artero-venous malformation in the parietal lobe. *Clin Neurol Neurosurg* 93:237–239, 1991.

157. Vincent FM: Hyperglycemia-induced hemichoreoathetosis: The presenting manifestation of a vascular malformation of the lenticular nucleus. *Neurosurgery* 18:787–790, 1986.

158. Carpay HA, Arts WF, Kloet A, et al: Hemichorea reversible after operation in a boy with cavernous angioma in the head of

the caudate nucleus. *J Neurol Neurosurg Psychiatry* 57:1547–1548, 1994.

159. Carella F, Caraceni T, Girotti F: Hemichorea due to a cavernous angioma of the caudate. Case report of an aged patient. *Ital J Neurol Sci* 13:783–785, 1992.

160. Linazasoro G, Urtasun M, Poza JJ, et al: Generalized chorea induced by nonketotic hyperglycemia. *Mov Disord* 8:119–120, 1993.

161. Lin JJ, Chang MK: Hemiballism-hemichorea and non-ketotic hyperglycaemia. *J Neurol Neurosurg Psychiatry* 57:748–750, 1994.

162. Nakagawa T, Mitani K, Nagura H, et al: Chorea-ballism associated with nonketotic hyperglycemia and presenting with bilateral hyperintensity of the putamen on MR T1-weighted images: A case report. *Clin Neurol* 34:52–55, 1994.

163. Shimomura T, Nozaki Y, Tamura K. Hemichorea-hemiballism associated with nonketotic hyperglycemia and presenting with unilateral hyperintensity of the putamen on MRI T_1-weighted images: A case report. *Brain Nerve* 47:557–561, 1995.

164. Broderick JP, Hagen T, Brott T, Tomsick T: Hyperglycemia and hemorrhagic transformation of cerebral infarcts. *Stroke* 26:484–487, 1995.

165. Hefter H, Mayer P, Benecke R: Persistent chorea after recurrent hypoglycemia. *Eur Neurol* 33:244–247, 1993.

166. Newman RP, Kinkel WR: Paroxysmal choreoathetosis due to hypoglycemia. *Arch Neurol* 41:341–342, 1984.

167. Sethi KD, Allen M, Sethi RK, McCord JW: Chorea in hypoglycemia and hyperglycemia. *Neurology* 40(suppl 1):337, 1990 (abstract).

168. Stone LA, Armstrong RM: An unusual presentation of diabetes: Hyperglycemia inducing hemiballismus. *Ann Neurol* 26:164, 1989 (abstract).

169. Haan J, Kremer HPH, Padberg G: Paroxysmal choreoathetosis as presenting symptom of diabetes mellitus. *J Neurol Neurosurg Psychiatry* 52:133, 1989.

170. Crossman AR, Sambrook MA, Jackson A: Experimental hemichorea/hemiballismus: Studies on the intracerebral site of action in a drug-induced dyskinesia. *Brain* 107:579–596, 1984.

171. Mitchell IJ, Jackson A, Sambrook MA, Crossman AR: Common neurological mechanism in experimental chorea and hemiballismus in the monkey. Evidence from 2-deoxyglucose autoradiography. *Brain Res* 339:346–350, 1985.

172. Mitchell IJ, Jackson A, Sambrook MA, Crossman AR: The role of the subthalamic nucleus in experimental chorea. Evidence from 2-deoxyglucose metabolic mapping and horseradish peroxidase tracing studies. *Brain* 112:1533–1548, 1989.

173. Crossman AR, Mitchell IJ, Sambrook MA, Jackson A: Chorea and myoclonus in the monkey induced by gamma-aminobutyric acid antagonism in the lentiform complex. The site of drug action and a hypothesis for the neural mechanisms of chorea. *Brain* 111:1211–1233, 1988.

174. Bashir K, Manyam BV: Clozapine for the control of hemiballismus. *Clin Neuropharmacol* 17:477–480, 1994.

175. Safirstein B, Shulman LM, Weiner WJ: Successful treatment of hemichorea with olanzapine. *Mov Disord* 14:532–533, 1999.

176. Evidente VG, Gwinn-Hardy K, Caviness JN, Alder CH: Risperidone is effective in severe hemichorea/hemiballismus. *Mov Disord* 14:377–379, 1999.

177. Erdinc OO, Ozdemir G, Uysal S, et al: Improvement of hemichorea with ondansetron. *Postgrad Med J* 73:127, 1997.

178. Chandra V, Wharton S, Spunt AL: Amelioration of hemiballismus with sodium valproate. *Ann Neurol* 12:407, 1982.

179. Dewey RB Jr, Jankovic J: Hemiballism-hemichorea. Clinical and pharmacologic findings in 21 patients. *Arch Neurol* 46:862–867, 1989.

180. Sethi KD, Patel BP: Inconsistent response to divalproex sodium in hemichorea-hemiballism. *Neurology* 40:1630–1631, 1990.

181. Thompson TP, Kondziolka D, Albright AL: Thalamic stimulation for choreiform movement disorders in children. Report of two cases. *J Neurosurg* 92:718–721, 2000.

182. Otsuka M, Ichiya Y, Kuwabara Y, et al: Cerebral glucose metabolism and ^{18}F-dopa uptake by PET in cases of chorea with or without dementia. *J Neurol Sci* 115:153–157, 1993.

183. Lee EJ, Choi JY, Lee SH, et al: Hemichorea-hemiballism in primary diabetic patients: MR correlation. *J Comput Assist Tomogr* 26:905–911, 2002.

184. Logothetic J: Neurologic and muscular manifestations of hyperthyroidism. *Arch Neurol* 5:533–544, 1961.

185. Fidler SM, O'Rourke RA, Buchsbaum HM: Choreoathetosis as a manifestation of thyrotoxicosis. *Neurology* 21:55–57, 1971.

186. Delwaide PJ, Schoenen J: Hyperthyroidism as a cause of persistent choreic movements. *Acta Neurol Scand* 58:309–312, 1978.

187. Shahar E, Shapiro MS, Shenkman L: Hyperthyroid-induced chorea. Case report and review of the literature. *Isr J Med Sci* 24:264–266, 1988.

188. Ahronheim JC: Hyperthyroid chorea in an elderly woman associated with sole elevation of T3. *J Am Geriatr Soc* 36:242–244, 1988.

189. Lucantoni C, Grottoli S, Moretti A: Chorea due to hyperthyroidism in old age. A case report. *Acta Neurol* 16:129–133, 1994.

190. Baba M, Terada A, Hishida R, et al: Persistent hemichorea associated with thyrotoxicosis. *Intern Med* 31:1144–1146, 1992.

191. Pozzan GB, Battistella PA, Rigon F, et al: Hyperthyroid-induced chorea in an adolescent girl. *Brain Dev* 14:126–127, 1992.

192. Fischbeck KH, Layzer RB: Paroxysmal choreoathetosis associated with thyrotoxicosis. *Ann Neurol* 6:453–454, 1979.

193. Drake ME Jr: Paroxysmal kinesigenic choreoathetosis in hyperthyroidism. *Postgrad Med J* 63:1089–1090, 1987.

194. Klawans HL, Shenker DM, Weiner WJ: Observations on the dopaminergic nature of hyperthyroid chorea. *Adv Neurol* 1:543–549, 1973.

195. Bruyn GW, Padberg G: Chorea and polycythemia. *Eur Neurol* 23:26–33, 1984.

196. Mas JL, Guergen B, Bouche P, et al: Chorea and polycythaemia. *J Neurol* 232:168–171, 1985.

197. Rigon G, Baratti M, Quaini F, Calzetti S: Polycythemia chorea. Description of a clinical case. *Minerva Med* 78:1325–1329, 1987.

198. Cohen AM, Gelvan A, Yarmolovsky A, Djaldetti M: Chorea in polycythemia vera: A rare presentation of hyperviscosity. *Blut* 58:47–48, 1989.

199. Chamouard JM, Smagghe A, Malalanirina BH, et al: Chorea disclosing polycythemia and renal adenocarcinoma. *Rev Neurol* 148:380–382, 1992.

200. Tang WY, Gill DS, Chuan PS: Chorea, a manifestation of hyponatremia? *Singapore Med J* 22:92–93, 1981.

201. Sparacio RR, Anziska B, Schutta HS: Hypernatremia and chorea. *Neurology* 26:46–50, 1976.

202. Howdle PD, Bone I, Losowsky MS: Hypocalcemic chorea secondary to malabsorption. *Postgrad Med J* 55:560–563, 1979.

203. Greenhouse AH: On chorea, lupus erythematosus, and cerebral vasculitis. *Arch Intern Med* 117:389–393, 1966.

204. Tabee-Zadeh MJ, Frame B, Kapphahn K: Kinesiogenic choreoathetosis and idiopathic hypoparathyroidism. *N Engl J Med* 286:762–763, 1972.

205. Soffer D, Licht A, Yaar I, Abramsky O: Paroxysmal choreoathetosis as a presenting symptom in idiopathic hypoparathyroidism. *J Neurol Neurosurg Psychiatry* 40:692–694, 1977.

206. Kashihara K, Yabuki S: Unilateral choreic movements in idiopathic hypoparathyroidism. *Brain Nerve* 44:477–480, 1992.

207. Salti I, Paris A, Tannir N, Khouri K: Rapid correction by 1-alpha-hydroxycholecalciferol of hemichorea in surgical hypoparathyroidism. *J Neurol Neurosurg Psychiatry* 45:89–90, 1982.

208. Rizzo GN, Olanow CW, Roses AD: Chorea in hyperparathyroidism. Report of a case. *AMB Rev Assoc Med Bras* 27:155–156, 1981.

209. Hurwitz LJ, Montgomery AD: Persistent choreoathetotic movements in liver disease. *Arch Neurol* 13:421–426, 1965.

210. Toghill PJ, Johnston AW, Smith JF: Choreoathetosis in portosystemic encephalopathy. *J Neurol Neurosurg Psychiatry* 30:358–363, 1967.

211. Gerard JM, Vanderhaeghen JJ, Telerman-Toppet N, Coers C: Choreo-athetosis with hepato-cerebral degeneration in a patient with a portocaval shunt. *Acta Neurol Belg* 73:100–109, 1973.

212. Spitaleri DL, Vitolo S, Fasanaro AM, Valiani R: Choreoathetosis. Uncommon manifestation during chronic liver disease with portocaval shunt. *Riv Neurol* 53:293–299, 1983.

213. Yokota T, Tsuchiya K, Umetani K, et al: Choreoathetoid movements associated with a spleno-renal shunt. *J Neurol* 235:487–488, 1988.

214. Tison FX, Ferrer X, Julien J: Delayed onset movement disorders as a complication of central pontine myelinolysis. *Mov Disord* 6:171–173, 1991.

215. Tsutada T, Hayashi H, Kitano S, et al: A case report of central pontine and extrapontine myelinolysis which occurred during pregnancy and was accompanied by choreic movement. *Clin Neurol* 29:1294–1297, 1989.

216. Roos RA, Wintzen AR, Vielvoye G, Polder TW: Paroxysmal kinesigenic choreoathetosis as presenting symptom of multiple sclerosis. *J Neurol Neurosurg Psychiatry* 54:657–658, 1991.

217. Mouren P, Tatassian A, Toga M, et al: Etude critique du syndrome hémiballique. *Encéphale* 55:212–274, 1966.

218. Sarkari NBS: Involuntary movements in multiple sclerosis. *Br Med J* 2:738–740, 1968.

219. Bachman DS, Laó-Vélez C, Estanol B: Dystonia and choreoathetosis in multiple sclerosis. *Arch Neurol* 33:590, 1976.

220. Taff I, Sabato UC, Lehrer G: Choreoathetosis in multiple sclerosis. *Clin Neurol Neurosurg* 87:41–43, 1985.

221. Mao C-C, Gancher ST, Herndon RM: Movement disorders in multiple sclerosis. *Mov Disord* 3:109–116, 1988.

222. Björk VO, Hultquist G: Brain damage in children after deep hypothermia for open-heart surgery. *Thorax* 15:284–291, 1960.

223. Bergouignan M, Fontan F, Trarieux M, Julien J: Syndromes choreiformes de l'enfant au décours d'interventions cardio-chirurgicales sous hypothermie profonde. *Rev Neurol* 105:48–60, 1961.

224. Brunberg JA, Doty DB, Reilly EL: Choreoathetosis in infants following cardiac surgery with deep hypothermia and circulatory arrest. *J Pediatr* 84:232–235, 1974.

225. Robinson RO, Samuels M, Pohl KRE: Choreic syndrome after cardiac surgery. *Arch Dis Child* 63:1466–1469, 1988.

226. DeLeon S, Ilbawi M, Arcilla R, et al: Choreoathetosis after deep hypothermia without circulatory arrest. *Ann Thorac Surg* 50:714–719, 1990.

227. Barratt-Boyes BG: Choreoathetosis as a complication of cardiopulmonary bypass. *Ann Thorac Surg* 50:693–694, 1990.

228. Wical BS, Tomasi LG: A distinctive neurological syndrome after profound hypothermia. *Pediatr Neurol* 6:202–205, 1990.

229. Wong PC, Barlow CF, Hickey PR, et al: Factors associated with choreoathetosis after cardiopulmonary bypass in children with congenital heart disease. *Circulation* 86:118–126, 1992.

230. Medlock MD, Cruse RS, Winek SJ, et al: A 10-year experience with postpump chorea. *Ann Neurol* 34:820–826, 1993.

231. Yoshii S, Mohri N, Suzuki S, et al: Postoperative choreoathetosis in a case of tetralogy of Fallot. *J Jpn Assoc Thorac Surg* 43:109–112, 1995.

232. Curless RG, Katz DA, Perryman RA, et al: Choreoathetosis after surgery for congenital heart disease. *J Pediatr* 124:737–739, 1994.

233. du Plessis A, Bellinger DC, Gauvreau K, et al: Neurologic outcome of choreoathetoid encephalopathy after cardiac surgery. *Pediatr Neurol* 27:9–17, 2002.

234. Kupsky WJ, Drozd MA, Barlow CF: Selective injury of the globus pallidus in children with post-cardiac surgery choreic syndrome. *Dev Med Child Neurol* 37:135–144, 1995.

235. Blunt SB, Brooks DJ, Kennard C: Steroid-responsive chorea in childhood following cardiac transplantation. *Mov Disord* 9:112–114, 1994.

236. Duvoisin RC: Chorea. *Semin Neurol* 2:351–358, 1982.

237. Shoulson I: On chorea. *Clin Neuropharmacol* 9(suppl 2):S85–S99, 1986.

238. Nomoto M, Thompson PD, Sheehy MP, et al: Anticholinergic-induced chorea in the treatment of focal dystonia. *Mov Disord* 2:53–56, 1987.

239. Matsumoto K, Nogaki H, Morimatsu M: A case of choreoathetoid movements induced by anticholinergic drugs, trihexyphenidyl HCl and dosulepin HCl. *Jpn J Geriatr* 29:686–689, 1992.

240. Harrison MB, Lyons GR, Landow ER: Phenytoin and dyskinesias: A report of two cases and review of the literature. *Mov Disord* 8:19–27, 1993.

241. Lancman ME, Asconape JJ, Penry JK, et al: Choreiform movements associated with the use of valproate. *Arch Neurol* 51:702–704, 1994.

242. Zaatreh M, Tennison M, D'Cruz O, Beach RL: Anticonvulsants-induced chorea: A role for pharmacodynamic drug interaction? *Seizure* 10:596–599, 2001.

243. Chudnow RS, Dewey RB Jr, Lawson CR: Choreoathetosis as a side effect of gabapentin therapy in severely neurologically impaired patients. *Arch Neurol* 54:910–912, 1997.

244. Sperling LS, Horowitz JL: Methamphetamine-induced choreoathetosis and rhabdomyolysis. *Ann Intern Med* 121:986, 1994.

245. Rhee KJ, Albertson TE, Douglas JC: Choreoathetoid disorder associated with amphetamine-like drugs. *Am J Emerg Med* 6:131–133, 1988.

246. Daras M, Koppel BS, Atos-Radzion E: Cocaine-induced choreoathetoid movements ("crack dancing"). *Neurology* 44:751–752, 1994.

247. Stuart AM, Worley LM, Spillane J: Choreiform movements observed in an 8-year-old child following use of an oral theophylline preparation. *Clin Pediatr* 31:692–694, 1992.

248. Bonnet U, Banger M, Wolstein J, Gastpar M: Choreoathetoid movements associated with rapid adjustment to methadone. *Pharmacopsychiatry* 31:143–145, 1998.

249. Helmuth D, Ljaljevic Z, Ramirez L, Meltzer HY: Choreoathetosis induced by verapamil and lithium treatment. *J Clin Psychopharmacol* 9:454–455, 1989.

250. Nielsen AS, Mors O: Choreiform dyskinesia with acute onset and protracted course following fluoxetine treatment. *J Clin Psychiatry* 60:868–869, 1999.

251. Fox GC, Ebeid S, Vincenti G: Paroxetine-induced chorea. *Br J Psychiatry* 170:193–194, 1997.

252. Crystal HA: Baclofen therapy may be associated with chorea in Alzheimer's disease. *Ann Neurol* 28:839, 1990.

253. Combarros O, Fabrega E, Polo JM, Berciano J: Cyclosporine-induced chorea after liver transplantation for Wilson's disease. *Ann Neurol* 33:108–109, 1993.

254. Samie MR, Ashton AK: Choreoathetosis induced by cyproheptadine. *Mov Disord* 4:81–84, 1989.

255. Patrick SJ, Snelling LK, Ment LR: Infantile chorea following abrupt withdrawal of diazepam and pentobarbital therapy. *J Toxicol Clin Toxicol* 31:127–132, 1993.

256. Mulder LJ, van der Mast RC, Meerwaldt JD: Generalised chorea due to digoxin toxicity. *Br Med J Clin Res Ed* 296:1262, 1988.

257. Moulignier A, Allo S, Singer B, et al: Sub-cortico-frontal encephalopathy and choreic movements related to recombinant interferon-alpha 2β. *Rev Neurol* 158:567–572, 2002.

258. Matsis PP, Fisher RA, Tasman-Jones C: Acute lithium toxicity: Chorea, hypercalcemia and hyperamylasemia. *Aust N Z J Med* 19:718–720, 1989.

259. Reed SM, Wise MG, Timmerman I: Choreoathetosis: A sign of lithium toxicity. *J Neuropsychiatry Clin Neurosci* 1:57–60, 1989.

260. Sweeney BJ, Edgecombe J, Churchill DR, et al: Choreoathetosis/ballismus associated with pentamidine-induced hypoglycemia in a patient with the acquired immunodeficiency syndrome. *Arch Neurol* 51:723–725, 1994.

261. Lehmann AB: Reversible chorea due to ranitidine and cimetidine. *Lancet* 8603:158, 1988.

262. Clarke CE, Bamford JM, House A: Dyskinesia in Creutzfeld-Jakob disease precipitated by antidepressant therapy. *Mov Disord* 7:86–87, 1992.

263. Fukutani Y, Nakamura I, Kobayashi K, et al: A case of familial juvenile Alzheimer's disease with apallic state at the relatively early stage and various neurological features: A clinicopathological study. *Clin Neurol* 29:633–638, 1989.

264. Voll R, Hoffmann GF, Lipinski CG, et al: Glutaric acidemia/glutaric aciduria I as differential chorea minor diagnosis. *Klin Padiatrie* 205:124–126, 1993.

265. Sethi KD, Ray R, Roesel RA, et al: Adult-onset chorea and dementia with propionic acidemia. *Neurology* 39:1343–1345, 1989.

266. Wiltshire EJ, Poplawski NK, Harbord MG, et al: Ornithine carbamoyltransferase deficiency presenting with chorea in a female. *J Inher Metab Dis* 23:843–844, 2000.

267. Friedman JH, Weitberg A: Ataxia without telangiectasia. *Mov Disord* 8:223–226, 1993.

268. Hanna MG, Davis MB, Sweeney MG, et al: Generalized chorea in two patients harboring the Friedreich's ataxia gene trinucleotide repeat expansion. *Mov Disord* 13:339–340, 1998.

269. Zhu D, Burke C, Leslie A, Nicholson GA: Friedreich's ataxia with chorea and myoclonus caused by a compound heterozygosity for a novel deletion and the trinucleotide GAA expansion. *Mov Disord* 17:585–589, 2002.

270. Namekawa M, Takiyama Y, Ando Y: Choreiform movements in spinocerebellar ataxia type 1. *J Neurol Sci* 187:103–106, 2001.

271. Manyam BV, Walters AS, Narla KR: Bilateral striopallidodentate calcinosis: Clinical characteristics of patients seen in a registry. *Mov Disord* 16:258–264, 2001.

272. Nelson I, Hanna MG, Alsanjari N, et al: A new mitochondrial DNA mutation associated with progressive dementia and chorea: A clinical, pathological, and molecular genetic study. *Ann Neurol* 37:400–403, 1995.

273. Truong DD, Harding AE, Scaravilli F, et al: Movement disorders in mitochondrial myopathies: A study of nine cases with two autopsy studies. *Mov Disord* 5:109–117, 1990.

274. Steiger MJ, Pires M, Scaravilli F, et al: Hemiballism and chorea in a patient with parkinsonism due to a multisystem degeneration. *Mov Disord* 7:71–77, 1992.

275. Colosimo C, Rossi P, Elia M, et al: Transient alternating hemichorea as presenting sign of progressive supranuclear palsy. *Ital J Neurol Sci* 12:99–101, 1991.

276. Seijo Martinez M, Castro del Rio M, Losada Campa A, et al: Chorea as the presenting form of progressive systemic sclerosis. *Neurologia* 15:304–306, 2000.

277. Wright RA, Pollock M, Donaldson IM: Chorea and tuberous sclerosis. *Mov Disord* 7:87–89, 1992.

278. Kimura N, Sugihara R, Kimura A, et al: A case of neuro-Behçet's disease presenting with chorea. *Rinsho Shinkeigaku* 41:45–49, 2001.

279. Kok J, Bosseray A, Brion JP, et al: Chorea in a child with Churg-Straus syndrome. *Stroke* 24:1263–1264, 1993.

280. Taurin G, Golfier V, Pinel JF, et al: Choreic syndrome due to Hashimoto's encephalopathy. *Mov Disord* 17:1091–1092, 2002.

281. Jones AL, Bouchier IA: A patient with neurosyphilis presenting as chorea. *Scot Med J* 38:82–84, 1993.

282. Blakeley J, Jankovic J: Secondary paroxysmal dyskinesias. *Mov Disord* 17:726–734, 2002.

283. Beskind DL, Keim SM: Choreoathetotic movement disorder in a boy with *Mycoplasma pneumoniae* encephalitis. *Ann Emerg Med* 23:1375–1378, 1994.

284. Krauss JK, Mohadjer M, Nobbe F, Mundinger F: Bilateral ballismus in children. *Child Nerv Sys* 7:342–346, 1991.

285. Gascon GG, al-Jarallah AA, Okamoto E, et al: Chorea as a presentation of herpes simplex encephalitis relapse. *Brain Dev* 15:178–181, 1993.

286. Wang HS, Kuo MF, Huang SC, Chou ML: Choreoathetosis as an initial sign of relapsing of herpes simplex encephalitis. *Pediatr Neurol*, 11:341–345, 1994.

287. Bhigjee AI, Kemp T, Cosnett JE: Cerebral cysticercosis presenting with hemichorea. *J Neurol Neurosurg Psychiatry* 50:1561–1562, 1987.

288. Mirsattari SM, Berry ME, Holden JK, et al: Paroxysmal dyskinesias in patients with HIV infection. *Neurology* 52:109–114, 1999.

289. Piccolo I, Causarano R, Sterzi R, et al: Chorea in patients with AIDS. *Acta Neurol Scand* 100:332–336, 1999.

290. Gallo BV, Shulman LM, Weiner WJ, et al: HIV encephalitis presenting with severe generalized chorea. *Neurology* 46:1163–1165, 1996.

291. Teive HA, Troiano AR, Cabral NL, et al: Hemichorea-hemiballism associated to cryptococcal granuloma in a patient with AIDS: Case report. *Arq Neuropsiquiatr* 58:965–968, 2000.

292. Sanchez-Ramos JR, Factor SA, Weiner WJ, Marquez J: Hemichorea-hemiballismus associated with acquired immune deficiency syndrome and cerebral toxoplasmosis. *Mov Disord* 4:266–273, 1989.

293. Pestre P, Milandre L, Farnarier P, Gallais H: Hemichorea in acquired immunodeficiency syndrome. Toxoplasmosis abscess in the striatum. *Rev Neurol* 147:833–837, 1991.

294. Nath A, Hobson DE, Russell A: Movement disorders with cerebral toxoplasmosis and AIDS. *Mov Disord* 8:107–112, 1993.

295. Moodley R, Seebaran AR, Rajput MC: Dystonia and choreoathetosis in Wernicke's encephalopathy. A case report. *S Afr Med J* 75:543–544, 1989.

296. Pacchetti C, Cristina S, Nappi G: Reversible chorea and focal dystonia in vitamin B12 deficiency. *N Engl J Med* 347:295, 2002.

297. Meucci G, Rossi G, Mazzoni M: A case of transient choreoathetosis with amnesic syndrome after acute carbon monoxide poisoning. *Ital J Neurol Sci* 10:513–517, 1989.

298. de Krom MC, Boreas AM, Hardy EL: Manganese poisoning due to use of Chien Pu Wan tablets. *Ned Tijdschr Geneeskd* 138:2010–2012, 1994.

299. Joubert J, Joubert PH: Chorea and psychiatric changes in organophosphate poisoning. A report of 2 further cases. *S Afr Med J* 74:32–34, 1988.

300. Poewe WH, Kleedorfer B, Willeit J, Gerstenbrand F: Primary CNS lymphoma presenting as a choreic movement disorder followed by segmental dystonia. *Mov Disord* 3:320–325, 1988.

301. Sakai M, Hashizume Y, Yamamoto H, Kawakami A: An autopsy case of primary cerebral malignant lymphoma initiated with choreoathetosis. *Clin Neurol* 30:849–854, 1990.

302. Schiff DE, Ortega JA: Chorea, eosinophilia, and lupus anticoagulant associated with acute lymphoblastic leukemia. *Pediatr Neurol* 8:466–468, 1992.

303. Albin RL, Bromberg MB, Penney JB, Knapp R: Chorea and dystonia: A remote effect of carcinoma. *Mov Disord* 3:162–169, 1988.

304. Vernino S, Tuite P, Adler CH, et al: Paraneoplastic chorea associated with CRMP-5 neuronal antibody and lung carcinoma. *Ann Neurol* 51:625–630, 2002.

305. Itoh H, Shibata K, Nitta E, Takamori M: Hemiballism-hemichorea from marked hypotension during spinal anesthesia. *Acta Anaesthesiol Scand* 42:133–135, 1998.

306. Watanabe K, Negoro T, Maehara M, et al: Moyamoya disease presenting with chorea. *Pediatr Neurol* 6:40–42, 1990.

307. Pavlakis SG, Schneider S, Black K, Gould RJ: Steroid-responsive chorea in moyamoya disease. *Mov Disord* 6:347–349, 1991.

308. Takanashi J, Sugita K, Honda A, Niimi H: Moyamoya syndrome in a patient with Down's syndrome presenting with chorea. *Pediatr Neurol* 9:396–398, 1993.

309. Tan EK, Lo YL, Chan LL, et al: Cervical disc prolapse with cord compression presenting with choreoathetosis and dystonia. *Neurology* 58:661–662, 2002.

310. Masjuan J, Buisan J, Gimeno A, Alvarez-Cermeno JC: Paroxysmal dyskinesias as the initial manifestation of multiple sclerosis. *Neurologia* 13:45–48, 1998.

311. Fowler WE, Kriel RL, Krach LE: Movement disorders after status epilepticus and other brain injuries. *Pediatr Neurol* 8:281–284, 1992.

312. Hadders-Algra M, Bos AF, Martijn A, Prechtl HF: Infantile chorea in an infant with severe bronchopulmonary dysplasia: An EMG study. *Dev Med Child Neurol* 36:177–182, 1994.

313. Bhatia KP: The paroxysmal dyskinesias. *J Neurol* 246:149–155, 1999.

314. Bhatia KP: Familial (idiopathic) paroxysmal dyskinesias: An update. *Semin Neurol* 21:69–74, 2001.

315. Chatterjee A, Louis ED, Frucht S: Levetiracetam in the treatment of paroxysmal kinesiogenic choreoathetosis. *Mov Disord* 17:614–615, 2002.

316. Chudnow RS, Mimbela RA, Owen DB, Roach ES: Gabapentin for familial paroxysmal dystonic choreoathetosis. *Neurology* 49:1441–1442, 1997.

317. Lee WL, Tay A, Ong HT, et al: Association of infantile convulsions with paroxysmal dyskinesias (ICCA syndrome): Confirmation of linkage to human chromosome 16p12-q12 in a Chinese family. *Hum Genet* 103:608–612, 1998.

318. Tomita H, Nagamitsu S, Wakui K, et al: Paroxysmal kinesigenic choreoathetosis locus maps to chromosome 16p11.2-q12.1. *Am J Hum Genet* 65:1688–1697, 1999.

319. Caraballo R, Pavek S, Lemainque A, et al: Linkage of benign familial infantile convulsions to chromosome 16p12-q12 suggests allelism to the infantile convulsions and choreoathetosis syndrome. *Am J Hum Genet* 68:788–794, 2001.

320. Fouad GT, Servidei S, Durcan S, et al: A gene for familial paroxysmal dyskinesia (FPD1) maps to chromosome 2q. *Am J Hum Genet* 59:135–139, 1996.

321. Khan Z, Jinnah HA: Paroxysmal dyskinesias in the lethargic mouse mutant. *J Neurosci* 22:8193–8200, 2002.

322. Spillane JD, Nathan PW, Kelly RE, Marsden CD: Painful legs and moving toes. *Brain* 94:541–556, 1971.

323. Nathan PW: Painful legs and moving toes: Evidence on the site of the lesion. *J Neurol Neurosurg Psychiatry* 41:934–939, 1978.

324. Schott GD: Painful legs and moving toes: The role of trauma. *J Neurol Neurosurg Psychiatry* 44:344–346, 1981.

325. Barrett RE, Singh N, Fahn S: The syndrome of painful legs and moving toes. *Neurology* 31(suppl 1):79, 1981.

326. Wulff CH: Painful legs and moving toes: A report of 3 cases with neurophysiologic studies. *Acta Neurol Scand* 66:283–287, 1982.

327. Schoenen J, Gonce M, Delwaide PJ: Painful legs and moving toes: A syndrome with different pathophysiologic mechanisms. *Neurology* 34:1108–1112, 1984.

328. Funakawa I, Muno Y, Takayanagi T: Painful hand and moving fingers. *J Neurol* 234:342–343, 1987.

329. Verhagen WIM, Horstink WMIM, Notermans SLH: Painful arm and moving fingers. *J Neurol Neurosurg Psychiatry* 48:384–385, 1985.

330. Ebersbach G, Schelosky L, Schenkel A, et al: Unilateral painful legs and moving toes syndrome with moving fingers: Evidence for distinct oscillators. *Mov Disord* 13:965–968, 1998.

331. Okuda Y, Suzuki K, Kitajima T, et al: Lumbar epidural block for "painful legs and moving toes" syndrome: A report of three cases. *Pain* 78:145–147, 1998.

332. Takahashi H, Saitoh C, Iwata O, et al: Epidural spinal cord stimulation for the treatment of painful legs and moving toes syndrome. *Pain* 96:343–345, 2002.

333. Pitagoras de Mattos J, Oliveira M, Andre C: Painful legs and moving toes associated with neuropathy in HIV-infected patients. *Mov Disord* 14:1053–1054, 1999.

334. Mattos JP, Rosso AL, Correa RB, Novis SA: Movement disorders in 28 HIV-infected patients. *Arq Neuropsiquiatr* 60:525–530, 2002.

335. Dressler D, Thompson PD, Gledhill RF, Marsden CD: The syndrome of painful leg and moving toes. *Mov Disord* 9:13–21, 1994.

336. Walters AS, Hening WA, Shah SK, Chokroverty S: Painless legs and moving toes: A syndrome related to painful legs and moving toes? *Mov Disord* 8:377–379, 1993.

V. MYOCLONIC DISORDERS

_____

CLASSIFICATION, CLINICAL FEATURES, AND TREATMENT OF MYOCLONUS

JOSE A. OBESO and IVANA ZAMARBIDE

DIFFERENTIATION FROM OTHER MOVEMENT
   DISORDERS   659
CLINICAL PRESENTATION   660
   Reflex Myoclonus   660
   Action Myoclonus   660
   Negative Myoclonus   660
   Spontaneous Myoclonus   661
   Rhythmic Myoclonus   661
NEUROPHYSIOLOGICAL ORIGIN   661
   Cortical Myoclonus   662
   Subcortical Myoclonus   662
   Spinal Myoclonus   662
ETIOLOGY   662
   Etiologic Classification   662
   Major Diagnostic Categories   663
TREATMENT   667
   Multifocal Action Myoclonus   667
   Focal Myoclonus of Cortical Origin   668

Myoclonus is a brief muscle jerk caused by neuronal discharges. A sudden and short-lasting interruption of ongoing voluntary muscle contraction may produce a postural pause clinically very similar to myoclonus, hence the term "negative myoclonus." Both forms often share the same etiology, coincide in the same patients, and can even affect the same muscle group.[1]

Myoclonus can be classified from various points of view (Table 39-1). The major categories are clinical presentation, neurophysiological origin, and etiology. Myoclonus may occur spontaneously, may be triggered by external stimulation ("reflex"), or may be induced during voluntary muscle activation ("action"). According to its distribution, myoclonus may be focal, segmental, generalized, or multifocal. The timing of myoclonus can be rhythmic or irregular.

A myoclonic jerk consists of a single muscle discharge but can be repetitive, giving rise to a salvo of muscle activity (Fig. 39-1). The latter is particularly frequent in action myoclonus and interferes severely with the execution of even the most simple motor tasks. For this reason, action myoclonus (both positive and negative types) may be considered as the movement disorder that produces the greatest interference with voluntary movements.

Differentiation from Other Movement Disorders

Myoclonus must be differentiated from other dyskinesias, such as tics, chorea, postural tremor, dystonia, and hemifacial spasm.[2]

Tics, as present in Tourette's syndrome, are frequently as brief as myoclonus. The main elements to distinguish between these two categories of muscle jerks include the following. (1) Myoclonus usually interferes notably with voluntary movement and is aggravated by action, whereas tics almost never disrupt motor acts. (2) Tics can be voluntarily suppressed and myoclonus cannot. (3) A high proportion of patients will feel a somesthetic sensation preceding the tic or an internal urgency to produce the movement. Myoclonus is not accompanied by any special sensation. (4) Most forms of myoclonus stop during sleep whereas tics often persist.

Chorea is a flowing combination of irregular muscle activity. Some of the movements of chorea may look "myoclonic" if taken in isolation, but it is the unpredictable concatenation of different patterns of movement that typifies chorea.

Postural and action tremor, when very severe, may be associated with sudden changes in the amplitude and rhythmicity of the muscle activity, giving rise to a false impression of a myoclonic jerk. This problem is easily resolved, when in doubt, by electromyographic (EMG) recording.[3] Slow resting tremor or myorrhythmia is difficult to distinguish clinically from rhythmical segmental myoclonus. True myoclonus,

TABLE 39-1 Classification of Myoclonus

Clinical
  Presentation
    Spontaneous
    Action
    Reflex
  Distribution
    Generalized
    Multifocal
    Segmental
    Focal
Neurophysiological origin
  Cortical
  Subcortical (brainstem)
  Spinal
Etiology
  Physiological
  Essential
  Symptomatic
    Associated with epilepsy
    Associated with other causes

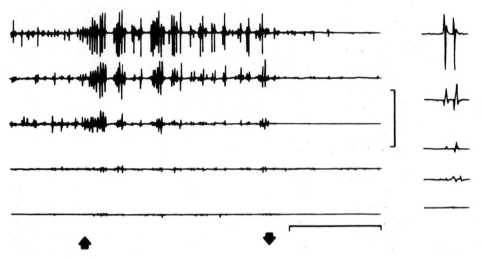

FIGURE 39-1 EMG recording from several muscles in the right arm of a patient with action myoclonus (Ramsay Hunt syndrome). From top to bottom are deltoid, biceps, triceps, finger extensors, and finger flexors. The horizontal scale bar indicates 2 s. The insert on the right shows the EMG discharges in more detail. Scale bar = 100 ms. The salvo of repetitive myoclonic discharges associated with silent periods is clearly seen in the proximal arm muscles. (*From Obeso et al.*[8] *Used with permission.*)

even when repetitive and rhythmical, must have a sudden and shock-like onset and end.

Dystonia consists of prolonged muscle spasms, which are longer than those of myoclonus and produce twisting, repetitive movements and abnormal postures.[4] Similarly, the muscle activity of hemifacial spasm lasts longer and provokes sustained, tonic contractions. However, such differentiation might not be so easy in early stages, when only clonic twitching of either the upper or lower facial musculature is present. In such instances, EMG studies are needed to clarify the diagnosis.

It should be kept in mind that myoclonus may coincide with other involuntary movement disorders in the same patients. For instance, some families with essential tremor and myoclonus have been described,[5] myoclonus and dystonia are combined in inherited myoclonic dystonia[6] (Fig. 39-2), and both action and reflex myoclonic jerks may be present in patients with Huntington's chorea.[7] These and other combinations also illustrate the point that the major motor manifestation of a given nosological entity does not imply that other movement disorders cannot be present in such diseases and syndromes. For example, not all the abnormal movements of Tourette's syndrome are tics, nor is chorea the only movement disorder present in Huntington's disease (HD).

Clinical Presentation

REFLEX MYOCLONUS

Somesthetic, visual, and auditory stimuli, independently and in combination, may trigger myoclonic jerking. Such myoclonus is focal or generalized in distribution. Pin-pricking the limbs distally (wrist and palmar surface of the upper limbs and the soles of the feet), as well as flicking the fingers and toes, are probably the most sensitive clinical methods of evoking reflex myoclonus limited to a body area.[8] In some

instances, the jerks are so sensitive to somesthetic stimuli that focal myoclonus may become self-perpetuated and simulate spontaneous myoclonus, as in epilepsia partialis continua, or even look like a tremor.

Generalized reflex myoclonus to somesthetic stimulation is more commonly obtained by touching or tapping the face, particularly the mentalis zone. Visually triggered reflex myoclonus may be evoked clinically by a threatening stimulus, but more often requires flash stimulation.[9] Auditory stimulation is not a frequent cause of myoclonus, except in children. Both visually and auditorily evoked myoclonus are always generalized. Generalized reflex myoclonus induced by unexpected sounds has to be distinguished from hyperekplexia, which is a pathological exaggeration of the startle response (see below).

ACTION MYOCLONUS

This occurs during active muscular contraction and affects both posturally acting muscles and prime movers. Action myoclonus may be focal or segmental, but the most common distribution is multifocal or generalized. This form is undoubtedly the one that produces the greatest disability. This is usually due to the concatenation of several brief EMG discharges (Fig. 39-1), which forces the limbs and trunk to move in unintended directions. The abnormal neuronal activity provoking action myoclonus probably arises from the same areas as those mediating normal motor control mechanisms. Thus, action myoclonus interferes with, prevents, and disrupts very gross voluntary movements to a much greater extent than other movement disorders such as dystonia and tics.

NEGATIVE MYOCLONUS

Negative myoclonus is by definition only present during active muscular contraction and in fact is almost always

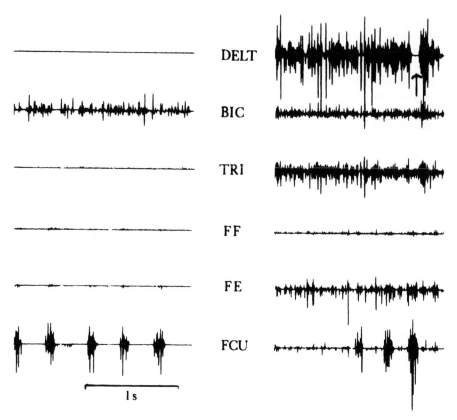

DELT

BIC

TRI

FF

FE

FCU

1 s

FIGURE 39-2 EMG recording from the right arm of a patient with myoclonic dystonia. On the *left*, spontaneous myoclonic activity is present in flexor carpi ulnaris (FCU) at rest. On the *right*, exaggerated EMG activity is seen in proximal arm muscles (deltoid, biceps, triceps) while the myoclonus persists in FCU. A brief negative myoclonus (asterixis) is indicated by the arrow in deltoid EMG (DELT). BIC, biceps; TRI, triceps; FF, finger flexor muscles; FE, finger extensor muscles. (*From Obeso et al.[17] Used with permission.*)

combined with positive action myoclonus. There are two major clinical presentations: asterixis and postural lapses.[1] Asterixis is the most common and best-characterized form of negative myoclonus. It consists of a silence of EMG discharges for a short period of time (50–200 ms), thus producing a brief loss of antigravitational activity and postural control (Fig. 39-2, arrow). Asterixis is usually multifocal in distribution but may affect a muscle group in isolation. Shibasaki et al.[10] have described reflex negative myoclonus limited to muscles of one limb. Postural lapses consist of a long-duration EMG silence (200–500 ms), usually occupying axial and proximal muscles of the lower limbs, with a tendency for repetitive appearance over a few seconds.[1] In patients with severe myoclonic encephalopathies, such as postanoxic myoclonus, these postural lapses may follow a myoclonic discharge and may actually lead to greater functional disability than the myoclonic discharge.

SPONTANEOUS MYOCLONUS

Spontaneous myoclonus may be focal, multifocal, or generalized, and have several presentations. It may be sporadic and occur unpredictably or coincide with specific moments, such as in normal people with nocturnal myoclonus or in patients with early morning myoclonic epilepsy. In other instances, it may be almost continuously present, as in patients

with metabolic encephalopathies or Creutzfeldt-Jakob disease (CJD).

RHYTHMIC MYOCLONUS

This is almost always spontaneous in presentation, with a focal or segmental distribution. The myoclonic discharge may persist during sleep and is little affected by sensory stimulation. The frequency is variable but usually slow (1–4 Hz). The most common type is spinal myoclonus. Palatal "myoclonus" is now considered a form of tremor and no longer included under the category of myoclonus.[11]

It is important to realize that different patterns are often combined in the same subject. For instance, reflex and action myoclonus may coincide and affect the same body region(s), multifocal spontaneous myoclonus, as seen in metabolic encephalopathies, is very commonly aggravated during action, and focal myoclonus may spread to become generalized.

Neurophysiological Origin

This topic is thoroughly covered in Chap. 40, but it will be briefly addressed here because it is important to understand some clinical and therapeutic aspects.

Electrophysiological analysis of myoclonus is mainly aimed at identifying the site of the discharges producing the jerks and the pathophysiological mechanisms involved in their origin. It should be noted that the origin of the discharges producing myoclonus does not necessarily coincide with the topography of the lesion(s) and that, on many occasions, the pathological basis cannot be determined.

Myoclonus can be divided into three major pathophysiological categories: cortical, subcortical, and spinal myoclonus.

CORTICAL MYOCLONUS

Cortical myoclonus results from abnormal activity arising in the sensorimotor cortex and spreading down via the corticospinal pathway. The EMG discharge is of short duration (usually 10–50 ms); the somatosensory evoked potentials (SEPs) are increased in amplitude (20–50 µV) and frequently associated with a reflex muscle response (C-wave) that follows the cortical potential by a short latency of 15–20 ms for the forearm muscles.[8] Back-averaging the EEG activity preceding the jerks reveals a biphasic potential over the contralateral sensorimotor cortex preceding the muscle discharge by some 20 ms in the arm and 35 ms in the leg (see Chap. 40).

SUBCORTICAL MYOCLONUS

Subcortical myoclonus indicates that the neuronal discharge originates in structures between the cortex and the spinal cord. The most common type is "reticular reflex myoclonus," characterized by generalized jerks, with predominant involvement of proximal limb and axial muscles provoked by sensory stimulation. EMG recording of the spreading of the jerk through different muscles is necessary to determine the brainstem origin (see Chap. 40).

SPINAL MYOCLONUS

Spinal myoclonus is secondary to abnormal neuronal discharge originating in the spinal cord. It is frequently rhythmical and only exceptionally stimuli-sensitive. A newly described form is propiospinal myoclonus,[13] in which spontaneous and stimuli-sensitive (tapping) jerks involve mainly the trunk and abdominal muscles. The EMG discharges consist of repetitive bursts with a frequency of 1–7 Hz.

Etiology

Myoclonus may occur in the setting of a wide variety of conditions. Indeed, a list of all causes of myoclonus could be almost as long as the index of a neurology textbook. However, in many instances, myoclonus is a nonspecific manifestation and is accompanied by many other neurological signs. In such cases, myoclonus is not a key clinical indicator.

The etiologic classification of myoclonus, as originally outlined by Marsden et al.,[14] is briefly summarized below; more detailed attention is given to those conditions in which myoclonus is a major complaint or the main clinical sign leading to a correct diagnosis.

ETIOLOGIC CLASSIFICATION

PHYSIOLOGICAL MYOCLONUS
This occurs in normal people in special circumstances and does not indicate an underlying abnormality. Nocturnal myoclonus of the legs is probably the most common type.

ESSENTIAL MYOCLONUS
This occurs in individuals in whom myoclonus is the only or most important neurological manifestation and the course is not progressive. It is now recognized that most cases are familial and frequently associated with dystonia (see below).

MYOCLONIC EPILEPSIES
Idiopathic epilepsy without any other neurological problem may have myoclonus as a major clinical expression. This includes entities such as benign myoclonus of infancy, myoclonic absences, juvenile myoclonic epilepsy of Janz, and photosensitive epileptic myoclonus. In such instances, the jerks are usually generalized and occur spontaneously, are frequently facilitated by lack of sleep, alcohol, etc., and may be triggered by visual stimuli.

Myoclonus may also be present in patients with generalized tonic-clonic epilepsy in the setting of a progressive encephalopathy (progressive myoclonic epilepsy), which will be discussed in detail below.

SECONDARY MYOCLONUS
As indicated above, any process causing central nervous system (CNS) damage or dysfunction may be associated with myoclonus. However, the list of conditions in which myoclonus is the only or major clinical manifestation is much less extensive. This includes anoxia (Lance-Adams syndrome), trauma, bismuth intoxication, and some metabolic problems such as renal failure, hyponatremia, hypokalemia, which may show myoclonus as an initial sign. More rarely, a late-onset degenerative disease such as progressive supranuclear palsy, olivopontocerebellar atrophy (OPCA), or HD may have action myoclonus as a major feature. Reflex myoclonus is a common feature of corticobasal degeneration (CBD) and OPCA, and may be a prominent feature in some rare families with HD. Focal lesion of the CNS may produce focal or segmental myoclonus (see below).

The list of drugs causing myoclonus is fairly long. Thus, the possibility of drug abuse should always be considered in any patient with a myoclonic encephalopathy of unknown origin.

MAJOR DIAGNOSTIC CATEGORIES

The principal clinical presentations and the most common etiologies of myoclonus as a movement disorder will be discussed in this section. Myoclonus in patients with epilepsy (i.e., myoclonic absences, juvenile myoclonic epilepsy, etc.) as the major clinical problem is not included here.

CAUSES OF SEVERE MULTIFOCAL OR GENERALIZED MYOCLONUS

This section deals with conditions in which myoclonus may be overt and a predominant clinical problem. The jerks usually have a multifocal distribution and appear spontaneously, but they may be aggravated by action and be stimulus sensitive.

Essential Myoclonus

In this condition the jerks are usually multifocal, extremely brief (hence the term "lightning"), and aggravated by action. The amplitude and intensity of the jerks are variable. In some patients the jerks are large and almost continuous, provoking severe disability, but in others the amplitude is so small that they interfere only minimally with routine motor acts. Essential myoclonus is a heterogeneous disorder, which may be sporadic but more often has a genetic basis (hereditary essential myoclonus). In familial cases, inheritance is autosomal-dominant with variable penetrance and expression, onset occurs in the first two decades of life, severity may be variable within the same family, and all routine laboratory tests and neuroimaging studies are normal.

While the existence of patients with myoclonus as the only manifestation must be admitted, recent observations indicate that essential myoclonus very often occurs in combination with dystonic postures and movements and shows an extreme sensitivity to alcohol ("alcohol-sensitive myoclonic dystonia").[6] Interestingly, none of the drugs commonly effective in other types of myoclonus has been capable of mimicking the dramatic antimyoclonic effect of alcohol.

The association of myoclonus and dystonia has been the subject of considerable debate and confusion.[15] The term "myoclonic dystonia" was actually used a long time ago by Davidenkow,[16] and refers to the association of two movement disorders: namely, brief (<100 ms) myoclonic jerking, and long-lasting (>500 ms) dystonic spasms, usually in different muscle groups (Fig. 39-2). This combination may occur in a low proportion of patients with idiopathic torsion dystonia,[15,17] and also in other clinical settings, such as after trauma and anoxia, or as part of the tardive dyskinesia syndrome. However, the most common, albeit infrequent, presentation is that of "inherited myoclonus-dystonia"(IMD) very often exhibiting a very dramatic response to alcohol.[15] Several families have been described in recent years.[6] The disease is autosomal-dominant, of early onset (<10 years), and has a relatively stereotyped clinical picture, characterized by predominance of dystonia in the neck and shoulder muscles, and very brief myoclonic jerking in the arms and hands.

Legs are rarely or minimally involved. The response to small amounts of alcohol is very impressive, with eradication of both myoclonus and dystonia. It is now clear that within the same family the presence and intensity of either myoclonus or dystonia are variable,[6,18] explaining the initial difficulties and uncertainties in understanding and accepting the existence of hereditary myoclonic dystonia as an entity. Considerable advance has occurred in recent years regarding the genetic basis of IMD.[19] In 6 German families, 5 independent mutations in the epsilon-sarcoglycan gene located in chromosome 7q21 have been identified, [20] and more recently a new locus has been linked to a 17-cM region on chromosome 18p11 in a large Canadian family.[21] To make the genetic basis of IMD more interesting but certainly more complicated, a missense change (Val > Ile) in the D2 dopamine receptor gene (DRD gene) on chromosome 11q23 and a deletion (Phe323-Tyr328del) in the DYT1 gene in chromosome 9q34 have been encountered in two different families.[19] In the same two families, however, a recent study found another mutation of the sarcoglycan gene.[20] The intriguing suggestion of all these ongoing findings is that each mutation could correspond and underlie a different clinical manifestation.

Progressive Myoclonic Encephalopathies

In patients with a progressive myoclonic encephalopathy, the features of myoclonus are not distinctive enough to enable the correct identification of the different entities under this title. The key to a correct diagnosis and understanding of the nosology of the progressive myoclonic encephalopathies is the predominant clinical signs associated with myoclonus.

PROGRESSIVE MYOCLONIC ENCEPHALOPATHIES WITH EPILEPSY AND DEMENTIA The major clinical features consist of action- and stimuli-sensitive multifocal and generalized myoclonus, tonic-clonic seizures that are difficult to control, and progressive dementia. Age of onset is usually in the first two decades of life, but patients with late onset are occasionally encountered. Other possible signs include ataxia, spasticity, or visual defects. In this setting, the diagnoses to consider are Lafora's disease, myoclonic epilepsy with ragged-red fibers (MERRF), lipofuscinosis (Kufs' disease), and sialidosis. In Japan, dentatorubralpallidoluysian atrophy (DRPLA) is probably the most common cause of the syndrome. [22] DRPLA is inherited with an autosomal-dominant, with incomplete penetrance, pattern. The recognition of a gene mutation (CTG-B37) in chromosome 12 producing a CAG triplet expansion has led to the recognition of various clinical presentations for DRPLA worldwide.[23] The phenotype of progressive myoclonus epilepsy is mainly observed in the young-onset (< 20 years) presentation. [22]

Electrophysiological analysis of patients with progressive myoclonus encephalopathies frequently indicates a cortical origin for the myoclonus, but this finding is not sufficiently specific to enable a definitive etiological diagnosis to be reached. Equally, neuroimaging studies often show brain atrophy but without any specific sign.

Lafora's disease has a mean age of onset of 14 years (ranging from 5 to 20) and consists of a rapidly progressing dementia, frequent grand mal seizures that are relatively difficult to control, and visual hallucinations. The disease is inherited by autosomal-recessive transmission. There are some 20 mutations reported in a gene coding for a protein known as laforin.[24] This is a tyrosine phosphatase regulatory protein localized in ribosomes in the endoplasmic reticulum. The linkage between laforin and the glucose polymers giving rise to the typical Lafora bodies has not yet been determined.[24]

A definitive diagnosis is established by skin and muscle biopsy that shows the characteristic inclusions bodies, but genetic testing will rapidly substitute pathological assessment for diagnostic purposes. The disease has a fatal evolution in less than 10 years from diagnosis, although more slowly evolving cases have been described.

MERRF is typically suspected in patients with a maternal inheritance pattern, and a clinical picture dominated by myoclonus, epilepsy, and ataxia, associated with other problems such as optic atrophy, deafness, peripheral neuropathy, myocardiopathy, diabetes, hypertension, short stature, and multiple lipomas.[25] Dementia is common, but early development is typically normal.[25] MERRF is a typical example of a respiratory chain/oxidative phosphorylation disease, causing lactic acidosis. Three mutations have been associated with MERFF. The A8344G mutation is present in about 90 percent of patients with MERFF.[25]

Neuronal storage diseases are the most frequent cause of progressive myoclonic encephalopathy in children. Tay-Sachs disease (hexosaminidase A deficiency), Sandhoff's disease (hexosaminidase A and B deficiency), infantile neuropathic Gaucher's disease, and the sialidosis are the most common diagnostic entities. Common to all is the generalized, stimuli-sensitive myoclonus and prominent photosensitivity. In the cherry-red-spot myoclonus syndrome (sialidosis type I), SEPs are giant, but the visual evoked potentials are decreased in amplitude, a rare combination which may have diagnostic value. In adults, Kufs' disease and sialidosis have been described, but are indeed very rare causes of progressive myoclonic encephalopathy.

SLOWLY PROGRESSIVE MYOCLONIC ENCEPHALOPATHIES WITH EPILEPSY This group is made up of patients with a slowly progressing disease with the combination of action myoclonus, epilepsy, and ataxia, in whom no evidence of mitochondrial or any other abnormality is found.[26] Dementia is not a feature, but mild cognitive impairment may be detected throughout evolution. Proper recognition of these patients has been marred by several factors, the least of which is semantic. Thus, such patients have been labeled as Unverricht-Lundborg's disease, Baltic myoclonus, and Ramsay Hunt syndrome. In fact, various types of neurodegenerations, most of which have cerebellar involvement in common, constitute the underlying pathology of the disease process in most cases. Two major clinical subgroups are now

recognized: (1) progressive myoclonic epilepsy (PME), and (2) progressive myoclonic ataxia (PMA).

The major cause of PME is Unverritch-Lundborg's disease. The disease has a worldwide spread, but it is more common in Finland where the incidence is 1:20,000 births.[27] A mutation in chromosome 21q22.3 leading to a marked reduction in cystatin B is the genetic cause of Unverricht-Lundborg's disease. Five other mutations affecting nucleotides in the cystatin B gene have been reported more recently.[27] How dysfunction in cystatin B causes neuronal degeneration in Unverricht-Lundborg's disease has not been precisely defined yet. In a mouse model, it has been shown that cerebellar granular cells die mainly by apopotosis, suggesting a neuroprotective mechanism for cystatin B.[27]

In most patients, symptoms begin in the first decade of life. Evolution is slow, with a marked variation within the same family as to the degree of progression and disability.[27] Action and stimuli-sensitive multifocal myoclonus is a major problem. Generalized tonic-clonic seizures are the initial manifestation in about 50 percent of patients and may become a practical management difficulty. Ataxia may be present but usually to a minor degree. Dementia is not a typical feature, but mild cognitive impairment becomes obvious on long-term evolution. Cortical SEPs are of large amplitude, photosensitivity is frequent, and the EEG is abnormal. Back-averaging the EEG activity preceding the myoclonus will often show a cortical potential antedating the jerks by a few milliseconds (e.g., 15–20 ms for the upper limb). Magnetic resonance imaging (MRI) and computed tomography (CT) brain scans are normal or show mild atrophy. In a few cases, atrophy of the cerebellum out of proportion with that present supratentorially can be encountered.

PMA is characterized by action myoclonus with multifocal and occasionally generalized distribution, variable presence of stimuli-induced myoclonus, and ataxia. The latter affects mainly gait in the early stage of evolution but evolves towards a widespread cerebellar syndrome. Clinical assessment of the ataxia is hampered by action myoclonus. It is only after proper drug control of the myoclonus that cerebellar signs may be properly evaluated. Epilepsy is absent or mild and almost always well controlled with the drugs used to treat the myoclonus.[26] Dementia is certainly not a feature of PMA, but changes in mood and depression are relatively common as disability increases due to disease progression. Many cases are sporadic, but familial forms have also been described.[2] Age at onset varies widely from the 1st to the 7th decade of life. A cortical origin for the myoclonus is demonstrated in about 70 percent of cases. It remains to be determined whether or not the same genetic defect may give rise to the clinical phenotype of PMA as well as PME.

Mitochondrial disease, MERRF in particular, may have a milder course and show the clinical picture of PMA, including late onset and absent cognitive deficit, but the notion that mitochondrial respiratory chain diseases are the most common etiology of progressive myoclonic syndromes with epilepsy or ataxia is erroneous. In fact, most patients have a neurodegeneration with variable pathological basis. This includes pure spinocerebellar degeneration, spinocerebellar plus dentatorubral degeneration, OPCA, and DRPLA.[2,26] A deficit of vitamin E (tocopherol) secondary to malabsorption is also a cause of Ramsay Hunt syndrome. Bhatia et al.[28] described 4 patients with sporadic celiac disease coursing without overt malabsorption or malnutritional symptoms with the typical clinical picture of PMA: action and stimuli-sensitive myoclonus, mild ataxia, and infrequent generalized seizures. The myoclonus has all of the electrophysiological characteristics of cortical myoclonus. Stressing a point we made in earlier writings,[8,10] the pathology of 1 case revealed Purkinje cell loss in the cerebellum but indemnity of the cortex, thus indicating that cortical myoclonus obeys a disinhibition mechanism.[28]

SLOWLY PROGRESSIVE MYOCLONIC ENCEPHALOPATHIES WITH DEMENTIA   Alzheimer's disease (AD) may have spontaneous and action-induced generalized myoclonus as a prominent and early sign. This form frequently courses clinically with the triad of myoclonus, dementia, and parkinsonism, and is a frequent cause of diagnostic confusion. In some of these patients, the typical physiological features of cortical myoclonus are present. More often, however, the jerks in AD consist of small amplitude, irregular twitching of the hand muscles, producing a pseudotremulous appearance called "polyminimyoclonus." A slow frontal cortical potential has been recorded preceding these small-amplitude jerks.[29,30]

CBD (see Chap. 45) is a progressive disorder of asymmetric onset, beginning in the 60s and 70s, and mainly characterized by limb apraxia, alien limb phenomenon, slowness and rigidity, cortical sensory defects, dysarthria and aphasia, hand dystonia, and stimuli-sensitive myoclonus. The evolution of CBD is slowly progressive. Most patients become bedridden over a period of 5–8 years. Severe cognitive deficit does not occur in the majority of patients, but in about 30 percent it appears late in the evolution.[31]

The myoclonus of CBD is a highly characteristic and very frequent (at least 50 percent),[32] although nonexclusive, feature of this condition. The affected limb, particularly the forearm and hand muscles, shows what appears to be spontaneous, irregular, and practically continuous jerking, aggravated by any attempt to move voluntarily. Careful observation indicates that the apparently spontaneous jerks are actually due to background ongoing muscle activity.[8] Thus, the myoclonic limb will stop moving when complete relaxation is achieved. The most notorious semiological feature of the myoclonus in CBD is the exquisite sensitivity to sensory stimuli such as light touching, stretching, or even air-puffing, the affected hand.[8] These will cause a salvo of muscle jerking that will continue indefinitely unless the explorer can obtain full relaxation of the limb. The extreme tendency for the affected limb to move continuously very often leads to the movement disorder being regarded as tremor,[32] which in addition to the clumsiness and rigidity may lead to an erroneous diagnosis of Parkinson's disease (PD) early in the

evolution of the illness. The features of myoclonus in CBD strongly suggest a cortical origin,[33] but the neurophysiological findings are not totally typical. SEPs are not enlarged, and back-averaging frequently fails to detect a potential preceding the jerks. A distinctive feature of the reflex myoclonus in CBD is that the latency of the jerks is very short (< 40 ms for the forearm and hand muscles).[33]

In HD, action myoclonus is a rare manifestation, but a few patients with genetic and autopsy-proven studies have been described in whom multifocal action myoclonus was the primary manifestation. In one such family,[34] electrophysiological studies showed large SEPs and reflex muscle responses typical of cortical myoclonus, and visual stimulation elicited an EEG pattern consistent with visual reflex myoclonus.[10]

Myoclonus is not a feature of PD, but it may be present in several parkinsonian syndromes, including Lewy body dementia. In this condition, myoclonus has been described in about 15 percent of patients, but this is in all probability an underestimation since the presence of stimulus-sensitive myoclonus is not generally included as part of the examination.[35] Indeed, focal reflex jerks induced by touching and particularly pin-pricking the wrist and hand ventral area are very frequent in patients with parkinsonism and dementia.[36]

Other causes of severe myoclonus associated with cognitive deficit are viral- or prion-related encephalopathies, particularly CJD, herpes simplex, and subacute sclerosing panencephalitis. The myoclonus in CJD is spontaneous, symmetrical, and generalized. The typical EEG triphasic waves are always present when myoclonus is clinically overt but their relationship is variable. EEG back-averaging shows a widespread negative potential preceding the jerks by some 60 ms. In a few patients, the typical features of cortical reflex myoclonus following somesthetic and photic stimulation have been reported.[33]

In patients with a subacute myoclonic encephalopathy of unknown cause accompanied by cognitive deficit associated or not with other neurological problems (ataxia, seizures, etc.), the diagnostic possibilities include metabolic derangements (renal and liver failure, hyperglycemia, hypokalemia, hyponatremia, etc.), toxic agents (bismuth, methyl bromide, heavy metals), and drugs (antidepressants, antibiotics, phenytoin, cocaine, amphetamine, etc.).

Static Myoclonic Encephalopathies

Action and spontaneous, multifocal, and/or generalized myoclonus may be extremely disabling in patients who have suffered severe anoxia or head trauma. Posthypoxic myoclonus was described by Lance and Adams in 1963[37] and received much attention after the discovery of its dramatic sensitivity to treatment with 5-hydroxytryptophan (5-HTP). However, a high proportion of patients show additional neurological deficits (ataxia, speech difficulties, memory loss, etc.), which reduce the chances of adequate therapeutic control. In their original article, Lance and Adams also described in detail the existence of long EMG silences following the myoclonic jerks. They recognized the importance of these silent periods as being responsible for the postural lapses (negative myoclonus) often seen in posthypoxic myoclonus. The long-term evolution of posthypoxic myoclonus is positive in a majority of patients, in keeping with the nonprogressive nature of the underlying pathology.

FOCAL MYOCLONUS

This section describes conditions characterized by focal or segmental myoclonus which may be spontaneous and rhythmical, may occur in response to sensory stimulation, and/or may occur during action.

Focal Myoclonus of the Limbs

A "jerking limb" may occur in a wide variety of clinical settings. Lesions located along the neuraxis, including the sensorimotor cerebral cortex, thalamus, mesencephalon, and spinal cord, may be associated with focal myoclonus. However, the major causes to consider here are those affecting the cortex or the spinal cord.

CORTICAL MYOCLONUS In general, cortical myoclonus must be used as a neurophysiological concept and not as a clinical entity. This is because there are many conditions that course with myoclonus of cortical origin but in which no pathological abnormality at the cortical level is found (e.g., see the description of celiac disease in Ref. 28). In this section, cortical myoclonus is used to refer to focal myoclonus associated with a lesion or functional alteration of the cerebral cortex.

In focal cortical myoclonus, the jerks are restricted to a few muscles with predominant activation of distal and flexor muscles. The most common presentation is during action and provoked by somesthetic stimulation. Stretching the fingers, delicate stimulation such as touching the hand or foot with a feather, and pin-pricking the wrist are all very effective in triggering a salvo of focal myoclonic jerking. In many patients the reflex myoclonus is modality-specific, and only one of the above stimuli is capable of eliciting the myoclonus. The condition most likely to be associated with cortical reflex myoclonus of one hand is CBD.[8,32,33]

Spontaneous and rhythmical presentation is the main characteristic of epilepsia partialis continua (EPC), which may also be stimuli-sensitive and aggravated by action.[8] The causes of EPC include tumors, arteriovenous malformations, focal encephalitis of Kozhevnikov, abscess, stroke, and disorders of neuronal migration. In a proportion of patients with EPC secondary to ischemia or tumors, the lesion is located subcortically.

Focal stimuli-sensitive myoclonus elicited by stimulation of any of the four limbs is very common in multiple-system atrophy with predominant OPCA.[35-38] However, the presence of reflex myoclonus may well pass unnoticed unless actively investigated. The best type of stimulus consists of pin-pricking the palmar surface of the wrist and the

metacarpal region of the index finger while the examiner extends the fingers and wrist. The rate of stimulation must be low (<1/s) to avoid habituation. Small jerks will be seen or felt in the forearm and intrinsic hand muscles. Occasionally, the same stimuli will induce a generalized jerk. SEPs are enhanced in amplitude and usually associated with a reflex muscle discharge, thus having the characteristics of cortical reflex myoclonus. Flash stimulation is also accompanied by reflex jerks in about 50 percent of patients with OPCA.[38] In contrast with the common photomyoclonic response more frequently found in patients with epilepsy, visual reflex myoclonus in OPCA is induced by low-frequency (<10 Hz) flash stimulation, each stimulus being accompanied by a cortical spike which antedates a myoclonic jerk.[10] The origin of the abnormal discharge is in the premotor and motor cortex.

The sensitivity to visual stimulus is blocked by L-dopa and dopamine agonists.[10] Because many patients with OPCA also have parkinsonian features, care must be taken to stop medication for at least 12 hours before conducting the electrophysiological evaluation.

SPINAL MYOCLONUS Spinal myoclonus is a typical, albeit rare, cause of focal and usually rhythmic myoclonus. The most frequent clinical presentation consists of spontaneous, repetitive jerks of one limb, sometimes spreading to adjacent neck and trunk muscles. The frequency of the myoclonus is very variable, from 10 to 50/min. In many reported cases the myoclonus persists during sleep. The most common etiologies are cervical myelopathy (including posttraumatic), tumors, multiple sclerosis, and infections.[39] A rather similar presentation may be observed in patients with evidence of peripheral nerve damage (nerve, plexus, root), with or without accompanying sympathetic changes (Sudeck's atrophy).

Facial Myoclonus

Twitching of some facial muscles may occur in normal people when tired or after excessive tobacco and alcohol consumption, in hemifacial spasm, and following focal brainstem lesions. In most instances, the EMG pattern is that of myokymia or spasms rather than truly myoclonic. Rhythmic slow movements of the orbicularis oris sometimes spreading to the adjacent musculature leads one to consider Whipple's disease. It may also occur in patients with a lesion of Mollaret triangle even without "palatal myoclonus."[40]

Authentic facial myoclonus without involvement of any other body part is actually rare. The most common condition associated with it is EPC (Epilepsia Partialis Continua).

Axial Myoclonus

Segmental and rhythmical myoclonus of the neck and trunk may rarely arise as a consequence of brainstem lesions, Arnold-Chiari malformation, and upper cervical cord damage. Nonrhythmic, repetitive axial flexion, and more rarely extension jerks, occurring spontaneously but aggravated by action and sensitive to stretching, are the major features of "propiospinal myoclonus."[12,13] The EMG shows irregular, brief bursts at a variable frequency of 1–7 Hz. Detailed neurophysiological analysis (see Chap. 40) is necessary to confirm the spinal origin of this uncommon presentation.

GENERALIZED, STIMULI-SENSITIVE MYOCLONUS

In a small proportion of all patients with myoclonus, the main problem consists in whole body jerks triggered by sensory stimuli (sound, touching, stretching, or visual threatening). This clinical presentation may correspond to three different mechanisms: (1) reticular reflex myoclonus, (2) hyperekplexia, and (3) psychogenic (also see Chap. 40).

Reticular reflex myoclonus (RRM) is a pathophysiological term describing the origin of myoclonus in the brainstem reticular formation. Anoxia, uremia, liver failure, drugs, and brainstem encephalitis are the major causes of RRM.

Hyperekplexia is the pathological manifestation of startle.[41] Clinical differences from RRM are that the latter may also occur during action whereas hyperekplexia is always stimuli-induced. Tonic spasms following stimulation may be present in hyperekplexia but are not associated with RRM. Otherwise, precise differentiation of the two conditions require electrophysiological assessment. Hyperekplexia may be symptomatic or inherited as an autosomal-dominant condition. The latter has been defined as a mutation in the alpha1-subunit of the glycine receptor.

Normal people may, for a variety of reasons, jump and jerk in response to external stimulation mimicking myoclonus and startle.[42] Clinical hints to the diagnosis are the acute onset, variability in the stimuli triggering the jerks, and variable recruitment of the muscles.[43] In such cases, the onset of the EMG discharge is always within the range of normal reaction time.[42]

Treatment

Myoclonus is a very disabling movement disorder because it utilizes the same motor control mechanisms that are necessary for normal voluntary movements. The treatment of myoclonus is largely empirical, because there has been little progress in understanding its biochemical basis. In this section, the therapeutic possibilities are discussed in accordance with the major clinical presentations, as described above, and the pathophysiological origin of myoclonus regardless of the etiology.

MULTIFOCAL ACTION MYOCLONUS

This is the most incapacitating form and the one requiring the major therapeutic effort. In around 70 percent of patients with action myoclonus, electrophysiological assessment indicates a cortical origin. This is a very important feature to consider when addressing the pharmacological approach. The initiation of drug treatments in action myoclonus occurred in the 1970s when 5-HTP, the precursor of serotonin, was given to a French patient with postanoxic action myoclonus[44] in whom a large number of drugs had been tried without success and a thalamotomy had also been performed with no benefit. Administration of 5-HTP with carbidopa to prevent peripheral decarboxylation produced a dramatic improvement in the patient. This result led to a number of studies on posthypoxic action myoclonus, which confirmed the therapeutic action of 5-HTP plus carbidopa (100–300/25 mg/day). It was found that the cerebrospinal fluid concentration of the major serotonin metabolite, 5-hydroxyindolacetic acid, was lowered in most of these patients.[45,46] Physiological analysis revealed that patients with postanoxic myoclonus with an excellent response to 5-HTP had reticular reflex myoclonus, whereas those with a moderate or no response had cortical reflex myoclonus.[46] The failure to control equally well all cases with 5-HTP and the associated side-effects (nausea, vomiting, diarrhea, hypotension, and gastrointestinal bleeding) led to the examination of other alternative drugs. Clonazepam, sodium valproate, and fluoxetine were found useful.[47] In later years, several patients with action myoclonus have been physiologically and pharmacologically studied, and a general picture of the treatment of severe action myoclonus has emerged.[48]

The major factor recognized as a predictor of the drug responsiveness is the neurophysiological origin. Cortical myoclonus responds exceedingly well to piracetam (8–20 g/day), clonazepam (2–15 mg/day), sodium valproate (1200–3000 mg/day), and primidone (500–1000 mg/day).[49] In the majority of patients with severe, highly disabling action myoclonus, these drugs have to be given in combination to achieve adequate control.[49,50] This is thought to be due to the various mechanisms implicated in the pathophysiology of cortical myoclonus.[8,49] Clonazepam is the most efficient antimyoclonic drug,[48] but piracetam is the first drug to be used because of its excellent tolerance up to 24 g/day.[50,51] All of these drugs are believed to act by increasing GABA (gamma-aminobutyric acid) activity in the cortex, but direct evidence of their mechanism of action against cortical myoclonus is still lacking. Surprisingly, the initial experience with other recently acquired anticonvulsant drugs such as vigabatrin and gabapentin has not been positive. In 2 patients with progressive myoclonic ataxia and cortical myoclonus, the addition of acetozalamide to the combination discussed above led to better control of the jerks.[52]

In the last 2 years, the newer antiepileptic agent levetiracetam, an analog of piracetam, has been tried in a few patients with myoclonus. The response is variable.[53] In our personal experience, not even patients with cortical myoclonus respond as well as to piracetam, but still a few patients may show a dramatic improvement.[53] Treatment with *N*-acetylcysteine (4–6 g/day) in 4 siblings with Unverricht-Lundborg disease was associated with dramatic improvement and excellent tolerance.[54] However, a more recent study[55] in 3 patients failed to support this claim and, in addition, found severe side-effects (sensorineural deafness in 1 patient, and nausea and gastric pain in another).

The degree of symptomatic control achieved in patients with action myoclonus of cortical origin is usually very striking at the beginning of treatment, but the long-term treatment response pattern is variable. This depends on several factors, the most important of which is the underlying disease. Patients with a static encephalopathy (e.g., posthypoxia), in whom myoclonus is the only or major clinical problem, achieve a very long-lasting and adequate control. On the other hand, patients with progressive illness (e.g., MERFF, sialidosis, neurodegenerations, etc.) are very difficult to control for any length of time. An important practical point in the management of such cases is the ease with which generalized seizures may occur when manipulating the drug regimen. Thus, when a given drug treatment is judged inefficient, its withdrawal must be achieved very carefully and slowly.

The above discussion relates to the treatment of action myoclonus understood to be a positive muscle discharge. However, in most patients the jerks are actually a combination of positive and negative (EMG silence) myoclonus.[1] The latter is as incapacitating as the former. However, there has not been any study specifically analyzing the effect of antimyoclonic drugs against negative myoclonus. In many patients, the postural lapses that affect the trunk and proximal leg muscles are the most difficult feature to keep under control.[48,50]

Patients with action myoclonus originating in the brainstem (reticular reflex myoclonus) or the spinal cord are much less frequent. Clonazepam is the drug of choice in such instances.

FOCAL MYOCLONUS OF CORTICAL ORIGIN

Focal myoclonus of cortical origin also responds very well to the drugs discussed above.[8] The only exception is CBD, but this is a very special pathophysiological type of cortical myoclonus and a rapidly evolving disease.[33,34] In extremely severe cases of cortical myoclonus producing epilepsia partialis continua, surgery may be considered after rigorous assessment.

Spinal myoclonus has no specific drug treatment. The best therapeutic approach is to treat the causative condition whenever this is possible. Drugs used with some benefit include clonazepam, carbamazepine, and tetrabenazine. Palatal myoclonus may respond to 5-HTP, trihexyphenidyl (up to 60 mg/day), carbamazepine, and piracetam.

Nocturnal myoclonus, usually involving the legs but occasionally the whole body, may require treatment when very frequent and so severe as to interfere with falling asleep. Clonazepam at a relatively low dose (1–3 mg at bedtime) is very effective for controlling this problem.

References

1. Obeso JA, Artieda J, Burleigh A: Clinical aspects of negative myoclonus. *Adv Neurol* 67:1–8, 1996.

2. Obeso JA, Artieda J, Marsden CD: Different clinical presentations of myoclonus, in Jankovic J, Tolosa E (eds): *Parkinson's Disease and Movement Disorders*, 2nd ed. Baltimore: Williams & Wilkins, 1993, pp 315–328.

3. Obeso JA, Narbona J: Post-traumatic tremor and myoclonic jerking. *J Neurol Neurosurg Psychiatry* 46:788, 1983.

4. Rothwell JC, Obeso JA: The anatomical and physiological basis of torsion dystonia, in Marsden CD, Fahn S (eds): *Movement Disorders 2*. London: Butterworth, 1987, pp 313–331.

5. Mahloudji M, Pikely RT: Hereditary essential myoclonus. *Brain* 90:669–674, 1967.

6. Quinn NP: Essential myoclonus and myoclonic dystonia: A review. *Mov Disord* 11:119–124, 1996.

7. Vogel CM, Drury I, Terry LC, Young AB: Myoclonus in adult Huntington's disease. *Ann Neurol* 29:213–215, 1991.

8. Obeso JA, Rothwell JC, Marsden CD: The spectrum of cortical myoclonus: from focal reflex jerks to spontaneous motor epilepsy. *Brain* 108:193–224, 1985.

9. Artieda J, Obeso JA: The pathophysiology and pharmacology of photic cortical reflex myoclonus. *Ann Neurol* 34:175–184, 1993.

10. Shibasaki H, Ikeda A, Nagamine T, et al: Cortical reflex negative myoclonus. *Brain* 117:477–486, 1994.

11. Deuschl G, Toro C, Valls-Sole J, et al: Symptomatic and essential palatal tremor 1. Clinical, physiological and MRI analysis. *Brain* 117:775–788, 1994.

12. Brown P, Thompson PD, Rothwell JC, et al: Axial myoclonus of propiospinal origin. *Brain* 114:197–214, 1991.

13. Brown P, Rothwell JC, Thompson PD, Marsden CD: Propiospinal myoclonus: "Pattern" generators in humans. *Mov Disord* 9:571–576, 1994.

14. Marsden CD, Hallett M, Fahn S: The nosology and pathophysiology of myoclonus, in *Movement Disorders 1*. London: Butterworth, pp 196–248, 1982.

15. Kurlan R, Berh J, Medved L, Shoulson I: Myoclonus and dystonia: A family study. *Adv Neurol* 50:385–389, 1988.

16. Davidenkow F: Auf hereditar-abiotrophischer Grundlage akut auf tretende, regressierende und episodische Erkrankungen des Nervensystems und Bemerkungen über die familäre subakute, myoklonische Dystonie. *Z Neurol Psychiatry* 104:596–622, 1926.

17. Obeso JA, Rothwell JC, Lang AE, Marsden CD: Myoclonic dystonia. *Neurology* 33:825–830, 1983.

18. Fahn S, Sjaastad O: Hereditary essential myoclonus in a large Norwegian family. *Mov Disord* 6:237–247, 1991.

19. Furukawa Y, Rajput AH: Inherited myoclonus-dystonia. *Neurology* 59:1130–1131, 2002.

20. Zimprich A, Grabowski M, Asmus F, et al: Mutations in the gene encoding ε-sarcoglycan cause myoclonus-dystonia syndrome. *Nat Genet* 29:66–69, 2001.

21. Grimes DA, Han F, Lang AE, et al: A novel locus for inherited myoclonus-dystonia on 18p11. *Neurology* 59:1183–1186, 2002.

22. Klein C, Liu L, Doheny D, et al: ε-Sarcoglycan mutations found in combination with other dystonia gene mutations. *Ann Neurol* 52:675–679, 2002.

23. Tsuji S: Dentatorubral-pallidoluysian atrophy: Clinical aspects and molecular genetics. *Adv Neurol* 89:231–239, 2002.

24. Minassian BA: Progressive myoclonus epilepsy with polyglucosan bodies: Lafora disease. *Adv Neurol* 89:199–210, 2002.

25. DiMauro S, Hirano M, Kaufmann P, et al: Clinical features and genetics of myoclonic epilepsy with ragged red fibres. *Adv Neurol* 89:217–229, 2002.

26. Marsden CD, Harding A, Obeso JA, Lu CS: Progressive myoclonic ataxia (the Ramsay Hunt syndrome). *Arch Neurol* 47:1121–1125, 1990.
27. Lehesjoki AE: Clinical features and genetics of Unverricht-Lundborg's disease. *Adv Neurol* 89:193–197, 2002.
28. Bhatia KP, Brown P, Gregory R, et al: Progressive myoclonic ataxia associated with coeliac disease. *Brain* 118:1087–1093, 1995.
29. Wilkins DE, Hallett M, Erba G: Primary generalized epileptic myoclonus: A frequent manifestation of minipolymyoclonus of central origin. *J Neurol Neurosurg Psychiatry* 48:506–516, 1985.
30. Wilkins DE, Hallett M, Berardelli A, et al: Physiological analysis of the myoclonus of Alzheimer's disease. *Neurology* 34:898–903, 1984.
31. Rinne JO, Lee MS, Thompson PD, Marsden CD: Corticobasal degeneration: A clinical study of 36 cases. *Brain* 117:1183–1196, 1994.
32. Thompson PD: Neurodegenerative causes of myoclonus. *Adv Neurol* 89:31–34, 2002.
33. Thompson PD, Day BL, Rothwell JC, et al: The myoclonus in corticobasal degeneration: Evidence for two forms of cortical reflex myoclonus. *Brain* 117:1197–1208, 1994.
34. Thompson PD, Bhatia KP, Brown P, et al: Cortical myoclonus in Huntington's disease. *Mov Disord* 9:633–641, 1994.
35. Shafiq M, Lang AE: Myoclonus in parkinsonian disorders. *Adv Neurol* 89:77–84, 2002.
36. Chen R, Ashby P, Lang AE: Stimulus-sensitive myoclonus in akinetic-rigid syndrome. *Brain* 115:1875–1888, 1992.
37. Lance JW, Adams RD: The syndrome of intention or action myoclonus as a sequel to hypoxic encephalopathy. *Brain* 86:111–136, 1963.
38. Rodriguez M, Artieda J, Zubieta JL, Obeso JA: Reflex myoclonus in olivopontocerebellar atrophy. *J Neurol Neurosurg Psychiatry* 57:316–319, 1994.
39. Jankovic J, Pardo R: Segmental myoclonus: Clinical and pharmacological study. *Arch Neurol* 43:1025–1031, 1986.
40. Lapresle J: Palatal myoclonus. *Adv Neurol* 43:265–274, 1986.
41. Brown P, Rothwell JC, Thompson PD, et al: The hyperekplexias and their relationship to a normal startle reflex. *Brain* 114:1903–1928, 1991.
42. Thompson PD, Colebatch JG, Rothwell JC, et al: Voluntary stimulus sensitive jerks and jumps mimicking myoclonus or pathological startle syndrome. *Mov Disord* 7:257–262, 1992.
43. Brown P: Neurophysiology of the startle syndrome and hyperekplexia. *Adv Neurol* 89:153–159, 2002.
44. Lhermitte F, Oeterfalvi M, Marteau R, et al: Analyse pharmacologique d'un cas de myoclonus d'intention et d'action postanoxique. *Rev Neurol (Paris)* 124:21–31, 1971.
45. Van Woert MH, Sethy VH: Therapy of intention myoclonus with l-5-hydroxytryptophan and a peripheral decarboxylase inhibitor, MK 486. *Neurology* 25:135–140, 1975.
46. Chadwick D, Hallett M, Harris R, et al: Clinical, biochemical and physiological features distinguishing myoclonus responsive to 5-hydroxytryptophan, tryptophan with a monoamine oxidase inhibitor and clonazepam. *Brain* 100:455–487, 1977.
47. Fahn S: Posthypoxic action myoclonus: Literature review update. *Adv Neurol* 43:157–169, 1986.
48. Frucht S: The clinical challenge of posthypoxic myoclonus. *Adv Neurol* 89:85–97, 2002.
49. Obeso JA, Artieda J, Rothwell JC, et al: The treatment of severe action myoclonus. *Brain* 112:765–777, 1989.
50. Obeso JA, Artieda J, Quinn NP, et al: Piracetam in the treatment of different types of myoclonus. *Clin Neuropharmacol* 11:529–536, 1988.
51. Brown P, Steiger MJ, Thompson PD, et al: Effectiveness of piracetam in cortical myoclonus. *Mov Disord* 8:63–68, 1993.
52. Vaamonde J, Legarda I, Jimenez-Jimenez J, Obeso JA: Acetazolamide improves action myoclonus in Ramsay Hunt syndrome. *Clin Neuropharmacol* 15:392–396, 1992.
53. Frucht S, Louis ED, Chuang C, et al: A pilot tolerability and efficacy study of levetiracetam in patients with chronic myoclonus. *Neurology* 57:1112–1114, 2001.
54. Hurd RW, Wilder BJ, Helvestn WR, Uthman BM: Treatment of four siblings with progressive myoclonus epilepsy of the Unverricht-Lundborg type with N-acetylcysteine. *Neurology* 47:1264–1268, 1996.
55. Edwards MJJ, Hargreaves IP, Heales SJR, et al: N-Acetylcysteine and Unverricht-Lundborg disease. *Neurology* 59:1447–1449, 2002.

Chapter 40 _____

PATHOPHYSIOLOGY OF MYOCLONIC DISORDERS

CAMILO TORO and MARK HALLETT

PHYSIOLOGICAL CLASSIFICATION OF
   MYOCLONUS   671
    Epileptic Myoclonus   672
    Nonepileptic Myoclonus   673
ELECTROPHYSIOLOGICAL EVALUATION OF
   MYOCLONUS   675
    Polygraphic EMG Studies   675
    Routine Electroencephalography (EEG)   675
    EEG Back-Averaging   676
    Somatosensory Evoked Potentials (SEPs)   677
    Reflex Studies   677
    Transcranial Magnetic Stimulation (TMS)   678
    Magnetoencephalography (MEG)   678
NEGATIVE MYOCLONUS   678

The electrophysiological study of myoclonic movements has interested clinical electrophysiologists, epileptologists, movement disorders specialists, and sleep medicine specialists. As early as 1935, Gibbs et al.[1] had described patients with spike-and-wave discharges in the electroencephalogram (EEG), with muscle jerking at the same rate as the EEG spikes. Grinker et al.[2] are credited with the first description of polyspike discharges in the EEG, with close association to myoclonic jerking in patients with progressive myoclonic epilepsy. In 1946, Dawson produced a detailed description of the relationship between EEG spikes and muscle jerks in patients with myoclonus, reporting also, in some of his patients, the possibility of inducing myoclonic jerks by tendon tapping.[3] One year later, Dawson himself not only demonstrated the first recording of somatosensory evoked potentials (SEPs) from the scalp in humans,[4] but also showed that SEPs in patients with myoclonus could be grossly exaggerated in amplitude.[5]

Electrophysiological studies aid in making the diagnosis and provide insight into the pathophysiology of myoclonus.[6–11] From a clinical perspective, myoclonus refers to quick muscle jerks, either irregular or rhythmic, and almost always arising from the central nervous system. This definition itself is quite nonspecific and is of little value in establishing a precise etiologic diagnosis or understanding of the basic pathophysiological mechanisms of the disorder. Myoclonus can be focal, involving only a few adjacent muscles, generalized, involving many or most of the muscles in the body, or multifocal, involving many muscles but in different jerks.[8] Myoclonus can be spontaneous, can be activated or accentuated by voluntary movement (action myoclonus), and can be activated or accentuated by sensory stimulation (reflex myoclonus).[9,11–13] In the differential diagnosis of myoclonus, the principal features that favor myoclonus are the quickness and fragmentary nature of the movement, and the absence of voluntary influence.[12] Some simple tics look identical to myoclonus and cannot be visually distinguished. Another disorder that could be confused with myoclonus is tremor, because some forms of myoclonus are rhythmic.[14] Conversely, some tremors, despite a regular frequency, have variable amplitude of the electromyogram (EMG), and present an irregular appearance that is not unlike that of myoclonus.[12]

Perhaps the only electrophysiological finding that can be generalized across the broad clinical definition of myoclonus is that myoclonus arises from abnormal muscle activation in the form of short (50–300 ms) EMG bursts (positive myoclonus).[6,7] Less often, myoclonus is the result of brief interruptions of ongoing tonic EMG (negative myoclonus).[15,16] In both instances, this abnormal EMG activity leads to a brief displacement of the involved body segment and/or disruption of posture. These features alone may aid in differentiating myoclonus from fragments of other movement disorders with more complex and lengthy patterns of muscle co-activation, such as chorea and dystonia.[6,7] Additional electrophysiological assessment can aid in deciding whether the movement disorder is indeed myoclonus, and, if so, which physiological type.[8]

Physiological Classification of Myoclonus

There are several useful schemes for classifying myoclonus.[8] For the purposes of therapy, it is valuable to consider both an etiologic classification and a physiological classification. The etiologic and physiological classifications of myoclonus often do not coincide. An etiologic classification of myoclonus provides guidance for treatment of the underlying metabolic, infectious, or toxic derangement, and it has clear implications in the prognosis and counseling of relatives of afflicted individuals. The physiological classification of myoclonus searches for the site and mechanism of origin of the symptoms, the precipitating factors, and the pathways of spread. Myoclonic disorders, with strikingly different etiologic, genetic, and prognostic implications, may fall into the same physiological group, sharing relatively homogeneous electrophysiological properties that usually point to common physiological derangement.[8–11,14] These findings, in turn, may aid the selection of the most appropriate symptomatic therapy, may serve as a quantitative tool for evaluating efficacy and mechanisms of action of antimyoclonic medications,[17–19] and may aid in the early recognition of patients at risk for some myoclonic disorders, even before clinically symptomatic, perhaps allowing for earlier interventions.[20,21]

Halliday[22] can be credited with the first comprehensive attempt to classify the myoclonias, based on their electrophysiological correlates. He divided myoclonus into three main groups: pyramidal, extrapyramidal, and segmental. Pyramidal myoclonus encompassed those myoclonic disorders characterized by a brief burst of EMG activity associated with an EEG correlate. Because of the short latency between the EEG event and the EMG burst (15–40 ms), he proposed an origin in the cortex propagated via the pyramidal tract. In extrapyramidal myoclonus, Halliday included those myoclonic movements in which the EEG events were less obvious and the EMG bursts were of longer duration. He considered the movements seen in subacute sclerosing panencephalitis as prototypical of this group. The loose association between EEG and EMG and the long and variable length of EMG bursts suggested to Halliday an extrapyramidal site of origin. Segmental myoclonus was used by Halliday to denote myoclonus, often symmetrical and rhythmic, confined to discrete brainstem segments or spinal cord myotomes, and arising from brainstem or spinal cord damage as a result of trauma, infection, or neoplasm.

We now classify myoclonus in two broad groups (Table 40-1). By defining epileptic myoclonus as myoclonus that is a fragment of epilepsy, myoclonus can be divided into epileptic and nonepileptic types.[23,24] The physiological characteristics of epileptic myoclonus are EMG burst length of 10–50 ms, synchronous antagonist activity, and an EEG correlate. Nonepileptic myoclonus shows EMG burst lengths of 50–300 ms, synchronous or asynchronous antagonist activity, and no EEG correlate. The classification of myoclonus into epileptic and nonepileptic groups has a value beyond simple taxonomic curiosity. Response to anticonvulsant agents and other antimyoclonic medications, such as piracetam, appears to be closely linked to the physiological features of the myoclonus.[17,18]

The terms cortical and subcortical myoclonus are used to classify myoclonus according to the location in the nervous system of the presumed generator of the myoclonus.[8] Cortical and subcortical myoclonus can be used almost interchangeably with epileptic and nonepileptic myoclonus, respectively. Reticular reflex myoclonus, classified as epileptic myoclonus, is the only form of myoclonus at odds with the overlap in the two classification schemes. Reticular reflex myoclonus originates from abnormal paroxysmal discharges in the brainstem reticular formation and thus has a subcortical origin.

EPILEPTIC MYOCLONUS

Cortical reflex myoclonus is a fragment of focal or partial epilepsy.[23] Each myoclonic jerk involves only a few adjacent muscles, but larger jerks with more muscles involved can be seen. The disorder is commonly multifocal and is accentuated by action and sensory stimulation. The EEG reveals a focal positive-negative event over the sensorimotor cortex contralateral to the jerk preceding both spontaneous and reflex-induced myoclonic jerks. With stimulus sensitivity, C-reflexes are seen and are correlated with giant SEPs. The EEG event associated with reflex jerks is a giant P1-N2 component of the SEP[19,23–26] (Fig. 40-1). Often, the P1-N2 has exactly the same topography as the positive-negative event preceding the spontaneous myoclonus, but at times there are some differences.[9,19,25,26] A final feature is that, when the cranial nerve muscles are involved, the timing of onset of activation follows a rostrocaudal sequence; that is, the masseter (5th cranial nerve) is active before the orbicularis oculi (7th cranial nerve), which is itself active before the sternocleidomastoid (11th cranial nerve)[23] (Fig. 40-2).

Reticular reflex myoclonus is a fragment of a type of generalized epilepsy.[27] These muscle jerks are usually generalized, with predominance that is proximal more than distal and flexor more than extensor. Voluntary action and sensory stimulation increase the jerking. This disorder has the following features. (1) There are brief generalized EMG bursts, lasting 10–30 ms and triggered by sensory stimulation, such as touch

TABLE 40-1 Physiological Classification of Myoclonus

Epileptic myoclonus
    Cortical reflex myoclonus
    Reticular reflex myoclonus
    Primary generalized epileptic myoclonus
    Photic cortical reflex myoclonus
Nonepileptic myoclonus
    Normal physiological phenomena (e.g., hypnic jerk)
    Essential myoclonus
    Palatal myoclonus (tremor)
    Spinal myoclonus, including propriospinal myoclonus
    Peripheral myoclonus
    Exaggerated startle
    Nocturnal myoclonus (e.g., periodic movements in sleep)
    Psychogenic myoclonus

Taps to left fingers

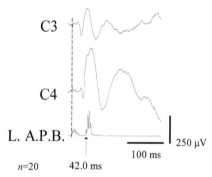

C3

C4

L. A.P.B.

250 μV

100 ms

n=20   42.0 ms

FIGURE 40-1 Giant SEPs in a patient with cortical sensory reflex myoclonus. Taps to the fingers on the left hand (indicated by the vertical dashed line) give rise to a giant SEP response, which is larger over the contralateral central regions (C4). There is a reflex EMG response (C-reflex) in the left abductor pollicis (L. A.P.B) at about 42.0 ms.

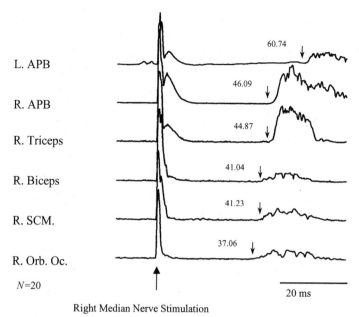

L. APB

R. APB

R. Triceps

R. Biceps

R. SCM.

R. Orb. Oc.

N=20

Right Median Nerve Stimulation

60.74
46.09
44.87
41.04
41.23
37.06

20 ms

FIGURE 40-2 Polygraphic average (*n* = 20) of rectified EMG reflex responses to stimulation of the right median nerve in a patient with cortical reflex myoclonus. In this patient, focal stimulation often resulted in generalized body twitches. The latency of activation of the different muscles is consistent with a rostrocaudal pattern of activation with muscles innervated by the highest cranial nerves activating first. R, right; L, left; APB, abductor pollicis brevis muscle; SCM, sternocleidomastoid muscle; Orb. Oc, orbicularis oculi. Activation of the L. APB follows activation of the R. APB by about 15 ms. This difference probably represents a delay related to transcallosal spread of the activation from the left to the right hemisphere.

or muscle stretch, or by action. (2) The EEG correlates, when present, are not time-locked to the muscle activation. (3) The pattern of EMG activation in cranial nerve muscles is with the sternocleidomastoid muscle activated first and the other cranial nerve muscles activated in reverse numerical order. It is as if the front of activation originates in proximity to the motor nucleus of the 11th cranial nerve and travels bidirectionally along the neuroaxis.[27] Reticular reflex myoclonus can be seen in patients with postanoxic myoclonus and in other toxic-metabolic encephalopathies associated with myoclonus, such as uremia.[28] In cats, urea infusions give rise to this form of myoclonus. Depth electrode recordings in these animals have defined the origin of the abnormal discharge in the nucleus reticularis gigantocellularis.[29]

Both cortical and reticular reflex myoclonus may be seen in the same patient.[23,30] Clinically, there will be both multifocal and generalized jerks, and physiological analysis will reveal features of both disorders.

Primary generalized epileptic myoclonus is a fragment of primary generalized epilepsy.[24] The most common clinical manifestation is small, focal jerks, often involving only the fingers; thus, the myoclonus is sometimes called minipolymyoclonus.[31] The term minipolymyoclonus was originally coined to refer to small jerks seen in patients with motor neuron disease. Minipolymyoclonus of central origin and minipolymyoclonus of peripheral origin have a similar clinical appearance, and they are most easily separated by the company they keep. One has associated seizures, while the other has progressive muscle weakness and denervation. A second clinical presentation of primary generalized epileptic myoclonus consists of generalized, synchronized whole-body jerks not unlike those seen with reticular reflex myoclonus.[31] The EEG correlate is a slow, bilateral

frontocentrally predominant negativity similar to the wave of a primary generalized paroxysm.

Detailed studies of photic cortical reflex myoclonus show that it has an origin in a hyperexcitable motor cortex and is driven by an occipital response of normal appearance.[32] There is a remarkable similarity in these findings and those of the myoclonus in the photosensitive baboon *Papio papio*.[33,34] Intermittent light stimulation in the photosensitive baboon gives rise to frontocentral paroxysmal discharges. The surface-positive component of the cortical discharge precedes activation of the orbicularis oculi by 4 ms, the masseter by 7 ms, the biceps by 8 ms, and the paraspinal muscles by 24 ms. These results are consistent with a pyramidal tract route of spread. Unit recordings indicate areas 4 and 6 of the cortex with the highest levels of activity.[35] Recordings from subcortical structures show that their involvement is always secondary to the cortical activation. A failure of intracortical recurrent inhibition seems to be responsible, at least in part, for these findings.[34]

Epileptic myoclonus has been recognized in several disease states not conventionally conceived of as part of the myoclonic syndromes. Cortical myoclonus has been reported in corticobasal degeneration (CBD),[36–38] Alzheimer's disease, Parkinson's disease,[39] Huntington's disease,[40] olivopontocerebellar atrophy,[41] progressive supranuclear palsy,[42] among others.

NONEPILEPTIC MYOCLONUS

Some myoclonic movements reflect normal physiological phenomena. One such phenomenon is the hypnic jerk experienced by all people at one time or another.[8]

Essential myoclonus is a term that is used for those patients whose sole neurological abnormality is myoclonus and who specifically do not have seizures, dementia, or ataxia.[8] The EEG and other laboratory investigations should be normal. Familial cases as well as sporadic cases are seen. Ballistic movement overflow myoclonus is one type of essential myoclonus that has been seen as an autosomal-dominant disorder.[8] The myoclonus is generalized, appears to occur seldom at rest, and is clearly induced by action. The EMG is characterized by the ballistic "triphasic" EMG pattern with alternating activity in antagonist muscles (although more tonic EMG patterns might also be seen).[43]

Palatal myoclonus, now preferentially called palatal tremor, is the prototypical rhythmic focal myoclonic disorder.[44–47] Palatal tremor has now been shown to consist of two separate disorders: essential palatal tremor (EPT), which manifests an ear click, and symptomatic palatal tremor (SPT), which is associated with cerebellar disturbances.[45–47] The palatal movements are consistent with activation of the tensor veli palatini muscle in EPT and of the levator veli palatini muscle in SPT.[47] Palatal movements, unilaterally or bilaterally, occur at 1.5–3 Hz and, in SPT, may be accompanied by synchronous movements of adjacent muscles, such as the external ocular muscles, tongue, larynx, face, neck, diaphragm, or even limb muscles. During sleep, EPT stops, whereas SPT continues, with only slight variations in the tremor rate. The palatal tremor cycle exerts remote effects on the tonic EMG activity of the upper and lower extremities only in patients with SPT. In SPT, cerebellar dysfunction ipsilateral to the palatal tremor may be a result in part of abnormal function of the contralateral hypertrophic inferior olive, but the pathophysiological basis of EPT remains unknown.[45–47] Focal movements of tongue or neck can occur without palatal movement and have been called bulbar myoclonus or branchial myoclonus.[44]

Spinal myoclonus is more commonly rhythmic than arrhythmic.[8,22] Involved regions can be one limb, one limb and adjacent trunk, or both legs. Lesions of the spinal cord giving rise to focal movements include infection, degenerative disease, tumor, cervical myelopathy, and demyelinating disease, and it may follow spinal anesthesia or the introduction of contrast media into the cerebrospinal fluid. Unlike palatal myoclonus, spinal myoclonus is only rarely idiopathic. Spinal myoclonus usually occurs spontaneously and may persist during sleep.

Another form of spinal myoclonus is propriospinal myoclonus.[48,49] This is clinically characterized by axial jerks that are nonrhythmic and that lead to symmetric flexion of neck, trunk, hips, and knees. Jerks can be spontaneous or stimulus-induced. By EMG studies, the myoclonus starts in the midthoracic region and propagates slowly, about 5 m/s, both rostrally and caudally.

Peripheral myoclonus has been reported, but it is not clear that this is always distinct from fasciculation or myokymia. Signs of acute or chronic denervation in the involved muscles characterize peripheral myoclonus. Cases have been reported with lesions of nerve, brachial plexus, and nerve root.[7,8]

Exaggerated startle is being increasingly recognized clinically as a form of myoclonus.[50,51] The normal startle consists of a quick muscular response to a surprise stimulus. An exaggerated startle consists of a response that is too large in magnitude, too widespread or too complex, but, most commonly, it is exaggerated because it appears when it is not expected to occur. For example, a normal startle response would not be expected when the stimulus is not a surprise, as normal human beings habituate fairly quickly to low-intensity or repeated stimuli. There has been considerable confusion in the literature as to which myoclonic phenomena are truly exaggerated startle reflexes. One source of confusion, for example, is stimulus-sensitive myoclonus, which might be difficult to distinguish purely on clinical grounds from exaggerated startle. Creutzfeldt-Jakob disease is commonly said to be characterized by an exaggerated startle, but the stimulus-induced response is a myoclonic jerk.[8,51] The normal features of the audiogenic startle response have been well characterized and enable proper recognition of this phenomenon.[52,53] There is a bilaterally symmetric pattern with an invariable blink; other craniocervical muscles almost always are activated, but recruitment in the limbs is variable. Onset latencies of EMG activity are 20–40 ms in the orbicularis oculi, 35–80 ms in masseter and sternocleidomastoid, 50–100 ms in biceps brachii, 100–125 ms in hamstrings and quadriceps, and 130–140 ms in tibialis anterior. The latency of the response in abductor pollicis brevis is much delayed, compared to what would be expected from the latency of the response in the biceps.[50,52] There is synchronous activation of antagonist muscles with an EMG burst duration of 50–400 ms, shortening with habituation. The response significantly habituates within a few trials.

Recent studies have shown that hyperekplexia or startle disease is characterized by a truly exaggerated startle.[50–52] Startle epilepsy is a disorder consisting of epilepsy after a startle. The interesting syndrome known by many names, including jumping or latah, appears also to be initiated with a startle, but its physiology has never been investigated in detail.

Nocturnal myoclonus includes several different phenomena, including the hypnic jerk, periodic movements in sleep, and excessive fragmentary myoclonus in non-rapid eye movement (NREM) sleep. Myoclonus associated with epilepsy, intention myoclonus associated with semivolitional movements, and segmental myoclonus also occur in sleep but are not primarily nocturnal.[8] Periodic movements of sleep are characterized by a pattern that is unmistakable. EMG bursts of tonic type, lasting 500–2000 ms (really out of the myoclonus range), come every 10–30 s, and are most prominent in the tibialis anterior muscles. The two sides of the body can be activated independently, simultaneously, or even alternately. They occur in NREM sleep but can occur also in drowsiness, when the patient can be fully conscious of their occurrence.[54]

These may be the result of disinhibition of spinal cord flexor reflexes.[55]

Myoclonus can also be psychogenic. Monday and Jankovic[56] reported on the clinical features of 18 such patients. The myoclonus was present for 1–110 months; it was segmental in 10 patients, generalized in 7 patients, and focal in 1 patient. Stress precipitated or exacerbated the myoclonic movements in 15 patients; 14 had a definite increase in myoclonic activity during periods of anxiety. The following findings helped to establish the psychogenic nature of the myoclonus: (1) clinical features incongruous with "organic" myoclonus, (2) evidence of underlying psychopathology, (3) an improvement with distraction or placebo, and (4) the presence of incongruous sensory loss or false weakness. More than one-half of all patients with adequate follow-up improved after gaining insight into the psychogenic mechanisms of their movement disorder. Physiological investigation in such cases is lacking. One single case report of a patient with a paroxysmal psychogenic movement disorder showed evidence of a "readiness" potential in relation to movement.[57]

Electrophysiological Evaluation of Myoclonus

POLYGRAPHIC EMG STUDIES

Because EMG is a direct measure of alpha motor neuron activity, it provides information about the central nervous system command that generates the movement. Numerous muscles act on each joint, and it is usually necessary to record from at least two muscles with antagonist actions. EMG is mainly used for the purpose of timing information and in most cases can be collected from surface electrodes.[6]

Inspection of the EMG signal of an involuntary movement reveals, first, whether the movement is regular (usually a tremor) or irregular. Irregular EMG activity will sometimes clinically appear rhythmic if it is rapid. The duration of the EMG burst correlating with an involuntary movement can be measured; specific ranges of duration are associated with different types of movements. Specification of duration in the range from 30 to 300 ms merely by clinical inspection is virtually impossible as a result of the relative slowness of the mechanical events, compared to that of the electrical events. Antagonist muscle relationships also can be specified as synchronous or asynchronous (reciprocal). In a tremor, asynchronous activity is described as alternating. It is important to keep in mind that some disorders of the peripheral nervous system can also give rise to involuntary movements. These include fasciculations, tetany, myokymia, and neuromyotonic discharges and, generally, they can be recognized with needle EMG.[7]

The polygraphic study of the EMG activity alone can provide useful information in classifying and understanding the pathophysiology of myoclonus. EMG bursts of brief duration (50 ms or less) are almost exclusively seen in epileptic myoclonus. Discharges approaching 150 ms are typical of nonepileptic myoclonus. Rapid movements with EMG bursts lasting between 150 and 300 ms are often seen as fragments of other movement disorders, such as dystonia. The time relation of activation of different muscles involved in a generalized twitch also provides information on the type of myoclonus. A rostrocaudal "wave" of activation, beginning with the uppermost motor cranial nerves and progressing in a descending fashion along the neuroaxis with a conduction velocity appropriate for the pyramidal tract, is typical of epileptic myoclonus originating in the cortex[23] (Fig. 40-2). A pattern of activation initiating with the sternocleidomastoid muscle and progressing with the activation of both rostrally and caudally innervated muscles is typical for reticular reflex myoclonus. Proximal muscles are most often involved in nonepileptic myoclonus. Synchronous activation of distal antagonist muscles is usually the rule in epileptic myoclonus.

The latency differences between homologous muscles in the upper and lower extremities and among muscles innervated by different segments along the neuroaxis may also provide insight into intracortical and transcallosal spread of activation[58,59] (Fig. 40-2).

ROUTINE ELECTROENCEPHALOGRAPHY (EEG)

The most common encounter of the neurologist with the electrophysiology of myoclonus occurs in the setting of studies involving a routine EEG, using additional EMG monitoring leads. A similar procedure is routinely used in polygraphic sleep recordings when sleep-related movement disorders are suspected. The presence of well-defined spike, spike-wave, or polyspike discharges in close association with the bursts of EMG activation may indicate an epileptic mechanism. Other encephalopathies not necessarily regarded as epileptic in nature may also show EEG events time-locked to myoclonus, as is the case in Creutzfeldt-Jakob disease.[60] In some patients, despite an obvious epileptic disorder, the routine EEG may not reveal a distinct abnormality associated with myoclonic movements. Many patients with epilepsia partialis continua may not have a distinct EEG/EMG correlation.[11,61,62] This may be related in part to the specific three-dimensional arrangement of the involved cortical ribbon generating tangential dipoles, or to involvement of a relatively small area of cortical area lacking the "critical mass" necessary to project an abnormality to the scalp with an amplitude discernible from the background EEG signal. Under these circumstances, back-averaging of EEG to the EMG burst may help identify the location and characteristics of EEG abnormalities related to the movements.

The EEG itself is also of value in the diagnosis and follow-up of patients with metabolic or degenerative forms of myoclonic disorders.[10,63] Occipital and rolandic spikes, as well as paroxysms of generalized spikes and polyspikes, are often seen in the setting of the syndrome of progressive myoclonic epilepsy.[10] Progressive deterioration of background rhythms parallels disease progression.[10,63]

EEG BACK-AVERAGING

Averaging of EEG activity time-locked to the onset of myoclonic EMG bursts, known as EEG back-averaging or "jerk-locked" averaging, is used to establish the presence, location, and characteristics of cortical activity that is correlated (time-locked) to the onset of the positive myoclonic event.[8,9,11,23] A similar averaging procedure but one that is time-locked to the onset of EMG silent periods can be applied to the study of negative myoclonus (silent period-locked averaging).[16,64,65] These techniques can be performed "on-line," using most conventional evoked potential equipment driving the triggering of an averager with a threshold trigger set to fire at myoclonic EMG burst onset. The sampled EEG epochs should include at least 100 ms of data before EMG onset. The exact number of averaged epochs may vary, depending on the signal-to-noise ratio. Most laboratories studying myoclonus electrophysiologically record the EEG and EMG data using magnetic or digital media and conduct the analysis "off-line." This offers the advantage of post hoc sorting of different myoclonic events and better control of artifact rejection. Multiple scalp and EMG leads are desirable. The use of back-averaging may not be necessary with patients whose clear-cut spikes time-locked to myoclonic EMG burst can be seen in the raw EEG. Even in this situation, however, back-averaging may provide more detailed information on the topography and components of the epileptiform paroxysms that best correlate with the myoclonic movements.[7]

A cortical participation in the genesis of myoclonus is indicated by the presence of a reproducible EEG potential that precedes the onset of the myoclonic EMG activity. The prototypical finding is the presence of a myoclonus-related cortical spike.[9,11,23] This is usually a positive-negative, biphasic sharp EEG potential time-locked to the myoclonus. In most cases, the spike is located over the central region contralateral to the upper extremity muscle used to drive the averaging when the myoclonus is focal or multifocal. The early positive peak of the spike precedes the EMG onset in upper extremity muscles by about 15–25 ms and for the lower extremity by about 40 ms[9] (Fig. 40-3). These latencies are compatible with the corticospinal conduction times for the hand and foot muscles, respectively. Other patterns of myoclonus-related EEG activity have been described. These include monophasic and triphasic EEG potentials, or even more complex sets of wavelets time-locked to the myoclonus.[14]

The discharge is maximal over the vertex when myoclonus is recorded from the lower extremities, in keeping with the homuncular organization of the motor cortex. When the myoclonic movements are generalized or bilaterally synchronous, the EEG discharge is widespread with a vertex maximum.[14] In some patients with cortical myoclonus, the initial cortical discharge, spontaneous or reflex, spreads to adjacent motor cortical areas or to homologous areas in the other hemisphere. A high degree of spread characterizes subjects with a tendency to experience generalized myoclonic twitches and frequent seizures.[58] Increased coherency between EEG and EMG activity in patients with epileptic

A

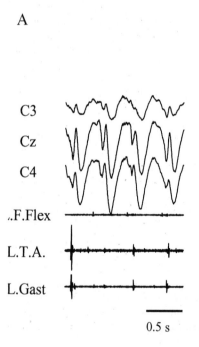

C3
Cz
C4
..F.Flex
L.T.A.
L.Gast

0.5 s

B

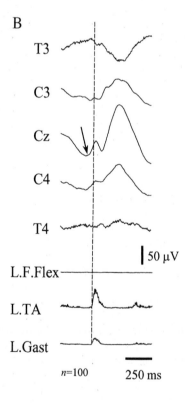

T3
C3
Cz
C4
T4

| 50 μV

L.F.Flex
L.TA
L.Gast

n=100   250 ms

FIGURE 40-3 (*A*) Polygraphic EEG and EMG recording in a patient with epilepsia partialis continua manifested as irregular twitching of the left leg and nearly continuous spike/wave discharges over the right central and vertex area. (*B*) Back-averaging of 100 EEG epochs aligned to the onset of myoclonic twitches of the left tibialis anterior muscle (L.TA). Compared to the raw recordings, a much more discrete surface positive potential emerges over the vertex area (indicated by the arrow) with a latency of 40 ms preceding the EMG twitches. Recording of the left gastrocnemius muscle (L. Gast.) shows a synchronous activation to that of the L.TA muscle. Abnormal myoclonic activity did not spread to the left finger flexors (L.F. Flex).

myoclonus indicates an abnormally enhanced coupling of motor cortical neurons and spinal motor neurons, most likely as a result of deficient inhibition.[59]

SOMATOSENSORY EVOKED POTENTIALS (SEPs)

Since Dawson's initial observations in 1947,[5] it is well known that a subgroup of patients with myoclonus have a grossly enhanced SEP amplitude.[9,19,25] "Giant SEP" is the term generally used to describe this abnormality in patients with cortical myoclonus.[9] Giant SEPs deviate from normal SEPs not only in their amplitude but also in the distortion of the waveform components (Fig. 40-1). The waveform morphology in giant SEPs is usually "simplified" into three large amplitude peaks. Naming the waveforms according to their polarity and sequence (N1, P1, N2, etc.), rather than according to the more conventional terminology (N20, P25/P30, N35, etc.) is favored by some authors.[19] When labeled by its polarity, the N1 component is usually normal in amplitude and has a latency comparable to that of the N20 component of regular SEPs. In contrast, the P1 and N2 components are enlarged in magnitude and usually are delayed, when compared to those of normal SEPs.[9,19] A N1/P1 or a P1/N2 amplitude greater than 10 μV and measured at the contralateral central region in ear-referenced recordings is considered a giant response.[9] In many patients, giant SEPs resemble typical spike-wave paroxysms (Figs. 40-1 and 40-4). Giant SEPs are often associated with a reflex myoclonic jerk at a latency of approximately 45 ms in hand muscles after median nerve stimulation (C-reflex).[9,19,66,67] The concomitant presence of these two is the hallmark of sensory-reflex cortical myoclonus. The striking resemblance in latency and morphology of the giant SEP-C-reflex complex to the myoclonus-related cortical spike suggests that both originate from common cortical mechanisms.[9,19,23]

The generator of the giant SEP resides in, or in close proximity to, the central sulcus.[25,26,68,69] Because the subcortical components and the first cortical component (N1) are usually normal in amplitude, it can be suggested that an abnormality in intracortical inhibition after the arrival of the first volley of thalamocortical activity might be responsible for the abnormal activation of surrounding cortex which, in turn, leads to enlargement of both the giant SEP responses and activation of descending motor outputs leading to the C-reflex.[9,19]

The use of paired somatosensory stimuli at variable intervals has been used to trace the excitability cycle of the sensorimotor cortex in cortical myoclonus.[70,71] Patients with cortical myoclonus tend to show a "triphasic" cycle of initial depression of cortical excitability, followed within 20–80 ms by a period of increased excitability and a subsequent period of depression with recovery of the baseline excitability after 300 ms.[71] There is evidence suggesting that this cycle may be heavily weighted towards inhibition in patients presenting with epileptic negative myoclonus.[72]

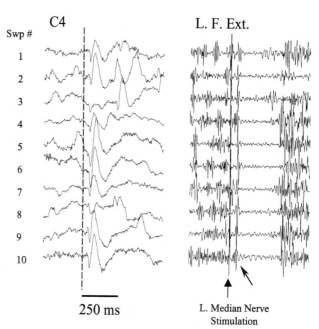

FIGURE 40-4 Ten epochs of EEG activity recorded from the right central region (C4) and surface EMG activity recorded from the left finger extensor muscles (L. F. Ext.) in a patient with sensory-reflex asterixis. The patient has been asked to hold her hands outstretched in the air against gravity while the left median nerve was electrically stimulated at motor threshold at 0.2-Hz frequency. Epochs were aligned to electrical stimulation. Electrical stimulation produces in most epochs a large-amplitude response (giant SEP), which resembles an epileptic spike. Median nerve stimulation induces a brief myoclonic burst consistent with a C-reflex (oblique arrow) followed by a 250–300-ms period of EMG suppression clinically associated with a postural lapse typical for asterixis.

REFLEX STUDIES

In some patients with myoclonus, certain types of stimulation will produce a reflex response that is not present in normal subjects. This was named the C-reflex by Sutton and Mayer,[66] who thought it was the result of an abnormal cortically mediated reflex. The latency of the C-reflex in upper extremity muscles is approximately 36–50 ms after the stimulus given to the hand and 60–70 ms when the reflex is elicited and recorded in lower extremities. These latencies are about twice those of the first cortical component of the SEPs (18–25 ms in upper limb and 30–35 ms in lower limb)[9] (Fig. 40-1). In cases of cortical reflex myoclonus, the C-reflex is the result of abnormal activity in a cortical loop. This loop would involve fast-conducting tracts up to the sensory cortex, using the posterior column, lemniscal, and thalamocortical pathways. The events in the cortex that lead to large SEPs may in parallel activate the motor cortex via corticocortical connections, generating a rapid descending discharge to the anterior horn motor neurons. In rare patients, the reflex may only occur in response to cutaneous stimuli, whereas in others it occurs in response only to passive stretch.[66,67] A direct relationship is most often seen between the amplitude of the giant SEP and the presence of a reflex myoclonic jerk.[19] These two events, however, appear to be differentially affected by pharmacological interventions such as lisuride or clonazepam.[19]

Care should be exerted not to confuse the C-reflex with normal reflex EMG responses. For example, electrical stimulation of a mixed nerve gives rise to an F-wave. In normal individuals, some degree of voluntary activation of the recorded muscle results in several responses after the direct muscle response.[73] There are also late responses after stimulation of a cutaneous nerve when the recorded muscle is not at rest. One of these responses, the E2 response, is mediated via a long-loop pathway. The use of the reflex responses to differentiate different types of myoclonus has been demonstrated by Chen et al.[74] They studied the responses to cutaneous stimulation in patients with Parkinson's disease and other akinetic-rigid syndromes. In patients with myoclonus in the setting of Parkinson's disease or multiple-system atrophy, there was facilitation of the E2 component of the response. In patients with corticobasal degeneration, there was a response at a shorter latency than E2.[36,38,74] The pathways for these responses are not completely clear, but they do differ, and the physiological test can be used clinically for differential diagnosis.[36,38,74]

TRANSCRANIAL MAGNETIC STIMULATION (TMS)

Motor thresholds to magnetic stimulation are low in those myoclonic patients with a tendency to experience generalized twitches and seizures and are high, even higher than in normal subjects, in those with only focal twitches.[75] Cortical excitability is also enhanced in cortical myoclonus when TMS is presented with a concomitant somatosensory stimulus.[75,76] After TMS there is a brief period of cortical inhibition in which the cortex is relatively refractory to a second stimulus. In normal subjects, this phenomenon relies on intact intracortical inhibition. The recovery of cortical excitability can be probed with the use of pairs of cortical stimuli, and it has been shown to be abnormally modulated in patients with cortical myoclonus as a result of abnormal intracortical inhibition.[75,76] Patients with cortical myoclonus and the tendency to have generalized and multifocal twitches and frequent seizures exhibit a deficient intra- and transcortical inhibition to paired stimuli[75] and a tendency for spread of their cortical EEG discharges.[58]

MAGNETOENCEPHALOGRAPHY (MEG)

Magnetoencephalography (MEG) offers several advantages over conventional EEG recordings in the study of myoclonus. MEG recordings are "reference-independent," and are clear of the troublesome "smearing" effect of the skull and scalp on electrical fields. These factors simplify the process of localizing the neuronal sources implicated in the generation of cortical myoclonus. Furthermore, MEG information complements information derived from EEG recordings, as neuronal populations producing electrical fields oriented parallel to the surface of the scalp, typically under-represented in the surface EEG recordings, are better represented in MEG recordings.

MEG has proven valuable in pinpointing the critical role of the motor cortex in the generation of the giant SEP response in cortical myoclonus.[77] It may further clarify the contribution of other cortical generators to myoclonic phenomena.[77–79] Magnetic rhythmic oscillations over the motor cortex exhibit distinctly abnormal reactivity to stimulation,[80,81] and reproduce the EEG finding of marked level of coherency with EMG activity indicative of impaired inhibitory mechanisms.[59,82]

Negative Myoclonus

Asterixis, a form of negative myoclonus, was the name given to brief postural lapses associated with cessation of tonic EMG activity. Asterixis was first described by Adams and Foley[83] in patients with hepatic encephalopathy, but it is known now to represent a nonspecific neurological finding associated with multiple forms of toxic and metabolic encephalophathies. Asterixis has been reported to arise from subcortical and brainstem lesions,[15] but physiological studies in these cases are lacking. EEG abnormalities similar to those of epileptic cortical myoclonus can also present in the setting of negative myoclonus. In fact, positive and negative myoclonus often coexist. The classification scheme and the electrophysiological methods proposed for positive myoclonus can be identically applied to negative myoclonus.

Ugawa et al.[64,84] have evaluated the EEG correlates of asterixis, using the silent period-locked averaging technique in patients with well-defined postural lapses associated with EMG silent periods. The silent periods in these patients were classified in two forms. In type I, silent periods were associated with a complete cessation of background EMG activity, lasting for 50–100 ms. The second form, type II, was characterized by a primarily negative event that was associated with a brief and discrete but definite burst of EMG activity that occurred before the silence. Only type II silent periods were preceded by well-defined EEG discharges. The discharges were localized to the contralateral central regions and preceded the event by 20–30 ms. Similar findings have been reported in other patients.[16,64]

Epileptiform discharges preceding negative myoclonus have been reported in children with epilepsy.[85–87] The presenting symptoms in these patients were tremulousness or postural lapses of tonically activated muscles and rare convulsions. The EEG showed focal epileptiform discharges on average 30–50 ms before the onset of the EMG silence. It remains undetermined as to when the EEG discharge of positive and negative myoclonus is consistently different. Giant SEPs are variably present in patients with negative myoclonus. The recovery curve of SEP amplitude to paired somatosensory stimuli in patients with epileptic negative myoclonus shows a more prominent inhibition, compared to that of patients with positive myoclonus.[72]

The C-reflex elicited by electrical stimulation of the median nerve is sometimes present in patients with negative myoclonus. Rare patients may show negative myoclonus in response to sensory stimulation (sensory-reflex asterixis)[16,72] (Fig. 40-4).

It can be postulated that epileptic negative and positive myoclonus are parts of the same phenomenon. During the abnormal cortical discharge, positive and negative influences on motor activity are generated. These influences may differ in their time of maximal expression, threshold for clinical manifestation, their time course, pathways of spread, their sensitivity to medications, and sensitivity to different physiological states such as sleep-wake cycles and fatigue.[16]

Negative myoclonus of subcortical origin may have a completely different pathophysiology. Type I silent periods, without an EEG correlate, may originate primarily from subcortical structures. The high coexistence of type I and type II silent periods in the same patient population may indicate that important cortical-subcortical interactions are operative in the genesis of negative myoclonus.[16]

References

1. Gibbs FA, Davis H, Lennox WG: The electro-encephalogram in epilepsy and in conditions of impaired conciousness. *Arch Neurol Psychiatry* 34:1133–1148, 1935.

2. Grinker RR, Serota H, Stein SI: Myoclonic epilepsy. *Arch Neurol Psychiatry* 40:968–980, 1938.

3. Dawson GD: The relation between the electroencephalogram and muscle action potentials in certain convulsive states. *J Neurol Neurosurg Psychiatry* 9:5–22, 1946.

4. Dawson GD: Cerebral responses to electrical stimulation of peripheral nerve in man. *J Neurol Neurosurg Psychiatry* 10:134–140, 1947.

5. Dawson GD: Investigations on a patient subject to myoclonic seizures after sensory stimulation. *J Neurol Neurosurg Psychiatry* 10:141–162, 1947.

6. Hallett M: Analysis of abnormal voluntary and involuntary movements with surface electromyography, in Desmedt JE (ed): *Motor Control Mechanisms in Health and Disease.* New York: Raven Press, 1983, pp 907–914.

7. Hallett M: Electrophysiologic evaluation of movement disorders, in Aminoff MJ (ed): *Electrodiagnosis in Clinical Neurology,* 3rd ed. New York: Churchill Livingstone, 1992, pp 403–419.

8. Marsden CD, Hallett M, Fahn S: The nosology and pathophysiology of myoclonus, in Marsden CD, Fahn S (eds): *Neurology 2: Movement Disorders.* London: Butterworths, 1982, pp 196–248.

9. Shibasaki H, Yamashita Y, Kuroiwa Y: Electroencephalographic studies of myoclonus: Myoclonus-related cortical spikes in progressive myoclonic epilepsy. *Brain* 108:225–240, 1978.

10. So N, Berkovic S, Andermann F, et al: Myoclonus epilepsy and ragged red fibres (MERRF). 2. Electrophysiological studies and comparison with other progressive myoclonus epilepsies. *Brain* 112:1261–1276, 1989.

11. Obeso JA, Rothwell JC, Marsden CD: The spectrum of cortical myoclonus. *Brain* 108:193–224, 1985.

12. Hallett M, Topka H: Myoclonus (Chapter 85). In: Brandt T, Caplan LR, Dichgans J, Diener HC, Kennard C (eds). *Neurological Disorders: Course and Treatment,* Second Edition, Academic Press, San Diego, 2003, pp. 1221–1231.

13. Lance JW, Adams RD: The syndrome of intention or action myoclonus as a sequel to hypoxic encephalopathy. *Brain* 86:111–136, 1963.

14. Toro C, Pascual-Leone A, Deuschl G, et al: Cortical tremor: A common manifestation of cortical myoclonus. *Neurology* 43:2346–2353, 1993.

15. Shahani BT, Young RR: Asterixis: A disorder of the neural mechanisms underlying sustained muscle contraction, in Shahani M (ed): *The Motor System: Neurophysiological and Muscle Mechanisms.* Amsterdam: Elsevier, 1976, pp 301–306.

16. Toro C, Hallett M, Rothwell JC, et al: Physiology of negative myoclonus, in Fahn S, Hallett M, Luders HO, Marsden CD (eds): *Negative Motor Phenomena.* New York: Raven Press, 1995, pp 211–217.

17. Brown P, Steiger MJ, Thompson PD, et al: Effectiveness of piracetam in cortical myoclonus. *Mov Disord* 8:63–68, 1993.

18. Chadwick D, Hallett M, Harris R, et al: Clinical, biochemical and physiologic features distinguishing myoclonus responsive to 5-hydroxytryptophan, tryptophan with monoamine oxidase inhibitor and clonazepam. *Brain* 100:455–487, 1977.

19. Rothwell JC, Obeso JA, Marsden CD: On the significance of giant somatosensory evoked potentials in cortical myoclonus. *J Neurol Neurosurg Psychiatry* 47:33–42, 1984.

20. Garvey MA, Toro C, Goldstein S, et al: Somatosensory evoked potentials as a marker of disease burden in type 3 Gaucher disease. *Neurology* 56:391–394, 2001.

21. Liepert J, Haueisen J, Hegemann S, et al: Disinhibition of somatosensory and motor cortex in mitochondriopathy without myoclonus. *Clin Neurophysiol* 112:917–922, 2001.

22. Halliday AM: The electrophysiological study of myoclonus in man. *Brain* 90:241–284, 1967.

23. Hallett M, Chadwick D, Marsden CD: Cortical reflex myoclonus. *Neurology* 29:1107–1125, 1979.

24. Hallett M: Myoclonus: Relation to epilepsy. *Epilepsia* 26 (suppl):s67–s77, 1985.

25. Shibasaki H, Yamashita Y, Neshige R, et al: Pathogenesis of giant somatosensory evoked potentials in progressive myoclonic epilepsy. *Brain* 108:225–240, 1985.

26. Shibasaki H, Kakigi R, Ikeda A: Scalp topography of giant SEP and pre-myoclonus spike in cortical reflex myoclonus. *Electroencephalogr Clin Neurophysiol* 81:31–37, 1991.

27. Hallett M, Chadwick D, Adam J, Marsden CD: Reticular reflex myoclonus: A physiological type of human post-hypoxic myoclonus. *J Neurol Neurosurg Psychiatry* 40:253–264, 1977.

28. Chadwick D, French AT: Uraemic myoclonus: An example of reticular reflex myoclonus? *J Neurol Neurosurg Psychiatry* 42:52–55, 1979.

29. Zuckerman EG, Glasser GH: Urea-induced myoclonic seizures. *Arch Neurol* 27:14–28, 1972.

30. Thompson PD, Maertens de Noordhout A, Day BL, et al: Clinical and electrophysiological observations in post-anoxic myoclonus, in Crossman AR, Sambrook MA (eds): *Current Problems in Neurology 9: Neuronal Mechanisms in Disorders of Movement.* London: John Libbey, 1989, pp 375–381.

31. Wilkins DE, Hallett M, Erba G: Primary generalized epileptic myoclonus: A frequent manifestation of minipolymyoclonus of central origin. *J Neurol Neurosurg Psychiatry* 48:506–516, 1985.

32. Artieda J, Obeso JA: The pathophysiology and pharmacology of photic cortical reflex myoclonus. *Ann Neurol* 34:175–184, 1993.

33. Brailowsky S: Myoclonus in *Papio papio. Mov Disord* 6:98–104, 1991.

34. Naquet R, Meldrum BS: Myoclonus induced by intermittent light stimulation in the baboon: Neurophysiological and neuropharmacological approaches. *Adv Neurol* 43:611–627, 1986.

35. Fischer-Williams M, Poncet M, Riche D, Naquet R: Light induced epilepsy in the baboon *Papio papio*: Cortical and depth recordings. *Electroencephalogr Clin Neurophysiol* 25:557–569, 1968.

36. Thomson PD, Day BL, Rothwell JC, et al: The myoclonus in corticobasal degeneration: Evidence for two forms of cortical reflex myoclonus. *Brain* 117:1197–1207, 1994.

37. Brunt ER, van Weerden TW, Pruim J, Lakke JW: Unique myoclonic pattern in corticobasal degeneration. *Mov Disord* 10:132–142, 1995.

38. Lu CS, Ikeda A, Terada K, et al: Electrophysiological studies of early stage corticobasal degeneration. *Mov Disord* 13:140–146, 1998.

39. Caviness JN, Adler CH, Beach TG, et al: Small-amplitude cortical myoclonus in Parkinson's disease: Physiology and clinical observations. *Mov Disord* 17:657–662, 2002.

40. Caviness JN, Kurth M: Cortical myoclonus in Huntington's disease associated with an enlarged somatosensory evoked potential. *Mov Disord* 12:1046–1051, 1997.

41. Rodriguez ME, Artieda J, Zubieta JL, et al: Reflex myoclonus in olivopontocerebellar atrophy. *J Neurol Neurosurg Psychiatry* 57:316–319, 1994.

42. Kofler M, Muller J, Reggiani L, et al: Somatosensory evoked potentials in progressive supranuclear palsy. *J Neurol Sci* 179(S1–2):85–91, 2000.

43. Hallett M, Chadwick D, Marsden CD: Ballistic movement overflow myoclonus. *Brain* 100:299–312, 1977.

44. Dubinsky RM, Hallett M: Palatal myoclonus and facial involvement in other types of myoclonus. *Adv Neurol* 49:263–278, 1988.

45. Deuschl G, Mischke G, Schenck E, et al: Symptomatic and essential rhythmic palatal myoclonus. *Brain* 113:1645–1672, 1990.

46. Deuschl G, Toro C, Valls-Sole J, et al: Symptomatic and essential palatal tremor. 1. Clinical, physiological, and MRI analysis. *Brain* 117:775–788, 1994.

47. Deuschl G, Toro C, Hallett M: Symptomatic and essential palatal tremor. 2. Differences in palatal movements. *Mov Disord* 9:676–678, 1994.

48. Brown P, Thompson PD, Rothwell JC, et al: Axial myoclonus of propriospinal origin. *Brain* 114:197–214, 1991.

49. Chokroverty S, Walters A, Zimmerman T, Picone M: Propriospinal myoclonus: A neurophysiologic analysis. *Neurology* 42:1591–1595, 1992.

50. Brown P, Rothwell JC, Thompson PD, et al: The hyperekplexias and their relationship to the normal startle reflex. *Brain* 114:1903–1928, 1991.

51. Thompson PD, Colebatch JG, Brown P, et al: Voluntary stimulus sensitive jerks and jumps mimicking myoclonus or pathological startle syndromes. *Mov Disord* 7:257–262, 1992.

52. Matsumoto J, Fuhr P, Nigro M, Hallett M: Physiological abnormalities in hereditary hyperekplexia. *Ann Neurol* 32:41–50, 1992.

53. Wilkins DE, Hallett M, Wess MM: Audiogenic startle reflex of man and its relationship to startle syndromes: A review. *Brain* 109:561–573, 1986.

54. Hening WA, Walters AS, Chokroverty S: Movement disorders and sleep, in Chokroverty S (ed): *Movement Disorders*. Great Neck, NY: PMA Publishing, 1990, pp 127–157.

55. Bara-Jimenez W, Aksu M, Graham B, et al: Periodic limb movements in sleep: State-dependent excitability of the spinal flexor reflex. *Neurology* 54:1609–1616, 2000.

56. Monday K, Jankovic J: Psychogenic myoclonus. *Neurology* 43:349–352, 1993.

57. Toro C, Torres F: Electrophysiological correlates of a paroxysmal movement disorder. *Ann Neurol* 20:731–734, 1986.

58. Brown P, Day BL, Rothwell JC, et al: Interhemispheric and intrahemispheric spread of cerebral cortical myoclonic activity and its relevance to epilepsy. *Brain* 114:2333–2352, 1991.

59. Brown P, Farmer SF, Halliday DM, et al: Coherent cortical and muscle discharge in cortical myoclonus. *Brain* 122:461–472, 1999.

60. Shibasaki H, Motomura S, Yamashita Y, et al: Periodic synchronous discharge and myoclonus in Creutzfeldt-Jacob disease: Diagnostic application of jerk-locked averaging method. *Ann Neurol* 9:150–156, 1981.

61. Kugelberg E, Widen L: Epilepsia partialis continua. *Electroencephalogr Clin Neurophysiol* 6:503–506, 1954.

62. Thomas JE, Reagan TJ, Klass DW: Epilepsia partialis continua: A review of 32 cases. *Arch Neurol* 34:266–275, 1977.

63. Reese K, Toro C, Malow B, Sato S: Progression of the EEG in Lafora-body disease. *Am J EEG Tech* 33:229–235, 1993.

64. Ugawa Y, Shimpo T, Mannen T: Physiological analysis of asterixis: Silent period locked averaging. *J Neurol Neurosurg Psychiatry* 52:89–93, 1989.

65. Artieda J, Muruzabal J, Larumbe R, et al: Cortical mechanisms mediating asterixis. *Mov Disord* 7:209–216, 1992.

66. Sutton GG, Mayer RF: Focal reflex myoclonus. *J Neurol Neurosurg Psychiatry* 37:207–217, 1974.

67. Sutton GG: Receptors in focal reflex myoclonus. *J Neurol Neurosurg Psychiatry* 38:505–507, 1975.

68. Cowan JMA, Rothwell JC, Wise RJS, Marsden CD: Electrophysiological and positron emission studies in a patient with cortical myoclonus, epilepsia partialis continua and motor epilepsy. *J Neurol Neurosurg Psychiatry* 49:796–807, 1986.

69. Kakigi R, Shibasaki H: Generator mechanisms of giant somatosensory evoked potentials in cortical reflex myoclonus. *Brain* 110:1359–1373, 1987.

70. Shibasaki H, Neshige R, Hashiba Y: Cortical excitability after myoclonus: Jerk-locked somatosensory evoked potentials. *Neurology* 35:36–41, 1985.

71. Ugawa Y, Gemba K, Shimpo T, Mannen T: Somatosensory evoked potential recovery (SEP-R) in myoclonic patients. *Electroencephalogr Clin Neurophysiol* 80:21–25, 1991.

72. Shibasaki H, Ikeda A, Nagamine T, et al: Cortical reflex negative myoclonus. *Brain* 117:477–486, 1994.

73. Deuschl G, Lucking CH: Physiological and clinical application of hand muscle reflexes, in Rossini PM, Mauguiere F (eds): *New Trends and Advanced Techniques in Clinical Neurophysiology*. Amsterdam: Elsevier, 1990, pp 84–101.

74. Chen R, Ashby P, Lang AE: Stimulus-sensitive myoclonus in akinetic-rigid syndromes. *Brain* 115:1875–1888, 1992.

75. Reutens DC, Puce A, Berkovic SF: Cortical hyperexcitability in progressive myoclonic epilepsy: A study with transcranial magnetic stimulation. *Neurology* 43:186–192, 1993.

76. Manganotti P, Tamburin S, Zanette G, et al: Hyperexcitable cortical responses in progressive myoclonic epilepsy: A TMS study. *Neurology* 57:1793–1799, 2001.

77. Mima T, Nagamine T, Ikeda A, et al: Pathogenesis of cortical myoclonus studied by magnetoencephalopathy. *Ann Neurol* 43:598–607, 1998.

78. Mima T, Nagamine T, Nishitani N, et al: Cortical myoclonus: sensorimotor hyperexcitability. *Neurology* 50:933–942, 1998.

79. Uesaka Y, Terao Y, Ugawa Y, et al: Magnetoencephalographic analysis of cortical myoclonic jerks. *Electroencephalogr Clin Neurophysiol* 99:141–148, 1996.

80. Silen T, Forss N, Jensen O, et al: Abnormal reactivity of the approximately 20-Hz motor cortex rhythm in Unverricht Lundborg type progressive myoclonus epilepsy. *Neuroimage* 12:707–712, 2000.

81. Karhu J, Hari R, Paetau R, et al: Cortical reactivity in progressive myoclonus epilepsy. *Electroencephalogr Clin Neurophysiol* 90:93–102, 1994.

82. Silen T, Forss N, Salenius S, et al: Oscillatory cortical drive to isometrically contracting muscle in Unverricht-Lundborg type progressive myoclonus epilepsy (ULD). *Clin Neurophysiol* 113:1973–1979, 2002.

83. Adams RD, Foley JM: The neurological changes in the more common types of severe liver disease. *Trans Neurol Assoc* 74:217–219, 1949.

84. Ugawa Y, Genba K, Shimpo T, Mannen T: Onset and offset of electromyographic (EMG) silence in asterixis. *J Neurol Neurosurg Psychiatry* 53:260–262, 1990.

85. Cirignotta F, Lugaresi E: Partial motor epilepsy with "negative myoclonus". *Epilepsia* 32:54–58, 1991.

86. Guerrini R, Dravet C, Genton P, et al: Epileptic negative myoclonus. *Neurology* 43:1078–1083, 1993.

87. Takanori Y, Tsukagoshi H: Cortical activity-associated negative myoclonus. *J Neural Sci* 111:77–81, 1992.

VI. TIC DISORDERS

TOURETTE'S SYNDROME

ROGER KURLAN

CLINICAL FEATURES   685
    The Tic Disorder   685
    Behavioral Features   686
NATURAL COURSE   686
EPIDEMIOLOGY   687
DIFFERENTIAL DIAGNOSIS   687
    Distinguishing Tics from Other Movement
        Disorders   687
    Primary and Secondary Tic Disorders   688
ETIOLOGY/PATHOGENESIS   689
    Genetics   689
    Neurobiology   689
THERAPY   689
    Treatment of Tics   689
    Treatment of Attention Deficit Hyperactivity
        Disorder (ADHD)   690
    Treatment of Obsessive-Compulsive
        Disorder (OCD)   690
    Non-Medication Therapies   690

In his now famous publication of 1885 where he described the illness that now bears his name, George Gilles de la Tourette reported 9 patients with motor and vocal tics some of whom had echophenomena and coprolalia. Since that time, Tourette's syndrome (TS) has been generally viewed as a rare, severe, and disabling condition with bizarre symptoms and an unknown etiology. However, notions concerning TS and related disorders have undergone a dramatic evolution in recent years[1] and will serve as the focus for this chapter.

Clinical Features

The fourth (1994) version of the *Diagnostic and Statistical Manual of Psychiatry (DSM-IV)* lists the following diagnostic criteria for TS:[2]

1. Both multiple motor and one or more vocal tics have been present at some time during the illness, although not necessarily concurrently.
2. The tics occur many times a day (usually in bouts) nearly every day or intermittently throughout a period of more than 1 year, and during this period there was never a tic-free period of more than 3 consecutive months.
3. The disturbance causes marked distress or significant impairment in social, occupational, or other important areas of functioning.
4. The onset is before age 18 years.
5. The disturbance is not due to the direct physiological effects of a substance (e.g., stimulants) or a general medical condition (e.g., Huntington's disease or postviral encephalitis).

The formulation of such criteria, however, fails to convey the very heterogeneous clinical characteristics of the condition. The clinical manifestations of TS can best be viewed as a spectrum that includes both tics and associated behavioral features (Table 41-1).

THE TIC DISORDER

Tics are recurrent, nonrhythmic, stereotyped movements (motor tics) or sounds produced by moving air through the nose, mouth, or throat (vocal tics).[3] In contrast to most other types of involuntary movements, tics are not constantly present (except when extremely severe) and occur out of a background of normal motor activity. Motor and vocal tics may take a variety of forms and can be divided conceptually into simple and complex types. Simple motor tics are sudden, brief, isolated movements such as an eye blink, a shoulder shrug or a head jerk. Although most simple motor tics are fast and abrupt, some may appear as slower, sustained, tonic movements (e.g., neck twisting, abdominal or buttock tightening) that resemble dystonia and are therefore termed "dystonic tics."[4] Complex motor tics consist of more coordinated and complicated movements that may appear purposeful, as if performing a voluntary motor act. Examples include touching, smelling, jumping, copropraxia (obscene gestures), and echopraxia (mimicking movements performed by others). Motor tics usually recur in the same part of the

TABLE 41-1 Clinical Heterogeneity of TS

I. The Tic Disorder
  A. Tic types
    1. Simple motor tics
    2. Simple vocal tics
    3. Complex motor tics
    4. Complex vocal tics
    5. Tic variants
      a. Dystonic tics
      b. Sensory tics
  B. Primary tic disorder syndromes
    1. Tourette's syndrome
    2. Chronic tic disorder (motor or vocal)
    3. Transient tic disorder
  C. Tic severity
II. The Behavioral Disorder
  A. Obsessive-compulsive behavior
  B. Attention deficit hyperactivity disorder
  C. Anxiety disorders
  D. Other behavioral disturbances

body and multiple body regions can be involved. Over time, tics often recede from one body part and evolve elsewhere.

Simple vocal tics include a variety of inarticulate noises and sounds, such as throat clearing, sniffling and grunting. Complex vocal tics have linguistic meaning and consist of full or truncated words, such as echolalia (repeating the words of others), palilalia (repeating the individual's own words), and coprolalia (obscene words). Although coprolalia has been the symptom perhaps most responsible for the public notoriety of TS, the presence of this symptom is certainly not required for diagnosis. It is now clear that this symptom may be mild and transient, and occurs in only a minority of cases. Some patients experience the obscene words only internally in thought (mental coprolalia).

Tics may manifest themselves by virtually any body movement or noise. Thus, the tic disorder of TS represents a wide spectrum of involuntary movements and noises, some of which may appear quite bizarre (e.g., throwing objects, pulling down pants) and be misinterpreted as manifestations of psychological illness.

The patient often experiences an irresistible urge to tic. This urge can usually be suppressed temporarily, but at the expense of a build-up of psychic tension which can be relieved only by the production of a tic. Recent attention has focused on sensory symptoms that may occur in TS. "Sensory tics" are patterns of uncomfortable somatic sensations, such as pressure, tickle or warmth, that are localized to specific body regions, such as face, shoulder or neck.[5,6] Patients attempt to relieve the uncomfortable sensations with movements often interpreted as voluntary, usually tonic tightening or stretching of muscles indicative of a dystonic tic. Relief is temporary, however, and the movements are repeated. Some patients produce vocalizations that are responses to a sensory stimulus in the larynx or throat. Sensory tics, reported by about 40 percent of surveyed TS patients, may be the most prominent feature of illness for some patients and are often misdiagnosed.

The motor and vocal tics of TS characteristically follow a waxing and waning pattern, such that there are periods lasting days or weeks during which tics worsen, followed by other periods during which tics are less severe. The tics also characteristically occur in "waves," with a certain combination of tic types being present, only to eventually resolve and be replaced by another group of tics.

BEHAVIORAL FEATURES

Although chronic, multiple motor and vocal tics are usually the most prominent clinical features of TS and represent the signs upon which the diagnosis of the disorder is currently based, tics may also be accompanied by a variety of behavioral disturbances. Studies have demonstrated a high incidence of obsessive-compulsive disorder (OCD), generally about 50 percent, in TS patients.[7–9] Common examples of such symptoms include compulsive checking, counting and perfectionism, and obsessive worries or fears. About half of

patients with TS will also show evidence of attention deficit hyperactivity disorder (ADHD), manifested by inattention, distractibility, impulsivity, and hyperactivity.[10] TS has been reported to have a close clinical association with a variety of other behavioral disturbances, including anxiety disorders, conduct disorder, depression, mania, stuttering, obesity, and alcoholism.[11] At present, however, the full spectrum of the TS behavioral disorder has not been accurately delineated and remains an area of controversy.[12–14]

A number of distinctive personality traits, such as argumentativeness, defensiveness, negativism, and impulsiveness, are seen commonly among TS patients. It is unclear whether these behavioral traits are specific for TS, reflect associated behavioral disorders (e.g., ADHD), or result from the peculiar social and emotional difficulties associated with living with the illness. Disturbed interpersonal relationships with parents, siblings, peers, teachers, and others may underlie some of the observed problems.

Self-injurious behavior occurs occasionally in patients with TS.[15] This type of behavior has been linked to high levels of obsessionality and hostility. Other socially inappropriate behavior may accompany TS, such as verbalizing insults and other derogatory remarks or destroying personal property.[16] Such behavior may have a substantial functional impact on patients with TS and may contribute to social difficulties and isolation.

It is not uncommon to encounter difficulties with reading, writing, and arithmetic, including specific learning disabilities, in children with TS.[17] Patients with TS usually have normal intelligence, as their IQ distribution parallels that of the general population.[18]

Natural Course

The onset of tics occurs between the ages of 2 and 15 years in most cases, with the mean age at onset being 7 years.[19] The initial tics usually occur in the upper body, commonly involving the eyes (e.g., eye blinking) or other parts of the face. Vocal tics represent the initial manifestation of illness for a minority of patients.

Over the short term, tics characteristically change in type and wax and wane in severity. The longer-term, lifelong course of the TS tic disorder has been investigated in several studies. Erenberg found that 73 percent of adult TS subjects reported that over a period of years their tics had either lessened considerably or almost disappeared.[20] Bruun followed 136 TS patients from 5 to 15 years and found that tic severity lessened over time, with 59 percent rated mild-moderate initially and 91 percent rated so at follow-up.[21] Over time, 28 percent came off medications and 52 percent reported spontaneous improvement. Shapiro and Shapiro observed that 5–8 percent of TS patients recover completely and permanently in adolescence; tics become less severe in 35 percent of cases during adolescence, and less severe in "most patients" in adulthood.[22] Thus, many patients with TS experience an improvement or resolution of tics after adolescence.

While the natural course of the tic disorder in TS has received considerable attention, little investigative work has focused on the behavioral components. Comings and Comings have suggested that, for many children with TS, symptoms of ADHD antedate the appearance of tics by an average of 2.5 years.[23] Park et al. found it unusual for ADHD or OCD to be absent at the time of initial diagnosis of TS and then to appear later on, with only 4–6 percent of patients following this course.[24] On the other hand, disruptive behaviors (20 percent) and school problems (13 percent) more likely appeared over time.

Epidemiology

There is a 3:1 male predominance among patients with TS.[19] However, if one considers OCD to be an alternative clinical expression of the condition (see below), the gender ratio is nearly equal.[25] The disorder has been identified in all races and appears to be uniformly distributed across socioeconomic classes.[19] The clinical features appear to be uniform among different cultural groups, except that coprolalia is particularly uncommon in Japanese patients.[19] Traditionally, TS has been viewed as a rare disorder. However, recent evidence suggests that it is much more common than generally appreciated. An accurate lifetime prevalence rate for TS has not been established. Past estimates, ranging from 0.03 percent to 1.6 percent,[26] have been based largely on case series of patients referred for medical evaluation, or on data obtained from questionnaires without direct clinical examinations. For example, in estimating the prevalence of TS in North Dakota adults and children, Burd et al. included only subjects on a state-wide list of medical diagnoses.[27,28] The epidemiologic survey of TS in Monroe County, New York, by Caine et al. involved only children referred by school and health personnel following an extensive informational campaign in the local news media.[29] Several lines of evidence suggest that these approaches are likely to be inaccurate and lead to gross underestimates of disease prevalence. Systematic analysis of large TS kindreds using a family study method in which all available members are directly interviewed and examined indicates that most cases of TS are mild and do not come to medical attention, and that the disorder is often unrecognized and misdiagnosed by physicians.[26,30] Furthermore, studies of the prevalence of TS have been restricted to an analysis of the tic disorder, and mounting evidence (see below) indicates that behavioral disorders, including OCD and ADHD, may be the only clinical manifestations of illness for some individuals.[8,25] Thus, the prevalence of the disorder may be much higher than current estimates, particularly if behavioral manifestations are included. Although his conclusions have been challenged,[12,14] Comings has estimated that, if one accepts TS as a broadly based behavioral disorder, up to 1 in

100 individuals may manifest one or more clinical aspects of the TS genetic trait, making it one of the most common neurobehavioral disorders affecting man.[11]

Further support for a high prevalence for tic disorders comes from epidemiologic surveys of school-age children that have identified tic rates ranging from 4 percent to 50 percent.[31–33] Although such studies identified a high rate of tics during the course of childhood development, the authors did not examine the clinical characteristics of tics (e.g., presence of motor and vocal types, duration of at least 1 year) which are necessary to determine whether or not they satisfy criteria for TS. More recent studies that employed modern diagnostic criteria have identified TS fairly commonly in studied school populations. Mason et al. studied all grade 9 pupils in a single school and found that 2.9 percent met criteria for TS (excluding the impairment criterion).[34] A school-based study in Sweden assessed children at age 7 who were followed for up to 4 years and found a 1 percent prevalence for TS.[35] Interestingly, a series of studies have consistently found a high rate of tic disorders of about 25 percent in school children requiring special educational services, suggesting that the presence of tics might be a sign of an underlying subtle brain developmental disorder that contributes to problems in school.[36–38] For most subjects identified with tics in these community-based surveys, the severity of tics observed has generally been quite mild.

Taken together, current evidence suggests that TS and related tic disorders are quite common in the general childhood population. For the most part, they appear to represent mild, nondisabling conditions which do not lead to medical attention or therapy, although they do appear to be linked to childhood school problems. It remains unclear whether all cases of chronic motor and vocal tics represent TS. DSM-IV added the diagnostic criteria for TS that tics must cause marked distress or a significant impairment in daily functioning (see above). It has not been established, however, that such functional criteria are truly valid for making diagnostic distinctions and this criterion has been removed in the new, revised DSM-IV version.

Differential Diagnosis

DISTINGUISHING TICS FROM OTHER MOVEMENT DISORDERS

Simple motor tics may resemble the rapid muscle jerks of myoclonus. However, even when most tics are simple jerks, more complex forms of motor tics or more sustained dystonic tics may also be present, allowing one to establish the diagnosis by association with these other forms of motor tics. Moreover, simple motor tics tend to have a less random, more predictable body distribution and a wider range of amplitude and forcefulness when compared with myoclonus. The characteristic voluntary suppressibility of tics and the tendency of myoclonus to increase with intentional acts may also help distinguish between the conditions. It is important to recognize, however, that voluntary suppressibility is a feature that is not specific for tics, but can be seen to at least some degree in virtually all hyperkinetic movement disorders (see Chap. 1).

Repetitive eye blinking and forceful eye closures from tics and from blepharospasm, a form of focal cranial dystonia, can usually be differentiated by the presence of other tics or dystonic movements at other sites. In addition, while tics typically begin in childhood, blepharospasm is predominantly a disorder with onset in later adult life. Dystonic tics may be differentiated from torsion dystonia in that the latter is a continual movement that can result in a sustained abnormal posture, whereas dystonic tics usually cause an abnormal posture that is present for only a short period of time. The presence of more typical jerk-like tics in other body regions would favor that the sustained contractions could be dystonic tics rather than torsion dystonia. In addition, dystonic tics are often preceded by localized uncomfortable sensations (sensory tics) which may be relieved by the movement.[5] Such sensory experiences are typically absent in torsion dystonia.

It may be difficult to distinguish complex motor tics and compulsions. In contrast to tics, compulsions are closely associated with obsessions, are often performed in response to an obsessive thought pattern and may be performed according to certain rules (rituals), such as a specified number of times, in a specified order, or at a particular time of day (e.g., bedtime rituals). In addition, compulsive rituals may be performed with the thought of preventing discomfort or a future dreaded event. Response to drug therapy (see below) may be helpful for differential diagnosis as well. For example, while tics usually predictably respond to dopamine antagonist drugs, compulsions do not. Rather, antidepressant drugs which selectively inhibit serotonin reuptake (e.g., fluoxetine, fluvoxamine) may be quite effective for compulsions. The repetitive complex motor acts, known as stereotypies, of patients with mental retardation, psychosis, autism, or congenital blindness of deafness, may also be difficult to distinguish from motor tics. The correct diagnosis of tics is usually made by excluding conditions known to be associated with stereotypies or by identifying associated simple motor or vocal tics.

PRIMARY AND SECONDARY TIC DISORDERS

A variety of primary tic disorders are now recognized and TS can be considered to represent one member of a family of tic disorders.[1] Chronic motor tic disorder and chronic vocal tic disorder differ from TS in that motor or vocal tics, but not both, are present. Transient tic disorder differs from the others by having a duration of less than 1 year. Chronic motor and vocal tic disorder and transient tic disorder are now generally viewed as clinical variants of TS.[39,40]

It is now generally believed that the primary tic disorders occur on an hereditary basis.[41] Occasional cases of acute or chronic tics may represent phenocopies of the genetic disorder;[42] examples include chronic neuroleptic exposure (tardive TS),[43] viral encephalitis,[44] head trauma,[45] carbon monoxide intoxication,[46] and Sydenham's chorea[47] (Table 41-2). A recently proposed and controversial hypothesis suggests that some cases of TS occur on the basis of an autoimmune process following streptococcal infection as part of a spectrum of neurobehavioral symptoms termed "pediatric autoimmune neuropsychiatric disorders associated with streptococcal infection (PANDAS)."[48] Tics may also occur in a number of neurologic disorders, including Huntington's disease, Parkinson's disease, progressive supranuclear palsy, neuroacanthocytosis, Meige's syndrome, and startle disorders.[42] The excessive startle syndromes may be associated with echolalia, coprolalia, and echopraxia. For these secondary tic disorders, tics are usually combined with other disorders of movement (e.g., with chorea in Huntington's disease and neuroacanthocytosis).[42] In our experience, it is common to find a clinical syndrome resembling TS, including tics, obsessive-compulsive behavior, inattention, and impulsivity, in children with an array of developmental disorders that are often difficult to characterize. The Tourette-like features, which we have termed the "developmental basal ganglia syndrome,"[49] are often associated with developmental delays (motor, cognitive, social/emotional), learning disabilities, other involuntary movements (dystonia, chorea, stereotypies), and other movement disturbances (handwriting difficulties, clumsiness, stuttering, speech articulation disorders). We have observed this constellation of symptoms in children with pervasive developmental disorders, fetal-alcohol syndrome, intrauterine exposure to illicit drugs, and other perinatal insults, and we suspect that it reflects a disruption of normal basal ganglia developmental processes which can occur from a variety of causes.

TABLE 41-2 Secondary Tic Disorders

Inherited
  Huntington's disease
  Neuroacanthocytosis
  Torsion dystonia
  Chromosomal abnormalities
  Other

Acquired
  Drugs: neuroleptics (tardive tics), stimulants, anticonvulsants,
    L-dopa
  Trauma
  Infectious/immune: encephalitis, Creutzfeldt-Jakob disease,
    Sydenham's chorea, pediatric autoimmune neuropsychiatric
    disorders associated with streptococcal infection (PANDAS)
  Developmental: static encephalopathy, mental retardation,
    autism, pervasive developmental disorder
  Stroke
  Degenerative: Parkinson's disease, progressive supranuclear palsy
  Toxic: carbon monoxide

Etiology/Pathogenesis

GENETICS

Although Gilles de la Tourette himself stated that the disorder was hereditary in nature, for many years the etiology of TS was ascribed to psychogenic causes and the importance of genetic factors was overlooked. It was not until the late 1970s that investigators demonstrated a familial concentration for TS and found that susceptibility to the illness is transmitted vertically from generation to generation, indicating a genetic trait. Studies of monozygotic twins have confirmed a genetic influence.[50] Today, hereditary factors are thought to be responsible for most cases of TS. Single major locus, polygenic and multifactorial patterns of transmission within families have been proposed.[25,41,51] Current evidence points to a complex transmission pattern that involves a major gene influence, contributions from other loci, incomplete and sex-specific penetrances (affected males are more common that affected females), and variable clinical expression, which includes TS, chronic tic disorder, OCD, and possibly ADHD.[25,52] There is a high frequency of bilineal transmission (from maternal and paternal sides) in studied TS families.[53] Environmental factors may also be involved in the ultimate clinical expression of the illness.

NEUROBIOLOGY

While genetic factors are now recognized as those most important for the development of TS and related tic disorders, investigators continue to search for underlying neuroanatomic and neurochemical disturbances that may be manifestations of the gene defect and involved in the pathogenesis of the disorder. Several lines of evidence have supported the notion that striatal dopamine receptor supersensitivity at least partly underlies the tic disorder: (1) dopamine receptor antagonists are the most effective drugs for suppressing tics, (2) tics may be exacerbated by dopaminergic medications such as amphetamines, (3) reduced levels of the dopamine metabolite homovanillic acid have been identified in the cerebrospinal fluid of patients with TS,[54] and (4) the phenomenon of tardive tics following chronic dopamine antagonist therapy.[43] More recent observations, however, that the dopamine agonist pergolide,[55] the dopaminergic agent L-dopa,[56] and the psychostimulant methylphenidate[57] all lessen tics have challenged this hypothesis. The reported absence of staining for dynorphin in the globus pallidus of a postmortem brain from a patient with TS[58] and clinical observations that drugs affecting the endogenous opioid system may influence the symptoms of TS[59–61] have focused attention on the role of this neurochemical system in the pathogenesis of the disorder. Another study of postmortem TS brains revealed reduced concentrations of adenosine 3′,5′-monophosphate (cyclic AMP) in the cerebral cortex and suggests a possible dysfunction of secondary neurochemical messengers.[62] Other authors have suggested that sex hormone influences on brain development and function may be important in the pathogenesis of TS.[63,64] Recent studies involving cerebral magnetic resonance imaging have revealed that the basal ganglia in patients with TS do not have the volumetric asymmetry (left greater than right) seen in normal controls.[65,66]

Therapy

The management of patients with TS can be both challenging and rewarding. The initial step is to identify the clinical features that are interfering most with daily activities and direct initial therapy at this "target" symptom (Table 41-3). The target symptom is not always tics; it may be ADHD, OCD, or other behavior problems (e.g., depression, anxiety).

TREATMENT OF TICS

Most patients with mild tics who have made a good adaptation in their lives can avoid the use of any medications. Educating patients, family members, peers, and school personnel regarding the nature of TS, restructuring the educational environment, and supportive counseling are measures that may be sufficient to avoid drug therapy. Pharmacotherapy should be considered once it is determined that the tics are functionally disabling and not remediable to psychosocial interventions. The goal in treating tics is generally to achieve "satisfactory" suppression or control rather than to attempt to make the patient completely free of tics. For the patient with mild or moderate tics, treatment is usually initiated with an alpha-agonist. Clonidine is initiated at 0.05 mg at bedtime, and the dosage is increased by 0.05 mg every few days until satisfactory control of tics is achieved or unacceptable side-effects are encountered. Most patients

---

TABLE 41-3 Pharmacologic Treatment of TS

Tics
    Alpha agonists: clonidine (oral, transdermal), guanfacine
    Atypical antipsychotics: risperidal, olanzapine, ziprasidone
    Classical neuroleptic antipsychotics: haloperidol, pimozide,
       fluphenazine, others
    Tetrabenazine
    Clonazepam
    Calcium channel antagonists
    Botulinum toxin (dystonic tics)

Attention Deficit Hyperactivity Disorder
    Alpha agonists: clonidine (oral, transdermal), guanfacine
    Stimulants: methylphenidate (Ritalin, Concerta, Metadate CR),
       Adderal

Obsessive-Compulsive Behavior
    Serotonin reuptake inhibitors: fluoxetine, fluvoxamine,
       paroxetine, clomipramine, others

respond to 1 tablet (0.1 mg) 3 times per day (before and after school and at bedtime for children), but the maintenance dose should be the lowest one that gives satisfactory suppression of tics. Due to a short duration of action, particularly in children, 4 times daily dosing may be required. When necessary, higher doses of clonidine (generally up to 0.6 mg/day) can be used, letting adverse effects (usually sedation) be the dose-limiting factor. Transdermal clonidine is an alternative dosing form, particularly for children who cannot swallow pills, but this formulation often causes skin irritation and may fall off. Guanfacine is a newer alpha-agonist that has the advantages of single daily dosing and causing less sedation than clonidine.[67] This drug has become the first-choice alpha-agonist for many clinicians. It is initiated at 0.5–1 mg at bedtime and gradually titrated as needed to a maximum dosage of 4 mg.

If an alpha-agonist alone is insufficient, one can add an antipsychotic drug (if partial relief with an alpha-agonist was observed) or replace the alpha-agonist with an antipsychotic (if no benefit was perceived). If clonidine or guanfacine are to be discontinued, the drug should be tapered over 7–10 days in order to avoid potential withdrawal phenomena, usually tachycardia and hypertension.

The newer so-called atypical antipsychotics have generally supplanted the traditional neuroleptic antipsychotics as second-line tic suppressants (after the alpha-agonists) due to better side-effect profiles. The atypical agents can generally be given in a single bedtime dose. Those atypical antipsychotics with reported tic-suppressing actions include risperidone (0.25–16 mg/day), olanzapine (2.5–15 mg/day), and ziprasidone (20–200 mg/day). If the atypical antipsychotics are ineffective or not tolerated, a trial of a classical neuroleptic antipsychotic is indicated. Haloperidol remains one of the most commonly used classical antipsychotics neuroleptics for treating tics. The drug is initiated at 0.25 mg at bedtime, increasing as necessary; most patients have a favorable response to 2 mg/day or less, given at bedtime. If haloperidol is unsuccessful or produces unacceptable side-effects, one can then switch to pimozide, fluphenazine, or another neuroleptic. For patients with very severe tics that are extremely problematic, one can initiate therapy with an antipsychotic, rather than an alpha-agonist. Local intramuscular injections of botulinum toxin have been used to treat patients with painful dystonic tics.[68]

Other medications that have been reported to improve tics include tetrabenazine, clonazepam, and calcium channel antagonists.

TREATMENT OF ATTENTION DEFICIT HYPERACTIVITY DISORDER (ADHD)

When ADHD is the target symptom, clonidine or guanfacine is a useful starting medication. If symptoms are not adequately controlled, one can switch to a stimulant, such as methylphenidate or one of its long-acting forms. Although treatment with stimulants may exacerbate tics in some patients, the occasional worsening of tics may be tolerable when these medications are effective in improving attentional abilities and alleviating hyperactivity.[69] If tics are significantly worsened by stimulant therapy, an alpha-agonist or an antipsychotic can be added.

TREATMENT OF OBSESSIVE-COMPULSIVE DISORDER (OCD)

Antidepressant drugs that inhibit serotonin reuptake, including fluoxetine, fluvoxamine, paroxetine, clomipramine, and others, may be effective for the treatment of OCD associated with TS.[70,71] Cognitive-behavioral therapy by an experienced therapist is also often very helpful. Psychosurgical approaches have been used for rare patients severely disabled by OCD who had inadequate responses to psychotherapy and medications.[72,73]

NON-MEDICATION THERAPIES

One of the most important aspects of treating TS is educating the patient and family members about tic disorders, ADHD, OCD, and other behavioral disturbances. A variety of educational brochures, videotapes, and other materials are available from the Tourette Syndrome Association (4240 Bell Boulevard, Bayside, NY 11361). A local TS support group may be of great benefit to patients and family members. Individual, group, or family counseling may be helpful in facilitating a healthy adaptation to the illness. Specific psychoeducational assessments and therapy are often needed for children with school problems.

References

1. Kurlan R: Tourette's syndrome: current concepts. *Neurology* 39:1625–1630, 1989.
2. American Psychiatric Association: *Diagnostic and Statistical Manual of Mental Disorders*, 4th ed. Washington, DC: American Psychiatric Association, 1994.
3. The Tourette Syndrome Classification Study Group: Definitions and classification of tic disorders. *Arch Neurol* 50:1013–1016, 1993.
4. Jankovic J, Stone L: Dystonic tics in patients with Tourette's syndrome. *Mov Disord* 6:248–252, 1991.
5. Kurlan R, Lichter D, Hewitt D: Sensory tics in Tourette's syndrome. *Neurology* 39:731–734, 1989.
6. Scahill LD, Leckman JF, Marek KL: Sensory phenomena in Tourette's syndrome. *Adv Neurol* 65:273–280, 1995.
7. Frankel M, Cummings JL, Robertson MM, et al: Obsessions and compulsions in Gilles de la Tourette's syndrome. *Neurology* 36:378–382, 1986.
8. Pauls DL, Towbin KE, Leckman JF, et al: Gilles de la Tourette's syndrome and obsessive-compulsive disorder: Evidence supporting a genetic relationship. *Arch Gen Psychiatry* 43:1180–1182, 1986.
9. Como PG: Obsessive-compulsive disorder in Tourette's syndrome. *Adv Neurol* 65:281–291, 1995.

10. Comings DE, Comings BG: Tourette's syndrome and attention deficit disorder with hyperactivity: Are they genetically related? *J Am Acad Child Psychiatry* 23:138–146, 1984.

11. Comings DE: A controlled study of Tourette's syndrome. VII. Summary: A common genetic disorder causing disinhibition of the limbic system. *Am J Hum Genet* 41: 839–866, 1987.

12. Cohen DJ: Gilles de la Tourette's syndrome and attention deficit disorder with hyperactivity: Evidence against a genetic relationship. *Arch Gen Psychiatry* 43:1177–1179, 1986.

13. Pauls DL, Cohen DJ, Kidd KK, Leckman JR: Tourette's syndrome and neuropsychiatric disorders: Is there a genetic relationship? *Am J Hum Genet* 43:206–209, 1988.

14. Kurlan R: What is the spectrum of Tourette's syndrome? *Curr Opin Neurol Neurosurg* 1:294–298, 1988.

15. Robertson MM, Yakeley JW: Obsessive-compulsive disorder and self-injurious behavior, in Kurlan R (ed): *Handbook of Tourette's Syndrome and Related Tic and Behavioral Disorders.* New York: Marcel Dekker, 1993, pp 45–87.

16. Kurlan R, Daragjati C, Como PG, et al: Non-obscene, complex, socially inappropriate behavior in Tourette's syndrome. *J Neuropsychiatry Clin Neurosci* 8:311–317, 1996.

17. Walkup JT, Scahill LD, Riddle MA: Disruptive behavior, hyperactivity, and learning disabilities in Tourette's syndrome. *Adv Neurol* 65:259–272, 1995.

18. Como PG: Neuropsychological testing, in Kurlan R (ed): *Handbook of Tourette's Syndrome and Related Tic and Behavioral Disorders.* New York: Marcel Dekker, 1993, pp 221–239.

19. *Gilles de la Tourette Syndrome,* 2nd edition, Shapiro AK, Shapiro ES, Young JG, Feinberg TE (eds), Raven Press, NY 1988, pp 61–193.

20. Erenberg G, Cruse RP, Rothner AD: The natural history of Tourette syndrome. A follow-up study. *Ann Neurol* 22:383–385, 1987.

21. Bruun RD: The natural history of Tourette's syndrome, in Cohen DJ, Bruun RD, Leckman (eds): *Tourette's Syndrome and Tic Disorders: Clinical Understanding and Treatment.* New York: Wiley, 1988, pp 21–39.

22. Shapiro ES, Shapiro AK: Gilles de la Tourette syndrome and tic disorders. *The Harvard Medical School Mental Health Letter* 5, May 1989.

23. Comings DE, Comings BG: Tourette syndrome: Clinical and psychological aspects of 250 cases. *Am J Hum Genet* 37:435–450, 1985.

24. Park S, Como PG, Cui L, Kurlan R: The early course of the Tourette's syndrome clinical spectrum. *Neurology* 43:1712–1715, 1993.

25. Pauls DL, Leckman JF: The inheritance of Gilles de la Tourette's syndrome and associated behaviors: Evidence for autosomal dominant transmission. *N Engl J Med* 315:993–997, 1986.

26. Kurlan R, Behr J, Medved L, et al: Severity of Tourette's syndrome in one large kindred: Implication for determination of disease prevalence rate. *Arch Neurol* 44:268–269, 1987.

27. Burd L, Kerbeshian J, Wikenheiser M, et al: Prevalence of Gilles de la Tourette's syndrome in North Dakota adults. *Am J Psychiatry* 143:787–788, 1986.

28. Burd L, Kerbeshian J, Wikenheiser M, Fisher W: A prevalence study of Gilles de la Tourette syndrome in North Dakota school-age children. *J Am Acad Child Psychiatry* 4:552–555, 1986.

29. Caine ED, McBride MC, Chiverton P, et al: Tourette's syndrome in Monroe County school children. *Neurology* 38:472–475, 1988.

30. McMahon WM, Leppert M, Filloux F, et al: Tourette symptoms in 161 related family members. *Adv Neurol* 58:159–165, 1992.

31. Kellmer Pringle ML, Butler NR, Davie R: 1st report of national child development study, in *11,000 Seven-Year-Olds.* Long: National Bureau for Co-operation in Child Care, London 1967, p 185.

32. MacFarlane JW, Honzik MP, Allen L: in *Behavior Problems in Normal Children.* University of California Publications in Child Development, Berkeley 1954.

33. Lapouse R, Monk M: Behavior deviations in a representative sample of children: Variation by sex, age, race, social class and family size. *Am J Orthopsychiatry* 34:436–446, 1964.

34. Mason A, Banerjee S, Eapen V, et al: The prevalence of Tourette syndrome in a mainstream school population. *Dev Med Child Neurol* 40:292–296, 1998.

35. Kadesjoe B, Gilbert C: Tourette's disorder: Epidemiology and comorbidity in primary school children. *J Am Acad Child Adolesc Psychiatry* 39:548–555, 2000.

36. Comings DE, Himes JA, Comings BG: An epidemiologic study of Tourette's syndrome in a single school district. *J Clin Psychiatry* 51:463–469, 1990.

37. Kurlan R, Whitmore D, Irvine C, et al: Tourette's syndrome in a special education population: A pilot study involving a single school district. *Neurology* 44:699–702, 1994.

38. Kurlan R, McDermott MP, Deeley C, et al: Prevalence of tics in school children and association with placement in special education. *Neurology* 57:1383–1388, 2001.

39. Golden GS: Tics and Tourette's syndrome: A continuum of symptoms? *Ann Neurol* 4:145–148, 1978.

40. Kurlan R, Behr J, Medved L, Como P: Transient tic disorder and the clinical spectrum of Tourette's syndrome. *Arch Neurol* 45:1200–1201, 1988.

41. Pauls DL: The inheritance pattern, in Kurlan R (ed): *Handbook of Tourette's Syndrome and Related Tic and Behavioral Disorders.* New York: Marcel Dekker 1993, pp 307–315.

42. Jankovic J: Tics in other neurological disorders, in Kurlan R (ed): *Handbook of Tourette's Syndrome and Related Tic and Behavioral Disorders.* New York: Marcel Dekker, 1993, pp 167–182.

43. Klawans HL, Falk DK, Nausieda PA, Weiner WJ: Gilles de la Tourette's syndrome after long-term chlorpromazine therapy. *Neurology* 28:1064–1068, 1978.

44. Sacks OW: Acquired tourettism in adult life, in Friedhoff AJ, Chase TN (eds): *Gilles de la Tourette's Syndrome.* New York: Raven Press, 1982, pp 89–92.

45. Fahn S: A case of post-traumatic tic syndrome, in Friedhoff AJ, Chase TN (eds): *Gilles de la Tourette's Syndrome.* New York: Raven Press, 1982, pp 349–350.

46. Pulst SM, Walshe TM, Romero JA: Carbon monoxide poisoning with features of Gilles de la Tourette's syndrome. *Arch Neurol* 40:443–444, 1983.

47. Cardoso F, Eduardo C, Silva AP, et al: Chorea in fifty consecutive patients with rheumatic fever. *Mov Disord* 12:701–703, 1997.

48. Swedo SE, Leonard HL, Garvey M, et al: Pediatric autoimmune neuropsychiatric disorders associated with streptococcal infections: Clinical description of the first 50 cases. *Am J Psychiatry* 155:264–271, 1998.

49. Palumbo D, Maughan A, Kurlan R: Hypothesis III: Tourette's syndrome is only one of several causes of a developmental basal ganglia syndrome. *Arch Neurol* 54:475–483, 1997.

50. Price RA, Kidd KK, Cohen DJ, et al: A twin study of Tourette's syndrome. *Arch Gen Psychiatry* 42:815–820, 1985.

51. Pauls DL: Issues in genetic linkage studies of Tourette syndrome: Phenotypic spectrum and genetic model parameters. *Adv Neurol* 58:151–157, 1992.

52. Knell ER, Comings DE: Tourette's syndrome and attention-deficit hyperactivity disorder: Evidence for a genetic relationship. *J Clin Psychiatry* 54:331–337, 1993.

53. Kurlan R, Eapen V, Stern T, et al: Bilineal transmission in Tourette's syndrome families. *Neurology* 44:2336–2342, 1994.

54. Singer HS, Butler IJ, Tune LE, et al: Dopaminergic dysfunction in Tourette's syndrome. *Ann Neurol* 12:361–366, 1982.

55. Gilbert DL, Sethuraman G, Sine L, et al: Tourette's syndrome improvement with pergolide in a randomized, double-blind, crossover trial. *Neurology* 54:1310–1315, 2000.

56. Black KJ, Mink JW: Response to levodopa challenge in Tourette syndrome. *Mov Disord* 15:1194–1198, 2000.

57. Kurlan R, and the Tourette Syndrome Study Group: Treatment of attention-deficit hyperactivity disorder in children with Tourette's syndrome (TACT Trial). *Ann Neurol* 48:953, 2000 (abstract).

58. Haber SN, Kowell NW, Vonsattel JP, et al: Gilles de la Tourette's syndrome: A postmortem neuropathological and immunohistochemical study. *J Neurol Sci* 75:225–241, 1986.

59. Gilman MA, Sandyk R: The endogenous opioid system in Gilles de la Tourette's syndrome. *Med Hypotheses* 19:371–378, 1986.

60. Lichter D, Majumdar L, Kurlan R: Opiate withdrawal unmasks Tourette's syndrome. *Clin Neuropharmacol* 11:559–564, 1988.

61. Kurlan R, Majumdar L, Deeley C, et al: A controlled trial of propoxyphene and naltrexone in Tourette's syndrome. *Ann Neurol* 30:19–23, 1991.

62. Singer HS, Hahn I-H, Krowiak E, et al: Tourette's syndrome: A neurochemical analysis of postmortem cortical brain tissue. *Ann Neurol* 27:443–446, 1990.

63. Kurlan R: The pathogenesis of Tourette's syndrome: A possible role for hormonal and excitatory neurotransmitter influences in brain development. *Arch Neurol* 49:874–876, 1992.

64. Peterson BS, Leckman JF, Scahill L, et al: Steroid hormones and CNS sexual dimorphisms modulate symptom expression in Tourette's syndrome. *Psychoneuroendocrinology* 17:553–563, 1993.

65. Peterson B, Riddle MA, Cohen DJ, et al: Reduced basal ganglia volume in Tourette's syndrome using three-dimensional reconstruction technique from magnetic resonance images. *Neurology* 43:941–949, 1993.

66. Singer HS, Reiss AL, Brown JE, et al: Volumetric MRI changes in basal ganglia of children with Tourette's syndrome. *Neurology* 43:950–956, 1993.

67. Chappell PB, Riddle MA, Scahill L, et al: Guanfacine treatment of comorbid attention-deficit hyperactivity disorder in Tourette's syndrome: Preliminary clinical experience. *J Am Acad Child Adolesc Psychiatry* 34:1140–1146, 1995.

68. Jankovic J: Botulinum toxin in the treatment of tics associated with Tourette's syndrome. *Neurology* 43(suppl 2):A310, 1993 (abstract).

69. Robertson MM, Eapen V: Pharmacologic controversy of CNS stimulants in Gilles de la Tourette's syndrome. *Clin Neuropharmacol* 15:408–425, 1992.

70. Como PG, Kurlan R: An open-label trial of fluoxetine for obsessive-compulsive disorder in Gilles de la Tourette's syndrome. *Neurology* 41:872, 1991.

71. Kurlan R, Como PG, Deeley C, et al: A pilot controlled study of fluoxetine for obsessive-compulsive symptoms in children with Tourette's syndrome. *Clin Neuropharmacol* 16:167, 1993.

72. Kurlan R, Kersun J, Ballentine HT Jr, et al: Neurosurgical treatment of severe obsessive-compulsive disorder associated with Tourette's syndrome. *Mov Disord* 5:152, 1990.

73. Robertson M, Doran M, Trimble M, et al: The treatment of Gilles de la Tourette syndrome by limbic leucotomy. *J Neurol Neurosurg Psychiatry* 53:691, 1990.

Chapter 42

PATHOPHYSIOLOGY AND DIFFERENTIAL DIAGNOSIS OF TICS

JORGE L. JUNCOS

CLINICAL PRESENTATION AND COURSE   693
    Abnormal Sensory Experiences in Tic Disorders   693
    Are Tics Voluntary or Involuntary?   694
PATHOPHYSIOLOGY   694
DIFFERENTIAL DIAGNOSIS   696
ETIOLOGIES   698
    Primary Tic Disorders   698
    Secondary Tic Disorders   699
TREATMENT   699

A tic is a brief, rapid, repetitive, and seemingly purposeless stereotyped action that may involve a single muscle or multiple muscle groups. Its hyperkinetic properties may make it difficult to distinguish from other fast "jerky" movements, such as chorea and myoclonus. The most common and best-studied disorder characterized by tics is Tourette's syndrome (TS) (discussed in more detail in Chap. 41). This chapter focuses on what is known about the phenomenology, pathophysiology, and differential diagnosis of tics.

Clinical Presentation and Course

Tics typically present in childhood or adolescence and may be transient or last a lifetime. With aging, most tics tend to reach a stable plateau or disappear altogether.[1–3] Traditionally, tics are divided into motor or vocal, depending on the affected muscle group, and into simple or complex, depending on the intricacy of their phenomenology (Table 42-1). Motor tics have a wide spectrum of severity, ranging from the barely detectable and easily rationalized "nervous habits," to the complex, emotionally laden gestures. Similarly, vocal tics can range from throat clearing or sniffing sounds, to other simple sounds or words, to the sometimes offensive utterances found in a minority of patients with TS, sometimes termed coprolalia.

Motor tics can affect any part of the body but they typically begin in the eyelids or face and, over time, involve other muscle groups, spreading to the neck, shoulders, trunk, legs, and feet with an apparent rostrocaudal migration.[4] Phenomenologically, motor tics may be fast or clonic, or slower and more sustained dystonic tics.[5] Typical clonic tics include repetitive and persisting blinking, nose twitching, shoulder shrugging and head jerking. In contrast, dystonic tics are characterized by sustained twisting, pulling, or squeezing movements, producing a briefly maintained body posture. Examples include painless oculogyric eye movements, blepharospasm, and dystonic neck movements.[6,7] Clonic tics respond to selected dopamine blockers and other therapies, as discussed in Chap. 41. In our experience, dystonic tics may be more difficult to control with conventional pharmacotherapy.

ABNORMAL SENSORY EXPERIENCES IN TIC DISORDERS

Tics can be associated with a surprisingly broad array of sensory experiences. First, external and internal sensory experiences, if intense enough, can aggravate tics. These experiences can range from any event leading to excitation or distress, to anxiety to pain. Brief focal sensory experiences (e.g., tightness, numbness, tingling, pain, or even pleasant sensations) may precede, accompany or follow the movements or vocalization.[8,9] Sensory experiences preceding tics, so called premonitory experiences, are reported by 41–92 percent of patients.[10,11] In this setting, the sensory experience or "urges" have been termed a "sensory tic." These are described by patients as an "urge to move," a "pent-up feeling," or a tension in the underlying muscle group affected by the motor tic. In the case of vocal tics, in our experience, sensory experiences are commonly complex, bordering on obsessions, with muscle tensions around the neck or pharynx being less common.

The term "sensory tic" was introduced by Shapiro et al. in 1988.[12] It refers to recurrent involuntary somatic sensations in various parts of the body that evoke a dysphoric feeling, sometimes causing the patient to respond intentionally with a movement of vocalization that can partially and temporarily alleviate the abnormal sensation.[12] Sensory tics commonly affect the face, head, and neck areas, with the limbs being less often involved.[9] Rarely, sensory tics can occur in the absence of a motor or vocal tic; in such instances, they tend to be less responsive to traditional therapies for motor tics. In a case followed by the author for more than 12 years, the patient presented at age 12 with "arm claudication" during swimming practice. This sensation was not associated with a corresponding motor tic in that limb, although she did have facial and neck motor tics. These and her vocal tics were otherwise controlled with dopamine blockers. After an extensive negative vascular workup, the arm claudication finally responded by ≤ 30 percent to higher doses of the same dopamine agents. After 7 years this symptom gradually subsided and finally disappeared.

Shapiro suggested that, when tics occur in response to a sensory tic, the motor or vocal tic tends to be more prolonged (several seconds or more), and often consists of squeezing, stretching or tightening of the corresponding body part.[12] In our experience, the more complex the sensory experience,

TABLE 42-1 Classification of Tic Phenomenology

	Motor	Vocal	Sensory
Simple	Frequent blinking	Sniffing	Burning sensations
	Blepharospasm	Grunting	Tightness
	Grimacing	Throat clearing	Muscle heaviness
	Pouting	Barking	Tingling
	Jaw opening	Growling	Itching
	Head jerking	Coughing	Impulsions
	Shoulder shrugging	Moaning	
	Fist clenching	Humming	
Complex	Head twisting or shaking	Panting	Inner tension
	Spitting	Belching	Pain syndromes
	Hitting (self, others)	Stuttering	• Premonitory
	Jumping, kicking	Echolalia	• Exertional
	Squatting	Coprolalia	• Secondary to prolonged voluntary tic suppression
	Pelvic/abdominal thrusting	Palilalia	"Phantom tics"

the more its phenotype begins to suggest an obsession followed by a compulsion or impulsion. This would explain the relatively poor response of sensory tics to conventional therapy used for the treatment of motor tics. In any event, it remains unclear whether these sensory experiences are independent of the motor tics, or subjective components of the more readily recognized motor or vocal tic.

From the standpoint of differential diagnosis, these premonitory sensory phenomena are occasionally reported by patients with cranial dystonia (Meige's syndrome) and tics, and by patients with hemifacial spasms. In the latter case, the complaints are often described as persistent dullness, heaviness or aching in the affected muscle.

ARE TICS VOLUNTARY OR INVOLUNTARY?

Motor tics have traditionally been interpreted as involuntary, because they are not associated with the negative premotor electroencephalographic (EEG) potential (Bereitschaftspotential) normally linked to voluntary movement.[13] However, more recently, it has been reported that not all voluntary movements are necessarily preceded by these potentials.[14] Furthermore, when patients are asked directly, many of them report that the tics are under "voluntary control."[15] More specifically, motor tics that occur in response to premonitory urges are interpreted by patients as a voluntary act to relieve the often-uncomfortable sensation.[15] The term "unvoluntary" was recently coined in an effort to reconcile this dichotomy that underlies the terms voluntary and involuntary when referring to tics.[16] Unvoluntary refers to an "automatic movement performed without conscious effort," such as scratching in response to an itch.[16]

In contrast to motor and vocal tics, sensory tics are interpreted by patients as involuntary.[9] More complex sensations or affects associated with tics have been referred to as "complex sensory tics."[5] It is unclear, however, whether these complex phenomena are themselves related to the more

involved comorbid conditions associated with tic disorders, such as obsessions and compulsions (see Chap. 41). For instance, Karp and Hallett recently described a patient whose tics were associated with out-of-body sensations that were relieved by intentional movements, or tics, directed at the object in question.[17] These "phantom tics" may represent a continuum with obsession and compulsions that are common in primary tic disorders (see Chap. 41). Previous authors have used the term "impulsion" to refer to similar actions that fall between the spectrum of compulsions and tics.[18]

Finally, motor tics, although conspicuous, are seldom the most disabling feature of a chronic tic disorder. Vocal tics can be more socially incapacitating than motor tics, especially the complex utterances and the coprolalia seen in TS. Sensory tics are highly variable but can be distressing, particularly when they present as pain syndromes.[11] In our experience, they are less responsive than the above tics to dopamine blockers and other therapies. Furthermore, in TS, comorbid entities such as obsessions, compulsions, learning disabilities, attention deficit disorder (ADD), and its associated behaviors, when present, are more disabling than the tics themselves. Much like stressors from any source, poor control of these comorbid entities will aggravate the tics.

Pathophysiology

The neurobiological substrate of tics is unknown, but is thought to involve abnormalities in corticostriatothalamic circuits modulated by ascending monoaminergic pathways.[19] Evidence for this has been obtained in part from autopsies in neurological conditions in which tics are a secondary manifestation. For instance, tics have been described as late sequelae of encephalitis lethargica (i.e., postencephalitic parkinsonism), in which there is extensive pathological involvement of the ascending monoaminergic pathways, the midbrain tegmentum, and the periaqueductal gray.[20,21] Presumably, the resulting dopaminergic denervation of basal ganglia leads to "postsynaptic dopamine hypersensitivity," which can lead to tics when combined with the extensive midbrain pathology found in postencephalitic parkinsonism.[21]

Striatal regions forming part of the above circuits, such as the caudate and putamen, are thought to be involved in the generation of motor tics. Vocal tics may involve nonmotor circuits such as those projecting to the prefrontal and limbic cortices.[22,23] Unlike the striatum, which receives dopaminergic innervation from the pars compacta of the substantia nigra, these nonmotor circuits receive dopaminergic projections from the ventral tegmental area of the midbrain.[23] The cortical projection regions of these circuits include the prefrontal cortex, the cingulate gyrus, the entorhinal cortex, the olfactory tubercle, the amygdala, and selected regions of the midbrain tegmentum. Experiments in primates indicate that manipulations of the cingulate gyrus and other limbic forebrain regions can lead to changes in vocalization that depend on the nature of the perturbation and the testing conditions.[24,25] The cingulate gyrus is of particular interest in that it connects cortical and limbic structures involved in vocalization.[24] Other limbic structures have also been associated with obsessions and compulsions, in primary tic disorders, and postencephalitic parkinsonism.[21]

Morphometric neuroanatomic studies of these structures, using high-resolution magnetic resonance imaging with volumetric analysis, support the view that there are basal ganglia abnormalities in TS.[26,27] The studies indicate that children and adults with TS have reduced volumes in the region of the left lenticular nucleus (globus pallidus and putamen), compared to those of age-matched controls.[26,27] Because the left hemisphere is typically larger than the right, TS subjects also exhibit significant attenuation in the normal interhemispheric asymmetries seen in controls. In one study this lack of asymmetry was particularly striking in individuals with comorbid TS and ADD.[27,28]

Positron emission tomography studies using ^{18}F-fluorodeoxyglucose suggest that, in TS, there is decreased metabolic activity in subcortical regions, including basal ganglia and limbic cortices, and increased normalized metabolic activity in overlying cortex.[29] These regions are connected by the motor/limbic striatothalamic circuitry described above.[23] Areas that exhibit decreased metabolic rates include the orbital, frontal, and superior insular cortices, the mesial temporal regions, and the striatum. Regions exhibiting increased metabolic rate include the premotor regions (lateral premotor, and supplementary motor areas), the rolandic cortices, and the postrolandic sensory association areas.[29] More importantly, it seems that the functional metabolic relationship between these regions is altered in TS, compared to that of controls.

Much like the morphometric studies discussed above, these altered relationships gravitate around the ventral striatum, including the globus pallidus. In TS, striatal metabolic changes are positively coupled to the metabolic rates in overlying cortical regions.[29] In normal subjects, this relationship is negatively correlated; that is, if the metabolic activity in the ventral striatum increases, it is expected to decrease in the corresponding target cortical regions. This has led to speculation that, in TS, there is functional cortical-subcortical "short-circuiting" between these regions, leading to failure of "gating mechanisms" responsible for the coupling of motor and limbic cortical regions through the ventral striatum.[29] Clinically, this may lead to inability to suppress activity generated somewhere within the motor/limbic striatothalamic circuitry. Depending on where in the circuitry this activity originates, the patient may present with inability to control motor impulses (tics, compulsions), failure to control sensory overload (ADD), or intrusive thoughts and impulsions (obsessive-compulsive disorder, OCD). Using auditory and visual startle responses as a model of sensorimotor "gating" by striatal outflow, animal experiments have produced evidence that indirectly support this hypothesis.[30] Startle responses are profoundly affected by dopaminergic transmission in the basal ganglia, thereby tying this model to what is known about the pharmacology of tics and TS (see below).

Key questions for which there are still only speculative answers are: Where in the supposedly abnormal motor/limbic striatothalamic circuits is the abnormal activity generated? What sustains, and at the same time makes so variable, the clinical course of TS? These questions force us again to examine the key role that the ventral striatum may play in transforming motivation into action by serving as an interface between the above motor circuits, the limbic system, and the hypothalamus.[31] However, if tics are viewed as involuntary (or "unvoluntary," as discussed above) phenomena, then theories regarding motivation, decision-making, and action would be only of limited value in explaining tics.

Gedye has proposed a theory that incorporates the involuntary quality of tics.[32] He theorized that "abnormal discharges in the frontal lobes" mediate the numerous phenomena that constitute TS.[32] He suggests that the phenomenology of tics is similar to that of the motor and vocal manifestations of frontal lobe seizures. Frontal cortical dysfunction resulting from abnormal electrical activity may help to explain the neuropsychological abnormalities described in some cases of TS (e.g., inattention, difficulties with planning, sequencing, and with shifting mental sets).[32] He tries to dispel skepticism regarding this theory by pointing out that: (1) frontal lobe epileptiform discharges are often missed on surface EEG; (2) frontal seizures are not necessarily associated with loss of consciousness; (3) frontal seizures are less responsive to anticonvulsants than the more common seizures originating from other brain regions. Presumably, this would explain the lack of response of tics to anticonvulsants. The author's view is that this theory is weakened by several observations. Although patients with frontal seizures do not necessarily lose consciousness during an event, they frequently exhibit subtle and not-so-subtle alterations of consciousness not seen in TS. Although anticonvulsants have been used to treat several aspects of TS, they are typically not very effective at treating the tics.[5]

Detailed electrophysiological studies also fail to support the above theory. The contribution of electrophysiological studies to the understanding of the involuntary ("unvoluntary") nature of tics was discussed above. Beyond this, they provide little insight into the pathogenesis of tics. A number of EEG studies have failed to document consistent abnormalities in subjects with TS.[33,34] Bergen et al. reported a 34 percent incidence of nonspecific EEG abnormalities in a random selection of 38 TS patients, most of which could be attributed to coexisting signs of neurological dysfunction (so-called "soft neurologic signs").[33] Only 2 patients exhibited EEG epileptiform activity, and none reported seizures.[33] Neufeld et al. examined quantitative EEGs in 48 consecutive patients with TS and concluded that "there was no significant difference between TS patients and matched controls."[34] Krumholz et al. examined the EEG ($n = 40$), and the visual, brainstem, and auditory-evoked responses ($n = 17$) in TS and found no "diagnostic or therapeutic value to justify their routine use in this syndrome."[35]

Polysomnographic contributions to the study of TS are limited, even though insomnia and other sleep-related complaints are not uncommon in TS.[36] In selected cases, polysomnographic studies have shown a higher percentage of stage III/IV sleep and decreased rapid eye movement sleep in patients with TS, compared to that of controls.[36] Although these findings fail to explain the frequent sleep disruption in TS, they suggest that disordered arousal may be playing a role in TS. Two tantalizing studies suggest that disorders of arousal, such as somnambulism and night terrors, are more common in TS than in controls.[37,38] It can be speculated that disordered arousal may be the sleep cycle equivalent of the "gating" abnormalities postulated above. This hypothesis predicts that, just as tics do not disappear during sleep, TS patients are more likely than controls to "be driven" by urges associated with dreaming (e.g., sleep walking or somnambulism). In the case of night terrors, the subject is unable to suppress the energy typically generated by nightmares and, as a result, awakes in a panic. The mechanisms for these intrusions into normal sleep have yet to be defined.

Based in part on the above findings and on speculations regarding the neural circuitry involved in tic disorders, several neurosurgical procedures have been proposed for the treatment of TS.[39] These include stereotactic coagulation of the rostral intralaminar and medial thalamic nuclei, lesions of the cerebellar dentate nucleus, and frontal lobotomies.[39] These procedures have remained unpopular because of their limited and inconsistent results and their considerable morbidity. Leckman et al. recently reported a case in which bilateral anterior cingulotomy was followed by bilateral infrathalamic lesions for the treatment of severe TS. The patient's tics and obsessive-compulsive symptoms improved. However, the patient developed marked dysarthria, dysphasia, and a lasting parkinsonian syndrome.[40] Limbic leukotomies and isolated lesions of the cingulate gyrus carry much less morbidity than the above combined procedures and may be effective in the treatment of OCD and selected cases of TS.[39,41]

Dysfunction of central dopaminergic pathways is suspected as playing a role in the pathophysiology of tic disorders, in particular TS.[19,42] This suspicion is based on indirect clinical and pharmacological evidence discussed in detail in Chap. 41. An alternative hypothesis is that tics may result in part from dysfunction in cerebral cholinergic systems.[43,44] According to this hypothesis, evidence for central dopaminergic "hyperfunction" in tic disorders could be interpreted instead as indirect evidence of cerebral cholinergic "hypofunction." In experimental animals, dopamine and acetylcholine play complementary and often reciprocal roles.[45] In man, clinical evidence suggests dopaminergic transmission can be enhanced by cholinergic antagonists.[45] Examples of this include the response of hypodopaminergic states, such as neuroleptic-induced extrapyramidal syndromes and Parkinson's disease, to cholinergic antagonists. Conversely, cholinergic agonists may alleviate hyperdopaminergic states, such as tics and chorea.[46]

Indirect evidence for abnormal cholinergic transmission in TS has been obtained through a series of pharmacological experiments. For instance, oral anticholinergic agents have a definite but variable effect on tics.[47] Most studies support the view that augmentation of central cholinergic transmission relieves tics and possibly other symptoms of TS.[43,44,47] Accordingly, several purported cholinomimetics have been investigated as possible alternatives to the standard dopamine-blocking strategies in TS.[46] The results have been limited by the agents used which, like choline and lecithin, are poorly tolerated and poorly penetrate the central nervous system.[43,48] Further work on this hypothesis will have to await the availability of new cholinergic agents with better therapeutic profiles that are now being tested for Alzheimer's disease.

Serotonin is another potentially important neurotransmitter in the pathogenesis of tic disorders and, in particular, TS. Most of its relevance to TS appears to be in its relationship to OCD symptomatology, for which serotonin reuptake inhibitors (SSRIs) have proven moderately effective,[46,49,50] (see Chap. 41 for detailed discussion). It has been our experience, however, that the SSRIs, which are normally tolerated in OCD patients without TS, not infrequently aggravate tics, limiting their use in some patients with TS.

Differential Diagnosis

The clinical features of tics have been extensively studied in primary tic disorders such as TS, but not in other conditions in which tics are a secondary manifestation. For the purposes of this chapter, we will discuss primary and secondary tics together because, phenomenologically, there is no evidence that there are significant differences between them.

TABLE 42-2 Response of Patients with Selected Movement Disorders to Questions Regarding Subjective Perception and Other Maneuvers[a]

	Subjective Perception	Premonitory Urges	Distraction	Suppression	Effect of Selected Movements
Tics	Vol or Invol	Yes	↓		Usually ↓
Myoclonus	Invol	No	0 or ↑	0	Commonly ↑
Chorea	Invol	No	0 or ↑	±	Variable
Akathitic movements	Vol	Yes	↓	++	↓
Orofacial tardive dyskinesia	Invol	No	↑	++	Commonly ↑
Drug-induced dyskinesia	Invol	No	↑	++	Commonly ↑
Psychogenic movements	Invol	± Yes[b]	↓	±	Usually ↓[b]
Tremors	Invol	No	0 or ↑	In PD: ++ In others: 0	± ↑
Dystonia	Invol	No	0 or ↑	±	Commonly ↑

[a]This important information should be elicited in the course of the history. "Vol" and "Invol" refer to the patients' interpretation of the activity as voluntary or not. The direction of the arrow refers to an increase or a decrease in movement; the thickness of the arrow is an arbitrary representation of the intensity of this change. 0, no change; ±, variable change; +, ++, + + +, mild, moderate, or marked suppressibility, respectively.
[b]This is highly variable from patient to patient.
SOURCE: Modified from Lang AE: Clinical phenomenology of tic disorders: Selected aspects. *Adv Neurol* 58:27, 1992.

Tics can be differentiated from hyperkinesias by their suppressibility, distractability, suggestibility, by their tendency to persist during sleep, and by the associated premonitory symptoms mentioned above (see Table 42-2). Unlike tics, and perhaps chorea, other movement disorders are seldom suppressible or perceived by patients as "voluntary." In particular, motor or vocal tics occurring in response to a premonitory urge are often perceived by patients as voluntary. Note that voluntary control may be difficult to assess in children. Table 42-2 also illustrates other aspects of the history and the physical examination that may help differentiate tics from other movement disorders.

Other features that help differentiate tics from hyperkinesias are their onset, their rostrocaudal spread as noted above, their variability, course, and, to some extent, the company they keep in terms of associated comorbidities. For instance, over the course of primary tic disorders, the severity of tics typically waxes and wanes, with predictable crises during adolescence. Tics may temporarily "disappear" or, more likely, become barely noticeable for extended periods, only to recur unprovoked, or triggered by nonspecific stressors. The character of the tics can also change from time to time, more typically over the course of years. For example, excessive blinking or grimacing in childhood may transform into intermittent nose flaring and grunting in adolescence or into neck jerking in adulthood. Compounding this intrinsic variability are the profound effects that stress, stimulants, and other drugs can have on tics. Sensitivity to drugs, unfortunately, does not help differentiate tics from any other movement disorders.

Dyskinesias (hyperkinesias) that may be difficult to differentiate from tics include myoclonus, chorea, akathisia, tardive dyskinesia, L-dopa-induced dyskinesia, the nonspecific movements (stereotypies) encountered in psychotic patients, and psychogenic movement disorders. Dystonic tics can be differentiated from dystonia by the company they keep; that is, they seldom occur in the absence of clonic or tonic tics. Compared to other tics, dystonic tics are more commonly associated with uncomfortable sensations that are relieved by movements.[6,11] Unlike myoclonus, a patient with tics would not be expected to lose motor control while executing a task such as holding a glass.

Chorea and tics are hard to differentiate phenomenologically, because both are quick, involuntary movements. However, chorea is less suppressible and is not associated with premonitory urges. Chorea, unlike tics, consists of a dance-like flow of "irregularly irregular" finger, limb, trunk, or facial movements that ebb or cease during sleep. L-Dopa-induced dyskinesia occurs in association with the treatment of Parkinson's disease. Tics are seldom mistaken for tremors, which are, in contrast to tics, regular and oscillatory in nature. Tardive dyskinesia can be distinguished from tics by drug history and a typical pattern of predominant orobuccolingual involvement. Interestingly, in TS, tardive dyskinesia in response to chronic neuroleptic therapy appears to be exceedingly rare.

Other movements superficially resembling tics include mannerisms, disorders of excessive startle, and hyperekplexia. Mannerisms are physiological tics or patterned, sequential movements that are commonly outgrown during childhood. Although they appear in normal children, they are more commonly associated with mental subnormality.

Comorbidities often associated with TS, or primary tic disorder, include attention deficit hyperactivity disorder (ADHD), OCD and learning disabilities. The presence of these comorbidities in secondary tic disorders is largely unknown, and their presence is not specific to primary tic disorders. Nonetheless, their association with tics would suggest a primary tic disorder, by virtue of how often they are encountered as comorbid conditions in TS.

Table 42-3 is a guide to the differential diagnosis of disorders associated with tics.

Etiologies

PRIMARY TIC DISORDERS

In tic disorders, the terms primary and secondary are again arbitrary, because we are uncertain of their pathophysiology and mechanisms. Transient tic disorder, by definition, lasts more than 1 month but less than 1 year. This diagnosis is made retrospectively, because there is no way to predict the course of tics when they first appear. The age of onset is always in childhood or early adolescence. For a tic to qualify as a chronic motor tic disorder, it must be present for more than 1 year. This entity presents in childhood and is frequently encountered in an individual from a family with TS; hence, it may be a variant of TS. Adult-onset tic disorders are rare and are frequently associated with other neurological disorders (discussed below).

NEURODEGENERATIVE DISORDERS

Neuroacanthocytosis is a rare inherited neurodegenerative syndrome characterized by acanthocytosis in the peripheral blood smear and progressive neurological dysfunction. Associated neurological findings not encountered in primary tic disorders include orofacial dyskinesia, chorea, lip and tongue biting, hypertonia, and hyporeflexia. Spitz et al. recently described a neuroacanthotic syndrome in which tics are the predominant movement disorder.[51]

MISCELLANEOUS NEUROLOGIC CONDITIONS

Hyperekplexias represent a group of disorders of unknown etiology that can superficially mimic tics. Clinical manifestations consist of an exaggerated startle response sometimes accompanied by congenital hypertonia and prominent nocturnal myoclonus.[52] Clusters of familial cases have been described in the literature under the rubrics of "jumping Frenchman of Maine" and "latah," with the latter cases being limited to certain Malaysian and Indonesian cultures.[53] Symptoms usually present in childhood and persist into adulthood, yet the course of the illness is relatively benign. Typically, the patients have a tendency to drop things or fall in response to a startling stimulus.

Hyperekplexia can be differentiated from tics by the following: it causes loss of postural tone, cannot be suppressed, is stimulus-sensitive, and is devoid of vocalizations. Hyperekplexia can be treated with clonazepam or methysergide;[54,55] anticonvulsants, such as phenobarbital, are of only partial or inconsistent benefit. Recently, a mutation in the alpha1-subunit of inhibitory glycine receptor was

TABLE 42-3 Etiologies of Tics and Tic-Like Disorders

Primary
    Acute transient tic of childhood
    Chronic motor tic disorder[a]
    Tourette's syndrome[a]
    Adult-onset tic disorder
    Senile tic disorder
Secondary
    Hereditary
      • Chromosomal abnormalities
      • Down syndrome
      • Fragile X, others (e.g., XXY)
      • Huntington's disease
      • Dystonia (e.g., Meige's syndrome)
      • Hyperekplexias (see text)
    Developmental
      • Autistic syndromes
          Rett syndrome
      • Static encephalopathy (anoxic, etc.)
      • Pervasive developmental delay
    Degenerative
      • Neuroacanthocytosis
      • Progressive supranuclear palsy
    Psychiatric
      • Schizophrenia
      • Obsessive-compulsive disorder
    Toxic-metabolic
      • Carbon monoxide poisoning
      • Hypoglycemia
    Drug-induced
      • Neuroleptics (tardive tics)
      • Stimulants
      • Anticonvulsants
      • L-Dopa (in parkinsonism)
    Infectious
      • Sydenham's chorea
      • Encephalitis
      • Postencephalitic parkinsonism
      • Creutzfeldt-Jakob disease
      • Rubella syndrome
Habitual Body Manipulations[b]
    ○ Finger sucking
    ○ Nail biting, trichtilomania[c]
    ○ Eye rubbing, ear touching
    ○ Genital manipulation
    ○ Nose picking
Stereotypies[d]
    ○ Head nodding or banging
    ○ Body rocking
    ○ Arm jerking

[a]Discussed in Chap. 41. Chronic motor tic disorder is now considered part of the clinical spectrum of TS.
[b]May be nonspecially associated with emotional disturbance.
[c]May be seen in obsessive-compulsive disorders.
[d]Most commonly seen with pervasive developmental delay and mental retardation.
SOURCE: Modified from Lees AJ, Tolosa E: Tics, in Jankovic J, Tolosa E (eds): *Parkinson's Disease and Movement Disorders.* Baltimore: Urban & Schwarzenberg, 1988.

described in one of the familial pedigrees.[56] There is now evidence that abnormalities in spinal reciprocal inhibitory mechanisms modulated by glycine receptors may be abnormal in patients with hereditary hyperekplexia.[57]

SECONDARY TIC DISORDERS

Secondary tics are associated with a variety of systemic and iatrogenic conditions not primarily related to the nervous system. The tics themselves may be indistinguishable from those in TS, but the neurological signs associated with these conditions are not features of TS. Table 42-3 lists most medical and neurological conditions in which tics have been described. A detailed description of each one is beyond the scope of this chapter, but many are discussed elsewhere in this book.

POSTTRAUMATIC

Rarely, secondary tics disorders have been reported as a sequelae of head and peripheral trauma.[58,59] The latency from the time of the trauma to the first tic manifestation has ranged from 1 day to several months, making a link based on causality difficult to establish. The distribution of tics typically coincides with the region that sustained the traumatic injury.

TOXIC

Tic-like phenomena have been described after episodes of hypoglycemia and after carbon monoxide poisoning.[60] These cases are associated with a monophasic insult, typically have a subacute onset and may remain static or evolve over time. These patients generally tolerate dopamine blockers poorly and exhibit a limited to nil response to such therapy.

VASCULAR ETIOLOGIES

Tics may also be secondary to hypertensive or lacunar states or systemic vasculitides involving the basal ganglia.[53] When these disorders are complicated by hyperkinesia, typically chorea which may obscure the tics. Again these cases are accompanied by signs of long-tract dysfunction, nonspecific parkinsonism, dementing features, or focal neurologic finding. Tolerance to traditional medications for tics is also limited.

INFECTIOUS, PARAINFECTIOUS, AND IMMUNOLOGIC DISORDERS

Infections and parainfectious processes, including selected viral encephalitides, Sydenham's chorea and cerebral malaria, may be associated with tic-like movements.[20,53,61,62] The most notable of these entities was that caused by the 1916–1927 pandemic of viral encephalitis, a major sequelae of which was parkinsonism often accompanied by tics. In this and other postinfectious encephalitides, the tics are rarely pure and are often missed clinically due to coexisting choreiform or myoclonic movements. In the acute setting, tics

associated with viral encephalitis, may be obscured by the otherwise critical state of the patient.

More recently, there have been reports of cases of obsessions and compulsions with and without tics associated with recent beta-streptococcal infection. The term used for these entities is pediatric autoimmune neurologic disorders or PANDAS. These cases are described in more detail in Chap. 41 and probably represent a subset of cases carrying the diagnosis of OCD and TS. Kiessling and Swedo have hypothesized that circulating antineuronal antibodies resulting from the primary infection crossreact with neuronal elements causing dysfunction in these circuits, and the above symptoms. Evidence for such crossreactivity has been identified in the caudate and subthalamic nuclei.[63] Some of these cases have improved subacutely following treatment with penicillin or plasma exchange.[64] These results are limited by the probably heterogeneous population being treated and the lack of consensus over the relationship of the circulating antibodies and the neurologic picture. Nonetheless they support the view that this is an autoimmune-mediated disorder.

The above entities should be sought in individuals with tics and systemic symptoms, or in individuals with prior history of systemic medical problems that occasionally affect the central nervous system, and in individuals presenting with tics above age 21, the arbitrary upper age of onset of TS.

DRUG-INDUCED TIC DISORDERS

Tics may be aggravated by psychostimulants, any agent that produces akathisia, and drugs that may cause excitation and anxiety, including steroids, bronchodilators and SSRIs. Examples of stimulants are methylphenidate, dexedrine, pemoline, decongestants, and illicit substances such as amphetamine, cocaine, or their derivatives.[65] Other agents that can induce or aggravate tics include anticonvulsants,[66–68] L-dopa, tricyclic antidepressants, and birth control pills.[37] Neuroleptics can paradoxically aggravate tics when they provoke motor restlessness or akathisia.[69] Except for tardive (neuroleptic-induced) tics, most cases of drug-induced tic disorders are readily reversible when the offending agent is withdrawn. In cases where the tic problem persists longer than a few weeks, the suspicion has been that the drug may have unmasked an underlying primary tic disorder.

Carbamazepine-induced tics constitute an idiosyncratic reaction that can occur at therapeutic blood levels and without signs of toxicity.[66] Neuroleptics can produce transient tics when abruptly withdrawn ("emergence" hyperkinesis), or chronic tics secondary to long-term neuroleptic exposure (i.e., "tardive tics").[69] L-Dopa-induced tics have been reported with the treatment of Parkinson's disease but are an exceedingly rare complication of this disorder.

Treatment

Pharmacological and nonpharmacological management of tics is covered with the treatment of TS (see Chap. 41).

There are very few data on the course and treatment of tics secondary to neurologic conditions other than TS. The first goal is to treat the primary condition whenever possible, or to eliminate the agent thought to be mediating the symptoms. Examples include the use immune modulators in the treatment of poststreptococcal tics/chorea/OCS, and the judicious substitution or elimination of the suspected agent (see Table 42-3). The limited literature and our cumulative experience suggest that the results of pharmacotherapy in the treatment of tics in neurologic conditions other than TS and in secondary tic disorders is variable and in general inferior to the results obtained in TS. In neurologically impaired individuals, we favor the use of low doses of dopamine blockers with low potential for sedation. Recent reports suggest that clonic and dystonic motor tics refractory to pharmacotherapy may respond to local injections of botulinum toxin.[70,71] In carefully selected patients with severe vocal tics (including coprolalia), botulinum toxin injections have been shown to significantly improve these symptoms.[72,73]

References

1. Erenberg G, Cruse RP, Rothner AD: The natural history of Tourette syndrome: A follow-up study. *Ann Neurol* 22:383–385, 1987.
2. Goetz CG, Tanner CM, Stebbin GT, et al: Adult ticks in Gilles de la Tourette's syndrome: Description and risk factors. *Neurology* 42:784–788, 1992.
3. Leckman JF, Zhang H, Vitale A, et al: Course of tic severity in Tourette syndrome: The first two decades. *Pediatrics* 102:14–19, 1998.
4. Leckman JF, Cohen AJ (eds): *Tourette's Syndrome: Developmental Psychopathology and Clinical Care.* New York: Wiley, 1999.
5. Jankovic J: The neurology of tics. *Mov Disord* 383–405, 1987.
6. Jankovic J, Stone L: Dystonic tics in patients with Tourette's syndrome. *Mov Disord* 6:248–252, 1991.
7. Stone L, Jankovic J: The coexistence of tics and dystonia. *Arch Neurol* 48:862–865, 1991.
8. Cohen AJ, Leckman JF: Sensory phenomena associated with Gilles de la Tourette's syndrome. *J Clin Psychiatry* 53:319–323, 1992.
9. Leckman JF, Walker DE, Cohen DJ: Premonitory urges in Tourette's syndrome. *Am J Psychiatry* 150:98–102, 1993.
10. Bliss J: Sensory experiences of Gilles de la Tourette syndrome. *Arch Gen Psychiatry* 37:1343–1347, 1980.
11. Kurlan R, Lichter D, Hewitt D: Sensory tics in Tourette's syndrome. *Neurology* 39:731–734, 1989.
12. Shapiro AK, Shapiro ES, Young YB, Feinber TE (eds): *Gilles de la Tourette Syndrome.* New York: Raven Press, 1088.
13. Obeso JA, Rothwell JC, Marsden CD: Simple tics in Gilles de la Tourette's syndrome are not prefaced by a normal premovement EEG potential. *J Neurol Neurosurg Psychiatry* 14:735–738, 1981.
14. Papa SM, Artieda J, Obeso JA: Cortical activity preceding self-initiated and externally triggered voluntary movement. *Mov Disord* 6:217–224, 1991.
15. Lang A: Patient perception of tics and other movement disorders. *Neurology* 41:223–238, 1991.
16. Fahn S: Motor and vocal tics, in *Handbook of Tourette Syndrome and Related Tic and Behavioral Disorders.* 1993, pp 3–16.
17. Karp BI, Hallet M: Extracorporeal "phantom tics" in Tourette's syndrome. *Neurology* 46:38–40, 1996.
18. Green RC, Pitman RK: Tourette syndrome and obsessive-compulsive disorder: Clinical relationship, in *Obsessive Compulsive Disorders: Theory and Management.* 1990.
19. Singer HS: Neurobiological issues in Tourette syndrome. *Brain Dev* 16:353–364, 1994.
20. Sacks OW: Acquired tourettism in adult life. *Adv Neurol* 35:89–92, 1982.
21. Devinsky O: Neuroanatomy of Gilles de la Tourette's syndrome: Possible midbrain involvement. *Arch Neurol* 40:508–514, 1983.
22. Alexander GE, DeLong MR, Strick PL: Parallel organization of functionally segregated circuits linking basal ganglia and cortex. *Annu Rev Neurosci* 9:357–381, 1986.
23. Alexander GE, Crutcher MD, DeLong MR: Basal ganglia-thalamocortical circuits: Parallel substrates for motor, oculomotor, "prefrontal" and "limbic" functions. *Prog Brain Res* 85:119–146, 1990.
24. Muller-Perus P, Jurgens U: Projections from the "cingular" vocalization area in the squirrel monkey. *Brain Res* 103:29–43, 1976.
25. Baleydier C, Mauquierre F: The duality of the cingulate gyrus in monkey. *Brain* 103:525–554, 1980.
26. Peterson B, Riddle MA, Cohen DJ, et al: Reduced basal ganglia volumes in Tourette's syndrome using three dimensional reconstruction techniques from magnetic resonance images. *Neurology* 43:941–948, 1993.
27. Singer HS, Reiss AL, Brown JE, et al: Volumetric MRI changes in basal ganglia of children with Tourette's syndrome. *Neurology* 43:950–956, 1993.
28. Witelson SF: Clinical neurology as data for basic neuroscience: Tourette's syndrome and the human motor system. *Neurology* 43:859–861, 1993.
29. Stoetter B, Braun AR, Randolpf C, et al: Functional neuroanatomy of Tourette's syndrome limbic-motor interactions studied with FDG PET. *Adv Neurol* 58:213–226, 1992.
30. Swerdlow NB, Caine SB, Geyer MA: Regionally selective effects of intracerebral dopamine infusion on sensorimotor gating of the startle reflex in rats. *Psychopharmacology* 108:189–195, 1992.
31. Mogenson GJ, Jones DL, Chi YY: From motivation to action: Functional interface between the limbic system and the motor system. *Prog Neurobiol* 14:69–97, 1980.
32. Gedye A: Tourette syndrome attributed to frontal lobe dysfunction: Numerous etiologies involved. *J Clin Psychol* 47:233–252, 1991.
33. Bergen D, Tanner C, Wilson R: The electroencephalogram in Tourette syndrome. *Ann Neurol* 11:382–385, 1982.
34. Neufeld MY, Berger Y, Chapman J, Korcyzn A: Routine and quantitative EEG analysis in Gilles de la Tourette's syndrome. *Neurology* 40:1837–1839, 1990.
35. Krumholz A, Singer HS, Niedermyer E, et al: Electrophysiological studies in Tourette's syndrome. *Ann Neurol* 14:638–641, 1983.
36. Glaze DG, Frost JD, Jankovic J: Sleep in Gilles de la Tourette's syndrome. *Neurology* 33:586–592, 1983.
37. Gabor B, Matthewes WS, Ferrari M: Disorders of arousal in Gilles de la Tourette's syndrome. *Neurology* 33:586–592, 1984.
38. Bock RD, Goldberger L: Tonic, phasic and cortical arousal in Gilles de la Tourette's syndrome. *J Neurol Neurosurg Psychiatry* 48:535–544, 1985.

39. Robertson M, Doran M, Trimble M, Less AJ: The treatment of Gilles de la Tourette syndrome by limbic leucotomy. *J Neurol Neurosurg Psychiatry* 53:691–694, 1990.

40. Leckman JF, Lotbiniere D, Marek K, et al: Severe disturbances in speech, swallowing and gait following stereotactic infrathalamic lesions in Gilles de la Tourette's syndrome. *Neurology* 43:890–893, 1993.

41. Kurlan JF, Kersun J, Ballantine J, et al: Neurosurgical treatment of severe obsessive-compulsive disorder associated with Tourette's syndrome. *Mov Disord* 5:152–155, 1990.

42. Messiha FS: Biochemical pharmacology of Gilles de la Tourette's syndrome. *Neurosci Biobehav Rev* 12:295–305, 1988.

43. Barbeau A: Cholinergic treatment in Tourette syndrome. *N Engl J Med* 302:1310–1311, 1980.

44. Sandyk R: Cholinergic mechanisms in Gilles de la Tourette's syndrome. *Int J Neurosci* 81:95–100, 1995.

45. Guyenet PG, Agid Y, Javoy F, et al: Effects of dopaminergic receptor agonists and antagonists on the activity of neostriatal cholinergic system. *Brain Res* 84:227–244, 1975.

46. Jankovic J, Rohaidy H: Motor, behavioral and pharmacologic findings in Tourette's syndrome. *Can J Neurol Sci* 14:541–546, 1987.

47. Tanner CM, Goetz CG, Klawans HL: Cholinergic mechanisms in Tourette's syndrome. *Neurology* 32:1315–1317, 1982.

48. Polinsky RJ, Ebert MH, Caine ED, et al: Cholinergic treatment in the Tourette's syndrome. *N Engl J Med* 302:1310–1311, 1980.

49. Comings DE (ed): *Tourette Syndrome and Human Behavior.* Duarte, CA: Hope Press, 1990.

50. Charney DS, Goodman WK, Price LH, et al: Serotonin function in obsessive-compulsive disorder. *Arch Gen Psychiatry* 45:177–185, 1988.

51. Spitz MC, Jancovic J, Killian JM: Familial tic disorder, parkinsonism, motor neuron disease, and acanthocytosis: A new syndrome. *Neurology* 35:366–370, 1985.

52. Kurczynski TW: Hyperekplexia. *Arch Neurol* 40:246–248, 1983.

53. Lees AJ (ed): *Ticks and Related Disorders.* London: Churchil Livingstone, 1985.

54. Andermann F, Keene DL, Andermann E, Quesney LF: Startle disease or hyperekplexia: Further delineation of the syndrome. *Brain* 103:985–997, 1980.

55. Saenz-Lope E, Herran-Tanarro FJ, Masdeu JC, Chacon-Pena JR: Hyperplexia: A syndrome of pathologic startle responses. *Ann Neurol* 15:36–41, 1984.

56. Milani N, Dalpra L, del Prete A, et al: A novel mutation (Gln266→His) in the alpha 1 subunit of the inhibitory glycine receptor gene (GLRA1) in the hereditary hyperekplexia [letter]. *Am J Hum Genet* 58:420–422, 1996.

57. Floeter MK, Andermann F, Andermann E, et al: Physiological studies of spinal inhibitory pathways in patients with hereditary hyperekplexia. *Neurology* 46:766–772, 1996.

58. Fahn S: A case of post-traumatic tic syndrome. *Adv Neurol* 35:349–350, 1982.

59. Gaul JJ: Posttraumatic tic disorder. *Mov Disord* 9:121, 1994.

60. Pulst SM, Walshe TM, Romero JA: Carbon monoxide poisoning with features of Gilles de la Tourette's syndrome. *Arch Neurol* 40:443–444, 1983.

61. Northam RS, Singer HS: Postencephalitic acquired Tourette's-like syndrome in a child. *Neurology* 41:592–593, 1991.

62. Davis TME, Knezevick W: Multiple tics following cerebral malaria. *Med J Aust* 160:307–308, 1994.

63. Husby G, Van De Rijn I, Zabriskie JB, et al: Antibodies reacting with cytoplasm of subthalamic and caudate nuclei neurons in chorea and acute rheumatic fever. *J Exp Med* 144:1094, 1976.

64. Kiessling LS, Marcotte AC, Culpepper L: Antineuronal antibodies in movement disorders. *Pediatrics* 92:39–43, 1993.

65. Pasqual-Leone A, Dhuna A: Cocaine associated multifacial tics. *Neurology* 40:999–1000, 1990.

66. Robertson PL, Garofalo AG, Silverstein FS, Komarynski MA: Carbamazepine induced tics. *Epilepsia* 34:965–968, 1993.

67. Howrie DL, Crumrine PK: Phenytoin-induced movement disorder associated with intravenous administration for status epilepticus. *Clin Pediatr* 24:467–469, 1985.

68. Burd L, Kerbeshian J, Fisher W, Gascon G: Anticonvulsant medications: An iatrogenic cause of tic disorder. *Can J Psychiatry* 31:419–423, 1986.

69. Klawans H, Nausieda P, Goetz C, et al: Tourette-like symptoms following chronic neuroleptic therapy. *Gilles de la Tourette Syndrome* 35:415–418, 1982.

70. Kwak CH, Hanna PA, Jankovic J: Botulinum toxin in the treatment of tics. *Arch Neurol* 57:1190–1193, 2000.

71. Marras C, Andrews D, Sime E, Lang AE: Botulinum toxin for simple motor tics: A randomized, double-blind, controlled clinical trial. *Neurology* 56:605–610, 2001.

72. Trimble MR, Whurr R, Brookes G, Robertson MM: Vocal tics in Gilles de la Tourette syndrome treated with botulinum toxin injections. *Mov Disord* 13:617–619, 1998.

73. Scott BL, Jankovic J, Donovan DT: Botulinum toxin injection into vocal cord in the treatment of malignant coprolalia associated with Tourette's syndrome. *Mov Disord* 11:431–433, 1996.

VII. ATAXIAS

Chapter 43

THE MOLECULAR GENETICS OF THE ATAXIAS

GEORGE R. WILMOT and S.H. SUBRAMONY

CLINICAL APPROACH 705
   Diagnosis 705
   Symptomatic Treatment 707
   Supportive Care and Rehabilitation 707
   Counseling 708
AUTOSOMAL-DOMINANT ATAXIAS 708
   Spinocerebellar Ataxia Type 1 (SCA1) 708
   Spinocerebellar Ataxia Type 2 (SCA2) 709
   Spinocerebellar Ataxia Type 3 (SCA3)/
     Machado-Joseph Disease (MJD) 709
   Spinocerebellar Ataxia Type 4 (SCA4) 710
   Spinocerebellar Ataxia Type 5 (SCA5) 710
   Spinocerebellar Ataxia Type 6 (SCA6) 710
   Spinocerebellar Ataxia Type 7 (SCA7) 711
   Spinocerebellar Ataxia Type 8 (SCA8) 711
   Spinocerebellar Ataxia Type 10 (SCA10) 711
   Spinocerebellar Ataxia Type 11 (SCA11) 711
   Spinocerebellar Ataxia Type 12 (SCA12) 712
   Spinocerebellar Ataxia Types 13–16 (SCA13–16) 712
   Spinocerebellar Ataxia Type 17 (SCA17) 712
   Dentatorubropallidoluysian Atrophy (DRPLA) 712
   Episodic Ataxia Type 1 (EA1) 712
   Episodic Ataxia Type 2 (EA2) 712
   Other Autosomal-Dominant Ataxias 713
AUTOSOMAL-RECESSIVE ATAXIAS 713
   Friedreich's Ataxia (FRDA) 713
   Ataxia Telangiectasia (AT) 713
   Ataxias Associated with Vitamin E Deficiency 714
   Ataxia with Oculomotor Apraxia-1 (AOA1) 714
   Autosomal-Recessive Spastic Ataxia of
     Charlevoix-Saguenay 715
   Spinocerebellar Ataxia with Axonal
     Neuropathy (SCAN) 715
   Inborn Errors of Metabolism 715
   Other Autosomal-Recessive Ataxias 715
X-LINKED ATAXIAS 715
MITOCHONDRIAL ATAXIAS 715
SUMMARY 716

The inherited ataxias are a group of disorders that are characterized by incoordination and loss of balance and are often accompanied by other neurological symptoms depending on the extent that pathology extends beyond cerebellar circuitry. They are usually progressive, neurodegenerative disorders and can lead to significant debilitation and death.

Recent years have seen dramatic advances in our understanding of the genetic causes of the inherited ataxias, and with that our ability to diagnose and classify specific genetic conditions has greatly increased. But the rapid rate of new discoveries also makes it quite difficult to keep abreast of the current "state of the art" in diagnosis, much less the myriad scientific advances in the field. In Summer 2002, a search of Online Mendelian Inheritance in Man (OMIM) returned 487 entries (including both diseases and genes) for the search word "ataxia." Clearly, this massive amount of information must be prioritized in order to more efficiently understand it. As with other recent reviews,[1–3] we have tried to address here the diseases that are most clinically relevant by virtue of their prevalence, predominance of ataxia among other neurological symptoms, ease of diagnosis, or response to treatment. Because this list is not exhaustive, other sources of information should be sought when necessary. Three very good online sources of frequently updated information are OMIM (http://www.ncbi.nlm.nih.gov/Omim/), Genetests/Geneclinics (http://genetests.org/), and the website of the Neuromuscular Disease Center at Washington University (http://www.neuro.wustl.edu/neuromuscular/ataxia/aindex.html).

Clinical Approach

Although there is no set clinical approach to the inherited ataxias, most specialists tend to use similar strategies when evaluating and treating someone who presents with a gait disorder that might fall into this category of disease (see Fig. 43-1). As with most clinical algorithms, the approach outlined in Fig. 43-1 represents a post-hoc conceptualization of these strategies rather than a rigid procedural prescription.

DIAGNOSIS

After ensuring that the patient truly suffers from ataxia, diagnostic considerations turn to separating the inherited ataxias from acquired conditions that are potentially treatable. If there is a clear family history of the disease, an inherited cause can be assumed and then investigated after considering the inheritance pattern. Acquired causes include a number of structural, nutritional, endocrine, toxic, paraneoplastic, and inflammatory conditions, some of which can be easily identified and possibly treated (e.g., vitamin E deficiency). Of particular interest are those that are hard to distinguish from some of the inherited ataxias. Patients in this subgroup of acquired ataxia tend to have slowly developing symptoms, nonspecific magnetic resonance imaging (MRI) changes (e.g., cerebellar atrophy), and normal routine laboratory values. In this subgroup, it is often prudent to consider toxic causes, to look for "gluten ataxia" with antigliadin and antiendomyseal antibodies,[4,5] and to check anti-glutamic acid decarboxylase

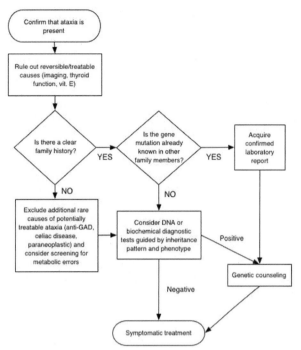

FIGURE 43-1 General clinical approach to the ataxic patient. GAD, glutamic acid decarboxylase.

TABLE 43-1 Reasons for a Negative Family History in Hereditary Disorders

Inadequately obtained family history
Autosomal-recessive or X-linked inheritance
Reduced penetrance
Genetic anticipation
Phenotypic variability
New mutation
False paternity
Early death of affected relative

antibodies, which can be associated with cerebellar degeneration even without symptoms of stiff-person syndrome.[6] If there is no family history and the onset of symptoms is subacute, inherited causes are unlikely and consideration should turn towards paraneoplastic and other inflammatory conditions.

Is the patient's disease inherited? The answer to this important question is obvious when a strong family history is present, but what about the patients who have a negative family history? In this case, it is important to keep in mind the potential explanations for genetic etiologies presenting with a negative family history (Table 43-1). In taking a good family history, accurate information should be obtained on all relatives (alive and dead) in three generations; this should include questions about age at symptom onset and age at death, consanguinity, spontaneous abortions, ethnic origin, and of course inquiries into relevant symptoms. Broad-based questioning is best (i.e., asking about walking or balance or coordination rather than "ataxia"). Even within individual families, many inherited ataxias have significant phenotypic variation that can make detection of a positive family history difficult, so careful, detailed questioning is required.

One source of phenotypic variation that applies particularly to the inherited ataxias is genetic anticipation, which refers to a feature of inheritance in which successive generations become increasingly affected either through higher penetrance (the likelihood that a person possessing the mutation will have the disease) or higher expressivity (earlier age of onset or more severe disease). The molecular basis of genetic anticipation involves the dynamic mutational mechanism of polynucleotide repeat instability. In most diseases, the mutation is an enlarged trinucleotide repeat that expands further upon germline transmission. A high degree of anticipation can lead to a false negative family history when a child is affected before the onset of symptoms in their parents or grandparents. This has been noted particularly in spinocerebellar ataxia type 7 (SCA7) and dentatorubropallidoluysian atrophy (DRPLA).

Since only 1 out of 4 offspring will inherit an autosomal-recessive disease from their heterozygous carrier parents, we frequently see no obvious family history in recessive disorders. By expanding the pedigree over many generations the likelihood of identifying other family members with the disease increases, but practical limitations come into play and evidence of familial involvement can therefore be hard to find.

Accurately diagnosing a progressive ataxia can be beneficial by leading to specific therapy (if not presently, then perhaps in the future), by allowing for accurate counseling (genetic, psychiatric, and prognostic) and by providing a greater peace of mind for the patient. These patients may see many physicians who have been unable to establish a diagnosis, and the patients may become extremely frustrated, sometimes fearing the unknown (e.g., is this life-threatening?) more than the actual disease itself. The value of accurate diagnosis should not be underestimated, even when no specific therapies exist for the potential diseases.[7]

Should all patients with a progressive ataxic syndrome be genetically screened for known ataxia mutations? Opinions differ among ataxia experts, but one reasonable approach is outlined in Fig. 43-2. One of the factors driving these decisions is that a number of studies have screened patients with sporadic ataxia and found that 5–15 percent actually have one of the known ataxia-associated mutations, most typically Friedreich's ataxia (FRDA) or SCA6.[8–12] The outcomes of these studies may be biased by referral patterns and the skill and knowledge of the examining neurologists, but the point that some patients with apparently sporadic ataxia actually have an inherited disease cannot be denied.

Diseases for which commercial DNA tests are available are outlined in Table 43-2.

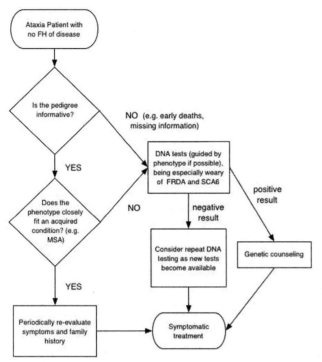

FIGURE 43-2 Strategy for DNA testing in ataxia patients without a family history of ataxia. MSA, multiple-system atrophy; FRDA, Friedreich's ataxia.

SYMPTOMATIC TREATMENT

Unlike extrapyramidal symptoms, ataxia rarely responds to any pharmacological intervention. This should not be surprising, since motor coordination is dependent on the precise integration of multiple neural events that encompass a variety of neurochemical systems. The few reports that show benefit of a particular agent[13–18] should be interpreted cautiously, taking into account the difficulties in accurately quantifying ataxia and the limited reproducibility of their findings.[19–21]

Unlike ataxia, some of the associated neurological symptoms may respond well to currently available medications. Extrapyramidal symptoms accompany ataxia in a variety of ataxic syndromes, and these may respond to standard treatment with dopaminergic agents, anticholinergic medications, or botox injections.[22–24] Neurogenic urinary dysfunction occurs often and typically responds well to treatment with oxybutynin or tolterodine.[25] Sleep disturbances, particularly restless legs syndrome, are common in the SCAs and usually respond to conventional treatment.[26–28]

Psychiatric disturbances should be sought in all ataxic patients and treated appropriately. Depression is common and often contributes significantly to lowered quality of life. Depending on the degree of disability, social difficulties may be significant and contribute markedly to affective dysfunction, so it is often imperative to include psychiatric counseling as part of the treatment. Psychosis and anxiety are less common, but when present should be treated as in any other patient.

SUPPORTIVE CARE AND REHABILITATION

Many different approaches may be required to maximize the daily functioning of an ataxic patient. Mobility is usually the prime issue, but swallowing function is often disturbed as well and requires careful monitoring and potentially intervention with a feeding tube. Evaluation and training for canes, walkers, and/or wheelchairs become necessary in most patients. Orthotics may be required, particularly in patients with superimposed weakness. Balance rehabilitation has been used successfully for vestibular disorders and may benefit ataxia as well.[29] It is unfortunate that so few studies

TABLE 43-2 Commercially Available DNA Tests for Ataxia

Disease	Repeat Type	Normal Alleles	Disease-Causing Alleles	Comments
SCA1	Coding CAG	6–44	38–81	Intermediate alleles 36–44 should be tested for CAA interruptions
SCA2	Coding CAG	14–31	36–>400	Intermediate alleles of 32–35 repeats have reduced penetrance
SCA3	Coding CAG	12–43	53–86	The low end of the pathogenic range may not be associated with ataxia
SCA6	Coding CAG	4–16	20–33	
SCA7	Coding CAG	4–19	37–>300	
SCA8	Noncoding CTG	16–34	~100–250	Variable penetrance, especially with large expansions
SCA10	Intronic ATTCT	10–22	800–4500	
SCA17	Coding CAG	30–42	45–63	
DRPLA	Coding CAG	3–36	49–88	
FRDA	Intronic GAA	5–33	66–>1700	~95 percent of cases will have expansions on each allele; the remainder are likely to be compound heterozygotes with an expansion on one allele and a point mutation on the other. Testing for point mutations is not routinely done but may be arranged through some laboratories

have been published on balance rehabilitation in ataxia, especially in light of the dearth of pharmacological treatment options.

COUNSELING

In addition to the general benefit of psychiatric counseling, genetic counseling can specifically address issues related to the inherited ataxias. Many patients do not understand the genetic probabilities of passing on the disease and want to know more for family planning purposes. Should they adopt? Should their spouse be tested? Is prenatal diagnosis available? These are all important questions that can be addressed by a genetic counselor. One of the most confusing topics is whether or not presymptomatic testing should be sought in at-risk family members. Many of the issues are nearly identical between Huntington's disease (HD) and the autosomal-dominant ataxias, since they share the molecular pathogenic mechanism of expanded CAG repeats, and an extensive literature exists on this topic in HD.[30,31]

Autosomal-Dominant Ataxias

Many years prior to the discovery of any causative gene mutation, Harding coined the term "autosomal-dominant cerebellar ataxia" (ADCA), and defined ADCA subtypes based on clinical criteria (type I, cerebellar signs with additional neurological features; type II, with visual loss; type III, pure cerebellar dysfunction).[32] Although the ADCA classification of dominant ataxias is still sometimes seen in the literature, the current scheme of classification by genotype is much more informative and practical and should be used in lieu of the ADCA classification.

Within the ataxia field, the term "spinocerebellar ataxia" (SCA) is usually reserved for the nonepisodic autosomal-dominant ataxias. We still do not know how many different gene mutations cause SCA, but at present more than 20 loci and 10 genes (DRPLA) have been found. In most populations, the known gene mutations account for the majority of cases of SCA,[8,10,12,33–37] so it is likely that additional genes and loci will represent relatively rare causes of SCA. The relative prevalence of each type of SCA varies in different ethnic populations; for example, among SCA patients, SCA1 and SCA2 are seen much more frequently in the UK[34] than in Japan.[35] Recent evidence suggests that the relative prevalence of some of the SCAs among different populations may be explained by the rates of large normal alleles, which presumably are more likely to expand into the pathogenic range.[37,38]

The high degree of phenotypic overlap between the SCAs limits the clinician's ability to predict genotype based on phenotype. Some clinical features tend to suggest specific SCAs (Table 43-3) and can be used to guide DNA testing, but the accuracy of this approach is currently limited.

TABLE 43-3 Clinical Features Suggesting Specific SCA Genotypes

Genotype	Phenotype
SCA1	Pyramidal signs, hypermetric saccades
SCA2	Slow saccades, hyporeflexia, tremor, occasional dementia
SCA3	High intrafamilial variability, extrapyramidal signs, gaze-evoked nystagmus, hypometric saccades, peripheral neuropathy
SCA4	Sensory neuropathy, slow course
SCA5	Mild, slow progression, pure cerebellar
SCA6	Downbeat nystagmus, episodic symptoms, slow progression
SCA7	Visual loss, slow saccades, dramatic anticipation
SCA8	Dorsal column sensation loss, pyramidal signs
SCA10	Seizures, dementia
SCA11	Mild ataxia
SCA12	Early tremor, dementia
SCA13	Short stature, mild mental retardation
SCA14	Myoclonus
SCA15	Mild, slow progression
SCA16	Tremor
SCA17	Dementia, extrapyramidal signs
DRPLA	Seizures, myoclonus, chorea, dementia, dramatic anticipation
EA1	Episodic ataxia (seconds to minutes), myokymia, no vertigo
EA2	Episodic ataxia and vertigo (minutes to hours), response to acetazolamide

Continued systematic acquisition of detailed clinical features may eventually lead to increased accuracy.[39]

Among the nonepisodic dominant ataxias, gene mutations have been identified for SCA1–3, 6–8, 10, 12, 17, and DRPLA. Perhaps remarkably, every one of these mutations is an expansion of a normally repetitive stretch of DNA, a mutational mechanism that was first described less than 10 years ago. Almost all are trinucleotide repeat expansions; only the SCA10 mutation is a different repeat unit (a pentanucleotide). Both episodic ataxias are caused by point mutations in ion channel genes and share many characteristics with other channelopathies.

SPINOCEREBELLAR ATAXIA TYPE 1 (SCA1)

Patients with this disorder most often present in the 3rd or 4th decades of life, but a wide variation in age of onset may be seen, including juvenile-onset.[40] At the very earliest stages, there may be only a mild gait imbalance, but, with time, progressive gait and limb ataxia, dysarthria, and bulbar dysfunction ensue.[41] Nystagmus is often present early in the disease, but eventually saccadic slowing and gaze palsies may develop and nystagmus may then diminish.[42] Likewise, hyperreflexia is most common early in the course of the disease and then may turn to hyporeflexia in later stages due to the development of peripheral neuropathy.[42–45]

Mild extrapyramidal features such as chorea[46] may develop in advanced, typically wheelchair-dependent patients, but these finding are usually less common and less severe than with SCA2 or SCA3. Cognitive impairment may also occur late in the disease.[47] Weakness and atrophy of the face and tongue occur along with severe dysphagia,[48] and reflect a progressive bulbar dysfunction that is associated with significant morbidity and mortality, most often by way of respiratory failure. The duration of the disease from onset until death is usually expected to range from ~10–15 years.

In the past decade there have been amazing strides in our scientific understanding of the SCAs, with Orr, Zhogbi and their colleagues leading the way with their studies on SCA1. In 1993, Orr et al. identified an expansion of a normally polymorphic CAG repeat within the SCA1 gene as the disease-causing mutation in this disorder.[40] Because the CAG triplet codes for glutamine, the crucial molecular defect appears to be a toxic gain-of-function caused by an enlarged tract of glutamine residues within the coded protein. SCA1 and other diseases with coding CAG expansions are therefore sometimes referred to as "polyglutamine diseases."

The SCA1 gene codes for ataxin-1, a protein with unknown cellular function that is largely localized to the cell nucleus.[49] Normal individuals have CAG lengths of 6–44 repeats, and in normal alleles with 21 or more repeats the CAG tract is interrupted 1–3 times by CAT triplets that code for histidine rather than glutamine.[50] In contrast, affected individuals have uninterrupted repeat sizes of 39–81 repeats.[40,51,52] As with the other inherited ataxias caused by repeat expansions, the relatively inexpensive DNA test for SCA1 utilizes the polymerase chain reaction (PCR) to amplify the repeat and determine its size. For individuals with intermediate-sized repeats (36–44), a specific restriction digestion of the PCR product can be utilized to test for the presence of CAA interruptions, thereby distinguishing normal from disease-associated alleles in this size range.[50] Uninterrupted repeat lengths of 36–38 have not yet been reported to cause the disease, but on transmission to offspring they may expand into the disease-causing range.

While the details of SCA1 pathophysiology continue to be elucidated, work to this point has shown that the mutant protein is likely to aggregate with itself and with other proteins, particularly within the nucleus, and that nuclear localization is critical for pathogenesis.[53] In animal models, changes in the expression of specific genes occur early in the disease process[54] and may eventually be a target for therapeutic intervention.

SPINOCEREBELLAR ATAXIA TYPE 2 (SCA2)

This disease was first identified in the Cuban population,[55] but has subsequently been described in a variety of populations. SCA2 has been found to be the most common autosomal-dominant ataxia in Italy,[56] the UK, and India;[57] in other populations it is less common.[33] Clinical variability is somewhat higher than with SCA1 but the clinical presentations often overlap.[43] Age of onset is centered around

the 4th decade, but a wide variation occurs. Ataxia and dysarthria are always present, but in addition dramatically slowed saccadic velocities, tremor, chorea/dystonia, hyporeflexia, and dementia may occur, particularly later in the course of the disease.[58]

SCA2 is caused by an expansion of a CAG repeat within the SCA2 gene.[59–61] Unlike most of the other triplet repeat diseases, the size of normal alleles is not very polymorphic; although normal alleles range from 14 to 31 repeats, approximately 95 percent of the normal alleles have either 22 or 23.[61]

Intermediate-sized alleles (32–35 repeats) may or may not be pathogenic, and the factors that may promote penetrance are not known. CAA interruptions of the repeat occur, but for SCA2 these interruptions do not clearly distinguish normal and disease-associated alleles from within the intermediate range. This makes sense since the interruptions are with CAA triplets, which, like CAG, code for glutamine and therefore will not affect the protein sequence. Uninterrupted repeats are likely to be more prone to expansion upon transmission to offspring, however.[62]

The mutant ataxin-2 protein has been shown to be cytoplasmic, and early studies failed to find evidence of nuclear inclusions that are found in many of the other polyglutamine diseases.[63,64] More recent experiments with a polyglutamine-specific antibody has provided evidence of nuclear accumulation, however.[65] Nonubiquinated microaggregates are also found in the cytoplasm.[64]

Expansions of 36 or more repeats are disease-causing, and most often occur as uninterrupted repeats of 36–64 units long. Recently there have been descriptions of very large expansions (200–500) associated with severe early-onset disease. These very large expansions are difficult to detect with the standard SCA2 PCR test, but they are identifiable with a PCR-blot assay.[66]

SPINOCEREBELLAR ATAXIA TYPE 3 (SCA3)/ MACHADO-JOSEPH DISEASE (MJD)

MJD was initially described among Portuguese Azorean families as an autosomal-dominant degenerative ataxia with an extremely wide phenotypic variability.[67] After the identification of the responsible genetic mutation[68] it became clear that this disorder is in fact the same as SCA3, a separately described dominant ataxia originally thought to have less phenotypic variability.

In the early clinical descriptions of Portuguese MJD patients three general phenotypes were identified: type I (spastic-rigid syndrome with bradykinesia and dystonia and relatively little ataxia), type II (the most common type, with ataxia and upper motor neuron signs), and type III (ataxia and peripheral neuropathy). More recently a type IV (relatively pure parkinsonism) has also been described.[23] In general, type I is more typical of early-onset patients and type III of later-onset patients. The usefulness of these distinctions is debatable since all types can occur within a single family and individuals may progress from one type to another, but their recognition does highlight the significant clinical variability that is seen in this disease, often much more than in SCA1 or SCA2.

The age of onset and disease duration of SCA3/MJD are similar to that of SCA1 and SCA2, although usually with more variability.[69] Most SCA3/MJD patients present with early gait ataxia and dysarthria and progressively lose ambulation, eventually dying from respiratory problems related to their severe debilitation. Although SCA3/MJD cannot be definitely distinguished from other SCAs on clinical grounds alone,[43] certain features tend to be more prominent in this subtype, including nystagmus and ophthalmoplegia,[39] facial fasciculations, blepharospasm and other facial dystonias,[24] a "bulging eyes" facies caused by lid retraction and decreased blinking, and prominent parkinsonism.[24]

SCA3/MJD is caused by a CAG repeat expansion in the MJD1 gene which results in a longer glutamine tract within the ataxin-3 protein. Unlike some of the other SCAs, there is no overlap in normal and disease-causing alleles; normal individuals have 12–43 repeats, and affected individuals possess repeat lengths from ~60 to 86.[70–73] The smallest abnormal expansions reported to date are 53 and 54 repeat units; these were associated with a variant phenotype consisting of restless legs syndrome and polyneuropathy.[28] Disease severity, as reflected by both age of onset and clinical symptoms, is clearly correlated with repeat size.

The function of ataxin-3 is unknown. It is normally found predominantly in the cytoplasm,[74] but expanded ataxin-3 occurs within intranuclear inclusions found mostly in areas of the brain affected by the disease.[75] Whether these inclusions are a key causative factor in the cellular pathophysiology of SCA3/MJD or simply a by-product of the cellular pathological process is not currently known but is under active investigation.[76–78]

SPINOCEREBELLAR ATAXIA TYPE 4 (SCA4)

This rare SCA subtype follows a relatively benign course and is characterized by ataxia and sensory loss due to a sensory axonal neuropathy.[79,80] Pyramidal signs may also occasionally be present. As with other inherited neuropathies, patients will often have minimal symptoms despite significant EMG/NCS abnormalities and physical examination findings of sensory loss. The responsible gene is unknown but has been localized to 16q22.1 by linkage analysis in a large Utah kindred.[80] Since the causative gene mutation has not yet been found, the only way to confirm a diagnosis of SCA4 is through linkage analysis. Recently, a Japanese family with a pure cerebellar syndrome localizing to the same region has been reported,[81,82] so sensory neuropathy may not be universal in this disease.

SPINOCEREBELLAR ATAXIA TYPE 5 (SCA5)

This ataxia has previously been referred to as "Lincoln ataxia" because it was described in a family descended from the grandparents of President Lincoln.[83] It appears to be rare, but has been described in an additional French family.[84] The onset of SCA5 is usually in the 3rd to 4th decade and the clinical course is typically slow, with relatively pure cerebellar dysfunction being the rule in all but a few patients with juvenile onset. In adult-onset cases there is no limitation of lifespan, perhaps owing to the paucity of bulbar dysfunction that otherwise may predispose patients to recurrent pneumonia.

The Lincoln family appears to display anticipation, indicating that a repeat expansion may be the genetic basis of this disorder. The SCA5 locus has been localized to a 3-cM region on 11q13,[83] and repeat expansions have been sought in order to identify the disease-causing gene. To date, none of these efforts has been successful, and positional cloning efforts are ongoing.

SPINOCEREBELLAR ATAXIA TYPE 6 (SCA6)

SCA6 is one of three allelic disorders that have been linked to mutations in the CACNA1A gene that codes for the alpha1A-subunit of the voltage-gated calcium channel. Whereas the other two diseases, familial hemiplegic migraine and episodic ataxia type 2 (EA2), are caused by point mutations, SCA6 is caused by a CAG repeat expansion. But, as might be expected, some clinical overlap occurs within this group of disorders and as a result the genotype-phenotype correlations are not as rigid as once thought. For instance, some patients with SCA6 appear to go through an early phase of episodic symptoms that can include tinnitus, nausea, vertigo, ataxia, dysarthria, and visual disturbances prior to the development of progressive ataxia.[85,86] Episodic symptoms may persist into this progressive phase. In addition, EA2 patients often have interictal signs of cerebellar dysfunction that may worsen over time.

The progressive ataxia of SCA6 is usually a rather pure cerebellar syndrome, but more widespread dysfunction can also occur, especially in patients with long-standing disease.[87,88] Therefore findings such as ophthalmoplegia, sensory disturbances, reflex changes, and extrapyramidal features do not exclude a diagnosis of SCA6. Although there is some overlap between the SCAs, the eye movement abnormalities of SCA6 include prominent nystagmus (often downbeat) and saccadic pursuits[89] and may help suggest a diagnosis of SCA6. SCA6 is probably significantly more common than SCA4 or SAC5 and therefore is more likely to be the correct diagnosis in patients with pure cerebellar features.

Aside from FRDA, SCA6 is the most commonly found gene mutation when apparently sporadic ataxia cases are genetically screened (~5 percent of cases).[88,90–92] This is most likely a result of its mild features, episodic tendencies, and late onset, all of which can allow a positive family history to go unnoticed. Bona fide incomplete penetrance may also occur. New mutations are probably not a strong contributor to the prevalence of SCA6 among sporadic cases; only 1 case of a new mutation has been found.[93]

SCA6 differs from the other SCAs in a number of ways. Clinically, the age of onset in SCA6 is later and the course is more benign. In addition, since the affected gene is an ion channel subunit and the polyglutamine expansion may affect channel function,[94-96] clinical features of a channelopathy (e.g., episodic symptoms) make up part of the phenotype. With regard to the molecular features, the SCA6 gene product is membrane-bound rather than cytoplasmic or nuclear as in all other SCAs. Cytoplasmic aggregates of the alpha1A-subunit have been reported, but they are not ubiquitinated as seen in other SCAs and their role in the disease process is even more obscure than the aggregates from the other SCAs.[97,98] Recently, small nuclear aggregates have also been detected.[99] The pathologically expanded CAG repeat is also shorter than other SCA gene expansions and tends to be much more stably transmitted between generations.[98,100]

SPINOCEREBELLAR ATAXIA TYPE 7 (SCA7)

The distinguishing feature of SCA7 is a progressive retinopathy that leads irreversibly to bilateral blindness. The process starts as degeneration of the macula with a pigmented central core and extends into the periphery with time. Dyschromotopsia in the blue-yellow axis can be found years before symptomatic visual failure. When it does begin, visual failure is in the central field and night vision is spared.

Other than the retinopathy, the neurological features of SCA7 overlap those of the other SCAs. In one series of 69 SCA7 patients, ataxia, dysarthria, decreased visual acuity, upper motor neuron signs, vibratory sensory loss, and eye movement abnormalities (typically slowed saccades, and ophthalmoplegia) were seen in the majority of patients.[101] Axonal neuropathy, auditory impairment, rigidity, and dementia were also present in at least 10 percent of the patients. Interestingly, both nystagmus and hyporeflexia were seen in less than 5 percent of cases.

The CAG repeat in SCA7 displays more meiotic instability than any other polyglutamine disease.[102] With paternal transmission, an average gain of more than 20 repeats occurs between generations and there is a gain of more than 10 repeats per generation overall.[101] Very large expansions can occur through paternal transmission, causing severe infantile disease with cardiac involvement and early death.[103] Survival can range from a few months in these cases, to over 30 years in patients with small expansions.[102]

The SCA7 gene encodes ataxin-7,[104] a protein with unknown function that has primarily a nuclear localization in patients[105] and transfected cell lines. As with many of the other polyglutamine diseases, nuclear inclusion bodies have been observed, but their role in pathogenesis is unclear.

SPINOCEREBELLAR ATAXIA TYPE 8 (SCA8)

Quite a bit of controversy surrounds SCA8, largely due to the unusual molecular features of the mutation and its variable penetrance.[106,107] The disorder usually does not limit lifespan, and patients often exhibit upper motor neuron signs and vibration sense loss in addition to ataxia and dysarthria.[108,109]

The mutation associated with SCA8 is an extremely unstable CTG repeat that occurs at the 3' end of a fully processed RNA transcript that does not code for a protein due to the lack of extended open reading frames.[110] The repeat is very unstable upon intergenerational transmission and can expand by hundreds of repeats when maternally inherited.[109] Paternal transmission tends to result in contractions. RNA is transcribed only from the strand that codes for CTG, and not from the complementary strand that codes for a CAG repeat.

How can an RNA transcript that is never translated into protein cause disease? This is a crucial question for which there is currently only speculation. Perhaps the mechanism is similar to that of other diseases in which the implicated repeats occur in untranslated regions of the RNA transcripts (myotonic dystrophy types 1 and 2, SCA10, late-onset neurodegeneration in males carrying a fragile X premutation). Another intriguing possibility specific for SCA8 is that the transcript functions as a regulatory antisense RNA for a recently identified protein-coding gene on the other strand.[111]

A number of studies have now shown that large SCA8 expansions can occur in unaffected controls as well as in unaffected family members of ataxia patients harboring SCA8 expansions.[109,111,112] This nonabsolute segregation of the expansion with the disease implies either that the SCA8 repeat is not itself pathogenic or that there are other factors that affect its penetrance. Haplotype analysis seems to favor the latter interpretation,[113] although controversy will probably remain until those factors are more clearly defined.

SPINOCEREBELLAR ATAXIA TYPE 10 (SCA10)

SCA9 has not been assigned, so the next dominant ataxia is SCA10. Published reports have thus far only found SCA10 in the Mexican population.[114,115] This ataxia has been considered to cause a pure cerebellar syndrome with seizures, but recently pyramidal signs, ocular dyskinesia, cognitive impairment, and polyneuropathy have also been described.[116] In addition, affected members of one family had cardiac, hepatic, and hematological manifestations in addition to ataxia. The responsible mutation is an ATTCT pentanucleotide repeat expansion that occurs in the intron of the SCA10 gene.[115] The mutation can reach phenomenally large lengths (>4000 units), larger than any other known microsatellite expansion. The pathophysiology of the disorder may relate to other disorders in which the repeat expansions reside in nontranslated portions of the transcript.

SPINOCEREBELLAR ATAXIA TYPE 11 (SCA11)

A mild ataxia with hyperreflexia has been described in 2 British families and localized to chromosome 15q14-21.3. The gene is not yet known.[117]

SPINOCEREBELLAR ATAXIA TYPE 12 (SCA12)

Patients with SCA12 typically present with limb tremor in their 4th decade and then progress to develop cerebellar dysfunction and ultimately dementia.[118,119] The responsible mutation has been identified as a CAG repeat expansion in the 5' region of the gene PPP2R2B, which encodes a brain-specific regulatory subunit of the protein phosphatase PP2A.[118] Nonaffected control alleles possess 9–31 repeats, and pathogenic alleles range from 55 to 78 repeats. This mutation has been found to be very rare in many populations;[62,120–122] however, a recent report from India found the mutation in 5 of 77 autosomal-dominant ataxia families.[123]

SPINOCEREBELLAR ATAXIA TYPES 13–16 (SCA13–16)

SCA13 has been described in a large French family and is characterized by childhood-onset ataxia and moderate mental retardation.[124] The gene has been localized to chromosome 19q13.3-13.4 but not yet identified. SCA14 is a pure, slowly progressive ataxia in older-onset patients, but early-onset cases of SCA14 may present with axial myoclonus and tremor. It has been linked to chromosome 19q13.4-qter.[125,126] A genetic locus for SCA15 has not yet been identified. The disease was described in an Australian family and is characterized by pure ataxia that is mild and slowly progressive, rarely limiting ambulation.[127] SCA16 has been localized to a large region on chromosome 8q22.1-24.1, SCA16 has been described in a single Japanese family. All patients had progressive ataxia and 15 percent had head tremor.[128]

SPINOCEREBELLAR ATAXIA TYPE 17 (SCA17)

Even in the early days of the polyglutamine disease story it was recognized that certain proteins, mainly transcription factors, normally possess large tracts of polyglutamine. In fact, an antibody raised to one of these proteins, TATA-binding protein (TBP), was found to recognize the expanded polyglutamine tracts in many of the SCA mutant proteins[129] and has been utilized for many purposes within the literature, including the discovery of new SCA genes.[59,65] As might be expected, the TBP gene was kept in mind as candidate genes for new SCAs were being sought, and in 1999 the first patient was described in which a polyglutamine expansion in TBP appeared to be the causative mutation.[130] Additional families in Japan and other countries have now been described with this mutation.[37,131,132] Along with ataxia, the disease frequently manifests extrapyramidal features and cognitive decline.

DENTATORUBROPALLIDOLUYSIAN ATROPHY (DRPLA)

DRPLA is characterized by wide phenotypic variability encompassing ataxia, myoclonus, choreoathetosis, psychiatric disturbances, epilepsy, and dementia.[133] The age of presentation correlates with the clinical features; patients with onset prior to the age of 20 almost always have seizures, often with a progressive myoclonus epilepsy phenotype, whereas seizures are rare in patients with onset after age 40. In patients with onset later than age 20, choreoathetosis is commonly seen and may mask ataxia, making the distinction from HD difficult, particularly when dementia is present.

The disease is most commonly seen in Japan, but rare cases are seen in other populations.[134–137] Like SCA7, DRPLA shows a large degree of anticipation, particularly with paternal transmission.[138,139] This anticipation is consistent with the DRPLA mutation, an unstable CAG expansion that results in a polyglutamine expansion in the atrophin-1 protein.[140,141] Atrophin-1 contains a nuclear localization sequence, and ubiquitinated neuronal intranuclear inclusions containing the mutant protein are seen in the disease.[142] Recent work has documented additional abnormalities of nuclear structure and mutant atrophin-1 accumulation,[143] illustrating the fact that intranuclear inclusions may be only part of the story explaining pathogenesis.[144]

EPISODIC ATAXIA TYPE 1 (EA1)

EA1 typically presents during childhood or adolescence and is characterized by brief attacks of ataxia lasting seconds to minutes that are often precipitated by startle or exercise.[145,146] Vertigo is not present. Interictal continuous myokymia is also a feature of the disease, which is caused by mutations (usually missense) in the voltage-gated potassium channel gene KCNA1.[147] Mutations in this gene can also cause isolated myokymia, myokymia with partial epilepsy,[148] and EA with partial epilepsy.[149] Some patients with EA1 benefit from treatment with acetozolamide, phenytoin, or carbamazepine.[150]

EPISODIC ATAXIA TYPE 2 (EA2)

EA2 is caused by mutations in the CACNA1A gene encoding the alpha1A voltage-dependent calcium channel subunit,[151] and is clearly distinguished from EA1 by longer episodes of ataxia and dysarthria that can also include vertigo, nausea, oscillopsia, and diplopia. Mild interictal abnormalities in cerebellar function exist and usually progress with time in accord with the progressive midline cerebellar atrophy that occurs in the disease. Although startle does not precipitate attacks, physical and emotional stress may do so, and alcohol and caffeine can increase the likelihood that an attack will occur. Acetozolamide is helpful in reducing the frequency and severity of attacks.[152]

Two other disorders are caused by mutations in the CACNA1A gene: SCA6, and familial hemiplegic migraine (FHM). EA2 mutations appear to cause a loss of P/Q-type calcium channel activity,[153] usually by truncation,[154] FHM mutations are missense, and SCA6 is caused by a polyglutamine expansion. The distinction between these disorders is somewhat blurred by clinical overlap; i.e., FHM patients often have mild cerebellar atrophy, EA2 patients often have migraines, and SCA6 patients often have episodic symptoms.[150,155]

OTHER AUTOSOMAL-DOMINANT ATAXIAS

Ataxia may be a prominent feature of other autosomal-dominant diseases. Among these, neurodegenerative causes that must be kept in mind include certain prion mutations[156,157] and hereditary spastic paraparesis subtypes.[158,159] Nondegenerative dominant diseases (e.g., Von Hippel-Lindau syndrome) may also present with ataxia.

Autosomal-Recessive Ataxias

FRIEDREICH'S ATAXIA (FRDA)

FRDA is probably the most common inherited ataxia, with a prevalence estimated at approximately 1:30,000–50,000 among Caucasians.[160] Due to a founder effect of the ancestral mutation, the disease is almost exclusively found amongst people of European, North African, Middle Eastern, and Indian descent.[161] Prior to the discovery of the FRDA gene mutation the clinical features of the disease were believed to be rather homogeneous: progressive ataxia with onset before age 25, dysarthria within 5 years from onset, areflexia in lower limbs, extensor plantar responses, and neurophysiological evidence of an axonal sensory neuropathy, often with vibration and/or proprioceptive sensation loss.[162] While these features are still found in the majority of FRDA patients, the availability of a specific gene test has allowed the phenotype to be extended to include unusual features such as late onset (even up to the 6th and 7th decades), hyperreflexia, and spastic ataxia.[163,164] Because of this widened phenotype, genetic testing for FRDA should not be reserved for early-onset classic cases, but rather should be performed in most cases of otherwise unexplained ataxia.

Extraneuronal manifestations of FRDA include cardiomyopathy, diabetes, and scoliosis. The extent of cardiomyopathy varies greatly from patient to patient, but it is likely that virtually every patient with FRDA has microscopic cardiac pathology. Electrocardiographic (ECG) changes (most often aberrant repolarization) are common but not universal and do not correlate well with cardiac hypertrophy, the most common form of cardiomyopathy.[165] Although symptoms of overt heart failure are seen in only ~10–15 percent of patients,[166] a higher percentage would likely be seen if it were not for the limited mobility of patients with advanced FRDA. Long-standing disease is clearly associated with more severe cardiac involvement.[167] At the time of diagnosis, all FRDA patients should have an ECG and echocardiogram, and these should be repeated every few months to few years depending on the extent of disease. Mild glucose intolerance has been reported in approximately 50 percent of FRDA patients and diabetes in 20 percent, but these percentages are likely to be overestimates because ascertainment of atypically mild or late-onset FRDA was impossible prior to the gene test.[168] Interestingly, carriers of the FRDA gene mutation show increased incidence of glucose intolerance,[169,170] although they have no neurological or cardiac abnormalities.[162]

The mutation implicated in FRDA is a GAA expansion in intron 1 of the FRDA gene.[171] This gene codes for the mitochondrial protein frataxin, and as a consequence of the GAA expansion FRDA patients produce less frataxin.[172,173] Most patients are homozygous for the GAA expansion, but a small percentage of patients (~3–4 percent) are compound heterozygotes with the expansion on one allele and a point mutation on the other allele.[174] The commercially available FRDA gene tests utilize PCR to check for the expansion and therefore cannot distinguish between unaffected carriers of the expansion and affected compound heterozygotes.

A great deal of research has been directed at understanding the pathophysiology of FRDA.[175–178] Studies in patients and in model systems have shown that the reduction of frataxin leads to abnormal intracellular iron metabolism, defects in oxidative phosphorylation, increased oxidant stress, and alterations in the synthesis of iron-sulfur cluster proteins[179–186] that function as key components in intracellular energy production. Which of these alterations is primary is the subject of scientific debate, as is the normal role of frataxin in cellular function.[178,187,188] But, given the biochemical alterations noted above, it should not be surprising that attempts at treatment have focused on antioxidant therapy. Idebenone, an antioxidant analogue of coenzyme Q_{10}, has been tried in small European and Canadian trials and may offer some benefit for the cardiomyopathy.[185,189–191] No consistent neurological benefit has been observed, but it should be noted that a large randomized, blinded study that is adequately powered to detect a neuroprotective effect has not yet been performed. A combination of coenzyme Q_{10} (400 mg/day) and vitamin E (2100 mg/day) has been shown to reduce the metabolic abnormalities present in the muscles of FRDA patients,[192] but whether or not treatment with these agents could result in clinically significant benefit is not yet known.

ATAXIA TELANGIECTASIA (AT)

Ataxia telangiectasia (AT) is probably the second most common cause of childhood progressive ataxia. The disease usually presents early in childhood and is characterized by telangiectasias, immune deficiencies, and a predisposition to malignancy, in addition to the progressive neurological deficits.[193] The disease usually results in wheelchair dependence by the 2nd decade and death by early adulthood, most often by recurrent sinopulmonary infections and/or lymphoreticular malignancy.[194] Survival into mid- to late adulthood can occur in rare instances.

Neurologically, patients usually present with progressive ataxia and dysarthria with facial hypotonia and drooling. Oculomotor abnormalities occur relatively early and are characterized by difficulties in initiating voluntary eye movements (oculomotor apraxia) and fixation instability. Other abnormalities may then develop such as myoclonic jerking, dystonia and/or choreoathetosis, upgoing toes, and dorsal column sensory loss. Later signs may also include areflexia and muscle atrophy, indicating peripheral nerve and lower motor neuron involvement. Cognitive function appears to be minimally affected.[195]

The nonneurological features of AT can aid greatly in the diagnosis of this disorder. Oculocutaneous telangiectasias occur in over 95 percent of patients, typically 2–4 years after the onset of ataxia. Alpha-fetoprotein (AFP) levels are usually elevated and variable immunodeficiencies occur as a result of incomplete development of the thymus.[195] Recurrent sinopulmonary infections commonly result from the immunodeficiency. Malignancies occur in almost 40 percent of AT patients, of which 85 percent are leukemia or lymphoma.[194] Endocrine defects, including gonadal abnormalities and insulin-resistant diabetes, may be seen, and signs of accelerated aging ("progeria") can also be present. Radiation sensitivity occurs and can be assayed in cell culture.[196] These clinical features, supported by laboratory evaluation of AFP levels, immunodeficiency, and sometimes characteristic chromosomal abnormalities,[197] are relied upon to establish the diagnosis. Due to the large size of the affected gene and the large number of known mutations, direct genetic testing is not routinely performed except in certain populations that have high probability of founder mutations.

The occurrence of these disease manifestations is a consequence of the inherent cellular and molecular defects that exist in patients with loss-of-function mutations in the ATM gene. The ATM gene product is a protein kinase with complex interactions with many proteins involved in cell cycle control, apoptosis, and DNA double-strand break repair.[198] AT cells appear to be defective in recognizing double-strand breaks and therefore do not adequately initiate their repair. As a result, problems with DNA replication, altered cell cycle checkpoints, and abnormalities in apoptosis may lead to the malignant transformation and neurodegeneration seen in the disease. Heterozygote carriers may be at increased risk for solid tumors even though they display no neurological phenotype.[199]

There is no specific treatment for the primary abnormality of AT, but many of the secondary clinical features will respond to conventional therapy. Because of the fundamental cellular and molecular defects of the disease, special care needs to be taken in these patients (e.g., immunization with killed vaccines, limiting radiation exposure, and reducing chemotherapy doses). Treatment by physicians who are very familiar with AT patients is therefore highly recommended.

ATAXIAS ASSOCIATED WITH VITAMIN E DEFICIENCY

Mutations in the alpha-tocopherol transfer protein (alpha-TTP) gene are responsible for ataxia with vitamin E deficiency (AVED), a syndrome with clinical manifestations that are similar to those of FRDA,[200] but with a lower incidence of cardiomyopathy.[201] Alpha-TTP is synthesized in the liver and normally functions to transfer vitamin E to a circulating plasma lipoprotein. AVED mutations lead to a loss of alpha-TTP activity; this results in reduced plasma vitamin E levels, which appears to be the crucial metabolic abnormality that leads to disease. Plasma levels of vitamin E can be used as a screen for AVED, and replacement of vitamin E by oral administration may lead to clinical stabilization and perhaps mild improvement, at least early in the disease process.[202]

The neurological features of abetalipoproteinemia (ABL, Bassen-Kornzweig syndrome) also resemble those of FRDA. The underlying defect appears to be genetically heterogeneous, but one mutation that has been identified occurs in the larger subunit of the microsomal triglyceride transfer protein.[203] Physiologically, ABL is characterized by the absence of plasma lipoproteins containing apolipoprotein B, and this results in fat malabsorption and therefore decreased levels of the fat-soluble vitamins. Vitamin E deficiency probably contributes to the progressive neurodegeneration, and likely plays a role in the development of pigmentary retinal degeneration. Additional diagnostic clues include the presence of acanthocytes in a peripheral blood smear and low serum cholesterol.[2] The diagnosis can be established by a characteristic abnormality on serum protein electrophoresis.

ATAXIA WITH OCULOMOTOR APRAXIA-1 (AOA1)

The phenotype of this disorder resembles AT but without the extraneuronal features.[204] There are also similarities with SCAN1 described below. The incidence and phenotypic spectrum of this mutation are not yet fully known, but in some populations (e.g., Portugal and Japan) it may be one of the most prevalent autosomal-recessive ataxias.[205,206] Patients present in childhood with slowly progressive ataxia, oculomotor apraxia, and areflexia progressing to severe axonal neuropathy. Chorea may be present, but tends to diminish with disease duration.[207] The gene associated with this disorder (APTX) has recently been found at chromosome 9p13.3 and codes for aprataxin, a protein that appears to be involved in DNA repair.[205,208] Analysis of additional pedigrees with mutations localized to the same chromosomal region has suggested that another disorder that had been described in Japanese patients, early-onset cerebellar ataxia with hypoalbuminemia (EOA-HA), is caused by mutations in the same gene,[205,208] and that the phenotypic differences of EOA-HA (mental retardation, less oculomotor apraxia) may be explained by different APTX mutations.[205] Hypoalbuminemia and hypercholesterolemia occur late in the disease and are not universally present in these disorders, but their presence in a patient with early-onset ataxia strongly suggests AOA1 or SCNA1.[209] DNA testing is not yet available commercially but may be obtained through a research laboratory.

AUTOSOMAL-RECESSIVE SPASTIC ATAXIA OF CHARLEVOIX-SAGUENAY

This is a rare cause of ataxia outside of the Charlevoix-Saguenay region of Quebec, but within this isolated area the incidence is quite high.[210,211] Cases from other populations have now been reported.[212] Clinically, the disease manifests as an early-onset ataxia with spasticity and later development of distal amyotrophy. Marked saccadic breakdown occurs on horizontal smooth pursuit eye movements. Nerve conduction velocities are low, indicating myelination abnormalities, and on fundoscopy myelinated fibers can be seen in the nerve fiber layer of the retina. The associated gene has been identified and is termed "sacsin." The encoded protein contains heat-shock protein domains and may function in protein folding.[213]

SPINOCEREBELLAR ATAXIA WITH AXONAL NEUROPATHY (SCAN)

This disease is the newest member of a group of disorders that feature ataxia as a prominent clinical feature and are caused by mutations in genes involved in DNA repair. SCAN1 is characterized by early-onset ataxia, axonal neuropathy, mild hypercholesterolemia, borderline hypoalbuminemia, and spared intellectual functioning, and has not been associated with malignancies or with oculomotor apraxia. The mutation that causes this disease occurs in the gene encoding tyrosyl-DNA phosphodiesterase I (TDP1), and appears to cause a loss of function.[214] Many of the details of pathogenesis need to be elucidated, but the association of ataxia with alterations in DNA repair pathways (seen in AT, ataxia with oculomotor apraxia, Cockayne syndrome, xeroderma pigmentosum, and now SCAN1) seems likely to be more than an intriguing coincidence.

INBORN ERRORS OF METABOLISM

Table 44-4 lists some of the inborn errors of metabolism that may have ataxia as one of their neurological features. In addition to the disorders listed in that table, cerebrotendinous xanthomatosis should be mentioned because of the readily identifiable association of xanthomatous swelling of tendons (particularly the Achilles) with ataxia and the ease of diagnostic confirmation by documenting elevated cholestanol levels. In general, ataxia is rarely seen in isolation in the inborn metabolic errors, and often there are systemic features that suggest a metabolic workup may be indicated, but these clues cannot always be counted on. Adult-onset metabolic errors are particularly difficult to diagnose because they are often not considered in the differential diagnosis. Broad-based metabolic screening of lysosomal enzymes, organic and amino acids, mucopolysaccharides, and oligosaccharides may pick up many of these disorders.

DiMauro and colleagues have reported a small series of ataxia patients that have very low levels of coenzyme Q_{10} in muscle biopsy specimens, and some of these patients responded to coenzyme Q_{10} replacement therapy.[215] In most instances, the genetic basis of the deficiency was not known. Seizures and cognitive impairment accompanied the ataxia in most patients.

OTHER AUTOSOMAL-RECESSIVE ATAXIAS

Clinical descriptions of many other recessive ataxias have appeared in the literature under the description "early-onset inherited ataxias."[216] Many of these disorders are described in only a few patients and have not been linked to specific chromosomal loci, and therefore may represent phenotypes rather than actual diseases. Congenital cerebellar ataxia would be classified as an early-onset inherited ataxia and includes a number of specific syndromes of cerebellar hypoplasia. Early-onset ataxia with retained reflexes is another example and is a heterogeneous grouping of multiple disorders (mainly atypical FRDA cases) rather than an individual disease. Finally, progressive myoclonus epilepsies such as EPM1 (also known as Baltic myoclonus or Undverricht-Lundborg disease) and EPM2 (Lafora disease) often present with ataxia late in their course.

X-Linked Ataxias

Sideroblastic anemia with ataxia is caused by mutations in the ABC7 gene, which encodes a putative mitochondrial iron transporter.[217] Patients usually present early in life with ataxia and a microcytic, hypochromic anemia. Usually there is little progression of their ataxia.

Fragile X syndrome is one of the most common causes of inherited mental retardation and is caused by a CGG repeat in the 5' untranslated region of the FMR1 gene that is located on the X chromosome. Recent reports have delineated a late-onset neurodegenerative disease characterized by tremor, ataxia, and mild parkinsonism that occurs in some males that carry small "premutation" expansions.[218] Pathologically, ubiquitin-positive inclusion bodies are seen in neurons and glia.[219] The pathophysiological mechanism that results in neurodegeneration is not well understood, but it may relate to abnormalities in protein binding to the transcribed CGG repeat. These patients are completely unaffected by the fragile X syndrome phenotype but may transmit a larger expansion to their daughters; they therefore may have grandchildren or other family members with mental retardation. Although more research is needed to determine the prevalence, phenotypic boundaries, and pathophysiology of this condition, the current clinical description is convincing enough to stress the importance of inquiring about a family history of mental retardation in late-onset male ataxia patients.

Mitochondrial Ataxias

Mutations within the mitochondrial DNA can cause diseases with prominent ataxia.[220] Mutations in the ATPase 6 gene can cause different mitochondrial diseases: neurogenic weakness, ataxia, and retinitis pigmentosa, and maternally inherited Leigh syndrome (MILS). These disorders span a broad spectrum of phenotypes according to the degree of heteroplasmy (the relative mix of mutated and normal mitochondria), from infantile-onset MILS with very severe neurological abnormalities to an adult-onset disorder with mild ataxia and retinitis pigmentosa. Patients may also complain of intermittent lethargy and nausea related to changing metabolic demands. Ragged-red fibers are absent on muscle biopsy and there may be no elevations in serum lactate or pyruvate. Patients with other mitochondrial diseases such as Kearns-Sayre syndrome and mitochondrial encephalopathy, lactic acidosis, and stroke-like episodes may also have ataxia, but the primary clinical features of these disorders usually predominate over the ataxia.[220]

Summary

Single gene defects that cause ataxia have been clinically characterized and molecularly defined at an unbelievably quick pace over the past decade. Each new description adds to the complexity of the field even as it clarifies previous assumptions, and can paradoxically add to our uncertainty. For example, when shouldn't we test for FRDA now that we know that it can present in middle age and with spasticity? Diagnostically, the description of new syndromes quickly outpaces our ability to test for them. Advances in molecular genetics will continue to benefit this situation, but only to a point. DNA tests for disorders that are caused by a variety of mutations in a large gene will continue to be difficult to perform and largely relegated to the research laboratory. Thus, we are left with our clinical acumen as a vital ally.

The rapid identification of gene mutations that cause Mendelian disorders is an exciting manifestation of our early "postgenomic" era of genetics. But many diseases are not inherited in a Mendelian fashion from a single gene, but rather are affected in complex and subtle ways by multiple genes. Complex genetic mechanisms may explain features of many of the ataxias: the increased intrafamilial incidence of gluten sensitivity and other autoimmune-mediated ataxias, the variation in disease severity and age of onset in the single gene ataxias, disease penetrance in disorders such as SCA8. The real value of our recent advances in molecular genetics may truly lie in defining complex genetic influences such as these.

Therapeutically, many strides still need to be made as we pursue a treatment for ataxia. Symptomatic improvement (e.g., increasing coordination) is simply not a reasonable goal for the ataxias as it is for many of the extrapyramidal disorders. On the other hand, neuroprotection may be achievable, and a concerted effort must be made in that direction.

References

1. Evidente VG, Gwinn-Hardy KA, Caviness JN, et al: Hereditary ataxias. *Mayo Clin Proc* 75:475–490, 2000.
2. Di Donato S, Gellera C, Mariotti C: The complex clinical and genetic classification of inherited ataxias. II. Autosomal recessive ataxias. *Neurol Sci* 22:219–228, 2001.
3. Durr A, Brice A: Clinical and genetic aspects of spinocerebellar degeneration. *Curr Opin Neurol* 13:407–413, 2000.
4. Burk K, Bosch S, Muller CA, et al: Sporadic cerebellar ataxia associated with gluten sensitivity. *Brain* 124:1013–1019, 2001.
5. Hadjivassiliou M, Grunewald RA, Davies-Jones GA: Gluten sensitivity as a neurological illness. *J Neurol Neurosurg Psychiatry* 72:560–563, 2002.
6. Honnorat J, Saiz A, Giometto B, et al: Cerebellar ataxia with anti-glutamic acid decarboxylase antibodies: Study of 14 patients. *Arch Neurol* 58:225–230, 2001.
7. Perlman SL: Cerebellar ataxia. *Curr Treat Options Neurol* 2: 215–224, 2000.
8. Moseley ML, Benzow KA, Schut LJ, et al: Incidence of dominant spinocerebellar and Friedreich triplet repeats among 361 ataxia families. *Neurology* 51:1666–1671, 1998.
9. Futamura N, Matsumura R, Fujimoto Y, et al: CAG repeat expansions in patients with sporadic cerebellar ataxia. *Acta Neurol Scand* 98:55–59, 1998.
10. Kim JY, Park SS, Joo SI, et al: Molecular analysis of spinocerebellar ataxias in Koreans: Frequencies and reference ranges of SCA1, SCA2, SCA3, SCA6, and SCA7. *Mol Cells* 12:336–341, 2001.
11. Mori M, Adachi Y, Kusumi M, et al: A genetic epidemiological study of spinocerebellar ataxias in Tottori prefecture, Japan. *Neuroepidemiology* 20:144–149, 2001.
12. Soong BW, Lu YC, Choo KB, et al: Frequency analysis of autosomal dominant cerebellar ataxias in Taiwanese patients and clinical and molecular characterization of spinocerebellar ataxia type 6. *Arch Neurol* 58:1105–1109, 2001.
13. Botez MI, Young SN, Rotez T, et al: Treatment of Friedreich's ataxia with amantadine. *Neurology* 39:749–750, 1989.
14. Lou JS, Goldfarb L, McShane L, et al: Use of buspirone for treatment of cerebellar ataxia. An open-label study. *Arch Neurol* 52:982–988, 1995.
15. Trouillas P, Xie J, Adeleine P: Treatment of cerebellar ataxia with buspirone: A double-blind study. *Lancet* 348:759, 1996.
16. Trouillas P, Xie J, Adeleine P, et al: Buspirone, a 5-hydroxytryptamine 1A agonist, is active in cerebellar ataxia. Results of a double-blind drug placebo study in patients with cerebellar cortical atrophy. *Arch Neurol* 54:749–752, 1997.
17. Sorbi S, Forleo P, Fani C, et al: Double-blind, crossover, placebo-controlled clinical trial with L-acetylcarnitine in patients with degenerative cerebellar ataxia. *Clin Neuropharmacol* 23:114–118, 2000.
18. Takei A, Honma S, Kawashima A, et al: Beneficial effects of tandospirone on ataxia of a patient with Machado-Joseph disease. *Psychiatry Clin Neurosci* 56:181–185, 2002.
19. Filla A, De Michele G, Orefice G, et al: A double-blind cross-over trial of amantadine hydrochloride in Friedreich's ataxia. *Can J Neurol Sci* 20:52–55, 1993.
20. Schulte T, Mattern R, Berger K, et al: Double-blind crossover trial of trimethoprim-sulfamethoxazole in spinocerebellar ataxia type 3/Machado-Joseph disease. *Arch Neurol* 58:1451–1457, 2001.

21. Hassin-Baer S, Korczyn AD, Giladi N: An open trial of amantadine and buspirone for cerebellar ataxia: A disappointment. *J Neural Transm* 107:1187–1189, 2000.

22. Gwinn-Hardy K, Chen JY, Liu HC, et al: Spinocerebellar ataxia type 2 with parkinsonism in ethnic Chinese. *Neurology* 55:800–805, 2000.

23. Gwinn-Hardy K, Singleton A, O'Suilleabhain P, et al: Spinocerebellar ataxia type 3 phenotypically resembling Parkinson disease in a black family. *Arch Neurol* 58:296–299, 2001.

24. Schols L, Peters S, Szymanski S, et al: Extrapyramidal motor signs in degenerative ataxias. *Arch Neurol* 57:1495–1500, 2000.

25. Watanabe M, Abe K, Aoki M, et al: Analysis of CAG trinucleotide expansion associated with Machado-Joseph disease. *J Neurol Sci* 136:101–107, 1996.

26. Schols L, Haan J, Riess O, et al: Sleep disturbance in spinocerebellar ataxias: Is the SCA3 mutation a cause of restless legs syndrome? *Neurology* 51:1603–1607, 1998.

27. Abele M, Burk K, Laccone F, et al: Restless legs syndrome in spinocerebellar ataxia types 1, 2, and 3. *J Neurol* 248:311–314, 2001.

28. van Alfen N, Sinke RJ, Zwarts MJ, et al: Intermediate CAG repeat lengths (53, 54) for MJD/SCA3 are associated with an abnormal phenotype. *Ann Neurol* 49:805–807, 2001.

29. Krebs DE, McGibbon CA, Goldvasser D: Analysis of postural perturbation responses. *IEEE Trans Neural Syst Rehabil Eng* 9:76–80, 2001.

30. Visintainer CL, Matthias-Hagen V, Nance MA: Anonymous predictive testing for Huntington's disease in the United States. *Genet Test* 5:213–218, 2001.

31. Evers-Kiebooms G, Nys K, Harper P, et al: Predictive DNA-testing for Huntington's disease and reproductive decision making: A European collaborative study. *Eur J Hum Genet* 10:167–176, 2002.

32. Harding AE: The clinical features and classification of the late onset autosomal dominant cerebellar ataxias. A study of 11 families, including descendants of the 'the Drew family of Walworth'. *Brain* 105:1–28, 1982.

33. Storey E, du Sart D, Shaw JH, et al: Frequency of spinocerebellar ataxia types 1, 2, 3, 6, and 7 in Australian patients with spinocerebellar ataxia. *Am J Med Genet* 95:351–357, 2000.

34. Giunti P, Sabbadini G, Sweeney MG, et al: The role of the SCA2 trinucleotide repeat expansion in 89 autosomal dominant cerebellar ataxia families. Frequency, clinical and genetic correlates. *Brain* 121:459–467, 1998.

35. Watanabe H, Tanaka F, Matsumoto M, et al: Frequency analysis of autosomal dominant cerebellar ataxias in Japanese patients and clinical characterization of spinocerebellar ataxia type 6. *Clin Genet* 53:13–19, 1998.

36. Lopes-Cendes I, Teive HG, Calcagnotto ME, et al: Frequency of the different mutations causing spinocerebellar ataxia (SCA1, SCA2, MJD/SCA3 and DRPLA) in a large group of Brazilian patients. *Arq Neuropsiquiatr* 55:519–529, 1997.

37. Silveira I, Miranda C, Guimaraes L, et al: Trinucleotide repeats in 202 families with ataxia: A small expanded (CAG)n allele at the SCA17 locus. *Arch Neurol* 59:623–629, 2002.

38. Takano H, Cancel G, Ikeuchi T, et al: Close associations between prevalences of dominantly inherited spinocerebellar ataxias with CAG-repeat expansions and frequencies of large normal CAG alleles in Japanese and Caucasian populations. *Am J Hum Genet* 63:1060–1066, 1998.

39. Rivaud-Pechoux S, Durr A, Gaymard B, et al: Eye movement abnormalities correlate with genotype in autosomal dominant cerebellar ataxia type I. *Ann Neurol* 43:297–302, 1998.

40. Orr HT, Chung MY, Banfi S, et al: Expansion of an unstable trinucleotide CAG repeat in spinocerebellar ataxia type 1. *Nat Genet* 4:221–226, 1993.

41. Genis D, Matilla T, Volpini V, et al: Clinical, neuropathologic, and genetic studies of a large spinocerebellar ataxia type 1 (SCA1) kindred: (CAG)n expansion and early premonitory signs and symptoms. *Neurology* 45:24–30, 1995.

42. Sasaki H, Fukazawa T, Yanagihara T, et al: Clinical features and natural history of spinocerebellar ataxia type 1. *Acta Neurol Scand* 93:64–71, 1996.

43. Burk K, Abele M, Fetter M, et al: Autosomal dominant cerebellar ataxia type I clinical features and MRI in families with SCA1, SCA2 and SCA3. *Brain* 119:1497–1505, 1996.

44. Schols L, Riess O, Schols S, et al: Spinocerebellar ataxia type 1: Clinical and neurophysiological characteristics in German kindreds. *Acta Neurol Scand* 92:478–485, 1995.

45. Schols L, Amoiridis G, Buttner T, et al: Autosomal dominant cerebellar ataxia: Phenotypic differences in genetically defined subtypes? *Ann Neurol* 42:924–932, 1997.

46. Namekawa M, Takiyama Y, Ando Y, et al: Choreiform movements in spinocerebellar ataxia type 1. *J Neurol Sci* 187:103–106, 2001.

47. Burk K, Bosch S, Globas C, et al: Executive dysfunction in spinocerebellar ataxia type 1. *Eur Neurol* 46:43–48, 2001.

48. Goldfarb LG, Vasconcelos O, Platonov FA, et al: Unstable triplet repeat and phenotypic variability of spinocerebellar ataxia type 1. *Ann Neurol* 39:500–506, 1996.

49. Servadio A, Koshy B, Armstrong D, et al: Expression analysis of the ataxin-1 protein in tissues from normal and spinocerebellar ataxia type 1 individuals. *Nat Genet* 10:94–98, 1995.

50. Zuhlke C, Dalski A, Hellenbroich Y, et al: Spinocerebellar ataxia type 1 (SCA1): phenotype-genotype correlation studies in intermediate alleles. *Eur J Hum Genet* 10:204–209, 2002.

51. Limprasert P, Nouri N, Nopparatana C, et al: Comparative studies of the CAG repeats in the spinocerebellar ataxia type 1 (SCA1) gene. *Am J Med Genet* 74:488–493, 1997.

52. Ranum LP, Chung MY, Banfi S, et al: Molecular and clinical correlations in spinocerebellar ataxia type I: Evidence for familial effects on the age at onset. *Am J Hum Genet* 55:244–252, 1994.

53. Klement IA, Skinner PJ, Kaytor MD, et al: Ataxin-1 nuclear localization and aggregation: Role in polyglutamine-induced disease in SCA1 transgenic mice. *Cell* 95:41–53, 1998.

54. Lin X, Antalffy B, Kang D, et al: Polyglutamine expansion downregulates specific neuronal genes before pathologic changes in SCA1. *Nat Neurosci* 3:157–163, 2000.

55. Orozco G, Estrada R, Perry TL, et al: Dominantly inherited olivopontocerebellar atrophy from eastern Cuba. Clinical, neuropathological, and biochemical findings. *J Neurol Sci* 93:37–50, 1989.

56. Filla A, Mariotti C, Caruso G, et al: Relative frequencies of CAG expansions in spinocerebellar ataxia and dentatorubropallidoluysian atrophy in 116 Italian families. *Eur Neurol* 44:31–36, 2000.

57. Saleem Q, Choudhry S, Mukerji M, et al: Molecular analysis of autosomal dominant hereditary ataxias in the Indian population: High frequency of SCA2 and evidence for a common founder mutation. *Hum Genet* 106:179–187, 2000.

58. Geschwind DH, Perlman S, Figueroa CP, et al: The prevalence and wide clinical spectrum of the spinocerebellar ataxia type 2 trinucleotide repeat in patients with autosomal dominant cerebellar ataxia. *Am J Hum Genet* 60:842–850, 1997.

59. Imbert G, Saudou F, Yvert G, et al: Cloning of the gene for spinocerebellar ataxia 2 reveals a locus with high sensitivity to expanded CAG/glutamine repeats. *Nat Genet* 14:285–291, 1996.

60. Sanpei K, Takano H, Igarashi S, et al: Identification of the spinocerebellar ataxia type 2 gene using a direct identification of repeat expansion and cloning technique, DIRECT. *Nat Genet* 14:277–284, 1996.

61. Pulst SM, Nechiporuk A, Nechiporuk T, et al: Moderate expansion of a normally biallelic trinucleotide repeat in spinocerebellar ataxia type 2. *Nat Genet* 14:269–276, 1996.

62. Schols L, Szymanski S, Peters S, et al: Genetic background of apparently idiopathic sporadic cerebellar ataxia. *Hum Genet* 107:132–137, 2000.

63. Huynh DP, Del Bigio MR, Ho DH, et al: Expression of ataxin-2 in brains from normal individuals and patients with Alzheimer's disease and spinocerebellar ataxia 2. *Ann Neurol* 45:232–241, 1999.

64. Huynh DP, Figueroa K, Hoang N, et al: Nuclear localization or inclusion body formation of ataxin-2 are not necessary for SCA2 pathogenesis in mouse or human. *Nat Genet* 26:44–50, 2000.

65. Pang JT, Giunti P, Chamberlain S, et al: Neuronal intranuclear inclusions in SCA2: A genetic, morphological and immunohistochemical study of two cases. *Brain* 125:656–663, 2002.

66. Mao R, Aylsworth AS, Potter N, et al: Childhood-onset ataxia: Testing for large CAG-repeats in SCA2 and SCA7. *Am J Med Genet* 110:338–345, 2002.

67. Nakano KK, Dawson DM, Spence A: Machado disease. A hereditary ataxia in Portuguese emigrants to Massachusetts. *Neurology* 22:49–55, 1972.

68. Kawaguchi Y, Okamoto T, Taniwaki M, et al: CAG expansions in a novel gene for Machado-Joseph disease at chromosome 14q32.1. *Nat Genet* 8:221–228, 1994.

69. Landau WM, Schmidt RE, McGlennen RC, et al: Hereditary spastic paraplegia and hereditary ataxia, Part 2: A family demonstrating various phenotypic manifestations with the SCA3 genotype. *Arch Neurol* 57:733–739, 2000.

70. Cancel G, Abbas N, Stevanin G, et al: Marked phenotypic heterogeneity associated with expansion of a CAG repeat sequence at the spinocerebellar ataxia 3/Machado-Joseph disease locus. *Am J Hum Genet* 57:809–816, 1995.

71. Silveira I, Lopes-Cendes I, Kish S, et al: Frequency of spinocerebellar ataxia type 1, dentatorubropallidoluysian atrophy, and Machado-Joseph disease mutations in a large group of spinocerebellar ataxia patients. *Neurology* 46:214–218, 1996.

72. Silveira I, Coutinho P, Maciel P, et al: Analysis of SCA1, DRPLA, MJD, SCA2, and SCA6 CAG repeats in 48 Portuguese ataxia families. *Am J Med Genet* 81:134–138, 1998.

73. Matsumura R, Takayanagi T, Murata K, et al: Autosomal dominant cerebellar ataxias in the Kinki area of Japan. *Jpn J Hum Genet* 41:399–406, 1996.

74. Trottier Y, Cancel G, An-Gourfinkel I, et al: Heterogeneous intracellular localization and expression of ataxin-3. *Neurobiol Dis* 5:335–347, 1998.

75. Fujigasaki H, Uchihara T, Koyano S, et al: Ataxin-3 is translocated into the nucleus for the formation of intranuclear inclusions in normal and Machado-Joseph disease brains. *Exp Neurol* 165:248–256, 2000.

76. Chai Y, Koppenhafer SL, Bonini NM, et al: Analysis of the role of heat shock protein (Hsp) molecular chaperones in polyglutamine disease. *J Neurosci* 19:10338–10347, 1999.

77. Evert BO, Wullner U, Schulz JB, et al: High level expression of expanded full-length ataxin-3 in vitro causes cell death and formation of intranuclear inclusions in neuronal cells. *Hum Mol Genet* 8:1169–1176, 1999.

78. Uchihara T, Fujigasaki H, Koyano S, et al: Non-expanded polyglutamine proteins in intranuclear inclusions of hereditary ataxias: Triple-labeling immunofluorescence study. *Acta Neuropathol* 102:149–152, 2001.

79. Nachmanoff DB, Segal RA, Dawson DM, et al: Hereditary ataxia with sensory neuronopathy: Biemond's ataxia. *Neurology* 48:273–275, 1997.

80. Flanigan K, Gardner K, Alderson K, et al: Autosomal dominant spinocerebellar ataxia with sensory axonal neuropathy (SCA4): Clinical description and genetic localization to chromosome 16q22.1. *Am J Hum Genet* 59:392–399, 1996.

81. Nagaoka U, Takashima M, Ishikawa K, et al: A gene on SCA4 locus causes dominantly inherited pure cerebellar ataxia. *Neurology* 54:1971–1975, 2000.

82. Takashima M, Ishikawa K, Nagaoka U, et al: A linkage disequilibrium at the candidate gene locus for 16q-linked autosomal dominant cerebellar ataxia type III in Japan. *J Hum Genet* 46:167–171, 2001.

83. Ranum LP, Schut LJ, Lundgren JK, et al: Spinocerebellar ataxia type 5 in a family descended from the grandparents of President Lincoln maps to chromosome 11. *Nat Genet* 8:280–284, 1994.

84. Stevanin G, Herman A, Brice A, et al: Clinical and MRI findings in spinocerebellar ataxia type 5. *Neurology* 53:1355–1357, 1999.

85. Yabe I, Sasaki H, Yamashita I, et al: Initial symptoms and mode of neurological progression in spinocerebellar ataxia type 6 (SCA6). *Rinsho Shinkeigaku* 38:489–494, 1998.

86. Geschwind DH, Perlman S, Figueroa KP, et al: Spinocerebellar ataxia type 6. Frequency of the mutation and genotype-phenotype correlations. *Neurology* 49:1247–1251, 1997.

87. Geschwind DH, Perlman S, Figueroa KP, et al: Spinocerebellar ataxia type 6. Frequency of the mutation and genotype-phenotype correlations. *Neurology* 49:1247–1251, 1997.

88. Ikeuchi T, Takano H, Koide R, et al: Spinocerebellar ataxia type 6: CAG repeat expansion in alpha 1A voltage-dependent calcium channel gene and clinical variations in Japanese population. *Ann Neurol* 42:879–884, 1997.

89. Buttner N, Geschwind D, Jen JC, et al: Oculomotor phenotypes in autosomal dominant ataxias. *Arch Neurol* 55:1353–1357, 1998.

90. Riess O, Schols L, Bottger H, et al: SCA6 is caused by moderate CAG expansion in the alpha1A-voltage-dependent calcium channel gene. *Hum Mol Genet* 6:1289–1293, 1997.

91. Zhuchenko O, Bailey J, Bonnen P, et al: Autosomal dominant cerebellar ataxia (SCA6) associated with small polyglutamine expansions in the alpha 1A-voltage-dependent calcium channel. *Nat Genet* 15:62–69, 1997.

92. Matsumura R, Futamura N, Fujimoto Y, et al: Spinocerebellar ataxia type 6. Molecular and clinical features of 35 Japanese patients including one homozygous for the CAG repeat expansion. *Neurology* 49:1238–1243, 1997.

93. Shizuka M, Watanabe M, Ikeda Y, et al: Molecular analysis of a de novo mutation for spinocerebellar ataxia type 6 and (CAG)*n* repeat units in normal elder controls. *J Neurol Sci* 161:85–87, 1998.

94. Restituito S, Thompson RM, Eliet J, et al: The polyglutamine expansion in spinocerebellar ataxia type 6 causes a beta subunit-specific enhanced activation of P/Q-type calcium channels in *Xenopus* oocytes. *J Neurosci* 20:6394–6403, 2000.

95. Matsuyama Z, Wakamori M, Mori Y, et al: Direct alteration of the P/Q-type Ca2+ channel property by polyglutamine expansion in spinocerebellar ataxia 6. *J Neurosci* 19:RC14, 1999.

96. Piedras-Renteria ES, Watase K, Harata N, et al: Increased expression of alpha 1A Ca2+ channel currents arising from expanded trinucleotide repeats in spinocerebellar ataxia type 6. *J Neurosci* 21:9185–9193, 2001.

97. Ishikawa K, Fujigasaki H, Saegusa H, et al: Abundant expression and cytoplasmic aggregations of [alpha]1A voltage-dependent calcium channel protein associated with neurodegeneration in spinocerebellar ataxia type 6. *Hum Mol Genet* 8:1185–1193, 1999.

98. Ishikawa K, Watanabe M, Yoshizawa K, et al: Clinical, neuropathological, and molecular study in two families with spinocerebellar ataxia type 6 (SCA6). *J Neurol Neurosurg Psychiatry* 67:86–89, 1999.

99. Ishikawa K, Owada K, Ishida K, et al: Cytoplasmic and nuclear polyglutamine aggregates in SCA6 Purkinje cells. *Neurology* 56:1753–1756, 2001.

100. Ishikawa K, Tanaka H, Saito M, et al: Japanese families with autosomal dominant pure cerebellar ataxia map to chromosome 19p13.1-p13.2 and are strongly associated with mild CAG expansions in the spinocerebellar ataxia type 6 gene in chromosome 19p13.1. *Am J Hum Genet* 61:336–346, 1997.

101. Stevanin G, Lebre AS, Zander C, et al: Autosomal dominant cerebellar ataxia with progressive pigmentary macular dystrophy, in Manto MU, Pandolfo M (eds): *The Cerebellum and Its Disorders.* Cambridge: Cambridge University Press, 2002, pp 459–468.

102. David G, Durr A, Stevanin G, et al: Molecular and clinical correlations in autosomal dominant cerebellar ataxia with progressive macular dystrophy (SCA7). *Hum Mol Genet* 7:165–170, 1998.

103. Hsieh M, Lin SJ, Chen JF, et al: Identification of the spinocerebellar ataxia type 7 mutation in Taiwan: Application of PCR-based Southern blot. *J Neurol* 247:623–629, 2000.

104. David G, Abbas N, Stevanin G, et al: Cloning of the SCA7 gene reveals a highly unstable CAG repeat expansion. *Nat Genet* 17:65–70, 1997.

105. Einum DD, Townsend JJ, Ptacek LJ, et al: Ataxin-7 expression analysis in controls and spinocerebellar ataxia type 7 patients. *Neurogenetics* 3:83–90, 2001.

106. Vincent JB, Neves-Pereira ML, Paterson AD, et al: An unstable trinucleotide-repeat region on chromosome 13 implicated in spinocerebellar ataxia: A common expansion locus. *Am J Hum Genet* 66:819–829, 2000.

107. Sobrido MJ, Cholfin JA, Perlman S, et al: SCA8 repeat expansions in ataxia: A controversial association. *Neurology* 57:1310–1312, 2001.

108. Juvonen V, Hietala M, Paivarinta M, et al: Clinical and genetic findings in Finnish ataxia patients with the spinocerebellar ataxia 8 repeat expansion. *Ann Neurol* 48:354–361, 2000.

109. Day JW, Schut LJ, Moseley ML, et al: Spinocerebellar ataxia type 8: Clinical features in a large family. *Neurology* 55:649–657, 2000.

110. Koob MD, Moseley ML, Schut LJ, et al: An untranslated CTG expansion causes a novel form of spinocerebellar ataxia (SCA8). *Nat Genet* 21:379–384, 1999.

111. Nemes JP, Benzow KA, Moseley ML, et al: The SCA8 transcript is an antisense RNA to a brain-specific transcript encoding a novel actin-binding protein (KLHL1). *Hum Mol Genet* 9:1543–1551, 2000.

112. Worth PF, Houlden H, Giunti P, et al: Large, expanded repeats in SCA8 are not confined to patients with cerebellar ataxia. *Nat Genet* 24:214–215, 2000.

113. Moseley ML, Schut LJ, Day JW, et al: Spinocerebellar ataxia type 8, in Manto MU, Pandolfo M (eds): *The Cerebellum and Its Disorders.* Cambridge: Cambridge University Press, 2002, pp 469–480.

114. Zu L, Figueroa KP, Grewal R, et al: Mapping of a new autosomal dominant spinocerebellar ataxia to chromosome 22. *Am J Hum Genet* 64:594–599, 1999.

115. Matsuura T, Yamagata T, Burgess DL, et al: Large expansion of the ATTCT pentanucleotide repeat in spinocerebellar ataxia type 10. *Nat Genet* 26:191–194, 2000.

116. Rasmussen A, Matsuura T, Ruano L, et al: Clinical and genetic analysis of four Mexican families with spinocerebellar ataxia type 10. *Ann Neurol* 50:234–239, 2001.

117. Worth PF, Giunti P, Gardner-Thorpe C, et al: Autosomal dominant cerebellar ataxia type III: Linkage in a large British family to a 7.6-cM region on chromosome 15q14–21.3. *Am J Hum Genet* 65:420–426, 1999.

118. Holmes SE, O'Hearn EE, McInnis MG, et al: Expansion of a novel CAG trinucleotide repeat in the 5′ region of PPP2R2B is associated with SCA12. *Nat Genet* 23:391–392, 1999.

119. Holmes SE, Hearn EO, Ross CA, et al: SCA12: An unusual mutation leads to an unusual spinocerebellar ataxia. *Brain Res Bull* 56:397–403, 2001.

120. Cholfin JA, Sobrido MJ, Perlman S, et al: The SCA12 mutation as a rare cause of spinocerebellar ataxia. *Arch Neurol* 58:1833–1835, 2001.

121. Maruyama H, Izumi Y, Morino H, et al: Difference in disease-free survival curve and regional distribution according to subtype of spinocerebellar ataxia: A study of 1,286 Japanese patients. *Am J Med Genet* 114:578–583, 2002.

122. Brusco A, Cagnoli C, Franco A, et al: Analysis of SCA8 and SCA12 loci in 134 Italian ataxic patients negative for SCA1–3, 6 and 7 CAG expansions. *J Neurol* 249:923–929, 2002.

123. Srivastava AK, Choudhry S, Gopinath MS, et al: Molecular and clinical correlation in five Indian families with spinocerebellar ataxia 12. *Ann Neurol* 50:796–800, 2001.

124. Herman-Bert A, Stevanin G, Netter JC, et al: Mapping of spinocerebellar ataxia 13 to chromosome 19q13.3-q13.4 in a family with autosomal dominant cerebellar ataxia and mental retardation. *Am J Hum Genet* 67:229–235, 2000.

125. Yamashita I, Sasaki H, Yabe I, et al: A novel locus for dominant cerebellar ataxia (SCA14) maps to a 10.2-cM interval flanked by D19S206 and D19S605 on chromosome 19q13.4-qter. *Ann Neurol* 48:156–163, 2000.

126. Brkanac Z, Bylenok L, Fernandez M, et al: A new dominant spinocerebellar ataxia linked to chromosome 19q13.4-qter. *Arch Neurol* 59:1291–1295, 2002.

127. Storey E, Gardner RJ, Knight MA, et al: A new autosomal dominant pure cerebellar ataxia. *Neurology* 57:1913–1915, 2001.

128. Miyoshi Y, Yamada T, Tanimura M, et al: A novel autosomal dominant spinocerebellar ataxia (SCA16) linked to chromosome 8q22.1–24.1. *Neurology* 57:96–100, 2001.

129. Trottier Y, Lutz Y, Stevanin G, et al: Polyglutamine expansion as a pathological epitope in Huntington's disease

and four dominant cerebellar ataxias. *Nature* 378:403–406, 1995.

130. Koide R, Kobayashi S, Shimohata T, et al: A neurological disease caused by an expanded CAG trinucleotide repeat in the TATA-binding protein gene: A new polyglutamine disease? *Hum Mol Genet* 8:2047–2053, 1999.

131. Nakamura K, Jeong SY, Uchihara T, et al: SCA17, a novel autosomal dominant cerebellar ataxia caused by an expanded polyglutamine in TATA-binding protein. *Hum Mol Genet* 10:1441–1448, 2001.

132. Zulke C, Hellenbroich Y, Dalski A, et al: Different types of reeat expansion in the TATA-binding protein gene are associated with a new form of inherited ataxia. *Eur J Hum Genet* 9:160–164, 2001.

133. Naito H, Oyanagi K: Familial myoclonus epilepsy and choreoathetosis: Hereditary dentatorubral-pallidoluysian atrophy. *Neurology* 32:789–817, 1982.

134. Watanabe H, Tanaka F, Matsumoto M, et al: Frequency analysis of autosomal dominant cerebellar ataxias in Japanese patients and clinical characterization of spinocerebellar ataxia type 6. *Clin Genet* 53:13–19, 1998.

135. Takano H, Cancel G, Ikeuchi T, et al: Close associations between prevalences of dominantly inherited spinocerebellar ataxias with CAG-repeat expansions and frequencies of large normal CAG alleles in Japanese and Caucasian populations. *Am J Hum Genet* 63:1060–1066, 1998.

136. Burke JR, Wingfield MS, Lewis KE, et al: The Haw River syndrome: Dentatorubropallidoluysian atrophy (DRPLA) in an African-American family. *Nat Genet* 7:521–524, 1994.

137. Destee A, Delalande I, Vuillaume I, et al: The first identified French family with dentatorubral-pallidoluysian atrophy. *Mov Disord* 15:996–999, 2000.

138. Ikeuchi T, Koide R, Onodera O, et al: Dentatorubral-pallidoluysian atrophy (DRPLA). Molecular basis for wide clinical features of DRPLA. *Clin Neurosci* 3:23–27, 1995.

139. Komure O, Sano A, Nishino N, et al: DNA analysis in hereditary dentatorubral-pallidoluysian atrophy: Correlation between CAG repeat length and phenotypic variation and the molecular basis of anticipation. *Neurology* 45:143–149, 1995.

140. Koide R, Ikeuchi T, Onodera O, et al: Unstable expansion of CAG repeat in hereditary dentatorubral-pallidoluysian atrophy (DRPLA). *Nat Genet* 6:9–13, 1994.

141. Nagafuchi S, Yanagisawa H, Sato K, et al: Dentatorubral and pallidoluysian atrophy expansion of an unstable CAG trinucleotide on chromosome 12p. *Nat Genet* 6:14–18, 1994.

142. Hayashi Y, Kakita A, Yamada M, et al: Hereditary dentatorubral-pallidoluysian atrophy: Detection of widespread ubiquitinated neuronal and glial intranuclear inclusions in the brain. *Acta Neuropathol (Berl)* 96:547–552, 1998.

143. Takahashi H, Egawa S, Piao YS, et al: Neuronal nuclear alterations in dentatorubral-pallidoluysian atrophy: Ultrastructural and morphometric studies of the cerebellar granule cells. *Brain Res* 919:12–19, 2001.

144. Sisodia SS: Nuclear inclusions in glutamine repeat disorders: Are they pernicious, coincidental, or beneficial? *Cell* 95:1–4, 1998.

145. Brandt T, Strupp M: Episodic ataxia type 1 and 2 (familial periodic ataxia/vertigo). *Audiol Neurootol* 2:373–383, 1997.

146. Surtees R: Inherited ion channel disorders. *Eur J Pediatr* 159(suppl 3):S199–203, 2000.

147. Browne DL, Gancher ST, Nutt JG, et al: Episodic ataxia/myokymia syndrome is associated with point mutations in the human potassium channel gene, KCNA1. *Nat Genet* 8:136–140, 1994.

148. Eunson LH, Rea R, Zuberi SM, et al: Clinical, genetic, and expression studies of mutations in the potassium channel gene KCNA1 reveal new phenotypic variability. *Ann Neurol* 48:647–656, 2000.

149. Zuberi SM, Eunson LH, Spauschus A, et al: A novel mutation in the human voltage-gated potassium channel gene (Kv1.1) associates with episodic ataxia type 1 and sometimes with partial epilepsy. *Brain* 122:817–825, 1999.

150. D'Adamo MC, Imbrici P, Pessia M: Episodic ataxias as ion channel diseases, in Manto MU, Pandolfo M (eds): *The Cerebellum and Its Disorders.* Cambridge: Cambridge University Press, 2002, pp 562–572.

151. Ophoff RA, Terwindt GM, Vergouwe MN, et al: Familial hemiplegic migraine and episodic ataxia type-2 are caused by mutations in the Ca2+ channel gene CACNL1A4. *Cell* 87:543–552, 1996.

152. Zasorin NL, Baloh RW, Myers LB: Acetazolamide-responsive episodic ataxia syndrome. *Neurology* 33:1212–1214, 1983.

153. Guida S, Trettel F, Pagnutti S, et al: Complete loss of P/Q calcium channel activity caused by a CACNA1A missense mutation carried by patients with episodic ataxia type 2. *Am J Hum Genet* 68:759–764, 2001.

154. Denier C, Ducros A, Vahedi K, et al: High prevalence of CACNA1A truncations and broader clinical spectrum in episodic ataxia type 2. *Neurology* 52:1816–1821, 1999.

155. Terwindt GM, Ophoff RA, Haan J, et al: Migraine, ataxia and epilepsy: A challenging spectrum of genetically determined calcium channelopathies. Dutch Migraine Genetics Research Group. *Eur J Hum Genet* 6:297–307, 1998.

156. Liou HH, Jeng JS, Chang YC, et al: Is ataxic gait the predominant presenting manifestation of Creutzfeldt-Jakob disease? Experience of 14 Chinese cases from Taiwan. *J Neurol Sci* 140:53–60, 1996.

157. Berciano J, Pascual J, Polo JM, et al: Ataxic type of Creutzfeldt-Jakob disease with disproportionate enlargement of the fourth ventricle: A serial CT study. *J Neurol Neurosurg Psychiatry* 62:295–297, 1997.

158. Hedera P, Rainier S, Zhao XP, et al: Spastic paraplegia, ataxia, mental retardation (SPAR): A novel genetic disorder. *Neurology* 58:411–416, 2002.

159. Fink JK: Hereditary spastic paraplegia: The pace quickens. *Ann Neurol* 51:669–672, 2002.

160. Lopez-Arlandis JM, Vilchez JJ, Palau F, et al: Friedreich's ataxia: An epidemiological study in Valencia, Spain, based on consanguinity analysis. *Neuroepidemiology* 14:14–19, 1995.

161. Labuda M, Labuda D, Miranda C, et al: Unique origin and specific ethnic distribution of the Friedreich ataxia GAA expansion. *Neurology* 54:2322–2324, 2000.

162. Harding AE: Friedreich's ataxia: A clinical and genetic study of 90 families with an analysis of early diagnostic criteria and intrafamilial clustering of clinical features. *Brain* 104:589–620, 1981.

163. Ragno M, De Michele G, Cavalcanti F, et al: Broadened Friedreich's ataxia phenotype after gene cloning. Minimal GAA expansion causes late-onset spastic ataxia. *Neurology* 49:1617–1620, 1997.

164. Schols L, Amoiridis G, Przuntek H, et al: Friedreich's ataxia. Revision of the phenotype according to molecular genetics. *Brain* 120:2131–2140, 1997.

165. Dutka DP, Donnelly JE, Nihoyannopoulos P, et al: Marked variation in the cardiomyopathy associated with Friedreich's ataxia. *Heart* 81:141–147, 1999.

166. Alboliras ET, Shub C, Gomez MR, et al: Spectrum of cardiac involvement in Friedreich's ataxia: Clinical, electrocardiographic and echocardiographic observations. *Am J Cardiol* 58:518–524, 1986.

167. Harding AE, Hewer RL: The heart disease of Friedreich's ataxia: A clinical and electrocardiographic study of 115 patients, with an analysis of serial electrocardiographic changes in 30 cases. *Q J Med* 52:489–502, 1983.

168. Finocchiaro G, Baio G, Micossi P, et al: Glucose metabolism alterations in Friedreich's ataxia. *Neurology* 38:1292–1296, 1988.

169. Ristow M, Giannakidou E, Hebinck J, et al: An association between NIDDM and a GAA trinucleotide repeat polymorphism in the X25/frataxin (Friedreich's ataxia) gene. *Diabetes* 47:851–854, 1998.

170. Hebinck J, Hardt C, Schols L, et al: Heterozygous expansion of the GAA tract of the X25/frataxin gene is associated with insulin resistance in humans. *Diabetes* 49:1604–1607, 2000.

171. Campuzano V, Montermini L, Molto MD, et al: Friedreich's ataxia: Autosomal recessive disease caused by an intronic GAA triplet repeat expansion. *Science* 271:1423–1427, 1996.

172. Campuzano V, Montermini L, Lutz Y, et al: Frataxin is reduced in Friedreich ataxia patients and is associated with mitochondrial membranes. *Hum Mol Genet* 6:1771–1780, 1997.

173. Bidichandani SI, Ashizawa T, Patel PI: The GAA triplet-repeat expansion in Friedreich ataxia interferes with transcription and may be associated with an unusual DNA structure. *Am J Hum Genet* 62:111–121, 1998.

174. Cossee M, Durr A, Schmitt M, et al: Friedreich's ataxia: Point mutations and clinical presentation of compound heterozygotes. *Ann Neurol* 45:200–206, 1999.

175. Patel PI, Isaya G: Friedreich ataxia: From GAA triplet-repeat expansion to frataxin deficiency. *Am J Hum Genet* 69:15–24, 2001.

176. Bradley JL, Blake JC, Chamberlain S, et al: Clinical, biochemical and molecular genetic correlations in Friedreich's ataxia. *Hum Mol Genet* 9:275–282, 2000.

177. Puccio H, Koenig M: Recent advances in the molecular pathogenesis of Friedreich ataxia. *Hum Mol Genet* 9:887–892, 2000.

178. Pandolfo M: Molecular basis of Friedreich ataxia. *Mov Disord* 16:815–821, 2001.

179. Babcock M, de Silva D, Oaks R, et al: Regulation of mitochondrial iron accumulation by Yfh1p, a putative homolog of frataxin. *Science* 276:1709–1712, 1997.

180. Cavadini P, Gellera C, Patel PI, et al: Human frataxin maintains mitochondrial iron homeostasis in *Saccharomyces cerevisiae*. *Hum Mol Genet* 9:2523–2530, 2000.

181. Gordon N: Friedreich's ataxia and iron metabolism. *Brain Dev* 22:465–468, 2000.

182. Lodi R, Cooper JM, Bradley JL, et al: Deficit of in vivo mitochondrial ATP production in patients with Friedreich ataxia. *Proc Natl Acad Sci U S A* 96:11492–11495, 1999.

183. Rotig A, de Lonlay P, Chretien D, et al: Aconitase and mitochondrial iron-sulphur protein deficiency in Friedreich ataxia. *Nat Genet* 17:215–217, 1997.

184. Wong A, Yang J, Cavadini P, et al: The Friedreich's ataxia mutation confers cellular sensitivity to oxidant stress which is rescued by chelators of iron and calcium and inhibitors of apoptosis. *Hum Mol Genet* 8:425–430, 1999.

185. Schulz JB, Dehmer T, Schols L, et al: Oxidative stress in patients with Friedreich ataxia. *Neurology* 55:1719–1721, 2000.

186. Emond M, Lepage G, Vanasse M, et al: Increased levels of plasma malondialdehyde in Friedreich ataxia. *Neurology* 55:1752–1753, 2000.

187. Adamec J, Rusnak F, Owen WG, et al: Iron-dependent self-assembly of recombinant yeast frataxin: Implications for Friedreich ataxia. *Am J Hum Genet* 67:549–562, 2000.

188. Lodi R, Taylor DJ, Schapira AH: Mitochondrial dysfunction in Friedreich's ataxia. *Biol Signals Recept* 10:263–270, 2001.

189. Lerman-Sagie T, Rustin P, Lev D, et al: Dramatic improvement in mitochondrial cardiomyopathy following treatment with idebenone. *J Inherit Metab Dis* 24:28–34, 2001.

190. Rustin P, von Kleist-Retzow JC, Chantrel-Groussard K, et al: Effect of idebenone on cardiomyopathy in Friedreich's ataxia: A preliminary study. *Lancet* 354:477–479, 1999.

191. Schols L, Vorgerd M, Schillings M, et al: Idebenone in patients with Friedreich ataxia. *Neurosci Lett* 306:169–172, 2001.

192. Lodi R, Hart PE, Rajagopalan B, et al: Antioxidant treatment improves in vivo cardiac and skeletal muscle bioenergetics in patients with Friedreich's ataxia. *Ann Neurol* 49:590–596, 2001.

193. Woods CG, Taylor AMR: Ataxia telangiectasia in the British Isles: The clinical and laboratory features of 70 affected individuals. *Q J Med* 82:169–179, 1992.

194. Morrell D, Cromartie E, Swift M: Mortality and cancer incidence in 263 patients with ataxia-telangiectasia. *J Natl Cancer Inst* 77:89–92, 1986.

195. Perlman S, Bay JO, Uhrhammer N, Gatti, RA: Ataxia telangiectasia and its variants, in Manto MU, Pandolfo M (eds): *The Cerebellum and Its Disorders*. Cambridge: Cambridge University Press, 2002, pp 531–547.

196. Sun X, Becker-Catania SG, Chun HH, et al: Early diagnosis of ataxia-telangiectasia using radiosensitivity testing. *J Pediatr* 140:724–731, 2002.

197. Stumm M, Neubauer S, Keindorff S, et al: High frequency of spontaneous translocations revealed by FISH in cells from patients with the cancer-prone syndromes ataxia telangiectasia and Nijmegen breakage syndrome. *Cytogenet Cell Genet* 92:186–191, 2001.

198. Khanna KK, Lavin MF, Jackson SP, et al: ATM, a central controller of cellular responses to DNA damage. *Cell Death Differ* 8:1052–1065, 2001.

199. Concannon P: ATM heterozygosity and cancer risk. *Nat Genet* 32:89–90, 2002.

200. Ouahchi K, Arita M, Kayden H, et al: Ataxia with isolated vitamin E deficiency is caused by mutations in the alpha-tocopherol transfer protein. *Nat Genet* 9:141–145, 1995.

201. Cavalier L, Ouahchi K, Kayden HJ, et al: Ataxia with isolated vitamin E deficiency: Heterogeneity of mutations and phenotypic variability in a large number of families. *Am J Hum Genet* 62:301–310, 1998.

202. Gabsi S, Gouider-Khouja N, Belal S, et al: Effect of vitamin E supplementation in patients with ataxia with vitamin E deficiency. *Eur J Neurol* 8:477–481, 2001.

203. Sharp D, Blinderman L, Combs KA, et al: Cloning and gene defects in microsomal triglyceride transfer protein associated with abetalipoproteinemia. *Nature* 365:65–69, 1993.

204. Nemeth AH, Bochukova E, Dunne E, et al: Autosomal recessive cerebellar ataxia with oculomotor apraxia

(ataxia-telangiectasia-like syndrome) is linked to chromosome 9q34. *Am J Hum Genet* 67:1320–1326, 2000.

205. Moreira MC, Barbot C, Tachi N, et al: The gene mutated in ataxia-ocular apraxia 1 encodes the new HIT/Zn-finger protein aprataxin. *Nat Genet* 29:189–193, 2001.

206. Barbot C, Coutinho P, Chorao R, et al: Recessive ataxia with ocular apraxia: Review of 22 Portuguese patients. *Arch Neurol* 58:201–205, 2001.

207. Shimazaki H, Takiyama Y, Sakoe K, et al: Early-onset ataxia with ocular motor apraxia and hypoalbuminemia: The aprataxin gene mutations. *Neurology* 59:590–595, 2002.

208. Date H, Onodera O, Tanaka H, et al: Early-onset ataxia with ocular motor apraxia and hypoalbuminemia is caused by mutations in a new HIT superfamily gene. *Nat Genet* 29:184–188, 2001.

209. Moreira MC, Barbot C, Tachi N, et al: Homozygosity mapping of Portuguese and Japanese forms of ataxia-oculomotor apraxia to 9p13, and evidence for genetic heterogeneity. *Am J Hum Genet* 68:501–508, 2001.

210. Bouchard JP, Richter A, Mathieu J, et al: Autosomal recessive spastic ataxia of Charlevoix-Saguenay. *Neuromuscul Disord* 8:474–479, 1998.

211. Scriver CR: Human genetics: Lessons from Quebec populations. *Annu Rev Genomics Hum Genet* 2:69–101, 2001.

212. Gucuyener K, Ozgul K, Paternotte C, et al: Autosomal recessive spastic ataxia of Charlevoix-Saguenay in two unrelated Turkish families. *Neuropediatrics* 32:142–146, 2001.

213. Engert JC, Berube P, Mercier J, et al: ARSACS, a spastic ataxia common in northeastern Quebec, is caused by mutations in a new gene encoding an 11.5-kb ORF. *Nat Genet* 24:120–125, 2000.

214. Takashima H, Boerkoel C, Joy J, et al: Mutation of TDP1, encoding a topoisomerase I-dependent DNA damage repair enzyme, in spinocerebellar ataxia with axonal neuropathy. *Nat Genet* 32:267–272, 2002.

215. Musumeci O, Naini A, Slonim AE, et al: Familial cerebellar ataxia with muscle coenzyme Q10 deficiency. *Neurology* 56: 849–855, 2001.

216. De Michele G, Filla A: Early-onset inherited ataxias, in Manto MU, Pandolfo M (eds): *The Cerebellum and Its Disorders.* Cambridge: Cambridge University Press, 2002, pp 519–530.

217. Allikmets R, Raskind WH, Hutchinson A, et al: Mutation of a putative mitochondrial iron transporter gene (ABC7) in X-linked sideroblastic anemia and ataxia (XLSA/A). *Hum Mol Genet* 8:743–749, 1999.

218. Hagerman RJ, Leehey M, Heinrichs W, et al: Intention tremor, parkinsonism, and generalized atrophy in male carriers of fragile X. *Neurology* 57:127–130, 2001.

219. Greco CM, Hagerman RJ, Tassone F, et al: Neuronal intranuclear inclusions in a new cerebellar tremor/ataxia syndrome among fragile X carriers. *Brain* 125:1760–1771, 2002.

220. Zeviani M, Antozzi C, Savoiardo M, et al: Ataxia in mitochondrial disorders, in Manto MU, Pandolfo M (eds): *The Cerebellum and Its Disorders.* Cambridge: Cambridge University Press, 2002, pp 548–561.

Chapter 44

CLINICAL FEATURES AND TREATMENT OF CEREBELLAR DISORDERS

SID GILMAN

FUNCTIONS OF THE CEREBELLUM 723
    Control of Posture and Movement 723
    Motor Learning 723
    Cognitive Functions 724
    A Cerebellar Cognitive Affective Syndrome 724
CLINICALLY RELEVANT CEREBELLAR
    ANATOMY 724
CLINICAL SIGNS OF CEREBELLAR
    DISORDERS 726
    Abnormalities of Stance and Gait 726
    Titubation 726
    Rotated or Tilted Postures of the Head 726
    Disturbances of Extraocular Movements 726
    Decomposition of Movement 727
    Dysmetria 727
    Dysdiadochokinesis and Dysrhythmokinesis 727
    Ataxia 727
    Abnormal Check and Rebound 727
    Tremor 728
    Ataxic Dysarthria 728
    Abnormalities of Muscle Tone 728
TREATMENT OF CEREBELLAR DISORDERS 729

Functions of the Cerebellum

CONTROL OF POSTURE AND MOVEMENT

Studies in experimental animals beginning early in the last century demonstrated that a key function of the cerebellum pertains to the control of motor function.[1,2] Observations of patients with disorders of cerebellar structure and function dating to the turn of the century buttressed this view.[3,4] These observations demonstrated that cerebellar lesions disturb posture and gait, and the smoothly integrated coordination of movements, both simple and compound. Disturbed cerebellar function disrupts movements that require an accurate estimate of the goal in time and space. Lesions of the cerebellum delay movement initiation and cause movements to be clumsy; however, these lesions do not prevent movement execution. With cerebellar injury, muscles that normally act together lose their capacity to do so. Movements then deteriorate into incomplete or inaccurate forms, producing errors of force, velocity, and timing. Muscle strength may be diminished somewhat, but usually cerebellar disease does not cause marked weakness. Cerebellar lesions affect essentially all movements coordinated by the somatic musculature, including extraocular movements and speech.

Evidence gathered over the past three decades suggests that several mechanisms underlie the functions of the cerebellum. Through its deep nuclei, the cerebellum tonically activates vestibulospinal, reticulospinal, and corticospinal influences upon both fusimotor[5] and alpha motor neurons[6] in both the brainstem and spinal cord. The cerebellar cortex maintains inhibitory control over the excitatory effects of the nuclei. The interactions of the cerebellar cortex and deep nuclei change constantly to provide fine control to posture and movement.[6] The cerebellum also performs timing functions that are critical to exquisite motor performance.[7] The cerebellum serves a combining and coordinating function essential to the development of complex compound movements.[8,9] The cerebellum monitors information gathered through essentially all sensory receptors, presumably to provide this information to motor structures.[10–12] This function does not include the conscious awareness of sensory experiences, as cerebellar lesions alone do not disrupt sensation, except possibly for weight discrimination.[13]

The cerebellum controls specific components of posture and movement through functions localized in a series of sagittal zones. These zones include the overlying cerebellar cortex and the cerebellar nuclei, which consist of three groups organized from medial to lateral: fastigial, interposed, and dentate. Discrete lesions of the cerebellar nuclei in experimental animals cause specific disorders of motor control that reflect the functions of the three sagittal zones. Ablation of the fastigial nucleus results in disorders of sitting, standing, and walking.[14,15] Injury to the portions of cerebellar cortex projecting to these nuclei, the vermal and paravermal regions, causes similar disorders in humans.[16,17] Ablation of the interpositus nucleus leads to limb tremor,[14,18] suggesting that this nucleus balances agonist with antagonist muscle activity of limbs during movement.[15] Interpositus lesions also impair the control of limb placement during reaching and locomotion.[19] In addition, ablation of the anterior interpositus nucleus affects grasping, whereas posterior interpositus lesions affect reaching movements, suggesting that these components coordinate distal with proximal musculature.[20] Dentate nucleus lesions delay the reaction times for limb movements, affect the accuracy of reaching movements, and impair movements requiring the use of multiple joints more than movements involving a single joint.[14,15,21,22]

MOTOR LEARNING

The cerebellum participates in motor tasks by learning new movements and by adapting already learned movements to a new task. Evidence for this comes from theoretical considerations,[23–25] anatomical observations in animals,[26,27] physiological studies in animals,[28–33] observations with positron emission tomography (PET) in normal humans,[34–41] and clinical/physiological testing of humans with cerebellar lesions.[42-47] Taken together, these observations indicate that the initial learning of skilled motor acts begins consciously under the control of the cerebral cortex. From the very start of the learning situation, the cerebellum participates in the control of the task and, as learning proceeds, the cerebellum assumes increasing responsibility until it gains essentially complete control of the task. The cerebellum comes to recognize the context requiring the movement, links together each component of the movement, and automatically triggers the movement upon presentation of the appropriate stimulus in the correct context. Through the cerebellum, the nervous system controls the sequence of many complex movements automatically, without the need for conscious awareness of the planning, execution, and termination required. Thus, movements programmed by the cerebellum can combine muscular actions, prevent movement errors, and develop complex movement sequences involving both single joints and multiple joints.

COGNITIVE FUNCTIONS

The observation that memory and intellect remain preserved in humans with large volumes of cerebellar tissue destroyed[4] led to the conclusion that the cerebellum does not participate in cognitive functions. Recently, however, growing evidence has linked the cerebellum to at least certain aspects of cognition. The initial interest in this idea came from the observation that the lateral cerebellum and the cognitively important structures of the forebrain developed phylogenetically in parallel.[48-50] Recent anatomical studies have begun to demonstrate linkages of the cerebellum with the motor association areas of the cerebral cortex that participate in motor planning, including premotor cortex, primary and secondary frontal eye fields, and areas 44, 45, and 46 of Brodmann.[51-54] These association areas include regions important in the motor components of speech in humans (areas 44, and 45 of Brodmann). The motor association areas receive projections from regions of the brain associated with perception and awareness. Studies in experimental animals utilizing single neuronal unit recordings and in humans using PET have shown that these areas become active with anticipation of a movement or rehearsal of a movement, even without actual performance of the movement.[35] Moreover, both the left frontal lobe of the cerebrum and the right cerebellar hemisphere become active when human subjects generate a word in an association task.[55] With repetition of the same task to the point of familiarity, frontal activity declines and cerebellar activity decreases,[56] suggesting that the cerebellum becomes responsible for execution of the task. Support for the idea that the cerebellum functions in this fashion came from the demonstration of impaired word production in an association task after a vascular insult of the right cerebellar hemisphere in one report,[57] and agrammatic speech after a similar lesion in another.[58] Observations in patients with cerebellar degenerations and focal lesions suggest other high-level

functions for the cerebellum, including cognitive planning,[59] associative learning,[60] classical conditioning,[61] instrumental learning,[62] and voluntary shifts of selective attention between sensory modalities.[63,64] Synaptic plasticity has been cited as a mechanism accounting for motor and cognitive learning in the cerebellum.[65]

A CEREBELLAR COGNITIVE AFFECTIVE SYNDROME

A cerebellar "cognitive affective syndrome" has been hypothesized based upon reports of patients with cerebellar lesions.[66] Many deficits have been described, including abnormalities of abstract reasoning, language, working memory, other components of memory, visuospatial functions, personality structure, planning, and set shifting. The cerebellar structures involved consist of those connecting to association areas of the frontal, parietal, and occipital lobes.[67] Also, a recent case report implicated the cerebellum in pathological laughter and crying.[68] Anatomical abnormalities of the cerebellum, particularly hypoplasia of the vermis, have been found in the cerebellum in autism, a developmental disorder that results in severe deficits of language and social and cognitive function.[69-72] Cerebellar vermal hypoplasia has been described in schizophrenia as well;[73-75] however, two PET studies have reported opposite results, with *decreased* cerebellar metabolic rates in medicated patients in one study[76] and *increased* rates in nonmedicated patients in another.[77] Decreased size of vermal lobules has been described in children with attention deficit hyperactivity disorder[78] and fragile X syndrome.[79] All of these interesting and provocative observations require follow-up and replication, but currently it seems premature to conclude that a cause-and-effect relationship exists between these complex disorders and anatomical changes in the cerebellum.

Clinically Relevant Cerebellar Anatomy

The cerebellum consists of a central longitudinal structure, the vermis, and two hemispheres.[80] A zone termed the "paravermis" lies between the vermis and the lateral part of the hemisphere on each side. Fissures divide the cerebellar cortex into three major lobes, the anterior, posterior, and flocculonodular. The primary fissure separates the anterior and posterior lobes, and the postnodular fissure divides the posterior and flocculonodular lobes. Additional shallow fissures subdivide the anterior and posterior lobes into a series of transverse lobules.

Comparative anatomic studies led to the division of the cerebellum into the archicerebellum, paleocerebellum, and neocerebellum[81] (Table 44-1). The archicerebellum consists of the flocculonodular lobe, the paleocerebellum includes the vermis of the anterior lobe and the pyramis, uvula, and paraflocculus, and the neocerebellum involves the lateral parts of the cerebellum, including most of the hemispheres

TABLE 44-1 Anatomic and Phylogenetic Organization of the Cerebellum

Structure	Phylogenetic Designation	Afferent Projections	Current Designation
Flocculonodular lobe	Archicerebellum	Vestibular receptors and nuclei	Vestibulocerebellum
Vermis of anterior lobe, pyramis, uvula, paraflocculus	Paleocerebellum	Spinal cord	Spinocerebellum
Cerebellar hemispheres, middle portions of vermis	Neocerebellum	Pons	Pontocerebellum

TABLE 44-2 Sagittal Organization of the Cerebellum

Zone	Principal Afferent Projections	Associated Deep Cerebellar Nuclei	Efferent Projections of Cerebellar Nuclei
Vermal	Spinal cord, reticular and vestibular nuclei	Fastigial	Vestibulospinal tract, reticulospinal tract
Intermediate (paravermal)	Spinal cord, brainstem, cerebral cortex	Interposed	Red nucleus, thalamus
Lateral	Pons, cerebral cortex	Dentate	Thalamus, cerebral cortex

and the middle portion of the vermis. These divisions correspond moderately well to the sites of afferent projections to the cerebellum.[81] Vestibular fibers project densely into the flocculonodular lobe (the archicerebellum), and correspondingly the term "vestibulocerebellum" has been applied to this lobe. The major projections from the spinal cord[82] terminate in the vermis (the paleocerebellum), leading to the designation "spinocerebellum" for this region. The projections from the pons, which are connected principally with the cerebral cortex, terminate in the cerebellar hemispheres, and the term "pontocerebellum" is used for the hemispheres. This system of nomenclature has been useful, but it provides only approximate localization since the locations of the termination sites describe only partially the regions activated physiologically.[80,83–85]

Clinically, the organization of the cerebellum can be viewed as a series of sagittal zones, including a vermal zone, a paravermal zone, and a lateral zone[80] (Table 44-2). The vermal zone contains cerebellar cortical efferent neurons projecting to the fastigial nucleus. The paravermal or intermediate zone contains cerebellar cortical efferents projecting to the interposed nuclei. The lateral zone, which includes the most lateral region of the anterior lobe and the lateral portion of the hemispheres, contains cerebellar cortical efferents projecting to the lateral (dentate) nucleus.[86–88] Many more sagittal zones have been identified,[89,90] but have not proved helpful clinically. Three additional anatomical sites have been identified as important clinically for eye movement abnormalities.[91,92] These include the flocculus and paraflocculus, the nodulus and ventral uvula, and the dorsal vermis and fastigial nucleus. The cerebellar hemispheres also contribute to the control of eye movements, and lesions restricted to one cerebellar hemisphere impair ipsilateral smooth pursuit movements.[93]

The midline zone of the cerebellum receives most afferents from the spinal cord and the brainstem reticular and vestibular nuclei and projects most efferents via the fastigial nucleus to vestibulospinal and reticulospinal neurons.

These connections participate in posture, locomotion, the position of the head in relation to the trunk, and the control of extraocular movements.[80] Correspondingly, the clinical signs resulting from midline cerebellar disease consist of disordered stance and gait,[94] truncal titubation,[80] rotated postures of the head,[95] and disturbances of extraocular movements[91] (Table 44-3). Some authors consider disorders of the flocculus, nodules, and uvula as a separate group, comprising the "vestibulocerebellum."[96–98] In the past, dysarthria has been considered a sign of midline cerebellar disease, but this disorder may be linked to several sites in the cerebellum, including the hemispheres.[57,58,99]

The intermediate zone of the cerebellum consists of the paravermal region of the cerebellar cortex and the interposed nuclei on each side. Major afferents to this zone arise in many structures, including the spinal cord, brainstem, and cerebral cortex, with cerebral cortical projections mediated through synapses in the brainstem. Similarly, efferent projections reach both rostral and caudal regions of the nervous system. Diseases strictly limited to the intermediate zone appear to be rare, and consequently the clinical disorders from injury to this zone have been linked with those due to disease of the midline zone or the lateral zone.

TABLE 44-3 Principal Clinical Signs Linked to the Sagittal Organization of the Cerebellum

Zone	Clinical Signs
Vermal	Abnormal stance and gait, truncal titubation, rotated postures of the head, disturbances of extraocular movements
Lateral	Abnormal stance and gait, disturbances of extraocular movements, decomposition of movement, dysmetria, dysdiadochokinesis, dysrhythmokinesis, ataxia, impaired check, excessive rebound, kinetic and static tremor, dysarthria, hypotonia

The lateral zone includes the cerebellar hemisphere and the dentate nucleus of each side. This zone receives afferent projections heavily from the cerebral cortex through relay nuclei in the pons and brainstem reticular nuclei. The lateral zone sends projections to brainstem and thalamic structures that make connections with both forebrain and spinal levels of the nervous system. The abnormalities resulting from lesions of the lateral zone are related chiefly to voluntary movements and consist of abnormalities of stance and gait, disturbances of extraocular movements, decomposition of movement, dysmetria, dysdiadochokinesis, dysrhythmokinesis, ataxia, impaired check, excessive rebound, kinetic and static tremor, dysarthria, and hypotonia[80] (Table 44-3).

Clinical Signs of Cerebellar Disorders

Clinical signs of cerebellar disease commonly reflect disease processes directly involving the cerebellum; however, similar signs can result from disorders of structures separate from the cerebellum. These structures include the spinal cord, usually from involvement of the spinocerebellar pathways, the pons, the midbrain, the thalamus,[100–102] the internal capsule,[103,104] and the parietal cortex.[105]

ABNORMALITIES OF STANCE AND GAIT

The most common clinical signs of cerebellar disease consist of abnormalities of standing and walking.[95,106] With disease restricted to the midline zone, these abnormalities usually appear with minimal disturbances in the coordinated movements of the limbs when tested separately. Anterior superior and intermediate vermal lesions lead to prominent body sway in the anterior-posterior direction, whereas posterior vermal lesions cause body sway in multiple directions.[107,108] With disease of the lateral zone, difficulty in standing and walking accompanies cerebellar movement disorders of the other limbs. The patient with a gait disorder from cerebellar disease usually stands on a wide base and may develop a severe truncal tremor. Closing the eyes worsens the unsteadiness.[109,110] With walking, truncal instability causes falls to the right, left, forwards, or backwards[4,111] and coordination of postural control with voluntary movement becomes difficult.[112] The gait disorder of cerebellar disease results from the same fundamental disturbances that are associated with other multijoint movements.[113] Thus, walking consists of a series of steps irregularly placed, some too far forwards, some not far enough forwards, and some too far to the sides. The patient often lifts the legs excessively during ambulation. Gait deficits can be enhanced by various maneuvers, including walking in tandem (heel-to-toe) or walking on the heels, the toes, or backwards. The side towards which a patient falls, swerves, drifts, or leans does not necessarily indicate the side of the cerebellar lesion. Ataxia of gait with unimpaired limb coordination occurs with injury to the anterior superior portion of the cerebellar vermis and frequently results from nutritional and alcoholic damage to the nervous system.[114] Lesions of the flocculonodular lobe also cause disorders of stance and gait, often in association with multidirectional nystagmus and head rotation.[80] Children in whom the posterior cerebellar vermis had been transected became severely impaired in attempting to walk in tandem, although they could stand, hop, and walk with only mild abnormalities.[115]

TITUBATION

This consists of a rhythmic tremor of the body or head, with a rocking motion forward and backward, from side to side, or in a rotatory movement, usually occurring several times per second.[80,107,108] The onset of the tremor requires no attempt at precision movement, only sitting or standing.[108] It occurs in any posture, varies in frequency, and can be found without associated kinetic tremor.[108] A distal static tremor of the fingers and wrist can accompany the body or head movements.

ROTATED OR TILTED POSTURES OF THE HEAD

Abnormal postures of the head are associated with disease of the vermis or the flocculonodular lobule. The direction of head tilt has no localizing significance with respect to the side of the cerebellar pathology.[80]

DISTURBANCES OF EXTRAOCULAR MOVEMENTS

Based upon experimental work in animals and correlation with neurological disorders in humans, three principal sites in the cerebellum are associated with distinctive disorders of extraocular movement.[91,92,116–118] The sites include (1) the flocculus and paraflocculus, (2) the nodulus and ventral uvula, and (3) the dorsal vermis and underlying caudal fastigial nucleus. Lesions of the flocculus and paraflocculus cause gaze-evoked nystagmus, rebound nystagmus, and downbeat nystagmus, impaired smooth tracking with the eyes alone or with the eyes and head, postsaccadic drift, and impaired ability to adapt the vestibulo-ocular response to changing visual needs.[93,119–124] Lesions of the nodulus and ventral uvula increase the duration of vestibular responses, predisposing to periodic alternating nystagmus.[91] These lesions also cause failure of tilt-suppression of postrotatory nystagmus, loss of habituation, and development of positional nystagmus and downbeat nystagmus.[125] Lesions of the dorsal vermis and fastigial nucleus result in saccadic dysmetria.[91] Typically, saccadic movements appear hypometric if the lesion affects only the vermis and hypermetric if the lesion affects the fastigial nucleus as well.[91] Fastigial nucleus lesions alone can result in saccadic hypermetria. Dorsal vermal lesions also cause defects of pursuit and of motion perception.[126]

In addition to the disturbances of extraocular movements associated with the three sites described above, many other disorders occur with cerebellar diseases, but have not as yet become associated with specific known sites. These include disorders of ocular alignment, fixation, smooth pursuit, vestibular function, and adaptive functions.[91] Disorders of ocular alignment include esotropia, alternating skew deviations, disconjugate saccades, and disconjugate gaze-evoked nystagmus.[118,127] Disturbances of fixation consist of nystagmus and saccadic intrusions. The varieties of nystagmus include divergent nystagmus, centripetal nystagmus, upbeating nystagmus, and acquired pendular nystagmus.[91] Square-wave jerks are examples of saccadic intrusions. The disorder of smooth pursuit consists of torsional nystagmus during vertical tracking.[128] Other vestibular disturbances include excessive responsiveness to vestibular stimulation and to the cervico-ocular reflex, abnormalities of off-vertical axis rotation, and impaired responses to linear translation.[91] Impairment of the adaptive properties of the vestibulo-ocular reflex exemplifies the disorder of adaptive functions from cerebellar disease.[91]

DECOMPOSITION OF MOVEMENT

Disease in the lateral zone of the cerebellum results in abnormalities of both simple and compound movements.[22,80,129] Simple movements consist of changes of posture or movements restricted to one joint or plane and can be slow or rapid. Compound movements involve a change of posture at two or more joints. The lateral zone of the cerebellum participates in many aspects of the control of both types of movements.[130–133] Cerebellar lesions impair the control of simple movements, both slow[134–136] and rapid.[4,132,137,138] Clinically, movement abnormalities appear more prominently during rapid than slow movement, probably owing to difficulty in generating muscle forces rapidly.[9,139,140] Cerebellar disorders impair muscular contractions under both isotonic and isometric conditions,[141–143] and disturb the execution of serial movements.[144,145] Self-terminated simple movements become abnormal, with delayed movement initiation[129] and abnormal braking.[146] Ballistic movements also become abnormal after cerebellar lesions.[147]

Injury to the cerebellar hemispheres results in deterioration of compound arm movements with decomposition into their constituent parts. This leads to errors of direction, delay in the initiation of one portion of the compound movement, and an excessive trajectory with movement.[148,149] Dysfunction of the lateral zone of the cerebellum also influences long-latency stretch reflexes.[150–152] The disorders of movement with cerebellar disease result from a variety of abnormalities, including disturbances in the central commands that initiate movements and in the regulation of sensory feedback.[142,153]

DYSMETRIA

This consists of a disturbance of the trajectory or placement of a body part during active movements. It affects proximal and distal joints essentially equally.[154] Hypometria refers to

a trajectory in which the body part falls short of its goal, and hypermetria indicates a trajectory in which the body part extends beyond its goal. Dysmetria can be detected by increasing the inertial load of the moving limb in patients with cerebellar lesions who otherwise do not have clinically apparent dysmetria.[155,156]

DYSDIADOCHOKINESIS AND DYSRHYTHMOKINESIS

Dysdiadochokinesis refers to abnormalities of alternating or fine repetitive movements. When the patient taps one hand with the other, rapidly placing the palmar and dorsal surfaces alternately upwards, deficits appear in the rate of alternation and in the completeness of the sequence.[110] The patient cannot produce rhythmic movements and the hand becomes supinated or pronated incompletely. Opposing each finger in rapid succession against the thumb of the same hand reveals finer deficits in coordination. Alternate tapping of the heel and toe on the floor also demonstrates deficits in movements of the feet. Dysrhythmokinesis refers to a disorder of the rhythm of rapidly alternating movements and can be demonstrated when patients attempt to tap out a rhythm such as three rapid beats followed by one delayed beat. The rhythm becomes abnormal and irregular with cerebellar lesions. These deficits stem in part from deficiencies in the timing functions of the cerebellum.[157,158]

ATAXIA

The term ataxia describes multiple simultaneous problems with movement, including delay in movement initiation, disorders of movement termination (dysmetria), disturbances of velocity and acceleration, and difficulty applying constant force.[159] These abnormalities result in decomposition of movement so that errors occur in the sequence and speed of the component parts of a movement. The consequences include a lack of speed and skill in acts requiring the smoothly coordinated activity of several muscles. Another term for the abnormalities of movement with cerebellar disease is asynergia or dyssynergia. These terms indicate that the patient cannot perform the various components of a movement at the right time in the appropriate space.

ABNORMAL CHECK AND REBOUND

Impaired check and excessive rebound are related signs of cerebellar injury. To examine for abnormal check, the examiner asks the patient to maintain the limbs extended forward in space while the examiner taps the wrists strongly enough to displace the arms. The patient keeps the eyes shut and the hands pronated. A small displacement should result in a rapid, accurate return to the original position in a normal subject. With injury to the cerebellum, a light tap to the wrist causes a large displacement of the affected limb followed by an overshoot beyond the original position. The limb returns to the original position after oscillating around its initial position. Wide excursion of the affected limb, which is termed excessive rebound, results from impaired check. Excessive rebound results in overshoot beyond the original position. Impaired check can be assessed also by forcefully pulling on the patient's forearm while the patient flexes the elbow. On releasing the forearm abruptly, the examiner will evoke an unchecked contraction of the arm and the hand will strike the patient's chest. The basic phenomenon underlying impaired check and excessive rebound is the inability to stop abruptly an ongoing movement.

TREMOR

Cerebellar dysfunction results in static and kinetic tremors.[22,80,160,161] The term "intention tremor" is a widely used but ambiguous term, usually referring to the tremor that occurs with voluntary (intentional) limb movement. The term "kinetic tremor" is preferable, as it refers to a tremor occurring during movement, whether voluntary or not. Static tremor can be demonstrated by observing a patient with the arms extended parallel to the floor with the hands open. Often this position can be sustained steadily for several seconds, but then a rhythmic oscillation occurs, generated at the shoulder. Kinetic tremor, usually affecting the proximal musculature exclusively in cerebellar disease, can be brought out by having the patient perform the finger-to-nose and heel-knee-shin tests. Stretch-evoked peripheral feedback to the cerebral cortex contributes to static tremor,[160,162] and deficient limb stabilization during maintained postures or after brisk voluntary movements contributes to both static and kinetic tremor.[22,160] Other mechanisms contributing to tremor include deficiency of suppressive bursts,[22,160] transcortical reflex activity,[163] and enhancement of long-loop stretch reflexes.[164]

ATAXIC DYSARTHRIA

The cerebellar contribution to speech concerns articulation and not cognitive processing.[165] Disease restricted to the cerebellum causes an ataxia of speech characterized by imprecise consonants, excessive and equalized stress patterns, irregular articulatory breakdowns, distorted vowels, prolonged phonemes, prolonged intervals, and slowness of rate, as well as excessive loudness variations, pitch breaks, and voice tremor.[166,167] Temporal dysregulation contributes to these disturbances.[168] Cerebellar disease alone does not lead to spastic (i.e., strained, strangled) speech, which appears to result from corticobulbar disease.[169] Although injury to several parts of the cerebellum has been associated with speech disorders, several studies have localized a region critical for ataxic dysarthria to the paravermal aspect of the left superior cerebellar hemisphere.[99,170,171] In a single case report, agrammatic speech resulted from a right cerebellar lesion, linking dominant hemisphere speech function to the cerebellum.[172]

A transient loss of speech termed "cerebellar mutism" can affect children after posterior fossa surgery.[173-178] The disorder occurs following manipulation of structures in the posterior fossa, including the cerebellum and the dorsal brainstem. The disorder appears to result from an interaction of trauma to the brainstem and cerebellum coupled with hydrocephalus.[177]

ABNORMALITIES OF MUSCLE TONE

Hypotonia (decreased resistance to passive muscular extension) can result from lateral cerebellar lesions, usually occurring acutely after cerebellar injury, and decreasing progressively over time.[4] Pendular deep tendon reflexes accompany cerebellar hypotonia. Tonic stretch reflexes induced by muscle vibration[179] become abnormal with cerebellar disorders and appear to be related to hypotonia. Hypotonia has been found in monkeys after complete cerebellar ablation,[180] in the ipsilateral limbs after unilateral cerebellar ablation,[180] and after lesions of the cerebellar nuclei.[181] Hypotonia occurs maximally in the extensor muscles of monkeys with cerebellar lesions, but decreases with time and gives way to tonic flexion of the affected limbs.[80] Hypotonia does not appear in subprimate mammals such as cats and dogs after cerebellar ablation; these animals develop marked extensor rigidity with opisthotonos. Termed alpha rigidity, the extensor rigidity in these animals persists after section of the dorsal roots, which abolishes decerebrate gamma rigidity.[80]

The cerebellum manipulates the linkage of alpha and gamma motoneurons in the performance of movements. Inactivation of the cerebellar cortex in the cat by cooling decreases the excitability of muscle spindle afferents.[80] In the monkey after surgical extirpation of the cerebellum, muscle spindle primary afferents become defective in function, showing raised thresholds and decreased static and dynamic sensitivity.[180] Muscle spindle secondary afferents, however, show essentially normal responses. Hypotonia appears to be related to the muscle spindle abnormalities. Cerebellar ablation in the cat reduces muscle spindle sensitivity to static extension and a variety of natural external inputs,[182] with greater abnormalities affecting afferents with high rather than low conduction velocity,[183] along with low baseline rates of alpha motoneuron firing.[184] The reason for this is that cerebellar lesions result in defective gamma motoneuron regulation of muscle spindle output.[80] Thus, alpha motoneurons having synaptic connection with spindle receptors innervated by afferent fibers of high conduction velocity receive a falsely low indication of static muscle length. The decrease of fusimotor activity leading to abnormalities in muscle spindle function is an important factor in the pathogenesis of cerebellar hypotonia. Although the decrease of fusimotor activity after cerebellar lesions results from abnormal function of a long reflex loop through the precentral cortex,[185,186] vestibulospinal and reticulospinal pathways also appear to be involved since lesions of the fastigial nucleus markedly decrease muscle spindle activity.[187]

Treatment of Cerebellar Disorders

Medical treatment of the symptoms of cerebellar disorders is limited at best. Despite the appearance periodically of enthusiastic claims for therapeutic benefits from administration of isoniazid, physostigmine, L-5-hydroxytryptophan, thyrotropin-releasing hormone, vitamin E, amantadine, and propranolol, most clinicians have found that these medications provide little or no benefit. Thyrotropin-releasing hormone appears to have the greatest efficacy in double-blind placebo-controlled studies, but the medication must be given by injection, limiting its clinical utility.[188] I have found oral administration of clonazepam 1.5–5 mg daily in divided doses to have limited benefit in some patients. I usually begin treatment with one-half of a 0.5-mg tablet at bedtime, and then gradually escalate the dose over many weeks, depending upon patient tolerance of the side-effects, which include drowsiness, lethargy, and worsening of ataxia. I have also found gabapentin to provide minimal to moderate improvement of ataxia. I use 100 mg three times daily, with a gradually increasing dose to as high as 1200 mg daily.

The key to treatment of cerebellar disorders is an accurate diagnosis, so that the appropriate therapeutic intervention can be made. Disorders of cerebellar function can arise from degenerative, demyelinating, neoplastic, paraneoplastic, vascular, and infectious diseases, and from drug effects, heavy metal intoxications, malformations, inherited metabolic diseases, and endocrinopathies.[80] Table 44-4 provides a summary of the common disorders affecting cerebellar function, the laboratory tests helpful in the diagnosis, and the specific treatments available. Recent publications provide lists of the inherited ataxias of infancy, childhood and adulthood, the patterns of inheritance, the appropriate laboratory tests, and the specific treatment available.[189–192]

TABLE 44-4 Differential Diagnosis and Treatment of Cerebellar Disorders

Disorders	Laboratory Tests	Specific Treatment
Degenerative		
Sporadic olivopontocerebellar atrophy	MRI, CT, PET	None
Multiple-system atrophy	MRI, CT, PET	Fludrocortisone, oxybutynin, tolterodine
Deficiency		
Alcoholic cerebellar degeneration	MRI, CT, PET	Thiamine and proper nutrition
Vitamin E deficiency, recessively inherited or secondary	Serum vitamin E level	Vitamin E
Demyelinating		
Multiple sclerosis	MRI, CSF evaluation, evoked potential studies	Interferon beta-1b, interferon beta-1a, glatiramer acetate, mitoxantrone
Neoplastic		
Primary neoplasms	CT, MRI, angiogram, ophthalmoscopic examination of the retina for von Hippel-Lindau syndrome	Surgery, chemotherapy, radiation therapy
Medulloblastoma		
Astrocytoma		
Ependymoma		
Meningioma		
Acoustic schwannoma		
Hemangioma (von Hippel-Lindau syndrome)		
Secondary neoplasms		
Lung, breast, skin (melanoma), kidney, lymphoma	CT, MRI, angiogram, CBC, X-rays, bone marrow, bone scan	Surgery, chemotherapy, radiation therapy
Paraneoplastic		
Paraneoplastic cerebellar degeneration	Search for primary neoplasm (ovarian, lung, breast, uterine, sarcomatous neoplasms in adults; neuroblastoma in children)	Surgery, chemotherapy, radiation therapy of the primary neoplasm
Vascular		
Infarction	MRI, CT, angiogram	Surgical and medical management
Hemorrhage	MRI, CT, angiogram	Surgical and medical management
Arteriovenous malformation	MRI, CT, angiogram	Surgical and medical management

(continued)

TABLE 44-4—*(continued)*

Disorders	Laboratory Tests	Specific Treatment
Infectious		
Bacterial abscess	MRI, CT, angiogram	Surgery, antibiotics
Creutzfeldt-Jakob disease	EEG	None
Acute cerebellar ataxia in children	CSF evaluation, viral studies, search for neuroblastoma	None
Drugs		
Anticonvulsants: phenytoin, valproate, carbamazepine, clonazepam, phenobarbital	Serum anticonvulsant drug levels	Decrease anticonvulsant drug intake
Psychotropic medications: neuroleptics, antidepressants	Serum levels if available	Decrease psychotropic medication intake
Lithium	Serum level of lithium	Decrease lithium intake
Heavy metals		
Thallium	Urinalysis for thallium, nerve conduction velocity	Chelating agents, hemodialysis
Lead (children)	Serum and urine levels of lead	Chelating agents, hemodialysis
Malformations		
Dandy-Walker	CT, MRI, angiogram	Surgery if indicated
Chiari malformations	MRI, angiogram, myelogram, skull and spine films	Surgery if indicated
Endocrine		
Myxedema	T3, T4, TSH	Thyroid-replacement medications
Dominantly inherited ataxias		
Spinocerebellar ataxia types 1–16	Laboratory testing for mutation (expanded CAG repeats in most)	None
Dentatorubropallidoluysian atrophy	Laboratory testing for mutation (expanded CAG repeats)	None
Recessively inherited ataxias		
Friedreich's ataxia	Laboratory testing for GAA repeats	None
Abetalipoproteinemia (Bassen-Kornzweig syndrome)	Red blood cell examination for acanthocytes, beta-lipoprotein screen	Vitamin E
Ataxia telangiectasia	Serum IgA, IgG, alpha-fetoprotein	Antibiotics for intercurrent infections
Neuronal ceroid lipofuscinosis	EEG, visual-evoked potentials, biopsy of skin, sweat glands, conjunctiva	Antioxidant medications, anticonvulsants if indicated
Niemann-Pick type C	Bone marrow, sphingomyelin	None
Juvenile GM1 gangliosidosis	Beta-galactosidase	None
Juvenile GM2 gangliosidosis	Hexosaminidase A	None
Metachromatic leukodystrophy	Urine arylsulfatase A	None
Adrenoleukodystrophy	Very long chain fatty acids	None
Late-onset globoid cell	Galactocerebroside	None
Sialidosis	Neuraminidase	None
Carbohydrate-deficient glycoprotein syndrome	Tetrasialotransferrin, asialotransferrin, MRI	None
Mitochondrial disorders (MERRF, KSS, NARP)	Muscle biopsy, retinal examination	None
Leigh's syndrome	Lactate, pyruvate, alanine	None

MRI, magnetic resonance imaging; CT, computed tomographic scanning; PET, positron emission tomography; CSF, cerebrospinal fluid; CBC, complete blood count; AVM, arteriovenous malformation; EEG, electroencephalogram; T3, T4, TSH, specific serum tests of thyroid function; MERRF, myoclonus epilepsy with ragged red fibers; KSS, Kearns-Sayer syndrome; NARP, neuropathy, ataxia, retinitis pigmentosum.

References

1. Fluorens P: *Recherches Expérimentales sur les Propriétés et les Fonctions du Système Nerveux dans les Animaux Vertébrés*. Paris: Crevot, 1824.

2. Luciani L: *Il Cervelletto: Nuovi Studi di Fisiologia Normale e Pathologica*. Florence: LeMonnier, 1891.

3. André-Thomas: *Le Cervelet: Etude Anatomique, Clinique, et Physiologique*. Paris: Steinheil, 1897.

4. Holmes G: The Croonian lectures on the clinical symptoms of cerebellar disease and their interpretation. *Lancet* i:1177–1182, 1231–1237; ii:59–65, 111–115, 1922.

5. Gilman S: The mechanism of cerebellar hypotonia. *Brain* 92: 621–638, 1969.

6. Bloedel JR: Functional heterogeneity with structural homogeneity: How does the cerebellum operate? *Behav Brain Sci* 3:1–39, 1992.

7. Ivry RB, Keele SW, Diener HC: Dissociation of the lateral and medial cerebellum in movement timing and movement execution. *Exp Brain Res* 73:167–180, 1988.

8. Bastian AJ, Martin TA, Keating JK, Thach WT: Cerebellar ataxia: Abnormal control of interaction torques across multiple joints. *J Neurophysiol* 76:492–509, 1996.

9. Topka H, Konczak J, Schneider K, et al: Multi-joint arm movements in cerebellar ataxia: Abnormal control of movement dynamics. *Exp Brain Res* 119:493–503, 1998.

10. Gao JH, Parsons LM, Bower JM, et al: Cerebellum implicated in sensory acquisition and discrimination rather than motor control. *Science* 26:545–547, 1996.

11. Bower JM: Control of sensory data acquisition. *Int Rev Neurobiol* 41:489–513, 1997.

12. Paulin MG: The role of the cerebellum in motor control and perception. *Brain Behav Evol* 41:39–50, 1993.

13. Angel RW: Barognosis in a patient with hemiataxia. *Ann Neurol* 7:73–77, 1980.

14. Thach WT, Goodkin HG, Keating JG: Cerebellum and the adaptive coordination of movement. *Annu Rev Neurosci* 15: 403–442, 1992.

15. Thach WT, Kane SA, Mink JW, Goodkin HP: Cerebellar output: Multiple maps and motor modes in movement coordination, in Llinas R, Sotelo C (eds): *The Cerebellum Revisited*. New York: Springer-Verlag, 1992, pp 283–300.

16. Mauritz KH, Dichgans J, Hufschmidt A: Quantitative analysis of stance in late cortical cerebellar atrophy of the anterior lobe and other forms of cerebellar ataxia. *Brain* 102:461–482, 1979.

17. Horak EB, Diener HC: Cerebellar control of postural scaling and central set. *J Neurophysiol* 72:479–493, 1993.

18. Villis T, Hore J: Central neuronal mechanisms contributing to cerebellar tremor produced by limb perturbations. *J Neurophysiol* 43:279–291, 1980.

19. Bracha V, Kolb FP, Irwin KB, Bloedel JR: Inactivation of interposed nuclei in the cat: Classically conditioned. *Exp Brain Res* 126:77–92, 1999.

20. Mason CR, Miller LE, Baker JF, Houk JC: Organization of reaching and grasping movements in the primate cerebellum. *J Neurophysiol* 79:537–554, 1998.

21. Spidalieri HJ, Busby L, Lamarre Y: Fast ballistic arm movements triggered by visual, auditory, and somesthetic stimuli in the monkey. II. Effects of unilateral dentate lesion on discharge of precentral cortical neurons and reaction. *J Neurophysiol* 50:1359–1379, 1983.

22. Flament D, Hore J: Movement and electromyographic disorders associated with cerebellar dysmetria. *J Neurophysiol* 55: 1221–1233, 1986.

23. Brindley GS: The use made by the cerebellum of the information that it receives from the sense organs. *Int Brain Res Organ Bull* 3:80, 1964.

24. Marr D: A theory of cerebellar cortex. *J Physiol (Lond)* 202: 437–470, 1969.

25. Albus JS: A theory of cerebellar function. *Math Biosci* 10:25–61, 1971.

26. Brand S, Dahl A-L, Mugnaini E: The length of parallel fibers in the cat cerebellar cortex. An experimental light and electron microscopic study. *Exp Brain Res* 26:39–58, 1976.

27. Mugnaini E: The length of cerebellar parallel fibers in chicken and rhesus monkey. *J Comp Neurol* 220:7–15, 1983.

28. Ito M, Shiida N, Yagi N, Yamamoto M: The cerebellar modification of rabbit's horizontal vestibulo-ocular reflex induced by sustained head rotation combined with visual stimulation. *Proc Jpn Acad* 50:85–89, 1974.

29. Robinson DA: Adaptive gain control of the vestibulo-ocular reflex by the cerebellum. *J Neurophysiol* 39:954–969, 1976.

30. Yeo CH, Hardiman MJ, Glickstein M: Discrete lesions of the cerebellar cortex abolish classically conditioned nictitating membrane response of the rabbit. *Behav Brain Res* 13:261–266, 1989.

31. Thompson RF: The neurobiology of learning and memory. *Science* 233:941–947, 1986.

32. Thompson RF: Neural mechanisms of classial conditioning in mammals. *Philos Trans R Soc Lond B* 329:161–170, 1990.

33. Thompson RF, Krupa DJ: Origin of memory traces in the mammalian brain. *Annu Rev Neurosci* 17:519–549, 1994.

34. Roland PE: Metabolic mapping of sensorimotor integration in the human brain. *Ciba Found Symp* 132:251–268, 1987.

35. Roland PE, Eriksson L, Widen L, Stone-Elander S: Changes in regional cerebral oxidative metabolism induced by tactile learning and recognition in man. *Eur J Neurosci* 1:3–17, 1988.

36. Seitz RJ, Roland PE, Bohm C, et al: Motor learning in man: A positron emission tomography study. *Neuroreport* 1:57–66, 1990.

37. Haier RJ, Siegel BV Jr, MacLachlan A, et al: Regional glucose metabolic changes after learning a complex visuospatial motor task: A positron emission tomography study. *Brain Res* 570: 134–143, 1991.

38. Mazziotta JC, Grafton ST, Woods RC: The human motor system studied with PET measurements of cerebral blood flow: Topography and motor learning, in Lassen NA, Ingvar DH, Raichle ME, Friberg L (eds): *Brain Work and Mental Activity, Alfred Benzen Symposium 31*. Copenhagen: Munksgaard, 1991, pp 280–290.

39. Friston KJ, Frith CD, Passingham RE, et al: Motor practice and neurophysiological adaptation in the cerebellum: A positron emission tomography study. *Proc R Soc Lond* 248:223–228, 1992.

40. Grafton ST, Mazziotta JC, Presty S, et al: Functional anatomy of human procedural learning determined with regional cerebral blood flow and PET. *J Neurosci* 12:2542–2548, 1992.

41. Jenkins IH, Brooks DJ, Nixon PD, et al: Motor sequence learning: A study with positron emission tomography. *J Neurosci* 14:3775–3790, 1994.

42. Horak FB, Diener HC: Cerebellar control of postural scaling and central set in stance. *J Neurophysiol* 72:479–493, 1994.

43. Horak FB: Comparison of cerebellar and vestibular loss on scaling of postural responses, in Brandt T, Paulus W, Bles W, et al (eds): *Disorders of Posture and Gait*. Stuttgart: Georg Thieme Verlag, 1990, pp 370–373.

44. Gautier GM, Hofferer J-M, Hoyt WF, Stark L: Visual-motor adaptation: Quantitative demonstration in patients with posterior fossa involvement. *Arch Neurol* 36:155–160, 1979.

45. Baizer JS, Glickstein M: Role of cerebellum in prism adaptation. *J Physiol* 23:34–35, 1974.

46. Weiner MJ, Hallett M, Funkenstein HH: Adaptation to lateral displacement of vision in patients with lesions of the central nervous system. *Neurology* 33:766–772, 1983.

47. Sanes JN, Dimitrov B, Hallett M: Motor learning in patients with cerebellar dysfunction. *Brain* 113:103–120, 1990.

48. Leiner HC, Leiner AL, Dow RS: Does the cerebellum contribute to mental skills? *Behav Neurosci* 100:443–453, 1986.

49. Leiner HC, Leiner Al, Dow RS: Cerebro-cerebellar learning loops in apes and humans. *Ital J Neurol Sci* 8:425–436, 1987.

50. Leiner HC, Leiner AL, Dow RS: The human cerebro-cerebellar system: its computing, cognitive, and language skills. *Behav Brain Res* 44:113–128, 1991.

51. Schell GR, Strick PL: The origin of thalamic inputs to the arcuate premotor and supplementary motor areas. *J Neurosci* 4:539–560, 1983.

52. Orioli PJ, Strick PL: Cerebellar connections with the motor cortex and the arcuate premotor area: An analysis employing retrograde transneuronal transport of WGA-HRP. *J Comp Neurol* 288:612–626, 1989.

53. Yamamoto T, Yoshida K, Yoshikawa H, et al: The medial dorsal nucleus is one of the thalamic relays of the cerebellocerebral responses to the frontal association cortex in the monkey: Horseradish peroxidase and fluorescent dye double staining study. *Brain Res* 579:315–320, 1992.

54. Middleton FA, Strick PL: Anatomic evidence for cerebellar and basal ganglia involvement in higher cognitive functions. *Science* 266:458–461, 1994.

55. Petersen SE, Fox PT, Posner MI, et al: Positron emission tomographic studies of the processing of single words. *J Cogn Neurosci* 1:153–170, 1989.

56. Raichle ME, Fiez JA, Videen TO, et al: Practice-related changes in human brain functional anatomy during nonmotor learning. *Cereb Cortex* 4:8–26, 1994.

57. Fiez JA, Petersen SE, Cheney MK, Raichle ME: Impaired nonmotor learning and error detection associated with cerebellar damage. *Brain* 115:155–178, 1992.

58. Silveri MC, Leggio MG, Molinari M: The cerebellum contributes to linguistic production: A case of agrammatic speech following a right cerebellar lesion. *Neurology* 44:2047–2050, 1994.

59. Grafman J, Litvan I, Massaquoi S, et al: Cognitive planning deficit in patients with cerebellar atrophy. *Neurology* 42:1493–1496, 1992.

60. Bracke-Tolkmitt R, Linden A, Canavan AGM, et al: The cerebellum contributes to mental skills. *Behav Neurosci* 103:442–446, 1989.

61. Topka H, Valls-Solé J, Massaquoi SG, Hallett M: Deficit in classical conditioning in patients with cerebellar degeneration. *Brain* 116:961–969, 1993.

62. Lalonde R: Cerebellar contributions to instrumental learning. *Neurosci Biobehav Rev* 18:161–170, 1994.

63. Akshoomoff NA, Courchesne E: A new role for the cerebellum in cognitive operations. *Behav Neurosci* 106:731–738, 1992.

64. Akshoomoff NA, Courchesne E: ERP evidence for a shifting attention deficit in patients with damage to the cerebellum. *J Cogn Neurosci* 6:388–399, 1994.

65. Ito M: Synaptic plasticity in the cerebellar cortex and its role in motor learning. *Can J Neurol Sci* 20:S70–S74, 1993.

66. Schmahmann JD, Sherman JC: The cerebellar cognitive affective syndrome. *Brain* 121:561–579, 1998.

67. Schmahmann JD, Pandya DN: The cerebrocerebellar system, in Schmahmann JD (ed): *The Cerebellum and Cognition*. San Diego: Academic Press, 1997, pp 31–60.

68. Parvizi J, Anderson SW, Martin CO, et al: Pathological laughter and crying. A link to the cerebellum. *Brain* 124:1708–1719, 2001.

69. Courchesne E, Yeung-Courchesne R, Press GA, et al: Hypoplasia of cerebellar vermal lobules VI and VII in autism. *N Engl J Med* 318:1349–1354, 1988.

70. Murakami JW, Courchesne E, Press GA, et al: Reduced cerebellar hemisphere size and its relationship to vermal hypoplasia in autism. *Arch Neurol* 46:689–694, 1989.

71. Holroyd S, Reiss AL, Bryan RN: Autistic features in Joubert syndrome: A genetic disorder with agenesis of the cerebellar vermis. *Biol Psychiatry* 29:287–294, 1991.

72. Ciesielski KT, Knight JE: Cerebellar abnormality in autism: A nonspecific effect of early brain damage? *Acta Neurobiol Exp* 54:151–154, 1994.

73. Weinberger D, Kleinman J, Luchins D, et al: Cerebellar pathology in schizophrenia. A controlled post-mortem study. *Am J Psychiatry* 137:359–361, 1980.

74. Nopoulos PC, Ceilley JW, Gailis EA, Andreasen NC: An MRI study of cerebellar vermis morphology in patients with schizophrenia: Evidence in support of the cognitive dysmetria concept. *Biol Psychiatry* 46:703–711, 1999.

75. Wassink TH, Andreasen NC, Nopoulos P, Flaum N: Cerebellar morphology as a predictor of symptom and psychosocial outcome in schizophrenia. *Biol Psychiatry* 45:41–48, 1999.

76. Volkow ND, Levy A, Brodie JD, et al: Low cerebellar metabolism in medicated patients with chronic schizophrenia. *Am J Psychiatry* 149:686–688, 1992.

77. Andreasen NC, O'Leary DS, Flaum M, et al: Hypofrontality in schizophrenia: distributed dysfunctional circuits in neuroleptic-naïve patients. *Lancet* 349:1730–1734, 1997.

78. Berquin PC, Giedd JM, Jacobsen LK, et al: Cerebellum in attention-deficit hyperactivity disorder: A morphometric MRI study. *Neurology* 50:1087–1093, 1998.

79. Mostofsky SH, Mazzocco MM, Aakaly G, et al: Decreased cerebellar posterior vermis size in fragile X syndrome: Correlation with neurocognitive performance. *Neurology* 50:121–130, 1998.

80. Gilman S, Bloedel JR, Lechtenberg R: *Disorders of the Cerebellum*. Philadelphia: Davis, 1981.

81. Brodal A: *Neurological Anatomy in Relation to Clinical Medicine*, 3rd ed. New York: Oxford University Press, 1981.

82. Kitamura T, Yamada J: Spinocerebellar tract neurons with axons passing through the inferior or superior cerebellar peduncles. *Brain Behav Evol* 34:133–142, 1989.

83. Brodal A, Brodal P: Observations on the secondary vestibulo-cerebellar projections in the macaque monkey. *Exp Brain Res* 58:62–74, 1985.

84. Suzuki DA, Keller EL: The role of the posterior vermis of monkey cerebellum in smooth-pursuit eye movement control. I. Eye and head movement-related activity. *J Neurophysiol* 59:1–18, 1988.

85. Suzuki DA, Keller EL: The role of the posterior vermis of monkey cerebellum in smooth-pursuit eye movement control. II. Target velocity-related Purkinje cell activity. *J Neurophysiol* 59:19–40, 1988.

86. Hoover JE, Strick PL: The organization of cerebellar and basal ganglia outputs to primary motor cortex as revealed by retrograde transneuronal transport of herpes simplex virus type 1. *J Neurosci* 19:1446–1463, 1999.

87. Middleton FA, Strick PL: Anatomical evidence for cerebellar and basal ganglia involvement in higher cognitive function. *Science* 266:458–461, 1994.

88. Middleton FA, Strick PL: Cerebellar output channels, in Schmahmann JD (ed): *The Cerebellum and Cognition.* San Diego: Academic Press, 1997, pp 61–82.

89. Voogd J: The importance of fibre connections in the comparative anatomy of the mammalian cerebellum, in Llinas R (ed): *Neurobiology of Cerebellar Evolution and Development.* Chicago: American Medical Association, 1969, pp 493–519.

90. Voogd J: The olivocerebellar projection in the cat. *Exp Brain Res* 6(suppl):134–161, 1982.

91. Leigh RJ, Zee DS: *The Neurology of Eye Movements,* 3rd ed. New York: Oxford University Press, 1999.

92. Baloh RW, Honrubia V: *Clinical Neurophysiology of the Vestibular System,* 3rd ed. New York: Oxford University Press, 2001.

93. Straube A, Scheuerer W, Eggert T: Unilateral cerebellar lesions affect initiation of ipsilateral smooth pursuit eye movements in humans. *Ann Neurol* 42:891–898, 1997.

94. Maurice-Williams RS: Mechanisms of production of gait unsteadiness by tumors of the posterior fossa. *J Neurol Neurosurg Psychiatry* 38:143–148, 1975.

95. Amici R, Avanzini G, Pacini L: Cerebellar tumors. *Monogr Neural Sci* 4:1–112, 1976.

96. Dichgans J: Clinical symptoms of cerebellar dysfunction and their topodiagnostical significance. *Hum Neurobiol* 2:269–279, 1984.

97. Dichgans J, Diener HC: Clinical evidence for functional compartmentalization of the cerebellum, in Bloedel JR, Dichgans J, Precht W (eds): *Cerebellar Functions.* Berlin: Springer, 1984, pp 126–147.

98. Dichgans J, Diener HC: Different forms of postural ataxia in patients with cerebellar diseases, in Bles W, Brandt T (eds): *Disorders of Posture and Gait.* Amsterdam: Elsevier, 1986, 207–215.

99. Lechtenberg R, Gilman S: Speech disorders in cerebellar disease. *Ann Neurol* 3:285–290, 1978.

100. Melo TP, Bogousslavsky J: Hemiataxia-hypesthesia: A thalamic stroke syndrome. *J Neurol Neurosurg Psychiatry* 55:581–584, 1992.

101. Melo TP, Bogousslavsky J, Moulin T, et al: Thalamic ataxia. *J Neurol* 239:331–337, 1992.

102. Solomon DH, Barohn RJ, Bazan C, Grissom J: The thalamic ataxia syndrome. *Neurology* 44:810–814, 1994.

103. Fisher CM, Cole M: Homolateral ataxia and crural paresis: A vascular syndrome. *J Neurol Neurosurg Psychiatry* 28:45–55, 1965.

104. Giroud M, Creisson E, Fayolle H, et al: Homolateral ataxia and crural paresis: A crossed cerebral-cerebellar diaschisis. *J Neurol Neurosurg Psychiatry* 57:221–222, 1994.

105. Yagnik PM, Dhaduk V, Huen L: Parietal ataxic hemiparesis. *Eur Neurol* 28:164–166, 1988.

106. Klockgether T, Ludtke R, Kramer B, et al: The natural history of degenerative ataxia: A retrospective study in 466 patients. *Brain* 121:589–600, 1998.

107. Dichgans J, Fetter M: Compartmentalized cerebellar functions upon the stabilization of body posture. *Rev Neurol (Paris)* 149:654–664, 1993.

108. Brown P, Rothwell JC, Stevens JM, et al: Cerebellar axial postural tremor. *Mov Disord* 12:977–984, 1997.

109. Diener HC, Dichgans J, Bacher M, Gompf B: Quantification of postural sway in normals and patients with cerebellar disease. *Clin Neurophysiol* 57:134–142, 1984.

110. Trouillas P, Takayanagi T, Hallett M, et al: International cooperative ataxia rating scale for pharmacological assessment of the cerebellar syndrome. *J Neurol Sci* 145:205–211, 1997.

111. Shan DE, Wang V, Chen JT: Isolated lateropulsion of the trunk in cerebellar infarct. *Clin Neurol Neurosurg* 97:195–198, 1995.

112. Diener HC, Dichgans J, Guschlbauer B, et al: The coordination of posture and voluntary movement in patients with cerebellar dysfunction. *Mov Disord* 7:14–22, 1992.

113. Palliyath S, Hallett M, Thomas SL, Lebiedowska MK: Gait in patients with cerebellar ataxia. *Mov Disord* 13:958–964, 1998.

114. Victor M, Adams RD, Collins GC: *The Wernicke-Korsakoff Syndrome and Related Neurologic Disorders Due to Alcoholism and Malnutrition,* 2nd ed. Philadelphia: Davis, 1989.

115. Bastian AJ, Mink JW, Kaufman BA, Thach WT: Posterior vermal split syndrome. *Ann Neurol* 44:601–610, 1998.

116. Lewis RF, Zee DS: Ocular motor disorders associated with cerebellar lesions: pathophysiology and topical localization. *Rev Neurol (Paris)* 149:665–677, 1993.

117. Raymond JL, Lisberger SG, Mauk MD: The cerebellum: A neuronal learning machine? *Science* 272:1126–1131, 1996.

118. Versino M, Hurko O, Zee DS: Disorders of binocular control of eye movements in patients with cerebellar dysfunction. *Brain* 119:1933–1950, 1996.

119. Helmchen C, Straube A, Büttner U: Saccadic lateropulsion in Wallenberg's syndrome may be caused by a functional lesion of the fastigial nucleus. *J Neurol* 241:421–426, 1994.

120. Waterson JA, Barnes GR, Grealy MA: A quantitative study of eye and head movements during smooth pursuit in patients with cerebellar disease. *Brain* 115:1343–1358, 1992.

121. Grant MP, Leigh RJ, Seidman SH, et al: Comparison of predictable smooth ocular and combined eye-head tracking behaviour in patients with lesions affecting the brainstem and cerebellum. *Brain* 115:1323–1342, 1992.

122. Vahedi K, Rivaud S, Amarenco P, Pierrot-Deseilligny C: Horizontal eye movement disorders after posterior vermis infarctions. *J Neurol Neurosurg Psychiatry* 58:91–94, 1995.

123. Waespe W: Deficits of smooth-pursuit eye movements in two patients with a lesion in the (para) floccular or dorsolateral pontine region. *Neuroophthalmology* 12:91–96, 1992.

124. Büttner U, Grundei T: Gaze-evoked nystagmus and smooth pursuit deficits: Their relationship studied in 52 patients. *J Neurol* 242:384–389, 1995.

125. Hain TC, Zee DS, Maria B: Tilt-suppression of the vestibulo-ocular reflex in patients with cerebellar lesions. *Acta Otolaryngol (Stockh)* 105:13–20, 1988.

126. Vahedi K, Rivaud S, Amarenco P, Pierrot-Deseilligny C: Horizontal eye movement disorders after posterior vermis infarctions. *J Neurol Neurosurg Psychiatry* 58:91–94, 1995.

127. Zee DS: Considerations on the mechanisms of alternating skew deviation in patients with cerebellar lesions. *J Vestibul Res* 6:1–7, 1996.

128. FitzGibbon EJ, Calvert PC, Dieterich MD, et al: Torsional nystagmus during vertical pursuit. *J Neuroophthalmol* 16:79–90, 1996.

129. Hallett M, Shahani BT, Young RR: EMG analysis of patients with cerebellar deficits. *J Neurol Neurosurg Psychiatry* 38:1163–1169, 1975.

130. Brown SH, Hefter H, Mertens M, Freund H-J: Disturbances in human arm movement trajectory due to mild cerebellar dysfunction. *J Neurol Neurosurg Psychiatry* 53:306–313, 1990.

131. Morrice B-L, Becker WJ, Hoffer JA, Lee RG: Manual tracking performance in patients with cerebellar incoordination: Effects of mechanical loading. *Can J Neurol Sci* 17:275–285, 1990.

132. Becker WJ, Kunesch E, Freund H-J: Coordination of a multi-joint movement in normal humans and in patients with cerebellar dysfunction. *Can J Neurol Sci* 17:264–274, 1990.

133. Thach WT, Perry JG, Kane SA, Goodkin HP: Cerebellar nuclei: rapid alternating movement, motor somatotopy, and a mechanism for the control of motor synergy. *Rev Neurol (Paris)* 149:607–628, 1993.

134. Beppu H, Suda M, Tanaka R: Analysis of cerebellar motor disorders by visually guided elbow tracking movements. *Brain* 107:787–809, 1984.

135. Hermsdörfer J, Wessel K, Mai N, Marquardt C: Perturbation of precision grip in Friedreich's ataxia and late-onset cerebellar ataxia. *Mov Disord* 9:650–654, 1994.

136. Müller F, Dichgans J: Dyscoordination of pinch and lift forces during grasp in patients with cerebellar lesions. *Exp Brain Res* 101:485–492, 1994.

137. Bonnefoi-Kyriacou B, Trouche E, Legallet E, Viallet F: Planning and execution of pointing movements in cerebellar patients. *Mov Disord* 10:171–178, 1995.

138. Tsujimoto T, Gemba H, Sasaki K: Effect of cooling the dentate nucleus of the cerebellum on hand movement of the monkey. *Brain Res* 629:1–9, 1993.

139. Massaquoi SG, Hallett M: Kinematics of initiating a two-joint arm movement in patients with cerebellar ataxia. *Can J Neurol Sci* 23:3–14, 1996.

140. Boose A, Dichgans J, Topka H: Deficits in phasic muscle force generation explain insufficient compensation for interaction torque in cerebellar patients. *Neurosci Lett* 261:53–56, 1999.

141. Mai N, Bolsinger P, Avarello M, et al: Control of isometric finger force in patients with cerebellar disease. *Brain* 111:973–998, 1988.

142. Flament D, Hore J: Comparison of cerebellar intention tremor under isotonic and isometric conditions. *Brain Res* 439:179–186, 1988.

143. Virji-Babul N, Cooke JD: Influence of joint interactional effects on the coordination of planar two-joint arm movements. *Exp Brain Res* 103:451–459, 1995.

144. Inhoff AW, Diener HC, Rafal RD, Ivry R: The role of cerebellar structures in the execution of serial movements. *Brain* 112:565–581, 1989.

145. Lu X, Hikosaka O, Miyachi S: Role of monkey cerebellar nuclei in skill for sequential movement. *J Neurophysiol* 79:2245–2254, 1998.

146. Vilis T, Hore J: Central neural mechanisms contributing to cerebellar tremor produced by limb perturbations. *J Neurophysiol* 43:279–291, 1980.

147. Spidalieri G, Busby L, Lamarre Y: Fast ballistic arm movements triggered by visual, auditory, and somesthetic stimuli in the monkey. II. Effects of unilateral dentate lesion on discharge of precentral cortical neurons and reaction time. *J Neurophysiol* 50:1359–1379, 1983.

148. Brooks VB, Thach WT: Cerebellar control of posture and movement, in Brooks VB (ed): *Handbook of Physiology Neurophysiology: Motor Control*. Bethesda: American Physiological Society, 1981, sect 1, vol 2, part 2, pp 877–946.

149. Miall RC, Weir DJ, Stein JF: Visuo-motor tracking during reversible inactivation of the cerebellum. *Exp Brain Res* 65:455–464, 1987.

150. Diener HC, Dichgans J: Long loop reflexes and posture, in Bles W, Brandt T (eds): *Disorders of Posture and Gait*. Amsterdam: Elsevier, 1986, Ch. 3, pp 41–51.

151. Diener HC, Dichgans J, Bacher M, Guschlbauer B: Characteristic alterations of long-loop 'reflexes' in patients with Friedreich's disease and late atrophy of the cerebellar anterior lobe. *J Neurol Neurosurg Psychiatry* 47:679–685, 1984.

152. Tokuda T, Tako K, Hayashi R, Yanagisawa N: Disturbed modulation of the stretch reflex gain during standing in cerebellar ataxia. *EEG Clin Neurophysiol* 81:421–426, 1991.

153. Grill SE, Hallett M, Marcus C, McShane L: Disturbances of kinaesthesia in patients with cerebellar disorders. *Brain* 117:1433–1447, 1994.

154. Hore J, Wild B, Diener HC: Cerebellar dysmetria at the elbow, wrist, and fingers. *J Neurophysiol* 65:563–571, 1991.

155. Manto M, Godaux E, Jacquy J: Cerebellar hypermetria is larger when the inertial load is artificially increased. *Ann Neurol* 35:45–52, 1994.

156. Manto M, Godaux E, Jacquy J: Detection of silent cerebellar lesions by increasing the inertial load of the moving hand. *Ann Neurol* 37:344–350, 1995.

157. Ivry R, Keele SW: Timing functions of the cerebellum. *J Cogn Neurosci* 1:136–152, 1989.

158. Ivry R: Cerebellar timing systems. *Int Rev Neurobiol* 41:555–573, 1997.

159. Diener HC, Dichgans J: Pathophysiology of cerebellar ataxia. *Mov Disord* 7:95–109, 1992.

160. Hore J, Flament D: Evidence that a disordered servo-like mechanism contributes to tremor in movements during cerebellar dysfunction. *J Neurophysiol* 56:123–136, 1986.

161. Cole JD, Philip HI, Sedgwick EM: Stability and tremor in the fingers associated with cerebellar hemisphere and cerebellar tract lesions in man. *J Neurol Neurosurg Psychiatry* 51:1558–1568, 1988.

162. Flament D, Vilis T, Hore J: Dependence of cerebellar tremor on proprioceptive but not visual feedback. *Exp Neurol* 84:314–325, 1984.

163. Topka H, Mescheriakov S, Boose A, et al: A cerebellar-like terminal and postural tremor induced in normal man by transcranial magnetic stimulation. *Brain* 122:1551–1562, 1999.

164. Friedemann HH, Noth J, Diener HC, Bacher M: Long latency EMG responses in hand and leg muscles: Cerebellar disorders. *J Neurol Neurosurg Psychiatry* 50:71–77, 1987.

165. Ackermann H, Wildgruber D, Daum I, Grodd W: Does the cerebellum contribute to cognitive aspects of speech production? A functional magnetic resonance imaging (fMRI) study in humans. *Neurosci Lett* 247:187–190, 1998.

166. Kluin KJ, Gilman S, Markel DS, et al: Speech disorders in olivopontocerebellar atrophy correlate with positron emission tomography findings. *Ann Neurol* 23:547–554, 1988.

167. Ackermann H, Ziegler W: Cerebellar voice tremor: an acoustic analysis. *J Neurol Neurosurg Psychiatry* 54:74–76, 1991.

168. Kent RD, Kent JF, Rosenbek JC, et al: A speaking task analysis of the dysarthria in cerebellar disease. *Folia Phoniatr Logop* 49: 63–82, 1997.

169. Gilman S, Kluin K: Perceptual analysis of speech disorders in Friedreich disease and olivopontocerebellar atrophy, in Bloedel JR, Dichgans J, Precht W (eds): *Cerebellar Functions*. Berlin: Springer, 1984, pp 148–163.

170. Ackermann H, Vogel M, Petersen D, Poremba M: Speech deficits in ischaemic cerebellar lesions. *J Neurol* 239:223–227, 1992.

171. Amarenco P, Chevrie MC, Roullet E, Bousser MG: Paravermal infarct and isolated cerebellar dysarthria. *Ann Neurol* 30:211–213, 1991.

172. Silveri MC, Leggio MG, Molinari M: The cerebellum contributes to linguistic production: A case of agrammatic speech following a right cerebellar lesion. *Neurology* 44:2047–2050, 1994.

173. Ammirati M, Mirzai S, Samii M: Transient mutism following removal of a cerebellar tumor. *Childs Nerv Syst* 5:12–14, 1989.

174. Dietze DD, Mickle JP: Cerebellar mutism after posterior fossa surgery. *Pediatr Neurosurg* 16:25–31, 1990.

175. Ferrante L, Mastronardi L, Acqui M, Fortuna A: Mutism after posterior fossa surgery in children. *J Neurosurg* 72:959–963, 1990.

176. Catsman-Berrevoets CE, van Dongen HR, Zwetsloot CP: Transient loss of speech followed by dysarthria after removal of posterior fossa tumour. *Dev Med Child Neurol* 34:1102–1117, 1992.

177. van Dongen HR, Catsman-Berrevoets CE, van Mourik M: The syndrome of "cerebellar" mutism and subsequent dysarthria. *Neurology* 44:2040–2046, 1994.

178. Cole M: The foreign policy of the cerebellum. *Neurology* 44: 2001–2005, 1994.

179. Lance JW, Degail P, Nielson PD: Tonic and phasic spinal cord mechanisms in man. *J Neurol Neurosurg Psychiatry* 29:535–544, 1966.

180. Gilman S: The mechanism of cerebellar hypotonia. An experimental study in the monkey. *Brain* 92:621–638, 1969.

181. Growdon JH, Chambers WW, Liu CN: An experimental study of cerebellar dyskinesia in the rhesus monkey. *Brain* 90:603–632, 1967.

182. Gilman S, McDonald WI: Cerebellar facilitation of muscle spindle activity. *J Neurophysiol* 30:1495–1512, 1967.

183. Gilman S, McDonald WI: Relation of afferent fiber conduction velocity to reactivity of muscle spindle receptors after cerebellectomy. *J Neurophysiol* 30:1513–1522, 1967.

184. Gilman S, Ebel HC: Fusimotor neuron responses to natural stimuli as a function of prestimulus fusimotor activity in decerebellate cats. *Brain Res* 21:367–384, 1970.

185. Gilman S, Marco LA, Ebel HC: Effects of medullary pryamidotomy in the monkey. II. Abnormalities of muscle spindle afferent responses. *Brain* 94:515–530, 1971.

186. Gilman S, Lieberman JS, Marco LA: Spinal mechanism underlying the effects of unilateral ablation of areas 4 and 6 in monkeys. *Brain* 97:49–64, 1974.

187. Kornhauser D, Bromberg MB, Gilman S: Effects of lesions of fastigial nucleus on static and dynamic responses of muscle spindle primary afferents in the cat. *J Neurophysiol* 47:977–986, 1982.

188. Sobue I, Takayanagi T, Nakanishi T, et al: Controlled trial of thyrotropin releasing hormone tartrate in ataxia of spinocerebellar degenerations. *J Neurol Sci* 61:235–248, 1983.

189. Gilman S: Inherited ataxia, in Johnson RT (ed): *Current Therapy in Neurologic Disease*, 2d ed. Toronto: Decker, 1987, pp 224–232.

190. Hurko O: Hereditary cerebellar ataxia, in Johnson RT, Griffin JW (eds): *Current Therapy in Neurologic Disease*, 4th ed. St. Louis: Decker, 1993, pp 254–261.

191. Klockgether T: *Handbook of Ataxia Disorders*. New York: Decker, 2000.

192. Paulson H, Ammache Z: Ataxia and hereditary disorders. *Neurol Clin* 19:759–782, 2001.

Chapter 45 _____

PATHOPHYSIOLOGY OF CEREBELLAR DISORDERS

SCOTT E. COOPER, DARRY S. JOHNSON,
and ERWIN B. MONTGOMERY Jr

CEREBELLAR SYMPTOMS AND SIGNS AND
   UNDERLYING MECHANISMS 737
     Dysmetria 737
     Tremor 738
     Dysdiadochokinesia 739
     Dysarthria 739
     Hypotonia 739
     Abnormalities of Eye Movements 740
     Gait Ataxia 740
     Limb Ataxia/Decomposition of Movement/
       Asynergia 740
     Is There a Common Fundamental Underlying
       Mechanism? 741
     Mechanisms of Dysmetria 741
ORGANIZATION OF THE CEREBELLUM 741
     Macroscopic View 741
     Microscopic View 746
CEREBELLAR SYNDROMES 748
     Vermal Syndrome 748
     Paravermal and Lateral Zone Syndrome 748
     Abnormal Eye Movements 749
     Dysarthria 750
THEORIES OF CEREBELLAR FUNCTION 750
     Theories Involving the Timing of Movement
       Components 750
     Cerebellar Effects on the Gamma Motor System ... 751
     Feedforward, Feedback, and Coordination 752
     Learning- and Plasticity-Based Theories 753
     Timing Theories 753
     Non-motor Functions of the Cerebellum 754
MECHANISMS OF DYSFUNCTION 756
SUMMARY 757

The concept of the cerebellum as being responsible only for the smooth coordination of motor acts has undergone a dramatic transformation since the work of the Italian neurophysiologist, Luigi Luciani, who described the effects of ablation experiments in dogs in 1891. Later, in 1917, Gordon Holmes produced what may still be considered the gold standard description of cerebellar signs and symptoms in soldiers with gunshot and shrapnel wounds during World War I. Since the descriptions of Holmes much has been discovered about cerebellar physiology via such techniques as selective ablation, electrical stimulation, reversible cooling, and functional imaging with single-photon emission computed tomography (SPECT) and positron emission tomography (PET). However, there remains much to be discovered. The objective of this chapter is to summarize what has been learned to date in regard to cerebellar pathophysiology and to give the clinician a useful background of information on which to base decisions when treating a patient with cerebellar disease.

The various symptoms and signs associated with disorders of the cerebellum will be described first. This is done so that there is an understanding of what the possible pathophysiological mechanisms are to explain. Then the symptoms and signs, explicated in terms of possible mechanisms, will be related to the macroscopic and microscopic anatomy of the cerebellum and various theories of cerebellar function.

Cerebellar Symptoms and Signs and Underlying Mechanisms

DYSMETRIA

Dysmetria is one of the cardinal signs of cerebellar disease. Holmes, in 1917, described dysmetria in terms of abnormal range and force of movement.[1] There appears to be an abnormality in bringing the limb to the appropriate endpoint. The movement either falls short or goes past the intended target, resulting in the sign of past pointing. Hypometria is a premature arrest of movement, whereas hypermetria is a result of excessive range of movement. Dysmetria is best seen in the finger-to-nose test, or, in the case of the lower extremity, great toe-to-examiner's finger test, provided that the patient has movement only at the hip. During these tests the arm (or foot) typically overshoots or undershoots the target. This can result in an abnormal movement trajectory, which may be manifested as ataxia or decomposition of movement (Fig. 45-1).

There are at least two possible mechanisms underlying dysmetria. First, dysmetria may result from an error in programming the precise patterns of muscle activity that initiate and execute a movement. It is a "disturbance of the trajectory or placement of a body part during active movements."[2] It often takes longer than normal to initiate and to stop voluntary movements, and there is a lack of uniform velocity.[3]

Alternatively, a second mechanism may be a failure to stop the movement. This could be because of the lack of an appropriately timed "braking" muscle contraction, or because of a delay and slowness in arresting muscle contraction,[4] or because the body part in movement is literally too floppy (meaning decreased resistance to passive movement) as a result of decreased muscle tone. Stopping the movement uses passive and active elements. The elastic properties of the limb resist movement and may help in stopping a movement. Muscle tone is an important contributor to elastic limb resistance, and is reduced in patients with cerebellar disease (see section on hypotonia below) (Fig. 45-2).

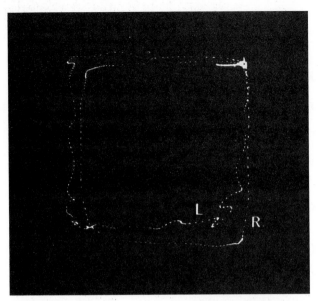

FIGURE 45-1 The patient has a lesion of the left cerebellar hemisphere. The patient is asked to outline the square end of a room with the normal (*right*) and affected (*left*) forefingers. Holmes secured a light to the end of the forefingers, and subsequent recordings were made; each flash of light represents 0.04 s of finger movement. (*From Holmes.*[7] *Used with permission.*)

The role of the cerebellum in controlling the trajectory of movements is reflected in the patterns of neuronal activities in the cerebellum. Laboratory animals can be trained to perform specific movements in response to cues. Simultaneously, neuronal activities in various parts of the cerebellum can be recorded and changes in neuronal activities correlated with the behaviors. Such studies have shown that changes in cerebellar neuronal activities correlate with the direction, magnitude, and velocity of the movements.[5] Alternatively, various parts of the cerebellum can be reversibly inactivated, causing abnormalities of magnitude, velocity, and coordination of movements.[6]

TREMOR

A tremor is a rhythmic, involuntary, oscillatory movement. Although tremors can be classified in numerous ways, perhaps the best way is to characterize them by their relationship to rest, movement, and maintenance of a particular posture. Rest tremor, also known as static tremor, can vary in amplitude and frequency. In Parkinson's disease, rest tremor is the typical slow and coarse tremor. It typically has a frequency of 4–6 Hz. Postural tremor is that seen when a limb is maintained in a position against gravity, as when outstretched. One example is the physiological tremor seen when the hands are held outstretched, with a frequency of about 8–12 Hz. This tremor is accentuated with such stressors as fear, anxiety, or fatigue. Subsets of this type of tremor include benign essential tremor (idiopathic) or familial tremor (autosomal-dominant). The toxic tremor resulting from thyrotoxicosis, uremia, drug toxins (e.g., bronchodilators, tricyclic antidepressants, and lithium), carbon monoxide poisoning, heavy metal poisoning (mercury, arsenic, or lead), or from withdrawal from alcohol or sedative drugs is another type of postural tremor. The third tremor type, known as intention, action, motor, or (preferably) kinetic tremor, occurs during activity. This type of tremor is most frequently associated with disorders of the cerebellum.

Holmes described the tremor seen in patients with cerebellar injuries as irregular oscillations in the intended direction that result from failure of uniform deceleration, complicated by secondary or correcting jerks when the object has not been accurately reached in the first attempt.[7] Holmes also said that "the tremulousness usually increases towards its completion when accuracy is most essential."[1] He described a static tremor as well: titubation (shaking of the head and trunk) increases when one is fatigued, and the body as a whole tends to sway with standing. He observed slow displacements by gravity and quicker voluntary jerks back towards the original position. Many recent authors, however, have indicated that static tremor that accompanies posture maintenance rarely occurs and has poor localizing value.[3,4]

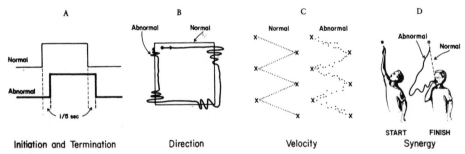

FIGURE 45-2 Cerebellar dysmetria and associated patterns of movement abnormalities. *A.* Delay of initiation and termination of movement. The delay may be 0.1–0.2 s of both start and stop. *B.* Abnormal change of direction as evidenced by increased oscillations during attempt to trace a square. (See original work from Holmes.) *C.* Irregular velocity when attempting to touch objects sequentially. *D.* Lack of synergy between muscles upon attempting to touch the nose with the tip of a finger, an example of dysmetria. (*From Pearlman, et al: Neurological Pathophysiology, 3rd ed. New York: Oxford University Press, 1984. Used with permission.*)

Having the patient do finger-to-nose testing as well as heel-to-knee testing can reveal kinetic tremor. Tremor appears when movement is initiated, during the course of the movement, or when the limb approaches the target. The amplitude of the tremor is especially prominent as the target is approached. Static tremor is demonstrated by having the patient extend the arms parallel to the floor with hands open. After several seconds, the arms will begin to oscillate rhythmically at the shoulder. This can also be demonstrated in the lower limb by asking the patient to extend one leg and hold the great toe close to, but not touching, the examiner's index finger. This posture, in a few seconds, will produce oscillations at the hip joint.[2]

Gilman et al.[2] emphasize, as do other authors, that the term "intention tremor" is a poor one and has often been misused, because it lumps together postural and kinetic tremor. Also, it is pointed out that kinetic tremor tends to involve primarily proximal limb muscles, in contradistinction to distal tremor, as seen in patients with parkinsonism.

DYSDIADOCHOKINESIA

First described by Babinski in 1902, dysdiadochokinesia is a disturbance in the patient's ability to perform rapid alternating movements. This is most easily demonstrated in the clinical setting by having the patient perform rapid supination-pronation of the forearms on a tabletop or on his or her lap[8] (Fig. 45-3). Holmes said that this was a very persistent sign, unlike that of hypotonia[1,7] (see below). In 1929, Wertham described a related abnormality, arrhythmokinesis,

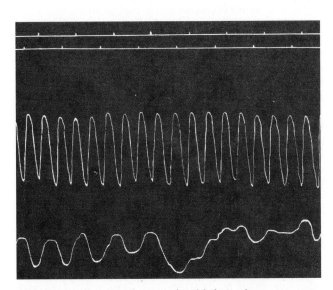

FIGURE 45-3 These tracings are of rapid alternating movements of the affected arm (*below*) and the unaffected arm (*above*). Note the slower velocity and smaller amplitude of the affected arm; notice how it becomes more irregular as the arm becomes almost locked in supination. This is dysdiadochokinesis. (*From Holmes.*[7] *Used with permission.*)

which is a disturbance in tapping out a definite rhythmic pattern; the two sides are then compared.[9]

DYSARTHRIA

Holmes described the speech pattern of patients with cerebellar disease as "slow, drawling, and monotonous, but at the same time [it] tends to be staccato and scanning."[1] The dysarthric speech of a patient with cerebellar disease typically has a sing-song character. Syllables can be explosive intermittently and at incorrect points of emphasis. This type of speech has also been described as having a nasal character. Production can be labored with excessive facial grimacing. Zentay described the speech by way of four components: (1) ataxic speech (interference of articulation, respiration, and phonation); (2) adiadochokinesis of speech (slowness of speech); (3) explosive-hesitant speech; and (4) scanning speech (stretching of the syllables, which are sharply cut off from one another).[10,11] Comprehension and grammar remain intact.

In the work by Amici et al., studying more than 250 patients with cerebellar tumors, the authors described the speech as "scanning and explosive against a background of monotony" (quoted from Lhermitte in 1958[4]). Brown et al. studied 30 patients with cerebellar ataxia without other neurological disturbances.[11] They analyzed the speech patterns of these patients and characterized ataxic dysarthria on the basis of 10 "deviant dimensions." Of the 10 dimensions, they discovered that excess and equal stress were prominent; that is, a prosodic disorder of speech in which magnified vocal emphasis is issued to normally unstressed words and syllables. The second dimension that was specific for cerebellar disease was irregular articulatory breakdown, which is recognized by sudden, intermittent telescoping (running together) of one or more syllables.

HYPOTONIA

Hypotonia is a decreased resistance to passive limb manipulation.[11,12] Limbs on the affected side show greater range of motion than normal when shaken passively; this tends to occur acutely after cerebellar injury and usually resolves within 1 week to 10 days. It is less apparent and less easy to detect in chronic cerebellar disease (Fig. 45-4).[7] Holmes defined tone as "the constant slight tension characteristic of healthy muscle, which offers a steadily maintained resistance to stretching." He also attributed to hypotonia the phenomenon of "rebound." This is tested clinically by asking the patient to maintain a limb in a fixed position. When the examiner displaces it with a brisk tap or shove, the normal limb returns quickly to its original position. In cerebellar disease, the displaced limb overshoots its original position, and may then continue to oscillate around that position, giving rise to a tremor, generally at a proximal joint. Such oscillations can also be precipitated by the jerk elicited by tapping the patellar tendon.

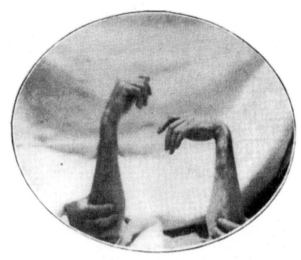

FIGURE 45-4 This is an extreme example of the hypotonia that can be seen following an acute cerebellar injury. In this case, the left cerebellar hemisphere has been injured, leading to the dramatic decrease in tone of the left wrist. (The photo was taken 1 week after the lesion occurred.) (*From Holmes.*[1] *Used with permission.*)

ABNORMALITIES OF EYE MOVEMENTS

Perhaps Miller made the most insightful statement concerning eye movements associated with cerebellar disease when he said, "many patients with cerebellar disease also have involvement of the brainstem as well. Thus, it is often unwarranted to attribute associated ocular motor abnormalities to cerebellar dysfunction."[13] This, for the majority of cases, seems to be intuitive. Mass lesions of the cerebellum usually compress the adjoining brainstem. The most commonly encountered lesions involving the cerebellum, such as those produced by stroke, multiple sclerosis, or the spinocerebellar degenerations, commonly affect the brainstem as well. Even so, years of clinical and experimental work have shown some ocular motor signs to be associated with cerebellar disease. These include: (1) different types of nystagmus, such as gaze-evoked, rebound, downbeat, or positional; (2) skew deviation; (3) saccadic dysmetria; (4) impairments in smooth pursuit, optokinetic nystagmus, or fixation suppression of caloric-induced nystagmus; (5) fixation abnormalities; (6) post-saccadic drift (glissades); and (7) increased gain in the vestibulo-ocular (VOR) reflex.[13]

GAIT ATAXIA

Patients with ataxia resulting from cerebellar disease walk with a wide base and tend to stagger, as if intoxicated. Their gait may be stiff-legged because of disturbed postural reflexes.[8] It has been described as "drunken reeling." Patients walk with their legs apart, trunk swaying, with a tendency to "veer" to one or the other side.[4] They generally fall to the side of the lesion when only one cerebellar hemisphere is affected.

Similar gait disorder can be seen with loss of tactile and/or proprioceptive sensation from the feet and legs. This can sometimes be distinguished from gait ataxia of cerebellar origin by Romberg's maneuver, in which the patient is asked to stand with feet together and eyes closed. Classically, the patient with sensory loss in the legs will be more unsteady with eyes closed, because of increased dependence on visual information; the patient with imbalance of cerebellar origin will be equally unsteady whether eyes are open or closed.

Gait ataxia can also arise from lesions in the frontal lobe and is known as Bruns' ataxia.[14] Before the invention of modern neuroimaging, neurosurgeons knew that if they did not find a lesion in the cerebellum during a suboccipital exploration, they would then have to look in the contralateral frontal lobe.[15,16]

LIMB ATAXIA/DECOMPOSITION OF MOVEMENT/ASYNERGIA

In cerebellar disease, limb movements, particularly those directed to a target, often have a jerky, irregular, wavering appearance different from the smooth, fluid character of normal movements. This is called limb ataxia. While limb ataxia is easy to recognize, it is difficult to say specifically what is wrong with the movements.

Holmes considered the problem to be "decomposition of movement," in which complex movements are broken down into their elemental components,[1] and performed serially, rather than simultaneously. Babinski[17] coined the term asynergia,[18] meaning the inability to orchestrate all the different movements necessary to accomplish an act smoothly.

Disrupted proprioceptive pathways cause ataxia. Disturbances can be either in the periphery in sensory nerves, sensory roots, in dorsal columns in the spinal cord, in the parietal cortex (Brodman areas 3, 1, 2, and 5), or in the occipital cortex.[14,19] This ataxia is known as sensory ataxia, and often it is indistinguishable from ataxia of cerebellar origin. The characteristics that delineate sensory ataxia from that resulting from cerebellar disease include absence of other cerebellar signs, such as nystagmus or dysarthria. With dorsal column involvement, vibratory and position sense are commonly impaired as well, leading to Romberg's sign. This sign is usually absent in cerebellar disease.[14]

Ataxias can be associated also with lesions of the internal capsule, and the middle and superior cerebellar peduncles (input and output pathways to and from the cerebellum, respectively). One theory as to why such diverse noncerebellar lesions cause symptoms virtually identical to those associated with direct cerebellar lesions is that these noncerebellar lesions still produce cerebellar dysfunction. Lesions of input systems, such as the frontopontocerebellar pathways in the internal capsule, the pontocerebellar fibers in the middle cerebellar peduncle, or the sensory system, result in failure to provide the cerebellum with information necessary for the normal successful programming of movement.[19]

IS THERE A COMMON FUNDAMENTAL UNDERLYING MECHANISM?

Some of the classical symptoms and signs of cerebellar dysfunction can be considered special cases of other, more fundamental symptoms and signs. For example, kinetic tremor can be considered a special case of dysmetria. Ataxia may be seen as a combination of kinetic tremor and dysmetria, particularly when it occurs in the context of walking or balance. The dysarthric speech could also be considered a form of dysmetria in which articulatory targets are under- or overshot, leading to abnormal intonations and inflections.

One argument that kinetic tremor is a special case of dysmetria is that it does not occur unless there is an initial error in the original movement. Subsequent correcting movements are dysmetric also, leading to another error requiring further correcting movements that also are dysmetric. These dysmetric correcting movements are most likely to occur towards the end of the movement. These oscillating movements at the end explain why kinetic tremor is sometimes described as terminal tremor. Vilis and Hore showed that monkeys whose dentate nucleus of the cerebellum is rendered inactive by cooling will not have tremor during movements unless there is an error. In the case of these experiments, error was introduced into the movements by injecting a brief resistance. In the normal monkey, such perturbations produced a rapid oscillation (or tremor) that dampened quickly. When the dentate nucleus was cooled, the tremor was slower and of much longer duration.[20]

It is possible that dysdiadochokinesia also may be a special case of dysmetria. In this case, the dysmetria of the component sequential movements may have an additive effect, thereby easily disrupting rapidly alternating movements. Alternatively, rapidly alternating movements may be physiologically distinct types of movements, thereby having their own unique pathophysiology.

It is possible that decomposition of movement is a learned response used to simplify the movement task. Breaking down complex synergistic movements reduces the degrees of freedom, thereby reducing the possibilities of error. This may be analogous to patients with ataxic gait who learn to walk with a wide-based gait to provide a better base of support, thereby reducing the risk of a fall.

It is unclear as to how dysmetria can explain static or positional tremor and nystagmus. It could be argued that maintenance of limb or eye position is an active process requiring continuous corrections. Dysmetria affecting these corrections could result in an inability to maintain position and errors in attempting to return to the intended position. These repetitive errors and corrections then lead to oscillation that appears as tremor and nystagmus. Clearly, dysmetria cannot explain hypotonia.

MECHANISMS OF DYSMETRIA

Dysmetria appears to be a fundamental abnormality associated with cerebellar dysfunction. Most of the symptoms and signs of cerebellar disease can be interpreted as special cases of dysmetria. The question now becomes: What is the nature of dysmetria? There are several possibilities that relate to abnormalities manifested through either the alpha motor system or the gamma motor system. The alpha motor system is that which drives the limb musculature directly. The gamma motor system may drive the musculature indirectly by first affecting the muscle spindle fibers. This changes the excitability of the muscle spindle which reflexively, through muscle spindle afferents, drives the alpha motor neurons.

Organization of the Cerebellum

MACROSCOPIC VIEW

Located in the posterior fossa, the cerebellum is a derivative of the metencephalon, or pons. It is attached to the dorsum of the pons by three sets of paired peduncles that transmit afferent and efferent signals. The cerebellum is separated from the cerebrum by the tentorium cerebelli. Grossly, the cerebellum is composed of the cortex (made up of folia), the internal white matter or medullary substance, four paired deep nuclei, and three paired peduncles. Folia represent a series of (mostly) transversely oriented cortical ridges or folds. When sectioned sagittally, the white matter of the cerebellum gives the appearance of tree-like branching, thus called the "arbor vitae" (tree of life). On the surface of the arbor vitae rests each folium (which is Latin for leaf).[21,22]

Anatomists have observed that the cerebellar cortex contains five deeper clefts than the folia, running in a transverse manner and separating the groups of folia into ten named lobules and three named lobes (Fig. 45-5). Two of the transverse clefts between lobules are especially deep, grouping the lobules into three lobes: anteriorly, the primary fissure separates the anterior from the posterior lobe, while, posteriorly, the posterolateral fissure separates the posterior lobe from the flocculonodular lobe. Two shallower clefts run anteroposteriorly on either side of the midline, separating all three lobes into the midline vermis (Latin for worm) and the lateral hemispheres. Numbering lobules from anterior to posterior, numbers I–V comprise the anterior lobe, numbers VI–IX comprise the posterior lobe, and the flocculonodular lobe consists of number X only. Most folia can be said to have a vermal (medial) and a hemispheral (lateral) part (e.g., the flocculonodular lobe consists of the midline nodulus and the paired lateral flocculi). In the vicinity of lobule IX, however, this classification breaks down (Fig. 45-5).

This division into lobes and lobules is based purely on gross morphology. The cerebellum can also be divided into four major divisions according to phylogeny and connectivity: (1) archicerebellum, (2) paleocerebellum, (3) spinocerebellum, (4) neocerebellum.

The archicerebellum is the flocculonodular lobe. Phylogenetically, it is the oldest division and is related to the

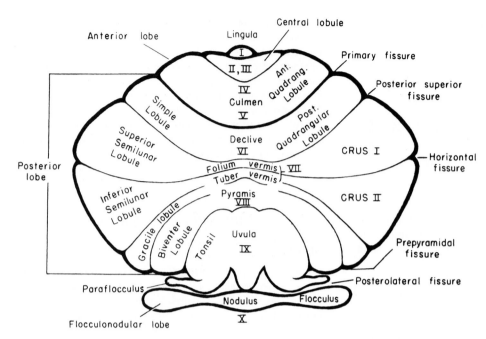

FIGURE 45-5 Classic neuroanatomic description of the fissures and lobules of the cerebellum. The anterior lobe, or paleocerebellum, is located rostral to the primary fissure. The posterior lobe, or neocerebellum, lies between the primary and posterolateral fissures. The flocculonodular lobe, or archicerebellum, lies caudal to the posterolateral fissure. Lobules are labeled with roman numerals. (*From Carpenter.*[22] *Used with permission.*)

vestibular system and to phylogenetically old types of eye movement, such as the VOR.

The paleocerebellum consists of the vermis and the medial part of the hemispheres (the "intermediate" zone). In humans, it is largely coextensive with the anterior lobe. The paleocerebellum is also called the spinocerebellum because it receives extensive afferents from ascending spinocerebellar pathways, carrying tactile and proprioceptive information and also information about the state of spinal interneuronal networks.

The spinocerebellum is conventionally supposed to be involved in the control of ongoing movement: the vermis with control of axial muscles, and the intermediate zone with control of the limbs. The vermis is also involved with control of phylogenetically newer types of eye movement such as saccades.

The neocerebellum, which is the largest and newest part of the cerebellum, is the most prominent in primates.[23] It occupies the most lateral part of the cerebellar hemispheres, mainly in the posterior lobe. It is phylogenetically the newest, being enormously enlarged in primates. It is often called the cerebrocerebellum because of its extensive connections with the cerebral hemispheres. It is conventionally supposed to play a role in higher-order planning of movements and perhaps even cognition.

The cells of the four paired deep cerebellar nuclei lie within the medullary substance of the cerebellum proper. From medial to lateral these nuclei are the fastigial, globose, emboliform, and dentate. The globose and emboliform nuclei are known collectively as the interpositus nucleus, with the emboliform situated more anteriorly than the globose. Output from cells of these nuclei is excitatory,

in contradistinction to the output of the cerebellar cortex via the Purkinje cells, which is entirely inhibitory.

AFFERENT CONNECTIONS TO THE CEREBELLUM

All afferent information that goes into the cerebellum, whether motor or sensory, courses through one of the three paired peduncles. Afferents to the cerebellum come from a wide range of sources at all levels of the nervous system: cerebral cortex, brainstem, and spinal cord. They are relayed in a variety of "precerebellar" nuclei located in the brainstem. From there, they pass through one of the three paired peduncles. Information then proceeds through the deep white medullary substance, ultimately to terminate in the cerebellar cortex. Collateral information is sent to deep cerebellar nuclei.

The inferior cerebellar peduncle carries ascending afferents from spinal cord and brainstem. It also carries a special class of afferents called climbing fibers originating in the inferior olive in the pons (see below). Climbing fibers relay descending afferents from cerebral cortex as well as ascending spinocerebellar afferents. Afferent connections to the cerebellum via the inferior peduncle include a relay to the fastigial nucleus from fibers of the vestibular nucleus. A structure known as the restiform body is entirely concerned with afferent information, whereas a juxtarestiform body contains both afferent and efferent information. In addition to fibers from the vestibular nucleus, fibers from the posterior spinocerebellar tract, accessory cuneate nucleus, olivocerebellar tract (from the contralateral inferior olive), and reticular formation in the brainstem are also relayed by way of the inferior peduncle to cerebellar cortex.[21,22,24]

The middle cerebellar peduncle carries afferents from cerebral cortex, relayed in the pontine nuclei. The primary projections from the cerebral cortex that form the corticopontocerebellar tracts include the premotor cortex and supplementary motor area (Brodman's area 6), the primary motor cortex (area 4), and the primary sensory cortex (areas 1, 2, and 3). It is of interest to note that the number of fibers involved in input from the cerebral cortex is on the order of 20 million, compared to that of the pyramidal tract, which is made up of only 1 million or so fibers.[23] In fact, the ratio of afferent to efferent connections is approximately 40:1 leading theorists to surmise that the cerebellum is involved with higher cognitive functions.[23,25,26]

The superior cerebellar peduncle carries mainly efferents, but also afferents from the ventral spinocerebellar tract.[21,22,24] As mentioned before, information from muscle spindles is transmitted to the cerebellum through spinocerebellar tracts. Vestibular end-organ information is also relayed, as is information from joint proprioreceptors.

EFFERENT CONNECTIONS FROM THE CEREBELLUM

The efferent output of the cerebellum goes by way of both the superior cerebellar peduncle and the fastigial nucleus fibers in the inferior peduncle. Almost all efferents from cerebellum originate in the deep cerebellar nuclei. These consist of the medial fastigial nucleus, the intermediate interpositus nucleus (composed of globose and emboliform nuclei), and the lateral dentate nucleus. Efferents from the vermis are relayed in the fastigial nucleus, efferents from the intermediate zone are relayed in the interpositus, and efferents from the cerebrocerebellum are relayed in the dentate. Efferents from the paleocerebellum, and from part of the vermis, are relayed in the vestibular nuclei.

Superior cerebellar peduncle fibers enter the brainstem and divide into an ascending and descending branch. Fibers in the ascending branch cross the midline in the tegmentum at the junction of the pons and midbrain and ascend to the contralateral red nucleus. Some fibers, predominantly from the interpositus nuclei, synapse on neurons in the magnocellular division of the red nucleus. Those from dentate synapse in parvocellular red nucleus, which projects, via inferior olive, back to the cerebellum.

Most of the fibers continue on to the thalamus, specifically to the ventral lateral pars caudalis and ventral posterolateral pars oralis nuclei, which project to the primary motor cortex (area 4). This fiber tract bundle is known as the dentatorubrothalamic tract, also called the brachium conjunctivum. The descending division of the superior cerebellar peduncle travels to the reticular nuclei and the inferior olive. Olivary fibers project back to the contralateral cerebellar cortex and nuclei.[21,22,24]

Classically, the interpositus has been thought of as a single nucleus, although it is anatomically divided into globose and emboliform nuclei (called anterior and posterior interpositus in nonprimate mammals). However, the two subdivisions of the interpositus are quite different in the source of some of their afferents and in the parts of cerebellar cortex with which they interconnect. Moreover, lesions of these two nuclei produce very different effects.[27] The fastigial efferent fibers are both crossed and uncrossed. The crossed fibers from the fastigial nucleus travel in the uncinate fasciculus, arching around the superior cerebellar peduncle, projecting bilaterally and symmetrically to both lateral and inferior vestibular nuclei, as well as to upper cervical cord motor neurons. A small number of fibers also ascend in the superior cerebellar peduncle to reach the ventral lateral and ventral posterolateral thalamus. Similarly, the uncrossed, smaller juxtarestiform body projects to the vestibular nuclei, as well as to lower brainstem structures.[21,22,24]

The modern concept of functional organization is quite different from the anatomic organization described above. The functional organization is divided into zones based on behavioral observation in ablation experiments[28–30] and anatomic connectivity (Fig. 45-6). This organization originated with Jansen and Brodal in 1940.[31] Their general concept stated

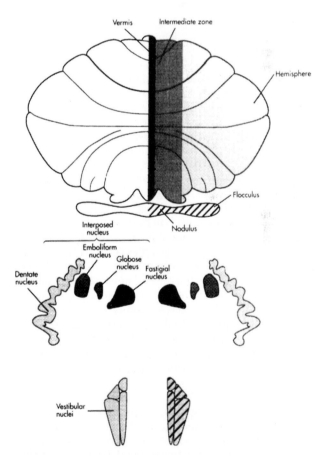

FIGURE 45-6 This shows that the cerebellar cortex is divided into three longitudinal zones with its subsequent projections to the four-paired cerebellar nuclei. (*From Nolte.*[21] *Used with permission.*)

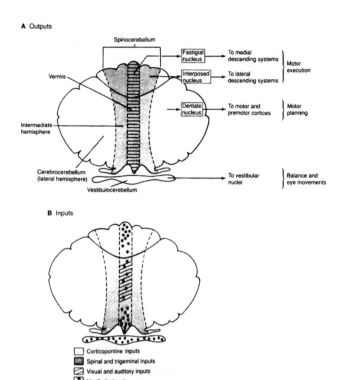

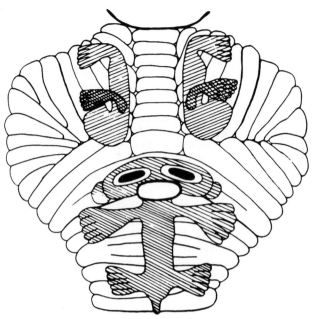

FIGURE 45-8 Homunculus of the cerebellum of the macaque. Note the two different representations of the somatotopic map, bilateral in paramedian lobules and ipsilateral in the anterior lobe. (*From Pearlman, et al: Neurological Pathophysiology, 3rd ed. New York: Oxford University Press, 1984. Used with permission.*)

FIGURE 45-7 Schematic representation of the outputs (*A*) and inputs (*B*) of the cerebellum. (*From Kandel et al.*[83] *Used with permission.*)

that the cerebellar cortex is anatomically organized into longitudinal corticonuclear zones.

The midline, or vermal, zone is made up of the cerebellar cortex of the vermis and the unpaired fastigial nucleus. The cerebellar cortex in this region projects primarily to the fastigial nuclei. This part of the cerebellum receives input primarily from the periphery, in contrast to the lateral zone, which receives very little input directly from the periphery. The outputs of the vermal zone project directly to brainstem structures or to the spinal cord, with very little going directly to the thalamus and cerebral cortex. The lateral cerebellum, in contrast, sends most of its output to the cerebral cortex via the thalamus.[22] The fastigial nucleus and its efferent target, the vestibular nuclei, are involved in limb extension to maintain posture. The human cerebellar stimulation and ablation studies of Nashold and Slaughter, in 1969, confirmed this. Nuchal and truncal postural mechanisms are under fastigial control as well[32] (Fig. 45-7).

The cerebellar cortex has a somatotopic arrangement, as well as a functional zone arrangement. A somatotopic organization has been described for cerebellar cortex (Fig. 45-8). There are actually two somatotopic maps, both with the body axis medial and the limbs lateral. One is in the anterior lobe with feet anterior and head posterior; the other is in the posterior lobe intermediate zone with head anterior and feet posterior. However, it does appear to be less discrete

and less acutely outlined than that of the cerebral cortex homunculus.[8]

The cerebellar homunculi delineated with surface recording and stimulation techniques are only a coarse representation of cerebellar somatotopic organization. Microelectrode recording from local groups of granule cells has revealed a fine grained organization of a very unusual kind. The granule cell layer is broken up into patches. Each patch receives sensory input from a particular portion of body surface. Adjacent patches receive input from nonadjacent portions of the body surface. The spatial arrangement of patches appears remarkably consistent from side to side and across individuals of a given species (Fig. 45-9).[33]

From numerous animal experiments, most notably those performed by Chambers and Sprague in 1955, the head and truncal regions occupy the vermis of the anterior lobe with the representation of the limbs extending into the paravermal zone.[29,30] Ablations of the vermal region in experimental animals produce abnormalities of gait and posture. In humans, lesions of this region most often produce gait and truncal ataxia without producing symptoms in the extremities during volitional movement. Consequently, the vermal region of the cerebellum is thought to be concerned primarily with modifying muscle tone, and controlling posture, locomotion, and whole-body equilibrium.

The lateral zone, made up of the dentate nucleus and its overlying cerebellar cortex, is involved with the coordination of ipsilateral somatic motor activity and preprogramming

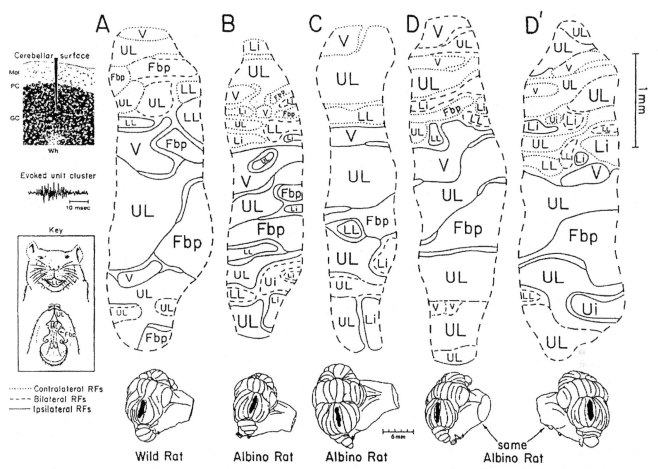

FIGURE 45-9 Cerebellar homunculi delineated with surface recording from local groups of granule cells revealing a fine grained organization broken up into patches. (*From Bower and Kassel.*[33] *Used with permission.*)

of learned volitional movements. The dentate is the largest cerebellar nucleus in man; it relays chiefly the efferent outflow from the lateral hemispheric area of the cerebellum, exerting its influence on tone and movement of ipsilateral limbs. Nashold and Slaughter, in 1969, showed that stimulation within the lateral interpositus nucleus or dentate nucleus results in facilitation of ipsilateral flexor tone.[32]

The paravermal zone comprises the interpositus nucleus and the overlying cerebellar cortex, which projects to the interpositus nucleus. The interpositus receives input from the motor cortex, as well as from the periphery. The interpositus nucleus projects to both the cerebral cortex and to the brainstem. Lesions of the interpositus in experimental animals cause postural defects in the ipsilateral limbs, as well as difficulties with locomotion and the righting postural response.[29] Animal experiments suggest that the interpositus nucleus and its efferent target, the red nucleus, are concerned more with flexor mechanisms.[29,34] Consequently, the paravermal zone of the cerebellum is thought to facilitate ipsilateral flexor muscle tone, via the rubrospinal tract.

Evarts and Thach, in 1969, stated that almost all of the cerebellar cortex receives at least some input from the cerebral cortex.[35] Somatotopic projections from sensory and motor areas of the cerebral cortex have been mapped to medial and intermediate zones of the cerebellar cortex. In the intermediate zone, both motor and sensory areas of the cerebral cortex project to the contralateral anterior lobe in the sagittal dimension as well, so that the head is oriented posteriorly, the legs are represented anteriorly, and the arms are in between[36] (Fig. 45-8). Even auditory and visual receiving areas project medially, overlapping the two head regions from cerebral cortex.

These different zones also differ in the timing of the neuronal activity changes associated with the generation of movement. Neurons in the dentate nucleus tend to become active before those of the motor cortex.[37] Neurons in the interpositus become active later, at approximately the same time as those of the motor cortex.[38] Neurons in the fastigial nucleus change activity latest and usually after the movement has been initiated.[39]

More recent research has revealed a finer-grained subdivision of the sagittal zones originally described by Jansen and Brodal.[31] The cerebellar cortex is divided into thin strips running approximately anterior to posterior. Starting at the midline these are designated A, B, C1, C2, C3, D1, and D2. A and B are in the vermis; C1-3 are in the intermediate zone, and D1-2 are in the lateral hemisphere. Each receives climbing fibers from a different, distinct part of the inferior olivary complex, and each projects to a different deep cerebellar nucleus. For example, area C2 receives climbing fibers from the rostral part of the medial accessory olive, while areas C1 and C3 receive climbing fibers from the rostral part of the dorsal accessory olive. C2 projects to the emboliform (posterior interpositus) nucleus, while C1 and C3 project to the globose (anterior interpositus).[40] Individual axons of inferior olivary neurons branch in the parasagittal plane to synapse at multiple different points along the same parasagittal strip.[41,42]

THE FLOCCULONODULAR LOBE

As previously mentioned, the flocculonodular lobe is phylogenetically the oldest, most primitive portion of the cerebellum and arises from the vestibular nuclei. As such, it retains direct afferent and efferent connections with the vestibular apparatus. The tract that carries such information is the juxtarestiform body. It conveys both afferent signals via direct and secondary vestibulocerebellar tracts and efferent signals via cerebellovestibular tracts. This vast amount of information comes and goes through the inferior cerebellar peduncle.

Lesions of the nodulus, flocculus, and uvula cause the flocculonodular syndrome. The hallmarks seen are poor equilibrium, during both standing and walking, nystagmus, and, sometimes, a rotated posture of the head.[8] Dow and Moruzzi stated that "when the body as a whole is at rest, individual movements, especially of the hand, can be carried out without evidence of locomotor disturbance; the heel-to-knee test can be performed without tremor, etc. Only when the body is propelled through space are difficulties encountered."[8] The basic mechanism of dysfunction is believed to result from the patient being unable to access vestibular information needed to coordinate movements of either the body or the eyes (see below).

MICROSCOPIC VIEW

To better understand how lesions in certain zones of the cerebellum produce the signs described above, it is essential to have a clear understanding of the circuitry involved, in both cerebellar cortical function and cerebrocerebellar and spinocerebellar loops. In contrast to cerebral cortex, where cytoarchitecture varies from region to region, the cellular organization of cerebellar cortex is extremely uniform. A single neuronal "circuit" is repeated throughout the cerebellum. Much of this has been described elegantly in the text by Eccles et al.[43] A brief description is given here.

CEREBELLAR CORTEX CIRCUITRY

The cerebellar cortex is divided into three layers (Fig. 45-10). From the outside towards the medullary white matter, these layers are the molecular, Purkinje, and granular layers. These cortical layers contain five types of neurons. The molecular layer contains stellate and basket cells. The Purkinje layer contains Purkinje cells. The granule layer contains granule and Golgi type II cells. The focal point of the cerebellar cortex is the Purkinje cell, from which the entire output of the cerebellar cortex originates.[44] As noted above, this output is almost entirely to the deep cerebellar nuclei, the exception being a small component from the flocculonodular lobe, which projects to the vestibular nuclei. The following discussion will focus on the relationship of the other neuron types to the Purkinje cell.

Purkinje cells receive input from two sources of fibers, mossy and climbing, both of which exert excitatory action. The climbing fibers originate from the inferior olivary complex and make monosynaptic connections with Purkinje cells. Each Purkinje cell receives afferent information from a single climbing fiber, but multiple synaptic connections are made. This is perhaps one of the strongest excitatory synapses found in the central nervous system. Mossy fibers are the primary afferent input into the cerebellar cortex, originating from spinocerebellar, pontocerebellar, and vestibulocerebellar systems.

Mossy fibers originate from spinocerebellar, pontocerebellar, and vestibulocerebellar systems. Mossy fibers do not make direct synapses on Purkinje cells but rather synapse on granule and Golgi cells. The cell bodies of the granule cells are located in the granular layer, whereas their axons ascend through the Purkinje layer to the molecular layer, where they bifurcate into parallel fibers, so named because these axons run parallel to each other and to the long axis of the folia. These axons run for 1–2 mm in both directions, synapsing on Purkinje cells. Each parallel fiber will make synaptic connection with thousands of Purkinje cells, but only a few synapses will be made with each individual Purkinje cell (in contrast to the climbing fibers). Each Purkinje cell, in turn, receives synapses from thousands of parallel axons.

Granule cells also send processes to stellate and basket cells, located in the molecular layer, as well as to those parts of the Golgi II neuron dendrites that penetrate the molecular layer. The postsynaptic action of granule cells, and thus of parallel fibers, is excitatory, although it is not as strong as that exhibited by climbing fibers.

When parallel fibers were first discovered, it was found that electrical stimulation activated a transverse "beam" of parallel fibers, which in turn excited a beam of Purkinje cells. For decades, physiologists were captivated by the concept of a parallel fiber beam, until Brown and Bower[45] pointed out that the ascending axon of the granule cell exerts a much stronger influence over Purkinje cell firing than parallel fibers do. Purkinje cell activity (and therefore cerebellar output) is thus dominated by the activity of adjacent granule cells, and

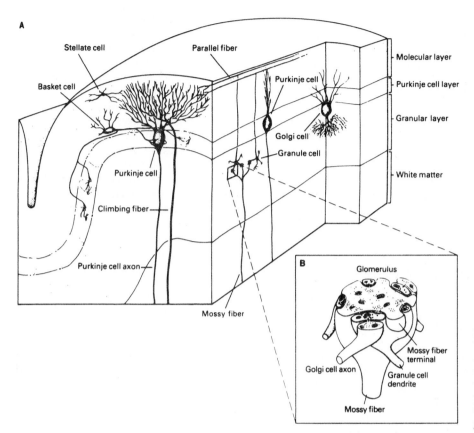

FIGURE 45-10 Diagram of the three layers of the cerebellar cortex. *A.* This shows the transverse and longitudinal planes of a single cerebellar folium, with the five types of neurons. *B.* Detailed drawing of a glomerulus, a clear space in the granular layer where terminals of mossy fibers synapse with Golgi cell axons and granule cell axons. (*From Kandel et al.*[83] *Used with permission.*)

only weakly influenced[46] by granule cells further out along the beam.[47]

The parallel fiber-Purkinje cell synapse is subject to a form of plasticity called "long-term depression." This occurs when excitation at a parallel fiber synapse is quickly followed by excitation of the same Purkinje cell by a climbing fiber. When this happens, the strength of that particular parallel fiber-Purkinje cell synapse is weakened. The climbing fiber thus represents a "teaching input." It has been postulated that climbing fiber activity is an "error signal" and that long-term depression results in selective weakening of synaptic inputs correlated with (and therefore presumably contributing to) erroneous behavior or inaccurate movement. Extensive evidence has been adduced for this mechanism in one particular case (gain adaptation in the VOR).[48]

As mentioned earlier, parallel fibers also synapse on stellate and basket cells. Some authors define these as the outer and inner stellate cells, respectively. These are cerebellar cortical interneurons located in the molecular layer. Both cells produce inhibitory input to the Purkinje cell, although basket cell inhibition is much stronger, owing to its synapse directly onto the Purkinje cell body. The stellate cells, on the other hand, send their axons to synapse on the distal dendrites of the Purkinje cell.

The last type of neuron is the Golgi neuron, located in the granule cell layer. It receives excitatory synapses both from granule cells and parallel fibers; it makes inhibitory synapses on granule cells. In fact, it synapses on the synapse between mossy fibers and granule cells, forming a complex called a glomerulus (Fig. 45-10B). Golgi cells also receive inhibitory synapses from recurrent collaterals of Purkinje cell axons.

The Golgi cell's main mode of action is the inhibition of up to 10,000 granule cells.[49] In addition to the two "classical" afferents (mossy fibers and climbing fibers), cerebellar cortex also receives serotonergic fibers from the raphe nuclei and noradrenergic fibers from locus ceruleus.[50] These terminate in a diffuse fashion in all three layers of cerebellar cortex, and historically have been ignored in theories of cerebellar physiology and pathophysiology. However, a recent report suggests that abnormal noradrenergic innervation of cerebellum may play a role in essential tremor, so it may no longer be possible to ignore these afferents.[51]

As mentioned previously, the entire output from the cerebellar cortex is via the Purkinje cell discharges.[44] They exert inhibitory synaptic action on their target neurons, the deep cerebellar nuclei. Eccles calls this sculpturing, in that the cerebellar nuclei also receive constant excitatory discharges from axon collaterals of mossy and climbing fibers.[52] Thus the cerebellar nuclei, which are in a state of background excitation from mossy and climbing collateral input, are subjected to changing inhibitory input from the cerebellar cortex via Purkinje cells.

Cerebellar Syndromes

Are there clear definable syndromes related to differences in anatomy and physiology? How do the basic mechanisms described above produce these syndromes when applied to specific regions of the cerebellum? What is the relation to the input and output connections of the cerebellum?

The concept of cerebellar syndromes has been classified in a variety of ways. Some authors have discussed it both based on classic anatomy and on the basis of functional zones, as described earlier. There is considerable overlap, because some of the descriptions ascribed to the lobe approach of classical anatomy correlate with the modern longitudinal organizations based on zones. For example, much of the anterior lobe of the cerebellum corresponds to the paravermal zone. Therefore, descriptions of symptoms and signs previously ascribed to the paleocerebellar syndromes are very similar to those described with lesions of the paravermal zone. In addition, much of the neocerebellum is correlated with the lateral zone. Descriptions of the neocerebellar syndromes then share significant similarities to the lesions of the lateral zone. With time, there should be less reference to paleo-, neo-, and archicerebellar syndromes, which will be replaced by vermal, paravermal, and lateral syndromes.

Much of what is known about the cerebellar syndromes stems from animal ablation studies, begun by Luciani in 1891, when he studied the effects in dogs.[12,18] Chambers and Sprague helped to define the concept of functional zones in their ablation studies in cats.[29,30] Other authors have added important data in primate studies.[8,28,53]

The effects in man were analyzed with great insight by the work of Holmes, who described the signs and symptoms in soldiers who suffered gunshot and shrapnel wounds (mostly to the lateral cerebellum) in World War I.[1,7] Later, effects of surgical manipulation were noted.[32] The accumulated evidence amassed from these and other studies allows for the categorization of cerebellar syndromes.

VERMAL SYNDROME

The midline of the cerebellum, consisting of the vermis of the cortex and fastigial nucleus, regulates posture, locomotion, tone, and equilibrium of the entire body.[29,30] An ataxic, titubating gait (a stumbling, staggering gait with shaking of the head and trunk), oscillations of the head and neck, and frequent falling have been observed in ablation studies in primates.[8] No tremor of the limbs and no change in reflexes or tone are seen. This part of the cerebellum is relatively independent from the rest of the cerebrum, lacking substantial cerebral cortical input.[35] However, it does have close connections with the vestibular system, both sensory and motor components. Thus, it is involved in the automatic regulation of whole body position (i.e., posture).[54] It has been called "a closed-loop system that regulates the segmental reflexes important in postural fixation or truncal movement."[2]

This section of the cerebellum is involved in phasic eye and head movements as well. In addition to the ocular motor aberrancies produced with lesions in this area, humans with lesions of the cerebellar vermis will tend to have a wide-based, ataxic gait, reeling and staggering as if drunk. When the lesion is in one cerebellar hemisphere, patients may tend to fall to the side of the lesion, but this is secondary to defective control of the affected leg, not weakness.

Balance in hemispheric (lateral) lesions is often surprisingly well maintained in distinction to vermal lesions. Victor et al., in 1959, showed a clinical correlation with the somatotopic map namely, that the marked and disproportionate gait disturbance in alcoholic cerebellar degeneration is related to the earliest and most marked degeneration in the most anterior folia of the vermis, associated with control of the lower extremities.[57] In this condition, marked ataxia during standing and ambulation is observed, as well as dysmetric heel-to-shin maneuver of the legs. The arms are relatively spared, however. Patients walk with a staggering, wide-based gait. Some authors believe that gait ataxia is the only sign that can be ascribed to anterior lobe lesions in man, but that, in order to use gait ataxia as a sign indicating involvement of the anterior vermis, there must be few or no signs of involvement of the posterior vermis or neocerebellum.[3] Lesions restricted to the neocerebellum produce no equilibrium disturbances or primary gait ataxia. Dow and Moruzzi pointed out that, with the patient lying in bed, the movement abnormalities so easily seen during ambulation could not be appreciated with volitional movements of the lower extremities.[8]

Another interesting phenomenon that has been described is the evanescent character of some cerebellar signs. Isolated unilateral lesions in the fastigial nucleus of the monkey produced equilibrium disturbances with a staggering gait and falling to the side of the lesion, whereas bilateral lesions produced the same but more pronounced errors in coordination of gait and in equilibrium.[8] However, these lasted only briefly and became attenuated and subsequently resolved in as little as 2 weeks. In regard to human clinical relevance, this "extraordinary capacity for compensation" may be the reason why isolated lesions restricted to cerebellar parenchyma that are slow growing, such as some tumors, can become quite substantial in size before any deficit in cerebellar function is appreciated.[8]

PARAVERMAL AND LATERAL ZONE SYNDROME

There do not seem to be discrete intermediate and lateral cerebellar syndromes in humans, because of the unlikelihood of lesions restricted to only one or the other area. Patients with lateral cerebellar lesions (generally also involving the intermediate cerebellum) have severe inaccuracy of limb movements, such as when reaching to grasp an object. Lesions are manifested by the signs of dysmetria, tremor, dysdiadochokinesia, hypotonia, and decomposition of movement (see below). Lesions restricted to the lateral cerebellum in humans produce no equilibrium or balance disturbances or primary gait disorders.

The intermediate portion of the cerebellum is believed to regulate the spatially organized and skilled movements of ipsilateral limbs, according to the ablation experiments done in cats by Chambers and Sprague,[29,30] and the reversible inactivation experiments of Martin et al.[27] and Brodal et al.[6] Recent studies of movement-related mossy fiber discharges in nonhuman primates reveal that the intermediate cerebellum receives information regarding velocity, position, and direction of movement from individual forelimb muscles. In turn, these interpositus neurons incorporate this information and help coordinate movement of the whole limb, with an emphasis on hand and finger joint manipulation.[58] In animal ablation studies, lesions in the lateral zone or neocerebellum produce no lasting changes in postural tone or in deep tendon reflexes.[29,30] Tremor was mainly attributed to dentate nucleus lesioning. Dentate lesions appear to have very little effect on simple one-joint movements, but severe ataxia of multijoint movements.[59]

ABNORMAL EYE MOVEMENTS

Before describing the eye findings in cerebellar disease, definitions of different types of eye movements will be provided to serve as a basis for the discussion. Nystagmus is a rhythmic back-and-forth oscillation of the eyes. Pendular nystagmus has smooth, equal velocity in both directions of gaze, whereas a slow drift, followed by a quick corrective phase in the opposite direction characterizes jerk nystagmus. Saccades are rapid eye movements, bringing the fovea to bear almost immediately on the target. They quickly change visual fixation. Pursuit refers to slow eye movements. Convergence refers to slow movements that bring both eyes onto a close target. The VOR is visual when eye deviation or nystagmus occurs in response to vestibular system stimulation by caloric testing (irrigation of the ears with either warm or cold water) or by angular acceleration or deceleration. (Caloric stimulation with cold water causes nystagmus with the fast component to the opposite side, whereas warm water produces nystagmus with the fast component to the same side in a normally functioning brain.)

In regard to nystagmus, the first report to document ocular motor abnormalities was published in 1973, when Westheimer and Blair described findings in monkeys after total cerebellectomy.[60] These included defects in holding eccentric positions of gaze, smooth pursuit, convergence, and optokinetic nystagmus. It was reported soon thereafter that hemicerebellectomy produced the same defects on the ipsilateral side of the lesion.[60,61] A persistent saccadic dysmetria is also seen after complete cerebellectomy in the monkey.[62] Their report and others revealed that the dorsal cerebellar vermis, paravermis, and fastigial nuclei are necessary for

proper placement of saccades.[63] These lesions of the cerebellar vermis also tend to affect the magnitude of ipsilateral saccades.[64] Selhorst et al., in 1976, revealed similar findings in humans with cerebellar lesions and reported that lesions of the dorsal vermis and underlying fastigial nucleus lead to abnormally large saccades or hypermetria of saccades.[65,66] It is postulated that the cerebellar vermis acts as a calibrator organ by constantly adjusting the gain of the direct visual motor pathway without actually being in the direct loop. With a cerebellar lesion (vermian lesion), this control is lost, and the gain subsequently increases, leading to overshoot of saccades or dysmetria of saccades. In fact, the authors propose that "saccadic overshoot dysmetria is a specific ocular motor sign occurring only in patients with cerebellar disease."[65]

Lesions of the deep cerebellar nuclei have been shown to cause saccadic oscillations, defined as horizontal clusters of saccades that reverberate about the intended fixation point and take the fovea off the target.[66] At the bedside, patients will often report a blurring of vision attempting to fixate on the intended target because of inability to keep the visual image on the fovea. Another proposed function, then, of this part of the cerebellum is to provide long-term adaptation functions that correlate eye movements correctly to the visual stimulus or target, thereby correcting for ocular motor dysmetria and ensuring accuracy of saccades.[13]

In addition to the vermis and fastigial nuclei, the flocculus and paraflocculus are important in coordinating eye movement. Ablation studies of this part of the cerebellum in monkeys has led to impaired smooth pursuit, whether the head is still or moving.[67] Furthermore, rebound nystagmus, downbeat nystagmus, and horizontal gaze-evoked nystagmus were shown to result from such ablations. These observations are evidence that the flocculus is important in preventing retinal slip and in stabilizing gaze holding.[64] The flocculus has also been implicated in the control of VOR gain (see below).

Kornhuber, in 1973, categorized the eye findings in cerebellar pathology differently.[68] He dichotomized the aberrant eye movements on the basis of cortical versus nuclear disease. With lesions of the vermis near the primary fissure, he found that dysmetria of saccadic eye movements usually occurred, with preservation of smooth pursuit. The dysmetria was usually of the hypometric form, in which the patient initiated eye movement in the correct direction but failed to reach the target, resulting in many smaller saccades, rather than in one single large movement.

Thus, the cerebellum plays an integral role in maintaining both adequate visual fixation and stabilization during eye movements. Saccadic overshoot dysmetria is considered consistent with a lesion in the vermis, whereas retinal slip is found with flocculus lesions. Other categories of nystagmus are not as specific, owing to the degree of complexity and integration of the structures involved. Only one type of nystagmus, saccadic overshoot dysmetria, appears to be specific to the cerebellum.

DYSARTHRIA

Speech disturbances are most often seen in patients with bilateral or diffuse cerebellar lesions. Some studies have shown pathologically that the midportion of the vermis and adjacent paravermian regions are likely to produce such dysfuction.[3,57] In contrast, Dow and Moruzzi localized cerebellar dysarthria to the lateral zones.[8] This was also the finding of Amici et al., who found that the cerebellar dysarthric pattern was more common in lesions of the lateral and intermediate cerebellar zones in their group of approximately 250 patients.[4] In agreement with this, Lechtenberg and Gilman found a correlation between dysarthria and focal left cerebellar hemisphere disease; in fact, 22 of 31 patients with dysarthria had mainly or exclusively left cerebellar hemisphere disease, whereas only 2 patients had vermal disease.[69] This report is not as clear-cut as it seems, however, because of the patient population studied. Most of the lesions were tumors, producing mass effect and most likely affecting other nearby structures. Possibly, the contralateral connections with the nondominant right cerebral hemisphere help to explain the qualities of cerebellar speech.

Grammar, per se, is not affected in cerebellar speech disorders. Rather, prosody and intonation are affected. It has been proposed that the right hemisphere is concerned with the perception of harmony and melody.[70] This holds true, except for professional musicians.[71] This might explain why predominantly left cerebellar hemisphere lesions are involved in dysarthric speech. Certainly, more work needs to be done to better elucidate the anatomic substrate for cerebellar dysarthria.

Theories of Cerebellar Function

As the preceding sections show, we possess a vast amount of detailed information about the cerebellum, its structure, its connectivity, and the effects of injuring it. At the same time, we do not know its function. This paradox has lead most researchers who have studied the cerebellum to propose general theories of cerebellar function. As a result, there are many such theories. Some have fallen by the wayside and been abandoned, while others have accumulated evidence and attracted supporters. None has approached universal acceptance, however. In this section, we present theories that have achieved a high degree of currency and which in our judgment show promise of containing at least a part of the truth.

We group these theories into six categories: (1) theories that emphasize the role of the cerebellum in controlling timing of movement components, (2) theories that emphasize gamma motor efferents, (3) theories that view the cerebellum essentially from an engineering point of view, emphasizing concepts from control systems theory (feedforward and feedback) and mechanical engineering (control of interjoint interactions), (4) theories that emphasize the role of the cerebellum in learning and behavioral plasticity, (5) theories

that relate the cerebellum to generation and estimation of time intervals, and (6) theories that challenge the traditional view of the cerebellum as concerned primarily with movement.

THEORIES INVOLVING THE TIMING OF MOVEMENT COMPONENTS

Normal movement requires the precise control of muscles that facilitate the movement (agonist muscles) and of those that oppose the movement (antagonist muscles). The precise control of these muscles includes which muscles are affected and the timing of those effects.

The control mechanisms are complex. For example, the antagonist muscles that oppose the intended movement are often activated during movement. Although this seems counterintuitive, activation of the antagonist muscles is necessary to brake the movement so that it does not overshoot. An abnormality in muscle selection and timing of activation leads to abnormal movements. Actual movements have separate components, each of which has to be precisely controlled. Mechanisms that initiate a movement are separate from those that control the final trajectory of the movement.[72]

Even at a single joint, there is a complex pattern of activation. Rapid single-joint movements are associated with a triphasic pattern of muscle activation. There is an initial agonist burst of electromyographic (EMG) activity, followed by an agonist pause during which there is a burst of EMG activity in the antagonist muscle. This is then followed by a third burst of EMG activity, this time occurring in the agonist. The first burst of EMG activity is thought to control movement initiation and is used to overcome the initial inertial load that would resist movement. The second burst, occurring in the antagonist muscle, acts as a brake on the inertia so that the movement does not overshoot. The function of the third and final agonist burst is less clear, but probably prevents the limb from oscillating about its final position.[73]

EMG studies in nonhuman primates suggest an explanation for cerebellar dysmetria. Lateral cerebellar lesions (affecting the lateral cerebellar hemisphere and/or the dentate nucleus) prolonged the agonist burst and delayed the antagonist burst.[74] The disorder in acceleration showed agonist EMG activity that was less abrupt in onset, smaller in magnitude, and longer in duration. EMG studies in humans with cerebellar disease, compared to those with normal subjects, confirmed the observation.[75–77]

Dysdiadochokinesia has been studied with similar techniques. Normally, during rapid alternating movements, the antagonistic activity decreases during the 50 ms or so before the initiation of biceps activity, and it always ends before that point.[77] The clinical sign of rebound may be a result of failure to reduce activity in the tonically active agonist muscle.

Hallett et al. concluded that the cerebellum plays a role in the organization of the relationship between agonists and antagonists in successive movements.[75] The distortion of the initial part of the motor pattern was a consistent finding in their EMG analysis. They surmised, then, that the deficit must be in the supraspinal segment, even before the program reaching the anterior horn cells. This is consistent with the view that the cerebellum normally contributes to the generation of the agonist burst that initiates learned movements.

Studies such as these, which examine laboratory examples of single-joint, single degree-of-freedom movements, must be interpreted with caution, however, when applied to limb movements in ordinary life, which typically involve multiple joints. Holmes noted that the latter type of movement is much more impaired by cerebellar lesions than the former.[1,7]

This concept of inappropriate timing of EMG bursts can be used to help explain the sign of dysdiadochokinesia, because it is an inability of the patient to time the onset and offset of agonist and antagonist muscles accurately. Tremor is likewise related, if it is postulated that the intention tremor seen in cerebellar disease involves an error in this braking system. Because the patient is unable to predict when braking should be initiated, the patient depends on external cues, or afferent input, in order to engage the antagonist. This explains the worsening seen as the target is approached, and it can be postulated to be a result of the patient trying to correct the movement by relying on external cues. The complexity of motor programs generated in the cerebellum may vary according to the complexity of the intended movement. For example, a complex movement may be made up of a learned sequence of simpler movements. Robertson and Grimm, in 1975, in their studies of dentate recordings in monkeys, showed that some dentate neurons fire before movement that involves a sequenced (not just a simple) response.[78] This suggests that the cerebellum may be involved in planning the whole sequence beforehand, prior to movement initiation.

Human subjects with moderate cerebellar deficiency were tested, along with controls, in executing a single-, two-, or three-keypress command in a certain sequence.[79] In patients with cerebellar disease there were negligible or no effects of sequence length on response time, whereas normal control subjects showed the expected increase in response onset time with an increase in sequence length. This observation suggests that patients with cerebellar disease are slow in their reaction times and cannot modify those times according to the complexity of the required task. A breakdown of the sequence into functional independent elements was also noted, correlating with Holmes' "decomposition of movement."[1,7] The authors concluded that the translation of a programmed sequence of responses into action involves cerebellar structures that schedule a sequence of ordered responses before movement onset. These results offered evidence for the theory that cerebellar integrity is critical for timing of the elements of a complex movement.

CEREBELLAR EFFECTS ON THE GAMMA MOTOR SYSTEM

The descriptions above clearly demonstrate that the timing and patterns of muscle activity are abnormal in patients with cerebellar pathology. Because the muscles are driven directly by alpha motor neurons, the activities of these neurons must also be abnormal in cerebellar disease. The question then becomes: Is the abnormality of the alpha motor system a direct or indirect consequence of cerebellar disease? The links from the cerebellum through the motor cortex to the alpha motor system at least provide a pathway for a direct effect of the cerebellum on the alpha motor system. However, what is anatomically possible may not be physiologically relevant.

The gamma motor system has an effect on the alpha motor system through a reflex mechanism involving the muscle spindles. If the cerebellum were to have an effect on the gamma motor system that affects the function of the muscle spindles, it could be another means by which the cerebellum affects movement. To this extent, it has been theorized that this association extends to the skeletal muscle level, involving alpha-gamma co-activation (i.e., the process that acts to maintain muscle spindle sensitivity during muscle contraction). This produces appropriate tone and, hence, hypothetically, smooth and coordinated movements. Thus, the cerebellum acts as the "head ganglion of the proprioceptive system," as Sherrington stated earlier in this century.[80]

To better understand how the cerebellum can influence muscle tone via its effects on the gamma motor system, it is necessary first to summarize the basic structures of skeletal muscle involved. The two types of nerve fibers that innervate skeletal muscle are the alpha motor neurons and the gamma motor neurons, both arising from the anterior horn cells in the spinal cord. The alpha motor neurons are fibers large in diameter (9–20 μm) that innervate extrafusal muscle fibers and which produce muscle tension, contraction, and movement. Gamma motor neurons average 5 μm in diameter and innervate the small, specialized intrafusal muscle fibers, which are contained within muscle spindles, constituting approximately 30 percent of the motor nerve fibers.[81] (For a more in-depth review, see the work of Granit[82] and Kandel et al.[83])

Two receptors in skeletal muscle exist that are necessary for motor control. Muscle spindles respond to stretch and signal changes in muscle length. The sensory input from the spindles is used by the brain to determine the relative attitudes (positions) of the limb portion in question. This system is extremely sensitive to very small changes in length and may be used by the brain to compensate and to correct for disturbances in movement. This sensitivity of Ia afferent discharge (from the muscle spindles) to small changes in velocity relies upon the co-activation of alpha-gamma motor neurons.[84] According to Granit, this co-activation may be important, because the responses by the spinal cord to changes of muscle length are made more symmetrical by the summed action of muscle spindles and extrafusal fibers.

The intrafusal fibers are specialized muscle fibers that make up part of the muscle spindle. Gamma motor neurons innervate the contractile polar regions of these fibers. The gamma motor neurons that innervate the muscle spindles are also known as the fusimotor system. Gamma motor neurons regulate and modulate spindle afferent discharge according to the following scheme: activation of a gamma efferent leads to shortening and contraction of the polar regions of the intrafusal fibers. This stretches the noncontractile region, leading to increased sensitivity and firing of the sensory endings.[81–83]

To better understand how the cerebellum relates to muscle tone, one must understand the ascending and descending pathways that affect the gamma motor system. Information from muscle spindles from the legs and trunk is transmitted via the dorsal spinocerebellar tract, keeping the cerebellum updated regarding evolving movement in terms of tension, position, force, and rate of movement. The cuneocerebellar tract subserves the upper extremity in the same manner. These tracts enter the cerebellum through the inferior cerebellar peduncle, ending on the same side as their origin. The ventral spinocerebellar tract, however, conveys different information. These tracts are mainly concerned with the information from segmental interneurons, that synthesize input from the periphery with descending commands through the corticospinal and rubrospinal tracts.[84] These tracts enter the cerebellum through the superior cerebellar peduncle, terminating mostly in the ipsilateral medial and intermediate zones. The function of this pathway is to keep the cerebellum updated regarding the ongoing execution of movement and regulation of muscle tone.

Gilman, in 1969, showed that cerebellar ablation (specifically of the interpositus and fastigial nucleus) in the monkey led to hypotonia, defined as decreased resistance to passive limb manipulation.[84] By deactivating cerebellar influence, stretch responses of muscle spindle afferents are decreased, possibly by decreasing the tonic facilitation of fusimotor activity. This decrease of spindle primary afferent input would then be expected to affect homonymous alpha motor neurons, in turn decreasing their facilitatory drive, and hence leading to a decrease of tonic extrafusal motor activity. He proposed that this might be the cause of cerebellar dysmetria. In summary, he concluded that a decrease in fusimotor activity, leading to abnormalities in muscle spindle function, is an important factor in the pathogenesis of cerebellar hypotonia.[84]

IS IT ALPHA OR GAMMA?

More recent data conflict somewhat with Gilman's hypothesis, however. Experiments in deafferentated primates abolish the influence of the gamma motor system. Liu and Chambers, in 1971, demonstrated that monkeys with lesioned cerebellar nuclei and deafferentated by dorsal rhizotomy showed marked cerebellar ataxia, in contradistinction to those monkeys that were deafferentated only.[85] Gilman et al., in 1976, found that cerebellar ablation in deafferentated monkeys resulted in a worse motor performance.[86] This led Flament and Hore, in 1986, to suggest that cerebellar movement deficits are a result of disordered central commands rather than primarily of the influence of the gamma motor

system.[74] Holmes himself postulated that hypermetria was related to decreased tone of the antagonist,[1,7] whereas other authors showed that, instead of decreased tone, prolonged, or delayed, antagonistic tone during movements accounted for the dysmetria.[74,77] Thus, the theory that dysmetria is caused by decreased fusimotor activity to antagonist muscle does not explain the disorders seen involving the antagonistic muscles in these studies.[84]

FEEDFORWARD, FEEDBACK, AND COORDINATION

The task of the nervous system in controlling movement is complicated by the mechanical complexity of the body part being moved. For example, a human arm exclusive of the fingers has three joints moving on seven axes, controlled by well over 20 muscles. A key concept in managing such complexity is coordination. For example, the large number of muscles contributing to a movement may be reduced to a smaller, more manageable number of elements to be controlled by grouping the muscles into synergies. It has been proposed that the cerebellum creates synergies appropriate to a given movement by imposing a coordinated pattern of activity on a group of muscles.

Coordination is also fundamental to the control of multijoint limbs because of the phenomenon of interjoint inertial interactions. This means that, as one joint moves, it may generate forces at another joint, which may help or hinder intended movements at that joint. Accurate movement thus requires coordinating muscle contraction in one part of the body with movement at another part. Studies of multijoint limb movements by patients with cerebellar disease suggest that lack of coordination between different joints of a limb contributes to clinical ataxia in those patients.[87] In engineering terms, the nervous system is a control system, and the body part is the physical plant. Engineering techniques are available by which a control system can cope with mechanical complexity in the physical plant. Some theories of cerebellar function propose that it implements such techniques.

One technique is feedforward control. With this technique, the nervous system "plans ahead," taking into account the mechanical properties of the plant to program a pattern of muscle contractions that will produce the desired movement. Evarts and Thach, in 1969, postulated that this indeed was the case, that the lateral part of the cerebellum influenced motor output by means of a feedforward mechanism.[35] Allen and Tsukahara theorize that the dentate is well suited for the preprogramming of movements.[54] This requires that plant properties such as inertial interactions be represented within the nervous system as "plant model." Some authors have found that interjoint inertial interactions are not appropriately compensated for in patients with cerebellar ataxia.[87,88] Ito proposed that the cerebellum, through a process of learning, comes to provide a model of the peripheral plant as well as the external world with which it interacts.[89] Others have constructed computer models of limb control in which the cerebellum plays the role of a plant model.[90]

Another technique is feedback control in which movements are continually monitored, by tactile, proprioceptive, or visual receptors, and errors are detected during movement execution. Corrections are then generated "on-line" or "in-flight" as the movement unfolds. With this technique, the nervous system can ignore some of the plant's complexity in planning movements; errors resulting from this simplified view will be corrected during the movement. Eccles et al. suggested that the cerebellum performs this function.[91] Some authors have suggested that the cerebellum serves this function either by adjusting the gain of spinal reflexes or by directly comparing actual to intended movement.[92,93]

Feedback need not originate outside the nervous system. The cerebellum may receive a copy ("efference copy") of output from other parts of the brain involved in controlling movement. For example, spinocerebellar pathways projecting to cerebellum reflect the activity in spinal interneuronal networks, which the cerebellum, in turn, can influence through its various direct and indirect descending projections.[94] Likewise, the cerebellum both receives information from cerebral cortex via the pontine nuclei, and projects to cerebral cortex via thalamus.

An intermediate sort of control has been proposed for the cerebellum on the basis of experiments in which a maintained posture is subjected to a perturbation whose timing is unpredictable. Compensation for the perturbation is necessarily by feedback control, and typically accomplished by short-latency reflexes. However, when information is available in advance about the character of the perturbation (e.g., direction or duration), the reflex response is "set" appropriately to the type of perturbation. Some authors have found that this predictive "set" is impaired by lesions of the cerebellum.[95,96]

LEARNING- AND PLASTICITY-BASED THEORIES

Whether learning or plasticity is central to the function of the cerebellum has been debated for the past 20 years. Recent studies on cerebellar learning has lead to another possible mechanism by which the cerebellum organizes the precise spatial and temporal actions of muscles for smooth and complex movements. In this case, sensory feedback is utilized in learning-coordinated movements by shaping the patterns of responses presumably in the mossy fibers.[97] Thus, when appropriate sensory cues are encountered, the cerebellum responses with the appropriate patterns and timings of muscle responses. Errors encountered during execution result in further learning to correct the responses. This theory builds on the observations of the role of the cerebellum in classical conditioning. A more detailed discussion of the role of the cerebellum in learning is given below.

The two most extensively studied cases are the classically conditioned rabbit nictitating membrane response, and VOR gain adaptation. The nictitating membrane response is a protective eyeblink with the rabbit's third, horizontal eyelid, in response to corneal stimulation with a puff of air.

In classical conditioning, the air-puff is paired with a conditioned stimulus such as a tone; the rabbit then associates the tone with the air-puff, and learns to blink to tone alone. Thompson reported that cerebellar lesions selectively abolished the classically conditioned blink, without impairing the response to air-puff.[99] Subsequent experiments suggested that the association between tone and air-puff actually took place in the cerebellum, with mossy fibers conveying the conditioned stimulus and climbing fibers the unconditioned stimulus. Some reports indicate that the actual site of plasticity is the cerebellar cortex, giving rise to the suggestion that the mechanism of plasticity is long-term depression at the parallel fiber-Purkinje cell synapse (see above).[98] Others, however, locate the site of plasticity in the deep cerebellar nuclei.[99,100] Furthermore, the idea that any part of the cerebellum is required for the classically conditioned nictitating membrane response has been disputed.[101]

A second case in which the cerebellum seems to contribute to learning is in adapting the gain of the VOR. When the head rotates, the semicircular canals (the afferent limb of the reflex) projecting to oculomotor nuclei via vestibular nuclei cause a compensatory counter-rotation of the eyes, keeping the visual image stable on the retina. If the counter-rotation were exactly of an amplitude to keep the eyes fixed on a stationary point in the environment, then the gain of the reflex would be said to be 1. With techniques such as magnifying lenses, the "optimal" gain can be changed, so that a stationary image on the retina is achieved with a gain greater or less than 1. Under these circumstances, the gain alters gradually in the appropriate direction. Lesion experiments suggest that the cerebellar flocculus is required for this adaptation. Moreover, microelectrode recording experiments suggest that mossy fibers convey to the flocculus information from the semicircular canals, while climbing fibers convey a retinal slip error signal, reflecting faulty reflex gain. This suggests that long-term depression might be the mechanism of gain plasticity, and, indeed, pharmacological manipulations aimed at inhibiting long-term depression in the flocculus prevent vestibulo-ocular gain adaptation.[89]

TIMING THEORIES

Several theories have attributed to the cerebellum a role in specifically temporal aspects of motor control. Experiments and computer simulations by Medina et al. suggest that, in the classically conditioned rabbit nictitating membrane response, long-term depression in the cerebellar cortex is responsible not for the conditioned response per se but for adjusting its timing relative to the conditioned stimulus in an adaptive way (i.e., to coincide with the anticipated timing of the unconditioned stimulus).[102,103] In human patients, cerebellar lesions disrupt timing of rhythmical movements.[104] Welsh and Llinas have proposed that the cerebellum generates control signals not continuously but in discrete time steps determined by an olivocerebellar (climbing fiber) clock.[105]

More recent research, however, suggests that the cerebellum has a role in processing of time intervals per se, not necessarily for purposes of controlling movement. Studies of patients with cerebellar lesions show deficits in estimation of time intervals in the absence of any overt movement.[106,107] Functional imaging and magnetoencephalographic (MEG) studies also suggest a cerebellar role in time perception in normal subjects.[108,109]

NON-MOTOR FUNCTIONS OF THE CEREBELLUM

THE CEREBELLUM AS A SENSORY ORGAN

Historically, most authors have regarded the cerebellum as having primarily a motor function, based on the clinical observation that a movement disorder is the most prominent symptom in cerebellar disease. Looked at from a neuroanatomical perspective, however, the cerebellum looks at least as much a sensory as a motor organ, since it receives a very extensive range of direct sensory afferents. A novel hypothesis, cogently argued by Bower, is that the cerebellum is "motor for sensory's sake," optimizing movements whose function is to orient sensory receptors optimally for acquiring sensory information.[110] For example, cerebellar metabolic activity, as assessed by functional magnetic resonance imaging (MRI), is greatest when manipulating an object in the fingers to judge its shape, less when performing a similar tactile discrimination task without finger movement, and least when manipulating the object without performing any sensory discrimination task.[111]

Recent research has increasingly demonstrated a role of sensory processing in cerebellar function. Electrical activity detected by MEG showed very different responses to sensory stimuli than occurs in the somatosensory cortex.[109] The timing and the expectation or anticipation of the sensory stimuli had marked effects on the cerebellar response.

A SYNTHETIC THEORY

Thach has attempted to synthesize several lines of research into a comprehensive theory of cerebellar function. He proposed that mossy fibers carry information about the "context" of a movement to Purkinje cells.[112] Context could include both proprioceptive information via spinocerebellar pathways, and information about movement planning relayed from cerebral cortex via pontine nuclei. In this theory, parallel fiber beams provide a mechanism for wide distribution of such information; for example, proprioceptive signals from the shoulder might reach Purkinje cells controlling wrist muscles. In movements where, for example, wrist muscles needed to compensate for inertial forces resulting from shoulder movements, strength of synapses by those parallel fibers on that Purkinje cell would be modulated by long-term depression. Appropriate selective modulation of synaptic strength would be ensured by climbing fibers whose firing reported movement errors. In this way, the next attempt at that movement would be more accurate, and, with

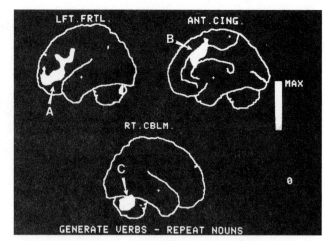

FIGURE 45-11 Sagittal slices through averaged subtraction images (utilizing PET technology) are shown of subjects asked to think of a verb associated with a noun. Note the activation in several prefrontal regions (*A*), in the anterior cingulate (*B*), and in the contralateral cerebellar hemisphere (*C*). Note the difference between this and the paramedian activation of the cerebellum during motor tasks. (*From Peterson and Fiez et al.*[114] *Used with permission.*)

practice, the cerebellum would learn an appropriate pattern of shoulder-wrist coordination.

In another example, subjects perform a task that requires two different patterns of motor coordination, depending on context (e.g., throwing darts accurately with and without prism glasses). In Thach's theory, parallel fibers would provide information about the presence or absence of the prisms, permitting differently directed dart-throws.

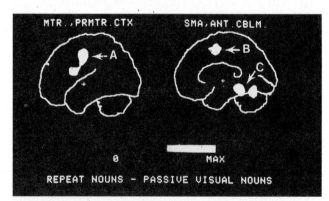

FIGURE 45-12 Sagittal slices through averaged subtraction images are displayed of subjects asked to repeat nouns aloud that were visually presented. Note the activation in the left motor (*upper*) and premotor (*lower*) cortex (*A*). The image on the *right* shows supplementary motor cortex activation (*upper, B*) and midline cerebellum activation (*lower, C*). Notice the difference in the areas of cerebellar activation between this task and the verb-generation task. (*From Petersen and Fiez et al.*[114] *Used with permission.*)

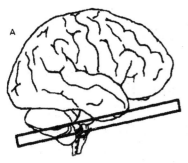

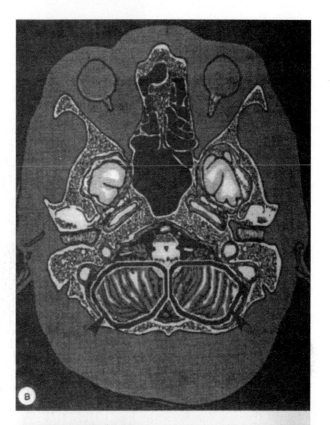

FIGURE 45-13 Area of increased regional cerebral blood flow (rCBF) during mental imagery. *A.* Lateral view of the brain; the boxed area is that corresponding to the orbitomeatal line. *B.* Anatomic model of the area of interest, 1 cm below the orbitomeatal line, where the thick black lines encircle the area affected. *C.* A rCBF image where regions of higher blood flow are indicated by the darkened "bulls-eye"-shaped areas within each cerebellar hemisphere (lateral cerebellum). (*From Ryding et al.*[115] *Used with permission.*)

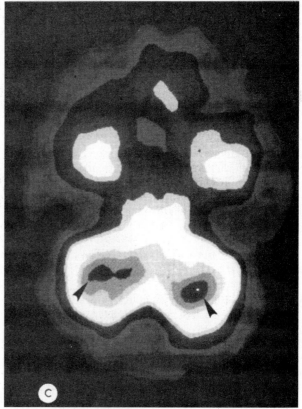

A remarkable finding is that the adaptation was specific to the arm used to throw and the method of throwing. Thus, adaptation to the optical prisms for throwing with the right hand did not carry over to throwing with the left hand. Similarly, for some subjects, adaptation to throwing underhand did not carry over to throwing overhand with the same arm. Thus, the adaptation was not to the change in sensory information alone but to the combination of specific sensory information and specific movement.

THE CEREBELLUM AND COGNITION

By far the largest part of the human cerebellum is the lateral portion (dentate nucleus, and lateral cerebellar cortex). Since afferent and efferent connections of this part of the cerebellum are primarily with cerebral cortex, it has been argued that the increased size of the dentate paralleling the increased size of the frontal cortex is evidence for the dentate influencing the frontal cortex. The ventrolateral dentate ("neodentate") projects to frontal lobe, motor areas 4 and 6, as well as prefrontal areas 44 and 45, area 8, and Broca's area 54, and to dorsolateral prefrontal cortex.[113] This suggests that the cerebellum may be involved in cognitive, and even language, processing.

Support for this hypothesis comes from functional imaging studies. In a study by Petersen and Fiez in 1993, normal human subjects were required to generate a cognitive association between words.[114] They were presented a noun and were asked to think (not speak) of a verb associated with that noun (e.g., "dog" and "bark"). During this rule-based word-generation task, it was found, using PET, that the right lateral-inferior portion of the cerebellum was metabolically active. This was anatomically distinct from the paramedian cerebellar activation that occurred during motor tasks, including speech (Figs. 45-11 and 45-12, respectively).

Another study, using SPECT, required 17 normal human subjects to count silently and to imagine certain movement sequences via motor imagery, both purely cognitive tasks. Again, the inferior lateral part of the cerebellum was markedly metabolically active during both cognitive tasks, supporting the notion that temporally organized planning of future motor acts depends on the integrity of the lateral inferior cerebellum. This is not identical to those parts of the cerebellum that are activated during actual voluntary motor movement—namely, the superior part of the vermis (Fig. 45-13).[115] A third line of evidence for cerebellar cognitive processing, obtained by way of neuroimaging, is from the recent work of Kim et al.[116] In this study, humans were imaged in a 4-Tesla MRI device while performing two tasks. The first task involved a visually guided task, moving pegs from one end of a pegboard to another. The other task involved solving a puzzle, a sort of brainteaser requiring cognitive processing (Fig. 45-14). During attempts to solve the puzzle, a dramatic bilateral activation was seen in the dentate nucleus in all 7 participants, with an intensity 3–4 times greater than that seen during the visually guided movement of pegs (Figs. 45-15 and 45-16). Again, the conclusion was reached that the dentate is involved in cognitive processing and that the specific regions responsible are distinct from those activated during eye and limb movement control.

A different approach was used by Middleton and Strick in 1994, when they examined the retrograde transneuronal transport of herpes simplex virus type I (HSV-1).[113] The HSV-1 was injected into area 46 (the dorsolateral prefrontal cortex), which is known to be involved in spatial working memory, and in planning the order and timing of future behavior. Retrograde transneuronal transport of the virus was noted to occur in many neurons of the dentate nucleus, mostly contralateral to the injection site and mostly in the ventral portion, concentrated there primarily in the middle third of the dentate. The authors pointed out that this region of the dentate differs considerably from more dorsal nucleus regions, which have been labeled in other experiments from motor and premotor areas, and from more caudal nucleus regions, which have been labeled from frontal eye fields. The results provide evidence that the dorsolateral prefrontal cortex is one of the targets of dentate nucleus output, separate from those with connections to cerebral cortex motor areas.[113]

Mechanisms of Dysfunction

Typically, when cerebellar symptomatology is evident in a patient, it is because of a lesion in the cerebellum due to ischemia, stroke, demyelination, tumor, mass effect, degeneration, or other such pathology. These lesions also may involve any one or more of the numerous inputs to, or outputs from, the cerebellum. Another possibility exists, however, whereby a remote area of pathology leads to secondary cerebellar dysfunction. One example is known as crossed cerebellar

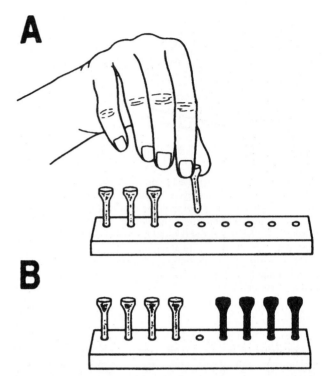

FIGURE 45-14 Sketch of the tasks performed in the work by Kim et al.[116] (see text). *A.* For the visually guided task, pegs were moved one at a time from one end of the pegboard to another. *B.* The brainteaser task involved moving the four pegs of each color from one end to the other. Three rules existed: only one peg could be moved at a time; a peg could only be moved forwards, never backwards; and a peg could be moved to an adjacent open space or could jump an adjacent peg of a different color. (*From Kim et al.[116] Used with permission.*)

diaschisis; examples of this phenomenon have already been described.[14–16,19]

Originally defined by von Monakow in the early part of this century, diaschisis is a potentially reversible functional hypometabolism. The first description relating the cerebellum with the cerebrum in terms of this concept was provided by Baron et al., in 1980, who presented cases in which there was a matched decrease in cerebral blood flow and oxygen metabolism in the cerebellar hemisphere contralateral to a cerebral infarct, ipsilateral to clinical symptoms (typically, hemiparesis).[117] Of interest is the finding that the diaschisis appears to be reversible, in that the phenomenon was not observed for more than 2 months after cerebral infarct. Another study of 55 patients with a single infarct in the distribution of the internal carotid artery revealed crossed cerebellar diaschisis in 58 percent of the patients.[118] Two processes may be suggested by this finding, according to the authors: (1) that transient hypometabolism could indeed represent true diaschisis or that persistent contralateral cerebellar degeneration may represent corticopontocerebellar transsynaptic degeneration; (2) that the association of

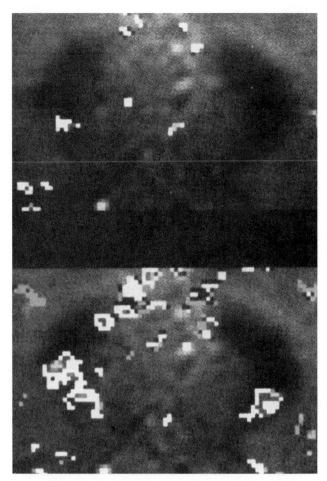

FIGURE 45-15 Functional maps of dentate nucleus during activation for one patient during the visually guided task (*top*) and during the brainteaser task (*bottom*). The dentate nuclei are the dark crescent-shaped areas with decreased signal intensity. Note the dramatic increase in dentate activation during the brainteaser task as opposed to the visually guided movement task. (See Fig. 45-16 for structure identification.) (*From Kim et al.[116] Used with permission.*)

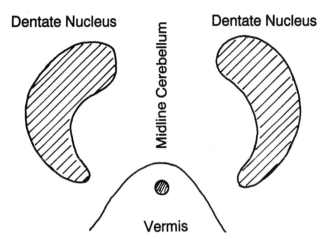

FIGURE 45-16 Line drawing corresponding to the functional maps of dentate nucleus (see Fig. 45-15).

Summary

The functions of the cerebellum and the pathophysiology of the symptoms and signs of cerebellar dysfunction have become more understood and, at the same time, more complex. The myriad abnormalities of movements and EMG patterns disordered by cerebellar disease may be accounted for by a relatively limited set of fundamental mechanisms. One of these mechanisms seems to be dysmetria, due to abnormal amplitude and timing of muscle contractions. Many of the classical symptoms and signs of cerebellar disease can be interpreted as manifestations of dysmetria. Abnormal coordination among the different parts of a complex movement may be another fundamental mechanism. Hypotonia is a third fundamental abnormality, but its contributions to the classical symptoms and signs of cerebellar disease are unclear.

Although there may be only a few fundamental mechanisms underlying the symptoms and signs of cerebellar disease, the manifestations of this mechanism differ according to the region of the cerebellum affected. Thus, there is a regional differentiation. Modern concepts of functional organization are now based on longitudinal zones. These zones are consistent with the anatomic connections between the deep cerebellar nuclei and the cerebellar cortex projecting to the nuclei. This longitudinal organization is also consistent with efferent and afferent connections to and from the cerebellum and the timing of activity changes relative to movement generation. These concepts have heuristic value in increasing the understanding of how cerebellar disorders present clinically. These concepts aid in differential diagnosis.

Until recently, the primary, if not the only, role of the cerebellum was the control of movement. Recent studies have now shown a possible role of the cerebellum, particularly the dentate nucleus, in cognitive functions including language. Although the clinical syndromes typically identified today do not include symptoms and signs of cognitive

cerebellar hypometabolism was more prominent with involvement of the cortex or the internal capsule lends support to the latter hypothesis.

Cerebellar glucose metabolism has also been studied in relation to patients with aphasia.[119] Of 37 patients with aphasia resulting from left cerebral infarcts or hemorrhages, 21 were found to have contralateral cerebellar hypometabolism; interestingly, all of the patients with Broca's aphasia (8 of 37) were found to have decreased right cerebellar glucose metabolic rates. The significance of this finding may not be fully appreciated; suffice it to say that this and other studies revealing contralateral cerebellar hypometabolism in PET studies highlight the importance of the association of cortex, cerebellum, and the connections in between for motor, and perhaps language, system integrity.

dysfunction, better understanding of these functions, as well as improved testing instruments, may identify abnormalities in these domains.

Although much has been learned about the function and dysfunction of the cerebellum, much more remains to be done. Compared to our understanding of the basal ganglia, less is known about the cerebellum. Consequently, the development of therapeutics for cerebellar diseases has lagged far behind those for basal ganglia diseases. Yet, cerebellar disorders are a common and important source of disability and suffering. It is to be hoped that scientists and clinicians in the future will narrow this knowledge gap.

References

1. Holmes G: The symptoms of acute cerebellar injuries due to gunshot injuries. *Brain* 40:461–535, 1917.
2. Gilman S, Bloedel JR, Lechtenberg R: *Disorders of the Cerebellum.* Philadelphia: FA Davis, 1981.
3. Nyberg-Hansen R, Horn J: Functional aspects of cerebellar signs in clinical neurology. *Acta Neurol Scand Suppl* 51:219–245, 1972.
4. Amici R, Avanzini G, Pacini L: Cerebellar tumors: Clinical analysis and physiopathologic correlations. *Monogr Neural Sci* 4:1976.
5. Ebner TJ: A role of the cerebellum in the control of limb movement velocity. *Curr Opin Neurobiol* 8:762–769, 1998.
6. Goodkin HP, Thach WT: Cerebellar control of constrained and unconstrained movements. I. Nuclear inactivation. *J Neurophysiol* 89(2):884–895, 2003.
7. Holmes G: The cerebellum of man. *Brain* 62:1–30, 1939.
8. Dow RS, Moruzzi G: *The Physiology and Pathology of the Cerebellum.* Minneapolis: The University of Minneapolis Press, 1958.
9. Wertham FI: A new sign of cerebellar disease. *J Nerv Ment Dis* 69:486–493, 1929.
10. Zentay PJ: Motor disorders of the central nervous system and their significance for speech: Cerebral and cerebellar dysarthrias (part I). *Laryngoscope* 47:147–156, 1937.
11. Brown JR, Darley FL, Aronson AE: Ataxic dysarthria. *Int J Neurol* 7:302–318, 1970.
12. Luciani L: *Il Cervelletto: Nuori Studi de Fisiologia Normale e Patologica.* Florence: Le Monnier, 1891.
13. Miller NR: *Walsh and Hoyt's Clinical Neuro-Ophthalmology*, 4th ed. Baltimore: Williams & Wilkins, 1988, pp 618–746.
14. Garcin R: The ataxias: Disturbances of nervous function, in Vinken PJ, Bruyn GW (eds): *Handbook of Clinical Neurology.* Amsterdam: North-Holland, 1969, vol 1, pp 309–355.
15. Grant FC: Cerebellar symptoms produced by supratentorial tumors. *AMA Arch Neurol* 20:292–308, 1928.
16. Frazier CH: Tumor involving the frontal lobe alone. *AMA Arch Neurol* 35:525–571, 1936.
17. Babinski J: De l'asynergie cérébelleuse. *Rev Neurol (Paris)* 7:806–816, 1899.
18. Luciani L: *Muscular and Nervous System*, translated by FA Welby. London: Macmillan, 1915, vol 3.
19. Montgomery EBM Jr: Signs and symptoms from a cerebral lesion that suggest cerebellar dysfunction. *Arch Neurol* 40:422–423, 1983.
20. Vilis T, Hore J: Central neural mechanisms contributing to cerebellar tremor produced by limb perturbations. *J Neurophysiol* 43:279–291, 1980.
21. Nolte J: *The Human Brain.* St. Louis: Mosby-Year Book, 1993, pp 337–359.
22. Carpenter MB: *Core Text of Neuroanatomy.* Baltimore: Williams & Wilkins, 1991, pp 224–249.
23. Leiner HC, Leiner AL, Dow RS: Cognitive and language functions of the human cerebellum. *Trends Neurosci* 16:444–447, 1993.
24. DeMyer W: *Neuroanatomy.* New York: J Wiley, 1988, pp 187–206.
25. Marr, D: A theory of cerebellar cortex. *J Physiol* 202:437–470, 1969.
26. Albus JS: A theory of cerebellar function. *Math Biosci* 10:25–61, 1971.
27. Martin JH, Cooper SE, Ghez C: Differential effects of deep cerebellar nuclei inactivation on reaching and adaptive control. *J Neurophysiol* 83:1886–1899, 2000.
28. Carrea RME, Mettler FA: Physiologic consequences following extensive removals of the cerebellar cortex and deep cerebellar nuclei and effect of secondary cerebral ablations in the primate. *J Comp Neurol* 87:169–288, 1947.
29. Chambers WW, Sprague JM: Functional localization in the cerebellum. I: Organization in longitudinal cortico-nuclear zones and their contribution to the control of posture, both extrapyramidal and pyramidal. *J Comp Neurol* 103:105–129, 1955.
30. Chambers WW, Sprague JM: Functional localization in the cerebellum. II: Somatotopic organization in cortex and nuclei. *AMA Arch Neurol Psychiatry* 74:653–680, 1955.
31. Jansen J, Brodal A: Experimental studies on the intrinsic fibers of the cerebellum. II: The cortico-nuclear projection. *J Comp Neurol* 73:267–321, 1940.
32. Nashold BS Jr, Slaughter DG: Effects of stimulating or destroying the deep cerebellar regions in man. *J Neurosurg* 31:172–186, 1969.
33. Bower JM, Kassel J: Variability in tactile projection patterns to cerebellar folia crus IIA of the Norway rat. *J Comp Neurol* 302:768–778, 1990.
34. Dow RS: Some aspects of cerebellar physiology. *J Neurosurg* 18:512–530, 1961.
35. Evarts EV, Thach WT: Motor mechanisms of the CNS: Cerebrocerebellar interrelations. *Annu Rev Physiol* 31:451–498, 1969.
36. Snider RS: The cerebellum. *Sci Am* 199:84–90, 1958.
37. Thach WT: Timing of activity in cerebellar dentate nucleus and cerebral motor cortex during prompt volitional movement. *Brain Res* 88:233–241, 1975.
38. Thach W: Correlation of neural discharge with pattern and force of muscular activity, joint position, and direction of the intended movement in motor cortex and cerebellum. *J Neurophysiol* 41:654–676, 1978.
39. Bava A, Grimm R, Rushmer D: Fastigial unit activity during voluntary movement in primates. *Brain Res* 288:371–374, 1983.
40. Niewenhuys, Voogd, Van Huijzen: *The Human Central Nervous System*, 3rd rev ed. Springer-Verlag, 1988.
41. Sugihara I, Wu HS, et al: The entire trajectories of single olivocerebellar axons in the cerebellar cortex and their contribution to cerebellar compartmentalization. *J Neurosci* 21:7715–7723, 2001.
42. Sugihara I, Lang EJ, et al: Uniform olivocerebellar conduction time underlies Purkinje cell complex spike synchronicity in the rat cerebellum. *J Physiol* 470:243–271, 1993.

43. Eccles JC, Ito M, Szentagothai J: *The Cerebellum as a Neuronal Machine.* New York: Springer-Verlag, 1967.

44. Ito M: Neurophysiological aspects of the cerebellar motor control system. *Int J Neurol* 7:162–176, 1970.

45. Brown IE, Bower JM: Congruence of mossy fiber and climbing fiber tactile projections in the lateral hemispheres of the rat cerebellum. *J Comp Neurol* 429:59–70, 2001.

46. Gundappa-Sulur G, De Schutter E, et al: Ascending granule cell axon: An important component of cerebellar cortical circuitry. *J Comp Neurol* 408:580–596, 1999.

47. LaMonte Hanson C: Functional mapping of the cerebellar cortex using pH sensitive dyes: an optical approach. *Doctoral Thesis.* University of Minnesota, 2001.

48. Ito M: Historical review of the significance of the cerebellum and the role of Purkinje cells in motor learning. *Ann N Y Acad Sci* 978:273–288, 2002.

49. Eccles JC: The cerebellum as a computer: Patterns in space and time. *J Physiol* 229:1–32, 1973.

50. Dieudonne S: Serotonergic neuromodulation in the cerebellar cortex: cellular, synaptic, and molecular basis. *Neuroscientist* 7:207–219, 2001.

51. Rajput A, Hornykiewicz O, Deng Y, et al: *Neurology* 56(suppl 3):A302, 2001.

52. Eccles JC: The role of the cerebellum in controlling movement, in Downman CBB (ed): *Modern Trends in Physiology.* London: Butterworth, 1972, vol 1, pp 86–111.

53. Botterell EH, Fulton JF: Functional localization in the cerebellum of primates. III: Lesions of hemispheres (neocerebellum). *J Comp Neurol* 69:63–87, 1938.

54. Allen GI, Tsukahara N: Cerebrocerebellar communication systems. *Physiol Rev* 54:957–1006, 1974.

55. Adrian ED: Afferent areas in the cerebellum connected with the limbs. *Brain* 66:289–315, 1943.

56. Snider RS, Eldred E: Cerebro-cerebellar relationships in the monkey. *J Neurophysiol* 15:27–40, 1952.

57. Victor M, Adams RD, Mancall EL: A restricted form of cerebellar cortical degeneration occurring in alcohol patients. *AMA Arch Neurol* 1:579–688, 1959.

58. van Kan PLE, Gibson AR, Houk JC: Movement-related inputs to intermediate cerebellum of the monkey. *J Neurophysiol* 69:74–94, 1993.

59. Goodkin HP, Keating JG, et al: Preserved simple and impaired compound movement after infarction in the territory of the superior cerebellar artery. *Can J Neurol Sci* 20(suppl 3):S93–104, 1993.

60. Westheimer G, Blair SM: Oculomotor defects in cerebellec-tomized monkeys. *Invest Ophthalmol* 12:618–621, 1973.

61. Westheimer G, Blair SM: Functional organization of primate oculomotor system revealed by cerebellectomy. *Exp Brain Res* 21:463–472, 1974.

62. Optican LM, Robinson DA: Cerebellar-dependent adaptive control of primate saccadic system. *J Neurophysiol* 44:1058–1076, 1980.

63. Ritchie L: Effects of cerebellar lesions on saccadic eye movements. *J Neurophysiol* 39:1246–1256, 1976.

64. Ito M: Neural design of the cerebellar motor control system. *Brain Res* 40:81–84, 1972.

65. Selhorst JB, Stark L, Ochs AL, Hoyt WF: Disorders in cerebellar ocular motor control. I. Saccadic overshoot dysmetria: An oculographic, control system and clinico-anatomical analysis. *Brain* 99:497–508, 1976.

66. Selhorst JB, Stark L, Ochs AL, Hoyt WF: Disorders in cerebellar ocular motor control. II. Macrosaccadic oscillation: An oculographic, control system and clinico-anatomical analysis. *Brain* 99:509–522, 1976.

67. Zee DS, Yamazaki A, Butler PH, Gucer G: Effects of ablation of flocculus and paraflocculus on eye movements in primate. *J Neurophysiol* 46:878–899, 1981.

68. Kornhuber HH: Cerebellar control of eye movements. *Adv Otorhinolaryngol* 19:241–253, 1973.

69. Lechtenberg R, Gilman S: Speech disorders in cerebellar disease. *Ann Neurol* 3:285–290, 1978.

70. Shankweiler D: Effects of temporal lobe lesions on recognition of dichotically presented melodies. *J Comp Physiol Psychol* 62:115–119, 1966.

71. Bever TG, Chiariello RJ: Cerebral dominance in musicians. *Science* 185:537–539, 1974.

72. Montgomery EBM Jr, Gorman DS, Nuessen J: Motor initiation versus execution in normal and Parkinson's disease subjects. *Neurology* 41:1469–1475, 1991.

73. Hallett M, Shahani BT, Young RR: EMG analysis of stereotyped voluntary movements in man. *J Neurol Neurosurg Psychiatry* 38:1154–1162, 1975.

74. Flament D, Hore J: Movement and electromyographic disorders associated with cerebellar dysmetria. *J Neurophysiol* 55:1221–1233, 1986.

75. Hallett M, Shahani BT, Young RR: EMG analysis of patients with cerebellar deficits. *J Neurol Neurosurg Psychiatry* 38:1163–1169, 1975.

76. Hore J, Wild B, Diener HC: Cerebellar dysmetria at the elbow, wrist, and fingers. *J Neurophysiol* 65:563–571, 1991.

77. Hallett M, Berardelli A, Matheson J, et al: Physiological analysis of simple rapid movements in patients with cerebellar deficits. *J Neurol Neurosurg Psychiatry* 53:124–133, 1991.

78. Robertson LT, Grimm RJ: Responses of primate dentate neurons to different trajectories of the limb. *Exp Brain Res* 23:447–462, 1975.

79. Inhoff AW, Diener HC, Rafal RD, Ivry R: The role of cerebellar structures in the execution of serial movements. *Brain* 112:565–581, 1989.

80. Sherrington CS: *The Integrative Action of the Nervous System.* New York: Charles Scribner's Sons, 1906.

81. Guyton AC: *Textbook of Medical Physiology.* Philadelphia: WB Saunders, 1986.

82. Granit R: *The Basis of Motor Control.* London: Academic Press, 1970.

83. Kandel ER, Schwartz JH, Jessell TM (eds): *Principles of Neural Science.* Norwalk, CT: Appleton & Lange, 1991.

84. Gilman S: The mechanism of cerebellar hypotonia. *Brain* 92:621–638, 1969.

85. Liu CN, Chambers WW: A study of cerebellar dyskinesia in the bilaterally deafferented forelimbs of the monkey (*Macaca mulatta* and *Macaca speciosa*). *Acta Neurobiol Exp* 31:263–289, 1971.

86. Gilman S, Carr D, Hollenberg J: Kinematic effects of deafferenta-tion and cerebellar ablation. *Brain* 99:311–330, 1976.

87. Bastian A, Martin T, Keating J, Thach W: Cerebellar ataxia: Abnormal control of interaction torques across multiple joints. *J Neurophysiol* 76:492–509, 1996.

88. Topka H, Konczak J, Schneider K, et al: Multijoint arm movements in cerebellar ataxia: Abnormal control of movement dynamics. *Exp Brain Res* 119:493–503, 1998.

89. Ito M: Mechanisms of motor learning in the cerebellum. *Brain Res* 886:237–245, 2000.

90. Schweighofer N, Doya K, Lay F: Unsupervised learning of granule cell sparse codes hances cerebellar adaptive control. *Neurosci* 103:35–50, 2001.

91. Eccles JC, Ito M, Szentagothai J: *The Cerebellum as a Neuronal Machine*. New York: Springer-Verlag, 1967.

92. MacKay WA, Murphy JT: Cerebellar modulation of reflex gain. *Prog Neurobiol* 13:361–417, 1979.

93. Jueptner M, Jenkins I, Brooks D, et al: The sensory guidance of movement: A comparison of the cerebellum and basal ganglia. *Exp Brain Res* 112:462–474, 1996.

94. Arshavsky YI, Gelfand IM, Orlovsky GN, et al: Messages conveyed by spinocerebellar pathways during scratching in the cat. II. Activity of neurons of the ventral spinocerebellar tract. *Brain Res* 151:493–506, 1978.

95. Hore J, Villis T: Loss of set in muscle responses to limb perturbations during cerebellar dysfunction. *J Neurophysiol* 51:1137–1148, 1984.

96. Timmann D, Horak FB: Prediction and set-dependent scaling of early postural sponses in cerebellar patients. *Brain* 120(Pt 2): 327–337, 1997.

97. Mauk MD, Medina JF, Nores WL, Ohyama T: Cerebellar function: Coordination, learning or timing. *Curr Biol* 10:R622–R525, 2000.

98. Attwell PJ, Rahman S, Yeo CH: Acquisition of eyeblink conditioning is critically dependent on normal function in cerebellar cortical lobule HVI. *J Neurosci* 21:5715–5722, 2001.

99. Krupa DJ, Thompson JK, Thompson RE: Localization of a memory trace in the mammalian brain. *Science* 260:989–991, 1993.

100. Bao S, Chen L, Kim JJ, et al: Cerebellar cortical inhibition and classical eyeblink conditioning. *Proc Natl Acad Sci U S A* 99:1592–1597, 2002.

101. Bracha V, Webster ML, Winters NK, et al: Effects of muscimol inactivation of the cerebellar interposed-dentate nuclear complex on the performance of the nictitating membrane response in the rabbit. *Exp Brain Res* 100:453–468, 1994.

102. Medina JF, Garcia KS, Nores WL, et al: Timing mechanisms in the cerebellum: Testing predictions of a large-scale computer simulation. *J Neurosci* 20:5516–5525, 2000.

103. Medina JF, Nores WL, Ohyama T, Mauk MD: Mechanisms of cerebellar learning suggested by eyelid conditioning. *Curr Opin Neurobiol* 10:717–724, 2000.

104. Ivry RB, Keele SW, Diener HC: Dissociation of the lateral and medial cerebellum in movement timing and movement execution. *Exp Brain Res* 73:167–180, 1988.

105. Welsh J, Llinas R: Some organizing principles for the control of movement based on olivocerebellar physiology. *Prog Brain Res* 114:449–461, 1997.

106. Malapani C, Dubois B, Rancurel G, Gibbon J: Cerebellar dysfunctions of temporal processing in the seconds range in humans. *Neuroreport* 9:3907–3912, 1998.

107. Mangels JA, Ivry RB, Shimizu N: Dissociable contributions of the prefrontal and neocerebellar cortex to time perception. *Brain Res Cogn Brain Res* 7:15–39,1998.

108. Tracy JI, Faro SH, Mohamed FB, et al: Functional localization of a "Time Keeper" function separate from attentional resources and task strategy. *Neuroimage* 11:228–242, 2000.

109. Tesche CD, Karhu JJ: Anticipatory cerebellar responses during somatosensory omission in man. *Hum Brain Mapping* 9:119–142, 2000.

110. Bower J: Is the cerebellum sensory for motor's sake or motor for sensory's sake: The view from the whiskers of a rat. *Prog Brain Res* 114:463–496, 1997.

111. Gao JH, Parsons LM, Bower JM, et al: Cerebellum implicated in sensory acquisition and discrimination rather than motor control. *Science* 272:545–547, 1996.

112. Thach W: What is the role of the cerebellum in motor learning and cognition? *Trends in Cogn Sci* 2:331–337, 1998.

113. Middleton FA, Strick PL: Anatomical evidence for cerebellar and basal ganglia involvement in higher cognitive function. *Science* 266:458–461, 1994.

114. Petersen SE, Fiez JA: The processing of single words studied with positron emission tomography. *Annu Rev Neurosci* 16:509–530, 1993.

115. Ryding E, Decety J, Sjoholm H, et al: Motor imagery activates the cerebellum regionally. A SPECT rCBF study with TcHMPAO. *Cogn Brain Res* 1:94–99, 1993.

116. Kim SG, Ugurbil K, Strick PL: Activation of a cerebellar output nucleus during cognitive processing. *Science* 265:949–951, 1994.

117. Baron JC, Bousser MG, Comar D, Castaigne P: "Crossed cerebellar diaschisis" in human supratentorial brain infarction. *Trans Am Neurol Assoc* 105:459–461, 1980.

118. Pantano P, Baron JC, Samson Y, et al: Crossed cerebellar diaschisis: Further studies. *Brain* 109:677–694, 1986.

119. Metter EJ, Kempler D, Jackson CA, et al: Cerebellar glucose metabolism in chronic aphasia. *Neurology* 37:1599–1606, 1987.

VIII. OTHER MOVEMENT DISORDERS

Chapter 46 _____

CORTICOBASAL DEGENERATION

NATIVIDAD P. STOVER, BRUCE H. WAINER, and RAY L. WATTS

SYNOPSIS OF THREE EARLY PATIENTS 763
EPIDEMIOLOGY 764
CLINICAL FEATURES 764
DIAGNOSIS 766
LABORATORY STUDIES 766
IMAGING STUDIES 766
ELECTROPHYSIOLOGIC STUDIES 767
NEUROPATHOLOGY 768
    Gross Findings 768
    General Microscopic Findings 769
    Tau-Associated Changes 770
    Tau Biochemistry and Genetic Analysis 771
    Heterogeneity and Overlap in Neurodegenerative
        Diseases 771
CLINICAL DIFFERENTIAL DIAGNOSIS 772
THERAPY 772
    Treatment of Motor Dysfunction 772
    Treatment of Cognitive and Neuropsychiatric
        Symptoms 773
    Treatment of Other Symptoms 773

Interest in corticobasal degeneration (CBD) has expanded exponentially in recent years and, as a result, our understanding of this disorder continues to evolve. This is largely due to the recognition of its clinical and neuropathological features, as well as the further characterization of CBD, using modern clinical and laboratory approaches. The clinical diagnosis is probably underestimated because of the heterogeneity of clinical features, overlap with symptoms of other neurodegenerative diseases, and the lack of biomarkers for the clinical diagnosis of CBD. Until recently, many questions were unresolved: Is CBD a movement disorder or a cognitive disorder, or both in some situations? Is CBD a distinctive nosological entity or a syndrome? Are there molecular and neuropathological changes unique to CBD? What is the relationship between CBD and other neurodegenerative disorders that cause abnormalities of movement and cognition, such as progressive supranuclear palsy (PSP), multiple-system atrophy (MSA), Pick's disease (PiD), Alzheimer's disease (AD), Parkinson's disease (PD) with dementia, dementia with Lewy bodies (DLB), frontotemporal dementia (FTD)? It is now appreciated that many of the neurodegenerative diseases share a common theme, which consists of the generation of abnormal protein aggregations that are toxic to vulnerable populations of neurons. CBD falls within the spectrum of diseases involving a primary defect in the processing of the microtubule-associated protein, tau. These diseases are referred to as tauopathies and include CBD, FTD, PiD and PSP. Similarly, abnormalities of the vesicle-associated protein, alpha-synuclein, are now known to underlie the pathogenesis of PD and MSA and comprise the synucleinopathies. It is common to encounter cases of CBD with features that may suggest PiD, FTD or PSP due to the overlap in disease phenotype. The appropriate neuropathologic examination can help to clarify the diagnosis. In this chapter we describe our current understanding of CBD and its place in the spectrum of neurodegenerative disorders, based on our experience and work of others over recent years. However, before we embark on a formal delineation of current concepts, a brief review of the original three reported cases is warranted.

Synopsis of Three Early Patients

Rebeiz et al. described 3 patients in 1967 with a unique pattern of progressive motor impairment in later adult life.[1,2] The disorder was characterized by slow, awkward voluntary limb movements accompanied by tremor and dystonic posturing. In all 3 patients, dysfunction began and remained most prominent in the left limbs; stiffness, lack of dexterity, and "numbness" or "deadness" were the initial symptoms. The gradual progression included gait impairment, with particular difficulty initiating steps, marked limb rigidity, loss of dexterity, impaired position and other sensory functions of the left limbs, as well as interference with attempted movements from involuntary synkinesia of the contralateral limbs. Although motor impairment progressed, intellectual function was said to remain relatively intact. Motor disability progressed, and the illness terminated in death 6–8 years after the onset of the neurological disease.

The pathological findings in all 3 patients were distinctive, with an unusual pattern of frontoparietal cortical neuronal loss. The asymmetrical presentation of signs and symptoms correlated with the corresponding atrophy in the contralateral frontal and parietal cortex in 2 of the 3 patients. The atrophic cortex showed extensive neuronal loss, with associated gliosis. Some of the pyramidal neurons, in the third and fifth layers, were swollen, with an eosinophilic hyaline appearance with hematoxylin-eosin staining. The swollen neurons often had eccentric nuclei, were devoid of Nissl substance, thus prompting the use of the terms "achromatic" or "ballooned neurons."

These striking pathological findings were not accompanied by features typical of other neurodegenerative conditions, such as Pick bodies, senile plaques, or Lewy bodies. The topography of neuronal loss in the cortex coincided with sites of the distribution of the achromatic neurons, mostly in the frontal, rolandic, and parietal regions. Although neuronal loss and gliosis were also observed elsewhere in cerebral cortex, the hippocampal formation, occipital cortex, and inferior and medial temporal cortex were spared in the original cases. Considerable loss of pigmented neurons in the substantia nigra was observed in the 3 patients. The medial portion of the subthalamic nucleus also showed gliosis and swollen neurons. In 2 patients, there were similar neuronal changes in the dentate and deep nuclei of the cerebellum; the cerebellar cortex was also intact. Evidence of secondary corticospinal tract degeneration was present in 2 of the 3 patients. In each case, the general autopsy, including examination of the circulatory system, as well as other organ systems, gave no clues concerning the pathogenesis of the intriguing neuropathological findings. With this historical backdrop, we will now address current knowledge of epidemiology, clinical features, laboratory and imaging studies, neuropathological findings, and differential diagnosis of CBD.

Epidemiology

The incidence and prevalence of CBD are unknown and most likely underestimated. CBD cases present in middle-to-late adult life with a mean onset of symptoms at 63 ($\pm$ 7.7) years.[3,4] Clinical cases consistent with CBD have been reported as early as age 40 years, and the youngest case with pathological confirmation was 45 years old. Some authors have observed predominance in women.[5-7] Current understanding suggests that it is a sporadic disease with negative family history of affected patients in most of the cases. Cases that were reported originally as familial CBD have been recently shown to be frontotemporal dementia with parkinsonism linked to chromosome 17 (FTDP-17).[8-10] However, some have suggested that a certain genetic background may be a risk factor.[11] Other risk factors such as toxic exposures or infectious agents have not been implicated in the pathogenesis of CBD thus far.[12]

Clinical Features

The most common initial motor symptom reported is limb clumsiness with or without rigidity, and it is observed in 50 percent of patients at the first visit in some studies. An asymmetrical, insidiously progressive parkinsonism usually of the akinetic-rigid type, with or without tremor, is also typical.[13-17] The symptoms respond poorly to L-dopa treatment, and this represents an early important characteristic clue that suggests an atypical parkinsonian condition.[18,19] Akinesia, rigidity, and apraxia are the most common findings during the course of CBD, occurring in over 90 percent of cases within the first 3 years of illness. Signs of cortical impairment develop within 1–3 years of onset, but in some series dementia was the most frequent presenting syndrome in patients with pathologic confirmation of CBD.[20] Riley and Lang[21] set practical criteria for the clinical

diagnosis of CBD with manifestations reflecting dysfunction of cerebral cortex (corticosensory loss, apraxia, frontal lobe reflexes, hyperreflexia, Babinski sign), and basal ganglia (akinesia, rigidity, limb dystonia, postural instability). There were also findings that did not clearly localize to either of these regions (action tremor, alien limb phenomenon, oculomotor impairment, dysarthria, dysphagia). Rinne et al.[5] analyzed the clinical features of 36 cases (6 with pathological confirmation of CBD). Of the 36 patients, 20 presented with symptoms related to a jerky, stiff, or clumsy upper extremity and 10 patients began with the symptom of difficulty walking (stiffness, jerking, or clumsiness of a leg or "unsteadiness"). Other less common presentations include combined arm and leg involvement with motor dysfunction, unilateral painful paresthesias, behavioral problems, and orofacial dyspraxia.[22,23] Gradual extension of the symptoms to contralateral limbs, postural instability, loss of facial expression, dysphagia, dysarthria, and other signs of midline or generalized motor impairment of extrapyramidal type also develop within 1 or more years. Litvan et al. published the statistical analysis of 105 clinical cases with known neuropathologic diagnosis of different neurodegenerative diseases presented to a group of neurologists trained in movement disorders in order to approach the accuracy of the clinical diagnosis of CBD.[24] The specialists then provided clinical diagnosis that was correlated with the pathologic findings. In this study, the best predictors for the diagnosis of CBD during the first visit of the patient included limb dystonia, asymmetric parkinsonism, ideomotor apraxia, and absence of balance or gait disturbances. There are, however, a few cases of limb dystonia with pathological diagnosis of PSP.[25-27] The absence of gait disturbances is a key feature for differentiating CBD from PSP and striatonigral degeneration (SND). Other clinical features commonly seen are: (1) an irregular, jerky action/postural tremor and myoclonus, (2) asymmetric limb dystonia and choreoathetoid involuntary movements, (3) the alien limb phenomenon, (4) eye movement abnormalities and blepharospasm, (5) cortical signs and neuropsychological symptoms, and (7) speech and swallowing problems[28-30] (Table 46-1).

The tremor in CBD differs from the typical resting or postural tremor seen in PD. It is a faster (6–8 Hz) action and postural tremor, more irregular and jerky. Myoclonus develops in approximately half of patients with CBD during the course of the illness.[31,32] Focal myoclonus may be superimposed upon the tremor in advanced stages of the disease and it tends to be present, at least initially, to a greater extent in the most affected limb(s). Myoclonus, like tremor, is best seen during action or maintenance of a posture; it is also stimulus-sensitive in many cases, elicited by cutaneous stimuli and may be masked by the presence of increased muscle tone.[33-36]

Asymmetric limb dystonia is observed frequently in patients with CBD.[21,24] The arm is the most frequently affected region. Usually the hand and forearm are flexed and the arm is adducted at the shoulder. The fingers are typically flexed at the metacarpophalangeal joints, extended

TABLE 46-1 Clinical Features of CBD

Nature of symptoms
 Insidious, chronic, progressive
 Asymmetric onset
 Unresponsive to L-dopa

Motor dysfunction
 Limb clumsiness, bradykinesia, akinesia, rigidity
 Action/postural tremor/focal myoclonus
 Limb dystonia (asymmetric)
 Eye movement difficulties; supranuclear gaze abnormalities
  (voluntary saccades affected more than smooth pursuit)
 Blepharospasm
 Orolingual dyskinesias
 Choreoathetoid movements
 Speech problems (monotonous, dysarthria, anarthria late)
 Gait disorder, postural instability, falls
 Upper motor neuron syndrome/corticospinal signs
 Swallowing disorder

Higher cortical dysfunction
 Limb apraxia (ideomotor, ideational, limb kinetic)
 Orofacial apraxia
 Eyelid opening apraxia
 Cortical sensory abnormalities (extinction to double simultaneous
  somatosensory stimulation, agraphesthesia, astereognosis)
 Alien limb phenomenon
 Aphasia
 Frontal lobe release signs
 Dementia

Neuropsychiatric abnormalities
 Depression
 Apathy
 Anxiety
 Irritability
 Agitation
 Disinhibition
 Delusions
 Obsessive-compulsive disorder

or flexed at the proximal and distal interphalangeal joints, and show variable degrees of fixed postures with or without associated contractures. Head, neck, trunk, leg, foot, and toe dystonia are less common. Dystonia is often associated with rigidity, bradykinesia, myoclonus, tremor, apraxia, alien limb phenomenon, and cortical sensory abnormality in the affected limb and, as dystonia progresses, patients may develop rigid postures. Pain accompanying dystonia is described in over 40 percent of cases; it can be very intense and is usually associated with contractures.[37] Spontaneous onset of choreoathetoid movements involving the limbs and facial muscles may be present, usually associated with a dystonic extremity.

The alien limb phenomenon is a failure to recognize ownership of an extremity in the absence of visual cues.[38,39] It is associated with autonomous activity of the affected extremity, which may be perceived by the subject as outside his or her control. Half of patients with CBD develop the alien limb

phenomenon, often with coexisting dystonia, myoclonus, apraxia, and cortical sensory loss. Posturing and levitation are associated with alien limb phenomenon in CBD more commonly than in other etiologies.[40,41] However, alien limb is rare on initial presentation.[42,43]

Differences in eye movement abnormalities in CBD are distinctive from other movement disorders frequently misdiagnosed as CBD, and this symptom may help to improve the diagnostic accuracy in the early stages of the disease.[44] In patients with CBD, there is a significantly increased latency bilaterally of horizontal saccades compared with PSP patients, who manifest a decreased velocity of movements. Vertical saccades may be slightly impaired in patients with CBD compared with PSP patients. Smooth pursuit eye movements in early stages of CBD may be slow and exhibit saccadic breakdown, but the range of movements is generally full (except for upgaze in elderly patients). As the illness progresses, patients with CBD gradually lose the ability to make rapid saccades to verbal command, with retained spontaneous saccades and optokinetic nystagmus.[45–48] Blepharospasm and eyelid opening apraxia are also reported.

The most frequent cortical signs are apraxia, cortical sensory loss, and dementia. Different types of apraxia can be appreciated, depending not only on the initial affected areas but also on the patterns of disease progression.[49] Ideomotor apraxia occurred most frequently in patients with CBD in several studies. Ideomotor apraxia is manifested by impairment of timing, sequencing, spatial organization, and mimicking of movements.[50] The patients with ideomotor apraxia commit mainly temporal (irregular speed and sequencing) and spatial errors (abnormal amplitude, orientation of objects and movements, and abnormal use of body parts as objects). The patients with CBD may also demonstrate ideational and "limb kinetic" apraxia. Ideational apraxia is a dysfunction of the praxis conceptual system.[51,52] The performance in ideational apraxia is abnormal in the content and tool selection (including perseverations and pantomime-related errors), and it may be observed in later stages of the disease or in patients with dementia and language dysfunction at presentation.[53,54] In limb kinetic apraxia, the manipulative behavior is affected with a decrease in dexterity and fine movements in the affected limb.[55,56] Rosenfield et al. presented 2 patients (1 with pathological confirmation of CBD) with speech apraxia as a presenting sign in the evolution of the classical clinical motor syndrome.[57] Truncal and limb apraxia have been described in patients with clinical diagnosis of CBD.[58] Orofacial apraxia with dysarthria was also reported in a series of ten patients.[59] Abnormalities of two-point discrimination and somatosensory extinction to double simultaneous stimulation may be present several years before apraxia and other symptoms are evident.[56]

Patients with CBD frequently show abnormal cognitive and neuropsychological profiles in association with motor and praxis disorders. Although many cases show little cognitive dysfunction, varying degrees of intellectual, memory, and language impairment may develop; furthermore, cognitive impairment may be the presenting or even sole feature in some cases.[20,60] In our study of 11 cases of neuropathologically confirmed CBD, all patients eventually developed cognitive deficits; the onset, nature, and severity of the impairment, however, varied widely. Cognitive disturbances preceded or accompanied the onset of the movement disorder in 4 patients; an additional 3 patients developed memory loss, progressing to more global dementia, within 2–3 years of the onset of neurological symptoms. Another patient displayed mild early memory impairment and, in 3 individuals, dementia was a late feature.[6]

Memory disorder in cases of CBD may result from the disruption of the subcorticofrontal circuits, as well as executive dysfunction as described in PSP and other disorders involving predominantly subcortical structures, that can be assessed by word fluency and switching between different tasks sets and activities.[61] Temporospatial orientation and recent and remote memories are usually preserved in early stages of the disease. In a study comparing clinically diagnosed CBD and AD patients with extrapyramidal features, CBD patients displayed better performance on tests of immediate recall and attention, whereas they performed significantly worse on tests of praxis, digit span, and uni- and bimanual motor series examinations.[62,63] Naming may be impaired in CBD patients, although their naming ability often benefits from phonemic cuing, unlike that of AD patients. Recognition memory may be preserved, but encoding and recall strategies are dysfunctional. A frontosubcortical pattern of dementia associated with gesture disorders may be very suggestive of CBD.

The neuropsychological features most frequently described in patients with CBD include depression, apathy, irritability, anxiety, disinhibition, and agitation. It was found that CBD patients with left-sided symptoms (as a result of right hemisphere involvement) manifested greater disinhibition, apathy, and irritability and lower depression scores than patients with predominantly right-sided symptoms (secondary to left hemisphere involvement). Manifestations of obsessive-compulsive disorder, including recurrent thoughts, repetitive acts, indecisiveness, checking behaviors, and preoccupation with perfectionism, are also included in the neuropsychological profile.[64–66] Compared with AD, patients with CBD have less apathy, agitation, anxiety, and delusions.[66–67] Patients with frontotemporal cortical degeneration usually manifest more disinhibition and euphoria. CBD patients manifest rates of depression similar to PD but lower rates of anxiety. DLB has a high rate of visual hallucinations, a phenomenon never described in CBD patients.[70–72]

Eventually, most patients exhibit signs of corticospinal dysfunction, with extensor plantar responses and hyperreflexia. The differentiation of spasticity from rigidity in these patients is clinically very difficult, but the loss of voluntary movement is almost certainly related in part to degeneration of primary and secondary motor cortical regions that contribute to the corticospinal tracts. In fairly advanced stages, frontal release signs (grasp, glabellar, and exaggerated facial and palmomental reflexes) may become prominent.

The majority of patients with CBD have speech changes, including slowness of speech production, monotonous voice, dysphonia, echolalia, or palilalia. The difficulties may evolve to include paraphasic errors with aphasia, and patients may later become anarthric and aphonic in advanced stages. Swallowing disorders are very common, especially in later phases of the disease.[73–75]

Symptoms associated with shorter survival in CBD patients are early onset of bilateral parkinsonism and the presence of a frontal lobe syndrome. The motor symptoms usually progress to a state of bilateral rigid immobility, and death ensues 5–10 years after disease onset.

Diagnosis

In summary, based on current evidence, CBD appears to be a distinctive nosological entity. When fully developed and observed over time, the motoric presentation is sufficiently characteristic to allow correct diagnosis during life with a relatively high accuracy. Additional studies, summarized below, including laboratory, imaging, and electrophysiologic studies, although not diagnostic, can provide supportive data. Neuropsychological tests and evaluation of the apraxia may be helpful when patients do not have the typical motor presentation. The ultimate confirmation, however, still depends on the neuropathological findings in concert with the clinical picture.

Laboratory Studies

Routine laboratory studies of blood, urine, and cerebrospinal fluid (CSF) are normal. Serum copper and ceruloplasmin levels are normal. Heavy metal toxic screens of urine have been negative. Watts et al. found that CSF levels of somatostatin were significantly decreased in all 3 patients assayed, 2 of whom had autopsy confirmation of CBD.[76]

Imaging Studies

The radiologist must be aware of the importance of observing cortical asymmetries when evaluating brain images of patients with suspected CBD. Radiographic evaluation with brain computed tomography (CT) scans and magnetic resonance imaging (MRI) are usually normal in the early stages of the disease, but, as the disease progresses, a pattern of asymmetric frontoparietal cortical atrophy (greatest contralateral to the most severely affected limbs) is frequently observed. The areas most affected are usually the posterior frontal and parietal regions. The cortex may appear thin and frequently with slight increase in signal intensity in proton density images. Abnormalities of the cortex are more easily detectable with fluid-attenuated inversion recovery

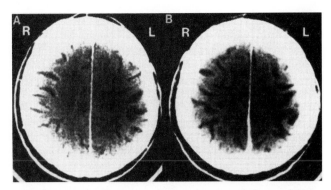

FIGURE 46-1 Cranial CT images from the autopsied case of Watts et al. in 1985, in the fifth year of the patient's illness. There is asymmetrical (left greater than right) frontoparietal cortical atrophy, which is most prominent in the perirolandic regions. Note the attenuation of subcortical white matter underlying the central sulcus in *A*.

sequences in the MRI.[77,78] As the atrophy becomes more prominent, abnormal signal attenuation is seen in the underlying subcortical white matter. Atrophy and abnormal signal in the corpus callosum are characteristic as a result of the cortical degeneration, as can be dilatation of the ipsilateral ventricle in cases with marked asymmetry. The degree of cognitive impairment shows a strong correlation with the severity of callosal atrophy and ventricular dilatation[79] (Fig. 46-1).

MRI can provide strong support for the diagnosis of CBD and may be helpful in distinguishing CBD from other neurodegenerative disorders. Savoiardo et al. addressed the role of MRI in various parkinsonian syndromes.[80,81] Compared with CBD, MRI in patients with PSP shows atrophy in the midbrain without asymmetrical cortical atrophy. Patients with AD may be differentiated from CBD by observing diffuse temporal and hippocampal atrophy in the MRI of AD cases. MRI in patients with SND demonstrates T_2 hypointensities in the posterior lateral putamen. In patients with MSA of the olivopontocerebellar atrophy (OPCA) type, the atrophy is more evident in the pons and cerebellum.[82,83] Cases of clinical diagnosis of FTD and PiD have MRI findings consistent with marked brain atrophy in frontal and temporal regions in a symmetrical or slightly asymmetrical way, the supratentorial ventricles enlarge and the caudate nucleus can be atrophic.[77] Another characteristic feature in cases of FTD is the widening of the interpeduncular fossa secondary to degeneration of frontopontine fibers. Serial evaluation of CT or MRI scans over time at 6–12 month intervals is generally more useful than one isolated study.

Functional imaging with positron emission tomography (PET), single-photon emission computed tomography (SPECT) and proton magnetic resonance spectroscopy (PMRS) have been used in suspected CBD cases to study changes in regional cerebral blood flow (CBF), cerebral metabolism (oxygen or glucose) and dopamine receptor binding. CBD patients show an asymmetrical global reduction of cortical oxygen metabolism and side-to-side regional glucose

metabolism (fluorodeoxyglucose, FDG), most prominent in the cerebral hemisphere contralateral to the most affected limbs and more evident in the inferior parietal, posterior frontal and superior temporal cortex. There is a corresponding reduction of CBF in the frontoparietal, medial frontal, and temporal cortical regions.[84–87] The only significantly affected subcortical area in CBD cases is the thalamus, where glucose metabolism can be asymmetrically reduced by 15 percent.[83] Dysfunction of the nigrostriatal dopaminergic system has been demonstrated by decreased PET tracer 6-fluorodopa (FD) uptake in the caudate and putamen, and moderately reduced postsynaptic striatal D2 receptor binding of ^{123}I-iodobenzamide on SPECT scanning, both in an asymmetric fashion.[88,89] SPECT labeling of the dopamine transporter by 2β-carboxymethoxy-3β(4-iodophenyl)-tropane (^{123}I-β-CIT) has demonstrated homogeneous reduction in caudate and putamen to as low as 25 percent of normal values in clinically diagnosed CBD, PSP, and MSA cases, compared with an asymmetric reduction in PD patients, where binding is selectively reduced in the putamen.[90–103] The characteristic pattern of asymmetrically reduced frontoparietal cerebral cortical metabolism and/or CBF coupled with equal reduction of FD uptake in the caudate and putamen provides strong supportive evidence in a patient with a clinical diagnosis of possible CBD.

Electrophysiologic Studies

Electrophysiologic studies can be useful in the evaluation of patients with CBD. The electroencephalogram (EEG) is usually normal on initial presentation of symptoms. As the disease progresses, the EEG may reveal asymmetric slowing, most prominent over the cerebral hemisphere contralateral to the most affected limb. Spike discharges are not present usually. In later stages, the EEG may show nonspecific bilateral slowing, so the time reference of the EEG in the serial evaluation of an individual patient can be very important. When correlated with asymmetric radiographic changes in a similar distribution and a typical clinical picture of CBD, this finding further supports the diagnosis. Electrophysiologic studies of the tremor with accelerometric and electromyographic (EMG) recording techniques demonstrate that the tremor present in CBD clearly differs from the classic parkinsonian tremor; it is more rapid, most evident during action, and the amplitude may vary, giving a more irregular appearance. Electrophysiologic studies of the myoclonus seen in CBD patients demonstrate that it is a reflex myoclonus and there is not a preceding cortical discharge. The myoclonus is best recorded using provocative maneuvers such as intentional movements of the limb, startle, or tactile stimulation of the affected limb(s). Cortical activity preceding myoclonus can be detected on back-averaged magnetoencephalography but is not evident on EEG. Pathophysiologically, reflex myoclonus in CBD may be caused by enhancement of the response to direct sensory input or by exaggeration of inputs in motor cortical areas due to increased cortical excitability.[34,35]

Somatosensory evoked potentials (SEP) are of minimal utility in evaluating patients with suspected CBD. Thalamocortical potentials of the SEP are occasionally prolonged. Brainstem auditory evoked potentials are also usually normal, but significant prolongation of the N200 and P300 latencies may be found occasionally in patients with both CBD and PSP.[104–106] Visual evoked potentials are normal in almost all cases, but prolonged P100 latencies can be seen. Abnormalities on electro-oculography may be evident early in the disease and may help to improve the diagnostic accuracy.[24] Routine EMG and nerve conduction studies show occasional focal or generalized neuropathies that are usually subclinical.

Neuropathology

The neuropathologic criteria for the diagnosis of CBD require careful gross and microscopic examination. Use of appropriate histochemical/immunohistochemical stains identifies the underlying tau pathology, and rules out other neurodegenerative processes (Table 46-2).

GROSS FINDINGS

The typical gross finding is atrophy of the frontoparietal cortex, which usually exhibits asymmetry correlating with the laterality of the clinical manifestations. Atrophy is usually most marked in the medial perirolandic superior frontal

TABLE 46-2 Neuropathological Features of CBD

Gross findings
   Superior frontoparietal and perirolandic cerebral cortical
      atrophy—asymmetric
   Atrophy of caudate and thalamus
   Thinning of corpus callosum
   Enlargement of lateral ventricles—asymmetric
   Atrophy of white matter, internal capsules, and cerebral
      peduncles—asymmetric
   Pallor of substantia nigra
Microscopic findings
   Neuronal loss, gliosis of cortical sections
   Spongiosis and ballooned achromatic neurons in cerebral cortex,
      especially frontoparietal
   Neurofibrillary tangles
   Abnormal cerebral white matter: swollen axons, demyelination of
      axons, spongiform appearance of neuropil in regions
      underlying heavy neuronal loss
   Pigmented nerve cell loss and gliosis in substantia nigra
   Variable neuronal loss and gliosis in locus ceruleus, raphe nuclei,
      tegmental gray matter, and thalamic and subthalamic nuclei

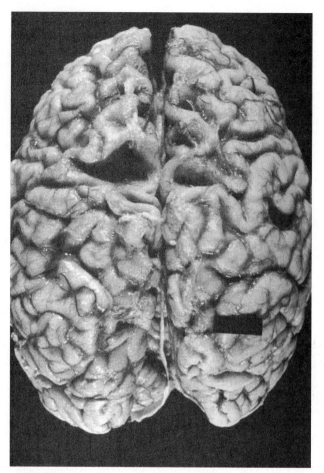

FIGURE 46-2 The convexity of the brain of a 75-year-old man with CBD exhibits striking asymmetric perirolandic cortical atrophy, which is greater on the left, where the sulcus is gaping. (*From Watts et al.[4] Used with permission.*)

gyrus, the parasagittal pre- and postcentral gyri, and the superior parietal lobule[107–110] (see Figs. 46-2 and 46-3). The distribution of the atrophy may be more generalized and involve the inferior frontal and temporal lobes in cases presenting with dementia or progressive aphasia.[111,112] Cingulate and insular cortical regions exhibit variable involvement. The occipital lobe, hippocampus and parahippocampal gyrus are usually spared. In cases where marked atrophy of the amygdala/hippocampus and adjacent entorhinal/perirhinal cortex is observed, the diagnosis of CBD should be questioned.

Atrophy of the white matter may be severe, particularly in regions underlying extensively involved cortex. Associated hydrocephalus ex vacuo, dilatation of the cerebral aqueduct, and thinning of the corpus callosum may also be seen. The anterior limb of the internal capsule may show attenuation, but other white matter pathways, such as the optic tract, anterior commissure, and fornix, are usually unaffected. The cerebral peduncles may show atrophy of quadrants containing corticospinal (middle) and frontopontine (medial) tracts.

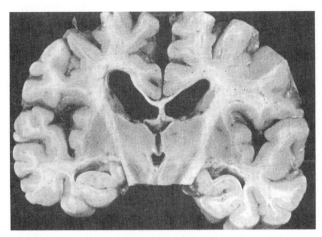

FIGURE 46-3 Coronal section through the cerebrum reveals asymmetric cortical atrophy (L > R) with thinning of the corpus callosum, loss of cerebral white matter, and resulting dilatation of the lateral ventricles (hydrocephalus ex vacuo). Note, too, the asymmetric narrowing predominantly involving the left posterior limb of the internal capsule and left cerebral peduncle. (*From Watts et al.*[4] *Used with permission.*)

There may also be atrophy of corticospinal fascicles within the base of the pons and the medullary pyramids (Fig. 46-3).

Involvement of subcortical nuclei varies widely from case to case in both severity and topography. The head of the caudate may have a flattened appearance, and the thalamus in CBD cases tends to be smaller than normal. Transverse sections of the brainstem show severe loss of neuromelanin pigment in the substantia nigra (Fig. 46-5); however, neuromelanin within the locus ceruleus is usually preserved. These findings may also be seen in PD, but in AD there is usually marked pallor of the locus ceruleus and preservation of the substantia nigra. Marked atrophy of the pons, inferior olivary nuclei, and cerebellar dentate nucleus suggests an alternative diagnosis such as MSA.

GENERAL MICROSCOPIC FINDINGS

Microscopic examination of cortical sections stained with hematoxylin-eosin show a variable amount of neuronal loss and gliosis. The most typical finding is vacuolar change or spongiosis of the upper cortical layers. This finding is in no way specific for CBD but is seen in a wide spectrum of neurodegenerative processes. In cases where there is marked neuronal loss and gliosis, the underlying white matter typically shows myelin pallor and vacuolar change. One of the characteristic cortical findings in hematoxylin-eosin preparations is the ballooned neuron (BN), which is indicative of central chromatolysis, representing a general reactive change of neurons with axonal damage[107,113] (Fig. 46-4). These cells typically appear as swollen perikarya with eccentrically placed nuclei and loss of Nissl substance, giving the cytoplasm a pale glassy eosinophilic or basophilic appearance. Immunocytochemistry for phosphorylated neurofilament proteins is

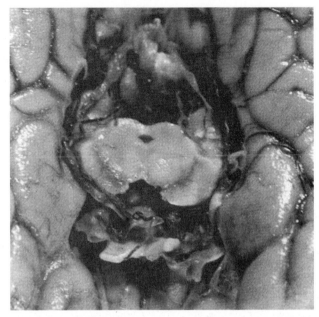

FIGURE 46-4 Pallor of the substantia nigra is seen, along with reduction in size of the left cerebral peduncle, as a result of degeneration of subcortical white matter. (*From Watts et al.*[4] *Used with permission.*)

positive in these cells as well as α-β-crystallin and sometimes ubiquitin. Tau and alpha-synuclein immunoreactivity are negative. BN can be seen in limbic and neocortical areas in CBD and other neurodegenerative processes. Their presence in the perirolandic region is considered to be of important

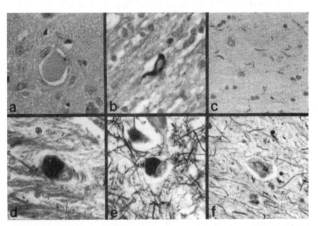

FIGURE 46-5 Cytoskeletal pathology in corticobasal degeneration *a*, ballooned neuron, perirolandic cortex; *b*, glial inclusion, white matter; *c*, neuropil threads, perirolandic cortex; *d*, globose-type tangle, globus pallidus; *e*, globular tangle or Pick-like inclusion, basis pontis; *f*, thread-like tangle, subthalamic nucleus. Stains used were as follows: hematoxylin-eosin (*a*); tau immunostain (*b* and *c*); modified Bielschowsky silver stain (*d–f*); Magnifications: 450× (*a*); 730× (*b*); 440× (*c*); 730× (*d*); 600× (*e* and *f*). (*From Schneider et al.*[6] *Used with permission.*)

diagnostic significance for CBD. BN can also be found in other tauopathies, AD, Creutzfeldt-Jakob disease (CJD), and amyotrophic lateral sclerosis (ALS).[114–116] Silver-stain preparations typically show the presence of neurofibrillary tangles (NFT) in affected areas. The tangles vary in configuration from delicate thread-like structures to compact globoid morphologies.[107,109,117,118] The typical flame-like appearance of NFT in AD is less frequent. Neuropil threads, indicative of dystrophic axonal and glial processes in gray and white matter areas, may also be present, but neuritic threads, as opposed to glial, are less common than in AD. A key distinguishing feature of CBD versus AD is the lack of either diffuse or neuritic plaques in silver-stained material. Conversely, AD does not exhibit the tau-positive glial inclusions observed in CBD, as discussed below. Cell loss in the substantia nigra is almost uniformly severe, with extraneuronal neuromelanin in phagocytes (melanophagia), and residual neurons containing NFT. The locus ceruleus, raphe nuclei, tegmental gray matter, and thalamic nuclei, mainly the ventrolateral nucleus and subthalamic nuclei, may also have NFT. The cerebellar dentate nucleus, inferior olivary nuclei, red nucleus, oculomotor complex, and colliculi are relatively spared, but may show a variable degree of neuronal loss and gliosis. The cerebellar cortex may also show focal Purkinje cell axonal torpedoes and Bergmann gliosis.

TAU-ASSOCIATED CHANGES

Tau is a microtubule-associated protein that promotes tubulin polymerization and stabilization of microtubules.[119] It is present mainly in axons and can also be expressed in glial cells. Tau protein undergoes selective phosphorylation, which controls its functional state. Tau is soluble and heat-stable, but, under pathological conditions, it forms aggregates and becomes "detergent-insoluble." Insoluble tau aggregates result either from abnormal ratios of the different isoforms, or abnormal phosphorylation, as discussed below.

The most important diagnostic finding in CBD and other tauopathies is the presence of abnormal deposits of tau immunoreactivity.[117,120–122] Tau pathology is present within neurons and glia of the cortex, subcortical nuclei, and brainstem, and these lesions are more widespread than the gross findings. Tau immunocytochemistry is more sensitive for detecting dystrophic neuronal and glial processes. In most affected neurons, the abnormal tau immunoreactivity is present as diffuse or granular cytoplasmic deposits, called pretangles.[122,123] The NFT are highly organized deposits which appear similar to the thread-like or globoid inclusions seen on silver stains.[107,117] The ultrastructure of tangles in CBD consists of paired helical filaments or "twisted filaments."[118] They have a wider diameter and longer periodicity than filaments present in AD. The tangles in PSP are more uniformly compact and globoid and consist of straight filaments at the ultrastructural level.[124]

A characteristic feature of CBD and other tauopathies, but distinct from AD, is the presence of tau-immunoreactive

glial inclusions. These inclusions are present in cell bodies and processes. In the latter instance, the inclusions can appear thread-like. In tauopathies the neuropil threads are believed to be present mainly in glial processes, while in AD the threads are localized to neuronal processes. The most characteristic astrocytic lesion in CBD, located mainly in the neocortex, is an annular cluster of short, stubby processes that resemble a neuritic plaque of AD. However, these "astrocytic plaques"[118] do not contain amyloid or dystrophic neurites (Fig. 46-6). Another lesion is the so-called "tufted astrocytes," which consist of fibrillary accumulations of tau within cell bodies and processes, and is believed to be more characteristic of PSP than of CBD.[125] Tau-positive inclusions in oligodendroglia, called "coiled bodies," are argyrophilic and frequently present in CBD as well as in other tauopathies. These inclusions are distinct from the oligodendroglial inclusions that are the hallmark of MSA, called "glial cytoplasmic inclusions," and which are immunoreactive for ubiquitin and alpha-synuclein but negative for tau.[107,117,126] The caudate and putamen have tau-immunoreactive lesions, most frequently pretangles, and the globus pallidus and putamen show variable nerve cell depletion with gliosis and NFT. The ventrolateral nucleus of the thalamus, subthalamic nucleus, red nucleus, raphe nuclei, and tegmental gray matter may have similar lesions but are usually less severely involved. Fibrillary gliosis typical of PSP is not seen in the subthalamic nucleus in CBD; the pontine base is usually free of NFT, but they are common in the locus ceruleus and substantia nigra. The latter structure, as well as the basal nucleus of Meynert, may have tau-immunoreactive pretangles.

White matter areas not contiguous with cortical atrophy may also contain tau-immunoreactive thread-like lesions and coiled bodies. The internal capsule and thalamic fasciculus often have many thread-like processes.

The minimal features for the pathologic diagnosis of CBD are cortical and striatal tau-positive neuronal and glial lesions, especially astrocytic plaques and thread-like lesions in white and gray matter, along with neuronal loss in focal cortical

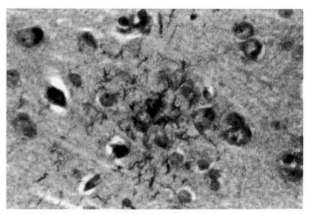

FIGURE 46-6 "Astrocytic plaque" seen on tau immunostain. Magnification: 450×.

regions and in the substantia nigra. BN have been considered of significant diagnostic value, but CBD can be diagnosed without BN if there is clear evidence of characteristic tau-positive neuronal and glial lesions in typical locations.

TAU BIOCHEMISTRY AND GENETIC ANALYSIS

It is now appreciated that the presence of widespread tau-positive inclusions in CBD links it to other disorders exhibiting tau-associated cytopathology, including PiD, PSP, argyrophilic grain disease (AGD) and FTDP-17.[120,121,127–130] AD is not considered in this group since tau pathology in AD is thought to arise secondary to the beta-amyloid pathology.

Tau is present in six different isoforms that are generated through alternative splicing of transcripts from a single gene on chromosome 17.[120,121] Three of these isoforms contain 3 microtubule binding domains (3-repeat, 3R) and three contain 4 microtubule binding domains (4-repeat, 4R). The abnormal protein aggregates can be isolated from brain tissue as detergent-insoluble tau fractions and analyzed for isoform composition and phosphorylation state. The insoluble tau of AD exhibits ratios of 4R:3R, which are not different from age-matched control brains. However, this tau is abnormally phosphorylated as well as hyperphosphorylated. The mechanisms that lead to these tau abnormalities in AD are still not well understood. Insoluble tau from CBD, PSP and AGD show elevated 4R:3R ratios relative to AD and controls. The isoforms, which form insoluble aggregates, are also hyperphosphorylated. In contrast, PiD insoluble tau consists of elevated levels of 3R tau. Therefore, in these disorders, there appears to be a fundamental abnormality in tau processing leading to an abnormal isoform composition, hyperphosphorylation, and aggregation. In FTDP-17 two major types of mutations may occur. Missense mutations of exon 10 may lead to mutant proteins that exhibit diminished affinity for microtubules. Alternatively, intronic mutations (and some exon 10 mutations) stabilize the splicing site so that higher levels of 4R tau are generated. This latter situation is similar to what occurs in PSP, CBD and AGD.

The factors adversely affecting tau processing in sporadic cases are not well understood. However, genetic analysis of the tau gene has revealed several polymorphisms in the coding and noncoding regions that represent two ancestral haplotypes, referred to as H1 and H2. In PSP and CBD, H1 homozygosity (H1/H1) is overexpressed and found in close to 90 percent of patients.[131,132] In contrast, 60 percent of normal controls are H1/H1. These findings suggest that genetic polymorphisms of the tau gene, in some way, influence the risk for developing the sporadic 4R diseases, CBD and PSP.

HETEROGENEITY AND OVERLAP IN NEURODEGENERATIVE DISEASES

Issues of overlap between various neurodegenerative disorders are well known to neurologists and neuropathologists.

In this regard we can identify three general types of diagnostic situations that may be encountered. First, there are situations where two different diseases may be present concomitantly. A common example is AD and PD. In this case the simplest explanation is that these are the two most common age-associated neurodegenerative diseases and a certain coincidence would be expected on a statistical basis. However, several recent studies have suggested that the development of dementia in PD is much more likely to result from progression of Lewy body pathology of the cortex than from coexistent AD pathology.[133–137] A very different observation has been made when Lewy body pathology has been studied in cases of AD. In these series Lewy bodies have been found in 20–40 percent of cases with a higher frequency in limbic areas as opposed to the brainstem.[133,138–141] These findings suggest that amyloid and perhaps tau pathology may somehow trigger abnormalities in alpha-synuclein processing. Experimental support for this hypothesis was provided by Masliah et al.[142] when beta-amyloid pathology was shown to facilitate alpha-synuclein accumulation and neuronal deficits in a transgenic mouse model of AD and PD.

Second, there are cases where related diseases have overlapping pathology. This is particularly relevant to CBD when there may be overlapping features with other forms of tauopathy. Another example are cases where pathologic changes of PiD coexist with CBD pathology. In these cases, each of the changes is reported and a determination, if possible, is made of the predominant pathological phenotype.

Finally, there are situations when different disease processes may present with a very similar clinical picture. Examples of this situation would be AD and CBD, or PSP and MSA. In these cases the neuropathology most often provides a definitive answer.

There is substantial neuropathological overlap between PiD and CBD. BN, variable degeneration of the substantia nigra and basal ganglia, and tau-positive inclusions occur in both disorders. However, Pick bodies, a characteristic feature of PiD, are rarely observed in CBD. Although both disorders exhibit cortical atrophy, the temporal cortex, as well as the hippocampus, are usually involved in PiD but are relatively spared in CBD. In PiD the perirolandic sensorimotor cortex is often spared but affected in CBD. CBD and PiD can also have overlapping clinical features, and CBD patients may manifest behavioral changes and language disturbances. The main features to determine the pathological diagnosis in PiD are related to the presence of Pick bodies and involvement of the limbic and neocortices with less subcortical involvement. The substantia nigra and brainstem nuclei are only mildly affected in PiD, and tau-immunoreactive lesions are located mainly in the neurons. PiD and CBD may have numerous BN in cortex but, in the CBD cases, this pathology usually extends outside the limbic cortices.

The pathological differentiation between CBD and FTDP-17 was not possible to establish by the study reported by Dickson et al.[107] Both disorders have widespread cortical and subcortical tau pathology and BN. Family history and genetic studies were crucial to make the diagnosis of these cases.

AGD is a newly recognized tauopathy with neuronal and glial tau-positive lesions and BN.[128,143,144] AGD pathology is mainly restricted to the medial temporal lobe and hypothalamus. Recent studies have provided evidence that AGD is a tauopathy involving an elevation of 4R:3R tau isoform ratios. Frontotemporal lobar degeneration (FTLD) does not have visible tau pathology and should be easy to differentiate from CBD. FTLD shows cortical atrophy, spongiosis, and gliosis, and BN may be present.[145,146] One finding that may be present in this disorder is ubiquitin-positive/tau-negative inclusions. These patients may also have concomitant motor neuron disease with the same inclusions and chromosome-17 linked familial cases have been identified. There is no evidence to date of tau abnormalities and the current thinking points to an as yet unidentified ubiquitinated protein aggregate.

Links among these disorders may occur also at a genetic level. The apolipoprotein ε4 allele is recognized as a major risk factor for familial and sporadic AD.[147,148] However, some studies observed an increased frequency of the ε4 allele in CBD, PiD and PSP, compared to that of control populations.

Clinical Differential Diagnosis

The different phenotypes of CBD reflect the variability of distribution and severity of lesions found in the pathology and it suggests that CBD should be considered in the presence of a parkinsonian or a cognitive disorder with atypical features.[5,6] The pattern of CBD presenting mainly with motor deficits is usually sufficiently distinctive such that, when fully developed, it generally would allow a confident clinical diagnosis and not be confused with PD. However, this is the most common misdiagnosis early in the course of the disease. The best early clues that can help to distinguish CBD from idiopathic PD are the lack of beneficial response to dopaminergic medication and the signs of cortical dysfunction, most notably apraxia and/or cortical sensory impairment. The differential diagnosis list of the motoric presentation of CBD includes PSP,[149] SND,[150,151], MSA,[151–153] atypical PiD,[154–157] diffuse Lewy body disease,[136] PD with dementia, AD with extrapyramidal features,[158] FTDP-17, Braack AGD,[159] the parkinsonism-dementia-ALS complex,[160,161] FTLD, Wilson's disease,[162] the rigid form of Huntington's disease,[163] hemiatrophy-hemiparkinson syndrome,[164] widespread cerebrovascular disease and variants of Binswanger's disease,[165] leukodystrophies,[166–169] variants of Azorean disease,[170–172] late-onset Hallervorden-Spatz disease,[173,174] and adult neuronal ceroid lipofuscinosis,[175] all of which typically differ in several clinical and pathological features.

PSP is the Parkinson-plus disorder most likely to be confused with CBD. PSP classically presents with prominent axial rigidity, postural instability with frequent early falls, and abnormal vertical eye movements. Several cases of "atypical PSP" have been reported, with clinical features similar to those of CBD. Atypical features such as asymmetric onset, oculomotor impairment that is only mild, focal dystonia, and involuntary limb levitation resembling the alien limb phenomenon are the most frequent features that may cause confusion with CBD.

Asymmetric cortical degenerations including PiD, primary progressive aphasia and FTDP-17 may present with features resembling early CBD, such as focal myoclonus, apraxia, alien limb phenomenon, and asymmetric rigidity. In FTDP-17 there are usually several family members affected. These syndromes, in general, lack the prominent and progressive extrapyramidal dysfunction characteristic of the typical motoric presentation of CBD. If a patient presents with a rapidly progressive CBD-like picture, a prion-related disease should be considered.[176]

There is significant overlap of these disorders with CBD, not only at the clinical presentation, but also at pathological and molecular levels as discussed above. The delineation of specific molecular and genetic markers for each disorder will help to further characterize the different diseases.

Table 46-3 summarizes the differential clinical features which are helpful in the evaluation of patients with combined parkinsonism and cognitive dysfunction.

Therapy

Pharmacotherapy for CBD has generally been of limited benefit, and this can best be ascribed to the widespread pathological involvement of cortical and subcortical neuronal systems as well as the lack of knowledge of the full biochemical and molecular background to explain the pathophysiology of the different manifestations. There is little or no beneficial response to dopaminergic medication; indeed, this is a characteristic feature. The treatment is symptomatic and the efforts are focused on alleviating the rigidity, dystonia, tremor, myoclonus, and neuropsychiatric manifestations.

TREATMENT OF MOTOR DYSFUNCTION

Improvement was reported in 24 percent of clinically diagnosed CBD patients with carbidopa/L-dopa treatment in one report.[177] The rest of the dopaminergic agents (bromocriptine, pergolide, pramipexole, ropinirole) produce more side-effects with less clinical benefit. Clonazepam has been the most beneficial agent for action tremor and myoclonus, but other benzodiazepines may be used. Baclofen and tizanidine may improve rigidity and tremor also but to a lesser degree. Anticholinergics have not been beneficial, and they have been tolerated poorly. Amantadine is of little or no benefit. Botulinum toxin injections may be useful in the treatment of painful focal dystonias as well as in blepharospasm.[177–179] Stereotactic surgeries for relief of

TABLE 46-3 Clinical Differential Diagnosis in Patients with Overlap Features of Motor and Cognitive Dysfunctions

Diagnosis	Principal Clinical Features	Features Suggesting Another Disorder or Concurrent Pathology
CBD	Apraxia, cortical sensory loss, unilateral or asymmetric rigidity and dystonia, action tremor superimposed myoclonus, alien limb phenomenon, lack of response to L-dopa	Prominent ocular impairment, axial rigidity or dystonia out of proportion to limb involvement, rest tremor, autonomic dysfunction, aphasia
PSP	Supranuclear ophthalmoplegia (especially vertical), axial dystonia, early gait impairment and frequent falls, dysarthria and pseudobulbar palsy, executive dysfunction, lack of or suboptimal response to L-dopa therapy, difficulties swallowing	Lack of or minimal ocular impairment, asymmetric rigidity, prominent dementia early in course, alien limb phenomenon-type behavior, apraxia, cortical sensory loss
MSA	Symmetric rigidity (less commonly asymmetric), lack of rest tremor, cerebellar and autonomic dysfunction, choreoathetosis, rapid course, lack of or suboptimal response to L-dopa therapy	Early and prominent ocular impairment, apraxia, cortical sensory loss
PD with dementia	Rest tremor, bradykinesia, asymmetric rigidity, gait impairment, memory loss, dementia, L-dopa-responsiveness	Symmetric rigidity, lack of rest tremor, axial dystonia, early ocular impairment, early myoclonus, apraxia, cortical sensory loss, lack of or suboptimal response to L-dopa therapy
DLBD	Early cognitive dysfunction (especially with fluctuating features), dopaminergic medication-induced psychosis, mild parkinsonism (initially)	Isolated cortical dysfunction (memory loss, aphasia, apraxia, cortical sensory loss, frontal lobe dementia), axial rigidity and dystonia, ophthalmoplegia
AD with parkinsonism	Early cognitive impairment (especially memory loss), cortical dysfunction (visuospatial, language, praxis), mild bradykinesia and rigidity	Parkinsonism before memory loss, progressive frontal lobe dysfunction, aphasia or apraxia without significant memory loss, early gait impairment, axial rigidity, ophthalmoplegia, alien limb phenomenon
PiD	Prominent frontal lobe dementia with personality changes (disinhibition or apathy, aphasia, memory loss)	Progressive aphasia or apraxia without dementia, prominent extrapyramidal features, rest tremor, L-dopa-responsiveness, ophthalmoplegia
CJD	Rapid course of dementia, personality changes, myoclonus, upper motor neuron, cerebellar and/or extrapyramidal signs	Protracted course, isolated parkinsonism or cortical dysfunction (apraxia, cortical sensory loss), rest tremor, L-dopa-responsiveness

CBD, corticobasal degeneration; PSP, progressive supranuclear palsy; MSA, multiple-system atrophy; PD, Parkinson's disease; PiD, Pick's disease; DLBD, diffuse Lewy body disease; AD, Alzheimer's disease; CJD, Creutzfeldt-Jakob disease.

severe painful limb dystonia and parkinsonism have little or no benefit, and they are not indicated in the treatment of this disorder.[180]

TREATMENT OF COGNITIVE AND NEUROPSYCHIATRIC SYMPTOMS

Treatment of cognitive dysfunction with medications that enhance cholinergic neurotransmitters have not been studied well but probably have limited benefit. Depression and obsessive-compulsive symptomatology may be treated effectively with selective serotonin reuptake inhibitors, but caution and low doses are recommended because these medications can exacerbate agitation. Antidepressants with anticholinergic side-effects, including tricyclic compounds, may exacerbate confusion. Small doses of atypical neuroleptic medications such as quetiapine, olanzapine, or clozapine may be considered if paranoid delusions, psychotic behavior,

agitation, irritability, and sleep problems emerge. The use of typical antipsychotic medications such as haloperidol may worsen parkinsonian motor symptoms and are not recommended. Small doses of sedative hypnotic agents may be helpful for sleep problems, but they also may exacerbate confusion and agitation. Clonazepam is usually helpful, and agents such as diphenhydramine, chloral hydrate and zolpidem may be useful. Small doses of an atypical antipsychotic, as mentioned above, decrease sleep-onset latency and increase overall sleep time. The use of transcranial magnetic stimulation for treatment of depression and other symptoms is still in experimental phases.[181]

TREATMENT OF OTHER SYMPTOMS

Gastrointestinal symptoms in CBD patients include hypersalivation, dysphagia, nausea, and constipation. Excessive salivation may respond to small doses of anticholinergic therapy, but side-effects are a limiting factor in most cases.

The goal of treatment of the dysphagia is to maintain safe and efficient nutrition and hydration. Evaluation with a barium swallow study may be necessary. Treatment includes dietary modifications, postural changes, swallowing maneuvers and exercises, and surgical interventions. Selection of foods with a consistency that facilitates swallowing is a critical aspect. Some patients may require thickened liquids. If they are not able to ingest enough food to meet nutritional requirements, placement of a percutaneous feeding gastrostomy tube may be necessary. The decision to place a gastrostomy in a patient with a chronically progressive neurodegenerative disease must be handled on an individual basis.

Constipation in parkinsonism is due to colonic hypomotility, outlet dysfunction, or both. Constipation also has been associated with pelvic floor dystonia. The use of stool softeners, increased fluid intake, food rich in fiber, and laxatives may be beneficial. Polyethylene glycol is another alternative for the treatment of severe constipation.

The urinary symptoms in CBD patients include urgency and frequency, and they may improve with the use of hyoscyamine, tolterodine or oxybutynin. Close observation for central and peripheral side-effects is warranted when using these or related medications.

Symptomatic orthostatic hypotension, although more frequently seen in MSA, may be treated with fludrocortisone or midodrine.

Other aspects of patient care, not involving pharmacotherapy, can be of special importance for these patients and their families. Physiotherapy is very helpful for maintenance of mobility and prevention of contractures. Pain related to dystonic posturing can be lessened by maintenance of good range of motion, and occasionally splinting can be helpful. Occupational therapy can help patients maintain some degree of functional independence by providing specially made devices such as eating utensils with large handles. Speech therapy may offer practical suggestions and exercises to optimize speech function and guard against aspiration secondary to swallowing difficulty. Good home care assistance can help prolong the time a patient can remain at home before requiring nursing home placement.

Despite all our best therapeutic efforts, the disease in patients with predominantly motor symptoms generally progresses to a state of bilateral rigid immobility and the patients usually die from aspiration pneumonia or urosepsis.

Acknowledgments

Suzanne S. Mirra, Randall P. Brewer, and Julie A. Schnneider contributed to this chapter in the first edition. This work was supported in part by the Emory University Parkinson Research Fund, the Sartain Lanier Family Foundation, the Mary Louise Morris Brown Foundation, the Francis Hollis Brain Foundation, and the American Parkinson Disease Association.

References

1. Rebeiz JJ, Kolodny EH, Richardson EP: Corticodentatonigral degeneration with neuronal achromasia: A progressive disorder of late adult life. *Trans Am Neurol Assoc* 92:23–26, 1967.

2. Rebeiz JJ, Kolodny EH, Richardson EP: Corticodentatonigral degeneration with neuronal achromasia. *Arch Neurol* 18:20–33, 1968.

3. Wenning GK, Litvan I, Jankovic J, et al: Natural history and survival of 14 patients with corticobasal degeneration confirmed at postmortem examination. *J Neurol Neurosurg Psychiatry* 64:184–189, 1998.

4. Watts RL, Mirra SS, Richardson EP: Corticobasal ganglionic degeneration, in Marsden CD, Fahn S (eds): *Movement Disorders 3*. London: Butterworths, 1994, pp 282–299.

5. Rinne JO, Lee MS, Thompson PD, Marsden CD: Corticobasal degeneration: A clinical study of 36 cases. *Brain* 117:1183–1196, 1994.

6. Schneider JA, Watts RL, Gearing M, et al: Corticobasal degeneration: Neuropathological and clinical heterogeneity. *Neurology* 48:959–989, 1994.

7. Stover NP, Watts RL: Corticobasal degeneration. *Semin Neurol* 21:49–58, 2001.

8. Brown J, Lantos PL, Rossor MN: Familial dementia lacking specific pathological features presenting with clinical features of corticobasal degeneration. *J Neurol Neurosurg Psychiatry* 65:600–603, 1998.

9. Verin M, Rancurel G, De Marco O, Edan G: First familial cases of corticobasal degeneration. *Mov Disord* 12:55, 1997.

10. Brown J, Lantos PL, Roques P, et al: Familial dementia with swollen achromatic neurons and corticobasal inclusion bodies: A clinical and pathological study. *J Neurol Sci* 135:21–30, 1996.

11. Di Maria E, Tabaton M, Vigo T, et al: Corticobasal degeneration shares a common genetic background with progressive supranuclear palsy. *Ann Neurol* 47:374–377, 2000.

12. Tanner CM: Epidemiologic approaches to cortical-basal ganglionic degeneration. *Mov Disord* 11:346–357, 1996.

13. Riley DE, Lang AE: Cortical-basal ganglionic degeneration, in Appel SH (ed): *Current Neurology (12)*. St. Louis: Mosby, 1992, pp 155–171.

14. Case Records of the Massachusetts General Hospital (Case 38-1985) (Case of corticonigral degeneration with neuronal achromasia). *N Engl J Med* 313:739–748, 1985.

15. Greene PE, Fahn S, Lang AE, et al: Progressive unilateral rigidity, bradykinesia, tremulousness, and apraxia, leading to fixed postural deformity of the involved limb. *Mov Disord* 5:341–351, 1990.

16. Lang AE: Parkinsonism in corticobasal degeneration. *Adv Neurol* 82:83–89, 2000.

17. Riley DE, Lang AE, Lewis A, et al: Cortical-basal ganglionic degeneration. *Neurology* 40:1203–1212, 1990.

18. Riley DE, Lang AE: Cortical-basal ganglionic degeneration, in Stern MB, Koller WC (eds): *Parkinsonian Syndromes*. New York: Marcel Dekker, 1993, pp 379–392.

19. Caselli RJ: Asymmetric cortical degeneration syndromes. *Curr Opin Neurol* 9:276–280, 1996.

20. Grimes DA, Lang AE, Bergeron CB: Dementia as the most common presentation of cortical-basal ganglionic degeneration. *Neurology* 53:1969–1974, 1999.

21. Riley DE, Lang AE: Clinical diagnostic criteria. *Adv Neurol* 82:29–34, 2000.

22. Lang AE: Corticobasal ganglionic degeneration presenting with "progressive loss of speech output and orofacial dyspraxia". *J Neurol Neurosurg Psychiatry* 55:1101, 1992.

23. Maraganore DM, Ahlskog JE, Petersen RC: Progressive asymmetric rigidity with apraxia: A distinctive clinical entity. *Mov Disord* 7:80, 1992.

24. Litvan I, Agid Y, Goetz CG, et al: Accuracy of the clinical diagnosis of corticobasal degeneration: A clinicopathologic study. *Neurology* 48:119–125, 1997.

25. Litvan I, Agid Y, Jankovic J, et al: Accuracy of clinical criteria for the diagnosis of progressive supranuclear palsy (Steele-Richardson-Olszewski syndrome). *Neurology* 46:922–930, 1996.

26. Rivest J, Quinn N, Marsden CD: Dystonia in Parkinson's disease, multiple system atrophy, and progressive supranuclear palsy. *Neurology* 40:1571–1578, 1990.

27. Collins SJ, Ahlskog JE, Parisi JE, Maraganore DM: Progressive supranuclear palsy: Neuropathologically based diagnostic clinical criteria. *J Neurol Neurosurg Psychiatry* 58:167–173, 1995.

28. Gibb WRG, Luthert PJ, Marsden CD: Corticobasal degeneration. *Brain* 112:1171–1192, 1989.

29. Case records of the Massachusetts General Hospital. Case 16-1986. *N Engl J Med* 314:1101–1111, 1986.

30. Lang AE, Riley DE, Bergeron C: Cortical-basal ganglionic degeneration, in Calne DB (ed): *Neurodegenerative Diseases*. Philadelphia: WB Saunders, 1994, pp 877–894.

31. Brunt ERP, van Weerden TW, Pruim J, Lakke JWPF: Unique myoclonic pattern in corticobasal degeneration. *Mov Disord* 10:132–142, 1995.

32. Thompson PD, Shibasaki H: Myoclonus in corticobasal degeneration and other neurodegenerations. *Adv Neurol* 82:69–81, 2000.

33. Carella F, Scaioli V, Franceschetti S, et al: Focal reflex myoclonus in corticobasal degeneration. *Funct Neurol* 6:165–170, 1991.

34. Chen R, Ashby P, Lang AE: Stimulus sensitive myoclonus in akinetic-rigid syndromes. *Brain* 115:1875–1888, 1992.

35. Thompson PD, Day BL, Rothwell JC, et al: The myoclonus of corticobasal degeneration: Evidence of two forms of corticobasal reflex myoclonus. *Brain* 117:1197–1207, 1994.

36. Piccione F, Meneghello F, Priftis K, et al: Masked myoclonus in corticobasal degeneration: Neurophysiological study of a case. *Electromyogr Clin Neurophysiol* 42:57–63, 2002.

37. Vanek ZF, Jankovic J: Dystonia in corticobasal degeneration. *Adv Neurol* 82:61–67, 2000.

38. Doody RS, Jankovic J: The alien hand and related signs. *J Neurol Neurosurg Psychiatry* 55:806–810, 1992.

39. Bogen JE: The callosal syndromes, in Heilman KM, Valenstein E (eds): *Clinical Neuropsychology*, 3rd ed. New York: Oxford University Press, 1993, pp 337–407.

40. Banks G, Short P, Martinez J, et al: The alien hand syndrome. Clinical and postmortem findings. *Arch Neurol* 46:456–459, 1989.

41. Goldberg G, Bloom KK: The alien hand sign. Localization, lateralization and recovery. *Am J Physical Med Rehab* 69:228–238, 1990.

42. Ay H, Buonanno FS, Price BH, et al: Sensory alien hand syndrome: Case report and review of the literature. *J Neurol Neurosurg Psychiatry* 65:366–369, 1998.

43. Ball JA, Lantos PL, Jackson M, et al: Alien hand sign in association with Alzheimer's histopathology. *J Neurol Neurosurg Psychiatry* 56:1020–1023, 1993.

44. Vidailhet M, Rivaud-Pechoux S: Eye movement disorders in corticobasal degeneration. *Adv Neurol* 82:161–167, 2000.

45. Rivaud-Pechoux S, Vidailhet M, Gallouedec G, et al: Longitudinal ocular motor study in corticobasal degeneration and progressive supranuclear palsy. *Neurology* 54:1029–1032, 2000.

46. Vidailhet M, Rivaud S, Gouider-Khouja N, et al: Eye movements in parkinsonian syndromes. *Ann Neurol* 35:420–426, 1994.

47. Rottach KG, Riley DE, Di Scenna AO, et al: Dynamic properties of horizontal and vertical eye movements in parkinsonian syndromes. *Ann Neurol* 39:368–377, 1996.

48. Pierrot-Deseilligny C, Rivaud S, Pillon B, et al: Lateral visually-guided saccades in progressive supranuclear palsy. *Brain* 112:471–487, 1989.

49. Jacobs DH, Boston MA, Adair JC, et al: Apraxia in corticobasal degeneration. *Neurology* 45:A266–A267, 1995.

50. Rothi LJG, Mack L, Verfaellie M, et al: Ideomotor apraxia: Error pattern analysis. *Aphasiology* 2:381–388, 1988.

51. De Renzi E, Lucchelli F: Ideational apraxia. *Brain* 111:1173–1185, 1988.

52. Poeck K: Ideational apraxia. *J Neurol* 230:1–5, 1983.

53. Okuda B, Tachibana H: The nature of apraxia in corticobasal degeneration. *J Neurol Neurosurg Psychiatry* 57:1548–1549, 1994.

54. Leiguarda R, Lees AJ, Merello M, et al: The nature of apraxia in corticobasal degeneration. *J Neurol Neurosurg Psychiatry* 57:455–459, 1994.

55. Okuda B, Tachibana H, Kawabata K, et al: Slowly progressive limb-kinetic apraxia with a decrease in unilateral cerebral blood flow. *Acta Neurol Scand* 86:76–81, 1992.

56. Otsuki M, Soma Y, Yoshimura N, Tsuji S: Slowly progressive limb-kinetic apraxia. *Eur Neurol* 37:100–103, 1997.

57. Rosenfield DB, Bogatka CJ, Viswanath NS, et al: Speech apraxia in corticobasal ganglionic degeneration. *Ann Neurol* 30:296–297, 1991.

58. Okuda B, Tanaka H, Kawabata K, et al: Truncal and limb apraxia in corticobasal degeneration. *Mov Disord* 16:760–762, 2001.

59. Ozsancak C, Auzou P, Hannequin D: Dysarthria and orofacial apraxia in corticobasal degeneration. *Mov Disord* 15:905–910, 2000.

60. Lerner A, Friedland R, Riley D, et al: Dementia with pathological findings of corticobasal ganglionic degeneration. *Ann Neurol* 32:271, 1992.

61. Green J: Neuropsychological profiles in corticobasal degeneration, in Green J (ed): *Neuropsychological Evaluation of the Older Adult*. New York: Academic Press, 2000, pp 142–143.

62. Massman PJ, Kreiter KT, Jankovic J, Doody RS: Neuropsychological distinction between corticobasal ganglionic degeneration and Alzheimer's disease with extrapyramidal signs. *Neurology* 44:194–195, 1994.

63. Massman PJ, Kreiter KT, Jankovic J, Doody RS: Neuropsychological functioning in cortical-basal ganglionic degeneration: Differentiation from Alzheimer's disease. *Neurology* 46:720–726, 1996.

64. Dubois B, Pillon B: Cognitive and behavioral aspects of movement disorders, in Jankovic J, Tolosa E (eds): *Parkinson's Disease and Movement Disorders*, 3rd ed. Baltimore: Williams & Wilkins, 1998, pp 837–858.

65. Litvan I, Cummings JL, Mega M: Neuropsychiatric features of corticobasal degeneration. *J Neurol Neurosurg Psychiatry* 65:717–721, 1998.

66. Cummings JL, Litvan I: Neuropsychiatric aspects of corticobasal degeneration. *Adv Neurol* 82:147–152, 2000.

67. Pillon B, Blin J, Vidailhet M, et al: The neuropsychological pattern of corticobasal degeneration: Comparison with progressive

supranuclear palsy and Alzheimer's disease. *Neurology* 45:1477–1483, 1995.

68. Bergeron C, Davis A, Lang AE: Corticobasal ganglionic degeneration and progressive supranuclear palsy presenting with cognitive decline. *Brain Pathol* 8:355–365, 1998.

69. Beatty WW, Scott JG, Wilson DA, et al: Memory deficits in a demented patient with probable corticobasal degeneration. *J Geriatr Psychiatry Neurol* 8:132–136, 1995.

70. Cummings JL, Mega M, Gray K, et al: The Neuropsychiatric Inventory: Comprehensive assessment of psychopathology in dementia. *Neurology* 44:2308–2314, 1994.

71. Levy ML, Miller BL, Cummings JL, et al: Alzheimer disease and frontotemporal dementias. Behavioral distinctions. *Arch Neurol* 53:687–690, 1996.

72. Mega MS, Cummings JL, Fiorello T, Gornbein J: The spectrum of behavioral changes in Alzheimer's disease. *Neurology* 46:130–135, 1996.

73. Frattali CM, Sonies BC: Speech and swallowing disturbances in corticobasal degeneration. *Adv Neurol* 82:153–160, 2000.

74. Duffy J: *Motor Speech Disorders: Substrates, Differential Diagnosis, and Management.* St. Louis: Mosby, 1995.

75. Darley FL, Aronson AE, Brown JR: *Motor Speech Disorders.* Philadelphia: WB Saunders, 1975.

76. Watts RL, William RS, Growdon JH, et al: Corticobasal ganglionic degeneration. *Neurology* 35:178, 1985.

77. Savoiardo M, Grisoli M, Girotti F: Magnetic resonance imaging in CBD, related atypical parkinsonian disorders, and dementias. *Adv Neurol* 82:197–208, 2000.

78. Schrag A, Good CD, Miszkiel K, et al: Differentiation of atypical parkinsonian syndromes with routine MRI. *Neurology* 54:697–702, 2000.

79. Yamauchi H, Fukuyama H, Nagahama Y, et al: Atrophy of the corpus callosum, cortical hypometabolism, and cognitive impairment in corticobasal degeneration. *Arch Neurol* 55:609–614, 1998.

80. Savoiardo M, Girotti F, Strada L, et al: Magnetic resonance imaging in progressive supranuclear palsy and other parkinsonian disorders. *J Neural Transm* 42:93–110, 1994.

81. Savoiardo M, Strada L, Girotti F, et al: MR imaging in progressive supranuclear palsy and Shy-Drager syndrome. *J Comput Assist Tomogr* 13:555–560, 1989.

82. Schonfeld SM, Golbe LI, Sage JI, et al: Computed tomographic findings in progressive supranuclear palsy: Correlation with clinical grade. *Mov Disord* 2:263–278, 1987.

83. Brooks DJ: Functional imaging studies in corticobasal degeneration. *Adv Neurol* 82:209–215, 2000.

84. Nagahama Y, Fukuyama H, Turjanski N, et al: Cerebral glucose metabolism in corticobasal degeneration: Comparison with progressive supranuclear palsy and normal controls. *Mov Disord* 12:691–696, 1997.

85. Sawle GV, Brooks DJ, Marsden CD, Frackowiak RS: Corticobasal degeneration. A unique pattern of regional cortical oxygen hypometabolism and striatal fluorodopa uptake demonstrated by positron emission tomography. *Brain* 114:541–556, 1991.

86. Okuda B, Tachibana H, Kawabata K, et al: Cerebral blood flow correlates of higher brain dysfunctions in corticobasal degeneration. *J Geriatr Psychiatry Neurol* 12:189–193, 1999.

87. Laureys S, Salmon E, Garraux G, et al: Fluorodopa uptake and glucose metabolism in early stages of corticobasal degeneration. *J Neurol* 246:1151–1158, 1999.

88. Blin J, Vidailhet MJ, Pillon B, et al: Corticobasal degeneration: Decreased and asymmetrical glucose consumption as studied with PET. *Mov Disord* 7:348–354, 1992.

89. Nagasawa H, Tanji H, Nomura H, et al: PET study of cerebral glucose metabolism and fluorodopa uptake in patients with corticobasal degeneration. *J Neurol Sci* 139:210–217, 1996.

90. Schwarz J, Tatsch K, Gasser T, et al: 123I-IBZM binding compared with long-term clinical follow up in patients with de novo parkinsonism. *Mov Disord* 13:16–19, 1998.

91. Sawle GV, Brooks DJ, Thompson PD, et al: PET studies on the dopaminergic system and regional cortical metabolism in corticobasal degeneration. *Neurology* 39:163, 1989.

92. Eidelberg D, Moeller JR, Sidtis JJ, et al: Corticodentatonigral degeneration: Metabolic asymmetries studied with 18F-fluorodeoxyglucose and positron emission tomography. *Neurology* 39:164, 1989.

93. Eidelberg D, Dhawan V, Moeller JR, et al: The metabolic landscape of corticobasal ganglionic degeneration: Regional asymmetries studied with positron emission tomography. *J Neurol Neurosurg Psychiatry* 54:856–862, 1991.

94. Blin J, Vidailhet M, Bonnet AM, et al: PET study in corticobasal degeneration. *Mov Disord* 5:19, 1990.

95. Brooks DJ: PET studies on the early and differential diagnosis of Parkinson's disease. *Neurology* 43:S6–16, 1993.

96. Marek K, Seibyl J, Fussell B, et al: Dopamine transporter imaging in Parkinson disease and Parkinson plus syndromes. *Mov Disord* 10:3, 1995.

97. Frisoni GB, Pizzolato G, Zanetti O, et al: Corticobasal degeneration: Neuropsychological assessment and dopamine D2 receptor SPECT analysis. *Eur Neurol* 35:50–54, 1995.

98. Turjanski N, Lees AJ, Brooks DJ: In vivo studies on striatal dopamine D1 and D2 site binding in l-dopa-treated Parkinson's disease patients with and without dyskinesias. *Neurology* 49:717–723, 1997.

99. Kish SJ, Shannak K, Hornykiewicz O: Uneven pattern of dopamine loss in the striatum of patients with idiopathic Parkinson's disease. Pathophysiologic and clinical implications. *N Engl J Med* 318:876–880, 1988.

100. Burn DJ, Sawle GV, Brooks DJ: Differential diagnosis of Parkinson's disease, multiple system atrophy, and Steele-Richardson-Olszewski syndrome: discriminant analysis of striatal 18F-dopa PET data. *J Neurol Neurosurg Psychiatry* 57:278–284, 1994.

101. Brooks DJ: Functional imaging in relation to parkinsonian syndromes. *J Neurol Sci* 115:1–17, 1993.

102. Markus HS, Lees AJ, Lennox G, et al: Patterns of regional cerebral blood flow in corticobasal degeneration studied using HMPAO SPECT: Comparison with Parkinson's disease and normal controls. *Mov Disord* 10:179–187, 1995.

103. Tedeschi G, Litvan I, Bonavita S, et al: Proton magnetic resonance spectroscopic imaging in progressive supranuclear palsy, Parkinson's disease and corticobasal degeneration. *Brain* 120:1541–1552, 1997.

104. Takeda M, Tachibana H, Okuda B, et al: Electrophysiological comparison between corticobasal degeneration and progressive supranuclear palsy. *Clin Neurol Neurosurg* 100:94–98, 1998.

105. Okuda B, Tachibana H, Takeda M, et al: Asymmetric changes in somatosensory evoked potentials correlate with limb apraxia in corticobasal degeneration. *Acta Neurol Scand* 97:409–412, 1998.

106. Homma A, Harayama H, Kondo H, et al: P300 findings in patients with corticobasal degeneration. *Brain Nerve* 48:925–929, 1996.

107. Dickson DW, Bergeron C, Chin SS, et al: Office of Rare Diseases of the National Institutes of Health, Office of Rare Diseases neuropathologic criteria for corticobasal degeneration. *J Neuropathol Exp Neurol* 61:935–946, 2002.

108. Dickson DW, Litvan I: Corticobasal degeneration, in Dickson DW (ed): *Neurodegeneration: The Molecular Pathology of Dementia and Movement Disorder.* Neuropath Press, 2003, pp 115–123.

109. Lowe J, Leigh N: Disorders of movement and system degenerations, in Graham D, Lantos P (eds): *Greenfield's Neuropathology.* New York: Gray Publishing, 2002, pp 325–430.

110. Feany MB, Dickson DW: Widespread cytoskeletal pathology characterizes corticobasal degeneration. *Am J Pathol* 146:1388–1396, 1995.

111. Bergeron C, Pollanen MS, Weyer L, et al: Unusual clinical presentations of cortico-basal ganglionic degeneration. *Ann Neurol* 40:893–900, 1996.

112. Ikeda K, Akiyama H, Iritani S, et al: Corticobasal degeneration with primary progressive aphasia and accentuated cortical lesion in superior temporal gyrus: Case report and review. *Act Neuropathol* 92:534–539, 1996.

113. Mirra SS, Hyman B: Aging and dementia, in Graham D, Lantos P (eds): *Greenfield's Neuropathology.* New York: Gray Publishing, 2002, pp 195–271.

114. Nakazato Y, Hirato J, Ishida Y, et al: Swollen cortical neurons in Creutzfeldt-Jakob disease contain a phosphorylated neuro-filament epitope. *J Neuropathol Exp Neurol* 49:197–205, 1990.

115. Mackenzie IRA, Hudson LP: Achromatic neurons in the cortex of progressive supranuclear palsy. *Acta Neuropathol* 90:615–619, 1995.

116. Manetto V, Sternberger NH, Perry G, et al: Phosphorylation of neurofilaments is altered in amyotrophic lateral sclerosis. *J Neuropathol Exp Neurol* 47:642–653, 1988.

117. Dickson DW: Neuropathology of Parkinsonism, in Pahwa R, Lyons KE, Koller WC (eds): *Handbook of Parkinson's Disease.* New York: Marcel Dekker, 2003, pp 203–220.

118. Ksiezak-Reding H, Morgan K, Mattiace LA, et al: Ultrastructure and biochemical composition of paired helical filaments in corticobasal degeneration. *Am J Pathol* 145:1496–1508, 1994.

119. Delacourte A, Buee L: Normal and pathological tau proteins as factors for microtubule assembly. *Int Rev Cytol* 171:167–224, 1997.

120. Buee L, Delacourte A: Comparative biochemistry of tau in progressive supranuclear palsy, corticobasal degeneration, FTDP-17 and Pick's disease. *Brain Pathol* 9:681–693, 1999.

121. Arvanitakis Z, Wszolek ZK: Recent advances in the understanding of tau protein and movement disorders. *Curr Opin Neurol* 14:491–497, 2001.

122. Dickson DW: Tau and synuclein and their role in neuropathology. *Brain Pathol* 9:657–661, 1999.

123. Bancher C, Brunner C, Lassmann H, et al: Accumulation of abnormally phosphorylated tau precedes the formation of neurofibrillary tangles in Alzheimer's disease. *Brain Res* 477:90–99, 1989.

124. Tellez-Nagel I, Wisniewski H: Ultrastructure of neurofibrillary tangles in Steele Richardson-Olszewski syndrome. *Arch Neurol* 29:324–327, 1973.

125. Komori T: Tau-positive glial inclusions in progressive supranuclear palsy, corticobasal degeneration and Pick's disease. *Brain Pathol* 9:663–679, 1999.

126. Wakabayashi K, Yoshimoto M, Tsuji S, et al: Alpha-synuclein immunoreactivity in glial cytoplasmic inclusions in multiple system atrophy. *Neurosci Lett* 249:180–182, 1998.

127. Rosso SM, van Swieten JC: New developments in frontotemporal dementia and parkinsonism linked to chromosome 17. *Curr Opin Neurol* 15:423–428, 2002.

128. Togo T, Sahara N, Yen SH, et al: Argyrophilic grain disease is a sporadic 4-repeat tauopathy. *J Neuropathol Exp Neurol* 61:547–556, 2002.

129. Dickson DW: Neuropathologic differentiation of progressive supranuclear palsy and corticobasal degeneration. *J Neurol* 246:II6–15, 1999.

130. Matsusaka H, Ikeda K, Akiyama H, et al: Astrocytic pathology in progressive supranuclear palsy: Significance for neuropathological diagnosis. *Acta Neuropathol* 96:248–252, 1998.

131. Baker M, Litvan I, Houlden H, et al: Association of an extended haplotype in the tau gene with progressive supranuclear palsy. *Hum Mol Genet* 8:711–715, 1999.

132. Houlden H, Baker M, Morris HR, et al: Corticobasal degeneration and progressive supranuclear palsy share a common tau haplotype. *Neurology* 56:1702–1706, 2001.

133. Pollanen MS, Dickson DW, Bergeron C: Pathology and biology of the Lewy body. *J Neuropathol Exp Neurol* 52:183–191, 1993.

134. Mattila PM, Rinne JO, Helenius H, et al: Alpha-synuclein-immunoreactive cortical Lewy bodies are associated with cognitive impairment in Parkinson's disease. *Acta Neuropathol* 100:285–290, 2000.

135. Hurtig HI, Trojanowski JQ, Galvin J, et al: Alpha-synuclein cortical Lewy bodies correlate with dementia in Parkinson's disease. *Neurology* 54:1916–1921, 2000.

136. Haroutunian V, Serby M, Purohit DP, et al: Contribution of Lewy body inclusions to dementia in patients with and without Alzheimer disease neuropathological conditions. *Arch Neurol* 57:1145–1150, 2000.

137. Dickson DW: Alzheimer-Parkinson disease overlap: neuropathology, in Clark CM, Trojanowski JQ (eds): *Neurodegenerative Dementias: Clinical Features and Pathological Mechanism.* New York: McGraw-Hill, 2000, pp 247–259.

138. Hamilton RL: Lewy bodies in Alzheimer's disease: A neuropathological review of 145 cases using alpha-synuclein immunohistochemistry. *Brain Pathol* 10:378–384, 2000.

139. Dickson DW, Corral A, Lin W: Alzheimer's disease with amygdaloid Lewy bodies: A form of Lewy body disease distinct from AD and diffuse Lewy body disease. *Neurology* 54:A451, 2000.

140. Arai Y, Yamazaki M, Mori O, et al: Alpha-synuclein-positive structures in cases with sporadic Alzheimer's disease: Morphology and its relationship to tau aggregation. *Brain Res* 888:287–296, 2001.

141. Marui W, Iseki E, Ueda K, et al: Occurrence of human alpha-synuclein immunoreactive neurons with neurofibrillary tangle formation in the limbic areas of patients with Alzheimer's disease. *J Neurol Sci* 174:81–84, 2000.

142. Masliah E, Rockenstein E, Veinbergs I, et al: Beta-amyloid peptides enhance alpha-synuclein accumulation and neuronal deficits in a transgenic mouse model linking Alzheimer's disease and Parkinson's disease. *Proc Natl Acad Sci U S A* 98:12245–12250, 2001.

143. Braak H, Braak E: Cortical and subcortical argyrophilic grains characterize a disease associated with adult onset dementia. *Neuropathol Appl Neurobiol* 15:13–26, 1989.

144. Jellinger KA: Dementia with grains (argyrophilic grain disease). *Brain Pathol* 8:377–386, 1998.

145. Trojanowski JQ, Dickson D: Update on the neuropathological diagnosis of frontotemporal dementias. *J Neuropathol Exp Neurol* 60:1123–1126, 2001.

146. Giannakopoulos P, Hof PR, Bouras C: Dementia lacking distinctive histopathology: Clinicopathological evaluation of 32 cases. *Act Neuropathol* 89:346–355, 1995.

147. Strittmatter WJ, Saunders AM, Schmechel D, et al: Apolipoprotein E: High avidity binding to beta-amyloid and increased frequency of type 4 allele in late onset familial Alzheimer's disease. *Proc Natl Acad Sci U S A* 90:1977–1981, 1993.

148. Corder EH, Saunders AM, Strittmatter WJ, et al: Gene dose of apolipoprotein E type 4 allele and the risk of Alzheimer's disease in late onset families. *Science* 261:921–923, 1993.

149. Steele JC, Richardson JC, Olszewski J: Progressive supranuclear palsy. *Arch Neurol* 10:333–358, 1964.

150. Adams RD, Van Bogaert L, Vander Eecken H: Striatonigral degeneration. *J Neuropathol Exp Neurol* 23:584–608, 1964.

151. Takei Y, Mirra SS: Striatonigral degeneration: A form of multiple system atrophy with clinical parkinsonism. *Prog Neuropathol* 2:217–251, 1973.

152. Spokes EGS, Bannister R, Oppenheimer DR: Multiple system atrophy with autonomic failure. *J Neurol Sci* 43:59–82, 1979.

153. Wenning GK, Ben Shlomo Y, Magalhaes M, et al: Clinical features and natural history of multiple system atrophy. An analysis of 100 cases. *Brain* 117:835–845, 1994.

154. Jendroska K, Rossor MN, Mathias CJ, Daniel SE: Morphological overlap between corticobasal degeneration and Pick's disease: A clinicopathological report. *Mov Disord* 10:111–114, 1995.

155. Lang AE, Bergeron C, Pollanen MS, Ashby P: Parietal Pick's disease mimicking cortical-basal ganglionic degeneration. *Neurology* 44:1436–1440, 1994.

156. Cole M, Wright D, Banker BQ: Familial aphasia due to Pick's disease. *Ann Neurol* 6:158, 1979.

157. Wojcieszek J, Lang AE, Jankovic J, et al: Rapidly progressive aphasia, apraxia, dementia, myoclonus and parkinsonism. *Mov Disord* 9:358–366, 1994.

158. Molsa PK, Marttila RJ, Rinne UK: Extrapyramidal signs in Alzheimer's disease. *Neurology* 34:1114–1116, 1984.

159. Chui HC, Teng EL, Henderson VW, Moy AC: Clinical subtypes of dementia of the Alzheimer type. *Neurology* 35:1544–1550, 1985.

160. Hirano A, Kurland LT, Krooth RS, et al: Parkinsonism-dementia complex, an endemic disease on the Island of Guam. I. Clinical features. *Brain* 84:642–661, 1961.

161. Hirano A, Malamud M, Kurland LT: Parkinsonism-dementia complex on the Island of Guam. II. Pathological features. *Brain* 84:662–679, 1961.

162. Wilson SAK: Lenticular degeneration. *Brain* 34:295–321, 1912.

163. Bruyn GW: The Westphal variant and juvenile type of Huntington's chorea, in Barbeau A, Brunette JR (eds): *Progress in Neurogenetics*. Amsterdam: Excerpta Medica, 1967, pp 666–673.

164. Giladi N, Fahn S: Hemiparkinsonism-hemiatrophy syndrome may mimic early-stage cortical-basal ganglionic degeneration. *Mov Disord* 7:384–385, 1992.

165. Zimmerman RD, Fleming CA, Lee BC, et al: Periventricular hyperintensity as seen by magnetic resonance: Prevalence and significance. *Am J Roentgenol* 146:443–450, 1986.

166. Okeda R, Matsuo T, Kawahara Y, et al: Adult pigment type (Pfeiffer) of sudanophilic leukodystrophy. Pathological and morphometrical studies on two autopsy cases of siblings. *Acta Neuropathol* 78:533–542, 1989.

167. Gray F, Destee A, Bourre JM, et al: Pigmentary type of orthochromatic leukodystrophy (OLD): A new case with ultrastructural and biochemical study. *J Neuropathol Exp Neurol* 46:585–596, 1987.

168. Pietrini V, Tagliavini F, Pilleri G, et al: Orthochromatic leukodystrophy with pigmented glial cells. An adult case with clinical-anatomical study. *Acta Neurol Scand* 59:140–147, 1979.

169. Bhatia KP, Morris JH, Frackowiak RS: Primary progressive multifocal leukoencephalopathy presenting as an extrapyramidal syndrome. *J Neurol* 243:91–95, 1996.

170. Nakano KK, Dawson DM, Spence A: Machado disease: A hereditary ataxia in Portuese emigrants to Massachusetts. *Neurology* 22:49–55, 1972.

171. Romanul FCA, Fowler HL, Radvany J, et al: Azorean disease of the nervous system. *N Engl J Med* 296:1505–1508, 1977.

172. Sachdev HS, Forno LS, Kane CA: Joseph disease: A multisystem degenerative disorder of the nervous system. *Neurology* 32:192–195, 1982.

173. Jankovic J, Kirkpatrick JB, Blonquist KA, et al: Late onset Halloverden-Spatz disease presenting as familial parkinsonism. *Neurology* 35:227–234, 1985.

174. Kritchevsky N, Hansen LA, Deteresa R, et al: Slowly progressive ideomotor apraxia: A presentation of adult onset Halloverden-Spatz disease. *Neurology* 39:237, 1989.

175. Martin JJ: Adult type of neuronal ceroid lipofuscinosis. *Dev Neurosci* 13:331–338, 1991.

176. Cannard KR, Galvez-Jimenez N, Watts RL: Creutzfeldt-Jakob disease presenting and evolving as rapidly progressive corticobasal degeneration. *Neurology* 50:A95, 1998.

177. Kompoliti K, Goetz CG, Boeve BF, et al: Clinical presentation and pharmacological therapy in corticobasal degeneration. *Arch Neurol* 55:957–961, 1998.

178. Parati EA, Fetoni V, Geminiani GC, et al: Response to L-DOPA in multiple system atrophy. *Clin Neuropharmacol* 16:139–144, 1993.

179. Hughes AJ, Colosimo C, Kleedorfer B, et al: The dopaminergic response in multiple system atrophy. *J Neurol Neurosurg Psychiatry* 55:1009–1013, 1992.

180. Fazzini E, Dogali M, Beric A, et al: The effects of unilateral ventral posterior medial pallidotomy in patients with Parkinson's disease and Parkinson's plus syndromes, in Koller WC, Paulson G (eds): *Therapy of Parkinson's Disease*. New York: Marcel Dekker, 1995, pp 353–379.

181. Cantello R: Applications of transcranial magnetic stimulation in movement disorders. *J Clin Neurophysiol* 19:272–293, 2002.

WILSON'S DISEASE

RONALD F. PFEIFFER

EPIDEMIOLOGY AND GENETICS 779
PATHOPHYSIOLOGY 780
CLINICAL FEATURES 780
   Hepatic Manifestations 780
   Neurological Manifestations 781
   Psychiatric Manifestations 782
   Ophthalmologic Manifestations 783
   Musculoskeletal Manifestations 783
   Other Manifestations 784
DIAGNOSIS 784
   Liver Biopsy 785
   Slit-Lamp Examination 786
   Ceruloplasmin 786
   24-Hour Urinary Copper Excretion 786
   Serum Copper 786
   Free (Nonceruloplasmin-Bound) Copper 786
   Radiocopper Incorporation 786
   CSF Copper 787
   Neuroimaging Studies 787
TESTING GUIDELINES 787
TREATMENT 787
   Dietary Therapy 787
   Inhibition of Intestinal Copper Absorption 788
   Copper-Chelation Therapy 789
   Liver Transplantation 790
TREATMENT GUIDELINES 791
SUMMARY 791

In 1912, Wilson penned, as his doctoral thesis, his now classic treatise describing the clinical and pathological features of the disease he labeled progressive hepatolenticular degeneration.[1] He was not, however, the first to describe the illness that now bears his name. Case descriptions of what likely was Wilson's disease (WD) were published by Frerichs in 1860,[2] Westphal in 1885,[3] Gowers in 1888,[4] Ormerod in 1890,[5] Homen in 1892,[6] and Strümpell in 1898,[7] but it was Wilson who accurately and in exhausting detail delineated the characteristics of this illness and distilled the information into a coherent clinical picture.

Since Wilson's description, our present-day understanding of WD has evolved and matured, with contributions from many individuals. Kayser in 1902[8] and Fleischer in 1903 and 1912[9,10] first described the rings of corneal pigmentation that are now so firmly linked with WD. Although Rumpel first described increased hepatic copper content in WD in 1913,[11] it was not until 1948, when Mandelbrote et al.[12] noted increased urinary excretion of copper and Cumings[13]

documented copper deposits in both liver and brain, that WD was finally recognized as a disturbance of copper metabolism. Ceruloplasmin deficiency was subsequently documented independently by Scheinberg and Gitlin[14] and by Bearn and Kunkel[15] in 1952. The presence of impaired biliary excretion of copper in WD was first reported by Frommer in 1974.[16] The last 5 decades have been marked by dramatic advances in our ability to treat WD, and the last 10 years have witnessed the identification and characterization of the genetic abnormality responsible for WD.

Epidemiology and Genetics

Although not recognized by Wilson himself—he noted it to be familial but believed that a toxin was the likely cause—WD was identified as an hereditary process by Hall in 1921.[17] It is an autosomal-recessive disease. Estimates of prevalence vary widely, but WD is by all accounts a rare disorder. A prevalence rate of 30 cases per million is often quoted,[18] but other lower estimates have also been published. A birth incidence rate of 17 per million (1 per 59,000) was reported in Ireland for the years 1950–1969;[19] others report incidence rates in the range of 1 per 30,000–40,000.[20,21] It has been estimated that there are approximately 6000 cases of WD in the US and that approximately 1 percent of the population are carriers.[20]

In 1985, Frydman et al. proposed chromosome 13 as the location of the mutation responsible for WD.[22] This was subsequently confirmed in 1993, when several groups of investigators specifically localized, identified, and characterized the gene, now labeled the WND or ATP7B gene, which maps to 13q14.3 and covers a region of almost 100 kilobase (kb), with 22 exons.[23–26] The protein encoded by the gene, also known as ATP7B or WNDP, has been identified as a copper-transporting ATPase that binds 6 copper molecules[27,28] and is expressed primarily in liver and kidney. Two specific functions have been proposed for ATP7B (WNDP). Under basal or steady-state conditions the protein is found primarily in the trans-Golgi network in hepatocytes, where it transports copper across organelle membranes so that the copper can be incorporated into ceruloplasmin.[29] Under high copper conditions, however, ATP7B is redistributed to cytoplasmic vesicles where it transports excess copper across the hepatocyte apical membrane into the bile canaliculus for subsequent biliary excretion.[30,31] In WD, mutation at the ATP7B locus results in defective ATP7B protein that is not capable of performing these functions.

WD is an autosomal-recessive disorder in which the affected individual must receive a defective copy of the gene from each parent. It has become abundantly clear, however, that no single mutation of the ATP7B gene is responsible for all cases of WD. In fact, over 200 different mutations have now been documented in WD patients and it is likely that this number will continue to grow. While missense mutations are most frequent, deletions, insertions, nonsense, and splice-site mutations all occur.[32] Most individuals with WD are actually compound heterozygotes, having inherited different mutations from each parent. In the US and in individuals of northern European origin, the most frequent mutation appears to be the H1069Q mutation in exon 14 in which glutamine is substituted for histidine, but this mutation accounts for only 28–45 percent of the identified mutations in these groups.[20,33,34] It is this mutational heterogeneity that has made the development of commercially viable genetic testing for WD impractical at this time.

It has been speculated that the genotypic variability in WD may also play a role in the phenotypic variability so characteristic of WD, but studies have not clearly borne this out. It appears that additional factors must also be operative, since even individuals with the same mutation may vary widely in age of symptom onset and clinical presentation.[35]

Pathophysiology

As a vital component of enzyme systems such as cytochrome c oxidase, dopamine beta-hydroxylase, superoxide dismutase and tyrosinase, copper is an essential element for cellular functioning.[36] On its own, however, free copper is an extremely toxic substance that can produce irreversible cellular damage and death. To protect against such injury, elegant systems have evolved that bind the copper molecule so that it can be safely absorbed, proper amounts can be transported to required sites, and excess copper can be eliminated from the body. When these delivery systems malfunction, cellular damage and death can result, either from too much or too little copper.

First isolated in 1948, ceruloplasmin is an α2-glycoprotein that binds and transports 6 copper molecules.[37] It also has ferroxidase activity and may play a role in iron metabolism.[36,38] There are actually multiple forms of ceruloplasmin, with molecular weights varying from 115,000 to 200,000.[39] Although ceruloplasmin is characteristically decreased in WD, this is not absolute and WD is not, in its essence, a disease of ceruloplasmin deficiency. In fact, 5–15 percent of individuals with WD may have normal or only slightly reduced ceruloplasmin, whereas 10–20 percent of heterozygotes who are clinically asymptomatic may have reduced ceruloplasmin.[40] Ceruloplasmin deficiency in WD is probably the consequence of reduced copper availability during ceruloplasmin synthesis because of reduced or defective ATP7B. The ceruloplasmin gene itself is on chromosome 3[41] and is normal in WD.

Ceruloplasmin deficiency is not unique to WD. It is also characteristic of Menkes' disease. An hereditary ceruloplasmin deficiency, now labeled aceruloplasminemia, has also been described and is characterized by only modest hepatic copper accumulation, but dramatic iron deposition in liver, pancreas, and brain.[42,43] Transient ceruloplasmin deficiency may occur in a variety of conditions, including protein-losing enteropathy, nephrotic syndrome, sprue, as well as other situations in which both protein and calorie intake are deficient.[40] Ceruloplasmin deficiency also can be found in patients with chronic liver disease of any cause, including hepatitis C infection.[44]

The primary route of elimination of copper is the gastrointestinal tract.[45] Copper is also excreted in the urine, but this is normally only a secondary route. It has been firmly established that impairment of gastrointestinal elimination of copper is the fundamental basis of copper accumulation in WD. Copper is routinely secreted in saliva, gastric juice, and bile, but the copper from salivary and gastric sources is reabsorbed more distally in the gut, leaving biliary excretion as the primary source of copper elimination.[46,47] As noted above, the fundamental abnormality that characterizes WD is impaired biliary excretion of copper because of the genetically determined deficiency or defective function of ATP7B. This defect in biliary excretion of copper results in slow, but steady accumulation of copper in the body. Initially, the copper is stored in the liver, but eventually the storage capacity of the liver is exceeded and unbound copper spills out of the liver and finds its way to other organs and tissues, where it also begins to accumulate. As the excess copper escapes from the liver, urinary copper excretion markedly increases but is not able to fully compensate for the defect in biliary excretion. This results in a positive copper balance, with consequent relentless deposition of copper in other tissues.

Clinical Features

Although the fundamental pathogenetic defect in WD has its source in the hepatobiliary system, the consequences of the defect play themselves out in multiple organs and systems. This multisystem involvement lends itself to an extremely diverse clinical picture that, at times, presents a formidable diagnostic challenge for even the most astute clinician.

HEPATIC MANIFESTATIONS

Hepatic symptoms or signs of hepatic dysfunction are the most frequent mode of clinical presentation of WD, representing the initial feature in approximately 40–50 percent of cases (Table 47-1).[20,48] This percentage is even higher in Asian populations.[49] The average age of onset for individuals with WD who present with hepatic symptoms is 11.4 years.[50]

TABLE 47-1 Hepatic Manifestations of WD

Asymptomatic spleen and liver enlargement
Acute transient hepatitis
Chronic hepatitis
Acute fulminant hepatitis
Progressive cirrhosis

It is rare for hepatic symptoms to appear before age 6; hepatic presentation beyond age 40 is unusual, but in one center's experience 17 percent of patients were over age 40 at the time of diagnosis.[51]

Hepatic dysfunction in WD can follow one of several routes in its evolution. There may simply be asymptomatic enlargement of both liver and spleen. Liver function tests, however, may be elevated and spider angiomata may appear.

Acute transient hepatitis is a second, more common, mode of presentation. This occurs in 25 percent of individuals and is typically characterized by jaundice, anorexia, and easy fatigability with a reduced sense of energy. This may be all too easily passed off as a viral-induced hepatitis or infectious mononucleosis, especially when family history is silent. However, the concomitant presence of a hemolytic anemia should serve as an important portent of the presence of WD.[20] Other abnormalities that may also be clues to a diagnosis of WD in this setting include elevated unconjugated (indirect) bilirubin and reduced uric acid.

A picture indistinguishable from autoimmune hepatitis (chronic active hepatitis) occurs in 10–30 percent of individuals with WD.[52,53] One diagnostically treacherous aspect of this presentation of WD is the potential for the serum ceruloplasmin, as an acute-phase reactant, to become "elevated" into the low normal range.[20,52]

Acute, fulminant hepatitis, with rapidly progressive liver failure, encephalopathy, and coagulopathy is yet another potential mode of hepatic presentation of WD. It carries with it an extremely high mortality rate. Individuals presenting in this fashion typically are younger than age 30, often in their teens; two-thirds are female.[54] A severe Coombs-negative hemolytic anemia, presumably as a result of intravascular hemolysis precipitated by the sudden release of hepatic copper into the bloodstream, is often present.[55] In contrast to fulminant hepatic failure in the setting of viral hepatitis, alkaline phosphatase and even aminotransferase levels are often disproportionately low, while bilirubin may be disproportionately elevated because of the hemolysis.[20,56,57]

The most frequent hepatic manifestation of WD is the development of progressive cirrhosis. Individuals typically develop slowly progressive hepatic failure with splenomegaly (with or without hepatomegaly), ascites, esophageal varices, and encephalopathy. There are no specific identifying characteristics of the cirrhosis.

Because of the absence of any pathognomonic clinical characteristics of hepatic dysfunction due to WD, any individual under age 50 with unexplained liver disease, whether viral negative hepatitis, chronic hepatitis, cirrhosis or acute fulminant hepatic failure, should be screened for WD.[20]

NEUROLOGICAL MANIFESTATIONS

Left untreated, most individuals with WD will eventually develop symptoms or signs of neurological dysfunction (Table 47-2). In 40–60 percent of affected persons, however, neurological symptoms are actually the initially recognized

TABLE 47-2 Neurological Manifestations of WD

Frequently present
  Tremor
  Dysarthria
  Cerebellar dysfunction
  Dystonia
  Gait abnormality
Occasionally present
  Autonomic dysfunction
  Headache
  Seizures
  Sleep disturbances
  Muscle cramps
  Pseudobulbar emotional lability
Typically absent
  Upper motor neuron dysfunction
    Weakness
    Spasticity
    Hyperreflexia
    Babinski response
  Lower motor neuron dysfunction
    Hyporeflexia
  Sensory loss
  Sphincter dysfunction

clinical feature.[20,48] As might be suspected from the pathophysiology of WD, the average age at which neurological features appear is significantly later than the average age of onset of hepatic WD manifestations (18.9 years versus 11.4 years), although neurological symptoms have been reported as early as age 6.[58] Although it is also infrequent, onset of neurological dysfunction after age 50 may also occur.[20,59]

Tremor is the most frequent neurological presenting feature in WD, occurring in approximately 50 percent of individuals.[60] The tremor may be resting, postural or kinetic in character. Asymmetry is the rule. The tremor may be fine or coarse, proximal or distal. A proximal component of tremor in the arms can endow the tremor with a "wing-beating" appearance. Head titubation may also be present. An unusual presentation of tremor in WD is isolated tongue tremor.[61,62] The importance of considering WD in the differential diagnosis of tremor presenting in young persons, even when the family history does not seem to be compatible with a recessive disorder, has recently been stressed.[63]

Dysarthria is another common feature of neurological WD, eventually developing in the vast majority of patients. Two broad categories of dysarthria have been described.[43] A hypokinetic dysarthria resulting from extrapyramidal dysfunction, particularly dystonia, affecting the tongue, face, and pharynx, commonly occurs. Speech can be severely compromised. The dysarthria can become so severe that the patient becomes virtually mute. Drooling, another frequent feature of WD, is also a consequence of the dystonia, as is the "risus sardonicus," or fixed grimace-smile, seen in some individuals with WD. An unusual "whispering dysphonia" has also been described in WD,[64] as has a very unusual laugh in which most of the sound is generated during inspiration.[65] The second type of dysarthria observed in WD is cerebellar in character, typified by scanning, explosive speech. It is the result of cerebellar and brainstem involvement.

Cerebellar dysfunction, which initially gave rise to the term "pseudosclerotic" as a type of WD, is seen in approximately 25 percent of WD patients with neurological dysfunction.[66] In addition to the scanning speech described above, individuals may display impaired coordination and kinetic (intention) tremor as part of the clinical picture. Deterioration of handwriting is often evident.

Dystonia, which can involve limbs and trunk in addition to the facial and pharyngeal muscles noted above, is seen quite frequently in WD, affecting 37 percent of patients in one series.[67] Chorea is uncommon in WD; both tics and myoclonus are very unusual.

Gait abnormalities are another hallmark of WD. As with dysarthria, both extrapyramidal and cerebellar patterns of impairment have been described. An individual with WD may display a parkinsonian gait, a wide-based ataxic gait, or a combination of the two.

Seizures have been reported in up to 6 percent of patients with WD, especially in younger individuals.[68] The combination of seizures and psychiatric disturbances may indicate the presence of frontal white matter lesions.[69] Pseudobulbar emotional lability,[70] hypersomnia,[71] altered REM (rapid eye movement) sleep function,[72] and even priapism[73] have been reported in WD. Muscle cramps can be a source of discomfort for some individuals. Headache can be the presenting neurological symptom, according to some investigators, in approximately 10 percent of patients with WD.[18] Although often not mentioned in reviews of WD clinical features, autonomic dysfunction, presumably due to central mechanisms, has been reported to be present in 26–30 percent of persons with WD.[74,75]

Neither upper motor neuron signs (weakness, spasticity, hyperreflexia, Babinski responses) nor lower motor neuron signs (hyporeflexia) are typically seen in WD. Sensory loss and sphincter dysfunction are also unusual.

Historically, neurological WD has been separated into two types, the classic (dystonic) and the pseudosclerotic (Westphal) forms, with the former characterized primarily by extrapyramidal dysfunction and the latter by cerebellar dysfunction. A more recent classification scheme has included pseudoparkinsonian, pseudosclerotic, and dyskinetic categories. However, these attempts at classification are of limited practical value, since considerable variability and overlap exist.

PSYCHIATRIC MANIFESTATIONS

The psychiatric features of WD are often underappreciated and underdiagnosed. Most reports indicate that psychiatric symptoms are the presenting clinical feature in approximately 20 percent of individuals with WD. However, some

TABLE 47-3 Psychiatric Manifestations of WD

Frequent
  Personality changes
    Emotional lability
    Irritability
    Impulsiveness
    Childishness
    Reduced anger threshold
    Aggressiveness
    Recklessness
    Disinhibition
  Mood disturbances
    Depression
    Mania
Infrequent
  Psychosis
  Dementia

investigators have reported that psychiatric symptoms were evident at the time of initial presentation in 65 percent of individuals with WD, and that these symptoms were sufficiently severe to warrant psychiatric intervention in almost 50 percent before the diagnosis of WD was ever made.[76]

Most individuals with WD will experience psychiatric symptomatology at some point during the course of their illness (Table 47-3). Not surprisingly, psychiatric manifestations of WD are most frequently present in individuals who also display neurological dysfunction. Therefore, WD should be considered and excluded in any young person, at least up to age 50, who develops otherwise unexplained psychiatric dysfunction, especially when signs of associated neurological impairment are also evident.[77] Brewer has also observed that it is important to consider the possibility of WD in young persons suspected of drug abuse, since the symptoms can be very similar.[20,77]

As with the neurological picture of WD, there is no archetypal psychiatric WD presentation. Subtle changes in personality and behavior may develop, including emotional lability, irritability, impulsiveness, childishness, reduced anger threshold, aggressiveness, recklessness, and disinhibition.[78,79] Deterioration in school or work performance may be an early clue of developing symptomatic WD.[20,79] Disturbances in mood, especially depression, are reported in 27 percent of patients[80] and may be unrecognized in many more. In one alarming study, almost 16 percent of patients had a history of suicide attempts.[80] Mania may also occur. Circadian rhythm abnormalities, with disturbances in temperature, pulse and blood pressure, have been noted in WD patients with psychiatric symptoms, suggesting hypothalamic dysfunction.[81]

Although clear-cut dementia is uncommon in WD, it may develop in patients with advanced WD, where structural central nervous system (CNS) damage has occurred. Patients with neurological symptoms of WD do, however, demonstrate a range of cognitive impairments that can involve frontal executive ability, visuospatial processing, and some aspects of memory.[82] Formal neuropsychological testing may demonstrate a spectrum of abnormalities.[83–86] It has been suggested that cognitive impairment in WD is a result of subclinical hepatic encephalopathy,[87] but this assessment is controversial.[79] The appearance of an individual with WD, who may display dysarthria, drooling, impaired coordination, and bradykinesia, can also be mistakenly perceived as indicative of cognitive impairment when, in fact, intellect is intact.

Psychosis, although unusual in WD, may occur and be characterized by paranoid thinking, delusional thoughts, hallucinations, and even catatonia.[88–90] These psychiatric features often respond poorly to conventional psychiatric medical management. Antisocial or criminal behavior has also been reported in individuals with WD.[91] Sexual preoccupation and disinhibition may develop in WD,[18,76] as may anorexia nervosa.[92]

Psychiatric symptoms often improve with appropriate treatment of WD, but the improvement may be delayed for as long as 6–18 months. Permanent psychiatric impairment may persist, despite adequate treatment, especially if diagnosis and appropriate treatment have been delayed.

OPHTHALMOLOGIC MANIFESTATIONS

As noted earlier, Kayser's initial description of the pigmented corneal rings that now bear his name was published in 1902, fully 10 years before Wilson's clinical compilation. Kayser's patient was believed at the time to be suffering from multiple sclerosis.[8] Fleischer described similar ocular changes in 1903, and in 1912 connected the corneal pigmented rings with the neurological picture of "pseudosclerosis."[9,10]

Kayser-Fleischer rings (KFRs) are formed by the deposition of copper in Descemet's membrane (See Table 47-4). The excess copper is actually deposited throughout the cornea, but it is only in Descemet's membrane that sulfur-copper complexes are formed, producing the visible copper deposits.[93,94] They are almost always bilateral, but unilateral KFRs have been described.[95] Vision is neither obstructed nor impaired by the KFRs. Their color is quite variable and can range from gold to brown to green. Because of their color composition, fully developed KFRs are often quite readily seen in blue eyes, but can be very difficult to discern when the iris is brown. The visible KFR pigment appears first in the periphery of the cornea at the limbus and then spreads centrally. In some individuals a clear area between the pigment and the corneoscleral junction may be present.[96] The superior aspect of the cornea is involved initially, followed by the inferior aspect and then, finally, the medial and lateral regions of the cornea fill in.

Because of this pattern of evolution, it is important always to lift the eyelid when examining for KFRs, so that the entire cornea is exposed and inspected, lest an incomplete KFR be overlooked.[97] Furthermore, in many individuals, especially those with brown eyes or in whom the KFRs are not mature, it may be impossible to see the KFRs under routine

ophthalmological examination. This mandates that slit-lamp examination by a neuro-ophthalmologist or experienced ophthalmologist be the routine, rather than the exception, in the evaluation of the patient with neurological or psychiatric features suspected of WD. (See Table 47-4.)

Corneal pigment deposition can occur in conditions other than WD. Copper-containing corneal rings indistinguishable from KFRs on slit-lamp examination have been described in a variety of hepatic conditions, including primary biliary cirrhosis,[96,98] autoimmune (chronic active) hepatitis,[99] possible partial biliary atresia,[99] cirrhosis, and chronic cholestatic jaundice.[100] Intraocular copper-containing foreign bodies, or "grinders," can stain the iris and cornea (chalcosis) and mimic KFRs.[93] Copper sulfate-containing ophthalmic solutions, used to treat trachoma, can also stain the cornea.[101] In some individuals with multiple myeloma,[102,103] and in others with pulmonary carcinoma,[104] marked elevations of gamma-globulin and copper have led to corneal ring formation, but in a central rather than a peripheral pattern.

In several other situations, corneal staining unrelated to copper deposition can occur. Arcus senilis is usually easily distinguishable from KFRs by its whitish color, even though its location coincides with KFR territory. However, if an individual has superimposed carotenemia, the arcus senilis may assume a yellowish tint or cast and can be mistaken for KFRs.[105] Corneal heme staining following cataract removal may also transiently mimic KFRs.[99]

KFRs are virtually always present in patients with WD who have developed neurological or psychiatric dysfunction, but they may not yet be apparent in persons with only hepatic symptoms or in presymptomatic individuals. There are case reports documenting the absence of KFRs in WD patients with neurological symptoms, but this must be an exceedingly rare occurrence.[59]

Another ocular manifestation of WD is the sunflower cataract, which was first described by Siemerling and Oloff in 1922.[106] The sunflower cataract is much less common than KFRs, occurring in only 17 percent of untreated individuals.[93] It consists of copper deposits in the lens that have a green, gold, brown or grey coloration and a sunburst or sunflower-like appearance, with a central powder-like disc and radiating petal-like spokes.[93,107] The sunflower cataract typically does not interfere with vision and in most instances can only be seen during slit-lamp examination.

Other ophthalmologic abnormalities may also be seen in WD. Eye movement abnormalities,[108] white retinal spot formation,[109] night blindness,[110] rapidly progressive visual loss due to optic neuropathy,[111] difficulty with gaze fixation,[112] eyelid-opening apraxia,[113] and oculogyric crisis[114] have all been described in WD, but whether they are rare features of WD or simply coincidental findings is uncertain.

MUSCULOSKELETAL MANIFESTATIONS

Joint and bone involvement is an under-recognized component of WD. (See Table 47-4) It has been reported with especially high frequency in Asian populations,[49] and the term "osteomuscular type" has been employed to describe such individuals with skeletal involvement and additional muscle weakness and wasting.[49,115] This higher frequency of musculoskeletal manifestations has been noted in Chinese,[116,117] Japanese,[118] and Indian[115] populations.

Osteoporosis, characterized by radiographic evidence of decreased bone density, may develop in up to 88 percent of persons with WD.[119,120] Osteomalacia, rickets, and localized bone demineralization all may occur.[121] These bone changes may lead to frequent, sometimes spontaneous, fractures.

Joint involvement, especially at the knees, may lead to joint hypermobility or, alternatively, to joint stiffness and pain suggesting premature osteoarthritis.[119,120,122,123] Periarticular and intra-articular calcifications can also develop.[121] Joint pain can be the presenting symptom of WD.[120] A variety of vertebral column abnormalities have also been described in WD patients, with radiological evidence of this in 20–33 percent.[119,124]

The mechanism of bone and joint damage in WD is not clear. With the use of X-ray microprobe spectrometry, synovial copper and iron deposition have been documented in WD, and it has been suggested that tissue destruction, mediated by free radical formation, may be responsible for the cartilage and synovial damage.[125]

OTHER MANIFESTATIONS

Hemolytic anemia may be the initial manifestation of WD in 10–15 percent of cases.[121,126,127] (See Table 47-4) The hemolysis is probably a result of free copper-induced oxidative injury to erythrocytes.[126,128,129] In the setting of transient hepatitis, the hemolytic anemia may also be transient. However, severe hemolytic anemia can develop in patients with WD who develop fulminant hepatic failure.[20,121,130] Additional complications, such as acute renal failure and pancreatitis, have also been reported in WD patients who develop severe hemolytic anemia.[131] Brewer stresses that the concomitant occurrence of hemolysis and liver disease, especially in the setting of fulminant hepatic failure, is a very useful diagnostic clue to the presence of WD.[20] Furthermore, any young person with an otherwise-unexplained nonspherocytic, Coombs-negative hemolytic anemia should also be investigated for possible WD. Thrombocytopenia may develop in conjunction with hemolytic anemia, but isolated thrombocytopenia has also been reported.[132,133]

Renal involvement may also be part of the WD clinical spectrum. Excessive amounts of copper in the urine induce renal tubular dysfunction, which, in turn, can produce hypercalciuria and hyperphosphaturia with consequent nephrocalcinosis.[134] Hypercalciuria and nephrocalcinosis may even be the presenting features of WD.[135] Aminoaciduria and total proteinuria may also be present in WD.[58,136]

Wilson mentioned the presence of hyperpigmentation of the legs and a dark complexion in his initial description

TABLE 47-4 Ophthalmological, Musculoskeletal, and Other Systemic Manifestations of WD

Ophthalmological features
  Kayser-Fleischer rings
  Sunflower cataracts
Musculoskeletal features
  Osteoporosis
  Joint involvement
  Vertebral column abnormalities
Hematologic features
  Hemolytic anemia
  Thrombocytopenia
Renal features
  Nephrocalcinosis
  Hypercalciuria
  Hyperphosphaturia
  Aminoaciduria
  Proteinuria
Dermatological features
  Hyperpigmentation
  Azure lunulae

of WD.[1] Skin changes seem to develop with particular frequency in Chinese WD patients,[49] with anterior lower leg hyperpigmentation noted in 60 percent of patients in one series.[137] These changes can be misinterpreted as Addison's disease by the unwary. Bluish discoloration of the lunulae of the nails[36,138] and acanthosis nigricans[139] have also been reported in WD.

Menstrual irregularity,[140–142] delayed puberty,[143] and gynecomastia have all been reported in WD, as have congestive heart failure, cardiac arrhythmia, glucose intolerance, and parathyroid insufficiency.[121]

Diagnosis

McIntyre has aptly stated, "the most important single factor in early diagnosis [of WD] is suspicion of the disease."[144] When the diagnosis is not considered, the diagnosis will not be made. WD should be considered and excluded in any "young" person (certainly up to age 50, but perhaps even to age 60) who develops unexplained neurological dysfunction, especially if the basal ganglia or cerebellum are involved. Moreover, because of its protean manifestations, similar consideration and exclusion of WD are equally important in similarly "young" individuals presenting with unexplained hepatic, psychiatric, and even other symptoms.

There presently is no single fail-safe diagnostic test for WD. The large numbers of mutations that occur in WD make genetic testing impractical as a screening tool at the present time, although advances in technology may lead to this capability in the future. For the present, certain identification of WD can only be reached with judicious use of a combination

TABLE 47-5 Diagnostic Testing for WD

Diagnostic Test	Advantages	Disadvantages
Liver biopsy	The diagnostic gold standard Virtually always diagnostically elevated in WD	Potential morbidity May be elevated in other long-standing liver diseases
Ceruloplasmin	Readily available Abnormal in presymptomatic patients	Normal in 10–20 percent of WD patients Abnormal in 20 percent of carriers Is acute-phase reactant
24-hour urinary copper	Virtually always elevated in untreated symptomatic patients	Cumbersome to collect Not always elevated in presymptomatic patients May be mildly elevated in carriers May be elevated in long-standing liver disease Chelation therapy complicates interpretation
Kayser-Fleischer rings (slit-lamp exam)	Virtually always present in patients with CNS symptoms (neurologic and psychiatric)	Requires referral to ophthalmologist Not reliably present in presymptomatic patients Not always present in hepatic WD
Free (unbound) copper	Measures potentially toxic portion of serum copper Typically elevated in symptomatic WD Useful for monitoring treatment compliance	Laboratories often unfamiliar with test Not reliably elevated in presymptomatic WD
Radiocopper incorporation	Useful when other tests show conflicting or nondiagnostic results	Somewhat complex to perform Can be abnormal in carriers
DNA analysis	Would be diagnostic in all patients	Vast number of potential mutations make it impractical

of studies, the most important of which include serum ceruloplasmin, 24-hour urinary copper determination, slit-lamp examination for KFRs, and liver biopsy for determination of hepatic copper content (Table 47-5). Additional studies, such as determination of the rate of incorporation of radiocopper into ceruloplasmin, neuroimaging studies, neurophysiological studies, serum free (nonceruloplasmin bound) copper levels, and even cerebrospinal fluid (CSF) copper levels, may be useful in some situations. However, it is not necessary to obtain each of the studies in every patient, and the testing typically necessary to diagnose the patient who presents with hepatic disease is different from that necessary in the individual with a neurological or psychiatric presentation.

It is important to perform the necessary studies in laboratories where the procedures are run frequently and the reported values are reliable. Care must be taken in collecting samples for analysis. Urine collections should always be in copper-free jugs supplied by the laboratory. Precautions must also be taken to avoid specimen contamination by the biopsy needle when performing liver biopsy.

LIVER BIOPSY

Determination of hepatic copper content via liver biopsy is the single most sensitive and accurate test for WD. Hepatic copper content will be significantly elevated in virtually all individuals with WD, even those who are clinically asymptomatic. Some investigators suggest that, because copper is not uniformly distributed in the liver, it is possible for a

sampling error to give a falsely low copper level when a sufficiently sized biopsy (1–2 cm of tissue) is not obtained,[145] although Brewer believes such findings are more probably the consequence of inadequate laboratory technique.[20] Hepatic copper elevation in WD is typically quite striking, generally greater than 250 µg/g dry tissue, compared to normal values of 15–55 µg/g.

Hepatic copper elevation is not, by itself, pathognomonic for WD and can develop in obstructive liver diseases such as primary biliary cirrhosis, biliary atresia, extrahepatic biliary obstruction, primary sclerosing cholangitis, intrahepatic cholestasis of childhood, Indian childhood cirrhosis (Brewer[20] has postulated that this entity actually occurs in WD heterozygotes exposed to excess dietary copper), and autoimmune (chronic active) hepatitis.[146–150]

Deceptively low hepatic copper levels may also be found in individuals with WD if the biopsy is performed just as copper is being mobilized from the liver and released into the general circulation. In this situation, the hepatic copper content is still elevated, but levels in the range of "only" 100 µg/g may be recorded.[151]

Although measurement of hepatic copper content is the most sensitive and accurate diagnostic study for WD, its invasiveness and small, but definite, risk of complication dictate that this study not be used as a universal screening procedure, but only when simpler approaches have not yielded a definitive diagnosis. This is unlikely to be necessary in persons presenting with neurological or psychiatric dysfunction, but is usually required in diagnosing those presenting with hepatic symptoms.

SLIT-LAMP EXAMINATION

Slit-lamp examination by a neuro-ophthalmologist or experienced ophthalmologist to look for KFRs is a vital part of the diagnostic evaluation for suspected WD. The presence of KFRs, although not absolutely specific for WD, is strong supportive evidence of the diagnosis in an individual with neurological or psychiatric features suggesting WD. It has been stated that the absence of KFRs in a patient with CNS symptoms or signs excludes the diagnosis of WD,[18] but exceptions to this doctrine have been reported and individuals with neurological WD but no KFRs described.[59,80,152,153] In persons with only hepatic symptoms or signs, where copper deposition may not yet have overwhelmed the storage capacity of the liver and systemic release of copper may not yet have occurred, KFRs are often absent. The same is true for presymptomatic individuals. It is worth repeating that KFRs can be difficult, and sometimes impossible, to see during routine office examination, especially if the patient has brown eyes, which makes it vital that slit-lamp examination be performed to accurately assess the presence or absence of KFRs.

CERULOPLASMIN

As a screening test for WD, assay of serum ceruloplasmin is both simple and practical, but not sufficient by itself. While it should be obtained on every individual in whom the diagnosis of WD is being considered, it is important to recognize that both false positive and false negative values may occur.

Ceruloplasmin may fall within or only slightly below the normal range in 5–15 percent of persons with WD.[18,20] Moreover, 10–20 percent of WD heterozygotes, who have only one defective copy of the WD gene and do not develop symptomatic WD or require WD treatment, may have ceruloplasmin levels that fall into the subnormal range.[18,20] Serum ceruloplasmin may also be reduced in a number of other conditions, as mentioned earlier. Because it is an acute-phase reactant, ceruloplasmin may increase in pregnancy, while taking birth control pills, during estrogen or steroid administration, or with infection or inflammation (including hepatitis).[20,40] It is possible, therefore, for ceruloplasmin to transiently reach normal or near-normal levels in persons with WD who also develop these conditions.[52] However, Yarze et al. believe that a serum ceruloplasmin level greater than 30 mg/dL virtually excludes the possibility of WD,[121] while Snow chooses a level of 40.[145]

24-HOUR URINARY COPPER EXCRETION

Urinary copper excretion rises dramatically in symptomatic WD, even though the increase is never sufficient to establish a negative copper balance. Urinary copper levels in symptomatic WD typically exceed 100 µg/day, but in presymptomatic individuals, where copper is still accumulating in the liver, urinary copper may still be in the normal range. Heterozygous carriers of WD may have modestly elevated urinary copper levels, but still less than 100 µg/day.[20] Moreover, obstructive liver disease, such as primary biliary cirrhosis, can also produce elevation of urinary copper.[150,154] Despite these caveats, a 24-hour urinary copper determination is, perhaps, the single best screening test for WD. The 24-hour nature of the test is a somewhat limiting factor in the use of the test as a screening tool, but the information obtained makes the test worth the trouble. Brewer routinely obtains two separate 24-hour urinary copper determinations and maintains that the 24-hour urinary copper will always be elevated in individuals with symptomatic WD; he believes that reports to the contrary [51,155] reflect laboratory error.[20]

SERUM COPPER

Routine serum copper levels, which measure total serum copper, are frequently obtained as a screening test for WD, but are actually of little real value. Copper bound to ceruloplasmin normally represents approximately 90 percent of total serum copper.[20] Even though this percentage is lower in WD, total serum copper is usually reduced in WD simply as a reflection of reduced ceruloplasmin, and thus provides no additional useful diagnostic information.[20,121,131,156]

FREE (NONCERULOPLASMIN-BOUND) COPPER

Determination of nonceruloplasmin-bound (free) serum copper directly measures the unbound (actually loosely albumin-complexed) copper in the blood.[121] It is this component that is free to be deposited in tissue and, thus, is potentially toxic. This copper fraction is typically elevated in symptomatic WD and may be used as another screening test for WD.[157] Its greater value, however, may be in monitoring response to and compliance with therapy. Brewer notes that the nonceruloplasmin serum copper level can be calculated by determining total serum copper and ceruloplasmin on the same blood sample. The number for the ceruloplasmin level (reported in mg/dL) is then multiplied by 3 and subtracted from the total serum copper level (reported in µg/dL), giving the serum free copper level, which is 10–15 µg/dL in normal individuals.[20]

RADIOCOPPER INCORPORATION

Measurement of the incorporation of radioactive copper (^{64}Cu) into ceruloplasmin may also be of value in selected situations in the diagnostic evaluation of suspected WD, but is not used as a screening test. In the normal individual there is an initial rise in ^{64}Cu after its oral or intravenous administration as it enters the blood and is complexed with albumin and amino acids. Serum ^{64}Cu levels then drop as the copper is cleared by the liver, only to show a secondary rise, peaking at 48 hours, as the ^{64}Cu is incorporated into newly synthesized ceruloplasmin by the liver and released into the circulation. This secondary rise in ^{64}Cu does not occur in

WD because of defective ATP7B function, as described above. This defect will be evident even in individuals with normal or near-normal ceruloplasmin. Thus, this study can be useful in identifying such "covert" WD patients,[158] although some overlap between persons with WD and heterozygous carriers can exist.[20]

CSF COPPER

CSF copper levels have been measured in WD and found to be elevated in persons with neurological symptoms.[159] Levels also may decline in concert with symptomatic neurological improvement, leading some to suggest that CSF copper levels may be the most accurate reflection of the brain copper load.[160] In one study, the average treatment time necessary to normalize CSF copper content (<20 μg/L) was 47 months.[161] However, this method of copper monitoring is not performed on a routine clinical basis, and such use would require extensive additional validation.

NEUROIMAGING STUDIES

Neuroimaging studies frequently demonstrate abnormalities in WD. The changes are not specific for WD, but characteristic patterns of abnormality have been identified. As might be expected, magnetic resonance imaging (MRI) is a more sensitive indicator of brain involvement in WD than is computed tomography (CT). Recent reports, in fact, have demonstrated MRI abnormalities in 100 percent of individuals with WD who have neurological dysfunction.[162,163] The most consistent abnormalities are found in the basal ganglia; thalamus and brainstem are also frequently affected.[164,165] Increased signal intensity on T_2-weighted images is the characteristic abnormality; the increased signal intensity sometimes surrounds an area of decreased signal intensity.[165] It has been suggested that either edema or demyelination may account for the increased signal intensity, whereas either iron or copper deposition (both are paramagnetic substances) may produce the area of reduced signal intensity.[165,166] Certain abnormalities, such as the "face of the giant panda" midbrain sign[167,168] and the "bright claustrum" sign,[169] have been suggested to be characteristic of WD, but are not consistently present. Abnormalities on diffusion MRI[170] and proton MR spectroscopy[171] have recently been described in WD, although an earlier study did not find the latter procedure to be useful in either diagnosis or follow-up of WD patients.[166]

Positron emission tomography (PET) scanning, both with ^{18}F-deoxyglucose[172,173] and ^{18}F-dopa,[174] typically demonstrates abnormalities in persons with WD, but PET still is not routinely available and, therefore, not part of the standard evaluation of the patient with suspected WD. Evoked potentials of various types may be abnormal in many patients with WD, often early in the course of the disease,[175] but are nonspecific and of no definitive diagnostic value.[176]

Testing Guidelines

In persons with WD presenting with hepatic dysfunction, KFRs are not consistently present, but 24-hour urinary copper content is usually elevated and serum ceruloplasmin often reduced. Liver biopsy is generally used to confirm the diagnosis by measurement of hepatic copper content and to assess the degree of hepatic injury. Individuals with long-standing hepatic failure or obstruction, regardless of cause, can demonstrate hepatic copper content that is elevated into the WD range. In these individuals radiocopper assay can be important in confirming or refuting the diagnosis of WD.

In individuals with suspected WD presenting with neurological or psychiatric dysfunction, the presence of KFRs on slit-lamp examination, coupled with appropriately elevated 24-hour urinary copper and reduced serum ceruloplasmin, virtually confirms the diagnosis and obviates the need for liver biopsy. There may be instances, such as when KFRs are present and 24-hour urinary copper elevated but ceruloplasmin is not markedly reduced, that liver biopsy is still necessary.

Treatment

Treatment strategies in WD center on restoring and maintaining appropriate copper balance within body tissues. With the exception of liver transplantation, treatment of WD is palliative rather than curative; the underlying defect that produces WD is not corrected, and treatment must be continued for the individual's lifetime. Four approaches to WD treatment have been employed, as discussed below.

DIETARY THERAPY

Limitation of dietary copper intake would seem, on the surface, to be a prudent and sensible maneuver in treating WD. In practice, however, it is difficult to achieve and has not been demonstrated to confer significant benefit. Brewer suggests that only shellfish and liver, both of which are especially high in copper content, be eliminated from the diet of WD patients.[20]

In contrast to the general ineffectiveness of dietary therapy in WD, there have been anecdotal descriptions in which a strict lactovegetarian diet seemed to control WD adequately without other therapy,[177] presumably because the bioavailability of dietary copper was sufficiently reduced by the dietary fiber and phytate in these individuals. For most individuals, however, such a restrictive diet is not feasible.

Copper content in the primary drinking sources (home, work, school) of an individual with WD should be measured, and if the level is above 0.1 ppm alternative water sources, such as bottled water, should be used.[20] Such elevations are likely to be found for approximately 10 percent of WD patients.[20] It should also be remembered that domestic water softeners increase the copper content of water.[121] Copper content in any vitamin/mineral supplements that the WD patient might be taking should also be scrutinized.

INHIBITION OF INTESTINAL COPPER ABSORPTION

POTASSIUM

Potassium iodide or potassium sulfide has been advocated in the past as a means of decreasing dietary copper absorption by interacting with copper to form insoluble copper iodide or copper sulfide. However, this approach is of no proven practical value and is not typically used in the treatment of WD.

ZINC

Zinc, administered either as acetate, sulfate or gluconate, provides another mechanism to limit gastrointestinal copper absorption in WD. The effect of zinc is mediated through the cysteine-rich 61-amino acid protein, metallothionein, which is present in many body tissues including brain, liver, and intestinal cells.[178,179] The presumed primary role of metallothionein in the body is as a zinc-binding ligand that is important for zinc homeostasis and transport.[179] Metallothionein has a high affinity for zinc, but an even higher affinity for copper.[180] When given on an empty stomach, supplemental oral zinc administration induces metallothionein formation in the intestinal enterocytes. The increased metallothionein then binds zinc and limits zinc absorption,[181] but it also binds dietary copper.[182] The bound copper, like the bound zinc, is then trapped and stored within the intestinal mucosal cells until the cells are eventually sloughed and excreted in the feces.[181,183] Reabsorption of copper that has been secreted into the gastrointestinal tract via saliva and gastric juices is also blocked by this mechanism. The net result of these actions is the induction of a small, but real, negative copper balance.

The role of zinc administration in the treatment of WD has become more clearly defined in recent years.[184] It is generally well tolerated, and this scant toxicity makes zinc very appealing as primary therapy of WD in the presymptomatic individual.[183–185] Its place in the treatment of the symptomatic patient has also been clarified. The effect of zinc administration on copper absorption does not become evident for 1–2 weeks because the induction of metallothionein is a rather slow process. Moreover, the negative copper balance induced by zinc is relatively small. In the eyes of most investigators these characteristics make zinc monotherapy unsuitable as initial therapy in the individual with WD who is already experiencing neurological symptoms,[20,184,186] although not all agree and zinc monotherapy has actually been used successfully in this clinical situation.[187,188] There is growing support for the use of zinc as "maintenance" therapy following (or in conjunction with) initial treatment with other more potent decoppering agents in neurologically symptomatic individuals, and extensive favorable experience is accumulating.[20,188] Zinc therapy has also been reported to be safe and effective as maintenance management in both children and pregnant women.[189,190] It should be noted, however, that some investigators still view the use of zinc as monotherapy in WD as controversial.[191]

A dosage regimen of 50 mg of elemental zinc three times daily is generally employed. Dosage designation can be confusing, however. Zinc sulfate tablets, which are readily available without prescription in the US, are listed as containing 220 mg of zinc sulfate salt, but this translates to 50 mg of elemental zinc. Zinc acetate, which is available by prescription, is labeled by its elemental zinc content.

Although zinc is almost always well tolerated, adverse effects may occur. Gastric irritation, typically with the morning dose, is more frequent with zinc sulfate than with zinc acetate.[183] For patients who are experiencing gastric discomfort with zinc administration, concomitant consumption of a small amount of a protein-containing snack (Jell-O, luncheon meat) often obviates the problem without significantly compromising efficacy.[20] Sideroblastic anemia resulting from impaired iron utilization has been reported with zinc therapy.[192] Zinc can lower high-density lipoprotein (HDL) cholesterol in both men and women by about 10 percent.[193,194] Serum amylase and lipase may increase early in the course of zinc therapy, later returning to normal.[195] The same phenomenon may be noted with alkaline phosphatase.[195] Whether neurological deterioration can develop as a direct result of initiating zinc therapy, as can occur with penicillamine, is disputed.[196–198]

TETRATHIOMOLYBDATE

Ammonium tetrathiomolybdate (TM), although first tested in the treatment of WD in 1984,[196] has only in recent years received sustained attention[20] as potential WD therapy, and still remains an experimental agent that is not available for general use. Nevertheless, available evidence is sufficiently encouraging that inclusion of TM, despite its experimental status, seems warranted in a review such as this.

TM has a distinct, dual mechanism of action that distinguishes it from other available treatment modalities. It is able to reduce the copper load in WD by working at two distinct sites.[20,199] TM, like zinc, is able to limit gastrointestinal absorption of copper, but it does so by an entirely different mechanism of action. In the gut lumen TM forms a tripartite complex with copper and albumin; the complexed copper cannot be absorbed by the intestinal mucosal cells and is excreted in the feces.[20,199] Both food-derived and endogenously secreted copper are complexed by TM. Unlike zinc, the negative copper balance produced by TM is present immediately because metallothionein induction is not necessary.

Inhibition of copper absorption, however, is not the only weapon that TM possesses in opposing copper toxicity. When TM is given without food it is readily absorbed into the bloodstream. Once absorbed, it forms the same tripartite complex with albumin and unbound (free) copper in the blood, which renders the copper unavailable for cellular uptake and, therefore, nontoxic.[20,199] Thus, TM can reduce the copper load in the WD patient systemically, in addition to its action in the gut lumen.

Unlike other available medications for WD, TM has not thus far been evaluated for chronic, or maintenance, therapy, but solely as an induction agent that is employed for an 8-week course of treatment and then discontinued and replaced with another agent, such as zinc, for chronic treatment. It is administered in a rather complex dosage regimen that is designed to maximize its effectiveness both in the gut and in the bloodstream. Six daily doses of 20 mg each are employed: three at mealtimes to reduce copper absorption via the gut, and three between mealtimes to enhance TM absorption and maximize its action in the bloodstream.[20]

When administered as the initial therapy in the fashion described above to individuals with neurologically symptomatic WD, prompt and significant reduction in unbound (free) copper has been documented in open-label studies.[20,199–201] In Brewer's experience, neurological deterioration has occurred in less than 4 percent (2/56) of patients to whom TM has been administered.[20] Although generally tolerated quite well, several potential complications have been recognized. Bone marrow depression, with resultant anemia and occasional leukopenia, has occurred and is presumed to be a consequence of copper depletion in the marrow; it resolves with drug discontinuation.[20] Mild transaminase elevations have also been noted.[20] In rats, TM has also been shown to damage epiphyses in growing bone,[202] leading Walshe and Yealland to suggest that TM not be used for more than short courses in children or adolescents with unfused epiphyses.[203]

COPPER-CHELATION THERAPY

BRITISH ANTI-LEWISITE (BAL)
Dimercaprol, or British anti-Lewisite (BAL), was the initial copper-chelating agent used in the treatment of WD, but has now been virtually abandoned because of the necessity to administer it parenterally and because of its proclivity to produce a plethora of adverse effects such as headache, nausea, dizziness, and pain at the injection site.

PENICILLAMINE
Penicillamine (dimethylcysteine) is a metabolic by-product of penicillin that avidly chelates copper; the resulting complexed copper is then excreted in the urine. Although it has generally been accepted that penicillamine produces its primary effect by copper chelation and subsequent cupriuresis, additional actions, including induction of metallothionein, have been proposed.[121] Following its introduction by Walshe in 1956 as a treatment for WD,[204] the consistent efficacy of penicillamine in inducing a negative copper balance and reducing the body's copper load was quickly recognized and penicillamine became the mainstay of WD treatment.

Improvement in function may begin within 2 weeks of initiating penicillamine therapy, but more typically it is delayed for 2–3 months.[205] With continued therapy, gradual improvement may continue for up to 1–2 years.[183] Improvement in virtually all facets of clinical dysfunction may occur. From a neurological standpoint, tremor and cerebellar signs seem to improve more readily than dystonia, whereas the fixed smile and dysarthria may show no improvement at all. KFRs recede gradually in a sequence inverse to their appearance.[97] Sunflower cataracts also clear, often more rapidly than KFRs.[93,97] Psychiatric symptoms improve with penicillamine therapy, although not as fully or as consistently as neurological symptoms and signs.[43,79] The same is true of psychometric testing.[206] Neuroimaging abnormalities, both on CT[207] and MRI,[162,163,208] may improve on penicillamine.

Penicillamine should always be given on an empty stomach. The traditionally recommended initial dose is 1–2 g daily, divided into four doses, but lower doses are recommended by some. Concomitant administration of pyridoxine has also been recommended by some because penicillamine is a pyridoxine antagonist;[121,209] however, others believe that penicillamine-induced pyridoxine deficiency only occurs in special circumstances, such as during pregnancy, during a growth spurt, or with dietary pyridoxine deficiency.[203,210]

A troublesome aspect of penicillamine is its propensity to produce initial deterioration in neurological function as treatment is initiated. The frequency with which this occurs is the subject of some dispute.[196–198] Walshe and Yealland[203] noted it in 22 percent (30 of 137) of patients that they treated, while Brewer et al.[20,211] reported it in 52 percent (13 of 25) in a retrospective survey. More ominously, Brewer adds that 50 percent of those in whom neurological deterioration occurred upon initiation of penicillamine therapy did not fully recover to their baseline level of functioning.[20,211] Lethal status dystonicus has recently been reported following initiation of penicillamine treatment.[212] Emergence of neurological dysfunction in previously neurologically asymptomatic individuals has also been described after starting penicillamine.[213,214] The reason for this deterioration is not absolutely certain. Mobilization of copper from the liver with subsequent redistribution to the brain has been suggested,[211] but studies of CSF copper levels during this deterioration do not support this hypothesis.[160]

This potential for neurological deterioration has led some investigators to propose more gentle initiation of penicillamine therapy, with lower doses, and others to advocate induction of therapy with zinc or TM instead of penicillamine. Brewer et al. have been most vocal in their opposition to the use of penicillamine in the treatment of WD, and strongly advocate that it not be used at all, with the possible exception of the patient with fulminant hepatic failure awaiting liver transplantation, since safer alternatives are available.[20,197] Walshe, on the other hand, believes that a place for penicillamine still exists.[196] Thus, the controversy continues.[191,198]

A variety of other problems may also attend penicillamine therapy. Acute sensitivity reactions develop in 20–30 percent of individuals on penicillamine in conventional doses.[215,216] Consisting of skin rash, fever, eosinophilia, thrombocytopenia, leukopenia, and lymphadenopathy, these reactions typically develop within 2 weeks of initiation of treatment. Even in the face of a severe reaction, however, it is not always necessary to abandon penicillamine therapy permanently. Therapy can often be reinstituted at a reduced dose following resolution of the symptoms, initially with steroid co-administration.[217] Despite such measures, 5–20 percent of patients are ultimately unable to tolerate penicillamine at all.[183] Agranulocytosis induced by penicillamine can be fatal.[218]

With chronic penicillamine administration a variety of other adverse effects may occur. Nephrotic syndrome,[219] Goodpasture's syndrome,[220] a lupus-like syndrome,[221] a myasthenia-like syndrome,[222] acute polyarthritis,[119] thrombocytopenia,[18] and retinal hemorrhages[223] have all been reported. Loss of the sense of taste may also occur with penicillamine therapy; a favorable response of this dysgeusia to zinc administration has been demonstrated.[224,225] Serum IgA deficiency has been noted with penicillamine.[226] Adverse reactions to penicillamine may still develop after prolonged therapy. There is a report of lupus developing after 30 years of therapy.[203]

Dermatologic problems may also develop with chronic penicillamine treatment. Penicillamine dermatopathy is characterized by brownish skin discoloration, which develops as a consequence of recurrent subcutaneous bleeding during incidental trauma.[227] The bleeding is attributed to penicillamine-induced inhibition of collagen and elastin cross linking.[228] Penicillamine can also impair wound healing,[229] which has led to the recommendation that penicillamine dosage should be reduced to 250–500 mg daily during perioperative periods.[18] Elastosis perforans serpiginosa,[230,231] pemphigus,[232] and aphthous stomatitis[233] are other reported penicillamine-induced dermatologic processes.

TRIENTINE

Triethylene tetramine dihydrochloride, or trientine, is a copper-chelating agent with a mechanism of action similar to that of penicillamine.[234–237] Trientine appears to be somewhat less potent than penicillamine and, thus, does not induce as vigorous decoppering, which may make it less likely to provoke the initial neurological deterioration that penicillamine can invoke, and thus safer to use.

As with penicillamine, trientine should be taken on an empty stomach; a typical daily dose is 750–2000 mg, divided into three doses.[121] Experience with trientine has been much less extensive than with penicillamine, but trientine appears to be a less toxic compound. Both lupus nephritis[236] and sideroblastic anemia[238] have been reported with trientine.

In the past, trientine was primarily used as an alternative copper-chelation therapy when penicillamine was not tolerated. With increasing recognition of the potential for initial neurological deterioration with the use of penicillamine, however, trientine has been increasingly advocated as a first line of treatment in the WD patient with neurological symptoms,[20,186,239] with subsequent switching to zinc for maintenance therapy.

LIVER TRANSPLANTATION

The most dreaded complication of WD is the development of fulminant hepatic failure. When treatment of Wilsonian fulminant hepatic failure is confined to medical management, the mortality rate is virtually 100 percent.[240–242] Because of this ghastly statistic, orthotopic liver transplantation (OLT) has been used with increasing frequency in this desperate situation. Chronic, severe hepatic insufficiency unresponsive to medical treatment measures is also seen as an appropriate indication for OLT in WD.[240]

A serious impediment to the employment of OLT in the setting of liver failure is the limited availability of donor organs, and it is not uncommon for patients to succumb, especially in the setting of fulminant hepatic failure, before a donor organ becomes available. Recent reports of the use of albumin dialysis[243,244] and extracorporeal perfusion through porcine liver cells[245] as a bridge to buy time while awaiting OLT, with reported improvement in encephalopathy and reduction in copper, provide some encouragement in this situation.

Schilsky et al. have reviewed the experience with OLT in the treatment of WD at 15 transplant centers in the US and three in Europe.[240] Data on 55 patients were reviewed. The survival rate at 1 year was 79 percent. Similar survival rates have been noted by other investigators.[241,246] More recently, a 1-year patient survival rate of 87.5 percent and a graft survival rate of 62.5 percent in 17 patients undergoing OLT at a single center have been reported.[247]

In addition to correction of hepatic dysfunction, improvement has been observed in the neurological, psychiatric, and ophthalmological features of WD following OLT.[240] Because the transplanted liver is free of the genetic defect responsible for WD, copper metabolism normalizes after OLT and continued chelation or other WD therapy is generally not necessary.[20,240,241] Although OLT may thus be viewed as curative therapy, it should be remembered that, if the transplant is received from a living related donor, such as a parent, the transplanted liver will carry the features of a heterozygote and, thus, may not have completely normal liver function.[248] Moreover, transplanted individuals still retain the genetic abnormality in other body tissues and will pass on the trait to all children.

Because of the success of OLT in treating WD patients with hepatic failure, the question as to whether patients with stable hepatic function but severe neurological dysfunction not responding to medical therapy should also be considered for OLT has been raised. There have been case reports of OLT performed in this situation,[249,250] but most investigators view such a treatment approach as experimental and not as the current standard of therapy. Brewer makes the point that improvement in neurological function following OLT is the result of normalized copper excretion with reduced brain copper load, which is also accomplished by medical management, and advocates that OLT be reserved for treatment of hepatic, not neurological, indications.[20]

A possible glimpse into the future may have been provided by recent reports of the success of hepatocyte transplantation with subsequent hepatic repopulation in the Long-Evans rat model of WD.[251] Adenovirus-mediated gene transfer therapy has also been transiently effective in the same rat model.[252]

Treatment Guidelines

In the individual with WD who is still asymptomatic (presymptomatic), most investigators recommend that therapy be initiated and maintained with zinc alone.

In the individual who has hepatic, but not neurological or psychiatric, symptoms, introduction of both a chelating agent and zinc may be ideal. Penicillamine has been the standard chelating agent in this situation in the past, but trientine is receiving increased attention because of the perception that it is less likely than penicillamine to induce neurological deterioration upon initiation of treatment.

It is in the individual who has developed neurological dysfunction that the most controversy regarding treatment choice has been evident. Available evidence suggests that TM may be the ideal treatment for initiation of treatment in this situation, but, until formal approval from regulatory agencies is granted, its availability will remain limited. Thus, for most clinicians the choice for initial therapy will be between trientine and penicillamine. Both have their advocates, but a shift toward the use of trientine, because of its perceived lesser potential for inducing neurological deterioration, seems apparent in the literature. Zinc is recommended by some investigators for initiation of therapy in neurologically symptomatic individuals, but most reserve its use for maintenance therapy after initial decoppering.

For the individual with fulminant or severe, chronic hepatic failure, OLT may be the only viable treatment option.

Adequate monitoring of patients following initiation of treatment is an extremely important and often neglected aspect of WD management. Assuring patient compliance in taking prescribed medication is vital for successful outcome. Even with close, dedicated follow-up of patients and extensive educational measures, intermittent compliance problems become evident in 30 percent of WD patients, and severe compliance problems are noted in approximately 10 percent. Compliance with zinc therapy can be assessed by measurement of 24-hour urinary zinc and copper levels. A 24-hour urinary zinc level of less than 2 mg indicates inadequate compliance.[20] Monitoring compliance with trientine or penicillamine therapy is a bit more difficult, but a spike in a previously gradually decreasing 24-hour urinary copper level

may indicate inadequate compliance.[20] Monitoring serum nonceruloplasmin (free) copper can also be used as a monitoring tool; a significant increase in this level suggests inadequate compliance.[20]

It should also be remembered that prolonged treatment, both with zinc and with chelating agents, can actually induce copper deficiency in patients with WD. Anemia, sometimes with associated leukopenia, may be the initial sign of copper deficiency.[20] In patients on zinc maintenance therapy, a 24-hour urinary copper level below 35 μg is suggestive of copper deficiency due to overtreatment.[20] For individuals on trientine or penicillamine, a serum nonceruloplasmin (free) copper level below 5 μg suggests overtreatment.[20]

Summary

In the near-century since Wilson's seminal description, our understanding of and ability to effectively treat WD has dramatically advanced. Nevertheless, because of its protean clinical features, WD remains a tremendous diagnostic and therapeutic challenge to the clinician. The palliative nature of most WD therapy dictates constant vigilance on the part of the treating physician to ensure ongoing patient compliance and to watch closely for treatment complications. The reward, however, of prompt diagnosis and attentive therapy can be an asymptomatic and healthy individual faced with an otherwise fatal disease.

References

1. Wilson SAK: Progressive lenticular degeneration: A familial nervous disease associated with cirrhosis of the liver. *Brain* 34:295–507, 1912.
2. Frerichs FT: *A Clinical Treatise on Diseases of the Liver.* London: The New Sydenham Society, 1860.
3. Westphal C: Über eine dem Bilde der cerebrospinalen grauen Degeneration ähnliche Erkrankung des centralen Nervensystems ohne anatomischen Befund, nebst einigen Bermerkungen über paradoxe Contraction. *Arch Psychiatr Nervenkrank* 14:87–134, 1883.
4. Gowers W: *A Manual of Diseases of the Nervous System.* London: J & A Churchill, 1988.
5. Ormerod JA: Cirrhosis of the liver in a boy, with obscure and fatal nervous symptoms. *St Bart Hosp Rep* XXVI:57, 1890.
6. Homen EA: Eine Eigenthümliche bei drei Geschwistern auftretende typische Krankheit unter der Form einer progressiven Dementia, in Verbindung mit ausgedehnten Gefässveränderungen (wohl lues hereditaria tarda). *Arch Psychiatr* XXIV:191–228, 1892.
7. Strümpell A: Über die Westphal'sche Pseudosklerose und über diffuse Hirnsklerose, inbesondere bei Kindern. *Dtsch Z Nervenheilk* 12:115–149, 1898.
8. Kayser B: Über einen Fall von angeborener grünlicher Verfärbung der Kornea. *Klin Monatsbl Augenheilkd* 40:22–25, 1902.

9. Fleischer B: Zwei weiterer Falle von grünlicher Verfärbung der Kornea. *Klin Monatsbl Augenheilkd* 41:489–491, 1903.

10. Fleischer B: Über eine der "Pseudosklerose" nahestehende, bisher unbekannte Krankheit (gekennzeichnet durch tremor, psychische storungen, braunliche Pigmentierung bestimmter gewebe, inbesondere auch der Hornhautperipherie, Lebercirrhose). *Dtsch Z Nervenheilkd* 44:179–201, 1912.

11. Rumpel A: Über das Wesen und die Bedeutung der Leberveränderungen und der Pigmentierunen bei den damit verbundenen Fällen von Pseudosklerose, zugleich ein Beitrag zur Lehre von der Pseudosklerose (Westphal-Strümpell). *Dtsch Z Nervenheilkd* 49:54–73, 1913.

12. Mandelbrote BM, Stanier MW, Thompson RHS, et al: Studies on copper metabolism in demyelinating diseases of the central nervous system. *Brain* 71:212–228, 1948.

13. Cumings JN: The copper and iron content of brain and liver in the normal and in hepato-lenticular degeneration. *Brain* 71:410–415, 1948.

14. Scheinberg IH, Gitlin D: Deficiency of ceruloplasmin in patients with hepatolenticular degeneration (Wilson's disease). *Science* 116:484–485, 1952.

15. Bearn AG, Kunkel HG: Biochemical abnormalities in Wilson's disease. *J Clin Invest* 31:616, 1952.

16. Frommer DJ: Defective biliary excretion of copper in Wilson's disease. *Gut* 15:125–129, 1974.

17. Hall HC: *La Dégénérescence Hépato-lenticulaire: Maladie de Wilson-Pseudosclérose*. Paris: Paul Masson, 1921.

18. Scheinberg IH, Sternlieb I: *Wilson's Disease*. Philadelphia: WB Saunders, 1984.

19. Reilly M, Daly L, Hutchinson M: An epidemiological study of Wilson's disease in the Republic of Ireland. *J Neurol Neurosurg Psychiatry* 56:298–300, 1993.

20. Brewer GJ: *Wilson's Disease: A Clinician's Guide to Recognition, Diagnosis, and Management.* Boston: Kluwer, 2001.

21. Olivarez L, Caggana M, Pass KA, et al: Estimate of the frequency of Wilson's disease in the US Caucasian population: A mutation analysis approach. *Ann Hum Genet* 65:459–463, 2001.

22. Frydman M, Bonné-Tamir B, Farrer LA, et al: Assignment of the gene for Wilson's disease to chromosome 13. *Proc Natl Acad Sci U S A* 82:1819–1821, 1985.

23. Bull PC, Thomas GR, Rommens JM, et al: The Wilson disease gene is a putative copper transporting P-type ATPase similar to the Menkes gene. *Nat Genet* 5:327–337, 1993.

24. Petrukhin K, Fischer SG, Piratsu M, et al: Mapping, cloning and genetic characterization of the region containing the Wilson disease gene. *Nat Genet* 5:338–343, 1993.

25. Yamaguchi Y, Heiny ME, Gitlin JD: Isolation and characterization of a human liver cDNA as a candidate gene for Wilson disease. *Biochem Biophys Res Commun* 197:271–277, 1993.

26. Petrukhin K, Lutsenko S, Chernov I, et al: Characterization of the Wilson's disease gene encoding a P-type copper transporting ATPase: Genomic organization, alternative splicing, and structure/function predictions. *Hum Mol Genet* 3:1647–1656, 1994.

27. Lutsenko S, Petrukhin K, Cooper MJ, et al: N-Terminal domains of human copper-transporting adenosine triphosphatases (the Wilson's and Menkes disease proteins) bind copper selectively *in vivo* and *in vitro* with stoichiometry of one copper per metal-binding repeat. *J Biol Chem* 272:18939–18944, 1997.

28. DiDonato M, Narindrasorasak S, Forbes JR, et al: Expression, purification, and metal binding properties of the N-terminal domain from the Wilson disease putative copper-transporting ATPase (ATP7B). *J Biol Chem* 272:33279–33282, 1997.

29. Hung IH, Suzuki M, Yamaguchi Y, et al: Biochemical characterization of the Wilson disease protein and functional expression in the yeast *Saccharomyces cerevisiae. J Biol Chem* 272:21461–21466, 1997.

30. La Fontaine S, Theophilos MB, Firth SD, et al: Effect of the toxic milk mutation (tx) on the function and intracellular localization of Wnd, the murine homologue of the Wilson copper ATPase. *Hum Mol Genet* 10:361–370, 2001.

31. Forbes JR, Cox DW: Copper-dependent trafficking of Wilson disease mutant ATP7B proteins. *Hum Mol Genet* 9:1927–1935, 2000.

32. Loudianos G, Lovicu M, Dessi V, et al: Abnormal mRNA splicing resulting from consensus sequence splicing mutations of ATP7B. *Hum Mutat* 20:260–266, 2002.

33. Tanzi RE, Petrukhin K, Chernov I, et al: The Wilson disease gene is a copper transporting ATPase with homology to the Menkes disease gene. *Nat Genet* 5:44–50, 1993.

34. Thomas GR, Forbes JR, Roberts EA, et al: The Wilson disease gene: Spectrum of mutations and their consequences. *Nat Genet* 9:210–217, 1999.

35. Shah AB, Chernov I, Zhang HT, et al: Identification and analysis of mutations in the Wilson disease gene (ATP7B): Population frequencies, genotype-phenotype correlation, and functional analyses. *Am J Hum Genet* 61:317–328, 1997.

36. Peña MMO, Lee J, Thiele DJ: A delicate balance: Homeostatic control of copper uptake and distribution. *J Nutr* 129:1251–1260, 1999.

37. Holmberg CG, Laurell CB: Investigations in serum copper. II. Isolation of the copper containing protein and a description of some of its properties. *Acta Chem Scand* 2:550–556, 1948.

38. Shiono Y, Wakusawa S, Hayashi H, et al: Iron accumulation in the liver of male patients with Wilson's disease. *Am J Gastroenterol* 96:3147–3151, 2001.

39. Sato M, Schilsky ML, Stockert RJ, et al: Detection of multiple forms of human ceruloplasmin: A novel Mr 2,000,000 form. *J Biol Chem* 265:2533–2537, 1990.

40. Gibbs K, Walshe JM: A study of the ceruloplasmin concentrations found in 75 patients with Wilson's disease, their kinships and various control groups. *Q J Med* 48:447–463, 1979.

41. Yang F, Naylor SL, Lum JB, et al: Characterization, mapping, and expression of the human ceruloplasmin gene. *Proc Natl Acad Sci U S A* 83:3257–3261, 1986.

42. Morita H, Ikeda S, Yamamoto K, et al: Hereditary ceruloplasmin deficiency with hemosiderosis: A clinicopathological study of a Japanese family. *Ann Neurol* 37:646–656, 1995.

43. Hellman NE, Gitlin JD: Ceruloplasmin metabolism and function. *Annu Rev Nutr* 22:439–458, 2002.

44. Jones RJ, Lewis SJ, Smith JM, et al: Undetectable serum ceruloplasmin in a woman with chronic hepatitis C infection. *J Hepatol* 32:703–704, 2000.

45. van Berge Henegouwen GP, Tangedahl TN, Hofman AF, et al: Biliary secretion of copper in healthy man. *Gastroenterology* 72:1228–1231, 1977.

46. O'Reilly S, Weber PM, Oswald H, et al: Abnormalities of the physiology of copper in Wilson's disease. *Arch Neurol* 25:28–32, 1971.

47. Owen CA Jr: Absorption and excretion of Cu^{64}-labeled copper by the rat. *Am J Physiol* 207:1203–1206, 1964.

48. Walshe JM: Wilson's disease: The presenting symptoms. *Arch Dis Child* 37:253–256, 1962.

49. Chu N-S, Hung T-P: Geographic variations in Wilson's disease. *J Neurol Sci* 117:1–7, 1993.

50. Walshe JM: Wilson's disease (HLD), in Vinken PJ, Bruyn GW (eds): *Handbook of Clinical Neurology*. Amsterdam: North-Holland, 1976, vol 27, pp 379–414.

51. Gow PJ, Smallwood RA, Angus PW, et al: Diagnosis of Wilson's disease: An experience over three decades. *Gut* 46:415–419, 2000.

52. Sternlieb I, Scheinberg IH: Chronic hepatitis as a first manifestation of Wilson's disease. *Ann Intern Med* 76:59–64, 1972.

53. Scott J, Gollan JL, Samourian S, et al: Wilson's disease presenting as chronic active hepatitis. *Gastroenterology* 74:645–651, 1978.

54. Schilsky ML, Scheinberg IH, Sternlieb I: Liver transplantation for Wilson's disease: Indications and outcome. *Hepatology* 19:583–587, 1994.

55. Roche-Sicot J, Benhamou J-P: Acute intravascular hemolysis and acute liver failure associated as a first manifestation of Wilson's disease. *Ann Intern Med* 86:301–303, 1977.

56. Hoshino T, Kumasaka K, Kawano K, et al: Low serum alkaline phosphatase activity associated with severe Wilson's disease. Is the breakdown of alkaline phosphatase molecules caused by reactive oxygen species? *Clin Chim Acta* 238:91–100, 1995.

57. Kenngott S, Bilzer M: Inverse correlation of serum bilirubin and alkaline phosphatase in fulminant Wilson's disease. *J Hepatol* 29:683, 1998.

58. Strickland GT, Leu ML: Wilson's disease: Clinical and laboratory manifestations in 40 patients. *Medicine* 54:113–137, 1975.

59. Ross E, Jacobson IM, Dienstag JL, et al: Late onset Wilson's disease with neurologic involvement in the absence of Kayser-Fleischer rings. *Ann Neurol* 17:411–413, 1985.

60. Walshe JM: Wilson's disease, in Vinken PJ, Bruyn GW, Klawans HL (eds): *Handbook of Clinical Neurology*. New York: Elsevier, 1986, vol 49, pp 223–238.

61. Topaloglu H, Renda Y: Tongue dyskinesia in Wilson disease. *Brain Dev* 14:128, 1992.

62. Topaloglu H, Gucuyener K, Orkun C, et al: Tremor of tongue and dysarthria as the sole manifestation of Wilson disease. *Clin Neurol Neurosurg* 92:295–296, 1990.

63. Nicholl DJ, Ferenci P, Polli C, et al: Wilson's disease presenting in a family with an apparent dominant history of tremor. *J Neurol Neurosurg Psychiatry* 70:514–516, 2001.

64. Parker N: Hereditary whispering dysphonia. *J Neurol Neurosurg Psychiatry* 48:218–224, 1985.

65. Cartwright GE: Diagnosis of treatable Wilson's disease. *N Engl J Med* 298:1347–1350, 1978.

66. Walshe JM, Yealland M: Wilson's disease: The problem of delayed diagnosis. *J Neurol Neurosurg Psychiatry* 55:692–696, 1992.

67. Svetel M, Kozic D, Stefanova E, et al: Dystonia in Wilson's disease. *Mov Disord* 16:719–723, 2001.

68. Dening TR, Berrios GE, Walshe JM: Wilson disease and epilepsy. *Brain* 111:1139–1155, 1988.

69. Huang C-C, Chu N-S: Psychosis and epileptic seizures in Wilson's disease with predominantly white matter lesions in the frontal lobe. *Parkinsonism Relat Disord* 1:53–58, 1995.

70. Mingazzini G: Über das Zwangsweinen und-lachen. *Klin Wochenschr (Wien)* 41:998–1002, 1928.

71. Firneisz G, Szalay F, Halasz P, et al: Hypersomnia in Wilson's disease: an unusual symptom in an unusual case. *Acta Neurol Scand* 101:286–288, 2000.

72. Portala K, Westermark K, Ekselius L, et al: Sleep in patients with treated Wilson's disease. A questionnaire study. *Nord J Psychiatry* 56:291–297, 2002.

73. Nair KR, Pillai PG: Trunkal myoclonus with spontaneous priapism and seminal ejaculation in Wilson's disease. *J Neurol Neurosurg Psychiatry* 53:174, 1990.

74. Bhattacharya K, Velickovic M, Schilsky M, et al: Autonomic cardiovascular reflexes in Wilson's disease. *Clin Auton Res* 12:190–192, 2002.

75. Meenakshi-Sundaram S, Taly AB, Kamath V, et al: Autonomic dysfunction in Wilson's disease: A clinical and electrophysiological study. *Clin Auton Res* 12:185–189, 2002.

76. Akil M, Schwartz JA, Dutchak D, et al: The psychiatric presentations of Wilson's disease. *J Neuropsychiatry Clin Neurosci* 3:377–382, 1991.

77. Brewer GJ: Recognition, diagnosis, and management of Wilson's disease. *Proc Soc Exp Biol Med* 223:39–46, 2000.

78. Walshe JM: Missed Wilson's disease. *Lancet* ii:405–406, 1975.

79. Akil M, Brewer GJ: Psychiatric and behavioral abnormalities in Wilson's disease. *Adv Neurol* 65:171–178, 1995.

80. Oder W, Grimm G, Kollegger H, et al: Neurological and neuropsychiatric spectrum of Wilson's disease: A prospective study of 45 cases. *J Neurol* 238:281–287, 1991.

81. Matarazzo EB: Psychiatric features and disturbance of circadian rhythm of temperature, pulse, and blood pressure in Wilson's disease. *J Neuropsychiatry Clin Neurosci* 14:335–339, 2002.

82. Seniow J, Bak T, Gajda J, et al: Cognitive functioning in neurologically symptomatic and asymptomatic forms of Wilson's disease. *Mov Disord* 17:1077–1083, 2002.

83. Portala K, Westermark K, von Knorring L, et al: Psychopathology in treated Wilson's disease determined by means of CPRS expert and self-ratings. *Acta Psychiatr Scand* 101:104–109, 2000.

84. Portala K, Levander S, Westermark K, et al: Pattern of neuropsychological deficits in patients with treated Wilson's disease. *Eur Arch Psychiatry Clin Neurosci* 251:262–268, 2001.

85. Portala K, Westermark K, Ekselius L, et al: Personality traits in treated Wilson's disease determined by means of the Karolinska Scales of Personality (KSP). *Eur Psychiatry* 16:362–371, 2001.

86. Rathbun JK: Neuropsychological aspects of Wilson's disease. *Int J Neurosci* 85:221–229, 1996.

87. Tarter RE, Switala J, Carra J, et al: Neuropsychological impairment associated with hepatolenticular degeneration (Wilson's disease) in the absence of overt encephalopathy. *Int J Neurosci* 37:67–71, 1987.

88. Scheinberg IH, Sternlieb I, Richman J: Psychiatric manifestations in patients with Wilson's disease, in Bergsma D, Scheinberg IH, Sternlieb I (eds): *Wilson's Disease: Birth Defects, Original Article Series*. New York: The National Foundation—March of Dimes, 1968, vol 4, pp 85–87.

89. Dening TR: Psychiatric aspects of Wilson's disease. *Br J Psychiatry* 147:677–682, 1985.

90. Davis EJ, Borde M: Wilson's disease and catatonia. *Br J Psychiatry* 162:256–259, 1993.

91. Kaul A, McMahon D: Wilson's disease and offending behavior: A case report. *Med Sci Law* 33:353–358, 1993.

92. Gwirtsman HE, Prager J, Henkin R: Case report of anorexia nervosa associated with Wilson's disease. *Int J Eat Disord* 13:241–244, 1993.

93. Wiebers DO, Hollenhorst RW, Goldstein NP: The ophthalmologic manifestations of Wilson's disease. *Mayo Clin Proc* 52:409–416, 1977.

94. Johnson RD, Campbell RJ: Wilson's disease: Electron microscopic, X-ray energy spectroscopic and atomic absorption spectroscopic studies of corneal copper deposition and distribution. *Lab Invest* 46:546–569, 1982.

95. Innes JR, Strachan IM, Triger DR: Unilateral Kayser-Fleischer ring. *Br J Ophthalmol* 70:469–470, 1979.

96. Tauber J, Steinert RF: Pseudo-Kayser-Fleischer ring of the cornea associated with non-Wilsonian liver disease: A case report and literature review. *Cornea* 12:74–77, 1993.

97. Sussman W, Scheinberg IH: Disappearance of Kayser-Fleischer rings. Effects of penicillamine. *Arch Ophthalmol* 82:738–741, 1969.

98. Fleming CR, Dickson ER, Wahner HW, et al: Pigmented corneal rings in non-Wilsonian liver disease. *Ann Intern Med* 86:285–288, 1977.

99. Frommer D, Morris J, Sherlock S, et al: Kayser-Fleischer-like rings in patients without Wilson's disease. *Gastroenterology* 72:1331–1335, 1977.

100. Kaplinsky C, Sternlieb I, Javitt N, et al: Familial cholestatic cirrhosis associated with Kayser-Fleischer rings. *Pediatrics* 65:782–788, 1980.

101. Stephenson S: Cases illustrating an unusual form of corneal opacity due to the long-continued application of copper sulphate to the palpebral conjunctiva. *Trans Ophthalmol Soc UK* 23:25–27, 1902.

102. Goodman SI, Rodgerson DO, Kaufman J: Hypercupremia in a patient with multiple myeloma. *J Lab Clin Med* 70:57–62, 1967.

103. Lewis RA, Falls HF, Troyer DO: Ocular manifestations of hypercupremia associated with multiple myeloma. *Arch Ophthalmol* 93:1050–1053, 1995.

104. Martin NF, Kincaid MC, Stark WJ, et al: Ocular copper deposition associated with pulmonary carcinoma, IgG monoclonal gammopathy and hypercupremia: A clinicopathologic correlation. *Ophthalmology* 90:110–116, 1983.

105. Giorgio AJ, Cartwright GE, Wintrobe MM: Pseudo-Kayser-Fleischer rings. *Arch Intern Med* 113:817–818, 1964.

106. Siemerling E, Oloff H: Pseudosklerose (Westphal-Strümpell) mit Cornealring (Kayser-Fleischer) und doppelseitiger Scheinkatarakt, die nur bei seitlicher Beleuchtung sichtbar ist und die der nach Verletzung durch Kupfersplitter entstehenden Katarakt ähnlich ist. *Klin Wochenschr* 1:1087–1089, 1922.

107. Cairns JE, Williams HP, Walshe JM: "Sunflower cataract" in Wilson's disease. *Br Med J* 3:95–96, 1969.

108. Goldberg MF, von Noorden GK: Ophthalmologic findings in Wilson's hepatolenticular degeneration: With emphasis on ocular motility. *Arch Ophthalmol* 75:162–170, 1966.

109. Pillat A: Changes in the eyegrounds in Wilson's disease (pseudosclerosis). *Am J Ophthalmol* 16:1–6, 1933.

110. Walsh FB, Hoyt WF: *Clinical Neuroophthalmology*, 3rd ed. Baltimore: Williams & Wilkins, 1969, vol 2, p 1140.

111. Gow PJ, Peacock SE, Chapman RW: Wilson's disease presenting with rapidly progressive visual loss: another neurologic manifestation of Wilson's disease? *J Gastroenterol Hepatol* 16:699–701, 2001.

112. Lennox G, Jones R: Gaze distractibility in Wilson's disease. *Ann Neurol* 25:415–417, 1989.

113. Keane JR: Lid-opening apraxia in Wilson's disease. *J Clin Neuroophthalmol* 8:31–33, 1988.

114. Lee MS, Kim YD, Lyoo CH: Oculogyric crisis as an initial manifestation of Wilson's disease. *Neurology* 52:1714–1715, 1999.

115. Dastur DK, Manghani DK, Wadia NH: Wilson's disease in India. I. Geographic, genetic, and clinical aspects in 16 families. *Neurology* 18:21–31, 1968.

116. Tu JB: A genetic, biochemical and clinical study of Wilson's disease among Chinese in Taiwan. *Acta Paediatr Sin* 4:81–84, 1963.

117. Xu XH, Yang BX, Feng YK: Wilson's disease (hepatolenticular degeneration): Clinical analysis of 80 cases. *Chin Med J* 94:673–678, 1981.

118. Saito T: Presenting symptoms and natural history of Wilson's disease. *Eur J Pediatr* 146:261–265, 1987.

119. Golding DN, Walshe JM: Arthropathy of Wilson's disease: Study of clinical and radiological features in 32 patients. *Ann Rheum Dis* 36:99–111, 1977.

120. Canelas HM, Carvalho N, Scaff M, et al: Osteoarthropathy of hepatolenticular degeneration. *Acta Neurol Scand* 57:481–487, 1978.

121. Yarze JC, Martin P, Munoz SJ, et al: Wilson's disease: Current status. *Am J Med* 92:643–654, 1992.

122. Feller E, Schumacher HR: Osteoarticular changes in Wilson's disease. *Arthritis Rheum* 15:259–266, 1972.

123. Balint G, Szebenyi B: Hereditary disorders mimicking and/or causing premature osteoarthritis. *Baillieres Best Pract Res Clin Rheumatol* 14:219–250, 2000.

124. Mindelzun R, Elkin M, Scheinberg IH, et al: Skeletal changes in Wilson's disease: A radiological study. *Radiology* 94:127–132, 1970.

125. Kramer U, Weinberger A, Yarom R, et al: Synovial copper deposition as a possible explanation of arthropathy in Wilson's disease. *Bull Hosp Jt Dis* 52:46–49, 1993.

126. McIntyre N, Clink HM, Levi AJ, et al: Hemolytic anemia in Wilson's disease. *N Engl J Med* 276:439–444, 1967.

127. Sternlieb I: Wilson's disease: Indications for liver transplants. *Hepatology* 4:15S–17S, 1984.

128. Meyer RJ, Zalusky R: The mechanisms of hemolysis in Wilson's disease: Study of a case and review of the literature. *Mt Sinai J Med* 44:530–538, 1977.

129. Forman SJ, Kumar KS, Redeker AG, et al: Hemolytic anemia in Wilson disease: Clinical findings and biochemical mechanisms. *Am J Hematol* 9:269–275, 1980.

130. Lee JJ, Kim HJ, Chung IJ, et al: Acute hemolytic crisis with fulminant hepatic failure as the first manifestation of Wilson's disease: A case report. *J Korean Med Sci* 13:548–550, 1998.

131. Druml W, Laggner AN, Lenz K, et al: Pancreatitis in acute hemolysis. *Ann Hematol* 63:39–41, 1991.

132. Prella M, Baccala R, Horisberger JD, et al: Haemolytic onset of Wilson disease in a patient with homozygous truncation of ATP7B at Arg1319. *Br J Haematol* 114:230–232, 2001.

133. Donfrid M, Jankovic G, Strahinja R, et al: Idiopathic thrombocytopenia associated with Wilson's disease. *Hepatogastroenterology* 45:1774–1776, 1998.

134. Wiebers DO, Wilson DM, McLeod RA, et al: Renal stones in Wilson's disease. *Am J Med* 67:249–254, 1979.

135. Hoppe B, Neuhaus T, Superti-Furga A, et al: Hypercalciuria and nephrocalcinosis, a feature of Wilson's disease. *Nephron* 65:460–462, 1993.

136. Sozeri E, Feist D, Ruder H, et al: Proteinuria and other renal functions in Wilson's disease. *Pediatr Nephrol* 11:307–311, 1997.

137. Leu ML, Strickland GT, Wang CC, et al: Skin pigmentation in Wilson's disease. *J Am Med Assoc* 211:1542–1543, 1970.

138. Bearn AG, McKusick VA: Azure lunulae: An unusual change in the fingernails in two patients with hepatolenticular degeneration (Wilson's disease). *J Am Med Assoc* 166:904–906, 1958.

139. Ezzo JA, Rowley JF, Finnegin JV: Hepatolenticular degeneration associated with acanthosis nigricans. *Arch Intern Med* 100:827–832, 1957.

140. Scheinberg IH, Sternlieb I: Wilson's disease. *Annu Rev Med* 16:119–134, 1965.

141. Lau JY, Lai CL, Wu PC, et al: Wilson's disease: 35 years' experience. *Q J Med* 75:597–605, 1990.

142. Erkan T, Aktuglu C, Gulcan EM, et al: Wilson disease manifested primarily as amenorrhea and accompanying thrombocytopenia. *J Adolesc Health* 31:378–380, 2002.

143. Sternlieb I, Scheinberg IH: Wilson's disease, in Wright R, Alberti KGM, Karran S, et al. (eds): *Liver and Biliary Disease*. London: Bailliere Tindall, 1985, pp 949–961.

144. McIntyre N: Neurological Wilson's disease. *Q J Med* 86:349–350, 1993.

145. Snow B: Laboratory diagnosis and monitoring of Wilson's disease, in *Neurological Aspects of Wilson's Disease, American Academy of Neurology Course 411*. 1995, pp 25–30.

146. Smallwood RA, Williams HA, Rosenauer VM: Liver copper levels in liver disease: Studies using neutron activation analysis. *Lancet* ii:1310–1313, 1968.

147. Benson GD: Hepatic copper accumulation in primary biliary cirrhosis. *Yale J Biol Med* 52:83–88, 1979.

148. Evans J, Newman S, Sherlock S: Liver copper levels in intrahepatic cholestasis of childhood. *Gastroenterology* 75:875–878, 1978.

149. Tanner MS, Portmann B, Mowat AP, et al: Increased hepatic copper concentration in Indian childhood cirrhosis. *Lancet* i:1203–1205, 1979.

150. LaRusso NF, Summerskill WH, McCall JT: Abnormalities of chemical tests for copper metabolism in chronic active liver disease: Differentiation from Wilson's disease. *Gastroenterology* 70:653–655, 1976.

151. Sternlieb I, Giblin DR, Scheinberg IH: Wilson's disease, in Marsden CD, Fahn S (eds): *Movement Disorders*. London: Butterworth, 1987, vol 2, pp 288–302.

152. Willeit J, Kiechl SG: Wilson's disease with neurologic impairment but no Kayser-Fleischer rings. *Lancet* 337:1426, 1991.

153. Vidaud D, Assouline B, Lecoz P, et al: Misdiagnosis revealed by genetic linkage analysis in a family with Wilson disease. *Neurology* 46:1485–1486, 1996.

154. Frommer DJ: Urinary copper excretion and hepatic copper concentrations in liver disease. *Digestion* 21:169–178, 1981.

155. Steindl P, Ferenci P, Dienes HP, et al: Wilson's disease in patients presenting with liver disease: A diagnostic challenge. *Gastroenterology* 113:212–218, 1997.

156. Cumings JN: Trace metals in the brain and in Wilson's disease. *J Clin Pathol* 21:1–7, 1968.

157. Stremmel W, Meyerrose K-W, Niederau C, et al: Wilson disease: Clinical presentation, treatment, and survival. *Ann Intern Med* 115:720–726, 1991.

158. Sternlieb I, Scheinberg IH: The role of radiocopper in the diagnosis of Wilson's disease. *Gastroenterology* 77:138–142, 1979.

159. Weisner B, Hartard C, Dieu C: CSF copper concentration: A new parameter for diagnosis and monitoring therapy of Wilson's disease with cerebral manifestation. *J Neurol Sci* 79: 229–237, 1987.

160. Hartard C, Weisner B, Dieu C, et al: Wilson's disease with cerebral manifestation: Monitoring therapy by CSF copper concentration. *J Neurol* 241:101–107, 1993.

161. Stuerenburg HJ: CSF copper concentrations, blood-brain barrier function, and coeruloplasmin synthesis during the treatment of Wilson's disease. *J Neural Transm* 107:321–329, 2000.

162. Thuomas KA, Aquilonius SM, Bergstrom K, et al: Magnetic resonance imaging of the brain in Wilson's disease. *Neuroradiology* 35:134–141, 1993.

163. Roh JK, Lee TG, Wie BA, et al: Initial and follow-up brain MRI findings and correlation with the clinical course in Wilson's disease. *Neurology* 44:1064–1068, 1994.

164. Selwa LM, Vanderzant CW, Brunberg JA, et al: Correlation of evoked potential and MRI findings in Wilson's disease. *Neurology* 43:2059–2064, 1993.

165. Magalhaes ACA, Caramelli P, Menezes JR, et al: Wilson's disease: MRI with clinical correlation. *Neuroradiology* 36:97–100, 1994.

166. Alanen A, Komu M, Penttinen M, et al: Magnetic resonance imaging and proton MR spectroscopy in Wilson disease. *Br J Radiol* 72:749–756, 1999.

167. Hitoshi S, Iwata M, Yoshikawa K: Midbrain pathology of Wilson's disease: MRI analysis of three cases. *J Neurol Neurosurg Psychiatry* 54:624–626, 1991.

168. Liebeskind DS, Wong S, Hamilton RH: Faces of the giant panda and her cub: MRI correlates of Wilson's disease. *J Neurol Neurosurg Psychiatry* 74:682, 2003.

169. Sener RN: The claustrum on MRI: Normal anatomy, and the bright claustrum as a new sign in Wilson's disease. *Pediatr Radiol* 23:594–596, 1993.

170. Sener RN: Diffusion MRI findings in Wilson's disease. *Comput Med Imaging Graph* 27:17–21, 2003.

171. Jayasundar R, Sahani AK, Gaikwad S, et al: Proton MR spectroscopy of basal ganglia in Wilson's disease: Case report and review of literature. *Magn Reson Imaging* 20:131–135, 2002.

172. Hawkins RA, Mazziotta JC, Phelps ME: Wilson's disease studied with FDG and positron emission tomography. *Neurology* 37:1707–1711, 1987.

173. Hefter H, Kuwert T, Herzog H, et al: Relationship between striatal glucose consumption and copper excretion in patients with Wilson's disease treated with D-penicillamine. *J Neurol* 241:49–53, 1993.

174. Snow BJ, Bhatt MH, Martin WRW, et al: The nigrostriatal dopaminergic pathway in Wilson's disease studied with positron emission tomography. *J Neurol Neurosurg Psychiatry* 54:12–17, 1991.

175. Topcu M, Topcuoglu MA, Kose G, et al: Evoked potentials in children with Wilson's disease. *Brain Dev* 24:276–280, 2002.

176. Grimm G, Madl C, Katzenschlager R, et al: Detailed evaluation of evoked potentials in Wilson's disease. *Electroencephalogr Clin Neurophysiol* 82:119–124, 1992.

177. Brewer GJ, Yuzbasiyan-Gurkan V, Dick R, et al: Does a vegetarian diet control Wilson's disease? *J Am Coll Nutr* 12:527–530, 1993.

178. Ebadi M, Paliwal VK, Takahashi T, et al: Zinc metallothionein in mammalian brain. *UCLA Symp Mol Cell Biol* 98:257–267, 1989.

179. Ebadi M: Metallothionein and other zinc-binding proteins in brain. *Methods Enzymol* 205:363–387, 1991.

180. Day FA, Panemangelore M, Brady FO: *In vivo* and *ex vivo* effects of copper on rat liver metallothionein. *Proc Soc Exp Biol Med* 168:306–310, 1981.

181. Brewer GJ, Hill GM, Prasad AS, et al: Oral zinc therapy for Wilson's disease. *Ann Intern Med* 99:314–320, 1983.

182. Hall AC, Young BW, Bremner I: Intestinal metallothionein and the mutual antagonism between copper and zinc in the rat. *J Inorg Biochem* 11:57–66, 1979.

183. Brewer GJ, Yuzbasiyan-Gurkan V: Wilson's disease, in Klawans HK, Goetz CG, Tanner CM (eds): *Textbook of Clinical Neuropharmacology and Therapeutics.* New York: Raven Press, 1992, pp 191–205.

184. Brewer GJ: Zinc acetate for the treatment of Wilson's disease. *Expert Opin Pharmacother* 2:1473–1477, 2001.

185. Brewer GJ, Yuzbasiyan-Gurkan V, Lee DY, et al: Treatment of Wilson's disease with zinc. VI. Initial treatment studies. *J Lab Clin Med* 114:633–638, 1989.

186. Schilsky ML: Treatment of Wilson's disease: What are the relative roles of penicillamine, trientine, and zinc supplementation? *Curr Gastroenterol Rep* 3:54–59, 2001.

187. Rossaro L, Sturniolo GC, Giacon G, et al: Zinc therapy in Wilson's disease: Observations in five patients. *Am J Gastroenterol* 85:665–668, 1990.

188. Hoogenraad T: *Wilson's Disease.* London: WB Saunders, 1996.

189. Brewer GJ, Dick RD, Johnson VD, et al: Treatment of Wilson's disease with zinc XVI: Treatment during the pediatric years. *J Lab Clin Med* 137:191–198, 2001.

190. Brewer GJ, Johnson VD, Dick RD, et al: Treatment of Wilson's disease with zinc XVII: Treatment during pregnancy. *Hepatology* 31:364–370, 2000.

191. Subramanian I, Vanek ZF, Bronstein JM: Diagnosis and treatment of Wilson's disease. *Curr Neurol Neurosci Rep* 2:317–323, 2002.

192. Simon SR, Branda RF, Tindle BH, et al: Copper deficiency and sideroblastic anemia associated with zinc ingestion. *Am J Hematol* 28:181–183, 1988.

193. Brewer GJ, Yuzbasiyan-Gurkan V, Lee D-Y: Molecular genetics and zinc-copper interactions in human Wilson's disease and canine copper toxicosis, in Prasad AS (ed): *Essential and Toxic Trace Elements in Human Health and Disease: An Update.* New York: Wiley-Liss, 1992, pp 129–145.

194. Hooper PL, Visconti L, Garry PJ, et al: Zinc lowers high-density lipoprotein-cholesterol levels. *J Am Med Assoc* 244:1960–1961, 1980.

195. Yuzbasiyan-Gurkan V, Brewer GJ, Abrams GD, et al: Treatment of Wilson's disease with zinc: V. Changes in serum levels of lipase, amylase and alkaline phosphatase in Wilson's disease patients. *J Lab Clin Med* 114:520–526, 1989.

196. Walshe JM: Penicillamine: The treatment of first choice for patients with Wilson's disease. *Mov Disord* 14:545–550, 1999.

197. Brewer GJ: Penicillamine should not be used as initial therapy in Wilson's disease. *Mov Disord* 14:551–554, 1999.

198. LeWitt PA: Penicillamine as a controversial treatment for Wilson's disease. *Mov Disord* 14:555–556, 1999.

199. Brewer GJ, Dick RD, Johnson V, et al: Treatment of Wilson's disease with ammonium tetrathiomolybdate. I. Initial therapy in 17 neurologically affected patients. *Arch Neurol* 51:545–554, 1994.

200. Brewer GJ, Dick RD, Yuzbasiyan-Gurkan V, et al: Initial therapy of patients with Wilson's disease with tetrathiomolybdate. *Arch Neurol* 48:42–47, 1991.

201. Brewer GJ, Johnson V, Dick RD, et al: Treatment of Wilson disease with ammonium tetrathiomolybdate. II. Initial therapy in 33 neurologically affected patients and follow-up with zinc therapy. *Arch Neurol* 53:1017–1025, 1996.

202. Spence JA, Suttle NF, Wenham G, et al: A sequential study of the skeletal abnormalities, which develop in rats given a small dietary supplement of ammonium tetrathiomolybdate. *J Comp Pathol* 90:139–153, 1980.

203. Walshe JM, Yealland M: Chelation treatment of neurological Wilson's disease. *Q J Med* 86:197–204, 1993.

204. Walshe JM: Penicillamine: A new oral therapy for Wilson's disease. *Am J Med* 21:487–495, 1956.

205. Deiss A: Treatment of Wilson's disease. *Ann Intern Med* 99:398–399, 1983.

206. Goldstein NP, Ewert JC, Randall RV, et al: Psychiatric aspects of Wilson's disease (hepatolenticular degeneration): Results of psychometric tests during long-term therapy. *Am J Psychiatry* 124:1555–1561, 1968.

207. Williams FJB, Walshe JM: Wilson's disease. An analysis of the cranial computerized tomographic appearances found in patients and the changes in response to treatment with chelating agents. *Brain* 104:735–752, 1981.

208. Nazer H, Brismar J, Al-Kawi MZ, et al: Magnetic resonance imaging of the brain in Wilson's disease. *Neuroradiology* 35:130–133, 1993.

209. Marsden CD: Wilson's disease. *Q J Med* 248:959–966, 1987.

210. Gibbs KR, Walshe JM: Interruption of the tryptophan-nicotinic acid pathway by penicillamine-induced pyridoxine deficiency in patients with Wilson's disease and in experimental animals. *Ann N Y Acad Sci* 111:158–169, 1969.

211. Brewer GJ, Terry CA, Aisen AM, et al: Worsening of neurological syndrome in patients with Wilson's disease with initial penicillamine therapy. *Arch Neurol* 44:490–493, 1987.

212. Svetel M, Sternic N, Pejovic S, et al: Penicillamine-induced lethal status dystonicus in a patient with Wilson's disease. *Mov Disord* 16:568–569, 2001.

213. Glass JD, Reich SG, DeLong MR: Wilson's disease: Development of neurological disease after beginning penicillamine therapy. *Arch Neurol* 47:595–596, 1990.

214. Brewer GJ, Turkay A, Yuzbasiyan-Gurkan V: Development of neurologic symptoms in a patient with asymptomatic Wilson's disease. *Arch Neurol* 51:304–305, 1994.

215. Sternlieb I, Scheinberg IH: Penicillamine therapy in hepatolenticular degeneration. *J Am Med Assoc* 189:748–754, 1964.

216. Haggstrom GC, Hirschowitz BI, Flint A: Long-term penicillamine therapy for Wilson's disease. *South Med J* 73:530–531, 1980.

217. Chan C-Y, Baker AL: Penicillamine hypersensitivity: Successful desensitization of a patient with severe hepatic Wilson's disease. *Am J Gastroenterol* 89:442–443, 1994.

218. Corcos JM, Soler-Bechera J, Mayer K, et al: Neutrophilic agranulocytosis during administration of penicillamine. *J Am Med Assoc* 189:265–268, 1964.

219. Hirschman SZ, Isselbacher KJ: The nephrotic syndrome as a complication of penicillamine therapy of hepatolenticular degeneration (Wilson's disease). *Ann Intern Med* 62:1297–1300, 1965.

220. Sternlieb I, Bennett B, Scheinberg IH: D-Penicillamine induced Goodpasture's syndrome in Wilson's disease. *Ann Intern Med* 82:673–675, 1975.

221. Walshe JM: Penicillamine and the SLE syndrome. *J Rheumatol* 8(suppl 7):155–160, 1981.

222. Czlonkowska A: Myasthenia syndrome during penicillamine treatment. *Br Med J* 2:726–727, 1975.

223. Bigger JF: Retinal hemorrhages during penicillamine therapy of cystinuria. *Am J Ophthalmol* 66:954–955, 1968.

224. Shoulson I, Goldblatt D, Plassche W, et al: Some therapeutic observations in Wilson's disease. *Adv Neurol* 37:239–246, 1983.

225. Henkin RI, Keiser HR, Jaffe IA, et al: Decreased taste sensitivity after D-penicillamine reversed by copper administration. *Lancet* ii:1268–1271, 1967.

226. Proesman W, Jaeken J, Eckels R: D-Penicillamine induced IgA deficiency in Wilson's disease. *Lancet* ii:804–805, 1976.

227. Sternlieb I, Fisher M, Scheinberg IH: Penicillamine-induced skin lesions. *J Rheumatol* 8(suppl 7):149–154, 1981.

228. Nimni ME: Mechanism of inhibition of collagen cross-linking by penicillamine. *Proc R Soc Med* 70(suppl 3):65–72, 1977.

229. Morris JJ, Seifter E, Rettura G, et al: Effect of penicillamine upon wound healing. *J Surg Res* 9:143–149, 1969.

230. Kirsch N, Hukill PB: Elastosis perforans serpiginosa by penicillamine. Electron microscopic observations. *Arch Dermatol* 113:630–635, 1977.

231. Pass F, Goldfischer S, Sternlieb I, et al: Elastosis perforans serpiginosa after penicillamine therapy for Wilson's disease. *Arch Dermatol* 108:713–715, 1973.

232. Eisenberg E, Ballow M, Wolfe SH, et al: Pemphigus-like mucosal lesions: A side effect of penicillamine therapy. *Oral Surg Oral Med Oral Pathol* 51:409–414, 1981.

233. Bennett RA, Harbilas E: Wilson's disease with aseptic meningitis and penicillamine-related cheilosis. *Arch Intern Med* 120:374–376, 1967.

234. Walshe JM: The management of penicillamine nephropathy in Wilson's disease: A new chelating agent. *Lancet* ii:1401–1402, 1969.

235. Walshe JM: Assessment of the treatment of Wilson's disease with triethylene tetramine 2HCl (Trien 2HCl), in Sarker B (ed): *Biological Aspects of Metal Related Diseases.* New York: Raven Press, 1983, pp 243–261.

236. Walshe JM: Treatment of Wilson's disease with trientine (triethylene tetramine) dihydrochloride. *Lancet* i:643–647, 1982.

237. Walshe JM: Copper chelation in patients with Wilson's disease: A comparison of penicillamine and triethylene tetramine hydrochloride. *Q J Med* 42:441–452, 1973.

238. Condamine L, Hermine O, Alvin P, et al: Acquired sideroblastic anaemia during treatment of Wilson's disease with triethylene tetramine dihydrochloride. *Br J Hematol* 83:166–168, 1993.

239. Brewer GJ: Wilson's disease. *Curr Treat Options Neurol* 2:193–204, 2000.

240. Schilsky ML, Scheinberg IH, Sternlieb I: Liver transplantation for Wilson's disease: Indications and outcome. *Hepatology* 19:583–587, 1994.

241. Rela M, Heaton ND, Vougas V, et al: Orthotopic liver transplantation for hepatic complications of Wilson's disease. *Br J Surg* 80:909–911, 1993.

242. Shafer DF, Shaw BW Jr: Fulminant hepatic failure and orthotopic liver transplantation. *Semin Liver Dis* 9:189–194, 1989.

243. Sen S, Felldin M, Steiner C, et al: Albumin dialysis and molecular adsorbents recirculating system (MARS) for acute Wilson's disease. *Liver Transpl* 8:962–967, 2002.

244. Kreymann B, Seige M, Schweigart U, et al: Albumin dialysis: Effective removal of copper in a patient with fulminant Wilson disease and successful bridging to liver transplantation: A new possibility for the elimination of protein-bound toxins. *J Hepatol* 31:1080–1085, 1999.

245. Mazariegos GV, Kramer DJ, Lopez RC, et al: Safety observations in phase I clinical evaluation of the Excorp Medical Bioartificial Liver Support System after the first four patients. *ASAIO J* 47:471–475, 2001.

246. Chen CL, Kuo YC: Metabolic effects of liver transplantation in Wilson's disease. *Transplant Proc* 25:2944–2947, 1993.

247. Emre S, Atillasoy EO, Ozdemir S, et al: Orthotopic liver transplantation for Wilson's disease: A single-center experience. *Transplantation* 72:1232–1236, 2001.

248. Komatsu H, Fujisawa T, Inui A, et al: Hepatic copper concentration in children undergoing living related liver transplantation due to Wilsonian fulminant hepatic failure. *Clin Transplant* 16:227–232, 2002.

249. Mason AL, Marsh W, Alpers DH: Intractable neurological Wilson's disease treated with orthotopic liver transplantation. *Dig Dis Sci* 38:1746–1750, 1993.

250. Stracciari A, Tempestini A, Borghi A, et al: Effect of liver transplantation on neurological manifestations in Wilson disease. *Arch Neurol* 57:384–386, 2000.

251. Malhi H, Irani AN, Volenberg I, et al: Early cell transplantation in LEC rats modeling Wilson's disease eliminates hepatic copper with reversal of liver disease. *Gastroenterology* 122:438–447, 2002.

252. Ha-Hao D, Merle U, Hofmann C, et al: Chances and shortcomings of adenovirus-mediated ATP7B gene transfer in Wilson disease: Proof of principle demonstrated in a pilot study with LEC rats. *Z Gastroenterol* 40:209–216, 2002.

Chapter 48

STIFF-PERSON SYNDROME

OSCAR S. GERSHANIK

HISTORICAL BACKGROUND   799
CLINICAL ASPECTS   800
    Physical Examination   801
    Laboratory   801
    Electromyography (EMG)   802
    Muscle Biopsy   802
    Imaging Studies   803
ASSOCIATED CONDITIONS   803
DIAGNOSIS   803
DIFFERENTIAL DIAGNOSIS   804
PATHOPHYSIOLOGY AND PATHOGENESIS   806
    Pathology   806
    Physiology   806
    Biochemistry and Pharmacology   807
    Immunology   807
    Etiology and Pathogenesis   809
TREATMENT   809

The stiff-person syndrome (SPS) is a rare neurologic disorder of uncertain cause, characterized by severe and incapacitating axial and proximal limb rigidity due to continuous motor unit activity. Rigidity is often enhanced by anxiety, sudden movements or external stimuli causing intermittent painful muscle spasms, often leading to skeletal deformity. Variants of this disorder include focal involvement of one limb ("stiff-limb syndrome"), or additional neurological symptoms suggestive of involvement of subcortical gray matter ("progressive encephalomyelitis with rigidity and myoclonus") and occasionally secondary to malignant disease (paraneoplastic SPS). Antineuronal antibodies often associated with other autoimmune diseases are characteristic features of this disorder. The disease follows a progressive, unremitting course, resulting in pronounced disability, if left untreated.

Historical Background

This unusual syndrome was first described by Moersch and Woltman in 1956.[1] The authors coined the term "stiff-man syndrome" in reporting 14 patients with clinical features of progressive fluctuating muscular rigidity and spasms. Their first case, a 49-year-old man, initially complained of a feeling of tightness of the neck musculature of variable occurrence. Over a period of 4 years this disorder progressively affected the muscles of the shoulder, back, abdomen, and thighs, causing the muscles to appear stiff and "board-like." Continuous muscle contraction causing pronounced stiffness of the axial and limb muscles forced the patient to walk in a peculiar way that was both slow and awkward. Voluntary movement or passive displacement of the limbs triggered prolonged and painful muscle spasms. If severe enough, the spasms caused postural instability and falls. In the words of the authors, the patient would fall like a "wooden man." The additional 13 patients in the original report were similar in all respects.

The clinical features of this previously unreported condition were described in detail in Moersch and Woltman's paper. No other signs of central or peripheral nervous system involvement were present in their 14 patients. The only additional clinical abnormality found in 4 of the 14 original patients was diabetes mellitus. Five of their 14 patients underwent electromyographic (EMG) studies, revealing motor unit activity resembling "that which accompanies contraction of voluntary muscle." In their 1967 review on the subject, Gordon et al.[2] summarized the EMG findings reported in the literature until then as "one of persistent tonic contraction reflected in constant firing even at rest." No attempt at relaxation could alter the continuous motor unit discharges according to these authors. Their observations provided the electrophysiological substrate of muscle stiffness in these patients.

Since the publication of Moersch and Woltman's description of the syndrome, more than 100 cases have been reported from different regions of the world.

The first successful attempt at treatment of this condition was that of Howard in 1963[3] with the use of diazepam to reduce stiffness and spasms.

A major breakthrough in the understanding of the pathogenesis of SPS came through the work of Solimena et al. in 1988,[4] who reported the presence of antibodies against glutamic acid decarboxylase (anti-GAD), an enzyme involved in the synthesis of gamma-aminobutyric acid (GABA) in a patient with SPS, diabetes mellitus, and evidence of additional immunological involvement. Since then, SPS has been postulated as an immunological disorder.

Gordon et al.[2] and later Lorish et al.[5] defined the clinical criteria necessary for the diagnosis of SPS. These criteria have been widely accepted and are currently used for the identification of cases of SPS. A significant number of patients fall outside these criteria, and are considered atypical SPS. In their recent review of cases seen at the National Hospital in London, Barker et al.[6] assigned cases into three distinct categories: SPS, progressive encephalomyelitis with rigidity (PEWR), and stiff-limb syndrome (a focal form of the disorder). Brown and Marsden,[7] in a follow-up, reviewed the clinical, immunological, and pathophysiological features of their own, and published cases presenting with features suggestive of SPS; they proposed a new classification, separating the classic form (stiff-man or stiff-person, SPS) from a distinct group designated the "stiff-man plus" syndrome, which includes both the clinically atypical presentations and the paraneoplastic forms of this disorder.

Numerous attempts at therapeutic intervention followed Howard's observation of clinical improvement with diazepam in patients with SPS. Benzodiazepines and baclofen have been recognized as the drugs of choice,[8] although reports of improvement with other drugs, such as sodium valproate, tizanidine, steroids, gabapentin, tiagabine, vigabatrin, immunoglobulin, and plasmapheresis, have been published in recent years.[6,9]

Clinical Aspects

The disease is sporadic, affecting individuals of both sexes in variable proportion. In their analysis of 34 "valid" cases, Gordon et al.[2] found a 2:1 male/female preponderance. This ratio, however, is not maintained in subsequent cases in the more recent literature; interestingly, in the recently published series from the National Institute of Neurological Disorders and Stroke (NINDS), up to 70 percent of the patients were female.[5,10,11] Although the age at onset varies considerably, the majority of those afflicted are adults ranging from 29 to 59 years of age. Both older and younger cases have been occasionally reported (extreme range 7–71 years).[12–14] Although families with "congenital" SPS have been described, doubts have been raised concerning their identity with sporadic SPS of later onset.[8,15,16] Mean age at onset in the original Mayo Clinic series was 45.5 ± 9.3 years.[5] In the series of Dalakas et al., the average age at symptom onset was 41.2 years. Time to diagnosis, however, was delayed from 1 year to 18 years.[10]

Symptoms usually start slowly and insidiously; patients often complaining of episodic aching and tightness of the axial musculature (neck, paraspinal, and abdominal muscles). Muscle tightness, stiffness, and rigidity become constant within several weeks or months. Involvement is usually symmetrical, spreading on to include proximal muscle groups in all four limbs,[5,8] although gross asymmetry is seen in 10 percent of cases according to Meinck.[9] Interestingly, this figure goes up to almost 70 percent in the series reported by Dalakas et al.,[10] taking into account all degrees of asymmetry. Sparing of distal muscles of the limbs and facial musculature is usually the rule in these patients; however, the hands or feet may be involved in up to 25 percent of cases,[9] and involvement of the cranial musculature has been reported occasionally (e.g., difficulty swallowing, dysphagia, changes in facial expression, pursing of the lips, etc.).[2] Stiffness due to involvement of antagonistic muscles causes significant restriction of voluntary movements. Patients are almost unable to bend over and find walking extremely difficult. They adopt a typical hyperlordotic lumbar posture, causing folding of the skin in that region; the neck is held in a somewhat extended position, and there is marked limitation of back and hip movement. Of importance is the fact that lumbar

hyperlordosis persists even when lying down on their back. This peculiar pattern of stiffness "has prompted patients and physicians to use such descriptions as 'stiff as a board' and 'he walks like a wooden man' or 'looks like a tin soldier...'" as it was colorfully reported by Lorish et al.[5] in their 1989 update on SPS. The rigidity or stiffness may fluctuate in intensity from hour to hour or from day to day, usually disappearing during sleep. Activities of daily living become severely impaired in these patients, as they find it extremely difficult to dress by themselves, leaning forward to tie their shoelaces or put on their socks. When severe rigidity of the cervical spine is present, patients must discontinue driving as they are limited in their capacity to rotate their head to look back or to the side.[5]

An additional incapacitating symptom is the occurrence of intermittent severe spasms in affected muscles.[1,2,5] Spasms are precipitated by a wide range of triggering factors. A sudden noise, an unexpected movement, a simple touch or just being gently nudged may often be the cause of severe spasmodic contraction of the affected muscles. Passive stretching of the muscles will also cause spasms. Emotional stimuli, as well as stress or fatigue may prompt a paroxysm. Spasms are short-lasting (minutes) and gradually disappear if the triggering stimulus is removed. Muscle spasms are often associated with pain. Painful sensation has been variably reported in the literature, either as an acute, sharp or excruciating pain, or more often as a dull, cramping feeling of fatigue.[1,2,5] Spasms may occur in rapid succession ("spasmodic storm") and the clinical picture may then resemble tetanus.[9] Patients experiencing a bout of spasms present a distressful picture, as they "appear to be in a shock-like state associated with sweating, tachycardia and restlessness."[2] An increase in blood pressure has been documented during these crises.[14] Spasms are a compounding factor of motor disability in these patients as they frequently are the cause of sudden falls. Anecdotal reports abound in the literature: patients complaining of spasmodic fits triggered by the ringing of the phone, being awaken in the middle of the night by a soft nudge by a spouse, being ejected from a chair while attempting to sit down.[5] The magnitude and intensity of the spasms is quite variable. In a few reported cases they became severe enough to cause fracture of long bones.[2]

In a recent analysis of clinical and laboratory findings in SPS patients, Meinck et al.[17] extended the repertoire of symptoms in this disorder, adding three new and distinct clinical features to those previously described. Five of their 8 patients reported an "aura"-like feeling preceding spontaneous spasmodic attacks. In the majority of their cases, spasmodic jerks adopted a stereotyped motor pattern, consisting of brief opisthotonos, stiffening of the slightly abducted legs and inversion of the plantar-flexed feet. In addition, their patients reported a feeling of paroxysmal fear invading them whenever they crossed an open space unaided. Moreover, even the thought of doing it would precipitate it. More than 50 percent of patients report a characteristic fear of open spaces which is frequently associated with spasms.[9]

Interestingly, the presence of excessive startle, space phobia, and spasms induced by emotional upset probably are the reasons behind almost 70 percent of initial misdiagnoses in SPS patients and a frequent label of hysteria that is attached to them.[9]

The illness follows a variable course, with a duration ranging from 6 to 28 years, measured from onset of symptoms to either death or last follow-up visit.[5] In the majority of cases, the disease slowly and steadily progresses over time. There are, however, some cases for which stabilization is achieved through medication. Lorish et al.[5] reported on the follow-up of 13 patients seen at the Mayo Clinic during the period 1955–1985. These patients had a disease duration ranging from 1 to 28 years. All 13 cases were under treatment with variable doses of diazepam and the great majority remained independently mobile in spite of the long duration of the disease in some of them. The rate of progression of the disease and the final outcome will depend in part on several factors: (1) whether the clinical presentation was typical and corresponded to classical SPS; (2) or belonged to the type of disorders grouped under the "stiff-man plus" rubric according to Brown and Marsden;[6] and (3) the conditions usually associated with these disorders (e.g., diabetes, malignancy, etc.). Unexpected sudden death has been reported in SPS cases.[18] Two patients carrying a diagnosis of SPS experienced sudden death, apparently secondary to autonomic instability. Of these two cases, however, 1 had atypical clinical signs and inflammatory changes in the basal ganglia, brainstem and spinal cord, more suggestive of encephalomyelitis.[19,20] Severe autonomic symptomatology may be precipitated in SPS patients by sudden withdrawal of medication. This contingency should always be entertained when making changes in medication in SPS patients.

PHYSICAL EXAMINATION

Neurologic examination is usually noncontributory except for those findings related to muscle rigidity. Palpatory examination of the affected muscles will reveal a "tight, rock-hard, board-like quality." Postural changes have been described in detail in the preceding paragraphs. Gait is slow and cautious to avoid precipitation of spasms and falls. Cognitive function, cranial nerves, muscle strength, sensory function and coordination are all normal; deep-tendon reflexes have often been found to be increased, without further evidence of pyramidal tract involvement. Some investigators have reported mild atrophy and weakness in the advanced stages of the disease. Studies of respiratory function may reveal in some cases a restrictive pattern due to involvement of the thoracic musculature.[1,2,5,8]

In the NINDS series,[10] the authors made an attempt to define the clinical presentation and physical findings of SPS patients on the basis of strict and homogeneous criteria. To that effect they studied 20 patients with SPS selected by the presence of anti-GAD antibody positivity in high titers. The neurologic signs in these 20 patients are summarized

TABLE 48-1 Neurologic Signs in 20 Patients with Stiff-Person Syndrome

Type	n (%)
Increased tone	
Paraspinal muscles	20 (100)
Face	13 (65)
Asymmetry with 1 leg predominant	15 (70)
Asymmetry with 1 arm predominant	7 (41)
Only in 1 leg (stiff-limb)	3 (17)
Prominent stiffness in the cervical paraspinal region	1 (6)
Mild proximal muscle weakness with coexisting signs of myopathy	1 (6)
Functional impairment resulting in:	
Stiff gait	20 (100)
Hyperlordosis	14 (65)
Need for cane	12 (65)
Need for walker	7 (35)
Inability to work	12 (65)
Shortness of breath	10 (50)
Task-specific phobias	10 (50)

SOURCE: Dalakas et al. (2000).[10]

in Table 48-1. In their conclusions these authors remarked that, although a hallmark diagnostic sign remains, the presence of hyperlordosis and axial rigidity and co-contractures, the presence of asymmetric involvement with predominant stiffness in one leg was very common in their patients. Moreover, all of their patients with initial asymmetric presentation progressed to generalized symptomatology. Another important finding was the presence of stiffness in the facial muscles in almost 70 percent of the patients, which could erroneously lead to the diagnosis of an akinetic-rigid syndrome in these cases.

The finding of central nervous system (CNS) involvement (myoclonus, brainstem signs, long tract signs, lower motor neuron signs, cognitive changes, autonomic failure/sphincter involvement) or rigidity not confined to the trunk but also involving the distal limbs, often exclusively, would be suggestive of the "stiff-man plus" syndrome (PEWR and related conditions).[7] Although exclusive involvement of one limb ("stiff-limb syndrome") is considered by some to be a separate entity from SPS, the findings of Dalakas et al.[10] would challenge this concept to some extent.

LABORATORY

Routine laboratory examinations are usually within normal limits, except in those cases in whom insulin-dependent diabetes mellitus (IDDM), thyroid disorders, malignancy, or other associated conditions are present (see associated conditions below).[1,2,5,8,11] Creatinuria is a rare finding in these patients, and is most probably linked to disuse atrophy.[2] Immunological determinations reveal the presence of antibodies directed against GABAergic neurons, more specifically to GAD in a large proportion of SPS patients (60–90 percent according to different authors;[4,6,9–11,21,22] autoantibodies directed against other cellular systems are also frequently found in these patients.[6,9–11,21] Oligoclonal IgG banding, both in serum and cerebrospinal fluid (CSF), had been reported as an occasional finding by several authors.[4,11,21,23–25] In a recent study including 18 patients, Dalakas et al.[26] found oligoclonal IgG bands in 67 percent of the cases, and an increased anti-GAD-65-specific IgG index in 85 percent; GABA was found to be lower in SPS patients than in controls. Similar findings regarding oligoclonal banding had been reported by Barker.[6] The presence of GAD autoantibodies in the CSF is indicative of de novo intrathecal antibody production,[9] which is important in the diagnosis of SPS. Elevated CSF IgG has been reported in isolated cases.[27] The presence of significant CSF abnormalities is, on the contrary, the rule in encephalomyelitis and related conditions ("stiff-man plus" syndrome) (see differential diagnosis below).[7,19,20] Certain human lymphocyte antigen (HLA) phenotypes appear to be more frequent than others in cases of SPS.[11,28–30] All of the above point in the direction of an immunological disorder as the underlying cause of SPS (see pathophysiology below).

ELECTROMYOGRAPHY (EMG)

The presence of continuous motor unit activity at rest and its persistence despite attempts at relaxation is a constant finding in SPS patients. There are no abnormalities in the morphology of motor units; peripheral nerve motor and sensory conduction velocities are normal, and no signs of denervation, such as fasciculations, fibrillations, and positive sharp waves, can be found. No evidence of grouping of rhythmic discharges or atypical high-frequency bursts are usually found. EMG recordings show this pattern of continuous motor unit activity to be more prominent in paraspinal muscles (thoracolumbar, and rectus abdominis), and proximal arm and leg muscles. Involvement of both agonist and antagonist muscle groups is common. Peripheral stimulation (gentle touching or stroking of the skin) of the muscles explored is followed by marked enhancement of motor unit activity, either continuous or intermittent (spasms) (Fig. 48-1). A stereotyped motor response to electrical stimulation of peripheral nerves is usually obtained when recording in the trunk muscles of all patients with SPS. This response is termed spasmodic reflex myoclonus or reflex-induced spasms.[31] Reflex-induced spasms have a short-onset latency (below 80 ms), are highly reproducible, and are composed of one or more hypersynchronous bursts of EMG activity. EMG bursting is interrupted by short pauses followed by slowly ceasing activity.[9]

The abnormal EMG activity is absent during sleep. Peripheral nerve or spinal nerve root block, spinal anesthesia and general anesthesia, or intravenous injection of diazepam can also abolish this pattern of motor unit activity.[2,5,8,32]

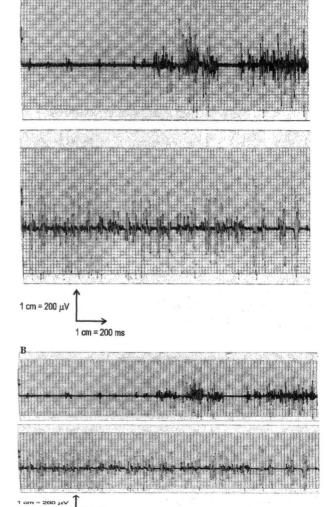

1 cm = 200 µV

1 cm = 200 ms

1 cm = 200 µV

1 cm = 200 ms

FIGURE 48-1 *A.* Simultaneous EMG recording of antagonist muscles of the upper extremity (biceps and triceps brachialis), showing bursts of motor unit discharges at rest. *B.* EMG recording of biceps brachialis, showing intermittent bursts of motor unit discharges after a mechanical stimulus (light tapping).

MUSCLE BIOPSY

Histologic study of muscle is usually noncontributory. Most studies performed have reported normal findings in muscle biopsy specimens. In some cases, nonspecific findings, such as minimal atrophy, slight fibrosis, occasional degeneration and regeneration of muscle fibers with associated sprouting of nerve terminals, edema, perivascular infiltration, and proliferation of connective tissue, have been described.[2] The majority of authors are in agreement in the interpretation of these findings as secondary to prolonged ischemia linked to intense muscular contraction.[2] However, in 2 cases that came to autopsy and were recently published,[33,34] microscopic examination of skeletal muscle showed signs of neurogenic atrophy.

IMAGING STUDIES

Plain X-ray films of the spine may reveal signs of spondylosis and ossification of spinal ligaments.[1] Although these findings have been reported in SPS patients, they probably represent common, nonspecific phenomena, equally present in the general population.[2] Cortical atrophy on computed tomography and white matter lesions on magnetic resonance imaging (MRI) have been reported in isolated cases of SPS, although its relevance to this condition has not been discussed.[8,23,27] It is indeed possible that the above-mentioned abnormalities would correspond to underlying encephalomyelitis. PEWR is often misdiagnosed as SPS (see differential diagnosis below). In cases with typical clinical presentation, positive for GAD autoantibodies, and typical neurophysiological findings, imaging studies might be dispensed with.[9]

Associated Conditions

A number of medical conditions are commonly associated with SPS and are useful in validating its diagnosis as well as providing clues concerning the pathogenesis of this disorder.

In Blum and Jankovic's review of reported cases until 1991,[11] of 84 patients fulfilling Gordon's criteria for SPS, 18 percent had definite clinical evidence of one or more organ-specific autoimmune diseases. These included pernicious anemia, vitiligo, myasthenia gravis, hypothyroidism, hyperthyroidism, and Hashimoto's thyroiditis. More recently, Dalakas et al.[10] in their review of 20 cases of SPS with anti-GAD positivity found that 8/20 had IDDM, 8/20 thyroid disease, 3/20 pernicious anemia, and 1/20 celiac disease. Moreover, family history in these patients was positive for IDDM in 7, thyroid disease in 4, and 1 each had family history of systemic lupus erythematosus, rheumatoid arthritis, myasthenia gravis, and vitiligo. A higher percentage of associated immune diseases (>50 percent) was reported by Meinck.[9]

Of special importance is the relationship of SPS and IDDM, not only because of the frequent association of these two conditions, but because the reason of its simultaneous occurrence may also bear upon the pathogenesis of SPS.[11] Four of the original 14 patients reported in Moersch and Woltman's paper,[1] and 8 out of 13 patients in Lorish et al.'s update on SPS published in 1989[5] had diabetes. The type of diabetes was not mentioned in these two reports. It is currently accepted that diabetes is present in one-third to two-thirds of patients with SPS. Blum and Jankovic's review of the literature[11] found that in 8 percent of the published cases IDDM was present,

while 13 additional patients had diabetes but without further characterization of its type. According to these authors, the frequency of IDDM in SPS patients is therefore more than 30 times that of the general population (0.25 percent). In recent years, this association has been further confirmed, and found to be more frequent than previously reported; 40 percent of the patients reported by Dalakas et al.[10] had IDDM, while in Meinck's series[9] the figure reached 41 percent. These findings are of relevance in the light of the current hypothesis on the pathogenesis of IDDM. It is presently accepted that an abnormal immune response directed against pancreatic islet cells is triggered by an exogenous agent, possibly a virus, causing the development of IDDM in genetically predisposed individuals.[11] A similar mechanism may be involved in the pathogenesis of SPS (see pathophysiology below).

Nocturnal myoclonus and epilepsy have also been reported in association with SPS. In their 1978 publication, Martinelli et al.[35] calculated, from a review of the literature, that the prevalence of epilepsy in SPS cases was close to 10 percent, which is exactly the figure reported recently by Dalakas et al.[10] in their own patients. They concluded that this figure was much higher than the prevalence of epilepsy in the general population, supporting the concept that this association was not by chance. However, this assertion has been contested by others, justifying the higher prevalence of epilepsy in SPS patients as a withdrawal phenomenon in individuals under diazepam therapy for extended periods.[36] Besides nocturnal myoclonus, other types of myoclonic jerks have been reported in cases diagnosed as SPS. Leigh et al.[37] published the clinical and electrophysiological findings in a 38-year-old patient with reflex myoclonus and muscle rigidity. The authors coined the term "jerking stiff-man syndrome" in view of the prominent jerking with similar characteristics to reticular reflex myoclonus, present in their patient. Although the patient had many of the clinical features necessary for the diagnosis of SPS, the presence of clinical and radiological signs of brainstem and cerebellar involvement would be more in favor of either encephalomyelitis or an atypical form of sporadic cerebellar system degeneration. An additional case reported by Alberca et al.[38] shares many of the clinical features described in the previous patient, although no evidence of structural involvement of the CNS was found. This concept has been more recently elaborated by Brown and Marsden,[7] who propose that the "jerking stiff-man syndrome" should be included as one of the variants of the "stiff-man plus syndrome" with prominent brainstem involvement, as opposed to the "stiff-limb syndrome" in which the spinal cord is primarily involved.

Diagnosis

Gordon et al.[2] were the first to establish a set of criteria for the diagnosis of SPS. They were based on the analysis of the original 14 cases of Moersch and Woltman and subsequent reports from the world literature. Their criteria included clinical and neurophysiologic findings, as well as a number of supportive tests. Clinical criteria were subdivided into six "key features" as follows:

1. *Prodromas* ("episodic aching and tightness of the axial musculature").
2. *Progression* (" … symmetrical, continuous stiffness characterized by tight, stony-hard, board-like muscles spreads to involve most of the limb, trunk and neck musculature").
3. *Painful spasms and precipitating factors* ("Superimposed upon this persistent rigidity of muscles, sudden stimuli often precipitate paroxysms of muscle spasm of such intensity as to lead, although not invariably, to excruciating pain").
4. *Sleep* ("In this state rigidity is abolished, … ").
5. *Neurologic findings* ("Normal motor and sensory examinations are the rule, except for the difficulty in active movement and the board-hard muscles referred to under 'Progression'").
6. *Intellect* ("Invariably intellect has been found intact, … ").

According to Gordon et al.'s criteria, the EMG "defines the peculiar state of voluntary muscle in stiff-man syndrome as one of persistent tonic contraction reflected in constant firing even 'at rest.'" Additional supportive tests included: (1) response to myoneural blocking agents, (2) effect of chemical block of peripheral motor fibers, and (3) response to general anesthesia. Furthermore, the beneficial effect of diazepam upon muscle stiffness was included as a final supportive criteria.

Thompson,[8] and more recently Dalakas,[39] modified and expanded the criteria for diagnosis proposed by Gordon et al.[2] and Lorish et al.[5] (Table 48-2).

Differential Diagnosis

Any patient presenting with muscle stiffness, rigidity, and cramps or muscle spasms may at one time be considered as a possible case of SPS. Moreover, there are several conditions with clinical features resembling SPS but with demonstrable CNS pathology that have been reported in the literature as atypical cases of this disorder. The list of conditions is long and includes disorders of muscle contraction of both central and peripheral origin (Table 48-3). Dealing with each of these disorders exceeds the scope of this chapter (for a review see Refs. 8 and 32).

Strict adherence to the criteria carefully delineated by Gordon et al.,[2] Lorish et al.,[5] and more recently Thompson[8] and Dalakas,[39] will help in identifying cases of SPS, differentiating them from the conditions listed in Table 48-3.

Some of the disorders included in Table 48-3 deserve special consideration because of the difficulties they may present in the differential diagnosis with SPS.

TABLE 48-2 Criteria for the Diagnosis of the Stiff-Man Syndrome

Clinical

Gradual and insidious onset of aching and tightness (rigidity) of limb and axial muscles

Slow progression; stiffness spreads from axial muscles to limbs (legs>arms) (according to Dalakas, a significant proportion may start with asymmetrical involvement of one limb and progressive generalization)

Continuous co-contraction of agonist and antagonist muscles with inability to relax, as confirmed clinically and electrophysiologically

Persistent contraction of thoracolumbar, paraspinal, and abdominal muscles

Abnormal hyperlordotic posture of lumbar spine

Board-like rigidity of abdominal muscles

Rigidity abolished by sleep

Stimulus-sensitive painful muscle spasms (precipitants: unexpected noises, tactile stimuli, or emotional upset)

No other abnormal neurological signs

Intellect normal

Cranial muscless rarely (if ever) involved (disputed by Dalakas)

Neurophysiological

Continuous motor unit activity

EMG activity abolished by sleep, peripheral nerve block, spinal or general anesthesia

Normal peripheral nerve conduction; normal motor unit morphology

Other observations that may be helpful but are of uncertain diagnostic specificity

Autoantibodies directed against GABAergic neurons, in particular to GAD

Association with autoimmune endocrine disease

SOURCE: Thompson,[8] with modifications according to Dalakas.[39]

PEWR is a rare, usually paraneoplastic, disorder featuring, in addition to the cardinal symptoms of SPS, evidence of brainstem and spinal cord involvement.[19,20,40] The latter may manifest by cranial nerve signs, segmental and long tract spinal cord symptomatology. Myoclonus and opsoclonus have also been reported in this disorder. Imaging studies may reveal cortical, brainstem, and cerebellar atrophy and sometimes hyperintense signals in the white matter on MRI examination. Abnormal findings in the CSF are frequent (lymphocytic pleocytosis, elevated protein levels, increased immunoglobulins and oligoclonal IgG bands). In a single case, diagnosed as having PEWR on the basis of a few atypical features (pattern of distribution of rigidity, loss of tendon jerks, nuclear and supranuclear gaze palsies, and reticular reflex myoclonus), GAD autoantibodies were detected.[41] However, no confirmation of an inflammatory process within the CNS was available. Results of biopsy or postmortem examination in PEWR cases show an inflammatory process, with perivascular lymphocytic infiltration, gliosis, and severe neuronal loss, involving mainly the lower brainstem and spinal cord (encephalomyelitis). In some cases there is a more widespread involvement, including brain cortical regions (hippocampus), and subcortical gray nuclei

TABLE 48-3 Differential Diagnosis of "Stiff-Person Syndrome"

Central	Peripheral	
	Nerve	Muscle

Encephalitis (including brainstem, spinal cord ["progressive encephalomyelitis with rigidity"])	Myokimia, neuromyotonia and pseudomyotonia
	    Idiopathic
	    Isaacs syndrome (continuous muscle fiber activity)
		Myotonic syndromes (channelopathies)
		    Myotonic dystrophy
		    Myotonia congenital
		    Paramyotonia

Dystonia
    Idiopathic
    Symptomatic
	Associated with neuropathy
	    Hereditary
	    Inflammatory
		Myopathies
		    Metabolic
		    Inflammatory

Akinetic-rigid syndromes
    Parkinson's disease
    Multiple-system atrophy
    Progressive supranuclear palsy
    Drug-induced parkinsonism
    Toxic parkinsonism (MPTP, carbon monoxide, manganese)
    Neuroleptic malignant syndrome
	Toxic
	    Radiation
	    Paraneoplastic
	
	Schwartz-Jampel syndrome
	
	Tetanus
	
	Cramps
		Endocrine
		    Congenital
		
		Contracture
		    Arthritis
		    Ankylosing spondylitis
		    Volkmann's ischemic contracture

Myelopathies (multiple sclerosis, infectious, trauma, ischemia, hemorrhage, spondylosis) Spinal cord tumor Spinal cord AVM Toxins (tetanus, strychnine, etc.) Motor neuron disease (primary lateral sclerosis, amyotrophic lateral sclerosis) Psychiatric illness (phobic neurosis, hysteria, malingering)		

MPTP, 1-methyl-4-phenyl-1,2,3,6-tetrahydropyridine; AVM, arteriovenous malformation.

(basal ganglia). The most striking pathological changes are usually restricted to the central gray zones of the spinal cord containing inhibitory interneurons. The disease follows a relentless course ending in death in a few months or years. This condition has been reported either as an isolated illness or more frequently associated with malignancy (oat-cell carcinoma of the lung, Hodgkin's disease).[6,42,43]

The question of SPS as a paraneoplastic autoimmune disorder in isolated cases has been raised in several publications. In 3 women with breast cancer, presenting with clinical features fulfilling the criteria necessary for the diagnosis of SPS, and in whom none of the conditions frequently associated with SPS (IDDM and other immunological disorders) and no GAD autoantibodies were detected, an extensive immunological screening detected the presence of a humoral autoimmune response against a neuronal protein of 128 kDa.[44] This antigen was found to be concentrated at synapses and its distribution outside the nervous system was highly restricted. Similar to GAD, the 128-kDa antigen is localized in the cytoplasmic compartment and is not a membrane surface protein. In a follow-up study, this 128-kDa antigen has been identified as the synaptic vesicle-associated

protein amphiphysin.[45] Both GAD and amphiphysin are concentrated in nerve terminals, associated to the cytoplasmic surface of synaptic vesicles. In a recently reported case of a patient who developed SPS, including disabling shoulder subluxation and wrist ankylosis, in association with breast cancer, immunologic investigations disclosed autoimmunity directed not only against amphiphysin but also GAD positivity. The patient improved after surgery and corticosteroid treatment and was reported to be stable for nearly 4 years on only antiestrogens. The triad of SPS, breast cancer, and autoantibodies against amphiphysin identifies a rather specific autoimmune paraneoplastic syndrome of the CNS in the view of these authors.[46] The presence of anti-amphiphysin antibodies is not specific to SPS as they have been detected in patients with various paraneoplastic neurological syndromes and tumors (e.g., sensory neuronopathy, encephalomyelitis, and breast cancer; limbic encephalitis, and small-cell lung cancer; encephalomyelitis and ovarian carcinoma; Lambert-Eaton myasthenic syndrome, and small cell lung cancer), and in association with other autoantibodies.[47] In addition to amphiphysin, Butler et al.[48] recently reported a patient with clinical features of SPS and mediastinal cancer in whom high-titer autoantibodies directed against gephyrin were detected. Gephyrin is a cytosolic protein selectively concentrated at the postsynaptic membrane of inhibitory synapses, associated with $GABA_A$ and glycine receptors. These findings suggest a possible link between the mechanism of autoimmunity in SPS and some paraneoplastic cases. It is also worth underlying that 40 percent of SPS cases lack autoantibodies directed against GAD and not all patients suffer from IDDM as an associated condition.

Therefore, it is possible that SPS be in fact a heterogeneous disorder in which different pathogenetic mechanisms, including a paraneoplastic immune response with or without inflammatory changes (PEWR), play a role.[41,42,49] As previously mentioned, Brown and Marsden,[7] in an analysis of their own and previously published cases, tried to sort out cases with typical presentation (axial stiffness, GAD positivity, and high incidence of IDDM) from those with atypical symptomatology, signs of CNS involvement, poor response to medication, and worse prognosis. To that effect they grouped together these atypical cases under the label of "stiff-man plus syndrome" or, more correctly, "stiff-person plus syndrome."

The first of the "plus" cases in the view of these authors corresponds to PEWR, running a subacute course and being pathologically characterized by subcortical demyelination (encephalomyelitis). Clinical features include widespread rigidity, painful myoclonus and spasms, and long tract and brainstem signs. Survival is short (less than 3 years), and its relentless progression and histological features are suggestive of a paraneoplastic etiology, which has been confirmed in occasional cases.

In contrast to PEWR, the remaining "plus" cases are chronic and, unlike the former, have a relative absence of long tract signs in the presence of significant rigidity. In cases where there is predominant brainstem involvement, the clinical picture is dominated by the presence of reflex myoclonus involving all four limbs ("jerking stiff-person syndrome"). The paroxysmal nature of the jerks may be so severe as to compromise respiration and lead to a fatal outcome. If properly treated (assisted ventilation, antimyoclonic agents) these patients may have a long survival (10 years or more), which makes a paraneoplastic etiology unlikely, at least in a large proportion of cases. In others, there are no signs of brainstem dysfunction and myoclonus is absent. The rigidity and painful spasms in these cases is restricted to the limbs, especially distally ("stiff-limb syndrome"), suggesting spinal involvement.[50] These cases have been found to have a particular pattern of EMG activity with an unusual segmented appearance due to an abnormally synchronous discharge of motor units, in contrast to the normal-looking interference pattern found in SPS. Only in 15 percent of these cases is there anti-GAD positivity, which has led some to consider these cases to be a "focal" form of SPS. However, in one reported case that came to autopsy, the pathological findings were consistent with an inflammatory process restricted to the spinal cord. This condition runs a protracted course, often measured in decades, and although many have

a variety of autoantibodies, the autoimmune profile in these patients is quite different from that usually observed in typical cases of SPS. Similar cases have been reported to be associated to breast or small-cell lung carcinoma and have antibodies against the presynaptic vesicle-associated protein amphiphysin.

Pathophysiology and Pathogenesis

PATHOLOGY

Postmortem examination of the CNS including the spinal cord, in patients with SPS has not yielded evidence of any significant abnormality in the majority of autopsied cases.[1,2,5,8,12] One exception is a case reported by Nakamura et al.,[51] showing involvement of the anterior columns of the spinal cord; an additional case was published by Warich-Kirches et al.,[34] who found a decrease of GABAergic cells in the cerebellar cortex, and a size reduction of Renshaw cells in the spinal cord. More recently, a case reported by Ishizawa et al.[33] showed reduction in the density of anterior horn neurons with somal areas up to 1500 μm^2 (corresponding to the smaller alpha motor neurons and gamma motor neurons) and relative sparing of the larger (>1500 μm^2) alpha motor neurons. Interestingly, GAD-like immunoreactivity in the spinal gray matter and density of GAD-containing Purkinje cells were not significantly reduced, in contrast to the observations of Warich-Kirches et al. No consistent macroscopic or microscopic changes have been found in the few remaining cases that underwent autopsy. The lack of pathological correlates to the marked derangement of motor unit activity and muscle contraction appears to indicate that SPS is a functional rather than a structural disorder.

PHYSIOLOGY

All evidence suggests a central origin for the spasms, rigidity, and continuous motor unit activity. This is substantiated by their disappearance with sleep, peripheral nerve block, general anesthesia, and systemic administration of diazepam.[1,2,5] Several hypotheses have been proposed to explain this enhancement of spinal motor neuron activity, including increased primary excitability of alpha motor neurons, a disorder of presynaptic inhibition of Ia terminals in the spinal cord, increased fusimotor activity, defective Renshaw cell function, and abnormalities in the suprasegmental descending pathways controlling spinal interneuronal systems. Several authors have addressed these hypotheses using different investigative techniques.

Monosynaptic stretch reflexes and F-waves are normal in SPS patients.[52] In addition, assessment of the ratio of the maximal H-reflex to M-wave size in the soleus muscle has failed to reveal any abnormality, excluding a primary enhancement of alpha motor neuron excitability.[52]

Evaluation of the recovery curve of the soleus H-reflex after a conditioning stimulus in patients with SPS yielded normal results, thus ruling out the Ia afferent system as the source of abnormal inputs to the motor neurons of the spinal cord.[35,53]

Although there is no conclusive evidence for or against the presence of increased gamma motor neuron (fusimotor) activity, most authors consider it unlikely in view of the normal tendon reflexes and particular pattern of distribution of muscle rigidity.[2,52]

Involvement of the recurrent inhibitory loop mediated by Renshaw cells has also been ruled out as the silent period following a supramaximal peripheral nerve stimulus was found to be normal in SPS patients.[52–55]

Evidence in favor of a disorder of presynaptic inhibition of Ia terminals in the spinal cord is based on the lack of depression in amplitude of the soleus H-reflex conditioned by tonic vibration applied to the Achilles tendon in SPS cases.[53] In a recent study, however, vibration-induced inhibition of H-reflexes was diminished in 8 of 9 patients tested, but the presynaptic period of reciprocal inhibition was found to be normal. Both neural circuits underlying these responses are presumed to involve presynaptic inhibition and GABAergic interneurons. In the same group of patients, occasional abnormalities were found in the first period of reciprocal inhibition and nonreciprocal (Ib) inhibition, which presumably involve glycinergic circuits. Recurrent inhibition was normal. The authors speculate that differences between the two presumptive GABAergic circuits may indicate that not all populations of GABAergic neurons are uniformly affected in SPS. On the other hand, the involvement of presumptive glycinergic circuits in some patients could point to impairment of non-GABAergic neurons, unrecognized involvement of GABAergic neurons in these inhibitory circuits, or, more likely, alterations of supraspinal systems that exert descending control over spinal circuits.[56] The finding of hyperexcitability of the motor cortex (decreased inhibition and markedly increased facilitation) in SPS patients, using transcranial magnetic stimulation, lends further support to this hypothesis.[57]

Another consistent abnormal finding in SPS patients is the presence of a widespread enhancement of exteroceptive reflexes, probably due to the proposed disorder of descending pathways controlling segmental interneuronal systems.[52,58] The responses to exteroceptive stimuli have been found to be grossly exaggerated, with abnormally short transmission times and the presence of abnormal excitatory reflex phases in face, arm and leg muscles. Both somatosensory and acoustic stimuli are the most effective in evoking an abnormal reflex response. The presence of an abnormally exaggerated blink reflex has also been noted in SPS cases.[52] A more prominent and persistent response of the acoustic startle reflex has been found in SPS patients in comparison to controls.[59] Most nonnociceptive reflexes have been found to behave abnormally, showing a low stimulation threshold, lacking habituation phenomena, and exhibiting co-contraction, suggesting nonspecific disturbances of the polysynaptic system.[35,52]

BIOCHEMISTRY AND PHARMACOLOGY

The existence of a disorder involving suprasegmental influences on inhibitory interneuronal systems at the spinal cord level is supported by a number of biochemical and pharmacological studies.

An increase in the severity of spasms induced by catecholamine precursors (e.g., L-dopa) or serotonin reuptake inhibitors (e.g., clorimipramine) has been reported.[13,52,58,60] On the contrary, opposite effects were observed with the use of drugs reducing aminergic activity within the CNS (e.g., clonidine and tizanidine),[52] or drugs that probably act by enhancing GABAergic transmission (e.g., diazepam and baclofen).[61] In addition, diazepam may also act indirectly through inhibition of catecholaminergic transmission.[13,52] These findings suggest an imbalance between noradrenergic and GABAergic neurotransmitter systems descending from the brainstem to the spinal cord.[13,52] The detection of reduced levels of GABA in the CSF of SPS patients would lend further support to this hypothesis.[11]

Neither physostigmine, a cholinergic drug, glycine, a putative inhibitory neurotransmitter at the spinal cord level, nor milacemide, a glycine precursor, produce any modification in the clinical status of SPS patients.[3,61,62] These observations lend little support to theories proposing a defective synaptic transmission either at the cholinergic synapse of recurrent axons of alpha motor neurons involving Renshaw cells or at the proposed glycinergic synapse between axons of spinal cord interneurons and cell bodies of alpha motor neurons.

The hypothesis of an imbalance between a descending excitatory catecholamine neuronal system and a GABAergic counterpart with net inhibitory effects on alpha motor neurons was further bolstered by findings of increased 3-methoxy-4-hydroxyphenylglycol (MHPG) excretion in a patient with SPS.[63] MHPG is the major metabolite of brain norepinephrine. Pharmacologic manipulations in this patient showed a direct correlation between clinical status and levels of MHPG in the urine, suggesting the presence of an overactive catecholamine system as one of the underlying mechanisms of rigidity and spasms.[13,52,63] However, a subsequent report failed to confirm these findings.[54] Nevertheless, the possibility that disturbances in the inhibitory descending GABAergic systems are indeed responsible for the development of rigidity and spasms is underscored by recent findings confirming the capacity of anti-GAD autoantibodies of inhibiting enzyme activity ("in vitro"), leading to reduced GABA synthesis.[64]

Although, on the basis of the therapeutic response to drugs, and additional experimental evidence, most authors agree on the possibility of such an imbalance, there is as yet no firm "in vivo" evidence to substantiate this.

IMMUNOLOGY

Young, in 1966,[65] was the first to advance the hypothesis of an autoimmune mechanism in the pathogenesis of SPS, based on the findings of pernicious anemia and possibly Hashimoto's thyroiditis in a patient with this disorder. The coexistence of diseases of autoimmune origin in patients with SPS is a consistent finding, suggesting a possibly common pathogenetic mechanism. As mentioned before, in Blum and Jankovic's review of 84 published cases, including 2 of their own, 18 percent had clinical evidence of one or more autoimmune diseases.[11]

A compelling argument in favor of the autoimmune origin of SPS came through the work of Solimena et al.[4] These authors detected the presence of autoantibodies against several nonneuronal tissues in the serum of a patient with SPS, epilepsy, and IDDM, carrying an autoimmunity predisposing HLA phenotype. These included complement-fixing islet-cell antibodies, gastric parietal-cell antibodies, and thyroglobulin and thyroid microsomal antibodies. In addition, both the serum and the CSF of the patient contained antibodies to mammalian CNS antigens. Antibodies were detected through immunocytochemistry and Western blot analysis. The cellular and subcellular distribution of immunoreactivity was identical to that of GAD, an enzyme involved in the synthesis of GABA. GAD is concentrated in GABAergic nerve terminals and, outside the CNS, in pancreatic beta cells. Cross-immunoreactivity was found in this patient. An important additional evidence in support of the hypothesis of an autoimmune process directed against the CNS was the finding of elevated levels of IgG with an oligoclonal pattern in the CSF of the patient.

In a subsequent publication, Solimena et al.[21] reported on the results of a systematic immunological study of patients with SPS. They studied the serum of 32 patients with an established diagnosis of SPS; in 24 of the cases the CSF was also available. Control serum samples of 218 individuals were used, including 16 healthy subjects, 111 patients with varied neurological disorders, 74 with IDDM, 20 with other organ-specific autoimmune disorders, and 3 with systemic autoimmune disease. The techniques used in the study included immunocytochemical assays to detect autoantibodies against GABAergic neurons, standard laboratory procedures to detect different organ-specific autoantibodies (islet-cell, gastric parietal-cell, thyroglobulin, and thyroid microsomal-fraction antibodies), immunoblotting, immunoprecipitation, and isoelectric focusing, and silver staining of serum and CSF to detect oligoclonal IgG bands. Sixty percent of the sera of SPS patients tested were positive for autoantibodies against GABAergic neurons, while 50 percent of the CSF samples were also positive. Twenty-seven percent of the CSF samples tested revealed the presence of oligoclonal IgG bands, including 2 patients negative for GABAergic neuron autoantibodies. In all patients that tested positive for GABAergic neuron antibodies there was cross-immunoreactivity directed against pancreatic beta cells. Other organ-specific autoantibodies that were positive in the same patient group included gastric parietal-cell antibodies (15/19), thyroid microsomal-fraction antibodies (9/19), and thyroglobulin antibodies (4/15). In the control population,

only 4 patients (1.8 percent) tested positive for GABAergic neuron autoantibodies. A Western blot assay was performed to investigate whether GAD was the autoantigen responsible for the positive immunoreactivity against brain and pancreas. A band comigrating with GAD was detected in the large majority of serum and CSF samples that were positive for autoantibodies against GABAergic neurons, confirming GAD as the antigen responsible for the autoimmune response.

More recent studies have attempted to better characterize the immunological response in both SPS and IDDM. GAD, the major autoantigen in both disorders, is present in two isoforms, GAD-65 and GAD-67; the isoforms have different molecular weights and are the products of two different genes.[66] The majority of SPS patients carry autoantibodies that react with the smaller isoform and specifically identify a dominant autoreactive target region (epitope) in the antigen.[67] The pattern of reactivity is somewhat different in IDDM, suggesting differences in epitope recognition in these two disorders.[68] These findings may indicate that, during the development of these diseases, the autoantigen is presented to the immune system through separate pathogenetic mechanisms.[69] The specificity of the immune response in SPS was further elaborated by Dalakas et al.[26] in a study of 18 patients with positive immunoreactivity to GABAergic neurons. Serum and CSF reactivity to purified GAD antigen was examined by Western blots, and the anti-GAD-65 antibody titers were quantified by ELISA and compared with 70 disease controls (11 patients with IDDM and 49 with other autoimmune disorders). In the serum of all patients with SPS there were significantly high anti-GAD-65 antibody titers (7.5–214 µg/mL), whereas in IDDM patients and in those carrying other autoimmune disorders the antibody titers were much lower. Moreover, only patients with SPS had detectable CSF anti-GAD-65 antibodies. Using immunoblotting techniques, both the serum and the CSF of SPS recognized a 65-kDa protein in brain homogenates corresponding to GAD-65, which was further confirmed with the monoclonal antibody against GAD-65. Epitope recognition of recombinant GAD-65 was specific for serum and CSF of SPS patients, while none of the patients with IDDM or other autoimmune disorders immunoreacted with purified GAD-65.

Moreover, there is other evidence indicating differences in the immune response between SPS and IDDM patients at both the cellular and the humoral level. Blood T-cells of SPS patients recognize different immunodominant epitopes of GAD-65 compared with T-cells from IDDM patients. Although IgG1 is dominant in both conditions, SPS patients, however, are more likely to have isotypes other than IgG1, in particular, IgG4 or IgE isotypes, which are not present in IDDM patients.[70]

Depending on the method of detection used, autoantibodies against the larger GAD-67 isoform and to an 80-kDa antigen can also be identified in SPS cases.[66,71] In a recent report, Johnstone and Nussey[25] detected the presence of autoantibodies reacting against the large isoform of human

GAD (GAD-67) using recombinant techniques, providing direct evidence for a clonally restricted response to GAD in SPS patients. These findings confirm previous observations suggesting immunological heterogeneity in SPS.[72] They also underline the need to perform different immunological techniques to identify the specific antigen involved in the production of anti-GABAergic autoantibodies in SPS cases.

The possibility of a genetically determined susceptibility to the development of SPS has been discussed by different authors. Several studies have reported on the detection of specific HLA haplotypes frequently linked to this disorder. The original patient of Solimena et al.[4] with autoantibodies to GAD was found to have the B44 and DR-3/4 antigens as major haplotypes. In the same year, Williams et al.[28] found that 4 of their 5 SPS patients, all suffering from autoimmune endocrinopathies, also typed to the B44 antigen, which is in linkage disequilibrium with DR4. HLA DR3 and DR4 are the alleles most commonly associated with IDDM in whites. Subsequently, Blum and Jankovic[11] speculated on the possibility that the specific organization of HLA-determined immunoregulatory molecules apparently involved in the development of IDDM possibly constitute the pathogenetic mechanism of autoimmunity to GABAergic cells in the CNS. The demonstration of HLA phenotypes common to both IDDM and SPS would lend further support to this hypothesis. In a more recent study on the genetics of susceptibility and resistance to IDDM in SPS, Pugliese et al.[29] found that, as in IDDM, SPS was associated with the allele DQB1*0201. In addition, the presence or absence of the related allele DQB1*0602 would in turn confer either a protective or a predisposing factor for the development of IDDM in SPS patients.[30] Although there is an overlap of the DQB1 allele between SPS and IDDM patients, the former are by themselves more frequently associated with the DRB1*0301 allele.[10] These findings are, according to the authors, further evidence of the importance of the HLA genetic background in the development of SPS and related autoimmune disorders.

ETIOLOGY AND PATHOGENESIS

Although as yet there is no definitive answer concerning the etiology and pathogenesis of SPS, all the available evidence, already discussed in previous paragraphs, suggests an autoimmune mechanism as responsible for its development. An unknown noxious stimulus would trigger the cascade of events leading to the exposure of intracellular GAD to the immune system causing the production of autoantibodies against this enzyme and GABA-containing neurons. This in turn would lead to a selective impairment of GABAergic transmission in suprasegmental systems influencing the inhibitory activity of spinal interneurons. The resulting imbalance between excitatory and inhibitory influences at the segmental level would be the cause of the enhancement of spinal motor neuron activity.

Treatment

Benzodiazepines have become the cornerstone of treatment of SPS, ever since Howard[3] first reported dramatic improvement of muscle spasms with diazepam in 3 patients with this disorder. The rationale behind Howard's approach was that, since diazepam blocked strychnine convulsions in mice and spinal reflexes in cats, he speculated that this drug would suppress the constant discharges originated in the motor neurons of the spinal cord believed to be the cause of rigidity and stiffness in individuals affected with this syndrome. His patients were treated with up to 60 mg/day of diazepam in four divided doses achieving significant functional improvement. Moreover, with the use of this drug, in addition to symptomatic benefit there were modifications in the EMG at rest. Unfortunately, the dose of diazepam usually needed to produce functional improvement is often associated with untoward side-effects, mainly profound sedation.[5,8] The dose range of diazepam presently used is between 10 and 100 mg daily in most cases. With this treatment regimen, patients tend to stabilize, and maintain some degree of functional capacity.[5] However, most patients experience their symptoms on a continued basis and some cases continue to deteriorate. Other benzodiazepines such as clonazepam have also been used in doses of 4–6 mg/day (1 mg of clonazepam is equivalent to 4–5 mg of diazepam) with apparent benefit in a few selected cases.[73] The second drug of choice according to several authors is baclofen in doses up to 100 mg/day in order to achieve maximum benefit.[54,61,74] A relative absence or unavailability of GABA, a putative inhibitory neurotransmitter at the level of the gamma motor neuron system in the spinal cord, had been proposed by Gordon[2] as the underlying mechanism for rigidity in SPS. The beneficial effects of baclofen would derive from its properties as a GABA analog (GABA$_B$ receptor agonist).[61,75] As with diazepam, the main side-effect observed with this drug is sedation. The administration of intrathecal baclofen through an infusion pump has been recently proposed.[75] The rationale behind this approach is to provide sufficiently high concentrations of the drug to the spinal cord receptors without the systemic side-effects usually seen with oral administration. Only a few patients have been treated with this method of drug delivery, and the results so far have been variable.[76] In a more recent double-blind, placebo-controlled trial of intrathecal baclofen, this approach resulted in significant improvement in reflex EMG activity compared to placebo that did not correlate with clinical improvement.[77] Special attention should be paid to the adequate operation of the drug-delivery system, as pump malfunctioning has been responsible for severe autonomic complications, delirium, and spasmodic storms.[78,79]

The standard treatment regimen in clinical practice today is a combination of diazepam and baclofen in lower doses than those used when each drug is given alone.[8] Furthermore, the best strategy is to gradually titrate the dosage of both to minimize the sedative effects of these drugs. The best results are obtained in the control of spontaneous and stimulus-sensitive muscle spasms, while axial rigidity, abnormal posturing, and limitations of mobility respond less well. Valproic acid has also been advocated, and anecdotal reports of marked benefit in some cases can be found in the literature.[80] As an anticonvulsant, valproic acid is thought to augment GABAergic transmission and perhaps its beneficial effect could be attributed to its ability to compensate a deficiency of GABA at the spinal cord level. Newly introduced anticonvulsants (gabapentin, tiagabine, vigabatrin) with proposed mechanism of action at the GABA level have been tried successfully in selected cases.[9,81,82] Several other drugs, including tizanidine, carbamazepine, sodium dantrolene, phenytoin, phenobarbital, cyclobenzaprine, mephenesin, L-dopa, 5-hydroxytryptophan, glycine, biperiden, dipropylacetate, gamma-hydroxybutyric acid, milacemide, have also been tried with inconsistent or detrimental results.[11,13,52,62,83]

Plasmapheresis became an obvious choice, after reports on the presence of antibodies reacting against GAD both in serum and CSF of patients with SPS and additional evidence of immunological involvement. The few cases undergoing this treatment obtained variable results. Two patients reported in separate papers had an excellent response to plasmapheresis; improvement was observed at variable times during the course of treatment in these 2 cases.[84,85] In 1 of them, clinical response was evident immediately after the second exchange, while subjective improvement lagged behind. Return to almost normal was reported by the patient almost 2 weeks after the end of plasmapheresis. Parallel to the reduction of rigidity and spasms there were signs of improvement in EMG studies and the areas of evoked exteroceptive reflex responses were dramatically reduced. In 1 of the cases, antibody levels remained unchanged, while, in the other, GAD-like immunoreactivity fell from 1:1280 to 1:80 during plasmapheresis. In contrast, in the 2 additional cases reported by Harding et al.,[24] results were disappointing, although the immunological markers in these patients were similar to the previous ones. In patients without anti-GAD positivity, plasma exchange has produced disappointing results according to a recent report.[86] Double filtration plasma exchange followed by immunoadsorption has been reported to be effective in another anti-GAD-negative SPS patient.[87] Plasmapheresis remains a promising therapeutic strategy, although controlled studies on the efficacy of this intervention have not been yet conducted.

The benefits of steroid treatment and immunosuppressive drugs have been reported on an anecdotal basis.[24,88,89] Most patients appear to require a daily dose of 30–60 mg of prednisone to achieve noticeable improvement; however, reappearance of symptoms develops whenever the steroid dosage is tapered.[89] The use of high-dose long-term steroids in the treatment of a chronic disorder, frequently associated with IDDM, does not seem convenient.

Several recent publications have reported on the beneficial effects of intravenous immunoglobulin (IVIg) in the treatment of SPS.[90,91,92] A total of 15 out of 17 cases showed significant subjective and functional improvement following treatment with IVIg, although this improvement has been reported to be sustained in only 3 cases. These results lend additional support to the hypothesis of an immune origin of SPS. As with other immune disorders, IVIg therapy could be effective through either neutralization of autoantibodies or downregulation of antibody production.

An anecdotal report on the benefits of paraspinal injection of botulinum toxin A in a patient with SPS has been recently published.[93] Significant reduction of rigidity at the paraspinal and thigh muscles, improvement of ambulation, and cessation of pain were obtained with the use of this medication.

In summary, present-day strategies for the treatment of SPS can be divided into two separate categories. The first category includes drugs known to interact with the pharmacological mechanisms underlying the production of muscle rigidity (diazepam, baclofen, valproic acid, clonidine, tizanidine, etc.) and the benefit derived from their use is purely symptomatic. On the other hand, the use of plasmapheresis, steroids and other immunomodulating agents (immunosuppressive drugs, IVIg) would be an attempt to modify or control the immunologic factors potentially involved in the pathogenesis of SPS.

References

1. Moersch FP, Woltman HW: Progressive fluctuating muscular rigidity and spasm ("stiff-man" syndrome): Report of a case and some observations in 13 other cases. *Mayo Clin Proc* 31:421–427, 1956.
2. Gordon EE, Januszko DM, Kaufman L: A critical survey of stiff-man syndrome. *Am J Med* 42:582–599, 1967.
3. Howard FM: A new and effective drug in the treatment of stiff-man syndrome: Preliminary report. *Mayo Clin Proc* 38:203–212, 1963.
4. Solimena M, Folli F, Denis-Donini S, et al: Autoantibodies to glutamic acid decarboxylase in a patient with stiff-man syndrome, epilepsy, and type I diabetes mellitus. *N Engl J Med* 318: 1012–1020, 1988.
5. Lorish TR, Thorsteinsson G, Howard FM: Stiff-man syndrome updated. *Mayo Clin Proc* 64:629–636, 1989.
6. Barker RA, Revesz T, Thom M, et al: Review of 23 patients affected by the stiff man syndrome: Clinical subdivision into stiff trunk (man) syndrome, stiff limb syndrome, and progressive encephalomyelitis with rigidity. *J Neurol Neurosurg Psychiatry* 65:633–640, 1998.
7. Brown P, Marsden CD: The stiff man and stiff man plus syndromes. *J Neurol* 246:648–652, 1999.
8. Thompson PD: Stiff people, in Marsden CD, Fahn S (eds): *Movement Disorders 3*. Oxford: Butterworth-Heinemann, 1994, pp 373–405.
9. Meinck HM: Stiff man syndrome. *CNS Drugs* 15:515–526, 2001.
10. Dalakas MC, Fujii M, Li M, McElroy B: The clinical spectrum of anti-GAD antibody-positive patients with stiff-person syndrome. *Neurology* 55:1531–1535, 2000.
11. Blum P, Jankovic J: Stiff-person syndrome: An autoimmune disease. *Mov Disord* 6:12–20, 1991.

12. Trethowan WH, Allsop JL, Turner B: The stiff-man syndrome. *Arch Neurol* 3:114–122, 1960.
13. Isaacs H: Stiff-man syndrome in a black girl. *J Neurol Neurosurg Psychiatry* 42:988–994, 1979.
14. Kugelmass N: Stiff-man syndrome in a child. *N Y State J Med* 61:2483–2487, 1961.
15. Klein R, Haddow JE, De Luca C: Familial congenital disorder resembling the stiff-man syndrome. *Am J Dis Child* 124:730–731, 1972.
16. Sander JE, Layzer RB, Goldsobel AB: Congenital stiff-man syndrome. *Ann Neurol* 8:195–197, 1979.
17. Meinck HM, Ricker K, Hulser PJ, et al: Stiff man syndrome: Clinical and laboratory findings in eight patients. *J Neurol* 241:157–166, 1994.
18. Schwartzman MJ, Mitsumoto H, Chou SM, et al: Sudden death in stiff-man syndrome with autonomic instability. *Ann Neurol* 26:166, 1989.
19. Kasperek S, Zebrowski S: Stiff-man syndrome and encephalomyelitis. *Arch Neurol* 24:22–31, 1971.
20. Whiteley AM, Swash M, Urich H: Progressive encephalomyelitis with rigidity. *Brain* 99:27–42, 1976.
21. Solimena M, Folli F, Morello F, et al: Autoantibodies to GABA-ergic neurones and pancreatic beta cells in stiff-man syndrome. *N Engl J Med* 322:1555–1560, 1990.
22. Baekkeskov S, Aanstoot H-J, Christgau S, et al: Identification of the 64K autoantigen in insulin dependent diabetes mellitus as the GABA-synthesizing enzyme glutamic acid decarboxylase. *Nature* 347:151–156, 1990.
23. Meinck HM, Ricker K: Long-standing "stiff-man" syndrome: A particular form of disseminated inflammatory CNS disease? *J Neurol Neurosurg Psychiatry* 50:1556–1557, 1987.
24. Harding AE, Thompson PD, Kocen RS, et al: Plasma exchange and immunosuppression in the stiff-man syndrome. *Lancet* ii:915, 1989.
25. Johnstone AP, Nussey SS: Direct evidence for limited clonality of antibodies to glutamic acid decarboxylase (GAD) in stiff-man syndrome using baculovirus expressed GAD. *J Neurol Neurosurg Psychiatry* 57:659, 1994.
26. Dalakas MC, Li M, Fujii M, Jacobowitz DM: Stiff person syndrome: Quantification, specificity, and intrathecal synthesis of GAD65 antibodies. *Neurology* 57:780–784, 2001.
27. Maida E, Reisner T, Summer K, Sandor-Eggerth H: Stiff-man syndrome with abnormalities in CSF and computerized tomography findings. *Arch Neurol* 37:182–183, 1980.
28. Williams AC, Nutt JG, Hare T: Autoimmunity in stiff-man syndrome. *Lancet* ii:22, 1988.
29. Pugliese A, Gianani R, Eisenbarth GS, et al: Genetics of susceptibility and resistance to insulin-dependent diabetes in stiff-man syndrome. *Lancet* 344:1027–1028, 1994.
30. Pugliese A, Solimena M, Awdeh ZL, et al: Association of HLA-DQB1*0201 with stiff-man syndrome. *J Clin Endocrinol Metab* 77:1550–1553, 1993.
31. Meinck HM, Ricker K, Hulser PJ, Solimena M: Stiff man syndrome: Neurophysiological findings in eight patients. *J Neurol* 242:134–142, 1995.
32. Auger RG: AAEM minimonograph 44: Diseases associated with excess motor unit activity. *Muscle Nerve* 17:1250–1263, 1994.
33. Ishizawa K, Komori T, Okayama K, et al: Large motor neuron involvement in stiff-man syndrome: A qualitative and quantitative study. *Acta Neuropathol (Berl)* 97:63–70, 1999.
34. Warich-Kirches M, Von Bossanyi P, Treuheit T, et al: Stiff-man syndrome: Possible autoimmune etiology targeted against GABA-ergic cells. *Clin Neuropathol* 16:214–219, 1997.
35. Martinelli P, Pazzaglia P, Montagna P, et al: Stiff-man syndrome associated with nocturnal myoclonus and epilepsy. *J Neurol Neurosurg Psychiatry* 41:458–462, 1978.
36. Meinck HM: Exteroceptive reflexes abnormalities in stiff-man syndrome. *J Neurol Neurosurg Psychiatry* 48:92–93, 1985.
37. Leigh PN, Rothwell JC, Traub M, Marsden CD: A patient with reflex myoclonus and muscle rigidity: "Jerking stiff-man syndrome". *J Neurol Neurosurg Psychiatry* 43:1125–1131, 1980.
38. Alberca R, Romero M, Chaparro J: Jerking stiff-man syndrome. *J Neurol Neurosurg Psychiatry* 45:1159–1160, 1982.
39. Dalakas MC: The stiff-person syndrome: An autoimmune disorder affecting neurotransmission of gamma-aminobutyric acid. *Ann Intern Med* 131:522–530, 1999.
40. McCombe PA, Chalk JB, Searle JW, et al: Progressive encephalomyelitis with rigidity: A case report with magnetic resonance imaging findings. *J Neurol Neurosurg Psychiatry* 52:1429–1431, 1989.
41. Burn DJ, Ball J, Lees AJ, et al: A case of progressive encephalomyelitis with rigidity and positive antiglutamic acid dehydrogenase antibodies. *J Neurol Neurosurg Psychiatry* 54:449–451, 1991.
42. Bateman DE, Weller RO, Kennedy P: Stiff-man syndrome. *J Neurol Neurosurg Psychiatry* 53:695–696, 1990.
43. Ferari P, Fedeico M, Grimaldi LME, Silingardi V: Stiff man syndrome in a patient with Hodgkin's disease: An unusual paraneoplastic syndrome. *Haematologica* 75:570–572, 1990.
44. Folli F, Solimena M, Cofiell R, et al: Autoantibodies to a 128-kd synaptic protein in three women with the stiff-man syndrome and breast cancer. *N Engl J Med* 328:546–551, 1993.
45. De Camilli P, Thomas A, Cofiell R, et al: The synaptic vesicle-associated protein amphiphysin is the 128-kD autoantigen of stiff-man syndrome with breast cancer. *J Exp Med* 178:2219–2223, 1993.
46. Rosin L, DeCamilli P, Butler M, et al: Stiff-man syndrome in a woman with breast cancer: An uncommon central nervous system paraneoplastic syndrome. *Neurology* 50:94–98, 1998.
47. Antoine JC, Absi L, Honnorat J, et al: Antiamphiphysin antibodies are associated with various paraneoplastic neurological syndromes and tumors. *Arch Neurol* 56:172–177, 1999.
48. Butler MH, Hayashi A, Ohkoshi N, et al: Autoimmunity to gephyrin in stiff-man syndrome. *Neuron* 26:307–312, 2000.
49. Piccolo G, Cosi V: Stiff-man syndrome, dysimmune disorder and cancer. *Ann Neurol* 25:105, 1989.
50. Brown P, Rothwell JC, Marsden CD: The stiff leg syndrome. *J Neurol Neurosurg Psychiatry* 62:31–37, 1997.
51. Nakamura N, Fujiya S, Yahara O, et al: Stiff-man syndrome with spinal cord lesion. *Clin Neuropathol* 5:40–46, 1986.
52. Meinck HM, Ricker K, Conrad B: The stiff-man syndrome: New pathophysiological aspects from abnormal exteroceptive reflexes and the response to clomipramine, clonidine and tizanidine. *J Neurol Neurosurg Psychiatry* 47:280–287, 1984.
53. Rossi B, Massetani R, Guidi M, et al: Electrophysiological findings in a case of stiff-man syndrome. *Electromyogr Clin Neurophysiol* 28:137–140, 1988.
54. Mamoli B, Heiss WD, Maida E, Podreka I: Electrophysiological studies on the stiff-man syndrome. *J Neurol* 217:111–121, 1977.

55. Boiardi A, Crenna P, Negri S, Merati B: Neurological and pharmacological evaluation of a case of stiff-man syndrome. *J Neurol* 223:127–133, 1980.

56. Floeter MK, Valls-Sole J, Toro C, et al: Physiologic studies of spinal inhibitory circuits in patients with stiff-person syndrome. *Neurology* 51:85–93, 1998.

57. Sandbrink F, Syed NA, Fujii MD, et al: Motor cortex excitability in stiff-person syndrome. *Brain* 123:2231–2239, 2000.

58. Meinck HM, Conrad B: Neuropharmacological investigations in the stiff-man syndrome. *J Neurol* 233:340–347, 1986.

59. Matsumoto JY, Caviness JN, McEvoy KM: The acoustic startle reflex in stiff-man syndrome. *Neurology* 44:1952–1955, 1994.

60. Guilleminault C, Sigwald J, Castaigne P: Sleep studies and therapeutic trial with L-dopa in a case of stiff-man syndrome. *Eur Neurol* 10:89–96, 1973.

61. Miller F, Korsvik H: Baclofen in the treatment of stiff-man syndrome. *Ann Neurol* 9:511–512, 1981.

62. Brown P, Thompson PD, Rothwell JC, et al: A therapeutic trial of milacemide in myoclonus and the stiff person syndrome. *Mov Disord* 6:73–75, 1991.

63. Schmidt RT, Stahl SM, Spehlmann R: A pharmacologic study of the stiff-man syndrome. *Neurology* 25:622–626, 1975.

64. Dinkel K, Meinck HM, Jury KM, et al: Inhibition of gamma-aminobutyric acid synthesis by glutamic acid decarboxylase autoantibodies in stiff-man syndrome. *Ann Neurol* 44:194–201, 1998.

65. Young W: The stiff-man syndrome. *Br J Clin Pract* 20:507–510, 1966.

66. Butler MH, Solimena M, Dirkx R Jr, et al: Identification of a dominant epitope of glutamic acid decarboxylase (GAD-65) recognized by autoantibodies in stiff-man syndrome. *J Exp Med* 178:2097–2106, 1993.

67. Li L, Hagopian WA, Brashear HR, et al: Identification of autoantibody epitopes of glutamic acid decarboxylase in stiff-man syndrome patients. *J Immunol* 152:930–934, 1994.

68. Kim J, Namchuk M, Bugawan T, et al: Higher autoantibody levels and recognition of a linear NH2-terminal epitope in the autoantigen GAD65, distinguish stiff-man syndrome from insulin-dependent diabetes mellitus. *J Exp Med* 180:595–606, 1994.

69. Bjork E, Velloso LA, Kampe O, Karlsson FA: GAD autoantibodies in IDDM, stiff-man syndrome, and autoimmune polyendocrine syndrome type I recognize different epitopes. *Diabetes* 43:161–165, 1994.

70. Lohmann T, Hawa M, Leslie RD, et al: Immune reactivity to glutamic acid decarboxylase 65 in stiffman syndrome and type 1 diabetes mellitus. *Lancet* 356:31–35, 2000.

71. Darnell RB, Victor J, Rubin M, et al: A novel antineuronal antibody in stiff-man syndrome. *Neurology* 43:114–120, 1993.

72. Gorin F, Baldwin B, Tait R, et al: Stiff-man syndrome: A disorder with autoantigenic heterogeneity. *Ann Neurol* 28:711–714, 1990.

73. Westblom U: Stiff-man syndrome and clonazepam. *JAMA* 237:1930, 1977.

74. Whelan JL: Baclofen in the treatment of the "stiff-man" syndrome. *Arch Neurol* 37:600–601, 1980.

75. Penn RD, Mangieri EA: Stiff-man syndrome treated with intrathecal baclofen. *Neurology* 43:2412, 1993.

76. Ford B, Fahn S: Intrathecal baclofen. *Neurology* 44:1367–1368, 1994.

77. Silbert PL, Matsumoto JY, McManis PG, et al: Intrathecal baclofen therapy in stiff-man syndrome: A double-blind, placebo-controlled trial. *Neurology* 45:1893–1897, 1995.

78. Meinck HM, Tronnier V, Rieke K, et al: Intrathecal baclofen treatment for stiff-man syndrome: Pump failure may be fatal. *Neurology* 44:2209–2210, 1994.

79. Stayer C, Tronnier V, Dressnandt J, et al: Intrathecal baclofen therapy for stiff-man syndrome and progressive encephalomyelopathy with rigidity and myoclonus. *Neurology* 49:1591–1597, 1997.

80. Spehlmann R, Norcross K, Rasmus SC, Schlageter NL: Improvement of stiff-man syndrome and sodium valproate. *Neurology* 31:1162–1163, 1981.

81. Sharoqi IA: Improvement of stiff-man syndrome with vigabatrin. *Neurology* 50:833–834, 1998.

82. Murinson BB, Rizzo M: Improvement of stiff-person syndrome with tiagabine. *Neurology* 57:366, 2001.

83. Gordon MF, Diaz Olivo R, Hunt AL, Fahn S: Therapeutic trial of milacemide in patients with myoclonus and other intractable movement disorders. *Mov Disord* 8:484–488, 1993.

84. Brashear HR, Phillips LH: Autoantibodies to GABAergic neurones and response to plasmapheresis in stiff-man syndrome. *Neurology* 41:1588–1592, 1991.

85. Vicari AM, Folli F, Pozza G, et al: Plasmapheresis in the treatment of stiff-man syndrome. *N Engl J Med* 320:1499, 1989.

86. Shariatmadar S, Noto TA: Plasma exchange in stiff-man syndrome. *Ther Apher* 5:64–67, 2001.

87. Hayashi A, Nakamagoe K, Ohkoshi N, et al: Double filtration plasma exchange and immunoadsorption therapy in a case of stiff-man syndrome with negative anti-GAD antibody. *J Med* 30:321–327, 1999.

88. George TM, Burke JM, Sobotak PA, et al: Resolution of stiff-man syndrome with cortisol replacement in a patient with deficiencies of ACTH, growth hormone, and prolactin. *N Engl J Med* 310:1511–1513, 1984.

89. Piccolo G, Cosi V, Zandrini C, Moglia A: Steroid-responsive and dependent stiff-man syndrome: A clinical and electrophysiological study of two cases. *Ital J Neurol Sci* 9:559–566, 1988.

90. Amato AA, Cornman EW, Kissel JT: Treatment of stiff-man syndrome with intravenous immunoglobulin. *Neurology* 44:1652–1654, 1994.

91. Karlson EW, Sudarsky L, Ruderman E, et al: Treatment of stiff-man syndrome with intravenous immune globulin. *Arthritis Rheum* 37:915–918, 1994.

92. Gerschlager W, Brown P: Effect of treatment with intravenous immunoglobulin on quality of life in patients with stiff-person syndrome. *Mov Dis* 17:590–593, 2002.

93. Davis D, Jabbari B: Significant improvement of stiff-person syndrome after paraspinal injection of botulinum toxin A. *Mov Disord* 8:371–373, 1993.

GAIT DISORDERS

LEWIS SUDARSKY

ANATOMY AND PHYSIOLOGY OF GAIT   813
    Neural Networks that Support Locomotion   813
    Cerebral Control of Walking   814
    Management of Dynamic Balance   814
CLASSIFICATION OF GAIT DISORDERS   815
COMMON PATTERNS OF GAIT DISORDER   815
    The Cautious Gait   815
    Stiff-Legged Gait   816
    Freezing Gait   816
    Frontal Gait (Marche à Petit Pas)   817
    Dystonic Gait   817
    Cerebellar Gait   817
    Sensory Ataxia   818
    Psychogenic Gait Disorders   818
LABORATORY TECHNIQUES FOR INVESTIGATION
    OF GAIT DISORDERS   819
    Laboratory Gait Analysis   819
    Observational Gait Analysis   819
    Imaging   819

Gait is an important motor function, which is unconscious and automatic. Gait is also a distinctive attribute; we can recognize people by their walk.[1] Disorders of gait are common, and may be the presenting feature of neurologic disease. Reliable estimates of prevalence are difficult to obtain, as there are no standard diagnostic criteria. In a study from Durham, North Carolina, 15 percent of volunteers over 60 were found to exhibit some abnormality of gait on neurologic examination.[2] In the East Boston Neighborhood Health Study, a degree of shuffling or difficulty with turns was noted in 15 percent of the population aged 67–74, 29 percent of those aged 75–84, and 49 percent of the population aged 85 and above.[3] Gait disorders are particularly important in the elderly because they compromise independence and contribute to the risk of falls and injury.[4,5] Our job as neurologists is not finished until the gait has been examined.

Anatomy and Physiology of Gait

Humans and other bipeds have two principal gaits: walking and running. Walking is our preferred mode. The biomechanical events of the gait cycle are illustrated with respect to time in Fig. 49-1. The stance phase begins as the right heel strikes the floor, where it remains for 60 percent of the gait cycle. The stance phase for the two legs overlap, such that 20 percent of the gait cycle is spent with both feet planted on the ground, while the center of mass continues its forward progression. Surface electromyographic (EMG) recorded from the leg muscles reveals an orderly, phasic pattern of activation: flexor muscles during the swing phase, extensor muscles during stance. There are two tasks that the nervous system must attend in order to initiate and maintain walking. (1) The brain and spinal cord generate a series of stepping movements; locomotor centers specify the timing, advance position, instructions for loading and unloading of the limbs. (2) At the same time, balance must be managed in order to maintain the upright posture and a stable progression.

NEURAL NETWORKS THAT SUPPORT LOCOMOTION

In quadrupedal animals, locomotion is produced by the activity of a spinal pattern generator. Cats and dogs with high spinal transection achieve a crude pattern of walking on the treadmill, provided their balance is supported. This "fictive locomotion" can be stimulated with L-dopa or clonidine, and occurs independent of sensory feedback.[6] In the spinal cord, central pattern generators for stepping are linked by the propriospinal tract. It is difficult to produce sustained spinal locomotion in primates,[7] although efforts have been made to harness spinal stepping in the rehabilitation of spinal injury patients.[8]

Primate bipedal locomotion depends on higher command and control centers in the brainstem and cerebellum.[9] Physiologists describe four areas where postural change and stepping can be evoked by electrical stimulation in animals: a subthalamic and a mesencephalic locomotor region, and a dorsal and ventral tegmental field in the caudal pons. The fastigial nucleus in the cerebellum can also induce expression of locomotor programs from the brainstem and spinal cord.[10,11] Eidelberg et al. evoked a form of "controlled locomotion," more natural than spinal stepping, by stimulation of the mesencephalic locomotor region (MLR) in primates. The animals swing their arms as they walk, and display a range of associated movements. With increasing stimulation, they pick up the pace of their walking, and ultimately shift into a running gait.[7] The MLR is an area near the nucleus cuneifomis, just below the superior cerebellar peduncle. The MLR is of particular interest as it includes the cholinergic neurons of the pedunculopontine nucleus (PPN).

There is a great deal of interest in the PPN as a locomotor center.[12] It sits at the convergence of important motor pathways. Afferents to the PPN come from the basal ganglia output (globus pallidus internal segment, substantia nigra pars reticulata) and motor cortex. The PPN projects to the brainstem reticular nuclei and spinal cord. In the cat, stimulation of the PPN produces stepping, and inhibition slows walking.[13] A complex pattern of activity is recorded from cells in the PPN during locomotor activity.[12] The dorsal midbrain (home of the PPN) is among the areas activated by walking in single-photon emission computed tomography (SPECT) imaging studies of human subjects.[14]

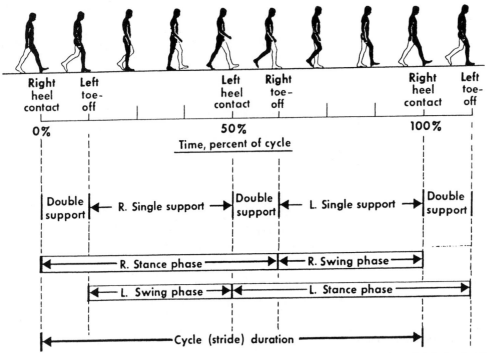

FIGURE 49-1 Events of the gait cycle are depicted with respect to time. From the point of right-heel strike, the right foot is in contact with the floor 60 percent of the time. This is the stance phase for the right leg. Roughly 20 percent of the gait cycle is spent in double limb support, during which forward motion of the center of mass continues. (*From Inman et al.[96] Used with permission.*)

Locomotor commands from the brainstem are passed along phylogenetically older, descending pathways in the spinal cord, including the reticulospinal and vestibulospinal tracts. Through a series of lesion experiments, Lawrence and Kuypers demonstrated that the ventromedial spinal pathways (reticulospinal, vestibulospinal) are necessary for recovery of postural control and locomotion in primates.[15] Eidelberg observed that primates with partial spinal transection can recover the capacity for locomotion, provided that one ventral quadrant of the spinal cord is preserved.[7]

CEREBRAL CONTROL OF WALKING

A clinician approaching the literature on gait physiology faces a paradox: an apparently natural locomotion can be expressed by a nervous system reduced to its fundamental elements (the brainstem, cerebellum, and spinal cord). Yet many of the gait disorders we struggle with in the clinic result from pathology in the forebrain (the basal ganglia, motor cortex, and frontal subcortical circuits). How does the cerebral control of locomotion operate and what does it contribute? Armstrong,[16] Garcia Rill,[17] and Mori[18] have reviewed this complex topic, and several elements stand out. The forebrain provides a *goal and purpose* for walking. It specifies when to start, when to stop, where to change direction, and it animates the performance. Cerebral control provides an element of *skill and finesse*. Cats with pyramidotomy recover an ability to walk on flat ground, but fail to walk on a narrow beam or across a ladder. Cerebral control is also involved in *context-dependent adaptation*, and *avoidance of obstacles*. Recording from awake behaving cats, Drew observed early and substantial changes in the discharge patterns of corticospinal tract neurons which occur as the animals respond to obstacles placed in their path.[19]

MANAGEMENT OF DYNAMIC BALANCE

An hierarchy of postural responses maintains balance in the upright posture during quiet stance and during locomotion. Standing balance requires that the center of mass be maintained over the base of support, an area defined by the foot floor contact. Unconscious postural adjustments are necessary to maintain this relationship. Long latency responses can be recorded from the trunk and leg muscles 110 ms after a perturbation in the support surface.[20–22] These responses provide a defense against slipping and tripping falls. While the physiology has been studied, the anatomic substrate for human postural control is not well defined. The vestibular nuclei and midline cerebellum are presumed to coordinate the motor response, and imbalance is evident if these systems are impaired.

Walking at a steady velocity along a flat surface poses little challenge, as the dynamics are inherently stable. The trajectory of the center of mass runs slightly ahead of the foot-floor contact, which helps maintain a propulsive force.[23]

Walking on uneven ground in a poorly illuminated area requires a greater degree of sensory-motor integration. Postural defense reactions (rescue response) and anticipatory postural responses are called as needed.

While step generation does not depend on sensory feedback, sensory information is critical for balance. Romberg observed the particular importance of dorsal column afferents from the lower limbs in maintenance of standing balance.[24] Sensory information from the vestibular system, the visual system, plantar touch, and musculoarticular proprioception are all utilized in dynamic balance during locomotion. There are some indications that muscle spindle afferents and cervical mechanoreceptors also play a role, particularly during more complex motor tasks.[25,26]

Classification of Gait Disorders

Because of the multiplicity of neural systems that support postural control and locomotion, there are many problems that can arise. Consequently, gait disorders encountered in clinical practice are heterogeneous and sometimes multifactorial. Neurologic disorders overlap with arthritic and antalgic gaits. Failing gaits may appear fundamentally similar even when they are mechanistically different. The disorder of gait we observe in the clinic is the product of a physiological abnormality and the compensatory response. Some of the salient features such as widened stance and increased double support time are nonspecific, and represent biomechanical adaptations to improve stability and efficiency. The classification and diagnosis of gait disorders based on observational gait analysis is thus a difficult challenge.

Neurologic disorders of gait can be classified based on (1) common clinical syndromes, (2) underlying physiologic mechanisms, or (3) etiologic factors. Each system has its proponents and its limitations. Nutt has proposed a classification of gait disorders into eight groups based on clinical characteristics: cautious, weak, stiff, ataxic, veering, freezing, marche à petit pas, and bizarre.[27,28] The advantage of this syndrome-based approach is that it lends itself to observational analysis, and is easily understood and applied. It tends to cluster together cases that share similar physiologic mechanism, although many complex cases are not easily handled.

A physiologic, systems-based approach was outlined by Nutt et al. in 1993.[29] The lowest level gait disorders include those due to arthritis, neuromuscular disease, and sensory loss. Middle level gait disorders include hemiplegic gait, cerebellar gait, and the extrapyramidal syndromes. The highest level gait disorders are the major focus of this review, and are subdivided further into five categories: cautious gait, subcortical disequilibrium, frontal disequilibrium, isolated gait ignition failure (i.e., pure freezing gait), and frontal gait. The major difficulty with this approach is that the criteria for the five highest level gait disorders are somewhat arbitrary and are not always uniformly applied. The categories do not correlate well with etiologic diagnosis, and may change in the

TABLE 49-1 Classification of Gait Disorder in 120 Patients, According to Etiologic Cause

	1980–1982	1990–1994	Total	Percent
Myelopathy	8	12	20	16.7
Parkinsonism	5	9	14	11.7
Hydrocephalus	2	6	8	6.7
Multiple infarcts	8	10	18	15.0
Cerebellar degeneration	4	4	8	6.7
Sensory deficits	9	13	22	18.3
Toxic/metabolic	3	0	3	2.5
Psychogenic	1	3	4	3.3
Other	3	3	6	5.0
Unknown cause	7	10	17	14.2
Total	50	70	120	100

The initial 50 patients are from Sudarsky and Ronthal.[31] (*From Masdeu et al.[97] with permission.*)

same patient over time. A patient with progressive supranuclear palsy, for example, might begin with a subcortical disequilibrium or freezing gait, and progress to a frontal gait with progression of the disease.

Classification of gait disorders based on etiology is practical.[30] Etiologic diagnosis is the first step in therapeutic intervention. Neurologic evaluation of 50 patients aged over 65 with an undiagnosed neurologic disorder of gait was successful at identifying the principal etiologic factor in 85 percent of cases. Treatable disorders were identified in 25 percent.[31] The categories of disease encountered are summarized in Table 49-1. Sometimes an etiology is not known and cannot be established, or the disorder is multifactorial. This system is not easily applied to older patients with higher level gait disorders, and patients with more advanced disability. Efforts have been made to incorporate the strengths of each system into a single framework, or to develop a hybrid system.[32]

Classification is useful as it facilitates communication among clinicians, and it helps focus clinical investigation. Literature from the late 19th and early 20th centuries can be more easily approached when older terms such as Bruns' ataxia, trepidant abasia, senile gait, and gait apraxia are placed in contemporary perspective. There is an evolving literature dealing with problem areas such as frontal gait disorder and freezing gait. Still none of these classifications is totally satisfactory, and they should not be considered the last word.

Common Patterns of Gait Disorder

THE CAUTIOUS GAIT

In their landmark paper on higher level gait disorders, Nutt et al. introduced the concept of the "cautious gait."[29] The pattern of reduced stride, wider base, shorter swing phase with preservation of rhythmic stepping is, in essence, an adaptation to perceived imbalance. Older people commonly adopt this guarded or cautious pattern of locomotion in order to achieve better stability.[33] While this pattern of gait is non-specific, there may be underlying neurologic deficits which pose a postural threat. As noted by Nutt et al., "Early in the course of such disorders, the cautious gait may dominate, but with progression of the condition, the characteristic gait disorder will emerge." The cautious gait was the most frequently observed higher level gait disorder, occurring in 16 of 43 patients in Nutt's series.

Despite a narrow intent, the designation cautious gait is often appropriated to include a variety of psychogenic gait disorders dominated by anxiety and fear of falling. Consider the older patient with apprehension and recent falls, who locomotes with the arms abducted, clutching at walls and furniture, as if walking on a slippery surface.[34] A better description for this phenomenon is inappropriately cautious or phobic gait. It is particularly amenable to rehabilitation therapies.

STIFF-LEGGED GAIT

A variety of stiff-legged gaits are observed among patients with cerebral palsy, demyelinating disease, and spinal disorders. The common denominator in these conditions is an element of spasticity, but there are several distinct patterns of abnormal locomotion, and "spastic gait" is not a unitary disorder.[35] There may be inappropriate flexion at the hip or knee. Some patients have adductor spasm, with circumduction and scissoring. Equinovarus is another common pattern. The shoes often reflect uneven wear, and with progression there may be a bouncy toe-walking. Intervention with botulinum toxin, nerve block or surgery will be successful only if the intervention is appropriately targeted.[36] It is not clear how much benefit oral spasticity medications provide for stiff-legged gait. There are no good randomized clinical trials, though patients report subjective benefits. Intrathecal baclofen has been used for treatment failures, particularly among the cerebral diplegia population.

A different stiff-legged gait is observed in patients with autoimmune stiffman syndrome. The disorder is characterized by anti-glutamic acid decarboxylase (GAD) antibodies, and a deficiency of gamma-aminobutyric acid (GABA)-mediated synaptic inhibition at a brain and spinal level.[37] There is spasm with hyperlordosis of the lumbar spine, and the patient walks as if the limbs and trunk were fused in a solid block. This "Frankenstein gait" improves with treatments that release muscle overactivity in the disorder, including high-dose benzodiazepines, intrathecal baclofen, and immunotherapy. There have been several reports of success with intravenous immunoglobulin (IVIg) in stiff-man syndrome.[38,39]

FREEZING GAIT

Charcot in the 19th century was the first to describe freezing of gait in patients with Parkinson's disease (PD).[40] It is a distinctive phenomenon. Arrests of movement (motor blocks) are usually brief, often occurring with gait initiation or when the patient turns to change direction. Motor blocks during gait initiation are sometimes termed start hesitation or "gait ignition failure." Patients report that their feet feel glued to the floor. There may be a series of quick, ineffective stepping movements with side-to-side shifting of weight, but no forward engagement ("slipping clutch syndrome"). Locomotor movements are then normal or near-normal once the patient is in motion, but freezing may return as the patient turns or attempts to navigate the door threshold. There is variability, in that the same doorway may be a problem on one occasion, but not the next. Freezing is often overcome with the aid of sensory cues; visual cues may be particularly effective.

Freezing of gait is particularly common in PD; the frequency increases with disease duration, motor disability, and duration of L-dopa treatment.[41] Freezing of gait was reported in 26 percent of Parkinson's patients at the 14-month endpoint of the DATATOP study, and in 25 percent of patients at 3–4 years in the ropinirole 056 study.[42] It is more common with advanced disease, and is correlated with dysarthria, axial rigidity, and postural instability. Pahapill and Lozano speculate about the role of cell loss in the pedunculopontine nucleus in the gait freezing of PD.[12] While motor fluctuations and dyskinesias are delayed by dopamine agonist treatment, gait freezing develops with similar frequency in L-dopa and agonist-treated patients.[43] In patients with motor fluctuations, gait freezing is most often observed during off-time. "Off-period" gait freezing may respond to an upward adjustment or redistribution of anti-parkinsonian medication. "On-period" gait freezing is more difficult to treat with medication, and responds best to rehabilitation-based interventions. Cueing to lengthen stride seems to be the most productive strategy.[44] Experience is variable with pallidotomy and deep brain stimulation surgical procedures, which may improve spatiotemporal characteristics of gait, but do not consistently help freezing.[45,46]

Gait freezing also occurs in patients with related neurodegenerative diseases such as progressive supranuclear palsy, multiple-system atrophy, corticobasal degeneration, and diffuse Lewy body disease. In one study, freezing of gait was present in 24 percent of patients with an atypical parkinsonian disorder at the time of presentation.[47] A syndrome of pure akinesia has been described, with dysarthria, gait freezing, postural instability, and a variable response to L-dopa. Some patients with pure akinesia have been found to exhibit the neuropathology of progressive supranuclear palsy at postmortem.[48] Primary progressive freezing gait ("pure gait ignition failure") may be a similar disorder with restricted expression.[49,50] Factor et al. reported on the natural history of 30 patients with primary progressive freezing gait who were not L-dopa-responsive. Most developed falls within 3 years and lost independent ambulation in 5 years.[51] Imaging studies in patients with primary progressive freezing gait do not show evidence of frontal hypometabolism[52] or dopamine cell loss.[53]

FRONTAL GAIT (MARCHE À PETIT PAS)

The frontal gait is a combination of impaired stepping (shuffling, freezing gait) and some degree of disequilibrium. The major cause of this phenomenon is cerebrovascular disease, particularly small-vessel disease involving the basal ganglia and periventricular white matter. In this context, the frontal gait is sometimes described as lower body parkinsonism,[54] although it is not a dopamine-deficiency disorder. The phenomenon has also been termed gait apraxia,[55] although it is really a higher-level motor control disorder as opposed to an apraxia. Walking depends on the successful integration of stepping with postural control, and these patients cannot achieve the objective consistently. The anatomic basis for the phenomenon is presumed to involve the disconnection of the cortical motor areas from the basal ganglia and brainstem locomotor centers. White matter lesions within this network produce a gait disorder in patients with hypertensive cerebrovascular disease and patients with hydrocephalus.

Thompson and Marsden characterized the gait disorder in 12 patients with subcortical arteriosclerotic encephalopathy (Binswanger's disease), based on observational analysis of the patients' chair rise and gait. Start and turn hesitation were salient features; festination was not observed.[56] Elble et al. studied the physiology of gait initiation in 5 patients with vascular disease (lower body parkinsonism). The basic architecture of the first step was preserved in these patients, though steps were irregular and sometimes aborted. Postural shifts necessary to initiate forward movement were not effectively generated.[57] Yanagisawa et al. captured episodes of gait freezing in the laboratory with surface EMG and analysis of ground reaction forces in patients with PD vascular parkinsonism. An increase in step frequency was observed prior to freezing. Co-contraction was observed in antagonist muscles in the legs, which interferes with phasic activation of locomotor movements and restrains forward motion.[58] Co-contraction has also been described in studies of patients with normal-pressure hydrocephalus.[59] Ebersbach et al. reported variability in the timing and size of stepping in patients with subcortical arteriosclerotic encephalopathy. They noted compensations for imbalance and some ataxic features, in addition to short steps and freezing.[60]

The major avenue of treatment for the frontal gait disorder of subcortical arteriosclerotic encephalopathy is physical therapy. Morris et al. trained patients with gait freezing using a paradigm of balance training, attentional cues, and stride lengthening.[61,62] Medications that promote the central nervous system (CNS) availability of monoamine neurotransmitters are often used (L-dopa, selegiline, L-threo-3,4-dihydroxyphenylserine), and some patients benefit.[63] Amantadine has also helped reduce unsteadiness and increase stride length.[64]

DYSTONIC GAIT

Dystonia may be focal or generalized. Whatever the cause, dystonia can produce unusual and sometimes bizarre disorders of gait. The two principal gaits (walking, and running) may be differentially affected. For many patients, dystonia may disappear when walking backwards. In patients with generalized dystonia, there may be torsion of the trunk, and the twisted posture of the lower body may make walking difficult altogether.

The most common focal disorder is dystonic inversion at the ankle, sometimes associated with extension of the great toe. Dystonic toe flexion also occurs, as do more complex proximal lower limb dystonias. Focal dystonia is generally amenable to botulinum toxin injection, provided that the active muscles can be successfully identified and targeted. Dynamic EMG or kinematic gait studies can sometimes be of help.[36] Dystonic flexion of the thoracolumbar spine (camptocormia) has been identified in patients with PD. It is activated as the patient stands to walk, and remits when lying supine, which helps distinguish the disorder from contracture.[65] Many patients with PD and related disorders have dystonic kyphoscoliosis caused by tone abnormalities from their extrapyramidal disease.

CEREBELLAR GAIT

Holmes characterized the gait ataxia in studies of patients with penetrating head injury.[66] Cerebellar disease produces imbalance (disequilibrium) and a distinct locomotor disorder. The gait is often slow and halting, with a widened base of support. Stepping is irregular, which results in a lurching quality as the upper body segments struggle to maintain alignment. The patient may stumble or veer off to the side. Truncal instability is more pronounced when attempting to walk on a narrow base, or tandem, heel-to-toe. Patients also exhibit imbalance when they turn or change direction. Control of gait and balance is localized within the cerebellum to the midline structures, including the efferent pathways of the interposed and fastigial nucleus.[67]

Kinematic studies in cerebellar patients confirm the features described above. The essential physiologic abnormality is irregular stepping: increased variability of timing, direction, and amplitude.[60] Palliyath et al. noted a reduced velocity and stride length in 10 patients with cerebellar degeneration.[68] While the gait was not wide-based in this study, other centers have demonstrated an increased base of support in cerebellar patients.[69] Analysis of moments about the knee and ankle joints revealed poor intralimb coordination, indicating a decomposition of multijoint movement. Other characteristic features included reduced dorsiflexion of the ankle at the onset of the swing phase, which might predispose to tripping.[68] Studies by Horak and Diener show that postural responses in cerebellar patients have a normal latency, but are hypermetric in force, contributing to truncal titubation. Patients often fall in a direction opposite to the force by which they were perturbed.[70]

Patients with alcoholic cerebellar degeneration, which affects primarily the midline vermis, often have a gait ataxia out of proportion to findings in the oculomotor system and limbs. Nearly half of patients with neurodegenerative ataxia have a form of hereditary cerebellar degeneration. There has been great progress over the last 10 years in understanding the hereditary ataxias, many of which can be identified through DNA diagnostic testing. The cost of genetic testing in ataxia patients is roughly comparable to the cost of one or two magnetic resonance imaging (MRI) scans, and the information is very helpful for prognosis and genetic counseling.

Pharmacotherapy of ataxia has not been a dramatic success to date. The neurodegenerative ataxias differ in how they prune the cerebellar circuit anatomy, and it is not apparent which neurotransmitter to replace. Buspirone and tandospirone have been explored, as these drugs stimulate $5-HT_{1A}$ receptors in the cerebellar cortex.[71,72] Individual patients may benefit, but randomized clinical trials do not show efficacy. Therapeutic trials are more informative when they are based on homogeneous, genetically defined subgroups of ataxia patients.

SENSORY ATAXIA

Locomotor ataxia was described in the 19th century in patients with tabetic neurosyphilis. There is excess motion of the center of mass and lateral path deviation, but patients tend to have a regular stride. Most patients are visually dependent in their walking, and do poorly in the dark. Features that distinguish sensory ataxia from cerebellar are summarized in Table 49-2. While there is a healthy redundancy of sensory information about the position of the body in space during locomotion, humans are particularly dependent on proprioception. Patients with peripheral neuropathy affecting large fibers are at a substantially increased risk for falls.[73] Causes of a predominantly ataxic neuropathy in clinical practice include vincristine and cisplatin chemotherapy, cobalamin deficiency, paraproteinemia, and subacute sensory neuropathy, which may be autoimmune or paraneoplastic.[74]

Several studies have examined the impact of proprioceptive deficits on postural control and gait. Horak has demonstrated increased body sway during stance, and displacement of the center of mass while walking in patients with diabetic neuropathy. In order to compensate for excess motion of the center of mass, patients alter lateral step placement. Somatosensory information derived from fingertip contact with a stable object (haptic information) can help with balance compensation.[75] Lajoie et al. reported kinematic studies in a patient with advanced sensory neuropathy, who had absent proprioception in the limbs by clinical measures. The focus of the discussion was on the compensatory strategies that enable locomotion to proceed in the absence of somatosensory feedback. This patient walked with a widened base of support and reduced stride, biomechanical adaptations to improve stability. A forward tilt was observed, with flexion of the neck such that the patient could monitor the performance visually. EMG demonstrated co-activation of the vastus lateralis and medial hamstring during weight acceptance, effectively bracing the leg during the stance phase. Although the gait appeared more mechanical, this strategy effectively reduces the number of degrees of freedom and simplifies the task of postural control.[76]

Vestibular deficits can also impair control of the head and center of mass during locomotion.[75] Fife and Baloh found bilateral vestibular deficits in 7 of 26 patients aged over 75 with disequilibrium of uncertain cause.[77] This syndrome is most often associated with a cautious gait and a feeling of unsteadiness, as opposed to a gross sensory ataxia.[78]

PSYCHOGENIC GAIT DISORDERS

Functional disorders of gait are well-described in the medical literature, dating back to the 19th century. A variety of psychogenic gait disorders were observed among combatants in the First World War, when astasia-abasia was the most common conversion disorder.[79] Psychogenic disorders of gait occur at all ages, although extra caution should be used in making this diagnosis in the elderly.[80] Older people often exhibit a combination of physical disability and an exaggerated compensatory response, particularly if there is apprehension and fear of falling.

Lempert et al. characterized the recognition features that help identify psychogenic disorders of gait, from a review of

TABLE 49-2 Clinical Distinction of Ataxic and Unsteady Gaits

	Cerebellar Ataxia	Sensory Ataxia	Frontal Gait
Stance	Wide-based	Looks down	Wide-based
Velocity	Variable	Slow	Very slow
Stride	Irregular, lurching	High-stepping	Short, shuffling
Romberg	+/−	Unsteady, falls	+/−
Heel-shin	Abnormal	+/−	Normal
Initiation	Normal	Normal	Hesitant
Turns	Veers away	+/−	Hesitant, fragmented
Postural instability	+	+ + +	+ + + +, poor postural synergies
Falls	Uncommon	Frequent	Frequent

video in 37 cases.[81] The abnormalities are often distinctive, and psychiatric history is sometimes revealing. Extreme slow motion may occur, as if the patient were walking through a viscous substance. Uneconomical postures with wastage of muscular effort are another classic example. Dramatic fluctuations may occur over minutes, which is unusual for patients with neurologic disease. Observation and distraction may activate and/or suppress the findings. A video atlas, published by Hayes et al., elaborates on these criteria and notes some diagnostic pitfalls.[80] Prognosis is often good for those patients in whom the history is recent and the decompensation of walking is acute. Dramatic cures are often possible in this setting.[82] When psychogenic disorders of gait persist for 6 months or more and become part of an established pattern of dependence and disability, it is often difficult to restore function.[83]

Laboratory Techniques for Investigation of Gait Disorders

LABORATORY GAIT ANALYSIS

In the 19th century, Eadweard Muybridge worked with a series of still cameras and a timing device to produce detailed kinematic studies of human walking. Laboratory gait analysis matured with the technology available in the late 20th century. Data captured by video camera are reconstructed on the computer to track trunk and limb movement in three dimensions. Some clinical gait laboratories and most research laboratories also provide information on ground reaction forces and surface EMG.

The principal strength of this technique is its ability to monitor the success of a specific therapeutic intervention. Kinematic studies document the efficacy of intrathecal baclofen for stiff-legged gait, and L-dopa and surgery for PD.[46,84] Gait analysis is also used to target therapeutic interventions such as botox and orthopedic surgery in patients with stiff-legged gait.[85,86] Clinical investigation has been done using kinematic data to help understand the pathophysiology of gait disorders.[87,88] Laboratory gait analysis is not always helpful with diagnostic problem cases and bizarre gaits that defy classification on clinical grounds. There is not yet enough sophisticated pattern recognition built into the software.

OBSERVATIONAL GAIT ANALYSIS

Observational gait analysis provides a less costly alternative to laboratory gait analysis.[89] With a stopwatch and a tape measure, the principal parameters of the gait can be recorded, including cadence, velocity, and stride. Videotape (or digital) replay provides an opportunity to slow down the performance, achieve objectivity, and look for subtle diagnostic clues. A timed test of walking is used as part of the CAPSIT

protocol for measuring the success of surgical interventions in PD.[90] Foot-switches can be affixed to the sole of the shoe, allowing an analysis of cadence and stride variability. Increased variability of stepping has been observed, particularly among those PD patients with a history of gait freezing.[91]

IMAGING

Imaging tests play an important role in the diagnostic evaluation of gait disorders, particularly higher-level gait disorders. MRI is often obtained in patients with gait problems to screen for vascular disease, demyelination, posterior fossa malformation, cerebellar degeneration, and hydrocephalus. The presence of white matter disease in the periventricular region or centrum semiovale on MRI has been correlated with gait and balance problems in numerous studies.[78,92] A modest amount of white matter change on MRI is not unusual in older patients, and careful clinical correlation is required. Brooks et al. used MR spectroscopy to distinguish symptomatic from incidental white matter lesions, and found abnormal spectra in those patients with white matter change and abnormal gait.[93] Walking is such a nested function that there is no critical localization for white matter stroke to produce an isolated gait impairment, but the entire burden of lesions needs to be considered.

Newer imaging techniques such as functional MRI, positron emission tomography (PET), and SPECT may be able to identify parts of the neural network active during integrative control of gait and balance. In PET studies, the anterior lobe of the cerebellum displays increased regional cerebral blood flow during quiet stance.[94] SPECT imaging has the advantage that the widely used radiopharmaceuticals have longer half-life, and subjects can walk for a few minutes outside of the machine in order to activate locomotor networks. Fukuyama et al. used SPECT imaging with ^{99}Tc-HMPAO to identify a number of structures active in normal subjects during locomotion, including supplementary motor area, primary sensorimotor cortex, striatum, and cerebellar vermis.[95] In a group of 10 PD patients studied with this technique, there was underactivation of the medial frontal area.[14] A study of 10 patients with primary freezing gait using SPECT imaging with xenon did not reveal measurable abnormalities of frontal lobe activation and perfusion.[52] Physiologic studies and imaging expand our toolkit as we explore complex phenomena such as freezing of gait, and try to come to terms with the decomposition of gait in neurologic patients.

References

1. www.sciencedaily.com/releases/2002/10/021015073446.htm.
2. Newman G, Dovermuehle RH, Busse EW: Alterations in neurologic status with age. *J Am Geriatr Soc* 8:915–917, 1960.

3. Odenheimer G, Funkenstein HH, Beckett L, et al: Comparison of neurologic changes in successfully aging persons vs the total aging population. *Arch Neurol* 51:573–580, 1994.

4. Tinetti ME, Speechley M, Ginter SF: Risk factors for falls among elderly persons living in the community. *N Engl J Med* 137:342–354, 1988.

5. Rubenstein L, Josephson KR: Interventions to reduce the multifactorial risks for falling, in Masdeu J, Sudarsky L, Wolfson L (eds): *Gait Disorders of Aging: Falls and Therapeutic Strategies*. Philadelphia: Lippincott-Raven, 1997, pp 13–36.

6. Grillner S, Wallen P: Central pattern generators for locomotion, with special reference to vertebrates. *Annu Rev Neurosci* 8:233–261, 1985.

7. Eidelberg E, Walden JG, Nguyen LH: Locomotor control in Macaque monkeys. *Brain* 104:647–663, 1981.

8. Dietz V, Colombo DM, Jensen DM, Baumgartner L: Locomotor capacity of spinal cord in paraplegic patients. *Ann Neurol* 37:574–582, 1995.

9. Orlovsky GN: The effect of different descending systems on flexor and extensor activity during locomotion. *Brain Res* 40:359–371, 1972.

10. Mori S, Matsui T, Mori F, et al: Instigation and control of treadmill locomotion in high decerebrate cats by stimulation of the hook bundle of Russell in the cerebellum. *Can J Physiol Pharmacol* 78:945–957, 2000.

11. Mori S, Matsuyama K, Mori F, Nakajima K: Supraspinal sites that induce locomotion in the vertebrate central nervous system. *Adv Neurol* 87:25–40, 2001.

12. Pahapill PA, Lozano AM: The pedunculopontine nucleus and Parkinson's disease. *Brain* 123:1767–1783, 2000.

13. Garcia-Rill E: The pedunculopontine nucleus. *Prog Neurobiol* 36:363–389, 1991.

14. Hanakawa T, Katsumi Y, Fukuyama H, et al: Mechanisms underlying gait disturbance in Parkinson's disease: A single photon emission computed tomography study. *Brain* 122:1271–1282, 1999.

15. Lawrence DG, Kuypers HGJM: The functional organization of the motor system in the monkey: II. The effects of lesions of the descending brain stem pathways. *Brain* 91:15–36, 1968.

16. Armstrong DM: The supraspinal control of mammalian locomotion. *J Physiol* 405:1–37, 1988.

17. Garcia-Rill E: The basal ganglia and the locomotor regions. *Brain Res Rev* 11:47–63, 1986.

18. Mori S: Neurophysiology of locomotion: Recent advances in the study of locomotion, in Masdeu J, Sudarsky L, Wolfson L (eds): *Gait Disorders of Aging: Falls and Therapeutic Strategies*. Philadelphia: Lippincott-Raven, 1997, 55–78.

19. Drew T: Discharge patterns of pyramidal tract neurons in motor cortex during a locomotion task requiring a precise control of limb trajectory. *Soc Neurosci Abstr* 72:17, 1987.

20. Horak FB, Nashner LM: Central programming of postural movements: Adaptation to altered support surface configurations. *J Neurophysiol* 55:1369–1381, 1986.

21. Nashner LM: Balance adjustments of humans perturbed while walking. *J Neurophysiol* 44:650–664, 1980.

22. Allum JHJ: Vestibulospinal and proprioceptive reflex assessment of balance control, in Bronstein AD, Brandt T, Woollacott M (eds): *Clinical Disorders of Balance Posture and Gait*. London: Arnold, 1996, pp 114–130.

23. Winter DA: *The Biomechanics and Motor Control of Human Gait*, 2nd ed. Waterloo: University of Waterloo Press, 1991.

24. Romberg MH: *Manual of the Nervous System of Man*, translated by Sieveking EH. London: Sydenham Society, vol 2, 1853.

25. Roll JP, Vedel JP, Roll R: Eye, head, and skeletal muscle spindle feedback in the elaboration of body references. *Prog Brain Res* 80:113–123, 1989.

26. Pozzo T, Berthoz A, Lefort L: Head stabilization during various locomotor tasks in humans. I. Normal subjects. *Exp Brain Res* 82:97–106, 1990.

27. Nutt JG: Gait and balance disorders, a syndrome approach, in Jankovic J, Tolosa E (eds): *Parkinson's Disease and Movement Disorders*, 3rd ed. Baltimore: Williams & Wilkins, 1998, pp 697–699.

28. Nutt JG: Classification of gait and balance disorders. *Adv Neurol* 87:135–141, 2001.

29. Nutt JG, Marsden CD, Thompson PD: Human walking and higher-level gait disorders, particularly in the elderly. *Neurology* 43:268–279, 1993.

30. Sudarsky L: Gait disorders: Prevalence, morbidity, and etiology. *Adv Neurol* 87:111–117, 2001.

31. Sudarsky L, Ronthal M: Gait disorders among elderly patients: a survey study of 50 patients. *Arch Neurol* 40:740–743, 1983.

32. Jankovic J, Nutt JG, Sudarsky LR: Classification, diagnosis, and etiology of gait disorders. *Adv Neurol* 87:119–134, 2001.

33. Murray MP, Kory RC, Clarkson BH: Walking patterns in healthy old men. *J Gerontol* 24:169–178, 1969.

34. Murphy J, Isaacs B: The post-fall syndrome: A study of 36 elderly patients. *Gerontology* 82:265–270, 1982.

35. Mayer NH, Esquenazi A, Keenan MA: Patterns of upper motoneuron dysfunction in the lower limb. *Adv Neurol* 87:311–320, 1999.

36. O'Brien CF: Chemodenervation with botulinum toxin for spasticity and dystonia: The effects on gait. *Adv Neurol* 87:265–270, 1999.

37. Levy LM, Dalakas MC, Floeter MK: The stiff-person syndrome: An autoimmune disorder affecting neurotransmission of GABA. *Ann Intern Med* 131:522–530, 1999.

38. Karlson EW, Sudarsky L, Ruderman E, et al: Treatment of stiff-man syndrome with intravenous immune globulin. *Arthritis Rheum* 37:915–918, 1994.

39. Souza-Lima CFL, Ferraz HB, Braz CA, et al: Marked improvement in a stiff-limb patient treated with intravenous immunoglobulin. *Mov Disord* 15:358–359, 2000.

40. Charcot JM, translated by G Sigerson: *Clinical Lectures on Disease of the Nervous System*. London: New Sydenham Society, 1877, vol 1, pp 145–146.

41. Giladi N, McDermott MP, Fahn S, et al: Freezing of gait in PD. *Neurology* 56:1712–1721, 2001.

42. Rascol O, Brooks DJ, Korczyn AD, et al: Five year study of the incidence of dyskinesia in patients with early Parkinson's disease who were treated with ropinerole or levodopa. *N Engl J Med* 342:1484–1491, 2000.

43. Parkinson Study Group: Pramipexole vs levodopa as initial treatment for Parkinson disease. *JAMA* 248:1931–1938, 2000.

44. Rubenstein TC, Giladi N, Hausdorff JM: The power of cueing to circumvent dopamine deficits: A review of physical therapy treatment of gait disturbances in Parkinson's disease. *Mov Disord* 17:1148–1160, 2002.

45. Allert N, Volkmann J, Dotse S, et al: Effects of bilateral pallidal or subthalamic stimulation on gait in advanced Parkinson's disease. *Mov Disord* 16:1076–1085, 2001.

46. Stolze H, Klebe S, Poepping M, et al: Effects of bilateral subthalamic nucleus stimulation on parkinsonian gait. *Neurology* 57:144–146, 2001.

47. Muller J, Seppi K, Stefanova N, et al: Freezing of gait in postmortem-confirmed atypical parkinsonism. *Mov Disord* 17:1041–1045, 2002.

48. Riley DE, Fogt N, Leigh RJ: The syndrome of "pure akinesia" and its relationship to progressive supranuclear palsy. *Neurology* 44:1025–1029, 1994.

49. Achiron A, Ziv I, Goren M, et al: Primary progressive freezing gait. *Mov Disord* 8:293–297, 1993.

50. Atchison PR, Thompson PD, Frackowiak RSJ, Marsden CD: The syndrome of gait ignition failure. *Mov Disord* 8:285–292, 1993.

51. Factor SA, Jennings DL, Molho ES, Marek KL: The natural history of the syndrome of primary progressive freezing gait. *Arch Neurol* 59:1778–1183, 2002.

52. Fabre N, Brefel C, Sabatini U, et al: Normal frontal perfusion in patients with frozen gait. *Mov Disord* 13:677–683, 1998.

53. Jennings DL, Factor SA, Molho ES, et al: Primary progressive freezing gait disorder: A neuroimaging study to evaluate dopamine transporter density. *Neurology* 54(suppl 3):A191, 2000.

54. Fitzgerald PM, Jankovic J: Lower body parkinsonism: Evidence for a vascular etiology. *Mov Disord* 4:249–260, 1989.

55. Meyer JS, Barron DW: Apraxia of gait: A clinicophysiologic study. *Brain* 83:261–284, 1960.

56. Thompson PD, Marsden CD: Gait disorder of subcortical arteriosclerotic encephalopathy: Binswanger's disease. *Mov Disord* 2:1–8, 1987.

57. Elble RJ, Cousins R, Leffler K, Hughes L: Gait initiation by patients with lower-half parkinsonism. *Brain* 119:1705–1716, 1996.

58. Yanagisawa N, Hayashi R, Mitoma H: Pathophysiology of frozen gait in parkinsonism. *Adv Neurol* 87:199–207, 2001.

59. Sudarsky L, Simon S: Gait disorder in late-life hydrocephalus. *Arch Neurol* 44:263–267, 1987.

60. Ebersbach G, Sojer M, Valldeoriola F, et al: Comparative analysis of gait in Parkinson's disease, cerebellar ataxia, and subcortical arteriosclerotic encephalopathy. *Brain* 122:1349–1355, 1999.

61. Morris ME, Iansek R, Matyas TA, Summers JJ: The pathogenesis of gait hypokinesia in Parkinson's disease. *Brain* 117:1169–1181, 1994.

62. Iansek R, Ismail NH, Bruce M, et al: Frontal gait apraxia: Pathophysiologic mechanisms and rehabilitation. *Adv Neurol* 87:363–374, 2001.

63. Narabayashi H, Kondo T, Yokochi F, Nagatsu T: Clinical effects of l-threo-3,4-dihydroxyphenylserine in cases of parkinsonism and pure akinesia. *Adv Neurol* 45:593–602, 1987.

64. Baezner H, Oster M, Henning O, et al: Amantadine increases gait steadiness in frontal gait disorder of subcortical vascular encephalopathy: A double-blind randomized placebo-controlled trial based on quantitative gait analysis. *Cerebrovasc Dis* 11:235–244, 2001.

65. Nieves AF, Miyasaki JM, Lang AE: Acute onset dystonic camptocormia caused by lenticular lesions. *Mov Disord* 16:177–180, 2001.

66. Holmes G: Clinical symptoms of cerebellar disease and their interpretation, the Croonian lectures. *Lancet* ii:59–65, 1922.

67. Lechtenberg R, Gilman S: Localization of function in the cerebellum. *Neurology* 28:376, 1978.

68. Palliyath S, Hallett M, Thomas SL, Lebiedowska MK: Gait in patients with cerebellar ataxia. *Mov Disord* 13:958–964, 1998.

69. Cueman-Hudson C, Krebs DE: Frontal plane dynamic stability and coordination in subjects with cerebellar degeneration. *Exp Brain Res* 132:103–113, 2000.

70. Horak FC, Diener HC: Cerebellar control of postural scaling and central set in stance. *J Neurophysiol* 72:479–493, 1994.

71. Trouillas P, Fuxe K: *Serotonin, the Cerebellum and Ataxia*. New York: Raven Press, 1993.

72. Lou J, Goldfarb L, McShane L, et al: Use of buspirone for treatment of cerebellar ataxia. *Arch Neurol* 52:982–988, 1995.

73. Richardson JK, Ching C, Hurvitz EA: The relationship between electromyographically documented peripheral neuropathy and falls. *J Am Geriatr Soc* 40:1008–1012, 1992.

74. Sabin TD: Peripheral neuropathy: Disorders of proprioception, in Masdeu J, Sudarsky L, Wolfson L (eds): *Gait Disorders of Aging: Falls and Therapeutic Strategies*. Lippincott-Raven, 1997, 273–282.

75. Horak F: Postural ataxia related to somatosensory loss. *Adv Neurol* 87:111–117, 2001.

76. Lajoie Y, Teasdale N, Cole JD, et al: Gait of a deafferented subject without large myelinated sensory fibers below the neck. *Neurology* 47:109–115, 1996.

77. Fife TD, Baloh RW: Disequilibrium of unknown cause in older people. *Ann Neurol* 34:694–702, 1993.

78. Kerber KA, Enrietto JA, Jacobson BA, Baloh RW: Disequilibrium in older people. *Neurology* 51:574–580, 1998.

79. Lhermitte JJ, Toussy G, translated by Christophersen W: *The Psychoneuroses of War*. London: University of London Press, 1918.

80. Hayes MW, Graham S, Heldorf P, et al: A video review of the diagnosis of psychogenic gait: Appendix and commentary. *Mov Disord* 14:914–921, 1999.

81. Lempert T, Brandt T, Dieterich M, Huppert D: How to identify psychogenic disorders of stance and gait. *J Neurol* 238:140–146, 1991.

82. Keane JR: Hysterical gait disorders: 60 cases. *Neurology* 39:586–589, 1989.

83. Bhatia K: Psychogenic gait disorders. *Adv Neurol* 87:251–254, 2001.

84. Dimanico U, Coletti Moja M, Knafitz M, et al: Role of gait analysis in decision making in long-term spasticity treatment by baclofen pump in de-ambulatory patients. *Mov Disord* 17(suppl 5):336, 2002.

85. Mayer NH, Esquenazi A, Keenan MA: Patterns of upper motoneuron dysfunction in the lower limb. *Adv Neurol* 87:311–320, 2001.

86. Wissel J, Muller J, Baldauf A, et al: Gait analysis to assess the effects of botulinum toxin A treatment in cerebral palsy. *Eur J Neurol* 6(suppl 4):63–68, 1999.

87. Stolze H, Kuhtz-Buschbeck JP, Drucke H, et al: Gait analysis in idiopathic normal pressure hydrocephalus: Which parameters respond to the CSF tap test. *Clin Neurophysiol* 111:1678–1686, 2000.

88. Stolze H, Kuhtz-Buschbeck JP, Drucke H, et al: Comparative analysis of the gait disorder of normal pressure hydrocephalus and Parkinson's disease. *J Neurol Neurosurg Psychiatry* 70:289–297, 2001.

89. Ebersbach G, Poewe W: Simple assessments of mobility: Methodology and clinical application of kinetic gait analysis. *Adv Neurol* 87:101–110, 2001.

90. Defer GL, Widner H, Marie RM, et al: Core assessment program for surgical interventional therapies in Parkinson's disease. *Mov Disord* 14:572–574, 1999.

91. Hausdorff JM, Schaafsma JM, Balash J, et al: Impaired regulation of stride variability in Parkinson's disease subjects with freezing of gait. *Exp Brain Res* 149:187–194, 2003.

92. Tell GS, Lefkowitz DS, Diehr P, et al: Relationship between balance and abnormalities in cerebral magnetic resonance imaging in older adults. *Arch Neurol* 55:73–79, 1998.

93. Brooks WM, Wesley MH, Kodituwakku PW, et al: 1H-MRS differentiates white matter hyperintensities in subcortical arteriosclerotic encephalopathy from those in normal elderly. *Stroke* 28:1940–1943, 1997.

94. Ouchi Y, Okada H, Yoshikawa E, et al: Brain activation during maintenance of standing postures in humans. *Brain* 122:329–338, 1999.

95. Fukuyama H, Ouchi Y, Matsuzaki S, et al: Brain functional activity during gait in normal subjects: A SPECT study. *Neurosci Lett* 228:183–186, 1997.

96. Inman VT, Ralston H, Todd F: *Human Walking*. Baltimore: Williams & Wilkins, 1981.

97. Sudarsky L: Clinical approach to gait disorders, in Masdeu J, Sudarsky L, Wolfson L (eds): *Gait Disorders of Aging: Falls and Therapeutic Strategies*. Lippincott-Raven, 1997, 147–157.

IX. SPECIAL CONSIDERATIONS

Chapter 50

MOVEMENT DISORDERS IN CHILDHOOD

LEON S. DURE IV

EPIDEMIOLOGY   825
APPROACH TO THE CHILD WITH A MOVEMENT
    DISORDER   826
TICS   826
TREMOR   827
    Clinical Characteristics   827
    Essential Tremor (ET)   827
    Other Tremors   828
DYSTONIA   828
    Clinical Issues   828
    Dystonic Conditions in Childhood 829
    Transient Dystonias   829
STEREOTYPIES   830
CHOREA   830
    Clinical Features   830
    Sydenham's Chorea (SC)   831
    Benign Hereditary Chorea   831
    Other Choreas   831
AKINETIC-RIGID SYNDROMES   831
CONCLUSION   832

Movement disorders in the pediatric age group appear phenomenologically the same as those in adults. The chorea seen in childhood looks essentially the same to an observer as that seen in an adult, and this is true for both hyperkinetic and bradykinetic conditions. Therefore, when considering the topic of pediatric movement disorders, a classification scheme based on the specific kinds of abnormality, whether they are tics, chorea, myoclonus, etc., has great utility in this patient population. However, when evaluating a child with a movement disorder, it is important to consider the inherent dynamism related to growth and development, and the contribution of this state to the presentation and evolution of various diseases. While children may manifest the gamut of dyskinetic conditions, whether bradykinetic or hyperkinetic, it must not be presumed that children are miniature adults, nor should it be expected that the course of a disorder will exactly parallel that seen in adults. Having introduced this element of uncertainty, which is familiar to all child neurologists, it is still worthwhile to try and formulate a cogent overview of childhood movement disorders. Indeed, a number of other chapters in this book deal with conditions that are primarily diseases of childhood (Tourette's syndrome, idiopathic torsion dystonia), and the reader is directed to these for comprehensive reviews. This chapter, however, will consider the various movement disorders that may present in childhood, with special emphasis on the more common presentations.

Epidemiology

Although medical centers specializing in movement disorders are not uncommon and have a worldwide distribution, clinics with a special emphasis on childhood conditions relating to movement are relatively rare. Thus, there are few reports in the literature that address the question of what the most common disorders might be in childhood. An exception has been the review of Fernandez-Alvarez and Aicardi,[1] who in a large series of children reported an incidence of tics (39 percent), dystonia (24 percent), tremor (19 percent), chorea (5 percent), myoclonus (3 percent), akinetic-rigid syndromes (2 percent), and mixed disorders (8 percent) out of a total of 684 patients (Fig. 50-1). These figures may not be representative of the general population, given that the source is a tertiary referral center, but no other broadly based data are currently available. It is striking, however, how these percentages differ from an adult movement disorder population, in which essential tremor and akinetic-rigid syndromes such as Parkinson's disease (PD) would certainly be more predominant.

Probably the most well-studied movement disorder to date in terms of epidemiology in childhood is that of tics. Large-scale studies of school-age children have estimated the prevalence at between 10 percent and 20 percent.[2,3] Studies of Tourette's syndrome (TS) have varied over the years in their estimations of prevalence, but recent reports indicate it to be as high as 3–4 percent in school-age children, with a much higher percentage in special needs populations.[4–9] While this may seem quite high, it is interesting to note that some of these estimates are of patients who met clinical criteria

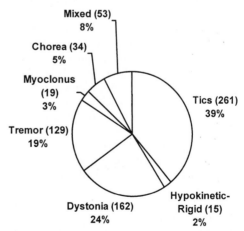

FIGURE 50-1 Distribution of movement disorders in 673 children seen in a tertiary referral center. (*Adapted from Fernandez Alvarez and Aicardi.*[1] *Used with permission.*)

for TS, but may never have received a diagnosis due to lack of impairment or disability. In any event, it would appear that tics would probably be the most frequently encountered childhood movement disorder, although characterization as a disease is not always true.

Among other disorders of movement, dystonia is a condition that may be seen in a number of contexts. The majority of epidemiologic studies of dystonia, however, primarily captures adult-onset focal or segmental dystonias, and do not report the incidence or prevalence of childhood-onset primary dystonia.[10] Moreover, dystonia in childhood may be seen in association with a variety of conditions, making ascertainment quite difficult. For example, dyskinetic cerebral palsy is thought to represent a subgroup of children who manifest a form of secondary dystonia. However, reports of the actual incidence of this form of movement disorder are quite disparate,[11–14] making any generalizations regarding frequency problematic.

The next most commonly encountered childhood movement disorder, tremor, has seldom been reported specifically in childhood.[15–18] This is despite the fact that essential tremor (ET) and tremor associated with other conditions are not uncommonly encountered in the clinical setting. Similarly, no data exist for chorea, myoclonus, or akinetic-rigid syndromes. Clearly, one area of potential research for the future will be to better examine and define the epidemiology of these disorders.

Approach to the Child with a Movement Disorder

As is true for most neurologic problems, when evaluating a child for a movement disorder, the history is of paramount importance. Unlike the evaluation of an adult, however, the complaint under scrutiny must be taken in the context of the child's stage of development.[19] For example, newborns and young infants may be described as manifesting myoclonus, which at that age and in many cases is a benign and transient finding.[20,21] This is also true for infants who may manifest chorea or dystonia.[22] Careful attention must be paid to the tempo of appearance of a movement disorder, the timing, and the course. Progression or worsening of symptoms or a loss of milestones certainly increases the likelihood of an active process, as opposed to the relatively unchanging features of a static motor encephalopathy. Family history is at times important, as are details regarding pregnancy, delivery, and developmental progress. Finally, it is important to ascertain any disability or impairment associated with the disorder, as well as any neurobehavioral correlates.

The examination of a child with a movement disorder can be quite challenging, and will often test the patience of the clinician. Perhaps one of the most profound advances in recent years has been the increasing popularity of affordable home video cameras. Indeed, sometimes the only way that a movement disorder can be witnessed by the clinician is for the family to provide a videotape demonstrating the child's movements. This is especially true for tics and stereotypies, which are often suppressible or state-dependent, and there are published recommendations on obtaining a home video assessment.[23] However, for many conditions, the movements are quite evident in the clinical setting. In all cases, a thorough neurologic examination is warranted, with the caveat that some parts of the examination are quite unreliable in many children (e.g., sensory testing, complex motor tasks, and some testing of higher cognitive function). Assessment of organomegaly, birthmarks, and occasionally detailed ophthalmologic examinations may be required in some cases.

Undoubtedly, the most important part of the assessment is to accurately designate the type of movement disorder. Definitions of tics, chorea, myoclonus, etc. are given elsewhere in this volume, but, despite the wealth of descriptive detail regarding the various disorders, practical determination of the type of movement can often be very difficult. Tics are often characterized by premonitory urges, suppressibility, and a sense of relief upon performance, but none of these features may be reported by young children who may exhibit frequent tics yet be oblivious to their presence. Hypertonic states such as spasticity, dystonia, and rigidity can at times be confusing for the less-experienced clinician, and, when occurring in the same patient, can engender disagreements even among those with significant expertise. Finally, disorders that may be difficult to differentiate upon observation, but are neurophysiologically distinct, such as rhythmic myoclonus and tremor, do not easily lend themselves to evaluation in the young child. Despite these difficulties, accurate characterization of movement disorders is usually possible, and serves as an adequate starting point to ultimate diagnosis and management. The subsequent discussion will be organized according to these standard categories of movement classification.

Tics

Probably the most common movement disorder of childhood, it must be stressed that not all tics are even worthy of the designation as a pathologic entity, and could even be considered a concomitant of normal development. Tics may be either motor or phonic, are involuntary, and may involve any part of the body.[24] One feature of tics that may distinguish them from other movement disorders is that they may be produced upon request, and can often be imitated by the examiner or a family member. Common motor manifestations include head shaking, eye blinking, facial grimacing, shoulder shrugging, mouth opening, and abdominal contractions. Phonic tics can be either simple sounds, such as sniffing or throat clearing, or take the form of more complex noises or utterances. Tics often occur in bouts, which in themselves may be the consequence of suppression.

As stated previously, tics have been observed in as many as 20 percent of school-age children, but the exact frequency is not known. When tics are diagnosed by primary care physicians, the recommended practice is to provide some education and reassurance to families, since it is felt that, in the majority of these children, the tics will resolve spontaneously and not recur.[25] It is for this reason that the evaluating physician must take into account the developmental context of the patient in question. A young child with a recent onset of tics does not necessarily need a comprehensive set of investigations, since there is probably some likelihood that the tics will resolve. The formal diagnosis for this entity would be most closely approximated by a transient tic disorder (DSM-IV 307.20),[26] with the exception that most children are not adversely affected by their tics, nor do they suffer significant impairment. For a more comprehensive discussion of chronic tic disorders, the reader is referred to Chap. 41.

Historical features of importance in the characterization of tics in childhood include the duration and repertoire of tics. Families often will relate that children with tic disorders have exhibited behavior in the past that would certainly be consistent with prior tics, even though the behavior contemporaneous to the evaluation may be thought of as the "first" episode of tics. Prior to the diagnosis, parents are usually unaware that sniffing, throat clearing, and blinking could be due to other processes than irritative or inflammatory conditions. Finally, a family history of tics, habits, or repetitive behaviors certainly points very strongly to a diagnosis within the spectrum of chronic tic disorders.

One issue relating to tic disorders and childhood that bears further discussion, though, is that of "tourettism." This term is used to describe patients who may meet criteria for TS or other chronic tic disorder, but within the context of some other disorder affecting the nervous system.[27–32] Tics that fluctuate over time both in location and intensity may be seen in the context of mental retardation and have been attributed to neuroleptic and anticonvulsant use. Although tempting to consider this association as somehow contributing to the pathophysiology of TS, it must be kept in mind that tics and TS are relatively common and a coincidental comorbidity is not unlikely. The answer to this question will await the development of a biological marker for TS.

Tremor

CLINICAL CHARACTERISTICS

The clinical phenotype of tremor in childhood is much the same as that in adults. Oscillatory movements about a joint or joints that may occur at rest or with action have a similar appearance in all ages, although rest tremor in children is quite uncommon because of the relative paucity of akinetic-rigid syndromes. Kinetic or postural tremors due to cerebellar disease, rubral lesions, or peripheral processes are rare in pediatrics, in parallel to the incidence of the underlying diseases that occur in this age group. Despite a dearth of research in this area, ET is probably the most common type seen in childhood.[1] In newborn infants, jitteriness is a rhythmic tremor that may be seen in up to 40 percent of children during the first few hours of life.[33] Although occasionally an accompaniment of central nervous system pathology such as hypoxic-ischemic encephalopathy or drug withdrawal, in normal full-term babies, jitteriness resolves in the vast majority of patients within the first year of life.[34] Tremor as a manifestation of a conversion reaction is also seen.

In a child with kinetic or postural tremor, it is important to determine if indeed the condition is monosymptomatic, with no other medical or neurologic history that could point towards a primary process that would cause tremor as part of another disorder. Family history of tremor may be helpful, but actual examination of the biological parents is often warranted. Assessment of exacerbating factors such as exercise or anxiety can help focus the diagnosis. Besides the routine neurologic examination, some specific techniques are necessary. Examination of tremor at rest, with the extremities held in a steady posture, or while reaching for an object, are maneuvers that, with encouragement, are tasks that most children can perform. In the reluctant child, observation as a tower of blocks is constructed, or the careful placement of an object by the child into the examiner's hand, can be informative. Children who are able to use a pen, pencil, or even a crayon can be encouraged to draw an Archimedes spiral, although in younger children a rather large drawing may be necessary. In cases where tremor is suspected to be the manifestation of a conversion disorder, examination for changes in frequency or amplitude of tremor by using a weight in the affected limb is useful.[35]

ESSENTIAL TREMOR (ET)

The most common type of tremor in adults is ET, and, in large retrospective studies of familial tremor, age of onset in childhood is certainly reported.[17,18,36] A case series of ET in 19 patients with a mean age of 12.7 years at the time of diagnosis has been described from a tertiary referral center specializing in childhood movement disorders. Although detailed neurophysiologic testing was not performed, the clinical course and examination of these patients suggests that childhood ET is very similar to the adult variety. What is not known, however, is if the long-term prognosis of ET differs if onset is in childhood. In adults, tremor severity has been reported to be independently associated with both age and duration of the illness.[37] It would be tempting to speculate that earlier-onset ET may lead to greater disability in adulthood. On the other hand, children with ET may avoid activities and tasks that prove to be too difficult, and thus significant impairment could be actually less in these patients. Anticipation has not been described in large family studies of adult ET, but the lack of continuing prospective follow-up in childhood ET makes counseling difficult.

There are two entities described in children that have been characterized as ET variants. These conditions are geniospasm (hereditary chin trembling),[38,39] and shuddering attacks.[40,41] Both of these conditions may present as early as infancy, and, in the case of geniospasm, most cases reported are within families and are consistent with autosomal-dominant inheritance. Geniospasm is a trembling of the chin that may be asymmetric, paroxysmal, and somewhat state-dependent, appearing more prominent with stress. It is seldom disabling and usually does not require attention. In the case of shuddering attacks, children will present with a history of paroxysms of fine shaking, as if they are experiencing a chill. The events are usually short-lived and are not associated with any change in level of consciousness. Shuddering attacks are quite difficult to diagnose by history alone, and it is rare that a child will manifest an attack during a clinic visit. Often, these patients undergo video electroencephalographic (EEG) monitoring to rule out epilepsy, but a home videotape of the events should suffice to make the diagnosis. Like geniospasm, shuddering attacks do not require any therapy. Moreover, they tend to disappear with time.

There are no published series of treatment strategies in childhood ET. In this author's experience, however, pharmacologic agents such as primidone, beta-adrenergic blockers, and topiramate have proven useful, as they have in adults.[42–44] Care should be taken, though, to assess treatment goals, as younger children seldom require more than education and perhaps modifications in school regarding handwriting. On the other hand, adolescents will often request a treatment trial in order to avoid exhibiting tremor in public.

OTHER TREMORS

Another tremor that is seldom described but is seen with some frequency is in the context of an underlying neurologic or developmental disorder. Tremor may accompany static encephalopathies such as cerebral palsy, and has been described in apraxic children.[45] Since these and other conditions are commonly seen by child neurologists, it is possible that they represent the occurrence of two diseases in the same child, similar to the situation described above regarding tourettism. However, until larger series are assembled for study, this issue remains unresolved.

In terms of tremors that are specific to childhood, spasmus nutans and the bobblehead doll syndrome must be considered. Spasmus nutans presents most commonly within the first year of life, and is usually described as the constellation of head tremor, nystagmus, and inconsistently with head tilt.[46] The tremor is usually slow (2–4 Hz), and is typically in a "no-no" direction. The nystagmus can be more clearly seen if the head is held still by the examiner. Since these symptoms have also been described with visual impairment and optic nerve tumors, imaging is usually necessary.[47] However, barring an abnormality of cranial imaging or vision, spasmus nutans almost always resolves spontaneously with no treatment. On the other hand, the bobblehead doll syndrome is an episodic head tremor in a "yes-yes" direction, associated with hydrocephalus.[48,49] When confronted with a child with this type of up-and-down tremor, the clinician should look for other signs of hydrocephalus or increased intracranial pressure. As opposed to spasmus nutans, a true bobblehead will not respond without alleviation of the ventricular obstruction.

Finally, tremor is a known side-effect of anticonvulsant drugs, lithium, and adrenergic agents, among others.[50,51] These drugs in particular are used with some frequency in children. A syndrome of transient tremor has been reported in infants who have received supplemental vitamin B_{12} for megaloblastic anemia.[52,53]

Dystonia

CLINICAL ISSUES

Defined as a condition in which there is an abnormality of posture that may be static or dynamic, dystonia in childhood is most frequently thought of as being synonymous with idiopathic torsion dystonia (ITD). This disorder is treated in detail in Chap. 32, and probably represents the most commonly diagnosed primary dystonia in childhood. The emphasis on "diagnosed" relates to the growing realization that dystonia is felt to be under-recognized, and may be part of the clinical phenotype of a number of childhood disorders. Family- and population-based studies have tended to focus on the typical adult forms of dystonia, such as blepharospasm, writer's cramp, and torticollis, which are certainly more common than ITD.[10] However, taking elements of the definition of dystonia (postural abnormalities, fluctuation of tone, a twisting quality), clinicians who take care of children with neurologic disorders can often detect this abnormality of movement.

As an example of the potential prevalence of dystonia in childhood, it is informative to consider the entity of static motor encephalopathy, or cerebral palsy (CP). There are a number of subtypes of CP based on the distribution and character of the clinical findings. These include: diplegic, triplegic, and quadriplegic, each of which is typically associated with spasticity; hypotonic; ataxic; dyskinetic; and mixed. Of these subtypes, dyskinetic CP has the appearance of what is typically referred to as a hyperkinetic movement disorder, and is often described as "choreic," "athetoid," or "choreoathetoid."[11–13,54,55] Population-based studies of the epidemiology of CP usually include any and all of these types as part of the analysis. The overall incidence of CP varies from study to study, but 1–2/1000 live births is a reasonable range. What is interesting, however, is the steadily increasing appreciation for mixed forms of CP (approaching 25 percent of cases), with the common feature of "dyskinesia." These dyskinetic patients often manifest some component of dystonia, although formal definitions of dystonia in this context are not necessarily well formulated. There are attempts being made to return to first principles and develop consensus guidelines for the characterization of these dyskinetic movements.[56] Should these movements be clearly accepted as dystonic, then incidence and prevalence rates of dystonia will clearly need to be re-evaluated.

When evaluating a child with dystonia, historical information relating to onset, course, distribution, and family history are necessary. Moreover, it is clear from the discussion above that the clinician needs to remain cognizant of the fact that dystonia may be a finding in other disorders, particularly CP. A list of other conditions in which dystonia may be present is described in Table 50-1. Examination of children for dystonia can be quite difficult, owing not so much to a lack of cooperation as much as to the fluctuating nature of the movement. Sometimes, the only way to appreciate subtle dystonias in childhood is to observe the child while playing or ambulating.

DYSTONIC CONDITIONS IN CHILDHOOD

The differential diagnosis and steps in evaluation are discussed in Chap. 32, but there is one entity that deserves some emphasis, if only because it is often unrecognized. Dystonia has been reported to develop in patients with a history of CP, sometimes years after what has been considered a stable clinical state.[57,58] Why this occurs is not known, although it is believed that maturational processes may result in an "evolving" motor disturbance in children, and does not necessarily indicate the development of a new disease. Another group of disorders that have been recently described as causing a dystonic phenotype are those of neurotransmitter synthesis and metabolism.[59–61] Deficiencies of tyrosine hydroxylase and aromatic acid decarboxylase have been described in infancy, and are characterized by abnormalities in cerebrospinal fluid neurotransmitter metabolites and documentation of enzyme hypoactivity. The incidence of these disorders is not known, but the index of suspicion should be high in infants with unexplained dystonic symptoms. Therapeutic trials of L-dopa can be quite helpful in these children, but not all, indicating that there may be other enzymatic or metabolic disturbances leading to this phenotype.

One of the more satisfying dystonias to diagnose and treat in childhood is that of dopa-responsive dystonia (DRD). In most cases due to a mutation affecting GTP cyclohydrolase I, an enzyme necessary for biopterin metabolism, DRD is characterized by limb dystonia that is often focal, bradykinesia, and sometimes postural tremor.[61–66] It has been reported in children mistakenly labeled as having CP, presenting with hypertonicity and developmental delay. In these cases, a family history of first-degree relatives with "cerebral palsy" and evidence of dystonia make DRD a possibility, and a trial of L-dopa/carbidopa is indicated. As opposed to most dystonias of childhood, DRD is exquisitely sensitive to treatment, with sometimes sensational reduction in symptoms. These treatment responses are apparently still present after as long as 20 years of therapy.[67,68]

The significance of the relationship between CP and dystonia has a clear therapeutic implication. Due to the desire to detect cases of DRD, it is generally recommended that all children with dystonia be given a therapeutic trial of L-dopa. Likewise, it is clear that the usual therapeutic interventions for CP may neither be beneficial nor indicated in children with significant dystonia. In some children, surgical or pharmacologic therapies directed at lessening spasticity may have a deleterious effect on children who are primarily dystonic. In conclusion, it is of paramount importance to recognize dystonia, keeping in mind that, unlike in adults, dystonia may be only one part of the neurologic process.

TABLE 50-1 Childhood Disorders Associated with Dystonia

Inherited dystonia (DYT1, DYT6, DRD)
Neurodegenerative diseases
    Juvenile Parkinson's disease
    Juvenile Huntington's disease
    Pantothenate kinase-associated neurodegeneration
    Rett's syndrome
    Ataxia telangiectasia
Metabolic disorders
    Glutaric acidemia type 1
    Methylmalonic acidemia
    Metachromatic leukodystrophy
    Niemann-Pick type C
    Aromatic amino acid decarboxylase deficiency
    Hypoparathyroidism
    Lesch-Nyhan disease
Perinatal injury (hypoxic-ischemic encephalopathy, kernicterus)
Infection
Drugs (dopamine receptor antagonists, anticonvulsants)
Toxins (manganese, mercury, carbon monoxide)

DRD, dopa-responsive dystonia.

TRANSIENT DYSTONIAS

Another type of presumably primary dystonia of childhood is that collection of entities with the common feature of transience. These include transient idiopathic dystonia of infancy, benign paroxysmal torticollis of infancy, and benign paroxysmal upgaze.[69] Transient idiopathic dystonia usually presents in the first year of life, resolving within some months.[22] Often unilateral, it has more of a focal or segmental distribution. The dystonia may fluctuate and be difficult to elicit in a clinical setting, but a home videotape will demonstrate dystonic posturing in the child that may or may not interfere with acquisition of developmental milestones. Little is known about this disorder from either an etiologic or pathologic perspective, because these children "outgrow" the dystonia, with complete resolution. A similar presentation and course has also been reported to occur in the setting of fever.[70] Infantile masturbation has been described as a transient or paroxysmal behavior that may appear dystonic, and some of these children have been evaluated for epileptic tonic spasms.[71,72] Dystonic posturing of the trunk and/or head has been seen in the setting of hiatal hernia or gastroesophageal reflux, the so-called Sandifer syndrome.[73–76]

Paroxysmal torticollis is usually thought of as an entity of little impact, hence the descriptor of "benign." Children will have episodes of torticollis and/or retrocollis, sometimes associated with significant discomfort, vomiting, and irritability.[77,78] Furthermore, episodes may last for days to weeks, and cause significant morbidity, suggesting that denoting this condition as "benign" may be inappropriate. Considered to be a migraine equivalent, benign paroxysmal torticollis has been described in families with familial hemiplegic migraine and a mutation of the CACNA1A gene.[79] There have been no comprehensive studies of treatment, although agents such as acetazolamide and calcium-channel blockers have been used.

Stereotypies

A clear definition of stereotypies can be somewhat difficult to elaborate, especially since elements of stereotypies are very similar to tics. It is perhaps more illustrative to describe them. Stereotypies are, as the name implies, stereotyped movements which most often involve the arms, head, and face, sometimes with a vocalization. They usually begin during infancy, and may evolve in their appearance over time. This is not the same as with tics, where there is a clear migration of tic behaviors from, for example, the eyes, to the mouth, to the head. By contrast, stereotypies tend to remain relatively constant in terms of the body parts involved, and, although they may vary in terms of intensity or frequency, the movements made by a child at 2 years will have a fundamental similarity to those the child makes at 5 years. Furthermore, stereotypies are often orchestrated movements that show a clear and relatively invariant pattern. A strong association with state is another feature of stereotypies, usually being most prominent with excitement, fatigue, anxiety, or boredom.

Most literature regarding stereotypies in children deals with repetitive behaviors in the setting of some form of sensory deprivation or developmental disability.[80–83] Stereotypies are seen commonly in children with autism, mental retardation, and visual impairment (blindisms), and are a hallmark of Rett's syndrome.[84–86] The etiology of these behaviors is unknown, and it has been implied that the movements are a form of self-stimulation, but this is nothing more than an inference.

Although the literature has dwelt on these behaviors in the disabled, stereotypies also occur in otherwise normal children.[87] In these children, a home video is often the only way that a clinician will have to actually determine the nature of the activity, owing to situation and state-sensitivity of stereotypies. Historically, it can be helpful to determine how easy or difficult it is to redirect a child who is engaged in stereotypic behavior, as well as to identify specific times and places in which they manifest.

In terms of an evaluation, the history and observation should be sufficient to make the diagnosis. Occasionally, if the events are suspicious, an EEG could be indicated to investigate the possibility of epilepsy. However, it must be kept in mind that, given the state sensitivity, a routine office EEG may be insufficient to capture a clinical event.

There is no proven therapy for stereotypies in the otherwise neurologically normal child, and it can be argued that one is seldom required. Typically, these are young children, and there are very few who persist with these behaviors in public into school age. However, in some cases, stereotypies have been felt to negatively impact on self-esteem and peer relationships. In these situations, habit reversal therapy may be of benefit.

Chorea

CLINICAL FEATURES

Chorea is defined as a hyperkinetic movement disorder that is rapid, nonrhythmic, unpredictable in amplitude with some dependence on state, and can be variable in terms of location. As is true in the case of tics, chorea is quite a common finding in early childhood, and "chorea minima," or a piano-playing movement seen with the arms outstretched, is present in many children in a general pediatrics setting.[88] Pathologic chorea, though, most often is described in the setting of rheumatic fever, or Sydenham's chorea (SC). In fact, other choreas being so unusual in childhood, a previously normal child who presents with chorea is considered to have SC until proven otherwise.

Examination of the child with chorea can be among the more difficult challenges facing a neurologist, because children are quite frequently reluctant to cooperate. Children with chorea often will not participate for a sufficient time in holding their hands outstretched, and it is sometimes easier to detect that a child with chorea will often sit on his/her hands in order to limit their movements. Likewise, motor impersistence seems to predominate, and maneuvers employed by the examiner to demonstrate this feature will prove more rewarding.

Chorea may be an accompaniment to the static motor encephalopathy that is a consequence of kernicterus, and this has been called choreoathetotic CP. However, the term "choreoathetosis" lends no further precision to the type of movements being described, and is essentially a vague means of conveying a dyskinesia that actually has elements of dystonia, athetosis, and chorea. The same is true for the word "choreiform," which has been used to describe adventitious movements in the context of the pediatric autoimmune neuropsychiatric disorder associated with streptococcus (PANDAS).[89] This illustrates the difficulty in recognition of chorea, however, since chorea can actually be thought of as the intrusion of fragments of movement into purposeful activity. Using this as a defining quality, then "choreiform" is less than informative.

SYDENHAM'S CHOREA (SC)

SC is one of the major criteria defining postinfectious rheumatic fever.[90,91] Usually presenting on the order of weeks to months after a group A beta-hemolytic streptococcus infection, SC is classically defined by the triad of chorea, emotional lability, and hypotonia. The abnormal movements may present as a hemichorea in almost 20 percent of patients. Due to more thorough investigations of these patients, the behavioral manifestations have been demonstrated to be quite striking, and at times are the main indication for therapy.[92–95] In most cases, SC resolves spontaneously over time, although there are reports of chronic and apparently permanent chorea associated with rheumatic fever.[96,97] Recrudescence of the chorea has been reported with reactivation of rheumatic fever and pregnancy (chorea gravidarum).[98]

The pathogenesis of SC is in all likelihood related to molecular mimicry and streptococcal antigens. Antibodies from the serum of patients with SC crossreact with human basal ganglia tissue.[99–103] Imaging studies in some patients with SC indicate the presence of an inflammatory process within caudate and putamen.[104] It is presumed that this immune process disrupts basal ganglia function in such a way as to produce choreic movements.

Although neuroleptic agents are quite effective in the treatment of SC, these agents are not often necessary for the chorea itself, as children are seldom debilitated significantly by the movements. On the other hand, the behavioral manifestations may be of such severity that neuroleptics make an excellent therapeutic intervention. Benzodiazepines, carbamazepine, and valproic acid have also been reported as useful for the movement disorder.[105,106] The role of immunosuppression has been examined, and there may be a role for steroids, intravenous gamma-globulin, and even plasmapheresis.[107] However, the possible side-effects of such therapies must be weighed carefully against the actual impairment.

BENIGN HEREDITARY CHOREA

Benign hereditary chorea is a relatively rare condition, unless the practitioner happens to live in some proximity to a family with the disorder. Most often autosomal-dominant, this is one occasion in which family history is of the utmost importance. Care must be taken to delineate the clinical features of the condition, as another autosomal-dominant chorea, Huntington's disease (HD), presents quite differently in childhood (see below). Nevertheless, due to lack of information or education about benign hereditary chorea, patients may believe that they are at risk for HD. The typical history is one of delayed motor development in childhood, with complaints consistent with chorea. Children may be reported to be clumsy, hyperactive, and slow to master fine motor skills. Examination reveals chorea that is diffuse in distribution. Some families have been reported who also manifest dystonia, myoclonus, or other features, and reassessment of these families has resulted in a substantial number of diagnostic revisions, leading some authors to put forward that benign hereditary chorea is not a disease but a collection of symptoms.[108] On the other hand, a mutation of the TITF-1 gene on chromosome 14 has been established in both an Alabama and a Dutch pedigree,[109,110] while excluded in other families. Interestingly, in the Alabama family, identification of affected patients by family members was remarkable due to the absence of any false positives or false negatives, suggesting that a specific phenotype does exist.

OTHER CHOREAS

Other choreas in childhood that may be encountered are seldom seen in the context of an otherwise normal child. Table 50-2 lists a number of potential etiologies for chorea. A secondary chorea which often has a poor outcome is that of "postpump" chorea, described in children who have undergone open-heart surgery with hypothermia.[111–113] Usually presenting within the first postoperative week, this disorder is characterized by chorea affecting the entire body, often so severe as to appear ballistic. Gaze abnormalities have been described as well. Factors associated with postpump chorea include surgery occurring in children past infancy and prolonged bypass times. The cause is not known, but microembolic phenomena have been suggested. Treatment is often unsuccessful, and long-term follow-up of patients indicates significant morbidity.[114,115]

Drug-induced choreas have been reported in childhood secondary to a variety of medications, including digoxin,[116] valproate,[117] and pemoline.[118] Chorea has also been described as part of the syndromes of moya-moya,[119] antiphospholipid antibodies,[120] and hypoparathyroidism.[121]

Akinetic-Rigid Syndromes

Hypokinetic or parkinsonian symptoms are rare in childhood. Primary causes of such a syndrome would include such

TABLE 50-2 Childhood Disorders Associated with Chorea

Sydenham's chorea
Benign hereditary chorea
Metabolic disorders
    Glutaric acidemia type 1
    Gangliosidosis (GM1, GM2)
    Ataxia telangiectasia
Drugs (anticonvulsants, neuroleptics)
Infections (viral encephalitis, bacterial meningitis)
Perinatal injury

entities as juvenile HD,[122–125] the juvenile form of neuronal ceroid lipofuscinosis (NCL-1, Batten's disease),[126] inherited forms of PD with juvenile onset,[127,128] and some cases of DRD.[62,63] Each of these disorders is relatively uncommon, thus emphasizing the exceptional circumstance of a child presenting with such features as a primary complaint. The hallmark features of parkinsonism, tremor at rest, bradykinesia, and postural instability are seldom seen in isolation in the pediatric age group. Each of the entities mentioned above will usually manifest other movement disorders, with the hypokinetic features being a part of a larger phenotype. For example, in juvenile HD, myoclonus, seizures, dystonia, and a rapidly progressive dementia are often more striking than the parkinsonism. Similarly, NCL-1 and DRD are accompanied by blindness and dementia in the former, and dystonia in the latter.

Secondary causes of parkinsonism are quite varied in scope,[129] but would of course include a variety of drug exposures. Neuroleptic use and acute or subacute parkinsonian symptoms are well described in adults and children, and a history of ingestion makes this a relatively simple diagnosis to make.[130–132] Interestingly, in children overmedicated with stimulants for the treatment of attention deficit hyperactivity disorder, hypomimia and bradykinesia can be seen, although a rest tremor has not been described. Other drugs reported to be associated with emergent parkinsonism include sodium valproate[133] and certain chemotherapeutic agents.[134] Hydrocephalus is another problem of childhood that unusually manifests as a parkinsonian phenotype.[135] Occasionally, the pseudodementia seen with untreated or refractory depression can certainly be associated with a masklike face, although again this is quite rare. Finally, parkinsonism continues to be seen rarely after encephalitis, but nowhere near to the extent of that described in the influenza epidemics of the early 1900s.[136–140]

Conclusion

As previously stated, movement disorders in childhood have significant phenomenologic similarities to those in adults. Although in the aggregate rarer than in adults, there are still a fairly large number of children, particularly those with other neurologic vulnerabilities, who may manifest a movement disorder at some time during their lives. What this chapter has endeavored to provide the reader is not an exhaustive list of those disorders that "can" be associated with dystonia, chorea, etc., since most of the clinical conditions causing movement pathology in adults have been described in children. The goal of this discussion is to emphasize conditions that are either unique to or have their typical onset in childhood, to better familiarize the readers with what they may encounter in clinical practice.

When considering a number of these disorders, it is apparent from the limited information that is available how incomplete is our understanding, and by extension how limited are the treatment options. What is clear, though, is the need for accurate classification of childhood movement disorders into well-defined categories. This task will not be without effort, since so many children seem to manifest mixed types of disorders. However, once there is consensus regarding phenotypic characterizations, the process of defining both pathophysiology and rational treatment strategies may begin.

References

1. Fernandez Alvarez E, Aicardi J: *Movement Disorders in Children*. London: MacKeith Press, 2001.
2. Scahill L, Tanner C, Dure L: The epidemiology of tics and Tourette syndrome in children and adolescents. *Adv Neurol* 85:261–271, 2001.
3. Costello EJ, Angold A, Burns BJ, et al: The Great Smoky Mountains Study of Youth. Goals, design, methods, and the prevalence of DSM-III-R disorders. *Arch Gen Psychiatry* 53:1129–1136, 1996.
4. Apter A, Pauls DL, Bleich A, et al: A population-based epidemiological study of Tourette syndrome among adolescents in Israel. *Adv Neurol* 58:61–65, 1992.
5. Eapen V, Robertson MM, Zeitlin H, et al: Gilles de la Tourette's syndrome in special education schools: A United Kingdom study. *J Neurol* 244:378–382, 1997.
6. Kurlan R, McDermott MP, Deeley C, et al: Prevalence of tics in schoolchildren and association with placement in special education. *Neurology* 57:1383–1388, 2001.
7. Mason A, Banerjee S, Eapen V, et al: The prevalence of Tourette syndrome in a mainstream school population. *Dev Med Child Neurol* 40:292–296, 1998.
8. Tanner CM, Goldman SM: Epidemiology of Tourette syndrome. *Neurol Clin* 15:395–402, 1997.
9. Kurlan R, Como PG, Miller B, et al: The behavioral spectrum of tic disorders: A community-based study. *Neurology* 59:414–420, 2002.
10. Epidemiological Study of Dystonia in Europe (ESDE) Collaborative Group: A prevalence study of primary dystonia in eight European countries. *J Neurol* 247:787–792, 2000.
11. Surveillance of Cerebral Palsy in Europe: Surveillance of cerebral palsy in Europe: A collaboration of cerebral palsy surveys and registers. *Dev Med Child Neurol* 42:816–824, 2000.
12. Albright L: Spasticity and movement disorders in cerebral palsy. *J Child Neurol* 11(suppl 1):S1–S4, 1996.
13. Pharoah P, Platt M, Cooke T: The changing epidemiology of cerebral palsy. *Arch Dis Child* 75:F169–F173, 1996.
14. Pharoah PO, Cooke T, Johnson MA, et al: Epidemiology of cerebral palsy in England and Scotland, 1984–9. *Arch Dis Child Fetal Neonatal Ed* 79:F21–25, 1998.
15. Paulson GW: Benign essential tremor in childhood: Symptoms, pathogenesis, treatment. *Clin Pediatr* 15:67–70, 1976.
16. Louis ED, Dure LSI, Pullman S: Essential tremor in childhood: A series of nineteen cases. *Mov Disord* 16:921–923, 2001.
17. Findley LJ, Koller WC: Essential tremor: A review. *Neurology* 37:1194–1197, 1987.
18. Bain PG, Findley LJ, Thompson PD, et al: A study of hereditary essential tremor. *Brain* 117(Pt 4):805–824, 1994.

19. Pranzatelli MR: An approach to movement disorders of childhood. *Pediatr Ann* 22:13–17, 1993.

20. Lombroso CT, Fejerman N: Benign myoclonus of early infancy. *Ann Neurol* 1:138–143, 1977.

21. Resnick TJ, Moshe SL, Perotta L, et al: Benign neonatal sleep myoclonus. Relationship to sleep states. *Arch Neurol* 43:266–268, 1986.

22. Rothfield K, Behr J, McBride M, et al: Developmental chorea and dystonia of infancy. *Neurology* 37:99, 1987.

23. Goetz CG, Leurgans S, Chmura TA: Home alone: methods to maximize tic expression for objective videotape assessments in Gilles de la Tourette syndrome. *Mov Disord* 16:693–697, 2001.

24. Leckman JF: Tourette's syndrome. *Lancet* 360:1577–1586, 2002.

25. Brett EM: Some syndromes of involuntary movements, in EM Brett (ed): *Paediatric Neurology*, 3rd ed. New York: Churchill Livingstone, 1997, pp 275–290.

26. American Psychiatric Association: *Diagnostic and Statistical Manual of Mental Disorders, Fourth Edition*. Washington, DC: American Psychiatric Association, 1994.

27. Angelini L, Sgro V, Erba A, et al: Tourettism as clinical presentation of Huntington's disease with onset in childhood. *Ital J Neurol Sci* 19:383–385, 1998.

28. Barabas G: Tourettism. *Pediatr Ann* 17:422–423, 1988.

29. Bharucha KJ, Sethi KD: Tardive tourettism after exposure to neuroleptic therapy. *Mov Disord* 10:791–793, 1995.

30. Collacott RA, Ismail IA: Tourettism in a patient with Down's syndrome. *J Ment Defic Research* 32(Pt 2):163–166, 1988.

31. Jankovic J, Ashizawa T: Tourettism associated with Huntington's disease. *Mov Disord* 10:103–105, 1995.

32. Kwak CH, Jankovic J: Tourettism and dystonia after subcortical stroke. *Mov Disord* 17:821–825, 2002.

33. Kramer U, Nevo Y, Harel S: Jittery babies: A short-term follow-up. *Brain Dev* 16:112–114, 1994.

34. Shuper A, Zalzberg J, Weitz R, et al: Jitteriness beyond the neonatal period: A benign pattern of movement in infancy. *J Child Neurol* 6:243–245, 1991.

35. Deuschl G, Koster B, Lucking CH, et al: Diagnostic and pathophysiological aspects of psychogenic tremors. *Mov Disord* 13:294–302, 1998.

36. Jankovic J, Beach J, Pandolfo M, et al: Familial essential tremor in 4 kindreds. Prospects for genetic mapping. *Arch Neurol* 54:289–294, 1997.

37. Louis ED, Jurewicz EC, Watner D: Community-based data on associations of disease duration and age with severity of essential tremor: implications for disease pathophysiology. *Mov Disord* 18:90–93, 2003.

38. Danek A: Geniospasm: Hereditary chin trembling. *Mov Disord* 8:335–338, 1993.

39. Soland VL, Bhatia KP, Sheean GL, et al: Hereditary geniospasm: Two new families. *Mov Disord* 11:744–746, 1996.

40. Holmes GL, Russman BS: Shuddering attacks. Evaluation using electroencephalographic frequency modulation radiotelemetry and videotape monitoring. *Am J Dis Child* 140:72–73, 1986.

41. Vanasse M, Bedard P, Andermann F: Shuddering attacks in children: An early clinical manifestation of essential tremor. *Neurology* 26:1027–1030, 1976.

42. Ondo W, Jankovic J: Essential tremor. *CNS Drugs* 6:178–191, 1996.

43. Galvez-Jimenez N: Topiramate and essential tremor. *Ann Neurol* 47:837–838, 2000.

44. Connor GS: A double-blind placebo-controlled trial of topiramate treatment for essential tremor. *Neurology* 59:132–134, 2002.

45. Gubbay SS, Ellis E, Walton JN, et al: Clumsy children. A study of apraxic and agnosic defects in 21 children. *Brain* 88:295–312, 1965.

46. Antony JH, Ouvrier RA, Wise G: Spasmus nutans: A mistaken identity. *Arch Neurol* 37:373–375, 1980.

47. Farmer J, Hoyt CS: Monocular nystagmus in infancy and early childhood. *Am J Ophthalmol* 98:504–509, 1984.

48. Benton JW, Nellhaus G, Huttenlocher PR: The bobblehead syndrome. Report of a unique truncal tremor associated with third ventricular cyst and hydrocephalus in children. *Neurology* 16:725–729, 1966.

49. Mussell HG, Dure LS, Percy AK, et al: Bobble-head doll syndrome: Report of a case and review of the literature. *Mov Disord* 12:810–814, 1997.

50. Zesiewicz TA, Hauser RA: Phenomenology and treatment of tremor disorders. *Neurol Clin* 19:651–680, 2001.

51. Deuschl G: Differential diagnosis of tremor. *J Neural Transm Suppl* 56:211–220, 1999.

52. Emery ES, Homans AC, Colletti RB: Vitamin B12 deficiency: A cause of abnormal movements in infants. *Pediatrics* 99:255–256, 1997.

53. Ozer EA, Turker M, Bakiler AR, et al: Involuntary movements in infantile cobalamin deficiency appearing after treatment. *Pediatr Neurol* 25:81–83, 2001.

54. Morris JG, Grattan-Smith P, Jankelowitz SK, et al: Athetosis II: The syndrome of mild athetoid cerebral palsy. *Mov Disord* 17:1281–1287, 2002.

55. Russman BS: Cerebral palsy. *Curr Treat Options Neurol* 2:97–108, 2000.

56. Sanger TD, Delgado MR, Gaebler-Spira D, et al: Classification and definition of disorders causing hypertonia in childhood. *Pediatrics* 111:e89–97, 2003.

57. Scott BL, Jankovic J: Delayed-onset progressive movement disorders after static brain lesions. *Neurology* 46:68–74, 1996.

58. Saint Hilaire MH, Burke RE, Bressman SB, et al: Delayed-onset dystonia due to perinatal or early childhood asphyxia. *Neurology* 41:216–222, 1991.

59. Hyland K, Surtees RA, Rodeck C, et al: Aromatic L-amino acid decarboxylase deficiency: Clinical features, diagnosis, and treatment of a new inborn error of neurotransmitter amine synthesis. *Neurology* 42:1980–1988, 1992.

60. Rondot P, Wevers RA: Dystonie dopa-sensible forme recessive mutation du gene de la tyrosine-hydroxylase. *Bull Acad Natl Med* 183:639–646, discussion 646–647, 1999.

61. Furukawa Y, Graf WD, Wong H, et al: Dopa-responsive dystonia simulating spastic paraplegia due to tyrosine hydroxylase (TH) gene mutations. *Neurology* 56:260–263, 2001.

62. Nagatsu T, Ichinose H: GTP cyclohydrolase I gene, dystonia, juvenile parkinsonism, and Parkinson's disease. *J Neural Transm Suppl* 49:203–209, 1997.

63. Nygaard TG, Trugman JM, de YJ, et al: Dopa-responsive dystonia: The spectrum of clinical manifestations in a large North American family. *Neurology* 40:66–69, 1990.

64. Steinberger D, Korinthenberg R, Topka H, et al: Dopa-responsive dystonia: Mutation analysis of GCH1 and analysis of therapeutic doses of L-dopa. German Dystonia Study Group. *Neurology* 55:1735–1737, 2000.

65. Nygaard TG, Wilhelmsen KC, Risch NJ, et al: Linkage mapping of dopa-responsive dystonia (DRD) to chromosome 14q. *Nat Genet* 5:386–390, 1993.

66. Muller U, Steinberger D, Topka H: Mutations of GCH1 in dopa-responsive dystonia. *J Neural Transm* 109:321–328, 2002.

67. Hwang WJ, Calne DB, Tsui JK, et al: The long-term response to levodopa in dopa-responsive dystonia. *Parkinsonism Relat Disord* 8:1–5, 2001.

68. Rajput AH: Levodopa prolongs life expectancy and is non-toxic to substantia nigra. *Parkinsonism Relat Disord* 8:95–100, 2001.

69. Fernandez Alvarez E: Transient movement disorders in children. *J Neurol* 245:1–5, 1998.

70. Dooley JM, Furey S, Gordon KE, et al: Fever-induced dystonia. *Pediatr Neurol* 28:149–150, 2003.

71. Deda G, Caksen H, Suskan E, et al: Masturbation mimicking seizure in an infant. *Indian J Pediatr* 68:779–781, 2001.

72. Wulff CH, Ostergaard JR, Storm K: Epileptic fits or infantile masturbation? *Seizure* 1:199–201, 1992.

73. O'Donnell JJ, Howard RO: Torticollis associated with hiatus hernia (Sandifer's syndrome). *Am J Ophthalmol* 71:1134–1137, 1971.

74. Kotagal P, Costa M, Wyllie E, et al: Paroxysmal nonepileptic events in children and adolescents. *Pediatrics* 110:e46, 2002.

75. Golden GS: Nonepileptic paroxysmal events in childhood. *Pediatr Clin North Am* 39:715–725, 1992.

76. Dias E, Ramachandra C, D'Cruz AJ, et al: An unusual presentation of gastro-oesophageal reflux: Sandifer's syndrome. *Trop Doct* 22:131, 1992.

77. Drigo P, Carli G, Laverda AM: Benign paroxysmal torticollis of infancy. *Brain Dev* 22:169–172, 2000.

78. Al-Twaijri WA, Shevell MI: Pediatric migraine equivalents: occurrence and clinical features in practice. *Pediatr Neurol* 26:365–368, 2002.

79. Giffin NJ, Benton S, Goadsby PJ: Benign paroxysmal torticollis of infancy: Four new cases and linkage to CACNA1A mutation. *Dev Med Child Neurol* 44:490–493, 2002.

80. Aichner F, Gerstenbrand F, Poewe W: Primitive motor patterns and stereotyped movements. A comparison of findings in early childhood and in the apallic syndrome. *Int J Neurol* 17:21–29, 1982.

81. MacLean WE Jr, Ellis DN, Galbreath HN, et al: Rhythmic motor behavior of preambulatory motor impaired, Down syndrome and nondisabled children: A comparative analysis. *J Abnorm Child Psychol* 19:319–330, 1991.

82. Rojahn J: Self-injurious and stereotypic behavior of noninstitutionalized mentally retarded people: prevalence and classification. *Am J Ment Defic* 91:268–276, 1986; published erratum appears in *Am J Ment Defic* 91:619, 1987.

83. Brown R, Hobson RP, Lee A, et al: Are there "autistic-like" features in congenitally blind children? *J Child Psychol Psychiatry* 38:693–703, 1997.

84. FitzGerald PM, Jankovic J, Percy AK: Rett syndrome and associated movement disorders. *Mov Disord* 5:195–202, 1990.

85. Nomura Y, Segawa M, Hasegawa M: Rett syndrome: Clinical studies and pathophysiological consideration. *Brain Dev* 6:475–486, 1984.

86. Nomura Y, Segawa M: Characteristics of motor disturbances of the Rett syndrome. *Brain Dev* 12:27–30, 1990.

87. Tan A, Salgado M, Fahn S: The characterization and outcome of stereotypic movements in nonautistic children. *Mov Disord* 12:47–52, 1997.

88. Swaiman KF: Movement disorders, in KF Swaiman (ed): *Pediatric Neurology Principles and Practice*, 1st ed. St. Louis: Mosby, 1989, vol 1, pp 205–218.

89. Swedo SE, Leonard HL, Garvey M, et al: Pediatric autoimmune neuropsychiatric disorders associated with streptococcal infections: Clinical description of the first 50 cases. *Am J Psychiatry* 155:264–271, 1998; published erratum appears in *Am J Psychiatry* 155:578, 1998.

90. Jummani R, Okun M: Sydenham chorea. *Arch Neurol* 58:311–313, 2001.

91. Marques-Dias MJ, Mercadante MT, Tucker D, et al: Sydenham's chorea. *Psychiatr Clin North Am* 20:809–820, 1997.

92. Freeman JM, Aron AM, Collard JE, et al: The emotional correlates of Sydenham's chorea. *Pediatrics* 35:42–49, 1965.

93. Swedo SE: Sydenham's chorea: A model for childhood autoimmune neuropsychiatric disorders. *JAMA* 272:1788–1791, 1994.

94. Bird MT, Palkes H, Prensky AL: A follow-up study of Sydenham's chorea. *Neurology* 26:601–606, 1976.

95. Swedo SE, Rapoport JL, Cheslow DL, et al: High prevalence of obsessive-compulsive symptoms in patients with Sydenham's chorea. *Am J Psychiatry* 146:246–249, 1989.

96. Berrios X, Quesney F, Morales A, et al: Are all recurrences of "pure" Sydenham chorea true recurrences of acute rheumatic fever? *J Pediatr* 107:867–872, 1985.

97. Cardoso F, Vargas AP, Oliveira LD, et al: Persistent Sydenham's chorea. *Mov Disord* 14:805–807, 1999.

98. Nausieda PA, Bieliauskas LA, Bacon LD, et al: Chronic dopaminergic sensitivity after Sydenham's chorea. *Neurology* 33:750–754, 1983.

99. Husby G, van de Rijn I, Zabriskie J, et al: Antibodies reacting with cytoplasm of subthalamic and caudate nuclei neurons in chorea and acute rheumatic fever. *J Exp Med* 144:1094–1110, 1976.

100. Singer HS, Loiselle CR, Lee O, et al: Anti-basal ganglia antibody abnormalities in Sydenham chorea. *J Neuroimmunol* 136:154–161, 2003.

101. Church AJ, Cardoso F, Dale RC, et al: Anti-basal ganglia antibodies in acute and persistent Sydenham's chorea. *Neurology* 59:227–231, 2002.

102. Church AJ, Dale RC, Cardoso F, et al: CSF and serum immune parameters in Sydenham's chorea: Evidence of an autoimmune syndrome? *J Neuroimmunol* 136:149–153, 2003.

103. Morshed SA, Parveen S, Leckman JF, et al: Antibodies against neural, nuclear, cytoskeletal, and streptococcal epitopes in children and adults with Tourette's syndrome, Sydenham's chorea, and autoimmune disorders. *Biol Psychiatry* 50:566–577, 2001.

104. Castillo M, Kwock L, Arbelaez A: Sydenham's chorea: MRI and proton spectroscopy. *Neuroradiology* 41:943–945, 1999.

105. Genel F, Arslanoglu S, Uran N, et al: Sydenham's chorea: clinical findings and comparison of the efficacies of sodium valproate and carbamazepine regimens. *Brain Dev* 24:73–76, 2002.

106. Harel L, Zecharia A, Straussberg R, et al: Successful treatment of rheumatic chorea with carbamazepine. *Pediatr Neurol* 23:147–151, 2000.

107. Garvey MA, Swedo SE: Sydenham's chorea. Clinical and therapeutic update. *Adv Exp Med Biol* 418:115–120, 1997.

108. Schrag A, Quinn NP, Bhatia KP, et al: Benign hereditary chorea: Entity or syndrome? *Mov Disord* 15:280–288, 2000.

109. Breedveld GJ, van Dongen JW, Danesino C, et al: Mutations in TITF-1 are associated with benign hereditary chorea. *Hum Mol Genet* 11:971–979, 2002.

110. Breedveld GJ, Percy AK, MacDonald ME, et al: Clinical and genetic heterogeneity in benign hereditary chorea. *Neurology* 59:579–584, 2002.

111. Ferry PC: Neurologic sequelae of open-heart surgery in children. An "irritating question." *Am J Dis Child* 144:369–373, 1990.

112. Robinson RO, Samuels M, Pohl KR: Choreic syndrome after cardiac surgery. *Arch Dis Child* 63:1466–1469, 1988.

113. Curless RG, Katz DA, Perryman RA, et al: Choreoathetosis after surgery for congenital heart disease. *J Pediatr* 124:737–739, 1994.

114. Wong PC, Barlow CF, Hickey PR, et al: Factors associated with choreoathetosis after cardiopulmonary bypass in children with congenital heart disease. *Circulation* 86:II118–126, 1992.

115. Medlock MD, Cruse RS, Winek SJ, et al: A 10-year experience with postpump chorea. *Ann Neurol* 34:820–826, 1993.

116. Sekul EA, Kaminer S, Sethi KD: Digoxin-induced chorea in a child. *Mov Disord* 14:877–879, 1999.

117. Lancman ME, Asconape JJ, Penry JK: Choreiform movements associated with the use of valproate. *Arch Neurol* 51:702–704, 1994.

118. Nausieda PA, Koller WC, Weiner WJ, et al: Pemoline-induced chorea. *Neurology* 31:356–360, 1981.

119. Watanabe K, Negoro T, Maehara M, et al: Moyamoya disease presenting with chorea. *Pediatr Neurol* 6:40–42, 1990.

120. Okun MS, Jummani RR, Carney PR: Antiphospholipid-associated recurrent chorea and ballism in a child with cerebral palsy. *Pediatr Neurol* 23:62–63, 2000.

121. Christiansen NJ, Hansen PF: Choreiform movements in hypoparathyroidism. *N Engl J Med* 287:569–570, 1972.

122. Bird MT, Paulson GW: The rigid form of Huntington's chorea. *Neurology* 21:271–276, 1971.

123. Byers RK, Gilles FH, Fung C: Huntington's disease in children. *Neurology* 23:561–569, 1973.

124. Jervis GA: Huntington's chorea in childhood. *Arch Neurol* 9:244–257, 1963.

125. Rasmussen A, Macias R, Yescas P, et al: Huntington disease in children: Genotype-phenotype correlation. *Neuropediatrics* 31:190–194, 2000.

126. Aberg LE, Rinne JO, Rajantie I, et al: A favorable response to antiparkinsonian treatment in juvenile neuronal ceroid lipofuscinosis. *Neurology* 56:1236–1239, 2001.

127. Golbe LI: Young-onset Parkinson's disease: A clinical review. *Neurology* 41:168–173, 1991.

128. Muthane UB, Swamy HS, Satishchandra P, et al: Early onset Parkinson's disease: Are juvenile- and young-onset different? *Mov Disord* 9:539–544, 1994.

129. Pranzatelli MR, Mott SH, Pavlakis SG, et al: Clinical spectrum of secondary parkinsonism in childhood: A reversible disorder. *Pediatr Neurol* 10:131–140, 1994.

130. Bateman DN, Darling WM, Boys R, et al: Extrapyramidal reactions to metoclopramide and prochlorperazine. *Q J Med* 71:307–311, 1989.

131. Richardson MA, Haugland G, Craig TJ: Neuroleptic use, parkinsonian symptoms, tardive dyskinesia, and associated factors in child and adolescent psychiatric patients. *Am J Psychiatry* 148:1322–1328, 1991.

132. Roberts MD: Risperdal and parkinsonian tremor. *J Am Acad Child Adolesc Psychiatry* 38:230, 1999.

133. Alvarez-Gomez MJ, Vaamonde J, Narbona J, et al: Parkinsonian syndrome in childhood after sodium valproate administration. *Clin Neuropharmacol* 16:451–455, 1993.

134. Boranic M, Raci F: A Parkinson-like syndrome as side effect of chemotherapy with vincristine and adriamycin in a child with acute leukaemia. *Biomedicine* 31:124–125, 1979.

135. Curran T, Lang AE: Parkinsonian syndromes associated with hydrocephalus: Case reports, a review of the literature, and pathophysiological hypotheses. *Mov Disord* 9:508–520, 1994.

136. Hsieh JC, Lue KH, Lee YL: Parkinson-like syndrome as the major presenting symptom of Epstein-Barr virus encephalitis. *Arch Dis Child* 87:358, 2002.

137. Mellon AF, Appleton RE, Gardner-Medwin D, et al: Encephalitis lethargica-like illness in a five-year-old. *Dev Med Child Neurol* 33:158–161, 1991.

138. Misra UK, Kalita J: Prognosis of Japanese encephalitis patients with dystonia compared to those with parkinsonian features only. *Postgrad Med J* 78:238–241, 2002.

139. Murgod UA, Muthane UB, Ravi V, et al: Persistent movement disorders following Japanese encephalitis. *Neurology* 57:2313–2315, 2001.

140. Ravenholt RT, Foege WH: 1918 influenza, encephalitis lethargica, parkinsonism. *Lancet* ii:860–864, 1982.

MOVEMENT DISORDERS AND AGING

ALI H. RAJPUT and ALEX RAJPUT

DISTINCTION BETWEEN NORMAL AGING
AND MOVEMENT DISORDER   837
  Akinesia-Hypokinesia-Bradykinesia and Old Age   837
  Tone Change and Old Age   838
  Hyperkinetic Disorders and Aging   839
  Station, Posture, Postural Reflexes, and Old Age   840
  Gait Abnormality and Old Age   840
  Gait Apraxia (GA)   841
  Ophthalmoplegia in the Elderly and in MD   842
  Primitive Reflexes in MD and the Elderly   842
CONSIDERATION OF MOVEMENT DISORDERS
THAT ARE CONCENTRATED IN OLD AGE   842
  Parkinsonism in the Elderly   842
  Drug-Induced Parkinsonism (DIP)   844
  Essential Tremor (ET) in the Elderly   844
  Stroke and Movement Disorders (MD)   845
  Hemiballismus (HB)   846
  Dystonia   846
  Stroke and Parkinsonism   846
  Orofacial Dyskinesias in the Elderly   846
MOVEMENT DISORDERS ASSOCIATED WITH
OTHER NEURODEGENERATIVE DISEASES
IN THE ELDERLY   847
SPECIAL CONSIDERATION OF MOVEMENT
DISORDER MANAGEMENT IN THE ELDERLY   848

There is no uniformly agreed definition of old age. For the purpose of this chapter we will use the commonly utilized retirement age of 65 years as the start of old age.[1-4] The proportion of the elderly in the general population has been steadily rising in western countries for several decades;[5] thus the prevalence of aging-related disorders has been increasing slowly but steadily. Some movement disorders (MD) are concentrated in old age and some manifestations of normal aging may resemble MD.

Posture and gait to a large extent depend on normal vestibular, visual, proprioceptive, postural sway adjustment, and motor functions. With advancing age there is decline in vestibular,[6] visual,[7,8] and proprioceptive[9] functions. The postural sway increases[10-13] and the muscle mass decreases progressively in old age.[14] Old age is also associated with slowed walking,[15] reduced motor velocity,[12] shortened stride,[15] reduced vibration sensation in the feet, reduced ankle jerks,[9] memory decline,[9,16] reduced upward gaze,[12,16] and emergence of primitive reflexes.[16-18] Positron emission tomography (PET) studies reveal that with normal aging there is hypometabolism in the frontal lobes.[19] Together, these anatomic and physiologic changes lead to alteration in station, posture, gait, postural reflexes, motor functions, and extraocular movements—all well known features in some movement disorders.

The elderly are more likely to have other systemic diseases,[5] and malnutrition,[20] and, therefore, take multiple prescription drugs.[1,5,21-23] The frequency and the severity of drug side-effects, including MD,[24-34] increase with advancing age.[5,35] Compared to younger adults, drug adverse effects occur twice as frequently in those over age 60 years. In those over age 80 years, there is a 25 percent risk of intoxication with some drugs.[5]

Several common MD are concentrated in the elderly,[2,3,24,36-38] and there is an increased concentration of other neurological illnesses, such as Alzheimer's disease (AD) and stroke, which may simulate or be associated with motor function abnormalities.[39-43]

The appropriate chapters in this volume cover MD in greater detail. We will concentrate on age-related changes that resemble MD and those aspects of MD that require special consideration in old age. This chapter is divided into:

(1) the distinction between normal aging and MD,
(2) the common MD that are concentrated in old age,
(3) movement abnormalities that are part of other illnesses in the elderly,
(4) special consideration of MD management in the elderly.

Distinction Between Normal Aging and Movement Disorder

MD can be broadly classified into hypokinetic and hyperkinetic disorders. The two clinical features tremor (hyperkinesia) and bradykinesia (hypokinesia) typically coexist in Parkinson syndrome (PS) and in dystonia, where tremor may be a part of the picture. Slowing of motor function, abnormalities of posture, gait and extraocular movements, and the presence of primitive reflexes which are characteristic of Parkinson's disease (PD) and progressive supranuclear palsy (PSP), may also be part of normal aging. Because there are no biological markers to distinguish between age-related findings and MD, their significance in the elderly is based on careful clinical assessment.[16,17,44-49]

AKINESIA-HYPOKINESIA-BRADYKINESIA AND OLD AGE

The akinesia-hypokinesia-bradykinesia complex is characterized by slowed initiation (akinesia), small-amplitude movements (hypokinesia), and reduced motor velocity (bradykinesia).[50] The term bradykinesia is often used to imply all three of these features. Bradykinesia is almost

TABLE 51-1 Normal Aging and Hypokinetic Disorders

	Normal Aging-Related Slowing	Focal Pathology Emulating Slowing	MD-Related Slowing (PS, Dystonia)	Other Nervous System (Central or Peripheral) Pathology Causing Slowing
Symmetry of findings	Symmetrical	Asymmetrical	Often asymmetrical	Frequently asymmetrical
Focal examination	Normal	Abnormal	Normal	Normal
Tone	Normal	Normal (discontinue if pain or joint movement restriction). Test at unaffected joint helpful to identify normal tone	Increased (rigidity or dystonia)	May have paratonia. Spasticity if corticospinal involvement. Decreased if lower motor pathology
Sensory function	Normal (except vibration reduction in feet)	As in normal aging	As in normal aging	May be impaired, depending on the nature of lesion
Reflexes	Normal symmetrical (ankle jerks may be hypoactive), plantars flexor	As in normal aging	As in normal aging	Hyperactive with extensor plantar or hypoactive depending on site of lesion. Frequently asymmetrical
Strength	Normal	Normal, but patient unable to fully exert due to pain or joint restriction	Normal in PS (if repeatedly tested). May appear reduced in dystonia	Reduced or inconsistent

invariably a feature of PS.[29,50,51] Slowed motor performance is also a part of normal aging.[9,52] Clinical assessment is the main tool to differentiate normal age-related slowing from MD-related bradykinesia. Table 51-1 summarizes the clinical features that are helpful in distinguishing age-related slowing from hypokinetic MD and some other disorders that may produce motor slowing.

Any focal process that produces pain or mechanical restriction at a joint would result in slowing of the movement at that site and may, therefore, be mistaken for bradykinesia. Careful examination of the suspected joint and testing for bradykinesia at an unaffected joint will help ascertain the true nature of the problem. Detailed assessment of sensory functions, tone, muscle strength, and reflexes, as noted in Table 51-1, are valuable adjuncts to distinguish hypokinetic MD from other neurological diseases and from normal age-related slowing. Age-related slowing is symmetrical and generalized, whereas hypokinesia due to a MD is more likely to be asymmetrical.

TONE CHANGE AND OLD AGE

Testing for tone is dependent on the patient's ability to comprehend command, follow instructions, and cooperate. In normal elderly, there is no change in muscle tone. In cognitively and language-impaired elderly there may be an apparent change in tone known as paratonia (Gegenhalten).[47] Paratonia is characterized by progressively increasing resistance to an attempted passive movement or to an irregular unpredictable opposition to the passive movement which may be mistaken as cogwheel rigidity.[16,26,47] Some of these patients may voluntarily move the body part in the same

direction as the examiner attempts to move it passively. In that event, the increase in tone may not be detected. This distinction is possible in most cases on careful clinical assessment (Table 51-2).

The two main forms of hypertonicity in MD are rigidity and dystonia. Rigidity is characterized by a sustained resistance through the range of passive movement. It is equally severe in opposite directions at a joint (i.e., flexor and extensor movements would have comparable resistance),[53] and is reproducible. The literature suggests that cogwheel rigidity is a characteristic feature of only those PS cases that have clinically evident tremor. Personal experience indicates that cogwheel rigidity can also be detected in PS cases with no visible tremor.

Dystonia is characterized by co-contraction of agonist and antagonist muscles. The force of muscle contraction, however, is unequal in the opposing groups of muscles, thereby resulting in dystonic movement or dystonic posture. Although the resistance to passive movement is increased in all directions, the degree of hypertonicity depends on the direction of the attempted passive movement. The resistance is more pronounced when the passive movement counteracts the dystonic posture than when the examiner moves the part in the same direction as the dystonic movement or posture. A passive movement away from the sustained dystonic posture may be interrupted by irregular jerks (dystonic tremor).

Increased tone is also a feature of corticospinal tract dysfunction and is known as spasticity. It is characterized by a velocity-dependent catch which is followed by a release without further increase in resistance through the remainder of the movement known as the "clasp knife" phenomenon. By contrast, the increased tone in rigidity is evident through the

TABLE 51-2 Tone Changes in Elderly MD and Selected Conditions

	Normal Elderly	(a) Rigidity (b) Dystonia	Spasticity (mild)	Paratonia (Gegenhalten)	Cogwheeling Froment Maneuver
Characteristic	Equal and normal resistance in all directions of movement	(a) Resistance sustained and equal in opposite directions of movement, reproducible (b) Increased tone different when passive movement is with than when against dystonic posture	Increased tone Velocity-dependent catch ("clasp-knife")	Irregular, unpredictable, intermittently increased tone or progressively greater resistance on attempted movement	Interruption of passive movement coinciding with tremor. Rhythmic resistance to passive movement seen only on reinforcement in tremor-producing conditions (Froment maneuver)
Symmetry	Symmetrical	Usually asymmetrical	Frequently asymmetrical	Usually symmetrical	May be symmetrical or asymmetrical depending on tremor location
Reflexes	Normal, reduced at ankles, plantars flexor	Normal (may be difficult to elicit when pronounced dystonia). Striatal toe	Hyper-reflexic, extensor plantar response	Usually normal	Normal
Tremor Reinforcement-related tone increase	Absent No significant change. Minimal if any, and is symmetrical	Frequently part of PD Usually asymmetrical increase	Absent May increase slightly asymmetrically	Absent Unpredictable change	Prominent feature Rhythmic symmetrical increase (Froment maneuver)

entire range of movement. In mild corticospinal dysfunction the tone abnormality may not be easily distinguishable from the rigidity. One helpful maneuver is to let an extended knee of the patient suddenly drop over the examiner's arm and observe the flexion pattern at the knee joint as the leg drops downwards. Spastic leg manifests as a single catch followed by the heel rapidly falling downwards. By contrast, the rigid leg falls slowly at a relatively steady velocity until the movement is completed.

For all practical purposes, the tendon reflexes are normal in the common MD, except they may be difficult to elicit when optimal positioning is prevented by dystonia. In some extrapyramidal disease patients there is spontaneous or gait-related extension of the big toe on the affected side. When the plantar reflex is attempted, that toe will either flex or its extended position will become less pronounced. Such toe abnormality is known as striatal toe.[54] The presence of hyper-reflexia and extensor-plantar response in the presence of increased tone indicates spasticity.

Any joint movement that produces pain will be involuntarily guarded and may, therefore, be mistaken as rigidity. Mechanical restriction to passive movement can also simulate hypertonicity. Examination of the affected joint for pain and the range of movement and tone assessment at a nonaffected joint will help clarify this.

Cogwheeling, which is characterized by rhythmic interruption of attempted passive movement,[53,55] is seen in patients with medium- to large-amplitude tremor. The cogwheel rigidity in PS typically lacks the rhythmicity that is characteristic of cogwheeling due to prominent tremor. Rhythmic resistance to passive movement, which is detected only with reinforcement (i.e., voluntary motor activity at a distant, noncontiguous part of body), is known as the Froment maneuver. It may be detected in a variety of disorders where tremor is the prominent feature (e.g., in essential tremor, ET). Table 51-2 summarizes tone in the normal elderly, in extrapyramidal hypertonicity, and in selected other conditions.

HYPERKINETIC DISORDERS AND AGING

The most common hyperkinetic disorder in adults is tremor.[48,56–58] Rautakorpi et al.[58] noted tremor in 25 percent of the general population of Finland over age 40 years. The most common tremor-associated movement disorders in adults are ET and PS,[56] both of which are concentrated in old age.[24,36–38,56,58,59] The elderly, in general, take a larger number of drugs than younger individuals. Tricyclics, monoamine-oxidase inhibitors, antihistamines, valproate, anticholinergics, corticosteroids, calcium-channel blockers, amiodarone, lithium, sympathomimetic drugs, drugs for asthma such as isoproterenol, terbutaline, methylxanthines (aminophylline, and theophylline), can all produce tremor.[1,49,60,61] Nutritional disorders, other systemic illnesses, and metabolic diseases (e.g., hyperthyroidism) that accentuate physiological tremor or produce pathological tremor are also more common in old age.[20,49,58,61] When all these are considered, the elderly would have a higher prevalence of tremor than the 25 percent reported in the population over age 40 years.[58] The high prevalence rate of tremor in old age has sometimes been erroneously interpreted as an indication that tremor is part of the normal aging phenomenon. There is no scientific evidence that old age by itself leads to tremor production.[16,49,51,52,55,62,63] All tremors in the elderly should be considered pathological or enhanced physiological tremor caused by drugs or other stress.

STATION, POSTURE, POSTURAL REFLEXES, AND OLD AGE

The manner or attitude of standing is known as station, and the position of the whole body and its different parts indicate the posture. As noted above, visual,[7,8] vestibular,[6] and proprioceptive[9] functions decline with age, and the normal postural sway in the standing position increases[10,11] with age. Dizziness, characterized by a sensation of instability, is a common symptom in the elderly.[6,64,65] By age 65 years 30 percent and by age 80 years approximately 66 percent of the general population have experienced dizziness at some time.[65] The sensation of stability in the standing position in general declines with old age. Consequently, the normal elderly have a slightly widened base when standing or walking.[9]

The body posture in the standing position in the elderly is slightly flexed at the neck and trunk while in the standing position, with the knees and elbows remaining straight. Flexion of neck, trunk, hips, knees, and elbows are features of PS, except in PSP, where the posture may be unduly erect. Advanced PS patients have difficulty maintaining an erect posture for more than several seconds, whereas normal elderly can do this easily.

The ability to regain balance in response to spontaneous body sway or following active perturbation depends on the integrity of the postural reflexes. Maki et al.[10] noted that both spontaneous and induced sway are exaggerated in the normal elderly. In old age there is significantly increased sway velocity both with eyes open and with eyes closed.[11] This is most pronounced in those who are afraid of falling.[11] Duncan et al.[66] noted that the elderly with poor balance have impairment of at least two of sensory, effector, and central processing. They concluded that cumulative, rather than a single, deficit is the basis of impaired mobility in old age.[66]

Postural stability is clinically tested as follows. The patient, while standing with eyes open and feet comfortably apart (approximately shoulder width), is asked to resist the examiner's pull. S/he is instructed to take one step if necessary to regain balance in response to the pull and is assured

that the examiner will prevent falling. Depending on the size of the patient and the force of the pull, any individual may be displaced. The examiner first applies a modest forward pull.[45,46,67] This is then followed by a similar backward pull.[45,46,67] If the patient takes one step, the postural reflexes are considered normal. When two or three steps are taken, the posture is considered as minimally abnormal: four or more steps indicate impaired postural reflexes.[45,46,67] If in response to the pull the patient makes no effort to regain balance and would fall like a solid object, it indicates even more pronounced impairment of postural reflexes.

Loss of postural reflexes is part of normal aging,[46,47,68] and its prevalence increases with advancing age. Between age 80 and 89 years the postural reflexes (tested as above) are impaired in 70 percent.[46] Loss of postural reflexes is a well-known feature of moderate and severe PS and is used to classify the degree of disability. A Hoehn and Yahr stage III or higher[67,69] is characterized by loss of postural reflexes. Duncan and Wilson noted bradykinesia in 37 percent of normal elderly community residents and in 76 percent of day-hospital cases.[52] Thus, if bradykinesia and loss of postural reflexes are used as the minimum requirement for the diagnosis of PS,[70] a large number of normal elderly would be erroneously diagnosed and treated unnecessarily.[29,46,47,68,71,72] It is, therefore, recommended that the diagnosis of PS be made when two of the three (bradykinesia, rigidity, and tremor) are present.[29,47,71,72] Resting tremor is perhaps the most reliable sign for the diagnosis of PS in the elderly. Impaired postural reflexes should only be used as an adjunct to other PS features when diagnosing PS in an elderly individual.[46,47]

GAIT ABNORMALITY AND OLD AGE

Human-beings learn to crawl on four limbs before standing or walking on two feet. Because standing and gait are more recently evolved functions with advancing age they decline before the upper limb motor functions do. The gait in normal elderly is slightly wide-based and has short, slow strides, but the heel strike and the armswing are normal and symmetrical.[9,47] The stride velocity declines by 10–20 percent by age 80 years.[45,73]

Those who have an excessively slowed or abnormal pattern of ambulation are classified as having a gait disorder. It is estimated that 15 percent of the general population 60 years and older have a gait abnormality.[45] In addition to the identifiable causes (e.g., arthritis, motor weakness, coordination difficulty, PS, etc.) in 10–20 percent of the elderly with gait abnormality (approximately 2.25 percent of the population over age 60) there is no identifiable cause for the gait difficulty.[45,74]

PS is the most common MD associated with gait abnormality in old age. Flexed posture, narrow base, delayed gait initiation, slow, short and shuffling steps, reduced armswing, and impaired postural reflexes are typical of PS.[47,69] Paradoxically, in the event of an emergency, a PD patient may walk or run as fast as a normal person. Another feature of PS gait is that, after the gait initiation, there may be an involuntary acceleration of the pace known as festination. Most PS patients do not lift their feet high enough to clear the ground but rather drag the feet, known as shuffling gait. Unlike most other PS variants, the PSP cases have an erect posture, broad base, and lift the feet high, striking the ground flat, giving the gait a mechanical (robotic) quality. Unlike PD, the parkinsonian features in PSP are often symmetrical.[75–78]

GAIT APRAXIA (GA)

In gait apraxia (GA), walking difficulty cannot be attributed to mechanical, motor, sensory, coordination, visual, or vestibular dysfunction.[47,79–81] These patients have normal lower limb functions when seated or lying flat.[79] The GA patient can tap normally, make a circle or simple drawings in the air or on the floor with the lower limbs, and can emulate complex actions such as riding a bicycle in the supine position.[46,47,51,74,79,80] On the other hand, leg functions in the weight-bearing position, such as would be necessary for walking, are impaired.[80,81] The posture is erect and the gait is typically broad-based with short, shuffling, hesitating steps as if the patient were "glued" to the floor.[74,81,82]

The gait abnormality is a result of impaired central sensorimotor integration. The gait in GA cases has some parkinsonian features. However, unlike PD, GA patients cannot copy steps or improve with visual guiding lines—features well known in PD.[82] The armswing, which is reduced in PS, is not significantly affected in GA, and the leg function dissociation between supine and standing positions that is characteristic of GA is not a prominent feature in PS. Similarly, normal upper limb function, but with marked walking-related leg dysfunction characteristic of GA, is not part of typical PD cases. In PD, some functional impairment would be seen in both the upper and lower limbs on the same side. Nearly all PD patients benefit from L-dopa,[29,83] but GA patients do not. Most GA patients have frontal lobe disease or normal pressure hydrocephalus.[47,79–81]

Table 51-3 compares the gait in the normal elderly, GA, and PD patients.

Another, less clearly understood, gait abnormality resembling PD is known as senile gait.[84] It is characterized by stooped posture, broad base, reduced armswing, stiff turns, and a tendency to fall.[84] These patients do not manifest other major parkinsonian features such as resting tremor,[62,63,85] upper limb bradykinesia or rigidity, and, unlike PD, they do not improve on L-dopa or other antiparkinsonian drugs.[84]

TABLE 51-3 Posture and Gait in Normal Elderly, Parkinson's Disease, and Gait Apraxia

Clinical Features	Normal Elderly	Parkinson's Disease	Gait Apraxia
Base (distance between feet)	Slightly wider than at younger age	Narrow	Broad
Symmetry of abnormality	Symmetrical	Usually asymmetrical	Symmetrical
Functions in the involved lower limb	Normal and symmetrical	Impaired regardless of weight-bearing or not (no dissociation)	Impaired only when weight-bearing, but normal when not weight-bearing (dissociation pronounced and early)
Upper limb motor function	Normal	Impaired on the involved side	Unimpaired
Armswing	Normal	Reduced on involved side	Normal on both sides
Posture	Minimal flexion at trunk	Generalized flexion (neck, trunk, hip, knee, elbow)	As in normal elderly
Postural reflexes	May be normal or impaired	Impaired in moderately advanced disease	Impaired early
Foot tapping in sitting or lying position	Normal	Affected side slow and progressively slowed	As in normal elderly
Gait abnormality	Uncommon, increases with advancing age	Late manifestation	Major problem, early manifestation
Stripes on the floor for visual guidance	No change in gait	Improve gait	No improvement in gait
Tremor	Absent	Frequently seen, typically resting	As in normal elderly
Dementia	Absent	In about one-third of cases	Common but not invariable
Reflexes	Normal (may be reduced at ankles)	As in normal (may have striatal toe)	May be brisk, may have Babinski sign
Grasp reflex	Normal	Usually negative	Usually positive
Bladder function	Normal	Normal or hypertonic or hypotonic bladder	Incontinence common
L-Dopa response	None	Improvement	None

OPHTHALMOPLEGIA IN THE ELDERLY AND IN MD

Supranuclear vertical gaze palsy is the characteristic manifestation of PSP.[75–77] In our autopsy-verified 16 cases, we noted that 50 percent did not have supranuclear ophthalmoplegia.[78] Early eye signs may be slowed horizontal saccades,[86] slowed vertical saccades,[87] or square-wave jerks.[88] Similar[77] gaze changes may be seen in rare cases of multiple-system atrophy (MSA),[89] PD,[90] Whipple's disease,[91] and other diseases. Some limitation of the upward vertical gaze may be also seen in normal elderly.[16] Jenkyn et al.[16] contend that an upward gaze deviation of 5 mm or less and a downward gaze deviation of 7 mm or less from the mid-position should be regarded as abnormal. Based on a study of more than 2000 normal volunteers between ages 50 and 93 years, they[16] observed that, in the 8th decade of life, upward gaze was impaired in 29 percent and downward gaze in 34 percent. The diagnostic significance of gaze restriction should, therefore, be interpreted in conjunction with other clinical features.[78,89]

PRIMITIVE REFLEXES IN MD AND THE ELDERLY

A sustained glabellar reflex (Myerson's sign) and a positive snout reflex are common features in PD. Jenkyn et al.[16] noted that 37 percent of normal elderly in the 8th decade had a persistent glabellar reflex and 26 percent had a positive snout reflex. Koller et al.[17] concluded that the frequency of positive snout reflex correlates with increasing age. Primitive reflexes are soft clinical signs which, when considered with other findings, strengthen the diagnosis, but in isolation have limited significance in the diagnosis of PS.

In summary, the distinction between normal elderly and MD may be difficult, as several features of MD are also present in the normal elderly. In this regard, tremor in general, and RT in particular, which is not a part of normal aging, strongly indicate MD. Since diagnosis of MD is based on clinical assessment, the global clinical picture should be considered in order to distinguish between normal aging and MD. If one is uncertain, a short (approximately 1 month) therapeutic trial on L-dopa (or another drug) is justifiable to be able to arrive at the correct diagnosis. Normal elderly would not benefit, but PD cases would improve on L-dopa.[29,83]

Consideration of Movement Disorders that Are Concentrated in Old Age

The common MD that are concentrated in old age include parkinsonism, ET, MD due to stroke, drug-induced MD, and orofacial dyskinesias.

PARKINSONISM IN THE ELDERLY

The onset of PS before age 40 is rare.[92] In a large series of PS patients the mean age of onset was in the early 60s.[92–94]

The incidence and prevalence rates of PS rise sharply after age 60 years.[24,37,38,69,92,94–98] In a door-to-door survey, the prevalence ratio of PD in those age 75 years and older was 7 times higher than in the 40–64-year age group.[38] In the population between ages 0 and 29 years, the annual incidence was 0.8/100,000, but it rose dramatically to 305/100,000 in those between ages 80 and 99 years. If there was no other cause of death, the cumulative incidence up to age 90 years was 7500/100,000[98] in Rochester, Minnesota (see Chaps. 12, 15 and 20).

We will focus on those aspects of PS that are pertinent to the elderly. A longitudinal survey of the Italian general population between ages 65 and 84 revealed an annual incidence of 530/100,000.[94] Men were twice as likely to develop PS as women.[99] Several other studies also indicate that men are at higher risk of parkinsonism.[98] Others detected no significant sex difference.[100,101]

Parkinsonism in the elderly can be divided into two subgroups: (1) onset at an early age and the patient surviving to old age; and (2) parkinsonism first manifesting in old age.[102] Both these categories increase with age.[98,103,104]

When the disease begins at a younger age, the patient is likely to have received antiparkinsonian drugs, including L-dopa, for several years before reaching old age.[103,105] Since the widespread use of L-dopa, the life-expectancy in PS has increased markedly.[103,104] The typical PD patient with onset at age 62 years is now expected to live a nearly normal lifespan, approximately 2–3 years less than expected compared to the general population. Most such cases would manifest chronic L-dopa side-effects, including dyskinesias, wearing-off, and on-off fluctuations.[83,104,106] The elderly with a long history of PS are at greater risk of freezing episodes and falls.[69]

When PS starts in old age, the distinction from normal aging may be difficult as some features of PS are also seen in the normal elderly. As noted above, a large number of normal elderly have motor slowing, primitive reflexes, vertical gaze palsy, and impaired postural reflexes.[16,17,45–47,51] A survey of 92 elderly community residents with no neurological disease revealed that nearly one-half of subjects had one manifestation (excluding postural instability) of PS,[52] and in day-hospital patients nearly everyone had at least one clinical feature of PS.[52] The normal elderly may therefore be mistakenly diagnosed as PS and treated with antiparkinsonian drugs which could result in side-effects in addition to the financial hardship. Conversely, PS features may be mistaken as part of normal aging and the individual deprived of the appropriate treatment. Careful population surveys indicate that between 35 percent and 41 percent of PS cases in the community are undiagnosed and hence untreated.[38,101] In a survey of persons 65 years and older in Saskatchewan, we detected that 50 percent of the PS cases in the community[2] and 25 percent in chronic care institutions were undiagnosed.[3] Missed diagnosis deprives these cases the opportunity to live an optimal quality of life. This is illustrated by following two examples. A family physician who looks after a chronic care facility reported excitedly, "With the impending influenza season, I gave amantadine to all the residents. Within days, one man who had been in the nursing home for several years, improved so dramatically that he was discharged to go home." The second such example is the case of a 60-year-old woman who had slowed down and could no longer live alone. Her 7 children (including a nurse) attributed that to "old age" and arranged admission to a private care home. While there, she deteriorated further as she was unable to get out of bed and go to the dining area to eat. Neurological examination after hospitalization revealed stage IV Hoehn and Yahr[69] akinetic-rigid PS. She had a remarkable improvement on L-dopa, regaining nearly full functional independence. When in doubt of the diagnosis of PS, a trial of antiparkinson drugs is justified.

In 1958, Kurland[97] estimated a 1 percent prevalence rate of PD in those aged 60 years and older, 2.6 percent in those aged 85 years and older, and a lifetime risk of PS at 2.4 percent. We have observed a PS prevalence rate of 3 percent in the community[2] and 6 percent in the institutionalized aged 65 years and older in a Saskatchewan population.[3] In a random sample study of the general population in 65 years and older, two of tremor, bradykinesia, rigidity, and impaired postural reflexes were noted in 15 percent between ages 65 and 74, 29.5 percent in those aged 75–84 years, and in 52 percent of those aged 85 and older.[107] The proportion of the North American population over ages 65 and 85 has increased substantially since 1958.[97] Thus the lifetime risk of PS in the contemporary population is greater than 1 in 40, and probably closer to 3 percent.[2,3] The akinetic-rigid PS cases are most likely to remain undiagnosed, however, and even those elderly who have classical PS features (including tremor) and advanced disability may be unrecognized as tremor may be erroneously interpreted as a sign of normal aging.

Tremor is the most common first manifestation of PS, ranging from 41 percent[108] to 70.5 percent[69] in different studies. In autopsy-verified PS cases, we noted that tremor alone was the first manifestation in 49 percent.[109] In 41 percent of PS cases, the initial tremor was restricted to the upper limbs.[109] By contrast, only 3 percent of cases first manifested as lower-limb tremor.[109] Other PS features, in conjunction with tremor, were the first manifestations in 53 percent cases.[109]

The akinetic-rigid PS onset cases are prone to developing gait abnormalities early[109,110] and are classified as postural instability and gait difficulty (PIGD) variant.[109–111] Onset in older age is more likely as akinesia-rigidity, while in the younger age tremor is the most common initial manifestation.[109,112] Other less dramatic presentations include upper or lower limb functional decline, handwriting deterioration, foot dragging when tired, difficulty with fine tasks such as doing up buttons or piano playing, loss of self-confidence, feeling of stiffness, decline in coordination, a sense of leg control loss, lack of energy, fatigue, general physical slowing,[109] and frozen shoulder.[113]

Because resting tremor (RT) is not a feature of normal aging, it is the most reliable distinguishing feature between normal aging and parkinsonism.[49,51,85,109,114,115] Isolated lower-limb

RT has even higher diagnostic value.[109,114] On fluorodopa PET scanning, isolated RT cases have the same profile as PD cases.[115]

The most common PS variant is that with marked loss of substantia nigra (SN) pigmented neurons and the presence of Lewy body inclusions,[24,29,70,116] known as idiopathic PD.[116] It is distinguished from other PS variants by the lack of history of a preceding insult and by the presence of associated other clinical features in other variants.[27,29,47,70] The other PS variants may never manifest tremor but all the PD cases have RT at some point.[85] Akinetic-rigid symmetrical onset and the presence of autonomic, corticospinal, or cerebellar dysfunction favor a diagnosis of MSA.[29,51,62,117] In general, the onset of MSA is at younger age compared to PD. Symmetrical neurological findings, vertical gaze palsy, slowed saccades, absence of tremor, and erect posture favor a diagnosis of PSP.[29,75–78] The onset age in PSP is similar to that in PD (early 60s), but, unlike PD, there is no evidence that PSP incidence continues to rise with age.

Clinical features in the PS cases depend on the anatomical site of lesion rather than the pathological process.[29,63,109,118,119] Like PD, other diseases focused on the SN lead to all the major parkinsonian features and respond to L-dopa.[29,83,118–121] Such entities include cases that may or may not have any inclusions.[29,118] Neurofibrillary tangle inclusions at the sites typically involved in PD result in clinical features indistinguishable from those of PD.[118] An autosomal-recessively inherited variant of PS which manifests neurofibrillary tangles but not Lewy body inclusions has onset at a younger age[122,123] than typical PD cases. Collectively, the SN-centered pathology as the basis of PS can be clinically distinguished from the other PS variants in 85 percent of cases.[29] Nearly all PD cases improve on L-dopa,[83] although isolated L-dopa-nonresponsive PD cases have been reported.[124,125] Approximately one-third of the other PS variant cases also improve on L-dopa, although the benefit in those is less dramatic and of shorter duration, usually less than 3 years.[78,83] In suspected PS cases, a trial on L-dopa is therefore justifiable. We have noted a beneficial effect with amantadine in some PSP and MSA cases that did not benefit from L-dopa.[126] When L-dopa/carbidopa and amantadine are initiated simultaneously, the onset of benefit is usually more rapid than on L-dopa/carbidopa alone. A positive response to L-dopa, although helpful, is not diagnostic of PD.[83]

Elderly PS patients, in general, have a more rapid functional decline than the younger-onset cases.[108,111,127,128] However, late-onset age by itself does not shorten survival when compared with age- and sex-matched populations.[93,129,130] The PIGD-onset mode in PD has been reported as more common in old age,[110] but one autopsy-confirmed study revealed no difference in onset age between PIGD and tremor-onset cases.[109] While 74 percent of the tremor-onset cases had Lewy body disease, only 27 percent of PIGD cases had the same pathology.[109] The PIGD cases have more widespread pathology, which accounts for the rapid progression of disability, less favorable drug response, and reduced survival.[109]

The accelerated disability in elderly PS patients may reflect additional functional decline related to the aging process, or concurrent senile gait,[84] or GA.[79]

Compared to the early-onset PS cases, dementia is nearly 10 times more frequent when the onset is in old age.[127,131,132] Dementia is more common in PD than would be expected in the age-matched general population. At any point, nearly one-third of PD cases have dementia,[133–136] and new dementia cases emerge 3–5 times more commonly in PD compared to age-matched normal controls during 5 years of follow-up.[131,134,136–138] Dementia is the presenting or major feature in PD when Lewy body inclusions are detected in the neocortex. This is discussed in Chapter 25 under dementia with Lewy bodies (DLB). Demented cases more often manifest psychiatric and other adverse effects on antiparkinsonian drugs,[102,127,129,130,139] thus making symptomatic control more difficult. Demented PS cases also have a significantly reduced life-expectancy.[93,103,104,127,129,130,137,138,140,141]

It has been suggested that elderly PD cases are resistant to developing L-dopa-induced dyskinesias. One study compared early-onset (mean 38 years) and late-onset (mean 73 years) cases on comparable L-dopa doses and there was no difference in the duration of L-dopa exposure before dyskinesia onset.[108] Another report which compared patients with onset before age 40 years and those with onset after age 40[142] noted a significantly lower incidence of dyskinesia in later-onset cases. We have noted a trend to lower incidence of dyskinesia in older-onset PD in a clinicopathological study.[105] However, elderly cases are not immune from developing dyskinesias. We have observed early and prominent dyskinesia on L-dopa in the elderly, and that age of onset by itself is not the major predictor of dyskinesia.

Approximately 25 percent of the elderly with dementia have Lewy body inclusions in the brainstem and neocortex.[143] The pathological diagnosis of DLB is based on the presence of cortical Lewy bodies. However, nearly half of such patients also have cortical pathology consistent with the diagnosis of AD.[144] There is still a debate as to how to classify DLB. While some classify DLB only when there are no neurofibrillary tangles in the neocortex, others include cases with cortical AD changes of minor severity in DLB.[143] Clinically, it is characterized by three main features: visual hallucinations, cognitive fluctuations (variations from one day to the next, and even from one time of day to another), and parkinsonism. These patients are unduly sensitive to neuroleptics, have less favorable response, and have more common hallucinations on L-dopa.

The DLB criteria[145] have either high specificity or high sensitivity but not both.[144] Impairment of attention and fluctuating attention seen in DLB are also present in AD.[146] Thus the clinical distinction between mild AD and DLB is difficult.[143] Clinical diagnosis of DLB in 96 pathologically confirmed DLB cases revealed that only 45 percent had a correct clinical diagnosis.[147] These indicate that DLB is an entity which needs further studies to distinguish it from PD and AD, AD alone, and other dementias.[147]

DRUG-INDUCED PARKINSONISM (DIP)

Neuroleptic use may produce an acute or chronic extrapyramidal syndrome (EPS). The prevalence of these adverse effects varies widely in different reports.[148] The elderly are more likely to develop chronic EPS on neuroleptics (see Chap. 25).

Drug-induced parkinsonism (DIP) has been well known since the 1960s.[27,30,31] There are very few reports on the incidence and prevalence of DIP in the general population. In community surveys of PS, DIP is second only to PD in both incidence and prevalence.[24,98] In a nursing home population over 65 years we noted a 3 percent prevalence of DIP.[3] In one study of 1559 psychiatric hospital patients, parkinsonism was noted in 19 percent of the cases.[148]

Use of multiple drugs is common in the elderly.[1] In a study of 100 consecutively hospitalized elderly, we noted an average of 5.15 drugs per patient, and 3 percent of the cases were receiving 12 or more drugs,[1] including drugs well known to cause DIP. Another reason for the exaggerated frequency of DIP in old age[27,28,32,102] is likely the age-related striatal dopamine deficiency.[28,149,150] In more than 90 percent of cases DIP emerges within 90 days of neuroleptic initiation.[27] Although akinesia and rigidity may be the prominent features in these patients, DIP is clinically indistinguishable from PD.[29,33,34,102] Theoretically, the DIP should be symmetrical; however, that is not always the case.[27,29] One reason is that some DIP cases may have an underlying PD pathology, and added dopaminergic stress precipitates asymmetrical PS.[28] The PS manifestations that are entirely due to drug-induced dopamine depletion or receptor block improve when the offending agent is discontinued.[34] When there is preclinical PD pathology, the drug-induced clinical features may continue or worsen slowly after the drug is discontinued.[33,34] Careful drug history in the elderly PS cases is vital, as discontinuing the unnecessary drug may be the only treatment required. The time for full recovery after discontinuing the neuroleptics may be as long as 6 months.

Theoretically, the best symptomatic drugs for DIP are the anticholinergics. Since only a small proportion of neuroleptic-treated cases develop DIP,[24] routine[27,30,32] prophylactic use of the anticholinergics (which the elderly tolerate poorly) is not justifiable.[32] Amantadine or L-dopa may be beneficial in some DIP cases.[32,33] When the antipsychotic agents cannot be withdrawn safely in DIP, they should be replaced with atypical antipsychotic agents[40] (clozapine, risperdal, olanzapine, or quetiapine). Because quetiapine is reported not to worsen parkinsonism[151] and does not require the monitoring necessary with clozapine, it should be the drug of choice in such individuals.

ESSENTIAL TREMOR (ET) IN THE ELDERLY

ET onset ranges from childhood to old age,[36,59,60] but the incidence and prevalence rates increase markedly in old age.[36,56,58,59,152–154] (see Chaps. 27 and 29). One-quarter of the

Finnish population over age 40 years are reported to have tremor.[58] The majority (55 percent; i.e., 14 percent of the population studied) had ET.[58] ET was the most common cause of tremor in the elderly community residents who reported "shaking."[155] We found ET prevalence rates of 14 percent in the community,[2] and 10 percent in the institutionalized[3] population 65 years and older in Saskatchewan, Canada.

The tremor frequency in ET varies from 4 to 12 Hz, and there is usually an inverse relationship between the frequency and tremor amplitude.[156,157] With advancing age, the tremor involves wider body areas, the amplitude increases,[156] and the frequency decreases in ET cases.[60,150,152,158] Functional disability in ET is mainly related to tremor amplitude which, as noted above, increases in old age.[150,152,156] Therefore, the tremor-related dysfunction is more common in the elderly than in younger ET patients.[150]

Because life-expectancy in ET is normal[36] and tremor is the only clinical abnormality in most cases, it was once known as "benign" ET. If we consider the psychological and functional handicap related to tremor, even at a young age there is a significant handicap.[36,154,159,160] One sickness profile study dealing with patients' own assessment of emotional behavior, work, communication, home management, recreation, and pastime, found that ET cases were significantly handicapped compared to controls in nearly every category.[160] In childhood, the ET patients are often embarrassed by the tremor and may be ridiculed by other children. These patients may experience anxiety which could lead to depression and, in rare cases, to suicide attempts.[150,160,161] These patients may have to settle for lesser social and employment opportunities than their abilities and qualifications warrant.[36,150,154,159–162] In old age, the exaggerated tremor makes these patients self-conscious, resulting in voluntary social isolation. The functional disability is usually due to the upper limb action tremor, including impaired writing, drinking from a cup, feeding, manipulating fine objects, etc.[36,152,154,159,160,162] Head and voice tremor each may interfere in the daily activities of elderly ET cases. Head tremor is reported to be more common among females than males.[163] One of our elderly patients had such pronounced head tremor that he could not get a haircut at a barber shop. He needed to consume several alcoholic drinks before the head tremor would subside sufficiently that a family member could give him a haircut. We have also seen some ET patients for whom the voice tremor was the main handicap in daily life.

In addition to the action tremor, in old age some ET patients may develop RT without evidence of bradykinesia or rigidity.[150] In an autopsy study of 9 cases, one-third of the ET cases developed RT at a later age.[150] We have now extended that study to include 21 autopsies: of these, 7 (33 percent) had additional RT in upper or lower limbs without evidence of other parkinsonian features. Therefore, the term senile tremor[49,60] is no longer justified. ET patients who first manifest in old age may develop RT and the action tremor typical of ET as the initial symptoms. However, RT alone should not be regarded as a manifestation of ET.[62,63,114] Leg RT alone at the onset without head or upper limb action tremor is against the diagnosis of ET.[114] The PET scan pattern in such patients is similar to that of parkinsonism.[115] The pathophysiological basis of the RT in ET is unknown. It has been postulated that the age-related decline in the striatal dopamine level[149] contributes to the emergence of RT in ET patients as RT is nearly always seen in older ET cases.[150]

Several clinical studies reported an increased risk of PS in ET cases,[164–166] but others found no such association.[36,59,167,168] In our autopsy series of 21 ET cases, the PS diagnosis was made only when all three of RT, bradykinesia, and rigidity were observed.[161] Six (29 percent) of the 21 ET patients also had PS. One such patient had Lewy body pathology, 2 had PSP, 2 had DIP, and 1 had basal ganglia ischemic lesions.[150,161] In addition to our observations, only 7 other ET autopsy cases have been reported since 1919 when the link between SN atrophy, Lewy body inclusions, and PD was first established. In our 21 ET autopsies, 6 had additional features of parkinsonism but only 1 of those had Lewy body disease, which was less frequent than the PSP pathology. Neither of our PSP cases was diagnosed with PSP during life. The biochemical abnormalities typical of PD[169] are not found in ET.[170] In summary, PS may be more common in ET cases referred to subspecialty clinics, but the risk of PD (Lewy body disease) in these patients is not different from that in the general population.[150,161]

Cogwheeling in ET cases may be mistaken for cogwheel rigidity,[53,55,171,172] in particular with the Froment maneuver, and RT, as noted above, is a natural evolution in some ET cases.[150,161] Considering these factors, the distinction between natural evolution of ET and superimposed PS may be difficult.[150] The additional diagnosis of PS is, therefore, justified only when there has been a distinct change in the classical ET profile, and bradykinesia, rigidity, and RT are all unequivocally detected.[150,161] Asymmetry of bradykinesia and rigidity, especially when more pronounced on the side least affected by tremor, is a valuable clue for making the additional diagnosis of PS in ET cases. Piano playing finger movements and rapid hand tapping, contrasted to pronation-supination movements, are better indicators of bradykinesia in ET cases. The distinction between cogwheeling and cogwheel rigidity is outlined in Table 51-2. An alcoholic beverage temporarily relieves symptoms in most, but not all, ET cases.[162,173] This effect is not specific for ET as other tremor variants may also improve with alcohol.[162] Based on the self-made patient observations that alcohol alleviates tremor, some ET patients come to rely on that and may progressively consume larger quantities.[36,161,162,174] With time, the benefit of alcohol declines, requiring larger quantities or producing no relief of the tremor.

STROKE AND MOVEMENT DISORDERS (MD)

Stroke is a common disorder in old age,[43] and some stroke patients may have abnormal movements (e.g., hemiballismus), dystonia, and PS. In one large study of 2500 first stroke patients, 1 percent of the cases had an acute or delayed MD.[175] The most common MD were hemichorea-hemiballismus (in 0.4 percent) and dystonia (in 0.2 percent). Ninety percent of acute-onset MD subsided within 6 months.[175] In most cases, the lesions are due to small-vessel disease in the middle or posterior cerebral artery area.[175] Stroke involving several different anatomical sites may lead to delayed onset of abnormal movement. In one study of 35 thalamic strokes with delayed onset of abnormal movement, the most frequent clinical combination was dystonia, athetosis, and chorea.[176] Those with hemorrhagic lesions are more likely to develop abnormal movements than those with ischemic lesions.[176] Delayed onset of dystonia-athetosis is more often associated with proprioceptive impairment.

HEMIBALLISMUS (HB)

HB is characterized by proximal large-amplitude, irregular, flinging, unilateral limb movements. Rarely, the ballistic movements involve only one limb[177–179] (monoballismus), or both sides (paraballismus or biballismus).[179–182] In one study of 25 ballismus patients, 19 had HB.[179] In only 2 of these 25 (8 percent) cases was the clinical picture that of pure ballismus; most cases had additional abnormalities such as dystonia or chorea.[179] In the vast majority of these cases the HB was due to ischemic pathology which may subsequently have had a hemorrhagic transformation.[179] The main site of pathology in HB is the subthalamic nucleus (STN). The lesion, however, may not be restricted to the STN, or the STN may be unaffected. A lesion of the caudate, putamen, or thalamus alone or in conjunction with an STN lesion can also produce hemiballismus.[179,183–185] A neuroimaging study[179] of 22 ballismus patients revealed that only 1 (4 percent) had a lesion restricted to the STN, and in 5 (23 percent) there were STN plus other basal ganglia, pontine or midbrain lesions. In 6 (27 percent) cases the lesion was restricted to other basal ganglia or the thalamus, without STN involvement, and in 3 (14 percent) cases there were parietal and/or temporal cortex lesions. In 7 (32 percent) cases no neuroimaging abnormality could be identified.[179]

The onset in HB is usually sudden, but in some cases it evolves over several days to weeks.[179] With time, the ballistic movements become less violent and acquire a choreic quality.[186,187] When the STN stroke is the basis of HB, there is usually a spontaneous recovery. In rare cases, multiple basal ganglia lacunar infarcts may produce generalized chorea.[188]

Symptomatic control of ballistic movements can be achieved with haloperidol or other neuroleptics within several days.[179,181] Valproate and sulpiride are also useful in some cases.[184,189]

DYSTONIA

In the elderly, both focal and hemidystonia (HD) are often due to a stroke in the basal ganglia.[190,191] In one study of 22 HD patients, 36 percent of cases of all ages and nearly all those over age 65 years had HD secondary to stroke.[190] Another study of 28 cases noted that 15 (56 percent) of the posthemiplegic dystonia cases were caused by stroke.[191] In general, HD in individuals aged 50 years and older is almost always secondary to stroke.[191] When there is only a discrete lesion as the basis of HD, it may be localized to the lentiform nucleus, head of the caudate, or the posterolateral thalamus,[191] but most HD cases have larger lesions or multiple sites of pathology.[191,192] Lesions of the putamen, globus pallidus, caudate (head), or thalamus (posterolateral) occurring in isolation or in different combinations can produce contralateral focal or hemidystonia.[190–192] The contralateral putamen is the most common isolated site of pathology in HD.[190] The onset of HD following stroke may be delayed for several weeks to years,[190,191] but in rare cases, depending on the site of pathology, dystonia may emerge within several days. In most stroke with HD cases, the dystonia emerges as the severity of the motor weakness declines.

The other forms of dystonia (blepharospasm and Meige's syndrome),[193] although common in the old age, are not related to stroke.

STROKE AND PARKINSONISM

Fully developed parkinsonism secondary to stroke is very rare, but one or more of bradykinesia, rigidity, tremor, and/or gait difficulty has been reported in nearly 1/3 of stroke patients, primarily with multiple lacunar strokes[194] (see Chap. 27). Such PS patients are more likely to have greater lower limb involvement, impaired postural reflexes, corticospinal signs, dementia, and pseudobulbar affect.[195] On the other hand, tremor is rare. In general, they do not improve on L-dopa.[194–196] Ischemic lesions in the basal ganglia, frontal lobe, or the deep subcortical white matter are most likely to produce a parkinson-like clinical picture.[194,196] Parkinsonism secondary to SN infarction is extremely rare. These cases would have associated features indicating damage to the adjoining structures (corticospinal tract, cerebellar outflow pathways, extra-ocular movement abnormalities, etc.). As in the nigral variants of PS,[83,105,118] the PS features may improve on L-dopa.[119] While some PS features are seen secondary to strokes, the PD cases have a reduced risk of stroke.[197,198] Because PD and stroke are both common in older age, at one time stroke was regarded as the basis of PD in a large proportion of cases;[95,97] further studies have excluded this as the cause of PD.

OROFACIAL DYSKINESIAS IN THE ELDERLY

Chronic neuroleptic-treated patients are prone to developing tardive dyskinesia (TD), the frequency of which rises with advancing age.[193,199–201] TD patients may have orobuccolingual-masticatory, cervical, truncal, or extremity stereotyped movements in different combinations (see Chap. 39). Orofacial dyskinesias are also reported in the elderly who have never used neuroleptics[148,201–203] (see Chap. 33). Wide variation in the prevalence rate of drug-induced and spontaneous orofacial dyskinesias (SOFD) has been reported.[193] One community-based survey of individuals aged 71 years and older reported a 0.22 percent prevalence of TD.[203] Khot and Wyatt[204] reviewed 9 TD studies conducted in psychiatric patient populations. The cumulative TD prevalence rate was approximately 20 percent in all ages, but increased markedly after age 40 years. Most of the TD cases had a history of neuroleptic usage.[204]

The existence of SOFD has been questioned by some experts.[205,206] Sweet et al.[205] studied 45 patients over age 60 years at a psychiatric hospital and detected neuroleptic-induced dyskinesias in 21 percent, but noted no instance of SOFD. Based on a survey of institutionalized elderly, Ticehurst[206] concluded that the presumed SOFD cases represent an incomplete history of neuroleptic usage. On the other hand, Chiu et al.[207] noted a 26 percent prevalence of neuroleptic-induced tardive dyskinesia and a 2.4 percent prevalence of SOFD in a psychogeriatric clinic population. Klawans and Barr[201] noted SOFD in 0.8 percent between ages 50 and 59 years, in 6 percent aged between 60 to 69 years, and in 7.8 percent of those between 70 and 79 years in the general population who had neither a neurological illness nor were receiving neuroleptics. Waddington and Youssef[202] reported 4 elderly schizophrenics with SOFD who had never received neuroleptics. On balance, the current evidence favors that rare elderly individuals suffer from orofacial dyskinesias of unknown etiology.

The pathogenesis of orofacial dyskinesia is unknown. It has been suggested that dental extraction and ill-fitting dentures may be contributory factors.[201,208–210] Sandyk and Kay[211] studied the role of edentulousness in neuroleptic-induced dyskinesias in 131 psychiatric patients. Dyskinesias of the tongue, face, or the extremities did not correlate with edentulous status.[211] Edentulous patients, on the other hand, were more liable to developing cervical and truncal dyskinesias.[211] In contrast to patients with limb TD, the patients with orofacial dyskinesia are less likely to have additional features of PD.[148]

Movement Disorders Associated with Other Neurodegenerative Diseases in the Elderly

The most common neurodegenerative disorder in the elderly population is AD.[4,39,40] Several forms of abnormal movements have been reported in AD cases, the most common being parkinsonism.[212–216] There is accumulating evidence that PS is more common in AD than expected in the general population.[217]

The reasons for PS manifestations in AD include neuroleptic usage,[212] concomitant PD,[139] diffuse Lewy body disease,[218,219] and extranigral pathology.[212] The clinical picture may be PS onset with dementia emerging several years later, or the simultaneous development of PS and dementia. When the PD features are later followed by AD, the early clinical picture is indistinguishable from that of PD.[139] As the AD evolves, RT becomes less prominent and an irregular small-amplitude kinetic tremor may emerge. Although there is motor function improvement on L-dopa, psychiatric side-effects are a common and early problem.[139] In those who manifest PD and AD simultaneously, the typical parkinsonian RT is less evident and the response to L-dopa is poor.[139] The AD cases who develop extrapyramidal features early have rapid progression of bradykinesia, rigidity, and gait abnormalities,[220] and global disability.[212,216,221]

Morris et al.[212] longitudinally studied 44 AD cases and 58 controls, none of whom had PS at entry point. At the end of a 66-month follow-up, based on the presence of two of bradykinesia, rigidity, and resting tremor, PS was detected in 16 (37 percent) cases. Six (14 percent) of those were on neuroleptics, and in 10 (23 percent) PS evolved spontaneously. By contrast, over the same interval, only 3 (5 percent) of the 58 controls developed PS.[212] Thus, the spontaneous emergence of new PS manifestations in AD cases over 66 months was nearly 5 times that expected in the general population of the same age.

Kischka et al.[222] conducted electrophysiological tests on AD patients and controls. Reaction time (bradykinesia) and muscle tone (rigidity) were significantly increased in AD patients compared to the normal controls, thus indicating that preclinical PS features are common in AD.[222] A 3-year follow-up of AD cases noted a progressively more common emergence of bradykinesia.[216] Bradykinesia was noted initially in 39 percent of untreated cases and in 72 percent of cases 3 years later. The prevalence of rigidity also increased from 11 percent in untreated cases to 61 percent in AD cases at the end of 3 years.[216] However, tremor was not evident in the early or late AD cases.[216] Nearly every AD patient treated with neuroleptics develops bradykinesia, rigidity, or orofacial dyskinesias when followed for a long time.[216] While tremor is rarely reported in AD-associated PS,[217,223] one study of untreated community residents with mild AD noted RT in 10 percent of cases.[214] Unlike PD, none of these cases improved on L-dopa.[214] On the other hand, Bennett et al.,[215] who studied a 235-bed nursing home patient population, noted some parkinsonian features in a large proportion of the AD cases, and some of them improved on antiparkinsonian drugs.[215] Personal experience indicates that some AD cases have tremor,[29] and in those with AD plus PD dual pathology parkinsonian features may improve on L-dopa.[139]

Myoclonus may be a feature in some AD patients,[221,224] and rare AD cases may have prominent chorea, thus resembling HD.[225]

Parkinsonism, chorea, and myoclonus in different combinations are also seen in Jakob-Creutzfeldt disease.[226] Corticobasal ganglionic degeneration patients typically present with unilateral dystonia, apraxia, and action tremor, and later develop stimulus-sensitive myoclonus.[227,228] In rare Pick's disease cases, the clinical picture is indistinguishable from that of corticobasal ganglionic degeneration.[229–231]

Special Consideration of Movement Disorder Management in the Elderly

The elderly are prone to having other systemic disorders[5] and consume large numbers of drugs.[1,5,232] Altered drug metabolism[21–23,233] predisposes them to drug toxicity and side-effects.[1,5] Drug-induced MD are more likely in the elderly than in younger subjects. Therefore, when considering the diagnosis and management of MD, a careful history of drug intake is necessary. The elderly are liable to have prostatic hypertrophy, glaucoma, age-related memory deficit, cardiac dysrhythmias, leg edema, etc., which are contraindications to the use of commonly prescribed drugs for movement disorders (anticholinergics, beta-adrenergic blockers, dopamine precursors, dopamine agonists, amantidine, etc.). Wherever possible, the first choice in the treatment of drug-induced MD should be to discontinue the offending agent.

The major functional goal of treatment in elderly retired individuals is self-sufficiency for personal, physical, and social needs, and physical safety. The expected survival in the elderly is naturally shortened. Therefore, drugs that may slow down the disease[234] need not be a significant consideration in the treatment of those aged over 75 years. When one drug is sufficient to control the symptoms, additional drugs should be avoided as they increase the risk of side-effects. Nonmedical supports such as physiotherapy, occupational therapy, home care, home safety measures, proper diet, and judicious physical and social activity are important adjuncts. Many elderly individuals suffering from MD are liable to isolate themselves socially. Nonprofit disease-specific organizations are highly valuable in providing social support and interaction among those suffering from similar diseases. Surgical procedures to treat movement disorders should be used with caution and only when noninvasive treatments do not produce sufficient benefit for the desired quality of life.

References

1. Desai T, Rajput AH, Desai HB: Use and abuse of drugs in the elderly. *Prog Neuropsychopharmacol Biol Psychiatry* 14:779–784, 1990.
2. Moghal S, Rajput AH, D'Arcy C, Rajput R: Prevalence of movement disorders in elderly community residents. *Neuroepidemiology* 13:175–178, 1994.
3. Moghal S, Rajput AH, Meleth R, et al: Prevalence of movement disorders in institutionalized elderly. *Neuroepidemiology* 14:297–300, 1995.
4. Canadian Study of Health and Aging Working Group: Canadian Study of Health and Aging. Study methods and prevalence of dementia. *Can Med Assoc J* 150:899–913, 1994.
5. Rowe JW: Aging and geriatric medicine, in Wyngaarden JB, Smith LH (eds): *Cecil Textbook of Medicine*. Philadelphia: WB Saunders, 1988, pp 21–27.
6. Parker SW: Dizziness in the elderly, in Albert ML, Knoefel JE (eds): *Clinical Neurology of Aging*, 2nd ed. New York: Oxford University Press, 1994, pp 569–579.
7. Matjucha ICA, Katz B: Neuro-ophthalmology of aging, in Albert ML, Knoefel JE (eds): *Clinical Neurology of Aging*, 2nd ed. New York: Oxford University Press, 1994, p 447.
8. Kline D, Sekuler R, Dismukes K: Social issues, human needs, and opportunities for research on the effects of age on vision: An over-view, in Sekuler R, Kline D, Dismukes K (eds): *Aging and Human Visual Function*. New York: Alan R Liss, 1982, pp 3–6.
9. Drachman DA, Long RR, Swearer JM: Neurological evaluation of the elderly patient, in Albert ML, Knoefel JE (eds): *Clinical Neurology of Aging*, 2nd ed. New York: Oxford University Press, 1994, pp 159–180.
10. Maki BE, Holliday PJ, Fernie GR: Aging and postural control. A comparison of spontaneous- and induced-sway balance tests. *J Am Geriatr Soc* 38:1–9, 1990.
11. Baloh RW, Fife TD, Zerling L, Socotch T: Comparison of static and dynamic posturography in young and older normal people. *J Am Geriatr Soc* 42:405–412, 1994.
12. Waite LM, Broe GA, Creasey H, et al: Neurological signs, aging, and the neurodegenerative syndromes. *Arch Neurol* 53:498–502, 1996.
13. Melzer I, Benjuya N, Kaplanski J: Age-related changes of postural control: Effect of cognitive tasks. *Gerontology* 47:189–194, 2001.
14. Lexell J, Taylor CC, Sjostrom M: What is the cause of the ageing atrophy? Total number, size and proportion of different fiber types studied in whole vastus lateralis muscle for 15- to 83-year-old men. *J Neurol Sci* 84:275–294, 1988.
15. Woo J, Ho SC, Lau J, et al: Age-associated gait changes in the elderly: Pathological or physiological? *Neuroepidemiology* 14:65–71, 1995.
16. Jenkyn LR, Reeves AG, Warren T, et al: Neurological signs in senescence. *Arch Neurol* 42:1154–1157, 1985.
17. Koller WC, Glatt S, Wilson RS, Fox JH: Primitive reflexes and cognitive function in the elderly. *Ann Neurol* 12:302–304, 1982.
18. Odenheimer G, Funkenstein HH, Beckett L, et al: Comparison of neurologic changes in "successfully aging" persons vs the total aging population. *Arch Neurol* 51:573–580, 1994.
19. Moeller JR, Ishikawa T, Dhawan V, et al: The metabolic topography of normal aging. *J Cereb Blood Flow Metab* 16:385–398, 1996.
20. Duckett S, Schoedler S: Nutritional disorders and alcoholism, in Duckett S (ed): *The Pathology of the Aging Human Nervous System*. Philadelphia: Lea & Febiger, 1991, pp 200–209.
21. Benet LZ, Sheiner LB: Pharmacokinetics: The dynamics of drug absorption, distribution, and elimination, in Gilman AG, Goodman LS, Rall TW, Murad F (eds): *The Pharmacological Basis of Therapeutics*, 7th ed. New York: Macmillan, 1985, pp 3–34.
22. Ross EM, Gilman AG: Pharmacodynamics: Mechanisms of drug action and the relationship between drug concentration and effect, in Gilman AG, Goodman LS, Rall TW, Murad F

(eds): *The Pharmacological Basis of Therapeutics,* 7th ed. New York: Macmillan, 1985, pp 35–48.

23. Blaschke TF, Nies AS, Mamelok RD: Principles of therapeutics, in Gilman AG, Goodman LS, Rall TW, Murad F (eds): *The Pharmacological Basis of Therapeutics,* 7th ed. New York: Macmillan, 1985, pp 49–65.

24. Rajput AH, Offord KP, Beard CM, Kurland LT: Epidemiology of parkinsonism: Incidence, classification, and mortality. *Ann Neurol* 16:278–282, 1984.

25. Lang AE: Lithium and parkinsonism. *Ann Neurol* 15:214, 1984.

26. Klawans HL: Abnormal movements in the elderly. *Sandorama* 15–18, 1981.

27. Friedman JH: Drug-induced parkinsonism, in Lang AE, Weiner WJ (eds): *Drug-Induced Movement Disorders.* Mt. Kisco: Futura, 1992, pp 41–83.

28. Rajput AH, Rozdilsky B, Hornykiewicz O, et al: Reversible drug-induced parkinsonism. Clinicopathologic study of two cases. *Arch Neurol* 39:644–646, 1982.

29. Rajput AH, Rozdilsky B, Rajput AH: Accuracy of clinical diagnosis in parkinsonism: A prospective study. *Can J Neurol Sci* 18:275–278, 1991.

30. Ayd FJ: A survey of drug-induced extrapyramidal reaction. *JAMA* 175:1054–1060, 1961.

31. Delay J, Deniker P: Drug-induced extrapyramidal syndromes, in Vinken PJ, Bruyn GW (eds): *Handbook of Clinical Neurology.* New York: Elsevier, 1968, vol 6, pp 248–266.

32. Rajput AH: Drug induced parkinsonism in the elderly. *Geriatr Med Today* 3:99–107, 1984.

33. Hardie RJ, Lees AJ: Neuroleptic-induced Parkinson's syndrome: Clinical features and results of treatment with levodopa. *J Neurol Neurosurg Psychiatry* 51:850–854, 1988.

34. Burn DJ, Brooks DJ: Nigral dysfunction in drug-induced parkinsonism: An ^{18}F-dopa PET study. *Neurology* 43:552–556, 1993.

35. Gordon M, Preiksaitis HG: Drugs and the aging brain, in Duckett S (ed): *The Pathology of the Aging Human Nervous System.* Philadelphia: Lea & Febiger, 1991, pp 443–448.

36. Rajput AH, Offord KP, Beard CM, Kurland LT: Essential tremor in Rochester, Minnesota: A 45-year study. *J Neurol Neurosurg Psychiatry* 47:466–470, 1984.

37. Bharucha NE, Bharucha EP, Bharucha AE, et al: Prevalence of Parkinson's disease in the Parsi community of Bombay, India. *Arch Neurol* 45:1321–1323, 1988.

38. Schoenberg BS, Anderson DW, Haerer AF: Prevalence of Parkinson's disease in the biracial population of Copiah County, Mississippi. *Neurology* 35:841–845, 1985.

39. Schoenberg BS, Kokmen E, Okazaki H: Alzheimer's disease and other dementing illnesses in a defined United States population: Incidence rates and clinical features. *Ann Neurol* 22:724–729, 1987.

40. Terry RD, Katzman R: Senile dementia of the Alzheimer type. *Ann Neurol* 14:497–506, 1983.

41. Boller F, Mizutani T, Roessmann U, et al: Parkinson's disease, dementia, and Alzheimer's disease: Clinicopathological correlations. *Ann Neurol* 7:329–335, 1980.

42. Hansen L, Salmon D, Galasko D, et al: The Lewy body variant of Alzheimer's disease: A clinical and pathological entity. *Neurology* 40:1–8, 1990.

43. Babikian VL, Kase CS, Wolf PA: Cerebrovascular disease in the elderly, in Albert ML, Knoefel JE (eds): *Clinical Neurology of Aging,* 2nd ed. New York: Oxford University Press, 1994, pp 548–568.

44. Sudarsky L: Gait disturbances in the elderly, in Albert ML, Knoefel JE (eds): *Clinical Neurology of Aging,* 2nd ed. New York: Oxford University Press, 1994, pp 483–492.

45. Sudarsky L: Geriatrics: Gait disorders in the elderly. *N Engl J Med* 322:1441–1446, 1990.

46. Weiner WJ, Nora LM, Glantz RH: Elderly inpatients: Postural reflex impairment. *Neurology* 34:945–947, 1984.

47. Rajput AH: Parkinsonism, aging and gait apraxia, in Stern MB, Koller WC (eds): *Parkinsonian Syndromes.* New York: Marcel Dekker, 1993, pp 511–532.

48. Jankovic J, Fahn S: Physiologic and pathologic tremors. Diagnosis, mechanism, and management. *Ann Intern Med* 93:460–465, 1980.

49. Kelly J, Taggart HM, McCullagh P: Normal and abnormal tremor in the elderly, in Findley LJ, Koller WC (eds): *Handbook of Tremor Disorders.* New York: Marcel Dekker, 1995, pp 351–370.

50. Marsden CD: Slowness of movement in Parkinson's disease. *Mov Disord* 4(suppl 1):S26–S37, 1989.

51. Rajput AH: Clinical features and natural history of Parkinson's disease (special consideration of aging), in Calne DB (ed): *Neurodegenerative Diseases.* Philadelphia: WB Saunders, 1994, pp 555–571.

52. Duncan G, Wilson JA: Normal elderly have some signs of PS. *Lancet* 2:1392, 1989.

53. Findley LJ, Koller WC: Definitions and behavioral classifications, in Koller WC, Findley LJ (eds): *Handbook of Tremor Disorders.* New York: Marcel Dekker, 1995, pp 1–5.

54. Duvoisin RG: The differential diagnosis of parkinsonism, in Stern GM (ed): *Parkinson's Disease.* Baltimore: Johns Hopkins University Press, 1990, pp 431–466.

55. Findley LJ, Gresty MA, Halmagyi GM: Tremor and cogwheel phenomena and clonus in Parkinson's disease. *J Neurol Neurosurg Psychiatry* 44:534–546, 1981.

56. Rautakorpi I, Takala J, Marttila RJ, et al: Essential tremor in a Finnish population. *Acta Neurol Scand* 66:58–67, 1982.

57. Findley LJ, Gresty MA: Tremor. *Br J Hosp Med* 26(1):16–32, 1981.

58. Rautakorpi I, Marttila RJ, Takala J, Rinne UK: Occurrences and causes of tremors. *Neuroepidemiology* 1:209–215, 1982.

59. Haerer AF, Anderson DW, Schoenberg BS: Prevalence of essential tremor: Results from the Copiah County Study. *Arch Neurol* 39:750–751, 1982.

60. Koller WC, Hubble JP, Busenbark KL: Essential tremor, in Calne DB (ed): *Neurodegenerative Diseases.* Philadelphia: WB Saunders, 1994, pp 717–742.

61. LeWitt PA: Tremor induced or enhanced by pharmacological means, in Findley LJ, Koller WC (eds): *Handbook of Tremor Disorders.* New York: Marcel Dekker, 1995, pp 473–481.

62. Rajput AH: Clinical features of tremor in extrapyramidal syndromes, in Findley LJ, Koller WC (eds): *Handbook of Tremor Disorders.* New York: Marcel Dekker, 1994, pp 275–291.

63. Rajput AH, Rozdilsky B, Ang L: Site(s) of lesion and resting tremor. *Ann Neurol* 28:296–297, 1990.

64. Koch H, Smith MC: Office-based ambulatory care for patients 75 years old and over. *National Ambulatory Medical Care Survey, 1980 and 1981.* Hyattsville, MD: National Center for Health Statistics, Public Health Service, 1985.

65. Luxon LM: A bit dizzy. *Br J Hosp Med* 32:315, 1984.

66. Duncan PW, Chandler J, Studenski S, et al: How do physiological components of balance affect mobility in elderly men? *Arch Phys Med Rehabil* 74:1343–1349, 1993.

67. Fahn S, Elton RL, UPDRS Development Committee: Unified Parkinson's disease rating scale, in Fahn S, Marsden CD, Calne D, Goldstein M (eds): *Recent Developments in Parkinson's Disease*, 2nd ed. Florham Park, NJ: Macmillan Healthcare Information, 1987, pp 153–305.

68. Tinetti ME, Speechley M, Ginter SF: Risk factors for falls among elderly persons living in the community. *N Engl J Med* 319:1701–1707, 1988.

69. Hoehn MM, Yahr MD: Parkinsonism: Onset, progression, and mortality. *Neurology* 17:427–442, 1967.

70. Hughes AJ, Daniel SE, Kilford L, Lees AJ: Accuracy of clinical diagnosis of idiopathic Parkinson's disease: A clinicopathological study of 100 cases. *J Neurol Neurosurg Psychiatry* 55:181–184, 1992.

71. Rajput AH: Diagnosis of PD [letter]. *Neurology* 43:1629–1630, 1993.

72. Rajput AH: Accuracy of clinical diagnosis of idiopathic Parkinson's disease. *J Neurol Neurosurg Psychiatry* 56:938–939, 1993.

73. Winter DA, Patla AE, Frank JS, Walt SE: Biomechanical walking pattern changes in the fit and healthy elderly. *Phys Ther* 70:340–347, 1990.

74. Sudarsky L, Ronthal M: Gait disorders among elderly patients. A survey study of 50 patients. *Arch Neurol* 40:740–743, 1983.

75. Rajput AH, Chornell G, Rozdilsky B: Progressive external ophthalmoplegia with parkinsonism and dementia treatment with L-dopa. *Can J Ophthalmol* 7:368–374, 1972.

76. Steele JC, Richardson JC, Olszewski J: Progressive supranuclear palsy: A heterogeneous degeneration involving the brain stem, ganglia and cerebellum with vertical gaze and pseudobulbar palsy, nuchal dystonia and dementia. *Arch Neurol* 10:333–359, 1964.

77. Jackson JA, Jankovic J, Ford J: Progressive supranuclear palsy: Clinical features and response to treatment in 16 patients. *Ann Neurol* 13:273–278, 1983.

78. Birdi S, Rajput AH, Fenton M, et al: Progressive supranuclear palsy diagnosis and confounding features: Report of 16 autopsied cases. *Mov Disord* 17(6):1255–1264, 2002.

79. Sudarsky L, Simon S: Gait disorder in late-life hydrocephalus. *Arch Neurol* 44:263–267, 1987.

80. Estanol BV: Gait apraxia in communicating hydrocephalus. *J Neurol Neurosurg Psychiatry* 44:305–308, 1981.

81. Fisher CM: Hydrocephalus as a cause of disturbances of gait in the elderly. *Neurology* 32:1358–1363, 1982.

82. Forssberg H, Johnels B, Steg G: Is parkinsonian gait caused by a regression to an immature walking pattern? *Adv Neurol* 375–379, 1984.

83. Rajput AH, Rozdilsky B, Rajput A, Ang L: Levodopa efficacy and pathological basis of Parkinson syndrome. *Clin Neuropharmacol* 13:553–558, 1990.

84. Koller W, Wilson R, Glatt S, et al: Senile gait: Correlation with computed tomographic scan. *Ann Neurol* 13:343–344, 1983.

85. Rajput AH, Rozdilsky B, Ang L: Occurrence of resting tremor in Parkinson's disease. *Neurology* 41:1298–1299, 1991.

86. Rivaud-Péchoux S, Vidailhet M, Gallouedec G, et al: Longitudinal ocular motor study in corticobasal degeneration and progressive supranuclear palsy. *Neurology* 54:1029–1032, 2000.

87. Leigh RJ, Riley DE: Eye movements in parkinsonism. It's saccadic speed that counts. *Neurology* 54:1018–1019, 2000.

88. Golbe LI, Davis PH: *Progressive Supranuclear Palsy*. Baltimore: Williams & Wilkins, 1993.

89. Jankovic J, Rajput AH, Golbe LI, Goodman JC: What is it? Case 1, 1993: Parkinsonism, dysautonomia, and ophthalmoparesis. *Mov Disord* 8:525–532, 1993.

90. Stewart BJ, Rajput AH, Ravindran J: Ophthalmoplegia in parkinsonism. *Can J Neurol Sci* 21:S27, 1994 (abstract).

91. Simpson DA, Wishnow R, Gargulinski RB, Pawlak AM: Oculofacial-skeletal myorhythmia in central nervous system Whipple's disease: Additional case and review of the literature. *Mov Disord* 10:195–200, 1995.

92. Rajput AH: Frequency and cause of Parkinson's disease. *Can J Neurol Sci* 19:103–107, 1992.

93. Rajput AH, Uitti RJ, Rajput AH, Basran P: Life expectancy in Parkinsonism today. *Mov Disord* 5(suppl 1):13, 1990 (abstract).

94. Marttila RJ: Epidemiology, in Koller WC (ed): *Handbook of Parkinson's Disease*. New York: Marcel Dekker, 1987, pp 35–50.

95. Nobrega FT, Glattre E, Kurland LT, Okazaki H: Comments on the epidemiology of parkinsonism including prevalence and incidence statistics for Rochester, Minnesota, 1935–1966, in Barbeau A, Brunette JR (eds): *Progress in Neurogenetics*. Amsterdam: Excerpta Medica, 1967, pp 474–485.

96. Schoenberg BS: Environmental risk factors for Parkinson's disease: The epidemiologic evidence. *Can J Neurol Sci* 14:407–413, 1987.

97. Kurland LT: Epidemiology: Incidence, geographic distribution and genetic considerations, in Fields WS (ed): *Pathogenesis and Treatment of Parkinsonism*. Springfield, IL: Charles C Thomas, 1958, pp 5–43.

98. Bower JH, Maraganore DM, McDonnell SK, Rocca WA: Incidence and distribution of parkinsonism in Olmsted County, Minnesota, 1976–1990. *Neurology* 52:1214–1220, 1999.

99. Baldereschi M, De Carlo A, Rocca WA, et al: Parkinson's disease and parkinsonism in a longitudinal study. Two-fold higher incidence in men. *Neurology* 55:1358–1363, 2000.

100. Hofman A, Collette HJA, Bartelds AIM: Incidence and risk factors of Parkinson's disease in The Netherlands. *Neuroepidemiology* 8:296–299, 1989.

101. Morgante L, Rocca WA, Di Rosa AE, et al: Prevalence of Parkinson's disease and other types of parkinsonism: A door-to-door survey in three Sicilian municipalities. *Neurology* 42:1901–1907, 1992.

102. Rajput AH: Parkinson's disease in the elderly. *Med North Am* 1:101–106, 1986.

103. Rajput AH, Uitti RJ, Rajput AH, Offord KP: Timely levodopa (LD) administration prolongs survival in Parkinson's disease. *Parkinsonism Relat Disord* 3:159–165, 1997.

104. Rajput AH: Levodopa prolongs life expectancy and is non-toxic to substantia nigra. *Parkinsonism Relat Disord* 8:95–100, 2001.

105. Rajput AH, Fenton ME, Birdi S, et al: A clinical-pathological study of levodopa complications. *Mov Disord* 17(2):289–296, 2002.

106. Rajput AH, Stern W, Laverty WH: Chronic low dose therapy in Parkinson's disease: An argument for delaying levodopa therapy. *Neurology* 34:991–996, 1984.

107. Bennett DA, Beckett LA, Murray AM, et al: Prevalence of Parkinsonian signs and associated mortality in a community population of older people. *N Engl J Med* 334:71–76, 1996.

108. Gibb WR, Lees AJ: A comparison of clinical and pathological features of young- and old-onset Parkinson's disease. *Neurology* 38:1402–1406, 1988.

109. Rajput AH, Pahwa R, Pahwa P, Rajput A: Prognostic significance of the onset mode in parkinsonism. *Neurology* 43:829–830, 1993.

110. Zetusky WJ, Jankovic J, Pirozzolo FJ: The heterogeneity of Parkinson's disease: Clinical and prognostic implications. *Neurology* 35:522–526, 1985.

111. Jankovic J, McDermott M, Carter J, et al: Variable expression of Parkinson's disease: A base-line analysis of the DATATOP cohort. *Neurology* 40:1529–1534, 1990.

112. Nagayama H, Hamamoto M, Nito C, et al: Initial symptoms of Parkinson's disease with elderly onset. *Gerontology* 46:129–132, 2000.

113. Riley D, Lang AE, Blair RDG, et al: Frozen shoulder and other shoulder disturbances in Parkinson's disease. *J Neurol Neurosurg Psychiatry* 52:63–66, 1989.

114. Rajput AH, Rozdilsky B, Rajput AH: Essential leg tremor. *Neurology* 40:1909, 1990.

115. Brooks DJ, Playford ED, Ibanez V, et al: Isolated tremor and disruption of the nigrostriatal dopaminergic system: An 18F-dopa PET study. *Neurology* 42:1554–1560, 1992.

116. Duvoisin R, Golbe LI: Toward a definition of Parkinson's disease. *Neurology* 39:746, 1989.

117. Rajput AH, Kazi KH, Rozdilsky B: Striatonigral degeneration response to levodopa therapy. *J Neurol Sci* 16:331–341, 1972.

118. Rajput AH, Uitti RJ, Sudhakar S, Rozdilsky B: Parkinsonism and neurofibrillary tangle pathology in pigmented nuclei. *Ann Neurol* 25:602–606, 1989.

119. Murrow RW, Schweiger GD, Kepes JJ, Koller WC: Parkinsonism due to a basal ganglia lacunar state: Clinicopathologic correlation. *Neurology* 40:897–900, 1990.

120. Langston JW, Ballard P: Parkinsonism induced by 1-methyl-4-phenyl-1,2,3,6-tetrahydropyridine (MPTP): Implications for treatment and the pathogenesis of Parkinson's disease. *Can J Neurol Sci* 11:160–165, 1984.

121. Langston JW, Quik M, Petzinger G, et al: Investigating levodopa-induced dyskinesias in the parkinsonian primate. *Ann Neurol* 47(4 suppl 1):S79–89, 2000.

122. Mori H, Yokochi M, Matsumine H, et al: Pathologic and biochemical studies of juvenile parkinsonism linked to chromosome 6q. *Neurology* 51:890–892, 1998.

123. Rajput AH: Pathologic and biochemical studies of juvenile parkinsonism linked to chromosome 6q [letter]. *Neurology* 53:1357, 2000.

124. Mark MH, Sage JI, Dickson DW, et al: Levodopa-nonresponsive Lewy body parkinsonism: Clinicopathologic study of two cases. *Neurology* 42:1323–1327, 1992.

125. Sage JI, Miller DC, Golbe LI, et al: Clinically atypical expression of pathologically typical Lewy-body parkinsonism. *Clin Neuropharmacol* 13:36–47, 1991.

126. Rajput AH, Uitti RJ, Fenton ME, George D: Amantadine effectiveness in multiple system atrophy and progressive supranuclear palsy. *Parkinsonism Relat Disord* 3:211–214, 1998.

127. Hietanen M, Teravainen H: The effect of age of disease onset on neuropsychological performance in Parkinson's disease. *J Neurol Neurosurg Psychiatry* 51:244–249, 1988.

128. Goetz CG, Tanner CM, Stebbins GT, Buchman AS: Risk factors for progression in Parkinson's disease. *Neurology* 38:1841–1844, 1988.

129. Uitti RJ, Rajput AH, Offord KP: Parkinsonism survival in the levodopa era. *Neurology* 41(suppl 1):190, 1991.

130. Rajput AH, Uitti RJ, Rajput AH, Basran P: Parkinsonism: Onset and mortality update. *Can J Neurol Sci* 16:241, 1989 (abstract).

131. Mayeux R, Stern Y, Rosenstein R, et al: An estimate of the prevalence of dementia in idiopathic Parkinson's disease. *Arch Neurol* 45:260–262, 1988.

132. Mayeux R, Chen J, Mirabello E, et al: An estimate of the incidence of dementia in idiopathic Parkinson's disease. *Neurology* 40:1513–1517, 1990.

133. Marttila RJ, Rinne UK: Dementia in Parkinson disease. *Acta Neurol Scand* 54:431–441, 1976.

134. Rajput AH: Prevalence of dementia in Parkinson's disease, in Huber SJ, Cummings JL (eds): *Parkinson's Disease. Neurobehavioral Aspects*. New York: Oxford University Press, 1992, pp 119–131.

135. Rajput AH, Rozdilsky B: Parkinsonism and dementia: Effects of L-dopa. *Lancet* i:1084–1084, 1975.

136. Rajput AH, Offord KP, Beard CM, Kurland LT: A case control study of smoking habits, dementia and other illnesses in idiopathic Parkinson's disease. *Neurology* 37:226–232, 1987.

137. Marder K, Leung D, Tang M, et al: Are demented patients with Parkinson's disease accurately reflected in prevalence surveys? A survival analysis. *Neurology* 41:1240–1243, 1991.

138. Mindham RHS, Ahmed SWA, Clough CG: A controlled study of dementia in Parkinson's disease. *J Neurol Neurosurg Psychiatry* 45:969–974, 1982.

139. Rajput AH, Rozdilsky B, Rajput A: Alzheimer's disease and idiopathic Parkinson's disease coexistence. *J Geriatr Psychiatry Neurol* 6:170–176, 1993.

140. Uitti RJ, Rajput AH, Ahlskog JE, et al: Amantadine treatment is an independent predictor of improved survival in Parkinson's disease. *Neurology* 46:1551–1556, 1996.

141. Marder K, Mirabello E, Chen J, et al: Death rates among demented and nondemented patients with Parkinson's disease. *Ann Neurol* 28:295, 1990.

142. Kostic V, Przedborski S, Flaster E, Sternic N: Early development of levodopa-induced dyskinesias and response fluctuations in young-onset Parkinson's disease. *Neurology* 41:202–205, 1991.

143. Lopez OL, Hamilton RL, Becker JT, et al: Severity of cognitive impairment and the clinical diagnosis of dementia with Lewy bodies. *Neurology* 54:1780–1797, 2000.

144. Verghese J, Crystal HA, Dickson DW, Lipton RB: Validity of clinical criteria for the diagnosis of dementia with Lewy bodies. *Neurology* 53:1974–1982, 1999.

145. McKeith IG, Galasko D, Kosaka K, et al: Consensus guidelines for the clinical and pathologic diagnosis of dementia with Lewy body (DLB): Report of the consortium on DLB international workshop. *Neurology* 47:1113–1124, 1996.

146. Ballard C, O'Brien J, Gray A, et al: Attention and fluctuating attention in patients with dementia with Lewy bodies and Alzheimer disease. *Arch Neurol* 58:977–982, 2001.

147. Merdes AR, Hansen LA, Ho G, et al: Diagnostic accuracy for dementia with Lewy bodies. *Proceedings of 126th Annual Meeting of the American Neurological Association* 2001, pp 30 (abstract).

148. Muscettola G, Barbato G, Pampallona S, et al: Extrapyramidal syndromes in neuroleptic-treated patients: Prevalence, risk factors, and association with tardive dyskinesia. *J Clin Psychopharmacol* 19:203–208, 1999.

149. Kish SJ, Shannak K, Rajput A, et al: Aging produces a specific pattern of striatal dopamine loss: Implications for the etiology of idiopathic Parkinson's disease. *J Neurochem* 58:642–648, 1992.

150. Rajput AH, Rozdilsky B, Ang L, Rajput A: Significance of parkinsonian manifestations in essential tremor. *Can J Neurol Sci* 20:114–117, 1993.

151. Korczyn AD: Hallucinations in Parkinson's disease. *Lancet* 358:1031–1032, 2001.

152. Louis ED: Samuel Adams' tremor. *Neurology* 56:1201–1205, 2001.

153. Salemi G, Savettieri G, Rocca WA, et al: Prevalence of essential tremor: A door-to-door survey in Terrasini, Sicily. *Neurology* 44:61–64, 1994.

154. Bain PG, Findley LJ, Thompson PD, et al: A study of hereditary essential tremor. *Brain* 117:805–824, 1994.

155. Louis ED, Marder K, Cote L, et al: Prevalence of a history of shaking in persons 65 years of age and older: Diagnostic and functional correlates. *Mov Disord* 11:63–69, 1996.

156. Elble RJ: Physiologic and essential tremor. *Neurology* 36:225–231, 1986.

157. Stiles RN: Frequency and displacement amplitude relations for normal hand tremor. *J Appl Physiol* 40:44–54, 1976.

158. Calzetti S, Baratti M, Findley LJ: Frequency/amplitude characteristic of postural tremor of the hands in a population of patients with bilateral essential tremor: Implications for the classification and mechanism of essential tremor. *J Neurol Neurosurg Psychiatry* 50:561–567, 1987.

159. Rajput AH: Essential tremor that is not "benign". *Trans Can Congr Neurol* 55:151, 1976 (abstract).

160. Busenbark KL, Nash J, Nash S, et al: Is essential tremor benign? *Neurology* 41:1982–1983, 1991.

161. Rajput AH: Pathological and neurochemical basis of essential tremor, in Koller WC, Findley LJ (eds): *Handbook of Tremor Disorders*. New York: Marcel Dekker, 1994, pp 233–244.

162. Rajput AH, Jamieson H, Hirsch S, Quraishi A: Relative efficacy of alcohol and propranolol in action tremor. *Can J Neurol Sci* 2:31–35, 1975.

163. Hubble JP, Busenbark KL, Pahwa R, et al: Clinical expression of essential tremor: Effects of gender and age. *Mov Disord* 12:969–972, 1997.

164. Geraghty JJ, Jankovic J, Zetusky WJ: Association between essential tremor and Parkinson's disease. *Ann Neurol* 17:329–333, 1985.

165. Barbeau A, Roy M: Familial subsets in idiopathic Parkinson's disease. *Can J Neurol Sci* 11:144–150, 1984.

166. Hornabrook RW, Nagurney JT: Essential tremor in Papua New Guinea. *Brain* 99:659–672, 1976.

167. Cleeves L, Findley LJ, Koller W: Lack of association between essential tremor and Parkinson's disease. *Ann Neurol* 24:23–26, 1988.

168. Marttila RJ, Rautakorpi I, Rinne UK: The relation of essential tremor to Parkinson's disease. *J Neurol Neurosurg Psychiatry* 47:734–735, 1984.

169. Ehringer H, Hornykiewicz O: Verteilung von Noradrenalin und Dopamin (3-Hydroxytyramin) im Gehirn des Menschen und ihr Verhalten bei Erkrankungen des extrapyramidalen Systems. *Klin Wochenschr* 38:1236–1239, 1960.

170. Rajput AH, Hornykiewicz O, Deng Y, et al: Increased noradrenaline levels in essential tremor brain. *Neurology* 56(suppl 3):A302, 2001 (abstract).

171. Findley LJ, Gresty MA: Tremor and rhythmical involuntary movements in Parkinson's disease, in Findley LJ, Capildeo R (eds): *Movement Disorders: Tremor*. Basingstoke: Macmillan, 1984, pp 295–304.

172. Salisachs P, Findley LJ: Problems in the differential diagnosis of essential tremor, in Findley LJ, Capildeo R (eds): *Movement Disorders: Tremor*. Basingstoke: Macmillan, 1984, pp 219–224.

173. Koller WC, Biary N: Effect of alcohol on tremors: Comparison with propranolol. *Neurology* 34:221–222, 1984.

174. Rajput AH, Rozdilsky B, Ang L, Rajput A: Clinicopathological observations in essential tremor. Report of 6 Cases. *Neurology* 41:1422–1424, 1991.

175. Ghika-Schmid F, Ghika J, Regli F, Bogousslavsky J: Hyperkinetic movement disorders and after acute stroke: The Lausanne Stroke Registry. *J Neurol Sci* 152:109–116, 1997.

176. Kim JS: Delayed onset mixed involuntary movements after thalamic stroke: Clinical, radiological and pathophysiological findings. *Brain* 124(Pt 2):299–309, 2001.

177. Maruyama T, Hasimoto T, Miyasaka M, Yanagisawa N: A case of thalamo-subthalamic hemorrhage presenting monoballism in the contralateral lower extremity. *Rinsho Shinkeigaku* 32:1022–1027, 1992.

178. Ikeda M, Tsukagoshi H: Monochorea caused by a striatal lesion. *Eur Neurol* 31:257–258, 1991.

179. Vidakovic A, Dragasevic N, Kostic VS: Hemiballism: report of 25 cases. *J Neurol Neurosurg Psychiatry* 57:945–949, 1994.

180. Nicolai A, Lazzarino LG: Paraballism associated with anterior opercular syndrome: A case report. *Clin Neurol Neurosurg* 96:145–147, 1994.

181. Caparros-Lefebvre D, Deleume JF, Bradaik N, Petit H: Biballism caused by bilateral infarction in the substantia nigra. *Mov Disord* 9:108–110, 1994.

182. Lodder J, Baard WC: Paraballism caused by bilateral hemorrhagic infarction in basal ganglia. *Neurology* 31:484–486, 1981.

183. Lazzarino LG, Nicolai A: Hemichorea-hemiballism and anosognosia following a contralateral infarction of the caudate nucleus and anterior limb of the internal capsule. *Riv Neurol* 61:9–11, 1991.

184. Hanaoka Y, Ohi T, Matsukura S: A case of hemiballism successfully treated by sulpiride, caused by lesions of the striatum. *Rinsho Shinkeigaku* 30:774–776, 1990.

185. Konagaya M, Nakamuro T, Sugata T, et al: MRI study of hemiballism. *Rinsho Shinkeigaku* 30:17–23, 1990.

186. Hyland HH, Forman DM: Prognosis in hemiballismus. *Neurology* 7:381–391, 1957.

187. Pappenheim E: Therapeutic response in hemiballismus. *Ann Neurol* 6:139, 1979.

188. Sethi KD, Nichols FT, Yaghmai F: Generalized chorea due to basal ganglia lacunar infarcts. *Mov Disord* 2:61–66, 1987.

189. Lenton RJ, Copti M, Smith RG: Hemiballismus treated with sodium valproate. *Br Med J* 283:17–18, 1981.

190. Pettigrew LC, Jankovic J: Hemidystonia: A report of 22 patients and a review of the literature. *J Neurol Neurosurg Psychiatry* 48:650–657, 1985.

191. Marsden CD, Obeso JA, Zarranz JJ, Lang AE: The anatomical basis of symptomatic hemidystonia. *Brain* 108:463–483, 1985.

192. Fross RD, Martin WRW, Li D, et al: Lesions of the putamen: Their relevance to dystonia. *Neurology* 37:1125–1129, 1987.

193. Comella CL, Klawans HL: Nonparkinsonian movement disorders in the elderly, in Albert ML, Knoefel JE (eds): *Clinical Neurology of Aging*, 2nd ed. New York: Oxford University Press, 1994, pp 502–520.

194. van Zagten M, Lodder J, Kessels F: Gait disorder and parkinsonian signs in patients with stroke related to small deep infarcts and white matter lesions. *Mov Disord* 13:89–95, 1998.

195. Winikates J, Jankovic J: Clinical correlates of vascular parkinsonism. *Arch Neurol* 56:98–102, 1999.

196. Chang CM, Yu UL, Ng HK, et al: Vascular pseudoparkinsonism. *Acta Neurol Scand* 86:588–592, 1991.

197. Korten A, Lodder J, Vreeling F, et al: Stroke and idiopathic Parkinson's disease: Does a shortage of dopamine offer protection against stroke? *Mov Disord* 16:119–123, 2001.

198. Struck LK, Rodnitzky RL, Dobson JK: Stroke and its modification in Parkinson's disease. *Stroke* 21:1395–1399, 1990.

199. Schwartz M, Silver H, Tal I, Sharf B: Tardive dyskinesia in northern Israel: Preliminary study. *Eur Neurol* 33:264–266, 1993.

200. Casey DE: Tardive dyskinesia. *West J Med* 153:535–541, 1990.

201. Klawans HL, Barr A: Prevalence of spontaneous lingual-facial-buccal dyskinesias in the elderly. *Neurology* 32:558–559, 1982.

202. Waddington JL, Youssef HA: The lifetime outcome and involuntary movements of schizophrenia never treated with neuroleptic drugs: Four rare cases in Ireland. *Br J Psychiatry* 156:106–108, 1990.

203. Green BH, Dewey ME, Copeland JR, et al: Prospective data on the prevalence of abnormal involuntary movements among elderly people living in the community. *Acta Psychiatr Scand* 87:418–421, 1993.

204. Khot V, Wyatt RJ: Not all that moves is tardive dyskinesia. *Am J Psychiatry* 148:661–666, 1991.

205. Sweet RA, Mulsant BH, Rifai AH, Zubenko GS: Dyskinesia and neuroleptic exposure in elderly psychiatric inpatients. *J Geriatr Psychiatry Neurol* 5:156–161, 1992.

206. Ticehurst SB: Is spontaneous orofacial dyskinesia an artefact due to incomplete drug history? *J Geriatr Psychiatry Neurol* 3:208–211, 1990.

207. Chiu HF, Wing YK, Kwong PK, et al: Prevalence of tardive dyskinesia in samples of elderly people in Hong Kong. *Acta Psychiatr Scand* 87:266–268, 1993.

208. Klawans HL, Bergen D, Bruyn GW, Paulson GW: Neuroleptic-induced tardive dyskinesias in nonpsychotic patients. *Arch Neurol* 30:338–339, 1974.

209. Koller WC: Edentulous orodyskinesia. *Ann Neurol* 13:97–99, 1983.

210. Kai S, Kai H, Tashiro H: Tardive dyskinesia affected by occlusal treatment: A case report. *Cranio* 12:199–203, 1994.

211. Sandyk R, Kay SR: Edentulousness and neuroleptic-induced neck and trunk dyskinesia. *Funct Neurol* 5:361–363, 1990.

212. Morris JC, Drazner M, Fulling K, et al: Clinical and pathological aspects of parkinsonism in Alzheimer's disease. *Arch Neurol* 46:651–657, 1989.

213. Molsa PK, Marttila RJ, Rinne UK: Extrapyramidal signs in Alzheimer's disease. *Neurology* 34:1114–1116, 1984.

214. Tyrrell PJ, Rossor MN: Extrapyramidal signs in dementia of Alzheimer type. *Lancet* 2(8668):920, 1989.

215. Bennett RG, Greenough WB, Gloth FMI, et al: Extrapyramidal signs in dementia of Alzheimer type. *Lancet* 2:1392, 1989.

216. Soininen H, Laulamaa V, Helkala EL, et al: Extrapyramidal signs in Alzheimer's disease: A 3-year follow-up study. *J Neural Transm* 4:107–119, 1992.

217. Lopez OL, Wisnieski SR, Becker JT, et al: Extrapyramidal signs in patients with probable Alzheimer disease. *Arch Neurol* 54:969–975, 1997.

218. Crystal HA, Dickson DW, Lizardi JE, et al: Antemortem diagnosis of diffuse Lewy body disease. *Neurology* 40:1523–1528, 1990.

219. Dickson DW, Ruan D, Crystal H, et al: Hippocampal degeneration differentiates diffuse Lewy body disease (DLBD) from Alzheimer's disease: Light and electron microscopic immunocytochemistry of CA2–3 neurites specific to DLBD. *Neurology* 41:1402–1409, 1991.

220. Wilson RS, Bennett DA, Gilley DW, et al: Progression of parkinsonian signs in Alzheimer's disease. *Neurology* 54:1284–1289, 2000.

221. Chui HC, Teng EL, Henderson VW, Moy AC: Clinical subtypes of dementia of the Alzheimer type. *Neurology* 35:1544–1550, 1985.

222. Kischka U, Mandir AS, Ghika J, Growdon JH: Electrophysiologic detection of extrapyramidal motor signs in Alzheimer's disease. *Neurology* 43:500–505, 1993.

223. Clark CM, Ewbank D, Lerner A, et al: The relationship between extrapyramidal signs and cognitive performance in patients with Alzheimer's disease enrolled in the CERAD Study. Consortium to Establish a Registry for Alzheimer's Disease. *Neurology* 49:70–75, 1997.

224. Mayeux R, Stern Y, Spanton S: Heterogeneity in dementia of the Alzheimer type: Evidence of subgroups. *Neurology* 35:453–461, 1985.

225. Ravindran J, Stewart BJ, Siemens P, et al: Chorea as a presenting feature of Alzheimer's disease. *Can J Neurol Sci* 21:S67, 1994 (abstract).

226. Weiner WJ, Lang AE: Other akinetic-rigid and related syndromes, in Weiner WJ, Lang AE (eds): *Movement Disorders: A Comprehensive Survey.* Mt. Kisco, NY: Futura, 1989, pp 192–195.

227. Lang AE, Riley DE, Bergeron C: Cortical-basal ganglionic degeneration, in Calne DB (ed): *Neurogenerative Diseases.* Philadelphia: WB Saunders, 1994, pp 877–894.

228. Brunt ER, van Weerden TW, Pruim J, Lakke JWPF: Unique myoclonic pattern in corticobasal degeneration. *Mov Disord* 10:132–142, 1995.

229. Lang AE, Bergeron C, Pollanen MS, Ashby P: Parietal Pick's disease mimicking cortical-basal ganglionic degeneration. *Neurology* 44:1436–1440, 1994.

230. Kertesz A, Hudson L, Mackenzie IRA, Munoz DG: The pathology and nosology of primary progressive aphasia. *Neurology* 44:2065–2072, 1994.

231. Jendroska K, Rossor MN, Mathias CJ, Daniel SE: Morphological overlap between corticobasal degeneration and Pick's disease: A clinicopathological report. *Mov Disord* 10:111–114, 1995.

232. McKim WA, Mishara BL: Prescription and over-the-counter drugs, in Hines L, Turner J, Kee L, et al (eds): *Drugs and Aging.* Toronto: Butterworths, 1987, pp 17–40.

233. McKim WA, Mishara BL: Age-related changes in absorption, distribution, excretion and sensitivity to drugs, in Hines L, Turner J, Kee L, et al (eds): *Drugs and Aging.* Toronto: Butterworths, 1987, pp 7–15.

234. The Parkinson Study Group: Effect of deprenyl on the progression of disability in early Parkinson's disease. *N Engl J Med* 321:1364–1371, 1989.

MOVEMENT DISORDERS SPECIFIC TO SLEEP AND THE NOCTURNAL MANIFESTATIONS OF WAKING MOVEMENT DISORDERS

DAVID B. RYE and DONALD L. BLIWISE

NORMAL MOVEMENT IN SLEEP   855
MOVEMENT DISORDERS SPECIFIC TO SLEEP   856
    Periodic Leg Movements in Sleep/Restless
      Legs Syndrome (PLMs/RLS)   856
    Rapid Eye Movement Sleep Behavior Disorder
      (RBD)   859
OTHER MOVEMENT DISORDERS SPECIFIC
  TO SLEEP   861
    Fragmentary NREM Sleep Myoclonus   861
    Paroxysmal Nocturnal Dystonia (PND)   861
    Head Banging (Jactatio Capitis Nocturna)
      and Body Rocking   862
    Bruxism   862
    Sleeptalking (Somniloquy)   862
    Sleepwalking (Somnambulism)   862
    Night Terrors (Pavor Nocturnus)   863
    Nocturnal Eating   863
    General Considerations on the Treatment of Other
      Movement Disorders Specific to Sleep   863
SLEEP IN WAKING MOVEMENT DISORDERS   863
    Sleep in Parkinson's Disease (PD)   863
    Treatment   867
    Sleep in Other Waking Movement Disorders   874
    Treatment of Disturbed Sleep in Waking
      Movement Disorders   875
MECHANISMS CONTRIBUTING TO DISTURBED
  SLEEP IN WAKING MOVEMENT DISORDERS   875
    Role of Dopamine in Behavioral State Control   875
    Significance of Extranigral Pathology, Including
      the Ascending Reticular Activating System, to
      Behavioral State Control Abnormalities in PD   876
    Role of the Basal Ganglia in Behavioral State
      Control   877

In this chapter we review nonepileptiform movement disorders in sleep. The disorders reviewed encompass an extraordinarily wide range of movements and behaviors. For ease of presentation, we have divided this review into movement disorders known to be specific to sleep versus those movement disorders that are characteristic of wakefulness but which may be modulated by sleep. Additionally, we focus on practical guidelines for treatment which are, in part, driven by anatomic and physiological considerations of movement in sleep, using Parkinson's disease (PD) as the prototypical disorder. The similarity of the sleep-related manifestations of many of these disorders and their assumed common underlying pathophysiology lead to treatment considerations that are parallel, despite heterogeneity of waking clinical disease. In fact, it is our belief that the various states of sleep may represent an exquisitely sensitive window on the functional anatomy and pharmacology of the basal ganglia and related structures, which may enhance our knowledge of the mechanisms underlying these conditions.

Much of our knowledge of sleep and movement disorders derives from studies on small groups of patients, including many reports of individual patients. There are sparingly few comprehensive studies that (1) evaluate the natural history of disordered sleep in various movement disorders; (2) control adequately for all variables that may confound clinical presentation, including aging, dementia, and affective state; and (3) evaluate response to treatment in a placebo-controlled fashion. This is not surprising, given the existence of multiple interacting variables that hinder identification of homogeneous patient populations. Moreover, complex combinations of pathology in brain regions such as the basal forebrain, raphe nuclei, locus ceruleus, and pedunculopontine nucleus occur in many movement disorders and would be expected to contribute appreciably to the manifestations of most of the conditions discussed below.

Normal Movement in Sleep

In order to define abnormal quantities or qualities of nocturnal movement, it is first necessary to establish the parameters of what constitutes normal movement during sleep. In some cases (e.g., paroxysmal nocturnal dystonia (PND) or rapid eye movement (REM) sleep behavior disorder, RBD), the pattern and amplitude of movement are clearly abnormal. Conversely, in other cases, either by virtue of the widespread prevalence of a condition (e.g., periodic leg movements in sleep, PLMs) or its transient expression during development (e.g., somnambulism), defining the limits of normality may be problematic. Undoubtedly, some of the complexity stems from the varying sensitivities of the techniques used to detect movements; that is, can they be documented videographically, or do they require more sophisticated detection methods, such as accelerometers (e.g., actigraphy), or surface, or even needle electromyography (EMG)? Muscle activity recorded from surface electrodes, as is used in most polysomnographic studies, for example, may reveal some information regarding individual motor units when those units are not deeply distributed, but, in other situations involving higher threshold force or when the muscle group of interest is further from skin, surface EMG may be insufficient.[1] Additionally, determining whether movement in sleep is focal or is a manifestation of a more complex pattern of movement adds another dimension of complexity. Polysomnographic studies often rely on surface EMG recordings of only several muscle groups (mentalis, anterior tibialis), which may show somewhat different patterns of activation relative to other muscles. Using actigraphic measures, for example, Van Hilten et al.[2] have shown that the upper limbs consistently reflect more movement during sleep relative to body trunk.

Although most skeletal muscles show reduced tonic activity during sleep,[3,4] it has long been known that the body of the sleeper is far from still throughout the night. Seminal studies from the first part of this century by Kleitman et al.[4] and Johnson et al.,[5] using primitive techniques, confirmed that the average sleeper exhibits from 40–50 movements during a night of sleep. Later work, using video time-lapse photography, confirmed these findings.[6] Gardner and Grossman[7] have maintained that gross body movements represent the endpoints of afferent stimulation as the sleeper adjusts position to maintain comfort. For example, a hard bed surface has been associated with a larger number of body movements relative to a more comfortable bed.[8] Generally, however, the characteristic number of such gross body movements during sleep has been demonstrated to be a relatively stable individual trait[9] that predicts change in sleep state,[10] decreases during postsleep deprivation recovery sleep,[11] and is often preceded by autonomic activation.[12]

In contrast to these gross body movements are brief twitches of distal limb muscles also known to occur during sleep. These were originally described in humans by De Lisi,[13] and have been associated with both sleep onset ("hypnic jerks" or "sleep starts")[14] and REM sleep, as recorded both in the finger,[15] in the leg,[16] and in the mimetic muscles.[17,18] Middle-ear muscle activity has been investigated extensively during sleep, and has been shown to relate at above chance levels with motor activity in the face, neck, and extremities.[19,20] Brief isolated twitches in REM sleep have also been described in normal animals, including the cat[21] and baboon.[22] In humans, they have been likened to fasciculations and are without pathological significance.[23] Fasciculations in patients with lower motor neuron disease appear unaffected by sleep.[24]

Although limb jerks and twitches can be seen in normal sleepers, an increasingly large body of evidence suggests that waking movement disorders in general and disorders of the basal ganglia specifically may be characterized by excessive amounts of such activity within sleep.[25–27] Parkinsonian patients undergoing long-term L-dopa therapy are known to demonstrate myoclonic-like limb activity.[28] Such activation of motor systems during sleep in basal ganglia disorders may be distinguished from the normal activity during sleep described above because of its duration, frequency, and/or widespread distribution across muscle groups.

A more complete description of these movements, as well as potential mechanisms underlying their occurrence, will be explored in greater detail below.

Movement Disorders Specific to Sleep

In recent years, the development of the multidisciplinary field of sleep disorders has led clinicians and researchers to examine movement patterns during sleep. In this section we briefly review many of the movement disorders confined to sleep or, in some cases, those exacerbated by sleep. The enormous range and rich panoply of movements observed in otherwise neurologically normal individuals challenges the assumption that human sleep is a period of virtual quiescence.

PERIODIC LEG MOVEMENTS IN SLEEP/RESTLESS LEGS SYNDROME (PLMs/RLS)

Originally coined "nocturnal myoclonus" by Symonds in 1953, periodic leg movements during sleep (PLMs) are repetitive, stereotypic, nonepileptiform movements of the lower limbs unique to sleep. The conventional definition requires that each movement lasts between 0.5 and 5.0 s, with a frequency of 1 every 20–40 s.[29] PLMs seldom occur in the upper limbs.[16,30–32] Movements typically consist of uni- or bilateral ankle dorsiflexion that occurs in clusters and can be followed by arousal on the electroencephalogram (EEG) as manifested by K-complexes, bursts of alpha activity or lightening of sleep stages. They are most common in light (stages 1 and 2) non-REM (NREM) sleep, when compared to deep (stages 3 and 4) NREM and REM sleep.[33] PLMs are clearly more prevalent in the aged population[34] without demonstrating a gender proclivity. Although PLMs are frequently associated with brief arousals from sleep that result in sleep fragmentation and, sometimes, profound excessive daytime sleepiness (EDS), the patient suffering with PLMs is just as likely to complain of insomnia.[35–37] Because the prevalence of PLMs approaches 50 percent of the geriatric population,[35,36] they may represent a common endpoint of many different medical conditions. For example, folate or iron deficiency and renal failure have been associated with PLMs, and a history of prior alcohol use may be a contributing factor.[38] Other etiologic factors potentially important in modulating PLMs include lumbosacral stenosis,[39] and limb position.[40]

The underlying neurophysiological mechanisms for PLMs remain enigmatic. Nerve conductions[32,41] and sensory-evoked potentials[42] are normal in patients with PLMs, suggesting that a primary afferent sensory disturbance is not at play. Cinematography has shown that PLMs resemble a Babinski response; however, during wakefulness this pathological response is generally absent.[43,44] Others have implicated brainstem dysfunction in noting a long-latency component of the blink reflex.[42,45] The remarkably constant 20–40-s periodicity of leg movements mimics and even coincides with alterations in blood pressure,[46,47] respiration, intraventricular pressure, pulse frequency and electroencephalogram (EEG) arousal, suggesting the presence of an underlying central nervous system pacemaker. Neuropharmacological hypotheses regarding the pathophysiological basis of PLMs derive in part from the observed therapeutic benefits of dopaminomimetics and opioids.[48] A recent study[49,50] has suggested that impaired dopaminergic neurotransmission underlying PLMs reflects a decreased density of D2 receptors in the basal ganglia. It is premature, however, to rule out other potential substrates as contributors to the pathophysiology of PLMs, because dopaminergic and opioid systems interact outside of the basal ganglia in the brainstem and spinal cord.

The restless legs syndrome (RLS) is a nosological entity distinct from PLMs that was first described by Ekbom.[51,52] A great majority (>90 percent)[53] of patients with RLS, however, also experience PLMs, and, because associated risk factors and treatment strategies are common to both conditions, they are commonly discussed together. The RLS manifests as a distressing urge to move the legs (akathisia), usually accompanied by disagreeable leg sensations. These sensations are perceived variably as "pins and needles," a "crawling sensation," and even as a deep-seated "fullness" in the calves. Additional clinical criteria for the diagnosis of RLS demand that the need to move/sensory disturbance are: (1) brought on by rest (sitting or lying down); (2) relieved by moving or walking; and (3) worse at night or in the evening (versus a "protected" window around 10 am). Because vigorous leg movements or walking bring some relief, sleep onset is markedly delayed. Symptoms may also occur after awakenings that are spontaneous or possibly precipitated by PLMs and, therefore, interfere with sleep continuity as well. RLS should be distinguished from nocturnal leg cramps (systremma), generalized or neuroleptic-induced anxiety/akithisia, and hypotensive akathisia manifesting as "leg fidgeting" in autonomic failure.[54] Nocturnal leg cramps are thought to reflect muscle spasms secondary to excessive muscular fatigue and salt loss, and are typically treated with quinine, electrolyte repletion, or skeletal muscle relaxants, more or less successfully.[55,56] Some patients with RLS have been reported to experience leg cramps as well.[57] Generalized akithisia can be differentiated from RLS as it is perceived of as an "inner," generalized, psychic sensation versus a focal, sensorimotor disturbance, and fails to demonstrate a circadian pattern of expression. Hypotensive akithisia typically only occurs while seated (versus lying), and fails to demonstrate a circadian pattern of expression. The International Classification of Sleep Disorders[58] schematizes the severity of RLS as: mild, if symptoms occur episodically and are associated with only mild sleep disruption; moderate, if symptoms occur less than twice a week and cause moderate sleep disruption and mild impairment of daytime functioning; and severe, if symptoms occur more than twice a week and result in severe disruption of sleep patterns and marked daytime symptoms.

RLS is common with estimated prevalences of 2–15 percent, and is slightly more common in women and probably in individuals of Northern European descent.[58,59] The disorder can occur at any age, but symptoms often begin in middle-age with the mean age of onset being between 27 and 41 years.[60,61] Approximately 40 percent of RLS patients first experience symptoms before the age of 20.[53,58,62] The condition has also been described in children.[63–65] A prominent familial component has been suspected ever since Ekbom's seminal description of RLS in 1945.[52] Positive family histories are obtainable in 40–60 percent of affected individuals,[53,61,62,66] with first-degree relatives afflicted 25–40 percent of the time. Several clinical features help distinguish individuals suffering with familial RLS, including: symptom onset before the age of 30; exacerbation during pregnancy; and sensitivity to alcohol.[66–68] The mode of inheritance in familial RLS seems to be autosomal-dominant with the causative factor appearing to be a single major gene.[68] This confirms and extends an earlier study revealing a high concordance rate for RLS between identical twins,[69] despite reports that expression of the full RLS spectrum (e.g., onset of symptoms) can vary between twins and within families.[69–71] Many other cases of RLS, best characterized as "sporadic," typically appear in later life (>50 years of age), cannot be as readily identified as familial, and often are termed "secondary" due to identifiable aggravating factors (see below).

The hunt for causative genes has been taken up within areas of four genetically distinct populations (Quebec, Northern Italy, Germany, and Iceland). A major susceptibility locus has been reported on a region on the long arm of chromosome 12 in French-Canadians.[72] The significance of this finding is unclear, however, because linkage required assumption of a recessive versus dominant mode of inheritance, linkage could not be confirmed in some kindreds, and the results could not be replicated in two large families from South Tyrol.[73,74] Genetic linkage of RLS to a region on the long arm of chromosome 14 has been demonstrated in a 30-member, three-generation Italian family with an autosomal-dominant mode of inheritance.[75] Of particular relevance in this study was characterization of RLS as a phenotypic spectrum including PLM lacking subjective appreciation of restless legs, and the fact that two additional large families lacked linkage to either the 12q or 14q loci. Thus, increasingly RLS appears to be a complex disorder likely to be influenced by many, rather than a single, genetic factors.

PLM disorder is also seen with other primary sleep disorders such as narcolepsy,[76] insomnia, hypersomnia, central[77] and obstructive sleep apnea[78] syndrome, REM behavior disorder,[79,80] and fibromyalgia.[81,82] There are three, well-accepted "secondary" forms of RLS/PLM that are reversible: (1) pregnancy; (2) renal failure; and (3) anemia.[83] Recently, RLS and PLM disorders in children have been associated with attention-deficit/hyperactivity disorder.[63–65]

It is likely that RLS and PLM disorders share a common pathophysiological basis as they frequently coexist and respond to the same medications. The final common pathway mediating PLM are neural elements intrinsic to the spinal cord given their unveiling below the level of pontine infarction,[84] or spinal cord transection or pathology.[85–88] A strict derivation from a spinal locomotor network common to many vertebrates is unlikely because leg movements detected by standard surface electrodes placed over both anterior tibialis muscles most often occur simultaneously (versus alternately), can exhibit co-contraction with antagonists (viz. gastrocnemius;[87] personal observations), and may coincide with changes in the activity of upper limb or bulbar musculature (personal observations). Identification of a single neurophysiological mechanism underlying PLM remains enigmatic although the principal deficit manifests as brainstem[42,89] and spinal reflex "hyperexcitability."[90] The origin of this enhancement of motoneuron output must ultimately derive from a source that can account for the circadian quality and state dependency of RLS/PLM. In this regard, the recent delineation of state-dependent changes in spinal cord excitability in RLS/PLM is of fundamental importance.[90] These changes manifest as: (1) decreased threshold of the flexor reflex; and (2) segmental spread of the flexor reflex (from distal to proximal muscles). The pathophysiology of RLS/PLM does not reside in the principal sensory and motor elements themselves, based upon observations that waking EMG activity, resting motoneuron excitability, simple reflexes, and sensory-evoked potentials are generally normal.[42,91] Diffuse peripheral nerve dysfunction is nonetheless common, and may be an important modifier of RLS/PLM expression.[61,92–94] The most powerful and consistent influences impacting upon RLS/PLM originate from outside the spinal cord, in supraspinal, premotor circuits. This is best exemplified in the setting of spinal cord injury, where pharmacologic agents effective in treating RLS/PLM and dampening flexor reflex responses via local spinal circuits (e.g., dopaminomimetics and opioids), are generally, but not universally, ineffective.[87,88] This argues that the primary benefit is mediated predominantly by alternate, dopaminergic or dopamine-sensitive pathways located supraspinally. Thus, imaging studies, clinical observations, and animal studies have focused principally upon the nigrostriatal component of the mesotelencephalic dopamine system as a potential key substrate in the pathogenesis of RLS/PLM. Reductions in dopamine uptake via the dopamine transporter into presynaptic axons,[95] and D2 receptor binding[49,95] seen in some imaging studies suggest a relative excess of extracellular dopamine. However, the magnitude of these changes is small and has not been confirmed.[96]

PLM also occur when the striatum is depleted of dopamine axons either in the experimental setting,[97] or in the face of neurodegeneration occurring with PD.[98,99] That RLS/PLM could be attributed to enhanced extracellular striatal dopamine, but also occur in the setting of striatal dopamine loss, is paradoxical. This might be reconciled if one posits that primary/idiopathic RLS/PLM reflects suboptimal striatal dopaminergic signaling at postsynaptic, rather than presynaptic, sites. This would account for observations that the prevalence of RLS in PD patients lacking intact nigrostriatal dopaminergic axons mirrors that observed in the general population.[100] Alternatively, this could point to the principal pathophysiology residing outside dopaminergic nigrostriatal pathways (e.g., in dopaminergic diencephalospinal pathways). As these pathways terminate largely in the dorsal horn where they likely inhibit superficial and deep tissue afferents, their dysfunction would provide the most parsimonious, unifying explanation for augmentation of the flexor reflex observed in RLS, and the occurrence of abnormal sensations. Only one very preliminary experimental study has tested whether dopaminergic diencephalospinal pathway lesions can induce RLS/PLM.[101] While the findings are suggestive, they lack adequate behavioral analysis and a comprehensive accounting of the synaptic, cellular, and network mechanisms responsible.

TREATMENT

Because PLMs/RLS is associated with a variety of other conditions, including myelopathies, neuropathies, anemia, uremia, and iron deficiency (even in the absence of anemia), these entities should be carefully screened for and properly treated, when present. Of these, increasing interest has focused on iron deficiency because iron deficiency occurs at a higher frequency among patients with later-life onset of RLS,[67,102] brain iron deficiency may be a critical factor in the pathology of RLS,[83,103] and iron repletion can lead to long-term clinical improvement.[51,104,105] Testing for iron deficiency should therefore be performed routinely, particularly in the patient with later-life onset of RLS/PLM. The single best assessment of iron "stores" is obtained with serum ferritin. Serum ferritin levels in the range of 20 μg/L and iron saturations of less than 16 percent are indicative of rather significant depletion of iron stores, with values under 50 μg/L still suggestive. When identified, iron deficiency is treated with 65 mg of elemental iron (e.g., 325 mg of ferrous sulfate) together with 100 mg of vitamin C on an empty stomach three to four times a day. Oral supplementation should be continued for 3–4 months until ferritin levels exceed 50 μg/L and iron saturations surpass 20 percent. Many patients will be able to discontinue symptomatic relief once iron has been repleted. Additional treatment strategies for RLS are generally the same as those for PLMs. Nonpharmacological approaches include encouraging abstinence from caffeine, an agent that reportedly worsens RLS but not PLMs.[106] Alcohol and a variety of antidepressants make the condition more severe and should also be avoided if possible. Our clinical impression that antidepressants with serotonin (5-hydroxytryptamine, 5-HT) and/or norepinephrine reuptake blocking activity demonstrate a proclivity to increase PLM has been confirmed by others;[107–109] yet it remains unclear how often exacerbation of RLS/PLM is encountered in the general neuropsychiatric patient population.

Symptomatic relief for the principal features of RLS/PLM is very much dependent upon the timing, frequency, severity, and quality of symptoms. There are four well-established treatments for PLMs/RLS: dopaminomimetics, gabapentin, opioid agonists, and benzodiazepines (Table 52-1). Dopaminomimetics are now widely considered the first line of treatment for RLS/PLM.[110] Gabapentin and opioids also suppress PLMs,[111–114] whereas benzodiazepines improve sleep continuity only by decreasing arousals without decreasing the number of PLMs.[48,115]

Regular (versus sustained-release) carbidopa/L-dopa is an excellent choice for patients with sporadic, infrequent symptoms given a short delay (15–20 minutes) to reach effectiveness when taken on an empty stomach. Chronic use of this medication should be avoided as worsening of symptoms occurs in approximately 80 percent of subjects at some interval after initial improvement (viz. "rebound" or "augmentation").[116] In patients with moderate-to-severe RLS/PLM, well-controlled clinical trials have demonstrated long-term efficacy of dopamine agonists such as pergolide (mean effective dose about 0.5 mg),[117–120] pramipexole (mean effective dose about 0.375 mg),[121,122] and ropinirole

TABLE 52-1 Treatment Regimens for PLMs/RLS

Medication	Dose
Dopamine precursors	
Levodopa/carbidopa	25/100, 50/200 CR before bedtime and during sleep
Dopamine Agonists	
Pergolide (Permax)	0.05–1.0 mg HS
Pramipexole (Mirapex)	0.125–1.5 mg HS
Ropinirole (Requip)	1–4 mg HS (taken in divided dosages at intervals before bedtime)
Anticonvulsants	
Gabapentin (Neurontin)	200–1800 mg HS (divided doses)
Carbamazepine (Tegretol)	200–400 mg HS
Opiods	
Oxycodone	5 mg HS
Codeine	15–60 mg HS
Propoxyphene (Darvon)	200 mg HS
Tramadol hydrochloride (Ultram)	50–200 mg HS
Benzodiazepines	
Clonazepam (Klonopin)	0.5–3.0 mg HS
Temazepam (Restoril)	15–30 mg HS
Triazolam (Halcion)	0.25 mg HS
Miscellaneous	
Clonidine (Catapres)	0.1–0.9 mg daily
Bromocriptine (Parodel)	5–15 mg
Iron	325 mg of ferrous sulfate 2–3 times/day
Vitamin B_{12}	100 μg/day for 6–7 days with follow-up doses
Folic acid	0.4–1.0 mg daily
Magnesium	100–840 mg/day

(mean effective dose about 1.5 mg).[123,124] We frequently recommend divided dosing (dinner and bedtime), or dosing several hours before typical symptom onset, because dopamine agonists take at least 2 hours to reach their peak effect. Dosing should be titrated to subjective relief, although increasingly it is recognized that some degree of PLM disorders may still exist (manifesting as fragmented sleep or daytime sleepiness), albeit significantly reduced from pretreatment levels. Common side-effects include nausea and orthostatic hypotension, with insomnia, nasal congestion, and peripheral edema encountered less frequently. Augmentation of RLS has been less frequently encountered with dopamine agonists (10–20 percent),[119,120] but this may simply reflect relatively recent changes in treatment patterns. In patients in whom pain is a predominant symptom, or who have neuropathy or parkinsonism, we advocate the use of gabapentin (600–1800 mg in divided doses) because it benefits both subjective and objective features of RLS/PLM.[114] We reserve the use of tramadol (50–200 mg), oxycodone (5–15 mg), or propoxyphene (65–100 mg) for patients with a prominent component of pain, or for those who are refractory to the above approaches in order to avoid the development of tolerance and dependence. We have also noted beneficial effects with other opioids, including hydrocodone, codeine, and methadone. Several other treatments have been proposed for PLMs, but few of them have been systematically evaluated (see Table 52-1). Successes have also been reported with valproate,[125] and gabapentin (200–1800 mg qhs).[114,126] We generally reserve use of benzodiazepines, such as clonazepam (0.5–2.0 mg), temazepam (15–30 mg) or triazolam (0.125–0.375 mg) at least 1 hour before bedtime, as adjuvant treatments. These agents have proven most useful in combination with other treatments in those patients who present with a component of psychophysiologic insomnia possibly reflecting years of inadequate treatment of RLS symptoms.

RAPID EYE MOVEMENT SLEEP BEHAVIOR DISORDER (RBD)

In the mid-1980s, Schenck et al. described patients (predominantly older males in their 50s and 60s) with purposeful nocturnal motor activity, often violent in nature, that resembled dream enactment.[127] This condition, now termed rapid eye movement behavior disorder (RBD), is "... characterized by the intermittent loss of REM sleep EMG atonia and by the appearance of elaborate motor activity associated with dream mentation."[64] The behaviors are nonstereotypic, emotionally laden, and semipurposeful. Frequently these are accompanied by vocalization and are violent in nature, appearing to correlate with defensive dream content. These behaviors are differentiated from other parasomnias by their nonstereotypy, coincidence with dream recall, restriction to REM sleep, and nonepileptiform nature. Differentiating RBD from panic attacks or nocturnal terrors by history alone can be problematic given variability in dream recall. Panic attacks and terrors, however, arise from stage 2 at the transition to stage 3 and from stage 3/4 sleep, respectively.[128] Nocturnal motor behavior with lack of dream recall, abrupt arousal accompanied by diffuse autonomic symptoms, and amnesia for the event suggest the diagnosis of panic attacks. Nocturnal terrors also manifest with extreme autonomic activation and retrograde amnesia; however, motor behaviors are usually more pronounced and marked by confusion and violence on attempted arousal.[75] There is a strong male predominance (at least 4:1) for RBD and relationship to neurodegenerative diseases,[129] particularly parkinsonian conditions such as idiopathic PD,[130,131] dementia with Lewy bodies (DLB),[132-135] multiple-system atrophy (MSA),[136] and olivopontocerebellar degeneration (OPCD),[137] more commonly than progressive supranuclear palsy (PSP),[138] corticobasal ganglionic[139] and striatonigral degenerations, and spinocerebellar ataxia type 3 (Machado-Joseph disease).[140-142] Nocturnal motor dyscontrol including RBD is also frequently encountered in narcolepsy-cataplexy,[80] and in many neurologic conditions that affect the brainstem.[130,137,143,144] Numerous pharmacological agents in humans have been associated with some loss of REM atonia, including tricyclic antidepressants, monoamine oxidase inhibitors, monoamine reuptake inhibitors, and alcohol.[145-149]

Diagnosis is often made through the clinical history and home videotapes because of intranight and internight variability in expression. A definitive diagnosis may necessitate video NPSG with an expanded EEG montage to rule out nocturnal frontal lobe epileptic variants. The polysomnogram (PSG) in the prototypical RBD patient demonstrates aperiodic and periodic movements in NREM sleep, and particularly elevated tonic and phasic EMG activity in REM sleep.[130,150-152] Elevated amounts of stages 3 and 4 NREM sleep have been noted in idiopathic RBD as well. Despite a compelling history, the NPSG may fail to capture the overt behavioral manifestations of RBD or even the heightened muscle activity in REM sleep because of variability in expression.

Pathophysiological insights have their origin in a feline disease model that predates clinical recognition of RBD. The dorsolateral pons inclusive of the subceruleal region has been the focus of much attention since bilateral lesions here release elaborate behavior suggestive of dream enactment in cats[153,154] (see Fig. 52-6). The absence of REM atonia in cats correlates best with degree of loss of glutamatergic versus cholinergic neurons in the subceruleal region.[155] The subceruleal region is extremely heterogeneous anatomically, neurochemically, and physiologically, with significant interspecies variability, making it difficult to confidently discern the substrates responsible for RBD with precision. It is tempting to implicate neurons intrinsic to this region as the ultimate mediators of RBD since they exhibit REM sleep-specific increases in discharge and descending pathways to ventromedial medullary regions essential in maintaining REM atonia. When these pathways are interrupted, REM sleep-specific motor behaviors can be seen in humans.[130,137,143,144] The most parsimonious explanation for RBD therefore posits that it derives from loss of REM sleep-specific glutamatergic

drive to atonia generating premotor, glycinergic elements in the ventromedial medulla. Alternatively, enhanced phasic and tonic REM sleep-specific motor activity and a continuum to dream enactment behaviors may reflect increased excitatory drive to motor circuits from supratentorial brain regions (e.g., the basal ganglia, and ventral forebrain) that modulate emotive behaviors and exhibit multisynaptic connections with the ventromedial medulla by way of the dorsolateral mesopontine tegmentum. This is supported by several observations, including: (1) cats with RBD exhibit significant increases in open field, exploratory activity in wake;[156] (2) drugs that enhance prolocomotor monoaminergic neurotransmission can release or exacerbate RBD[147-149] (personal observations); and (3) there is a paradoxically heightened REM sleep-specific, serotonergic neural activity in cats exhibiting RBD features.[157]

As RBD predates or accompanies diseases that share in common waking features of parkinsonism, it has been suggested that the pathophysiological basis of RBD may lie in loss of noradrenergic subceruleal or cholinergic pedunculopontine tegmental nucleus (PPN) region neurons given their frequent involvement by the primary pathology of many neurodegenerative conditions. This hypothesis, however, is inconsistent with experimental work. Loss of noradrenergic function, for example, might be expected to promote atonia rather than eliminate it,[158] whereas loss of cholinergic PPN neurons would be expected to result in loss, rather than enhancement, of phasic motor elements of REM sleep.[155] Alternatively, abnormal signals impinging upon the dorsolateral mesopontine tegmentum, including the subceruleal region, may alter neural responsivity, thereby releasing RBD. As the particular behavior released in REM sleep in cats depends upon the site and size of lesions[154,159] in a brain region exhibiting a wide array of forebrain afferents,[160] there are potentially numerous structures in the hypothalamus, amygdala or basal ganglia that might modify RBD. Of these structures that link themselves with lower motor centers via the dorsolateral pons, clinical and experimental evidence argues that the basal ganglia nuclei may be most relevant to the pathophysiology of "idiopathic" RBD. Each of the neurodegenerative conditions in which RBD is commonly observed, for example, share in common loss of nigrostriatal dopamine pathways, and imaging studies in "idiopathic" RBD demonstrate loss of dopamine transporter activity in nigrostriatal axons but no detectable alterations of D2 receptor density.[161,162] Rats[97] and nonhuman primates[163] depleted of striatal dopamine lack overt behavioral manifestations suggestive of RBD, but do exhibit heightened phasic and tonic somatomotor activity in REM sleep that predominates in limb versus axial musculature (personal observations). Enhancement of phasic motor phenomena of REM sleep ultimately derives from transient hyperpolarization of subpopulations of glutamatergic and cholinergic PPN region neurons that exhibit low-threshold calcium spikes, as might be expected given pathologically elevated phasic bursting of gamma-aminobutyric acid (GABA)ergic basal ganglia output nuclei in PD.[164,165] Enhancement of tonic EMG activity in REM sleep, on the other hand, may reflect excessive inhibition of alternate subpopulations of glutamatergic and cholinergic neurons whose REM sleep-specific activation is otherwise necessary for engaging REM atonia premotor elements in the ventromedial medulla. Thus, removal of excessive, inhibitory pallidal influences upon the upper brainstem by pallidotomy might account for reversal of REM sleep elevations in somatomotor activity observed in some PD patients[166] (personal observations). Pharmacologic dampening of pathologic pallidal firing with low doses of L-dopa/carbidopa may similarly account for the reported benefits of this agent in treating RBD.[130,167] Reversal of RBD by surgical and pharmacologic interventions is by no means universal, and is increasingly viewed as the exception rather than the rule. Bilateral subthalamic nucleus stimulation, for example, appears ineffective in reversing RBD[168,169] (A Iranzo, personal communication), while treatment with L-dopa/carbidopa may enhance rather than suppress REM sleep-specific EMG activity early in the course of PD.[170] These mixed experiences likely reflect the heterogeneous nature of parkinsonian pathologies, the complicated effects of dopamine upon behavioral state-related muscle activity (see below), and our relative lack of knowledge concerning the full spectrum of parkinsonian-related neuropathological alterations. The novel suggestion that disease burden in idiopathic PD progresses rostralward from the medulla[171] is particularly germaine to the clinicopathophysiology of parkinsonian-related RBD. Early involvement of REM atonia regions in the ventromedial medulla, for example, might account for the fact that RBD can presage overt waking manifestations of PD by years, and the ineffectiveness of surgical interventions in universally reversing RBD.

TREATMENT

Treatment of RBD needs to be highly individualized and includes avoidance of suspected aggravators such as caffeine, nicotine, alcohol, sleep deprivation, antidepressants with significant blockade of serotonin or norepinephrine reuptake, and traditional antidopaminergic compounds. Many patients' RBD symptoms are particularly negatively affected by D2 receptor dopamine agonists, but, somewhat counterintuitively, responsive to low doses of L-dopa/carbidopa (25/100–50/200 qhs) early in the disease course. Clonazepam (0.5–2.0 mg qhs), however, remains the mainstay of treatment as it is reportedly effective in 75–90 percent of patients.[129,130] Inadequate treatment responses may necessitate adjunctive treatment with low doses of L-dopa/carbidopa (25/100 qhs), or the atypical antipsychotic quetiapine (37.5–75 mg qhs). In DLB the quetiapine dose may need to be increased to 200 mg qhs. Improvement has been noted in a small experience with donepezil.[172] Limited experience with melatonin also suggests that it may be beneficial in some patients experiencing RBD.[173–175] Because RBD may result in serious injury to patients and bed partners, management should

also employ measures to insure safe sleeping arrangements, including: removal of objects from nightstands, placement of pillows on the bedside floor, alternative sleeping arrangements for the bed partner, and using beds with padded bedrails.

Other Movement Disorders Specific to Sleep

FRAGMENTARY NREM SLEEP MYOCLONUS

Broughton et al.[176] have reported on brief (150 ms) bursts of potentials of 50–250 mV amplitude occurring in seemingly random fashion throughout NREM sleep. Unlike PLMs, which are confined to the lower limbs,[32] these potentials are less prolonged and occur in widespread fashion in various limbs bilaterally and in different muscle groups. In most cases, visible movements are not noted. Fragmentary myoclonus is commonly noted as an incidental finding in patients diagnosed with other primary sleep disorders (e.g., sleep apnea, narcolepsy, insomnia), yet, since it does not systematically coincide with oxygen desaturations, appears to be a distinct entity. Fragmentary NREM sleep myoclonus is a disorder that may be associated with marked EDS.[176,177] There is insufficient information on the etiology and treatment of this specific disorder, although improvement has been noted with clonazepam (0.5–2.0 mg) at bedtime.

PAROXYSMAL NOCTURNAL DYSTONIA (PND)

Originally considered to be a movement disorder specific to sleep lacking an EEG correlate, it now appears that PND is caused by partial seizures of frontal lobe origin.[178,179] Patients experience spells that arise abruptly from NREM sleep and consist of uni- or bilateral dystonic posturing, and choreoathetoid or ballistic movements lasting 10–60 s. On some occasions, vocalizations occur.[180] Often these behaviors appear grossly "unusual" and may not suggest seizures to the inexperienced clinician despite their stereotypic quality and tendency to cluster. They may be only occasional, or recur 30–40 times nightly. A 10–40-s modal interval between attacks appears casually related to waxing and waning in thalamocortical arousability as manifest in the cyclic alternating pattern of normal NREM sleep.[181,182] In some patients, semipurposeful arm activity or even sexual automatisms may be seen. Thus, NPD patients share some features with RBD; however, the episodes in NPD clearly evolve from NREM (typically stage 4) sleep. Typical patients exhibit normal interictal EEG activity during both sleep and wakefulness.[183] Less often, spike wave complexes, often prominent in frontal regions, may be observed during a behavioral episode.[184] Diagnosis is therefore often made through the clinical history and home videotapes because localization of a frontal epileptic focus is difficult, particularly with the limited EEG montages employed by routine NPSG (nocturnal polysomnography).

A definitive diagnosis of PND (e.g., versus psychogenic seizures) may necessitate video NPSG with an expanded EEG montage, or even inpatient or outpatient video EEG monitoring. Treatment includes the use of carbamazepine (200–400 mg qhs) which seems to produce more effective results than other anticonvulsants. Treatment failures should alert one to the possibility of a primary sleep disorder, since for PND, as with any seizure disorder, sleep disruption or deprivation can increase seizure frequency.

HEAD BANGING (JACTATIO CAPITIS NOCTURNA) AND BODY ROCKING

These movement disorders may occur during NREM or REM sleep,[185,186] with more than 600 distinct movements observed on a given night. Head movements are typically anteroposterior. Occasionally head rolling, consisting of lateral movements, may also occur. Body rocking occurs with the sleeper often on his or her knees in bed with anteroposterior thrusting of the entire body into the pillow. These conditions are most typically seen in infants for whom, at the age of 9 months, a prevalence of 60 percent has been reported;[187] they are much less frequent in older children and adults. Spontaneous presentations in adults have been noted; one report implied that head banging may have resulted from closed-head injury.[188] Other variants may exist as well. A case of repetitive, nocturnal tongue biting in a 2-year-old child, occurring in slow-wave sleep and not associated with epileptiform activity in waking or sleep, has been reported by Tuxhorn and Hoppe.[189] There is no clear consensus on treatment. In severe cases with self-injurious behavior, the judicious use of clonazepam (0.5–2.0 mg) at bedtime seems warranted. In milder cases, behavioral modification that involves audio masking with a metronome may be of benefit. Overpracticing of rhythmic behavior in a rocking chair or more vigorous rhythmic exercises before retiring may be of additional benefit, and self-hypnosis has also been reported to be successful.[190]

BRUXISM

Excessively high masseter EMG activity during sleep, particularly when associated with tooth wear, temporomandibular joint pain, or destruction of dental restorations, is labeled bruxism (see Lavigne et al.[191] for a recent detailed review). Bruxism is reported by 8 percent of the adult population; it commonly occurs during both day and night, declines with age, and patients present an anxious personality (not an anxiety disorder), and are more task-oriented compared with normal controls.[192–194] Sleep duration and efficiency in bruxism patients is usually normal, with the vast majority of events (60–80 percent) occurring during light NREM sleep.[195,196] Of note, is that 75–85 percent of bruxing events co-occur with more generalized body movements, typically in the anterior tibialis.[197] Current literature supports the view that bruxism represents a terminal event in a sequence of repetitive brain

and autonomic activations termed "micro-arousal during sleep"[191,195,198] (not dissimilar from PLM).

Alcohol has been reported to increase bruxism.[199] Moreover, as for most other nocturnal movements, sleep bruxism has been associated with the use of agents that lead to excess amounts of prolocomotor monoamines, including serotonin reuptake inhibitors.[200,201] Antagonism[202] or enhancement[203,204] of dopaminergic neurotransmission has also been anecdotally noted to predispose to sleep bruxism. Lacking a comprehensive understanding of the pathophysiology of bruxism, there are no established direct treatments.[191,192] Measures should be taken to limit the morbidity associated with bruxism, such as use of mouth guards and nonsteroidal anti-inflammatory agents. Modest, but significant, reductions in sleep bruxism have recently been reported with L-dopa[205] and the beta-adrenergic receptor blocker propranolol.[206,207] These findings await confirmation with larger, double-blind studies before formal recommendation and widespread clinical use. Muscle relaxation, biofeedback, and psychotherapy may be of some benefit, but their effectiveness has not been further defined.[192]

SLEEPTALKING (SOMNILOQUY)

This phenomenon has been investigated extensively by Arkin,[208] who reported that episodes may arise from both NREM and REM sleep and have varying levels of complexity and semantic structure. There was little relationship to psychopathology. MacNeilage[209] reported that episodes of sleeptalking were preceded by an average of 10 s of muscle activity, as recorded in the genioglossus and other orobuccal muscles. Additionally, individuals who characteristically talked in their sleep showed a greater abundance of such activity, even during periods without vocalization. Vocalizations during sleep are also common during RBD and night terrors. Sleeptalking, when present without other associated parasomnic behaviors, is of unknown significance and has no known treatment.

SLEEPWALKING (SOMNAMBULISM)

Classic sleepwalking (somnambulism) was described polysomnographically in the 1960s,[210] and appears to occur largely in stage 4 sleep and not uncommonly in children. More recent reports have confirmed these findings.[211] Because the condition derives out of slow-wave sleep and often involves incomplete awakening, some have considered the condition as a disorder of arousal.[212] It is distinguished from complex partial seizures by a normal EEG during both waking and sleep. The subject remains amnestic during and after the event and, unlike the case of the complex, purposeful movements of RBD, the sleeper's movements are awkward and gangly. Somnambulism is common in children, with a prevalence as high as 39–48 percent in 4–6-year-olds noted in some epidemiological studies.[213] It is thought to be of little psychopathological consequence in childhood, although adults who sleepwalk have been reported to have schizoid tendencies.[214] Childhood trauma or posttraumatic stress disorder are risk factors. At all ages, the sleepwalker should be considered potentially dangerous to self and others. Adult sleepwalkers have been shown to have higher amounts of stages 3 and 4 sleep and have more spontaneously occurring disruptions of these stages as well.[215] There appears to be an hereditary component.[216] Somnambulism should be differentiated from the phenomenon of sundowning in geriatric patients.[217] Sleepwalking may respond to psychotherapy[218] and/or hypnosis.[211,219] Symptomatic treatment with clonazepam (0.5–2.0 mg qhs) is effective in about one-half of cases.

NIGHT TERRORS (PAVOR NOCTURNUS)

Often occurring with somnambulism with arousals from stage 4 sleep,[220] night terrors are characterized by dramatic awakenings, accompanied by extraordinarily loud vocalizations, screaming, and a heightened affective state. Tachycardia, tachypnea, sweating, and enlarged pupils have been described.[221] As is the case with somnambulism, this condition is usually seen in children rather than in adults, and may represent a transiently normal developmental event. More serious psychopathology may be implicated in adults.[222] Retrograde amnesia usually exists, although the sleeper may have a vague recollection of frightening experiences. Some potential overlap with RBD may exist. Night terrors frequently respond to diazepam or alprazolam alone or in combination with a tricyclic antidepressant, such as nortriptyline. In the elderly patient in whom benzodiazepines may induce confusion or disorientation, trazodone (25–150 mg), carbamazepine (200–300 mg), or valproate (125–500 mg) at bedtime may be of some benefit.

NOCTURNAL EATING

Of apparent similarity to RBD is a syndrome involving excessive night-time food consumption in patients without a comorbid eating disorder diagnosis in the waking state. Schenck et al.[223] and others[224,225] have described a dissociated state involving complex, purposeful motor behavior, specifically limited to eating, in several series of patients. Patients are usually amnestic for the experiences, which are identified by the patients by containers, etc., and food remnants in the morning. The few cases documented in the laboratory suggest that the awakenings may occur out of NREM, rather than REM, sleep.[225] The mainstays of treatment for nocturnal binge-eating include L-dopa/carbidopa alone or in combination with clonazepam.[224,226] Favorable response to L-dopa is thought, in part, to be related to the frequent coexistence of PLMs in these patients, so that treatments with opioids may also be indicated.[226] Favorable responses to serotonin reuptake inhibitors, representing a smaller subset of patients, have also been reported.[224,226]

GENERAL CONSIDERATIONS ON THE TREATMENT OF OTHER MOVEMENT DISORDERS SPECIFIC TO SLEEP

Historical or PSG identification of the specific form of nocturnal movement disorder will dictate the course of treatment. Once the proper diagnosis is established, the vast majority are treatable by either behavioral or pharmacological means. Because their etiologies are likely to be diverse, however, the proposed treatments are legion and usually lack validated objective results. The physician should first attempt to rule out any associated condition and/or medication that may account for nocturnal movements or parasomnic behaviors. Antidepressant medications, for example, may worsen fragmentary NREM myoclonus, whereas cardiac antiarrhythmic agents and some antidepressants may exacerbate nocturnal terrors.[227,228] Before pharmacological interventions, the physician should always council the patient and family on proper sleep hygiene, including: (1) avoidance of sleep deprivation; (2) maintenance of a strict sleep-wake schedule; and (3) avoidance of alcoholic and caffeinated beverages, as well as nicotine, secondary to their tendencies to worsen sleep fragmentation.

Sleeptalking, sleepwalking, night terrors, and nocturnal binge-eating comprise a group of parasomnias that frequently coexist.[229] One of the most important aspects of the treatment of these disorders is ruling out coexistent depression or other psychopathology, particularly in the elderly patient. A medication history is also important, because these parasomnias may be associated with long-term benzodiazepine use or withdrawal, as well as cardiac antiarrhythmic agents. A wide variety of stimuli, such as PLMs, apnea, and gastroesophageal reflux, may also present with complaints of parasomnic behavior, presumably secondary to their precipitating nocturnal arousals. PSG, therefore, is frequently indicated to consider these etiologies that demand distinct treatment strategies. Nocturnal seizures less commonly present with complaints simulating one of these parasomnias or head banging/body rocking. Video monitoring and PSG with EEG montages that are more elaborate than those typically used in routine studies are, therefore, only occasionally required for proper diagnosis.

Sleep in Waking Movement Disorders

SLEEP IN PARKINSON'S DISEASE (PD)

Disorders of sleep in patients with PD have long been recognized; however, their pathophysiological basis remains ill-defined, and universal treatment strategies have not been established. Reasons for these deficiencies are many, and they include the pathological heterogeneity of PD and coincident factors such as medication use, aging, dementia, and mood disturbances, each of which independently affect sleep parameters. The sleep of PD patients is profoundly disturbed, even relative to other neurodegenerative conditions. One survey placed the prevalence of sleep disturbance in PD at 98 percent.[230] PSG studies of PD patients, extending back into the 1960s, consistently demonstrate poor sleep efficiency, decreases in stages 3 and 4 sleep, and marked sleep fragmentation.[231–236] The sleep state-specific EEG also changes in PD, with sleep spindles being reduced during slow-wave sleep,[234,237,238] and alpha activity intruding into REM sleep.[231] Reported changes in REM sleep are variable across studies and appear highly dependent on dose and length of dopaminomimetic treatment and individual patient differences.[232–234,239–242] Given the REM sleep-suppressant effects of L-dopa,[243] many have hypothesized that REM sleep rebound underlies hallucinations experienced by many PD patients.[244–250] The recent demonstration of REM sleep intrusions into daytime naps in hallucinating and nonhallucinating patients provides electrophysiologic evidence supporting these conclusions.[251–253]

Disordered sleep in the form of excessive nocturnal movement in PD was first noted in Parkinson's 19th century *Essay on the Shaking Palsy*, and these findings have subsequently been confirmed and extended. A detailed account of previous studies and the development of this line of investigation is presented in the 1st edition of this book.[254] Despite the widely held belief that involuntary movements associated with disease of the extrapyramidal motor system disappear during sleep, motor dyscontrol in sleep in the form of tremor (Figs. 52-1 and 52-2), aperiodic (Fig. 52-3) and periodic leg movements (Fig. 52-4), increased phasic and tonic EMG activity in REM sleep (Fig. 52-3), and frank RBD predate or accompany neurodegenerative disease involving nuclei of the basal ganglia.

In summary:

1. Sleep can be punctuated by parkinsonian tremor (Figs. 52-1 and 52-2), although tremor may be preceded by microawakenings, and, during REM, isolated muscle contractions are common (Fig. 52-3).
2. NREM and REM sleep are characterized by large numbers of isolated and periodic limb movements (Fig. 52-4).
3. Stages 3 and 4 of NREM sleep are least likely to manifest movements.
4. Nocturnal movements are common in both upper and lower extremities.
5. Nocturnal movements are common in both flexor and extensor muscles.

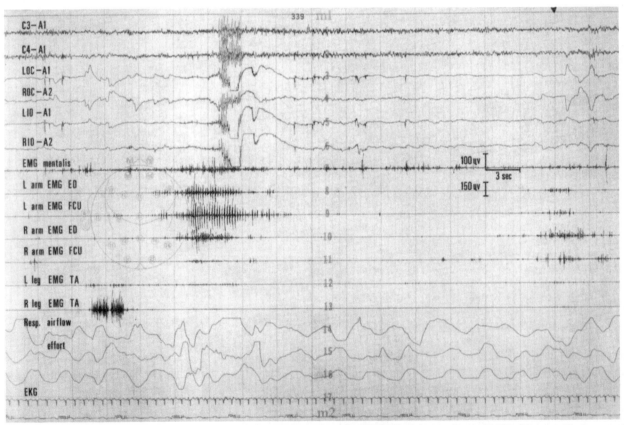

FIGURE 52-1 PSG recording of an episode of tremor intruding on an epoch of REM sleep in a patient with PD. Also note the increased level of tonic activity in the chin EMG (EMG mentalis). R, right; L, left; ED, extensor digitorum; FCU, flexor carpi ulnaris; TA, tibialis anterior.

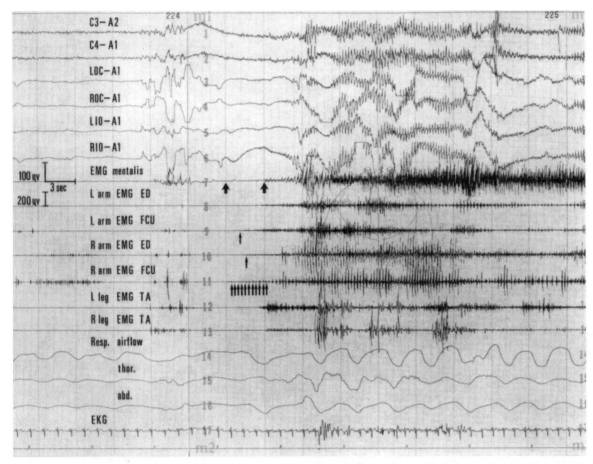

FIGURE 52-2 PSG recording of an episode of tremor intruding on REM sleep with subsequent arousal in a patient with PD. Multiple small arrows denote tremor that begins in the right flexor carpi ulnaris (FCU), coincident with the development of tonic activity in the right extensor digitorum (ED) and left flexor carpi ulnaris (small arrows). During this 3-s epoch there is no change in chin muscle activity, as detected by the mentalis EMG (two broad arrows) or in the cortical EEG. Arousal from REM sleep, therefore, clearly occurs after these EMG changes. Abbreviations are as designated in Fig. 52-1.

6. Nocturnal movements are generally best controlled when waking motor symptomatology is best treated, although movement may persist even in the presence of antiparkinsonian medication.

7. RBD can accompany and even precede waking signs of PD, as well as other degenerative conditions affecting the basal ganglia and/or brainstem.

The prevalence of nocturnal motor dyscontrol in PD is difficult to establish because most published data derive from PSG studies carried out at referral centers, thereby selecting for patients with disturbed sleep. PLMs lacking subjective RLS complaints are common in PD, occurring at a greater prevalence than in conditions lacking severe nigrostriatal dopamine neuron loss, such as aging and (AD),[98] and MSA.[99] Historical accounts from patients and their bed partners estimate that RBD in idiopathic PD is also relatively common, possibly reaching 15 percent.[151,255] The degree to which nocturnal movements contribute to sleep fragmentation, and whether these are disease-specific or treatment-related phenomena, remain controversial issues that are still to be resolved. The intrinsic pathology in PD itself is likely to be the major contributor, because early and/or untreated PD patients exhibit disturbed sleep that includes excessive nocturnal movement.[232–234,256] Moreover, rats[97] and nonhuman primates[163] depleted of striatal dopamine bilaterally exhibit excessive nocturnal movement, and sleep in the parkinsonian patient deteriorates with disease progression.[238,240,257] The fact that nocturnal movements are generally best controlled when waking motor symptomatology is best treated medically, argues further that their pathophysiological bases are firmly rooted in nigrostriatal dopaminergic neuron loss. Clinical improvements of PD seen with surgical interventions that restore balance in basal ganglia neurotransmission also improve sleep architecture.[160,168,169] A systematic analysis

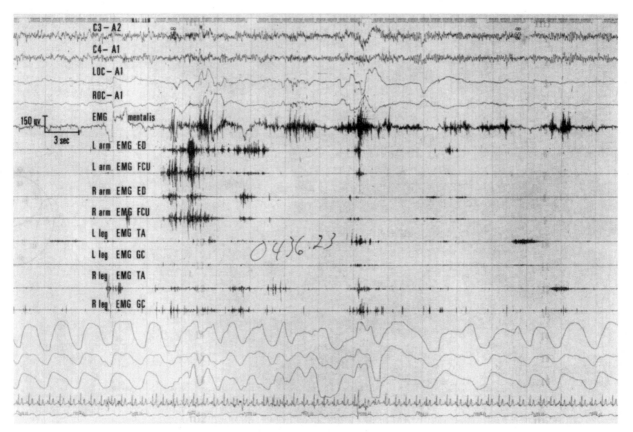

FIGURE 52-3 PSG recording of intermittent, phasic muscle activity during REM sleep in a patient with PD. It is not unusual to detect similar phasic muscle activity coincident with other phasic events of REM sleep (e.g., eye movements) in normals. Note, however, the occurrence of heightened phasic and tonic muscle activity in the chin (EMG mentalis) that occurs independent of eye movements in the parkinsonian patient. REM sleep appears to persist despite these EMG changes. Abbreviations as for Fig. 52-1; GC, gastrocnemius.

of this phenomenon is warranted given potential differential effects that pallidotomy[160] and bilateral subthalamic nucleus stimulation[168] have upon PLM and RBD. The precise substrates accounting for the detrimental effects of nigrostriatal dopamine loss upon nocturnal movement are ill-defined. It is tempting to speculate that dopamine modulates brainstem circuits effecting PLM and REM sleep atonia. This does not occur via direct dopaminergic innervation of the brainstem, but rather by indirect, multisynaptic routes linking the basal ganglia output nuclei with pontomedullary reticulospinal pathways via the dorsolateral pons, including the subceruleal region (see Fig. 52-6). Accentuated blink reflexes[258–260] and acoustic stimulation of spinal reflexes,[261,262] argue for the presence of heightened brainstem responsivity. Similar reflex pathway abnormalities in patients with PLM, but not suffering from PD, suggest that PLM in PD are modulated by the same neuropharmacologic substrates.

Other neuromodulatory systems are frequently involved by the neuropathology of PD, and may potentially account for alterations in sleep architecture. Neuronal degeneration in PD, for example, has been described in the serotonergic dorsal and median raphe, noradrenergic locus ceruleus, and

cholinergic PPN neurons.[263–266] Cell loss has been estimated at between 30 percent and 90 percent, and is proposed to underlie many of the functional waking deficits observed in PD, particularly akinesia, depression, and dementia.[263,267] Decrements in spinal norepinephrine and serotonin and their metabolites suggest additional degeneration of descending cerulospinal and raphespinal pathways, but quantitative estimates of death in the cells of origin are not available.[268] The significance of these alternate pathologies to the etiology of nocturnal movement disorders of PD is unknown. The majority of experimental findings argue against a significant role for serotonergic, noradrenergic or cholinergic pathologies in the nocturnal motor disturbances of PD. Loss of central and spinal monoamines, for example, might be expected to protect against, rather than increase, the incidence of PLM in NREM sleep given the prolocomotor effects of systemic serotonin and nornepinephrine during sleep.[269] With respect to REM sleep, lack of serotonergic and adrenergic innervation of the cholinergic PPN would diminish rather than enhance RBD-related phasic EMG events by removing sources of transient hyperpolarization necessary for a burst firing mode. Loss of cholinergic PPN neurons themselves

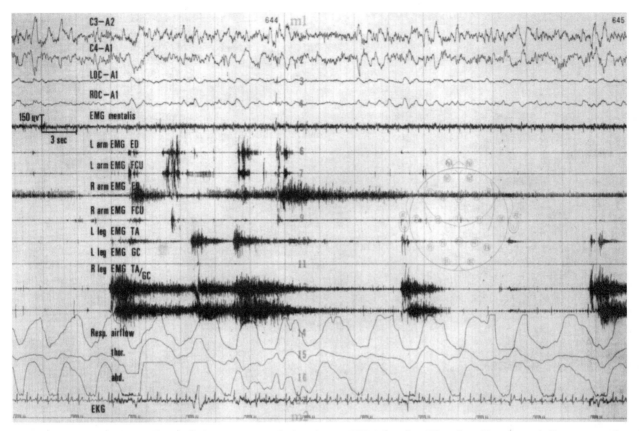

FIGURE 52-4 PSG recording of periodic leg movements during stage 2 NREM sleep in a PD patient. Note the periodic co-contraction of the right tibialis anterior (TA) and gastrocnemius (GC) indicative of PLMs. In the parkinsonian patient this is more likely to occur coincident with, as well as independent of, activity in several other upper- and lower-extremity muscle groups. Arousal from sleep clearly does not accompany these EMG changes.

would also favor less, rather than more, phasic EMG activity in REM sleep.[155] Extranigral, nondopaminergic pathology in sporadic PD is increasingly recognized to involve medullary and pontine regions containing multiple neuron types with presumed influences upon wake/sleep-related somatomotor activity.[270] The proposition that this pathology predates the extensive loss of midbrain dopaminergic neurons traditionally thought to underly PD[271,272] may account for the near ubiquitous occurrence of sleep-related movements in PD, and the experience that disturbed sleep, particularly RBD, can presage the development of the waking manifestations of parkinsonism.

The daytime consequences of sleep fragmentation have not been systematically investigated, although patients and their spouses frequently volunteer that activities of daily living are improved when sleep is undisturbed.[273] Sleep and levels of arousal have generally accepted benefits on mobility in parkinsonism and remain an area of active investigation.[250,273–277] An expected consequence of disturbed sleep in PD might be EDS, but the results of questionnaire-based surveys paint a conflicting picture,[278,279] and recent quantitative assessments argue that short,

fragmented sleep is less, rather than more, likely to be associated with EDS.[251,253] Our own and others' experiences with PD patients suggests a wide range of daytime sleep latencies between and within subjects that reflects principally the pathology in brain regions critical for maintaining arousal (see below), and also a complex interplay between medications, the "on-off" phenomenon (Fig. 52-5), disease-related sleep fragmentation, and disruption secondary to PLM or sleep apnea.

TREATMENT

Clinicians treating patients with PD and other neurodegenerative diseases of the basal ganglia should always carefully inquire about sleep quality, since disturbed sleep can presage the development of further more troublesome sleep disorders.[247] When sleep disturbances in patients with PD do occur, their management is highly individualized. In general, appropriate management of waking motor symptoms generally reduces nocturnal movement and improves sleep efficiency.[280] Although amelioration of waking motor symptoms is always the desired outcome, the fact that

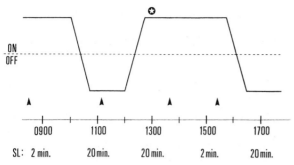

FIGURE 52-5 Multiple sleep latencies (SL) in a patient with PD demonstrate extreme variability across time of day and are likely to reflect complex inter-relationships among circadian factors, medications, and "on-off" status. Note sleep latencies of 2 minutes at 9 am (0900) and 3 pm (1500) while the patient was "on," versus no sleep (i.e., sleep latencies of 20 minutes) during "off"-periods or peak-dose dyskinesias (star). Arrowheads indicate times of dosing of one-half tablet of controlled-release carbidopa/L-dopa 50/200 (Sinemet-CR).

anywhere from 74 percent to 98 percent of medicated PD patients complain of sleep disturbances[230,247] suggests that suboptimal management may well be the rule rather than the exception. Because a typical pattern of disordered sleep has not been clearly delineated and etiology is generally unknown, no clear-cut algorithms exist for approaching the treatment of PD patients with disordered sleep. Specific treatments need to be customized to complaints only after an adequate sleep history and review of PSG findings, as discussed in detail below, have been completed. History should not rely on subjective reports of sleep alone, since reliability of personal assessments is well known to be poor secondary to sleep state misperception. Information from a caregiver and preferably a bed partner is a sine qua non to guide treatment decisions, as is historical information on the timing of medications and nocturnal symptoms, as well as the relationship of symptoms to any changes in medication. Whenever historical evidence exists for nocturnal motor behavior, abnormal respiratory patterns, or EDS, PSG should be performed. Before pharmacological interventions, the physician should always counsel the patient and family on proper sleep hygiene,

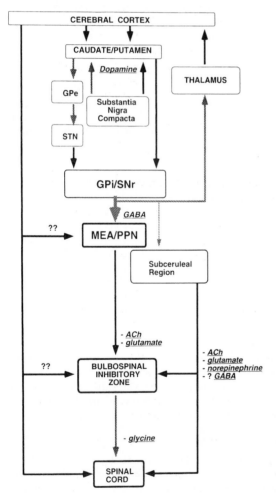

FIGURE 52-6 Schematic representation of established pathways linking dopamine-sensitive basal ganglia circuits with premotor elements in the brainstem and, in turn, to spinal motor circuits. The dorsolateral mesopontine tegmentum including the midbrain extrapyramidal area (MEA), adjacent pedunculopontine tegmental nucleus (PPN), and subceruleal region are key elements that can relay GABAergic influences from the internal segment of the globus pallidus (GPi) and substantia nigra pars reticulata (SNr) to the ventromedial medulla (i.e., the bulbospinal inhibitory zone of Magoun and Rhines). Descending pathways from these structures employ glutamate and/or acetylcholine and are ultimately responsible for REM sleep-specific tonic and phasic increases in ventromedial medullary neuronal activity. Because this increased neural activity is necessary to maintain atonia, any alterations in glutamatergic, cholinergic, or glycinergic influences on, or exiting from, the ventromedial medulla will impact upon EMG activity in REM sleep. These alterations may take the form of neuronal loss in the BIZ or MEA/PPN region that accompanies many neurodegenerative conditions, or alternatively, of abnormal modulation of these neurons by pathological influences originating in one of their many afferent sources (e.g., amygdala, hypothalamus, basal ganglia). As the pathophysiologic basis of many movement disorders specific to sleep are envisioned to lie in the basal ganglia, these brainstem pathways may also represent the substrates mediating many additional motor disturbances in sleep. ACH, acetylcholine; GPe, external segment of the globus pallidus; STN, subthalamic nucleus.

which includes, but is not restricted to, avoidance of alcoholic beverages, nicotine, and caffeine.

SLEEP-ONSET INSOMNIA

Sleep-onset insomnia appears to be no greater a problem in the PD patient than in the general aged population, based on questionnaire data.[230,249,278,279] In most instances, sleep-onset problems can be related to anxiety or to agitated depression, which should then be the focus of treatment. Additional contributors to sleep-onset insomnia in subpopulations of PD patients include RLS and akathisia, which are discussed in more detail below.

When treatment with L-dopa is instituted, some patients may experience sleep-onset insomnia that typically resolves with time.[281] Sleep-onset insomnia, at the outset of L-dopa therapy, is best treated by administering medications earlier and waiting patiently. When insomnia is severe enough to produce a significant and persistent phase delay in sleep onset, the use of fairly rapidly absorbed and/or short-acting benzodiazepines, such as temazepam (15–30 mg), alprazolam (0.125–0.25 mg), estazolam (1–2 mg) or triazolam (0.125–0.25 mg), seems warranted. In our own experience, we have been most satisfied with triazolam, with the comment that it should be used with caution in elderly and demented patients. Our own repeated attempts to treat advanced patients with zolpidem (5–10 mg), a very rapidly absorbed and short-acting benzodiazepine-like medication, as well as other sedative-hypnotics (chloral hydrate, pentobarbital), have met with limited success.

SLEEP-MAINTENANCE INSOMNIA

Sleep-maintenance insomnia (i.e., sleep fragmentation) is the most common nocturnal complaint in PD patients. It is of primary importance to first rule out, by history, other comorbid conditions that might present as a complaint of sleep-maintenance insomnia. For example, poor sleep characterized by early morning awakenings can signal the appearance of depression, the use of alcohol as a sedative, or the natural effect of aging in phase advancing the wake-sleep cycle. Having ruled out these possibilities, the clinician should recognize that the complaint of sleep fragmentation in PD manifests in PSG as a continuum from unexplained spontaneous awakenings to awakenings associated with quite specific nocturnal motor disturbances. Each of the latter conditions can be associated with either under- or overtreatment of the daytime symptoms of PD, or represent side-effects of adjunct medications and, therefore, require very different treatment strategies.

Clinical experience dictates that, early in the course of treatment with L-dopa, daytime administration improves motor symptoms and may not disrupt sleep. Frequent awakenings, for the most part unassociated with movements, are treated with sedating antidepressants, such as trazodone, nefazodone, nortriptyline, amitriptyline, or clomipramine. Some caution should be exercised in prescribing antidepressants,

because they may precipitate confusion/hallucinosis,[281] worsen PD,[282] or worsen PLMs (see above). Because the latter two side-effects appear related to serotonergic mechanisms, the antidepressants listed above are presented in order of preference, based on their increasing potencies in blocking serotonin reuptake.[283]

As PD progresses and/or L-dopa use becomes long-term, patients may experience "off" phenomena during the night. These patients, usually advanced in their disease, typically relate a history of marked interdose motor fluctuations during the day. Not only dyskinesia but also immobility with subsequent inability to turn over, or to rise to use the bathroom, may be troubling for the patient at night.[230] In this instance, historical documentation frequently uncovers the presence of nocturnal movements, severe akinesia, and/or prolonged awakenings that occur later in the night. This situation should be carefully distinguished, preferably by PSG, from nocturnal movements early in the night, which are more suggestive for nocturnal myoclonus secondary to overtreatment or PLMs. Treatment for PD patients with distinct nocturnal motor disabilities such as tremor, dyskinesias, akinesia, and prolonged awakenings should begin with dosing L-dopa closer to bedtime, particularly in sustained-release form, because this is felt to diminish sleep fragmentation by nocturnal movements.[284,285] Alternatively, selegiline and bromocriptine have been shown to improve sleep in patients with PD, even when L-dopa has minimal effect.[242,281] High evening doses, however, might increase sleep latency and disrupt sleep in the first half of the night, despite improving sleep continuity in the second half of the night.[233,234] When PSG-documented nocturnal movements persist, we complement treatment with benzodiazepines, which are known to attenuate phasic sleep events and small and large body movements.[286] We prefer the use of triazolam (0.125–0.25 mg qhs) in nondemented patients because of its documented benefit for elderly patients with PLMs, sleep fragmentation, and daytime sleepiness.[287]

Frequently encountered in our practice has been the worsening of nocturnal myoclonus and PLMs with antidepressants, particularly serotonin reuptake inhibitors, which is an infrequently recognized side-effect but is commonly accepted among sleep clinicians (see above).[107,288] This phenomenon is consistent with reports of benefits from methysergide, a serotonin antagonist, in alleviating the nocturnal myoclonus of PD (see below).[16,28,248] Treatment options include discontinuation of antidepressant medication or its substitution with an antidepressant, whose potency in blocking serotonin reuptake is less. We have also observed worsening of PLMs in PD, secondary to the inadvertent prescription of metaclopromide for the gastrointestinal symptoms of PD and presumably reflects its dopamine antagonist action.

FRAGMENTARY NOCTURNAL MYOCLONUS

The chronic administration of L-dopa can lead to the development of fragmentary nocturnal myoclonus during slow-wave sleep.[28,248] Historical data that may suggest the presence of nocturnal myoclonus include the complaint of troubling daytime dyskinesias related to L-dopa dosing,[28] or that of exaggerated axial myoclonus at sleep onset that may precipitate abrupt arousals from sleep. This phenomenon is thought to reflect L-dopa-induced upregulation of serotonergic neurotransmission, because it is alleviated by methysergide (2 mg), a serotonergic antagonist, and by discontinuing L-dopa but not by altering anticholinergic medications.[28] Treatment options include a reduction in night-time dosing of dopamine agonists, addition of a benzodiazepine such as temazepam, clonazepam, or triazolam, and possibly a trial with methysergide (2 mg) shortly before bedtime.

PERIODIC LEG MOVEMENTS OF SLEEP (PLMs)

PLMs are an entity distinct from fragmentary nocturnal myoclonus, although their presence early in NREM sleep disrupts sleep in a similar manner. They can be differentiated clinically from myoclonus, because they are more often unilateral and prolonged, spaced at very regular intervals, and characterized by a flexor withdrawal-type movement typically restricted to the lower extremities. Although a careful history from a spouse or bed partner may, therefore, distinguish between these two entities, PSG is sometimes required and warranted since treatment modalities are distinct. Although PLMs exhibit high prevalence rates in the general population over the age of,[42,45,289,290] they are more prevalent in PD patients.[98,99] Because the neurophysiological abnormalities delineated in patients with PLMs but not suffering from PD[42,43] approximate those seen in PD patients,[261,262] a common pathophysiology is suggested. In treating PD patients with coexistent PLMs, we follow the strategies outlined above for PLMs in the nonparkinsonian population. Given the decreased capacity of the pathologically effected substantia nigra to synthesize dopamine from L-dopa, trials with low doses of dopamine agonists seem particularly warranted. When dopaminomimetics are unsatisfactory, aggravate insomnia, produce troubling nocturnal myoclonus, or result in "rebound" leg movements in the early morning, we will substitute gabapentin (300–1800 mg in divided doses), oxycodone (5–15 mg) or propoxyphene (65–100 mg) at bedtime for the dopaminomimetics. We reserve the use of benzodiazepines for patients that are refractory to these approaches to avoid problems associated with the development of tolerance and possible worsening of coexistent depression.

RESTLESS LEGS SYNDROME (RLS)

Several investigators have failed to note the coincidence of RLS in patients with PD.[281,291] However, in our experience and that of others,[100] the two frequently coexist. Suspected RLS in a PD patient should be very carefully differentiated from akathisia, which is also encountered in PD patients.

An anecdotal report of alleviation of RLS in PD with pallidotomy is consistent with suggestions that the basal ganglia and their connections are intimately involved in the expression of RLS.[292]

AKATHISIA

Nocturnal akathisia is a reported problem in a small subgroup of PD patients and should be carefully differentiated from RLS. Akathisia is not associated with prominent paresthesias, and symptoms are not typically relieved by movements or pacing, unlike those of RLS. Moreover, there is no PSG-documented hallmark that has yet been defined in the PD patient experiencing akathisia. Akathisia is frequently described by the PD patient as a vague sensation of an "inner restlessness." Moreover, akathisia is thought to be precipitated by L-dopa,[293,294] whereas it would be expected to suppress the symptoms of RLS. While one report suggests that akathisia more commonly occurs in PD patients with bradykinesia and "stiffness,"[293] another notes that it is unrelated to motor or mental state or time of day.[294] Successful treatments include alterations in the timing or dosage of L-dopa[293] and bedtime dosing of clozapine, which has the added benefit of reducing night-time tremor.[294] Successful treatment of akathisia has also been reported, using fluoxetine alone or together with amitriptyline in 1 depressed PD patient.[295]

REM SLEEP BEHAVIOR DISORDER (RBD)

The recognition that RBD predates and is associated with neurodegenerative diseases that share waking manifestations of parkinsonism has captured considerable attention. This clinical entity is more frequently encountered in the male PD patient, as is the case with "idiopathic" RBD.[129] In MSA, the male/female ratio is closer to 1:1. Histories consistent with RBD can be obtained from nearly 1 in 6 patients with idiopathic PD.[151,255] PSG analysis reveals "subclinical" evidence of RBD in 50 percent of PD patients,[151] and this electrophysiologic correlate of RBD appears significantly specific in distinguishing parkinsonian subjects from age-matched controls and AD patients.[151,296] The waking EEG in these patients also demonstrates subtle abnormalities that distinguish them from control and PD patients lacking RBD.[297] The yield for elucidating a history of RBD seems particularly high in those suffering from L-dopa or dopamine agonist-induced hallucinations.[250] Nearly 65 percent of RBD cases presage the development of the waking motor manifestations of parkinsonian states by several to many years.[152] Several investigators have suggested that RBD is almost predictive of a synucleinopathy.[132,298] This has been confirmed in a recent neuropathologic investigation of RBD plus dementia or parkinsonism.[299] The clinicopathologic associations are so strong that the consensus criteria now include RBD as a core clinical feature strongly suggestive of a diagnosis of DLB.[300] The treatment of choice for RBD is clonazepam (0.5–2.0 mg qhs), which is effective in 75–90 percent of cases. Dopaminomimetics and/or antidepressants, which exhibit some ability to block dopamine reuptake (e.g., buproprion and sertraline), may theoretically, prove to be useful alternative or adjunct medications in the PD patient with RBD.

OTHER PARASOMNIAS

Parasomnia is a term that includes a variety of complex sleep-related behavioral phenomena in addition to RBD. In PD patients, these include sleeptalking, sleepwalking (i.e., somnambulism), altered dream content, nocturnal hallucinations, nocturnal terrors, and panic disorder. Difficulties in differentiating between parasomnias on the basis of history and the lack of specific PSG features in PD have precluded accurate delineation of their pathophysiology and treatment. Because many of these parasomnias have been reported as prodromes to the development of full-blown RBD,[79,301] they may describe a continuum reflecting a common pathophysiology. The sleep of patients experiencing nocturnal terrors, however, lacks any distinct alterations in sleep architecture,[281] whereas that of patients with nocturnal hallucinations is markedly fragmented and approximates that seen in RBD.[250] Although panic disorder could theoretically manifest nocturnally in PD, it is rarely encountered and typically occurs during the "off"-phase in depressed PD patients taking L-dopa but not direct agonists.[302] Most studies attribute parasomnias in PD to the long-term effects of L-dopa treatment.[245–247,281,291] Pathological differences between individual PD patients are as likely to contribute to parasomnias, because nocturnal hallucinations[250] and nocturnal wandering/disruptive behavior[303] in PD can be unrelated to medication type or dose. A greater prevalence of parasomnia-type behaviors in the subpopulation of PD patients with dementia further supports this contention.[291] There is little information on the treatment of patients with nocturnal terrors or panic attacks, particularly those with coexistent PD. Instruction on proper sleep hygiene, and sedating antidepressants, alone or together with an anxiolytic such as alprazolam, are the mainstays of treatment. The parasomnia condition most familiar to the clinician treating PD patients is that of nocturnal hallucinations/delirium, where pre-existing sleep complaints are more common,[247] sleep deprivation markedly aggravates the severity of symptoms,[304] and sleep efficiency, total REM sleep time, and percentage are significantly reduced.[250] Other than reducing the dosage of dopaminomimetics, the mainstays of treatment include clozapine (6.25–50 mg qhs),[305,306] risperidone (0.5–2.0 mg qhs),[307,308] or quetiapine (12.5–150 mg ghs). In our practice, we prefer quetiapine as it appears to exhibit less tendency for motor worsening.[309–311] The nature of the beneficial effects of atypical neuroleptics in the PD population has been attributed to antagonism of 5-HT$_{2A}$ receptors and may reflect their tendency to enhance sedation, improve sleep continuity, reduce gross body movements, and enhance REM sleep.[312–315] Sedating antidepressants such as amitriptyline or trazodone may be of additional added benefit.

SLEEP APNEA

Central or obstructive sleep apnea, hypoventilation, and irregular patterns of respiration likely contribute to sleep fragmentation in a small subpopulation of PD patients; however, few detailed studies have been reported.[316,317] With the possible exception of MSA, encompassing the Shy-Drager syndrome and OPCD, nocturnal respiratory disturbances probably are no more likely to occur in PD or other movement disorders, given their high prevalence in the normal adult population.[253,291,318] Increased tone or dyskinesias in the upper airway muscles, caused by either the disease itself or medications,[319] can predispose the PD patient to obstructive apneas. Dyscoordination of respiratory muscle activity and abnormalities in respiratory drive have also been observed that might contribute to nocturnal respiratory disturbances.[320–322] The severity of respiratory abnormalities is greater in patients with coincident autonomic dysfunction,[317] possibly accounting for the fact that EDS is more regularly present in patients with Shy-Drager and OPCD. Obstructive and central sleep apnea, respirations with variable amplitude, and arrhythmic respiration are commonly observed in such patients.[323–326] Although in PD it is generally felt that respiratory disturbances correlate with the severity of rigidity and tremor, they do not typically improve with administration of L-dopa.[291] Treatment of the sleep-related respiratory disturbances in PD and other neurodegenerative conditions is, therefore, similar to that when these problems are encountered in the normal adult population. For obstructive and central sleep apnea, treatment with continuous positive airway pressure (CPAP) offers the best chance of success and can be used effectively by most patients. In patients who cannot tolerate CPAP, we first explore the use of bilevel PAP before adding adjunct medications such as sedative antidepressants or the extremely short-acting sedative/hypnotic zolpidem (5–10 mg qhs). One anecdotal report notes successful treatment of central sleep apnea in OPCD using trazadone (50 mg qhs).[327]

EXCESSIVE DAYTIME SLEEPINESS (EDS)

Sleepiness in PD is common, very real, yet under-recognized. As captured by Oliver Sacks' familiar memoir *Awakenings*, the sleepiness of the parkinsonian patient transcends the metaphor. It is undeniably verifiable, and likely as much a consequence of the disease as its treatment. Treatment of PD with psychostimulants in the pre-L-dopa era, in fact, may owe its partial benefit to alleviation of sleepiness.[328–331] Intrinsic sleepiness therefore represents an important target in disease management, as much as a fear of pharmacologic intervention.

Dopamine cell death in PD profoundly alters not only nocturnal movement, but also thalamocortical arousal state. This manifests as daytime sleepiness, and intrusion of REM sleep into daytime naps (sleep-onset REM sleep (SOREM)).[253,332] The initial report of dose-related "sleep attacks" with pramipexole and ropinirole was interpreted as a novel, idiosyncratic response specific to the new nonergot D2/D3 receptor agonists.[333] Clinical experience and more comprehensive assessments agree that sleepiness has long been under-recognized in PD, but that it is a phenomenon not restricted to a specific class of dopaminomimetics.[100,334–336]

In community-based samples of PD patients, the rate of sleepiness ranges from 7 percent to 14 percent as compared to 1–2 percent in healthy, elderly controls,[337,338] and longitudinal studies have demonstrated that the rate increases by about 6 percent per year.[339] In clinic-based samples, the rate is much higher (20–50 percent).[100,336,340,341] Employing a standardized measure of physiological sleep tendency across five daytime nap opportunities, we and others have objectively documented "pathological" sleepiness in 30–50 percent of patients, and a narcolepsy-like phenotype in a similar number[251,253] (Fig. 52-5). Sleepiness bears little relationship to the primary motor manifestations of disease (e.g., disability scale, medication burden), or sleep architecture measures (e.g., total sleep time, stage, etc.). These findings argue that parkinsonism itself accounts for impairments in the expression of wake and REM sleep, an important concept that finds further support from animal models of parkinsonism. Remarkably, contrary to what one would expect based upon the demands of sleep homeostatic mechanisms, poor nocturnal sleep is generally associated with greater, rather than lesser, degrees of daytime alertness. The dissociation of arousal state from the motor manifestations of disease and homeostatic sleep drives (viz., sleep propensity should be inversely rather directly related to the quality and quantity of prior nights' sleep) in PD has several implications. First, it emphasizes that dopamine pathway integrity is critical for maintaining homeostatic sleep mechanisms. Second, it points to the pathophysiological basis of impaired thalamocortical arousal state residing outside of the sensorimotor subcircuit of nigrostriatal pathways traditionally thought to underlie parkinsonian motor disabilities. A threshold of 60–90 percent dopamine loss in the sensorimotor putamen is necessary for the emergence of waking clinical manifestations,[342] and then proceeds in an orderly fashion through associative (i.e., caudate), and eventually limbic (i.e., nucleus accumbens) striatal subcircuits. Thus, it is loss of dopamine in these latter circuits, most characteristic of advanced disease, that is a potential factor in the expression of sleepiness and SOREM in PD.

The objective findings in a small number of newly diagnosed, unmedicated or young PD patients[253,256] emphasize that the parkinsonian state itself is a major factor in the expression of sleepiness and SOREM. The point is best made in animal models of disease that control for potentially confounding variables such as age, comorbid conditions, and medications. Rats spend less of their subjective day awake following destruction of nigrostriatal pathways with bilateral, intrastriatal infusions of the dopamine toxin 6-hydroxydopamine.[97] Similarly, daytime sleepiness and SOREM have been reported in a single nonhuman primate following systemic delivery of the dopamine neurotoxin 1-methyl,4-phenyl-1,2,3,6-tetrahydropyridine (MPTP),[163] and

this has been confirmed in two additional animals (personal observations). The cellular and subcellular substrates underlying these disease related effects remain ill-defined. These phenomena may reflect loss of dopamine's effects upon neural excitability in any one of a number of brain regions necessary for maintaining normal states of thalamocortical excitability. One plausible substrate given the narcolepsy-like phenotype seen in nearly half of "sleepy" PD patients, are hypocretin-containing neurons in the lateral hypothalamus known to degenerate in primary narcolepsy/cataplexy.[343] Other plausible neural substrates that deserve future investigation include targets of ventral tegmental area (VTA) dopamine neurons, including the prefrontal cortex, the cholinergic magnocellular basal forebrain, and midline thalamic nuclei. This hypothesis is supported by the results of several studies, including one which demonstrated that D2 receptor antagonists microinjected into the VTA block the sedation seen with systemic administration of dopamine agonists,[344] and another which demonstrated that infusions of amphetamine directly into ventral forebrain targets of the VTA neurons both initiated and maintained alert wakefulness.[345] Alternatively, sleepiness and SOREM may reflect extranigral pathology[263] (e.g., in nuclei comprising the traditional ascending reticular activating system such as the dorsal raphe, locus ceruleus, and PPN). Dysregulation of the PPN region, an area known to promote thalamocortical arousal and REM sleep, may also be an important factor secondary to its position as a principal brainstem target of pathological basal ganglia outflow[160] (see Fig. 52-6).

Separate from the neurobiological substrates governing PD, other factors may influence expression of sleepiness and SOREM. Advanced disease or disease duration have been contributing factors noted in several studies.[100,253,335,339,341] Other potential risk factors include benzodiazepine use,[253] male sex,[100] comorbid dementia or psychosis,[339] and autonomic failure (e.g., orthostatic hypotension).[340] Many of these clinical features are also shared by patients exhibiting DLB,[346] suggesting that sleepiness may be a phenotypic characteristic of this subtype of parkinsonism. This is supported by a longitudinal study that found that nearly two-thirds of PD patients with sleepiness went on to develop dementia.[339]

There has been a recent explosion in the number of reports of sleepiness and sudden onset of sleep associated with dopaminomimetic use.[333,347–351] Sleepiness or "sleep attacks" associated with dopaminomimetics in a subset of PD patients appear to be dose-related, but are not clearly related to specific class of agent (e.g., L-dopa versus ergot- and nonergot-derived D2/D3 receptor-like agonists).[100,335,336,351] These reports are largely anecdotal and only a few have documented or investigated the nature of related sleep architecture changes.[352,353] While sleepiness observed with dopaminomimetic use in PD is now well recognized, it remains unresolved how often this use contributes and how much of a contributing factor it is. L-Dopa[354] and ropinirole,[355] for example, can exacerbate sleepiness even in drug-naïve controls. It has been suggested that obstructive sleep apnea and PLMs coexisting with PD may also contribute to sleepiness and SOREM.[251] Yet, this is controversial since sleepiness in nonparkinsonian patients is not completely explained by the severity of obstructive sleep apnea and PLMs. A final important determinant of sleepiness in PD is premorbid sleepiness level, which is increasingly recognized to be an heritable trait in the general population. One survey of sudden-onset sleep in a large number of movement disorder clinics, in fact, found that 20 percent of PD patients reporting sudden onset of sleep while driving experienced similar events prior to the diagnosis of PD being made.[336] In summary, the pathophysiological bases underlying the spectrum of PD-related changes in sleep-wake tendencies are complex and unique to the individual patient. Until more data are forthcoming, the most prudent clinical and experimental approaches should proceed from the assumption that the parkinsonian condition represents an underlying diathesis to sleepiness and SOREM expression that can be exaggerated by numerous coexistent factors, including use of dopamine agonists and L-dopa, sedative-hypnotic and potentially other medications, primary sleep disorders, and potentially comorbid conditions such as dementia and depression.

Daytime somnolence experienced by idiopathic PD patients is thus very real, common, and potentially as severe as that manifest by narcoleptics. Proper treatment can dramatically enhance quality of life and prevent the significant morbidity and mortality that attends pathological sleepiness. Physicians treating PD should therefore educate patients and their families on the potential detrimental effects of this disease and its treatment not only upon motor symptoms but also upon the ability to maintain an active, awake state. Patients should be informed about the potential dangers of driving. Administration of the Epworth Sleepiness Scale (ESS),[356] possibly completed by the caregiver or significant other, and queries about unintended sleep episodes, particularly while driving, should be routine. Anywhere from 11 percent to 22 percent of PD patients experience sleepiness while driving, and this risk tends to correlate with higher ESS scores.[100,336,357] The frequency of sudden-onset sleep while driving is reported to be about 3.8 percent,[336] with the majority of these preceded by drowsiness or warning signs (about 85 percent). If significant or unpredictable sleepiness is suspected, driving should be temporarily restricted until the sleepiness resolves.

The first step in effecting resolution of parkinsonian-related sleepiness demands a careful review of medications and defining any temporal relationship between dosing and symptoms, as dosage reduction or discontinuation of dopaminomimetics, particularly agonists, or long-lasting benzodiazepines might reverse sleepiness. Nightly benzodiazepine use intended to improve daytime alertness by lengthening total sleep time and preventing nocturnal arousals seems particularly unwarranted given the strong inverse correlation of parkinsonian sleepiness with the quantity or quality of prior nights' sleep. If medication adjustments are ineffectual, the diagnostic "yield" for routine PSG and mean

sleep latency evaluation of PD patients could be considerable (15 percent prevalence of PLMs, 20 percent prevalence of obstructive sleep apnea, 40 percent prevalence of "secondary" narcolepsy). Treatment strategies may then need to be targeted at alleviating PLMs and obstructive sleep apnea, if present. If sleepiness persists, treatments that until now have focused primarily on minimizing waking motor disability should include agents specifically designed to promote daytime alertness. Prescribing wake-promoting agents such as bupropion,[358] traditional psychostimulants,[329,330] and modafinil are justified upon identification of a narcolepsy-like phenotype or mean sleep latencies of <8 minutes. While the initial open-label experiences with modafinil in PD patients with drug-related drowsiness are encouraging, a double-blind, randomized, placebo-controlled study is needed to corroborate and extend the results.[359–362] The use of selegiline in treating the EDS in PD is also deserving of investigation, given its metabolization to amphetamine derivatives,[363] tendency to improve memory and learning of word associations in PD patients,[364,365] increased theta EEG frequency bands over delta activity,[366] and utility in treating the EDS accompanying other disorders such as narcolepsy.[367–369]

Selection of the most appropriate drug and its dosing for maximizing wakefulness in PD will require future clinical trials. As the problem of PD-related sleepiness has only recently been recognized, there are no comprehensive studies on how it might be best reversed. Pharmacologic treatment is employed only for those patients in whom identification and treatment of other causes of daytime sleepiness has proved ineffectual (Table 52-2). In the nonhuman MPTP primate model of PD, sleepiness and SOREM have been reversed with the dopamine precursor L-dopa, the dopamine reuptake blocker bupropion,[370] but not the D2-like receptor

TABLE 52-2 Treatment of Sleepiness in PD

Medication adjustments
   Reduce over-the-counter sleeping aids with antihistaminergic
     activity
   Minimize benzodiazepine use
   Minimize "sedating" antidepressant use
   Dopaminomimetic dose adjustment if dosing temporally
     associated with sleepiness
Treat documented sleep or other disturbance
   Continuous positive airway pressure for sleep apnea
   Night-time dosing of dopaminomimetics, opiates, or gabapentin
     for periodic leg movements of sleep
   Consider treatment of orthostatic hypotension
Treat "residual" daytime sleepiness
   Hygiene measures
     Scheduled naps
     More frequent, smaller meals
   Pharmacologic measures
     Bupropion (75–150 mg two or three times per day)
     Modafinil (100–200 mg each morning and noon)
     Dextroamphetamine sulfate (5–30 mg each morning and noon),
      combination of sustained-release and regular tablets

---

agonist pergolide.[163] L-Dopa and bupropion require presynaptic integrity to enhance synaptic availability of dopamine by promoting its synthesis, or by blockade of dopamine transporter, respectively. Thus, the abilities of these agents to reverse sleepiness and SOREM likely reflect actions upon surviving mesocorticolimbic dopamine circuits which are less vulnerable to MPTP and affected only later in the course of idiopathic PD. Enhancement of synaptic dopamine availability in mesocorticolimbic circuits, in fact, may underlie the success of amphetamines in the treatment of PD described nearly 30 years ago,[329,330] providing beneficial alerting effects in truly "sleepy" patients.

SLEEP IN OTHER WAKING MOVEMENT DISORDERS

HUNTINGTON'S DISEASE (HD)
PSG studies of Huntington's disease (HD) have demonstrated some disturbance of sleep architecture, including reduced sleep efficiency, prolonged sleep latency, and reduced slow-wave sleep.[371] Early studies claimed an absence of REM sleep in HD,[372] but this has not been confirmed by others.[371,373] Increased density of sleep spindle (12–14 Hz) activity has been noted in the stage 2 sleep of HD patients.

Dyskinesias have been reported to occur in sleep in HD,[374] with lowest frequency during slow-wave sleep (stages 3 and 4). REM sleep, by contrast, appeared to be a time of relative activation of the chorea. Fish et al.[375] reported that HD patients showed a larger number of movements across the entire sleep period relative to PD patients, although they contended that such apparent sleep-related movements were preceded by several seconds of EEG arousal before the movement itself. PLMs are sometimes noted in the sleep of HD patients.

PROGRESSIVE SUPRANUCLEAR PALSY (PSP)
The sleep of patients with PSP is characterized by a near absence of REM sleep.[376,377] This decrease may reflect selective cell loss within the PPN. Additionally, sleep efficiency and sleep fragmentation indicate severe sleep disturbance, and have been correlated with extent of dementia,[376] although body movement in these patients appears to be no more severe than in age-matched controls.

TORSION DYSTONIA
There is a general consensus that the elevated muscle tonus seen in many conditions characterized by dystonia, decreases in sleep.[374,378,379] Hemifacial spasm has been shown to be decreased during sleep, as well.[380] REM atonia is generally unchanged in both primary and secondary dystonia.[381]

Although Fish et al.[375] also contend that sleep-related movements during sleep, in both primary and secondary torsion dystonia, emerge only after brief awakenings, other investigators have noted that muscle tension in the affected sternocleidomastoid in spasmodic torticollis can appear as a specific sleep-related event.[257,382] Emser et al.[257] even

suggested a temporal linkage of such EMG activity with vertex sharp waves during stage 1 sleep. Mano et al.[374] also concluded that the long-lasting EMG discharges corresponding to the waking clinical dystonic condition can "... appear in any sleep stage with the same EMG characteristics as in wakefulness."

Segawa et al.[379] and others[383] have described diurnal variation in a juvenile form of dystonia, with symptoms greatly improved during and immediately subsequent to sleep. REM sleep deprivation has been shown to aggravate movement during sleep in these patients, and administration of L-dopa increased the number and frequency of movements in sleep.[379]

CREUTZFELDT-JAKOB DISEASE
In Creutzfeldt-Jakob disease, generalized paroxysmal spike activity precludes normal identification of NREM sleep stages. REM sleep is typically difficult to discern.[384] Diffuse myoclonus is seen in all limbs and is apparent throughout sleep and wakefulness.

OLIVOPONTOCEREBELLAR ATROPHY (OPCA)
Shimizu et al.[137] reported that patients with OPCA demonstrated RBD-like behaviors, with awakening from REM sleep characterized by dream-enactment behavior. Of note, however, were patients with late cerebellar cortical atrophy without brainstem involvement, who did not show such behavior.

HEMIFACIAL SPASM/BLEPHAROSPASM
Movements associated with blepharospasm and hemifacial spasm can occur at night and interfere with sleep continuity. Several studies have demonstrated that these movements decrease in amplitude and frequency through sleep stages, with the lowest values seen in REM sleep.[380,385]

HEMIBALLISMUS
A small number of cases of hemiballismus have been reported in the literature.[374] Results are similar to those seen in HD, in that movements are decreased in NREM sleep but continue to be detectable.

TOURETTE'S SYNDROME (TS)
Clinical data indicate that sleep disturbance is present in 62 percent (69/112) of TS patients, with tics during sleep reported in about one-third of these patients, and somnambulism and bruxism reported in a lower percentage of these.[386] Sandyk and Bamford[387] have suggested that decreases in tic frequency during sleep may be a useful indicator of improvement on waking clinical state in these patients.

Early PSG studies of TS patients did not report on movement during sleep,[388] but did note normalization of sleep architecture after haloperidol administration. Some studies have reported reduced REM sleep percentages or slow-wave sleep in these patients,[388] but these results may reflect the fact that the subjects in these studies were not drug-naive.[389] Among 34 patients studied by PSG, motor activity was reported to be present in 23,[386] although quantified PSG data were not presented. Numerous other studies have confirmed the persistence of PSG-defined movement during sleep in TS.[390–392] Movements were reported to decrease from wakefulness to sleep, although they re-occurred during the sleep period. As was the case for many movement disorders studied by Fish et al.,[375] these authors contend that most of the sleep-related movements in TS, although technically occurring during the "sleep period," actually represent events that are preceded by brief microawakenings or by lightening of sleep stages to stage 1. Movements were rare, according to these authors, during stages 2, 3, 4, or REM. Several recent studies, however, have noted an increased prevalence of PLMs in TS, which, by definition, occur from sleep and are not preceded by microarousals.[393,394]

Glaze et al.[389] noted "unusual" behavior episodes in TS which originated from stage 4 sleep and consisted of high-amplitude delta activity accompanied by disorientation, confusion, or combativeness. Unlike typical episodes of night terrors or somnambulism, there was no evidence of elevated heart rate or breathing rate during these episodes.

PALATAL MYOCLONUS

Chokroverty and Barron[395] first noted persistence of palatal myoclonus in sleep in patients with brainstem infarcts. Later, Kayed et al.[396] reported several cases of palatal myoclonus in patients without infarcts, which clearly persisted in sleep. Although rates of movement typically declined from high rates during wakefulness (120–200/min) to rates as low as 80/min, the data of Kayed et al. conclusively indicated continued presence of palatal myoclonus during EEG-defined sleep. Of particular interest was that, in REM sleep, the amplitude of the movements showed considerable clustering with 2–4 high-amplitude movements alternating with lower-amplitude movements. This did not appear to be related to bursting of eye movements. Yokota et al.[397] reported that palatal myoclonus was exacerbated in REM sleep.

TREATMENT OF DISTURBED SLEEP IN WAKING MOVEMENT DISORDERS

The nature and prevalence of disturbed sleep across the spectrum of waking movement disorders is complex, and their pathophysiologies are poorly defined. It is not, therefore, surprising that scientifically validated objective results documenting specific treatments of disturbed sleep in each waking movement disorder do not exist. Nonetheless, it has been our impression that effective treatment of the core symptoms of the underlying waking movement disorder will typically result in a corresponding improvement in any associated sleep disturbances. Difficulties with sleep onset and sleep maintenance seem to be the most frequent complaints

encountered in patients with waking movement disorders. As detailed above for patients with PD, sleep-maintenance problems can respond favorably to sedating antidepressants or the judicious use of benzodiazepines (e.g., clonazepam). Clozapine, risperidone, or quetiapine in low doses seem particularly useful in PSP. As is the case with the PD patient, we have also noted the worsening of nocturnal movements in many patients receiving tricyclic antidepressants and potent serotonin reuptake inhibitors, although the prevalence of this complication is unclear. When sleep complaints persist after the successful treatment of the core waking motor disturbance and/or the simple approaches outlined here, a re-evaluation of the patient for a possible underlying sleep disorder should be performed, including PSG.

Mechanisms Contributing to Disturbed Sleep in Waking Movement Disorders

The neural and pharmacological substrates underlying the disturbed sleep of PD patients remain poorly defined. Dopamine, serotonin, norepinephrine, and acetylcholine play critical roles in wake-sleep regulation and might be suspected to be primary contributors to the disturbed sleep of PD, given their depletion in PD (see Chap. 18).[263] An alternative heuristic model considers the sleep disturbances of PD to be secondary in character (i.e., directly related to impaired motor functions). It has been suggested, for example, that nocturnal motor dyscontrol in PD is mediated by the same neuroanatomic and neurochemical substrates responsible for bradykinesia/akinesia, tremor, rigidity, and other waking disturbances in PD.[280,398,399]

As reviewed in earlier chapters (see Chaps. 5–7, and 9), the neural and pharmacological substrates underlying the pathophysiology of waking movement disorders lie primarily in the basal ganglia. It is unclear, however, how this knowledge can be extrapolated to account for the sleep disturbances manifested in these disorders. What follows is a discussion of several neural and pharmacological factors that represent a framework from which the pathophysiology behind sleep disturbances in waking movement disorders and more rational treatment strategies might be derived. Because most of our knowledge concerning waking movement disorders derives from PD, we will focus this discussion around PD. It should be recognized that sleep disruption in other waking movement disorders and movement disorders specific to sleep may involve similar substrates.

ROLE OF DOPAMINE IN BEHAVIORAL STATE CONTROL

Dopamine, like other biogenic amines, has long been suspected of having important effects on the behavioral state,[400–403] and has recently been reviewed.[332] A parsimonious explanation for wake-sleep-related alterations in

PD might, therefore, relate directly to the pathological involvement of dopaminergic neurons, which is the hallmark of the disease (see Chaps. 12 and 19). The cellular and pharmacological substrates mediating dopamine's role in behavioral state control, however, are ill-defined and, therefore, preclude simple pathophysiological associations in PD. The mesocortical, mesolimbic, and mesostriatal systems are the most conspicuous of central pathways employing dopamine,[404] and are traditionally believed to govern cognitive, emotive, and motor behaviors, respectively. Midbrain dopamine neurons have the potential to modulate normal and pathological thalamocortical neuron excitability, and by inference sleep-wake state, not only through the traditional pathways to the striatum, but also by way of novel extensive axon collaterals to the thalamus.[405] Lack of changes in group mean firing rates across sleep-wake states in midbrain dopamine neurons, reported nearly 20 years ago,[406,407] has been interpreted to mean that dopamine must not modulate sleep-wake behaviors. Critical reappraisal of these experiments and recent findings, however, suggest that state-dependent alterations in dopamine neuron activity might manifest as changes in temporal pattern, rather than rate, of neural firing. Such "burst firing" drives synaptic dopamine release more efficiently,[408] and is modulated by glutamatergic inputs from subthalamic[409] and pedunculopontine tegmental[410] neurons whose firing rates and patterns themselves are intimately related to behavioral state.

The most compelling evidence that dopamine modulates the sleep-wake continuum has come from the clinical arena. Conditions such as atypical depression, narcolepsy, and PD, for example, are characterized by variable degrees of sleepiness, inappropriate intrusion of sleep-onset REM sleep into daytime naps (SOREM), hypoactivity responsive to dopaminomimetics, and alterations in markers of dopamine transmission in targets of dopamine neurons. Dopamine activity is in turn influenced by circadian and homeostatic factors. The rate-limiting enzyme in dopamine synthesis, tyrosine hydroxylase (TH), for example, falls several hours prior to wake, and mid-day peaks coincide with those of extracellular dopamine, dopamine metabolites, and motor activity.[411,412] The most critical determinant of synaptic dopamine levels, the dopamine transporter, is expressed inversely in relation to TH (personal observations). Sleep, and particularly REM sleep, deprivation induces plasticity in the mesostriatal dopamine system as manifest in enhanced striatal dopamine and metabolite levels.[413,414]

A principal problem in ascribing wake-sleep effects to dopamine has been the inability to distinguish its role from that of other monoamines. Psychomotor stimulants such as amphetamine facilitate locomotion and stereotypic movements, and coincidentally enhance wakefulness at the expense of slow-wave sleep and REM sleep.[415] The mechanisms underlying these effects have been difficult to dissect given that amphetamines increase dopamine and norepinephrine and serotonin neurotransmission. The development of more specific blockers of the dopamine transporter that inhibit dopamine reuptake has made it clear that stimulant-induced wake (i.e., a thalamocortical aroused state characterized by EEG desynchronization) is mediated principally by dopamine.[416] The effects of dopaminomimetics upon sleep-wake state are more complex. They are dose- and receptor-dependent due to regional differential expression, pre- versus postsynaptic localization, and differential affinities of two pharmacologically, and five molecularly, defined dopamine receptor subtypes.[254,417] Low doses promote sleep principally via D2-like pharmacologic receptors in healthy controls, as illustrated recently by Ferreira et al. with the D2/3 agonist ropinirole.[355] Low doses of the dopamine precursor L-dopa have a similar effect and habituate over 1 week of treatment.[354] Higher dopaminomimetic doses that are usually sufficient to increase locomotor activity enhance wakefulness and suppress slow-wave sleep and REM sleep, likely via D1-like postsynaptic receptors. The central locus mediating the soporific effects of low doses of dopaminomimetics appears to be D2-like inhibitory autoreceptors on the cell bodies or terminal axonal fields of dopamine VTA neurons (the origin of the mesolimbic and mesocortical dopamine pathways). Local applications of D2-like receptor antagonists in the VTA block sedation seen with systemic agonists,[344] while amphetamine administration into the ventromedial forebrain targets of VTA neurons initiates and maintains alert waking.[345] Blockade of dopamine transmission (D1- and/or D2 receptor-like antagonism at unknown pre- or postsynaptic sites) with classical or atypical neuroleptics can also induce sedation.

In addition to the potential direct role of the mesotelencephalic dopamine system in modulating behavioral state, some attention has been directed to the inverse relationship (i.e., how behavioral state may modulate the nigrostriatal pathway). TH activity in the striatum, for example, undergoes diurnal modulation.[411] Plasticity in the nigrostriatal system, governed by behavioral state, is also suggested by the downregulation of striatal dopamine receptor number and increased receptor affinity with REM sleep deprivation[418] and during hibernation.[419] In light of the known REM sleep-suppressant effects of L-dopa and decreased REM sleep in PD, these findings may be relevant to the morning/daytime motor fluctuations encountered in PD.[273,274,278–280,420]

SIGNIFICANCE OF EXTRANIGRAL PATHOLOGY, INCLUDING THE ASCENDING RETICULAR ACTIVATING SYSTEM, TO BEHAVIORAL STATE CONTROL ABNORMALITIES IN PD

It is plausible to postulate that extranigral dopaminergic neurons in the diencephalon and their innervation of the posterior pituitary, hypothalamus, and spinal cord might be implicated in behavioral state control, either directly or indirectly (e.g., by influencing PLMs);[269] however, they are rarely pathologically involved in idiopathic PD.[268,421] Rather, other, nondopaminergic, neural systems are involved by the neuropathology of PD and possibly relevant to the sleep-wake abnormalities observed in parkinsonian states. Of these nondopaminergic nuclei, those constituting the traditional ascending reticular activating system have attracted the most attention as they are conspicuous and included in routine neuropathologic sections. Cell loss in the ascending reticular activating system ranges from 30 percent to 90 percent and has been proposed to underlie many of the waking functional deficits observed in PD, particularly akinesia, depression, and dementia.[263,267] Neuronal degeneration has been described in the serotonergic dorsal and median raphe, the noradrenergic locus ceruleus, and the cholinergic pedunculopontine tegmental nucleus.[264-266] Pathological involvement of some of these same structures in PSP,[264,422] torsion dystonia,[423] and HD[424] may also be relevant to the pathological sleep observed in these diseases. Pathological involvement of the forebrain cholinergic magnocellular basal nucleus and its widespread connections to the cerebral cortex also occurs in some cases of PD (see Chap. 18) and might be expected to contribute to some of the observed behavioral state-related alterations. The significance of pathological involvement of the ascending reticular activating system to the etiology and treatment of state-specific disorders in PD is limited. Experimental studies of the effects of lesioning or stimulating these structures, and their wake-sleep-specific neural activity, however, is of some heuristic value in understanding their potential contributions to the disturbed wake-sleep observed in PD, and is reviewed in the 1st edition of this book.

The development of more sensitive tools with which to localize dopaminergic axons and parkinsonian pathology, and their systematic application to the entire neuroaxis, has revealed novel sites in the thalamus and brainstem to which sleep-wake abnormalities may arise in parkinsonian conditions. With respect to disruption of thalamocortical rhythms, two observations are particularly relevant: (1) that widespread thalamic regions receive direct dopaminergic innervation via collaterals of nigrostriatal neurons;[405] and (2) that midline thalamic nuclei sometimes recognized as components of the ascending reticular activating system exhibit extensive pathology in idiopathic PD.[425-428] As mentioned earlier, involvement of motor and premotor neurons in the pontine and medullary reticular formation by the primary pathology of PD is particularly relevant to understanding state-dependent alterations of somatomotor output in parkinsonism[270] (see above).

ROLE OF THE BASAL GANGLIA IN BEHAVIORAL STATE CONTROL

Considerable evidence suggests that the basal ganglia influence sleep. Although there are several plausible substrates that might mediate this effect, our present understanding of the contribution of the basal ganglia to normal and pathological sleep is limited. According to current concepts, the basal ganglia may be viewed as components of a family of segregated, cortical-subcortical re-entrant pathways centered upon thalamocortical relationships (see Chap. 5).

An extensive literature invokes basal ganglia-thalamocortical circuits in modulating sleep, particularly sleep spindling,[429] but a unifying picture has not emerged. Cortical synchronization and somnolence, followed by increased REM sleep, after the withdrawal of low-frequency caudate stimulation in rats, monkey, and man[430,431] has been attributed to inhibition of the ascending reticular activating system.[432,433] Furthermore, REM sleep is enhanced after bilateral caudate ablation in rats.[434] Dopamine infusions into the caudate produce frontal sleep spindling and somnolence that are antagonized by acetylcholine.[435] Also intriguing are the reductions of REM sleep reported in animals and schizophrenics after frontal lobotomy/leukotomy.[436-439] Bilateral thalamotomy in animals and PD results in marked insomnia.[439-441] In summary, lesions and stimulation of individual components of basal ganglia-thalamocortical circuits clearly influence sleep, but the neural and pharmacological bases are poorly understood.

Functional models of the basal ganglia focus themselves, therefore, on an accounting of many aspects of normal and pathological waking movement.[442-444] The emphasis of these models on basal ganglia-thalamocortical circuitry largely ignores two pathways through which the basal ganglia might have important effects on sleep. First, midbrain dopamine neuron axon collaterals to the entire thalamus, including the thalamic reticular nucleus,[405] whose inhibition of thalamocortical activity is critical for entering slow-wave sleep.[445] Second, the PPN and midbrain extrapyramidal area (MEA) (Fig. 52-6), located at the junction of the midbrain and pons, are in receipt of a wide array of forebrain afferents, including fibers from the internal segment of the globus pallidus (GPi) via collaterals of the pallidothalamic pathway.[160] The MEA/PPN and the subceruleal region, with which they merge imperceptibly, contain neurons characterized as either "REM-on" or "REM-off"[446] and project to ventromedullary reticulospinal neurons of the "bulbospinal inhibitory zone" (BIZ) of Magoun and Rhines (Fig. 51-6).[446-449] The BIZ contains neurons that display REM sleep-specific increases in discharge rates and are necessary for maintaining REM atonia via active, glycine-mediated inhibition of motor neurons.[450] The MEA/PPN region, therefore, is optimally situated to transfer a wide array of forebrain influences to more caudal, medullary structures that modulate somatomotor activity in a state-dependent fashion.[160] The most parsimonious explanation for loss of REM sleep somatomotor inhibition would be medullary pathology, which is increasingly recognized in PD.[270] In fact, the contention that this pathology occurs very early in parkinsonian conditions[171] may account for the recognition of RBD, years before waking manifestations of the disease. Brain pathologies centered upon the MEA/PPN, or on brain regions connected with the MEA/PPN region via multisynaptic circuits also are very relevant to discussions of the pathophysiological basis of nocturnal movements, including RBD, in numerous neurodegenerative conditions.[160,451]

The influence of basal ganglia on brainstem-reticulospinal pathways originating from the MEA/PPN/subceruleal

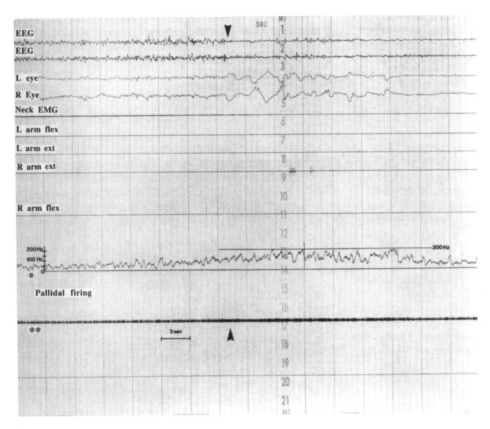

FIGURE 52-7 Enhanced neural discharge in the nonhuman primate globus pallidus (GPi) preceding and at transition (arrowheads) from stage 2 NREM to REM sleep. Phasic elevations of activity approaching 200 Hz coincide with bursts of rapid eye movements. In tonic REM sleep, for example, to the extreme right-hand side of the figure, GPi neural discharge decreases to near waking levels (35–45 Hz). This extracellular recording was from a neuron located in the sensorimotor portion of the GPi and was responsive to passive limb movement. An identical discharge pattern was observed in this unit during two subsequent transitions to REM sleep that occurred during 3 hours of continuous recording. *Single-unit activity in the GPi, expressed as a 200-ms moving average of frequency of firing. Ordinate divisions in increments of 50 Hz. **Single-unit activity in the GPi, recorded as acceptance pulse indicating time-discriminated spikes.

region has been inferred on the basis of accentuated blink reflexes[258–260] and acoustic facilitation of spinal reflexes in PD patients.[261,262] Similar reflex pathway abnormalities in patients with PLMs, but not suffering from PD, suggest modulation of PLMs by the same neuropharmacological substrates.[42,45]

The relevance of this multisynaptic pathway between the basal ganglia and lower neural axis to the modulation of normal and pathologic sleep-wake states remains ill-defined. The GABAergic output of the GPi to cholinergic PPN neurons has been proposed to play an active role in generating pontogeniculate-occipital waves that herald the onset of REM sleep and presumably correlate with dream imagery.[452,453] The MEA/PPN/subceruleal region and its potential modulation by output from the GPi may also play an important role in modulating motor activity in REM sleep. In both cats and humans, for example, lesions of the MEA/PPN/subceruleal region or interruption of their descending output tract (i.e., the central tegmental or reticulotegmental tracts) to the BIZ eliminate REM atonia[446,454–456] or result in RBD (see above). The occurrence of RBD in PD, therefore, suggests a disruption of midbrain-pontine-BIZ neural circuits manifesting as insufficient motor inhibition in REM sleep. The pathophysiological basis of RBD may lie in degeneration of the PPN itself, because this nucleus is involved in the primary pathology of PD in some cases;[264,265] however, recent studies

suggest that such pathology might result in decreased, rather than increased, phasic EMG activity in REM sleep.[456] The neural basis underlying REM-related myoclonus and RBD in PD could also reflect excessive GABAergic drive to the MEA/PPN/subceruleal region from the GPi. One might hypothesize that GABAergic basal ganglia output modulates midbrain-pontine REM sleep-related neural activity, which, in turn, would influence BIZ reticulospinal neuronal activity necessary for maintaining REM atonia. Phasic neural activity in nuclei implicated in waking movement, in fact, coincides with somato- and oculomotor activity during REM sleep; for example, in the GPi[457] (Fig. 52-7), reticulospinal neurons,[458] red nucleus,[459] and pyramidal cells in the motor cortex.[460] The excessive bursting of GPi neurons observed in PD[444,461] might therefore prove to be one of the underlying reasons why somatic motorneuron inhibition is overcome in REM sleep in parkinsonism.

Acknowledgments

The authors would like to extend their greatest appreciation to Drs. Dainis Irbe, Bhupesh Dihenia, Lisa Johnston, and Paul Gurecki for their assistance in performing and scoring polysomnographic records from a variety of movement disorder patients, as well as

Dr. Robert Turner for his critical help in recording sleep/wake-specific neuronal discharge in the primate globus pallidus. Supported in part by US Public Health Service grants NS-36697, NS-40221, NS-43374, and the Restless Legs Syndrome Foundation (DBR), and NS-35345 and AG-10643 to DLB.

References

1. Fujimoto T, Nishizono H: Muscle contractile properties by surface electrodes compared with those by needle electrodes. *Electroencephalogr Clin Neurophysiol* 89:247–251, 1993.

2. van Hilten J, Kabel J, Middelkoop H, et al: Assessment of response fluctuations in Parkinson's disease by ambulatory wrist activity monitoring. *Acta Neurol Scand* 87:171–177, 1993.

3. Jacobson A, Kales A, Lehmann D, Hoedemaker F: Muscle tonus in human subjects during sleep and dreaming. *Exp Neurol* 10:418–424, 1964.

4. Kleitman N, Cooperman N, Mullin F: Studies on the physiology of sleep IX. Motility and body temperature during sleep. *Am J Physiol* 105:574–584, 1933.

5. Johnson H, Swan T, Weigand G: In what positions do healthy people sleep? *J Am Med Assoc* 94:2058–2062, 1930.

6. Hobson J, Spagna T, Malenka R: Ethology of sleep studied with time-lapse photography: Postural immobility and sleep-cycle phase in humans. *Science* 204:251–253, 1978.

7. Gardner JR, Grossman W: Normal motor patterns in sleep in man, in *Advances in Sleep Research*. New York: Spectrum Publications, 1975, pp 67–107.

8. Suckling E, Koenig E, Hoffman B, Brooks C: The physiological effects of sleeping on hard or soft beds. *Hum Biol* 29:274–288, 1957.

9. Moses J, Lubin A, Naitoh P, Johnson L: Methodology: Reliability of sleep measures. *Psychophysiology* 9:78–82, 1972.

10. Muzet A, Naitoh P, Townsend R, Johnson L: Body movements during sleep as a predictor of stage change. *Psychon Sci* 29:7–10, 1972.

11. Naitoh P, Muzet A, Johnson L, Moses J: Body movements during sleep after sleep loss. *Psychophysiology* 10:363–368, 1973.

12. Townsend R, Johnson L, Naitoh P: Heart rate preceding motility in sleep. *Psychophysiology* 12:217–219, 1975.

13. De Lisi L: Su di un fenomeno motorio constate del sonno normale: Le mioclonie ipniche fisiologiche. *Riv Pat Nerv Ment* 39:481–496, 1932.

14. Oswald I: Sudden bodily jerks on falling asleep. *Brain* 82:92–103, 1959.

15. Stoyva J: Finger electromyographic activity during sleep: Its relation to dreaming in deaf and normal subjects. *J Abnorm Psychol* 70:343–349, 1965.

16. Askenasy J, Yahr M, Davidovitch S: Isolated phasic discharges in anterior tibial muscle: A stable feature of paradoxical sleep. *J Clin Neurophysiol* 5:175–181, 1988.

17. Chokroverty S: Phasic tongue movements in human rapid-eye-movement sleep. *Neurology* 30:665–668, 1980.

18. Bliwise D, Coleman R, Bergmann B, et al: Facial muscle tonus during REM and NREM sleep. *Psychophysiology* 11:447–508, 1974.

19. Slegel DE, Benson KL, Zarcone VPJ, et al: Middle-ear muscle activity (MEMA) and its association with motor activity in the extremities and head in sleep. *Sleep* 14:454–459, 1991.

20. Pessah M, Roffwarg H: Spontaneous middle ear muscle activity in man: A rapid eye movement sleep phenomenon. *Science* 178:773–776, 1972.

21. Gassel MM, Marchiafava PL, Pompeiano O: Phasic changes in muscular activity during desynchronized sleep in unrestrained cats. *Arch Ital Biol* 102:449–470, 1964.

22. Cepeda C, Naquet R: Physiological sleep myoclonus in baboons. *Electroencephalogr Clin Neurophysiol* 60:158–162, 1985.

23. Montagna P, Liguori R, Zucconi M, et al: Physiological hypnic myoclonus. *Electroencephalogr Clin Neurophysiol* 70:172–175, 1988.

24. Montagna P, Liguori R, Zucconi M, et al: Fasciculations during wakefulness and sleep. *Acta Neurol Scand* 76:152–154, 1987.

25. van Hilten B, Hoff J, Middelkoop H, et al: Sleep disruption in Parkinson's disease. Assessment by continuous activity monitoring. *Arch Neurol* 51:922–928, 1994.

26. Silber M, Dexter D, Ahlskog J, et al: Abnormal REM sleep motor activity in untreated Parkinson's disease. *Sleep Res* 22:274, 1993 (abstract).

27. Laihinen A, Alihanka J, Raitasuo S, Rinne U: Sleep movements and associated autonomic nervous activities in patients with Parkinson's disease. *Acta Neurol Scand* 76:64–68, 1987.

28. Klawans H, Goetz C, Bergen D: Levodopa-induced myoclonus. *Arch Neurol* 32:331–334, 1975.

29. Bliwise D, Keenan S, Burnburg D, et al: Inter-rater reliability for scoring periodic leg movements in sleep. *Sleep* 14:249–251, 1991.

30. Askenasy J, Yahr M: Different laws govern motor activity in sleep than in wakefulness. *J Neural Transm* 79:103–111, 1990.

31. Coleman R, Pollak C, Weitzman E: Periodic movements in sleep (nocturnal myoclonus): Relation to sleep disorders. *Ann Neurol* 8:416–421, 1980.

32. Bliwise D, Ingham R, Date E, Dement W: Nerve conduction and creatinine clearance in aged subjects with periodic movements in sleep. *J Gerontol A* 44:M164–M167, 1989.

33. Pollmächer T, Schulz H: Periodic leg movements (PLM): Their relationship to sleep stages. *Sleep* 16:572–577, 1993.

34. Bliwise D: Sleep in normal aging and dementia. *Sleep* 16:40–81, 1993.

35. Bliwise D, Petta D, Seidel W, Dement W: Periodic leg movements during sleep in the elderly. *Arch Gerontol Geriatr* 4:273–281, 1985.

36. Ancoli-Israel S, Martin J, Jones D, et al: Sleep-disordered breathing and periodic leg movements in sleep in older patients with schizophrenia. *Biol Psychiatry* 45:1426–1432, 1999.

37. Kales A, Bixler E, Soldatos C, et al: Biopsychobehavioral correlates of insomnia, part 1: Role of sleep apnea and nocturnal myoclonus. *Psychosomatics* 23:589–600, 1982.

38. Aldrich M, Shipley J: Alcohol use and periodic limb movements of sleep. *Alcohol Clin Exp Res* 17:192–196, 1993.

39. Shafor R: Prevalence of abnormal lumbo-sacral spine imaging in patients with insomnia associated restless legs, periodic movements in sleep. *Sleep Res* 20:396, 1991.

40. Dzvonik M, Kripke D, Klauber M, Ancoli-Israel S: Body position changes and periodic movements in sleep. *Sleep* 9:484–491, 1986.

41. Smith R, Gouin P, Minkley P, et al: Periodic limb movement disorder is associated with normal motor conduction latencies when studied by central magnetic stimulation: Successful use of a new technique. *Sleep* 15:312–318, 1992.

42. Wechsler L, Stakes J, Shahani B, Busis N: Periodic leg movements of sleep (nocturnal myoclonus): An electrophysiological study. *Ann Neurol* 19:168–173, 1986.

43. Smith R: Confirmation of Babinski-like response in periodic movements in sleep (nocturnal myoclonus). *Biol Psychiatry* 22:1271–1273, 1987.

44. Smith R: Relationship of periodic movements in sleep (nocturnal myoclonus) and the Babinski sign. *Sleep* 8:239–243, 1985.

45. Wechsler L, Stakes J, Shahani B, Busis N: Nocturnal myoclonus, restless legs syndrome, and abnormal electrophysiological findings. *Ann Neurol* 21:515, 1987.

46. Lugaresi E, Coccagna G, Mantovani M, Lebrun R: Some periodic phenomena arising during drowsiness and sleep in man. *Electroencephalogr Clin Neurophysiol* 32:701–705, 1972.

47. Ali N, Davies R, Fleetham J, Stradling J: Periodic movements of the legs during sleep associated with rises in systemic blood pressure. *Sleep* 14:163–165, 1991.

48. Montplaisir J, Godbout R: Restless legs syndrome and periodic movements during sleep, in Kryger M, Roth T, Dement W (eds): *Principles and Practice of Sleep Medicine*. Philadelphia: WB Saunders, 1994, pp 402–409.

49. Staedt J, Stoppe G, Kogler A, et al: Nocturnal myoclonus syndrome (periodic movements in sleep) related to central dopamine D2-receptor alteration. *Eur Arch Psychiatry Clin Neurosci* 245:8–10, 1995.

50. Staedt J, Stoppe G, Kogler A, et al: Dopamine D2 receptor alteration in patients with periodic movements in sleep (nocturnal myoclonus). *J Neural Transm* 93:71–74, 1993.

51. Ekbom K: Restless legs syndrome. *Neurology* 10:868–875, 1960.

52. Ekbom K: Restless legs. *Acta Med Scand Suppl* 158:1–123, 1945.

53. Montplaisir J, Boucher S, Poirier G, et al: Clinical, polysomnographic, and genetic characteristics of restless legs syndrome: A study of 133 patients diagnosed with new standard criteria. *Mov Disord* 12:61–65, 1997.

54. Cheshire WP Jr: Hypotensive akathisia: Autonomic failure associated with leg fidgeting while sitting. *Neurology* 55:1923–1926, 2000.

55. Jones K, Castleden C: A double-bind comparison of quinine sulphate and placebo in muscle cramps. *Age Ageing* 12:155–158, 1983.

56. Sidorov J: Quinine sulfate for leg cramps: Does it work? *J Am Geriatr Soc* 41:498–500, 1993.

57. Jacobsen J, Rosenberg R, Huttenlocher P, Spire J-P: Familial nocturnal cramping. *Sleep* 9:54–60, 1986.

58. American Sleep Disorders Association: *International Classification of Sleep Disorders. Diagnostic and Coding Manual, Revised*. Rochester, MN: 1997.

59. Lavigne G, Montplaisir J: Restless legs syndrome and sleep bruxism: Prevalence and association among Canadians. *Sleep* 17:739–743, 1994.

60. Tan E, Ondo W: Restless legs syndrome: Clinical features and treatment. *Am J Med Sci* 319:397–403, 2000.

61. Ondo W, Jankovic J: Restless legs syndrome: Clinicoetiologic correlates. *Neurology* 47:1435–1441, 1996.

62. Walters A, Hickey K, Maltzman J, et al: A questionnaire study of 138 patients with restless legs syndrome: The "Night-Walkers" survey. *Neurology* 46:92–95, 1996.

63. Picchietti D, Walters A: Severe periodic limb movement disorder in childhood and adolescence, in Chase M, Rosenthal L, O'Connor C (eds): *Sleep Research*. Los Angeles: Brain Information Service/Brain Research Institute, UCLA, 1996, p 333.

64. Picchietti D, Walters A: Moderate to severe periodic limb movement disorder in childhood and adolescence. *Sleep* 22:297–300, 1999.

65. Picchietti D, England S, Walters A, et al: Periodic leg movement disorder and restless legs syndrome in children with attention-deficit hyperactivity disorder. *J Child Neurol* 13:588–594, 1998.

66. Winkelmann J, Wetter T, Collado-Seidel V, et al: Clinical characteristics and frequency of the hereditary restless legs syndrome in a population of 300 patients. *Sleep* 23:597–602, 2000.

67. Allen R, Earley C: Defining the phenotype of the restless legs syndrome (RLS) using age-of-symptom-onset. *Sleep Med* 1:11–19, 2000.

68. Winkelmann J, Muller-Myshok B, Wittchen H, et al: Complex segregation analysis of restless legs syndrome provides evidence for an autosomal dominant mode of inheritance in early age at onset families. *Ann Neurol* 52:297–302, 2002.

69. Ondo WG, Vuong KD, Wang Q: Restless legs syndrome in monozygotic twins. *Neurology* 55:1404–1406, 2000.

70. Walters A, Picchietti D, Hening W, Lazzarini M: Variable expressivity in familial restless legs syndrome. *Arch Neurol* 47:1219–1220, 1990.

71. Lazzarini A, Walters AS, Hickey K, et al: Studies of penetrance and anticipation in five autosomal-dominant restless legs syndrome pedigrees. *Mov Disord* 14:111–116, 1999.

72. Desautels A, Turecki G, Montplaisir J, et al: Identification of a major susceptibility locus for restless legs syndrome on chromsome 12q. *Am J Hum Genet* 69:1266–1270, 2001.

73. Kock N, Culjkovic B, Maniak S, et al: Mode of inheritance and susceptibility locus for restless legs syndrome, on chromosome 12q. *Am J Hum Genet* 71:205–207, 2002.

74. Desautels A, Turecki G, Montplaisir J, Rouleau GA: Reply to Kock et al: *Am J Hum Genet* 71:208–209, 2002.

75. Bonati M, Ferini-Strambi L, Aridon P, et al: Autosomal dominant restless legs syndrome maps on chromosome 14q. *Brain* 126:1485–1492, 2003.

76. Wittig R, Zorick F, Piccione P, et al: Narcolepsy and disturbed nocturnal sleep. *Clin Electroencephalogr* 14:130–134, 1983.

77. Guilleminault C, Crowe C, Quera-Salva M, et al: Periodic leg movement, sleep fragmentation and central sleep apnoea in two cases: Reduction with clonazepam. *Eur Respir J* 1:762–765, 1988.

78. Fry J, DiPhillipo M, Pressman M: Periodic leg movements in sleep following treatment of obstructive sleep apnea with nasal continuous positive airway pressure (CPAP). *Chest* 96:89–91, 1989.

79. Mahowald M, Schenck C: REM sleep behavior disorder, in Kryger M, Roth T, Dement W (eds): *Principles and Practices of Sleep Medicine*. Philadelphia: WB Saunders, 1994, pp 574–588.

80. Schenck C, Mahowald M: Motor dyscontrol in narcolepsy: Rapid-eye-movement (REM) sleep without atonia and REM sleep behavior disorder. *Ann Neurol* 32:3–10, 1992.

81. Moldofsky H, Tullis C, Lue F: Sleep related myoclonus in rheumatic pain modulation disorder (fibrositis syndrome). *J Rheumatol* 13:614–617, 1986.

82. Moldofsky H, Tullis C, Lue F, et al: Sleep-related myoclonus in rheumatic pain modulation disorder (fibrositis syndrome) and in excessive daytime somnolence. *Psychosom Med* 46:145–151, 1984.

83. Allen R, Earley C: Restless legs syndrome: a review of clinical and pathophysiologic features. *J Clin Neurophysiol* 18:128–147, 2001.

84. Freeman A, Ranadive V, Rye D: Human forebrain devoid of brainstem influences exhibits EEG and neuroendocrine rhythms. *Sleep* 23(suppl 2):A347–A348, 2000.

85. Yokota T, Hirose K, Tanabe H, Tsukagoshi H: Sleep-related periodic leg movements (nocturnal myoclonus) due to spinal cord lesion. *J Neurol Sci* 104:13–18, 1991.

86. Dickel M, Renfrow S, Moore P, Berry R: Rapid eye movement sleep periodic leg movements in patients with spinal cord injury. *Sleep* 17:733–738, 1994.

87. Lee M, Choi Y, Lee S: Sleep-related periodic leg movements associated with spinal cord lesions. *Mov Disord* 11:719–722, 1996.

88. de Mello MT, Poyares DL, Tufik S: Treatment of periodic leg movements with a dopaminergic agonist in subjects with total spinal cord lesions. *Spinal Cord* 37:634–637, 1999.

89. Briellmann R, Rosler K, Hess C: Blink reflex excitability is abnormal in patients with periodic leg movements in sleep. *Mov Disord* 11:710–714, 1996.

90. Bara-Jimenez W, Aksu M, Graham B, et al: Periodic limb movements in sleep. State dependent excitability of the spinal flexor reflex. *Neurology* 54:1609–1615, 2000.

91. Montplaisir J, Godbout R, Boghen D, et al: Familial restless legs with periodic movements in sleep: Electrophysiologic, biochemical, and pharmacologic study. *Neurology* 35:130–134, 1985.

92. Iannaccone S, Zucconi M, Marchettini P, et al: Evidence of peripheral axonal neuropathy in primary restless legs syndrome. *Mov Disord* 10:2–9, 1995.

93. Rutkove S, Matheson J, Logigian E: Restless legs syndrome in patients with polyneuropathy. *Muscle Nerve* 19:670–672, 1996.

94. Gemignani F, Marbini A, Di Giovanni G, et al: Charcot-Marie-Tooth disease type 2 with restless legs syndrome. *Neurology* 52:1064–1066, 1999.

95. Turjanski N, Lees A, Brooks D: Striatal dopaminergic function in restless legs syndrome. *Neurology* 52:932–937, 1999.

96. Eisensehr I, Wetter TC, Linke R, et al: Normal IPT and IBZM SPECT in drug-naive and levodopa-treated idiopathic restless legs syndrome. *Neurology* 57:1307–1309, 2001.

97. Decker M, Keating G, Freeman A, Rye D: Parkinsonian-like sleep-wake architecture in rats with bilateral striatal 6-OHDA lesions. *Soc Neurosci Abstr* 26:1514, 2000.

98. Bliwise D, Rye D, Dihenia B, et al: Periodic leg movements in elderly patients with parkinsonism. *Sleep* 21(suppl):196, 1998.

99. Wetter T, Collado-Seidel V, Pollmacher T, et al: Sleep and periodic leg movement patterns in drug-free patients with Parkinson's disease and multiple system atrophy. *Sleep* 23:361–367, 2000.

100. Ondo WG, Vuong KV, Khan H, et al: Daytime sleepiness and other sleep disorders in Parkinson's disease. *Neurology* 57:1392–1396, 2001.

101. Ondo WG, He Y, Rajasekaran S, Le WD: Clinical correlates of 6-hydroxydopamine injections into A11 dopaminergic neurons in rats: A possible model for restless legs syndrome. *Mov Disord* 15:154–158, 2000.

102. O'Keeffe S, Gavin K, Lavan J: Iron status and restless legs syndrome in the elderly. *Age Ageing* 23:200–203, 1994.

103. Allen R, Barker P, Wehrl F, et al: MRI measurement of brain iron in patients with restless legs syndrome. *Neurology* 56:263–265, 2001.

104. Nordlander N: Therapy in restless legs. *Acta Med Scand* 145:453–457, 1953.

105. O'Keefe S, Noel J, Lavan J: Restless legs syndrome in the elderly. *Postgrad Med J* 69:701–703, 1993.

106. Brown T, Fleishman S: Caffeine consumption and periodic limb movements of sleep. *Sleep Res* 24:208, 1995.

107. Morgan J, Brown TM, Wallace ER 4th: Monoamine oxidase inhibitors and sleep movements. *Am J Psychiatry* 151:782–783, 1994.

108. Bakshi R: Fluoxetine and restless legs syndrome. *J Neurol Sci* 142:151–152, 1996.

109. Salin-Pascual R, Galicia-Polo L, Drucker-Colin R: Sleep changes after 4 consecutive days of venlafaxine administration in normal volunteers. *J Clin Psychiatry* 58:348–350, 1997.

110. Hening W, Allen R, Earley C, et al: The treatment of restless legs syndrome and periodic limb movement disorder: An American Academy of Sleep Medicine review. *Sleep* 22:970–999, 1999.

111. Hening W, Walters A, Kavey N, et al: Dyskinesias while awake and periodic movements in sleep in restless legs syndrome: Treatment with opioids. *Neurology* 36:1363–1366, 1986.

112. Kavey N, Walters AS, Hening W, Gidro-Frank S: Opioid treatment of periodic movements in sleep in patients without restless legs. *Neuropeptides* 11:181–184, 1988.

113. Kavey N, Whyte J, Gidro-Frank S, et al: Treatment of restless legs syndrome and periodic movements in sleep with propoxyphene. *Sleep Res* 16:367, 1987 (abstract).

114. Garcia-Borreguero D, Larrosa O, de la Llave Y, et al: Treatment of restless legs syndrome with gabapentin: A double-blind, cross-over study. *Neurology* 59:1573–1579, 2002.

115. Mitler M, Browman C, Menn S, et al: Nocturnal myoclonus: Treatment efficacy of clonazepam and temazepam. *Sleep* 9:385–392, 1986.

116. Allen R, Earley C: Augmentation of the restless legs syndrome with carbidopa/levodopa. *Sleep* 19:205–213, 1996.

117. Staedt J, Wassmuth F, Ziemann U, et al: Pergolide: Treatment of choice in restless legs syndrome (RLS) and nocturnal myoclonus syndrome (NMS). A double-blind randomized crossover trial of pergolide versus L-dopa. *J Neural Transm* 104:461–468, 1997.

118. Wetter T, Stiasny K, Winkelman J: A randomized controlled study of pergolide in patients with restless legs syndrome. *Neurology* 52:944–950, 1999.

119. Silber M, Shepard JJ, Wisbey J: Pergolide in the management of restless legs syndrome: An extended study. *Sleep* 20:878–882, 1997.

120. Stiasny K, Wetter T, Winkelman J, et al: Long-term effects of pergolide in the treatment of restless legs syndrome. *Neurology* 56:1399–1402, 2001.

121. Montplaisir J, Nicolas A, Denesle R, Gomez-Mancilla B: Restless legs syndrome improved by pramipexole: A double-blind randomized study. *Neurology* 52:938–943, 1999.

122. Montplaisir J, Denesle R, Petit D: Pramipexole in the treatment of restless legs syndrome: A follow-up study. *Eur J Neurol* 7; suppl 1:27–31, 2000.

123. Saletu B, Anderer P, Saletu B, et al: Sleep laboratory studies in restless legs syndrome patients as compared with normals and acute effects of ropinirole. 2. Findings on periodic leg movements, arousals and respiratory variables. *Neuropsychobiology* 41:190–199, 2000.

124. Ondo W: Ropinirole for restless legs syndrome. *Mov Disord* 14:138–140, 1999.

125. Ehrenberg B, Eisensehr I, Walters A: Influence of valproate on sleep and periodic limb movements disorder. *Sleep Res* 24:227, 1995.

126. Mellick G, Mellick L: Successful treatment of restless leg syndrome with gabapentin (Neurontin). *Sleep Res* 24:290, 1995.

127. Schenck C, Bundlie S, Ettinger M, Mahowald M: Chronic behavioral disorders of human REM sleep: A new category of parasomnia. *Sleep* 9:293–308, 1986.

128. Uhde T: The anxiety disorders, in Kryger M, Roth T, Dement W (eds): *Principles and Practice of Sleep Medicine*. Philadelphia: WB Saunders, 1994, pp 871–898.

129. Olson E, Boeve B, Silber M: Rapid eye movement sleep behaviour disorder: Demographic, clinical and laboratory findings in 93 cases. *Brain* 123:331–339, 2000.

130. Mahowald M, Schenck C: REM sleep parasomnias, in Kryger M, Roth T, Dement W (eds): *Principles and Practice of Sleep Medicine*, 3rd ed. St. Louis: WB Saunders, 2000, pp 724–743.

131. Schenck C, Bundlie S, Mahowald M: Delayed emergence of a parkinsonian disorder in 38% of 29 older men initially diagnosed with idiopathic rapid eye movement sleep behavior disorder. *Neurology* 46:388–393, 1996.

132. Boeve B, Silber M, Ferman T, et al: REM sleep behavior disorder and degenerative dementia: An association likely reflecting Lewy body disease. *Neurology* 51:363–370, 1998.

133. Boeve B, Silber M, Ferman T, et al: Association of REM sleep behavior disorder and neurodegenerative disease may reflect an underlying synucleinopathy. *Mov Disord* 16:622–630, 2001.

134. Turner R, Chervin R, Frey K, et al: Probable diffuse Lewy body disease presenting as REM sleep behavior disorder. *Neurology* 49:523–527, 1997.

135. Turner R: Idiopathic rapid eye movement sleep behavior disorder is a harbinger of dementia with Lewy bodies. *J Geriatr Psychiatry Neurol* 15:195–199, 2002.

136. Tison F, Wenning GK, Quinn NP, Smith SJ: REM sleep behaviour disorder as the presenting symptom of multiple system atrophy [letter]. *J Neurol Neurosurg Psychiatry* 58:379–380, 1995.

137. Shimizu T, Inami Y, Sugita Y, et al: REM sleep without muscle atonia (stage 1-REM) and its relation to delirious behavior during sleep in patients with degenerative diseases involving the brain stem. *Jpn J Psychiatry Neurol* 44:681–692, 1990.

138. Aldrich MS, Foster NL, White RF, et al: Sleep abnormalities in progressive supranuclear palsy. *Ann Neurol* 25:577–581, 1989.

139. Kimura K, Tachibana N, Aso T, et al: Subclinical REM sleep behavior disorder in a patient with corticobasal degeneration. *Sleep* 20:891–894, 1997.

140. Syed B, Rye D, Singh G: REM sleep behavior disorder and SCA-3 (Machado-Joseph disease). *Neurology* 14:148, 2003.

141. Iranzo A, Munoz E, Santamaria J, et al: REM sleep behavior disorder and vocal cord paralysis in Machado-Joseph disease. *Mov Disord* 18(10):1531–8257, 2003.

142. Friedman J: Presumed rapid eye movement behavior disorder in Machado-Joseph disease (spinocerebellar ataxia type 3). *Mov Disord* 17:1350–1353, 2002.

143. Culebras A, Moore J: Magnetic resonance findings in REM sleep behavior disorder. *Neurology* 39:1519–1523, 1989.

144. Kimura K, Tachibana N, Kohyama J, et al: A discrete pontine ischemic lesion could cause REM-sleep behavior disorder. *Neurology* 55:894–895, 2000.

145. Gross M, Goodenough D, Tobin M, et al: Sleep disturbances and hallucinations in the acute alcoholic psychoses. *J Nerv Ment Dis* 142:493–514, 1966.

146. Greenberg R, Pearlman C: Delirium tremens and dreaming. *Am J Psychiatry* 124:37–46, 1967.

147. Guilleminault C, Raynal D, Takahaski S, et al: Evaluation of short-term and long-term treatment of the narcolepsy syndrome with clomipramine hydrochloride. *Acta Neurol Scand* 54:71–87, 1976.

148. Akindele M, Evans J, Oswald I: Mono-amine oxidase inhibitors, sleep and mood. *Electroencephalogr Clin Neurophysiol* 29:47–56, 1970.

149. Schenck C, Mahowald M, Kim S, et al: Prominent eye movements during NREM sleep and REM sleep behavior disorder associated with fluoxetine treatment of depression and obsessive-compulsive disorder. *Sleep* 15:226–235, 1992.

150. Lapierre O, Montplaisir J: Polysomnographic features of REM sleep behavior disorder: Development of a scoring method. *Neurology* 42:1371–1374, 1992.

151. Gagnon J, Bedard M-A, Fantini M, et al: REM sleep behavior disorder and REM sleep without atonia in Parkinson's disease. *Neurology* 59:585–589, 2002.

152. Schenck C, Bundlie S, Mahowald M: REM behavior disorder (RBD): Delayed emergence of parkinsonism or dementia in 65% of older men initially diagnosed with idiopathic RBD, and an analysis of the minimum and maximum tonic and/or phasic electromyographic abnormalities found during REM sleep. *Sleep* 26 (suppl):A316, 2003.

153. Hendricks JC, Morrison AR, Mann GL: Different behaviors during paradoxical sleep without atonia depend on pontine lesion site. *Brain Res* 239:81–105, 1982.

154. Morrison A: Paradoxical sleep without atonia. *Arch Ital Biol* 126:275–289, 1988.

155. Shouse M, Siegel J: Pontine regulation of REM sleep components in cats: Integrity of the pedunculopontine tegmentum (PPT) is important for phasic events but unnecessary for atonia during REM sleep. *Brain Res* 571:50–63, 1992.

156. Morrison AR, Mann GL, Hendricks JC: The relationship of excessive exploratory behavior in wakefulness to paradoxical sleep without atonia. *Sleep* 4:247–257, 1981.

157. Trulson ME, Jacobs BL, Morrison AR: Raphe unit activity across the sleep-waking cycle in normal cats and in pontine lesioned cats displaying REM sleep without atonia. *Brain Res* 226:75–91, 1981.

158. Wu MF, Gulyani SA, Yau E, et al: Locus coeruleus neurons: Cessation of activity during cataplexy. *Neuroscience* 91:1389–1399, 1999.

159. Morrison A: The pathophysiology of REM-sleep behavior disorder. *Sleep* 21:446, 1998.

160. Rye D: Contributions of the pedunculopontine region to normal and altered REM sleep. *Sleep* 20:757–788, 1997.

161. Eisensehr I, Linke R, Noachtar S, et al: Reduced striatal dopamine transporters in idiopathic rapid eye movement behaviour disorder. Comparison with Parkinson's disease and controls. *Brain* 123:1155–1160, 2000.

162. Albin R, Koeppe R, Chervin R, et al: Decreased striatal dopaminergic innervation in REM sleep behavior disorder. *Neurology* 55:1410–1412, 2000.

163. Daley J, Turner R, Bliwise D, Rye D: Nocturnal sleep and daytime alertness in the MPTP-treated primate. *Sleep* 22 (suppl):S218–S219, 1999.

164. Vitek J, Kaneoke Y, Turner R, et al: Neuronal activity in the internal (GPi) and external (GPe) segments of the globus pallidus (GP) of parkinsonian patients is similar to that in the MPTP-treated primate model of parkinsonism. *Soc Neurosci Abstr* 19:1584, 1993.

165. Magnin M, Morel A, Jeanmonod D: Single-unit analysis of the pallidum, thalamus and subthalamic nucleus in parkinsonian patients. *Neuroscience* 96:549–564, 2000.

166. Rye D, Dempsay J, Dihenia B, et al: REM-sleep dyscontrol in Parkinson's disease: Case report of effects of elective pallidotomy. *Sleep Res* 26:591, 1997.

167. Tan A, Salgado M, Fahn S: Rapid eye movement sleep behavior disorder preceding Parkinson's disease with therapeutic response to levodopa. *Mov Disord* 11:214–216, 1996.

168. Arnulf I, Bejjani B, Garma L, et al: Improvement of sleep architecture in PD with subthalamic nucleus stimulation. *Neurology* 55:1732–1734, 2000.

169. Iranzo A, Valldeoriola F, Santamaria J, et al: Sleep symptoms and polysomnographic architecture in advanced Parkinson's disease after chronic bilateral subthalamic stimulation. *J Neurol Neurosurg Psychiatry* 72:661–664, 2002.

170. Garcia-Borreguero D, Caminero A, de la Llave Y, et al: Decreased phasic EMG activity during REM-sleep in treatment-naive Parkinson's disease: Effects of treatment with L-dopa and progression of illness. *Mov Disord* 17:934–941, 2002.

171. Braak H, Rub U, Gai W, Del Tredici K: Idiopathic Parkinson's disease: Possible routes by which vulnerable neuronal types may be subject to neuroinvasion by an unknown pathogen. *J Neural Transm* 110:517–536, 2003.

172. Ringman J, Simmons J: Treatment of REM sleep behavior disorder with donepezil: A report of three cases. *Neurology* 55:870–871, 2000.

173. Kunz D, Bes F: Melatonin restores REM-sleep muscle atonia in 5/6 RBD patients. *Sleep* 21:195, 1998.

174. Kunz D, Bes F: Melatonin as a therapy in REM sleep behavior disorder patients: An open-labeled pilot study on the possible influence of melatonin on REM-sleep regulation. *Mov Disord* 14:507–511, 1999.

175. Takeuchi N, Uchimura N, Hashimuze Y, et al: Melatonin therapy for REM sleep behavior disorder. *Psychiatry Clin Neurosci* 55:267–270, 2001.

176. Broughton R, Tolentino M, Krelina M: Excessive fragmentary myoclonus in NREM sleep: A report of 38 cases. *Electroencephalogr Clin Neurophysiol* 61:123–309, 1985.

177. Dagino N, Loeb C, Massazza G, Sacco G: Hypnic physiological myoclonus in man: An EEG-EMG study in normals and neurological patients. *Eur Neurol* 2:47–58, 1969.

178. Provini F, Plazzi G, Tinuper P, et al: Nocturnal frontal lobe epilepsy. A clinical and polygraphic overview of 100 consecutive cases. *Brain* 122:1017–1031, 1999.

179. Provini F, Plazzi G, Lugaresi E: From nocturnal paroxysmal dystonia to nocturnal frontal lobe epilepsy. *Clin Neurophysiol* 111 (suppl 2):S2–S8, 2000.

180. Sforza E, Montagna P, Rinaldi R, et al: Paroxysmal periodic motor attacks during sleep: Clinical and polygraphic features. *Electroencephalogr Clin Neurophysiol* 86:161–166, 1993.

181. Terzano M, Parrino L, Spaggiari M: The cyclic alternating pattern sequences in the dynamic organization of sleep. *Electroencephalogr Clin Neurophysiol* 69:437–447, 1988.

182. Terzano M, Monge-Strauss M, Mikol F, et al: Cyclic alternating pattern as a provocative factor in nocturnal paroxysmal dystonia. *Epilepsia* 38:1015–1025, 1997.

183. Lugaresi E, Cirignotta F: Hypnogenic paroxysmal dystonia: Epileptic seizure or a new syndrome? *Sleep* 4:129–138, 1981.

184. Tinuper P, Cerullo A, Cirignotta F, et al: Nocturnal paroxysmal dystonia with short-lasting attacks: Three cases with evidence for an epileptic frontal lobe origin of seizures. *Epilepsia* 31:549–556, 1990.

185. Regestein Q, Hartmann E, Reich P: A head movement disorder occurring in dreaming sleep. *J Nerv Ment Dis* 16:432–435, 1977.

186. Gagnon P, Koninck JD: Repetitive head movements during REM sleep. *Biol Psychiatry* 20:176–178, 1985.

187. Klackenberg G: Rhythmic movements in infancy and early childhood. *Acta Pediatr Scand* 224(suppl):74, 1971.

188. Drake ME Jr.: Jactatio nocturna after head injury. *Neurology* 36:867–868, 1986.

189. Tuxhorn I, Hoppe M: Parasomnia with rhythmic movements manifesting as nocturnal tongue biting. *Neuropediatrics* 24:167–168, 1993.

190. Rosenberg C: Elimination of a rhythmic movement disorder with hypnosis: A case report. *Sleep* 18:608–609, 1995.

191. Lavigne G, Kato T, Kolta A, Sessle B: Neurobiological mechanisms involved in sleep bruxism. *Crit Rev Oral Biol Med* 14:30–46, 2003.

192. Hartmann E: Bruxism, in Kryer M, Roth T, Dement W (eds): *Principles of Practice of Sleep Medicine*, 2nd ed. Philadelphia: WB Saunders, 1994, pp 598–601.

193. Glaros A, Rao S: Bruxism: A critical review. *Psychol Bull* 84:767–781, 1977.

194. Kampe T, Tagdae T, Bader G, et al: Reported symptoms and clinical findings in a group of subjects with longstanding bruxing behavior. *J Oral Rehabil* 24:581–587, 1997.

195. Macaluso G, Pavesi G, De Laat A: Sleep bruxism is a disorder related to periodic arousals during sleep. *J Dent Res* 77:565–573, 1998.

196. Saber M, Guitard F, Rompre P, et al: Distribution of rhythmic masticatory muscle activity across sleep stages and association with sleep stage shifts . *J Dent Res* 81 (special issue A):297, 2002.

197. Sjöholm T, Polo O, Alihanka J: Sleep movements in teeth-grinders. *J Craniomandib Disord Facial Oral Pain* 6:184–191, 1992.

198. Kato T, Rompre P, Montplaisir J, et al: Sleep bruxism: An oromotor activity secondary to microarousal. *J Dent Res* 80:1940–1944, 2001.

199. Hartmann E: Alcohol and bruxism. *N Engl J Med* 301:334, 1979.

200. Ellison J, Stanziani P: SSRI-associated nocturnal bruxism in four patients. *J Clin Psychiatry* 54:432–434, 1993.

201. Por C, Watson L, Doucette D, Dolovich L: Sertraline-associated bruxism. *Can J Clin Pharmacol* 3:123–125, 1996.

202. Kamen S: Tardive dyskinesia, a significant syndrome for geriatric dentistry. *Oral Surg Oral Med Oral Pathol* 39:52, 1975.

203. Pohto P: Experimental aggression and bruxism in rats. *Acta Odontol Scand* 37:117–126, 1979.

204. Magee K: Bruxism related to levodopa therapy. *J Am Med Assoc* 214:147, 1970.

205. Lobbezoo F, Lavigen G, Tanguay R, Montplaisir J: The effect of the catecholamine precursor L-dopa on sleep bruxism: A controlled clinical trial. *Mov Disord* 12:73–78, 1997.

206. Sjöholm T, Lehtinen I, Piha S: The effect of propranolol on sleep bruxism: Hypothetical considerations based on a case study. *Clin Autonom Res* 6:37–40, 1996.

207. Amir I, Hermesh H, Gavish A: Bruxism secondary to antipsychotic drug exposure: A positive response to propranolol. *Clin Neuropharmacol* 20:86–89, 1997.

208. Arkin A: *Sleep-Talking: Psychology and Psychophysiology*. Hillsdale, NJ: Lawrence Erlbaum, 1981.

209. MacNeilage L: Activity of the speech apparatus during sleep and its relation to dream reports. Unpublished doctoral dissertation, Columbia University, 1971.

210. Jacobson A, Kales A: Somnambulism: All-night EEG and related studies, in *Sleep And Altered States of Consciousness*. Baltimore: Williams & Wilkins, 1967, pp 424–455.

211. Kavey NB, Whyte J, Resor SR Jr., Gidro-Frank S: Somnambulism in adults. *Neurology* 40:749–752, 1990.

212. Broughton R: Sleep disorders: Disorders of arousal? *Science* 159:1070, 1968.

213. Cirignotta F, Zucconi M, Mondini S, et al: Enuresis, sleepwalking, and nightmares: An epidemiological survey in the Republic of San Marino, in Guilleminault C, Lugaresi E (eds): *Sleep/Wake Disorders: Natural History, Epidemiology, and Long-Term Evolution*. New York: Raven Press, 1983, pp 237–241.

214. Kales A, Soldatos C, Caldwell A, et al: Somnambulism. *Arch Gen Psychiatry* 37:1406–1410, 1980.

215. Blatt I, Peled R, Gadoth N, Lavie P: The value of sleep recording in evaluating somnambulism in young adults. *Electroencephalogr Clin Neurophysiol* 78:407–412, 1991.

216. Hublin C, Kaprio J, Partinen M, et al: Prevalence and genetics of sleepwalking: A population-based twin study. *Neurology* 48:177–181, 1997.

217. Bliwise D: What is sundowning? *J Am Geriatr Soc* 42:1009–1011, 1994.

218. Fisher C, Kahn E, Edwards A, Davis D: A psychophysiological study of nightmares and night terrors. *Psychoanal Contemp Sci* 3:317–398, 1974.

219. Reid W: Treatment of somnambulism in military trainees. *Am J Psychiatry* 29:101–105, 1975.

220. Kales J, Kales A, Soldatos C, et al: Night terrors. *Arch Gen Psychiatry* 37:1413–1417, 1980.

221. Rogozea R, Florea-Ciocoiu V: Orienting reaction in patients with night terrors. *Biol Psychiatry* 20:894–905, 1985.

222. Llorente M, Currier MB, Norman S, Mellman T: Night terrors in adults: Phenomenology and relationship to psychopathology. *J Clin Psychiatry* 53:392–394, 1992.

223. Schenck C, Hurwitz T, Bundlie S, Mahowald M: Sleep-related eating disorders: Polysomnographic correlates of a heterogeneous syndrome distinct from daytime eating disorders. *Sleep* 14:419–431, 1991.

224. Winkelman J, Dorsey C, Cunningham S, Lukas S: Nocturnal binge eating: Sleep disorder or eating disorder? *Sleep Res* 22:291, 1993.

225. Spaggiari M, Granella F, Parrino L, et al: Nocturnal eating syndrome in adults. *Sleep* 17:339–344, 1994.

226. Schenck C, Hurwitz T, O'Connor K, Mahowald M: Additional categories of sleep-related eating disorders and the current status of treatment. *Sleep* 16:457–466, 1993.

227. Huapaya L: Somnambulism and bedtime medication. *Am J Psychiatry* 133:1207, 1976.

228. Huapaya L: Seven cases of somnambulism induced by drugs. *Am J Psychiatry* 36:985, 1979.

229. Keefauver SP, Guilleminault C: Parasomnias. Sleep terrors and sleepwalking, in Kryger M, Roth T, Dement W (eds): *Principles and Practice of Sleep Medicine*, 2nd ed. Philadelphia: WB Saunders, 1994, pp 567–573.

230. Lees A, Blackburn N, Campbell V: The night-time problems of Parkinson's disease. *Clin Neuropharmacol* 11:512–519, 1988.

231. Mouret J: Differences in sleep in patients with Parkinson's disease. *Electroencephalogr Clin Neurophysiol* 38:653–657, 1975.

232. Kales A, Ansel R, Markham C, et al: Sleep in patients with Parkinson's disease and normal subjects prior to and following levodopa administration. *Clin Pharmacol Ther* 12:397–406, 1971.

233. Bergonzi P, Chiurulla C, Cianchetti C, et al: Clinical pharmacology as an approach to the study of biochemical sleep mechanisms: The action of L-dopa. *Confin Neurol* 36:5–22, 1974.

234. Bergonzi P, Chiurulla C, Gambi D, et al: L-Dopa plus dopa-decarboxylase inhibitor. Sleep organization in Parkinson's syndrome before and after treatment. *Acta Neurol Belg* 75:5–10, 1975.

235. Wilson W, Nashold B, Green R: Studies of the cortical and subcortical electrical activity during sleep of patients with dyskinesias. *Third Symp Park Dis* Edinburgh, Scotland: Livingstone, 1969:160–164.

236. Traczynska-Kubin D, Atef E, Petre-Quadens O: Le sommeil dans la maladie de Parkinson. *Acta Neurol Belg* 69:727–733, 1969.

237. Puca F, Bricolo A, Rurella G: Effect of L-dopa or amantadine therapy on sleep spindles in parkinsonism. *Electroencephalogr Clin Neurophysiol* 35:327–330, 1973.

238. Friedman A: Sleep pattern in Parkinson's disease. *Acta Med Pol* 21:193–199, 1980.

239. Rabey J, Vardi J, Glaubman H, Streifler M: EEG sleep: Study in parkinsonian patients under bromocryptine treatment. *Eur Neurol* 17:345–350, 1978.

240. Schneider E, Ziegler B, Maxion H, et al: Sleep in parkinsonian patients under levodopa. Results of a long-term follow-up study, in *3rd European Congress Sleep Research* Montpellier. Basel: Karger, 1976, pp 447–450.

241. Lavie P, Bental E, Goshen H, Sharf B: REM ocular activity in parkinsonian patients chronically treated with levodopa. *J Neural Transm* 47:61–67, 1980.

242. Lavie P, Wajsbort J, Youdim M: Deprenyl does not cause insomnia in parkinsonian patients. *Commun Psychopharmacol* 4:303–307, 1980.

243. Gillin J, Post R, Wyatt R, et al: REM inhibitory effect of L-dopa infusion during human sleep. *Electroencephalogr Clin Neurophysiol* 35:181–186, 1973.

244. Lesser R, Fahn S, Sniker S, et al: Analysis of the clinical problems in parkinsonism and the complications of long-term levodopa therapy. *Neurology* 29:1253–1260, 1979.

245. Moskovitz C, Moses H 3rd, Klawans HL: Levodopa-induced psychosis: A kindling phenomenon. *Am J Psychiatry* 135:669–675, 1978.

246. Sharf B, Moskovitz C, Lupton M, et al: Dream phenomena induced by chronic levodopa therapy. *J Neural Transm* 43:143–151, 1978.

247. Nausieda P, Weiner W, Kaplan L: Sleep disruption in the course of chronic levodopa therapy: An early feature of the levodopa psychosis. *Clin Neuropharmacol* 5:183–194, 1982.

248. Nausieda P, Tanner C, Klawans H. Serotonergically active agents in levodopa-induced psychiatric toxicity reactions. *Adv Neurol* 37:23–32, 1983.

249. Nausieda P, Glantz R, Weber S, et al: Psychiatric complications of levodopa therapy of Parkinson's disease. *Adv Neurol* 40:271–277, 1984.

250. Comella C, Tanner C, Ristanovic R: Polysomnographic sleep measures in Parkinson's disease patients with treatment-induced hallucinations. *Ann Neurol* 34:710–714, 1993.

251. Arnulf I, Konofal E, Merino-Andreu M, et al: Parkinson's disease a sleepiness: An integral part of PD. *Neurology* 58:1019–1024, 2002.

252. Arnulf I, Bonnet A, Damier P, et al: Hallucinations, REM sleep, and Parkinson's disease: A medical hypothesis. *Neurology* 55:281–288, 2000.

253. Rye DB, Bliwise DL, Dihenia B, Gurecki P: FAST TRACK: Daytime sleepiness in Parkinson's disease. *J Sleep Res* 9:63–69, 2000.

254. Rye D, Bliwise D: Movement disorders specific to sleep and the nocturnal manifestations of waking movement disorders, in Watts R, Koller W (eds): *Movement Disorders: Neurologic Principles and Practice*. New York: McGraw-Hill, 1997, pp 687–713.

255. Comella C, Nardine T, Diederich N, Stebbins G: Sleep-related violence, injury, and REM sleep behavior disorder in Parkinson's disease. *Neurology* 48:A539, 1997.

256. Rye D, Johnston L, Watts R, Bliwise D: Juvenile Parkinson's disease with REM behavior disorder, sleepiness and daytime REM-onsets. *Neurology* 53:1868–1870, 1999.

257. Emser W, Hoffmann K, Stolz T, et al: Sleep disorders in diseases of the basal ganglia, in *Interdisciplinary Topics in Gerontology*. Basel: Karger, 1987, pp 144–157.

258. Nakashima K, Shimoyama R, Yokoyama Y, Takahashi K: Auditory effects on the electrically elicited blink reflex in patients with Parkinson's disease. *Electroencephalogr Clin Neurophysiol* 89:108–112, 1993.

259. Penders C, Delwaide P: Blink reflex studies in patients with parkinsonism before and during therapy. *J Neurol Neurosurg Psychiatry* 34:674–678, 1971.

260. Kimura J: Disorder of interneurons in parkinsonism. The orbicularis oculi reflex to paired stimuli. *Brain* 96:87–96, 1973.

261. Delwaide PJ, Pepin JL, Maertens de Noordhout A: Short-latency autogenic inhibition in patients with parkinsonian ridigity. *Ann Neurol* 30:83–89, 1991.

262. Delwaide PJ, Pepin JL, Maertens de Noordhout A: The audiospinal reaction in parkinsonian patients reflects functional changes in reticular nuclei. *Ann Neurol* 33:63–69, 1993.

263. Jellinger K: Pathology of Parkinson's disease. Changes other than the nigrostriatal pathway. *Mol Chem Neuropathol* 14:153–197, 1991.

264. Jellinger K: The pedunculopontine nucleus in Parkinson's disease, progressive supranuclear palsy and Alzheimer's disease. *J Neurol Neurosurg Psychiatry* 51:540–543, 1988.

265. Hirsch E, Graybiel A, Duyckaerts C, Jovoy-Agid F: Neuronal loss in Parkinson's disease and in progressive supranuclear palsy. *Proc Natl Acad Sci U S A* 84:5976–5980, 1987.

266. Gai W, Halliday G, Blumbergs P, et al: Substance P-containing neurons in the mesopontine tegmentum are severely affected in Parkinson's disease. *Brain* 114:2253–2267, 1991.

267. Paulus W, Jellinger K: The neuropathologic basis of different clinical subgroups of Parkinson's disease. *J Neuropathol Exp Neurol* 50:743–755, 1991.

268. Scatton B, Dennis T, L'Heureux R, et al: Degeneration of noradrenergic and serotonergic but not dopaminergic neurones in the lumbar spinal cord of parkinsonian patients. *Brain Res* 380:181–185, 1986.

269. Rye D: Modulation of normal and pathologic motoneuron activity during sleep, in Chokroverty S, Hening W, Walters A (eds): *Sleep and Movement Disorders*. Philadelphia: Butterworth-Heinemann, 2003, pp 94–119.

270. Braak H, Rub U, Sandmann-Keil D, et al: Parkinson's disease: Affection of brain stem nuclei controlling premotor and motor neurons of the somatomotor system. *Acta Neuropathol (Berl)* 99:489–495, 2000.

271. Braak H, Tredici K, Bratzke H, et al: Staging of the intracerebral inclusion body pathology associated with idiopathic Parkinson's disease (preclinical and clinical stages). *J Neurol* 249 (suppl 3):III/1–IIII/5, 2002.

272. Braak H, Tredici K, Rub U, et al: Staging of brain pathology related to sporadic Parkinson's disease. *Neurobiol Aging* 24:197–211, 2003.

273. Marsden C, Parkes J, Quinn N: Fluctuations of disability in Parkinson's disease: Clinical aspects, in Marsden C, Fahn S (eds): *Movement Disorders*. London: Butterworth Scientific, 1982, pp 96–122.

274. Comella C, Bohmer J, Stebbins G: The frequency and factors associated with sleep benefit in Parkinson's disease. *Sleep Res* 24:386, 1995.

275. Schwab R, Zieper I: Effects of mood, motivation, stress and alertness on the performance in Parkinson's disease. *Psychiat Neurol Basel* 150:345–357, 1965.

276. Hogl BE, Gomez-Arevalo G, Garcia S, et al: A clinical, pharmacologic, and polysomnographic study of sleep benefit in Parkinson's disease. *Neurology* 50:1332–1339, 1998.

277. Ploski H, Levita E, Riklan M: Impairment of voluntary movement in Parkinson's disease in relation to activation level, autonomic malfunction, and personality rigidity. *Psychosom Med* 28:70–77, 1966.

278. Factor S, McAlarney T, Sanchez-Ramos J, Weiner W: Sleep disorders and sleep effect in Parkinson's disease. *Mov Disord* 5:280–285, 1990.

279. van Hilten J, Weggeman M, Velde E, et al: Sleep, excessive daytime sleepiness and fatigue in Parkinson's disease. *J Neural Transm* 5:235–244, 1993.

280. Askenasy J, Yahr M: Reversal of sleep disturbance in Parkinson's disease by antiparkinsonian therapy: A preliminary study. *Neurology* 35:527–532, 1985.

281. Nausieda P: Sleep in Parkinson disease, in Thorpy N (ed): *Handbook of Sleep Disorders*. New York: Marcel Dekker, 1990, pp 719–733.

282. Steur E: Increase of Parkinson disability after fluoxetine medication. *Neurology* 43:211–213, 1993.

283. Richelson E: Pharmacology of antidepressants: Characteristics of the ideal drug. *Mayo Clin Proc* 69:1069–1081, 1994.

284. Lees A: A sustained release formulation of L-dopa (Madopar HBS) in the treatment of nocturnal and early morning disabilities in Parkinson's disease. *Eur Neurol* 27(suppl 1):126–134, 1987.

285. Kerchove M Vd, Jacquy J, Gonce M, Deyn PD: Sustained-release levodopa in Parkinsonian patients with nocturnal disabilities. *Acta Neurol Belg* 93:32–39, 1993.

286. Gaillard J: Benzodiazepines and GABA-ergic transmission, in Kryger MH, Roth TS, Dement WC (eds): *Principles and Practice of Sleep Medicine*. Philadelphia: WB Saunders, 1994, pp 349–354.

287. Bonnet M, Arand D: The use of triazolam in older patients with periodic leg movements, fragmented sleep, and daytime sleepiness. *J Gerontol* 45:M139–144, 1990.

288. Ware J, Brown F, Moorad PJ, et al: Nocturnal myoclonus and tricyclic antidepressants. *Sleep Res* 13:72, 1984.

289. Ancoli-Israel S, Kripke D, Klauber M, et al: Periodic limb movements in sleep in community dwelling elderly. *Sleep* 14:496–500, 1991.

290. Roehrs T, Zorick F, Sicklesteel J, et al: Age-related sleep-wake disorders at a sleep disorder center. *J Am Geriatr Soc* 31:364–370, 1983.

291. Aldrich M: Parkinsonism, in MH Kryger TR, Dement WC, (ed): *Principles and Practice of Sleep Medicine*. Philadelphia: WB Saunders, 1994, pp 783–789.

292. Rye D, DeLong M: Amelioration of sensory limb discomfort of restless legs syndrome by pallidotomy. *Ann Neurol* 46:800–801, 1999.

293. Lang A, Johnson K: Akathisia in idiopathic Parkinson's disease. *Neurology* 37:477–481, 1987.

294. Linazasoro G, Masso JM, Suarez J: Nocturnal akathisia in Parkinson's disease: Treatment with clozapine. *Mov Disord* 8:171–174, 1993.

295. Fischer P, Naske R: Akathisia-like motor restlessness in major depression responding to serotonin-reuptake inhibition. *J Clin Psychopharmacol* 12:295–296, 1992.

296. Bliwise D, Rye D, He L, Ansari F: Influence of PLMs on scoring phasic leg muscle activity. *Sleep* 26:A344, 2003.

297. Lavia Fantini M, Gagnon J, Petit D, et al: Slowing of electroencephalogram in rapid eye movement sleep behavior disorder. *Ann Neurol* 53:774–780, 2003.

298. Turner R, D'Amato C, Chervin R, Blaivas M: The pathology of REM-sleep behavior disorder with comorbid Lewy body dementia. *Neurology* 55:1730–1732, 2000.

299. Boeve B, Silber M, Pirisi J, et al: Synucleinopathy pathology and REM sleep behavior disorder plus dementia or parkinsonism. *Neurology* 61:40–45, 2003.

300. McKeith IG, Ballard CG, Perry RH, et al: Prospective validation of consensus criteria for the diagnosis of dementia with Lewy bodies. *Neurology* 54:1050–1058, 2000.

301. Schenck C, Boyd J, Mahowald M: A parasomnia overlap disorder involving sleepwalking, sleep terrors, and REM sleep behavior disorder in 33 polysomnographically confirmed cases. *Sleep* 20:972–981, 1997.

302. Vazquez A, Jimenez-Jimenez F, Garcia-Ruiz P, Garcia-Urra D: "Panic attacks" in Parkinson's disease. A long-term complication of levodopa therapy. *Acta Neurol Scand* 87:14–18, 1993.

303. Bliwise D, Watts R, Watts N, et al: Disruptive nocturnal behavior in Parkinson's disease and Alzheimer's disease. *J Geriatr Psychiatry Neurol* 8:107–110, 1995.

304. Lauterbach E: Sleep benefit and sleep deprivation in subgroups of depressed patients with Parkinson's disease. *Am J Psychiatry* 151:782–783, 1994.

305. Friedman J, Lannon M: Clozapine in the treatment of psychosis in Parkinson's disease. *Neurology* 39:1219–1221, 1989.

306. Wolters E, Hurwitz T, Mak E, et al: Clozapine in the treatment of parkinsonian patients with dopaminomimetic psychosis. *Neurology* 40:832–834, 1990.

307. Meco G, Alessandria A, Bonifati V, Giustini P: Risperidone for hallucinations in levodopa-treated Parkinson's disease patients. *Lancet* 343:1370–1371, 1994.

308. Tavares AR Jr.: Risperidone in Parkinson's disease. *J Neurol Neurosurg Psychiatry* 58:521, 1995.

309. Morgante L, Epifanio A, Spina E, et al: Quetiapine versus clozapine: A preliminary report of comparative effects on dopaminergic psychosis in patients with Parkinson's disease. *Neurol Sci* 23(suppl 2):S89–90, 2002.

310. Fernandez H, Trieschmann M, Burke M, Friedman J: Quetiapine for psychosis in Parkinson's disease versus dementia with Lewy bodies. *J Clin Pyschiatry* 63:513–515, 2002.

311. Menza M, Palermo B, Mark M: Quetiapine as an alternative to clozapine in the treatment of dopamimetic psychosis in patients with Parkinson's disease. *Ann Clin Psychiatry* 11:141–144, 1999.

312. Touyz S, Beumont P, Saayman G, Zabow T: A psychophysiological investigation of the short-term effects of clozapine upon sleep parameters of normal young adults. *Biol Psychiatry* 12:801–822, 1977.

313. Touyz S, Saayman G, Zabow T: A psychophysiological investigation of the long-term effects of clozapine upon sleep patterns of normal young adults. *Psychopharmacology* 56:69–73, 1978.

314. Blum A: Triad of hyperthermia, increased REM sleep, and cataplexy during clozapine treatment? *J Clin Psychiatry* 51:259–260, 1990.

315. Blum A, Girke W: Marked increase in REM sleep produced by a new antipsychotic compound. *Clin Electroencephalogr* 4:80–84, 1973.

316. Hardie R, Efthimiou J, Stern G: Respiration and sleep in Parkinson's disease [letter]. *J Neurol Neurosurg Psychiatry* 49:1326, 1986.

317. Apps M, Sheaff P, Ingram D, et al: Respiration and sleep in Parkinson's disease. *J Neurol Neurosurg Psychiatry* 48:1240–1245, 1985.

318. Bliwise D, Watts R, Watts N, Rye D: Nocturnal behavior disruption in Parkinson's disease and Alzheimer's disease. *Sleep Res* 23:352, 1994 (abstract).

319. Vincken W, Gauthier S, Dollfuss R, et al: Involvement of upper-airway muscles in extrapyramidal disorders. *N Engl J Med* 311:438–442, 1984.

320. Hovestadt A, Bogaard J, Meerwaldt J, et al: Pulmonary function in Parkinson's disease. *J Neurol Neurosurg Psychiatry* 52:329–333, 1989.

321. Rosen J, Feinsilver S, Friedman J: Increased CO_2 responsiveness in Parkinson's disease: Evidence for a role of dopamine in respiratory control. *Am Rev Respir Dis* 131:A297, 1985.

322. Feinsilver S, Friedman J, Rosen J: Respiration and sleep in Parkinson's disease. *J Neurol Neurosurg Psychiatry* 49:964, 1986.

323. Guilleminault C, Briskin J, Greenfield M, Silvestri R. The impact of autonomic nervous system dysfunction on breathing during sleep. *Sleep* 4:263–278, 1981.

324. McNicholas W, Rutherford R, Grossman R, et al: Abnormal respiratory pattern generation during sleep in patients with autonomic dysfunction. *Am Rev Respir Dis* 128:429–433, 1983.

325. Bergonzi P, Gigli G, Laudisio A, et al: Sleep and human cerebellar pathology. *Int J Neurosci* 15:159–163, 1981.

326. Chokroverty S, Sachdeo R, Masdeu J: Autonomic dysfunction and sleep apnea in olivopontocerebellar degeneration. *Arch Neurol* 41:926–931, 1984.

327. Salazar-Grueso E, Rosenberg R, Roos R: Sleep apnea in olivopontocerebellar degeneration: Treatment with trazodone. *Ann Neurol* 23:399–401, 1988.

328. Nakano K, Hasegawa Y, Tokushige A, et al: Topographical projections from the thalamus, subthalamic nucleus and pedunculopontine tegmental nucleus to the striatum in the Japanese monkey, *Macaca fuscata*. *Brain Res* 537:54–68, 1990.

329. Miller E, Nieburg H: Amphetamines. Valuable adjunct in treatment of Parkinsonism. *N Y State J Med* 73:2657–2661, 1973.

330. Parkes JD, Tarsy D, Marsden CD, et al: Amphetamines in the treatment of Parkinson's disease. *J Neurol Neurosurg Psychiatry* 38:232–237, 1975.

331. Cantello R, Aguggia M, Gilli M, et al: Major depression in Parkinson's disease and the mood response to intravenous

methylphenidate: Possible role of the "hedoni" dopamine synapse. *J Neurol Neurosurg Psychiatry* 52:724–731, 1989.

332. Rye DB, Jankovic J: Emerging views of dopamine in modulating sleep/wake state from an unlikely source: PD. *Neurology* 58:341–346, 2002.

333. Frucht S, Rogers J, Greene P, et al: Falling asleep at the wheel: Motor vehicle mishaps in persons taking pramipexole and ropinirole. *Neurology* 52:1908–1910, 1999.

334. Sanjiv CC, Schulzer M, Mak E, et al: Daytime somnolence in patients with Parkinson's disease. *Park Rel Disord* 7:283–286, 2001.

335. O'Suilleabhain PE, Dewey RB: Contributions of dopaminergic drugs and disease severity to daytime sleepiness in Parkinson disease. *Arch Neurol* 59:986–989, 2002.

336. Hobson DE, Lang AE, Martin WRW, et al: Excessive daytime sleepiness and sudden-onset sleep in Parkinson disease. *JAMA* 287:455–463, 2002.

337. Tandberg E, Larsen J, Karlsen K: Excessive daytime sleepiness and sleep benefit in Parkinson's disease: A community based study. *Mov Disord* 14:922–927, 1999.

338. Tan EK, Lum SY, Fook-Chong SMC, et al: Evaluation of somnolence in Parkinson's disease: Comparison with age and sex matched controls. *Neurology* 58:465–468, 2002.

339. Gjerstad MD, Aarsland D, Larsen JP: Development of daytime somnolence over time in Parkinson's disease. *Neurology* 58:1544–1546, 2002.

340. Montastruc J-L, Brefel-Courbon C, Senard J-M, et al: Sleep attacks and antiparkinsonian drugs: A pilot prospective pharmacoepidemiologic study. *Clin Neuropharmacol* 24:181–183, 2001.

341. Kumar S, Bhatia M, Behari M: Sleep disorders in Parkinson's disease. *Mov Disord* 17:775–781, 2002.

342. Agid Y: Parkinson's disease: Pathophysiology. *Lancet* 337:1321–1324, 1991.

343. Silber MH, Rye DB: Solving the mysteries of narcolepsy. *Neurology* 56:1616–1618, 2001.

344. Bagetta G, Sarro GD, Priolo E, Nisticó G: Ventral tegmental area: Site through which dopamine D$_2$-receptor agonists evoke behavioral and electrocortical sleep in rats. *Br J Pharmacol* 95:860–866, 1988.

345. Berridge C, O'Neil J, Wifler K: Amphetamine acts within the medial basal forebrain to initiate and maintain alert waking. *Neuroscience* 93:885–896, 1999.

346. Mega M, Masterman D, Benson F, et al: Dementia with Lewy bodies: Reliability and validity of clinical and pathologic criteria. *Neurology* 47:1403–1409, 1996.

347. Frucht S, Rogers J, Greene P, et al: Falling asleep at the wheel: Motor vehicle mishaps in people taking pramipexole and ropinirole [letter]. *Neurology* 54:274–277, 2000.

348. Olanow CW, Schapira AHV, Roth T: Waking up to sleep episodes in Parkinson's disease. *Mov Disord* 15:212–215, 2000.

349. Ryan M, Slevin J, Wells A: Non-ergot dopamine agonist-induced sleep attacks. *Pharmacotherapy* 20:724–726, 2000.

350. Hauser RA, Gauger L, Anderson WM, Zesiewicz TA: Pramipexole-induced somnolence and episodes of daytime sleep. *Mov Disord* 15:658–663, 2000.

351. Ferreira J, Galitzky M, Montastruc J, Rascol O: Sleep attacks and Parkinson's disease treatment. *Lancet* 355:1333–1334, 2000.

352. Tracik F, Ebersbach G: Sudden daytime sleep onset in Parkinson's disease: Polysomnographic recordings. *Mov Disord* 16:500–506, 2001.

353. Ulivelli M, Rossi S, Lombard C, et al: Polysomnographic characterization of pergolide-induced "sleep attacks" in an idiopathic PD patient. *Neurology* 58:462–465, 2002.

354. Andreau N, Chale J, Senard J, et al: L-dopa induced sedation: A double-blind cross-over controlled study versus triazolam and placebo in healthy volunteers. *Clin Neuropharmacol* 22:15–23, 1999.

355. Ferreira JJ, Galitzky M, Thalamas C, et al: Effect of ropinirole on sleep onset: A randomized placebo controlled study in healthy volunteers. *Neurology* 58:460–462, 2002.

356. Johns M: A new method for measuring daytime sleepiness: The Epworth Sleepiness Scale. *Sleep* 14:540–545, 1991.

357. Moller JC, Stiasny K, Hargutt V, et al: Evaluation of sleep and driving performance in six patients with Parkinson's disease reporting sudden onset of sleep under dopaminergic medication: A pilot study. *Mov Disord* 17:474–481, 2002.

358. Goetz C, Tanner C, Klawans H: Bupropion for Parkinson's disease. *Neurology* 34:1092–1094, 1984.

359. Hauser RA, Wahba MN, Zesiewicz TA, Anderson WM: Modafinil treatment of pramipexole-associated somnolence. *Mov Disord* 15:1269–1271, 2000.

360. Rabinstein A, Shulman LM, Weiner WJ: Modafinil for the treatment of excessive daytime sleepiness in Parkinson's disease: A case report. *Park Rel Disord* 7:287–288, 2001.

361. Nieves AV, Lang AE: Treatment of excessive daytime sleepiness in patients with Parkinson's disease with modafinil. *Clin Neuropharmacol* 25:111–114, 2002.

362. Hogl B, Saletu M, Brandauer E, et al: Modafinil for the treatment of daytime sleepiness in Parkinson's disease: Double-blind, randomized, cross-over, placebo-controlled polygraph trial. *Sleep* 25:905–909, 2002.

363. Reynolds G, Elsworth J, Blau K, et al: Deprenyl is metabolized to methamphetamine and amphetamine in man. *Br J Clin Pharmacol* 6:542–544, 1978.

364. Hietanen M: Selegiline and cognitive function in Parkinson's disease. *Acta Neurol Scand* 84:407–410, 1991.

365. Portin R, Rinne U: The effect of deprenyl (selegiline) on cognition and emotion in parkinsonian patients undergoing long-term levodopa treatment. *Acta Neurol Scand* (suppl) 95:135–144, 1983.

366. Nickel B, Borbe H, Szelenyi I: Effect of selegiline and desmethylselegiline on cortical electric activity in rats. *J Neural Transm* (suppl) 32:139–144, 1990.

367. Hublin C, Partinen M, Heinonen E, et al: Selegiline in the treatment of narcolepsy. *Neurology* 44:2095–2101, 1994.

368. Reinish L, MacFarlane J, Sandor P, Shapiro C: REM changes in narcolepsy with selegiline. *Sleep* 18:362–367, 1995.

369. Mayer G, Meier K, Hephata K. Selegeline hydrochloride treatment in narcolepsy. A double-blind placebo-controlled study. *Clin Neuropharmacol* 18:306–319, 1995.

370. Cooper B, Wang C, Cox R, et al: Evidence that the acute behavioral and electrophysiological effects of bupropion (Wellbutrin) are mediated by a noradrenergic mechanism. *Neuropsychopharmacology* 11:133–141, 1994.

371. Wiegand M, Moller A, Lauer C-J, et al: Nocturnal sleep in Huntington's disease. *J Neurol* 238:203–208, 1991.

372. Starr A: A disorder of rapid eye movements in Huntington's chorea. *Brain* 90:545–564, 1967.

373. Emser W, Brenner M, Stober T, Schimrigk K: Changes in nocturnal sleep in Huntington's and Parkinson's disease. *J Neurol* 235:177–179, 1988.

374. Mano T, Shiozawa Z, Sobue I: Extrapyramidal involuntary movements during sleep, in Broughton R (ed): *Neurosciences.* Amsterdam: Elsevier Biomedical Press, 1982, pp 431–442.

375. Fish D, Sawyers D, Allen P, et al: The effect of sleep on the dyskinetic movements of Parkinson's disease, Gilles de la Tourette syndrome, Huntington's disease, and torsion dystonia. *Arch Neurol* 48:210–214, 1991.

376. Aldrich M, Foster N, White R, et al: Sleep abnormalities in progressive supranuclear palsy. *Ann Neurol* 25:577–581, 1989.

377. Gross R, Spehlmann R, Daniels J: Sleep disturbances in progressive supranuclear palsy. *Electroencephalogr Clin Neurophysiol* 45:16–25, 1978.

378. Jankel W, Allen R, Niedermeyer E, Kalsher M: Polysomnographic findings in dystonia musculorum deformans. *Sleep* 6:281–285, 1983.

379. Segawa M, Hosaka A, Miyagawa F, et al: Hereditary progressive dystonia with marked diurnal fluctuation *Adv Neurol* 14:215–233, 1976.

380. Montagna P, Imbriaco A, Zucconi M, et al: Hemifacial spasm in sleep. *Neurology* 36:270–273, 1986.

381. Fish D, Sawyers D, Smith S, et al: Motor inhibition from the brainstem is normal in torsion dystonia during REM sleep. *J Neurol Neurosurg Psychiatry* 54:140–144, 1991.

382. Forgach L, Eisen A, Fleetham J, Calne D: Studies on dystonic torticollis during sleep. *Neurology* 36(suppl 1):120, 1986.

383. Sunohara N, Mano Y, Ando K, Satoyoshi E: Idiopathic dystonia: Parkinsonism with marked diurnal fluctuation of symptoms. *Ann Neurol* 17:39–45, 1985.

384. Calleja J, Carpizo R, Berciano J, et al: Serial waking-sleep EEGs and evolution of somatosensory potentials in Creutzfeldt-Jakob disease. *Electroencephalogr Clin Neurophysiol* 60:504–508, 1985.

385. Silvestri R, Domenico PD, Rosa AD, et al: The effect of nocturnal physiological sleep on various movement disorders. *Mov Disord* 5:8–14, 1990.

386. Jankovic J, Rohaidy H: Motor, behavioral and pharmacologic findings in Tourette's syndrome. *Can J Neurol Sci* 14:541–546, 1987.

387. Sandyk R, Bamford C: Sleep disorders in Tourette's syndrome. *Int J Neurosci* 37:59–65, 1987.

388. Mendelson W, Caine E, Goyer P, et al: Sleep in Gilles de la Tourette syndrome. *Biol Psychiatry* 15:339–343, 1980.

389. Glaze D, Frost J, Jankovic J: Sleep in Gilles de la Tourette's syndrome: Disorder of arousal. *Neurology* 33:586–592, 1983.

390. Silvestri R, Domenico PD, Gugliotta M, et al: Gilles de la Tourette's syndrome: Arousal and sleep polygraphic findings. A case report. *Acta Neurol (Napoli)* 9:263–272, 1987.

391. Hashimoto T, Endo S, Fukuda K, et al: Increased body movements during sleep in Gilles de la Tourette syndrome. *Brain Dev* 3:31–35, 1981.

392. Drake ME Jr., Hietter SA, Bogner JE, et al: Cassette EEG sleep recordings in Gilles de la Tourette syndrome. *Clini Electroencephalogr* 23:142–146, 1992.

393. Voderholzer U, Muller N, Haag C, et al: Periodic limb movements during sleep are a frequent finding in patients with Gilles de la Tourette's syndrome. *J Neurol* 244:521–526, 1997.

394. Cohrs S, Rasch T, Altmeyer S, et al: Decreased sleep quality and increased sleep related movements in patients with Tourette's syndrome. *J Neurol Neurosurg Psychiatry* 70:192–197, 2001.

395. Chokroverty S, Barron K: Palatal myoclonus and rhythmic ocular movements: A polygraphic study. *Neurology* 19:975–982, 1969.

396. Kayed K, Sjaastad O, Magnussen I, Marvik R: Palatal myoclonus during sleep. *Sleep* 6:130–136, 1983.

397. Yokota T, Atsumi Y, Uchiyama M, et al: Electroencephalographic activity related to palatal myoclonus in REM sleep. *J Neurol* 237:290–294, 1990.

398. Askenasy J: Sleep patterns in extrapyramidal disorders. *Int J Neurol* 15:62–76, 1981.

399. Askenasy J, Weitzman E, Yahr M: Are periodic movements in sleep a basal ganglia dysfunction? *J Neural Transm* 70:337–347, 1987.

400. Jouvet M: Biogenic amines and the states of sleep. *Science* 163:32–41, 1963.

401. Wauquier A, Clincke G, van den Broek W, de Prins E: Active and permissive roles of dopamine in sleep-wakefulness regulation, in Wauquier A, Gaillard J, Monti J, Radulovacki M (eds): *Sleep: Neurotransmitters and Neuromodulators.* New York: Raven Press, 1985, pp 107–120.

402. Nicholson A, Pascoe P: Dopaminergic transmission and the sleep-wakefulness continuum in man. *Neuropharmacology* 29:411–417, 1990.

403. Cianchetti C: Dopamine agonists and sleep in man, in Wauquier A, Gaillard J, Monti J, Radulovacki M (eds): *Sleep: Neurotransmitters and Neuromodulators.* New York: Raven Press, 1989, pp 121–133.

404. Kandel ER, Schwartz JH, Jessell TM: *Principles of Neural Science.* 4th ed. New York: McGraw-Hill, 2000.

405. Freeman A, Ciliax B, Bakay R, et al: Nigrostriatal collaterals to thalamus degenerate in parkinsonian animal models. *Ann Neurol* 50:321–329, 2001.

406. Steinfels G, Heym J, Strecker R, Jacobs B: Behavioral correlates of dopaminergic unit activity in freely moving cats. *Brain Res* 258:217–228, 1983.

407. Miller J, Farber J, Gatz P, et al: Activity of mesencephalic dopamine and non-dopamine neurons across stages of sleep and waking in the rat. *Brain Res* 273:133–141, 1983.

408. Kitai S, Shepard P, Callaway J: Afferent modulation of dopamine neuron firing patterns. *Curr Opin Neurobiol* 9:690–697, 1999.

409. Urbain N, Gervasoni D, Souliere F, et al: Unrelated course of subthalamic nucleus of globus pallidus neuronal activities across vigilance states in the rat. *Eur J Neurosci* 12:3361–3374, 2000.

410. Steriade M, Paré D, Datta S, et al: Different cellular types in mesopontine cholinergic nuclei related to ponto-geniculo-occipital waves. *J Neurosci* 10:2560–2579, 1990.

411. McGeer E, McGeer P: Some characteristics of brain tyrosine hydroxylase, in Mandel A (ed): *New Concepts in Neurotransmitter Regulation.* New York: Plenum Press, 1973, pp 53–68.

412. Smith AD, Olson RJ, Justice JB Jr: Quantitative microdialysis of dopamine in the striatum: Effect of circadian variation. *J Neurosci Methods* 44:33–41, 1992.

413. Ghosh PK, Hrdina PD, Ling GM: Effects of REMS deprivation on striatal dopamine and acetylcholine in rats. *Pharmacol Biochem Behav* 4:401–405, 1976.

414. Farber J, Miller JD, Crawford KA, McMillen BA: Dopamine metabolism and receptor sensitivity in rat brain after REM sleep deprivation. *Pharmacol Biochem Behav* 18:509–513, 1983.

415. Edgar DM, Seidel WF: Modafinil induces wakefulness without intensifying motor activity or subsequent rebound hypersomnolence in the rat. *J Pharmacol Exp Ther* 283:757–769, 1997.

416. Wisor J, Nishino S, Sora I, et al: Dopaminergic role in stimulant-induced wakefulness. *J Neurosci* 21:1787–1794, 2001.

417. Gillin C, Kammen D v, Post R, et al: What is the role of dopamine in the regulation of sleep-wake activity? in Corsini G, Gessa G (eds): *Apomorphine and Other Dopaminomimetics*. New York: Raven Press, 1981, pp 157–164.

418. Zwicker A, Calil H: The effects of REM sleep deprivation on striatal dopamine receptor sites. *Pharmacol Biochem Behav* 24:809–812, 1986.

419. Kilduff T, Bowersox S, Faull K, et al: Modulation of the activity of the striatal dopaminergic system during the hibernation cycle. *Sleep Res* 16:63, 1987.

420. Askenasy J: Sleep in Parkinson's disease. *Acta Neurol Scand* 87:167–170, 1993.

421. Matzuk M, Saper C: Preservation of hypothalamic dopaminergic neurons in Parkinson's disease. *Ann Neurol* 18:552–555, 1985.

422. Zweig R, Whitehouse P, Casanova M, et al: Loss of pedunculopontine neurons in progressive supranuclear palsy. *Ann Neurol* 22:18–25, 1987.

423. Zweig R, Hedreen J, Jankel W, et al: Pathology in brainstem regions of individuals with primary dystonia. *Neurology* 38:702–706, 1988.

424. Zweig R, Ross C, Hedreen J, et al: Locus coeruleus involvement in Huntington's disease. *Arch Neurol* 49:152–156, 1992.

425. Xuereb JH, Perry RH, Candy JM, et al: Nerve cell loss in the thalamus in Alzheimer's disease and Parkinson's disease. *Brain* 114:1363–1379, 1991.

426. Henderson JM, Carpenter K, Cartwright H, Halliday GM: Degeneration of the centre median-parafascicular complex in Parkinson's disease. *Ann Neurol* 47:345–352, 2000.

427. Henderson J, Carpenter K, Cartwright H, Halliday G: Loss of thalamic intralaminar nuclei in progressive supranuclear palsy and Parkinson's disease: Clinical and therapeutic implications. *Brain* 123(Pt 7):1410–1421, 2000.

428. Rub U, Del Tredici K, Schultz C, et al: Parkinson's disease: The thalamic components of the limbic loop are severely impaired by alpha-synuclein immunopositive inclusion body pathology. *Neurobiol Aging* 23:245–254, 2002.

429. Villablanca J, Olmstead C: The striatum: A fine tuner of the brain. *Acta Neurobiol Exp* 42:227–299, 1982.

430. Oniani T, Keshelava-Gogiohadze M: Effect of low-frequency electrical stimulation of the caudate nucleus on cortical electrical activity and the waking-sleep cycle. *Fiziol Zh SSSR Imeni IM Sechenova* 62:29–37, 1976.

431. Heath R, Hodes R: Induction of sleep by stimulation of the caudate nucleus in macaqus rhesus and man. *Trans Am Neurol Assoc* 77:351–379, 1952.

432. Siegel J, Lineberry C: Caudate-capsular-induced modulation of single-unit activity in mesencephalic reticular formation. *Exp Neurol* 22:444–463, 1968.

433. Siegel J, Wang R: Electroencephalographic, behavioral, and single-unit effects produced by stimulation of forebrain inhibitory structure in cats. *Exp Neurol* 42:28–50, 1974.

434. Corsi-Cabrera M, Grinberg-Zylberbaum J, Arditti L: Caudate nucleus lesion selectively increases paradoxical sleep episodes in the rat. *Physiol Behav* 14:7–11, 1975.

435. Hall R, Keane P: Dopaminergic and cholinergic interactions in the caudate nucleus in relation to the induction of sleep in the cat, in Proceedings of the British Physiological Society. 1975, pp 247P–248P (abstract).

436. Hauri P, Hawkins D: Human sleep after leucotomy. *Arch Gen Psychiatry* 26:469–473, 1972.

437. Hosowaka K, Sawada J, Ohara J, Matsada K: Follow-up studies on the sleep EEG after prefrontal lobotomy. *Psychiatr Neurol Jpn* 22:233–243, 1968.

438. Ith T, Hsu W, Holden J, Gannon P: Digital computer sleep prints in lobotomized and nonlobotomized schizophrenics. *Biol Psychiatry* 2:141–152, 1970.

439. Villablanca J, Marcus R: Effects of caudate nuclei removal in cats. Comparison with effects of frontal cortex ablation. *UCLA Forum Med Sci* 18:273–311, 1975.

440. Bricolo A: Insomnia after bilateral sterotactic thalamotomy in man. *J Neurol Neurosurg Psychiatry* 30:154–158, 1967.

441. McGinty D, Sterman M, Iwamura Y: Activity and atonia in the decerebrate cat. *Sleep Study Abstr* 309, 1970.

442. Albin R, Young A, Penney J: The functional anatomy of basal ganglia disorders. *Trends Neurosci* 12:366–375, 1989.

443. Crossman A: Neural mechanisms in disorders of movement. *Comp Biochem Physiol* 93A:141–149, 1989.

444. Wichmann T, DeLong M: Physiology of the basal ganglia and pathophysiology of movement disorders of basal ganglia origin, in Watts R, Koller W (eds): *Movement Disorders: Neurologic Principles and Practice*. New York: McGraw-Hill, 1997, pp 87–98.

445. Steriade M, McCormick D, Sejnowski T: Thalamocortical oscillations in the sleeping and aroused brain. *Science* 262:679–684, 1993.

446. Sakai K: Some anatomical and physiological properties of ponto-mesencephalic tegmental neurons with special reference to the PGO waves and postural atonia during paradoxical sleep in the cat, in Hobson JA, Brazier MAB (eds): *The Reticular Formation Revisited: Specifying Function for a Nonspecific System*. New York: Raven Press, 1980, pp 427–447.

447. Magoun H, Rhines R: An inhibitory mechanism in the bulbar reticular formation. *J Neurophysiol* 9:165–171, 1946.

448. Lai Y, Siegel J: Medullary regions mediating atonia. *J Neurosci* 8:4790–4796, 1988.

449. Rye D, Lee H, Saper C, Wainer B: Medullary and spinal efferents of the pedunculopontine tegmental nucleus and adjacent mesopontine tegmentum in the rat. *J Comp Neurol* 269:315–341, 1988.

450. Chase M, Morales F: Control of motoneurons during sleep, in Kryger M, Roth T, Dement W (eds): *Principles and Practice of Sleep Medicine*, 3rd ed. St. Louis: WB Saunders, 2000, pp 155–168.

451. Rye D: The pathophysiology of REM-sleep behavior disorder [letter]. *Sleep* 21:446–449, 1998.

452. Steriade M: Basic mechanisms of sleep generation. *Neurology* 42(suppl 6):9–18, 1992.

453. Datta S, Dossi RC, Pare D, et al: Substantia nigra reticulata neurons during sleep-walking states: Relation with ponto-geniculo-occipital waves. *Brain Res* 566:344–347, 1991.

454. Sakai K: Anatomical and physiological basis of paradoxical sleep, in McGinty DJ, Drucker-Colin R, Morrison A, Parmeggiani PL (eds): *Brain Mechanisms of Sleep*. New York: Raven Press, 1985, pp 111–137.

455. Jones BE, Webster HH: Neurotoxic lesions of the dorsolateral pontomesencephalic tegmentum-cholinergic cell area in the cat. I. Effects upon the cholinergic innervation of the brain. *Brain Res* 451:13–32, 1988.

456. Shouse MN, Siegel JM: Pontine regulation of REM sleep components in cats: Integrity of the pedunculopontine tegmentum (PPT) is important for phasic events but unnecessary for atonia during REM sleep. *Brain Res* 571:50–63, 1992.

457. DeLong M: Activity of pallidal neurons in the monkey during movement and sleep. *Physiologist* 12:207, 1969 (abstract).

458. Wyzinski P, McCarley R, Hobson J: Discharge properties of pontine reticulospinal neurons during the sleep-waking cycle. *J Neurophysiol* 41:821–834, 1978.

459. Gassel M, Marchiafava P, Pompeiano O: Activity of the red nucleus during deep desynchronized sleep in unrestrained cats. *Arch Ital Biol* 103:369–396, 1965.

460. Evarts E: Temporal patterns of discharge of pyramidal tract neurons during sleep and waking in the monkey. *J Neurophysiol* 27:152–171, 1963.

461. Vitek J: Stereotaxic surgery and deep brain stimulation for Parkinson's disease and movement disorders, in Watts R, Koller W (eds): *Movement Disorders: Neurologic Principles and Practice*. New York: McGraw-Hill, 1997, pp 237–256.

Chapter 53

PSYCHOGENIC MOVEMENT DISORDERS

DANIEL S. SA, NÉSTOR GÁLVEZ-JIMÉNEZ,
and ANTHONY E. LANG

HISTORY	891
PSYCHIATRIC DEFINITIONS	892
EPIDEMIOLOGY	893
CLUES TO THE DIAGNOSIS	895
PSYCHOGENIC HYPERKINETIC MOVEMENT	
DISORDERS	896
Psychogenic Dystonia	896
Psychogenic Tremor	901
Psychogenic Myoclonus	902
Psychogenic Chorea/Ballism	904
Psychogenic Tics	904
PSYCHOGENIC PARKINSONISM	905
PSYCHOGENIC GAIT DISORDERS (INCLUDING	
PSYCHOGENIC ATAXIA)	906
ESTABLISHING A DIAGNOSIS	907
CATEGORIES OF DIAGNOSTIC CERTAINTY	909
APPROACH TO THERAPY OF PSYCHOGENIC	
MOVEMENT DISORDERS	909
PROGNOSIS	910

In 1922 Sir Henry Head wrote: "…Hysteria is sometimes said to imitate organic affections; but this is a highly misleading statement. The mimicry can only deceive an observer ignorant of the signs of hysteria or content with perfunctory examination."[1] Although in many cases of psychogenic movement disorders (PMDs) the nature of the problem is quite obvious from the first patient encounter, in the majority the diagnosis requires careful analysis of the history and the phenomenology of the abnormal movements, and occasionally prolonged periods of observation and assessment. In general, abnormal movements and postures due to primary psychiatric disease are among the most difficult diagnostic problems in neurology even for the most experienced neurologist. More recently, legal problems have increased the burden on such diagnoses. With the increasing risk of being sued for a mistake either way, either subjecting a patient to potentially dangerous diagnostic procedures and treatment options or denying potentially effective treatment options, the responsibility for accurate diagnosis has increased tremendously. Disputes involving work-related injuries and resulting compensation have become a major legal issue in most countries, and the increasing frequency of psychogenic or factitious disorders in these circumstances have taken the diagnosis of a PMD to a greater dimension

while we are still looking for good biological markers to aid us in the diagnosis of organic forms of movement disorders.

In this chapter we review the various manifestations of PMDs and provide guidelines for the diagnosis and approach to therapy of these patients.

History

In the 1880s Charcot was fascinated by "hysteria," directing much attention to its definition, analysis, treatment and research.[2] In one of his Tuesday lessons at the Salpêtrière, he presented a young woman who developed a contracture and deformity of her right foot 5 days following a fall. In his teachings, such a contracture should have been corrected as soon as it appeared. In this particular case he decided to watch the progression of the disorder over 4 days without interfering. He taught that in such cases the treatment involved inducing a second attack to make the "fixed" contracture completely disappear. He used "hysterogenic points" to provoke such a transient attack as a form of therapy in the treatment of static hysteric signs. From the patient description it appears that Charcot was dealing with a case of what we would now term "psychogenic dystonia."

According to Charcot, posttraumatic contractures were more frequently seen in hysterics. He concluded that hysteria was entirely in the mind. Charcot proposed that hysteria was not restricted to women but was also common in males, especially working-men,[3] children,[4] and effeminate men.[5] Freud[3] also reported Charcot's observations that many conditions previously ascribed to alcoholic or lead poisonings were, in fact, hysterical.

Charcot's approach to hysteria was criticized by many (among others, Paul Broca,[6] Sigmund Freud,[7] and later Gowers[8]), especially in regards to the therapeutic use of suggestion and hypnosis.[9] Freud in his writings on hypnosis and suggestion, said that "…if the supporters of the suggestion theory are right, all the observations made at the Salpêtrière are worthless" because there were many who believed (especially in Germany) that the power of suggestion was due to "…a combination of credulity on the part of the observers and of simulation on the part of the subjects of the experiments."[7] Charcot had the patients repeat their crises in front of physicians and medical students.[4] Furthermore, Charcot's experiments on hypnosis were performed by his chiefs of clinic, interns and other assistants but they were never personally checked, with the result that inadequacies and failures of this form of therapy were not known to him.[4] Because the majority of his hysterics were housed together with the epileptics ("…the old wards of the chronic patients"[7]), it was well known that many of the postures or attacks demonstrated by hysterics were nothing more than colorful imitations of real epileptic seizures, further reinforced by public demonstrations in his Tuesday clinics in front of, not only his pupils, but also society people, actors, writers, magistrates, and journalists.[4] Since then, the clinical manifestations and pathophysiological mechanisms underlying hysteria have been a matter of controversy.

Gowers[10] wrote, "there are few organic diseases of the brain that the great mimetic neurosis may not simulate. Palsy and spasm, coma … almost every symptom of positive disease find its counter part in the repertoire of … the nervous system." He insisted that "… given symptoms of hysteria, we must never infer that this is the primary disease until we have searched for, and excluded, the symptoms of organic disease."[10] He described "psychogenic laryngeal spasms" and "psychogenic pharyngeal spasms" in his writings on epilepsy and hysteria,[8] and used hypnosis to determine if these spasms could be altered during sleep, attempting to distinguish attacks due to hysteria from those due to real organic disease (although we now recognize that true organic dystonia can disappear during sleep or with hypnosis). Gowers believed that hysteria could occur in both sexes,[11] observing that "… hysteroid attacks are not very rare in lads and young men including transient paralysis, or contractures, of a limb, precisely similar to those met with in the female sex."[8]

In his address to the London Hospital Medical Society, Sir Henry Head[1] described a variety of PMDs. He described hysterical tremor as a positive repetitive movement of a high "voluntary" type, varying in rapidity, and ceasing with distraction: "… a soldier with a severe tremor of the right hand and arm was able to play the banjo perfectly and I used this musical aptitude for effecting his cure." He also described abnormal focal postures in a limb or a single joint, "… any attempt to break down a spasm of this kind, to open the closed hand, or to straighten the flexed knee, meets with intense resistance" and, in describing what he felt was "psychogenic torticollis," he stated that "… resistance may be experience not only in pushing the head towards the normal shoulder, but also in moving it farther in the direction of the affected side."[1] In the same address he referred to "psychogenic ataxia" which differs fundamentally from "ataxy of organic origin."[1] On attempting to touch the nose with the index finger, there was past-pointing "… to the same side of the head," but, if the head was pushed in the direction of the past-pointed finger as to make contact with it, the affected limb would deviate even further away from the head.

In general, many of the observations of these earlier writers have been corroborated with time as experience with specific psychogenic movement disorders has accumulated. However, older and even more modern medical literature contains many examples of organic movement disorders mistakenly attributed to primary psychological factors. Tourette's syndrome (TS) is possibly the best example of a condition once thought to have a psychological origin which is now accepted to be due to a disorder of the central nervous system (CNS). The same applies to the wide range of idiopathic dystonias, all of which at one time or another have been considered psychogenic. Reasons for this include the unusual nature of the movements, their appearance only on certain actions but not others using the same

muscles, their relief by certain peculiar "sensory tricks," the common worsening of the movements in response to mental or social stress, and until very recently the failure to find any underlying anatomical, physiological or biochemical abnormalities. These factors "supported" the common belief that such patients had an underlying psychiatric disturbance, which then encouraged the development of psychopathological hypotheses to explain the significance of the abnormal movements. Examples of these included the "turning away" from responsibilities or avoidance of conflict in the patient with dystonic head turning, or the phallic symbolism of a pen extruding ink causing writer's cramp. However, in recent years, several studies of patients with focal dystonias such as torticollis[12] and writer's cramp,[13,14] have failed to demonstrate evidence for abnormal premorbid personalities or an association with underlying causative psychopathology. Where abnormalities are found (e.g., depression, poor body-image and self-esteem), it is more likely that they are a result of the dystonia rather than the cause.

Psychiatric Definitions

It would be helpful to begin our review of PMDs with a brief discussion of the current terminology recommended by the American Psychiatric Association's *Diagnostic and Statistical Manual of Mental Disorders, Fourth Edition* (DSM-IV)[15] related to psychiatric disturbances that can be seen in such patients.

Somatoform disorders have as a feature the occurrence of symptoms suggesting a systemic medical condition, but these symptoms do not fit or cannot be fully explained by the presence of a known medical disorder, the exposure to a substance or drug, or by another psychiatric condition. These symptoms must cause significant distress or impairment in social, occupational or other areas of functioning. Somatoform disorders include somatization disorders, factitious disorders, malingering and conversion disorders. Somatization disorders (Table 53-1) were formerly referred to as hysteria or Briquet's syndrome. Somatization disorders begin before age 30 and consist of recurrent and multiple clinically significant

TABLE 53-1 Diagnostic Criteria for Somatization Disorder (DSM-IV)[15]

1. History of many physical complaints beginning before age 30 years occurring over a period of many years resulting in medical treatment or significant impairment in social, occupational or other areas of functioning
2. The following criteria must have been met, with the symptoms occurring any time during the course of the disturbance:

   A. Four pain symptoms in at least four different sites
   B. Two gastrointestinal symptoms other than pain
   C. One sexual symptom other than pain
   D. One pseudoneurological symptom suggesting a neurological condition not limited to pain

TABLE 53-2 Diagnostic Criteria for Factitious Disorder (DSM-IV)[15]

1. Intentional production or feigning of physical or psychological symptoms or signs (Münchausen syndrome)
2. The motivation for the behavior is to assume the sick role
3. External incentives for the behavior are absent (economic gain, avoidance of legal responsibilities, or improving physical well-being)

somatic complaints which result in medical intervention or social or occupational impairment. The differential diagnosis of these disorders must include major depressive, anxiety, and adjustment disorders.

Somatization disorders must be differentiated from factitious disorders, including Münchausen's syndrome (Table 53-2) and malingering (Table 53-3), where the symptoms are intentionally produced or feigned. The difference between these two is that in the former there is a motivation to assume a sick role to obtain medical evaluation and treatment, whereas in the latter there are external incentives such as financial gain or compensation, avoidance of duty, evasion of criminal prosecution, or obtaining drugs.

Conversion disorders (Table 53-4) are characterized by the presence of symptoms or signs affecting voluntary motor or sensory function suggesting a neurological deficit ("pseudoneurological") associated with psychological conflicts or other stressors, resulting in significant alterations in social or occupational functioning. These symptoms are not intentionally produced or feigned as in factitious disorders or malingering. Some patients with a histrionic personality disorder add to the clinical presentation a pattern of excessive emotionality and attention-seeking behavior (Table 53-5). Histrionic personality disorder occurs more frequently in women.[15,16]

Only recently have studies begun to assess the pathogenesis of the neurological dysfunction accompanying conversion disorders. For example, a recent imaging study in patients with hysterical unilateral sensorimotor loss demonstrated decreased regional cerebral blood flow in the contralateral

TABLE 53-3 Features Suggestive of Malingering

1. The essential feature is the intentional production of false or grossly exaggerated physical or psychological symptoms, motivated by external incentives (e.g., avoiding work, obtaining financial compensation)
2. Malingering may represent adaptive behavior
3. Malingering should be suspected if there is a medicolegal issue (e.g., the person has been referred by his/her attorney)
4. Marked discrepancy between the person's claimed stress and disability and the objective findings
5. Lack of cooperation during the diagnostic evaluation and in complying with the prescribed treatment
6. Presence of antisocial personality disorder

SOURCE: Modified from DSM-IV.[15]

TABLE 53-4 Diagnostic Criteria for Conversion Disorder (DSM-IV)[15]

1. One or more symptoms or deficits affecting voluntary motor or sensory functions that suggest a neurological or other general medical condition
2. Psychological factors judged to be associated with the symptom or deficit because the onset of symptoms is preceded by conflicts or other stressors
3. The symptom is not intentionally produced or feigned
4. The symptom cannot be explained by a general medical condition after a thorough medical and laboratory evaluation, or as a direct effect of a substance, or culturally sanctioned behavior or experience
5. The symptom causes significant distress or impairment in social, occupational, or other important areas of functioning or warrants medical evaluation
6. The symptom is not limited to pain or sexual dysfunction, does not occur exclusively during the course of somatization disorder, and is not better accounted for by another mental disorder

thalamus and basal ganglia which result after recovery. Lower activation of the caudate predicted a poorer outcome. The authors proposed the presence of a "functional disorder in striatothalamocortical circuits controlling sensorimotor function and voluntary motor behavior."[17] Similar studies in patients with PMDs will be exceedingly interesting, although, as discussed later in this chapter, it will be critical to control for the presence, nature, and duration of abnormal movements.

Epidemiology

Accurate epidemiological data are limited, but psychogenic disorders are relatively common. The Mannheim Cohort Project has estimated that up to 25 percent of the population at some time or other would fulfill criteria for psychogenic disorders.[18] Snyder and Strain, in a hospital-based study, found that somatoform disorders were responsible for

TABLE 53-5 Criteria for Histrionic Personality Disorder (DSM-IV)[15]

1. Constantly seeks or demands reassurance, approval, or praise
2. Is inappropriately sexually seductive in appearance or behavior
3. Overly concerned with physical attractiveness
4. Expresses emotion with inappropriate exaggeration (e.g., embraces casual acquaintances with excessive ardor, sobbing on minor sentimental occasions, or has temper tantrums)
5. Is uncomfortable in situations in which he or she is not the center of attention
6. Displays rapidly shifting and shallow expression of emotions
7. Is self-centered, actions being directed toward obtaining immediate satisfaction; has no tolerance for the frustration of delayed gratification
8. Has a style of speech that is exceedingly impressionistic and lacking in detail

2.6 percent of the main discharge diagnoses in a group of 1801 patients.[19] In patients with neurological signs and symptoms, psychogenic disorders are also relatively frequent, being estimated to account for 1–9 percent of all diagnoses.[20–22]

It has been reported that at Charcot's Tuesday clinic 7 percent (244 patients out of 3168) of the total population seen during one academic year were diagnosed as having hysteria.[4,5,23] This figure is probably influenced by ascertainment bias because Charcot's interest in hysteria was well known at the time. The extent of Charcot's overdiagnosis or false positive labeling of patients as hysterical is also uncertain.

Among the psychogenic neurological disorders that can be seen, movement disorders are not uncommon. In a group of 842 consecutive patients evaluated on a specialty clinic, 28 (3.3 percent) were ultimately diagnosed as having a PMD.[24] Phenomenologically, the most common movement disorders were tremor, dystonia, myoclonus, and parkinsonism, in that order. Fahn and Williams published a series of 131 patients, in which dystonia was the leading symptom.

In the Movement Disorders Clinic of The Toronto Western Hospital (TWH), between July 2000 and May 2002, 64 patients with a diagnosis of PMD were seen. Of these, tremor was the main abnormal movement in 21 (32.8 percent), dystonia in 16 (25 percent), myoclonus in 16 (25 percent), parkinsonism in 4 (6.1 percent), and a gait disorder in 7 (10.9 percent). Women predominated in this series as in most, accounting for 49 patients (76.5 percent). Interestingly, in reported patients with parkinsonism, there is a small preponderance of males (9:8).[24–26] In the movement disorders clinic of the Cleveland Clinic Florida (CCF), in a 5-year span between 1998 and 2002, 56 cases of PMDs were evaluated out of 2155 cases, accounting for 2.56 percent of the total diagnoses. The most common movement was tremor (18), followed by dystonia in 14, and myoclonus in 4. Combinations of movement disorders were also common, and movements resembling hemifacial spasms were seen in 4 cases, accounting for a 4 percent prevalence. Two of these had associated psychogenic blepharospasm.

A report from the movement disorders unit at Columbia-Presbyterian Medical Center (CPMC),[27] which houses a dystonia research center, described experience with 131 patients diagnosed as having PMDs. Many patients had more than one movement disorder subtype. Eighty-two (53 percent) had psychogenic dystonia, 21 (13 percent) psychogenic tremor, 14 (9 percent) psychogenic gait disturbances, 11 (7 percent) psychogenic myoclonus, 4 (2 percent) blepharospasm and facial movements, 3 (1.9 percent) parkinsonism, 2 (1.3 percent) tics, and stiff-person syndrome was seen in 1 case (0.6 percent). Nine percent of their cases (14) were categorized as having paroxysmal dyskinesias/shaking and undifferentiated movements. Better defined movements or postures (e.g., dystonia) occurring in a paroxysmal fashion is a relatively common manifestation of a PMD.

In one series of 405 patients with conversion disorders requiring admission to hospital, Lempert et al. found that the most common underlying psychiatric disorder was depression (38 percent), followed by "anxiety and compulsion" (13 percent), and hysterical personality disorders (9 percent).[22] The nature of the primary psychiatric abnormality did not predict the type of presenting neurological symptoms, although paroxysmal vertigo was seen more often in patients with anxiety and compulsion. In Marsden's experience, depression was present in 18 percent of the 34 "hysterical" patients admitted to hospital over a 5-year period, while 20 percent had Briquet's syndrome and 6 percent had anxiety.[21] Feinstein et al. (from our unit in Toronto), interviewing 42 patients with a diagnosis of documented or clinically established PMD (most often fulfilling criteria for a conversion disorder), found a variety of additional psychiatric disorders, including anxiety disorders in 16 (38.1 percent), major depression in 8 (19.1 percent), and a combination of the two in 5 (11.9 percent). Other lifetime psychiatric diagnoses included adjustment disorder in 9.5 percent (4), schizoaffective disorders in 2.4 percent (1), bipolar disorder in 2.4 percent (1), and alcohol or sedative abuse in 2.4 percent (1) each. This study was conducted an average of 3.2 years after the initial assessment, and therefore these disorders could also represent consequences of long-standing disability.[28]

Ford et al.[29] from the movement disorders unit at CPMC, found that the majority of patients with PMDs had no underlying organic neurological disorder. However, "... there are individuals who manifest psychogenic symptomatology that represents an exaggeration or elaboration of a neurological condition."[29] In this series of 24 patients with PMDs, the profile of a typical patient consisted of a young person (mean age 36 years, range 11–60), most often female (79 percent), of average or above-average intelligence (96 percent combined), with a mean duration of symptoms of 5 years (range <1 month to 23 years), unable to work, and on disability (70 percent of patients). The principal psychiatric diagnoses were conversion disorder (75 percent), followed by somatization (12.5 percent), factitious disorder (8 percent), and malingering (4 percent). Dysthymia, as a secondary psychiatric diagnosis, was present in 67 percent of patients. The rest included a variety of different psychiatric conditions such as major depression, adjustment disorder, organic mood or organic delusional disorders, obsessive-compulsive disorder, panic attacks, bipolar disorder, and others.

Therefore, it appears that the three most common psychiatric disturbances seen in patients presenting with psychogenic neurological disorders are depression, hysterical (somatization) personality disorders, and anxiety disorders.

Table 53-6 combines the data on a total of 272 PMDs from CPMC, CCF, and TWH. These figures give a rough guide to the relative frequencies of psychogenic movements; however, it is important to recognize that there are intrinsic biases in the reporting and pattern of referrals in these practices, and that the approach to classification was somewhat different (all subtypes versus predominant subtype). The combination of these experiences suggest that

TABLE 53-6 Combined Data on PMDs Seen at CPMC[123] and TWH

PMD	CPMC	TWH*	CCF*	Total**
Dystonia	82 (53%)	16 (25%)	14 (25%)	112 (41.8%)
Tremor	21 (13%)	21 (32.8%)	18 (32.1%)	60 (22%)
Gait	14 (9%)	7 (10.9%)	1 (1.8%)	22 (8.1%)
Myoclonus	11 (7%)	16 (25%)	4 (7.1%)	31 (11.4%)
Blepharospasm/facial movements	4 (2%)	–	4 (7.1%)	8 (2.9%)
Parkinsonism	3 (1.9%)	4 (6.3%)	0	7 (2.6%)
Tics	2 (1.3%)	–	2 (3.6%)	4 (1.5%)
Stiff-person syndrome	1 (0.6%)	–	–	1 (0.4%)
Other mixed/bizarre	14 (9%)	NL	13	27 (9.9%)
Total number	152	64	56	272

CPMC, Columbia-Presbyterian Medical Center (listed all types of PMD).[123] TWH, The Toronto Hospital (listed only the predominant PMD) (July 2000 to May 2002). CCF, Cleveland Clinic Florida (listed only the predominant PMD) (1998–2002).
*Despite the fact that combinations of movements are frequently seen, we listed only the predominant movement abnormality in these series.
**Totals represent types of PMDs. Some patients have more than one pattern of PMDs.
NL, not listed as separate diagnosis.

psychogenic dystonia is the most common psychogenic movement disorder (41.8 percent), followed by psychogenic tremor (22 percent), psychogenic myoclonus (11.4 percent), and other bizarre, mixed or difficult to classify movement disorders (9.9 percent). Dystonia predominates here largely due to the excess of these cases in the Columbia series which is almost certainly skewed by referral bias (a site of the dystonia research center). Other series suggest that psychogenic tremor is more common. In the study by Factor et al.,[30] involving 28 patients with PMDs, the most common PMDs were psychogenic tremor, followed by dystonia, myoclonus, and parkinsonism, more in keeping with our experience at TWH. On the other hand, in a review from Baylor College of Medicine Movement Disorders Center, psychogenic myoclonus predominated (8.5 percent of all patients with myoclonus, and 20.2 percent of all psychogenic movement disorders).[31] Unfortunately, no further data were given for the frequencies of other nonorganic movement disorders.

However, all these results must be considered cautiously, since referral bias is a likely consideration being these known referral centers. Another important confounding factor that cannot be overlooked is the possibility of an associated organic movement disorder along with the PMD. As in the case of pseudoseizures in known epileptic patients, patients with PMDs have been reported to have a concomitant organic disorder.[24,26,32–34] In the series of Factor et al., 25 percent of their patients with PMDs had a concomitant organic problem. In our series, however, this figure was much lower, being present in only 6 patients (9 percent).[24]

Clues to the Diagnosis

There are a number of important historical and clinical features that can give a clue to the psychogenic nature of a movement disorder (Table 53-7).[27,35,36] Many of these are generally applicable to all patients and others relate to a specific type of abnormal movement (e.g., tremor, dystonia). These clues may be evident on taking the patient's history, on clinical examination, or on assessment of response to therapeutic interventions. The general clues are listed in Table 53-7, while the more specific clues are considered in the sections dealing with specific disorders.

Most organic movement disorders have a relatively slow course; therefore, abrupt onset and rapid progression are suggestive of a PMD. Paroxysmal movements (i.e., attacks) are also strongly suggestive of a PMD, as well as spontaneous remissions, no progression, relationship to minor injury, and involvement in litigation. On the examination, selective disabilities, when a patient is unexpectedly able to do some tasks that would have been considered exceedingly difficult, if not impossible, on the basis of his alleged dysfunction and bizarre, mixed movement disorders should also suggest this possibility. Inconsistencies on the examination are also important, including variability, distractability, entrainability, and changes in pattern induced by suggestion or placebo. Additional atypical findings that can direct the attention to a PMD include "give-way" weakness, nonanatomical sensory disturbances, and extreme slowness or difficulty performing examination tasks along with excessive grimacing or sighing.

It should be noted, however, that, taken individually, most of these "clues" are no more than that; more substantive evidence is generally required before a diagnosis of a psychogenic disorder can be confirmed. All of the mentioned clues can be seen in organic disorders. Abrupt onset and rapid progression can occur in rapid-onset dystonia parkinsonism, Wilson's disease and some postlesional movement disorders. The same is true for paroxysmal movements, which can be due to a variety of relatively uncommon paroxysmal dyskinesias. Organic movement disorders, especially dystonia and tremor, can be task-specific. Although uncommon,

TABLE 53-7 General Clues Suggesting that a Movement Disorder may be Psychogenic[27,35,36]

A. Historical
 1. Abrupt onset
 2. Static course
 3. Spontaneous remissions (inconsistency over time)
 4. Obvious psychiatric disturbance
 5. Multiple somatizations
 6. Employed in a health profession
 7. Pending litigation or compensation
 8. Presence of secondary gain
 9. Young female
B. Clinical
 1. Inconsistent character of the movement (amplitude, frequency, distribution, selective disability)
 2. Paroxysmal movement disorder
 3. Movements increase with attention or decrease with distraction
 4. Ability to trigger or relieve the abnormal movements with unusual or nonphysiological interventions (e.g., trigger points on the body, tuning fork)
 5. False weakness
 6. False sensory complaints
 7. Self-inflicted injuries
 8. Deliberate slowness of movements
 9. Functional disability out of proportion to examination findings
 10. Movement abnormality that is bizarre, multiple or difficult to classify
C. Therapeutic responses
 1. Unresponsive to appropriate medications
 2. Response to placebos
 3. Remission with psychotherapy

spontaneous remissions may also occur in a number of organic disorders including idiopathic dystonias (especially cervical dystonia), and TS.

Other supportive evidence can be derived from the existence of multiple undiagnosed somatic complaints and known psychiatric disorders; however, it must be borne in mind that psychiatric patients frequently have an organic movement disorder, due to their medication side-effects or unrelated reasons. It is also important to remember the potential for an initial presentation with psychiatric alterations to be followed only later by abnormal movement disorders in a variety of diseases including Wilson's disease, Huntington's disease, dentatorubropallidoluysian atrophy, TS, and neuroacanthocytosis.

Obviously, surreptitious observation of a symptom-free period remains the most useful evidence for this diagnosis. Attempts to induce such periods utilizing placebo or suggestion can be extremely helpful, although it is known that patients with organic movement disorders can overcome the disability voluntarily and therefore this could happen during suggestion; placebo responses in organic movement disorders have been documented in the past.[37] The use of placebos in these circumstances is somewhat controversial, and will be discussed in detail in the diagnosis section.

Throughout these assessments, as mentioned earlier, it is important to remember that patients with organic neurological disorders can have hysterical or psychogenic dysfunction as well. Weir Mitchell is quoted by Gowers[8] as saying "... the symptoms of many organic diseases of the nervous system are pictures painted on an hysterical background." Gowers,[8] in his writings on epilepsy and hysteria, said "... hysteria, it must be remembered, is common not only as an isolated, but also as a conjoined, morbid state and that hysteria can be the consequence of organic disease. Striking symptoms of hysteria are often seen, for instance, in cases of tumors of the brain." The clinician should be cautious in attributing all symptoms to "hysteria" alone because up to 30 percent of patients thought to have a psychogenic disorder are eventually found to have a disease that could account for their symptoms.[36] Just as pseudoseizures often occur on a background of true epilepsy, PMDs may occur in patients with underlying organic movement disorders. For example, Ranawaya et al. reported 6 such cases.[34] The new movement disorders were considered psychogenic because of the historical, clinical, and behavioral features, and the responses to placebo and suggestion. Importantly, the PMD was typically the source of greater concern and disability than the pre-existing organic condition. In Fahn and Williams'[27] series of psychogenic dystonia, 1 patient developed "psychogenic worsening" of organic idiopathic familial dystonia due to his inability to compete with other students and teasing by his friends. Recently, psychogenic dystonia has been described in a nonmanifesting carrier of the DYT1 gene, the mother and caregiver of a child that is extremely disabled by DYT1 dystonia.[38]

"Pseudotics" have been reported in patients with Tourette's syndrome.[32] On the other hand, it is important to note that in patients who have been completely and adequately assessed and an underlying organic disorder has been excluded, it is rare for subsequent evaluation to uncover such an illness many months or years later.[39] This is important to note since failure to deal properly with a PMD and repeated investigations looking for an alternative explanation for the symptoms can be very detrimental to the long-term prognosis of these patients.

Psychogenic Hyperkinetic Movement Disorders

PSYCHOGENIC DYSTONIA

Dystonia refers to a syndrome dominated by sustained muscle contractions, frequently causing twisting and repetitive movements resulting in abnormal or dystonic postures.[40] Dystonias can be classified as primary or idiopathic if no

TABLE 53-8 Clinical Features of Organic Dystonias which Sometimes Encourage a Misdiagnosis of a Psychogenic Disorder[124-126]

1. The movements in dystonic syndromes can be quite varied, including prolonged spasms, sinuous writhing, brief myoclonic jerks, slow rhythmical movements, and faster tremors.	5. Occasional patients experience dystonia at rest with improvement on action ("paradoxical dystonia")
2. Dystonia can remit in up to 20 percent of patients, especially in those with cervical dystonia (spasmodic torticollis)	6. Dystonia can be relieved by "sensory tricks" (geste antagoniste). The best known of these occur in patients with cervical dystonia where light touch or pressure very often will correct the abnormal head position. Many other examples are seen in a variety of dystonias
3. Patients with idiopathic torsion dystonia (ITD) have no other neurological deficits and normal ancillary investigations	7. Organic dystonia can be relieved by relaxation and hypnosis and is typically worsened by emotional stress
4. Dystonia can be task-specific (e.g., writer's cramp), or may be purely action-induced (e.g., foot dystonia when walking forwards but not backwards, or oromandibular dystonia only when attempting to speak or alternatively only on eating)	8. Dystonia can be paroxysmal (e.g., paroxysmal kinesigenic choreoathetosis, paroxysmal nonkinesigenic choreoathetosis), or can show diurnal variation, as seen most prominently in dopa-responsive dystonia

cause can be found after exhaustive neurological evaluation, and secondary or symptomatic if a cause is evident. Dystonia can also be classified according to age of onset (childhood, adolescence, and adult) or by distribution (focal, segmental, multifocal, generalized, or hemidystonia).

Earlier we mentioned that certain symptoms and signs may occur in organic movement disorders which can encourage the misdiagnosis of a psychogenic cause. This error probably occurs more often in the case of dystonia, especially the idiopathic dystonias, than for other hyperkinesias. In fact, it is probably more common that an organic dystonia is misdiagnosed as psychogenic than the other way around, and this is certainly due in part to a lack of a biological marker (with increasing exceptions related to recognized gene mutations).[41] In his original description in 1908, Schwalbe considered dystonia as a psychogenic disorder.[42] Although a full discussion of dystonia and dystonic syndromes[35,43] is beyond the scope of this chapter, Table 53-8 outlines some of the features of dystonia which encourage this confusion by those unfamiliar with the disorder.

There are certain other clinical features of organic dystonias which can be extremely useful in raising the consideration of a psychogenic diagnosis. Idiopathic dystonia rarely begins in the lower limb in adult life. When this is a manifestation of a secondary dystonia, other neurological features (e.g., parkinsonism) or laboratory abnormalities (e.g. CT or MRI) regularly accompany the dystonia. The onset of organic dystonia is almost always gradual or slow. A notable but rare exception to these two rules is an autosomal-dominant disorder known as "rapid-onset dystonia-parkinsonism."[44] Idiopathic dystonia typically begins with action-induced movements (see Table 53-8), and only after a prolonged period (sometimes never) progresses to dystonia at rest. Secondary dystonia may present with rest dystonia; however, this is typically accompanied by other neurological dysfunction or abnormalities on investigation. Despite the extremely disfiguring postures, pain, other than muscle ache, is surprisingly uncommon in patients with dystonia. An important exception here is cervical dystonia where pain can be the principal source of disability. Finally, although primary sporadic forms of

paroxysmal nonkinesigenic dystonia do occur, psychogenic dystonia is a more common cause of this presentation. In a review of 25 patients with nonkinesigenic paroxysmal dystonia, 7 were found to have a definable symptomatic CNS cause, 7 were diagnosed as having primary sporadic paroxysmal dystonia, and 11 (44 percent) had PMD.[45] Response to medication is sometimes an important factor in the diagnosis of specific forms of dystonia, most notably dopa-responsive dystonia (DRD). However, as we have occasionally seen (including patients with a referral diagnosis of DRD on the basis of a marked response to L-dopa), placebo response to an active medication may result in the diagnosis of inorganic dystonia when in fact the problem is psychogenic.

It is also important to recognize that psychological and psychiatric disorders are not uncommon in patients with movement disorders, and this frequently is simply a consequence of the disability caused by it. In dystonia, this disability is not only physical, but also secondary to the social embarrassment related to the abnormal postures, and additional stressors related to delays in diagnosis and misdiagnosis, including labeling an organic disorder as psychogenic. It should also be noted that a number of neuropsychiatric dysfunctions can be secondary to basal ganglia abnormalities, and even some forms of hereditary dystonia such as myoclonus dystonia are associated with psychiatric disturbances. In these circumstances, a psychiatric diagnosis should be considered a comorbidity rather than an etiologic factor.[46]

Prior to the seminal paper of Fahn and Williams,[27] very few cases of true psychogenic dystonia had appeared in the literature. A critical review of most reports claiming a psychogenic origin in individual cases suggests that an organic source was in fact more likely. Indeed, because many patients with idiopathic torsion dystonia (ITD) had been misdiagnosed as hysterical and received years of unnecessary psychotherapy, it was generally emphasized by authorities in the field that psychogenic dystonia did not exist.[27] However, rare well-documented cases of psychogenic dystonia were occasionally reported.[41] Possibly the best known of these was a case of Münchausen syndrome simulating ITD reported by Batshaw et al.[47] This woman's symptoms began at age 29 with dystonia in the right foot accompanied by left-sided torticollis. Her symptoms progressed to generalized dystonia over a 7-year period despite aggressive medical therapy. The organic basis of her symptoms was questioned and a diagnosis of psychogenic dystonia was considered. Due to the bizarre and relentless progression of her disease despite aggressive psychotherapy, she underwent many consultations at centers with expertise in movement disorders, and many psychiatric evaluations and admissions to inpatient psychiatric units, all without benefit. She subsequently underwent bilateral thalamotomies in hopes of improving her limb dystonia. The thalamotomies were "complicated" by the onset of dysarthria progressing to aphonia 2 months after surgery. She had episodes of periodic breathing and acute opisthotonic posturing lasting up to 6 hours. During one of these episodes she had a "seizure" and had a respiratory arrest after intravenous diazepam, requiring subsequent tracheostomy. Trismus developed and she had to be fed by nasogastric and later gastrotomy tube-feedings. She lost 13.6 kg despite these procedures. It was not until nursing home placement became a consideration that one day the patient awoke with normal speech, volume, and articulation. She was transferred to a psychiatric unit where she appeared delusional, hallucinating and with features of a histrionic personality disorder. During behavioral modification therapy she sat up, began to use her arms normally and walked. Her psychotic symptoms disappeared and medications were discontinued. By the time of discharge, all symptoms of dystonia had resolved except for a 20-degree contracture of the right achilles tendon that had resulted from the volitional maintenance of an equino posture. Later, the patient admitted to have feigned all of her symptoms. It was also learned that she had previously feigned a number of disorders in order to gain sympathy and attention from her family and friends. This history had not been evident earlier because the patient had kept her family apart from her physicians. During subsequent psychiatric evaluations it was found that she was bisexual with difficulty maintaining long-term relationships and had difficulty communicating her needs. She had been abandoned by her father early in her life and had been diagnosed with a number of other medical disorders, including lymphoma and multiple sclerosis for which she claimed to have received therapy.

In 1988, Fahn and Williams[27] clearly defined the features of psychogenic dystonia, reviewing 39 patients, 21 of whom fulfilled their criteria for documented or clinically established psychogenic dystonia. The mean age of onset in these 21 patients was 26 years (ages ranging from 8 to 56 years). All patients but 2 were female (10.5:1). The duration of symptoms before a correct diagnosis of psychogenic dystonia varied between less than 1 month to 15 years. The most common clue suggesting psychogenic dystonia was the incongruity or inconsistency of the dystonic movements, which were present in 85 percent (18). Other clues included false weakness (14), onset of dystonia at rest (11), pain (9), multiple somatizations (8), bizarre nature of the movements (7), sudden weakness (6),

nonanatomic sensory changes (5), "seizures" (5), excessive slowness of movements (5), tenderness to light touch (4), and startle-induced "elaborate" movements (2). All patients except 2 had more than one such clue to the diagnosis. Fahn and Williams emphasized the presence of pain or tenderness in 62 percent (13/21), onset at rest in 11 out of the 15 patients who had continual instead of paroxysmal psychogenic dystonia, and onset in a lower limb, mostly the foot, in 66 percent (14). In this series, prior to the authors' diagnosis of psychogenic dystonia, all but 2 patients had a diagnosis of an organic movement disorder (12) or a combination of psychogenic and organic dystonia (7). None had been diagnosed as pure psychogenic dystonia.

Lang[48] reported his 10-year experience with 18 patients diagnosed as having clinically definite psychogenic dystonia, excluding cases with isolated paroxysmal movements. The clinical characteristics of the dystonia were inconsistent or incongruous with established forms of organic dystonia. The female/male ratio was 2.6:1. The mean age of onset was 35 years (range 17–59). The onset of dystonia was abrupt in half of the cases and progressed rapidly to fixed dystonic postures in 6. In 4 patients the dystonia progressed over a period of weeks up to 5 years. A known precipitant for the dystonic symptoms was evident in 14 cases, trauma being the most common (a motor vehicle accident in 5, and a local injury in 6, including hand surgery, a fall, a poorly described work injury, and a fractured patella with later surgery). The dystonia began in a leg in 7, and the upper extremity was initially affected in 4. Four had generalized dystonia from the onset and 3 had dystonia of the neck and shoulder. The dystonia was present at rest from the onset in 12, and 7 of these had persistent unchanging dystonia without spontaneous or action-induced changes in posturing. Five had periods in which they were free of dystonia; 11 had dystonia at least part of the time brought out or aggravated by action, with only 1 experiencing dystonia exclusively at these times (i.e., pure action-induced dystonia). Ten patients had paroxysmal symptoms superimposed upon the persistent dystonia. The final distribution of dystonia at time of diagnosis was segmental in 28 percent (5), focal in 22 percent (4), generalized in 44 percent (8), and 1 (6 percent) had hemidystonia. Pain was present in 88 percent (16) of patients, and was a prominent feature in 14 of the 18 patients. One of these had well-established reflex sympathetic dystrophy (RSD). Ten patients had accompanying other PMDs, including 3 with multiple forms (5 tremor, 2 myoclonus, and 6 miscellaneous). Other psychogenic neurological features included give-way weakness in 61 percent (11/18), excessive slowness in 28 percent (5/18), marked resistance to passive movements in 17 percent (3) and nonanatomic neurological changes in 44 percent (8/18). The primary psychiatric diagnosis most often was a conversion disorder, or somatoform disorder, and none had known factitious or malingering disorders.

Table 53-9 summarizes and combines the data from these two large series. As can be seen, psychogenic dystonia affects mostly young women, with abrupt "onset-at-rest" dystonia

TABLE 53-9 Clinical Features of Psychogenic Dystonia

	Fahn and Williams[27]	Lang[48]	Totals/means
Number of patients	21	18	39
Mean age of onset (years)	23	35	29
Female/male ratio	9.5:12	6:14	5:1
Duration between onset and diagnosis	<1 month to 15 years	2 months to 30 years	<1 month to 30 years
Onset-at-rest dystonia	11/14 (78%)	12/18 (66%)	23/39 (59%)
Pain/tenderness	13/21 (62%)	16/18 (88%)	29/39 (74%)
Distribution of dystonia at onset			
Upper limb	0	4 (22%)	4 (10%)
Neck/shoulder	4 (19%)	3 (17%)	7 (18%)
Trunk	1 (5%)	0	1 (2%)
Lower limb	14 (67%)	7 (39%)	21 (54%)
Hemidystonia	2 (9%)	0	2 (5%)
Generalized	0	4 (22%)	4 (10%)
Final distribution			
Focal	6 (28%)	4 (22%)	10 (26%)
Segmental	5 (24%)	5 (28%)	10 (26%)
Hemidystonia	0	1 (6%)	1 (3%)
Generalized	10 (48%)	8 (44%)	18 (46%)
Other psychogenic neurological findings			
Give-way weakness/paralysis	20/21 (95%)	11/18 (61%)	31/39 (79%)
Excessive slowness	5/21 (24%)	5/18 (28%)	10/39 (26%)
Marked resistance to passive movements	0	3 (17%)	3/39 (7.6%)
Nonanatomic sensory changes	5/21 (24%)	8/18 (44%)	13/39 (33%)
Multiple somatizations	8/21 (38%)	8/18 (14%)	16/39 (41%)

involving the lower limb, most often a foot, accompanied by excessive pain and tenderness with nonanatomic sensory dysfunction, give-way weakness or paralysis, excessive slowness of movement, and multiple somatizations. The dystonia will most often become generalized, followed in frequency by segmental or focal distribution. Rarely symptoms will begin as hemidystonia or progress to hemidystonia.

DYSTONIA WITH OR WITHOUT REFLEX SYMPATHETIC DYSTROPHY (RSD) FOLLOWING PERIPHERAL INJURY

In the past decade or so, there have been a number of reports describing a variety of movement disorders, most notably dystonia, following peripheral injury. When dystonia predominates it may occur in isolation, but it more often occurs in association with other movement disorders (particularly tremor), severe pain ("causalgia"), and sometimes full-blown RSD. A variety of case series of patients with typical idiopathic dystonia have mentioned the potential role of preceding local trauma in anywhere from 5 percent[49,50] to 16.4 percent.[51] However, in the only available case-control study, Fletcher et al. failed to show an association between idiopathic dystonia and a history of previous injury.[52] Importantly, if one reviews the descriptions of movement disorders following peripheral trauma, it is clear that the majority of patients have a clinical syndrome quite distinct from "classical"

movement disorder syndromes such as ITD. Bhatia et al.[74] outlined a number of clinical characteristics which distinguished "causalgia-dystonia" from primary torsion dystonia (Table 53-10). Importantly, many of the clinical characteristics

TABLE 53-10 Differences Between "Causalgia-Dystonia" and Primary Torsion Dystonia*

Causalgia-Dystonia	Idiopathic Dystonia
Clear preponderance of women	No preponderance of women
No family history	Positive family history not uncommon
Painful (causalgia)	Usually painless
Vasomotor, sudomotor, and trophic changes	Such changes not seen
Fixed spasm	Mobile spasms
Contractures common and early	Contractures uncommon and late
No geste antagoniste	Geste frequent
No improvement with sleep	Sleep often improves
Poor response to botulinum toxin and other therapy	Often responds to botulinum toxin, others
Onset in leg in adult	Adult leg-onset very rare
Rapid spread	Slow progression

*Adapted from Bhatia et al.[74]

of this form of dystonia are similar to those seen in patients with well-defined psychogenic dystonia (see above). This, then, represents one of the most problematic and controversial areas in movement disorders.

There is an extensive early literature on the role of trauma in a large number of neurological diseases.[54] With respect to modern movement disorder literature, Marsden et al. described 5 female patients developing dystonic posturing variably, combined with tremor and myoclonus associated with RSD.[55] This syndrome followed minor injury to the limb in 3 of the 5 patients. Schott in 1986 described a series of 10 patients with 6 demonstrating features of dystonia.[56] In 1988, Jankovic and Van der Linden described 23 patients with movement disorders following peripheral injury.[57] Ten of the 23 had reflex sympathetic dystrophy; 15 had dystonia as the primary movement disorder with 4 demonstrating additional tremor. In contrast to other studies of such patients, the authors felt that the movement disorders seen in their cases were "clinically similar to those typically seen in patients with ITD or ET [essential tremor]." Also in contrast to other studies, they found that fully 65 percent had evidence of "predisposing factors" such as a family history of a movement disorder or previous neuroleptic use. Although the authors felt that their patients represented examples of organic disorders, they admitted that "psychiatric disease may have contributed." In 1990, Schwartzman and Kerrigan described 43 of 200 RSD patients who demonstrated a movement disorder.[58] All 43 had dystonia, 10 of whom showed only "subtle features;" 31 of the 43 also had tremor. The features of dystonia were similar to those outlined in Table 53-7. In addition to the dystonia, all patients demonstrated "spasms" as well as difficulty initiating movement. Most demonstrated increased tone and reflexes. As in other reports, minor injuries were causative in most cases. No predisposing factors were mentioned in this report. Sympathetic blocks were said to improve the symptoms temporarily in 90 percent of patients. In 1993, Bhatia et al. coined the term "causalgia-dystonia syndrome," describing 18 patients who developed fixed dystonic postures, usually after minor injury.[74] In contrast to Schwartzman and Kerrigan's report, they found that sympathetic blockade, sympathectomies and a variety of medications were entirely unhelpful. These authors admitted the potential for psychogenic factors to have played an important role in the development of this problem, recognizing that the absence of overt psychopathology is not uncommon in isolated conversion reactions, contrary to the opinion of Schwartzman and Kerrigan.[59] More recently, Van Hilten et al. have reported a series of papers describing dystonia accompanying RSD.[60–62] Once again, many features, particularly the rapid onset, unusual progression (sometimes to generalized involvement), posturing at rest from the outset, and marked resistance to passive movement (indeed, increased resistance similar to that described by Head as quoted in the history section of this chapter), might suggest the alternative diagnosis of psychogenic dystonia. These authors described

a marked response to intrathecal infusion of baclofen.[61] Although this was a placebo-controlled study, we would argue that a placebo response is still a possible explanation for this benefit.

The movement disorders accompanying RSD, which recently has had its name changed to complex regional pain syndrome (CRPS) type I (clinical syndrome not limited to a peripheral nerve distribution) and type II (after documented damage to a particular nerve), has been the subject of an important study by Verdugo and Ochoa. In their group of 53 patients with an involuntary movement and CRPS, 74.2 percent had dystonia or some abnormal muscle spasm. The striking finding was that no patients with CRPS type II had an abnormal movement. All of their patients with movement disorders (100 percent had CRPS type I) had other signs of a psychogenic component, including "give-way" weakness, erratic fluctuations, distractability, response to placebo and psychotherapy, and nonanatomic sensory disturbances. Another important feature was a clear relationship to a minimal precipitating event, which was work-related in 81 percent of the cases.[63]

We have observed similar findings studying a group of patients with peripheral trauma-induced cervical "dystonia." In this group of 13 patients who developed muscle spasms with abnormal posturing of neck and shoulder soon after local injury, several characteristics were identified: (1) precipitants were always trivial with no serious injury detected, usually work-related, and frequently involving the neck/shoulder area; (2) abnormal movements developed quickly, with a fixed posture consisting of shoulder elevation and head tilt being present no later than 2 weeks after the inciting event; (3) pain was a prominent feature; (4) litigation or compensation were involved in the majority of patients; (5) psychological interview utilizing the Minnesota Multiphasic Personality Inventory was suggestive of conversion disorders; sodium amytal interview resulted in improvement of pain and posture in most patients; (6) other findings suggestive of a psychogenic disorder were frequent, including "give-way" weakness, nonanatomic sensory loss, distractability, improvement with sham botulinum toxin injections, symmetrical neck tan, and surreptitious observation of a symptom-free period.

Range of motion was affected in all of our patients. This finding raises concerns over "established" long-standing disability related to traumatic injuries; one recent study implicated impaired range of motion as a prognostic factor in whiplash injuries.[64] Even more important was the fact that, despite the clinical impression of the presence of muscle hypertrophy, this was excluded during amytal interview or general anesthesia in all but 1 patient.

It is important to realize that early medical visits, injury anatomically related to the site of dystonia, and the development of an abnormal (dystonic) posture within a year of the trauma are currently accepted criteria for the diagnosis of peripheral trauma-induced dystonia and these were evident in our patients.[65]

Various forms of evidence have been presented to support a causative role of peripheral trauma in dystonia suggesting a variety of pathophysiologic explanations mostly related to an aberrant response of the CNS to such traumatic injury.[56,65–71] However, given the frequent nature of traumatic injuries, it might be expected that we would encounter such patients extremely frequently in specialized clinics, which is not the case. Samii et al.[69] found a history of local injury within a year in 12 percent of their group of 114 consecutive patients with cervical dystonia, and recall bias was an important possible contribution to this figure. Furthermore, Jankovic and Van der Linden, from their highly specialized database of 3500 patients, found only 18 patients that could have a trauma-related dystonia, not limited to the neck.[57] In fact, that group of patients did not show any major clinical difference from idiopathic dystonia patients except for the temporal relationship to injury, pain, poor response to conventional treatment, and persistence of dystonic posturing at rest (all features strikingly similar to those found in psychogenic dystonia and in our patients with posttraumatic cervical posturing).

A genetic predisposition has been postulated to explain the relative rarity of the syndrome, when compared to the common occurrence of peripheral injury. Van Hilten et al. reported an association between dystonia complicating RSD and HLA-DR13.[62] Dryness of the eyes and mouth, and bladder and bowel disturbances, were also common in these patients. However, in a later paper they did not mention this finding (or some of the other accompanying symptoms)[60] and so it is unclear whether it was borne out in studying larger numbers of patients. Bressman et al.[72] and Gasser et al.[73] failed to find a correlation between the DYT1 founder mutation and dystonia in a group of patients with dystonia following peripheral trauma and repetitive stress, respectively.[72,73]

Based on the explanation of an aberrant CNS response to a peripheral injury, one might expect that, the more severe the nerve damage, the more likely aberrant responses and therefore abnormal movements would develop. However, Verdugo and Ochoa failed to identify involuntary movements in CRPS type II (evidence of nerve damage),[63] and Bhatia et al. found no overt nerve damage in their group of 18 patients with similar symptoms.[74]

The controversy surrounding this syndrome is not limited to the movement disorders aspect. Similar controversy flourishes in the field of CRPS, where some authors have argued that patients who lack clear evidence of nerve injury constitute a "pseudoneuropathy of psychogenic origin."[75] We would argue that an unquestioning acceptance of all cases of dystonia following injury as organic "peripheral trauma-induced dystonia" explaining them with a variety of peripheral and secondary suprasegmental pathophysiological mechanisms of unproven relevance legitimizes and intellectualizes the problem without sufficient justification. With respect to the acceptance of the diagnosis of RSD without nerve injury, Ochoa states "It is dangerous to diagnose RSD, because that term carries the illusion of pathophysiology and the illusion of efficacious treatment. These unfortunate patients are the pariahs of our incompetent health system. While they do carry a genuine health disorder, they have been cursed by diagnostic adjudication of a disease of medical understanding."[75] We would argue that a similar statement could be made of many patients who have been diagnosed as having "posttraumatic dystonia."

PSYCHOGENIC TREMOR

Tremor is defined as an involuntary, rhythmic, sinusoidal movement due in part to regular rhythmical contractions of reciprocally innervated muscles.[40,76] In the series presented in Table 53-6, it accounted for 22 percent of a total of 272 PMDs.

There is a long history of writing on this subject. For example, Charcot described proximal tremors (involving the shoulder or hip) as almost unique to hysterical disorders, referring to them (unfortunately) as "rhythmical chorea." Another variant was "hammering chorea," where the patient alternately flexed and extended the elbow as though using a hammer. We now recognize that both of these forms of tremor, although uncommon, may also be seen in organic neurological disease (e.g., the wing-beating tremor sometimes seen in Wilson's disease). Of the two, a rhythmic hammering movement is more characteristic of psychogenic tremor.

Gowers[10] described the presence of hysterical tremor in patients with hysterical paralysis. He stated that "... when the paralysis is incomplete, movement is slow, and is attended by characteristic irregular, ... coarser tremor than simple tremor." This is accompanied by interference of voluntary movements by the "... undue contractions in the opponents of the muscles that should effect the movement."

Wilson,[77] referring to hysterical tremors, said that "... they present no separate or contrasting features when set alongside those of so-called 'organic' type." He disagreed with Gowers, who firmly believed that hysterical tremor could be differentiated from organic tremor based on its variability, the influence of physical and emotional stimuli, and dependence on the attention paid to it because "... numerous organic tremors can be affected by a whole series of factors, exhibit marked fluctuations and fluidity, are highly irregular, shift their incidence and are aggravated when the subject is under observation." He considered both hysterical and organic tremors to be "escape phenomena of infracortical level," and, therefore, part of an individual's "physiologic" repertoire. This would explain why "... hysterical subjects exhibiting such movements do not complain of fatigue, or at least appear to be less conscious of it than does a normal subject who executes them intentionally." In the person who intentionally produces a tremor, fatigue sets in easily because the "artifactual" tremor forms no part of their habitual function.

More recently, Fahn reported 2 cases of psychogenic tremor;[78] subsequently, Koller et al.[79] described 24 patients with clinically established or documented psychogenic tremor. In this latter series the female/male ratio was 1.7:1.

The mean age was 43.4 years with a range of 15–78 years. The onset of tremor was abrupt in 87.5 percent of cases, and the duration of tremor ranged from 1 month to 10 years. The majority of patients showed no change in their tremors over time (45 percent), while 25 percent experienced improvement to complete resolution, 4 percent worsened, and 16 percent had a fluctuating course. Ninety-one percent of the patients had other features suggestive of a functional disorder such as nonphysiologic weakness, atypical gait disturbances, and nonanatomical sensory changes. The psychiatric diagnosis in order of frequency was a conversion reaction, depression, an anxiety disorder, and malingering. The tremors were characterized by resting, postural, and kinetic components. The postural component was the most prominent, followed by resting and action tremors (i.e., resting < postural > action). Twelve percent of patients had an associated head tremor. With distraction, all patients showed a reduction in the amplitude of tremor as well as variability in tremor frequency.

Our subsequent experience with psychogenic tremor continues to support these earlier observations.[80] The general historical and clinical features of PMDs all apply. Possibly more than in most forms of PMDs the abrupt onset and the early (sometimes immediate) attainment of maximal severity are very useful clues since these features are rarely if ever seen in organic tremors. As with other PMDs, abrupt onset often follows a known precipitant (e.g., minor trauma). Psychogenic tremors are often present equally at rest, with postural maintenance and during action, whereas organic tremors uncommonly persist in all states and, when they do, the tremor tends to increase in amplitude from one to another (i.e., rest < posture < intention). We would agree with Wilson's criticism of overemphasis on tremor variability given the pronounced variation seen in organic tremors. On the other hand, complete suppression with distraction is not seen in organic tremors. More often the opposite is seen; the tremor increases when the patient is concentrating on mental or physical tasks. Suppression with distraction is an especially useful sign when the movement disorder is continuous or constant, as are most examples of psychogenic tremor. Another extremely useful clinical sign is the entrainment of the tremor to a new frequency or pattern. When the patient is asked to beat out a slow rhythmical or complex irregular pattern with the uninvolved limb (or the opposite limb to that being observed in cases of bilateral psychogenic tremor), the tremor will often change frequency or character sometimes matching the imposed contralateral movement. Rarely organic mirror movements might be confused with this phenomenon, although these would not normally suppress the underlying tremor. Alternatively, the tremor continues unabated but the requested movement is performed poorly and incompletely. This is often seen when asking the patient to make a full, smooth, side-to-side movement with the tongue. Occasionally, forcefully restraining a tremulous limb will result in a tremor developing in a previously unaffected limb. Psychogenic tremor may affect a single limb or multiple limbs and axial structures. The arms are most often involved, followed by the head and then the legs. Interestingly, although arms are commonly affected, fingers are rarely involved;[81] it seems to depend on a clonus mechanism and therefore be mediated by reflex mechanisms.[82] Psychogenic tremor may be continuous or intermittent; in the upper limbs it is often continuous but it rarely if ever has this course in the legs, typically occurring intermittently or paroxysmally, often precipitated by attention, movement or some other activity.

The combination of general clues to psychogenicity with the specific features listed above permit the experienced clinician sufficient diagnostic certainty to categorize most typical cases as "clinically established" psychogenic tremor. In long-standing, well-established cases, it is remarkable how persistent and seemingly invariable the tremor is and, like Wilson, one cannot help remarking on the lack of an expected fatiguing component. However careful, sometimes prolonged or repeated assessments will demonstrate clinical inconsistencies or incongruities with organic tremors. These criteria must be reliably demonstrated and convincingly evident before accepting a psychogenic diagnosis.

Electrophysiological studies may be helpful in both diagnosing and understanding psychogenic tremor. These can evaluate the consistency of frequency and whether distractability is present. Increased amplitude with weighting of a limb and the "co-activation sign," whereby the tremor only persists while there is ongoing muscle contraction and immediately abates when this subsides, are two important features.[81] Deuschl et al. have also proposed, based on electrophysiological studies, that psychogenic tremor seems to depend on a clonus mechanism and is therefore mediated by reflex mechanisms.[82]

PSYCHOGENIC MYOCLONUS

Myoclonus is defined as brief, shock-like muscle contractions (positive myoclonus) or sudden lapses in tone (negative myoclonus) as exemplified by asterixis. Psychogenic myoclonus represented 11.4 percent of all PMDs seen in the combined New York, Fort Lauderdale, and Toronto data (Table 53-6), although, in Jankovic's series, it was the most common form of PMD, accounting for 8.5 percent of all patients with myoclonus and 20.2 percent of all PMDs.

The only reported series of psychogenic myoclonus is that of Monday and Jankovic,[31] who described 18 patients seen over a 10-year period. The female/male ratio was 2.6:1, with a mean age of 42.5 years (range 22–75 years). None had a family history of myoclonus. Eighty-three percent of patients (15/18) had a precipitating event; the abnormal involuntary movement began suddenly in 61 percent of patients (11), with gradual onset over several days in 38 percent. Eighty-three percent of patients (15) experienced exacerbations of the myoclonus with stress, and 77 percent (14) had definite worsening of the myoclonus during periods of anxiety. The most common distribution of the myoclonus was segmental in 10 (55 percent), followed by generalized in 39 percent and focal in 5 percent of patients. The myoclonus was present at rest in all and exacerbated by movement in 77 percent (14). Light and noise worsened myoclonus in 1 and 4 patients, respectively.

Other neurological findings included tremor (postural 3, kinetic 2, resting 1), focal (posttraumatic) dystonia in 1, and gait abnormalities in 6. In most, these neurological findings were believed to be also of psychogenic origin. Neurological evaluation showed no abnormalities except for these movement disorders. All patients had normal electroencephalography (EEG) and other neurological investigations were unrevealing.

Overt psychiatric disturbances were present in 55 percent of patients prior to the onset of myoclonus, and 61 percent had a demonstrable psychiatric pathology by psychiatric interview or neuropsychological testing. The most common diagnoses were depression in 4, anxiety disorder and panic attacks in 2, and personality disorders in 2. Eighty-eight percent of the patients had a variety of different predisposing factors. Six had trauma prior to the onset of myoclonus: 3 had "on-the-job"-related injuries, 1 slipped in a shopping mall, and 2 patients were involved in motor vehicle accidents. Only 1 had a worker's compensation suit.

Follow-up was available in 12/18 patients (67 percent). Fifty-eight percent reported improvement of the myoclonus over time, while 25 percent thought that the myoclonus was much worse after evaluation. The authors emphasized that spontaneous resolution of the myoclonus can be regarded as a strong indication of psychogenicity provided that reversible causes of myoclonus are ruled out, such as infections, metabolic encephalopathies or neurodegenerative disorders, and there is no family history of myoclonus. Reduction of myoclonus with distraction was found to be a very helpful finding in establishing the diagnosis. However, because psychogenic myoclonus is often intermittent or discontinuous, this sign is probably less useful than in cases of more persistent psychogenic movements (e.g., psychogenic tremor).

Electrophysiological testing may be very helpful in problematic cases. The temporal pattern of muscle activation in various forms of pathologic myoclonus is stereotypic and depends upon the location of the generator or origin of the myoclonus (e.g. cortex, brainstem, spinal cord). Myoclonic jerks originating in the cortex (electromyographic (EMG), burst of 10–50 ms[83]) and brainstem (EMG burst >100 ms[83]) induced by sensory input (i.e., reflex myoclonus) usually have a short latency (~60–70 ms[84]) between stimulus, and resulting jerk that is typically just long enough for the sensory input to reach the site of origin and for a return volley to travel down rapidly conducting descending pathways (e.g., the corticospinal tract) to the anterior horn cells and thence to the muscle. Less commonly, electrophysiological testing demonstrates evidence of much slower, presumably polysynaptic, propagation of the response, as in propriospinal myoclonus. Electrophysiological studies using EMG surface electrodes in patients with psychogenic myoclonus may show variable

and inconsistent muscle activation patterns, and, more importantly, the stimulus-induced responses tend to habituate as seen in the normal startle response.[85] More useful is the timing of responses (in stimulus-sensitive forms) where the latency from stimulus to jerk is much longer than that seen in pathological forms of myoclonus, and typically falls within the range of voluntary reaction time (~100–120 ms; P Ashby, personal communication). Terada et al.[86] reported an assessment of the readiness potential or Bereitschaftspotential (BP) in patients with psychogenic myoclonus. The BP is a negative shift in the EEG that occurs 1.5 s before a voluntary movement takes place.[87] Terada et al. hypothesized that an involuntary movement (such as that seen in pathological forms of myoclonus) would lack a preceding BP. They found that BPs preceded the jerks in patients with psychogenic myoclonus and concluded that this feature was consistent with the movements being generated through voluntary mechanisms. Although BPs can rarely be associated with involuntary movements due to neuroacanthocytosis[88] and mirror movements,[89,90] the presence of BP can be extremely useful in identifying a movement as psychogenic.

This same type of electrophysiological assessment is very helpful in cases where sound is the inducing stimulus (i.e., psychogenic startle). The normal startle response might be considered a form of physiological myoclonus which occurs in an exaggerated fashion in a familial disorder known as hyperekplexia or startle disease. Electrophysiological study[91–93] of a startle response demonstrates progression of muscle contraction, first involving closure of the eyes (onset latency of 30–40 ms), followed by facial grimacing and forward flexion of the head (55–85 ms), flexion of the elbows (85–100 ms), abduction of the shoulders, pronation of the forearms, and clenching of the fists. Onset latency of the muscle activity in hamstrings and quadriceps is about 100–125 ms and for the tibialis anterior 130–140 ms. Some patients only manifest closure of the eyes. The rostrocaudal progression of the muscle contraction follows a similar pattern to that seen in reticular reflex myoclonus or reflex myoclonus of brainstem origin.[85] The normal physiological behavior of the startle response includes sensitization (resulting in increased amplitude and/or shorter latency of a response) which is masked by the habituation resulting from several repetitive stimuli. In startle disease, patients have an exaggerated response and lack of habituation. Many patients with psychogenic myoclonus demonstrate an exaggerated response to startle. Typically this startle response habituates over several trials as expected in normal physiological startle. Simple visual analysis of the muscle contractions may show moment-to-moment variability (i.e., inconsistency) in the latency from stimulus to response and in the pattern of muscle activation; these inconsistencies can be confirmed by multichannel EMG assessment.

Brief mention should be made of three related disorders first described approximately 100 years ago in different populations. Latah, jumping Frenchmen of Maine and myriachit all variably demonstrate excessive startle, echolalia, echopraxia, and automatic obedience.[94] Considerable debate exists about the true origins of these disorders. Careful clinical and modern electrophysiological assessments of these uncommon conditions are lacking. Some authors believe that they are organically mediated neuropsychiatric disorders akin to TS.[95] In fact, Gilles de la Tourette himself thought of these disorders as part of the "syndrome of tic convulsive."[96,97] Others argue that they represent forms of "culturally mediated behavior,"[94,95,97,98] and as such might be considered types of "psychogenic movement disorders" in the broadest sense (Wilson called them "collective psychoneurosis"[97]). Having reviewed videotapes of latah patients from Indonesia[99] and cases from Louisiana with a disorder related to jumping Frenchmen of Maine ("ragin' Cajuns"),[100,101] the authors favor the latter opinion. However, further study of these unusual conditions is clearly required.

PSYCHOGENIC CHOREA/BALLISM

As mentioned in the section on psychogenic tremors, earlier medical writings used the term chorea to describe bizarre movement disorders, which would not be consistent with the current definition of chorea. Terms such as "rhythmical chorea," "hammering chorea," and "dancing chorea" were popularized by Charcot for very spectacular movements seen in hysterical patients. True chorea, defined as random fleeting movements which flow from one part of the body to another in an unpredictable fashion, is exceedingly rare in PMD patients. We have seen only 1 patient who could be considered as having psychogenic chorea. Importantly, unlike most cases of organic chorea, his movements were purely paroxysmal. There was a very clear psychiatric history and the patient lacked other features of organic paroxysmal dyskinesias. Given the exceedingly rare occurrence of psychogenic chorea, we would recommend caution in making this diagnosis even by clinicians with considerable experience in the field of movement disorders.

PSYCHOGENIC TICS

Little has been written about psychogenic tics. Psychogenic tics accounted for only 4 of 272 (1.5 percent) psychogenic movement disorders in the series of New York, Fort Lauderdale, and Toronto (Table 53-6).

Recently, Kurlan et al.[32] reported a young woman with long-standing TS and obsessive-compulsive disorder who developed complex movements such as slumping in a chair or to the floor or bed along with tonic-clonic-like movements suggestive of pseudoseizures. No alteration of consciousness or incontinence were noted. These episodes were referred to by the patient as "bad spells" and her physicians believed they represented poorly controlled tics. However, multiple adjustments of her anti-tic medications failed to improve the movements. After careful analysis it became clear that these "bad spells" were psychogenic in nature. The patient

received psychotherapy and was found to fulfill criteria for a borderline personality disorder. There were clear secondary "gains," such as the need for financial support from her parents and avoidance of social, educational, and domestic responsibilities.

What is not clear from the description of this case is whether the patient had any premonitory feelings or symptoms of an urge to perform her usual tics or the newly developed movements and, if in trying to control the movements, she had a build-up of tension with a subsequent worsening. The absence of this urge may have helped differentiate these "tics" from true tics. In our experience, a very high proportion of tic patients experience a subjective urge to perform the tics (at one time or another). The performance of the tic is commonly appreciated as a partially volitional capitulation to this urge.[102] In some of our tic patients who have had other concomitant movement disorders (e.g., dystonia, tardive dyskinesia), a similar subjective feeling has never been present, and the patient has always been able to distinguish between their tics and these other movements. In addition, none of our PMD patients have admitted to the "voluntary" performance of the movement (see below for a possible exception), and we are aware of only 1 patient in the literature with psychogenic tremor associated with posttraumatic stress disorder[103] who admitted to the purposeful performance of the movement. Thus, patients' responses to this line of questioning may be very helpful in defining bizarre or unusual movements as forms of tics or psychogenic movements.

Although Kurlan et al. chose to term the movements "psychogenic tics" based on the diagnostic confusion that had existed in their patient, it could be argued that the movements would be better classified as "pseudoseizures" or a mixed form of bizarre psychogenic movements given their paroxysmal nature and the complexity of the movements that did not conform to those usually seen in TS.

We have consulted on a 52-year-old man who, over a 2-week period after sustaining a minor injury to his lower back, developed paroxysmal episodes of flexion of shoulders and extension with twisting of the neck. These movements were associated with an inner urge and a preceding feeling of tightness in the neck that forced him to contract the shoulders and neck. The urges gradually disappeared but the movements continued to occur spontaneously in paroxysms with periods of remission. At this time the movements were described as "having a mind of their own" (in contrast to the purposeful or volitional performance of the same movements earlier in the course of his symptoms). There was a pronounced reduction in the frequency and severity of the movements after the patient's disability support was approved. He had been exposed to phentermine hydrochloride for appetite suppression but had only taken it intermittently for a total of 90 days over a 12-month period and had stopped taking the medication 2 months prior to the trauma and onset of the movements. He had no family history of neurological or psychiatric disorders and denied any tic-like symptomatology or obsessive-compulsive behavior at any time earlier in life. During the examination he demonstrated intermittent, abrupt, brief contraction of the trapezius muscle with "pulling" of the shoulders backwards, followed by extension of the neck and contraction of the platysma muscle. At times he had alternating contraction of the sternocleidomastoid muscles, giving a brief rotatory component to the neck movement. During the examination he sometimes stated that he needed to move his neck because of a "buildup" feeling in his neck. As with most cases of both tics and PMDs, distraction completely suppressed the movements. In contrast to tics, but like many psychogenic movements, the neck movements "entrained" with synkinetic and alternating finger-counting movements of his hands.

Although this may be an unusual case of trauma-induced adult-onset tics with the additional theoretic predisposition from prior stimulant use, some of the clinical features outlined above encourage a diagnosis of psychogenic tics. Without further support, one could only classify such a case as "probable" or "possible."

Psychogenic Parkinsonism

Walters et al.[25] described a case of psychogenic parkinsonism in a 64-year-old man with onset of symptoms in his lower limbs, later accompanied by stuttering, halting speech, and tremor over a 3-year period. His gait was slow and shuffling but atypical for parkinsonism. The patient would slide one foot "glued" to the floor a long distance and then would slide the other foot in the same manner to a point "equally" distant from the first foot. Finger tapping, alternating movements, and foot tapping were slowed. His speech was also very uncharacteristic of Parkinson's disease (PD). Tremor in his hands was equally prominent at rest, with postural maintenance and on action. The rest of the neurological examination was normal. The patient's symptoms did not respond to L-dopa therapy but resolved spontaneously 1 year after discontinuing L-dopa.

More recently, one of us reported 14 cases of psychogenic parkinsonism seen at three university movement disorders centers.[26] Thirteen had pure psychogenic parkinsonism and 1 had psychogenic parkinsonism superimposed on milder features of true parkinsonism. There was a 1:1 male/female ratio. The average age of the patients was 47 years, with a range of 21–63 years. The mean duration of symptoms before diagnosis was 5 years, with a range between 4 months and 13 years. In 71 percent (10), the symptoms of parkinsonism began suddenly after a minor work-related injury or motor vehicle accident, except in 1 case who had sustained a serious head injury 9 years earlier complicated by a subdural hematoma. Parkinsonian symptoms were bilateral in 57 percent of the patients and unilateral in the remainder, typically involving the dominant side. Reduced facial expression, probably related to depression in most, was present in 6 of the 14 patients. Tremor was present in 85 percent.

An isolated postural and action tremor was seen in only 1 case. More often, the tremor had characteristic features of a psychogenic tremor, as outlined earlier. It was typically present at rest and persisted in postures and with action, lacking the characteristic dampening of true parkinsonian rest tremor which occurs on adopting a new posture or with movement. In all cases the tremor dampened or disappeared with distraction. This is the opposite of what is usually seen in patients with true resting tremor of PD, where the performance of mental exercises typically accentuates or brings out the tremor. The entrainment of the tremor to the frequency of other repetitive movements performed in another limb (typical of psychogenic tremor) contrasts with what may be seen with true parkinsonian tremor, where it is the tremor that entrains the rate and rhythm of an attempted repetitive task (e.g., finger tapping). "Bradykinesia" was seen in all cases, but the marked degree of slowness seen in most was atypical for true parkinsonian bradykinesia. Movements were often performed painstakingly slowly. However, the fatigue with decremental amplitude and arrest in ongoing movement so common in organic bradykinesia were lacking. Rigidity was present in 42 percent of cases. This often had features of voluntary resistance or difficulty relaxing. Several patients complained of associated pain in the limb, which contributed to this increased resistance to passive movements. The increased tone usually diminished during the performance of synkinetic movements of an opposite limb in contrast to the normal accentuation of true parkinsonian rigidity (i.e., "activated rigidity"). No true cogwheeling was appreciated. Abnormal gait and postural instability were present in 85 percent of patients. Armswing was diminished or absent on the affected side. However, the arm might have been held stiffly extended and adducted at the side (even while running) or flexed across the chest rather than in the typical flexed posture with reduced swing characteristic of true PD. The gait also demonstrated a variety of other bizarre or atypical features, including a component of antalgia when pain was associated. Minimal force applied to the pull test often resulted in very exaggerated or extreme responses; however, no patient fell. The nature of this response often confirmed the psychogenicity of other features. For example, the distraction might have suppressed tremor. In 1 patient whose dominant arm was slow and stiff and held tightly at the side while walking and running, both arms flailed upwards equally rapidly in her extreme response to minimal posterior trunk displacements.

The 15 patients with psychogenic parkinsonism reported to date have demonstrated a combination of features (i.e., tremor, rigidity, bradykinesia, postural disturbances, and gait instability) which justify their classification as a form of parkinsonism. However, all of these features were somewhat atypical for PD and other akinetic-rigid syndromes. As with all PMDs, the recognition of the clinical incongruities with known disease required considerable experience in the assessment and management of the "organic" counterparts (i.e., parkinsonian disorders). Other important clues to the psychogenicity of the movement disorder (see Table 53-7) were present in all patients. Abrupt onset, inconsistencies in the character of the movements, alterations of the movements with attention or distraction and associated false neurological signs were characteristically present in all patients in different combinations. Disability from psychogenic parkinsonism was often considerable. Patients were either on full disability pensions or had been forced to take early retirement. Despite the recognition of a psychogenic cause in all 15 (documented in 9, 1 with additional mild organic parkinsonism, and clinically established in 6; see below for details on diagnostic categorization), outcome varied considerably. In some, the symptoms and signs resolved completely, either spontaneously or with psychiatric therapy; in others, symptoms and resulting disability persisted unabated.

In very difficult or questionable cases of psychogenic parkinsonism, PET or SPECT scanning of the presynaptic dopamine system or PET using fluorodeoxyglucose may provide useful supportive diagnostic information (see below).

Psychogenic Gait Disorders (Including Psychogenic Ataxia)

The French school, headed by Charcot, devoted some time to these disorders[104] (Table 53-11). In Woolsey's experience, the nature of the gait disturbance seen in hysteria related to the type of motor disability the patient imagined himself/herself to have.[23] For example, in the most common hysterical gait disorder observed by Woolsey, a supposed paretic limb was dragged behind, with the foot rotated outward contacting the floor on the medial aspect of the heel and the base of the great toe. Alternatively, if the patient believed himself to be unsteady or "ataxic," the gait would zig-zag from side-to-side with frequent lurches from one support to another "... making it in the nick of time to the next," but without falls or injuries.

TABLE 53-11 French-School Classification of Hysterical Gait Disorders at the Turn of the Century

Charcot and Tourette	Roussy and Lhermitte
Astasia-abasia	Astasia-abasia
Paralytic	Pseudotabetic
Ataxic	Pseudopolyneuritic
Choreiform	Tight-rope walker
Trepidant	Robot
	Habit limping
	Choreic
	Knock-kneed
	As on a sticky surface
	As through water

SOURCE: From Keane after Southard and Roussy and Lhermitte.[104]

In a recent review videotape, the most useful features to distinguish a psychogenic gait from organic causes included exaggerated effort or fatigue, excessive slowness, fluctuations, convulsive shaking, uneconomic postures such as camptocormia (discussed in more detail later), and a bizarre gait.[105]

Psychogenic gait disorders accounted for 8.1 percent of all PMDs reported in Table 53-6. At the Los Angeles County/University of Southern California Medical Center, of all patients admitted to a neurological service with "functional neurological disorders" over a 10-year period, 26 percent (60/228) of patients had hysterical gait disorders.[104] Hysterical gait disorders accounted for 1.5 percent (68/4470) of neurological admissions to the Munich University Clinic over a 3-year period.[106]

Keane[104] reported his experience with 60 patients with hysterical gait disorders seen over a 10-year period. There were 37 women and 23 males (1.6:1) with a mean age of 36.3 (range 19–80) years. He found that 43 percent (26/60) of patients had associated hysterical eye findings, including 13 with visual field cuts, 6 with decreased visual acuity, 4 with eye movement limitation, and 3 with monocular diplopia. Other "false" neurologic signs were present in 71 percent (43/60) of patients; motor abnormalities were the most common (hemiparesis in 12, quadriparesis in 7, paraparesis in 4, and triparesis in 1). Other findings included voice abnormalities, tremor, contractures, and abnormal finger-to-nose testing where 3 patients had either finger-to-eye or finger-to-cheek alterations. The most common gait abnormalities (some patients had more than one type of gait disturbance) included ataxia (38 percent), hemiparesis (20 percent), paraparesis (16 percent), and trembling gait (14 percent). Other unusual patterns seen included dystonic, myoclonic, stiff-legged, and slapping gaits, and 1 case of camptocormia (from the Greek for bent tree trunk). Camptocormia as a feature of "hysteria" has been emphasized previously, for example by Eames,[107] whose patient developed an hysterical gait after head trauma resulting in her walking around the hospital bent over with her palms down almost touching the floor. The term was first applied to a presumed hysterical gait in soldiers returning from the Balkan War and World Wars I and II. It is important to recognize that camptocormia may also occur in organic dystonia or parkinsonian disorders and we have seen 2 cases with unilateral basal ganglia infarcts in whom the onset of camptocormia was abrupt.[108]

Other associated features in Keane's series that were present in 23 of 60 patients included a scissoring gait, a knee giving-way with quick recovery, posturing of an "arm-above-head" while walking (however, we have patients with organic axial dystonia who hold the arm above the head as a trick to allow them to walk with a more upright posture), and ataxic (tandem) gaits that blended into trembling, although "tremblers" usually had additional arm or truncal tremors while lying in bed. Six patients in the ataxic group had a history of intentional overdose with phenytoin which had been prescribed for pseudoseizures.

In another series of psychogenic gait disturbances,[106] 37 patients seen at the Munich University Clinic over 9 years (1980–1989), were video analyzed (22 prospectively, and 15 retrospectively) for the purposes of establishing diagnostic criteria and to determine if a diagnosis of psychogenic gait disturbance was possible on phenomenological grounds alone. In this series, the most salient features seen included hesitation (16.2 percent), excessive slowness of movements (35 percent), fluctuations in the gait impairment with "uneconomic" postures and wasting of muscle energy (51 percent), a "walking-on-ice" gait pattern (30 percent), and a "psychogenic Romberg" test (32 percent). The authors concluded that, if one or more of these six features were present, a diagnosis of a psychogenic gait disturbance could be made on phenomenological grounds alone with over 90 percent certainty (97 percent of patients had one or more of these six characteristics).

Other features included sudden knee buckling in 27 percent; however, over 80 percent of patients did not fall despite this feature. Eleven percent of patients had astasia, and vertical shaking tremor was present in 8 percent of cases. A suffering or strained facial expression was seen in 19 patients, associated in all with moaning, mannered posturing of hands and grasping of the leg, along with hyperventilation.

These 37 patients had a total of 116 associated hysterical findings. The most common abnormalities included other motor disturbances in 53 (45 percent), which often added to the gait disorder. These included hemiparesis (23 percent), quadriparesis (13 percent), scissoring (9 percent), knee give-way with recovery (9 percent), assuming a tandem gait (9 percent), dragging a leg (7.5 percent), paraparesis (7.5 percent), and flailing of the arms (5 percent). Other associated hysterical findings included eye movement abnormalities (22 percent), bizarre tremors (12 percent), pseudoataxia (8 percent), and voice abnormalities (7 percent).

In Keane's experience, the most common initial diagnostic error was in not insisting that the patient attempt to walk.[104] Wilson's disease and Huntington's disease were the most frequent neurological disorders where a misdiagnosis of an hysterical gait was made. In his experience, a few minutes of observation are sufficient to determine that the pattern of gait disturbance is psychogenic in origin provided that spontaneous gait, tandem, heel and toe walking are examined. This is in keeping with the finding of Lempert et al.[106] that the diagnosis of an hysterical gait disorder can reliably be made on phenomenological grounds if unusual postures and gait patterns, striking slowness of locomotion, momentary fluctuations, and a psychogenic Romberg test are seen. Other clues helpful in diagnosis are incongruities in the neurological examination (e.g., normal reflexes in a chronically paralysed leg), give-way weakness, and elimination of symptoms with suggestion or placebo. We agree with Lempert et al.'s[106] word of caution that the presence of muscle atrophy or joint contractures does not necessarily argue against a psychogenic disorder; they can represent secondary changes due to lack of use or prolonged maintenance of a tonic posture.

Establishing A Diagnosis

As discussed extensively so far, a diagnosis of PMD should be carefully established, since an incorrect classification either way will subject the patient to additional psychological stress, increased costs of further diagnostic tests, and possibly even denial of a potentially helpful treatment or untoward side-effects of a wrongly prescribed drug.

Clinical diagnosis, even in experienced hands, is extremely difficult and filled with pitfalls. It should be established by an experienced neurologist, or preferably by a movement disorders specialist since one of the most useful and important features is how the movement compares to the organic equivalent and therefore extensive experience in the field is required. The differential diagnosis of PMDs encompasses the entire field of movement disorders; therefore, the neurologist should be alert to these diagnostic possibilities in any patient who fulfills some of the characteristics mentioned above. Although it is important to keep an open mind to the possibility of an incorrect diagnosis, a protracted course, pronounced disability or resistance to therapy should never be used as criteria against a diagnosis of a PMD when all other historical and clinical criteria are satisfied.

Admission to hospital can prove beneficial in some cases, providing continuous observation, and sometimes video-monitoring can provide additional evidence. It can also provide ancillary tests to exclude organic diseases and convince the patient that a reasonable effort to exclude them was undertaken.[27,42] However, once the diagnosis is established, additional investigations should be avoided as it could convey the feeling of diagnostic uncertainty to the patient.

Ancillary tests can occasionally be helpful. In the specific case of parkinsonism, carefully evaluated and quantified SPECT or PET scans can be strongly supportive of a PMD diagnosis. However, some cases, including DRD, can have normal results; furthermore, we have seen a small number of unequivocal cases of parkinsonism in whom PET scans were reported as normal.

Electrophysiological studies can also be of help in evaluating PMD, especially myoclonus and tremor, as discussed previously.

A variety of findings have been described in organic dystonic syndromes, such as a recent suggestion by Tijssen et al. that a short-term synchronization between sternocleidomastoid and splenius capitis, along with a lack of phase differences, could help in this differentiation.[109]

In a recent review, Brown and Thompson[110] point out findings that potentially could be useful in the evaluation of organic versus psychogenic dystonia. Diminished reciprocal inhibition at intermediate and long latencies, as well as the absence of broad-peak synchronization of co-contracting antagonist muscles could be useful in supporting the diagnosis of organic dystonia.[109] However, the extent to which these are contributors or merely secondary to abnormal posturing remains unclear. Since these findings have generally not been assessed in individuals voluntarily mimicking dystonic postures nor formally use in an attempt to differentiate well-defined organic versus psychogenic movement disorders, it is unclear whether they will be clinically useful in the diagnosis of psychogenic dystonia.

In the case of ataxias, it has been suggested that kinematic differences between centripetal and centrifugal phases of movements in the vertical plane might be useful to diagnose a psychogenic condition.[111] These observations are subject to the same criticism as the previous ones.

Utilization of placebo or suggestion is a more controversial subject. Suggestion is a relatively benign approach; the reinforcement that there is no serious underlying degenerative disease coupled sometimes with directed physiotherapy training and biofeedback techniques can be extremely helpful.

The use of placebos can be hazardous. First, there are ethical and legal concerns about the use of nonactive drugs, negating the patient's autonomy. Second, it can endanger the physician-patient relationship, with the latter feeling deceived and therefore abandoning treatment.[112] This is particularly the case since most authorities do not inform the patient in advance of the possible "inactive" nature of the therapy because this clearly reduces the likelihood of a response. Patients are generally told that they are going to receive a drug that has the potential to markedly improve or ameliorate their symptoms. Sometimes, patients are told they will receive a drug which can worsen the symptoms (useful when the movements are exclusively paroxysmal) followed by another ("an antidote") which will have the opposite effect. Usually these challenges are given intravenously. An alternative (which we have not used) is a small alcohol swab or gauze patch soaked in a very mild chemical irritant which causes a slight tingling or burning sensation on the skin. One of the major concerns or criticisms of the use of placebo is that the patient may respond to being told (or especially if they learn "by accident" in some other way) of the nature of the placebo test with the conviction that they have been tricked by the medical profession.[113] The resulting resentment is very counterproductive to the therapeutic relationship necessary for ongoing management of these patients. However, when the nature and results of placebo testing are shared with the patient in a supportive milieu as part of the overall treatment program, this can be an extremely effective tool with both diagnostic and therapeutic effects.

Little has been written on the use of placebos in PMDs, possibly because there is no "gold standard" for the confirmation of diagnosis with which to compare the results of this testing, as in the case of EEG and epilepsy. Lancman et al.[114] have reported that in patients with psychogenic seizures an "induction test" had a sensitivity of 77.4 percent and a specificity of 100 percent with a positive predictive value of 100 percent. The negative predictive value was 48.7 percent. They used a "patch" placed on the skin and the patients were told that the medication would be absorbed into the circulation and reach the brain in 30 s. They were also told not to control the seizures and that removal of the patch would stop the

resulting seizure if one developed. Similar approaches,[115,116] usually using intravenous injections of saline, are considered safe and effective,[114] although Walczack et al.[117] found that, in a minority of patients, placebo injections produced atypical events or epileptic seizures which could lead to an incorrect diagnosis. There is also the potential for both severe psychogenic "reactions" upon the challenge and false positive responses in suggestible patients with organic disease. Placebo effects are widely recognized in a variety of diseases, including movement disorders.[37] On the other hand, the use of a placebo enables a direct observation and can establish a diagnosis and even a therapeutic approach. One must remember that, as soon as the diagnosis of a PMD can be established with a reasonable degree of certainty, it is possible to both withdraw and avoid therapies with potential harmful side-effects. As previously mentioned, patients have been subjected to hazardous treatments, including neurosurgical procedures, due to incorrect diagnoses.

In general, we reserve the use of placebo saline injections for patients in whom there remains diagnostic uncertainty after a full clinical assessment. This would include patients with a history of paroxysmal events that could not be triggered by simpler means such as the application of a tuning fork to the forehead or sternum combined with the suggestion that vibration often triggers such attacks in other patients. The use of pressure points in a somewhat similar fashion is effective in some patients. Attacks are sometimes precipitated by asking the patient to look up quickly. In others, applying pressure to the top of the head when the head is held steady for evaluation of eye movements is an effective precipitant. The results of these triggering or relieving maneuvers, including placebo challenges, should be incorporated in the presentation of the diagnosis to the patient.

As with placebo challenges, little has been written on the use of sodium amytal (or pentobarbital) testing in patients with PMDs. It is critical to remember that amytal may have a nonspecific but pronounced ameliorative effect on a variety of organic movement disorders. Alternatively, PMDs, especially when long-standing, may change little in response to this agent. When the diagnosis is confirmed by other means, amytal testing may provide useful insights into the psychodynamic factors causing the problem. However, caution must be exercised not to overinterpret information volunteered during this testing, especially if the diagnosis of a PMD is not supported or established by other evidence. Recently, symptom persistence during sodium amytal infusion test[118] has been reported useful in differentiating organic spasmodic dysphonia from psychogenic vocal cord dystonia where improvement in speech symptoms was commonly evident. Family history, neurological and psychiatric evaluations, electrical stimulation of the superior laryngeal nerve, and standard speech testing did not help in distinguishing these two conditions.

In our experience, the most difficult diagnostic problems arise in two situations: (1) when there is a clear evidence of a PMD but an underlying organic component cannot be excluded, and (2) when the movement disorder is an unchanging tonic ("dystonic") contraction of muscles usually precipitated by a seemingly inconsequential injury. In most examples of the former, it is the psychogenic movements that are the predominant complaint and the chief source of disability and concern.[34] We suggest dealing with these cases in a similar manner to other PMDs, keeping in mind the potential contribution (sometimes progressively so) of the underlying organic condition. This point was recently emphasized by Mai,[119] who stated that "…the diagnosis of conversion disorders and neurological disorders are not mutually exclusive; they may occur in the same patient either concurrently or consecutively and are particularly common in chronic relapsing diseases such as multiple sclerosis and epilepsy." In the second situation, the nature of tonic muscle contraction ("dystonia" or "spasm") occurring after injury represents a major source of controversy in the field of movement disorders, as discussed previously.

Psychiatric consultation should be obtained for assistance with primary diagnosis and therapy. An established psychiatric diagnosis is of paramount importance in both the diagnosis and the treatment of patients with PMDs; a positive response to psychotherapy lends further support to the PMD diagnosis. However, it is important to reiterate that patients with organic movement disorders may have additional coincident or secondary psychopathology.

It should also be noted that, in many patients with PMDs, the underlying psychopathology is not overt even after an extended psychiatric assessment. It is not uncommon for such patients to have received "psychiatric clearance" with the final opinion expressed that there is no underlying psychiatric problem and therefore an organic cause of the movement disorder must be present. This is comparable to a time when psychiatrists found evidence for psychopathology in patients with organic dystonia and blamed these "disturbances" for the movement disorder, whereas we would now either disregard this evidence or recognize it as a consequence rather than as a cause of the motor dysfunction. The diagnosis of a PMD is made by a neurologist with experience in the field of movement disorders and should not be made or refuted by a psychiatrist, especially one inexperienced with movement disorders. As Ford et al.[29] pointed out, there are three basic errors in dealing with such patients that can lead to devastating consequences: (1) the patient may be misdiagnosed as having a psychogenic disorder when in fact it is organic; (2) a truly psychogenic disorder can be misdiagnosed as organic; and (3) the clinician fails to provide the appropriate care and therapy for the patient.

The accuracy of diagnosis in psychogenic disorders seems to be improving. Compared to his original paper in 1965, when Slater found that over half of his patients were diagnosed with a major physical or psychiatric disease over time,[39] this only accounted for 3 out of 64 patients in a 1998 series, of which a good proportion were psychogenic gait disorders.[120]

Categories of Diagnostic Certainty

The level of diagnostic certainty that the physician has for a psychogenic cause of a movement disorder varies greatly, depending on the clinical features of the movement disorder and the accompanying symptoms and signs. The four degrees of certainty for the diagnosis of psychogenic dystonia developed by Fahn and Williams[27] are now commonly applied to all forms of PMDs. These degrees of certainty are divided into documented, clinically established, probable, and possible PMDs. In documented PMDs, the movements must be persistently relieved by psychotherapy, suggestion, administration of placebos, or the patient is witnessed as being free of symptoms when left alone unobserved. Clinically established PMDs are inconsistent over time or are incongruent with the classical definitions of movement disorders. For example, in the case of dystonia, the patient cannot move the limb on request and resists passive movements, but easily grooms him or herself in daily life. Along with these incongruities the patient must show additional features that suggest psychogenicity, such as other neurological signs that are definitely psychogenic (e.g., false weakness or false sensory findings or self-inflicted injuries, multiple somatizations, and an obvious psychiatric condition). Caution needs to be exercised in the case of self-inflicted injuries since these can occasionally be symptoms of an organic movement disorder such as TS or neuroacanthocytosis. Probable PMD applies to those patients that fall into the following categories: (1) the movement disorder is inconsistent or incongruent with classical definitions, but there are no other features suggesting psychogenicity; (2) the movement disorder is consistent and congruent with organic disease, but accompanying neurological signs are definitely psychogenic, such as false weakness or sensory findings; (3) the movement disorder is consistent with a classical condition, but multiple somatizations are present. In the case of the second and third categories, it is important to consider the diagnostic alternative of an organic movement disorder accompanied by coincidental or associated psychiatric disturbances (see below). Finally, the diagnosis of a PMD is possible when an obvious emotional disturbance is present in a patient with a movement disorder that is otherwise consistent with a known organic disease.

Approach to Therapy of Psychogenic Movements Disorders

When a diagnosis is firmly established, empathy and understanding on the part of the physician are of paramount importance. The diagnosis should be presented carefully, avoiding conveyance of uncertainty. We agree with Ford et al.[29] that the use of a neurobiological explanation for the patient's symptoms helps in establishing trust, acceptance, and understanding of their diagnosis, and will help in the recovery of the symptoms. The nature of the movement disorder should be confirmed (i.e., the patient is told he/she has a form of dystonia, tremor, myoclonus, etc.) but that the problem is not due to severe or permanent structural brain disease. A psychiatric consultation should be obtained if the patient is not already under a psychiatrist/psychologist's care, both to develop and assist in a long-term treatment program. The importance of working closely with a psychiatrist interested in the care and management of such patients cannot be overemphasized. Depending upon the circumstances, one may have to introduce the need for psychiatric consultation by stating that it is strictly for the purposes of evaluating and assisting the patient in their strategies of coping with the disability caused by the abnormal movements. This approach is often necessary in patients with long-standing symptoms who have had multiple investigations, have been given a diagnosis of an organic movement disorder, and have undergone extensive therapeutic trials. In others, it may be possible to introduce the concept of a psychological cause even before obtaining the psychiatric consultation. In both circumstances, we eventually emphasize a neurobiological explanation for the movement disorder, stressing the notion that many underlying stressors or conflicts can result in CNS dysfunction and unequivocal disability, in the same fashion as stress is commonly believed to contribute to such better known (to the public) conditions as hypertension, peptic ulcer disease, coronary artery disease, irritable bowel syndrome, and neurodermatitis. This is done in a nonjudgmental fashion, reassuring the patient that it is not believed that they are "crazy" or that they are purposefully feigning or causing the movements to occur.

The patient should be reassured and counseled to the effect that there is a strong possibility of improvement. Further management approaches depend largely upon the nature and severity of the underlying psychopathology. Treatment may require the variable combination of physiotherapy, biofeedback, and other motor retraining paradigms, psychotherapy, suggestion, psychopharmacology, and at times even coercion and placebo treatments. Hypnosis might be considered; however, this had no additional benefit on treatment outcome of conversion disorders of the motor type in a recent study of 45 patients.[121]

Some patients with acute short-lived symptoms may only require reassurance, support, and active follow-up. Further discussion of the management of the causative psychiatric disorders is beyond the scope of this text.

Prognosis

Despite the reassurance given to patients suffering from PMDs, it should be emphasized that the prognosis must be guarded. Some patients will remain refractory to all treatment. However, a systematic approach involving a team composed of a neurologist, psychiatrist, nurses, physiotherapists, and others may be rewarded with striking successes even in long-lasting, extremely disabled cases. Very little is formally known about the long-term prognosis of these patients, both with respect to the movement disorders and the psychiatric features. Despite the suggestion that settlement resolves the problem in patients involved in legal or compensation issues, the natural intuitive thinking that abnormal movements of psychogenic origin will eventually settle, and previous uncontrolled findings that 25 percent of these patients improve spontaneously, it now seems that quite a high proportion of patients will have long-standing or persistent disability.[28,42]

Feinstein et al. have attempted to shed some light on this issue, interviewing 42 patients out of a group of 88 subjects seen in our unit in Toronto with either documented or clinically established PMD.[28] At the time of the study interview, on average 3.2 years after the initial assessment, all but 4 patients still had the abnormal movement (90.5 percent). Of these 4 patients, 2 had replaced the abnormal movement by a different somatoform disorder. Although there was no formal assessment at baseline, the psychiatric status showed a significant array of disorders; only 2 patients did not have a psychiatric diagnosis at follow-up (4.8 percent). Diagnosis at the time of interview included anxiety disorders in 16 patients (38.1 percent), major depression in 8 (19.1 percent) and a combination of the two in 5 (11.9 percent). A schizoaffective disorder was diagnosed in 1 patient (2.4 percent).

Twenty-three of our previously diagnosed PMD patients (most of them participating in the study of Feinstein described above) agreed to a follow-up detailed neurological examination (J Fine, A Nieves, and A Lang, unpublished observations). In this subset, all patients were still manifesting PMD at the time of follow-up, with a mean duration of symptoms of 8.6 ± 8.5 years. Activities of daily living such as eating, dressing, and hygiene were reported impaired in 19 of the examined patients (82.6 percent). Of the patients whose symptoms had improved or stabilized, 66.6 percent experienced this change within the first year of illness. This overall poor prognosis for recovery and substantial disability has been reported by other groups, for example studying psychogenic tremor.[81]

The outcome of PMDs depends greatly upon the underlying psychiatric basis. One study evaluating conversion disorders showed that patients with a conversion disorder admitted to hospital who were young (<40 years) and, similar to the case in pseudoepileptic disorders, had a recent onset of symptoms (usually a few days before admission to hospital) generally had a good prognosis.[122] The strongest predictive factor was found to be the condition of the patient upon discharge. If the symptoms improved while in hospital, a good outcome was observed in up to 96 percent of patients. In this study, only 2 patients mistakenly diagnosed as having a conversion disorder were later found to develop an organic neurological disease (left middle cerebral artery territory infarct, and multiple sclerosis, respectively). The authors concluded that neurological disease will emerge only rarely in patients with conversion disorders and although neuroimaging is helpful in difficult cases, it can also be a source of confusion by "...showing harmless anatomical variants." They found that apraxia, focal dystonia, and the combination of organic deficits with a conversion disorder are areas of most frequent diagnostic error and confusion. Finally, it was emphasized that recovery of a conversion disorder is rare if improvement does not occur during the initial hospital evaluation.

Thus, in summary, PMDs seem to carry a poor prognosis, both for psychiatric and motor function. Patients who fare better seem to be the ones whose symptoms improve and stabilize within the first year, suggesting that long-standing disease when first assessed carries a particularly poor prognosis. Other studies have suggested that additional features that may predict a good outcome in psychogenic neurological syndromes include a clear emotional trigger or precipitant, and lack of long-standing psychopathology.[122]

As expected, factitious disorders and malingering respond poorly. When litigation or compensation issues are pending, it is important to resolve them as quickly as possible. However, response to this approach is often disappointing or unpredictable. Malingerers may either keep up the act in order to justify the settlement or will have a striking improvement once a settlement has been reached. In our experience, although somatoform disorders less commonly improve in response to a financial settlement, spontaneous or therapeutically induced remissions are much less likely to occur while economic issues remain unresolved.

The experience of Ford et al.[29] contrasts with the rather negative impressions outlined above. They found that age, gender, intelligence, chronicity of illness, and PMD symptomatology had no influence on outcome. In PMD patients with either a conversion or somatoform disorder, the response to treatment was considered "successful" in all (except in 3 patients with either malingering or a factitious disorder), and they concluded that "... patients with many years of established psychogenic symptomatology were able to make full recoveries."[29] However, their treatment often entailed intensive, extended hospitalization (which is now rather impractical or even impossible in the era of managed-care) and long-term follow-up documenting sustained improvement once the patient left the intensive therapeutic milieu was generally not available. This highlights an urgent need for accurate outcome data documenting long-term prognosis in patients managed with a variety of treatment approaches. As emphasized previously, PMDs are common and frequently result in pronounced disability, with consequent impact on both the individual and society. Future research must be directed at advancing our understanding of the pathogenesis of these disorders and improving their management.

References

1. Head H: The diagnosis of hysteria. *Br Med J* 1:827–829, 1922.
2. Charcot J-M: Hystero-epilepsy: A young woman with a convulsive attack in the auditorium, in Goetz CG (ed): *Charcot The Clinician. The Tuesday Lessons.* New York: Raven Press, 1987, pp 102–122.
3. Freud S: Charcot, in Sutherland JD (ed): *Collected Papers.* London: The Hogarth Press, 1957, vol 1, pp 9–23.
4. Guillain G: *JM Charcot, 1825–1893, His Life—His Work.* New York: Paul B Hoeber, 1959.
5. Havens LL: Charcot and hysteria. *J Nerv Ment Dis* 141:505–516, 1966.
6. Schiller F: *Paul Broca: Founder of French Anthropology, Explorer of the Brain.* New York: Oxford University Press, 1992.
7. Freud S: Hypnotism and suggestion (1888), in Strachey J (ed): *Collected Papers.* London: Hogarth Press, 1957, pp 11–24.
8. Gowers WR: *Epilepsy and Other Chronic Convulsive Diseases: Their Causes, Symptoms and Treatment.* New York: Dover Publications, 1964.
9. Lecrubier Y: Images in psychiatry: Jean-Martin Charcot, 1825–1893. *Am J Psychiatry* 151:121, 1995.
10. Gowers WR: *A Manual of Diseases of the Nervous System.* Philadelphia: Blakiston, 1888.
11. Walshe SF: Diagnosis of hysteria. *Br Med J* 2:1451–1454, 1965.
12. Cockburn JJ: Spasmodic torticollis: A psychogenic condition? *J Psychosom Res* 15:471–477, 1971.
13. Harrington RC, Wieck A, Marks IM, Marsden CD: Writer's cramp: Not Associated with Anxiety. *Mov Disord* 3:195–200, 1988.
14. Grafman J, Cohen LG, Hallett M: Is focal hand dystonia associated with psychopathology? *Mov Disord* 6:29–35, 1991.
15. American Psychiatric Association: *Diagnostic and Statistical Manual of Mental Disorders, 4th edition (DSM-IV).* Washington: American Psychiatric Association, 1994.
16. Thompson DJ, Goldberg D: Hysterical personality disorder. *Br J Psychiatry* 150:241–245, 1987.
17. Vuilleumier P, Chicherio C, Assal F, et al: Functional neuroanatomical correlates of hysterical sensorimotor loss. *Brain* 124:1077–1090, 2001.
18. Schepank H, Hilpert H, Honmann H, et al: The Mannheim Cohort Project: Prevalence of psychogenic diseases in cities. *Z Psychosom Med Psychoanal* 30:43–61, 1984.
19. Snyder S, Strain JJ: Somatoform disorders in the general hospital inpatient setting. *Gen Hosp Psychiatry* 11:288–293, 1989.
20. Franz M, Schellberg D, Reister G, Schepank H: Incidence and follow-up characteristics of neurologically relevant psychogenic symptoms. *Nervenarzt* 64:369–376, 1993.
21. Marsden CD: Hysteria: A neurologist's view. *Psychol Med* 16:277–288, 1986.
22. Lempert T, Dieterich M, Huppert D, Brandt T: Psychogenic disorders in neurology: Frequency and clinical spectrum. *Acta Neurol Scand* 82:335–340, 1990.
23. Woolsey RM: Hysteria: 1875 to 1975. *Dis Nerv Syst* 37:379–386, 1976.
24. Factor SA, Podshalny GD, Molho ES: Psychogenic movement disorders: Frequency, clinical profile and characteristics. *J Neurol Neurosurg Psychiatry* 59:406–412, 1995.
25. Walters AS, Boudwin J, Wright D, Jones K: Three hysterical movement disorders. *Psychol Rep* 62:979–985, 1988.
26. Lang AE, Koller WC, Fahn S: Psychogenic parkinsonism. *Arch Neurol* 52:802–810, 1995.
27. Fahn S, Williams PJ: Psychogenic dystonia. *Adv Neurol* 50:431–455, 1988.
28. Feinstein A, Stergiopoulos V, Fine J, Lang AE: Psychiatric outcome in patients with a psychogenic movement disorder: A prospective study. *Neuropsychiatry Neuropsychol Behav Neurol* 14:169–176, 2001.

29. Ford B, Williams DT, Fahn S: Treatment of psychogenic movement disorders, in Kurlan R (ed): *Treatment of Movement Disorders*. JB Lippincott, 1995, pp 475–485.

30. Factor SA, Podskalny GD, Molho ES: Psychogenic movement disorders: Frequency, clinical profile, and characteristics. *J Neurol Neurosurg Psychiatry* 59:406–412, 1995.

31. Monday K, Jankovic J: Psychogenic myoclonus. *Neurology* 43:349–352, 1993.

32. Kurlan R, Deeley C, Comon PG: Psychogenic movement disorder (pseudo-tics) in a patient with Tourette's syndrome. *J Neuropsychiatry Clin Neurosci* 4:347–348, 1992.

33. Kanner AM, Parra J, Frey M, et al: Psychiatric and neurologic predictors of psychogenic pseudoseizure outcome. *Neurology* 53:933–938, 1999.

34. Ranawaya R, Riley D, Lang AE: Psychogenic dyskinesias in patients with organic movement disorders. *Mov Disord* 5:127–133, 1990.

35. Barclay CL, Lang AE: Other secondary dystonias, in Tsui J, Calne DB (eds): *Handbook of Dystonia*. New York: Marcel Dekker, 1995, pp 267–305.

36. Koller W: Movement disorders: Which ones are real? Malingering and conversion reactions. Washington, DC: American Academy of Neurology Annual Meeting, 1994, 222-3–225-25.

37. Goetz CG, Leurgans S, Raman R, Stebbins GT: Objective changes in motor function during placebo treatment in PD. *Neurology* 54:710–714, 2000.

38. Bentivoglio AR, Loi M, Valente EM, et al: Phenotypic variability of DYTI-PTD: Does the clinical spectrum include psychogenic dystonia? *Mov Disord* 17:1058–1063, 2002.

39. Crimlisk HL, Bhatia K, Cope H, et al: Slater revisited: 6 year follow up study of patients with medically unexplained motor symptoms. *BMJ* 316:582–586, 1998.

40. Weiner WJ, Lang AE: *Movement Disorders: A Comprehensive Survey*. New York: Futura Publishing, 1989.

41. Lesser RP, Fahn S: Dystonia: A disorder often misdiagnosed as a conversion reaction. *Am J Psychiatry* 153:349–352, 1978.

42. Marsden CD: Psychogenic problems associated with dystonia. *Adv Neurol* 65:319–326, 1995.

43. Weiner WJ, Lang AE: Idiopathic torsion dystonia, in Weiner WJ, Lang AE (eds): *Movement Disorders: A Comprehensive Survey*. Mt. Kisco, NY: Future Publishing, 1989, pp 1–725.

44. Dobyns WB, Ozelius LJ, Kramer PL, et al: Rapid-onset dystonia-parkinsonism. *Neurology* 43:2596–2602, 1993.

45. Bressman SB, Fahn S, Burke RE: Paroxysmal non-kinesigenic dystonia. *Adv Neurol* 50:403–413, 1998.

46. Saint-Cyr JA, Taylor AE, Nicholson K: Behavior and the basal ganglia. *Adv Neurol* 65:1–28, 1995.

47. Batshaw ML, Wachtel RC, Deckel AW, et al: Munchausen's syndrome simulating torsion dystonia. *N Engl J Med* 312:1437–1439, 1985.

48. Lang AE: Psychogenic dystonia: A review of 18 cases. *Can J Neurol Sci* 22:136–143, 1995.

49. Sheehy MP, Marsden CD: Writer's cramp: A focal dystonia. *Brain* 461:480, 1982.

50. Sheehy MP, Marsden CD: Trauma and pain in spasmodic torticollis. *Lancet* 1:777–778, 1980.

51. Fletcher NA, Harding AE, Marsden CD: The relationship between trauma and idiopathic torsion dystonia. *J Neurol Neurosurg Psychiatry* 54:713–717, 1991.

52. Fletcher NA, Harding AE, Marsden CD: A case-control study of idiopathic torsion dystonia. *Mov Disord* 6:304–309, 1991.

53. Bhatia KP, Bhatt MH, Marsden CD: The causalgia-dystonia syndrome. *Brain* 116:843–851, 1993.

54. Koller WC, Wong GF, Lang A: Posttraumatic movement disorders: A review. *Mov Disord* 4:20–36, 1989.

55. Marsden CD, Obeso JA, Traub MM, et al: Muscle spasms associated with Sudeck's atrophy after injury. *BMJ* 288:173–176, 1984.

56. Schott GD: The relationship of peripheral trauma and pain to dystonia. *J Neurol Neurosurg Psychiatry* 48:698–701, 1985.

57. Jankovic J, Van der Linden C: Dystonia and tremor induced by peripheral trauma: Predisposing factors. *J Neurol Neurosurg Psychiatry* 51:1512–1519, 1988.

58. Schwartzman RJ, Kerrigan J: The movement disorder of reflex sympathetic dystrophy. *Neurology* 40:57–61, 1990.

59. Schwartzman RJ: Movement disorder of RSD [letter]. *Neurology* 40:1477–1478, 1990.

60. Van Hilten JJ, Van de Beek WJT, Vein AA, et al: Clinical aspects of multifocal or generalized tonic dystonia in reflex sympathetic dystrophy. *Neurology* 56:1762–1765, 2001.

61. Van Hilten BJ, Van de Beek WJT, Hoff JI, et al: Intrathecal baclofen for the treatment of dystonia in patients with reflex sympathetic dystrophy. *N Engl J Med* 343:625–630, 2000.

62. Van Hilten JJ, Van de Beek WJT, Roep BO: Multifocal or generalized tonic dystonia of complex regional pain syndrome: A distinct clinical entity associated with HLA-DR13. *Ann Neurol* 48:113–116, 2000.

63. Verdugo RJ, Ochoa JL: Abnormal movements in complex regional pain syndrome: Assessment of their nature. *Muscle Nerve* 23:198–205, 2000.

64. Kasch H, Bach FW, Jensen TS: Handicap after acute whiplash injury: A 1-year prospective study of risk factors. *Neurology* 56:1637–1643, 2001.

65. Jankovic J: Post-traumatic movement disorders: Central and peripheral mechanisms. *Neurology* 44:2006–2014, 1994.

66. Tarsy D: Comparison of acute- and delayed-onset posttraumatic cervical dystonia. *Mov Disord* 13:481–485, 1998.

67. Truong DD, Dubinsky R, Hermanowicz N, et al: Posttraumatic torticollis. *Arch Neurol* 48:221–223, 1991.

68. Goldman S, Ahlskog JE: Posttraumatic cervical dystonia. *Mayo Clin Proc* 68:443–448, 1993.

69. Samii A, Pal PK, Schulzer M, et al: Post-traumatic cervical dystonia: A distinct entity? *Can J Neurol Sci* 27:55–59, 2000.

70. Wright RA, Ahlskog JE: Focal shoulder-elevation dystonia. *Mov Disord* 15:709–713, 2000.

71. Höllinger P, Burgunder JM: Posttraumatic focal dystonia of the shoulder. *Eur Neurol* 44:153–155, 2000.

72. Bressman SB, De Leon D, Raymond D, et al: Secondary dystonia and the DYTI gene. *Neurology* 48:1571–1577, 1997.

73. Gasser T, Bove CM, Ozelius LJ, et al: Haplotype analysis at the DYT1 locus in Ashkenazi Jewish patients with occupational hand dystonia. *Mov Disord* 11:163–166, 1996.

74. Bhatia KP, Bhatt MH, Marsden CD: The Causalgia-Dystonia Syndrome. *Brain* 116:843–851, 1993.

75. Ochoa J: Reflex sympathetic dystrophy: Fact or fiction. Malingering and conversion reactions. Washington: American Academy of Neurology Annual Meeting, 1994, 222-41–222-56.

76. Elble RJ, Koller WC: The definition and classification of tremor, in *Tremor*. Baltimore: Johns Hopkins University Press, 1990, pp 1–9.

77. Wilson SAK: The approach to the study of hysteria. *J Neurol Psychopathol* 11:193–206, 1931.

78. Fahn S: Atypical tremors, rare tremors and unclassified tremors, in Findley LJ, Capildeo R (eds): *Movement Disorders*. London: Macmillan Press, 1984, pp 431–443.

79. Koller W, Lang AE, Vetere-Overfield B, et al: Psychogenic tremors. *Neurology* 39:1094–1099, 1989.

80. Kim YJ, Pakiam AS, Lang AE: Historical and clinical features of psychogenic tremor: A review of 70 cases. *Can J Neurol Sci* 26:190–195, 1999.

81. Deuschl G, Köster B, Lücking CH, Scheidt C: Diagnostic and pathophysiological aspects of psychogenic tremors. *Mov Disord* 13:294–302, 1998.

82. Deuschl G, Raethjen J, Lindemann M, Krack P: The pathophysiology of tremor. *Muscle Nerve* 24:716–735, 2001.

83. Obeso JA, Artieda J, Martinez-Lage JM: The physiology of myoclonus in man, in Quinn NP, Jenner PG (eds): *Disorders of Movement. Clinical, Pharmacological and Physiological Aspects*. London: Academic Press, 1989, pp 437–444.

84. Hallett M, Chadwick D, Marsden CD: Cortical reflex myoclonus. *Neurology* 29:1107–1125, 1979.

85. Thompson PD, Colebatch JG, Brown P, et al: Voluntary stimulus-sensitive jerks and jumps mimicking myoclonus or pathological startle syndromes. *Mov Disord* 7:257–262, 1992.

86. Terada K, Ikeda A, Van Ness PC, et al: Presence of Bereitschaftspotential preceding psychogenic myoclonus: Clinical application of jerk-locked back averaging. *J Neurol Neurosurg Psychiatry* 58:745–747, 1995.

87. Rothwell J: *Cerebral Cortex. Control of Human Voluntary Movement*. London: Chapman & Hall, 1994, pp 293–386.

88. Shibasaki H, Sakai T, Nishimura H, et al: Involuntary movements in chorea-acanthocytosis: A comparison with Huntington's chorea. *Ann Neurol* 12:311–314, 1982.

89. Shibasaki H, Nagae K: Mirror movement: Application of movement-related cortical potentials. *Ann Neurol* 15:299–302, 1984.

90. Cohen LG, Meer J, Tarkka I, et al: Congenital mirror movements: Abnormal organization of motor pathways in two patients. *Brain* 114:381–403, 1991.

91. Hallett MD: *The Pathophysiology of Tics, Startle Reactions, and Other Complex Involuntary Movements*. Motor Control Course Notes: American Academy of Neurology Annual Meeting, Seattle, 1995, pp 77–92.

92. Matsumoto J, Hallett M: Startle syndromes, in Marsden CD, Fahn S (eds): *Movement Disorders 3*. Oxford: Butterworth-Heinemann, 1994, pp 418–433.

93. Matsumoto J, Fuhr P, Nigro M, Hallett M: Physiological abnormalities in hereditary hyperekplexia. *Ann Neurol* 32:41–50, 1992.

94. Chapel JL: Latah, myriachit, and jumpers revisited. *N Y State J Med* 70:2201–2204, 1970.

95. Andermann F, Andermann E: Excessive startle syndromes: Startle disease, jumping and startle epilepsy. *Adv Neurol* 43:321–338, 1986.

96. Stevens H: "Jumping Frenchmen of Maine." *Arch Neurol* 12:311–314, 1965.

97. Kunkle EC: The "jumpers" of Maine: A reappraisal. *Arch Intern Med* 119:355–358, 1967.

98. Saint-Hilaire MH, Saint-Hilaire JM, Granger L: Jumping Frenchmen of Maine. *Neurology* 36:1269–1271, 1986.

99. Tanner CM, Chamberland J: Latah in Jakarta, Indonesia. *Mov Disord* 16:526–529, 2001.

100. Saint-Hilaire M-H, Saint-Hilaire JM: Jumping Frenchmen of Maine. *Mov Disord* 16:530, 2001.

101. McFarling DA: The "Ragin' Cajuns" of Louisiana. *Mov Disord* 16:531–532, 2002.

102. Lang AE: Patient perception of tics and other movement disorders. *Neurology* 41:223–228, 1991.

103. Walters AS, Hening WA: Noise-induced psychogenic tremor associated with post-traumatic stress disorder. *Mov Disord* 7:333–338, 1992.

104. Keane JR: Hysterical gait disorders: 60 cases. *Neurology* 39:586–589, 1989.

105. Hayes MW, Graham S, Heldorf P, et al: A video review of the diagnosis of psychogenic gait. *Mov Disord* 14:914–921, 1999.

106. Lempert T, Brandt T, Dieterich M, Huppert D: How to identify psychogenic disorders of stance and gait. *J Neurol* 238:140–146, 1991.

107. Eames P: Hysteria following brain injury. *J Neurol Neurosurg Psychiatry* 55:1046–1053, 1992.

108. Nieves AV, Miyasaki JM, Lang AE: Acute onset dystonic camptocormia caused by lenticular lesions. *Mov Disord* 16:177–180, 2001.

109. Tijssen MA, Marsden JF, Brown P: Frequency analysis of EMG activity in patients with idiopathic torticollis. *Brain* 123:677–686, 2000.

110. Brown P, Thompson PD: Electrophysiological aids to the diagnosis of psychogenic jerks, spasms, and tremor. *Mov Disord* 16:595–599, 2001.

111. Manto MU: Discrepancy between dysmetric centrifugal movements and normometric centripetal movements in psychogenic ataxia. *Eur Neurol* 45:261–265, 2001.

112. Markus AC: The ethics of placebo prescribing. *Mt Sinai J Med* 67:140–143, 2000.

113. Bok S: The ethics of giving placebos. *Sci Am* 231:17–23, 1974.

114. Lancman ME, Asconape JJ, Craven WJ, et al: Predictive value of induction of psychogenic seizures by suggestion. *Ann Neurol* 35:359–361, 1994.

115. Levy RS, Jankovic J: Placebo-induced conversion reaction: A neurobehavioural and EEG study of hysterical aphasia, seizure, and coma. *J Abnorm Psychol* 92:243–249, 1983.

116. Friedman WE, Rothner AD, Luders H, et al: Psychogenic seizures in children and adolescents. Outcome after diagnosis by ictal video and electroencephalographic recording. *Pediatrics* 85:480–484, 1990.

117. Walczak TS, Williams DT, Berten W: Utility and reliability of placebo infusion in the evaluation of patients with seizures. *Neurology* 44:394–399, 1994.

118. Ludlow CL, Martinez P, Braun AR, et al: Differential diagnosis between psychogenic and neurogenic dysphonias. *Neurology* 45:A393, 1995.

119. Mai FM. "Hysteria" in clinical neurology. *Can J Neurol Sci* 22:101–110, 1995.

120. Slater E: Diagnosis of "hysteria." *Br Med J* 1:1395–1399, 1965.

121. Moene FC, Spinhoven P, Hoogduin KAL, Van Dyck R: A randomised controlled clinical trial on the additional effect of hypnosis in a comprehensive treatment programme for in-patients with conversion disorder of the motor type. *Psychother Psychosom* 71:66–76, 2002.

122. Couprie W, Wijdicks EFM, Rooijmans HGM, van Gijn J: Outcome in conversion disorder: A follow up study. *J Neurol Neurosurg Psychiatry* 58:750–752, 1995.

123. Williams DT, Ford B, Fahn S: Phenomenology and psychopathology related to psychogenic movement disorders, in Weiner WJ, Lang AE (eds): *Behavioural Neurology in Movement Disorders*. New York: Raven Press, 1994, pp 231–257.

124. Verma A, Berger JR, Bowen BC, Sanchez-Ramos J: Reversible parkinsonian syndrome complicating cysticercus midbrain encephalitis. *Mov Disord* 10:215–219, 1995.

125. Herz E: Dystonia II: Clinical classification. *Arch Neurol Psychiat (Chicago)* 51:319–355, 1944.

126. Marsden CD, Harrison MJG: Idiopathic torsion dystonia (dystonia musculorum deformans). A review of forty-two patients. *Brain* 97:793–810, 1974.

Chapter 54

SYSTEMIC ILLNESSES THAT CAUSE MOVEMENT DISORDERS

AMY COLCHER and HOWARD I. HURTIG

ENDOCRINE DISORDERS — 915
    Hyperthyroidism — 915
    Hypothyroidism — 916
    Diabetes — 916
    Hypoparathyroidism — 916
METABOLIC/NUTRITIONAL DISORDERS — 916
    Tetrahydrobiopterin (BH$_4$) deficiency — 916
    Malabsorption syndromes — 917
    Hepatic failure — 917
    Kwashiorkor — 917
    Alcoholism — 917
    Kernicterus — 917
    Homocystinuria — 918
HEMATOLOGIC DISORDERS — 918
    Polycythemia — 918
    Mastocytosis — 918
INFECTION — 918
    Sydenham's Chorea (SC) — 918
    Lyme disease — 919
    HIV-1 — 919
    Encephalitis — 920
    Whipple's disease (WD) — 920
    Hemolytic-uremic syndrome (Hus) — 920
    Sarcoidosis — 921
AUTOIMMUNE DISORDERS — 921
    Autoimmune disease — 921
    Sjögren's syndrome (SS) — 921
    Systemic Lupus Erythematosus (SLE) — 921
    Antiphospholipid Antibody Syndrome — 922
    Gluten enteropathy — 922
PREGNANCY — 922
NEOPLASMS — 922

Movement disorders often complicate systemic illnesses. They occur in conjunction with metabolic encephalopathy, infection, neoplasms, and disorders of the endocrine, immune, and hematologic systems. Movement disorders associated with systemic illness run the gamut from an exaggerated physiologic tremor to hemiballismus, and also include the akinetic-rigid syndromes. In some cases, the movement disorder is what causes the patient to consult a physician. The underlying disorder may or may not be known at the time the movement disorder becomes obvious. In some cases, the pathophysiology of the systemic disorder causing the movement disorder is known. In some cases, there is a structural lesion in the brain responsible for the neurologic problem. In other cases, there is no clear explanation for the movement disorder in the context of the systemic disease.

Endocrine Disorders

HYPERTHYROIDISM

Endocrine abnormalities are commonly recognized causes of hyperkinetic movement disorders. Hyperthyroidism is associated with an exaggerated physiologic tremor. Up to 97 percent of patients with hyperthyroidism will exhibit a tremor,[1] the oscillatory frequency of which is the same as a physiologic tremor, but the amplitude is greater. The hands are predominantly affected, although the feet, tongue, and eyelids can be affected as well. The pathophysiology is thought to be mediated by changes in peripheral beta-adrenergic receptor tone. This theory is supported by the fact that beta-blockers, including propranolol, will dampen the tremor. It is unclear whether there is a central generator for tremor. Positron emission tomography (PET) studies of patients with essential tremor reveal abnormal bilateral cerebellar, red nuclear, and thalamic activation.[2] When thyrotoxicosis is the etiology of the tremor, the tremor is reversible by returning thyroid function to normal.

Chorea is a rare complication of hyperthyroidism, occurring in less than 2 percent of patients with thyrotoxicosis.[1] The pathophysiology is not well understood, but the chorea is reversible with treatment of the hyperthyroidism.[1,3-5] Baba described a young woman with unilateral chorea and thyrotoxicosis with normal computed tomography (CT), magnetic resonance imaging (MRI), and single-photon emission CT (SPECT) scans.[3] Autopsy studies of patients with hyperthyroid chorea reveal no pathologic lesion within the basal ganglia.[16] Measurements of dopamine metabolites in the cerebrospinal fluid (CSF) of patients with and without hyperthyroidism reveal lower levels of homovanillic acid (HVA) in patients with hyperthyroidism than in normals.[6] Decreased HVA levels suggest an alteration in dopamine metabolism in hyperthyroid individuals.[6] Thyroid abnormalities may alter the sensitivity of dopaminergic receptors.[1,6] An alteration in basal ganglia metabolism or function, such as heightened sensitivity of dopamine receptors in the basal ganglia of hyperthyroid individuals, is one postulated mechanism for the chorea.[6] It is possible that there may need to be pre-existing damage to the basal ganglia to predispose a hyperthyroid individual to develop chorea. Fischbeck and Layzer described a patient who had an anoxic event prior to the development of hyperthyroidism and later developed chorea.[7] The initial insult may have made the basal ganglia more susceptible to the altered receptor sensitivity induced by the change in thyroid function.[6] The chorea of hyperthyroidism is responsive to dopamine receptor blocking agents such as haloperidol.

HYPOTHYROIDISM

Myxedema is associated with cerebellar dysfunction in a percentage of patients,[1] most of whom complain of unsteadiness,[8] difficulty walking, and incoordination. Examination of patients with these complaints reveals a truncal ataxia, although appendicular ataxia is also seen. Rare patients will exhibit dysarthria. A 3-Hz body oscillation has been described.[8] Dysfunction of the cerebellum or cerebellar connections is a postulated mechanism for the ataxia seen with myxedema. Autopsy of patients with myxedema and alcoholism reveal degeneration of the cerebellar cortex and glycogen-containing inclusions within cerebellar cortical neurons.[1] It is not clear that the pathology is related purely to the thyroid disorder. The ataxia improves as the patient becomes euthyroid.

DIABETES

Both hyper- and hypoglycemia have been reported as uncommon causes of choreoathetosis.[9,10] SPECT studies on a patient with hemichorea/hemiballism secondary to hyperglycemia reveal increased blood flow in the contralateral striatum and thalamus.[11] Haan's description of an 80-year-old woman who had paroxysmal choreoathetosis when her blood sugar was both high and low raises interesting questions about pathogenesis. A possible theory is that a prolonged blood glucose level resets the osmoreceptors in the brain and any rapid change from that level is poorly tolerated.[12] Hyperglycemia without ketosis is a recognized cause of chorea. The chorea associated with blood sugar abnormalities may resolve with correction of the blood sugar, or it may be slow, taking months to resolve,[13] or it may be permanent.[14] The patients described with chorea associated with abnormal blood sugar have, for the most part, been elderly. A multifactorial etiology may play a role here in that some pre-existing structural damage such as lacunar infarction or hemorrhage may be necessary to make the striatum more susceptible to the effects of hyperglycemia,[15] or an ischemic episode in small arterioles occurring at the time of the hyperglycemia may contribute.

HYPOPARATHYROIDISM

Hypoparathyroidism results in hypocalcemia, hypophosphatemia, and hypomagnesemia. Metabolic derangements, primarily hypocalcemia, are responsible for the frequently encountered neurologic complications such as tetany, neuromuscular irritability, and seizures. Pseudohypoparathyroidism is an hereditary parathyroid resistance syndrome caused by a defect in the parathyroid hormone (PTH) receptor. Pseudohypoparathyroidism produces the same metabolic abnormalities in association with pathognomonic phenotypic changes such as short metacarpal bones, short stature, round face, mental retardation, dental abnormalities, and obesity. Inheritance is X-linked or autosomal-dominant. Most patients have a defect of the PTH receptor-adenylate cyclase system.[16] Calcifications of the basal ganglia are seen in the majority of patients with primary hypoparathyroidism.[17] Calcification, described as early as 1855, is not limited to the basal ganglia. It can be present in the cerebral hemispheres and in the dentate nucleus of the cerebellum.[16] Basal ganglia calcification does not correlate with the presence of movement disorders.[18] Chorea is a described complication of both hypoparathyroidism[19] and pseudohypoparathyroidism.[18]

Paroxysmal dystonias are seen in some metabolic disorders, including hypoparathyroidism and hyperthyroidism. Hypoparathyroidism with basal ganglia calcification has been associated with paroxysmal dystonic choreoathetosis.[20] This has been described infrequently, but seems to represent basal ganglia dysfunction secondary to disordered calcium metabolism.[21] The movement disorder responds to treatment of the underlying disorder with calciferol. The structural alterations in the basal ganglia from the calcification do not seem to be responsible for the dystonic syndrome, as the calcifications do not resolve with treatment of the hypoparathyroidism.

Parkinsonism can occur in the setting of hypoparathyroidism[22] and pseudohypoparathyroidism (4–12 percent of patients) with or without basal ganglia calcifications.[23] It has been reported to occur at ages ranging from 20 to 73 years. The pathogenesis of parkinsonism in these patients initially was presumed to result in some way from calcification in the basal ganglia, although cases without basal ganglia calcification have been reported. Evans and Donley hypothesize that parkinsonism may be related to a defect of G protein,[23] intermediaries in neurotransmission as well as hormonal neuromodulation. An alteration in G protein function could impair neurotransmission in the striatum and produce parkinsonism. Untreated hypoparathyroidism often results in basal ganglia calcification, but it is rare that it is associated with parkinsonism. When the two occur together it is usually in the setting of symptomatic hypocalcemia. In this setting, the parkinsonism is slowly progressive, as in idiopathic Parkinson's disease (PD), and is responsive to L-dopa therapy. Cases have been described without symptomatic hypocalcemia in which the parkinsonism was responsive to vitamin D, calcium, and magnesium replacement.[22]

Metabolic/Nutritional Disorders

TETRAHYDROBIOPTERIN (BH$_4$) DEFICIENCY

Tetrahydrobiopterin (BH$_4$) is a cofactor necessary for the enzymatic synthesis of biogenic amines. Deficiency states lead to defective production of serotonin and catecholamines in addition to hyperphenylalaninemia. Symptoms occur in infancy and include developmental delay, seizures, hypotonia, and dystonia. Three patients have been reported with tremor and orofacial dyskinesias as presenting symptoms. In the case described by Factor et al. an episodic high-amplitude coarse flapping tremor initially appeared at 3 months of age and recurred twice before 6 months.[24] Each episode lasted several hours and improved with sedation. The tremor was present both at rest and with action. The child was also found to be hypotonic. Treatment with L-dopa led to cessation of the movements. Improvement was seen within 24 hours, and further development was normal when followed up at 18 months. The significant improvement with L-dopa implies that the pathogenesis of movement disorders associated with BH_4 deficiency relates to insufficient dopamine synthesis.

MALABSORPTION SYNDROMES

Any disease that causes fat malabsorption or steatorrhea has the potential to cause tocopherol (vitamin E) deficiency. Deficiency of tocopherol must be present for years before neurologic sequelae are evident. The associated syndrome of spinocerebellar ataxia and peripheral neuropathy may resemble B_{12} deficiency. Patients are dysarthric with oculomotor abnormalities, ataxia, and position and vibratory sense loss. Pathologically there is a loss of myelinated nerve fibers in the posterior columns and central nervous system (CNS). Ataxia has been reported in patients with cystic fibrosis, chronic cholestasis, after small bowel resection, blind loop syndromes, and intestinal lymphangiectasia in addition to other malabsorption syndromes.[25]

HEPATIC FAILURE

Hepatic failure is a well-known cause of tremor, asterixis, and other involuntary movements. Asterixis is seen in the setting of an underlying encephalopathy and can be associated with metabolic derangements secondary to failure of various organ systems. It is encountered in hepatic encephalopathy, uremia, hypercarbia, alcohol withdrawal, cardiac failure, sepsis, and sometimes as a result of the treatment used for these disorders, such as hemodialysis.[26] The mechanism of pathogenesis is unknown. Asterixis can be caused by a variety of focal lesions in the thalamus (especially the ventrolateral portion), midbrain, parietal cortex, and medial frontal cortex,[26] but in cases of encephalopathy no structural lesion is evident on imaging studies. In most cases, EEG reveals diffuse rather than focal brain disturbance.[27] MRI scans can show increased signal on T_1-weighted images of the caudate. Generalized myoclonus, ataxia, and chorea can be seen in the setting of hepatic or renal failure.[27]

KWASHIORKOR

Kwashiorkor is a nutritional deficiency of protein and calories, which can produce movement disorders. Kwashiorkor can produce a combination of myoclonus, rigidity, and bradykinesia.[28] Tremors are also apparent in children when they are treated for malnutrition.[28,29]

ALCOHOLISM

A tremor can be prominent among alcoholics when they are not actively drinking or are withdrawing from alcohol. The alcoholic tremor is postural, usually mild, and it causes little if any functional limitation. It is often of a higher frequency than essential tremor, the majority of patients having a tremor frequency of less than 7 Hz,[30] although patterns similar to those seen with essential tremor are described. Postural tremor with a frequency of 6–11-Hz can be seen. The tremor of chronic alcoholism has two components. There is a 4–7-Hz peak and a 9.4–9.6-Hz peak. Increasing the speed of movement of the arm decreases the low-frequency peak without changing the high-frequency peak. Increasing effort increases the amplitude of the low-frequency peak.[31] The tremor of chronic alcoholism is usually asymmetric and can persist for years during complete abstinence. Treatment with beta-blockers is usually effective.

A second type of tremor that is seen in alcoholics is a 3-Hz tremor of the legs. The tremor is slow and rhythmic, involves flexion and extension of the muscles of the hip girdle, and can affect the gait. It does not disappear with cessation of alcohol consumption.[32]

Transient parkinsonism has been described in intoxicated patients or within days of the last drink.[33,34] Symptoms include bradykinesia, shuffling gait, stooped posture, cogwheel rigidity, and resting tremor. The condition is self-limited and usually resolves within a few weeks.[32] Alcohol causes decreased dopamine release, and this may explain the parkinsonism.[35]

Alcoholic cerebellar degeneration is a well-known complication of alcohol abuse. It is postulated to be nutritional in origin. PET scans of ataxic patients reveal hypometabolism in the superior vermis.[36] MRI reveals atrophy of the cerebellar vermis, and, when severe, the cerebellar hemispheres. Pathologically, there is degeneration of the anterior superior aspect of the cerebellar vermis, and, when severe, atrophy of the cerebellar hemispheres. There is a striking loss of Purkinje cells as well as other neural cells.

KERNICTERUS

Prolonged untreated hyperbilirubinemia in the perinatal period damages nuclei of the basal ganglia, especially the globus pallidus and subthalamic nucleus. The cerebellum and the auditory and vestibular pathways are also involved. Children may show signs of damage early with high-tone hearing loss, dysarthria, and athetosis. Usually symptomatic children will have delayed motor development and show signs of dystonia, choreoathetosis, tremor, and rigidity by the time they are 10 years old.[37] Other children may be asymptomatic, and dystonia can occur up to 20 years after the initial insult.[38] In children who die early in the course of the disease, pathologic findings reveal yellow staining of the subthalamic nucleus, Ammon's horn, globus pallidus, dentate nucleus, and olives. In children who live longer these areas reveal cell loss, demyelination, and gliosis.[37]

TABLE 54-1 Metabolic Disorders of Childhood that Cause Dystonia

Hexosaminidase A and B deficiency
GM1 and GM2 gangliosidosis
Phenylketonuria
Triose phosphate isomerase deficiency
Tetrahydrobiopterin deficiency
Metachromatic leukodystrophy
Glutaric acidemia
Methylmalonic acidemia
Wilson's disease
Homocystinuria
Pyruvate decarboxylase deficiency
D-Glyceric acidemia
Lesch-Nyhan syndrome
Ceroid lipofuscinosis
Hartnup's disease

HOMOCYSTINURIA

Many metabolic disorders of childhood have dystonia as a prominent symptom. These will not all be discussed here but are listed in Table 54-1.

Homocystinuria is not commonly associated with dystonia, but the combination has been described. A deficiency of cystathione synthetase leads to a build-up of homocysteine and methionine. Patients generally are mentally retarded, have lens dislocations, seizures, bony abnormalities, and are predisposed to strokes. In a report of 2 sisters, symptoms began at ages 3 and 4, with dysarthria in one and foot inversion in the other.[39] Dystonia progressed over the next few years until it was generalized and both girls severely disabled. MRI studies revealed bilateral low-intensity lesions in the basal ganglia on T_2 imaging. Other patients with dystonia had later onset of dystonic symptoms, starting in the teenage years.[38] Other patients described had typical features of homocystinuria, which the 2 sisters did not. As homocystinuria is associated with thromboembolic events, it is possible that the dystonia is secondary to basal ganglia infarcts.[38] Others postulate that a neurochemical derangement (i.e., a defect in sulfur amino acid metabolism) is responsible.[39]

Hematologic Disorders

POLYCYTHEMIA

Polycythemia vera usually has its onset in middle age. There is an increase in all myeloid elements, although the increase in hemoglobin concentration is the primary hematologic manifestation of this disease. Neurologic symptoms are primarily related to increased blood volume and viscosity. These include headache, dizziness, visual changes, and syncope.[40] Chorea occurs in less than 1 percent of patients with polycythemia vera, and is more common in females than males.[6]

It is usually bilaterally symmetrical and can be short-lived, lasting only weeks, or persistent. Two-thirds of patients who have chorea in the setting of polycythemia do not know that they have polycythemia when the chorea is initially evaluated, although the associated symptoms of a ruddy complexion and splenomegaly are often seen.

The pathophysiology of polycythemic chorea is unclear. Some patients have a history of rheumatic fever in childhood, which may in some way predispose them to the development of chorea later on. Hyperviscosity due to the polycythemia can lead to small infarctions or hemorrhage in the basal ganglia, especially the caudate and putamen. Neuropathologic specimens support this, although demyelination in the interior globus pallidus has also been reported.[3] Treatment of the polycythemia is not always correlated with amelioration of the chorea. A presynaptic catechol-depleting drug such as reserpine or tetrabenazine is the treatment of choice, although dopamine receptor-blocking agents (neuroleptics) may be required in resistant cases.

MASTOCYTOSIS

Mastocytosis is a hematologic disorder in which mast cells proliferate and deposit themselves in various tissues in the body. Most often their distribution is limited to cutaneous structures. CNS dysfunction has been reported with systemic mastocytosis, but usually takes the form of headache, seizures, and encephalopathy. One case of chorea has been described in association with this disorder in a 13-year-old girl.[41] The chorea resolved spontaneously within 5 days and did not recur. According to one theory of pathogenesis, mast cells release various substances (histamine, prostaglandins, and other peptide mediators), which induce alterations in the basal ganglia neurotransmission. This may be responsible for the chorea.

Infection

SYDENHAM'S CHOREA (SC)

SC, a sequela of infection with group A streptococcus, is the most celebrated example of a movement disorder resulting from an infection. Chorea occurs 1–6 months after the initial febrile illness, which most often presents with pharyngitis. The onset is usually insidious, progressing over weeks to months. Women are more often affected than men. The movements are usually bilateral, but can be unilateral, and the face is usually involved. Dysarthria and hypotonia are frequently seen. Behavioral changes include psychosis, irritability, confusion, and obsessive-compulsive disorder (OCD).[42] These symptoms usually begin several days to weeks before the onset of the chorea. The behavioral as well as the motoric symptoms can wax and wane during the course of the syndrome.[42] Antineuronal antibodies are present in the majority of children affected. The initial bout of chorea is self-limiting, but recurrences are well documented, independent of the natural history of rheumatic fever, which is, for the most part, a monophasic illness. Recurrences usually occur within 2 years of the initial chorea.[43] SC is known to recur during pregnancy in women who have had rheumatic fever as a child,[43] and in patients who later take medications such as oral contraceptives and phenytoin.[43]

Few PET studies have been done on patients with SC. Weindl et al., using 2 patients, found increased striatal regional cerebral glucose consumption in both patients.[44] This study was done without age-matched controls.

Circulating antibodies to brain and cardiolipin have been described in association with SC. Streptococcal proteins can induce antibodies that will crossreact with human brain.[45] Others have reported finding IgG antibodies that crossreact with nuclear protein of caudate and subthalamus.[46] This may begin to explain the pathophysiology of SC. Figueroa found that 80 percent of patients with acute rheumatic fever had anticardiolipin antibodies during an acute attack.[47] There was no difference in the percentage of patients with antibodies when comparing those with SC (76 percent) and those without chorea (83 percent). All patients with cardiac valvular abnormalities had antibodies.

The neuropathology in patients with SC is not specific. There are reports of a broad spectrum of abnormalities, including hemorrhage, inflammation, and vasculopathy.[6]

SC is self-limited in most cases. Therefore, treatment with dopamine blockers, which may have permanent tardive sequelae, should be avoided unless the chorea is incapacitating. Presynaptic dopamine-depleting agents (reserpine and tetrabenazine) can be used. There is no treatment that has been proven to shorten the course of the chorea.

Poststreptococcal autoimmune movement disorders have also been described. The most controversial of these is PANDAS (pediatric autoimmune neuropsychiatric disorders associated with streptococcal infection).[48] Symptoms of PANDAS closely resemble Tourette's syndrome (see Chap. 41). Children develop complex motor and vocal tics associated with behavioral abnormalities, weeks to months after a streptococcal infection. Behavioral abnormalities include OCD, ritualistic behaviors, ADHD (attention deficit hyperactivity disorders), oppositional behavior, nightmares, sleep disturbance. The onset of symptoms is acute, and the symptoms follow a relapsing remitting course. More recently, a case of paroxysmal dystonic choreoathetosis has been described in a poststreptococcal setting.[49] Symptoms in this case were the acute onset of dystonic posturing, choreoathetosis, visual hallucinations, and behavioral disturbance. Episodes lasted from 10 minutes to 4 hours. Symptoms continued with variable severity for 6 months. MRI of the brain was normal. Antibodies to basal ganglia structures were detected.

LYME DISEASE

Lyme disease, which in the last decade has become the great imitator, can produce chorea along with a myriad of other neurologic abnormalities.[50] The disease is transmitted through the bite of the deer tick *Ixodes damani*. The causative organism is a spirochete, *Borrelia burgdorferi*. The initial manifestation is usually an expanding red rash (erythema chronicum migrans). As the rash expands, the center clears, creating the appearance of a target. The rash occurs most commonly 1–3 weeks after the tick bite. At the time of the rash, constitutional symptoms, headache, fever, arthralgias, and myalgias may occur. Secondary Lyme disease causes myocarditis, cranial neuritis, and myositis. Stage 3 or chronic Lyme disease occurs months after the initial onset and may persist for years. Clinical findings associated with this stage are arthritis, myositis, peripheral neuropathies, chronic meningitis, and acrodermatitis chronica atrophicans. Cranial nerve palsies are common, including facial diplegia. Patients with meningitis will have positive CSF antibody to *B. burgdorferi*.[51] Serologic testing for Lyme disease (ELISA and indirect fluorescent antibody staining) should be positive in most cases of disseminated Lyme infection.[52] False positive tests do occur in patients with other infections (syphilis), autoimmune disorders (systemic lupus erythematosus, SLE), and some malignancies.[51] A Western blot analysis should be done to confirm the diagnosis before therapy is initiated. MRI findings in patients with focal CNS findings reveal white matter changes representing leukoencephalitis, which can improve with antibiotic therapy.[53] Movement disorders have been reported in the setting of Lyme disease.[50] Chorea and synkinesis are associated with encephalitis.[53] Cerebellar ataxia also has been described.[53] These symptoms usually improve with treatment of the underlying infection and/or with steroids.

HIV-1

A tremor at rest resembling a parkinsonian tremor is seen in the HIV-1 associated cognitive motor complex. The resting tremor and slowness of movement parallel the slowness in thought processing associated with HIV-1 dementia. Pathologic studies reveal white matter pallor, reactive gliosis, and microglial nodules. The caudate, putamen, and pons are involved early, and cortical structures later.[54] Parkinsonism is seen as part of the HIV-cognitive-motor complex. Patients manifest psychomotor slowing, bradykinesia, bradyphrenia, stooped posture, shuffling gait, and postural instability clinically similar to that seen in PD.[55] It appears from primate models that there is early dopaminergic cell loss in HIV-infected patients.[56] Highly active antiretroviral therapy may improve symptoms.[57,58] Imaging should be performed on patients presenting with parkinsonism as structural lesions need to be excluded. Cerebral toxoplasmosis in combination with HIV infection is another rare cause of parkinsonism. A woman with enhancing lesions in the anterior limb of both internal capsules was found to have decreased facial expression, cogwheel rigidity, monotone speech, and drooling.[59] Toxoplasmosis was found in these lesions. Neither anti-toxoplasmosis therapy nor L-dopa/carbidopa combinations improved her condition. Bradykinesia, rigidity, facial masking and grimacing, and gait instability were described in a young girl with HIV and progressive multifocal leukoencephalopathy (PML).[60] MRI lesions involved the basal ganglia and deep white matter, centrum semiovale, and corona radiata and enhanced slightly with the administration of gadolinium. Brain biopsy in this case revealed demyelination, Alzheimer type 1 astrocytes, and intranuclear eosinophilic inclusions within oligodendroglial cells. The biopsy as well as the CSF and blood were positive for JC virus by PCR (polymerase chain reaction). A patient with granulomas in the basal ganglia was also described.[61]

HIV can cause movement disorders, as can the opportunistic infections associated with it. Toxoplasmosis, the most common opportunistic infection causing neurologic symptoms in HIV-positive patients, has been associated with akathisia, chorea, athetosis, and hemiballism, especially when the lesions are in the basal ganglia.[59] When ring-enhancing lesions are seen on CT or MRI, empiric antitoxoplasmosis therapy is indicated. If treatment causes resolution of the lesions on imaging studies, but the movement disorder persists, treatment with dopamine-depleting or -blocking agents may become necessary. In general, patients without HIV infection who have cerebral toxoplasmosis do not have movement disorders associated with it.[59] There may be an interaction between the two infections, making HIV-positive patients more susceptible to developing a movement disorder when they are coinfected with toxoplasmosis.

Cerebral toxoplasmosis has also been associated with dystonia. Nath et al. described a man with HIV and toxoplasmosis who presented with dystonic posturing of the left arm.[59] An enhancing lesion was seen on CT scan in the right globus pallidus and right thalamus. In this case, the dystonia was not improved by treatment of the toxoplasmosis.

Paroxysmal dyskinesias have been reported in association with HIV infection.[62] Both kinesogenic and nonkinesogenic chorea have been described. Associated myoclonus, tremor, and dysarthria were seen. In some patients dystonic posturing was evident. Gliosis and neuronal loss in the subcortical gray matter was found on autopsy of 1 patient with nonkinesogenic dyskinesia. Chorea itself can be the result of structural lesions such as PML or toxoplasmosis, bacterial encephalitis, or direct HIV infection.[63]

ENCEPHALITIS

Mycoplasma is a microorganism that accounts for a large number of cases of pneumonia each year. Uncommon complications of infection with this organism include myopathy and encephalitis. Beskind and Keim described a boy with encephalitis who presented with acute choreoathetosis, dysarthria, and fever who was found to have serologic evidence of *Mycoplasma pneumoniae* infection.[64] Choreoathetosis and hemiballismus are rarely associated with encephalitis of viral etiology. This may be a direct result of the infection or a postinfectious phenomenon.[65] The movements may

be difficult to control, necessitating the use of dopamine-depleting agents (reserpine).

WHIPPLE'S DISEASE (WD)

WD is an infectious disease of the small intestine, causing malabsorption, lymphadenopathy, arthritis, and neurologic symptoms. Gastrointestinal manifestations usually bring the patient to medical attention. These include diarrhea, steatorrhea, abdominal pain, and weight loss. WD and its symptoms respond to antibiotics if therapy is initiated early in the course of the illness. The pathology in the small intestine reveals PAS (periodic acid-Schiff)-positive macrophages and Gram-positive bacilli. Neurologic complications of WD occur in 10 percent of patients,[66] including encephalopathy, myoclonus, seizures, tremor, and ophthalmoplegia. A dystonic syndrome characterized by involuntary bruxism[67] and abnormalities of extraocular movement has been designated an oculomasticatory myorhythmia (OMM).[36] Myorhythmia is a repetitive, regular 2–4-Hz involuntary movement affecting the face (lips, chin, jaw) and neck. Myorhythmia in WD occurs in conjunction with cognitive deterioration and ophthalmoparesis. Neurologic symptoms occur late in the disease and generally indicate a poor prognosis. OMM can improve with antibiotic therapy. Neurologic sequelae can occur even after successful treatment of the gastrointestinal symptoms with antibiotics. This may be due to poor CNS penetration of some antibiotics. Penicillin, trimethoprim-sulfamethoxazole, and streptomycin should be used. There is a high incidence of CNS relapse, so antibiotic therapy should be continued for a prolonged course of many months.[25] Patients have been reported with neurologic symptoms and no gastrointestinal complaints.[69] In patients with OMM, WD should be suspected with or without gastrointestinal symptoms.

Pathological studies of patients with WD affecting the nervous system have revealed nodules and granulomas throughout the brain. Locations include the cortex, basal ganglia, cerebellum, hypothalamus. Cases of WD with myorhythmia are rare and consistent clinicopathologic correlation has not been done.

Eye movement abnormalities in the form of supranuclear gaze palsies without myorhythmia have been described in patients with WD.[70] One patient described had rigidity and bradykinesia similar to that seen in progressive supranuclear palsy.[71]

HEMOLYTIC-UREMIC SYNDROME (HUS)

HUS is a postviral illness causing acute renal failure in children and adults. Hemolytic anemia, thrombocytopenic purpura, and oliguric renal failure are the major components of the illness, which mimics thrombocytopenic thrombotic purpura. CNS involvement in HUS is uncommon and can cause seizures, encephalopathy, and stroke. Pathologic studies in these patients reveal multiple small infarctions secondary to the ischemic effect of small arteriolar thrombi. Dystonia has been described in association with seizures in HUS.[72]

SARCOIDOSIS

Sarcoidosis is a systemic granulomatous disease without known etiology. Granulomas form in various organ systems, resulting in a varied clinical picture. CNS involvement is rare. Most patients with neurologic symptoms have evidence of sarcoidosis in other organ systems (i.e., hilar adenopathy, hypercalcemia, or anergy). As in polycythemia, neurologic symptoms can be the reason the patient seeks medical attention. Sarcoid most often causes meningitis, primarily at the base of the brain, affecting cranial nerves, hypothalamus, and the pituitary.[73] Facial nerve palsies and optic neuritis are the most common cranial neuropathies. Movement disorders can take the form of chorea and hemiballismus if granulomas infiltrate the basal ganglia.[73] Myelopathy and myopathy can also occur.

Neurosarcoid can produce akinetic-rigid syndromes or parkinsonism. Schlegel et al. reported a case of cerebral sarcoidosis that presented with vertical gaze palsy, bradykinesia, and rest tremors.[74] The patient had had systemic sarcoidosis for 11 years before these symptoms became apparent. The parkinsonism and gaze palsy resolved with the use of corticosteroids and antiparkinson medications. Treatment of neurosarcoidosis usually requires the temporary use of corticosteroids. The response of the movement disorder to this treatment is variable.

One concept of pathogenesis is that basilar meningitis leads to obstructive hydrocephalus, which compresses the tectal region of the brainstem and nuclei in the basal ganglia causing upgaze palsy and parkinsonism, respectively. This is a rare complication of neurosarcoidosis. Other reports of sarcoidosis causing parkinsonism have noted granulomatous infiltration of the basal ganglia.[73]

Autoimmune Disorders

AUTOIMMUNE DISEASE

Autoimmune diseases have also been reported to cause dystonic syndromes. Craniocervical dystonia (Meige's syndrome) was described in a patient with rheumatoid arthritis and Sjögren's syndrome. Other combinations of autoimmune disease and cranial dystonia have been described.[75] Patients with myasthenia gravis have been reported to have coexistent dystonic syndromes.[76] Autoimmune thyroid disease also has an unusually high association with dystonia.[77] In 2 cases of blepharospasm described by Jankovic and Patten, 1 with SLE and 1 with myasthenia, both cases responded to immunosuppressive therapy.[78] The mechanism underlying blepharospasm and other dystonic disorders in the setting of autoimmune disease is unclear.

SJÖGREN'S SYNDROME (SS)

SS is an immune-mediated disorder in which salivary and lacrimal glands are destroyed, resulting in mucosal and conjunctival dryness (the sicca syndrome). Xerostomia, xerophthalmia, and conjunctivitis are the principal manifestations. Other organs can be involved, including kidney, lungs, and blood vessels. SS is often associated with other autoimmune diseases. The most common neurologic manifestations are mononeuritis multiplex, peripheral neuropathy, and myositis. CNS dysfunction has been reported and can be either focal or diffuse. Some patients have anti-Ro (SS-A) antibodies that are directed against a 60-kDa peptide, and may be implicated in the production of a small vessel angiitis.[79] Cerebellar degeneration has been described in association with SS. In one reported case of SS, antineuronal antibodies were found.[80] These antibodies stained cytoplasmic elements in the cerebellum and hippocampus primarily. The antibodies found in this patient were not anti-Yo or anti-Hu antibodies, although they were similarly immunoreactive. The patient described improved after immunosuppression with corticosteroids. Parkinsonism has also been described in association with SS.[81] MRI in this case showed increased signal on T_2-weighted images in the pons and basal ganglia. The parkinsonism did not respond to treatment with L-dopa, but did respond to immunosuppression with corticosteroids.

SYSTEMIC LUPUS ERYTHEMATOSUS (SLE)

SLE is an autoimmune disease that affects multiple organ systems, including both the CNS and the peripheral nervous system. Chorea is by far the most common movement disorder associated with SLE[5] (see Chap. 38). Involuntary movements account for 2 percent of all neurologic symptoms in SLE and frequently precede the diagnosis of lupus. The patients who develop chorea are usually young and female. Chorea may be intermittent or persistent and is usually unilateral, although it can be generalized. The pathology is inconsistent, although widespread microinfarcts are the classic pathologic hallmark of CNS SLE. There is no consistent change in the basal ganglia. PET scans do not reveal any change in striatal glucose metabolism that could be responsible for the chorea. Antiphospholipid antibodies are seen in 45–70 percent of patients with SLE, but they can occur without other findings of lupus in primary antiphospholipid antibody syndrome[82] (see below). The lupus anticoagulant is any phospholipid antibody that prolongs the phospholipid-dependent coagulation steps when there is not a coagulation factor deficiency. The antiphospholipid antibody reacts with the platelet membrane and leads to recurrent thrombotic events. Blepharospasm and torticollis have been described in the setting of SLE.[83] The clinicopathologic correlation is not known, but vasculitis involving the brainstem and diencephalon is one postulated mechanism.[78] As in SC, another postulated mechanism is the crossreactivity of antibodies with neurons.[83]

ANTIPHOSPHOLIPID ANTIBODY SYNDROME

Antiphospholipid antibody syndrome is a condition in which antibodies that bind to the negatively charged phospholipids in the membrane of endothelial cells somehow cause recurrent arterial and venous thrombotic and embolic events. The syndrome is clinically expressed by thrombocytopenia, spontaneous abortion, thromboembolism, and chorea.[82] In SLE, imaging studies of the brain do not reveal infarcts in the basal ganglia in patients with chorea in spite of the frequency of infarction in this patient population as a whole. In some cases, an embolic source is identified, such as a cardiac valvular vegetation, and an infarct can be demonstrated on brain imaging studies. Kirk and Harding reported a patient with antiphospholipid antibody and chorea who had an infarct in the head of the caudate.[84] Recent PET studies in patients with antiphospholipid antibody syndrome using ^{18}F-fluorodeoxyglucose revealed contralateral striatal hypermetabolism.[85] Scans were done when the patient had chorea and later when the chorea had resolved. The hypermetabolism was present regardless of the presence of chorea. Chorea can occur in association with anticardiolipin antibodies with or without the associated thromboembolic events.

GLUTEN ENTEROPATHY

Gluten ataxia is now recognized as a form of episodic ataxia.[86,87] Testing patients with genetically confirmed or familial ataxias also yields 14 percent serum positivity for antigliadin antibodies.[88] Only 1 in 8 patients with gluten sensitivity will present with gastrointestinal symptomatology. A rash, dermatitis herpetiformis, or neurologic symptoms, most commonly ataxia, may be the presenting complaints. The mean age of onset is 48 years. Symptoms include eye movement disturbance, slow saccades or gaze-evoked nystagmus, dysarthria, limb ataxia, and gait disorder. MRI reveals cerebellar atrophy in most patients and white matter hyperintensity in a few patients. Sensorimotor axonal neuropathy was found on EMG (electromyography) evaluation in 45 percent of patients. Duodenal biopsy yields the typical pathology of celiac disease in less than a quarter of patients. Antigliadin antibodies are seen in 12 percent of the population at large. Pathologic specimens show perivascular cuffing with both CD4 and CD8 cells in the white matter of the cerebellum. There was also significant Purkinje cell loss. This does have implications for treatment.[89] Ataxia for the most part is not amenable to therapeutic intervention. Patients with antigliadin antibodies may benefit from a gluten-free diet with resultant improvement in their symptoms. Further study is needed.

Pregnancy

This heading does not imply that pregnancy is a systemic illness; rather, it is a systemic change from a woman's usual state that makes a woman susceptible to particular illnesses. Chorea gravidarum (CG) is a rare example of a movement disorder that occurs during pregnancy. The term does not specify etiology and is clinically indistinguishable from any other kind of chorea. CG occurs most frequently in young women during first pregnancies. Half of the cases will start in the first trimester and one-third in the second trimester.[90] The majority of women with CG have previously had chorea due to SC prior to pregnancy; it spontaneously remits in about a third. In the rest, the chorea will last until the child is born. In about one-fifth of patients, the chorea will recur with subsequent pregnancies. SLE, which can also be worsened by pregnancy, can be responsible for CG in some cases.

Neoplasms

Cerebellar dysfunction is seen in systemic illness, most commonly in the form of pancerebellar degeneration, one of the paraneoplastic syndromes. This syndrome can occur with any malignancy, but is most often associated with small cell lung cancer, ovarian cancer, and Hodgkin's lymphoma. The paraneoplastic cerebellar syndrome frequently precedes the diagnosis of cancer.

The ataxia in this syndrome usually has a subacute onset that may begin with dizziness, nausea, and vomiting, and progress to truncal and gait ataxia to dysarthria, diplopia, dysphagia, and limb ataxia over a few months. Frequently the neurologic deficit stabilizes, but the patient may remain significantly impaired. Treatment of the underlying malignancy is rarely helpful.

Pathologically there is cerebellar atrophy with almost total loss of Purkinje cells in the cerebellum. There is thinning of the molecular layer with gliosis, and mild thinning of the granular layer. The deep cerebellar nuclei show inflammatory infiltrates and gliosis. Other areas of the CNS may be affected, including the corticospinal tracts, dorsal columns, and spinocerebellar tracts, which show varying degrees of degeneration. Patchy demyelination is seen in the brainstem, spinal cord, and dorsal root ganglia.[91]

In some patients, antibodies associated with the underlying malignancy crossreact with Purkinje cells and result in their destruction.[92,93] These antibodies bind to membrane-bound and free ribosomes within the Purkinje cell.[94] A putative protein kinase C substrate protein has been detected in some patients with paraneoplastic cerebellar degeneration.[95] Anti-Yo antibodies are present in the serum and CSF of some patients.[96] The onset of this syndrome is similar to patients without antibodies in that the syndrome is subacute, progressing over a few weeks. These patients typically have ataxia of the trunk and limbs, dysarthric speech, and nystagmus.[96] Common malignancies associated with the anti-Yo antibody are, in order of frequency, ovarian, breast, endometrial, and adenocarcinoma with unknown primary. In the majority of patients, the neurologic symptoms precede the diagnosis of cancer. Neuropathologic findings in these patients reveal critical atrophy of the cerebellum with reduction in the number of Purkinje cells as in antibody-negative cases.

Treatment of the underlying malignancy rarely will improve the ataxia. Plasmapheresis to remove the anti-Yo antibody does not usually improve the ataxia.[96] Corticosteroids and immunosuppression have not been beneficial. It is not clear how the anti-Yo antibody causes cerebellar disease.

Hodgkin's disease is also associated with cerebellar degeneration.[97] In most of these patients, the cerebellar syndrome begins after the diagnosis of lymphoma. The onset of the ataxia is sudden or subacute. Gait instability is the most common complaint, followed by limb ataxia and truncal ataxia. Nystagmus and dysarthria are frequently present in this syndrome, especially downbeat nystagmus. Some of these patients have anti-Purkinje cell antibodies.[97] Anti-Tr antibodies have been detected in some patients.[98] This adds support to an autoimmune mechanism as there are similar antigens in both Purkinje cells and T-lymphocytes.[97] The patients with Hodgkin's disease have had more variable responses to treatment of their malignancies. Some patients will stabilize, some recover, and some recover and then remit.

Opsoclonus-myoclonus syndrome associated with malignancies is more commonly seen in children, but has been described in adults. Opsoclonus, or rapid multidirectional saccades, is associated with ataxia and myoclonus. Associated adult malignancies include lung and breast cancer.[99] Anti-Ri antibodies are associated with breast and gynecologic malignancies. Anti-Hu, anti-Yo, and anti-Ma2 antibodies have also been described. Pathology is variable, with some specimens showing normal findings and others with Purkinje cell loss and degeneration with inflammatory infiltrates in the brainstem and basilar meninges. The prognosis in adults is poor if the tumor is untreated. Patients progress to encephalopathy, coma, and death. The syndrome itself may respond to treatment with steroids or intravenous Ig.

In children, the most frequent associate malignancy is neuroblastoma; 50 percent of children with opsoclonus myoclonus have neuroblastoma. Median age of onset of symptoms is 18 months. The syndrome is seen in conjunction with hypotonia, ataxia, and irritability. Treatment of the underlying malignancy is helpful as are immunosuppressive therapies including ACTH (adrenocortico trophic hormone), steroids, and intravenous Ig. Unfortunately, even though the opsoclonus and myoclonus may resolve, the majority of children are left with psychomotor retardation, behavioral difficulties, and sleep disturbance. Relapses of the opsoclonus-myoclonus syndrome have been reported in 68 percent of patients in one study.[100]

Stiff-man syndrome presents as severe rigidity affecting the axial muscles, as well as spasms triggered by sensory and emotional stimuli. The spasms can be severe and painful. Most commonly the symptoms affect the leg and lower trunk, but neck and arm symptoms have been reported. EMG studies are helpful, demonstrating continuous motor unit activity. Antibodies have been described to cytoplasmic proteins that are associated with GABA (gamma-aminobutyric acid)-glycine synapses.[101] Most common are anti-amphiphysin antibodies, but anti-gephyrin antibodies have been described.[102] The most common associated malignancies are breast, lung, colon, and Hodgkin's lymphoma. The pathology in this disorder involves inhibitory interneurons in the spinal cord, vacuolar degeneration or motor neurons, and inflammatory infiltrates.[103] Treatment includes benzodiazepines, baclofen, valproate, steroids, and treatment of the underlying malignancy.

References

1. Swanson JW KJ, McConahey WM: Neurologic aspects of thyroid dysfunction. *Mayo Clin Proc* 56:504, 1981.
2. Wills AJ, Jenkins IH, Thompson PD, et al: A positron emission tomography study of cerebral activation associated with essential and writing tremor. *Arch Neurol* 52:299, 1995.
3. Baba M, Terada A, Hishida R, et al: Persistent hemichorea associated with thyrotoxicosis. *Intern Med* 31:1144, 1992.
4. Lucantoni C, Grottoli S, Moretti A: Chorea due to hyperthyroidism in old age. A case report. *Acta Neurol (Napoli)* 16:129, 1994.
5. Pozzan GB, Battistella PA, Rigon F, et al: Hyperthyroid-induced chorea in an adolescent girl. *Brain Dev* 14:126, 1992.
6. Weiner WJ: *Movement Disorders: A Comprehensive Survey.* Mt. Kisco: Futura, 1989.
7. Fischbeck KH, Layzer RB: Paroxysmal choreoathetosis associated with thyrotoxicosis. *Ann Neurol* 6:453, 1979.
8. Harayama H, Ohno T, Miyatake T: Quantitative analysis of stance in ataxic myxoedema. *J Neurol Neurosurg Psychiatry* 46:579, 1983.
9. Newman RP, Kinkel WR: Paroxysmal choreoathetosis due to hypoglycemia. *Arch Neurol* 41:341, 1984.
10. Rector WG Jr, Herlong HF, Moses H 3rd: Nonketotic hyperglycemia appearing as choreoathetosis or ballism. *Arch Intern Med* 142:154, 1982.
11. Nabatame H, Nakamura K, Matsuda M, et al: Hemichorea in hyperglycemia associated with increased blood flow in the contralateral striatum and thalamus. *Intern Med* 33:472, 1994.
12. Haan J, Kremer HP, Padberg GW: Paroxysmal choreoathetosis as presenting symptom of diabetes mellitus. *J Neurol Neurosurg Psychiatry* 52:133, 1989.
13. Linazasoro G, Urtasun M, Poza JJ, et al: Generalized chorea induced by nonketotic hyperglycemia. *Mov Disord* 8:119, 1993.
14. Hefter H, Mayer P, Benecke R: Persistent chorea after recurrent hypoglycemia. A case report. *Eur Neurol* 33:244, 1993.
15. Lin JJ, Chang MK: Hemiballism-hemichorea and non-ketotic hyperglycaemia. *J Neurol Neurosurg Psychiatry* 57:748, 1994.
16. O'Doherty DS CJ: Neurologic aspects of endocrine disturbances, in RI J (ed): *Clinical Neurology.* Philadelphia: JB Lippincott, 1990, Vol 4.
17. Sachs C, Sjoberg HE, Ericson K: Basal ganglia calcifications on CT: Relation to hypoparathyroidism. *Neurology* 32:779, 1982.
18. Kaminski HJ, Ruff RL: Neurologic complications of endocrine diseases. *Neurol Clin* 7:489, 1989.

19. Salti I, Faris A, Tannir N, et al: Rapid correction by 1-alpha-hydroxycholecalciferol of hemichorea in surgical hypoparathyroidism. *J Neurol Neurosurg Psychiatry* 45:89, 1982.

20. Barabas G, Tucker SM: Idiopathic hypoparathyroidism and paroxysmal dystonic choreoathetosis. *Ann Neurol* 24:585, 1988.

21. Yamamoto K, Kawazawa S: Basal ganglion calcification in paroxysmal dystonic choreoathetosis. *Ann Neurol* 22:556, 1987.

22. Tambyah PA, Ong BK, Lee KO: Reversible parkinsonism and asymptomatic hypocalcemia with basal ganglia calcification from hypoparathyroidism 26 years after thyroid surgery. *Am J Med* 94:444, 1993.

23. Evans BK, Donley DK: Pseudohypoparathyroidism, parkinsonism syndrome, with no basal ganglia calcification. *J Neurol Neurosurg Psychiatry* 51:709, 1988.

24. Factor SA, Coni RJ, Cowger M, et al: Paroxysmal tremor and orofacial dyskinesia secondary to a biopterin synthesis defect. *Neurology* 41:930, 1991.

25. Albers JW, Nostrant TT, Riggs JE: Neurologic manifestations of gastrointestinal disease. *Neurol Clin* 7:525, 1989.

26. Young RR, Shahani BT: Asterixis: One type of negative myoclonus. *Adv Neurol* 43:137, 1986.

27. Rothstein JD, Herlong HF: Neurologic manifestations of hepatic disease. *Neurol Clin* 7:563, 1989.

28. Swaiman: Disorders of the basal ganglia, in KF S (ed): *Pediatric Neurology: Principles and Practice*. St. Louis: CV Mosby, 1989, p 819.

29. Thame M, Gray R, Forrester T: Parkinsonian-like tremors in the recovery phase of kwashiorkor. *West Indian Med J* 43:102, 1994.

30. Koller WC, Busenbark K, Gray C, et al: Classification of essential tremor. *Clin Neuropharmacol* 15:81, 1992.

31. Aisen ML, Adelstein BD, Romero J, et al: Peripheral mechanical loading and the mechanism of the tremor of chronic alcoholism. *Arch Neurol* 49:740, 1992.

32. Neiman J, Lang AE, Fornazzari L, et al: Movement disorders in alcoholism: A review. *Neurology* 40:741, 1990.

33. Carlen PL, Lee MA, Jacob M, et al: Parkinsonism provoked by alcoholism. *Ann Neurol* 9:84, 1981.

34. Shandling M, Carlen PL, Lang AE: Parkinsonism in alcohol withdrawal: A follow-up study. *Mov Disord* 5:36, 1990.

35. Brust A: *Neurologic Aspects of Substance Abuse*. Stoneham: Butterworth-Heinemann, 1993.

36. Gilman S, Adams K, Koeppe RA, et al: Cerebellar and frontal hypometabolism in alcoholic cerebellar degeneration studied with positron emission tomography. *Ann Neurol* 28:775, 1990.

37. Swaiman KF JR: Developmental abnormalities of the central nervous system, in RI J (ed): *Clinical Neurology*. Philadelphia: JB Lippincott, 1988.

38. Calne DB, Lang AE: Secondary dystonia. *Adv Neurol* 50:9, 1988.

39. Berardelli A, Thompson PD, Zaccagnini M, et al: Two sisters with generalized dystonia associated with homocystinuria. *Mov Disord* 6:163, 1991.

40. Massey EW, Riggs JE: Neurologic manifestations of hematologic disease. *Neurol Clin* 7:549, 1989.

41. Iriarte LM, Mateu J, Cruz G, et al: Chorea: A new manifestation of mastocytosis. *J Neurol Neurosurg Psychiatry* 51:1457, 1988.

42. Swedo SE, Leonard HL, Schapiro MB, et al: Sydenham's chorea: Physical and psychological symptoms of St Vitus dance. *Pediatrics* 91:706, 1993.

43. Riley DE LA: Movement disorders, in Bradley WG DR, Fenichel GM, Marsden CD (eds): *Neurology in Clinical Practice*. Stoneham, England: Butterworth-Heinemann, 1991, Vol 2, p 1584.

44. Weindl A, Kuwert T, Leenders KL, et al: Increased striatal glucose consumption in Sydenham's chorea. *Mov Disord* 8:437, 1993.

45. Bronze MS, Dale JB: Epitopes of streptococcal M proteins that evoke antibodies that cross-react with human brain. *J Immunol* 151:2820, 1993.

46. Husby G, van de Rijn I, Zabriskie JB, et al: Antibodies reacting with cytoplasm of subthalamic and caudate nuclei neurons in chorea and acute rheumatic fever. *J Exp Med* 144:1094, 1976.

47. Figueroa F, Berrios X, Gutierrez M, et al: Anticardiolipin antibodies in acute rheumatic fever. *J Rheumatol* 19:1175, 1992.

48. Swedo SE, Leonard HL, Garvey M, et al: Pediatric autoimmune neuropsychiatric disorders associated with streptococcal infections: Clinical description of the first 50 cases. *Am J Psychiatry* 155:264, 1998.

49. Dale RC, Church AJ, Surtees RA, et al: Post-streptococcal autoimmune neuropsychiatric disease presenting as paroxysmal dystonic choreoathetosis. *Mov Disord* 17:817, 2002.

50. Reik L, Steere AC, Bartenhagen NH, et al: Neurologic abnormalities of Lyme disease. *Medicine (Baltimore)* 58:281, 1979.

51. Pachner AR: Early disseminated Lyme disease: Lyme meningitis. *Am J Med* 98:30S, 1995.

52. Magnarelli LA: Current status of laboratory diagnosis for Lyme disease. *Am J Med* 98:10S, 1995.

53. Garcia-Monco JC, Benach JL: Lyme neuroborreliosis. *Ann Neurol* 37:691, 1995.

54. Kieburtz K, Schiffer RB: Neurologic manifestations of human immunodeficiency virus infections. *Neurol Clin* 7:447, 1989.

55. Mirsattari SM, Power C, Nath A: Parkinsonism with HIV infection. *Mov Disord* 13:684, 1998.

56. Koutsilieri E, Sopper S, Scheller C, et al: Parkinsonism in HIV dementia. *J Neural Transm* 109:767, 2002.

57. Hersh BP, Rajendran PR, Battinelli D: Parkinsonism as the presenting manifestation of HIV infection: Improvement on HAART. *Neurology* 56:278, 2001.

58. Sacktor NC, Skolasky RL, Lyles RH, et al: Improvement in HIV-associated motor slowing after antiretroviral therapy including protease inhibitors. *J Neurovirol* 6:84, 2000.

59. Nath A, Hobson DE, Russell A: Movement disorders with cerebral toxoplasmosis and AIDS. *Mov Disord* 8:107, 1993.

60. Singer C, Berger JR, Bowen BC, et al: Akinetic-rigid syndrome in a 13-year-old girl with HIV-related progressive multifocal leukoencephalopathy. *Mov Disord* 8:113, 1993.

61. Maggi P, de Mari M, Moramarco A, et al: Parkinsonism in a patient with AIDS and cerebral opportunistic granulomatous lesions. *Neurol Sci* 21:173, 2000.

62. Mirsattari SM, Berry ME, Holden JK, et al: Paroxysmal dyskinesias in patients with HIV infection. *Neurology* 52:109, 1999.

63. Piccolo I, Causarano R, Sterzi R, et al: Chorea in patients with AIDS. *Acta Neurol Scand* 100:332, 1999.

64. Beskind DL, Keim SM: Choreoathetotic movement disorder in a boy with *Mycoplasma pneumoniae* encephalitis. *Ann Emerg Med* 23:1375, 1994.

65. Thiele EA SM, Siffert JO: Severe choreoathetosis associated with presumed encephalitis: A series of five cases. *Ann Neurol* 36:541, 1994.

66. Weiner SR, Utsinger P: Whipple disease. *Semin Arthritis Rheum* 15:157, 1986.

67. Tison F, Louvet-Giendaj C, Henry P, et al: Permanent bruxism as a manifestation of the oculo-facial syndrome related to systemic Whipple's disease. *Mov Disord* 7:82, 1992.

68. Hausser-Hauw C, Roullet E, Robert R, et al: Oculo-facio-skeletal myorhythmia as a cerebral complication of systemic Whipple's disease. *Mov Disord* 3:179, 1988.

69. Adams M, Rhyner PA, Day J, et al: Whipple's disease confined to the central nervous system. *Ann Neurol* 21:104, 1987.

70. Lee AG: Whipple disease with supranuclear ophthalmoplegia diagnosed by polymerase chain reaction of cerebrospinal fluid. *J Neuroophthalmol* 22:18, 2002.

71. Averbuch-Heller L, Paulson GW, Daroff RB, et al: Whipple's disease mimicking progressive supranuclear palsy: The diagnostic value of eye movement recording. *J Neurol Neurosurg Psychiatry* 66:532, 1999.

72. Whiting S FK, McCormic AQ, Carter JEJ: Retinal and neurologic involvement in the hemolytic uremic syndrome (HUS). *Neurology* 35:248, 1985.

73. Delaney P: Neurologic manifestations in sarcoidosis: review of the literature, with a report of 23 cases. *Ann Intern Med* 87:336, 1977.

74. Schlegel U, Clarenbach P, Cordt A, et al: Cerebral sarcoidosis presenting as supranuclear gaze palsy with hypokinetic rigid syndrome. *Mov Disord* 4:274, 1989.

75. Jankovic J, Ford J: Blepharospasm and orofacial-cervical dystonia: Clinical and pharmacological findings in 100 patients. *Ann Neurol* 13:402, 1983.

76. Jankovic J: Etiology and differential diagnosis of blepharospasm and oromandibular dystonia. *Adv Neurol* 49:103, 1988.

77. Nutt JG CJ, DeGarmo, Hammerstad JP: Meige syndrome and thyroid dysfunction. *Neurology* 34:222, 1984.

78. Jankovic J, Patten BM: Blepharospasm and autoimmune diseases. *Mov Disord* 2:159, 1987.

79. Alexander EL, Ranzenbach MR, Kumar AJ, et al: Anti-Ro (SS-A) autoantibodies in central nervous system disease associated with Sjögren's syndrome (CNS-SS): Clinical, neuroimaging, and angiographic correlates. *Neurology* 44:899, 1994.

80. Terao Y, Sakai K, Kato S, et al: Antineuronal antibody in Sjögren's syndrome masquerading as paraneoplastic cerebellar degeneration. *Lancet* 343:790, 1994.

81. Nishimura H, Tachibana H, Makiura N, et al: Corticosteroid-responsive parkinsonism associated with primary Sjögren's syndrome. *Clin Neurol Neurosurg* 96:327, 1994.

82. Coull BM, Levine SR, Brey RL: The role of antiphospholipid antibodies in stroke. *Neurol Clin* 10:125, 1992.

83. Rajagopalan N, Humphrey PR, Bucknall RC: Torticollis and blepharospasm in systemic lupus erythematosus. *Mov Disord* 4:345, 1989.

84. Kirk A, Harding SR: Cardioembolic caudate infarction as a cause of hemichorea in lupus anticoagulant syndrome. *Can J Neurol Sci* 20:162, 1993.

85. Furie R, Ishikawa T, Dhawan V, et al: Alternating hemichorea in primary antiphospholipid syndrome: Evidence for contralateral striatal hypermetabolism. *Neurology* 44:2197, 1994.

86. Burk K, Bosch S, Muller CA, et al: Sporadic cerebellar ataxia associated with gluten sensitivity. *Brain* 124:1013, 2001.

87. Luostarinen LK, Collin PO, Peraaho MJ, et al: Coeliac disease in patients with cerebellar ataxia of unknown origin. *Ann Med* 33:445, 2001.

88. Hadjivassiliou M, Grunewald R, Sharrack B, et al: Gluten ataxia in perspective: Epidemiology, genetic susceptibility and clinical characteristics. *Brain* 126:685, 2003.

89. Bushara KO, Goebel SU, Shill H, et al: Gluten sensitivity in sporadic and hereditary cerebellar ataxia. *Ann Neurol* 49:540, 2001.

90. Donaldson J: *Neurology of Pregnancy*, 2nd ed. London: WB Saunders, 1989.

91. Posner JB: Paraneoplastic syndromes. *Neurol Clin* 9:919, 1991.

92. Furneaux HM, Rosenblum MK, Dalmau J, et al: Selective expression of Purkinje-cell antigens in tumor tissue from patients with paraneoplastic cerebellar degeneration. *N Engl J Med* 322:1844, 1990.

93. Hetzel DJ, Stanhope CR, O'Neill BP, et al: Gynecologic cancer in patients with subacute cerebellar degeneration predicted by anti-Purkinje cell antibodies and limited in metastatic volume. *Mayo Clin Proc* 65:1558, 1990.

94. Hida C, Tsukamoto T, Awano H, et al: Ultrastructural localization of anti-Purkinje cell antibody-binding sites in paraneoplastic cerebellar degeneration. *Arch Neurol* 51:555, 1994.

95. Gandy SE, Grebb JA, Rosen N, et al: General assay for phosphoproteins in cerebrospinal fluid: A candidate marker for paraneoplastic cerebellar degeneration. *Ann Neurol* 28:829, 1990.

96. Peterson K, Rosenblum MK, Kotanides H, et al: Paraneoplastic cerebellar degeneration. I. A clinical analysis of 55 anti-Yo antibody-positive patients. *Neurology* 42:1931, 1992.

97. Hammack J, Kotanides H, Rosenblum MK, et al: Paraneoplastic cerebellar degeneration. II. Clinical and immunologic findings in 21 patients with Hodgkin's disease. *Neurology* 42:1938, 1992.

98. Graus F, Gultekin SH, Ferrer I, et al: Localization of the neuronal antigen recognized by anti-Tr antibodies from patients with paraneoplastic cerebellar degeneration and Hodgkin's disease in the rat nervous system. *Acta Neuropathol (Berl)* 96:1, 1998.

99. Wirtz PW, Sillevis Smitt PA, Hoff JI, et al: Anti-Ri antibody positive opsoclonus-myoclonus in a male patient with breast carcinoma. *J Neurol* 249:1710, 2002.

100. Pranzatelli MR, Tate ED, Wheeler A, et al: Screening for autoantibodies in children with opsoclonus-myoclonus-ataxia. *Pediatr Neurol* 27:384, 2002.

101. Bataller LDJ: Paraneoplastic neurologic syndromes. *Neurol Clin North Am* 21:221, 2003.

102. Butler MH, Hayashi A, Ohkoshi N, et al: Autoimmunity to gephyrin in stiff-man syndrome. *Neuron* 26:307, 2000.

103. Saiz A, Minguez A, Graus F, et al: Stiff-man syndrome with vacuolar degeneration of anterior horn motor neurons. *J Neurol* 246:858, 1999.

Appendix _____

PATIENT SUPPORT ORGANIZATIONS

Parkinson's Disease

ARGENTINA
Grupo de Autoayuda Parkinson Argentina
Fundacion Alfredo Thomson,
La Rioja 951,
1221-Buenos Aires, Argentina

Vivencias Self Support Group
Sarah Sidoti (Coordinadora),
Arroyo 980, 4th Floor,
(1007) Buenos Aires,
Tel. (54) 11 4393 9422
Fax (54) 11 4393 9422
E-mail: estem@datamarkets.com.ar

AUSTRALIA
National Australian Parkinson's Association, Inc
PO Box 363
Newtown
NSW 2042

Parkinson's Syndrome Society of NSW, Inc
Level 3, Roon 316
Community Health Services Building
Crn George Street & Marsden Street
Paramatta
NSW 2150 Suite 1, 82 Stud Road
Dandenong
Victoria 3175

Parkinson's Australian Capital Territory
Shout Office, The Pearce Centre
Collett Place, Pearce ACT 2607
PO Box 717, Mawson ACT 2607
Tel. (06) 290 1984
Fax (06) 286 4475

Parkinson's Australia
22 The Crescent,
Annandale, NSW 2038
E-mail: Parkinsonsaus@bigpond.com
Website: http://www.parkinsons.org.au/

Parkinson's Disease Society of the ACT Inc
PO Box 717, Mawson,
Australian Capital Territory 2607
Website:
http://www.parkinsons.org.au/document/
    about_parkinsons_act.html

Parkinson's New South Wales Inc
Concord RG Hospital,
Building 64, Hospital Road,
Concord NSW 2139
Tel. (02) 9767 7881
Fax (02) 9767 7882
E-mail: pdawkins@OZEMAIL.com.au
Website: http://www.parkinsonsnsw.org.au/

Parkinson's Queensland Inc
120 Main Street
Kangaroo Point QLD 4169
PO Box 8075
Woolloongabba QLD 4102
Tel. (07) 3391 3877
Fax (07) 3391 3398
E-mail: pqi@parkinsons-qld.org
Website: http://www.parkinsons-qld.org.au/

Parkinson's Society of the Gold Coast
P.O. Box 6096, Gold Coast Mail Centre,
Bundall, Queensland 4217
E-mail: Parkie@fan.net.au

Parkinson's South Australia Inc
Neurological Resource Centre,
23a King William Road,
Unley, South Australia, 5061
Tel. (61) 8 8357 8909
Fax (61) 8 8357 8876
E-mail: nrc@camtech.net.au

Parkinson's Association of Tasmania Inc.
Locked Bag 4,
Sandy Bay, Tasmania 7006
Tel. (03) 6224 4111
Fax (03) 6224 4222
E-mail: aboutus@mstas.org.au
Website:
http://www.parkinsons.org.au/document/
    about_parkinsons_tas.html

Parkinson's (Victoria) Inc
20 Kingston Road,
Cheltenham, Victoria 3192
Tel. (03) 955 11122
Fax (03) 613 955 11310
E-mail: parksvic@satlink.com.au
Website: http://www.parkinsons-vic.org.au/

**Parkinson's Association of Western
    Australia (Inc.)**
The Niche, Suite B
11 Aberdare Road, Nedlands, Western
    Australia 6009
Tel. (08) 9346 7373

Fax (08) 9346 7374
E-mail: pawa@cnswa.com
Website: http://www.quartec.com.au/parkinsons/

Parkinson's Australia
Bldg. 64 Hospital Road
Concord NSW 2139
Tel. (61) 2 9736 7881
Fax (61) 2 9736 7882

Parkinson's Australian Capital Territory
Shout Office, The Pearce Centre
Collett Place, Pearce ACT 2607
PO Box 717, Mawson ACT 2607
Tel. (06) 290 1984
Fax (06) 286 4475

AUSTRIA
Austrian Parkinson Patients Association
MarzstraBe 49
A-1150 Wien
Tel. (43) 1 9837383
Fax (43) 1 9837383

Parkinson Selbsthilfeverein Oberosterreich
Contact: Reinhard Hinterleitner
Bindergraben 4
Katsdorf 4223 Austria
Tel. (43) 7235 82 84

**Osterreichische Parkinson Gesellschaft
Univ.-Klinik für Neurologie**
Anichstrasse 35
A-6020 Innsbruck
Tel. (43) 512 504 3850
Fax (43) 512 504 3852
E-mail: werner.poewe@uibk.ac.at
E-mail: gerhard.ransmayr@akh.linz.at

Parkinson Selbsthilfe Osterreich
Staudgasse 75/2/1 45, A-1180 Wien
Tel. (43) 1 402 94 27
E-mail: sekretariat@parkinson-sh.at

BELGIUM
Belgische Parkinson Vereniging
J. Stobbaertslaan 43
1030 Brussels
Tel. (32) 2 2455945

BRAZIL
Associacao Brasil Parkinson
Contact: Dr. Wagner Horta
PO Box 3168, Fortaleza
Ceara 60431-970 Brazil

Tel. (55) 852 573 011
Fax (55) 852 617 822

CANADA
British Columbia Parkinson Disease Association
British Columbia Parkinson Disease Association
Suite 600-890 West Pender Street
Vancouver, British Columbia
CANADA V6C-1K4
Tel. (604) 662 3240
Toll free: B.C. only 1 800 668 3330
Fax (604) 687 1327

Parkinson's Society of Ottawa-Carleton
Ottawa Civic Hospital
1052 Carling Avenue
Ottawa
Ontario
K1Y 4E9
Tel. (613) 722 9238
Fax (613) 722 3241
E-mail: psoc@lri.ca

The Parkinson's Society Southern Alberta
600 Sloane Square
5920 - IA Street, SW
Clagary
Alberta T2H OG3
Tel. (416) 258 2595

Parkinson Foundation of Canada-National Office
Contact: Mary Jardine
4211 Yonge Street, Suite 316
Toronto, Ontario M2P 2A9 Canada
Tel. (416) 227 9700 or (800) 565 3000
Fax (416) 227 9600
Website: http://www.parkinson.ca

**Parkinson Foundation of Canada
 Newfoundland**
Provincial Resource Centre
P.O. Box 2568, Station C
St John's NF A1C 6K1

Parkinson's Society of Alberta
Room 3Y18, Edmonton General
11111 Jasper Avenue
Edmonton AB T5K 0L4
Tel. (403) 482 8993
Fax (403) 482 8969
1 888 873 9801
E-mail: psa@compusmart.ab.ca

The Parkinson's Society of Southern Alberta
480-d 36th Avenue S.E
Calgary, Alberta T2G1W4

Victoria Chapter/BC Parkinson's Disease Association
1740 Richmond Avenue
Victoria
BC V8R 4P8
Tel. (604) 370 2211

Victoria Epilepsy and Parkinson's Center Society
813 Darwin Avenue
Victoria, British Columbia
Canada V8X-2X7
Tel. (250) 475 6677
Fax (250) 475 6619
http://www.vepc.bc.ca/

CHILE
Liga Chilena Contra el Mal de Parkinson
Contact: Dr. Pedro Chana
Arturo Prat 1341
Santiago Chile
Tel. (55) 2555 7716
Fax (55) 2555 7716
E-mail: pchana@itn.cl
Website: http://www.andronet.cl/parkinson

COLOMBIA
**Asocicion Colobiana de la Enfermedad
   de Parkinson**
Calle 106 #31 - 45
Santefe de Bogota

CYPRUS
Cyprus Parkinson's Disease Association
Contact: Marios Tannousis
PO BOX 27653,
Nicosia 2431 Cyprus
Tel. (357) 99 678445
Fax (357) 22 371425
E-mail: info@cyprusparkinson.org
Website: www.cyprusparkinson.org

CZECH REPUBLIC
Spolecnost Parkinson
Czech Parkinson's Disease Society
Contact: Irena Rektorova
Volynska 20
Prague 10 100 00 Czech Republic
Tel. (42) 02 7273 9222
Fax (42) 02 7273 9222
E-mail: irena.rektorova@fnusa.cz

DENMARK
Dansk Parkinsonforening
Contact: Vibeke Joergensen
Hornemansgade 36
Koebenhavn, OE DK2100 Denmark
Tel. (45) 3927 1555

Fax (45) 3918 2075
E-mail: dansk@parkinson.dk

ESTONIA
Estonian Parkinson's Society
Sole 15-1
Tallinn EE0006
Tel. (3722) 49 15 03
Fax (3722) 49 68 15

EUROPE
European Parkinson's Disease Association
Contact: Lizzie Graham, EPDA Liason/Project Manager
4 Golding Road
Sevenoaks
Kent TN13 3NJ UK
Tel. (44) 1732 457683
Fax (44) 1732 457683
E-mail: Lizzie@epda.demon.co.uk
Website: http://www.epda.eu.com

FINLAND
Finlands Parkinsonforbund
Contact: Brita Nybom
Suomen Parkinson-litto, PB 905
Turku 20101 Finland
Tel. (358) 2 2740 400
Fax (358) 2 2740 444
E-mail: Brita.Nybom@parkinson.fi
Website: http://www.parkinson.fi

FRANCE
Association de Groupments de Parkinsoniens
Contact: Marcel Besnard
3 Chemin du Grand Fosse
St. Nazaire 44600 France
Tel. (33) 4022 00 84

Association France Parkinson
Contact: Alain Honorat
37 bis rue la Fontaine
Paris 75016 France
Tel. (33) 145 202 220
Fax (33) 140 501 644

Federation des Groupements de Parkinsoniens
2 Rue du Portgal
Malakoff 44000 Nantes
Tel. (33) 2 4048 2330
Fax (33) 2 4072 8877

GERMANY
Deutsche Parkinson Vereinigung Bundesverband e.V.
Contact: Friedrich Mehrhoff
Moselstrasse 31
Neuss 41464 Germany

Tel. (49) 213 141 016/7
Fax (49) 213 145 445

HONG KONG
The Parkinson's Disease Society of Hong Kong
703 East Town Building
41 Lockhart Road
Wanchai

ICELAND
Parkinsonsamtokin a Islandi
The Parkinson Association of Iceland
Contact: Þorvaldur Þorvaldsson, Chairman
Hatun 10b, 9th floor
Reykjavik IS-105 Iceland
Tel. (354) 5524440
E-mail: parkinson@parkinson.is
Website: http://www.parkinson.is

INDIA
Parkinson's Disease Society of Karnataka
Contact: Mr. Arun Kumar
No. 633, 3rd Cross, HMT Layout, RT Nagar
Bangalore 50032 India
Tel. (91) 80 3439038

Parkinson's Foundation of Bombay
Contact: Dr. Mohit Bhatt
Jaslok Hospital & Research Ctr. 12th Floor,
    Pedder Road (Bulbhai)
Bombay (Mumbai), Maharashtra 400 026 India
Tel. (91) 22 493 3333 (x340)
Fax (91) 22 494 8008

Parkinsons Disease Foundation and Research Association
Contact: Mr. C. R. DAS
214-A, Talwandi
Kota, Rajasthan India
Tel. (92) 744 421 966
Fax (92) 744 427 759
E-mail: iaaskot@jpl.dot.net.in

IRELAND
Parkinson's Association of Ireland
Carmichael House, North Brunswick St.
Dublin 7 Ireland
Tel. (353) 187 222 34
Fax (353) 187 354 34

ISRAEL
Israel Parkinson Group
P.O. Box 635
27100 Kiryat Bialik
Israel

ITALY
Associazione Italiana Parkinsoniani
Contact: Marzio Piccinini
Via Zuretti 35
Milano 20125 Italy
Tel. (39) 266 671 31111
Fax (39) 267 05283
E-mail: aip@planet.it
Website: http://www.acme.it/aip

**Centro per la Malattia di Parkinson e i
    Disturbi del Movimento**
Istituti Clinici di Perfezionamento
sede di Via Bignami, 1
20126 MILANO
Tel. (02) 5799 3353

Parkinson Italia
Italian Parkinson's Association
Contact: Lucilla Bossi
Piazza IV Novembre, 6
Milano 20124 Italy
Tel. (39) 02 669 79 85
Fax (39) 02 67 07 00 73
E-mail: lu.bossi@libero.it
Website: http://www.parkinson-italia.it

Azione Parkinson
Via Sesto Celere 6
00152 Roma
Tel. (39) 6 58330678/5819183
Fax (39) 6 58330678

JAMAICA
Parkinson's Society of Jamaica
Contact: David Mostyn
7 Glendon Circle, Hope Pastures
Kingston 6 Jamaica
Tel. (809) 972 2236

JAPAN
Japan Parkinson Disease Association
Contact: Hiro Sekine
1-9-13-812, Akasaka, Minato-ku
Tokyo Japan
Tel. (3) 3560 3355
Fax (3) 3560 3356
E-mail: jpda@mud.biglobe.ne.jp

LUXEMBURG
**Association Luxembourgeoise de la Maladie
    de Parkinson**
Contact: Junker Jean
169 Avenue de la Liberation
Schifflange 3850 Luxembourg
Tel. (352) 546 221

LIBYA
Libyan Parkinson's Association
Nijila City
Building No. 115, FLat No. 5
P.O. Box 81891
Tripoli - Libya
Tel. (00218) 21 4862093

MALAYSIA
Asia Pacific Parkinson's Disease Association
RMS Consultancy Sdn. Bhd.
F45, first floor, Plaza Ampang
Jalan Tun Razak
50400 Kuala Lumpur - Malaysia.
Tel. (603) 2454648
Fax (603) 2454649

MEXICO
Mexican Parkinson Disease Association
AMPAC, Apdo. Postal 27003
Col. Roma Sur D.F. 06761 Mexico
Website: http://www.ampacparkinson.org.mx

NEW ZEALAND
Parkinson's Society of New Zealand, Inc.
Contact: Bruce J. Cutfield
PO Box 10 392
Wellington New Zealand
Tel. (64) 4 472 2796
Fax (64) 4 472 2162
E-mail: parkinsonsnz@xtra.co.nz

NORWAY
Norges Parkinsonforbund
Norwegian Parkinson's Disease Association
Contact: Knut Johan Onarheim
Schweigaardsgt. 34, bygg F, oppg. 2
Oslo 0191 Norway
Tel. (47) 22 175 861
Fax (47) 22 175 862
Website: http://www.parkinson.no

PERU
Asociacion Peruana Para La Enfermedad De Parkinson
Contact: Dr. Carlos Cosentino
Rousseau 488
Lima 41 Peru
Tel. (511) 4361113
E-mail: cosenti@terra.com.pe

PUERTO RICO
Asociacion Puertorriquena de Parkinson, Inc.
Contact: Iris Sanchez
PO Box 66
Carolina 00986-0066 Puerto Rico
Tel. (246) 5000

SINGAPORE
Parkinson's Disease Society of Singapore
Counseling and Care Centre
536 Upper Cross St.
#05-241
Hong Lim Complex
Singapore 050536
Tel. (65) 536 6366

SLOVENIA
Parkinson's Disease Association of Slovenia
Contact: c/o Dr. Zvezdan Pirtosek
Institute of Clinical Neurophysiology,
   University Medical Centre
Ljubljana 1525 Slovenia
Tel. (38) 661 316 152
Fax (38) 661 302 771

SPAIN
Federación Española de Parkinson
Parkinson Federation of Spain
Contact: Ms. Yolanda Rueda
c/o Padilla, 235 1°1ª
Barcelona 08013 Spain
Tel. (34) 93 232 91 94
Fax (34) 93 232 91 94
E-mail: fedesparkinson@wanadoo.es

SWEDEN
Swedish Parkinson's Disease Association
Contact: Susanna Lindvall
Nybrokajen 7, 3 tr
Stockholm 111 48 Sweden
Tel. (46) 8 611 93 31
Fax (46) 8 583 515 44
E-mail: susanna.lindvall@swipnet.se

SWITZERLAND
Schweizerische Parkinsonvereinigung
Swiss Parkinson Association
Contact: Lydia Schiratzki
gewerbestrasse 12a, postfach 123
Zurich, CH-8132 Egg Switzerland
Tel. (41) 1984 01 69
Fax (41) 1984 03 93
E-mail: info@parkinson.ch
Website: http://www.parkinson.ch

THAILAND
Thai Parkinson's Disease Society
Pramongkutklao Army Hospital,
   315 Rajvithee Rd.
Phyathai, Bangkok 10400 Thailand
Tel. (662) 245 5526
Fax (662) 245 5526

THE NETHERLANDS
Parkinson Patienten Vereniging
Contact: Aaron Heijman
Postbus 46
Bunnik 3980 CA The Netherlands
Tel. (31) 340 561 369
Fax (31) 340 571 306

TURKEY
Turkish Parkinson's Disease Society
Contact: Prof. Dr. Sibel Ozekmekci
Istanbul Univ., Cerrahpasa Med. School,
    Dept. of Neurology
Istanbul 34303 Turkey
Tel. (90) 212 588 3770
Fax (90) 212 588 3770
E-mail: sibeloz@superonline.com

Parkinson's Disease Society of Turkey
c/o Bilim Sok Doost Apt No. 8 D. 8
Erenköy
81070 Istanbul
Tel. (90) 212 588 3770
Fax (90) 212 588 3770

UNITED KINGDOM
EKBOM Support Group
Contact: Eileen Gill
18 Rodbridge Drive
Thorpe Bay, Essex SS1 3DF UK
Tel. (44) 01702 582 002
E-mail: gill@ekbom-88.demon.co.uk
Website: http://welcome.to/ekbom

Parkinson's Disease Society of the UK
Contact: Robert Meadowcroft, Director, Policy,
    Research and Information
215 Vauxhall Bridge Road
London SW1V 1EJ UK
Tel. (44) 207 931 8080
Fax (44) 207 233 9226
E-mail: rmeadowcroft@parkinsons.org.uk

Parkinson's Disease Society of UK
22 Upper Woburn Place
LONDON WG1H 0RA
Tel. (44) 171 383 3513

UNITED STATES
**American Parkinson's Disease Association
    (APDA)**
NATIONAL OFFICE
1250 Hylan Boulevard, Suite 4B
Staten Island, NY 10305
Tel. (800) 223 2732 or (718) 981 8001
Fax (718) 981 4399

WEST COAST REGIONAL OFFICE
1500 Ventura Blvd. #384
Sherman Oaks, CA 91403
Tel. (800) 908 2732
Tel. (818) 916 7108
Fax (818) 906 4331

WASHINGTON D.C. OFFICE
807 South Alfred Street #2
Alexandria, VA 22314
Tel. (800) 684 2732
Tel. (703) 684 1108
Fax (703) 684 1109
E-mail: APDA@ADMIN.CON2.COM

**The Bachmann-Strauss Dystonia & Parkinson
    Foundation, Inc.**
One Gustave L. Levy Place, Box 1490
New York, NY 10029 USA
Tel. (212) 241 5614
Fax (212) 987 0662
E-mail: Bachmann.Strauss@mssm.edu
Website: http://www.dystonia-parkinsons.org

Central Ohio Parkinson Society
3166 Redding Road,
Columbus OH 43221
Tel. (614) 481 8829

Michael J. Fox Foundation for Parkinson's Research
381 Park Avenue South, Suite 820
New York, NY 10016 USA
Tel. (212) 213 3525
Fax (212) 213 3523
Website: http://www.michaeljfox.org

Michigan Parkinson Foundation
3990 John Road
Detroit MI48201
Tel. (313) 745 2000

National Parkinson's Foundation, Inc.
Bob Hope Parkinson Research Center
1501 N.W. 9th Avenue
Bob Hope Road
Miami, Florida 33136-1494
Tel. (305) 547 6666
Toll Free National: 1-800-327-4545
Fax (305) 243 4403
E-mail: mailbox@npf.med.miami.edu
Internet E-mail: mailbox@parkinson.org
World Wide Web: http://www.parkinson.org

Parkinson's Disease Foundation
Contact: Robin Elliott
710 West 168th Street 3rd floor

New York, NY 10032 USA
Tel. (800) 457 6676 or (212) 923 4700
Fax (212) 923 4778
E-mail: pdfcpmc@aol.co
Website: http://www.pdf.org

Parkinson's Action Network
822 College Avenue, Ste. C
Santa Rosa, CA 95404
Tel. (707) 544 1994
Tel. (800) 820 4716
Fax (707) 544 2363
E-mail: ParkActNet@AOL.com

Parkinson's Action Network (PAN)
Contact: Steven McClintock
300 N. Lee Street
Alexandria, VA 22314 USA
Tel. (703) 518 8877 or (800) 850 4726
Fax (703) 518 0673
E-mail: info@parkinsonsaction.org
Website: http://www.parkinsonsaction.org

The Parkinson's Institute (California)
1170 Morse Ave.
Sunnyvale CA 94089
Tel. (408) 734 2800

The United Parkinson Foundation
The United Parkinson's Foundation
   and the International Tremor Foundation
833 West Washington Boulevard
Chicago, IL 60607
Tel. (312) 733 1893

Young Parkinson's Support Network of California.
APDA Young Parkinson's I & R Center
1041 Foxenwood Drive
Santa Maria, CA 93455
Tel. (800) 223 9776, (805) 934 2216

World Parkinson's Disease Association
www.wpda.org

Huntington's Disease

AUSTRALIA
Australian Huntington's Disease Association (NSW) Inc.
21 Chatham Road, West Ryde NSW 2114, Australia
PO Box 178, West Ryde NSW 1685, Australia
E-mail: hdassoc@ahdansw.bu.aust.com

Huntington's Disease Association WA (Inc.)
439 Vincent Street West
Leederville WA 6007, Australia

Tel. (61 8) 9388 3200
Fax (61 8) 9388 3344
E-mail: huntingt@cygnus.uwa.edu.au
Australian Huntington's disease Associtation (Vic.) Inc.
   home page

AUSTRIA
Oesterreichische Huntington Hilfe
Hasnerstrasse 88/23, Vienna 1160,Austria
Tel. (43) 1 4929 153

BELGIUM
Huntington Liga
Krijkelberg 1 B 3360 Leuven, Belgium
Tel. (32) 16 452 759
Fax (32) 16 463 079

Ligue Huntington Francophone Belge
Rue de Brouckere 19
6150 Anderlues, Belgium
Tel. (32) 87 675 408

BRAZIL
Dr. Francisco Salzano
Departamento de Genetica
Instituto de Biociencias, UFRGS
Caixa psta; 15053
91501-970 Porto Aelegere RS, Brazil
Tel. (55) 51 316 6747
Fax (55) 51 319 3011
E-mail: salzano@ifl.if.ufrgs.br

Association Brasil Huntington
Rua Das Camelias, 38
Jardim Imperial
Atibai - SP
Brazil
ZIP CODE 12940-000
Tel. (55) 11 8963892
E-mail: hdbr@latinmail.com

CANADA
Huntington Society of Canada
(HSC)
Huntington Society of Canada
151 Federick Street
Suite 400
Kitchener, ON, Canada
N2H 2M2
Tel. (519) 749 7063
Fax (519) 749 8965
E-mail: info@hsc-ca.org

Huntington Society of Quebec
505 de Miasonneuve West, Suite 300
Montreal, Quebec, Canada H3A 3C2

Tel. (514) 282 4272
Fax (514) 282 4242

CZECH REPUBLIC
Spolecnost Pro Pomoc Pri Hintingtonove Chorobe
Dolní Brezany 153
25241 Dolní Brezany, Czech Republic
Tel. (42) 2 2490 4261/2490 4269
Fax (42) 2 294 905

DENMARK
**Landsforeningen mod Huntingtons
   Chorea**
Havnøvej 38
DK-9560 Hadsund
Denmark
Tel. (45) 9857 5323
Fax (45) 9857 3496

ECUADOR
Dr. Nelson Penafiel-Revelo
Toledo 1233 Y Luis Cordero
Quito, Ecuador
Tel. (593) 2 526 230
Fax (593) 2 503 575

Mrs. Monica Naranjo
Bristol Laboratories
Diguja 198 Y Voz Andes
Quito, Ecuador

FINLAND
Huntington Association of Finland
Meriraumantie 21 AS6
SF 26200 Rauma
Finland
Tel. (358) 2 821 1632
Fax (358) 2 822 404

FRANCE
Association Huntington France
42,44 Rue du Chateau Des Rentiers
75013 Paris, France
Tel. (33) 1 6986 9047
Fax (33) 1 6986 6050

GERMANY
Deutsche Huntington-Hilfe e.V.
Geschaefts- und Beratungsstelle
Boersenstr. 10
D-47051 Duisburg
Germany
Tel. *49 (0)203/22915
Fax *49 (0)203/22925
E-mail: dhh@dhh-ev.de
Website: www.dhh-ev.de
Website: www.selbsthilfenetz.de

HUNGARY
Dr. Bela Csala
Budal Nagy A.U. 14
7624 PACS, Hungary
Tel. (36) 72 314 344
Fax (36) 72 326 715

INDIA
Ms. Mano Singh
K 18/7 DLF Qutub Enclave Phase II
35-66-77 Gurgaon Haryana, India
Tel. c/o (91) 646 4544
Fax (91) 644 4221

IRELAND
Huntington's Disease Association of Ireland
Carmichael House, N. Brunswick St.
Dublin 7, Ireland
Tel. (44) 1 872 1303
Fax (44) 1 873 5737
E-mail:hdai@indigo.ie

ISRAEL
Amita Huntington Israel
3 Lubezky Street
Gedera 70700, Israel
Tel. (972) 8 859 8573
Fax (972) 2 670 8387
E-mail: farkash@netvision.net.il

ITALY
Associazione Italiana Corea Di Huntington
Via L. Ariosto 19
20145 Milano, Italy
Tel. (39) 2 4801 5529
Fax (39) 2 239 4448

JAPAN
Japan Huntington Disease Network
c/o Akutsu
5-29-6, Minami-senju, Arakawa-ku,
Tokyo 116-0003, JAPAN
http://homepage1.nifty.com/JHDN/index.html
E-mail: jhdn@mbd.nifty.com

LITHUANIA
Prof. Valius Pauza, MD, Ph.D.
Chair, Neurological Department and Clinic
Kaunas Medical Academy
Vmickevicuaus 9, Kaunas 3000, Lithuania
Tel. (370) 7 792 627/733 849
Fax (370) 7 220 733

MALTA
Prof. Alfred Cuschiari
Dept. of Anatomy

University of Malta
Msida MSD 06, Malta
Tel. (356) 336 451
Fax (356) 336 450/319 527

MEXICO
**Assocacion Mexicana de la Enfermedad de
  Huntington A.C.**
San Carlos #51
San Angel Inn, Mexico D.F.CP 0001060
Tel. (52) 5 550 76 26

THE NETHERLANDS
Vereniging Van Huntington
Post Box 30470
2500 Gl Den Haag, The Netherlands
Tel. (31) 70 314 8888
Fax (31) 70 314 8880
E-mail: iha-huntington@tip.nl

International Huntington Association (IHA)
Gerrit Dommerholt
Development Officer
Callunahof 8
7217 St. Harfsen
The Netherlands
Tel. (31) 573 431 595
Fax (31) 573 431719
E-mail: iha@huntington-assoc.com

NEW ZEALAND
Huntington's Disease Association of New Zealand
Post Box 78
Cust, Nort Canterbury, New Zealand
Tel. (64) 3 3125 612
Fax (64) 4 232 5365

NORTHERN IRELAND
**Huntington's Disease Association of
  Northern Ireland**
Dept. of Medical Genetics
Belfast BT9 7AB, Northern Ireland
Tel. (353) 232 653826

NORWAY
Landsforeningen for Huntington's Sykdom
Post Box 103
N 1415 Oppegard, Norway
Tel. (66) 992 477
Fax (66) 992 477
E-mail: astrid.jenssen@vist.v10.no

OMAN
Dr. Euan Scrimgeour
Dept. of Medicine, College of Medicine

Sultan Qaboos University
Post Box 35
Al-Khod 123, Sultanate of Oman
Tel. (968) 513 333
Fax (968) 513 419

PAKISTAN
**Huntington Disease Care and Cure
  Society of Pakistan**
2 Sawati gate
Peshawar Cantt
Pakistan
Tel. (92) 521 275 471
Fax (92) 521 273 900

PARAGUAY
Prof. Carlo Todisco
Dr. Hassler 5738 C. Ala Paraguayas
Asuncion, Paraguay

POLAND
Prof. Jacek Zaremba BR Insitute Psychiatry/Neurology
1/0 Sobieskiego Str.
02-957 Warsaw, Poland
Tel. (48) 22 642 6611 ext. 248
Fax (48) 22 642 5375

PORTUGAL
Mrs. Ursula-Anna Kleinbrink
Rue Dr. Afonso Cossta 30
P 8500 Alvor-Portimao, Portugal
Tel. (351) 82 459 337
Fax (351) 82 459 337

RUSSIA
Huntington Association of Russia
Institute of Neurology, AC Science
Volokolamskoye Shosse 80
123367 Moscow, Russia
Tel. (7) 95 490 2103/490 2039/490 2506
Fax (7) 95 490 2210

SCOTLAND
Scottish Huntington's Disease Association
Thistle House, 61 Main Road
Ederslie, Jonstone, PA5 9BA, Scotland
Tel. (44) 1505 3222 45
Fax (44) 1505 3829 80
E-mail: ronald.livingstone@virgin.net

SLOVAKIA
**Spolecnost Pre Pomoc Pri Huntingtonovej Chorobe V
  Slovenskej Republike**
Oddelinie Lekarskej Genetiky
97517 Banska Bystrica, Slovakia

Tel. (42) 88 713 380
Fax (42) 88 320 65

SOUTH AFRICA
Huntington's Society of South Africa
Post Box 44501
Claremonte, Cape Town, South Africa
Tel. (27) 21 938 4911
Fax (27) 21 761 4438
E-mail: jschron@iafrica.com

SPAIN
**Associacon de Corea de Huntington
  Española**
Fund Jimenez Diaz. Serv/Neurologia
Avda Reyes Catolicos 2
28040 Madrid 28040, Spain
Tel. (34) 1 544 9008
Fax (34) 1 549 7381

**Associacion Catalna de Malalts de Huntingon
  (ACMAH)**
Av. Pere Verges s/n Despatx 7.1
(08020 Barcelona) Espana
Tel. and Fax (93) 314 56 57
E-mail: acmah.b@suport.org

SWEDEN
Huntington Foreningen I Sverige
C/o NHR Post Box 3284
Kungsgatan 32, 10365 Stockholm, Sweden
Tel. (46) 8 140 320
Fax (46) 8 241 315/677 7010

SWITZERLAND
Schweizerische Huntington Vereinigung
Heidy Moser-Welti, Presdient
Bahnweg 4
CH 8156 Oberhasli, Switzerland
Tel. (41) 1 885 1941
Fax (41) 1 885 1844
E-mail: shv@swissonline.ch

UNITED KINGDOM
UK Huntington's Disease Association
108 Battersea High St.
London SW11 3HP, United Kingdom
Tel. (44) 171 223 7000
Fax (44) 171 223 9489

UNITED STATES
Hereditary Disease Foundation
1303 Pico Boulevard
Santa Monica, California 90405
Tel. (310) 450 9913
Fax (310) 450 9532

New York Office:
Hereditary Disease Foundation
3960 Broadway, 6th Floor
New York, NY 10032
Tel. (212) 928 2121
Fax (212) 928 2172
E-mail: cures@hdfoundation.org
http://www.hdfoundation.org

Huntington's Disease Society of America
158 West 29th Street, 7th Floor
New York, N.Y. 10001-5300
Tel. (800) 345-HDSA
Fax (212) 239 3430

Dystonia

AUSTRALIA
Spasmodic Dysphonia Support Group
Contact: Cynthia Turner
8 Corona Avenue
Roseville, New South Wales 2069 Australia
Tel. (61) 294 112 424
Fax (61) 294 112 424

AUSTRIA
Österreichische Dystonie Gesellschaft
Austrian Dystonia Society
Contact: Christa HAFENSCHER
Vorgartenstraße 140 - 142 / 5 / 12
Vienna, Austria 1020 Austria
Tel. (43) 1 2197161
Fax (43) 1 2197161
E-mail: oesterreichische,dystonie@mcnon.com
Website: www.dystonie.at

BELGIUM
**Belgische Zelphulpgroep Voor Dystonie
  Patiënten**
Belgian Dystonia Association
Contact: Christine Wauters
Blokmakerstraat 6
Haasdonk 9120 Belgium
Tel. (32) 3 7755125
Fax (32) 3 7755125

BRAZIL
**Associacao Brasileira dos Portadores
  de Distonias**
Brazilian Dystonia Society
Contact: Elenita Ferreira de Macedo
Al. Joaquim Eugenio de Lima, 870 apto. 41
Sao Paolo, SP Cep: 01403-000 Brazil
Tel. (55) 11 288 7032
Fax (55) 11 228 7032

CHILE
Fundacion Distonia
Dystonia Foundation of Chile
Contact: Benedicte De Pauw
Av. Irarrazaral 5185, Of. 311
Nunoa, Santiago Chile
Tel. (56) 22268874
Fax (56) 22267346

CROATIA
Hrvatska Grupa Za Istrazivanje Distonije
Croatia Dystonia Association
Contact: Prof. Maja Relja
University of Zagreb, Kispaticeva 12
Zagreb 10000 Croatia
Tel. (385) 1 2388 377
Fax (385) 1 7345 595

DENMARK
Dansk Dystoniforening
Danish Dystonia Association
Contact: Ulla Balser Poulsen
Solhojpark 16
Farum DK - 3520 Denmark
Tel. (45) 4495 5165
Fax (45) 4495 5165
E-mail: ullafarum@teliamail.dk
Website: http://www.dystoni.dk

EUROPE
European Dystonia Federation
Contact: Secretariat
69 East King Street
Helensburgh G84 7RE UK
Tel. 44 (0) 1436 678799
Fax 44 (0) 1436 678799
E-mail: alistair@newton1.co.uk
Website: http://www.dystonia-europe.org

FINLAND
Finnish Dystonia Association
Contact: Liisi Niemi
Ostjakinkatu 5 as 29
Turku 20750 Finland
Tel. (358) 92 792 738
E-mail: liisi.niemi@iki.fi
Website: http://www.dystoniayhdistys.com

FRANCE
**Association de Malades atteints de Dystonie
   (AMADYS)**
Contact: Robert Perbet
Le Lac
Saint-Paulien 43350 France
Tel. (33) 4 71 00 46 15
Fax (33) 4 71 00 45 49

E-mail: contact@amadys.net
Website: http://www.amadys.net

Ligue Francaise contre la Dystonie
Contact: Secrétariat
Chemin le Chatelard; Lot. La Tour 38190
Champ-près-Froges 91210 France
Tel. (33) 4 76 71 31 83
Fax (33) 4 76 71 31 83
E-mail: secretariat@lfcdystonie.org
Website: http://www.lfcdystonie.org

GERMANY
Deutsche Dystonie Gesellschaft e. V.
German Dystonia Association
Contact: Didi Jackson
Bockhorst 45 A
22589 Hamburg Germany
Tel. (49) 40 87 56 02
Fax (49) 40 87 08 28 04
E-mail: Deutsche-Dystonie@t-online.de
Website: http://www.dystonie.de

INDIA
Writers Cramp Research Foundation
Contact: Gursharan Singh
25 A Adarsh Vihar; Raipur Road
Dehradun 248001 India
Tel. (91) 135 788 147
E-mail: writerscramp_foundation@yahoo.co.in

IRELAND
Dystonia Ireland
Contact: Maria Hickey
33, Larkfield Grove-Harold's Cross
Dublin 6W Ireland
Tel. (353) 1 4922514
Fax (353) 1 4922565
E-mail: info@dystonia.ie
Website: http://www.dystonia.ie

ITALY
Assoc. Italiana per la Ricerca Sulla Distonia
Italian Dystonia Association
Contact: Nadia Trinci
Via Arturo Colautti 28
Rome 00152 Italy
Tel. (39) 06 589 8727
Fax (39) 06 580 3940
E-mail: info@distonia.it
Website: http://www.distonia.it

NEW ZEALAND
NZ Spasmodic Dysphonia Patients' Network
Contact: David Barton
15 Pluto Place

North Shore City, Auckland 1310 New Zealand
Tel. (64) 9 482 1567
Fax (64) 9 482 284
E-mail: dsbarton@ihug.co.nz

NORWAY
Norwegian Dystonia Association
Contact: Norwegian Dystonia Association
Kastellveien 10 B
Oslo N -1170 Norway
Tel. (47) 22 28 58 02
Fax (47) 22 28 03 81
E-mail: kontakt@dystoniforeningen.no
Website: http://www.dystoniforeningen.no

SERBIA
Yugoslav Dystonia Association
Contact: Dr. Marina Svetel
Institute of Neurology, Dr. Subotica Nr. 6
Belgrade 11000 Serbia
Tel. (381) 11 689 554
Fax (381) 11 684 577
E-mail: marinas@imi.bg.ac.yu

SLOVENIA
Dystonia Association of Slovenia
Contact: Dr. Zvezdan Pirtosek
Institute of Clinical Neurophysiology,
    University Medical Centre
Ljubljana 1525 Slovenia
Tel. (38) 661 316 152
Fax (38) 661 302 771

SOUTH AFRICA
Dystonia Association South Africa
Contact: Maureen Langford
PO Box 3160
Pinegowrie 2123 South Africa
Tel. (27) 11 787 8792
Fax (27) 11 787 2047
E-mail: dystonia@global.co.za

SPAIN
Asoc. de Lucha contra la Distonia en España
Spainish Dystonia Society
Contact: Begoña Paris
c/o Galileo, 69-1
Madrid 28015 Spain
Tel. (34) 91 5940066
Fax (34) 91 5940066
E-mail: alde@distonia.org
Website: http://www.distonia.org

SWEDEN
Svensk Dystoni Forening
Swedish Dystonia Society

Contact: Anders Silfors
Stjarngossevagen 108
Alvsjo 125 35 Sweden
Tel. (46) 89 99 956
Fax (46) 89 99 956
Website: http://www.dystoni.com

SWITZERLAND
Schweizerische Dystonie Gesellschaft
Swiss Dystonia Association
Contact: Dr. Brigitte Gygli
Tramstrasse 39
Muttenz CH - 4131 Switzerland
Tel. (41) 614 616 993
Fax (41) 614 616 993

THE NETHERLANDS
Nederlanse Verening van Dystoniepatienten
Netherlands Dystonia Association
Contact: Louis Beduwe
Postbus 9345
Breda 4801 LH The Netherlands
Tel. (31) 76 514 0765
Fax (31) 76 521 6495

UNITED KINGDOM
The Dystonia Society
46/47 Britton Street
London EC1M 5UJ UK
Tel. (44) 20 7490 5671
Fax (44) 20 7490 5672
Website: http://www.dystonia.org.uk

UNITED STATES
**The Bachmann-Strauss Dystonia & Parkinson
    Foundation, Inc.**
One Gustave L. Levy Place, Box 1490
New York, NY 10029 USA
Tel. (212) 241 5614
Fax (212) 987 0662
E-mail: Bachmann.Strauss@mssm.edu
Website: http://www.dystonia-parkinsons.org

Dystonia Medical Research Foundation
One East Wacker Drive, Suite
2430, Chicago, IL 60601-1905.
Tel. (312) 755 0198

Care4Dystonia, Inc.
Contact: Beka Serdans, RN
440 East 78 th Street
New York, NY 10021 USA
Tel. (800) C4D-INFO
E-mail: infoc4d@aol.com
Website: http://www.care4dystonia.org

Dystonia Medical Research Foundation
One East Wacker Drive, Suite 2430
Chicago, IL 60601-1905 USA
Tel. (312) 755 0198 in Canada (800) 361-8061
Fax (312) 803 0138
E-mail: dystonia@dystonia-foundation.org
Website: http://www.dystonia-foundation.org

National Spasmodic Dysphonia Association
Contact: Dysphonia Association
One E. Wacker Drive, Suite 2430
Chicago, IL 60601-1905 USA
Tel. (800) 795-NSDA
Fax (312) 803 0138
E-mail: NSDA@dysphonia.org
Website: http://www.dysphonia.org

Blepharospasm

AUSTRALIA
Blepharospasm Support Group
Contact: Marisa Nowak
Royal Victorian Eye & Ear Hospital, 32 Gisborne Street
East Melbourne, Victoria 3002 Australia
Tel. (61) 3 9929 8666
Fax (61) 3 9663 7203
E-mail: mnowak@rveeh.vic.gov.au

UNITED STATES
Benign Essential Blepharospasm Research Foundation, Inc.
Contact: Mary Lou Thompson
PO Box 12468
Beaumont, Texas 77726-2468 USA
Tel. (409) 832 0788
Fax (409) 832 0890
E-mail: bebrf@sbcglobal.net
Website: http://www.blepharospasm.org/

Spasmodic Troticollis

AUSTRALIA
Australian Spasmodic Torticollis Association
Contact: Annette Walker
PO Box 133
Westmead, New South Wales 2145 Australia
Tel. (61) 296 859 020
Fax (61) 296 859 599
E-mail: a.walker@uws.edu.au

GERMANY
Bundesverband Torticollis e. V.
Contact: Helga Weber
Eckernkamp 39
Hamm 59077 Germany
Tel. (49) 2389 53 69 88

Fax (49) 2389 53 62 89
E-mail: BVTorti@aol.com
Website: http://www.schiefhals.de

UNITED STATES
National Spasmodic Torticollis Association
9920 Talbert Avenue #233
Fountain Valley, CA 92708 USA
Tel. (800) HURTFUL
E-mail: nstamail@aol.com
Website: http://www.torticollis.org

Spasmodic Torticollis/Dystonia, Inc.
Contact: Howard Thiel
P.O. Box 28
Mukwonago, WI 53149 USA
Tel. (888) 445 4598
E-mail: info@spasmodictorticollis.org
Website: http://www.spasmodictorticollis.org

Tardive Dyskinesia

Tardive Dyskinesia/Tardive Dystonia National Association
4424 University Way NE
P.O. Box 45732
Seattle, WA 98145-0732
Tel. (206)522 3166

Tourettes Syndrome

ARGENTINA
Tourette Syndrome Association of Argentina
Contact: Stella Ortiz
Segurola 483, V.Sarmiento (1706)
Buenos Aires Argentina

AUSTRALIA
Tourette Syndrome Association of Victoria Inc.
Contact: Debbie Redelman
The Nerve Centre; 54 Railway Road
Blackburn, Victoria 3130 Australia
Tel. (03) 9845 2700
Fax (03) 9845 2777
E-mail: info@tourette.org.au
Website: http://www.tourette.org.au

TSA of Queensland
20 Balfour Street
Newfarm 4007 Australia
Tel. (61) 7 3358 4988

TSA of South Australia
23a King William Street
Unley 5061 Australia

Tel. (61) 8 8357 8909
Fax (61) 8 8357 8876
E-mail: nrc@camtech.net.au

TSA of Victoria, Inc.
Contact: Tim Morrissey
34 Jackson Street
Toorak 3142 Australia
Tel. (61) 3 9828 7218
Fax (61) 3 9826 9054
E-mail: tourettes@mssociety.com.au
Website: http://www.devolution.com.au/tourette

Western Australia TS Organisation
320 Rokeby Road
Sabiaco 6008 Australia
Tel. (61) 9388 3486
Fax (61) 9382 1149

AUSTRIA
Öestereichische Tourette Geselschaft
Contact: Maria Stamenkovic
Wien Universitat Hospital vor Psykiatrie,
    Wahringergutrel 18-20
Wien A 1090 Austria
Tel. (43)140 400 3526
Fax (43) 140 400 3560

BELGIUM
Vlaamse Vereniging Gilles de la Tourette
Contact: Vera Casier Cassimon Jozet
Nauwelaertstraat 7
Wynegem 2210 Belgium
Tel. (32) 33 54 3669
Fax (32) 35 53 6791
E-mail: vera@glo.be

BRAZIL
**Associaco de Pacientes com Sindrome de Tourette
    Tiques e transformos Obsessivo-compulsivo
    (ASTOC)**
R. Bras Cardoso 201
Sao Paulo Brazil
Tel. (55) 11 822 0023
Fax (55) 11 822 0023

CANADA
Tourette Syndrome Foundation of Canada
Contact: Rosie Wartecker
206-194 Jarvis Street
Toronto, Ontario M5B 2B7 Canada
Tel. (416) 861 8398 or (800) 361 3120
Fax (416) 861 2472
E-mail: tsfc.org@sympatico.ca
Website: http://www.tourette.ca

DENMARK
Dansk Tourette Forening
Contact: Kjeld Christensen
Søllerødvej 76
Holte DK 2840 Denmark
Tel. (45) 45 80 07 53
Fax (45) 45 80 32 16
E-mail: tdc@post8.tele.de
Website: http://www.tourette.dk

FINLAND
Suomen Tourette Yhdistys
Finnish Tourette Association
Contact: Mika Marjalaakso
E-mail: mika.marjalaakso@tourette.fi

GERMANY
Tourette-Gesellschaft Deutschland E.V.
Contact: Tourette Gesellschaft Deutschland e.V.
c/o Prof. Dr. A. Rothen Von Siebold Str. 5
Gottingen 37015 Germany
Tel. (49) 551 396727
Fax (49) 551 398120
E-mail: info@tourette.de
Website: http://www.tourette.de

ICELAND
Tourette Samtokin a Islandi
Contact: Eliz. Magrusdottir
Postholf 3128
Reykjavik 123 Iceland
Tel. (354) 588 8581
Fax (354) 551 4580
E-mail: emagn@islandia.is

IRELAND
Tourette Syndrome Association of Ireland
Contact: Una Finucane
29 Granville Road
Dun Laoghair, Dublin Ireland
Tel. (353) 1 623 0500
Fax (353) 1 623 0500

ISRAEL
Yirgoon Syndrome Tourette Israel (ESTI)
Contact: Anat Imber
PO Box 7018
Ramat Gan 52170 Israel
Tel. (03) 9012956

ITALY
Associazione Italiana Sindrome Tourette
Tourette Syndrome Association of Italy
Contact: Mauro Porta, MD
Policlinico San Marco; Corso Europa, 7

Bergamo-Zingonia 24040 Italy
Tel. (39) 035 886298
Fax (39) 035 885789

NEW ZEALAND
TSA of New Zealand
Contact: Carol Bridle
146 Weymouth Road, Manurowa
South Auckland New Zealand

NORWAY
INTERNATIONAL ASSOCIATION
Tourette Syndrome Global Awareness Program
Contact: Christian Melbye
Munkerudasen 33
Oslo N-1165 Norway
Fax (47) 22 28 67 52
E-mail: melbye@intertourette.com
Website: http://www.intertourette.com

Norsk Tourette Forening
Contact: Tom A. Wulff, President
Brolandsveien 19 B
Oslo N-0980 Norway
Tel. (47) 2221 6506
Fax (47) 2210 9921

PERU
Asociaocion Sindrome de Tourette del Peru
Contact: Luisa Fernanda L. Romana
Las Golondras no. 390
Lima 27 Peru

POLAND
Polskie Stowarzyszenie Syndrom Tourette's
Contact: Ewa Boguszewska
c/o Osrodek Informacij TOPOS
38/40 ul.Dulga
Warsaw 00-238 Poland
Tel. (48) 22 831 22 12 (Tuesdays from 17:00 - 18:30hrs)
Fax (48) 22 831 47 12
E-mail: aboguszewski@poczta.onet.pl

SPAIN
Asociacion Espanola para Tics y Tourette
Gran Via de les Corts Catalanes, 562 pral. 2a
Barcelona 08011 Spain
Tel. (34) 451 5550

SWEDEN
Svensk Tourette Forening
St Johannesgatan 28
Uppsala S 752 33 Sweden
Tel. (46) 18 56 09 04
Fax (46) 18 56 09 01
E-mail: info@tourette.se

SWITZERLAND
Tourette Gesellschaft Schweiz Burozentrum
Gibraltarstrasse 34, Postfach 7147
600 Luzern 7 Switzerland
Tel. (41) 1 760 0265

THE NETHERLANDS
Stiching Gilles de la tourette
Post bus 925
Rhoon 3160 AC The Netherlands
Tel. (31) 10 501 3043
Fax (31) 10 591 5278

UNITED KINGDOM
Tourette Syndrome (UK) Association
Contact: Tourette Syndrome (UK) Association
PO Box 26149
Dunfermline KW12 9WT UK
Tel. (44) 845 458 1252
Fax (44) 845 458 1252
E-mail: enquiries@tsa.org.uk
Website: http://www.tsa.org.uk

UNITED STATES
Tourette Syndrome Association, Inc.
Contact: Sue Levi-Pearl or Mary Lilly
42-40 Bell Boulevard
Bayside, NY 11361 USA
Tel. (718) 224 2999/(800) 237 0717
Fax (718) 279 9596
E-mail: ts@tsa-usa.org
Website: http://tsa-usa.org

Ataxia

AUSTRALIA
Friedreich's Ataxia Association of New South Wales
Chisholm Street 31a
Turramurra 2074 Australia
Tel. (61) 2 94408233
Website: http://www.faa.org.au

**Spino Cerebellar Ataxia Resources &
   Support (SCARS)**
7 Robilliard Street
Mays Hill 2145 Australia
E-mail: michelle@bmu.net.au
Website: http://www.backmeup.net.au

BELGIUM
**Association Belge de l'Ataxie de Friedreich et des autres
   Ataxies Hereditaires**
Contact: Madeline Pelousse
Rue Longe 68
Bouffioulx B-6200 Belgium

Tel. (32) 71 50 42 48
Fax (32) 71 50 42 48

CANADA
Canadian Assoc. of Friedrich's Ataxia
Contact: Claude St-John
5620 C.A. Jobin Street
Montreal, Quebec H1P 1H8 Canada
Tel. (514) 321 8684
Fax (514) 321 9257

EUROPE
European Federation of Hereditary Ataxias
Contact: Dagmar Kroebel
Haagwindelaan 19
Overijse B-3090 Belgium
Tel. (32) 2 657 1510
Fax (32) 2 657 6176
E-mail: dagmar.kroebel@euro-ataxia.org
Website: http://www.euro-ataxia.org

FINLAND
Rare Neurological Disabilities Group
Suomen MS-Liitto - Finlands MS-Förbund
Seppalantie 90
Masku FIN-21251 Finland
Tel. (358) 2 4392111
Fax (358) 2 4392133
Website: http://www.ms-liitto.fi

FRANCE
Association Strumpell-Lorrain
9 bis, rue Fabre
Besancon F-25000 France
Tel. (33) 3 81502391
Fax (33) 3 81502391
E-mail: asl.spastic@wanadoo.fr
Website: http://www.afaf.ree.fr

GERMANY
**Deutsche Heredo-Ataxie Gesellschaft
Bundesverband e.v.**
Haussmannstrasse 6
Stuttgart D-70188 Germany
Tel. (49) 711 2155114
Fax (49) 711 2155214
Website: http://www.ataxie.de

IRELAND
Friedrich's Ataxia Society of Ireland
Contact: Clare Creedon, San Martin
Mart Lane, San Martin
Dublin 18 Ireland
Tel. (353) 1289 47 88
Website: http://www.fasi.ie

ITALY
**Associazione Italiana per la lotta alle Sindromi
Atassiche**
Via Cattaneo 22
Magenta (MI) I-20013 Italy
Tel. (39) 2 9792271
E-mail: aisa@iol.it
Website: http://www.hosting.iol.it/aisa

THE NETHERLANDS
ADCA-Vereniging Nederland
Contact: Marco Meinders
Fazantenkamp 839
Maarssen NL-3607 EC The Netherlands
Tel. (31) 346 563913
Fax (31) 346 580417
E-mail: ataxie@ataxie.nl
Website: http://www.ataxie.nl

UNITED STATES
A-T Children's Project
Contact: Jennifer Thornton, Executive Director
668 S. Military Trail
Deerfield Beach, FL 33442 USA
Tel. (800) 5-HELP-A-T
E-mail: info@atcp.org
Website: www.atcp.org

Ataxia MJD Research Project, Inc.
Contact: Laura Denning
875 Mahler Road, Ste 161
Burlingame, CA 94010-1621 USA
Tel. (650) 373 0674
Fax (650) 342 8741
E-mail: LDenning@ataxiamjd.org
Website: http://www.ataxiamjd.org

National Ataxia Foundation
Contact: Donna Gruetzmacher
2600 Fernbrook Lane, Suite 119
Minneapolis, MN 55447-4752 USA
Tel. (763) 553 0020
Fax (763) 553 0167
E-mail: naf@mr.net
Website: http://www.ataxia.org

Myolclonus

UNITED STATES
Moving Forward
Contact: Pauline Dill
2934 Glenmore Avenue
Kettering, OH 45409 USA
Tel. (513) 293 0409

Myoclonus Families United
Contact: Sharon Dobkin
155 E. 35th Street
Brooklyn, NY 11234 USA
Tel. (718) 252 2133

Myoclonus Research Foundation
Contact: Theodora Mason
200 Old Palisade Road, Suite 17D
Fort Lee, NJ 07024 USA
Tel. (201) 585 0770
Fax (201) 585 8114
Website: http://www.myoclonus.com

Progressive Supranuclear Palsy

UNITED KINGDOM
PSP Europe Association
Contact: The Old Rectory
Wappenham
Towchester, Northants NN12 85Q UK
Tel. (44) 1327 860 299
Fax (44) 1327 861 007
E-mail: psp.eur@virgin.net
Website: http://www.pspeur.org

UNITED STATES
Society for PSP, Inc.
Contact: Ellen Pam Katz
Woodholme Medical Bldg., Ste. #515, 1838 Greene Tree Road
Baltimore, MD 21208 USA
Tel. (410) 486 3330
Fax (410) 486 4283
E-mail: SPSP@psp.org
Website: http://www.psp.org

Restless Legs Syndrome

GERMANY
Deutsche Restless Legs Vereinigung
Contact: Claudia Trenkwalder, MD
Max Planck Institute
Munich Germany
Tel. (49) 89 30 62 2585

UNITED STATES
Restless Legs Syndrome Foundation
819 Second Street SW
Rochester, MN 55902 USA
Tel. (507) 287 6465
Fax (507) 287 6312

E-mail: rlsfoundation@rls.org
Website: http://www.rls.org

Tremor

UNITED KINGDOM
International Essential Tremor Foundation
Contact: International Essential Tremor Foundation
PO Box 14005
Lenexa, KS 66285-4005 USA
Tel. (913) 341 3880
Fax (913) 341 1296
E-mail: Staff@essentialtremor.org
Website: http://www.essentialtremor.org

UNITED STATES
International Tremor Foundation
Contact: Karen Walsh
Disablement Services Center, Harold Wood Hospital
Rumford, Essex RM3 OBE UK
Tel. (44) 1708 386399
Fax (44) 1708 378032

Educational Organizations for Physicians

The Movement Disorder Society Secretariat
Milwaukee Secretariat
611 East Wells Street
Milwaukee, WI 53202, USA
Tel. (1) 414 276 2145
Fax (1) 414 276 3349
E-mail: info@movementdisorders.org

NIH/National Institute of Neurological Disorders and Stroke
"Brain Resources and Information Network" (BRAIN)
Bethesda MD 20824 USA
Tel. (301) 496 5751
Fax (800) 352 9424
E-mail: N/A
Home Page: http://www.ninds.nih.gov

WE MOVE (Worldwide Education and Awareness for Movement Disorders)
Mt. Sinai Medical Center
One Gustave L. Levy Place Box 1052
New York, NY 10029 USA
Tel. (212) 241 8567
Fax (800) 437 6682
E-mail: wemove@wemove.org
Home Page: http://www.wemove.org

INDEX

Note: Please note that page numbers followed by *f* or *t* indicate figures and tables respectively. Abbreviations used in subentries are defined as main entries.

A

Abdominal wall dystonia, 516
Abortion, tissue acquisition guidelines, 276
Acanthocytes, 410, 639
Acetazolamide, essential tremor therapy, 447
Acetylcholine
  see also Cholinergic neurons
  basal ganglia role, 94–95, 120–123
  cognitive dysfunction and, 262
  Parkinson's disease, 201, 257, 262
  receptors
    basal ganglia, 121–123, 122f
    types, 121, 121t
  tic pathophysiology, 694
Acetylcholinesterase, Huntington's disease, 607f
Achromatic neurons *see* Balloon (achromatic) neurons
Action myoclonus, 657
  clinical features, 658
  cortical tremor, 461, 488
  EMG, 658, 658f
  treatment, 665–666
Action tremor *see* Kinetic tremor
AD *see* Alzheimer's disease (AD)
Adenosine triphosphate (ATP) synthesis, 68, 68f,
    69, 70
Adenoviral vectors, GDNF expression in PD, 138
ADHD *see* Attention deficit hyperactivity disorder
    (ADHD)
Adrenergic receptor antagonists
  alpha-blockers, ET treatment, 448
  beta-blockers
    essential tremor treatment, 445–446, 451, 485
    tremor induction, 464
Aging, 837–853
  see also individual disorders
  dopaminergic system, 198–199
  drug-induced disorders, 839–840, 844, 846, 848
  essential tremor, 431, 433, 436, 844–845
  gait disorders, 840–841, 841t
  hemiballismus, 846
  hypokinetic disorders, 837–838, 838t
  mitochondria, 73–74
  movement disorder management, 848
  muscle tone, 838–839, 838t, 839t, 846
  neurodegenerative disease and, 847–848
    see also Alzheimer's disease (AD)
  normal
    gait, 840, 841t
    motor performance, 838
    movement disorders *vs.*, 837–842
  old age, definitions, 837
  ophthalmoplegia, 842
  Parkinson's disease/parkinsonism, 73–74
    drug-induced, 844
    epidemiology, 184, 186, 842, 843
    gait, 840–841, 841t
    stroke and, 846
  postural changes, 840
  primitive reflexes, 842
  senile chorea, 641
  stroke-related conditions, 845–846
  systemic disease in, 837
  tics and, 691
Agitation, corticobasal degeneration, 764
AIDS *see* HIV infection/AIDS
Akathisia, 9–10, 242
  nocturnal in PD, 870
  "tardive," 627, 633
Akinesia
  aging and, 837–838
  corticobasal degeneration, 762
  pallidonigroluysian degeneration, 413
  parkinsonism, 106, 236, 236t
    neuropathology, 107–108
  PPN lesion, 96
Akinetic-rigid syndromes *see* Parkinsonism
Alcohol
  cerebellar degeneration and, 917
    gait, 815–816
  essential myoclonus effects, 661
  essential tremor effects, 4, 436, 444, 485
  nocturnal bruxism, 862
  withdrawal, 425
    tremor induction, 462–463, 917
Alien limb, 11, 763

α-Antichymotrypsin (ACT), PD gene association studies, 216

Alprazolam, essential tremor therapy, 447

Alzheimer's disease (AD)
apolipoprotein E ε4 link, 156–157
gross examination, 147, 148
movement disorders in, 847
myoclonus, 663
neurofibrillary tangles, 342
Parkinson's disease and, 150, 771t, 847
pathogenesis, 327
progressive supranuclear palsy and, 154, 343

Amantadine, 258, 259, 261
essential tremor therapy, 447–448
hemiparkinsonism-hemiatrophy, 408

Ambulation *see* Gait

American Psychiatric Association Task Force, tardive dyskinesia definition, 627

Amino acid metabolism disorders, dystonia, 554–555

Amiodarone
drug-induced parkinsonism, 399
tremor induction, 463

Amitriptyline, progressive supranuclear palsy, 350–351

AMPA/kainate receptors, 124
basal ganglia distribution, 122f, 125, 125f, 126f, 126t
functions, 126–127

Amphetamines, postencephalitic parkinsonism, 376

Amputation, phantom dyskinesia, 10

Amygdala, 148

Amyotrophic lateral sclerosis (ALS), antioxidants and, 78–79

Amyotrophy
chorea *see* Choreoacanthocytosis (CHAC)
parkinsonism-plus syndrome, 164

Anterior cervical rhizotomy, dystonia treatment, 535

Anterior cingulate circuit, behavior role, 18, 18f

Antiasthma drugs, tremor induction, 464

Anti-cardiolipin antibodies, Sydenham's chorea, 919

Anticholinergic drugs
see also individual drugs
carbon monoxide poisoning, 387
cyanide poisoning, 388
dystonia treatment, 504, 529–530, 632
hemiparkinsonism-hemiatrophy, 408
multisystem atrophy, 368
Parkinson's disease, 257, 257t, 259–260
postencephalitic parkinsonism, 376
progressive supranuclear palsy, 350
side-effects, 257, 529
use in drug-induced parkinsonism, 398

Anticonvulsant drugs *see* Antiepileptic drugs

Antidepressant drugs, 262, 320
see also individual drugs/drug types
Huntington's disease, 594
obsessive-compulsive disorder therapy, 688, 771

progressive supranuclear palsy, 350–351
tremor induction, 463

Antidopaminergic drugs *see* Antipsychotic drugs

Antiepileptic drugs
see also individual drugs
dystonia treatment, 531
myoclonus treatment, 665–666
PLMS and RLS treatment, 859, 859t
tremor induction, 463

Anti-GAD antibodies
progressive encephalomyelitis with rigidity, 802
stiff-person syndrome, 797, 800, 806–807

Anti-Hu antibodies, 923

Anti-Ma2 antibodies, 923

Antioxidants, 77–80
see also Oxidative stress; *specific molecules*
aging and, 74
ALS, therapy, 78–79
cellular, 72, 72f, 202–203
coenzyme Q₁₀, 77–79, 259, 594
enzymes, 79–80
general features, 77
Huntington's disease therapy, 78, 79, 590
nutrients/diet, 79
Parkinson's disease, 219
prevention, 189–190
therapy, 78, 79, 189–190, 259
problems with therapy, 77
tardive dyskinesia treatment, 79, 632

Antiparkinsonian drugs, 199, 247–271
see also individual drugs/drug types
dopaminergic agents *see* Dopaminergic agents
fluctuations, 43–44, 242, 249–250, 250t
management, 260–261
non-dopaminergic agents, 257–258
anticholinergics, 257, 257t
glutamate antagonists, 77, 78, 257–258
motor symptom control, 259–260
post-fetal transplantation, 281
side-effects, 43–44, 45f, 242–243, 249–250, 257, 258, 275
management, 260–264
prevention, 260
treatment decisions, 258–264
advanced PD, 260–264
early monotherapy, 258–260, 259t
motor symptom control, 259–260
neuroprotective intervention, 258–259
use in drug-induced parkinsonism, 398

Antiphospholipid antibody syndrome, 922
chorea, 638–639, 922

Antipsychotic drugs, 263, 263t, 323–324, 395, 395t
see also individual drugs
atypical, 323–324, 396, 688
reduced side-effects, 630
conventional, 396

dopamine, effects on, 397
drug choice, 630
drug switching, 398
guidelines on use, 629–630, 630t
non-psychiatric use, 396
   dystonia, 504, 529
   Sydenham's chorea, 638
   tic treatment, 688
side-effects, 323, 398
   dyskinesia see Tardive dyskinesia
   dystonia, 520, 556, 556f, 556t
   neuroleptic malignant syndrome, 424–425
   parkinsonism see Drug-induced parkinsonism
   preventing/treating, 629–630
   tics, 687
   tremor, 464, 627
Antiretroviral therapy, HIV-related parkinsonism, 377–378
Anti-Ri antibodies, 923
Anti-Ro antibodies, 921
Anti-Yo antibodies, 922–923
Anxiety, 23–24
  ataxias, 705
  Parkinson's disease, 23–24, 243, 320
  stiff-person (man) syndrome, 798–799
  tremor induction, 463
Apathy, 22
  corticobasal degeneration, 764
  Huntington's disease, 590
Aphasia, 26
Apolipoprotein E ε4
  Alzheimer's disease link, 156–157
  dementia with Lewy bodies (DLB), 408
  PD gene association studies, 216
Apomorphine
  effects, 46
  motor fluctuation management, 261
  multisystem atrophy, 368
  neuroleptic malignant syndrome treatment, 425
  pharmacology, 235t, 254–255
Apoptosis
  cascade, 221–223, 222f
  in disease, 70–71
    Huntington's disease, 605
    Parkinson's disease, 221–223
  endogenous neurotoxin-induced, 212
  mitochondria role, 69, 70
  MPTP-induced, 210
  as therapeutic target, 77
  TUNEL analysis, 221
Apraxia, 27
  corticobasal degeneration, 27, 762, 763
  gait, 841, 841t
  ideational, 763
  ideomotor, 27, 763
  limb kinetic, 763

APTX mutation, ataxia with oculomotor apraxia-1 (AOA-1), 712
Aqueduct of Sylvius, enlargement in PSP, 153
Archicerebellum, 722, 723t, 739–740
Argyrophilic grain disease (AGD), corticobasal degeneration vs., 770
Aromatic amino acid decarboxylase (AADC)
  deficiency, dystonia, 827
  levodopa (L-dopa) metabolism, 247, 248f
Arousal, progressive supranuclear palsy, 346–347
Artemin (neuroblastin/enovin), 137
Arteriosclerotic parkinsonism see Vascular parkinsonism
Ashkenazi Jews, primary torsion dystonia, 496, 497
Aspiny interneurons
  Huntington's disease, 604, 604f
  striatal motor circuitry, 94
Association studies
  dystonia, 517
  Parkinson's disease, 212–217, 213t
Asterixis see Negative myoclonus/asterixis
Astrocytes
  Huntington's disease, 609
  plaques, corticobasal degeneration, 155, 768, 768f
Ataxia
  see also individual disorders
  acquired conditions, 703–704
  cerebellar see Cerebellar ataxias
  clinical approach, 703–706, 704f
    counseling, 706
    diagnosis, 703–704, 705f, 705t
    genetic screening, 704, 705f, 705t
    support/rehabilitation, 705–706
    symptomatic treatment, 705
  differential diagnosis, 816t
  dystonia and, 551, 552f
  hereditary, 360, 551, 703–720
    see also molecular genetics (below)
  metabolic/nutritional diseases, 917
  molecular genetics, 703–720, 705t
    anticipation, 704, 708, 710
    autosomal-dominant, 706–711
    autosomal-recessive, 711–713
    family history and, 704, 704t
    mitochondrial, 74, 713–714
    phenotypic variation, 704
    repeat expansion see Repeat expansion diseases
    X-linked, 713
  neurological symptoms, 705
  neuropsychiatric disturbances, 705
  paraneoplastic, 922
  pathophysiology, 738
  progressive myoclonic, 662–663
  psychogenic, 705, 906, 907
  sensory, 816, 816t
  spinocerebellar see Spinocerebellar ataxias (SCAs)

Ataxia telangiectasia (AT), 711–712
  dystonia, 551, 552f
Ataxia with oculomotor apraxia-1 (AOA-1), 712
Ataxia with vitamin E deficiency (AVED), 712
Ataxin-1 gene, SCA1, 707
Ataxin-2 gene, SCA2, 707
Ataxin-3 gene, SCA3 (Machado-Joseph disease), 708
Ataxin-7 gene, SCA7, 709
Athetosis, 8
Athlete's cramp, 516
ATM gene, ataxia telangiectasia, 712
ATP7B (WNDP) gene, Wilson's disease, 777
Attention deficit hyperactivity disorder (ADHD)
  cerebellar dysfunction, 722
  Tourette's syndrome, 684, 693, 695–696
  treatment, 687t, 688
Autoantibodies
  see also Autoimmune disease; *specific antibodies*
  paraneoplastic, 922–923
  Sydenham's chorea, 919
Autoimmune disease, 921–922
  see also individual disorders
  chorea, 638–639, 644t
  dystonia in, 517
  paraneoplastic, 802–804, 923
  parkinsonism, 921
  postinfective, 919
  stiff-person (man) syndrome and, 797, 800, 801, 803–804, 805–807, 923
  tic disorders, 686
Autonomic dysfunction, 24
  failure in MSA, 359f, 360, 362–363
  hereditary choreas, 639
  management, 263, 264t
  neuroleptic malignant syndrome, 425
  Parkinson's disease, 24, 238–239, 263, 362
  progressive supranuclear palsy, 347
Autosomal recessive juvenile parkinsonism (ARJP), 166, 168–170
Autosomal recessive spastic ataxia of Charlevoix-Seguenay, 713
Axial dystonia, 547–548
Axial myoclonus, 664–665

B

Baclofen
  dystonia treatment, 504, 530–531
  stiff-person syndrome treatment, 807
  tardive dyskinesia treatment, 631
Bacterial infections, parkinsonism, 378
Balance *see* Postural control

Ballism, 7
  basal ganglia role, 109, 109f
  psychogenic, 904
Ballistic movement overflow myoclonus, 672
Balloon (achromatic) neurons, 156, 768
  corticobasal degeneration, 154, 155f, 767
Baltic myoclonus, 662
Basal forebrain, gait and, 812
Basal ganglia, 103–115
  see also Globus pallidus; Striatum; Substantia nigra; Subthalamic nucleus (STN)
  anatomy, 103, 104f, 117–118, 118f, 197–198, 197f
  BDNF role, 139
  disorders of *see* Basal ganglia disorders
  functional organization, 93–98, 94f, 103, 104–106
    see also motor circuitry (below)
    convergence, 105
    motor functions, 104, 105–106
    scaling *vs.* focusing, 105
    segregation, 96–97, 104–105
  HIV effects, 377
  imaging, 13t, 36
  motor circuitry, 89, 94–96, 94f, 95f, 103, 104, 117–118
    cortical inputs, 94, 103, 104f
    direct *vs.* indirect pathways, 95–96, 117, 499–500, 629
    dopamine role, 97
    globus pallidus, 95, 95f, 96
    lesions, 98
    models, 97–98
    PPN connections, 96
    striatum, 94–95
    subcircuits, 105–106
    substantia nigra, 95
    thalamic connections, 96
  neurochemistry, 117–134, 197f
    see also specific transmitters
    acetylcholine, 94–95, 120–123
    dopamine, 97, 103, 118–120
    glutamate, 123–127, 257
    in PD, 197–209
    serotonin, 127–129
  primary torsion dystonia and, 53
  procedural memory, 25–26
  sleep-wake role, 858, 877–878, 878f
Basal ganglia disorders, 3, 106–110
  see also individual symptoms/signs; specific disorders
  calcification, 550
    hypoparathyroidism, 916
    idiopathic *see* Idiopathic calcification of the basal ganglia (ICBG)
  chorea and, 109, 641, 642–643
  developmental, 686
  dystonia and, 109, 110, 499–500, 518–519, 544, 545t, 546, 549–551
  executive function, 25

frontal subcortical circuits and, 18
hyperintense MRI, 13t
hyperkinetic, 109–110
hypokinetic, 106–108
    akinesia, bradykinesia, rigidity, 107–108
    nonmotor phenomena, 108
    pathophysiological model, 106, 107f
    tremor, 108
motor control and, 104
Basic fibroblast growth factors (bFGF)
    neural transplantation and, 284
    Parkinson's disease, 220
Bassen-Kornzweig syndrome, 410, 548
BAX, apoptosis, 222–223
Bcl-2, apoptosis, 222–223
BDNF *see* Brain-derived neurotrophic factor (BDNF)
Behavior, 17
    changes *see* Neurobehavioral changes
    frontal subcortical circuits controlling, 17–18, 18f
    therapy, essential tremor (ET), 450–451
    Tourette's syndrome, 683t, 684
"Belly dancer's dyskinesia," 516
Benedikt's syndrome (Holmes' tremor), 466–467, 467t
    pathophysiology, 486–487
Benign hereditary chorea (BHC), 640, 829
Benign paroxysmal torticollis of infancy, 827, 828
Benign paroxysmal upgaze, 827
Benzodiazepines
    see also individual drugs
    drug-withdrawal syndromes, 425
    dystonia treatment, 504, 530
    essential tremor therapy, 446–447
    sleep disorder management
        PLMS and RLS, 859, 859t
        sleep-onset insomnia, 869
    stiff-person syndrome treatment, 797, 799, 807
    tardive dyskinesia treatment, 631–632
    tremor induction, 464
β-Carbolines, 211f
    Parkinson's disease etiology, 212
β-Carotene, as antioxidant treatment, 79
Beta-blockers *see* Adrenergic receptor antagonists
Bethanechol, drug-induced parkinsonism, 399
Binswanger's disease, 422, 815
Biochemistry
    chorea-acanthocytosis, 412
    Hallervorden-Spatz disease, 406
    hemiparkinsonism-hemiatrophy, 408
    Rett syndrome, 416
    stiff-person (man) syndrome, 805
    X-linked dystonia-parkinsonism syndrome, 410
Biopsy
    liver, Wilson's disease, 783, 783t
    muscle, stiff-person syndrome, 800–801
Bipolar disorder, Huntington's disease, 594

Bladder dysfunction
    ataxias, 705
    corticobasal degeneration, 772
    multisystem atrophy, 362–363
    Parkinson's disease, 238
    progressive supranuclear palsy, 347
Blepharospasm, 7, 513, 513t, 514f
    SLE and, 921
    sleep disturbance, 874
    tics *vs.*, 686
    treatment, 528t
        botulinum toxin, 532
Bobblehead doll syndrome, 826
"Bon-bon" sign, 521
Borna virus, Parkinson's disease etiology, 209
Borrelia burgdorferi, 919
BOTOX *see* Botulinum toxin
Botulinum toxin, 530–531
    antibody development, 531
    clinical applications, 530t
    corticobasal degeneration, 770
    dystonia treatment, 410, 502, 504, 527, 531–534
        blepharospasm, 532
        limb dystonias, 533–534
        oromandibular dystonia, 532
        peripheral surgery *vs.*, 535
        spasmodic dysphonia, 532–533
        spasmodic torticollis, 533
        tardive dystonia, 632
    essential tremor, 449
    FDA approval, 531
    neurotoxin types, 531t
    progressive supranuclear palsy, 351
    stiff-person syndrome, 808
    X-linked dystonia-parkinsonism syndrome, 410
Bowel problems
    COMT inhibitors, 252
    multisystem atrophy, 363
    Parkinson's disease, 238
Bradykinesia, 11
    aging and, 837–838
    Alzheimer's disease, 847
    encephalitis lethargica, 373–374
    parkinsonism, 106
        drug-induced, 396
        neuropathology, 107–108
        psychogenic, 905
    X-linked dystonia-parkinsonism syndrome, 410
Brain
    see also Neuropathology; *specific anatomical regions*
    activation in Parkinson's disease, 46–48, 47f
    gross examination, 147–148
    imaging *see* Neuroimaging

Brain (continued)
  injury
    see also Trauma
    diffuse, 545–546, 545t
    parkinsonism and, 422–423
    tremor and, 473
  metabolism see Brain metabolism
  structural lesions and parkinsonism, 424
Brain-derived neurotrophic factor (BDNF), 139–140
  neural transplantation and, 284
  Parkinson's disease, 220–221
    treatment, 139
Brain metabolism
  cerebellar hypometabolism, 754–755
  creatine role, 80
  Huntington's disease, 51
  hypermetabolism, choreas, 639
  Parkinson's disease, 45, 203–204
  primary torsion dystonia, 53
  progressive supranuclear palsy, 49
  Rett syndrome, 416
  striatonigral degeneration, 48
  Tourette's syndrome, 693
Brain parenchyma sonography (BPS), multisystem
    atrophy, 365
Brainstem
  see also specific regions/nuclei
  dystonia pathophysiology, 499, 519–520, 519f
    secondary lesions, 545, 545t
  focal myoclonus, 664–665
  gross examination, 147, 148, 327, 328f
  Huntington's disease, 611
  locomotion and, 811
  Parkinson's disease, 327, 328f, 329t
  progressive supranuclear palsy, 346–347
  sleep-wake role, 876–877
    basal ganglia and, 877–878
Briquet's syndrome, 892, 892t
British anti-lewisite (BAL), Wilson's disease
    management, 787
Bromocriptine mesylate
  neuroleptic malignant syndrome, 425
  pharmacology, 253–254, 253t
  sleep-maintenance insomnia treatment, 869
Bruxism, nocturnal, 862
Buproprion, sleepiness management, 874

C

Cabergoline, pharmacology, 253t, 254
Caffeine
  food-induced tremor, 462
  Parkinson's disease prevention, 189

Calcium channel blockers
  drug-induced parkinsonism, 399
  essential tremor therapy, 448
  tremor induction, 463–464
Calcium metabolism, parkinsonism and, 424, 916
Calcium regulation
  mitochondrial, 70
    disruption, 73
    therapeutic target, 77
  NMDA receptors, 126
Camptocormia, psychogenic gait, 906
Cancer see Malignancy
CAPIT (core assessment protocol for intracerebral
    transplantation), 280
Carbamazepine
  cerebellar tremor, 462
  dystonia treatment, 504
  tic induction, 697
Carbidopa (Lodosyn), 249
  cyanide poisoning, 388
  REM sleep behavior disorder treatment, 861
Carbon disulfide, parkinsonism, 387–388
Carbonic anhydrase inhibitors, essential tremor therapy,
    447
Carbon monoxide
  dystonia, 557
  free radical scavenger, 211
  mechanism of toxicity, 387
  parkinsonism, 386–387
Cardiac abnormalities
  Friedreich's ataxia, 711
  postpump chorea and, 642–643
  Rett syndrome, 415
Cardiac drugs, tremor induction, 463–464
Caspases, apoptosis, 223
Catalase, PD gene association studies, 215
Catechol-O-methyltransferase (COMT)
  dopamine metabolism, 198, 199f
  inhibitors, 248, 251–252, 261
  levodopa (L-dopa) metabolism, 247, 248f
  Parkinson's disease
    changes seen, 200, 200t
    gene association studies, 214
  Parkinson's disease changes, 200, 200t
Caudate nucleus, 117
  cholinergic neurons, 122
  dopaminergic inputs, 97
  Huntington's disease, 601, 602f, 603f
  serotonergic innervation, 127
Cautious gait, 813–814
CBD see Corticobasal degeneration (CBD)
Celiac disease, 922
Cell-based vectors, GDNF expression in PD, 138
Cell damage, oxidative see Oxidative stress

Cell death
    apoptosis *see* Apoptosis
    calcium-mediated, 73, 77
    excitotoxicity, 70, 77
    inclusions and, 204
    necrosis, 70
    polyglutamine toxicity, 76
Central oscillatory networks, essential tremor and, 441–442,
    442f
Cerebellar ataxias, 724, 725
    see also Spinocerebellar ataxias (SCAs); *individual*
        disorders
    congenital, 713
    differential diagnosis, 816t
    gait, 738, 815–816
    hereditary, 360, 551
        autosomal dominant (ADCA), 706–711, 728t
        autosomal recessive, 711–713, 728t
        episodic, 706, 706t, 710–711
        mitochondrial, 713–714
        X-linked, 713
    hypothyroidism and, 916
    limb, 738
    pharmacotherapy, 816
    vermal syndrome, 746
Cerebellar atrophy, paraneoplastic, 922
Cerebellar dysfunction
    see also specific disorders
    alcoholic, 815–816
    anatomical relationships, 722–724, 723t
    ataxia *see* Cerebellar ataxias
    cerebellar syndromes, 746–748
    clinical symptoms/signs, 724–726, 735–739
        see also specific symptoms/signs
        abnormal check/rebound, 725–726, 735–736
        dysarthria, 737, 748
        dysdiadochokinesia, 737, 737f, 739, 748–749
        dysmetria, 735–736, 736f, 739, 747
        hypotonia, 726, 737, 738f
        movement abnormalities, 725
        oculomotor abnormalities, 724–725, 738, 747
        stance/gait, 724, 815–816
        tremor *see* tremor *(below)*
    cognitive affective syndrome, 722
    diagnosis/differential diagnosis, 727t-728t
    Huntington's disease, 610–611, 611f
    laboratory tests, 727t-728t
    multisystem atrophy, 359f, 360, 363, 366f
    paraneoplastic disorders, 727t, 922–923
    pathophysiology, 735–758
        alpha *vs.* gamma motor systems, 739, 747–750
        common mechanisms?, 739
        coordination control, 750–751
        hypometabolism, 754–755
        lesions, 753–754

        secondary, 754–755
        tremor, 485–486, 486f
    treatment, 727, 727t-728t
    tremor, 461–462, 726, 736–737
        see also Tremor
        essential, 441, 442f
        kinetic, 736–737, 739
        pathophysiology, 485–486, 486f
        titubation, 724
        vocal, 474
    vestibular disturbances and, 725, 746
    Wilson's disease and, 780
Cerebellar gait, 815–816
Cerebellar homunculus, 742, 742f, 743f
"Cerebellar mutism," 726
Cerebellum
    anatomy/organization, 721, 722–724, 739–745
        afferent connections, 740–741, 742f
        archicerebellum, 722, 723t, 739–740
        cortex, 721, 739, 741f, 744–745, 745f
            glomeruli, 745f
            granule cell layer, 742, 744, 745f
            molecular layer, 744, 745f
            mossy fibers, 744
            parallel fibers, 744–745
            patches, 742, 743f
            Purkinje cell layer, 744–745, 745f
            somatotropic arrangement, 742, 742f, 743f
        deep nuclei, 721, 739, 740, 741
        efferent connections, 741–744, 742f
        folia, 739
        lobes/lobules, 739, 740f
            flocculonodular, 744
        neocerebellum, 722–723, 723t, 740
        paleocerebellum, 722, 723t, 740
        peduncles, 739, 740–741
        sagittal zones, 721, 723t, 741–744, 741f
            intermediate, 723, 741f
            lateral, 724, 742–743
            middle, 723, 742
            neuronal activity, 743
            subdivisions, 744
        spinocerebellum, 740
        vermis, 722
        vestibulocerebellum, 723
        white matter, 739
    circuitry, 744–745
        motor, 89, 726
    dysfunction *see* Cerebellar dysfunction
    functions, 721–722, 756
        cognitive, 722, 752–753
        coordination, 750–751
        locomotion, 811
        motor learning, 721–722, 751
        muscle tone, 726, 749

Cerebellum *(continued)*
  functions *(continued)*
    posture/movement control, 721, 724, 725, 748–750
    sensory, 752
    speech, 722, 726
    theories, 748–753
    timing, 751–752
  gross examination, 147, 148, 739–740
  phylogeny, 739–740
  plasticity, 746, 751
    long-term depression, 745
Cerebral abscess, parkinsonism, 424
Cerebral blood flow (CBF)
  see also Brain metabolism; *specific techniques*
  Parkinson's disease, 46–48
  voluntary movement, 92
Cerebral cortex
  see also entries beginning cerebral/cortical; specific
    anatomical areas
  atrophy *see* Cortical degeneration/atrophy
  cortical tremor, 461, 488
  efferents, cerebellar projections, 741
  histopathology, 148
    see also Neuropathology; *specific conditions*
  motor system, 90–93, 91f, 608
    basal ganglia circuits, 94, 103, 104f
  representational organization, 92
Cerebral palsy
  dystonia, 827
  hemidystonia, 545f
  symptomatic (secondary) dystonia, 541
Cerebral peduncles, gross examination, 148
Cerebral toxoplasmosis, 920
Cerebroside sulfatase, 553
Cerebrospinal fluid (CSF)
  chorea-acanthocytosis, 549
  corticobasal degeneration, 764
  encephalitis lethargica, 374
  HIV infection, 377
  hydrocephalus, 423
  progressive supranuclear palsy (PSP), 342
  Rett syndrome, 551
  Wilson's disease, copper levels, 783t, 785
Cerebrotendinous xanthamatosis, 713
Cerebrovascular disease
  see also Stroke-associated conditions
  chorea and, 645t
  parkinsonism due to *see* Vascular parkinsonism
  Parkinson's disease *vs.*, 240
Ceroid lipofuscinosis, dystonia, 553
Ceruloplasmin deficiency
  Menkes' disease, 778
  Wilson's disease, 777, 778
    diagnosis, 783t, 784
Cervical dystonia *see* Spasmodic torticollis

Charcot, Jean-Martin, 891–892, 894, 901
Charcot-Marie-Tooth disease (HMSN type I), tremor,
    440–441, 469
Charcot's sign, blepharospasm, 513
Chemical exposure
  see also Toxin-induced parkinsonism; *specific chemicals*
  Parkinson's disease, 74–75, 188
  toxin-induced dystonia, 556, 557t
  toxin-induced tremor, 466
Chemomyectomy, dystonia treatment, 531
Childhood movement disorders, 823–833
  see also specific disorders
  akinetic-rigid syndromes, 829–830
    juvenile familial parkinsonism, 166, 168–170, 830
  chorea, 640, 642–643, 828–829, 829t
  clinical approach, 824
  dystonia, 495–510, 511, 516, 824, 826–828
    conditions causing, 827, 827t
    metabolic disorders, 918t
    primary torsion *see* Primary torsion dystonia (PTD)
    transient, 827
  epidemiology, 823–824, 823f
  stereotypies, 828
  tics, 823–824, 824–825
  tremor, 825–826
Chlordecone (kepone), toxin-induced tremor, 466
Chlorpromazine, drug-induced parkinsonism, 395
Cholecystokinin (CCK), Parkinson's disease, 202
Choline acetyltransferase (ChAT), Parkinson's
    disease, 201
Cholinergic drugs
  drug-induced parkinsonism, 399
  Parkinson's disease, 262
  progressive supranuclear palsy, 350
Cholinergic neurons
  basal ganglia, 120–123, 122f
    striatal motor circuitry, 94–95
  Parkinson's disease, 201, 257
  tic pathophysiology, 694
Cholinesterase inhibitors, 262
  dementia with Lewy bodies, 409
Chorea, 6–7, 7t, 637–653
  see also individual disorders
  associated conditions, 643, 643t-645t
  ataxia with oculomotor apraxia-1 (AOA-1), 712
  childhood, 640, 642–643, 828–829, 829t
  clinical symptoms/signs, 6
    dystonia, 548–549
    obsessive-compulsive disorder, 23, 638
  definition, 6, 588, 637, 828
  degenerative conditions, 644t
  differential diagnosis
    myoclonus *vs.*, 657
    tics *vs.*, 695
  hereditary, 639–641, 644t

Huntington's *see* Huntington's disease (HD)
neuroimaging, 50–51
"painful legs and moving toes," 645–646
paroxysmal dyskinesias, 10, 643, 645
pathophysiology
    basal ganglia role, 109, 641, 642–643
    immune system, 639
psychogenic, 904
secondary disorders, 642–643
senile, 641
Sydenham's *see* Sydenham's chorea (St. Vitus dance)
systemic causes, 637–639, 644t, 915, 918, 921, 922
tardive dyskinesia and, 6–7, 50–51, 627, 630, 631–632
treatment, 593, 631–632
vascular, 641, 644t
Chorea gravidarum, 638, 922
"Chorea minima," 828
Chorein gene, 411
Choreoacanthocytosis (CHAC), 410–412, 639–640
acanthocytes, 410–411, 639
clinical features, 411
    cognitive, 639
    dystonia, 544–545
    neurological, 639
    tics, 696
diagnosis/differential diagnosis, 411–412, 592
molecular genetics, 639
pathology/pathogenesis, 411, 640
treatment, 640
Choreoathetosis, diabetes mellitus and, 916
Ciliary neurotrophic factor (CNTF), 141
    Parkinson's disease, 221
Cingulate motor areas, 90, 91f, 93
Cingulate nucleus, lesion in tic treatment, 694
Cinnarizine, drug-induced parkinsonism, 399
Circle of Willis, gross examination, 147
Cirrhosis, Wilson's disease, 779
Clinical assessment, 3, 5t
    depression, 19
Clinical trials
    coenzyme Q$_{10}$, 78, 259
    fetal cell transplantation in PD, 41–43, 281–283
    mitochondrial disorders, coenzyme Q$_{10}$, 78
Clomipramine, Huntington's disease, 594
Clonazepam
    corticobasal degeneration, 770, 771
    dystonia treatment, 530, 632
    essential tremor therapy, 447
    myoclonus management, 665, 666
    REM sleep behavior disorder treatment, 861, 870–871
    stiff-person syndrome treatment, 807
Clonic motor tics, 691
Clonidine
    ADHD treatment, 688
    essential tremor therapy, 448

neuroleptic malignant syndrome, 425
    tic treatment, 687–688
Clozapine, 263, 323, 398
    dystonia treatment, 529
    extrapyramidal side-effects, 395–396
        reduction, 630
Cocaine, catecholamine transport, 200
"Cock walk," manganese-induced parkinsonism, 385
Coenzyme Q$_{10}$, 77–79
    cellular antioxidant system, 72
    clinical trials in PD, 259
    Huntington's disease, 594
Cognitive-behavioral therapy, obsessive-compulsive
        disorder, 688
Cognitive dysfunction, 25–27, 237, 339, 363, 404
    see also Dementia; *specific disorders*
    assessment, 280
    corticobasal degeneration, 763–764, 771
    depression relationship, 19, 319
    executive functions, 25
    Huntington's disease, 25, 26, 27, 589–590
    management, 262–263
    memory *see* Memory impairment
    multisystem atrophy, 363
    Parkinson's disease *see under* Parkinson's disease
    praxis, 27
    speech/language, 26
    visuospatial function, 26–27
    Wilson's disease, 780–781
Cognitive function, cerebellum role, 722, 752–753
Cogwheeling
    aging and, 839, 839t
    essential tremor, 845
Cogwheel rigidity, 11, 236
    cogwheeling *vs.* in essential tremor, 845
Coiled bodies, corticobasal degeneration, 155
Columbia Presbyterian Medical Center, 894
Complex regional pain syndrome (CRPS), 900
Complex tics, 9, 683, 692t
Computed tomography (CT)
    chorea-acanthocytosis, 412
    corticobasal degeneration, 764, 765f
    dystonia, 503, 546f
    hemiparkinsonism-hemiatrophy, 408
    multisystem atrophy, 363–364
    pallidonigroluysian degeneration, 413
    pallidopyramidal disease, 414
    postpump chorea, 642
    progressive supranuclear palsy, 341–342
    Wilson's disease, 785
    X-linked dystonia-parkinsonism syndrome, 410
COMT *see* Catechol-*O*-methyltransferase (COMT)
Confusional states, 262
Congenital heart disease, postpump chorea and, 642–643

Constraint-induced movement therapy, dystonia treatment, 527–528
Conversion disorders, 893, 893t
    psychogenic dystonia, 557
Copper
    absorption inhibition, 786–787
    chelators, 787–788
    dietary sources, 785
    exposure/toxicity, dystonia, 557
    Wilson's disease, 777, 778, 783t, 784
        diagnosis, 783t, 784–785
Coprolalia, 691
Core assessment protocol for intracerebral transplantation (CAPIT), 280
Cornea, staining, 781
Corpora amylacea, pallidonigroluysian degeneration, 413
Corpus callosum lesion, alien limb, 11
Cortical degeneration/atrophy, 147
    see also specific disorders
    corticobasal degeneration, 766–767, 766f, 767f
    Huntington's disease, 602f, 608–610
        CAG repeats and, 609
        gross/regional pathology, 609
        laminar pathology, 609–610, 610f
        MRI, 611, 611f
        neurochemistry, 610
    PSP, 343–344
Cortical motor fields, 90, 91, 91f
    dopaminergic innervation, 97
    premotor, 92–93
Cortical myoclonus, 8, 660, 664, 665, 666, 670, 670t
    associated conditions, 671
    C-reflex, 670, 675–676, 677
    EMG/EEG, 670, 671f
    giant SEPs, 660, 664, 670, 670f, 675, 675f
    photic reflex, 671
Cortical tremor, 461, 488
Corticobasal degeneration (CBD), 12, 761–776
    clinical features, 49, 761, 762–764, 763t, 771t
        akinesia, 762
        alien limb, 11, 763
        aphasia, 26
        apraxia, 27, 762, 763
        cognitive/psychological, 763–764, 771
        dysphagia, 772
        dystonia, 548, 762–763
        gastrointestinal, 771–772
        myoclonus, 663
        oculomotor, 763
        rigidity, 762
        tremor, 762
    dementia in, 29, 155
    diagnosis, 155–156, 761, 764
        clinical criteria, 762
        pathologic, 768–769

differential diagnosis, 770, 771t
    disease overlap, 769–770
    FTDP-17 *vs.*, 762, 769–770
    MSA *vs.*, 367
    Parkinson's disease *vs.*, 240–241, 242
    Pick's disease *vs.*, 50, 155, 156, 769
    PSP *vs.*, 341, 341t, 762, 770
    SND *vs.*, 762
electrophysiology, 765–766
epidemiology, 762
genetics, 769
historical cases, 761–762
laboratory studies, 764
myoclonus in, 660
neuroimaging, 49–50, 764–765, 765f
neuropathology, 154–156, 155f, 761, 766–770, 766t
    atrophy, 766–767, 766f, 767f
    balloon (achromatic) neurons, 154, 155f, 767
    gliosis, 767
    histological, 767–768
    neurofibrillary tangles, 154–155, 342, 768
    neuronal loss, 761–762, 767
    subcortical involvement, 767
    tau pathology, 767f, 768–769
treatment, 770–772
    cognitive/psychological dysfunction, 771
    motor dysfunction, 770–771
    occupational therapy, 772
    physiotherapy, 772
Corticobasal ganglionic degeneration (CBGD) *see* Corticobasal degeneration (CBD)
Corticospinal tract, 90–92
    corticobasal degeneration, 762
    multisystem atrophy, 363
    spasticity, 838
Corticostriatothalamic circuits, tic pathophysiology, 692–693
Cranial dystonia
    Meige's syndrome, 513, 518, 547, 921
    tics *vs.*, 686, 692
Creatine
    as bioenergetic therapy, 80
        Huntington's disease, 594
    oxidative phoshorylation effects, 77, 80
C-reflex, 670, 675–676, 677
Creutzfeldt-Jakob disease (CJD), 847–848
    aphasia, 26
    apraxia, 27
    differential diagnosis, 771t
        dementia with Lewy bodies *vs.*, 151
        Parkinson's disease *vs.*, 241–242
    myoclonus, 659, 663
    parkinsonism, 378–379
    sleep disturbance, 874
Crossed cerebellar diaschisis, 754–755
Cryopreservation, embryonic tissue, 277, 277f

Cryptococcal infection, parkinsonism, 378
α-B-Crystallin, corticobasal degeneration, 155f
CT see Computed tomography (CT)
CTP2D6 (debrisoquin hydroxylase), Parkinson's disease
    etiology, 213
Cyanide poisoning
  dystonia, 557
  parkinsonism, 388
Cyclosporin A, fetal transplantation, 279–280
Cytochrome P450s, 213
Cytokines, Parkinson's disease and, 219–221, 220t
  gene association studies, 215

D

DDT (dichlorodiphenyltrichloroethane), toxin-induced
    tremor, 466
Deafness dystonia syndrome, 74
Debrisoquin hydroxylase (CTP2D6), Parkinson's disease
    etiology, 213
Declarative memory, impairment, 25
Deep brain stimulation (DBS)
  globus pallidus
    dystonia, 504, 534–535
    Parkinson's disease, 48
  subthalamic nucleus
    essential tremor, 485
    Parkinson's disease, 48
  thalamus
    essential tremor therapy, 449–450, 484–485
    pallidal vs. in dystonia, 535
Delusions, Huntington's disease, 590
Dementia, 12, 27–29
  see also Cognitive dysfunction; specific types
  clinical features, 27
  cortical vs. subcortical, 27, 28t
  corticobasal degeneration, 29, 155
  depression and, 20
  Huntington's disease, 28
  multisystem atrophy, 29
  neuroimaging, 45–46
  pallidonigroluysian degeneration, 413
  parkinsonism-plus syndromes, 164–165
  Parkinson's disease, 27–28, 45–46, 771t, 844
    differential diagnosis, 241–242
  progressive myoclonic encephalopathy with, 661–662, 663
  progressive supranuclear palsy, 28, 154
  Rett syndrome, 415
  Wilson's disease, 29
Dementia pugilistica, 423
Dementia with Lewy bodies (DLB), 12, 408–409, 844
  definition, 151, 408
  diagnosis/differential diagnosis, 409, 771t
    criteria, 150–151

Parkinson's disease vs., 241
  epidemiology, 408
  molecular genetics, 408
  myoclonus, 663
  neuroimaging, 409
  neuropathology, 150–152, 408
    gross examination, 148
    Lewy bodies, 151, 151f
    spongiform changes, 151–152, 151f
    α-synuclein, 151
    ubiquitin immunoreactivity, 151, 151f
  sleep disorders, 24
  therapy, 409
Demyelinating disorders
  cerebellar dysfunction, 727t
  multiple sclerosis, chorea, 642
  tremor, 469
Denatorubropallidoluysian atrophy (DRPLA), 640–641
  dystonia in, 549
  Huntington's disease vs., 592, 710
  molecular genetics, 710
    anticipation, 710
    DNA tests, 705t
    phenotype, 706t
    triplet repeat expansion, 577f, 641, 710
  myoclonic encephalopathies, 661
  pathology, 640
  subtypes, 640–641
Dendrites, Huntington's disease neuropathology,
    605–606, 605f
Dentate nucleus
  functional imaging, 755f
  neurosurgical lesion, tic treatment, 694
Deprenyl (Selegiline), 252
Deprenyl (Seligiline), 259, 260, 262, 869
Depression, 19–20, 19t
  assessment, 19
  ataxias, 705
  corticobasal degeneration, 764
  dementia and, 20
  Huntington's disease, 20, 590
  management, 262, 320
  neural substrates, 19
  Parkinson's disease, 19–20, 242, 262, 319–320
    cognitive decline and, 19, 319
    pathogenesis, 320
    risk factors, 319
  Wilson's disease, 20, 780
Dermatological features
  Parkinson's disease, 239
  Wilson's disease, 782
Development, dopaminergic system, 135–136, 276–277
Diabetes mellitus, 916
  choreoathetosis, 916
  stiff-person syndrome and, 799, 801, 806–807

Diagnostic and Statistical Manual of Mental Disorders, Fourth Edition (DSM-IV), psychogenic movement disorders, 892–893, 892t, 893t
Diarrhea, COMT inhibitors, 252
Diaschisis, crossed cerebellar, 754–755
Diazepam
    drug-induced parkinsonism, 399
    dystonia treatment, 530
    stiff-person syndrome treatment, 797, 799, 807
    X-linked dystonia-parkinsonism syndrome, 410
Dichlorodiphenyltrichloroethane (DDT), toxin-induced tremor, 466
Diet
    deficient *see* Nutritional deficiency
    Parkinson's disease
        etiology, 188
        prevention, 189–190
    supplements
        antioxidants, 77, 79
        creatine, 80
    Wilson's disease management, 785–786
Diffuse Lewy body disease (DLBD) *see* Dementia with Lewy bodies (DLB)
Dihydroergocriptine, pharmacology, 253t, 254
Dihydrolipoamide succinyltransferase, PD gene association studies, 216–217
Diphenhydramine
    dystonia treatment, 529–530
    X-linked dystonia-parkinsonism syndrome, 410
Disinhibition-dementia-parkinsonism-amyotrophy complex (DDPAC) *see* Frontotemporal dementia with parkinsonism linked to chromosome 17 (FTDP-17)
DLB *see* Dementia with Lewy bodies (DLB)
DNA
    mitochondrial *see* Mitochondrial genome (mtDNA)
    oxidative damage, 71
        Parkinson's disease, 219
    repair disorders, 551
DNA markers, *huntingtin* (HD) gene identification, 570, 571, 571f, 572
Domperidone, 249, 398
Donepezil, REM sleep behavior disorder treatment, 861
L-Dopa *see* Levodopa (L-dopa)
Dopamine
    see also Dopaminergic agents
    antipsychotic drugs and, 397
    basal ganglia, 97, 103, 118–120
    distribution in brain *see* Dopaminergic system
    as free radical generator, 202
    manganese and auto-oxidation, 386
    metabolism, 198, 199f, 248f
    motor control, 236
    pathological changes
        see also specific disorders
        dystonia, 499

    Huntington's disease, 603
    Parkinson's disease, 199–200, 199t, 200t, 202
    sleep disturbance, 858, 865–866
    tardive dyskinesia, 628–629
    receptors *see* Dopamine receptors
    release, 198
    sleep-wake role, 858, 865–866, 868f, 875–876
    storage inhibitors in drug-induced parkinsonism, 398–399
    structure, 211f
    transporter, 215, 398–399
Dopamine agonists, 253–257
    see also individual drugs
    comparative trials, 259
    effects of treatment, 46
    efficacy, 253
    functional imaging, 40–41, 46–48
    Huntington's disease treatment, 593
    indications, 249, 256, 261
    motor symptom control, 260
    multisystem atrophy, 367–368
    neuroprotective properties, 256
    pharmacology, 253–256, 253t
    PLMS and RLS treatment, 859, 859t
    side-effects, 256–257, 556
    tardive dyskinesia treatment, 631
Dopamine antagonists *see* Antipsychotic drugs
Dopamine D1 receptors, 119, 120t, 200
    basal ganglia distribution, 119, 122f, 125
    functions, 120
        sleep-wake role, 876
    progressive supranuclear palsy, 344
Dopamine D2–like receptors (D2–D5), 119, 120t, 200
    basal ganglia distribution, 119, 122f
        HD striatum, 603
    BDNF-induced D3 expression, 139
    dopamine agonists, 253
    functions, 120
        sleep-wake role, 876
    PD gene association studies, 214
    tardive dyskinesia, 628–629
Dopamine-depleting agents
    dystonia management, 632–633
    tardive dyskinesia treatment, 631–632
Dopamine receptors, 198, 200
    see also specific types
    agonists *see* Dopamine agonists
    antagonists *see* Antipsychotic drugs
    basal ganglia, 94, 103, 119, 122f
    estrogen-related blockade, 397
    functions, 119–120
    Parkinson's disease
        changes seen, 200
        gene association studies, 214
    subtypes, 119, 120t

Dopaminergic agents
  see also specific drugs
  agonists *see* Dopamine agonists
  COMT inhibitors, 251–252
    L-dopa combination, 248, 251, 261
  dystonia treatment, 528
  Huntington's disease treatment, 593
  L-dopa *see* Levodopa (L-dopa)
  MAO-B inhibitors, 252–253, 260
  motor symptom control, 260
  multisystem atrophy and, 362, 367–368
  Parkinson's disease, 247–257
  PLMS and RLS treatment, 859, 859t
  progressive supranuclear palsy, 350
  side-effects, 242–243, 249–250, 252, 256–257
    drug-induced dyskinesia, 44, 45f, 110
    drug-induced dystonia, 110
    dyskinesia, 43–44, 45f, 110, 242, 250, 250t, 252, 283
    dystonia, 110, 250, 547, 556–557, 556t
    management, 260–264
    neuroleptic malignant syndrome, 424–425
    neuropsychiatric, 24, 239, 242, 249, 252, 262–264, 320, 321–324
    sleep disorders, 24, 872–873
  use in drug-induced parkinsonism, 398
Dopaminergic system, 198–199
  see also specific components
  aging and, 198–199
  basal ganglia, 97, 103, 118–120, 122f
    source, 118–119
  development, 135–136, 276–277
  Parkinson's disease, 197, 198–200
    cell loss, 198–199
    dementia and, 45–46
    neuroimaging, 36–38, 37f, 45–46
    presynaptic, 36–38
  tic pathophysiology, 692–693, 694
  trophic factors and neuronal survival, 135–141
    see also specific factors
Dopamine transporter
  inhibitors in drug-induced parkinsonism, 398–399
  PD gene association studies, 215
Dopa-responsive dystonia (DRD), 7, 54, 504–505, 528
  childhood, 827
  epidemiology, 504–505
  genetics, 168, 504, 505
  neuroimaging, 54
  pathogenesis, 505
Dorsal raphe nucleus (DRN), basal ganglia innervation, 127, 129, 201
Dorsolateral prefrontal circuit
  behavior role, 17–18, 18f
  in Parkinson's disease, 46, 47f
Drawing, essential tremor assessment, 443–444
Dreams, levodopa side-effects, 321

Dressing, essential tremor assessment, 443
DRPLA *see* Denatorubropallidoluysian atrophy (DRPLA)
Drug-induced disorders
  see also Toxin-induced disorders; *specific drugs/drug types*
  aging and, 839–840, 844, 846, 848
  cerebellar dysfunction, 728t
  chorea, 643, 643t
  dyskinesias *see* Drug-induced dyskinesia
  dystonia, 110, 250, 520, 547, 556–557, 556t-557t
  neuroleptic malignant syndrome, 424–425
  neuropsychiatric disturbances, 21, 242–243, 250, 252, 257, 263t, 264t
  parkinsonism *see* Drug-induced parkinsonism
  tardive tics, 627, 687, 697
  tremor, 463–464, 489, 736, 826, 839–840
Drug-induced dyskinesia, 110, 250t, 283
  COMT inhibitors, 252
  dopamine agonist delay, 256, 260
  levodopa-induced *see* Levodopa-induced dyskinesia
  management, 261, 261t
  neuroleptic-induced *see* Tardive dyskinesia
Drug-induced parkinsonism, 395–402, 399t
  see also specific drugs
  aging and, 839–840, 844
  calcium channel blockers, 399
  clinical features, 396–397, 396t
  dopamine storage/transport inhibitors, 398–399
  MPTP *see* MPTP-induced parkinsonism
  pathogenesis, 397–398
  susceptibility, 397
  treatment, 398–400
DSM-IV criteria, psychogenic movement disorders, 892–893, 892t, 893t
Dynamic balance, gait, 812–813
Dysarthria
  see also Speech/speech disorders
  ataxic, cerebellar dysfunction, 726
  cerebellar dysfunction, 737, 748
  Huntington's disease, 589
  multisystem atrophy, 363
  progressive supranuclear palsy, 346t, 347, 351
  speech and, 26, 726
  Wilson's disease, 779
Dysdiadochokinesia, 725, 737, 737f, 739
  α control theories, 748–749
Dyskinesia
  definition, 3
  drug-induced *see* Drug-induced dyskinesia
  HIV infection and, 920
  neural substrates, 98
    basal ganglia pathology, 110
  neuroimaging, 43–44, 45f
  orofacial, 846–847
  Parkinson's disease, neuroimaging, 43–44, 45f
  paroxysmal, 10, 643, 920

Dyskinesia *(continued)*
  phantom, 10
  tardive *see* Tardive dyskinesia
Dysmetria, 725, 735–736
  see also Kinetic tremor; Muscle tone
  α control theories, 748
  mechanism, 739
  saccadic, 747
Dysphagia
  corticobasal degeneration, 772
  dystonic, 516
  Huntington's disease, 589
  multisystem atrophy, 363
  Parkinson's disease, 238
  progressive supranuclear palsy, 347
  Rett syndrome, 415
Dysphonia
  spasmodic (laryngeal dystonia), 514, 517
    treatment, 528t, 532–533
  "whispering," Wilson's disease, 779–780
Dysrhythmokinesis, 725
Dystonia, 7–8, 495–496, 511
  see also specific types
  activity relationship, 7–8
  adult-onset, 511–525
  aging and, 838, 838t, 839t, 846
  childhood (early-onset), 495–510, 511, 516, 824, 826–828
    clinical issues, 826–827, 827t
    transient, 827–828
  chorea-acanthocytosis, 411
  classification, 495–496, 511, 896–897
    distribution, 495, 495t
    etiological, 495, 496t, 541, 541t
  clinical features
    age at onset relationship, 500, 500t
    disease progression, 501–502
    early-onset, 500–502, 505
    early *vs.* late-onset, 511, 511t
    gait abnormalities, 502, 815
    genotype and, 501, 501t
    late-onset, 512–516, 512t
    myoclonus, 513
    neurological abnormalities, 520–521
    other hyperkinetic disorders *vs.*, 500
    "overflow," 501, 512
    remission, 512
    sleep disturbance, 874
    tremor, 462, 502, 513, 521
      essential, 440
      pathophysiology, 488
    X-linked dystonia-parkinsonism syndrome, 410
  in corticobasal degeneration, 762–763
  deafness dystonia syndrome, 74
  definitions, 541, 896

diagnosis, 503t, 544t
  early-onset, 502–503
  genetic testing, 502–503
  late-onset dystonia, 520–521
  misdiagnosis, 897, 897t
differential diagnosis, 542t–543t
  early-onset dystonia, 503, 827
  late-onset dystonia, 520–521
  myoclonus *vs.*, 658
  psychogenic dystonia, 558, 558t, 897
  tics *vs.*, 686, 695
epidemiology
  adult-onset, 511–512
  early-onset, 496, 504–505, 824
etiology, 495, 516–518, 556–557
  peripheral trauma and, 546–547, 899–901
factors affecting, 502
genetics
  early-onset, 496–499, 505
  late-onset, 517
  phenotype relationship, 501, 501t
hemiparkinsonism-hemiatrophy, 407
historical aspects, 495, 497
"myoclonic," 661
neuroimaging, 52–54, 500, 503
neuropathology
  early-onset, 499, 505
  late-onset, 518–519
pallidonigroluysian degeneration, 413
parkinsonism-plus syndromes, 165
paroxysmal nocturnal, 861–862
pathophysiology
  basal ganglia role, 109, 110, 499–500, 518–519, 544, 545t, 546
  brainstem role, 499, 519–520, 519f, 545, 545t
  early-onset, 499–500, 505
  late-onset, 518–520
  motor cortex, 519
  spinal cord role, 499, 520
  thalamus role, 518, 545, 545t, 546
patient organizations, 536t
primary/idiopathic *see* Primary torsion dystonia (PTD)
pseudopsychogenic, 558, 558t
psychogenic *see* Psychogenic movement disorders (PMDs)
secondary/symptomatic *see* Secondary (symptomatic) dystonia
treatment, 527–539, 528t
  see also individual drugs/treatments
  botulinum toxin, 410, 502, 504, 527, 531–534
  brain stimulation, 504, 527
  early-onset, 504, 535–536
  evaluation, 527
  guidelines, 535–536
  pharmacological, 504, 528–534, 529t
  physical/supportive therapy, 527–528

"sensory tricks," 512, 514–515
 surgical, 110, 504, 534–535
 Wilson's disease, 549, 549f, 779–780
DYT1 gene, 496, 511, 517
 GAG deletion, 498, 501
 genetic testing, 503
 identification, 498
 linkage disequilibrium, 497–498
 myoclonic, 661
 pathophysiological mechanism, 498–499
 phenotype relationship, 501, 501t
 torsin A gene product
  abnormal, 498–499
  normal, 498
DYT6 gene, 517
DYT7 gene, 517
DYT13 gene, 517

E

Eating/drinking, essential tremor assessment, 442–443
Echolalia, 26
Ekbom's syndrome *see* Restless legs syndrome (RLS)
Elderly *see* Aging
Electrochemical gradients, 69
Electroconvulsive therapy (ECT), 320
 progressive supranuclear palsy, 351
Electroencephalography (EEG)
 see also Somatosensory evoked potentials (SEPs)
 corticobasal degeneration, 765
 Huntington's disease, 592
 myoclonus, 669, 670, 673
  back-averaging, 674–675, 674f
  cortical, 660, 670
  EMG correlation, 673, 674f
  negative (asterixis), 676–677
  psychogenic, 903
 periodic leg movements in sleep, 856
 progressive myoclonic epilepsy, 662
 Sydenham's chorea, 638
 tics, 692, 694
Electromyography (EMG)
 cerebellar function, 748–749
 corticobasal degeneration, 765–766
 multisystem atrophy, 365
 myoclonus, 657–658, 658f, 659f, 660, 673
  cortical, 660, 670
  EEG correlation, 673, 674f
  epileptic, 670–671, 671f
  negative, 659f, 676
  non-epileptic, 672
  psychogenic, 903
 primary torsion dystonia, 499
 stiff-person syndrome (SPS), 797, 800, 800f

tremor
 cerebellar, 486, 486f
 cortical, 488
 essential, 435, 438–439, 484f
 orthostatic, 488
 physiological, 481, 482f
 psychogenic, 470, 902
Electron transport chain, 67–69, 68f
 see also Mitochondria
 components, 68–69
 MPP$^+$ effects, 74, 203, 210, 384
 PD gene association studies, 216
Embarrassment, essential tremor assessment, 443
Embryonic cell transplants *see* Fetal cell transplantation
Emotional state, dystonia effects, 502
Employment, essential tremor assessment, 442
Encephalitis, 920
 parkinsonism following *see* Postencephalitic parkinsonism (PEP)
Encephalitis lethargica, 209
 clinical features, 373–374
Encephalopathies
 see also specific disorders
 carbon monoxide poisoning, 387
 childhood chorea, 828
 childhood tremor, 826
 progressive myoclonic, 661–663
  with dementia, 663
  with epilepsy, 662–663
  with epilepsy and dementia, 661–662
 spontaneous myoclonus, 659
 static myoclonic, 663–664
 subacute necrotizing (Leigh's disease), 64, 67
 subcortical arteriosclerotic (Binswanger's disease), 422, 815
Endocrine disorders, 915–916
 see also specific disorders
 cerebellar dysfunction, 728t, 916
 chorea, 642, 644t, 915
 choreoathetosis, 916
 dystonia, 916
 parkinsonism, 424, 916
 tremor, 472, 915
Enkephalin, Parkinson's disease, 201–202
Enovin (artemin/neuroblastin), 137
Entacapone, 251
Entorhinal cortex, histopathology, 148
Enzymes, therapeutic antioxidants, 79–80
Epidermal growth factor (EGF), 141
 Parkinson's disease, 221
Epilepsia partialis continua (EPC), 664, 674f
Epilepsy
 myoclonus, 8, 660, 661–663, 664, 670–671, 670t
 progressive encephalopathies, 661–663
 stiff-person syndrome and, 801

Episodic ataxia type 1, 706t, 710
Episodic ataxia type 2, 706t, 710–711
Epworth Sleepiness Scale (ESS), 873
Ergotism, dystonia, 557, 557f
Erythrocytes, choreoacanthocytosis, 640
Essential myoclonus, 8, 660, 661, 672
Essential tremor (ET), 4, 6, 431–458
    age-association, 431, 433, 436, 844–845
    associated conditions, 439–441, 483
        dystonia, 440
        Klinefelter's syndrome, 441
        nonspecific neurological, 439
        PD relationship, 439–440
        peripheral neuropathies, 440–441
        writer's cramp, 440
    childhood, 825–826
    clinical manifestations, 434–439, 483, 825
        body regions affected, 436, 437, 438
        classification, 435
        cogwheeling, 845
        gait abnormalities, 434–435, 439
        kinetic tremor and, 438
        onset/progression, 436, 844–845
        orthostatic tremor and, 438–439, 488
        postural tremor and, 437, 438, 440
        psychological/behavioral, 435
        resting tremor and, 845
        tremor types, 437–438
        variants, 438–439
        vocal tremor, 437
    clinical rating scales, 442–444
    diagnosis, 437–438
    differential diagnosis
        Parkinson's tremor *vs.*, 240, 433
        primary orthostatic tremor *vs.*, 468, 468t
        primary writing tremor *vs.*, 438
    disability and, 436–437, 845
        assessment, 442–443
        objective quantification, 444
        writing skills, 438, 443, 473
    electromyography, 435, 438–439, 845
    epidemiology, 432–433, 432t, 439, 483
    factors influencing, 436
    familial factors/genetics, 432, 433–434, 825
        linkage studies, 434, 434t
    geniospasm, 826
    historical aspects, 431–432
    pathophysiology, 441–442, 442f, 483–485, 484f
        olivary hypothesis, 484
    shuddering attacks, 826
    treatment, 444–451
        see also specific drugs/treatments
        alcohol, 436, 444
        behavioral, 450–451
        botulinum toxin, 449
        children, 826
        gamma knife thalamotomy, 450
        pharmacological, 445–449, 451, 485, 826
        recommended schedule, 451
        thalamic stimulation, 449–450
        thalamotomy, 441, 449, 484–485
Estazolam, sleep-onset insomnia treatment, 869
Estrogen
    chorea gravidarum, 638
    dopamine receptors and, 397
ET *see* Essential tremor (ET)
Ethical issues, genetic testing in Huntington's
        disease, 580
Ethnic differences, Parkinson's disease epidemiology,
        184–185, 184t
Ethylenediamine tetraacetic acid (EDTA)
    lead poisoning management, 465
    manganese-induced parkinsonism, 386
Evolutionary conservation, huntingtin, 576
Exaggerated startle *see* Hyperekplexia (startle disease)
Excessive daytime somnolence (EDS)
    Parkinson's disease, 871–874
    treatment, 873–874, 873t
Executive dysfunction, 25
    progressive supranuclear palsy, 344
Extrapyramidal disorders, 3
    see also Dyskinesia; Parkinsonism
Extrapyramidal signs
    multisystem atrophy (MSA), 359, 359f, 360, 361–362
    postencephalitic parkinsonism, 374–375
Eye blinking, Parkinson's disease, 238
Eyelid(s)
    blepharospasm *see* Blepharospasm
    postencephalitic parkinsonism, 375
    progressive supranuclear palsy, 346
Eye movements, 747
    see also Oculomotor abnormalities; *specific movements*
    aging and, 842
    autosomal-recessive spastic ataxia of
            Charlevoix-Seguenay, 713
    celiac disease, 922
    cerebellum and, 738, 747
    corticobasal degeneration, 763
    Huntington's disease, 589
    paraneoplastic disorders, 923
    progressive supranuclear palsy, 346
    SCA1, 706
    Whipple's disease, 920

F

Facial dysfunction
    chorea-acanthocytosis (CHAC), 411
    chorea, grimacing, 6
    dystonia, 548

essential tremor and, 439
oromandibular dystonia, 513–514
Parkinson's disease, 238
Facial grimacing, chorea, 6
Facial myoclonus, 664
Factitious disorders, 893, 893t
Fahr's disease *see* Idiopathic calcification of the basal
 ganglia (ICBG)
Familial hyperbetalipoproteinemia, 410
Familial parkinsonism, 163–175, 234t
 classification, 163
 historical background, 164
 molecular genetics
  juvenile phenotype (type IV), 168–170, 170t
  neurodegenerative phenotype (type III), 168, 168t
  PD phenotype (type I), 166–167, 167t, 168t, 178, 204,
   217–218, 217t, 331–333, 332t
  PPS phenotype (type II), 166–167, 169t
 neuropathology, 164
 phenotypic characterization, 164–166
  juvenile phenotype (type IV), 166
  neurodegenerative phenotype (type III), 166
  PD phenotype (type I) *see* Familial Parkinson's disease
  PPS phenotype (type II), 163, 164–165
 risk, 186–187, 187t
Familial Parkinson's disease, 38, 163, 217–218, 331–333, 332t
 see also Genetics
 early-onset, 166, 168–170, 170t
 genetic analysis, 166–167, 167t, 168t, 217t
 historical background, 164
 neurotrophic factors, 135
 oxidative stress and, 75
 risk, 186–187, 187t
 symptoms, 163
Fas/Fas ligands, apoptosis, 221
Fatigue, dystonia effects, 502
Fear, stiff-person (man) syndrome, 798–799
Feeding, essential tremor assessment, 442
Festinating gait, Parkinson's disease, 237
Fetal cell transplantation
 graft rejection, 279, 282
 historical aspects, 275–276
 Huntington's disease, 51
 immunosuppression, 279–280
 MPTP-induced parkinsonism, 384–385
 Parkinson's disease, 46–47, 275–290
  adverse events, 281–282
  approaches, 41
  clinical evaluation, 280–281
  clinical issues, 279–281
  clinical trials, 41–43, 281–283
   double-blind, 282–283
   open-label, 281–282
  donor age effects, 276–277
  drug use after, 281

future directions, 284
implant site, 277–278, 278f
implant volume/distribution, 278–279
limitations, 284
neuroimaging, 41–43, 42f, 280–281, 280f
neuropathology, 281–282, 282f
patient selection, 279
preclinical issues, 276–279
progressive supranuclear palsy, 351
safety issues, 279
suspension *vs.* solid grafts, 277
tissue acquisition, 276
tissue storage, 277, 277f
trophic factors and, 284
xenografts, 283
Fetal tissue acquisition guidelines, 276
Fever
 encephalitis lethargica, 374
 neuroleptic malignant syndrome, 424–425
Fibroblast growth factor receptors (FGFRs), 140–141
Fibroblast growth factors (FGFs), 140–141
 neural transplantation and, 284
 Parkinson's disease, 220
Fine movements, essential tremor assessment, 443
Finger-to-nose test
 cerebellar tremor, 461
 dysmetria, 735
Flash stimulation, reflex myoclonus, 658
Flocculonodular lobe, 744
Fludrocortisone, multisystem atrophy, 368
Fluoxetine
 drug-induced parkinsonism, 399
 Huntington's disease, 594
Fluphenazine, tic treatment, 688
"Fly-catching tongue," 521
Focal dystonias, 7, 516
 see also Primary torsion dystonia (PTD); Secondary
  (symptomatic) dystonia; *individual types*
 classification, 495t
 diagnosis/differential diagnosis, 520–521, 542t-543t,
  544t
 familial, 517
 pathophysiology, 518–520, 544–546, 545t
 primary writing tremor, 472–473, 488
 symptomatic (secondary), 541–546
 treatment, 528t
 X-linked dystonia-parkinsonism syndrome, 410
Focal myoclonus, 664–665
Food-induced tremor, 462–463
Foot dystonia, 515–516
Forebrain, 200–201
Foundation for the Care and Cure of Huntington's
 Disease Inc., 593t
Fragile X syndrome, 713
 cerebellar dysfunction, 722

Fragmentary NREM sleep myoclonus, 861
    Parkinson's disease, 869–870
    treatment, 870
Free radicals
    see also Oxidative stress; Reactive oxygen species
            (ROS)
    aging role, 73–74
    mitochondrial production, 69–70
    Parkinson's disease, 75, 202–203, 218, 218f
    "scavenger" molecules *see* Antioxidants
    smoking and, 211
Free radical scavengers *see* Antioxidants
Freezing gait, 814
    Parkinson's disease, 237, 814
Friedreich's ataxia (FRDA), 711
    molecular genetics, 704, 705t, 711
        phenotype and, 706t
Froment's sign, 11
Frontal gait (*marche à petit pas*), 421, 815, 816t
Frontal lobes
    executive function, 25, 344
    progressive supranuclear palsy, 343–344
    tic pathophysiology, 693–694
Frontal subcortical circuits
    behavior, 17–18, 18f
    executive function, 25
Frontotemporal dementia with parkinsonism linked to
            chromosome 17 (FTDP-17), 12, 404–405
    clinical features, 404
    diagnosis/differential diagnosis, 405
        CBD *vs.*, 762, 769–770
    epidemiology, 404
    molecular genetics, 167, 168, 404
    neuropathology, 156, 404
    PSP and, 349–350
FTDP-17 *see* Frontotemporal dementia with parkinsonism
            linked to chromosome 17 (FTDP-17)
Fumerase deficiency, dystonia in, 555
Fungal infections, parkinsonism, 378

G

GABA, 201
    Huntington's disease, 594, 603, 607, 610
    Parkinson's disease, 201
    tardive dyskinesia, 629
GABAergic drugs
    see also individual drugs
    progressive supranuclear palsy, 351
    side-effects, 631
    tardive dyskinesia, 631–632
GABAergic neurons
    basal ganglia, motor circuitry, 94, 95
    stiff-person syndrome, 799–800

    autoimmunity, 797
    muscle spasm and, 805
Gabapentin
    PLMS and RLS treatment, 859, 859t
    tremor therapy, 447, 469
Gain of function mutations, *huntingtin* (HD) gene, 578, 619
Gait, 811–813
    disorders *see* Gait abnormalities/disorders
    dynamic balance, 812–813
    neural networks, 811–812
        see also Motor control
    normal aging, 840, 841t
    normal cycle, 812f
    senile, 841
Gait abnormalities/disorders, 811–820
    age-related, 840–841, 841t
    analysis, 817
    cerebellar dysfunction, 724
        see also Cerebellar ataxias
    classification, 813, 813t
    common patterns, 813–817
        ataxic *see* Ataxia
        cautious gait, 813–814
        cerebellar gait, 815–816
        dystonic gait, 815
        freezing gait, 237, 814
        frontal gait (*marche à petit pas*), 421, 815, 816t
        stiff-legged gait, 814
    essential tremor, 434–435, 439
    Hallervorden-Spatz disease, 405, 406
    multisystem atrophy, 363
    neuroimaging, 817
    paraneoplastic, 922, 923
    parkinsonism
        age-related, 840–841, 843
        drug-induced, 396
        manganese-induced, 385
        parkinsonian syndromes, 814
        psychogenic, 905
        vascular, 421, 815
    Parkinson's disease, 237, 814
        age-related, 840–841
    primary orthostatic tremor, 467–468
    primary torsion dystonia, 502
    progressive supranuclear palsy, 339
    psychogenic *see* Psychogenic movement
            disorders (PMDs)
    Wilson's disease, 780
Gait analysis, 817
Gait apraxia, 841, 841t
Gait ignition failure, Parkinson's disease (PD), 814
Gametogenesis, Huntington's disease (HD), 574
Gamma-aminobutyric acid *see* GABA
Gamma knife thalamotomy, essential tremor treatment, 450
Gamma-vinyl-GABA, tardive dyskinesia treatment, 631

Gangliosidoses, dystonia in, 552–553, 553f
Gastrointestinal dysfunction
    corticobasal degeneration, 771–772
    Rett syndrome, 415
Gaucher's disease, myoclonus, 662
Gaze
    cerebellum role, 747
    multisystem atrophy, 363
    Parkinson's disease, 238
    postencephalitic parkinsonism, 375
    progressive supranuclear palsy, 346
GDNF see Glial cell line-derived neurotrophic
        factor (GDNF)
Gegenhalten (paratonia), 236, 838, 839t
Gender differences
    essential tremor, 432–433
    Parkinson's disease epidemiology, 184, 184t, 186
    PSP epidemiology, 348
    spasmodic torticollis, 515
Gene mapping
    see also Association studies
    huntingtin (HD) gene, 570–572, 571f
    linkage analysis see Linkage studies
Generalized dystonia, 7
    AIDS, 546f
    classification, 495t
    essential tremor and, 440
    mitochondrial disorders, 554
    treatment, 528t
    Wilson's disease, 549, 549f, 779–780
    X-linked dystonia-parkinsonism syndrome,
        410
Gene therapy in Parkinson's disease, 285
    GDNF expression, 138, 285
Genetic anticipation
    see also Repeat expansion diseases
    essential tremor, 434
    hereditary ataxias, 704, 708, 710
Genetic counseling
    hereditary ataxias, 705
    Huntington's disease, 580
Genetic heterogeneity, essential tremor, 434
Genetics, 13t
    see also specific disorders
    ataxia see Ataxia
    chorea-acanthocytosis, 411
    dementia with Lewy bodies, 408
    dopa-responsive dystonia, 168
    essential tremor, 432, 433–434, 434t
    FTDP-17, 167, 168, 404
    genotype-phenotype relationship, 67, 501, 501t,
        578
    Hallervorden-Spatz disease, 405
    Huntington's disease see Huntington's disease (HD)
    mitochondrial, 64–67, 65f

    see also Mitochondria
    myoclonus, 661
    pallidonigroluysian degeneration, 412
    pallidopyramidal disease, 414
    parkinsonism see Familial parkinsonism
    Parkinson's disease, 163–175, 178, 212, 331–333
        see also Familial Parkinson's disease
        association studies, 212–217, 213t
        familial PD, 166–167, 167t, 168t, 217–218
        mitochondria and, 75, 168t
        PARK genes, 166–167, 167t, 168t, 217–218, 217t, 331–333,
            332t
        parkin (PARK2) mutation, 38, 168–170, 170t, 178, 204,
            216, 217t, 218, 332–333
        risk, 186–187, 187t
        risk/predisposition, 167, 186–187, 187t
        susceptibility gene (PARK3), 167
        a-synuclein (PARK1) mutation, 166, 204, 215–216, 217,
            217t, 331–332
        tau mutation, 167, 216
        twin studies, 38, 187, 212
        ubiquitin hydrolase (PARK5) mutation, 167
    primary torsion dystonia see Primary torsion
        dystonia (PTD)
    progressive supranuclear palsy, 348–349, 349–350
    restless legs syndrome, 857
    Rett syndrome, 415
    Tourette's syndrome, 686, 687
    Wilson's disease, 777–778
    X-linked dystonia-parkinsonism syndrome, 409
Genetic testing/screening
    ataxias, 704, 705f, 705t
    FTDP-17, 156
    Parkinson's disease, 178
    predictive, Huntington's disease, 579–581, 592
    primary torsion dystonia, 502–503
    Wilson's disease, impracticality, 782–783
Geniospasm, 826
Genitourinary dysfunction
    see also Bladder dysfunction
    multisystem atrophy, 362–363
    Parkinson's disease, 238
    progressive supranuclear palsy, 347
Genotype-phenotype relationship
    dystonias, 501, 501t
    huntingtin (HD) gene, 578
    mitochondrial function, 67
Genotyping, huntingtin (HD) gene mapping, 571
Geographic factors
    Parkinson's disease, 181t-183t, 185–186, 210
    progressive supranuclear palsy, 349
"Geste antagonistique", 514–515
Glabellar reflex
    aging and, 842
    Parkinson's disease, 238

Glial cell line-derived neurotrophic factor (GDNF), 135–136
  developmental expression, 136
  dopaminergic effects, 135–136
  neural transplantation and, 284
  Parkinson's disease etiology, 220
  Parkinson's disease treatment, 136, 284
    direct infusion, 43, 137–138
    gene therapy, 138, 285
    progenitor cell proliferation, 138–139
  related molecules, 136–137
Glial cytoplasmic inclusions (GCI)
  astrocytic plaques *vs.*, 768
  MSA, 152–153, 152f, 365, 366f
Glia, progressive supranuclear palsy, 153
Gliosis
  Huntington's disease (HD), 601, 606, 610
  progressive subcortical, 49
Globus pallidus, 93, 117–118
  carbon monoxide poisoning, 387
  cholinergic innervation, 121, 122, 123
  cyanide poisoning, 388
  dopamine, 118
  dystonia, 499–500, 550
  glutamatergic innervation, 125f
  gross examination, 148
  Hallervorden-Spatz disease, 405
  Huntington's disease, 109, 603, 606, 607f
  motor circuitry, 95, 95f, 96
  pallidonigroluysian degeneration, 412–413
  pallidotomy
    dystonia treatment, 110, 504, 534
    Parkinson's disease treatment, 48
  Parkinson's disease, 48, 201, 203–204
  postpump chorea, 642–643
  progressive supranuclear palsy, 153, 153f, 154f, 345
  serotonergic innervation, 127
  sleep role, 878, 878f
  stimulation
    dystonia treatment, 504, 534–535
    PD treatment, 48
Glutamate
  see also Glutamatergic neurons
  Huntington's disease, 608, 610, 613, 614
  mitochondrial dysfunction, 70, 73
    therapeutic target, 77
  Parkinson's disease, 221, 257–258
  receptors *see* Glutamate receptors
  tardive dyskinesia, 628
Glutamate receptors
  see also individual types
  antagonists, 77, 78, 257–258
    side-effects, 258
  basal ganglia distribution, 122f, 124–126, 125f, 126f, 126t
  functions, 126–127

hypothalamus, Huntington's disease, 608
  types, 124
Glutamatergic neurons
  basal ganglia, 123–127, 257
    cortical projections to, 608
    source, 123–124
  corticospinal tracts, 90
Glutamic acid decarboxylase (GAD)
  gene therapy, 285
  Parkinson's disease, 201
Glutaric aciduria type I, dystonia, 554–555
Glutaryl-CoA dehydrogenase deficiency, 554–555
Glutathione and GPX system
  cellular antioxidant system, 72, 72f
  Parkinson's disease, 215, 219
Glutathione S-transferase, PD gene association studies, 215
Gluten ataxia, 703–704, 922
Gowers, W.R., 892, 901
G protein-coupled receptors (GPCRs)
  dopamine, 119, 120t
  metabotropic glutamate receptors, 124
  muscarinic acetylcholine receptors (nAChRs), 121
  serotonin receptors, 127
Granule cells, cerebellar, 744, 745
Grumose degeneration, progressive supranuclear palsy, 153, 343
GTPCH I mutation
  dopa-responsive dystonia, 505
  familial parkinsonism genetics, 168
Guam, parkinsonism-dementia/ALS complex of, 29, 209, 463
Guanfacine
  ADHD treatment, 688
  tic treatment, 688

H

Hallervorden-Spatz disease, 405–406, 549–550
  clinical features, 406
    dementia in, 29
    dystonia, 549–550, 550f
  diagnosis/differential diagnosis, 406
    Parkinson's disease *vs.*, 240
  genetics, 405
  neuroimaging, 406
  neuropathology, 405
    gross examination, 148
Hallucinations, 21
  drug-induced, 242, 252, 262
  Parkinson's disease, 322
Haloperidol, tic treatment, 688
Hands, essential tremor, 436
Haplotype analysis, *huntingtin* (HD) gene identification, 572–573, 573f
Hartnup disease, dystonia in, 555

HD *see* Huntington's disease (HD)
Head
    abnormal posture, cerebellar dysfunction, 724
    essential tremor, 436, 845
Head banging, nocturnal *(jactatio capitis nocturna)*, 862
Head, Henry, 891, 892
Head injury *see* Brain, injury
HEAT motifs, huntingtin structure, 576–577
Heavy metals
    cerebellar dysfunction, 728t
    dystonia, 557
    Parkinson's disease, 188, 209
    tremor induction, 465–466
Heel-to-shin test, cerebellar tremor, 461
Hemiballismus
    aging and, 846
    basal ganglia role, 109, 109f, 846
    HIV infection, 377
    sleep disturbance, 874
    vascular, 641, 846
Hemichorea, vascular, 641
Hemidystonia, 7
    aging and, 846
    cerebral palsy, 545f
    pallidonigroluysian degeneration, 413
    putamen lesion, 545f
    stroke-associated, 846
Hemifacial spasm (HS), 11
    sleep disturbance, 874
Hemiparesis, psychogenic gait, 906
Hemiparkinsonism-hemiatrophy (HPHA), 242, 407–408
Hemolytic anemia, Wilson's disease, 782
Hemolytic-uremic syndrome, 920–921
Hepatic dysfunction *see* Liver
Hepatitis, Wilson's disease, 779
Hereditary Disease Foundation, 593t
Hereditary hemochromatosis, tremor, 472
Hereditary motor sensory neuropathy (HMSN), tremor,
        440–441, 469
Herpes simplex virus, Parkinson's disease etiology, 209
Heteroplasmy, mtDNA mutations, 66–67
Hexosaminidase deficiency, 552–553
Hippocampus
    declarative memory, 25
    gross examination, 147–148
    histopathology, 148
    Parkinson's disease, 201
    progressive supranuclear palsy, 344
Histopathology, 148–149
Histrionic personality disorder, 893, 893t
HIV infection/AIDS, 919–920
    encephalopathy, 377
    parkinsonism, 377–378, 919–920
    paroxysmal dyskinesia, 920
    tremor, 464, 472

Hodgkin's disease, 923
Hoehn and Yahr Staging Scale, Parkinson's disease, 243
Holmes' midbrain tremor, 466–467, 467t
    pathophysiology, 486–487
Homocystinuria, 918
    dystonia in, 555, 918
Homoplasmy, mtDNA mutations, 66
Homovanillic acid (HVA)
    dopa-responsive dystonia, 505
    Parkinson's disease, 199, 199t
    primary torsion dystonia, 499
    synthesis, 199f
Homunculi, cerebellar, 742, 742f, 743f
5–HTP, myoclonus management, 665
Huntingtin, 614
    abnormal function, 578
        aberrant interactions, 615, 618–619
        CAG repeat length and, 616–617
        conformational changes, 578–579, 614
        neuronal aggregation, 579, 614–618, 617f, 618f
        in vitro studies, 617–618
    evolutionary conservation, 576
    gene *see Huntingtin* (HD) gene
    normal function, 576, 614
        protein interactions, 618–619
    structure, 576–577
Huntingtin (HD) gene
    CAG repeats, 50, 75, 76, 573–574, 574f, 601
        clinical correlation, 574–576, 575f, 576f, 581, 588,
            588f
        cumulative distribution, 574, 574f
        gain of function, 578, 619
        huntingtin aggregation and, 616–617
    expression
        distribution, 576–577, 614
        levels, 578
    genetic testing, 579–581
    identification in HD, 569–585, 587
        chromosome 4 location, 570, 571, 571f, 601
        DNA markers, 570, 571, 571f, 572
        genetic/physical mapping, 570–572, 571f
        haplotype analysis, 572–573, 573f
        linkage analysis, 569–570, 570f
        problems, 572
        therapeutic consequences, 581
    penetrance, 569
    transgenic mice, 578, 579, 604, 618
Huntington-like disorders
    clinical features, dystonia, 548
    Wolf-Hirschhorn syndrome, 571
Huntington's disease (HD), 587–599, 601
    animal models, 76
        3–NP injection, 614, 615f, 616t
        neuroprotection in, 613
        transgenic mice, 578, 579, 604, 618

Huntington's disease (HD) *(continued)*
  clinical features, 588–591, 601
    cognitive, 589–590
    in "at risk" patients, 589
    executive function, 25
    memory impairment, 25, 589
    speech/language, 26
    visuospatial, 27
    dementia, 28, 589
    functional decline, 590–591, 591f
    movement, 588–589, 606–607
      chorea, 588
      dysarthria/dysphagia, 589
      dystonia, 548, 589
      myoclonus, 663
      oculomotor abnormalities, 589
      other hyperkinesias, 589
      parkinsonism, 589
    myoclonus in, 660
    neuropsychiatric, 590
      anxiety, 23
      depression, 20, 590
      mania, 20–21
      obsessive-compulsive, 590
      personality changes, 22
      psychosis, 21, 590, 594
      sexual disturbances, 24
      sleep disturbance, 590, 874
    terminal, 589
    variation, 575
  diagnosis, 575, 591–592
    family history, 591–592
    molecular, 580, 580f, 592
  differential diagnosis, 592
    chorea-acanthocytosis *vs.*, 412, 592
    denatorubropallidoluysian atrophy *vs.*, 592
    Parkinson's disease *vs.*, 240
  epidemiology, 569, 587
  genetic counseling, 580
  genetics, 50, 75, 76, 569–585, 587
    see also Huntingtin (HD) gene
    candidate genes, 573
    gametogenesis, 574
    idealized pedigree, 570f
    mouse models, 579
    sporadic mutations, 575
  historical perspective, 569, 587, 592–593
  juvenile, 569, 575–576, 587
  late-onset, 641
  natural history, 569, 587–588
    CAG repeat length and, 574–576, 575f, 576f, 581, 588, 588f
  neurochemistry, 603–605, 607, 608, 610
    GABA, 594, 603, 607, 610
    glutamate, 608, 610, 613, 614

    neuropeptides, 605
  neuroimaging, 50–51, 52f, 611–613, 611f, 612f, 613f
    see also specific techniques
  neuropathology, 50, 109, 575, 601–613
    see also specific regions
    brainstem, 611
    CAG repeats and, 609
    cerebellum, 610–611, 611f
    cortical, 602f, 608–610, 610f, 611, 611f
    gliosis, 601, 606, 610
    globus pallidus, 109, 603, 606, 607f
    grading, 601, 602f
    hypothalamus, 608
    striatum, 601–606, 602f, 603f, 604f, 605f, 606f, 607f, 611
    substantia nigra, 606–607, 608f
    subthalamic, 608
    thalamus, 607–608
  pathophysiology, 50, 75, 578–579, 613–619
    see also Huntingtin
    excitotoxicity, 613, 614
    mitochondrial dysfunction, 51, 75–77, 613–614
  patient groups/organizations, 593t
  predictive genetic testing, 579–581, 580f, 592
  suicide risk, 590
  treatment, 592–594
    antioxidants, 78, 79, 594
    antiparkinsonian/antichoreic, 593
    antipsychotic, 594
    experimental, 594
    fetal transplantation, 51, 594
    prospects, 581
    psychosocial, 593
    replacement strategies, 594
    symptomatic, 592–593
Huntington's Disease Society of America, 593t
Huntington's Disease Society of Canada, 593t
Hydrocarbons, Parkinson's disease etiology, 211
Hydrocephalus
  normal pressure, 423
    Parkinson's disease *vs.*, 241
  obstructive, 424
  parkinsonism, 241, 423
5–Hydroxytryptamine (5–HT) *see* Serotonin
Hygiene
  essential tremor assessment, 443
  sleep, Parkinson's disease, 871
Hyperammonemia, Rett syndrome, 416
Hyperbilirubinemia, 917
Hyperekplexia (startle disease), 11, 665, 672, 686, 695
  tics and, 696–697
Hyperkinetic disorders, 3–11, 837
  see also individual disorders
  aging and, 839–840
  basal ganglia role, 109–110, 109f
  diagnostic characteristics, 4

dystonia in, 548–549
  HIV-related, 377
  psychogenic, 896–905
  tics *vs.*, 695, 695t
Hyperlordosis, stiff-person (man) syndrome, 798
Hypermetabolism, choreas, 639
Hypermetria, cerebellar dysfunction, 725, 735
Hypersexuality, 24
Hypersomnia, 24
Hyperthyroidism
  chorea, 642, 915
  tremor, 472, 915
Hypertonia, 838
  see also Dystonia; Rigidity; Spasticity
Hypnic jerk, 671, 856
Hypobetalipoproteinemia, dystonia, 548
Hypokinetic disorders, 3, 11–12, 837–842
  see also individual disorders
  aging and, 837–838, 838t
  basal ganglia role, 106–108, 107f
  dystonia in, 547–548
Hypometria, cerebellar dysfunction, 725, 735
Hypoparathyroidism, 916
  dystonia, 916
  parkinsonism, 424, 916
Hypotension
  orthostatic, Parkinson's disease, 243
  tremor, 472
Hypothyroidism, 916
  ataxia, 916
  tremor, 472
Hypotonia
  cerebellar dysfunction, 726, 737, 738f
  multisystem atrophy, 363
Hypoxanthine-guanine phosphoribosyl transferase
    (HGPRT) deficiency, 555
Hypoxia
  ischemic damage, postpump chorea, 642
  tremor, 472
Hysteria *see* Psychogenic movement disorders (PMDs)

I

Ideational apraxia, 763
Ideomotor apraxia, 27, 763
Idiopathic calcification of the basal ganglia (ICBG), 13t
  dementia in, 29
  dystonia, 550
  neuropsychiatric aspects, 20, 21
  parkinsonism, 424
Idiopathic (essential) myoclonus, 8, 660, 661, 672
Idiopathic orthostatic hypotension, MSA and, 359f
Idiopathic parkinsonism *see* Parkinson's disease (PD)
Idiopathic torsion dystonia (ITD) *see* Primary torsion
    dystonia (PTD)

Immobilization, dystonia treatment, 527
Immune system
  see also Autoimmune disease
  chorea pathophysiology, 639
  postencephalitic parkinsonism, 375
  suppression *see* Immunosuppression
  tics and, 697
Immunohistochemistry, 148
  corticobasal degeneration, 155f
  Huntington's disease, 603–605, 603f
Immunosuppression
  fetal cell transplantation, 279–280
  stiff-person syndrome treatment, 808
  tremor induction, 464
Incertohypothalamic system, 198
Inclusion bodies
  see also Synucleinopathies; Tauopathies; *specific inclusions*
  cell death and, 204
  corticobasal degeneration, 768, 768f
  Huntington's disease, 50, 616–617
  intraneuronal inclusion disease, 550
  multisystem atrophy, 152–153, 365, 366f
  Parkinson's disease, 149–150, 150f, 201, 204–205, 330
  triplet expansion diseases, 617
Infantile neuroaxonal dystrophy (INAD), 549–550
Infection, 918–921
  see also specific infections
  cerebellar dysfunction, 728t
  chorea and, 637, 639, 644t, 918–919
  fetal cell transplantation, 279
  parkinsonism, 373–382
    bacterial, 378
    fungal/parasitic, 378
    non-encephalitic viral, 376–378
    postencephalitic *see* Postencephalitic
      parkinsonism (PEP)
    prion disease, 378–379
  Parkinson's disease etiology, 188–189, 209
  tics and, 686, 697
Inflammatory responses, postencephalitic parkinsonism, 375
Influenza virus
  encephalitis lethargica, 374
  Parkinson's disease etiology, 209
Inherited myoclonus-dystonia (IMD), 661
Insomnia, 24
  Parkinson's disease, 869
Insulin, trophic effects, 141
Intention tremor *see* Kinetic tremor
Interleukins, Parkinson's disease, 220
  gene association studies, 215
International Huntington Association (IHA), 593t
  genetic testing, 580, 592
Interneurons
  Huntington's disease, 604, 604f
  striatal motor circuitry, 94

Intraneuronal inclusion disease, dystonia, 550
Intrathecal baclofen (ITB), dystonia treatment, 504, 530–531
Intravenous immunoglobulin (IVIg), stiff-person syndrome
    treatment, 808
Involuntary movement disorders
    tics, 692
Iron
    Hallervorden-Spatz disease, 405
    metabolism, Parkinson's disease, 188, 202, 218

J

"Jack-in-the-box tongue," chorea, 6
Jactatio capitis nocturna (nocturnal head banging), 862
Japanese encephalitis, post-infection parkinsonism, 376–377
"Jerking stiff-man syndrome," 801
Jewish populations
    GM2 gangliosidosis, 552–553
    primary torsion dystonia, 496, 497
Joint disease, Wilson's disease, 781–782
Jumping Frenchmen of Maine, 903–904
Juvenile familial parkinsonism, 166, 830
    molecular genetics, 168–170

K

Kayser-Fleischer rings, Wilson's disease, 781, 783t, 784
Kelley-Seegmiller syndrome, dystonia in, 555
Kepone (chlordecone), toxin-induced tremor, 466
Kernicterus, 917
Kinesia paradoxica, Parkinson's disease, 237
Kinetic tremor, 4, 6, 240, 485–486, 488, 736
    cerebellar, 461, 485–486, 736–737, 739
    childhood, 825
    definition, 459
    essential tremor and, 437, 438
    multisystem atrophy, 363
    myoclonus *vs.*, 657
Klinefelter's syndrome, essential tremor and, 441
Kufor-Rakeb syndrome, 413
Kufs' disease, myoclonic encephalopathies, 661
Kwashiorkor, 917
Kyphosis, Parkinson's disease, 238

L

Lafora's disease, myoclonus, 661, 662
Lance-Adams syndrome, myoclonus, 9
Language disturbance, 26
    see also Speech/speech disorders
L-aromatic amino acid decarboxylase (L-AAD)
    dopamine metabolism, 198, 199f

Parkinson's disease changes, 199–200, 200t
Laryngeal dystonia *see* Spasmodic dysphonia (laryngeal
    dystonia)
Latah, 903–904
Lateral orbitofrontal circuit, behavior role, 18, 18f
L-dopa *see* Levodopa (L-dopa)
Lead pipe rigidity, 11, 236
Lead poisoning, tremor, 465–466
Learning, cerebellum and motor learning, 721–722
Leber's hereditary optic neuropathy (LHON), 67, 554
Leigh's disease, 64, 67, 714
    dystonia, 554
Lenticular nuclei, MSA, 152f
Lentiviral vectors, GDNF expression in PD, 138
Lesch-Nyhan syndrome, dystonia in, 555
Leukocytosis, neuroleptic malignant syndrome, 425
Leukodystrophy, metachromatic, 553
Levetiracetam, myoclonus management, 665
Levodopa (L-dopa)
    carbon monoxide poisoning, 387
    current indications, 248–249
    cyanide poisoning, 388
    dementia with Lewy bodies, 409
    dopamine agonists and, 249, 253
    dystonia responsive to *see* Dopa-responsive dystonia
    enzyme inhibitor co-administration, 247–248, 251, 261
    fluctuations (on-off phenomena), 43–44, 242, 249–250
        management, 260–261, 261t
    hemiparkinsonism-hemiatrophy, 408
    HIV-related parkinsonism, 377–378
    Huntington's disease treatment, 593
    mechanism of action, 248
    metabolism, 247, 248f
    methanol poisoning, 389
    motor symptom control, 260
    MSA and, 362, 367
    pallidonigroluysian degeneration, 413
    pallidopyramidal disease, 414
    Parkinson's disease treatment, 199, 247–251
        post-fetal transplantation, 281
    pharmacokinetics, 247–248, 248t
    PLMS and RLS treatment, 859, 859t
    postencephalitic parkinsonism, 376
    preparations, 249t
        new pharmacokinetic, 251
        slow release, 250–251
    progressive supranuclear palsy, 350
    REM sleep behavior disorder treatment, 861
    side-effects, 249–250, 249t, 260
        dyskinesia *see* Levodopa-induced dyskinesia
        dystonia, 110, 250, 547, 556
        nausea/vomiting, 249
        sleep disorders, 321, 869–870
    X-linked dystonia-parkinsonism syndrome, 410

Levodopa-induced dyskinesia, 43–44, 45f, 242, 250, 250t, 258, 261, 261t
  management, 261, 261t
  neuroimaging, 43–44, 44, 45f
  NMDA role, 258
Lewy bodies, 327–328
  apolipoprotein E ε4 link, 157
  dementia with *see* Dementia with Lewy bodies (DLB)
  Marinesco bodies *vs.*, 328
  occurrence, 329
  parkinsonism-plus syndrome, 164
  Parkinson's disease, 149–150, 150f, 201, 327–329, 423, 844
    see also α-Synuclein
    distribution, 328–329, 329f, 329t
    midbrain, 328f
    neurochemical analysis, 204–205
    postencephalitic parkinsonism, 375
    progressive supranuclear palsy, 154
Limb dystonia, 515–516
  botulinum toxin, 533–534
  essential tremor and, 440
Limbic system, tic pathophysiology, 693
Limb kinetic apraxia, 763
Limb myoclonus, 664
Lincoln ataxia (SCA5), 705t, 706t, 708
Linkage disequilibrium
  DYT1 gene, 497–498
  huntingtin (HD) gene, 574
Linkage studies
  dystonia
    adult-onset, 517
    early-onset, 497–498
  essential tremor, 434, 434t
  Huntington's disease, 569–570
  paroxysmal dyskinesias, 645
  spinocerebellar ataxia type 4, 708
Lipid metabolism disorders, dystonia and, 552–554
Lipid peroxidation, 71, 74
Lipofuscin
  age-effects, 74
  Huntington's disease, 76
  myoclonic encephalopathies, 661
Lisuride, pharmacology, 235t, 254
Lithium
  drug-induced parkinsonism, 399
  tremor induction, 463
Liver
  failure, 779, 917
  toxicity, COMT inhibitors, 252
  Wilson's disease, 778–779, 778t, 788
    biopsy, 783, 783t
    transplantation, 788–789
Locomotion *see* Gait
Locus ceruleus
  norepinephrine efferents, 200

progressive supranuclear palsy, 345
Lodosyn *see* Carbidopa (Lodosyn)
Long-term depression (LTD)
  cerebellar, 745
  dopamine role, 97
  glutamate receptors, 126, 127
Long-term potentiation (LTP)
  dopamine role, 97
  glutamate receptors, 126, 127
Lorazepam
  dystonia treatment, 530
  X-linked dystonia-parkinsonism syndrome, 410
"Lower body parkinsonism" *see* Vascular parkinsonism
Lubag syndrome (X-linked dystonia-parkinsonism), 409–410
Lyme disease, 919
Lymphomas, 923

M

Machado-Joseph disease (SCA3)
  clinical features, 708
    dystonia, 551
    sleep disorders, 24
  molecular genetics, 705t, 706t, 707–708
    repeat expansion, 708
  Parkinson's disease *vs.*, 240
  phenotypic variability, 707
Madopar CR, 250, 251
Magnetic resonance imaging (MRI), 14t, 35
  ataxia telangiectasia, 552f
  chorea-acanthocytosis, 412
  corticobasal degeneration, 764–765
  dystonia
    primary, 503
    symptomatic (secondary), 544t
    X-linked dystonia-parkinsonism syndrome, 410
  gait disorders, 817
  Huntington's disease, 611–612, 611f, 612f, 613
  hyperintense basal ganglia, 13t
  hypointense basal ganglia, 13t
  mitochondrial disorders, 554
  multisystem atrophy, 35f, 364, 364f
  pallidonigroluysian degeneration, 413
  pallidopyramidal disease, 414
  parkinsonism
    hemiparkinsonism-hemiatrophy (HPHA), 408
    vascular, 422
    X-linked dystonia-parkinsonism syndrome, 410
  postpump chorea, 642
  progressive supranuclear palsy, 341–342, 342t
  Rett syndrome, 416
  Sydenham's chorea, 638
  systemic lupus erythematosus, 639

Magnetic resonance imaging (MRI) *(continued)*
  tremor
    palatal, 469
    stroke-associated, 471
  Wilson's disease, 549, 785
Magnetic resonance spectroscopy (MRS), 36
  corticobasal degeneration, 765
  focal dystonia, 518–519
  gait disorders, 817
  Huntington's disease, 612, 612f
  multisystem atrophy, 48, 365
Magnetoencephalography (MEG), myoclonus
      studies, 676
Malabsorption syndromes, 917
Malignancy, 922–923
  see also specific types
  ataxia telangiectasia and, 711, 712
  cerebellar dysfunction, 727t
  chorea and, 645t
  parkinsonism, 424
Malingering, 893, 893t
  psychogenic dystonia, 557
Malondialdehyde, Parkinson's disease, 219
Manganese exposure
  dystonia, 557
  neuropathology, 385
  neuropsychiatric disturbances, 385
  parkinsonism, 188, 209, 385–386
  toxicity mechanism, 386
  treatment, 386
  tremor, 465
Mania, 20–21, 20t
Mannheim Cohort project, 893–894
Marche à petit pas (frontal gait), 421, 815
  ataxia *vs.*, 816t
Marinesco bodies, 328
Masked facies, Parkinson's disease, 238
Masseter muscle, nocturnal bruxism, 862
Mastocytosis, chorea, 918
Maternal mitochondrial inheritance, 64
McLeod syndrome, 410, 639–640
  dystonia, 548–549
Mechanical-reflex oscillation
  cerebellar tremor, 485, 486f
  essential tremor, 483–484, 484f
  physiological tremor, 481, 482f
Medium spiny neurons (MSNs)
  Huntington's disease, 603–605, 603f
    dendritic changes, 605f
  striatal motor circuitry, 94, 117, 122
  subpopulations, 603
Meige's syndrome, 513, 518, 921
  Parkinson's disease and, 547
Melanocyte-stimulating hormone-release-inhibiting factor
      (MIF), Parkinson's disease, 209

Melanophagia, Parkinson's disease, 327, 328f
Memory impairment, 25–26
  corticobasal degeneration, 764
  essential tremor, 435
  Huntington's disease, 25, 589
  Parkinson's disease, 25
Menkes' disease, ceruloplasmin deficiency, 778
Mephenesin, essential tremor therapy, 448
Mercury, Parkinson's disease risk factors, 188
Mercury poisoning
  dystonia, 557
  tremor, 465
MERRF *see* Myoclonic epilepsy with ragged-red fibers
      (MERRF)
Mesencephalic areas, progressive supranuclear palsy,
      345–346
Mesencephalic locomotor region (MLR), 811
Mesocortical system, 198
Mesotenecephalic dopamine group, 198
Metabolic disorders, 916–918
  see also Nutritional deficiency; *specific disorders*
  amino acid metabolism, 554–555
  ataxia and, 713
  chorea and, 642, 644t
  dystonia in, 552–555, 827, 918t
  Huntington's disease and, 75
  lipid metabolism disorders, 552–554
  mitochondrial *see* Mitochondrial dysfunction
  myoclonus, 662
  purine metabolism, 555
  tremor, 916–917
Metabotropic glutamate receptors (mGlurRs), 124
  basal ganglia distribution, 125–126, 126t
  functions, 127
Metachromatic leukodystrophy, dystonia, 553
Methanol, dystonia, 557
Methazolamide, essential tremor therapy, 447
1–Methyl-4–phenyl-1,2,3,6–tetrahydropyridine *see* MPTP
1–Methyl-4–phenylpyridinium *see* MPP$^+$
Methyl-CpG-binding protein (MeCP2), Rett syndrome,
      415, 550
α-Methyldopa, in drug-induced parkinsonism, 399
Methyl ethyl ketone, toxin-induced tremor, 466
Methylmalonic aciduria, dystonia in, 555
Methylmalonyl-CoA mutase mutations, 555
S-Methyltransferase, Parkinson's disease genetics, 213
Methysergide, fragmentary nocturnal myoclonus
      treatment, 870
Metoclopramide
  extrapyramidal side-effects, 396, 397
  side-effects, tardive dyskinesia, 627
  tremor induction, 464
Metoprolol, essential tremor therapy, 445
Mexiletine, dystonia treatment, 504
Microaggregates, huntingtin, 618, 618f

Microglial activation, Parkinson's disease (PD), 38–39
β2–Microglobulin, Parkinson's disease, 220
Microvascular decompression, dystonia treatment, 535
Midbrain
    gross examination, 148, 328f
    Parkinson's disease, 328f
    posttraumatic parkinsonism, 422–423
    posttraumatic tremor, 473
    tremor, 473
        Holmes', 466–467, 467t, 486–487
        stroke-induced, 487
Midodrine, multisystem atrophy, 368
MIF, Parkinson's disease etiology, 209
"Milkmaid grip," chorea, 6
Minipolymyoclonus, 671
Minocycline, 77
Mirtazapine, essential tremor therapy, 447
Mitochondria, 63–70
    age-effects, 73–74
    DNA *see* Mitochondrial genome (mtDNA)
    dysfunction *see* Mitochondrial dysfunction
    functions, 63–64, 69
        age-effects, 73
        apoptosis role, 69, 70
        calcium regulation, 70, 73
        oxidative phosphorylation *see* Oxidative
            phosphorylation
    oxidative damage, 71–72
    reactive oxygen species production, 69–70, 71
    structure, 63–64, 64f
    PT pore, 71, 76
Mitochondrial dysfunction, 63–88
    see also specific conditions
    ataxias and, 74, 713–714
    consequences, 70–73, 76
        see also Oxidative stress
        abnormal apoptosis, 70–71
        calcium dysregulation, 73
        decreased ATP synthesis, 70
        oxidative stress, 71–72
        PT pore and, 71, 76
    dystonia and, 554
    manganese toxicity, 386
    in movement disorders, 63, 74–77
        Huntington's disease, 51, 75–77, 613–614
        Parkinson's disease, 74–75, 203, 218
        progressive supranuclear palsy, 349
    MPTP/MPP$^+$ toxicity, 74, 203, 210, 384
    mtDNA mutation *see* Mitochondrial genome
        (mtDNA)
    myoclonus and, 661, 662–663
    therapeutics, 77–80
Mitochondrial genome (mtDNA), 63, 64–67, 65f
    genotype, 67
    inheritance, 64

mutations
    acquired, 64, 66
    ataxias, 713–714
    deletions, 76
    genotype to phenotype conversion, 67
    heteroplasmy, 66–67
    homoplasmy, 66
    inherited, 64
    multiple processes, 67
    somatic, 73
    threshold effects, 67
    PD gene association studies, 217
Mitochondrial mutation rate, 66
Mitochondrial respiratory chain, 67–69, 68f
Mobility aids, ataxias, 705
Moclobenide, 262
Mohr-Tranebjaerg syndrome, 554
Monoamine oxidase (MAO), 211f
    dopamine metabolism, 198, 199f
    inhibitors, tremor induction, 463
    MAO-A
        inhibitors, 262
        Parkinson's disease association, 213
    MAO-B
        inhibition by cigarette smoke, 211
        inhibitors, 252–253, 260, 262
        Parkinson's disease association, 213–214
    Parkinson's disease changes, 200, 200t
Morphine, dystonia treatment, 531
Morphometric studies, tic pathophysiology, 693
Mossy fibers, 744
Motor abnormalities
    block, Parkinson's disease, 237
    cerebellar, alpha *vs.* gamma motor systems, 739, 748–749
    dystonia, 499, 519–520
Motor assessment, post-fetal transplantation in PD, 280
Motor control
    see also Basal ganglia, motor circuits; Cerebellum; Motor
        system; Movement
    basal ganglia, 104
    cerebellar
        alpha motor systems, 739, 748–749
        feedback, 751
        feedforward, 750–751
        gamma motor systems, 739, 749–750
        temporal aspects, 751–752
        trajectory, 735–736, 736f
    PD pathophysiology, 236
Motor cortex, 90
    dystonia pathophysiology, 519
    functional anatomy, 91f, 92
    Huntington's disease, 610f
    in Parkinson's disease, 46, 47f
    primary torsion dystonia, 53
    tremor pathophysiology, 483, 483f

Motor learning, cerebellar control, 721–722, 751
Motor neurons, cerebellar control, 726
Motor performance, normal aging, 838
Motor planning, cerebellum role, 722
Motor signs
    FTDP-17, 404
    Parkinson's disease, 201, 234, 259–260
    progressive supranuclear palsy, 344
Motor system
    see also Basal ganglia, motor circuits; *specific components*
    component relationships, 89f
    cortical areas, 90–93, 91f
        see also Motor cortex; Premotor cortex
        association areas, cerebellar connections, 722
    functional anatomy, 89–102
    pathways
        corticospinal tracts, 90–92
        descending, 89, 89f, 812
        dystonia physiology, 499–500
        tremor physiology, 482–483, 483f
Motor tics, 9, 683–684, 683t, 686, 687, 691, 824
    clonic, 691
    complex, 9, 683, 692t
    drug-induced, 627, 687, 697
    dystonic, 686
    simple, 9, 683, 692t
    voluntary *vs.* involuntary, 692
Motor tremor *see* Kinetic tremor
Movement
    see also Motor system
    abnormal, 3, 725
    cerebellar control, 721, 725
    control *see* Motor control
    coordination, 750–751
    discontinuity/decomposition, 461, 725, 735–736, 736f, 738
    disorders *see* Movement disorders
    during normal sleep, 855–856
    sequential, control, 93, 104
    voluntary, rCBF, 92
Movement disorders, 3–16, 837
    see also individual disorders
    aging and *see* Aging
    childhood *see* Childhood movement disorders
    definition, 3
    diagnosis, 147
    genetics *see* Genetics
    HIV-related, 377–378
    hyperkinetic *see* Hyperkinetic disorders
    hypokinetic *see* Hypokinetic disorders
    imaging *see* Neuroimaging
    involuntary, 50–54, 411, 521
    neurobehavioral aspects *see* Neurobehavioral changes
    neuropathology *see* Neuropathology
    overlapping signs, 3, 4t
    patient approach, 5t, 12, 13t, 14t
    psychiatric/psychological comorbidity, 897
    psychogenic *see* Psychogenic movement disorders (PMDs)
    psychosocial aspects, 17
Movement Disorders Clinic of the Toronto Western Hospital, 894
MPP+, 74, 203, 210, 384
    structure, 211f
MPTP, 383
    metabolism, 210, 384
    parkinsonism *see* MPTP-induced parkinsonism
    related compounds, 211f
    structure, 211f
MPTP-induced parkinsonism, 188, 197, 209, 210, 331, 383–385
    clinical features, 383–384, 389t
    free radical generation, 202
    mitochondrial dysfunction, 74, 203
    neuropathology, 384
    treatment, 384–385
        fetal transplants, 384–385
        levodopa (L-dopa) response, 384
MRI *see* Magnetic resonance imaging (MRI)
MRS *see* Magnetic resonance spectroscopy (MRS)
MSA *see* Multisystem atrophy (MSA)
Multifocal dystonia, 7
    classification, 495t
Multiple sclerosis, chorea, 642
Multisystem atrophy (MSA), 12, 234t, 359–369
    see also Olivopontocerebellar atrophy (OPCA); Shy-Drager syndrome (SDS); Striatonigral degeneration (SND); *specific syndromes*
    clinical diagnosis, 360–363
        autonomic failure, 360, 362–363
        cerebellar dysfunction, 360, 363
        cognitive/behavioral signs, 363
        criteria, 360–361, 361t
        extrapyramidal signs, 359, 360, 361–362
        pyramidal signs, 360, 363
    clinical features, 48, 360, 361t, 771t
        dystonia, 548
        orthostatic hypotension, 359–360, 362
        overlapping symptoms/signs, 359f
        parkinsonism, 360
    differential diagnosis, 365, 367, 367t, 771t
        CBD *vs.*, 367
        Parkinson's disease *vs.*, 241, 361, 367
        PSP *vs.*, 341, 341t, 367
    epidemiology, 360
    familial, 360
    historical background, 359
    neuroimaging, 5–7, 35f, 48–49, 364f
    neuropathology, 152–153, 152f, 365, 366f

non-familial, 152
nosology, 359–360
pathogenesis, 327
treatment, 367–368
Munchausen's syndrome, psychogenic dystonia, 557
Muscarinic acetylcholine receptors (mAChRs), 121
    basal ganglia, 94–95
        distribution, 121–123, 122f
        functions, 123
    subtypes, 121t
Muscle(s)
    normal sleep activity, 856
    stiff-person syndrome
        biopsy, 800–801
        spasm, 798, 800, 800f, 804–805
    tone *see* Muscle tone
    wasting, chorea-acanthocytosis, 411
Muscle field, 91
Muscle spindles, motor control, 749–750
Muscle synergy, cerebellar dysfunction, 738
Muscle tone
    see also Dysmetria; Spasticity
    aging and, 838–839, 838t, 839t, 846
    cerebellar control, 749
    cerebellar disorders, 726, 735, 736f, 737
    hypertonia, 838
        see also Dystonia; Rigidity; Spasticity
    hypotonia, 363, 726, 737, 738f
Musculoskeletal deformity, Parkinson's disease, 238
Musician's cramp, 516
Mutation rate, mitochondrial, 66
Mutism
    "cerebellar," 726
    encephalitis lethargica, 373–374
Mycoplasma pneumoniae encephalitis, 920
Myerson's sign
    aging and, 842
    Parkinson's disease, 238
Myoclonic dystonia, 661
Myoclonic epilepsy, 660
Myoclonic epilepsy with ragged-red fibers (MERRF)
    with epilepsy, 662–663
    with epilepsy and dementia, 661, 662
Myoclonus, 8–9, 657–667
    see also specific types/causes
    action, 657, 658, 669
        cortical tremor, 461
        multifocal, 665–666
    alcohol-responsive, 661
    Alzheimer's disease, 847
    associated conditions, 658, 671
        dementias, 663
        idiopathic dystonias, 513, 661
        multisystem atrophy, 363
        parkinsonism-plus syndrome, 165, 663

axial, 664–665
classification, 657, 657t, 669
    etiological, 660, 669
    Halliday's, 670
    physiological, 669–673
clinical features, 658–659
definition, 8, 657, 902
diagnostic categories, 661–665
    focal, 664–665
    severe multifocal/generalized, 661–664
    stimuli-sensitive, 665
differential diagnosis, 657–658, 669, 685–686
epileptic, 670–671, 670t
    cortical myoclonus, 8, 660, 664, 665, 666, 670, 670f
    primary generalized, 671
    reflex myoclonus, 657, 658, 660, 665, 669, 670–671
    subcortical, 660, 677
etiology, 660–665
facial, 664
focal, 664–665, 669
genetic basis, 661
multifocal (generalized), 665–666, 669
negative *see* Negative myoclonus/asterixis
non-epileptic, 670t, 671–673
    essential (idiopathic) myoclonus, 8, 660, 661, 673
    hyperekplexia (startle disease), 11, 665, 672, 686, 695
    hypnic jerk, 671, 856
    nocturnal *see* Periodic leg movements in sleep (PLMS)
    palatal, 9, 468–469, 468t, 487, 672
    physiological, 660
    posthypoxic, 663–664
    propiospinal, 664–665, 672
    psychogenic, 673, 902–904
    spinal, 9, 660, 664, 666, 672
pathophysiology, 659–660, 669–679
    see also specific techniques
    EEG recording, 669, 670f, 673–675, 674f
    EMG recording, 657–658, 658f, 659f, 660, 669, 671f, 673
    MEG studies, 676
    reflex studies, 675–676
    SEPs, 660, 664, 670, 670f, 675, 675f
    TMS studies, 676
positive, 669, 902
progressive encephalopathies, 661–663
    with dementia, 663
    with epilepsy, 662–663
    with epilepsy and dementia, 661–662
rhythmic, 659
secondary, 660
spontaneous, 659, 669
static encephalopathies, 663–664
treatment, 665–666

Myorhythmia (Holmes' tremor), 466–467, 467t
    pathophysiology, 486–487
Myriachit, 903–904

N

N-acetyltransferase, PD gene association studies, 215
Nadolol, essential tremor therapy, 445
Naltrexone, Rett syndrome, 416
Nausea/vomiting
    COMT inhibitor side-effects, 252
    levodopa (L-dopa) side-effects, 249
Neck
    essential tremor, 436
    spasmodic torticollis *see* Spasmodic torticollis
Necrotic cell death, mitochondrial dysfunction, 70
Negative myoclonus/asterixis, 9, 657, 676–677, 902
    clinical features, 657–658, 658–659
    EEG, 676–677
    EMG, 659f, 676
    hepatic failure and, 917
Neocerebellum, 722–723, 723t, 740
Neocortex, dopaminergic innervation, 97
Neoplasms *see* Malignancy
Nerve conduction studies, multisystem atrophy, 365
Nerve growth factor (NGF), 135
    Parkinson's disease, 221
Neural transplantation
    fetal *see* Fetal cell transplantation
    Huntington's disease, 51
    neurotrophic factors and, 284
    Parkinson's disease, 275–290
        retinal epithelia, 283–284
        stem cells, 284–285
        xenografts, 283
    progressive supranuclear palsy, 351
Neuroacanthocytosis *see* Choreoacanthocytosis (CHAC)
Neuroaxonal dystrophies, 549–550
    see also Hallervorden-Spatz disease
Neurobehavioral changes, 17–34
    see also individual disorders; specific symptoms
    cognitive *see* Cognitive dysfunction
    dementia and, 27–29
    neural substrates, 17–18, 18f
    neuropsychiatric *see* Neuropsychiatric disturbances
    Parkinson's disease, 319–326
    poststreptococcal infection, 919
Neuroblastin (artemin/enovin), 137
Neuroblastoma, 923
Neurocysticercosis, parkinsonism, 378
Neurodegenerative disorders
    see also specific disorders
    aging and movement disorders, 847–848
    apoptosis role, 70

cerebellar, 727t
chorea and, 644t
dementia *see* Dementia
familial parkinsonism and, 166, 168
heterogeneity and overlap in, 769–770
mitochondria and, 63, 74
    see also Mitochondrial dysfunction
neurological signs, 367t
pathogenesis, 327
rare parkinsonism-associated syndromes,
        403–419
symptomatic (secondary) dystonia, 547–552
Neurofibrillary tangles
    Alzheimer's disease, 342
    corticobasal degeneration, 154–155, 342, 768
    Parkinson's disease, 328
    postencephalitic parkinsonism, 375–376
    progressive supranuclear palsy, 153, 154f, 342
Neuroimaging, 13t, 14t, 35–60
    see also individual techniques; specific disorders
    atypical parkinsonian syndromes, 48–50
    carbon monoxide poisoning, 386–387
    cerebellar dysfunction, 727t-728t
    functional, 35–36, 92, 613
    Hallervorden-Spatz disease, 406
    hemiparkinsonism-hemiatrophy, 408
    involuntary movement disorders, 50–54
    Parkinson's disease, 36–48, 203–204
Neuroleptic malignant syndrome (NMS), parkinsonism,
        424–425
Neuroleptics *see* Antipsychotic drugs
Neurological conditions
    dystonia, 520–521
    tics and, 696–697
    trauma role, 900
Neurological examination, stiff-person (man) syndrome
        (SPS), 799, 799t
Neuronal regeneration, GDNF effects, 136
Neuronal storage diseases, myoclonus, 662
Neurons
    see also individual types; specific neurotransmitters
    aspiny interneurons, 94, 604, 604f
    balloon *see* Balloon (achromatic) neurons
    decreased ATP synthesis, 70
    inclusions *see* Inclusion bodies
    medium spiny *see* Medium spiny neurons (MSNs)
    mtDNA mutation effects, 67
    trophic support, 135
Neuropathology, 147–162
    see also individual disorders
    gross examination, 147–148
    microscopic examination, 148–149
    parkinsonism, 106–108, 107f
    synucleinopathies, 149–153
    tauopathies, 153–156

Neuropeptides
  Huntington's disease, 605
  Parkinson's disease, 201–202
Neuropeptide Y, striatal preservation in HD, 605
Neuroprotection
  antioxidants *see* Antioxidants
  creatine, 80, 594
  Huntington's disease, 594
  Parkinson's disease, 258–259
    dopamine agonists, 256
    nicotine/smoking, 189, 211–212
Neuropsychiatric disturbances, 18–24
  see also specific disorders
  anxiety *see* Anxiety
  depression *see* Depression
  drug-induced, 21, 242–243, 250, 252, 257, 263t, 264t
    see also individual drugs
  management, 262–264, 594
  mania, 20–21, 20t
  obsessive-compulsive disorder *see* Obsessive-compulsive
    disorder
  personality changes *see* Personality
  premorbid personality and, 319
  psychosis *see* Psychosis
  sexual dysfunction, 24, 239, 257, 362
  sleep disturbance *see* Sleep disturbance in movement
    disorders
Neurotensin, Parkinson's disease, 201–202
Neurotoxins
  see also Toxin-induced disorders; *specific toxins*
  botulinum toxin *see* Botulinum toxin
  chorea and, 644t
  endogenous, Parkinson's disease etiology, 212
  environmental
    dystonia, 556–557, 557t
    Parkinson's disease etiology, 74–75, 188, 203, 209,
      210–211
    tremor, 465–466
  tics, 697
Neurotrophic factors, 135–146
  see also individual molecules
  pathology role, 135
  therapeutic role, 43, 135, 137–139
    neural transplantation and, 284
Neurotrophins, 139–140
  BDNF *see* Brain-derived neurotrophic factor (BDNF)
  neural transplantation and, 284
  NT-3, 140, 221
  NT-4/5, 140, 221
  Parkinson's disease, 220–221
Neurturin, 136–137
NFκB, apoptosis role, 221–222
Nicotine
  Parkinson's disease and, 211–212
  tremor induction, 463

Nicotinic acetylcholine receptors (nAChRs), 121, 123
Niemann-Pick disease, dystonia in, 553
Nifedipine, essential tremor therapy, 448
Night terrors *(pavor nocturnus)*, 863
  differential diagnosis, 859–860
  levodopa (L-dopa) side-effects, 321
  Parkinson's disease, 871
Nigrostriatal system, 198
  see also Dopamine; Striatum; Substantia nigra
  BDNF role, 139
  degeneration, 106
  FGF role, 141
  Parkinson's disease, 198, 205
  progressive supranuclear palsy, 344–345
NMDA receptors, 124
  basal ganglia distribution, 124–125, 125f, 126t
  functions, 126
  Huntington's disease, 608, 613, 614, 615f, 616t
  Parkinson's disease, 258
N-methyl-β-carboline
  Parkinson's disease etiology, 212
  structure, 211f
N-methyl-salsolinol
  Parkinson's disease etiology, 212
  structure, 211f
N-methyl-tetrahydroisoquinoline
  Parkinson's disease etiology, 212
  structure, 211f
N-methyltransferase, 211f
Nocardia asteroides infection, parkinsonism, 378
Nocturnal body rocking, 862
Nocturnal bruxism, 862
Nocturnal eating, 863
Nocturnal head banging *(jactatio capitis nocturna)*, 862
Nocturnal myoclonus *see* Periodic leg movements
    in sleep (PLMS)
Nocturnal tongue biting, 862
Norepinephrine
  Parkinson's disease (PD), 200–201
  sleep role, 866
Nucleus accumbens, 117, 118
Nucleus reticularis of thalamus (NRT), motor circuitry, 96
Nurr1 mutation, familial Parkinson's disease, 135
Nutrients, as antioxidant treatment, 79
Nutritional deficiency
  see also Metabolic disorders; *individual nutrients/vitamins*
  cerebellar dysfunction, 727t
  chorea and, 644t
  hyperkinetic disorders in elderly, 840
  tremor, 916–917
Nystagmus, 747
  cerebellar syndromes, 747
  Huntington's disease, 589
  progressive supranuclear palsy, 346
  SCA1, 706

O

Obsessive-compulsive disorder (OCD), 22–23, 23t
  choreas, 23
    Huntington's disease, 590
    Sydenham's chorea, 638, 918
  corticobasal degeneration, 764
  parkinsonism, 108
  Tourette's syndrome, 23, 684, 693, 695–696
  treatment, 687t, 688, 771
Occupational risk factors, Parkinson's disease
    etiology, 188, 189
Occupational therapy, corticobasal degeneration, 772
OCD *see* Obsessive-compulsive disorder (OCD)
Oculofacialcervical dystonia, 547
Oculogyric crisis (OGC), encephalitis lethargica, 374
Oculomasticatory myorhythmia (OMM), Whipple's disease,
    379, 920
Oculomotor abnormalities
  see also specific types
  ataxia with oculomotor apraxia-1, 712
  cerebellar dysfunction, 724–725, 738, 747
  corticobasal degeneration, 763
  encephalitis lethargica, 373
  Huntington's disease, 589
  multisystem atrophy, 363
  parkinsonism-plus syndrome, 165
  Parkinson's disease, 108, 237–238
  postencephalitic parkinsonism, 375
  progressive supranuclear palsy, 345–346
    management, 351
  SCA1, 706
Olanzapine, 263, 323
  extrapyramidal side-effects, 396
  tic treatment, 688
Olfactory dysfunction, Parkinson's disease, 238
Oligodendrocytes, Huntington's disease, 601, 609
Olivary nuclei
  essential tremor, 441, 442f, 484
  palatal tremor (myoclonus), 469
Olivopontocerebellar atrophy (OPCA)
  classification, 360
  dementia, 29
  dystonia in, 548
  familial, 360
  historical background, 359–360
  myoclonus in, 660, 664
  neuroimaging, 48, 49, 364, 364f
  neuropathology, 152, 366f
    gross examination, 147, 148
  Parkinson's disease *vs.*, 241
  sleep disturbance, 874
  symptom overlap with other MSA syndromes, 359f
  visuospatial disturbances, 27
Ondansetron, 324

Online Mendelian Inheritance in Man (OMIM), hereditary
    ataxias, 703
Ophthalmologic abnormalities
  paraneoplastic disorders, 923
  Wilson's disease, 781, 783t, 784
Ophthalmoplegia
  aging and, 842
  encephalitis lethargica, 373
Opiates/opioids
  agonists, PLMS and RLS treatment, 859, 859t
  dystonia treatment, 531
  endogenous, Parkinson's disease, 201–202
  tardive akathisia treatment, 633
Opsoclonus-myoclonus syndrome, paraneoplastic
    disorders, 923
Optokinetic nystagmus, Huntington's disease, 589
Orofacial dyskinesias, age-related, 846–847
Oromandibular dystonia (OMD), 513–514
  familial, 517
  in Hallervorden-Spatz disease, 550f
  treatment, 528t
    botulinum toxin, 532
Orthostatic hypotension
  idiopathic, MSA and, 359f
  management, 368
  MSA and, 359–360, 362, 368
  Parkinson's disease, 243
Orthostatic tremor
  essential tremor and, 438–439, 488
  essential tremor *vs.*, 468, 468t
  pathophysiology, 488
    frequency, 483, 488
    neural pathway, 483, 483f
  primary, 467–468
Orthotics, ataxias, 705
Oscillatory neural activity, 235
  see also Tremor
Osteoporosis, Wilson's disease, 782
"Overflow" dystonia, 501, 512
Over-the-counter drugs, antioxidants, 77
Overuse syndromes, 516, 518
Oxidative phosphorylation, 67–69, 68f, 70
  see also Mitochondrial dysfunction
  creatine effects, 77, 80
  defects and apoptosis, 70–71
  electron "leakage," 70
  inhibition in PD, 75, 203
  therapeutic target, 77, 80
Oxidative stress, 71–72
  see also Antioxidants; Free radicals; Mitochondrial
      dysfunction
  aging and, 73–74
  DNA damage, 71, 219
  Huntington's disease, 76, 613–614, 615f, 616t
  lipid peroxidation, 71, 74

Parkinson's disease, 75, 188, 202–203, 218–219, 218f, 218t, 331, 332f
    gene association studies, 215
    progressive supranuclear palsy, 349
    protein damage, 74, 219
    α-synuclein (PARK1) and, 217
8–Oxo-dGTPase MTH2, Parkinson's disease, 215, 219
Oxygen
    mitochondrial consumption, 69–70
    reactive species *see* Reactive oxygen species (ROS)

P

Pain
    Parkinson's disease, 238
    primary torsion dystonia, 502
    reflex sympathetic dystrophy (causalgia), 899–901
    spasmodic torticollis, 514
    stiff-person (man) syndrome, 798
"Painful legs and moving toes," 645–646
Palatal tremor (myoclonus), 9, 468–469
    EMG, 672
    MRI, 469
    pathophysiology, 487, 672
    sleep disturbance, 875
    symptomatic *vs.* essential, 468t, 487
Paleocerebellum, 722, 723t, 740
Palilalia, 26, 238
Pallidonigroluysian degeneration (PNLD), 412–413
Pallidopyramidal disease, 413–414
Pallidotomy
    dystonia treatment, 110, 504, 534
    Parkinson's disease treatment, 48
Panic attacks, Parkinson's disease, 243, 320, 871
Pantothenate kinase-associated neurodegeneration *see* Hallervorden-Spatz disease
"Paradoxical sleep," Parkinson's disease, 321
Parallel fibers, 744–745
Paralysis, psychogenic gait, 906
Paraneoplastic disorders, cerebellar dysfunction, 727t, 922–923
Paranoid delusions, Huntington's disease, 590
Paraparesis, psychogenic gait, 906
Paraquat
    MPP$^+$ similarity, 384
    Parkinson's disease, 74–75, 188, 211
Parasitic infections, parkinsonism, 378
Parasomnias, 24, 861–863
    see also specific disorders
    in Parkinson's disease, 871
Paratonia (Gegenhalten), 236, 838, 839t
Paravermal/lateral zone syndrome, 746–747
Paresthesia, Parkinson's disease, 238

Parietal cortex, activation in Parkinson's disease, 46, 47f
PARK genes, 166–167, 167t, 217–218, 217t, 331–333, 332t
    see also individual genes/proteins
Parkin (PARK2) mutation, 38, 178, 217t, 218, 332–333
    association studies, 216
    juvenile/early-onset phenotypes, 168–170, 170t
    Lewy bodies and, 204
    neurodegenerative phenotypes, 168
Parkinsonian tremor, 6, 106, 165, 235, 470, 471, 736
    aging and, 843
    atypical, 240–241
    definition, 459
    drug-induced, 396
    essential tremor *vs.*, 240
    MSA, 361
    neuropathology, 108
    pathophysiology, 485
    postencephalitic, 375
    psychogenic, 905
    treatment, 471
Parkinsonism, 11
    aging and, 842–844
        functional decline, 843–844
        gait abnormalities, 840–841, 843
        subgroups, 842
    childhood, 829–830
    classification, 234t
    clinical features, 8, 106, 107–108, 843
        see also specific symptoms/signs
        akinesia, 106, 107–108, 236, 236t
        atypical, 239t
        dopa-responsiveness, 233
        dystonia, 8, 547–548
        gait, 814, 840–841, 843
        obsessive-compulsive disorder in, 23
        rigidity, 106, 107–108, 235–236
        tremor *see* Parkinsonian tremor
    definitions, 233–234
    differential diagnosis, 239–242
    drug treatment *see* Antiparkinsonian drugs
    epidemiology, 842, 843
    etiology, 163, 233
        alcohol, 917
        autoimmune disease, 921
        calcium metabolism disorders, 424, 916
        cerebrovascular disease, 240, 367, 421–422, 846
        chemicals/toxins *see* Toxin-induced parkinsonism
        CNS conditions, 421–427
        drug-induced *see* Drug-induced parkinsonism
        genetic *see* Familial parkinsonism
        historical aspects, 209
        hydrocephalus, 241, 423–424
        infectious, 373–382, 919–920, 921
        neuroleptic malignant syndrome, 424–425

Parkinsonism (continued)
   etiology (continued)
      structural lesions, 424
      trauma, 422–423
   familial see Familial parkinsonism
   historical aspects, 421
   Huntington's disease and, 589, 830
   MPTP-induced see MPTP-induced parkinsonism
   parkinsonian syndromes see Parkinsonism-plus
         syndromes (PPS)
   pathophysiology, 106–108, 107f, 233, 485
   postencephalitic see Postencephalitic parkinsonism (PEP)
   postural instability and gait difficulty (PIGD), 843
   primary (idiopathic) see Parkinson's disease (PD)
   psychogenic, 905–906
   rare degenerative syndromes, 403–419
   vascular see Vascular parkinsonism
Parkinsonism-dementia/ALS complex of Guam, 209
   dementia in, 29
   tremor in, 463
Parkinsonism-hyperpyrexia syndrome, 424–425
Parkinsonism-plus syndromes (PPS), 11–12, 163,
         164–165, 234t
   amyotrophy, 164
   corticobasal degeneration see Corticobasal degeneration
         (CBD)
   dementia, 150, 164–165
      see also Dementia with Lewy bodies (DLB)
   dystonia, 165
   familial see Familial parkinsonism
   molecular genetics, 167–168, 169t
   multisystem atrophy see Multisystem atrophy (MSA)
   myoclonus, 165, 663
   neuroimaging, 48–50
   neuropathology, 152–156, 164
   neuropsychiatric disturbances, 165
   oculomotor abnormalities, 165
   parkinsonism-dementia/ALS complex of Guam, 29,
         209, 463
   Parkinson's disease vs., 240–241
   postural tremor, 165
   progressive supranuclear palsy see Progressive
         supranuclear palsy (PSP)
   respiratory abnormalities, 165
Parkinson's disease (PD), 12, 12t, 163, 275
   see also Parkinsonism-plus syndromes (PPS)
   animal models, 203, 210, 331
      transgenic, 333
   assessment, 280–281
      see also neuroimaging (below)
      clinical rating scales, 39, 243
      cognitive, 280
      fluctuations, 43–44
      motor, 280
      progression, 39–41
   associated conditions
      Alzheimer's disease and, 150, 847
      essential tremor and, 439–440
      progressive supranuclear palsy and, 154
   clinical features, 233–245, 235t
      see also individual symptoms/signs
      akinesia/bradykinesia, 106, 107–108, 236, 236t
      asymmetric, 242
      atypical, 239–242, 239t
      autonomic disturbances, 24, 238–239, 362
         management, 263, 264t
      cardinal, 235–237
      cognitive disturbances, 108, 237
         apraxia, 27
         depression relationship, 19, 242, 262, 319
         executive function, 25
         management, 262–263
         memory impairment, 25
         speech/language, 26, 238
         visuospatial, 26–27
      dermatological, 239
      dysphagia, 238
      dystonia, 547
      facial abnormalities, 238
      gait abnormalities, 237
         age-related, 840–841
         freezing, 237, 814
      motor signs, 201, 234
      musculoskeletal deformity, 238
      neuropsychiatric disturbances, 108, 242–243, 250,
            319–326, 319t
         anxiety, 23–24, 243, 320
         depression, 19–20, 242, 262, 319–320
         management, 262–264, 263t, 264t
         personality changes, 22
         psychosis, 21, 263, 321–324, 322t
         sexual disturbances, 24, 239
         sleep see Sleep disturbance in Parkinson's disease
      oculomotor abnormalities, 108, 237–238
      onset, 234
         young patients, 240
      postural instability, 233, 236–237
         predominant, 241
      rigidity, 106, 107–108, 235–236
      secondary, 237–239, 249t
      treatment-related, 242–243, 249–250, 252
         see also Levodopa (L-dopa)
         cognitive/behavioral, 242–243, 249, 252, 257, 263–264
         dyskinesias, 43–44, 45f, 242, 250, 250t, 252, 283
         motor fluctuations, 242, 249–250, 250t, 260–261
         orthostatic hypotension, 243
      tremor, 6, 106, 108, 235, 736
         atypical, 240–241
         vocal, 474
   definition, 233–234

dementia in, 27–28, 771t, 844
   differential diagnosis, 241–242, 771t
   imaging, 45–46
diagnosis, 177–178, 234
   dopa-responsiveness, 233, 248
   history taking, 239–240
   neuropathological, 150, 178
differential diagnosis, 239–242, 340, 341, 341t, 367, 367t
   drug-induced parkinsonism *vs.*, 396
   toxin-induced parkinsonism *vs.*, 389t
epidemiology, 177–195, 234
   age-specific distribution, 184, 186, 843
   gender-specific distribution, 184, 184t, 186
   geographic distribution, 181t-183t, 185–186
   incidence, 74, 178–179, 180t
   mortality rates, 179, 184
   prevalence, 179, 181t, 182t, 183t
   race-specific distribution, 181t-183t, 184–185, 184t
   temporal trends, 185
etiology/pathogenesis, 106–108, 107f, 163, 186–190, 209–231, 210f, 327, 330–331
   see also neurochemistry (below)
   aging, 73–74, 178, 843
   apoptosis, 221–223
   cytokines, 215, 219–221, 220t
   directly associated factors, 186–189
     see also Genetics; Toxin-induced parkinsonism
     chemicals/pesticides, 74–75, 188, 210–211
     demographic, 186, 210
     dietary, 188
     endogenous neurotoxins, 212
     infection, 188–189, 209
     metal exposure, 188, 209
   inversely associated factors, 189–190
     antioxidants, 189–190
     caffeine, 189
     smoking, 189, 211–212
   iron metabolism, 188, 202, 218
   methodological limitations, 186
   MIF deficiency, 209
   mitochondrial dysfunction, 74–75, 78, 203, 218
   oxidative stress, 75, 188, 202–203, 218–219, 218f, 218t, 331, 332f
   risk assessment, 178
   α-synuclein, 75, 149–150, 166–167, 204, 217, 330–331
familial *see* Familial Parkinson's disease
genetic factors *see* Genetics
historical aspects, 209, 233, 422
misdiagnosis/misclassification, 177, 178
neurochemistry, 197–209
   see also specific transmitters
   acetylcholine, 201, 257
   dopamine, 198–200, 202
   free radicals/scavengers, 202–203
   GABA, 201

glutamate, 221, 257–258
Lewy body analysis, 204–205
neuropeptides, 201–202
norepinephrine, 200–201
serotonin, 36, 38, 129, 201, 322–323
significance, 205
in vivo imaging, 203–204
neuroimaging, 36–48
   see also specific techniques
   brain activation, 46–48, 47f
   dementia, 45–46
   disease progression, 39–41
   dopaminergic function, 45–46
   dyskinesias, 43–44, 45f
   microglial activation, 38–39
   preclinical detection, 38, 39f
   presynaptic dopaminergic, 36–38, 37f
   restorative treatments, 41–43, 42f, 280–281, 280f
   treatment fluctuations, 43–44
   in vivo neurochemistry, 203–204
neuropathology, 36, 149–150, 178, 234, 275, 327–336
   diagnostic criteria, 329
   dystrophic neurites, 330, 330f
   extradopaminergic, 866–867
   familial disease, 164
   gross, 327, 328f
   Lewy bodies *see* Lewy bodies
   melanophagia, 327, 328f
   microscopic, 327–330, 328f, 329f, 330f
   neurofibrillary tangles, 328
   nigral pallor, 149, 149f
   post-fetal transplantation, 281–282, 282f
   spheroids, 330
   α-synuclein, 75, 149, 166, 167, 204–205, 328, 329, 329f
pathophysiology, 106–108, 107f
   see also Dopaminergic system; Substantia nigra
   mitochondrial dysfunction, 74–75, 78, 203
   oxidative stress, 75, 188, 202–203
   α-synuclein, 166–167
subtypes, 234
treatment, 275
   antioxidants, 78, 79, 259
   effects of, 46–48
   fetal nigral transplants *see* Fetal cell transplantation
   fluctuations, 43–44, 242, 249–250, 250t
     management, 260–261, 261t
   gene therapy, 138, 285
   neuroprotective interventions, 258–259
   pallidotomy, 48
   pharmacological *see* Antiparkinsonian drugs
   progenitor cell proliferation, 138–139
   stem cell transplants, 284–285
   STN lesion, 106
   STN stimulation, 48
   trophic factors, 43, 135, 136, 137–139

Paroxysmal dyskinesias, 10, 643, 645, 920
Paroxysmal exertional dyskinesia (PED), 10, 645
Paroxysmal kinesigenic dyskinesia (PKD), 10, 643
Paroxysmal nocturnal dystonia (PND), 861–862
Paroxysmal nonkinesigenic dyskinesia (PNKD), 10, 645
Patient organizations, dystonia, 536t
Pavor nocturnus see Night terrors (pavor nocturnus)
PD see Parkinson's disease (PD)
Pediatric disorders see Childhood movement disorders
Pedunculopontine nucleus (PPN)
    cholinergic projections, 96, 121
    gait/locomotion, 811
    motor circuitry, 96
    progressive supranuclear palsy, 345
    sleep role, 860, 866–867, 877
Pelizaeus-Merzbacher disease, dystonia, 553–554
Penicillamine
    adverse effects, 788
    Wilson's disease management, 787–788
Pentoxifylline, drug-induced parkinsonism, 399
Pergolide mesylate, pharmacology, 235t, 254
Perinatal trauma, secondary dystonia, 541, 545f, 546
Periodic leg movements in sleep (PLMS), 10, 672–673,
        856–859, 861, 869–870
    see also Restless legs syndrome (RLS)
    associated conditions, 857
    EEG, 856
    neurophysiology, 856–857
    Parkinson's disease, 864, 867f, 870
    pathophysiological mechanism, 857–858
    stiff-person syndrome and, 801
    treatment, 858–859, 859t
Peripheral deafferentation, dystonia treatment,
        531, 535
Peripheral nerve injury
    dystonia and, 546–547, 899–901
    tremor, 473
Peripheral neuropathies
    "painful legs and moving toes," 645–646
    tremor, 469, 469t
        essential tremor and, 440–441
        pathophysiology, 488
        physiological, 441, 469
Periventricular system, 198
Personality
    changes, 22
        chorea-acanthocytosis, 411
        Hallervorden-Spatz disease, 406
        multisystem atrophy, 363
        Parkinson's disease, 22
        progressive supranuclear palsy, 22
        PSP, 28
        Wilson's disease, 22, 780
    Parkinson's disease etiology, 189, 319
    Tourette's syndrome, 22, 684

Pesticides
    Parkinson's disease, 74–75, 188, 211
    tremor, 466
PET see Positron emission tomography (PET)
Phantom dyskinesia, 10
"Phantom" tics, 692
Phenobarbital, essential tremor therapy, 446
Phenol, dystonia treatment, 531
Phenylethylamine, structure, 211f
Phosphocreatine shuttle hypothesis, 80
Photosensitivity, myoclonus, 671
Physical mapping, huntingtin (HD) gene, 570–572, 571f
Physiological myoclonus, 660
Physiological tremor, 4, 459–461, 736
    etiological factors, 460
    functional significance, 460, 472
    hyperthyroidism, 915
    neuropathy and, 441, 469
    pathophysiology, 481–482
        8–12 Hz component, 481–482
        mechanical reflex component, 481, 482f
    postanesthetic, 461
    tetrahydrobiopterin deficiency, 916–917
Physiotherapy, corticobasal degeneration and, 772
Pick-like inclusions, corticobasal degeneration, 767f
Pick's disease, corticobasal degeneration vs., 50, 155, 156,
        769, 771t
"Pill-rolling" tremor, 235, 396
Pindolol
    essential tremor therapy, 445
    tremor induction, 464
Piperazine, drug-induced parkinsonism, 399
Piracetam, myoclonus management, 665
Piribedil, pharmacology, 235t, 255
Plasmapheresis, stiff-person syndrome treatment, 808
Polycythemia vera, 918
    chorea, 642, 918
Polyglutamine toxicity, 76
    see also Repeat expansion diseases
Polysomnography (PSG)
    Parkinson's disease, 864, 864f, 865f, 866f, 867f
    tic disorders, 694
Pons, progressive supranuclear palsy, 345–346
Porphyria, tremor, 472
Positron emission tomography (PET), 14t, 36
    cerebellar function, 721, 722, 752, 753f
    choreoacanthocytosis, 412, 640
    corticobasal degeneration, 49, 765
    dementia, 45
    differential diagnosis role, 204
    dystonia, 500, 503, 518
        primary torsion, 52–53
    gait disorders, 817
    hemiparkinsonism-hemiatrophy, 408
    Huntington's disease, 51, 52f, 612–613, 613f

MPTP-induced parkinsonism, 384
multisystem atrophy, 48, 49, 364–365
Parkinson's disease, 203–204
   brain activation, 46, 47, 47f
   dementia, 45
   dyskinesias, 43–44, 45f
   fetal transplants, 41, 42f, 280–281, 280f
   microglial activation, 39, 40f
   preclinical diagnosis, 38, 39f
   presynaptic dopaminergic system, 36–38, 37f
   progression analysis, 40–41
   treatment fluctuations, 43–44
postpump chorea, 642
progressive supranuclear palsy, 49, 50f, 341
psychogenic movement disorders, 907
resting brain metabolism, 45
Rett syndrome, 416
Sydenham's chorea, 638
tardive dyskinesia, 629
tic pathophysiology, 693
tremor, 483, 915
   stroke-associated, 471
vascular chorea, 641
Wilson's disease, 785
X-linked dystonia-parkinsonism syndrome, 410
Postanesthetic tremor, 461
Postencephalitic parkinsonism (PEP), 209, 374–376
   clinical features, 374–375
      extrapyramidal, 374–375
      obsessive-compulsive disorder, 23
      sleep disturbances, 24
   differential diagnosis, PSP *vs.*, 341
   historical aspects, 373
   neuropathology, 375–376
   pathophysiology, 375
   treatment, 376
Posterior fossa cysts, parkinsonism, 424
Posterior ramisectomy, dystonia treatment, 535
Posthypoxic myoclonus, 663–664
Postpump chorea, 642–643, 829
Posttraumatic parkinsonism, 422–423
Posttraumatic tics, 697
Posttraumatic tremor, 473
Postural control, 11
   see also Postural instability
   aging and, 840
   cerebellum role, 721, 724, 738
   gait and, 812–813
   Hallervorden-Spatz disease, 406
   muscle synergy, 738
   myoclonus, 659
   primary torsion dystonia, 502
Postural hypotension, multisystem atrophy, 362, 365
Postural instability, 11
   assessment, 840

Huntington's disease, 589
parkinsonism, 843
Parkinson's disease, 233, 236–237
   atypical presentation, 241
progressive supranuclear palsy, 345
Postural reflexes, aging and, 840
Postural tremor, 4, 6
   definition, 459
   differential diagnosis, myoclonus *vs.*, 657
   drug-induced parkinsonism, 396
   dystonia and, 462
   essential tremor and, 437, 438, 440
   parkinsonism-plus syndrome (PPS), 165
Potassium, Wilson's disease treatment, 786
Pramipexole
   functional imaging *vs.* clinical outcome, 41
   pharmacology, 235t, 255
Pregnancy, chorea gravidarum, 638, 922
Premotor cortex, 90
   functional anatomy, 91f, 92–93
   primary torsion dystonia, 53
Premotor fields, 92–93
Primary antiphospholipid syndrome (PAPS), chorea,
     638–639
Primary orthostatic tremor, 467–468
Primary torsion dystonia (PTD), 7, 52–54, 511–525, 541t
   see also individual types
   childhood, 495–511, 826–828
      clinical issues, 826–827, 827t
      transient, 827
   clinical features, 512–516
      see also individual disorders
      adult *vs.* childhood-onset, 511, 511t
      age at onset and, 500–501, 500t
      childhood, 500–502
      onset, 512
      progression, 501–502
      commonalities, 512t
      commonalities, 512–513
      neurological abnormalities, 520–521
      remission, 512
      sleep disturbances, 874
   definitions, 541, 896–897
   diagnosis/differential diagnosis
      adult-onset, 520–521
      "causalgia-dystonia" *vs.*, 899t
      genetic testing, 502–503
      misdiagnosis as psychogenic, 897–898
   epidemiology
      adult-onset, 511–512
      childhood, 496, 826–827
   etiology, 495, 516–518
      childhood disorders, 827t
   genetics, 52
      adult-onset, 511, 511t, 518

Primary torsion dystonia (PTD) *(continued)*
  genetics *(continued)*
    childhood, 496–499
    DYT1 gene, 496, 497–499, 503
    linkage studies, 497–498
    mode of inheritance, 496–497
    penetrance, 497
    phenotype relationship, 501, 501t
  neuroimaging, 53, 518–519
  neuropathology, 499
  pathophysiology
    adult-onset, 518–520, 519f
    childhood, 499–500
  secondary *vs.*, 8, 496t, 541
    see also Secondary (symptomatic) dystonia
  treatment, 527–539
    see also specific drugs/treatments
    childhood, 504
Primidone, essential tremor therapy, 446, 485
Primitive reflexes
  aging and, 842
  Parkinson's disease, 238
Primozide, tic treatment, 688
Procedural memory, impairment, 25–26
Progenitor cells, GDNF-mediated proliferation in PD,
    138–139
Progressive autonomic failure (PAF), 48
Progressive encephalomyelitis with rigidity (PEWR),
    802–803
Progressive myoclonic ataxia (PMA), 662–663
Progressive myoclonic epilepsy syndromes (PMEs), 8, 662
Progressive pallidal degeneration, dystonia in, 550
Progressive supranuclear palsy (PSP), 12, 49, 339–358
  assessment
    clinical evaluation, 341
    clinical rating scale, 340
    CSF evaluation, 342
    radiological evaluation, 341–342, 342t
  clinical features, 339–340, 771t
    atypical, 340
    autonomic dysfunction, 347
    dysarthria, 346t, 347
    dystonia, 547–548
    executive dysfunction, 25
    gait, 339
    neurobehavioral changes, 22, 28, 343, 346–347
    oculomotor, 346, 351
    postural instability, 345
    presentation/course, 339–340, 339t, 345
    sleep disturbances, 346–347, 874
  coexisting pathologies, 154
    Alzheimer's disease and, 343
  dementia in, 28, 154
  diagnostic criteria, 340–342, 340t, 341t
  differential diagnosis, 341, 341t, 771t

    corticobasal degeneration *vs.*, 341, 341t, 762, 770
    MSA *vs.*, 341, 341t, 367
    Parkinson's disease *vs.*, 241, 340
  epidemiology, 347–348
  etiology, 348–350
    demographic factors, 349
    familial factors, 348–349
    gene mutations, 349–350
    mitochondrial dysfunction, 349
    oxidative stress, 349
    transmissible agent?, 348
  neurochemistry, 342–343
    cortical changes, 344
  neuroimaging, 49, 50f
  neuropathology, 153–154, 153f, 154f, 342–343, 343–347
    basal ganglia, 153, 153f, 154f, 344–345
    brainstem, 346–347
    cortical distribution, 343–344
    grumose degeneration, 153, 343
    hippocampus, 344
    neurofibrillary tangles, 153, 154f, 342
    oculomotor, 345–346
    spinal/autonomic, 347
    tau inclusions, 153–154, 342–343
  patient resources, 351–352
  treatment, 350–351
    drugs, 347t, 350–351
    non-drug, 351
Progressive Supranuclear Palsy Association, 351, 352
Propanolol
  contraindications, 445
  essential tremor therapy, 445, 451
  tardive akathisia treatment, 633
Propiospinal myoclonus, 664–665, 672
Protein oxidation
  age-effects, 74
  Parkinson's disease, 219
Pseudoathetosis, 8
Pseudodementia, Parkinson's disease, 242
Pseudohypoparathyroidism, parkinsonism, 424
Pseudoseizures, 904
PSP *see* Progressive supranuclear palsy (PSP)
Psychiatric disorders
  see also Neuropsychiatric disturbances; Psychogenic
      movement disorders (PMDs); *specific conditions*
  ataxias, 705
  comorbid conditions
    movement disorders, 897
    psychogenic disorders, 900, 903
  somatoform, 892–893, 892t, 893t
Psychogenic movement disorders (PMDs)
  chorea/ballism, 904
  comorbidity
    organic disorders, 896, 908–909
    psychiatric disorders, 900, 902

diagnosis, 907–909
    accuracy, 909
    categories of certainty, 909
    clues to, 895–896, 896t
    criteria, 892–893, 892t, 893t
    difficulty, 908–909
    electrophysiology, 902, 903, 907
    misdiagnosis, 892, 897, 897t, 907
    placebo challenges, 908
differential diagnosis, 907
dystonia, 8, 521, 557–558, 558t, 896–901
    "causalgia-dystonia," 899–901, 899t
    clinical features, 898
    differential diagnosis, 907
    epidemiology, 898–899, 899t
    history, 891–892
    misdiagnosis, 897, 897t
epidemiological studies, 893–895, 895t
    psychogenic dystonia, 898–899, 899t
gait disorders, 814, 816–817, 906–907, 906t
    ataxia, 705, 906, 907, 908
    diagnosis/misdiagnosis, 907, 908
    epidemiology, 906
    parkinsonian, 905
historical aspects, 891–892
myoclonus, 673, 902–904
    comorbid conditions, 903
    epidemiology, 902
    related conditions, 903–904
parkinsonism, 905–906
prognosis/outcome, 909–910
psychiatric definitions, 892–893
tics, 904–905
treatment approach, 909–910
tremor, 6, 469–470, 470t, 901–902
    clinical features, 470t
    diagnosis, 902
    epidemiology, 901–902
Psychosis, 21–22, 21t
    ataxias, 705
    drug-induced, 21, 262–263
    Huntington's disease, 21, 590, 594
    management, 263, 263t, 323–324, 323t, 594
    neural substrates, 21
    Parkinson's disease, 21, 263, 321–324, 322t
        mechanisms, 322–323
    Wilson's disease, 781
Psychosocial issues, 17
    Huntington's disease, 593
PTD see Primary torsion dystonia (PTD)
"Pull test," 237
Purine metabolism, disorders, dystonia in,
        555
Purkinje cells, 744–745
    loss in HD, 610–611

Putamen, 117
    cholinergic inputs, 122
    dopamine, 97, 118
        loss in parkinsonism, 107
    fetal graft sites, 277–278, 278f
    focal dystonia, 518, 544, 545f, 546, 546f
    Huntington's disease, 601, 602f
    motor circuitry, 94
    Parkinson's disease, 201
    serotonergic innervation, 127
Pyramidal signs, multisystem atrophy, 360, 363
Pyramidal tract see Corticospinal tract
Pyridostigmine, drug-induced parkinsonism, 399
Pyridoxine (vitamin B₆), tardive dyskinesia treatment,
        398, 632

Q

Quetiapine, 263, 323
    extrapyramidal side-effects, 396
    REM sleep behavior disorder treatment, 861

R

Rabbit nictitating membrane response, 751
Rabbit syndrome, 6, 463, 464
Racial differences, Parkinson's disease epidemiology,
        184–185, 184t
Radiocopper incorporation, Wilson's disease diagnosis,
        783t, 784–785
Radiological evaluation, progressive supranuclear palsy,
        341–342
Ramisectomy, posterior, dystonia treatment, 535
Ramsay-Hunt syndrome, 662, 663
Rasageline mesylate, 252–253
Reactive oxygen species (ROS), 218f
    see also Antioxidants; Free radicals
    cellular antioxidant systems, 72, 72f
    mitochondrial production, 69–70, 71
    in Parkinson's disease, 75, 218, 218f, 331, 332f
    toxicity see Oxidative stress
Red nucleus, progressive supranuclear palsy, 345
Reflexes
    chorea-acanthocytosis, 411
    C-reflex, 670, 675–676, 677
    myoclonus studies, 675–676
    photic reflex, 671
    postural, aging and, 840
    primitive
        aging and, 842
        Parkinson's disease, 238
    startle see Startle reflex
    tendon, aging and, 839
    vestibuloocular, gain adaptation, 751

Reflex myoclonus, 657, 665
    clinical features, 658
    photic cortical, 671
    reticular, 660, 665, 670–671
Reflex sympathetic dystrophy (RSD), dystonia and, 518, 899–901, 899t
Remacemide, Huntington's disease trial, 78
REM sleep, 24
    mechanisms, 866–867, 878
        basal ganglia, 877
        glutamatergic drive, 860
    normal movements, 856
    Parkinson's disease, 239, 321
    progressive supranuclear palsy, 346–347
REM sleep behavior disorder (RBD), 859–861
    diagnosis, 860
    differential diagnosis, 859–860
    disease associations, 860
    epidemiology, 860
    Parkinson's disease, 870–871
    pathophysiology, 860–861
    treatment, 861, 870–871
Renal dysfunction, Wilson's disease, 782
Repeat expansion diseases
    see also specific disorders
    ataxias, 577f, 705t
        diagnostic tests, 705t
        DPLA, 641, 710
        fragile X, 713
        FRDA, 711
        SCAs, 707, 708, 709, 710
    essential tremor, 434
    Huntington's disease, 50, 75, 76, 574–576
        mechanism of action, 578
    pentanucleotide repeats, SCA10, 709
    protein inclusions, 617
    trinucleotide repeats, 577–578
Reserpine
    tardive dyskinesia treatment, 631
    tremor induction, 464
Respiratory abnormalities
    parkinsonism-plus syndromes, 165
    Rett syndrome, 415
Resting tremor, 4, 6, 235, 470–471
    aging and, 843
    conditions causing, 471t
    definition, 459, 736
    essential tremor and, 845
    monosynaptic, 470–471
    parkinsonian see Parkinsonian tremor
Restless legs syndrome (RLS), 10, 856–859
    see also Periodic leg movements in sleep (PLMS)
    clinical criteria, 857
    genetics, 857
    Parkinson's disease, 238, 870

pathophysiological mechanism, 857–858
    PLMS and, 857
    PND and, 861
    prevalence, 857
    treatment, 858–859, 859t
Restriction fragment-length polymorphisms (RFLPs), huntingtin, 570, 572
Reticular activating system, sleep-wake role, 876–877
Reticular reflex myoclonus, 660, 665, 670–671
Retroviral infections, encephalitis lethargica, 374
Rett syndrome, 414–416, 550–551
    cerebrospinal fluid analysis, 551
    clinical features, 415
        dystonia, 550–551
    definition, 414–415
    diagnosis/differential diagnosis, 416
    molecular genetics, 415
Rett Syndrome Diagnostic Criteria Work Group, 416
RFLPs, huntingtin identification, 570, 572
Rheumatic fever, chorea and, 828, 829
    see also Sydenham's chorea (St. Vitus dance)
Rhizotomy, dystonia treatment, 535
Richardson's disease see Progressive supranuclear palsy (PSP)
Rigidity, 11
    aging, 838, 839t
    Alzheimer's disease, 847
    corticobasal degeneration, 762
    drug-withdrawal syndromes, 425
    essential tremor and, 439
    Hallervorden-Spatz disease, 406
    neuroleptic malignant syndrome, 425
    pallidonigroluysian degeneration, 413
    Parkinson's disease/parkinsonism, 106, 235–236, 410
        drug-induced, 396
        neuropathology, 107–108
        postencephalitic, 375
        psychogenic, 905
    progressive encephalomyelitis with, 802–803
    stiff-person (man) syndrome, 798
    X-linked dystonia-parkinsonism syndrome, 410
Risperidone
    dystonia treatment, 529
    extrapyramidal side-effects, 396
    tic treatment, 688
RNA transcripts, SCA8 mutations, 709
Ropinirole
    functional imaging vs. clinical outcome, 41
    pharmacology, 235t, 255–256
Rotenone, parkinsonism, 74–75, 188, 203, 211
Roussy-Levy syndrome, essential tremor and, 440
Rubral (Holmes') tremor, 466–467, 467t
    pathophysiology, 486–487

S

Saccades, 747
  autosomal-recessive spastic ataxia of
      Charlevoix-Seguenay, 713
  cerebellar syndromes, 747
Safety issues, fetal cell transplantation, 279
Saint Vitus dance *see* Sydenham's chorea (St. Vitus dance)
Salsolinols
  Parkinson's disease etiology, 212
  structure, 211f
Sandhoff's disease, 552–553
  myoclonus, 662
Sarcoidosis, 921
Scaling, basal ganglia, 105
Schwab and England Capacity for Daily Living Scale, 243
Scoliosis
  Parkinson's disease, 238
  Rett syndrome, 415
SDS *see* Shy-Drager syndrome (SDS)
Seborrhea, Parkinson's disease, 239
Secondary (symptomatic) dystonia, 500–501, 500t, 503t, 541t
  chemical-induced, 556, 557t
  definition, 541, 897
  diagnosis, 544t
  differential diagnosis, 542t-543t
  drug-induced, 110, 250, 520, 547, 556–557, 556t-557t
  focal brain lesions, 541, 544–546, 545t
    anatomicoclinical correlation, 546
    basal ganglia, 544, 545t, 546
    brainstem, 545
    cerebral palsy, 541, 545f
    delayed onset, 546
    lesion type, 545–546
    thalamus, 545
  metabolic disorders, 552–555, 918t
    amino acid metabolism, 554–555
    hypoparathyroidism, 916
    lipid metabolism, 552–554, 553f
    mitochondrial, 554
    purine metabolism, 555
  neurodegenerative disorders, 547–552
    see also individual disorders
    akinetic-rigid syndromes, 8, 547–548
    basal ganglia disorders, 549–551, 549f
    choreic syndromes, 548–549
    frequency, 547
    hereditary ataxias, 551
    Wolfram's syndrome, 551–552
    xeroderma pigmentosum, 551
  neuroimaging, 544t
  primary *vs.*, 8, 496t, 541
  pseudopsychogenic, 558, 558t
  pyschogenic, 557–558

  trauma and, 556
    perinatal, 541, 545f, 546
    peripheral, 546–547, 899–901
Segmental dystonia, 7
  classification, 495t
  treatment, 528t
Seizures
  see also Myoclonus
  Hallervorden-Spatz disease, 406
  parkinsonism-plus syndromes, 165
  partial in PND, 861
  Wilson's disease, 780
Selective serotonin reuptake inhibitors (SSRIs), 262
Selegiline (deprenyl), 252, 259, 260, 262
  sleep-maintenance insomnia treatment, 869
Self-harm
  Huntington's disease, 590
  Tourette's syndrome, 684
Senile chorea, 641
Senile gait, 841
Senile plaques, progressive supranuclear palsy, 154
Sensorimotor cortex, primary torsion dystonia, 53
Sensory abnormalities
  dystonia, 499, 520
  Parkinson's disease, 238
Sensory ataxia, 816, 816t
Sensory system, cerebellum functions, 752
Sensory tics, 9, 691–692, 692t
SEPs *see* Somatosensory evoked potentials (SEPs)
Sequential movement, control, 93, 104
Serotonergic drugs, essential tremor therapy, 448
Serotonin, 201
  basal ganglia, 127–129, 128t
    sources, 127
  deficits
    depression relationship, 19–20
    Parkinson's disease, 36, 38, 129, 201, 322–323
  forebrain, 201
  receptors *see* Serotonin receptors
  sleep role, 866
  tic pathophysiology, 694
Serotonin receptors, 127
  antagonists, progressive supranuclear palsy, 350–351
  basal ganglia distribution, 127–128, 128t
  functions, 128–129
  knockout animals, 128
  types, 127
Serotonin syndrome, 262
Sexual deviation, 24
Sexual dysfunction, 24
  multisystem atrophy, 362
  Parkinson's disease, 239, 257
"Shaky leg syndrome," 467–468
Shuddering attacks, 826

Shy-Drager syndrome (SDS)
  dementia, 29
  dystonia in, 548
  historical background, 359–360
  neuropathology, 152
  Parkinson's disease *vs.*, 241
  symptom overlap with other MSA syndromes, 359f
Simple sequence repeats, *huntingtin* (HD) gene, 572
Simple tics, 9, 684, 692t
Sinemet CR, 250
Single photon emission tomography (SPECT), 36
  cognitive processes, cerebellum role, 752–753,
      753t–754t
  corticobasal degeneration, 49, 765
  gait disorders, 817
  multisystem atrophy, 48–49
  Parkinson's disease
    dopaminergic function in dementia, 46
    treatment effects, 46
    treatment fluctuations, 43
  postpump chorea, 642
  primary torsion dystonia, 53–54
  progressive supranuclear palsy, 342
  psychogenic movement disorders, 907
  Rett syndrome, 416
  Sydenham's chorea, 638
  vascular chorea, 641
Sjögren's syndrome, 921
Sleep
  disorders of *see* Sleep disorders
  myoclonus in, 10, 672–673
  neural substrates/mechanisms, 858, 860, 868f, 875–878
    basal ganglia, 877–878, 878f
    brainstem, 876–877, 877–878
    dopamine, 858, 865–866, 875–876
    extranigral systems, 876–877
    norepinephrine, 866
    PPN role, 860, 866–867, 877
    serotonin, 866
    VTA role, 872, 876
  non-REM (NREM), 861
  normal movement in, 855–856
  REM *see* REM sleep
Sleep apnea, Parkinson's disease, 871
Sleep disorders, 856–863
  see also specific disorders
  abnormal movement in, 856–861
    mechanisms, 857–858
    parasomnias, 24, 861–863, 871
    treatment considerations, 863
  sleep apnea, 871
  in waking movement disorders *see* Sleep disturbance in
      movement disorders
Sleep disturbance in movement disorders, 24, 863–875
  ataxias, 705

Creutzfeldt-Jakob disease, 874
dementia with Lewy bodies, 24
encephalitis lethargica, 373
hemiballismus, 874
hemifacial spasm/blepharospasm, 874
Huntington's disease, 590, 874
Machado-Joseph disease, 24
management, 263, 264t, 321
neural substrates/mechanisms, 875–878
olivopontocerebellar atrophy, 874
palatal tremor, 875
Parkinson's disease *see* Sleep disturbance in Parkinson's
    disease
progressive supranuclear palsy, 346–347, 874
Rett syndrome, 415
tic disorders, 694, 874–875
torsion dystonia, 874
treatment considerations, 875
Whipple's disease, 24
Sleep disturbance in Parkinson's disease, 24, 239, 242, 257,
    263, 321, 863–874
  akathisia, 870
  epidemiology, 865, 868
  excessive daytime somnolence, 871–874
    drug-induced, 872–873
    neural substrates, 872
    prevalence, 872
    treatment, 873–874, 873t
  fragmentary nocturnal myoclonus, 869–870
  limb movements, 864–865, 866f, 867f
  "on-off" phenomena and, 867, 868f, 869
  parasomnias, 871
  pathophysiology, 865–867
  periodic leg movements in sleep, 864, 867f, 870
  polysomnography, 864, 864f, 865f, 866f, 867f, 868
  REM sleep behavior disorder, 870–871
  restless legs syndrome, 238, 870
  sleep apnea, 871
  sleep fragmentation, 865
    daytime consequences, 867
  sleep-maintenance insomnia, 869
  sleep-onset insomnia, 869
  treatment, 867–874
  tremor, 864, 864f, 865f
Sleep hygiene, Parkinson's disease, 871
Sleep-maintenance insomnia, Parkinson's disease, 869
Sleep-onset insomnia, Parkinson's disease, 869
Sleeptalking (somniloquy), 862
Sleepwalking (somnambulism), 862–863
Slit-lamp examination, Wilson's disease, 783t, 784
S-methyltransferase, Parkinson's disease genetics, 213
Smoking, Parkinson's disease prevention, 189,
    211–212
Social phobia, essential tremor, 435
Society for Progressive Supranuclear Palsy, 351, 352

Solvents
  dystonia, 557
  parkinsonism and, 388–389
  toxin-induced tremor, 466
Soman, toxin-induced tremor, 466
Somatic cell hybrids, *huntingtin* (HD) gene mapping, 571
Somatic mutations, mitochondria, 73
Somatization disorder, 892, 892t
Somatoform disorders, 557, 892–893, 892t, 893t
  see also Psychogenic movement disorders (PMDs);
      individual disorders
  differential diagnosis, 893
Somatosensory cortex, in Parkinson's disease, 46, 47f
Somatosensory evoked potentials (SEPs)
  cortical myoclonus, 660, 664, 670, 670f
  corticobasal degeneration, 766
  Huntington's disease, 592
  myoclonus, 662
Somatostatin
  Parkinson's disease, 202
  striatal preservation in HD, 605
Somatotopic organization
  motor cortex, 92
  PPN, 96
Somnambulism (sleepwalking), 862–863
Somniloquy (sleeptalking), 862
Spasmodic dysphonia (laryngeal dystonia), 514, 517
  treatment, 528t, 532–533
Spasmodic torticollis, 495
  clinical features, 514–515
  familial, 517
  pathophysiology, 518–519
  patient examination, 533, 533t
  rating scale, 533
  remission, 512
  treatment, 528t
    botulinum toxin, 533
    immobilization, 527
Spasmus mutans, 826
Spasticity
  aging and, 838–839, 839t
  drug treatment, 504, 530–531
  Parkinson's disease *vs.*, 235
  stiff-legged gait, 814
SPECT *see* Single photon emission tomography (SPECT)
Speech/speech disorders, 26
  see also Dysarthria
  cerebellum role, 722, 726, 737, 738, 748
  corticobasal degeneration, 764
  essential tremor assessment, 442
  Huntington's disease, 589
  laryngeal dystonia (spasmodic dysphonia), 514
  multisystem atrophy, 363
  Parkinson's disease, 238
  progressive supranuclear palsy, 347, 351

somniloquy (sleeptalking), 862
  therapy, 351
Speech therapy, progressive supranuclear palsy, 351
Spheroid bodies
  Hallervorden-Spatz disease, 405
  Parkinson's disease, 330
Sphingomyelin accumulation, Niemann-Pick disease, 553
Spinal accessory nerve, microvascular decompression, 535
Spinal cord
  dystonia pathophysiology, 499, 520
  efferents, cerebellar projections, 740
  lesion, 672
  myoclonus, 9, 660, 664, 666, 672
  progressive supranuclear palsy, 347
  quadruped gait control, 811
  sleep movements pathophysiology, 858
  sleep-wake role, 858
Spinal pattern generators, 811
Spinobulbar muscular atrophy (SBMA), repeat expansion,
      577f
Spinocerebellar ataxias (SCAs), 706–711
  clinical features, 705, 706t
  definition, 706
  DNA tests, 705t
  DRPLA *see* Denatorubropallidoluysian atrophy (DRPLA)
  dystonia, 551
  Friedreich's ataxia (FRDA), 704, 705t, 706t, 711
  phenotypic overlap, 706
  repeat expansion, 577f, 641, 705t, 707, 708, 709, 710, 711
  SCA1, 705t, 706–707, 706t
  SCA2, 705t, 706t, 707
  SCA3 *see* Machado-Joseph disease
  SCA4, 706t, 708
  SCA5 (Lincoln ataxia), 705t, 706t, 708
  SCA6, 705t, 706t, 708–709
  SCA7, 705t, 706t, 709
  SCA8, 705t, 706t, 709
  SCA10, 705t, 706t
  SCA11, 706t, 709
  SCA12-16, 706t, 710
  SCA17, 705t, 710
Spinocerebellum, 740
Spongiform changes
  dementia with Lewy bodies, 151–152, 151f
  Rett syndrome, 415
Spontaneous orofacial dyskinesia (SOFD), 847
Staining, 148
Stance/station
  aging, 840
  cerebellar dysfunction, 724
Startle reflex, 672
  exaggerated (hyperekplexia), 11, 665, 672, 686
  tics and, 696–697
  tics *vs.*, 695
Static tremor *see* Resting tremor

Stem cell transplantation
  cell sources, 284
  Parkinson's disease, 284–285
Stereotypy, 9
  childhood, 828
  dystonia, 521
  tardive dyskinesia, 627, 631–632
  Tourette's syndrome *vs.*, 686, 828
Steroids, stiff-person syndrome treatment, 808
Stiff-legged gait, 814
"Stiff-limb syndrome," 804
Stiff-man plus syndrome, 797–798
Stiff-person (man) syndrome (SPS), 11, 797–810
  clinical course, 799
  clinical features, 797, 798–801
    fear/anxiety, 798–799
    hyperlordosis, 798
    muscle spasm, 798
    rigidity, 798
    stiff-legged gait, 814
  clinical presentation, 798
  diagnosis, 801–802
    clinical criteria, 797–798, 802, 802t
  differential diagnosis, 797–798, 802–804, 803t
    progressive encephalomyelitis with rigidity, 802–803
  disease associations, 801
    autoimmune diseases, 801
    diabetes, 799, 801, 806–807
    neoplasms, 923
  EMG studies, 797, 800, 800f
  epidemiology, 798
  etiology, 807
  historical background, 797
  laboratory tests, 799–800
  muscle biopsy, 800–801
  neurological examination, 799, 799t
  neuropathology, 804
  pathophysiology/pathogenesis, 804–807
    autoimmune mechanism, 797, 800, 805–807
    biochemistry, 805
    GABAergic neurons, 799–800, 805
    as paraneoplastic disorder, 803–804, 923
    physiology, 804–805
  treatment, 798, 807–808
    diazepam, 797, 799, 807
Stimulants
  ADHD treatment, 688
  tremor induction, 464
Streptococcal infections, Sydenham's chorea, 918, 919
Stress
  dystonia effects, 502
    blepharospasm, 513
  Parkinson's disease etiology, 189
  tremor induction, 463
Striatonigral degeneration (SND), 106

corticobasal degeneration *vs.*, 762
dementia, 29
dystonia in, 548
historical background, 359–360
neuroimaging, 48–49, 364
neuropathology, 152
  gross examination, 148
Parkinson's disease *vs.*, 240, 241
symptom overlap with other MSA syndromes, 359f
Striatum, 93, 117, 129, 129f, 198
  see also Caudate nucleus; Putamen
  abscess, 424
  cholinergic neurons, 94–95, 120–121, 122, 122f
  cyanide poisoning, 388
  development, 277
  dopamine, 97, 118–119, 122f
  dystonia, 110
  glutamatergic innervation, 123–124
    AMPA/kainate receptors, 122f, 125
    mGluR receptors, 125
    NMDA receptors, 124–125
  Huntington's disease, 601–606
    gross/histological pathology, 601–603, 602f
    huntingtin and, 614
    MRI, 611
    neurochemistry, 603–605
    neuronal degeneration, 605–606, 605f, 606f
    neuronal remodeling, 605, 605f
    selective neuronal loss, 603–605, 603f
    selective neuronal preservation, 604f, 605
    striosomes, 606, 607f
  motor circuitry, 94–95, 95f
  Parkinson's disease/parkinsonism, 201, 204, 424
    drug-induced, 397
  progressive supranuclear palsy, 344
  serotonin, 127
  tic pathophysiology, 692–693
  transplantation into
    sites, 277–278, 278f
    tissue distribution, 278–279
    volume, 278
Striosome, Huntington's disease, 606, 607f
Stroke-associated conditions, 845–846
  hemidystonia, 846
  parkinsonism, 846
    see also Vascular parkinsonism
  tremor, 471–472
    pathophysiology, 486f, 487
Subacute necrotizing encephalomyelopathy *see* Leigh's disease
Subcortical arteriosclerotic encephalopathy, 422
Subdural hematoma, parkinsonism, 424
Substance P
  Huntington's disease, 609
  Parkinson's disease, 201–202

Substantia nigra, 93, 198
    see also Dopamine
    BDNF effects, 140
    cholinergic innervation, 121, 123
    corticobasal degeneration, 762, 767f
    dopamine, 97, 118
    dystonia, 499–500
    glutamatergic innervation, 124, 125f
    gross examination, 148
    Hallervorden-Spatz disease, 405
    Huntington's disease, 606–607, 608f
    infarction, 846
    insulin receptors, 141
    motor circuitry, 95, 95f, 96
    MPTP-induced parkinsonism, 384
    pallor, 148, 149, 149f, 153, 327, 375, 384
    Parkinson's disease, 149, 149f, 201, 275, 327
        see also Parkinson's disease (PD)
        decreased free radical scavengers, 203
        iron content, 188, 327
        Lewy bodies, 150, 150f
        pathogenesis, 210f
    progressive supranuclear palsy, 153, 344
    serotonergic innervation, 127
Subthalamic nucleus (STN), 93
    cholinergic innervation, 121
    glutamatergic innervation, 124, 126f
    gross examination, 148
    hemiballism, 109, 109f, 846
    Huntington's disease, 608
    motor circuitry, 95f, 96
    Parkinson's disease treatment
        gene therapy, 285
        lesion, 106
        stimulation, 48
    progressive supranuclear palsy, 153, 345
    stimulation
        in ET treatment, 485
        in PD treatment, 48
Suicide risk, Huntington's disease, 590
Sunflower cataract, Wilson's disease, 781
Superoxide dismutase (SOD)
    boosting activity, 79–80
    cellular antioxidant system, 72, 72f
    Parkinson's disease, 219
        gene association studies, 215
Supplementary motor area (SMA), 90, 91f, 92–93
    lesion effects, 93
Surgical interventions
    see also Deep brain stimulation (DBS); Fetal cell
        transplantation; *specific procedures*
    dystonia treatment, 110, 504, 534–535
    Parkinson's disease
        fetal transplants *vs.*, 282
        neuropsychiatric management, 324

    pallidotomy, 48
    STN lesion, 106
    STN stimulation, 48
    tic treatment, 694
    tremor *see* Thalamotomy
    Wilson's disease, liver transplantation, 788–789
Swallowing
    difficulty *see* Dysphagia
    essential tremor assessment, 442–443
Sydenham's chorea (St. Vitus dance), 50, 637–638, 918–919
    childhood, 828, 829
    neuropathology, 919
Synaptic plasticity
    cerebellar LTD, 745
    dopamine role, 97
    glutamate receptors, 126, 127
    long-term depression/potentiation, 97, 126, 127, 745
Synphilin-1, Parkinson's disease, 204
α-Synuclein (PARK1 gene), 330
    dementia with Lewy bodies, 151
    multisystem atrophy, 152, 152f
    normal function, 204–205, 331
    oxidative stress and, 217
    Parkinson's disease, 75, 149–150, 166–167, 204, 328,
            329, 329f
        association studies, 215–216
        dystrophic neurites, 330, 330f
        mutation, 166, 167t, 168t, 217, 217t, 331–332
        role in pathogenesis, 330–331
Synucleinopathies
    see also α-Synuclein (PARK1 gene)
    dementia with Lewy bodies *see* Dementia with Lewy
            bodies (DLB)
    iron metabolism in, 202
    multisystem atrophy *see* Multisystem atrophy (MSA)
    neuropathology, 149–153
        immunohistochemistry, 148–149
    Parkinson's disease *see* Parkinson's disease (PD)
Syphilis, parkinsonism, 378
Systemic disease, 915–925
    see also individual diseases
    autoimmune *see* Autoimmune disease
    chorea, 637–639, 644t
    dystonia in, 517
    elderly, 837
    endocrine *see* Endocrine disorders
    hematological, 918
    infections *see* Infection
    metabolic *see* Metabolic disorders
    tremor in, 472
Systemic lupus erythematosus (SLE), 921
    blepharospasm, 921
    chorea, 50, 638–639, 921
    torticollis, 921

T

Tardive akathisia, 627, 633
Tardive dyskinesia, 398, 556, 846
  clinical features
    akathisia, 627, 633
    chorea/stereotypy, 6–7, 50–51, 627, 630, 631–632
    dystonia, 520, 627, 630, 632–633
    tics/myoclonus, 627, 687
    tremor, 464, 627
  definition, 3, 627
  differential diagnosis, 628
  epidemiology, 628
  natural history, 628
  neuroimaging, 629, 633
  neuropathology, 629
  pathophysiology, 628–629, 633
  phenomenology, 627
    treatment and, 630t
  prevention, 629–630
  risk factors, 628
  treatment, 630–633, 630t
    akathisia, 633
    antioxidants, 79, 632
    choreic movements, 631–632
    dopamine-depletion, 631, 632–633
    drug choice, 630
    dystonic movements, 632–633
    GABAergiuc drugs, 631–632
Tardive dystonia, 520, 627, 630, 632–633
Tardive tics, 627, 687, 697
Tardive tremor, 464, 627
Task-specific dystonia, 515–516
  primary torsion dystonia, 512
  treatment, 528t
    botulinum toxin, 533–534
Task-specific tremor, 472–473
  pathophysiology, 488
  writing tremor, 472–473
    essential tremor *vs.*, 438
TATA-binding protein, SCA17 mutation, 710
Tauopathies
  see also Tau protein
  Alzheimer's disease *see* Alzheimer's disease (AD)
  corticobasal degeneration *see* Corticobasal degeneration (CBD)
  FTDP-17 *see* Frontotemporal dementia with parkinsonism linked to chromosome 17 (FTDP-17)
  neuropathology, 153–156
    immunohistochemistry, 148
  progressive supranuclear palsy *see* Progressive supranuclear palsy (PSP)
Tau protein
  aggregate formation, 769
  familial parkinsonism genetics, 167–168, 168, 169t

FTDP-17, 404
  normal isoforms, 769
  pallidonigroluysian degeneration, 412
  PD gene association studies, 216
  postencephalitic parkinsonism, 376
  progressive supranuclear palsy, 349–350
Tay-Sachs disease, myoclonus, 662
Tendon reflexes, aging and, 839
Terminal tremor, 461
Tetrabenazine
  in drug-induced parkinsonism, 398–399
  dystonia treatment, 504, 529
  tardive dyskinesia treatment, 631
  tremor induction, 464
Tetrahydrobiopterin deficiency, 916–917
Tetrahydroisoquinolines (TIQs)
  Parkinson's disease etiology, 212
  structure, 211f
Tetrathiomolybdate, Wilson's disease treatment, 786–787
TGF-α, 141
TGF-β family *see* Transforming growth factor-β (TGF-β) family
Thalamic disinhibition theories, 98, 105
Thalamic reticular nucleus, motor circuitry, 96
Thalamic stimulation, essential tremor therapy, 449–450
Thalamic tremor (Holmes' tremor), 466–467, 467t
  pathophysiology, 486–487
Thalamotomy, 483
  cerebellar tremor, 461–462
  essential tremor, 441, 449
    DBS *vs.*, 450
    gamma knife, 450
    mechanism, 484–485
Thalamus
  basal ganglia motor circuitry, 96, 98, 105
    dystonia, 518, 545, 545t, 546
    in hypokinetic disorders, 106, 107–108
  degeneration in dementia, 29
  glutamatergic innervation, 124
  Huntington's disease, 607–608
  neurosurgical lesion, tic treatment, 694
  progressive supranuclear palsy, 345
  stimulation
    essential tremor therapy, 449–450, 484–485
    pallidal *vs.* in dystonia, 535
  stroke, 471–472, 846
  tremor, 235, 483
    see also Thalamotomy
    essential, 441, 442f, 449–450
    Holmes' tremor, 466–467, 467t, 486–487
    stroke-induced, 471–472
Theophyllines, essential tremor therapy, 448–449
Thioridazine
  drug-induced parkinsonism, 395
  tremor induction, 464

Thymoxamine, essential tremor therapy, 448
Thyroid disorders
    autoimmune, 921
    cerebellar ataxias, 916
    chorea, 642, 915
    tremor, 472, 915
Tics, 9, 691–699, 824–825
    associated conditions, 695–696
    characteristics, 9
    childhood, 824–825
    classification, 9, 692t
    clinical presentation/course, 691–692
    complex, 9, 683, 684, 692t
    differential diagnosis, 686–687, 694–696,
            696t
        chorea *vs.*, 695
        dystonia *vs.*, 686, 692, 695
        hyperkinesias vs, 695t
        hyperkinesias *vs..*, 695
        myoclonus *vs.*, 657, 685–686
    epidemiology, 823–824, 825
    etiologies, 696–697, 696t
        Huntington's disease and, 589
        neuroacanthocytosis, 696
        secondary, 697
    factors affecting, 691
    motor *see* Motor tics
    neurochemistry, 694
    pathophysiology, 692–694
        corticostriatothalamic circuits, 692–693
        electrophysiology, 692, 694
        frontal discharges, 693–694
        morphometric studies, 693
        neural substrates, 692–693
        PET studies, 693
    "phantom," 692
    primary *vs.* secondary, 686, 686t, 696–697, 696t
    psychogenic, 904–905
    sensory, 691–692, 692t
    simple, 9, 684, 692t
    sleep disturbance, 694, 874–875
    Tourette's syndrome *see* Tourette's syndrome (TS)
    treatment, 687–688, 687t, 697–698
        neurosurgical, 694
    vocal *see* Vocal tics
    voluntary *vs.* involuntary, 692
Tilt table, multisystem atrophy, 365
Timolol, essential tremor therapy, 445
Titubation, 724
Tizanidine hydrochloride (Zanaflex), dystonia
            treatment, 530
α-Tocopherol *see* Vitamin E (α-tocopherol)
α-Tocopherol transfer protein (α-TTP), ataxia, 712
Tolcapone, 251, 252
Toluene, toxin-induced tremor, 466

Tongue
    essential tremor, 436, 438
    nocturnal biting, 862
Topiramate, essential tremor therapy, 447
TOR1A gene *see* DYT1 gene
Toronto Western Spasmodic Torticollis Rating Scale
            (TWSTRS), 533
Torsin A (DYT1 gene product)
    abnormal in PTD, 498–499
    normal function, 498
Torticollis
    benign paroxysmal of infancy, 827, 828
    spasmodic (cervical dystonia) *see* Spasmodic torticollis
    systemic lupus erythematosus and, 921
Total functional capacity (TFC), Huntington's disease,
            590–591
Tourette's syndrome (TS), 683–690
    clinical features, 683–684, 683t
        behavioral abnormalities, 683t, 684, 685, 687
            ADHD, 684, 693, 695–696
            obsessive-compulsive disorder, 23, 684, 693, 695–696
            personality, 22, 684
            sexual disturbances, 24
            sleep disturbances, 694, 874–875
        speech/language disturbance, 26
        tics, 657, 683–684, 683t
        waxing/waning, 684
    differential diagnosis, 685–686
    DSM-IV diagnostic criteria, 683
    epidemiology, 685, 823–824
    etiology/pathogenesis, 687
    genetics, 686, 687
    historical aspects, 683
    Huntington's disease and, 589
    myoclonus *vs.*, 657
    natural history, 684–685
    neurobiology, 687, 693
    treatment, 687–688
        behavior disorders, 687t, 688
        non-drug, 688
        tics, 687–688, 687t
Tourette Syndrome Association, 688
Toxin-induced disorders
    see also Drug-induced disorders; *specific toxins*
    parkinsonism *see* Toxin-induced parkinsonism
    tics, 697
    tremor, 465–466, 736
        heavy metals, 465–466
        herbicides/insecticides, 466
        solvents, 466
Toxin-induced parkinsonism, 210–211, 383–393
    see also Drug-induced parkinsonism
    carbon disulfide, 387–388
    carbon monoxide, 386–387
    clinical features, 389t

Toxin-induced parkinsonism *(continued)*
  cyanide, 388
  manganese, 188, 209, 385–386
  methanol, 388–389
  MPTP *see* MPTP-induced parkinsonism
  pesticides, 74–75, 188, 211
Toxoplasmosis, 920
Tranquilizers, tremor induction, 464
Transcranial magnetic stimulation (TMS)
  dystonia treatment, 528
  myoclonus studies, 676
Transcription, huntingtin and, 618–619
Transforming growth factor-α (TGF-α), 141
Transforming growth factor-β (TGF-β) family, 135–139
  see also individual members
  GDNF family, 135–137
  Parkinson's disease, 220
  TGF-β, 137
  therapeutic use, 43, 135, 136, 137–139
Transgenic mice, *huntingtin* (HD) gene, 578
Trauma
  dystonia and, 515, 517–518, 556
    perinatal, 541, 545f, 546
    peripheral injury-induced, 546–547, 899–901
  neurological disease following, 900
  parkinsonism, 422–423
  spasmodic torticollis, 515
  tics and, 697
  tremor, 473
Trazodone, essential tremor therapy, 448
Trembling psychogenic gait, 906
Tremor, 4, 6, 459–480, 825
  see also specific types
  action *see* Kinetic tremor
  age-related, 840, 843
  childhood, 825–826
  clinical rating scales, 442
  corticobasal degeneration, 762
  definitions, 459, 481, 736, 901
  diagnosis, 460t
  differential diagnosis, 6
    myoclonus *vs.*, 657, 669
  drug-induced, 463–464, 489, 736, 839–840
  essential *see* Essential tremor
  food-induced, 462
  hemiparkinsonism-hemiatrophy, 407
  intentional *see* Kinetic tremor
  motor *see* Kinetic tremor
  multisystem atrophy, 363
  neural substrates, 441–442, 442f, 459
    cerebellum, 441, 461–462, 485–486, 724, 726, 736–737
    cerebral cortex, 461, 483, 488
    common pathways, 482–483, 483f
    midbrain, 466–467
    thalamus, 235, 441, 449–450, 483
  parkinsonism *see* Parkinsonian tremor
  pathophysiology, 481–492
  peripheral neuropathies, 440–441, 469
  physiological *see* Physiological tremor
  posttraumatic, 473
  psychogenic *see* Psychogenic movement disorders (PMDs)
  resting *see* Resting tremor
  systemic disease and, 472, 915, 916–917
    see also Physiological tremor
  titubation, 724
  toxin-induced, 465–466, 736
  Wilson's disease, 472, 779
Triazolam, sleep-onset insomnia treatment, 869
Tricyclic antidepressants (TCAs), 262
  Huntington's disease, 594
  tremor induction, 463
Trientine (triethylene tetramine dihydrochloride), Wilson's disease management, 788
Trigan (trimethobenzamide), 249
Trihexyphenidyl, X-linked dystonia-parkinsonism syndrome, 410
Trimethobenzamide (Trigan), 249
Trinucleotide repeat expansion *see* Repeat expansion diseases
Truncal tremor, essential tremor and, 438
Tryptamine, structure, 211f
Tuberohypophysial system, 198
Tufted astrocytes, progressive supranuclear palsy, 153, 154f
Tumor necrosis factor-α (TNF-α), Parkinson's disease, 220
Tumors *see* Malignancy
TUNEL method, 221
Twin studies
  essential tremor, 434
  Parkinson's disease (PD), 38, 187, 212
Typist's cramp, 516
Tyrosine hydroxylase (TH)
  deficiency, dystonia, 827
  dopamine synthesis, 198, 199f
  Parkinson's disease
    changes seen, 199–200, 200t
    gene association studies, 215

U

Ubiquitin C-terminal hydrolase (PARK5), Parkinson's disease genetics, 167
Ubiquitin immunoreactivity, dementia with Lewy bodies, 151, 151f
Ubiquitin protein ligase, 218
  gene mutation *see* *Parkin* (PARK2) mutation
Ultrasound, multisystem atrophy, 365
Unified Parkinson's Disease Rating Scale (UPDRS), 39, 243
  post-transplantation, 281
Unverricht-Lundborg's disease, 662, 665
Urinary dysfunction *see* Genitourinary dysfunction

V

Valproic acid (valproate)
  stiff-person syndrome treatment, 808
  tardive dyskinesia treatment, 631
  tremor induction, 463
Variable number tandem repeats (VNTRs), *huntingtin* (HD)
      gene mapping, 572
Vascular disease
  cerebellar dysfunction, 727t
  chorea, 641, 644t
  tics, 697
Vascular malformations
  cerebellar dysfunction, 728t
  parkinsonism, 424
Vascular parkinsonism, 240, 367, 421–422, 846
  diagnostic criteria, 422
  gait, 421, 815
  historical/nosological aspects, 421
Ventral tegmental area (VTA)
  dopaminergic pathways, 97, 872
  progressive supranuclear palsy, 345
  sleep role, 872, 876
Ventricles
  enlargement in HD, 609
  gross examination, 147
Verapamil, essential tremor therapy, 448
Vermal syndrome, 746
Vestibular disturbances, cerebellar dysfunction,
      725, 746
Vestibulocerebellum, 723
Vestibuloocular reflex (VOR), gain adaptation, 751
Viral infections
  see also specific infections
  encephalitis lethargica, 374
  fetal cell transplants, 279
  parkinsonism following, 376–378
  Parkinson's disease etiology, 209
Viral vectors, GDNF expression in PD, 138
Visual convergence, 747
Visual pursuit, 747
Visuospatial disturbances, 26–27
Vitamin B$_6$ (pyridoxine), tardive dyskinesia treatment,
      398, 632
Vitamin C (ascorbic acid), as antioxidant treatment, 79
Vitamin E (α-tocopherol)
  as antioxidant treatment, 79
  ataxia with vitamin E deficiency (AVED), 712
  cellular antioxidant system, 72
  deficiency, 917
  Parkinson's disease prevention, 189–190
  tardive dyskinesia treatment, 632
Vitamins, as antioxidant treatments, 79
Vocal tics, 9, 683t, 684, 691, 824
  complex, 9, 684, 692t

  simple, 9, 684, 692t
  voluntary *vs.* involuntary, 692
Vocal tremor, 459, 474
Voltage-gated calcium channels
  episodic ataxia type 2, 710–711
  spinocerebellar ataxia type 6, 708
Voluntary movement, rCBF, 92
Vomiting
  COMT inhibitor side-effects, 252
  levodopa (L-dopa) side-effects, 249
Von Economo's encephalitis *see* Encephalitis lethargica

W

Walking *see* Gait
Wechsler Adult Intelligence Scale-Revised (WAIS-R),
      Huntington's disease, 589
Western equine encephalitis, parkinsonism, 376–377
Whipple's disease, 920
  oculomasticatory myorhythmia, 379, 920
  parkinsonism, 379
  sleep disturbances, 24
"Whispering dysphonia," Wilson's disease, 779–780
White matter
  see also Encephalopathies
  Binswanger's disease, 422, 815
  carbon monoxide poisoning, 387
  corticobasal degeneration, 766, 768
Wilson's disease (WD), 777–795, 782t
  clinical features, 778–782
    cognitive impairment, 780–781
    dermatological, 782
    hemolytic anemia, 782
    hepatic, 778–779, 778t, 788
    musculoskeletal, 781–782
    neurological, 779–780, 779t
      cerebellar dysfunction, 780
      chorea, 637
      dysarthria, 779
      dystonia, 549, 549f, 779–780
      tremor, 472, 779
    neuropsychiatric, 780–781, 781t
      anxiety, 23
      depression, 20
      personality changes, 22, 780
      psychosis, 781
      sexual disturbances, 24
    ophthalmologic, 781
      Kayser-Fleischer rings, 781, 784
      sunflower cataract, 781
    renal, 782
  dementia in, 29, 780
  diagnosis, 782–785, 783t
    ceruloplasmin levels, 784
    copper levels/metabolism, 784–785

Wilson's disease (WD) (continued)
  diagnosis (continued)
    liver biopsy, 783, 783t
    radiocopper incorporation, 784–785
    slit-lamp examination, 784
    testing guidelines, 785
  differential diagnosis
    early-onset dystonia vs., 503
    Parkinson's disease vs., 240
  epidemiology, 777
  genetics, 777–778
  historical aspects, 777
  neuroimaging, 785
  pathophysiology, 549, 778
    ceruloplasmin deficiency, 777, 778
  treatment, 785–789
    copper absorption inhibition, 786–787
    copper chelation, 787–788
    dietary, 785–786
    guidelines, 789
    liver transplantation, 788–789
"Wing-beating" tremor, 6
WNDP (ATP7B) gene, Wilson's disease, 777
Wolf-Hirschhorn syndrome, 571
Wolfram's syndrome, dystonia, 551–552
World Federation of Neurology (WFN), genetic testing
    in HD, 580, 592

Writer's cramp, 515, 516
  botulinum toxin, 533–534
  essential tremor and, 440
  familial, 517
  pathophysiology, 519
Writing, essential tremor assessment, 443
Writing tremor, 472–473, 488
  essential tremor vs., 438

X

Xanthine derivatives, essential tremor therapy, 448–449
Xenografts, Parkinson's disease, 283
Xeroderma pigmentosum, dystonia, 551
X-linked ataxias, 713
X-linked dystonia-parkinsonism syndrome, 409–410

Z

Zanaflex (tizanidine hydrochloride), dystonia treatment, 530
Zinc, Wilson's disease treatment, 786
Ziprasidone, tic treatment, 688
Zolpidem
  progressive supranuclear palsy, 351
  X-linked dystonia-parkinsonism syndrome, 410